::

Management of

PERIPHERAL NERVE PROBLEMS

Editors

George E. Omer, Jr., M.D., M.S. (Orthopaedic Surgery), F.A.C.S.
Colonel, Medical Corps, U.S. Army (Ret)
Professor Emeritus of Orthopaedics and Chairman Emeritus
Department of Orthopaedics and Rehabilitation
Professor and Chief Emeritus, Division of Hand Surgery
Professor Emeritus of Anatomy and Surgery, University of New Mexico School of Medicine
Medical Director, Emeritus, School of Physical Therapy, The University of New Mexico Health Sciences Center
Consultant Hand Surgeon, The Carrie Tingley Childrens Hospital, Lovelace Hospital, Presbyterian Hospital,
    University Hospital, and the Veterans Administration Medical Center, Albuquerque, New Mexico
Past President, The Sunderland Peripheral Nerve Society
Past President, The American Society for Surgery of the Hand
Past President, The American Orthopaedic Association
Past President, The American Board of Orthopaedic Surgery
Past President, The Western Orthopaedic Association

Morton Spinner, M.D., F.A.C.S.
Clinical Professor of Orthopaedic Surgery
Albert Einstein College of Medicine
Bronx, New York
Consultant in Hand Surgery
South Nassau Community Hospital, Oceanside, New York
Brookdale Hospital Medical Center, Brooklyn, New York
North Shore University Hospital, Manhasset, New York
Past President, The Sunderland Peripheral Nerve Society

Allen L. Van Beek, M.D., F.A.C.S.
Clinical Associate Professor of Plastic Surgery
Department of Surgery
The University of Minnesota Hospital and Clinics
Minneapolis, Minnesota
Director, Plastic Surgery, North Memorial Medical Center, Robbinsdale, Minnesota
Past President, The American Society for Reconstructive Microsurgery
American Society of Peripheral Nerve
Director, Plastic Surgery Education Foundation
Past President, Minnesota Medical Society

Special Medical Illustrator

Miguel A. Pirela-Cruz, M.D., F.A.C.S.
Hand, Upper Extremity and Microsurgical Consultant for
Memorial Medical Center, Las Cruces, New Mexico

2nd Edition

Management of PERIPHERAL NERVE PROBLEMS

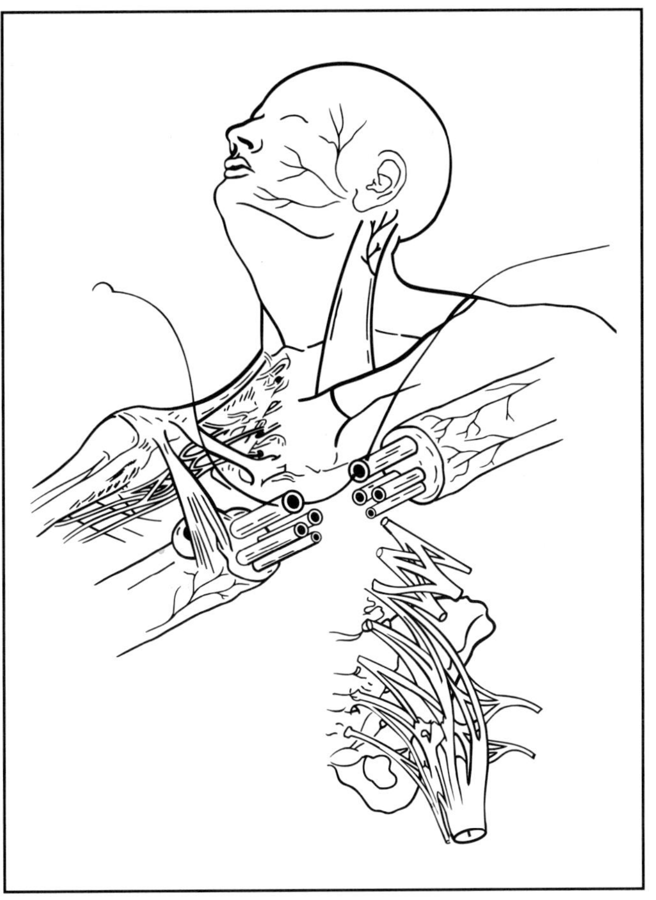

W.B. SAUNDERS COMPANY
A Division of Harcourt Brace & Company
Philadelphia   London   Toronto   Montreal   Sydney   Tokyo

W.B. SAUNDERS COMPANY
A Division of Harcourt Brace & Company

The Curtis Center
Independence Square West
Philadelphia, Pennsylvania 19106

Library of Congress Cataloging-in-Publication Data

Management of peripheral nerve problems / editors, George E. Omer, Jr., Morton Spinner, Allen L. Van Beek; special medical illustrator, Miguel A. Pirela-Cruz.—2nd ed.

p.   cm.

Includes bibliographical references and indexes.

ISBN 0–7216–4276–4

1. Nerves, Peripheral—Surgery.   2. Nerves, Peripheral—Wounds and injuries.   3. Nerves, Peripheral—Diseases.   I. Omer, George E.   II. Van Beek, Allen.   III. Spinner, Morton. [DNLM: 1. Peripheral Nervous System Diseases—therapy.   WL 500   M 266 1997]

RD595.M25   1998

617.4′83—dc20

DNLM/DLC   96-28473

MANAGEMENT OF PERIPHERAL NERVE PROBLEMS   ISBN 0–7216–4276–4

Dedicated to our wives,

Wendie, Paula, and Sharon

and to our children,

Eric, Michael,

Jeffrey, Robert, Stephen,

Troy, Greg, and Jeremy

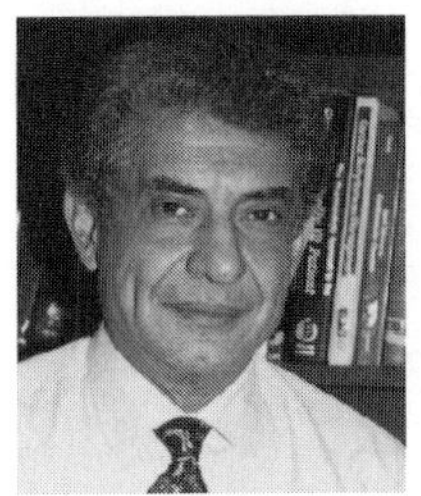

Dr. Abadir

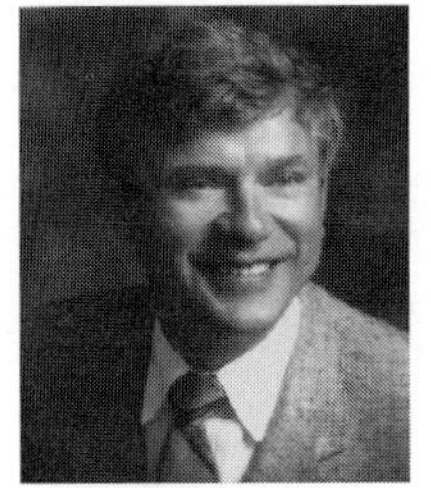

Dr. Almquist

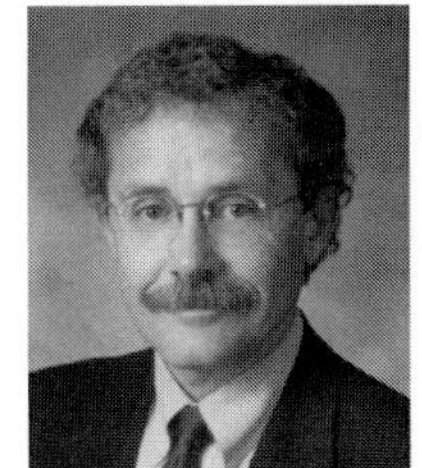

Dr. Anderson

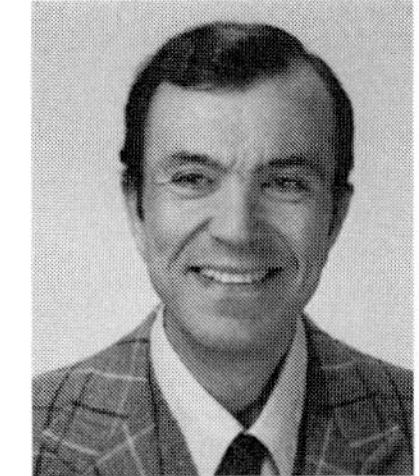

Dr. Atasoy

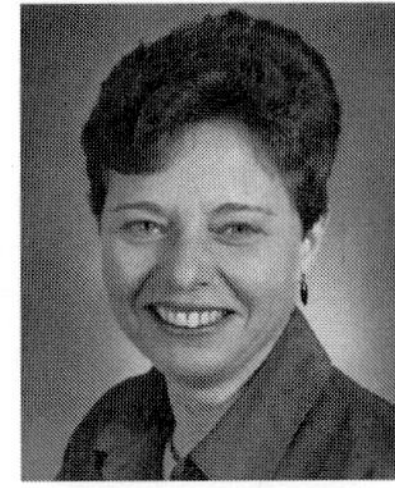

Dr. Badalamente

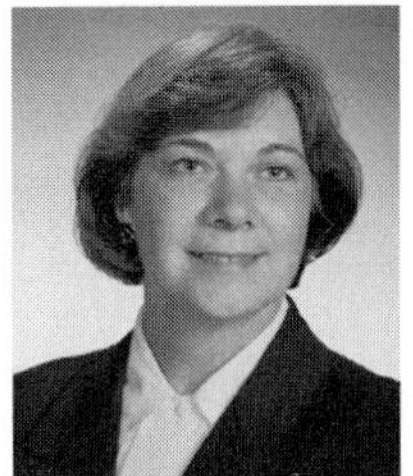

Capt. Bell-Krotoski

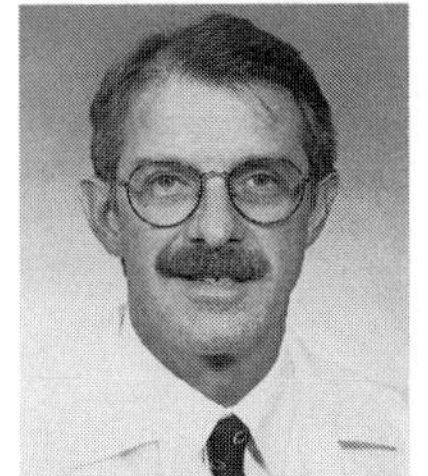

Dr. Blair

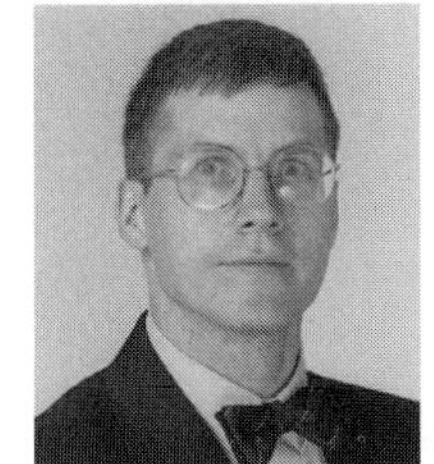

Dr. Bonatz

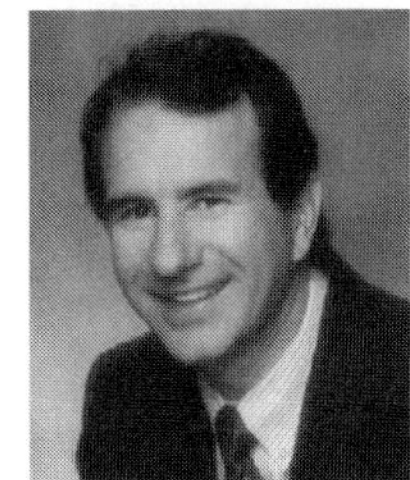

Dr. Botte

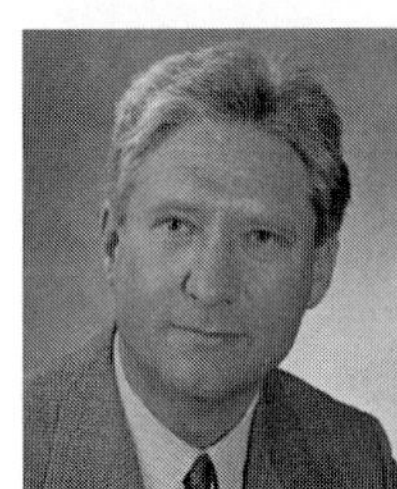

Dr. Boyd

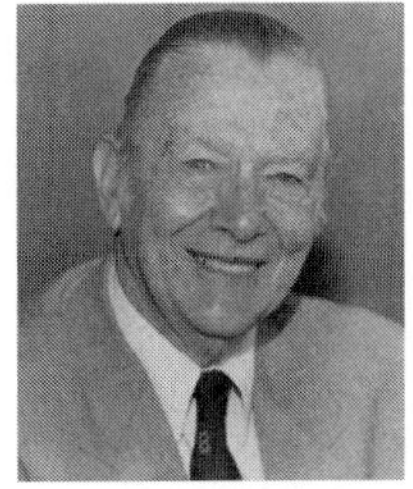

Dr. Brand

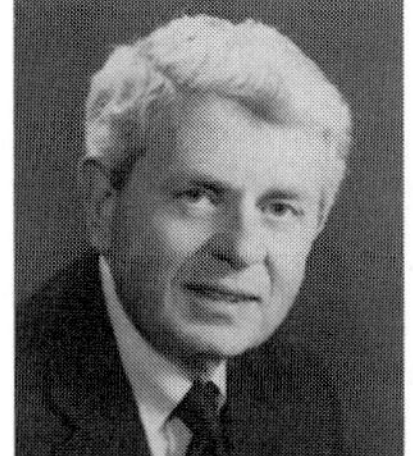

Dr. Braun

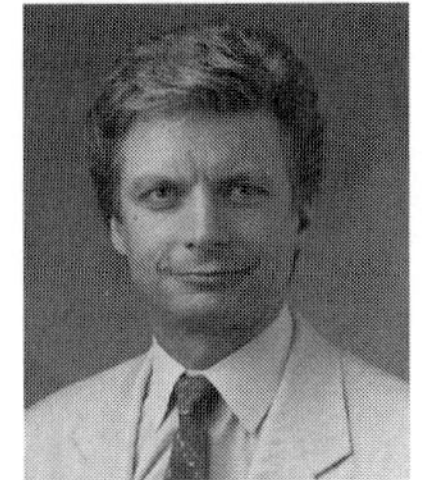

Dr. Breidenbach

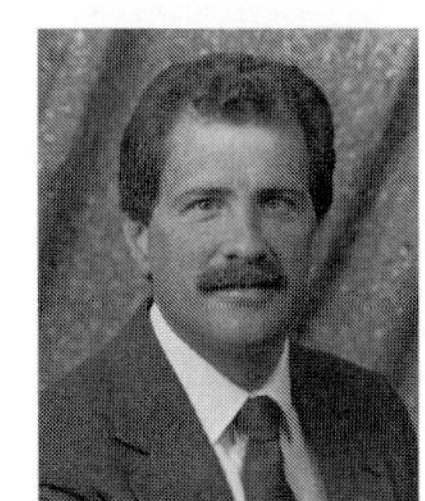

Dr. Brown

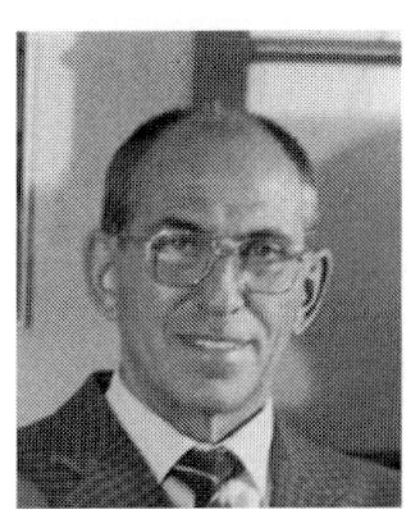

Dr. Giorgio Brunelli

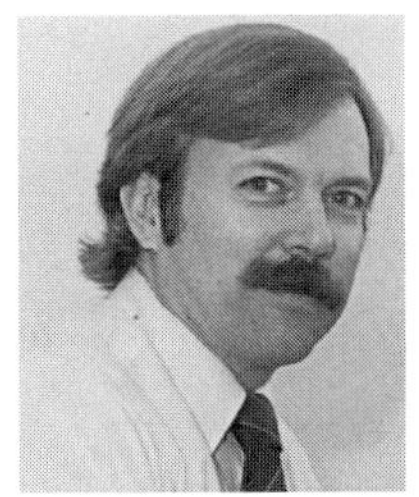

Dr. Brushart

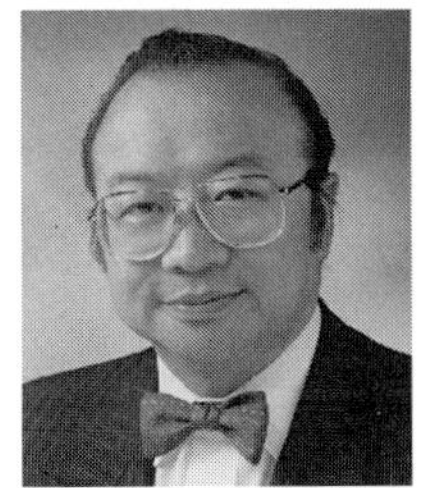

Dr. Chiu

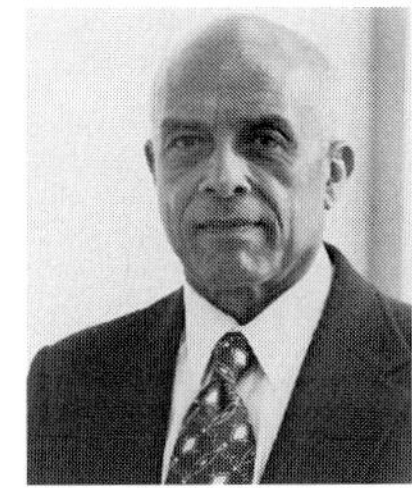

Dr. Collins

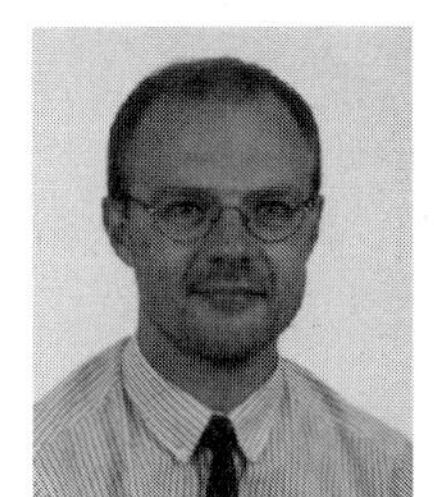

Dr. Dahlin

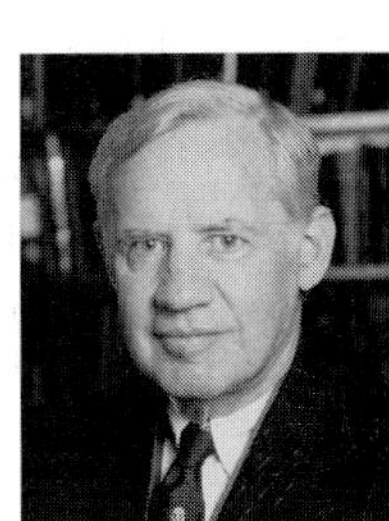

Dr. Dick

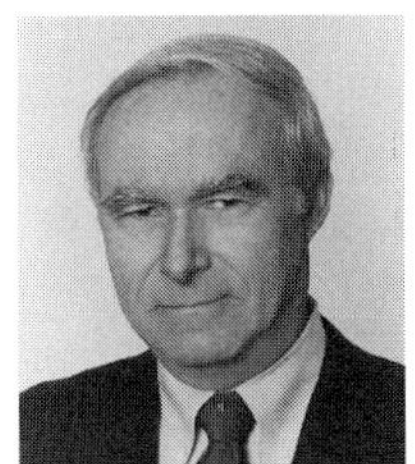

Dr. Eaton

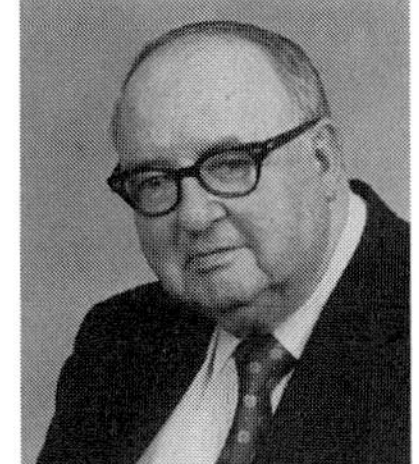

Dr. Enna

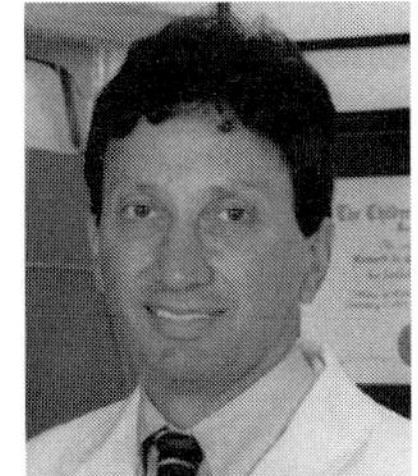

Dr. Gelberman

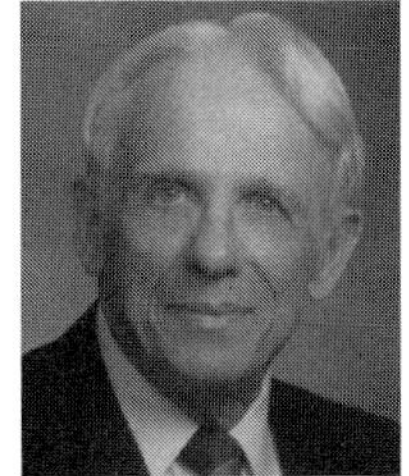

Dr. Goldner

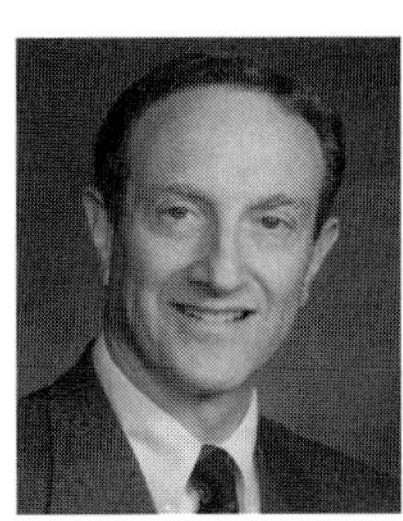

Dr. Gould

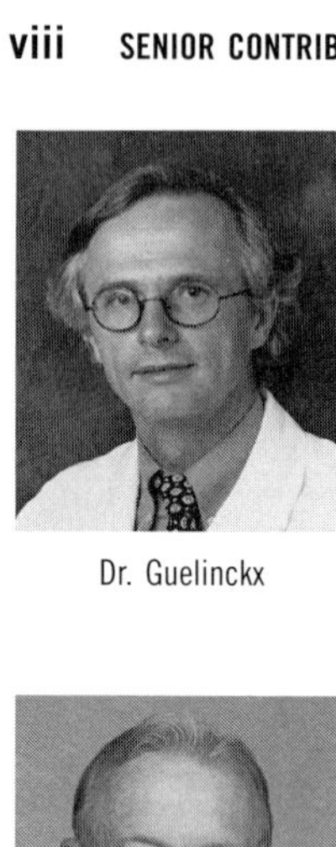

Dr. Guelinckx

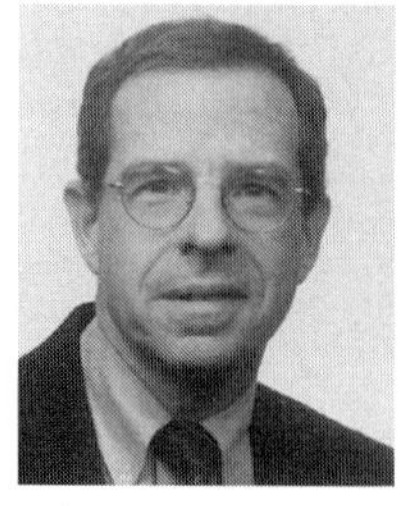

Dr. Hentz

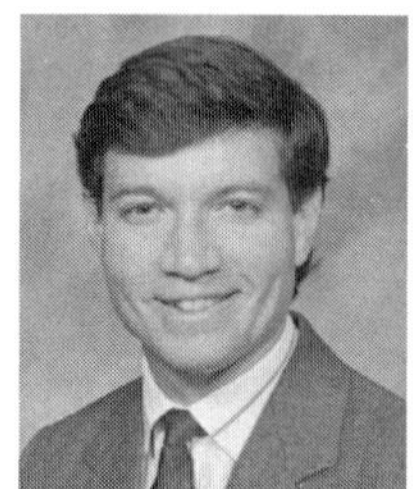

Dr. Hoffman

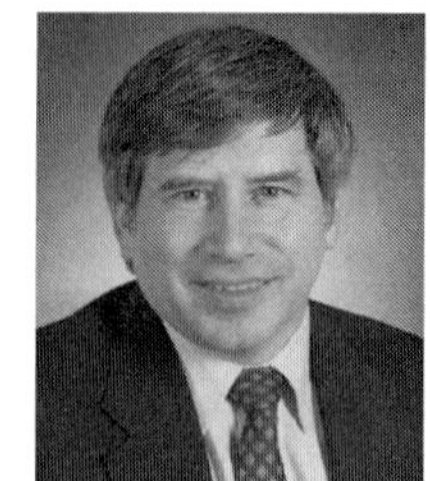

Dr. Hurst

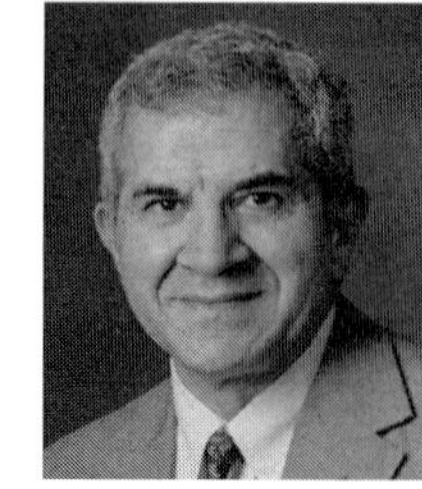

Dr. Jabaley

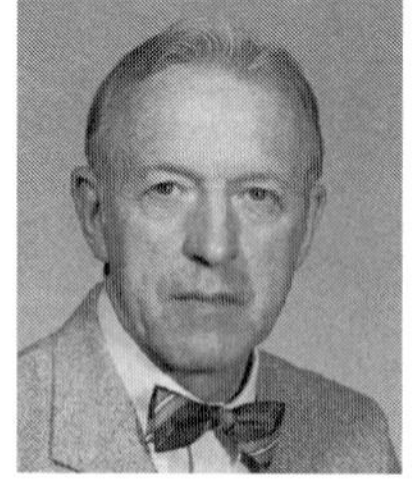

Dr. Kleinert

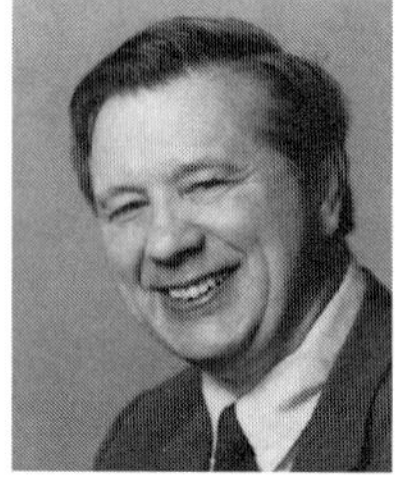

Dr. Kline

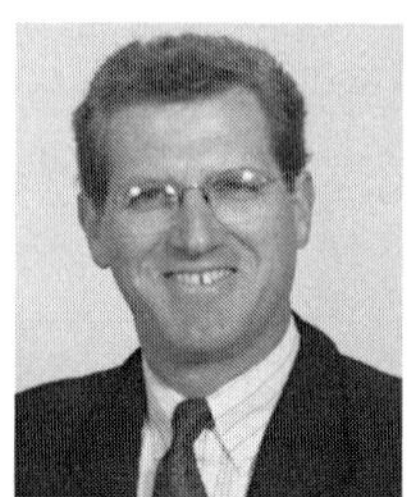

Dr. Koman

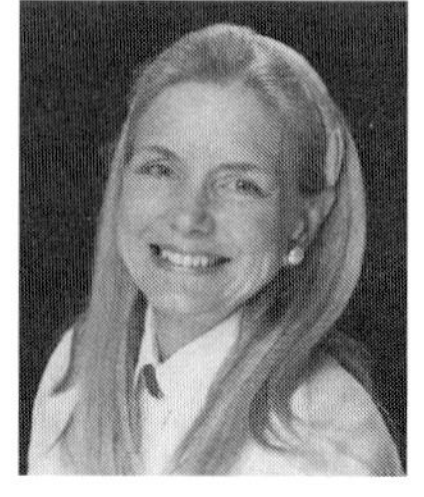

Ms. Lauckhardt
(From C. Christopher Semmes,
23 Pilgrim Drive, Greenwich,
Connecticut 06831-4925. ©
May 1, 1996, C.S. photo #
2¼-12. All rights reserved)

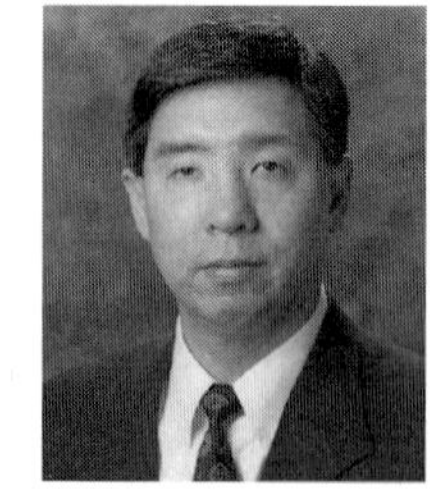

Dr. Lee

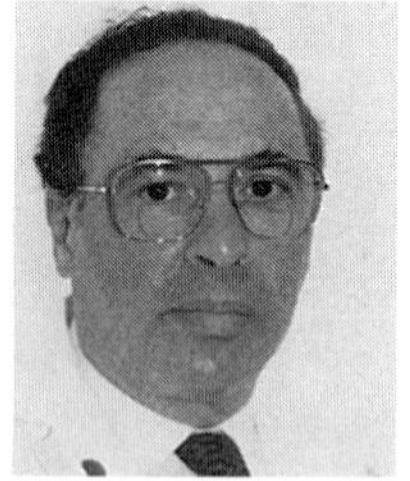

Dr. Leffert

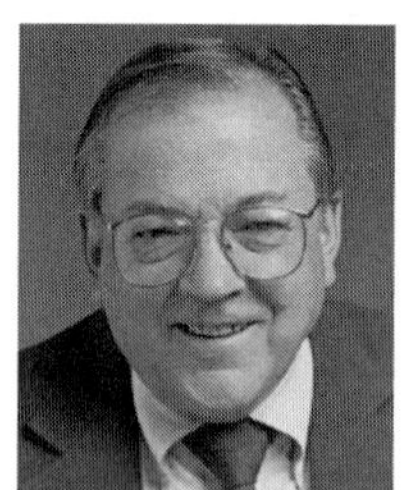

Dr. Louis

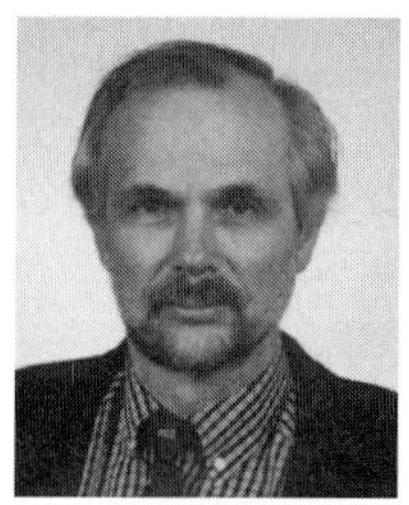

Dr. Lundborg

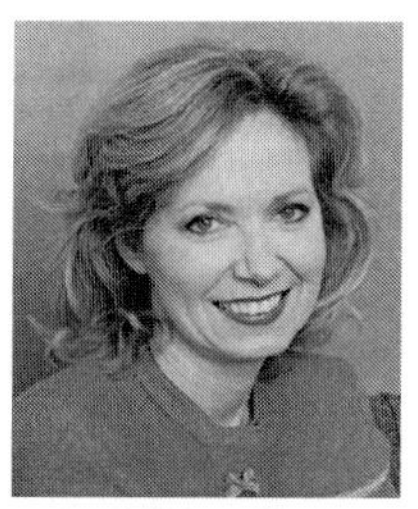

Dr. Mackinnon

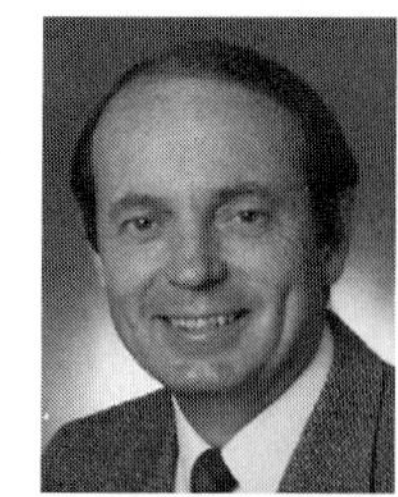

Dr. Manktelow

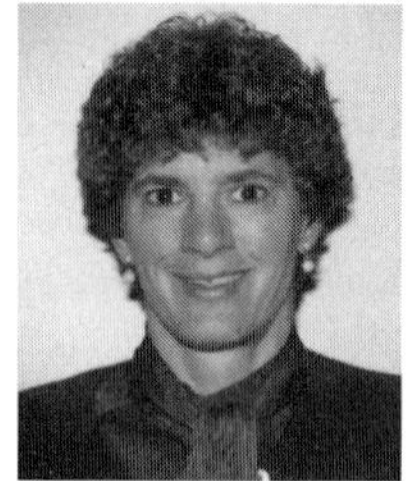

Dr. Masear

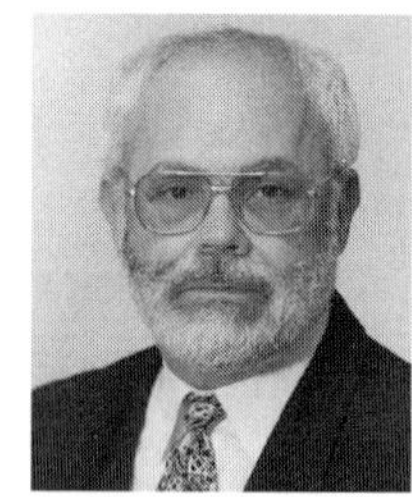

Dr. Meyer

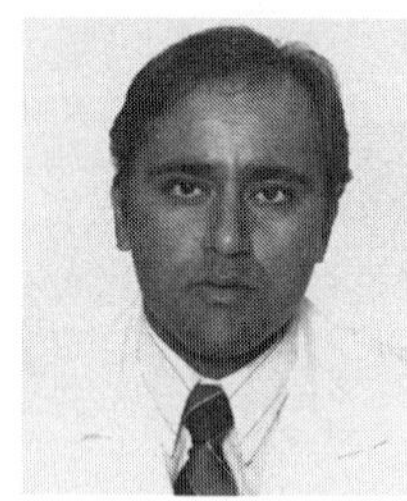

Dr. Midha

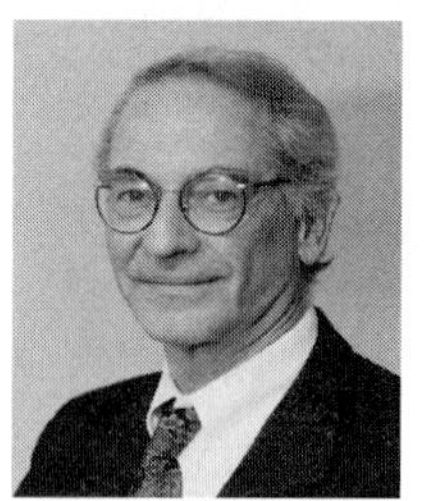

Dr. Millender

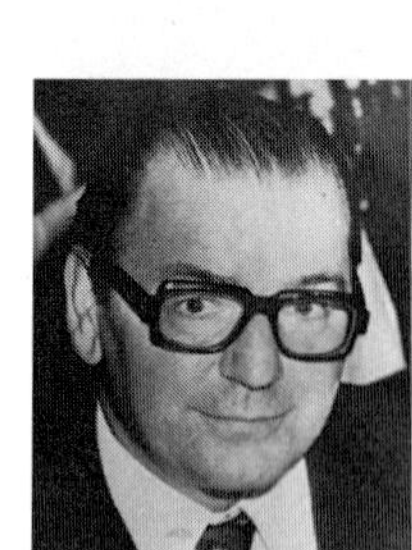

Dr. Millesi

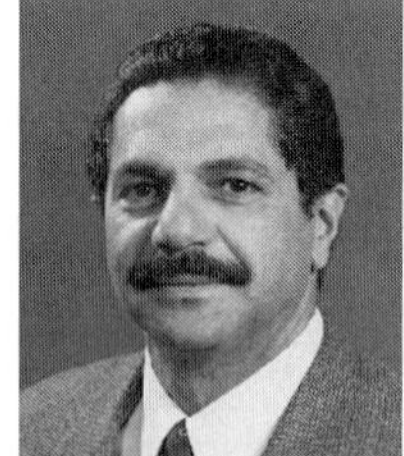

Dr. Moneim

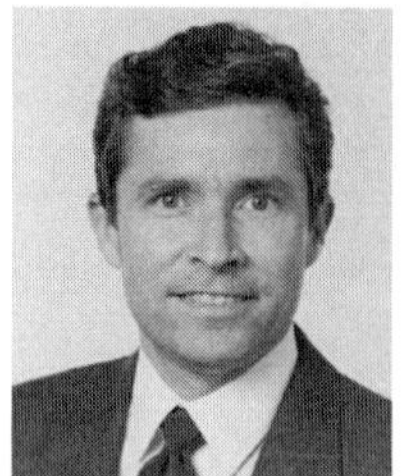

Dr. Nolan

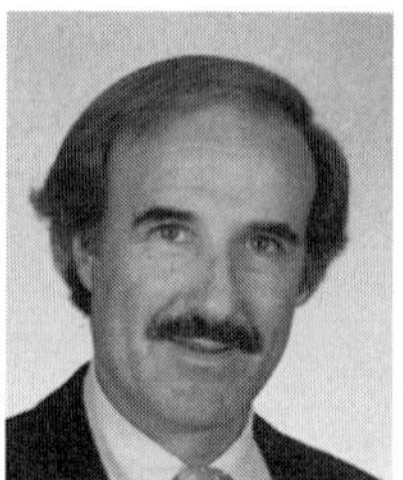

Dr. Ochoa

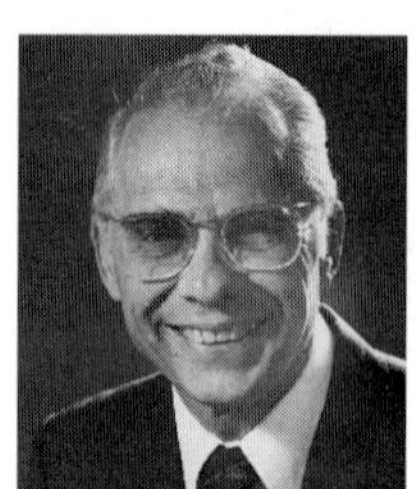

Dr. Omer

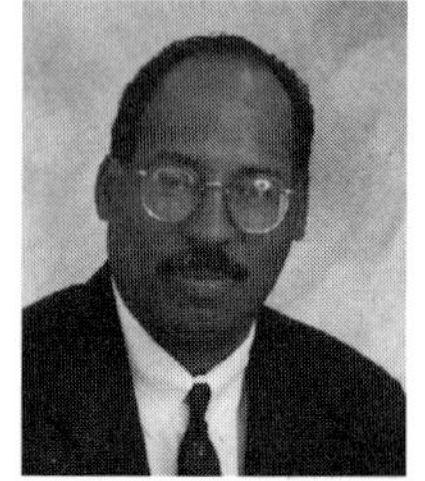

Dr. Pirela-Cruz

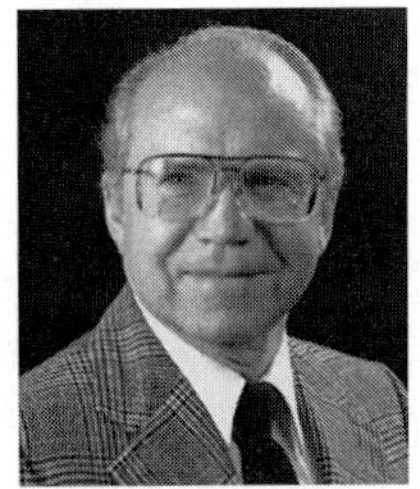

Dr. Ray

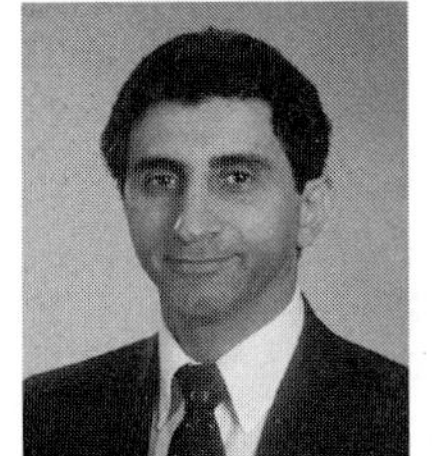

Dr. Rayan

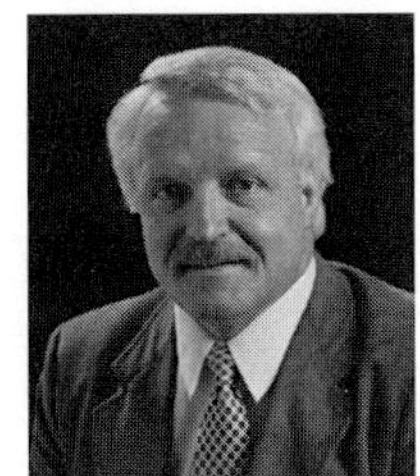

Dr. Russell

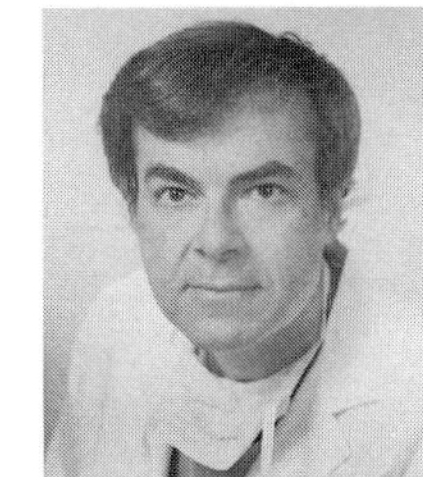

Dr. Salisbury

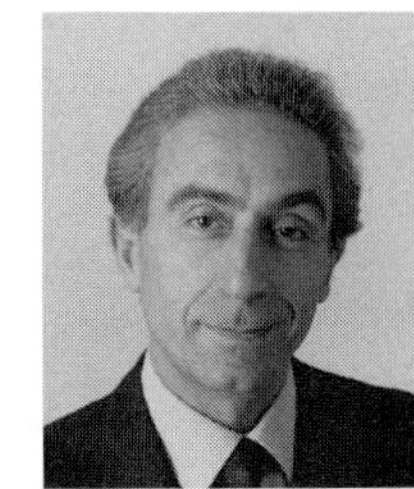

Dr. Samii

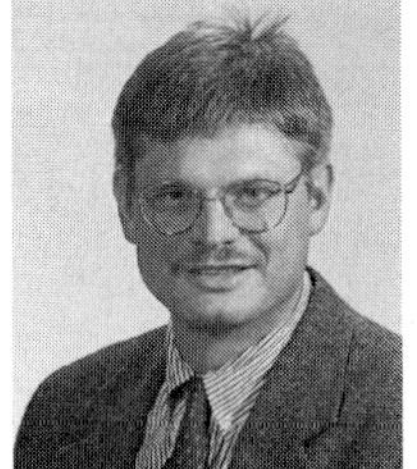

Dr. Schubert

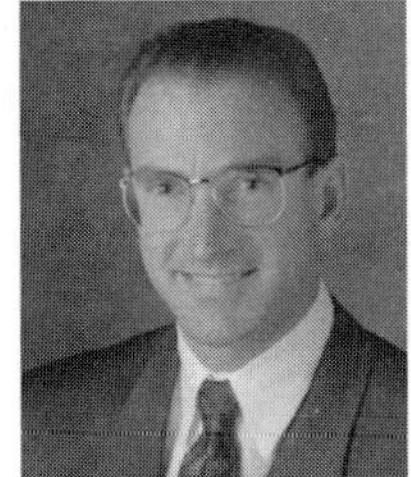

Dr. Schultz

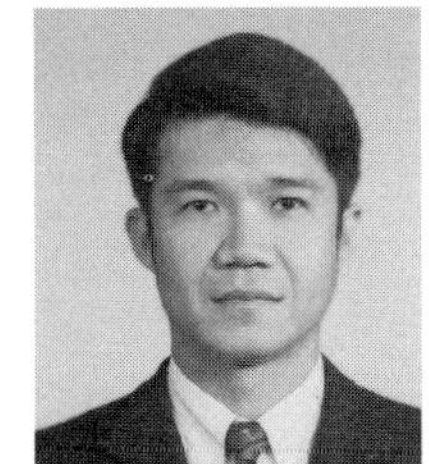

Dr. Songcharoen

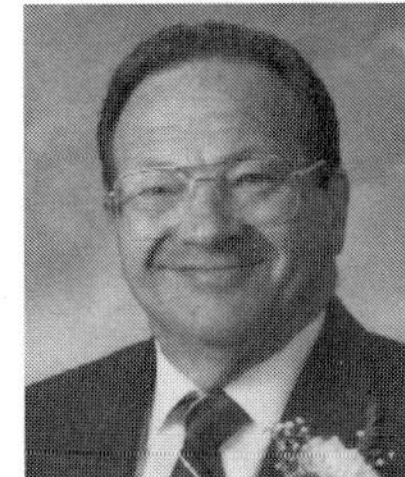

Dr. M. Spinner

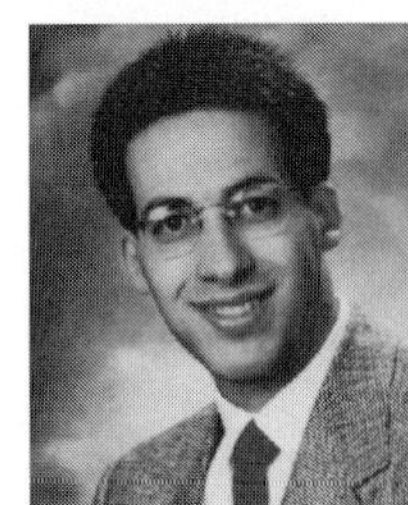

Dr. R. Spinner

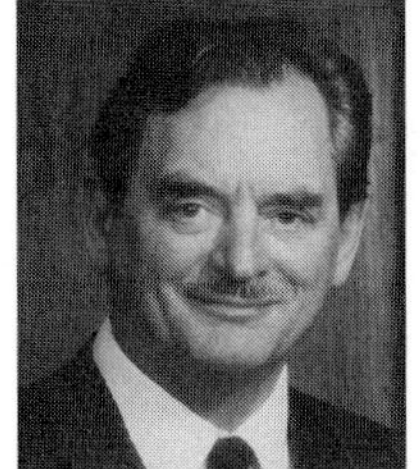

Dr. A. Swanson

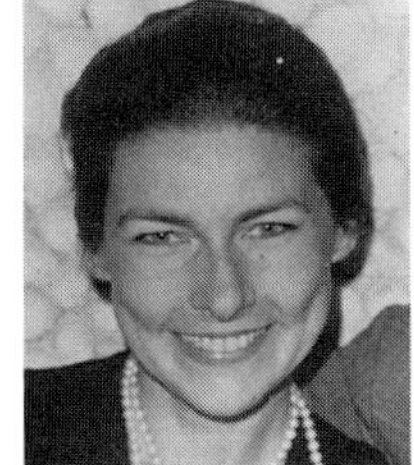

Dr. G. Swanson

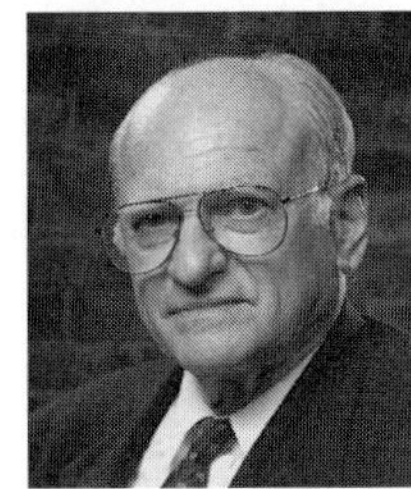

Dr. Tupper
(Photographed by G. Paul
Bishop, Jr., 2125 Durant Ave,
Berkeley, California 94704.)

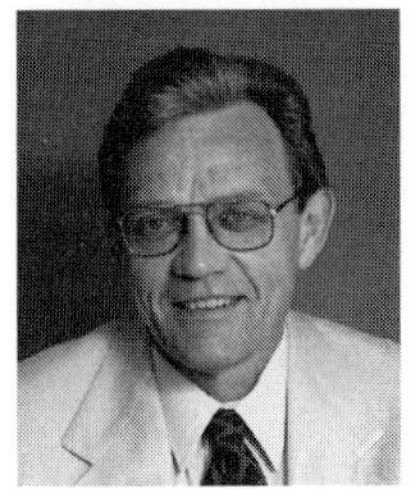

Dr. Van Beek

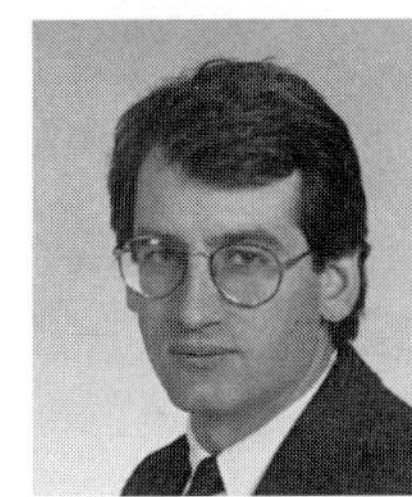

Dr. Watchmaker

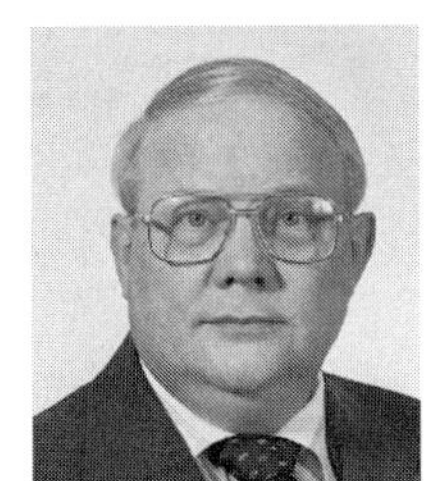

Dr. Wilbourn

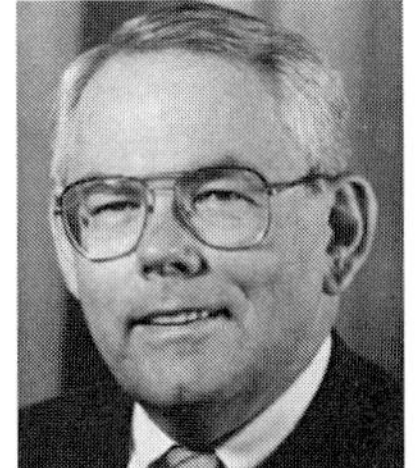

Dr. Wilgis

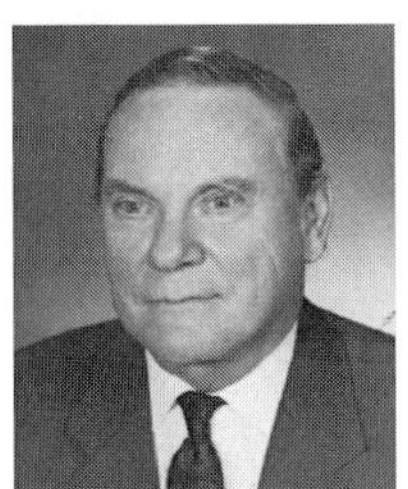

Dr. Williams

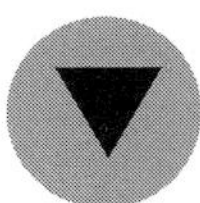

Contributors

Adel R. Abadir, M.D.
Clinical Professor of Anesthesia, New York University
Medical Center; Director, Department of Anesthesia,
Director, Residency Training Program, The Brookdale
University Hospital and Medical Center; Delegate, New
York Academy of Medicine, New York, New York
Diagnostic Nerve Blocks

Edward Almquist, M.D.
Clinical Professor, Department of Orthopedics, University
of Washington School of Medicine; Director, Hand Surgery,
Children's Hospital; Attending Physician, Swedish Hospital,
Seattle, Washington
*Adjuncts to Suture Repair of Peripheral Nerves: Laser, Glue,
and Other Techniques*

Robert G. Anderson, M.D., F.A.C.S.
Clinical Assistant Professor of Plastic Surgery, Department
of Plastic Surgery, University of Texas Southwestern
Medical School at Dallas, Dallas, Texas; Director, Facial
Paralysis Treatment Center, Fort Worth, Texas
*Normal and Anomalous Innervation Patterns of the Face and
Neck*

Nabih R. Asal, Ph.D.
David Ross Boyd Professor and Chair, Department of
Biostatistics and Epidemiology, College of Public Health,
University of Oklahoma, Health Sciences Center, Oklahoma
City, Oklahoma
*Epidemiology and Economic Impact of Compression
Neuropathy*

Erdoğan Atasoy, M.D.
Associate Clinical Professor of Surgery, University of
Louisville School of Medicine; Active Staff, Jewish
Hospital, Louisville, Kentucky
*Surgical Sympathectomy and Sympathetic Blocks for the
Upper and Lower Extremities, and Local and Plexus Levels*

Marie A. Badalamente, Ph.D.
Professor, Department of Orthopaedics, State University of
New York at Stony Brook, Stony Brook, New York
*Histochemical Aids to Control Specificity in Peripheral Nerve
Repair*

Janette T. Baker, B.S., O.T.R., C.H.T.
Clinical Specialist, Occupational Therapy, University of
Michigan Hospital, Ann Arbor, Michigan
*Rehabilitation Techniques for Patients with Occupational
Disorders*

Catherine E. Basil, B.S.
Occupational Therapist, Certified Hand Therapist, Clinical
Specialist, University of Michigan Hospital, Ann Arbor,
Michigan
*Rehabilitation Techniques for Patients with Occupational
Disorders*

Judith A. Bell-Krotoski, O.T.R., C.H.T., F.A.O.T.A.
Captain, Clinical Research Hand Therapist/Chief, Hand and
Occupational Therapy Department, Rehabilitation
Research Department, U.S. Public Health Service, Gillis W.
Long Hansen's Disease Center, Carville, Louisiana
*Sensibility Testing; Evaluation of Nerve Gaps: Upper and
Lower Extremities*

A. Griswold Bevin, M.D.
Professor of Surgery, Chief of Plastic and Reconstructive
Surgery (Retired), Department of Surgery, University of
North Carolina at Chapel Hill, School of Medicine, Chapel
Hill, North Carolina
Burn-Induced Peripheral Nerve Injury

William F. Blair, M.D.
Steindler Orthopaedic Clinic, Iowa City, Iowa
Clinical Motor Function Testing—Lower Extremity

Paula C. Bohr, Ph.D., O.T.R/C, F.A.O.T.A.
Instructor, Program in Occupational Therapy, Washington
University School of Medicine, St. Louis, Missouri
*Epidemiology and Economic Impact of Compression
Neuropathy*

Ekkehard Bonatz, M.D., F.A.C.S.
Assistant Professor of Surgery, Division of Orthopaedic
Surgery, University of Alabama, Birmingham, Alabama
*Painful Neuromas of the Lower Extremity and
Postneurectomy Pain*

Michael J. Botte, M.D.
Associate Professor of Orthopaedic Surgery, Director,
Hand and Foot Surgery Section, Department of
Orthopaedics, University of California, San Diego, School
of Medicine, San Diego, California
Management of the Cerebral Palsy Patient

J. Brian Boyd, M.B., Ch.B., M.D., F.R.C.S., F.R.C.S.C., F.A.C.S.
Chairman, Department of Plastic Surgery, Cleveland Clinic
Florida, Fort Lauderdale, Florida
Sensation-Bearing Flaps

Paul W. Brand, M.B., B.S. (Lond.) F.R.C.S. (Eng.)
Clinical Professor Emeritus, Department of Orthopedics,
University of Washington, Seattle, Washington
Management of Sensory Loss in the Extremities

Richard M. Braun, M.D.
Associate Clinical Professor of Orthopaedic Surgery, University of California, San Diego; Instructor in Orthopaedic Surgery, University of Southern California, Rancho Los Amigos Hospital, Downey; Consultant in Orthopaedic Surgery—Hand Surgery, U.S. Navy Medical Center—Balboa, San Diego; Active Staff, Sharp Memorial Hospital, Mercy Hospital, Alvarado Hospital, San Diego, California
Quantitative Measurement of Hand Function: Application to Medical Decision-Making and Return to the Workplace After Cumulative Nerve Trauma

Warren C. Breidenbach, M.D.
Assistant Clinical Professor of Surgery (Plastic and Reconstructive), University of Louisville, School of Medicine, Louisville, Kentucky
Vascularized Nerve Grafts

Richard E. Brown, M.D., F.A.C.S.
Associate Professor, Division of Plastic Surgery, Southern Illinois University School of Medicine, Springfield, Illinois
Endoscopic Carpal Tunnel Release

Giovanni R. Brunelli, M.D.
Senior Assistant, Department of Orthopaedics, Spedali Civili, Brescia, Italy
Lower Extremity Nerve Topography (Sciatic and Femoral Nerve); Direct Muscle Neurotization

Giorgio A. Brunelli, M.D.
Professor and Chairman, Department of Orthopaedics, Brescia University Medical School, Brescia, Italy
Lower Extremity Nerve Topography (Sciatic and Femoral Nerve); Direct Muscle Neurotization

Thomas Marshall Brushart, M.D.
Associate Professor of Orthopaedic Surgery, Plastic Surgery and Neurology, The Johns Hopkins University, Baltimore, Maryland
Trophic and Tropic Influences on Peripheral Nerve Regeneration

Mary Burns, O.T.R./L., C.H.T.
Assistant Professor, Department of Surgery, Southern Illinois University School of Medicine, Springfield, Illinois
Clinical Motor Function Testing—Upper Extremity

John J. Callaghan, M.D.
Professor, Department of Orthopaedic Surgery, University of Iowa Hospitals and Clinics, Iowa City, Iowa
Clinical Motor Function Testing—Lower Extremity

David T.W. Chiu, M.D., F.A.C.S.
Thomas S. Zimmer Professor of Surgery, Columbia University, College of Physicians and Surgeons; Director, Microsurgery Center, Columbia-Presbyterian Medical Center, New York, New York
Autogenous and Synthetic Conduits for Nerve Repair

James D. Collins, M.D., M.A.
Professor of Radiological Sciences, UCLA Medical School; UCLA Olive View Medical Center, American College of Radiology, Los Angeles, California
Bilateral Magnetic Resonance Imaging of the Brachial Plexus and Peripheral Nerve Imaging: Technique and Three-Dimensional Color

Eugene E. Curry, M.D.
W. D. Carrell Memorial Clinic, Dallas, Texas
Tendon Transfers as Reconstructive Procedures in the Leg and Foot Following Peripheral Nerve Injuries

Lars Dahlin, M.D., Ph.D.
Associate Professor, Department of Hand Surgery, Malmö University Hospital, Lund University, Malmö, Sweden
Pathophysiology of Peripheral Nerve Trauma

Harold M. Dick, M.D.
Frank E. Stinchfield Professor and Chairman, Department of Orthopaedic Surgery, Director of Services, Orthopaedic Surgery, Columbia-Presbyterian Medical Center, New York, New York
Management of Peripheral Nerve Tumors

Anthony C. Disher, M.D.
Assistant Professor, Charles R. Drew University of Medicine and Science, Physician Specialist, King/Drew Medical Center, Department of Radiology, Los Angeles, California
Bilateral Magnetic Resonance Imaging of the Brachial Plexus and Peripheral Nerve Imaging: Technique and Three-Dimensional Color

Sandra Doehr, M.S., O.T.R., C.H.T.
Hand Center, San Diego, California
Quantitative Measurement of Hand Function: Application to Medical Decision-Making and Return to the Workplace After Cumulative Nerve Trauma

René Dom, M.D., Ph.D.
Professor, Faculty of Medicine, Catholic University of Leuven, Belgium; Head of Clinic Department of Neurology; Director, Division of Neuropathology, University Hospital Gasthuisberg, Leuven, Belgium
Contemporary Muscle Morphology as Related to Nerve Pathology

Richard G. Eaton, M.D.
Associate Professor, Department of Surgery, Columbia University College of Physicians and Surgeons; Director, Hand Center, Roosevelt Hospital, New York, New York
Painful Neuromas of the Upper Extremity and Postneurectomy Pain

Carl Damian Enna, M.D., F.A.C.S., F.I.C.S.
Associate Clinical Professor of the Department of Anatomy, Louisiana State University School of Medicine, New Orleans; Chief, Department of Surgery and Clinical Branch (Retired), U.S.P.H.S. Hospital (National Leprosarium), Carville, Louisiana
The Management of Leprous Neuritis

Richard H. Gelberman, M.D.
Fred C. Reynolds Professor, Department of Orthopaedic Surgery, Washington University School of Medicine; Chairman, Orthopaedic Surgery, Barnes-Jewish-Christian Children's Hospital System, St. Louis, Missouri
Management of the Cerebral Palsy Patient

Fred Gentili, M.D., F.R.C.S.(C.), F.A.C.S.
Associate Professor, Department of Surgery, University of Toronto, Toronto, Ontario, Canada
Peripheral Nerve Injection Injury

J. Leonard Goldner, M.D.
James B. Duke Professor Emeritus, Department of Orthopaedic Surgery, Duke University Medical Center, Durham, North Carolina
The Effect of Extremity Blood Flow on Pain and Cold Tolerance; Nerve Entrapment Syndromes of the Low Back and Lower Extremities

John S. Gould, M.D.
Clinical Professor of Orthopaedic Surgery, University of Virginia School of Medicine, Charlottesville, Virginia; Director of Foot and Ankle Fellowship Program, American Sports Medicine Institute, Alabama Sports Medicine and Orthopaedic Center, Health South Medical Center, Birmingham, Alabama
Tendon Transfers as Reconstructive Procedures in the Leg and Foot Following Peripheral Nerve Injuries

Paul J. Guelinckx, M.D., Ph.D.
Professor of Plastic and Reconstructive Surgery, Faculty of Medicine, Catholic University of Leuven; Head of Clinic Department of Plastic and Reconstructive Surgery, Hand and Microsurgery, University Hospital Gasthuisberg, Leuven, Belgium
Contemporary Muscle Morphology as Related to Nerve Pathology

Abhijit Guha, M.D., F.R.C.S.(C.), F.A.C.S.
Associate Professor, Department of Surgery, University of Toronto, Toronto, Ontario, Canada
Peripheral Nerve Injection Injury

Reginald L. Hall, M.D.
Assistant Professor, Department of Orthopaedic Surgery, Duke University Medical Center, Durham, North Carolina
Nerve Entrapment Syndromes of the Low Back and Lower Extremities

Carter Harsh, B.A., M.D.
Active Staff, St. Vincent's Hospital, Birmingham, Alabama; Walker Baptist and Regional Medical Center, Jasper, Alabama
Lower Extremity Nerve Injuries

Vincent R. Hentz, M.D.
Professor of Functional Restoration (Hand Surgery), Stanford University; Chief of Division of Hand Surgery, Stanford University Health Services, Stanford, California
Brachial Plexus Injuries

Christine M. Hoban, B.S.
Hand Therapist, Occupational Therapy Department, Piedmont Therapy, Frye Regional Medical Center, Hickory, North Carolina
Rehabilitation Techniques for Patients with Occupational Disorders

James A. Hoffman, M.D., D.D.S.
Clinical Instructor, Plastic and Reconstructive Surgery, University of Minnesota Medical School, Division of Plastic and Reconstructive Surgery, Minneapolis, Minnesota
Nerve Lengthening Using Balloon Expansion

Alan R. Hudson, M.B., F.R.R.C.S.
Professor, Division of Neurosurgery; President and CEO, The Toronto Hospital, University of Toronto, Toronto, Ontario, Canada
Peripheral Nerve Injection Injury

Lawrence C. Hurst, M.D.
Professor and Chairman; Chief, Division of Hand Surgery and Microsurgery, Department of Orthopaedics, State University of New York at Stony Brook, Stony Brook, New York
Histochemical Aids to Control Specificity in Peripheral Nerve Repair

Jurgen Hussmann, M.D.
Chief, Division of Plastic Surgery and Hand Surgery, Park-Klinik Weissensee; Faculty of Charité University Hospital, Humboldt University, Berlin
Clinical Motor Function Testing—Upper Extremity

Michael E. Jabaley, M.D., F.A.C.S.
Professor (Clinical) of Plastic and Orthopaedic Surgery, University of Mississippi School of Medicine; Plastic Surgery Associates, Jackson, Mississippi
Pertinent Internal Topography of Peripheral Nerves

Daniel Kim, B.S., M.D.
Salem Hospital, Valley Community Hospital, Santiam Memorial Hospital, Salem, Oregon
Lower Extremity Nerve Injuries

Harold E. Kleinert, M.D.
Clinical Professor of Surgery, University of Louisville School of Medicine, Louisville, Kentucky; Clinical Professor of Surgery, Indiana University–Purdue University, School of Medicine, Indianapolis, Indiana
Surgical Sympathectomy and Sympathetic Blocks for the Upper and Lower Extremities, and Local and Plexus Levels

David G. Kline, A.B., M.D.
Boyd Professor and Chairman, Department of Neurosurgery, Louisiana State University Medical Center; Active Staff, Charity and University Hospitals (MCLNO); Academic Staff, Ochsner Hospital; Consultant, New Orleans Veterans Administration Hospital, Baptist, Tuoro, and New Orleans, Louisiana; Keesler Air Force Base Hospitals, Mississippi
Evaluation of the Neuroma in Continuity; Peripheral Nerve Injection Injury; Lower Extremity Nerve Injuries

L. Andrew Koman, M.D.
Professor and Vice Chairman, Department of Orthopaedic
Surgery, Bowman Gray School of Medicine of Wake Forest
University; Staff, North Carolina Baptist Hospital, Winston-
Salem, North Carolina
*The Effect of Extremity Blood Flow on Pain and Cold
Tolerance*

George H. Landis, M.D.
Assistant Professor, Division of Plastic & Reconstructive
Surgery, University of Minnesota; Chief of Plastic Surgery,
Minneapolis Veterans Affairs Medical Center, Minneapolis,
Minnesota
Reconstruction of the Replanted Upper Arm

Karen H. Prendergast Lauckhardt, M.A., P.T., C.H.T.
Attending Therapist, Greenwich Hand Therapy Center,
Greenwich, Connecticut
*Decision Pathways for the Therapist's Management of
Peripheral Nerve Injury*

Donald H. Lee, M.D.
Associate Professor, Hand Fellowship Director, Division of
Orthopaedic Surgery, University of Alabama at
Birmingham, Birmingham, Alabama
Management of Peripheral Nerve Tumors

Robert D. Leffert, M.D.
Professor of Orthopaedic Surgery, Harvard Medical
School; Chief of the Surgical Upper Extremity
Rehabilitation Unit and Visiting Orthopaedic Surgeon,
Massachusetts General Hospital, Boston, Massachusetts
*Reconstruction of the Shoulder and Elbow Following Brachial
Plexus Injury; Thoracic Outlet Syndrome*

Nancy Leonard, B.S.
San Diego, California
*Quantitative Management of Hand Function: Application to
Medical Decision-Making and Return to the Workplace After
Cumulative Nerve Trauma*

Robert E. Lins, M.D.
Hand Treatment Center, Atlanta, Georgia
Management of the Cerebral Palsy Patient

Aldo A. Lombardo, M.D.
Assistant Clinical Professor of Surgery, New York Medical
College; Attending Physician, Westchester County Medical
Center, Valhalla, New York
Burn-Induced Peripheral Nerve Injury

Dean S. Louis, M.D.
Professor of Surgery, University of Michigan Medical
Center; Chief, Orthopaedic Hand Service, University of
Michigan Hospitals, Ann Arbor, Michigan
*Rehabilitation Techniques for Patients with Occupational
Disorders*

Göran Lundborg, M.D., Ph.D.
Professor, Department of Hand Surgery, Malmö University
Hospital, Lund University, Malmö, Sweden
Pathophysiology of Peripheral Nerve Trauma

Susan E. Mackinnon, M.D.
Professor of Surgery, Chief, Division of Plastic Surgery,
Washington University School of Medicine; Barnes-Jewish
Hospital, St. Louis, Missouri
Evaluation of Nerve Gaps: Upper and Lower Extremities

Ralph T. Manktelow, M.D.
Professor, Department of Surgery, University of Toronto;
Chief of Hand Program, University of Toronto Hospital,
Toronto, Ontario, Canada
Microneurovascular Free Muscle Transfer

Victoria R. Masear, M.D.
Clinical Associate Professor of Orthopaedic Surgery,
University of Alabama, Birmingham, Alabama
*Painful Neuromas of the Lower Extremity and
Postneurectomy Pain*

Richard Meyer, M.D.
Associate Professor of Orthopaedics, Department of
Surgery; Staff Surgeon, University Hospital, The University
of Alabama at Birmingham, Birmingham, Alabama
Treatment of Obstetrical Palsy

Rajiv Midha, M.D., M.Sc., F.R.C.S.(C.)
Assistant Professor, Division of Neurosurgery, University of
Toronto; Staff Surgeon, Sunnybrook Health Sciences
Centre, North York, Toronto, Canada
*Evaluation of the Neuroma in Continuity; Peripheral Nerve
Injection Injury*

Lewis H. Millender, M.D.*
Late Clinical Professor, Department of Orthopaedic
Surgery, Tufts University, Boston, Massachusetts
*Neurological Involvement of the Extremities Associated with
Rheumatoid Arthritis*

Theodore Q. Miller, M.D.
Professor, Charles R. Drew University of Medicine and
Science; Senior Physician, King/Drew Medical Center,
Department of Radiology, Los Angeles, California
*Bilateral Magnetic Resonance Imaging of the Brachial Plexus
and Peripheral Nerve Imaging: Technique and Three-
Dimensional Color*

H. Millesi, M.D.
Professor Emeritus of Plastic Surgery, University of Vienna
Medical School; Medical Director, Vienna Private Hospital;
Chairman, Ludwig Boltzmann Institute for Experimental
Plastic Surgery, Vienna, Austria
*Nerve Grafts: Indications, Techniques, and Prognoses;
Trauma Involving the Brachial Plexus*

Moheb S. A. Moneim, M.D., F.R.C.S.(C.)
Professor and Chairman, Department of Orthopaedics and
Rehabilitation; Chief, Division of Hand Surgery and the
George E. Omer, Jr., M.D. Professor, The School of
Medicine, University of New Mexico; Medical Director,
School of Physical Therapy and School of Occupational
Therapy; Chief, Orthopaedics, University of New Mexico
Health Sciences Center, Albuquerque, New Mexico
*Clinical Outcome Following Acute Nerve Repair;
Conventional (Open) Carpal Tunnel Release*

---

*Deceased.

William B. Nolan, III, M.D.
Assistant Professor of Surgery; Director, New York Hospital—Cornell Hand Center, Cornell University, New York, New York
Painful Neuromas of the Upper Extremity and Postneurectomy Pain

José L. Ochoa, M.D., Ph.D., D.Sc. (London)
Professor of Neurology and Professor of Surgery (Neurology), Oregon Health Sciences University; Director, Neuromuscular Disease Unit, Good Samaritan Hospital and Medical Center, Portland, Oregon
Nerve Fiber Pathology in Acute and Chronic Compression

Martin J. O'Malley, M.D.
Assistant Professor of Surgery—Orthopaedic, Cornell University Medical College; Assistant Attending Surgeon, Orthopedic Hospital for Special Surgery, New York, New York
Neurological Involvement of the Extremities Associated with Rheumatoid Arthritis

George E. Omer, Jr., M.D., M.S., F.A.C.S.
Colonel, Medical Corps, U.S. Army (Ret), Professor Emeritus of Orthopaedics and Chairman Emeritus, Department of Orthopaedics and Rehabilitation, Professor and Chief Emeritus, Division of Hand Surgery, Professor Emeritus of Anatomy and Surgery, University of New Mexico School of Medicine, Medical Director, Emeritus, School of Physical Therapy, The University of New Mexico Health Sciences Center, Consultant Hand Surgeon, The Carrie Tingley Childrens Hospital, Lovelace Hospital, Presbyterian Hospital, University Hospital, and the Veterans Administration Medical Center, The University of New Mexico Health Sciences Center, Albuquerque, New Mexico; Past President, The Sunderland Peripheral Nerve Society; Past President, The American Society for Surgery of the Hand, Past President, The American Orthopaedic Association, Past President, The American Board of Orthopaedic Surgery, Past President, The Western Orthopaedic Association
Peripheral Nerve Injuries; Sensibility Testing; Continuous Peripheral Epineural Infusion for the Treatment of Acute Pain; The Evaluation of Clinical Results Following Peripheral Nerve Suture; The Prognosis for Untreated Traumatic Injuries; Peripheral Nerve Injuries and Gunshot Wounds; Clinical Outcome Following Acute Nerve Repair; Conventional (Open) Carpal Tunnel Release; Reconstruction of the Forearm and Hand After Peripheral Nerve Injuries; Reconstruction of the Replanted Upper Arm

Miguel A. Pirela-Cruz, M.D., F.A.C.S.
Medical Director, Orthopedic Center; Hand, Upper Extremity and Microsurgical Consultant for Memorial Medical Center, Las Cruces, New Mexico
Surgical Exposures of the Peripheral Nerves in the Extremities; Microsurgical Nerve Repairs

Charles D. Ray, M.D., F.A.C.S., F.R.S.H. (Lond.)
Director, Research and Development, Spinal Research and Education Foundation, Norfolk, Virginia
Spinal Cord and Peripheral Nerve Stimulation for Management of Peripheral Pain

Ghazi M. Rayan, M.D.
Clinical Professor of Orthopedic Surgery, University of Oklahoma Health Sciences Center; Director of Oklahoma Hand Surgery Fellowship Program, Chairman, Hand Surgery Division, Baptist Medical Center, Oklahoma City, Oklahoma
Epidemiology and Economic Impact of Compression Neuropathy

Robert C. Russell, M.D., F.R.A.C.S., F.A.C.S.
Professor of Surgery, Institute for Plastic and Reconstructive Surgery, Southern Illinois University School of Medicine, Springfield, Illinois; Medical Staff, Memorial Medical Center, Springfield, Illinois, St. John's Hospital, Springfield, Illinois, Illini Hospital, Pittsfield, Illinois
Clinical Motor Function Testing—Upper Extremity

Roger E. Salisbury, M.D.
Professor of Surgery; Chief, Plastic and Reconstructive Surgery, New York Medical College; Director, Burn Center; Chief, Plastic and Reconstructive Surgery, Westchester County Medical Center, Valhalla, New York
Burn-Induced Peripheral Nerve Injury

Madjid Samii, M.D.
Professor of Neurosurgery, Hannover Medical School; Professor and Chairman, Head of Department of Neurosurgery, Center of Neurology, Hannover Medical School Hospital; Head of Department of Neurosurgery, Nordstadt Hospital, Hannover, Germany
Diagnosis and Management of Intracranial Nerve Lesions

Warren Schubert, M.D.
Assistant Professor, University of Minnesota; Chairman, Department of Plastic and Reconstructive Surgery, St. Paul Ramsey Medical Center, St. Paul, Minnesota
Trauma Involving the Key Motor and Sensory Nerves of the Face

David Schultz, M.D., D.A.C.P.M.
Assistant Clinical Professor, Department of Anesthesiology, University of Minnesota; Medical Director, Medical Advanced Pain Specialists, Minneapolis, Minnesota
Indications for Utilization of a Pain Clinic

Marla L. Shaver, M.D.
Instructor, Charles R. Drew University School of Medicine and Science; Fellow, King/Drew Medical Center, Department of Radiology, Los Angeles, California
Bilateral Magnetic Resonance Imaging of the Brachial Plexus and Peripheral Nerve Imaging: Technique and Three-Dimensional Color

Robert W. Shields, Jr., M.D.
Staff Neurologist, Cleveland Clinic Foundation, Cleveland, Ohio
Generalized Polyneuropathies and Other Nonsurgical Peripheral Nervous System Disorders

Aamir Siddiqui, B.A., M.D.
Plastic Surgery Fellow, University of Minnesota, Minneapolis, Minnesota
Microneurovascular Free Muscle Transfer

Nadia K. Sinsel, M.D.
Research Fellowship of National Institute for Scientific Research (N.F.W.O.), Catholic University of Leuven Belgium; Assistant in Plastic and Reconstructive Surgery, Hand and Microsurgery, University Hospital Gasthuisberg, Leuven, Belgium
Contemporary Muscle Morphology as Related to Nerve Pathology

Thomas L. Smith, M.S., Ph.D.
Associate Professor, Department of Orthopaedic Surgery, Bowman Gray School of Medicine of Wake Forest University, Winston-Salem, North Carolina
The Effect of Extremity Blood Flow on Pain and Cold Tolerance

Panupan Songcharoen, M.D.
Associate Professor, Chief of Hand and Microsurgery Unit, Department of Orthopaedic Surgery, Faculty of Medicine, Siriraj Hospital, Mahidol University, Bangkok, Thailand
Neurotization in the Treatment of Brachial Plexus Injuries

Morton Spinner, M.D., F.A.C.S.
Clinical Professor of Orthopaedic Surgery, Albert Einstein College of Medicine, Bronx, New York; Consultant in Hand Surgery, South Nassau Community Hospital, Oceanside, New York; Brookdale Hospital Medical Center, Brooklyn, New York; North Shore University Hospital, Manhasset, New York; Past President, The Sunderland Peripheral Nerve Society
Peripheral Nerve Problems—Past, Present, and Future; Management of Nerve Compression Lesions of the Upper Extremity

Robert J. Spinner, M.D.
Department of Neurologic Surgery, Mayo Clinic, Rochester, Minnesota
Management of Nerve Compression Lesions of the Upper Extremity

Alfred B. Swanson, M.D.
Professor of Surgery, Michigan State University, East Lansing, Michigan; Director of Orthopaedic Surgery Residency Training Program of the Grand Rapids Hospitals, Director of Hand Surgery Fellowship and Orthopaedic Research, Blodgett Memorial Medical Center, Grand Rapids, Michigan
Impairment Evaluation of the Peripheral Nerve System of the Upper Extremity

Geneviève de Groot Swanson, M.D.
Assistant Clinical Professor of Surgery, Michigan State University, Lansing, Michigan; Coordinator, Orthopaedic Research Department, Blodgett Memorial Medical Center, Grand Rapids, Michigan
Impairment Evaluation of the Peripheral Nerve System of the Upper Extremity

Andrew L. Terrono
Assistant Clinical Professor, Department of Orthopaedic Surgery, Tufts University School of Medicine; Department of Orthopaedic Surgery, New England Baptist Hospital, Boston, Massachusetts
Neurological Involvement of the Extremities Associated with Rheumatoid Arthritis

Robert Tiel, M.D.
Assistant Professor, Louisiana State University Medical School; Charity & University Hospital (MCLNO), Academic Staff, Ochsner Hospital, New Orleans, Louisiana
Lower Extremity Nerve Injuries

Jack W. Tupper, M.D., B.S.
Clinical Professor, Department of Orthopaedic Surgery, University of California, San Francisco, California; Chief, Hand Surgery, Summit Hospital; Chief, Hand Surgery, Children's Hospital, Oakland, California
Fascicular Nerve Repair

Allen L. Van Beek, M.D., F.A.C.S.
Clinical Associate Professor of Plastic Surgery, Department of Surgery, The University of Minnesota Hospital and Clinics, Attending Plastic Surgeon, Fairview Southdale Hospital, Minneapolis, Minnesota; Director, Plastic Surgery, North Memorial Medical Center, Robbinsdale, Minnesota; Past President, The American Society for Reconstructive Microsurgery; Past President, Minnesota Medical Society; American Society of Peripheral Nerve; Director, Plastic Surgery Education Foundation
Peripheral Nerve Injuries of the Lower Extremity; Intraoperative Nerve Stimulation and Recording Techniques; Microsurgical Nerve Repairs; Nerve Lengthening Using Balloon Expansion; Reconstruction of the Replanted Upper Arm; Microneurovascular Free Muscle Transfer

Adolfo Vigasio, M.D.
AIUTO, Department of Orthopaedics, Spedali Civili, Brescia, Italy
Lower Extremity Nerve Topography (Sciatic and Femoral Nerve)

Greg P. Watchmaker, M.D.
Megan, Wisconsin
Pertinent Internal Topography of Peripheral Nerves

Asa J. Wilbourn, M.D.
Director, EMG Laboratory, Department of Neurology, Cleveland Clinic; Associate Clinical Professor of Neurology, Case Western Reserve University, School of Medicine, Cleveland, Ohio
Generalized Neuropathies and Other Nonsurgical Peripheral Nervous System Disorders

E. F. Shaw Wilgis, M.D.
Associate Professor of Plastic Surgery, Associate Professor of Orthopaedic Surgery, The Johns Hopkins School of Medicine; Director, Raymond Curtis Hand Center, Chief, Division of Hand Surgery, Union Memorial Hospital, Baltimore, Maryland
Special Diagnostic Studies; Epineurial Repair: Technique and Long-Term Results

H. Bruce Williams, M.D., F.A.C.S., F.R.C.S.(C.)
Professor of Surgery (Plastic Surgery), McGill University; Surgeon-in-chief, Montreal Children's Hospital, Montreal, Quebec, Canada
Electrical Stimulation of Denervated Muscles

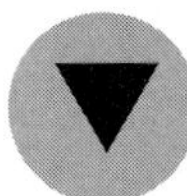

Foreword to the First Edition

The problems of management of peripheral nerve afflictions are complicated and require the participation of experts in a variety of fields. Clinical experience and a knowledge of precise morphological anatomy and physiology are essential.

The contributions of Sterling Bunnell, Sir Herbert Seddon, Sir Sydney Sunderland, and Erik Moberg in this century brought attention to the problems of peripheral nerve injuries. Their methods and techniques have spread throughout the world. They have encouraged others to investigate and study the application of the improved methods and principles which are developed in the present text.

The authors who have contributed to this edition have added distinct contributions to the surgery of peripheral nerves. It was not intended to present an encyclopaedic treatise but a practical and valuable text for general application and understanding. The purpose of this book is to indicate how to solve specific clinical problems. In addition, experimental methods to study particular aspects of the basic physiology and internal morphology of the peripheral nerves are presented. The book will be of great assistance to all who have taken up the challenge of the management of affictions of the peripheral nervous system.

I have known the editors, George Omer and Morton Spinner, for more than 25 years. I have encouraged and enjoyed their excellent progress and contributions in the area of understanding and treatment of the complicated problems that are observed in derangements of the peripheral nervous system, and I am pleased to have had a part in their development.

This work brings together experts with national and international reputations in this field. The contributors successfully present the contemporary status of the art of management of peripheral nerve problems.

EMANUEL B. KAPLAN, M.D.

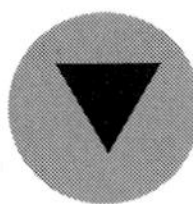

Preface to the First Edition

Peripheral nerve injuries are seen in large numbers, with major complications, during military campaigns. Our clinical interest in these devastating conditions was stimulated by surgical experience gained during the early 1950's in the Medical Corps of the United States Army. Military professional and administrative assignments during the 1960's provided an overview of the chronicity of these problems and the difficult rehabilitation process faced by these patients. The management of the civilian with a peripheral nerve injury should be individualized, but the basic professional principles remain the same during peace or war. During the 1970's, we have shared our continuing surgical experience through applied teaching, such as an ongoing Instructional Course on Peripheral Nerve Testing and Suture Techniques for the annual meetings of the American Academy of Orthopaedic Surgeons, and many Symposia on varied peripheral nerve conditions for the American Society for Sugery of the Hand. This book is the result of our accumulated experience and continuing interest in the complex clinical problems associated with peripheral nerve injury. We intend that this volume will present the current state of the art for those professionals actively involved with the management of these complex problems.

There has been a tremendous expansion in techniques and innovative concepts for the management of peripheral nerve problems that can be attributed to the practical use of microsurgery, computer technology, and the electron microscope. This makes it impossible for the individual surgeon to evaluate all available research and clinical studies; yet he must make practical decisions based on pertinent data from these sources. In an attempt to meet his need, we have selected a limited number of contributors who are recognized as being in the vanguard of research and clinical activities related to peripheral nerve disorders. We believe these contributors represent well the great number of specialists who have evolved in this complex field of medicine. We have limited the subjects for discussion to a representative cross section of the common peripheral nerve problems confronting the clinical surgeon.

For individualized reference, the book has been arranged into sections related to clinical problems. The laboratory section was designed to indicate the future for current clinical techniques and concepts.

We are indebted to our colleagues who have contributed to this book; and to Doctors Emanuel B. Kaplan, Leo Mayer, Erik Moberg, and Daniel Riordan, who have been our mentors in orthopaedics and hand surgery and peripheral nerve techniques and concepts. Our gratitude to Marleece Kendrick and Jean Fertel for their administrative assistance, and to Hugh Thomas and George Thomas for their artistic contributions. We extend credit to Doctors Mooyoung Jun and Irwin R. Cohen for editorial assistance with some specific chapters; and we recognize the research assistance of Mrs. Ada Gams and Mr. Denis Gafney of the Library of the New York Academy of Medicine. We are thankful to our wives and children for their encouragement and tolerance under the stress of many hours forfeited from family activities to this project. We also want to acknowledge the assistance and contributions of the editorial staff of W. B. Saunders Company, especially George Vilk, Carroll Cann, Charles Graham, and Andrew J. Piernock, Jr.

George E. Omer, Jr., M.D.
Morton Spinner, M.D.

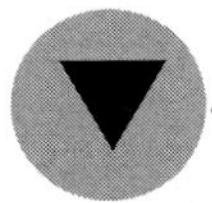

Preface to the Second Edition

This textbook is a comprehensive guide for surgeons managing peripheral nerve injuries in the upper extremity, lower extremity, face, or neck. Hand Surgeons, Orthopaedic Surgeons, Plastic Surgeons, Otolaryngologists, Microsurgeons, Neurosurgeons, and General Surgeons will find this book a useful addition to their library.

While I was working as a surgical intern at Brooke Army Medical Center in 1969, one of my rotations was on the Orthopaedic Hand Service. I first met Dr. George Omer there, and I still have a vivid memory of watching him evaluate the mutilating injuries of hundreds of Vietnam casualties. In 1969, he told me that if he was a young man, he would look into the prospects of using microscopic surgery to help reconstruct severe hand injuries. As he predicted and as a result of the development of microsurgical techniques, much has changed in the field of hand and peripheral nerve reconstruction since the Vietnam War.

I met Dr. Morton Spinner when I became a member of a peripheral nerve study group called the Sunderland Society, and I gained some insight into why Dr. Spinner has been able to delineate the nerve compression syndromes so vividly. Thorough anatomical understanding, thoughtful diagnosis, careful surgical planning, and accurate documentation are evident in all of his efforts and conversations.

Dr. Miguel Pirela-Cruz was formerly a Hunter Hand Fellow and is an accomplished medical illustrator. We are grateful for the many medical illustrations he has created for the textbook. His clinical understanding combined with the remarkable gift of being a skilled medical illustrator has provided the reader with interesting interpretations.

The opportunity to help edit this monumental text book has been both an exciting and rewarding experience. The first edition, which was published in 1980, has influenced surgeons throughout the world. The textbook had the unique perspective of outlining a method of care for nearly all of the major peripheral nerves of the body. However, some aspects of peripheral nerve surgery have changed significantly since 1980 because of the application of microsurgical principles to nerve repair and problems. Concurrent with these changes are the application of reconstructive microvascular surgery to enhance the surgeon's ability to reconstruct nerves or the deficit produced through the use of microvascular free flap transfers, microneurovascular muscle transfers, vascularized nerve transfers, and other adjunctive procedures. Readers will notice the addition of these important topics to the second edition.

Our profound gratitude to those authors who have contributed their experience and time to this book. The combined experience of our authors is daunting. Their contributions have created a book providing an experienced and knowledgeable perspective for the treatment of nerve injuries throughout the peripheral nervous system.

Our sincere thanks go to Mr. Richard Lampert and the editorial staff at W.B. Saunders Company for their advice, support, and perseverance.

For the Editors:
ALLEN L. VAN BEEK, MD

Introduction to the First Edition

Although Paul of Aegina (625–690) was the first to attempt nerve repair by approximation of the nerve stumps when closing a wound, for many centuries following, surgeons did not dare to touch the nerve stumps, being afraid that they would cause convulsions in the patient by such a maneuver. Approximation of nerve ends was achieved indirectly, *cum carne*, by approximation of the remaining soft tissue (Avicenna, 980–1037). These rules were obeyed even until the middle of the last century (Baudens, 1836; von Langenbeck, 1854).

With the introduction of the epineural nerve suture (Hueter, 1871, 1873), a new era began. Hueter suggested primary nerve repair, and Nelaton (1864) secondary nerve repair. The problem of tension at the suture site was recognized, and Mikulicz in 1882 introduced tension-relieving sutures. Loebke (1884) performed bone shortening by osteotomy to achieve coaptation without tension. Albert in 1876 grafted nerve defects, and Gluck (1880) and Büngner (1891) were pioneers in tubulization of the suture site.

The reader should be aware that all the problems discussed today had been perceived a century ago. The main contributions of modern times are microsurgery, which permits surgery within the nerve without too much punishment resulting from tissue reaction, and a more biologic approach rather than a mechanistic one. There is still no magic solution, and different situations require different attitudes and approaches. To help the practicing surgeon select the proper technique, a survey of the complete problem of peripheral nerve surgery is an ultimate necessity.

George Omer and Morton Spinner accepted the challenge to edit a volume that surveys the many problems facing the surgeon who deals with peripheral nerves. Both men are eminently qualified for this enterprise. Each is a distinguished surgeon with an outstanding scientific and professional career, and each has made remarkable contributions to the field of peripheral nerve surgery. They have succeeded in enlisting a large number of authors for the task who have risen to the challenge admirably. The 63 chapters in this book cover the problems of peripheral nerve surgery comprehensively and authoritatively.

The great experience of the editors, their excellent grasp of the subject matter, and their perceptive selection of contributors virtually ensure that the book will fulfill its task; that is, be a useful guide for the surgeon confronted with the problems of peripheral nerve surgery.

PROF. DR. HANNO MILLESI

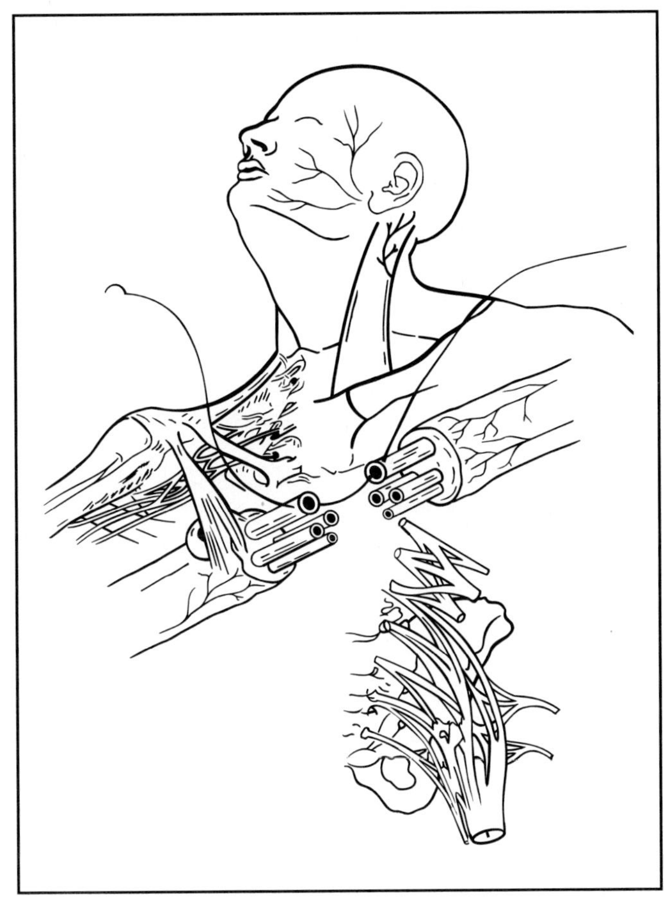

The logo on the book cover is a composite representation developed by Miguel A. Pirela-Cruz, with contributions from all the editors. Dr. Cruz combines the anatomical knowledge of an orthopaedic and hand surgeon with the conceptual abilities of a trained medical illustrator. In this logo, those peripheral nerves most subject to trauma and surgical reconstruction are illustrated. The nerves of the head and neck represent a new section of the text. Therefore, the motor and sensory nerves of the face and neck, the brachial plexus, and the lumbosacralcoccygeal plexus are outlined. An epineurial repair of a peripheral nerve is depicted, which is still the gold standard for the measurement of new techniques. All of these subjects are discussed in detail in the appropriate chapters of this text. Dr. Pirela-Cruz has illustrated several chapters on surgical approaches and specific nerve lesions.

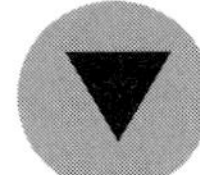

Contents

Color Plates follow page xxxii

PART I
PROLOGUE 1

Chapter 1
Peripheral Nerve Injuries: 45-Year Odyssey . . .
and the Quest Continues 3
George E. Omer, Jr

Chapter 2
Peripheral Nerve Problems—Past, Present,
and Future 7
Morton Spinner

PART II
INNERVATION PATTERNS AND DIAGNOSTIC
TECHNIQUES 9

Chapter 3
Sensibility Testing 11
George E. Omer, Jr • Judith Bell-Krotoski

Chapter 4
Trauma Involving the Key Motor and Sensory
Nerves of the Face 29
Warren Schubert

Chapter 5
Clinical Motor Function Testing—Upper
Extremity 39
Robert C. Russell • Jurgen Hussmann • Mary Burns

Chapter 6
Clinical Motor Function Testing—Lower
Extremity 50
William F. Blair • John J. Callaghan

Chapter 7
Peripheral Nerve Injuries of the Lower
Extremity 56
Allen L. Van Beek

Chapter 8
Diagnostic Nerve Blocks 65
Adel R. Abadir

Chapter 9
Special Diagnostic Studies 77
E. F. Shaw Wilgis

Chapter 10
Bilateral Magnetic Resonance Imaging of the
Brachial Plexus and Peripheral Nerve Imaging:
Technique and Three-Dimensional Color 82
James D. Collins • Marla L. Shaver • Anthony C. Disher •
Theodore Q. Miller

Chapter 11
Decision Pathways for the Therapist's
Management of Peripheral Nerve Injury 94
Karen H. Prendergast Lauckhardt

PART III
PAIN 105

Chapter 12
The Effect of Extremity Blood Flow on Pain
and Cold Tolerance 107
L. Andrew Koman • J. Leonard Goldner • Thomas L. Smith

Chapter 13
Continuous Peripheral Epineural Infusion for
the Treatment of Acute Pain 116
George E. Omer, Jr

Chapter 14
Indications for Utilization of a Pain Clinic 120
David Schultz

Chapter 15
Spinal Cord and Peripheral Nerve Stimulation
for Management of Peripheral Pain 135
Charles D. Ray

Chapter 16
Painful Neuromas of the Upper Extremity and
Postneurectomy Pain 146
William B. Nolan III • Richard G. Eaton

Chapter 17
Painful Neuromas of the Lower Extremity and
Postneurectomy Pain 151
Victoria R. Masear • Ekkehard Bonatz

Chapter 18
Surgical Sympathectomy and Sympathetic
Blocks for the Upper and Lower
Extremities, and Local and Plexus Levels 157
Erdoğan Atasoy • Harold E. Kleinert

PART IV
ANATOMICAL OVERVIEW **173**

Chapter 19
Surgical Exposures of the Peripheral
Nerves in the Extremities 175
Miguel A. Pirela-Cruz

Chapter 20
Pertinent Internal Topography of Peripheral
Nerves 210
Greg P. Watchmaker • Michael E. Jabaley

Chapter 21
Lower Extremity Nerve Topography
(Sciatic and Femoral Nerve) 217
Giorgio A. Brunelli • Adolfo Vigasio • Giovanni R. Brunelli

Chapter 22
Normal and Anomalous Innervation Patterns
of the Face and Neck 228
Robert G. Anderson

Chapter 23
Trophic and Tropic Influences on Peripheral
Nerve Regeneration 235
Thomas Marshall Brushart

Chapter 24
Histochemical Aids to Control Specificity in
Peripheral Nerve Repair 243
Lawrence C. Hurst • Marie A. Badalamente

PART V
SUTURE TECHNIQUES **249**

Chapter 25
Intraoperative Nerve Stimulation and
Recording Techniques 251
Allen L. Van Beek

Chapter 26
Microsurgical Nerve Repairs 260
Allen L. Van Beek • Miguel A. Pirela-Cruz

Chapter 27
Epineurial Repair: Technique and Long-Term
Results 271
E. F. Shaw Wilgis

Chapter 28
Fascicular Nerve Repair 274
Jack W. Tupper

Chapter 29
Nerve Grafts: Indications, Techniques,
and Prognoses 280
H. Millesi

Chapter 30
Nerve Lengthening Using Balloon Expansion 290
Allen L. Van Beek • James A. Hoffman

Chapter 31
Vascularized Nerve Grafts 295
Warren C. Breidenbach

Chapter 32
Autogenous and Synthetic Conduits For
Nerve Repair 305
David T. W. Chiu

Chapter 33
Adjuncts to Suture Repair of Peripheral
Nerves: Laser, Glue, and Other Techniques 311
Edward Almquist

Chapter 34
Evaluation of the Neuroma in Continuity 319
Rajiv Midha • David G. Kline

Chapter 35
Evaluation of Nerve Gaps: Upper and Lower
Extremities 328
Susan E. Mackinnon

Chapter 36
The Evaluation of Clinical Results Following
Peripheral Nerve Suture 340
George E. Omer, Jr • Judith Bell-Krotoski

PART VI
TRAUMA: MISSILES, LACERATIONS, TRACTION,
AND INJECTIONS **351**

Chapter 37
Pathophysiology of Peripheral Nerve Trauma 353
Göran Lundborg • Lars Dahlin

Chapter 38
The Prognosis for Untreated Traumatic
Injuries 365
George E. Omer, Jr

Chapter 39
Diagnosis and Management of Intracranial
Nerve Lesions 371
Madjid Samii

Chapter 40
Direct Muscle Neurotization 393
Giorgio A. Brunelli • Giovanni R. Brunelli

Chapter 41
Peripheral Nerve Injuries and Gunshot
Wounds 398
George E. Omer, Jr

Chapter 42
Peripheral Nerve Injection Injury 406
Rajiv Midha • Abhijit Guha • Fred Gentili •
David G. Kline • Alan R. Hudson

Chapter 43
Clinical Outcome Following Acute Nerve
Repair 414
Moheb S. A. Moneim • George E. Omer, Jr

Chapter 44
Lower Extremity Nerve Injuries 420
David G. Kline • Robert Tiel • Daniel Kim • Carter Harsh

**PART VII
BRACHIAL PLEXUS: TRAUMA AND RECONSTRUCTION 431**

Chapter 45
Trauma Involving the Brachial Plexus 433
H. Millesi

Chapter 46
Brachial Plexus Injuries 445
Vincent R. Hentz

Chapter 47
Treatment of Obstetrical Palsy 454
Richard Meyer

Chapter 48
Neurotization in the Treatment of Brachial
Plexus Injuries 459
Panupan Songcharoen

Chapter 49
Reconstruction of the Shoulder and Elbow
Following Brachial Plexus Injury 465
Robert D. Leffert

**PART VIII
COMPRESSION LESIONS 473**

Chapter 50
Nerve Fiber Pathology in Acute and Chronic
Compression 475
José L. Ochoa

Chapter 51
Epidemiology and Economic Impact of
Compression Neuropathy 484
Ghazi M. Rayan • Nabih R. Asal • Paula C. Bohr

Chapter 52
Thoracic Outlet Syndrome 494
Robert D. Leffert

Chapter 53
Management of Nerve Compression Lesions
of the Upper Extremity 501
Morton Spinner • Robert J. Spinner

Chapter 54
Conventional (Open) Carpal Tunnel Release 534
George E. Omer, Jr • Moheb S. A. Moneim

Chapter 55
Endoscopic Carpal Tunnel Release 538
Richard E. Brown

Chapter 56
Quantitative Management of Hand Function:
Application to Medical Decision-Making
and Return to the Workplace After
Cumulative Nerve Trauma 543
Richard M. Braun • Sandra Doehr • Nancy Leonard

Chapter 57
Rehabilitation Techniques for Patients with
Occupational Disorders 551
Dean S. Louis • Janette T. Baker • Christine M. Hoban •
Catherine E. Basil

Chapter 58
Nerve Entrapment Syndromes of the Low
Back and Lower Extremities 554
J. Leonard Goldner • Reginald L. Hall

PART IX
SPECIAL PROBLEMS **585**

Chapter 59
Neurological Involvement of the Extremities
Associated with Rheumatoid Arthritis 587
Lewis H. Millender (Deceased) • Andrew L. Terrono •
Martin J. O'Malley

Chapter 60
Management of Peripheral Nerve Tumors 597
Donald H. Lee • Harold M. Dick

Chapter 61
The Management of Leprous Neuritis 615
Carl Damian Enna

Chapter 62
Burn-Induced Peripheral Nerve Injury 623
Roger E. Salisbury • A. Griswold Bevin • Aldo A. Lombardo

Chapter 63
Management of the Cerebral Palsy Patient 630
Robert E. Lins • Michael J. Botte • Richard H. Gelberman

Chapter 64
Generalized Polyneuropathies and Other
Nonsurgical Peripheral Nervous
System Disorders 648
Asa J. Wilbourn • Robert W. Shields, Jr

PART X
RECONSTRUCTION **661**

Chapter 65
Contemporary Muscle Morphology as Related
to Nerve Pathology 663
Paul J. Guelinckx • Nadia K. Sinsel • René Dom

Chapter 66
Electrical Stimulation of Denervated Muscles 669
H. Bruce Williams

Chapter 67
Reconstruction of the Forearm and Hand After
Peripheral Nerve Injuries 675
George E. Omer, Jr

Chapter 68
Reconstruction of the Replanted Upper Arm 706
Allen L. Van Beek • George E. Omer, Jr • George L. Landis

Chapter 69
Tendon Transfers as Reconstructive Procedures
in the Leg and Foot Following Peripheral
Nerve Injuries 717
John S. Gould • Eugene E. Curry

Chapter 70
Microneurovascular Free Muscle Transfer 731
   Background and Clinical Application 731
   Ralph T. Manktelow

   Microvascular Fine Muscle Transfer Technique 734
   Aamir Siddiqui • Allen L. Van Beek

Chapter 71
Sensation-Bearing Flaps 745
J. Brian Boyd

Chapter 72
Management of Sensory Loss in the
Extremities 762
Paul W. Brand

Chapter 73
Impairment Evaluation of the Peripheral Nerve
System of the Upper Extremity 767
Alfred B. Swanson • Geneviève de Groot Swanson

Index 781

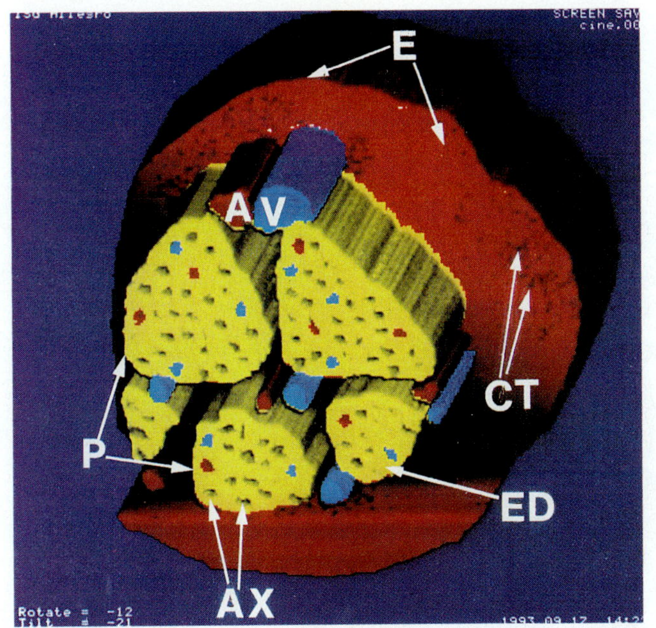

FIGURE 10–3. This is a three-dimensional, computer-generated transverse section of a peripheral nerve demonstrating the rich nutrient blood supply that Sunderland described in 1945. The collateral blood vessels have been omitted. Epineurium (E), small dark capillaries (*arrows*) in the red connective tissue (CT), rich nutrient supply to nerves. A, Artery; V, vein; P, perineurium; ED, endoneurium; and AX, axons.

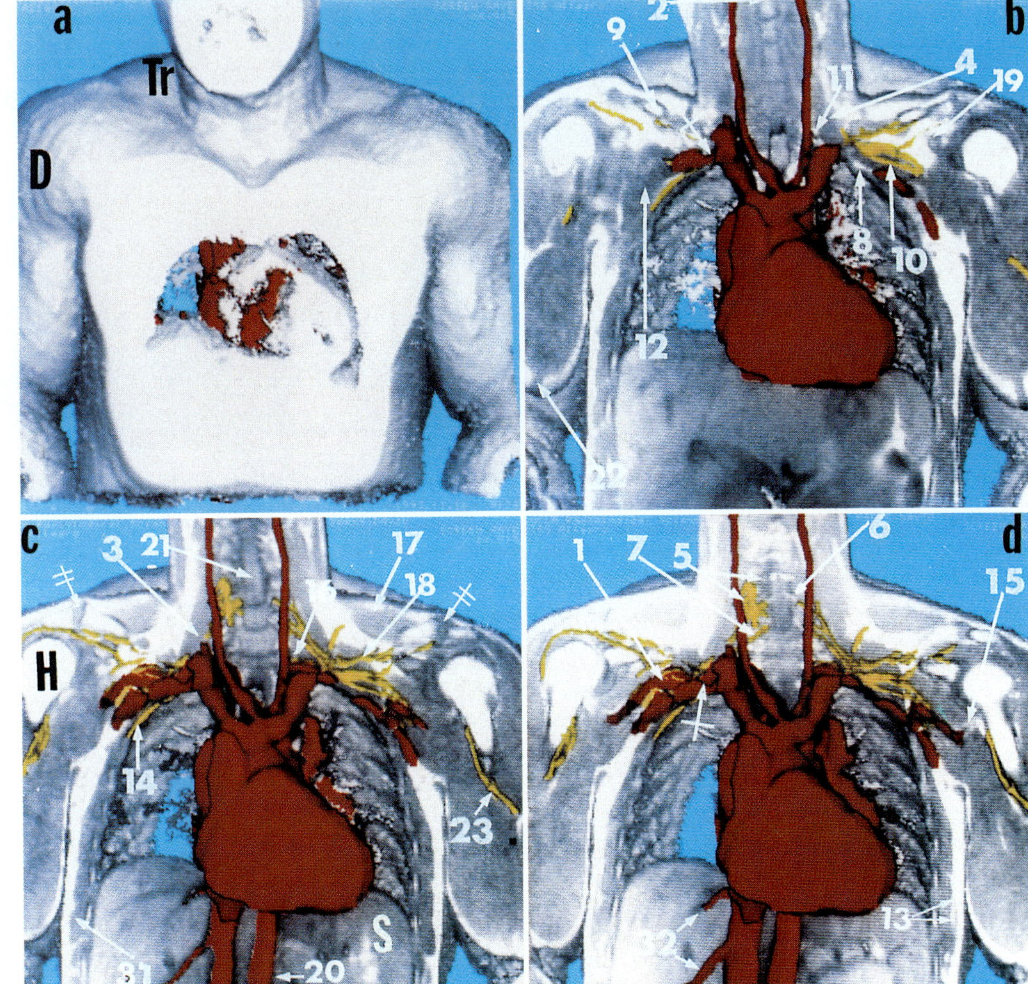

FIGURE 10–6. This figure demonstrates a computer-generated image (*A*) and three serial coronal three-dimensional color reconstructed images (*B*, *C*, and *D*) traced from the coronal gray scale sequential images. The shoulder girdle muscles are asymmetric (*A*), and there are compressive changes of the right neurovascular bundle (*bar arrows* below 9 in *B* to *D*) and a compressed flattened arch of the left subclavian artery and vein (inferior to the first thoracic nerve) in *D*. Poststenotic dilated axillary artery (1), second cervical vertebral body (2), anterior scalene muscle (3), middle scalene muscle (4), cervical nerve roots (5, 6, and 7), inferior trunk (8), clavicle (9), middle trunk (10), phrenic nerve (11), pectoralis minor muscle (12), left long thoracic nerve (13), right long thoracic nerve (14), axillary nerve (15), supraspinatus muscle (17), suprascapular nerve (18), coracoid process (19), abdominal aorta (20), spinal cord (21), fascicle of serratus anterior muscle (31), basilic vein (22), musculocutaneus nerve (23), hepatic veins (32), humerus (H), trapezius muscle (Tr), and spleen (S).

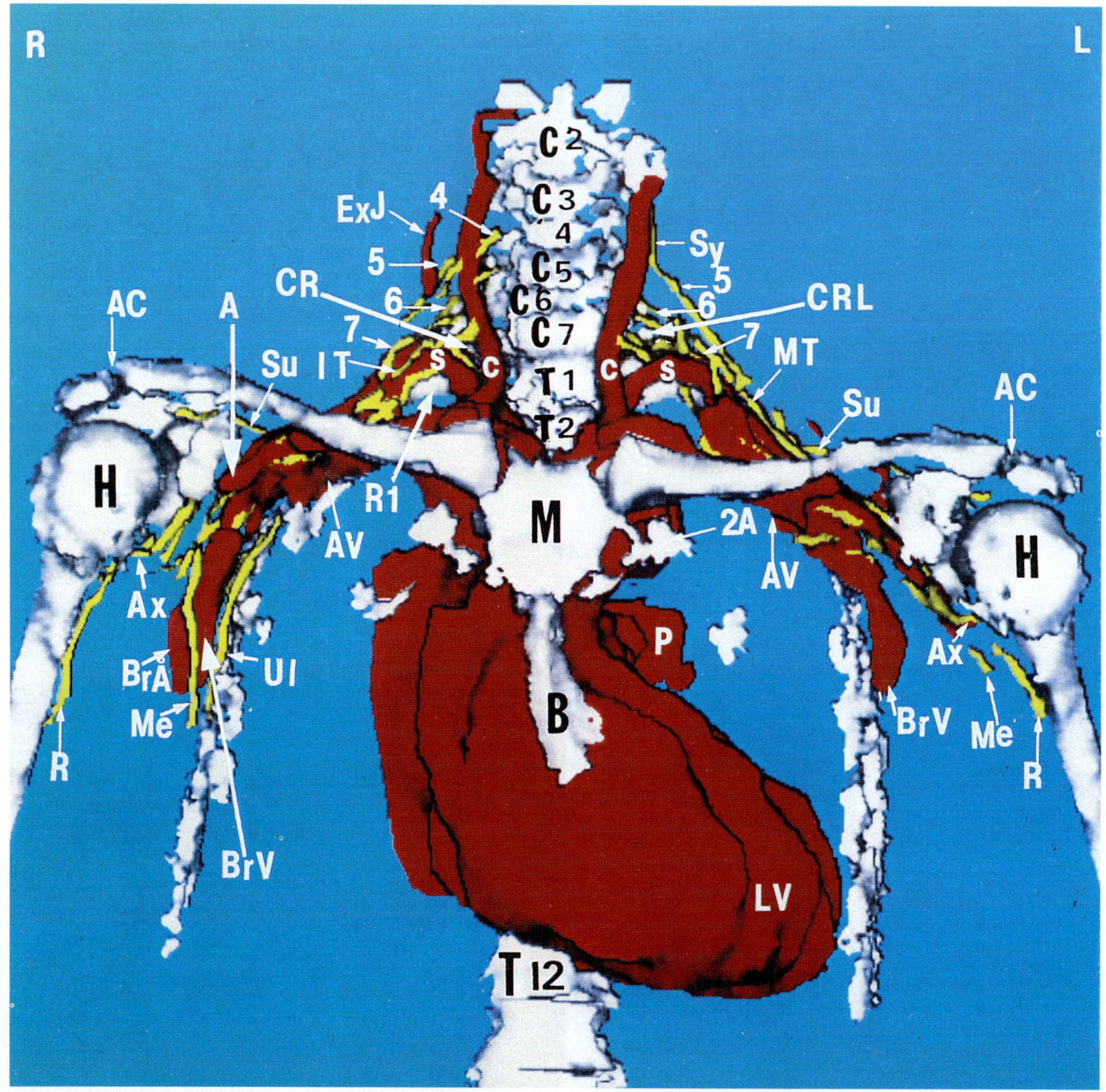

FIGURE 10–10. Three-dimensional image of osseous, neurovascular bundles, heart, and great vessels demonstrating the mild right convexed cervicothoracic scoliosis. Right (R); 1st Rib (R1); cervical rib (CR); C4–7 nerve roots; small left (L) cervical rib (CRL); manubrium sterni (M); anterior rib (2A); acromioclavicular joints (AC); humerus (H); 1st, 2nd and 12th thoracic (T1, T2, T12) and cervical (C2–7) vertebral bodies; body of the manubrium sternum (B); and middle (MT) and inferior (IT) trunks. Axillary (Ax), suprascapular (Su), radial (R), median (Me), ulnar (Ul), and long thoracic (LT) nerves. Pulmonary artery (P), left ventricle (LV). Axillary (A), subclavian (S), common carotid (C), and brachial (BrA) arteries. Brachial (BrV), axillary (AV), and external jugular (Ex J) veins. Sympathetic nerve (Sy).

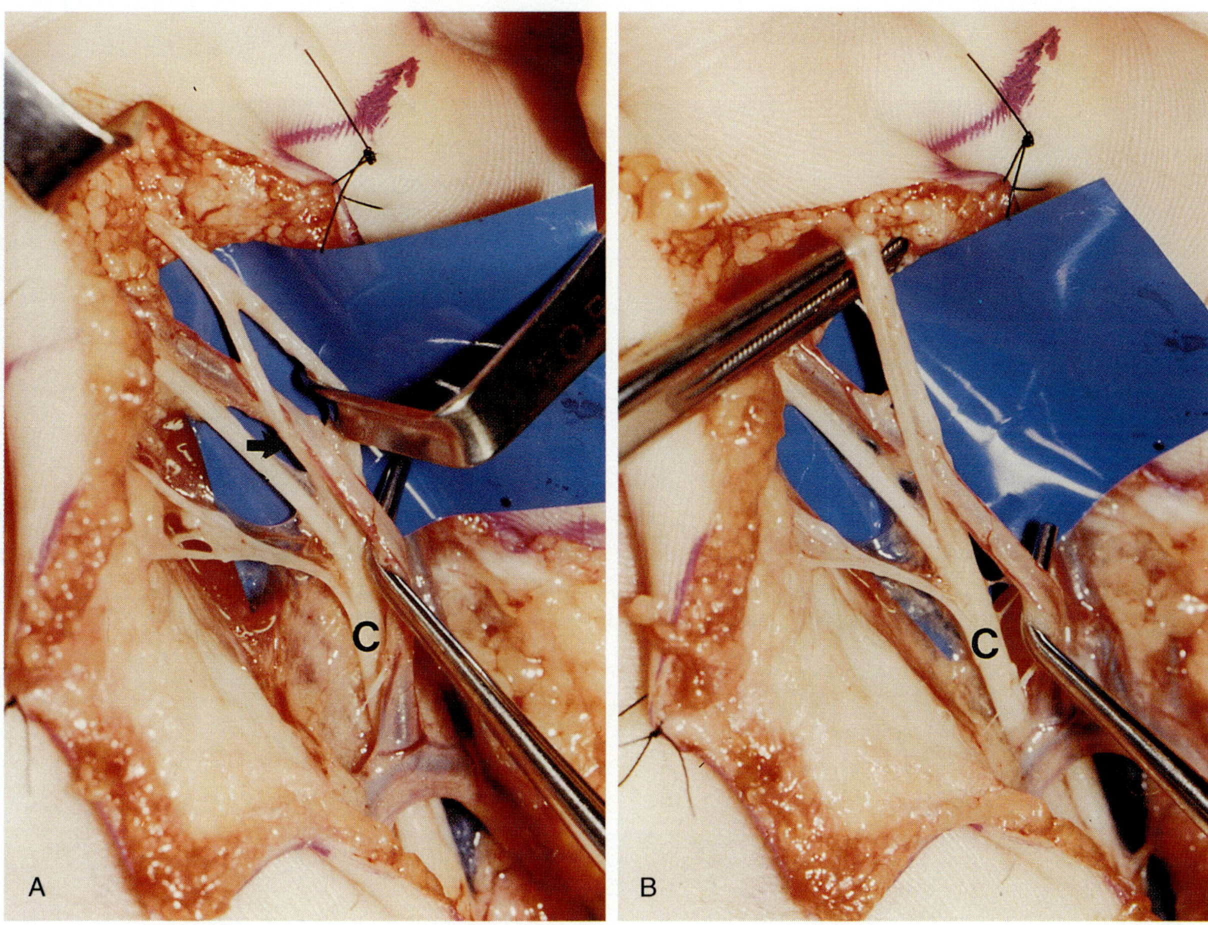

FIGURE 53–32. Neural penetration by an artery at the digital level. See other reports of similar neural penetration at other levels in the upper extremity in patients with evidence of nerve compression (Spinner, 1976; Gainor and Jeffries, 1987; Jones and Ming, 1988; Proudman and Menz, 1992). *A,* A 26-year-old man presented following a crush injury with palmar pain, intermittent numbness in the webspace between the index and long fingers and cold intolerance in the hand. He had diminished two-point discrimination in the ulnar aspect of the index finger and radial aspect of the long fingers. The sweat test showed decreased coloration in the common digital nerve distribution to the index and long fingers. The Digital Allen test filled normally. At surgery, the common digital artery was noted to penetrate the proper digital nerve to the radial aspect of the long finger. A portion of the proper digital nerve was compressed and was slightly discolored (*arrow*). The common digital nerve (C) and the superficial palmar arch can be seen. *B,* The tight "resting" relationship of the common digital artery (probe) and the two halves of the proper digital nerve to the long finger can be appreciated. Dynamic compression of the common digital artery probably also occurred. (From Spinner RJ, Varela CD, Urbaniak JR: Digital nerve penetration by a digital artery in a patient with neurovascular symptoms. Accepted, J Hand Surg, 1996.)

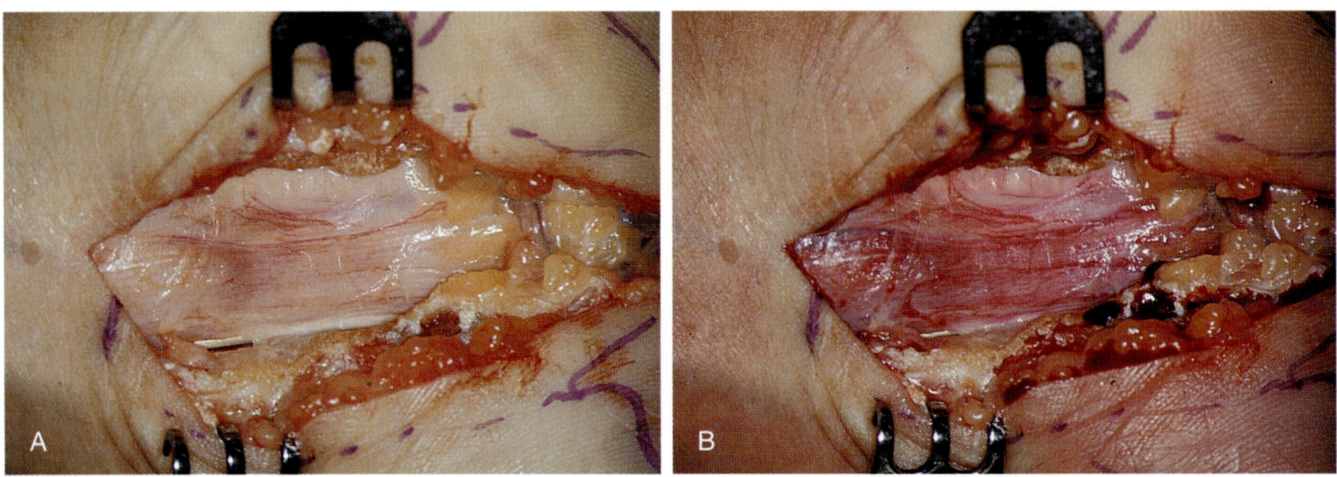

FIGURE 54–2. *A,* Compression of the median nerve under the proximal edge of the transverse carpal ligament, with discoloration and hourglass-shaped compression. *B,* Improved circulation usually occurs when the tourniquet is released for a short period (one minute) of time.

Part I

PROLOGUE

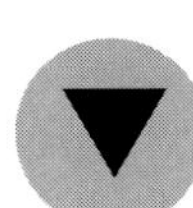

Chapter 1

• George E. Omer, Jr.

Peripheral Nerve Injuries: 45-Year Odyssey . . . and the Quest Continues

Sir Winston Churchill once said: "The further you look back, the further you can look forward" (Berry, 1965).

William A. Hammond, Surgeon General of the U.S. Army during the American Civil War, established special clinical services for problem cases. He requested S. Weir Mitchell, George R. Morehouse, and William W. Keen to establish a service for nervous diseases in a 400-bed hospital in Philadelphia. Mitchell and his colleagues contributed pioneer investigations in the diagnosis and treatment of nerve injuries, causalgia, hysteria, and malingering. In 1864, they published *Gunshot Wounds and Other Injuries of Nerves* that included 43 cases of wounds of large nerves. In 1895, Mitchell's son, John Kearsley Mitchell, published *Remote Consequences of Injuries to Nerves* that included a 27- to 28-year follow-up of 20 cases in his father's text (McHenry, 1965). This is one of the unique outcome investigations in the history of medicine.

Military neurosurgical centers for peripheral nerve injuries were established in World War I, and 3129 peripheral nerve injuries were registered (Woodhall and Beebe, 1956). Subsequently, the cases were examined by physicians of the Veterans Administration during the postwar period. The evaluation of 400 cases of nerve suture were reported only in terms of good, mediocre, or negative. Essentially, the patients with peripheral nerve injuries were absorbed into the veteran population without follow-up.

There were an estimated 25,000 peripheral nerve injuries during World War II that were distributed among 19 neurosurgical centers developed by the U.S. Army. Army Surgeon General Norman T. Kirk established a peripheral nerve registry for evaluation of peripheral nerve injuries, and a total of 7050 nerve sutures and 67 nerve grafts were registered by September 1945. Five follow-up centers were established under a Veterans Administration–National Research Council program with coordination by Barnes Woodhall at Duke University. Follow-up studies were begun in 1947 and published in 1956 as *Peripheral Nerve Regeneration: A follow-up study of 3,656 World War II injuries* (Woodhall and Beebe, 1956). The report included scales to grade the motor and sensory recovery of a peripheral nerve with total extremity function. The British Medical Research Council had introduced a very similar grading scale in 1954. More than 40 years later, these scales still are considered the most appropriate to assess the recovery of a peripheral nerve injury. However, the expertise gained was not utilized by the mainstream of surgery following World War II.

In addition to the neurosurgical centers, the U.S. Army established nine centers for surgery of the hand in Army General Hospitals in the United States. The consultant for the hand centers was Sterling Bunnell. Bunnell wrote: "It is impractical for three specialists (plastic, orthopaedic, and neurosurgery) to work together or in series. There is no shortcut. The surgeon must face the situation and equip himself to handle any and all of the tissues in a limb" (Newmeyer, 1995). Bunnell (1955) estimated that 22,000 injured hands were treated in the hand centers. Repair of motor nerves was given equal priority with most plastic and orthopaedic procedures, resulting in great improvement in reconstruction with less permanent disability (Bunnell, 1955).

Sterling Bunnell suggested that the military hand surgeons continue their interest and fellowship by means of a "round robin" letter (Barsky, 1977; Bell, 1970). At the Newton D. Baker Army Hospital in the fall of 1945, Major Joseph H. Boyes, Captains S. Benjamin Fowler, Robert L. Payne Jr, and Darrel T. Shaw were assigned to the hand service. Lt. Commander George V. Webster was visiting from the Bethesda Naval Medical Center. These five surgeons met in Major Boyes' quarters and formulated the basic plan for the American Society for Surgery of the Hand (ASSH) (Barsky, 1977; Bell, 1970). The hand surgeons organized the ASSH in January, 1946, and the concept of peripheral nerve repairs as an integrated part of reconstruction and functional rehabilitation of the upper extremity was accepted. In addition, hand surgeons had developed innovative reconstructive procedures, such as tendon transfers for reconstruction of the upper extremity following nerve loss. These techniques clearly improved functional activities.

The outbreak of the Korean War once again demonstrated the need for multidisciplinary care of the individual case. However, the military had closed its hand surgery centers and peripheral nerve injury centers. The solution was to appoint recognized civilians, many of whom had served during World War II, as consultants to the general hospitals (Berry, 1965). Conscripted physicians had the opportunity to note the value of multidisciplinary care only in the general hospitals. Two of the editors of this text (George Omer and Morton Spinner) were active in the Army Medical Corps during the Korean War. After the war, Morton Spinner returned to civilian practice to use his trauma experience and to continue research as a clinical professor at the Albert Einstein College of Medicine in New York, while George Omer elected to remain on active duty in the regular Army.

References from the peripheral nerve experience gained in World War II (Woodhall and Beebe, 1956) were not published until 1956. Medical libraries during the Korean

War included texts that had limited references to peripheral nerves: Allen B. Kanavel, *Infections of the Hand* (1925); Marc Iselin, *Surgery of the Hand,* (English edition, 1940); Condict W. Cutler Jr, *The Hand* (1942); and Sterling Bunnell, *Surgery of the Hand* (1944).

During the Vietnam conflict, most of the surgical lessons of the past were remembered when sophisticated medical facilities were used in the combat theater (Jacobsen and Suarez, 1960). Residency programs for orthopaedic and plastic surgery were continued at most military general hospitals in the United States. However, special clinical centers for peripheral nerves were not established by the U.S. Army Surgeon General. The majority of the patients with peripheral nerve injuries evacuated from Vietnam were seen in five hand surgery centers within the Brooke, Fitzsimons, Letterman, Tripler, and Walter Reed Army Medical Centers (Omer and Eversmann, 1994). Raymond M. Curtis, as consultant in hand surgery to the Army Surgeon General, had an active clinical role at Walter Reed Army Medical Center, and he established a 1-year fellowship in hand surgery. Sensibility re-education concepts were taken by Curtis's Military Fellows in Hand Surgery and the participating hand therapists to all Army Medical Centers (Omer and Graham, 1989).

In 1966, the hand surgery and the general orthopaedic sections of the Orthopaedic Service at Brooke Army Medical Center (BAMC) in San Antonio were designated a hand surgery center. George Omer was chief of the orthopaedic service and director of the hand surgery center; he was the first career military member of the ASSH from the Army, Navy, or Air Force. Allen Van Beek also was on active duty at BAMC in 1969 and worked in the hand surgery section before returning to a civilian academic practice. Peripheral nerve injuries of the lower extremity were seen on the general orthopaedic service, that is, in 1968, there were 166 lesions of lower extremity nerves and 262 lesions of upper extremity nerves seen at BAMC (Omer, 1968). Twenty-two percent of the patients with injuries of the upper extremity admitted to BAMC from Vietnam had lesions of major peripheral nerves (Omer, 1974). From May 1966 to July 1970, 917 peripheral nerves of the upper extremity were examined at the BAMC Hand Center (Omer, 1974). Surgical reconstruction techniques and prosthetic devices were innovative and evaluated appropriately, but there was inadequate follow-up of peripheral nerve repair. Only the hand center at Fitzsimons Army Medical Center had a planned long-term follow-up study from 1967 to 1983 (Omer and Eversmann, 1994). Significant findings included documented return of intrinsic function of the hand more than two years after above-elbow suture of the ulnar nerve (Omer and Eversmann, 1994). The Brooke and Walter Reed Army Medical Centers included many occupational and physical therapists, and provided a model for future organizational relationships in all extremity surgery as well as hand surgery.

Military general hospitals included residency programs with many consultants and visitors. At BAMC, Erik Moberg visited in both 1968 and 1969 to stimulate our interest in sensibility as well as motor function, and Bernard McC. O'Brien made surgical rounds, while Paul W. Brand presented a captivating lecture. A partial list of American hand surgery consultants and visitors in 1969 included John Boswick, Jr., Robert E. Carroll, Robert A. Chase, James H. Dobyns, Adrian E. Flatt, S. Benjamin Fowler, J. Leonard Goldner, David P. Green, Lot D. Howard, James M. Hunter, Emanuel B. Kaplan, Harold E. Kleinert, L. Lee Langford, Lee Milford, John J. Niebauer, George S. Phalen, Dan Riordan, Spencer Rowland, Frank H. Stelling III, and Alfred B. Swanson. BAMC hosted hand surgery educational symposia for the ASSH, the Riordan Hand Society, and The American Academy of Orthopaedic Surgeons (AAOS).

By the end of the Vietnam war, the medical libraries had added several texts pertinent to peripheral nerves: Sterling Bunnell, *Hand Surgery in World War II* (1955); Barnes Woodhall and Gilbert Beebe, *Peripheral Nerve Regeneration* (1956); James E. Bateman, *Trauma to Nerves in Limbs* (1962); Sydney Sunderland, *Nerves and Nerve Injuries* (1968), J. C. White and W. H. Sweet, *Pain and the Neurosurgeon: A Forty Year Experience* (1969); and H. Seddon, *Surgical Disorders of the Peripheral Nerves* (1972).

Our military experience from World War II through the Vietnam conflict was valuable in three major areas:

1. Development of a matrix of tests to evaluate sensibility; motor performance; sympathetic nerve activity, including pain syndromes; and total extremity function. At the BAMC hand surgery center, more than 26,900 separate tests were documented (Omer, 1974). In addition to assessing sensibility, techniques for retraining sensibility were developed (Omer, 1974; Omer and Eversmann, 1994).

2. Assessing the potential for spontaneous recovery. In a prospective study of 648 nerve lesions with the involved nerve in continuity, the authors found 69% spontaneous recovery for both low-velocity and high-velocity gunshot wounds within 3 to 9 months following injury (Omer, 1974). Similar findings were noted in smaller studies performed during World Wars I and II (Sunderland, 1978).

3. Accumulative and useful experience in reconstructive procedures following nerve loss. A great number of tendon transfers over a relatively short time frame provides reliable outcome studies for techniques and relates to long-term function (Ledford, 1994; Omer, 1968, 1974; Omer and Eversmann, 1994). Prosthetic devices were developed to avoid localized pressure and subsequent ulceration in insensitive extremities (Omer, 1968).

The military experience of World War II did not significantly enhance techniques for nerve suture and provided inadequate outcome studies for the results of nerve suture during the Korean and Vietnam conflicts (Omer and Eversmann, 1994). Sutures were too bulky, and loupe magnification was inadequate. Yet, in contrast to World War II, the experience gained in military hand centers stimulated a number of general, orthopaedic, and plastic surgeons to continue to work with peripheral nerve problems. After World War II, there was a massive shift toward specialization by physicians in the United States (Omer, 1989, 1990). The United States government funded several additional medical schools, and subspecialty surgery was developed by full-time faculty. The first formal Division of Hand Surgery in the United States was organized in 1970 at the University of New Mexico (Newmeyer, 1995; Omer, 1982), by George Omer, the first Professor and Chairman of the Department of Orthopaedics and Rehabilitation. In 1970, the ASSH identified 56 preceptor-type training programs for hand surgery in the United States and Canada (Omer, 1968). The ASSH provided a forum for their research in peripheral nerve problems as well as other clinical activities involving the upper extremity.

Subspecialization encouraged pertinent clinical research by peripheral nerve physicians. Erik Moberg demonstrated the importance of measuring sensibility. Sydney Sunderland supplied detailed information concerning the internal neuroanatomy of the peripheral nerves. Emanuel B. Kaplan enhanced the understanding of peripheral nerve anatomy; while in 1972, Morton Spinner presented significant anatomical variations and clinical applications in his text *Injuries to the Major Branches of Peripheral Nerves of the Forearm.*

But subspecialization was not enough. The renaissance of peripheral nerve surgical repair after injury was the advent of microsurgery for laboratory research. Jacobson and Suarez (1960) introduced the term microsurgery in 1960 while repairing small vessels in laboratory animals. The technique was applied to peripheral nerve surgery by Smith and Michon in 1964. Acland (1972) and Buncke (1971) were interested in instrumentation, and developed smaller needles and fine metallicized sutures for experimental replantation and transplantation. In 1972, Millesi, Meissl, and Berger introduced the concept of no-tension nerve repair with cable grafting and reported improved techniques with the operating microscope.

Organized replantation/microsurgical research centers appeared in the 1970s, such as Kleinert and Kutz in Louisville, Kentucky; O'Brien in Melbourne, Australia; and Tamai in Tokyo, Japan. Just as important, microscopic teaching laboratories were developed by recognized surgeons, such as Harry Buncke at the University of California in San Francisco, Berish Strauch at Albert Einstein College of Medicine, James R. Urbaniak at Duke University, and Victor E. Meyer at Zurich University in Switzerland. Microsurgery encouraged pertinent techniques other than nerve suture, such as vascularized nerve grafts and nerve lengthening procedures, as presented by Allen Van Beek, a former-president of the American Society for Reconstructive Microsurgery.

Many forums for microsurgery procedures were provided in the late 1970s and the 1980s by the American Society for Reconstructive Microsurgery, the American Society of Plastic and Reconstructive Surgeons (ASPRS), the ASSH, and the AAOS; these educational programs led to teaching laboratories at many universities in the United States for microsurgery instruction and development of surgical techniques. Microsurgery has developed on a worldwide scale, with the International Society of Reconstructive Microsurgery in a leadership role.

During the decade following the Vietnam War, peripheral nerve surgeons contributed to the ASSH, AAOS, and ASPRS Instructional Courses (Omer, 1975a, 1975b; Omer and Eversmann, 1994; Omer and Spinner, 1984; Spinner, 1976), and joined colleagues at university meetings on peripheral nerve problems. From 1977 to 1980, George Omer and Morton Spinner developed a book entitled *The Management of Peripheral Nerve Problems.* They discussed the concept of a peripheral nerve study group with several colleagues, including J. Leonard Goldner and Raymond Curtis, who were enthusiastic about the potential benefits for clinical practice.

In 1978, a group of surgeons interested in peripheral nerve pathology met at Duke University with J. Leonard Goldner as host. During this meeting, a biannual program was discussed. A preliminary society was formed, with Raymond Curtis, J. Leonard Goldner, David Kline, George Omer, and Morton Spinner as the founding senior members of this society (Goldner, 1995).

The concept was crystallized at the mid-year meeting of the ASSH in 1979, and The Peripheral Nerve Study Group was founded, with the purpose "to study in depth difficult problems and advances in peripheral nerve anatomy, physiology, and surgery." Present for that meeting were Ray Curtis, Mike Jabaley, Joseph Kutz, George Omer, Morton Spinner, Jack Tupper, Jim Urbaniak, and Shaw Wilgis. Leonard Goldner was absent but was aware of the meeting. Morton Spinner was elected president, and Shaw Wilgis served as secretary-treasurer.

The first formal program was held in New York City, in July 1980, with Morton Spinner as president. Sir Sydney Sunderland was a guest speaker. At this meeting, David Kline was elected president and George Omer was president-elect; Morton Spinner became past-president and Shaw Wilgis continued as secretary-treasurer. This was the first executive committee. It was determined that the "annual meetings" would be held approximately 18 months apart. The membership quickly expanded to include several more individuals from the United States, as well as members from Australia, Austria, Canada, France, Italy, Sweden, Switzerland, and West Germany. It became a forum for informal exchange of ideas and experiences in peripheral nerve problems.

In September 1980, David Kline proposed that the name of the group be changed because it was similar to The Neurologic Nerve Study Group, which had met for a number of years. David Kline's proposal was discussed by the executive committee. As the president of the ASSH from 1978 to 1979, George Omer had invited Sir Sydney Sunderland to be The Founders Lecturer at the annual meeting, and the members of the ASSH were well aware of Sir Sydney's professional contributions. In January 1981, David Kline wrote all members: "Morton Spinner and the executive committee have suggested Sunderland Club as our new name."

The second formal meeting was held in New Orleans, in November 1981, with David Kline as president. At the business meeting, the name of the group was changed from The Peripheral Nerve Study Group to The Sunderland Society.

The third meeting was held in Santa Fe, in May 1983, with George Omer as president. There were 22 members from six countries, as well as several guests in attendance. Sir Sydney was in attendance, with his wife Lady Gwen, and he subsequently attended every meeting until his death in 1993.

Our clinical experience from the Vietnam War till today has been valuable in three major areas:

1. The development of microsurgery has markedly increased the technical accuracy of nerve repair, and adjunctive reconstructive procedures such as microvascular free flap transfers and free muscle transfers.

2. Improved methods of electrophysiologic testing. These techniques are valuable in the diagnosis of the preoperative patient, more accurate assessment of the pathology in the intraoperative patient, improved spatial alignment of periph-

eral nerve repairs, and measurement of functional recovery in the postoperative patient.

3. Tropic and trophic influences on nerve regeneration are being investigated, as well as histochemical aids to control specificity. In addition, research in the past decade has varied widely from anatomical studies of the internal topography of peripheral nerves to comparative studies of different repair techniques.

Finally, there is much to do in this fascinating field of surgery. For example, more than 40 years later, there is consensus that the scales used to grade motor and sensory recovery after World War II are inadequate. We need correct testing to evaluate motor and sensibility recovery after nerve repair before we can develop appropriate outcome studies. How can we evaluate plasticity of central nervous mechanisms? All of us could add items to the list of things we need to know to improve end results following peripheral nerve repair, and the quest must continue. The editors have chosen authors in the vanguard of this field of surgery to present the second edition of this text.

References

Acland R: New instruments for microvascular surgery. Br J Surg 59:181–184, 1972.

Barsky AJ: History of the American Society for Surgery of the Hand. American Society for Surgery of the Hand, Chicago, September, 1977.

Bell JL: The American Society for Surgery of the Hand: 25 Years (1945–1970). American Society for Surgery of the Hand. Chicago, January, 1970.

Berry FB: Prologue. *In* Meirowsky AM (ed): Neurological Surgery of Trauma. Department of the Army, Washington, D.C., Office of the Surgeon General, 1965, pp xv–xvi.

Bunnell S (ed): Hand Surgery in World War II. Washington, D.C., Office of the Surgeon General, Department of the Army, 1955, pp 34–37, 300–302.

Buncke HJ, Murray DE: Autogenous arterial interposition graft of less than 1 mm in external diameter. Melbourne, Trans Int Congr Plast Reconstr Surg, 1971.

Buncke HJ: The development of microsurgery. *In* Daniller, A. I. and Strauch, B. (eds): Symposium on microsurgery, Vol 14. Educational Foundation of the American Society of Plastic and Reconstructive Surgery, C.V. Mosby, 1976.

Goldner JL: Sunderland Society—History. Letter dated 1 November 1995.

Jacobson JH II, Suarez EL: Microsurgery in anastomosis of small vessels. Surg Forum 11:243–245, 1960.

Ledford FF Jr: Foreword. *In* Burkhalter WE (ed): Orthopaedic Surgery in Vietnam. Washington, D.C., Office of the Surgeon General, U.S. Army and the Center of Military History, 1994

McHenry LC Jr: Introduction. *In* Weir MS: Injuries of Nerves and their Consequences. New York, American Academy of Neurology Reprint Series, Dover Publications, Inc., 1965.

Michon J, Masse P: Le moment optimum de la suture nerveuse dans les plaies du membre superior. Rev Chir Orthop 50:205–212, 1964.

Millesi H, Meissl G, Berger A: The interfascicular nerve grafting of the median and ulnar nerves. J Bone Joint Surg 54A:727–750, 1972.

Newmeyer WL (ed): American Society for Surgery of the Hand. The First Fifty Years. New York, Churchill Livingstone, 1995, pp 1–4.

Omer GE Jr: Annual Report, Orthopaedic Service. Fort Sam Houston, TX, Brooke Army Medical Center, 1968.

Omer GE Jr: Injuries to nerves of the upper extremity. J Bone Joint Surg 56A:1615–1624, 1974.

Omer GE Jr: Neurovascular sensory island transplants, 52–63; 100–107. *In* Fredricks S, Brody GS: Symposium on the neurologic aspects of plastic surgery. Educational Foundation, American Society for Plastic and Reconstructive Surgery, Vol 17. St. Louis, C.V. Mosby, 1975a, pp 52–63.

Omer JE Jr: Reflex sympathetic dystrophies. *In* Fredricks S, Brody GS (eds): Symposium on the Neurologic aspects of plastic surgery. Educational Foundation, American Society for Plastic and Reconstructive Surgery, Vol 17. St. Louis, C.V. Mosby, 1975b, pp 100–107.

Omer GE Jr: The Joint Committee for Surgery of the Hand. J Hand Surg 7:221–223, 1982.

Omer GE Jr, Graham WP III: Development of certification in hand surgery. J Hand Surg 14A:589–593, 1989.

Omer GE Jr: The development of orthopaedic certification in the United States. Clin Orthop 257:11–17, 1990.

Omer GE Jr, Eversmann WW Jr: Peripheral nerve problems. *In* Burkhalter WE (ed): Orthopaedic Surgery in Vietnam. Washington, D.C., Office of the Surgeon General, U.S. Army and the Center of Military History. 1994, pp 155–188.

Omer GE Jr, Spinner M: Peripheral nerve testing and suture techniques. *In* Amer. Acad. Orthop. Surg. Instr. Course Lect., Vol. 24, 1975. St. Louis, C.V. Mosby, pp 122–143.

Omer GE Jr, Spinner M: Management of peripheral nerve problems. *In* Amer. Acad. Orthop. Surg. Instr. Course Lect., Vol 33. St. Louis, C.V. Mosby, 1984, pp 461–530.

Smith JW: Microsurgery of peripheral nerves. Plast Reconstr Surg 33:317–329, 1964.

Spinner M: Injuries to the Major Branches of Peripheral Nerves of the Forearm. Philadelphia, W.B. Saunders Company, 1972.

Spinner M: Compression nerve injuries. *In* Daniller AI, Strauch B (eds): Symposium on microsurgery. Educational Foundation of the American Society for Plastic and Reconstructive Surgery, Vol 14. St. Louis, C.V. Mosby, 1976, pp 161–171.

Sunderland S: Nerves and Nerve Injuries, 2nd ed. Edinburgh, Churchill Livingstone, 1978, pp 505–507.

Woodhall B, Beebe GW (eds): Peripheral Nerve Regeneration. A Follow-Up Study of 3,656 World War II Injuries. Washington, D.C., V.A. Medical Monograph, U.S. Government Printing Office, 1956, pp xx–xxi.

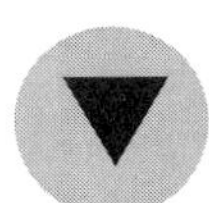

Chapter 2

• Morton Spinner

Peripheral Nerve Problems—Past, Present, and Future

The second edition of *Management of Peripheral Nerve Injuries* emerges after a hiatus of 16 years, its update dictated by the recent recognition of newer diagnostic methods and technical advances. The editors have wisely postponed premature publication until the test of time had clearly vindicated innovative developments described in the first edition—interfascicular nerve grafting and intraoperative electrical evaluation of neural lesions in continuity, for example, are now established techniques.

In this edition, fresh ideas from new faces have been amalgamated with neural dilettantes from all over our nation and the world. It is exciting to read the works of these shining stars of the younger generation. These contributions complement those of established neural masters. It is difficult for me to imagine that just 50 years ago, there were only a few experts in the field—Sir Herbert Seddon, Sir Sydney Sunderland, Sir James Learmonth, and Barnes Woodhall.

In the 40 years since I completed my orthopedic residency education, I have had an ongoing romance with peripheral nerve problems commencing with a child with a supracondylar fracture who could not flex the terminal phalanx of his thumb. Subsequently, a group of patients who were unable to extend spontaneously their fingers and thumb but could extend their wrist was described. During my career I have attempted to understand such problems and others on an anatomical basis, and this has been a joy to me. There has been a remarkable growth in the number of clinicians and basic scientists committed to all aspects of clinical evaluation, and optimal therapy and research in peripheral nerves.

As this current edition makes clear, the greatest advances in patient care have come from two factors—the intraoperative microscope and the ingenuity of the treating surgeon. The technical repair of a fourth or fifth degree nerve lesion has been improved most markedly by the enhanced visualization afforded by the microscope, coordinated with fine instrumentation and small caliber sutures and needles. Application of the internal neural topography has added greatly to the repair. In addition, when neural lesions cannot be repaired, there have been tremendous advances in the area of reconstruction now available with vascularized flaps and grafts.

Much basic information about the type and timing of peripheral nerve repair has been gleaned during the last generation. Serial examinations correlated with electrical studies have provided the best insight as to appropriate management. When spontaneous resolution of the problem does not occur in a timely manner and when surgical intervention is deemed necessary, my experience strongly suggests that *early* surgical intervention offers the best end result. Furthermore, the more proximal the lesion, the earlier accurate classification of injury is needed in order to obtain the best functional recovery.

I predict the next major movement in this field will come from information gained from the noninvasive positron emission tomography scan of the spinal cord. Knowledge of the physiological activity of the anterior horn and spinal ganglion cells would unquestionably aid the treating surgeon in deciding whether neural repair or reconstructive surgery is indicated following injury. In addition, the evolution of new basic scientific techniques at the molecular level offers great promise for future clinical application.

One of my fervent wishes for the future is the discovery of a neurotrophic substance that would encourage axon regeneration, especially in a proximal nerve lesion. One Nobel prize has already been awarded for a nerve growth factor; it is hoped that there is another on the way for solving this problem.

We, who care for patients afflicted with neural trauma, are on the horizon of a wonderful era.

Part II

INNERVATION PATTERNS AND DIAGNOSTIC TECHNIQUES

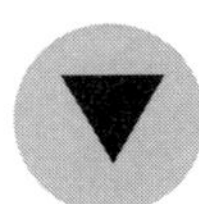

Chapter 3

• George E. Omer, Jr
• Judith Bell-Krotoski

Sensibility Testing

The human nervous system is bombarded simultaneously by a multitude of stimuli. The afferent input is limited by the inconstant threshold of the peripheral nerve endings and the specialized receptor organs associated with them. Sensation is the acceptance and activation of impulses in the afferent nerve fibers of the nervous system.

The brain receives and elaborates a continuously changing flood of sensations. Varied sensations are synthesized into three-dimensional experiences. Central neural mechanisms, such as memory storage and introspection, influence the conscious perception of the external and internal environment. Sensibility is the conscious appreciation and interpretation of the stimulus that produced sensation.

ANATOMICAL CONSIDERATIONS

A sensory unit is a single first-order afferent neuron, including all peripheral and central branches. Five elementary qualities of sensibility can be evoked: (1) touch-pressure, (2) warmth, (3) cold, (4) pain, and (5) movement and position. Sensation for these qualities depends upon many factors; some involving the sensory unit are (1) the diameter of the first-order afferent neuron, (2) the properties of the sensory receptors, (3) the size and population of the receptive field, and (4) the threshold for the entire sensory unit.

Axons are classified in three groups: A (with subgroups alpha, beta, and delta), B, and C. The A axons are the largest, up to 20 μ in diameter, while C axons may be less than 1 μ in diameter. The larger the diameter of an axon, the more rapid the conduction rate and the lower its threshold to electrical stimulation. The larger myelinated afferents (alpha and beta groups, A axons) are specialists in touch-pressure and movement-position. Small myelinated afferents (delta group, A axons) conduct acute pricking pain, cold and warmth, and deep pressure. Single unit analysis of unmyelinated afferents (C axons) reveals that they conduct the total range of qualitative sensations. All major somesthetic sensations (pressure, pain, cold, and warmth) are conducted by the small myelinated afferents (delta group, A axons) and the smaller unmyelinated afferents (C axons); these two systems indicate the multiple functional duplication in the peripheral nervous system. A property of any group of axons is that they transmit an identical impulse no matter how they are excited; different sensations occur through the combinations of axons transmitting impulses. The frequency and sequence of the impulses are determined by the peripheral receptors.

The peripheral branches of sensory units may terminate in complex receptor organs composed in part of non-neural tissue, such as the hair follicle or pacinian corpuscles (Table 3–1). These receptors initiate the depolarization of the afferent neuron through their generator potential. The generator potential is not conducted but can be increased both temporally and spatially to invade adjacent regions of the parent axon. Receptors vary in their rate of adaptation to continued stimuli. Most of the receptor organs with non-neural tissue are mechanoreceptive afferents. The form, number, and distribution of specialized receptor organs vary with age, region of the body, and occupation. Free nerve endings can be differentially sensitive in the absence of a specialized receptor organ.

The receptor fields of ectodermal sensory units vary greatly in population and size. The population of the isolated cutaneous spots for temperature sensitivity is an example: Cold spots are more numerous than warm spots by ratios of 4:1 to 10:1, and both types of cutaneous spots are more common on the hands and face than elsewhere on the body (Mountcastle, 1980). The smaller the receptive field is in size, the greater the number of sensory units in a given body area and the greater the representation of that body part at the cerebral cortex. The superficial tissues of the hand are densely innervated compared with more proximal cutaneous areas of the upper extremity and may have as many as 2500 nerve endings in one square millimeter of tissue (Mountcastle, 1980). The peripheral branches of one ectodermal sensory unit overlap with the branches of adjacent sensory units, so that the activity of sensory units gradually changes with a moving stimulus. Consequently, sensibility is very accurate for a light pressure or moving position stimulus to the volar tip of the fingers. Discrimination of light touch on the volar finger pulp, as two points and not one, is normally accurate between 3 to 5 mm. In contrast, two-point discrimination of light touch proximal to the elbow is between 65 and 75 mm (Werner and Omer, 1970).

Sensibility for body position and movement results from stimulation of proprioceptors in mesodermal tissues, such as muscles, tendons, joints, and periosteum, as well as of cutaneous receptors (Moberg, 1965). Impulses generated in muscle-tendon units and joints assist in guiding action in such diverse performances as hand grip, lever manipulation, estimating hardness of compliant materials, and spanning an object with the fingers. The preciseness of proprioception is the reverse of exteroception for the proximal and distal portions of the extremities. In the shoulder joint, less than 1 degree of passive movement can be recognized, and a given position can be reproduced within 2 degrees. An interphalangeal joint requires 5 to 10 degrees of movement for recognition (Cohen, 1958). The precise sense of position and direction of extremity movement is related to the receptors found about joints, and proximal joints are more densely populated than distal joints (Stopford, 1921/1922).

The mesodermal receptors with the highest threshold to stretch are the Golgi organs within tendons. These afferents

▼ TABLE 3–1
Sensibility and Receptor Organs

Stimulus of Sensation	Modality of Sensibility	Receptor Structure	Adaptability of Receptor
Mechanical force	Light touch and vibration	Free nerve endings (A and C)	Slow
		Pacinian corpuscles	Fast
		Meissner corpuscles	Fast
Mechanical force	Pressure	Free nerve endings (A and C)	Slow
		Merkel disk-hair follicles	Slow
Mechanical force	Deep pressure	Free nerve endings (A and C)	Slow
	Movement-rate direction	Cylinders of Ruffini	Fast
	Position-posture	Muscle spindles–flower spray annulospiral	Slow
Temperature change	Warmth (24°–45°C)	Golgi-Mazzoni corpuscles	Slow
	Cold (12°–37°C)	Free nerve endings (A and C)	Fast
		Arteriolar diameter change	Slow
Extremes of mechanical force or temperature change; presence of chemicals or electrical energy	Pain	Free nerve endings	Slow
		Pricking pain—delta group, A axons	Fast
		Burning pain—C axons	Slow

connect into a disynaptic reflex arc that influences both synergists and antagonists of the involved muscle (Omer and Vogel, 1965). The flower-spray nerve endings (beta and gamma groups, A axons) and the annulospiral nerve endings (alpha group, A axons) are afferents found in the muscle spindle. The annulospiral nerve endings have the lowest threshold to stretch. In addition to the afferent receptors, small motor nerves termed gamma efferents terminate in the muscle spindle. The gamma efferents can tense the muscle spindle even when the total muscle is relaxed. This causes the annulospiral alpha afferents to discharge even though the total muscle continues relaxed. This double stimulation mechanism maintains the myostatic reflex while the muscle is either contracted or relaxed. The motor neurons for these spinal reflex arcs come from a competing pool of afferent impulses that includes cutaneous and central stimulation. The central pathways are inhibitory to protect the muscle from overload by preventing damaging contraction against strong stretch. When central impulses are uncoordinated, as in cerebral palsy, the alpha afferents and gamma efferents are always imbalanced. As the afferent pool is increased, the sphere of influence involves additional synergistic and antagonistic muscles.

First-order sensory afferent impulses are conducted centrally by at least two systems. The larger myelinated afferents (alpha and beta groups, A axons) connect with large myelinated fibers in the dorsal horn of the spinal cord and traverse the ipsilateral dorsal column. The impulse is then projected, via the medial lemniscus, on the contralateral ventrobasal thalamic complex and finally to the postcentral gyrus of the sensory cortex. The distinguishing feature of this system is that information concerning location, shape, quality, and temporal sequence of stimuli is transmitted with great fidelity at each synaptic station (Mountcastle, 1980). Small myelinated afferents (delta group, A axons) and unmyelinated afferents (C axons) also connect by the interneuronal system of the dorsal horn. Some cross to the contralateral side in the spinothalamic tract, and others remain ipsilateral to continue centrally in the anterolateral columns. Compared with the lemniscal system, these tracts are phylogenetically older and less precise. Their cortical representation is less exact. Little is known about how messages coded by the activity of ensembles of peripheral neurons are integrated by centrally located neurons. However, it is the process that ultimately leads to the conscious recognition termed sensibility (Omer, 1974).

THRESHOLD FACTORS

The thresholds of sensory units vary for many reasons (Table 3–2). The sensorimotor system works best at the level to which it is adapted, and unexperienced variations in threshold will influence the interpretation by the individual. For example, a temperature change produces a mechanoreceptive illusion, in that weights feel heavier when cold than when warm. Sensibility is affected also by sensory cortex storage. Almost all patterns of information are converted into a recorded form that preserves the topographical representation of the periphery in the sensory cortex. One example is the reaction of patients with neurovascular cutaneous

▼ TABLE 3–2
Threshold Variables for Sensibility

A. Receptors: somatic, peripheral
 1. Age of individual
 2. Condition of overlying epithelium—occupation
 3. Circulation in area of receptor
 4. Intensity of stimulation energy
 5. Time (duration) of stimulation
 6. Number of receptors or receptive fields stimulated
  a. region of body
 7. Temperature in area of receptor
 8. Specific morphology and adaptability
 9. Central influence on receptor system
  a. spinal reflex arcs, such as muscle spindle
  b. activity facilitated by autonomic efferents
B. Afferent pathway systems
 1. Both inhibitory and facilitory effect on transmission and summation
C. Sensory cortex
 1. Attention and concentration of individual
 2. Spatial—temporal pattern of impulse input
 3. Stored memory and experience
 4. Coordination with vision, smell, hearing
 5. Selection and erasure of irrelevant information

island pedicle transfers. The patient can be trained to interpret a sensory experience into the spatial pattern of the recipient site of the pedicle transfer, but in an emergency, the training will be lost (Omer et al, 1970). Thus, a patient will first move the donor ring finger when a cigarette burns the thumb that is the recipient of the pedicle transfer.

MEASUREMENT CONSIDERATIONS

Two aspects of sensibility are important to consider in testing peripheral nerve function: (1) physiological status, and (2) functional accommodation. Current physiological status is critical for comparison with a physiological normal. This information determines severity of nerve involvement and establishes a baseline status that clearly can show the direction of change on subsequent testing. Functional accommodation addresses the patient's ability to function with a given physiological status, either normal or abnormal. Two patients with the same level of peripheral nerve injury can differ greatly in their adaptation to the dysfunction, retraining, and subsequent level of use.

Accommodation by the patient can be confounding to the determination of physiological nerve status, and it should be eliminated in absolute measures. It is doubtful that both acuity and functional accommodation can be measured precisely by the same test, just as visual acuity for refraction does not precisely correlate with a patient's skill at shooting. These are two entirely different questions, although one may be predictive of the other. They can often be found to correlate loosely but should at least be considered separately.

Future sensibility tests will have to be more precise in isolating physiological status from patient accommodation in order for differences to be clear. There is potential for precise imaging of damage and repair in the future with nuclear magnetic resonance spectroscopy (Sillerud et al, 1987). One needs to know (1) if the nerve is normal or not; (2) if it is abnormal, to what extent; and (3) how the nerve responds with treatment. Once these factors are determined, one needs to determine (4) how well the affected extremity can be functionally used, and (5) how important the dysfunction or restoration of function is to the patient's work and well-being. Accommodation is important to patient satisfaction outcomes, but testing also must include the physiological status so that direct comparison can be made with treatment.

No test can substitute for overall physical findings, and the surgeon obtains invaluable information from the patient history and direct examination of the involved extremity. But even patient history can be misleading. For example, the degree of pain cannot be used as a measure for outcome. One patient may experience a loss of nerve pain when the nerve has returned to normal, and another may experience a loss of pain when the nerve has died. Nerves can be painful and provide unusual and unexpected sensations to the patient when they are improving in function as well as when deteriorating. Nerve pain can be exquisite, alarming, and distracting to the patient, thus greatly magnifying the problem. Some patients with hand pain report little change when significant areas are involved, others report that their whole hand is numb when only a small area is involved. Of the many tests used for measuring peripheral nerve dysfunction, those that are the most useful are the ones that can help answer examiner, patient, and employer questions.

PATTERNS OF LOSS AND RECOVERY

Regardless of the measurement used, there are commonalities regarding the degree of damage and potential for improvement. Patients with neuropathy and neuritis from disease and compression/entrapment syndromes show different patterns of loss and recovery than do patients with lacerations.

Neuropathy and Neuritis

Healthy peripheral nerves usually do not exhibit abnormal signs and symptoms other than brief periods following stress. They respond quickly and adversely to ischemia. Measurement of change in sensibility is often measurement of the distal effect of an ischemic event (Szabo and Gelberman, 1987).

Diminution in sensibility in neuropathy and neuritis begins with slight changes and progresses as the nerve becomes more severely involved. Any change in sensibility requires evaluation. Duration and severity affect the ability of the nerve to repair and the response to treatment. A nerve that is mildly compressed for a prolonged period of time may be unable to return to normal, and a nerve severely compressed for a short period of time may be unable to return to normal.

Even a slight diminution in sensibility can be significant. The nerve has a natural tendency to heal itself after an insult, thus there can be periods of improvement but a gradual worsening over time. As long as the nerve continues to show change (improvement or loss), it is still acute and may respond to treatment. Sensibility testing to detect subtle changes can help determine the direction of change and indicate whether treatment has been effective. Measured diminution or loss of sensibility that has been unchanged for longer than 6 months is not as likely to improve with treatment.

If the patient has negligible complaints at rest but significant symptoms when the extremity is used, stress testing can be particularly helpful. In carpal tunnel syndrome, stress testing is helpful in the patient who has negligible complaints at rest but significant symptoms when the hand is used. These patients have been identified as having transient stress neuropathy (Bell, 1978; Szabo et al, 1984) or dynamic carpal tunnel syndrome. Measurements can be made before and after the patient assumes typical positions used for evaluating the effect of tension or compression. For example, Tinel's test can be performed before and after a Phalen's position at the wrist, or before and after full flexion of the elbow (Tinel, 1918). In turn, the activities and positions that cause the signs and symptoms can be specifically reproduced. A patient who complains of tingling and numbness when maintaining a supinated forearm position can be tested before and after assuming this position for a specified period of time. If it can be demonstrated that there is a change in sensibility, many examiners believe that this is an indication that the nerve is abnormal.

Other neuropathies may or may not respond to treatment with improvement in sensibility, depending on the underlying cause. Patients with syringomyelia show sensibility changes with sensitive testing. Patients with toxic neuropathies may or may not achieve some degree of recovery. Patients with congenital neuropathy may have variable sensibility patterns of loss, often limited to the extremities, that do not improve over time (Fig. 3–1).

Diabetic patients deserve special consideration. In diabetic neuropathy, patterns of sensibility diminution and loss begin distally and move more proximally as the disease progresses; the patterns of diminution and loss are more reflective of a dying back phenomenon from distal to proximal ischemia rather than involvement of specific innervation. For instance, instead of the loss affecting only the median or ulnar innervated areas, all of the fingertips may be involved with the same degree of loss. Loss of sensibility in diabetes is often permanent, and diminution of sensibility is often progressive. Attempts at maintaining or increasing the vascular supply to the extremity are important in minimizing peripheral nerve changes.

Sensibility testing in diabetic patients has often focused on the presence or absence of so-called protective sensation. Protective sensation is the recognition of pressure, pain, cold, or warmth before tissue damage results from the stimulus (von Prince and Butler, 1967; Wynn-Parry and Salter, 1976). Patients who lack protective sensation in their extremities are likely to develop ulcers and complications resulting in amputations. Diabetic patients with loss of protective sensation benefit from learning protective techniques for insensitive areas, such as wearing adaptive footwear in order to maintain functional extremities. Appropriate tests of sensibility facilitate recognition of subtle changes in early stages, with the potential for improved treatment (Griffey et al, 1988; Holewski et al, 1988).

Patients with Hansen's disease often have cutaneous end-organ involvement that may or may not be limited to specific nerve areas. The ulnar nerve is most often affected, followed by the median nerve, then the radial nerve in the upper extremity. When there is generalized sensory loss, areas of superficial nerve involvement can mask peripheral nerve branch involvement, particularly late in the disease. For example, the palms are spared superficial nerve involvement (Brand and Ebner, 1969). If the palms are involved, usually there is a specific ulnar or median nerve problem.

Patients with Hansen's disease can rapidly lose sensory or motor function or both. Occasionally, they can regain sensory and motor function if they are treated with corticosteroids or other anti-inflammatory agents while the nerve involvement is still acute and changing. Other patients seem to have a progressing silent neuropathy, which can easily be missed without routine testing. Peripheral nerve involvement is the primary impairment factor underlying deformity. Early diagnosis of Hansen's disease is important to minimize peripheral nerve complications; however, antimicrobial treatment of the disease does not completely prevent peripheral nerve branch involvement.

If insensitive digits are heavily used, injuries and tissue reabsorption can occur in the hands or feet of any patient with peripheral nerve involvement (see Fig. 3–1). The problem is largely mechanical. The result of insensitivity alone can be seen most clearly in patients with a congenital loss of pain, in whom, even with intact intrinsic musculature, there is damage and reabsorption of the digits. With loss of feedback, a patient will squeeze harder in order to ensure contact with an object and to simulate the feedback they once had.

Once nerve involvement is established from any disease or injury, recognition of areas with loss of protective sensation and the institution of protective techniques are critical to minimizing deformity from damage during use. Reconstructive surgery can help restore balance to grasp and prehension patterns, but once insensitivity is established and long-standing, no current treatment can restore sensibility to the extremities. Patients can be taught to use their eyes to protect their extremities, but this is only marginally effective in some cases. Early recognition through sensibility testing and prevention of functional loss is critical.

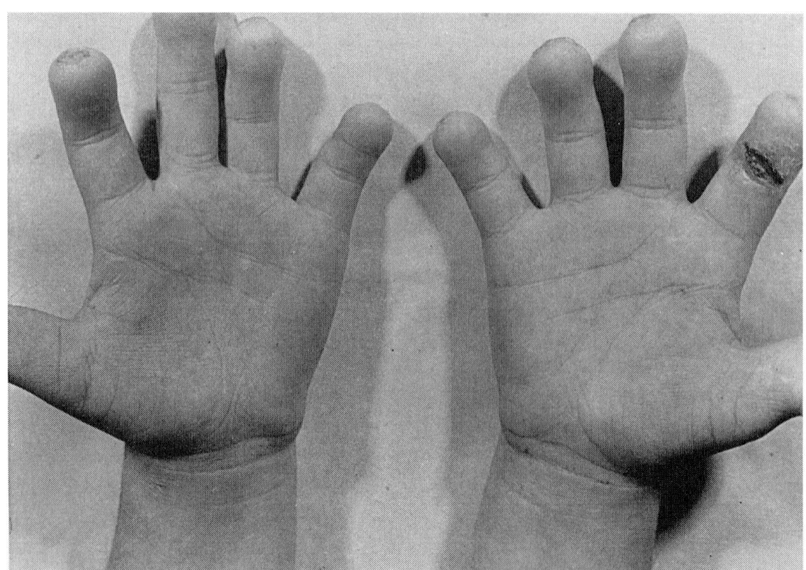

FIGURE 3–1. Child with hereditary sensory radicular neuropathy. There is finger absorption from the high concentration of pressure at fingertips secondary to absent sensibility. The intrinsic muscles of the hand are normal.

Trauma and Laceration

Patients with nerve lacerations exhibit loss of sensation consistent with the site and severity of injury. Some repaired peripheral nerves recover at a faster rate than others. Many digital nerves repair spontaneously. Some repaired peripheral nerves improve in a few months after suture and then worsen as they become trapped in reactive scar. Some nerves do not regain satisfactory sensory function; others quickly regain function from proximal to distal and return to near normal function. Serial evaluation demonstrates the course of the nerve improvement or loss (Fig. 3–2A and B).

The time from injury to recovery as well as the quality of recovery are indicative of how much sensibility will be restored. In general, the faster the rate of return and the better the early quality, the better the eventual result. Early mobilization of the nerve, within limits, is considered effec-

tive in reducing adhesions around the nerve. But adhesive traction on a repaired nerve can inhibit the return of function and should be eliminated or closely monitored (Hunter, 1991). In nerve repairs, it is most important to determine (1) when the nerve first begins to show restored function distal to suture and (2) the character and quality of nerve return as it attempts to heal. Much of the return of sensibility occurs in the year following the injury, although some patients have been observed to continue to experience improvement in motor function far beyond this period (Omer and Eversmann, 1994).

TEST SELECTION

Testing the skin with a pin for pain, with cotton wool for touch, or with test tube contact for warmth or cold is

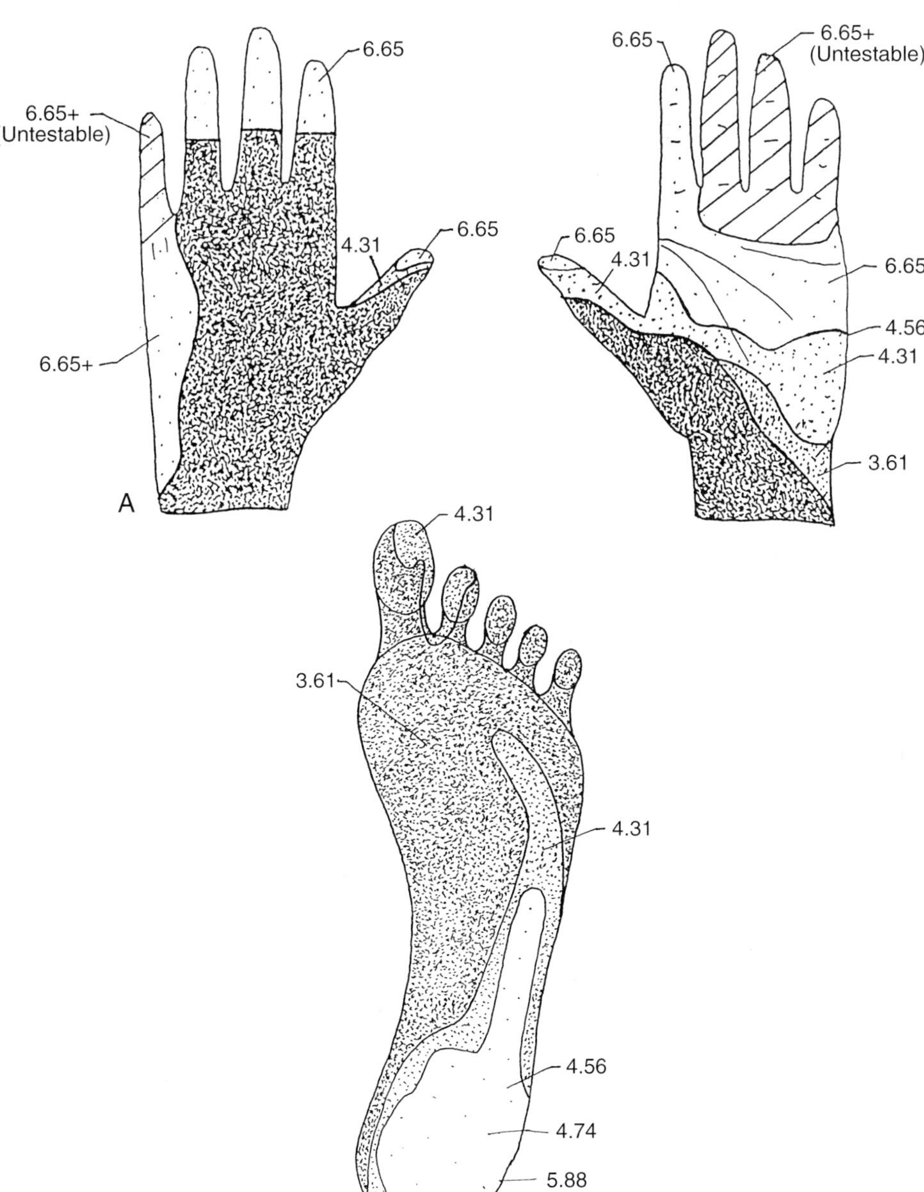

FIGURE 3–2. *A,* Semmes-Weinstein touch and pressure threshold map of child with axonotmesis after supracondylar fracture secondary to an automobile accident. Two-point discrimination is untestable at the fingertips and thumb. Sensibility returned to normal after 12 months. *B,* Threshold map of sural nerve abnormality secondary to subluxated spinal disc. In addition, there is a Morton's neuroma at the toes. Sensibility of either problem did not return with follow-up after more than 12 months.

unsatisfactory for estimating functional loss. It is impossible to duplicate these tests periodically with comparable quantitative results (Moberg, 1958, 1964). The modern von Frey (nylon filaments) test has quantifiable reproducibility (Table 3–3). In fact, most tests for sensibility cannot differentiate between paresthesia and good quality sensation (Brand and Ebner, 1969).

The usual pattern for recovery of sensibility in the hand after injury is pain, followed by higher orders of discrimination. Dellon and associates (1972) reported recovery in the following sequence: (1) pain, (2) flutter at 30 cycles per second (cps), (3) moving touch-pressure, (4) constant touch-pressure, and (5) vibration at 250 cps. However, that study included only 15 patients, and not all of those patients described the return of sensibility in the order specified. All clinical tests used to examine the degree of functional loss of sensibility are related to cutaneous touch-pressure sensation (Omer and Spinner, 1984). The sensation of touch is mediated through myelinated axons that are termed quickly adapting and slowly adapting in relation to their peripheral receptors (Dellon, 1978; Dellon et al, 1972, 1974; Mountcastle, 1980). Approximately 90% of A axons (tactile stimuli) are quickly adapting. Although there is some overlap and no clear distinction in receptor response, touch-pressure has been divided into moving touch and constant (static) pressure in relation to the receptors that are stimulated. Most clinical tests are not sensitive or specific enough to allow distinction between quickly and slowly adapting receptors (Bell-Krotoski and Buford, 1988).

The tests that are most useful to the examiner are those that are most frequently used and those that are objective. Those tests that are most frequently used provide a common language of understanding for measurement. Testing of sensibility is inherently subjective in that it requires the response of the patient (Omer, 1971). However, decisions based on uncontrolled tests are subject to error unless they are supported or followed by precise measurement (Buford, 1995; Fess, 1986). Objective tests provide data that can be depended on for repeatable information and impairment rating. Testing is more objective when variables that contribute to instrument error are controlled or eliminated and the procedure used is consistent in protocol.

The need for objective measurement is intuitively obvious in measuring a system that can be illusive to the eye but fundamental to the use of an extremity. It has been said that the hand without feeling is blind. The examiner is also blinded without the ability to visualize the system and image it for the patient and the employer as well as others with whom the patient comes in contact. As a group, patients with peripheral nerve problems are often defensive, having to explain why they are bothered by sensations and discomforts they cannot show and often do not understand. Many are relieved to know their problems are real, acknowledged, and recorded in a quantifiable way. It helps them allay real and subjective fears that others believe their problems are imaginary. Measurement helps others—those who otherwise often conclude that the patient is looking for excuses and wanting time off work—believe the patient. For both the patient and the employer, it is reassuring to know whether there is a measurable change in sensibility and whether a problem is relatively mild or severe. All involved stand to benefit when decision-making regarding projected use of the extremity can be based on absolute measures rather than conjecture.

Some test instruments are more objective than others. Problems in hand-held instruments were described by Dyck and associates (1979). Computerized instruments offer potential improvement in stimulus control, and instruments are now available for two-point discrimination and vibration testing. These devices do not adequately control the force applied by the examiner, or the force that can be added by the patient (Bell-Krotoski and Buford, 1988). When it is optimally controlled, computerized sensibility testing may add greatly to our knowledge of peripheral nerve impairment and response to treatment (Horch et al, 1992a, 1992b).

Computerized instruments need to demonstrate an advantage over simple hand-held instruments by comparison studies. A hand-held instrument, such as the Semmes-Weinstein monofilament pressure esthesiometer, that is controlled and designed to produce a specific stimulus may be found as sensitive at specific settings and may be more practical for many clinical situations. In either case, both hand-held and computerized test instruments need to be used with a full understanding of their strengths and weaknesses (Bell-Krotoski, 1991; Buford, 1995).

Level of the Lesion

Combined with the physical examination and educated judgment, electrical nerve conduction and electromyography testing are better at predicting the specific level of a lesion than sensibility tests. Sensibility tests alone do not predict the specific level of lesion.

Wallerian degeneration can be measured in the laboratory animal by using high-field proton nuclear magnetic resonance spectroscopy (Sillerud et al, 1987), but the electrical conduction velocity study for sensory nerves is the only quantitative clinical technique for measuring sensation. The range of conduction velocity is 45 to 75 meters per second

▼ **TABLE 3–3**
Quantitative Sensibility

Sensibility Modality	Technique and Normals
Touch-pressure	von Frey hair pressure, with point localization between 2.44 and 2.83*
	Weber two-point discrimination distance of 3 to 5 mm in the digital autonomous zone of cutaneous nerve in the hand
	Ridged esthesiometer, with recognition of keel depth at 3/8 mm or less
Body movement–position	5 to 10 degrees of movement at an interphalangeal joint, 1 degree at shoulder or hip joint
Pain	Algesimeter (5 gm pressure) should be localized within 2 cm
Temperature	Copper test tubes, with recognition between 20° and 35°C
Vibration	200 to 250 cps
Protective sensibility	Conscious appreciation of pain, cold, warmth, or pressure before tissue damage results from the stimulus

*Replaced in modern instruments with Semmes-Weinstein pressure esthesiometer.
cps = cycles per second.
Medical Research Council: Peripheral Nerve Injuries, Special Series No. 282. London, Her Majesty's Stationery Office, 1954.

(Juul-Jensen and Mayer, 1966). Regardless of the nature of the stimulus, the form of the action potential is remarkably constant. The combination of receptor organ and diameter of the myelinated afferent axon might provide some specificity to sensation, but this specificity cannot be expressed in the form of the action potential.

Nerve conduction is not totally objective, in that measurements can differ depending on time of day, temperature of the nerve tested, examiner conducting the test, instrument, and other variables (Kimura, 1984). Degrees of nerve slowing can be normal for some individuals but abnormal for others, and some abnormal nerve conduction studies are only suspect. Sensibility testing used in combination with other tests can also be extremely valuable for clustering of findings to support the belief that a specific peripheral nerve is abnormal.

Abnormal conduction does not mean that the patient has lost sensibility. Only a sensibility test can predict what a patient can feel. There is no direct correlation between the tests for nerve conduction and those for sensibility. For example, sensibility for light touch usually returns in the young patient after nerve suture, whereas sensory nerve conduction velocity may not recover (Almquist and Eeg-Olofsson, 1970). There is a loose correlation in that a positive test for abnormal nerve conduction will correlate with a positive change in sensibility if the tests used are sensitive enough or if the abnormality of the nerve is severe enough (Breger, 1987).

Greco noted in 1989 that nerve conduction is probably the most sensitive test for early detection of abnormal change, yet some patients without sensory nerve conduction have been found to have residual deep-pressure sensibility. Because abnormal values for nerve conduction are not always clear cut, with normal subjects sometimes showing mild slowing, intervention for treatment is usually delayed until there is a demonstrable change in sensibility.

Motor Function

Muscle testing should be conducted in combination with sensibility testing because the combination provides more information on the character and status of peripheral nerve abnormality (Fig. 3–3A to C).

SENSIBILITY TESTS

Touch-Pressure Threshold

In 1898, von Frey and Kiesow attempted to standardize the stimuli for testing the subjective sense of light touch by using a series of horsehairs of varying thickness and stiffness (von Frey, 1922). Semmes and Weinstein used nylon monofilaments mounted in Lucite rods as substitutes for the horsehairs (Weinstein, 1962). The Semmes-Weinstein monofilament system or pressure esthesiometer consists of a series of 20 probes marked 1.65 to 6.65. The number represents the logarithm of 10 times the force in milligrams required to bow the monofilament (Levin et al, 1978; Semmes et al, 1960). Clinical testing techniques for peripheral nerve abnormality were developed by von Prince and Butler

(1967), Werner and Omer (1970), and Bell (1978). Werner and Omer (1970) conducted more than 4000 tests of peripheral nerve injuries over a 2-year period in 787 patients. The original long kit consisted of 20 filaments that included threshold filaments and additional heavier filaments for testing the loss of protective sensation.

A reduced filament kit of five significant filaments is all that is needed in most cases to detect and map sensibility abnormality anywhere on the body. The five filaments in the minikit were selected to represent cut-off levels for significant sensibility function, based on a review of 150 patients given a battery of sensibility tests, which included tests for two-point discrimination, graphesthesia, texture discrimination, stereognosis, temperature, and proprioception (Bell, 1978). The use of fewer threshold filaments is an advantage because there is no possibility of filament application force overlap.

The 2.83 filament can be used to screen for sensory abnormality anywhere on the body. It is suprathreshold for the face and subthreshold for areas of the foot that contain callus (Bell-Krotoski et al, 1995). The filaments can be used to screen specific sites for particular nerves or to map an entire area or extremity, reflecting subtle and dramatic changes. The test yields reproducible components of sensibility that can be translated into levels of quality of sensibility (Werner and Omer, 1970) (Table 3–4).

The chemical name for the filament used is polyhexamethylene dodecandiamide, better known as nylon 612. Pure nylon has an indefinite shelf life and minimum humidity absorption (3% in 100% humidity) (Bell-Krotoski, 1990). The monofilaments have been used in psychophysiological studies to identify rapidly adapting fibers, although the literature describes them as only measuring the slowly adapting fiber system (Vallbo and Johansson, 1984). They have been found to produce both low and high frequency signals sufficient in strength to stimulate both slowly and rapidly adapting end-organs (Bell-Krotoski and Buford, 1988).

The Semmes-Weinstein pressure esthesiometer provides force control for damping the vibration of the examiner's hand and for repeated application, by bending at a peak force, and by maintaining a constant force while in contact with the skin. The elasticity of the nylon helps absorb the normal vibration of the examiner's hand, which otherwise introduces a large variable in testing at the lightest normal threshold sensitivities. The examiner and patient are prevented from adding any increase in the force, because the force is constant throughout the bend until severe bending results in lesser force, not greater (Fig. 3–4).

▼ TABLE 3–4
Scale of Interpretation of Monofilaments

		Filament Markings	Calculated Force (g)
Green	Normal	1.65–2.83	0.0045–0.068
Blue	Diminished light touch	3.22–3.61	0.166–0.408
Purple	Diminished protective sensation	3.84–4.31	0.697–2.06
Red	Loss of protective sensation	4.56–6.65	3.63–4.47
Red-lined	Untestable	Greater than 6.65	Greater than 4.47

From Bell JA: Sensibility evaluation. *In* Hunter J, Schneider L, Mackin E, Bell JA (eds): Rehabilitation of the Hand. Philadelphia, C.V. Mosby Company, 1978, pp 278–279.

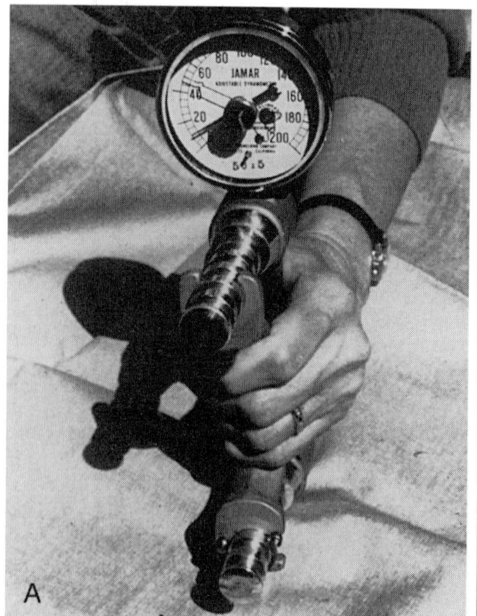

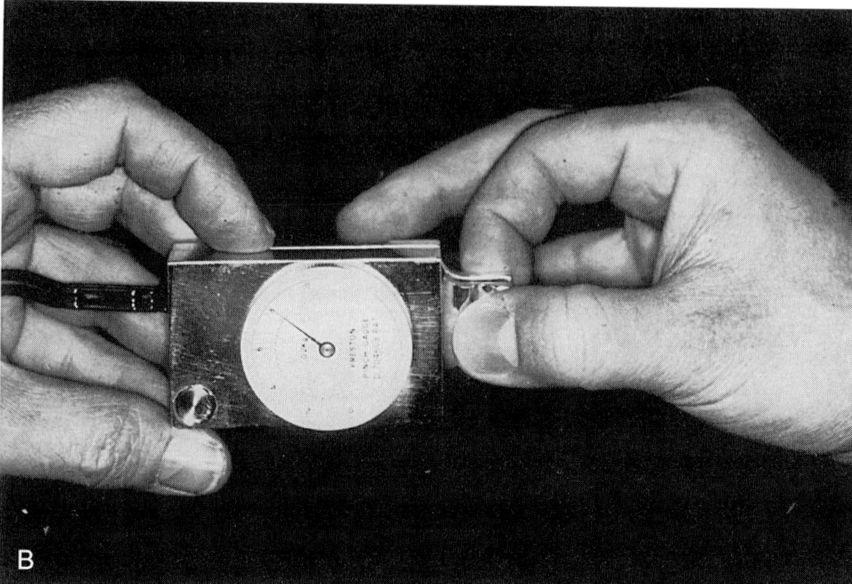

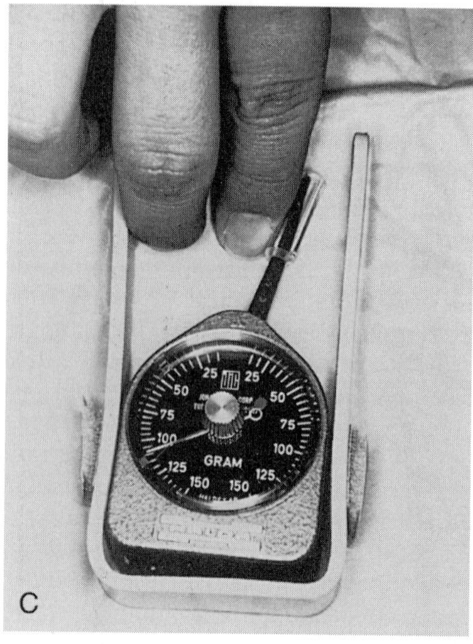

FIGURE 3–3. *A*, Technique to measure grasp strength. Notch used for crossbar should be recorded as well as strength reading. Best baseline comparison is grasp strength of contralateral hand. *B*, Technique to measure fingertip pinch strength. A pinch gauge can also measure key pinch. (*A* and *B*, From Omer GE Jr: Evaluation of the extremity with peripheral nerve injury and timing for nerve suture. Instr Course Lect Am Acad Orthop Surg *33:*480–481, 1984.) *C*, Technique to measure finger intrinsic muscle strength.

The filaments can be misapplied when applied too quickly, and they may exceed their peak force. Filaments should be applied in a smooth motion in about 1.5 seconds, held for 1.5 seconds, and lifted in 1.5 seconds. In 1979, Lamotte (Bell-Krotoski and Buford, 1988) noted that quick lifting elicits a burst of firing of mechanoreceptors, just as does a quick application, and the movement should be avoided. Peak force is achieved only when the filament is bent, and a crescent-shaped edge of the filament is in contact with the skin. It is impossible to calculate the area of the edge in contact precisely, and it is more important that it is constant from one application to another, while the force produced is controlled. Control of application force could easily be the single most important factor in sensibility testing with monofilaments.

If calibrated correctly, the Semmes-Weinstein pressure esthesiometer repeatedly determines light-touch and deep-pressure thresholds within a small range compared with the wide variation in uncontrolled tests (Bell-Krotoski and Tomancik, 1987). It is sensitive and is accurate enough at forces less than 1 g to produce the above- and below-threshold stimuli necessary for normative testing (Bell-Krotoski et al, 1993).

Measurement demonstrates both early diminution in sensibility and early return of sensibility, often demonstrating changes in a few weeks when patients are monitored serially. It can be the first quantifiable test that measures returning sensibility, often long before two-point discrimination is measurable.

There is no evidence that touch-pressure–threshold detection can be retrained or depends on cortical mediation. In experimental studies during brain surgery, the recognition of touch-pressure threshold could not be extinguished by stimulation of the sensory cortex, whereas recognition of difference between one and two points was totally extinguished (Weinstein, 1991).

PROCEDURE

The room temperature should be comfortable for the patient, and testing is performed in an area that is as quiet as

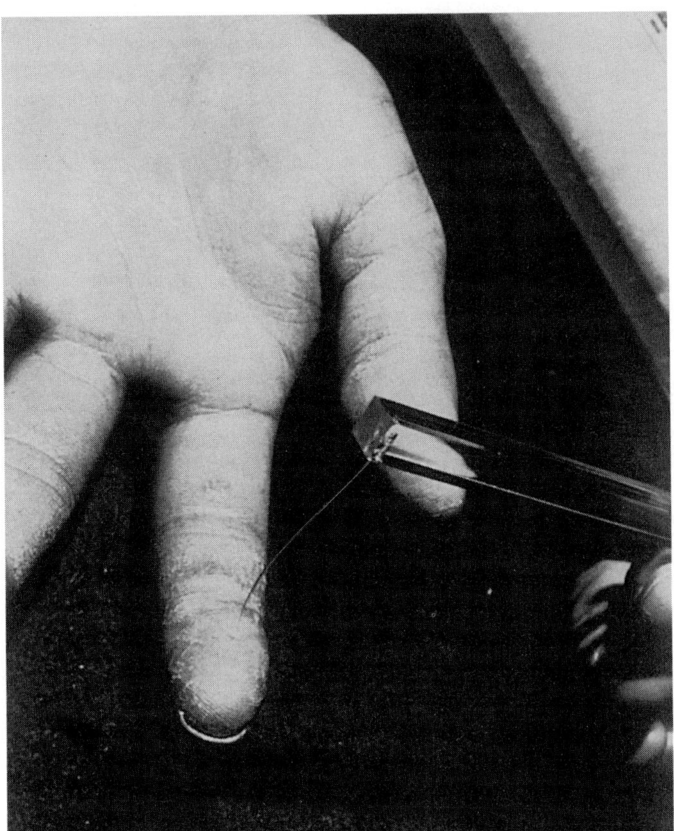

FIGURE 3–4. Technique for applying Semmes-Weinstein monofilaments. The monofilament should be perpendicular to the surface of the skin, and pressure should be increased until the monofilament bends. (Omer GE Jr: Physical diagnosis of peripheral nerve injuries. Orthop Clin North Am *12*:218, 1981.)

possible. Testing begins with the lightest filaments for screening normal areas. If these filaments are detected, it is not necessary to use heavier filaments. If they are not detected, progressively heavier filaments are used until a filament is recognized, or the patient does not respond to any filament.

The monofilament is applied perpendicular to the body surface, and pressure is increased until the monofilament bends. The monofilaments are applied at least three times to an unresponsive site. This is done to ensure delivery of desired threshold force, as the light filaments can sometimes be applied at an angle and result in too light a force. One response out of three is considered a correct response. The patient closes the eyes while the examiner touches the skin with the monofilament.

Testing begins by establishing an area that tests within normal limits. This allows the patient to become familiar with the testing procedure and the examiner to establish a normal sensibility site for reference (Fig. 3–5). This area can be revisited frequently in order to eliminate guessing, and to establish that what the subject cannot detect in a test site, he or she can detect at the control site. The contralateral extremity is not usually used as the control site, because peripheral nerve problems may be bilateral. However, higher values may be considered normal when the uninvolved extremity values are higher than established normals.

When an involved hand is tested, it should be marked off into theoretical zones of sensibility (Fig. 3–6). Usually, test-

ing proceeds from distal to proximal to avoid eliciting Tinel-type sensations, although these are not usually a problem. The examiner moves around on the hand or site tested, in order to eliminate anticipation of a particular sequence by the patient.

Localization has been both included and excluded in the test but is not used as a requirement of the test, because the examination is most repeatable if localization is not required. Generally, the patient should be able to indicate the site tested. Localization values are highly variable over the body and thus can alter the monofilament test, which is relatively constant (Weinstein, 1968). Localization can still be tested but is treated as a separate test.

Sensibility at level 4.56 and over is only protective and is lost when level 6.65 is unrecognized. Children recognize the same pressure as adults but will not localize as well, even when they cooperate. Judged by the Semmes-Weinstein test, some patients who do not regain motor function do develop minimal light touch several months after a traumatic nerve injury.

Two-Point Discrimination Sensibility

This test was introduced by Weber in 1835. The object is to determine whether the patient can discriminate between being touched with one or two points and the minimal distance at which two points touching the skin are recognized. Clinical testing techniques for the hand were developed by Moberg (1958, 1962).

The traditional two-point discrimination test became the static two-point discrimination test, when a "moving" two-point discrimination test was introduced by Dellon (1978). The term "static" refers only to one test relative to the other, because the static test is a dynamic stimulus as the instrument touches the hand and indents the skin, exciting mechanoreceptors.

PROCEDURE FOR THE TRADITIONAL OR STATIC TWO-POINT DISCRIMINATION TEST

Traditional testing instruments include a Boley gauge, a blunt eye caliper, or an ordinary paper clip (Moberg, 1965) (Fig. 3–7A and B). The test should be demonstrated while the patient is watching, so that he can anticipate the procedure. Several areas on the uninvolved hand should be checked because some patients have congenitally abnormal two-point discrimination. Testing is begun distally and proceeds proximally. The points of the caliper are set at 10 mm and are progressively brought together as accurate responses are obtained. The pressure from the testing instrument should not produce an ischemic area on the skin. When two points are applied, they make contact simultaneously, and the line between the points is in the longitudinal axis of the finger. The patient closes the eyes but indicates immediately if he feels one or two points. An interval of 3 to 5 seconds should be allowed between application of the points. A series of one or two points is applied with varied sequence in each finger zone (Fig. 3–8). The procedure is performed three times in each zone; if the patient does not record two of the three instances correctly, the result is considered a failure at that test distance. If the patient correctly identifies

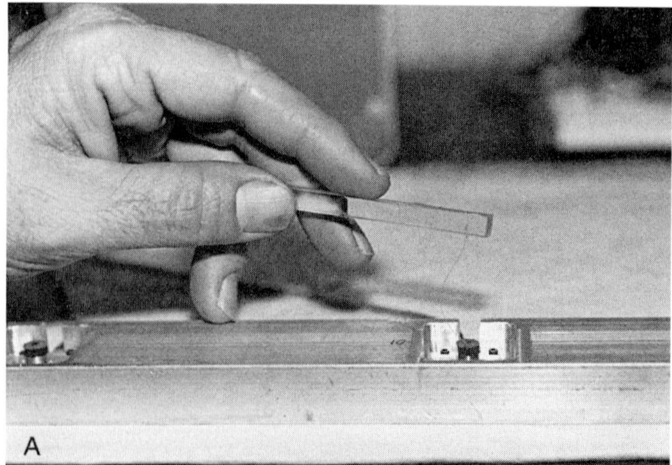
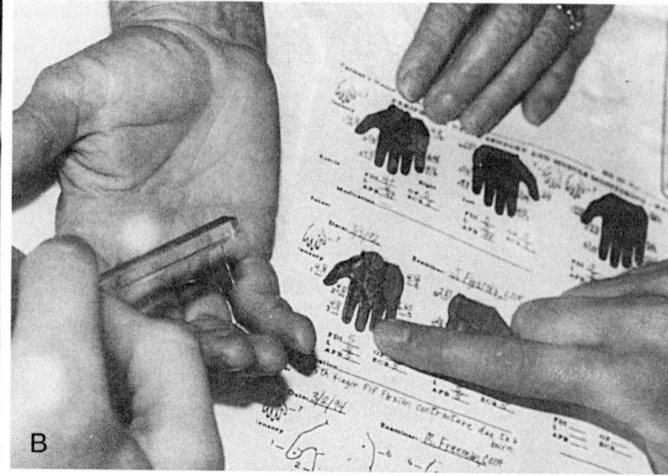

FIGURE 3–5. *A*, Semmes-Weinstein monofilament applied to a strain gauge to check calibration. A specific repeatable force is delivered when the filament bends and continues until the filament is lifted or is severely bent. The elastic nylon filament ensures a constant application force, prevents increase in the force by its bend, and absorbs vibrations of the examiner's hand. *B*, Application of Semmes-Weinstein monofilament and demonstration of mapping on a screening form.

the number of points applied, the testing distance is decreased by 5 mm. Omer uses this three-application technique throughout the extremity (Omer, 1968; Werner and Omer, 1970), but Moberg uses a different system in the hand; there are 10 applications of two points and 10 applications of one point at random. The total of incorrect one-point applications is subtracted from the total of correct two-point applications. An answer of five or more is considered a pass (Lister, 1977).

The normal threshold for two-point discrimination distance for the volar surface of the hand varies according to the zone being tested (see Fig. 3–6 and Table 3–5). The threshold for the dorsal surface is higher in all zones; the normal threshold is 7 to 12 mm, diminished is 13 to 20 mm, and absent is greater than 20 mm. Below-elbow and below-knee two-point discrimination distance is normal between 40 to 50 mm, diminished between 55 and 80 mm, and absent above 80 mm. Above-elbow and above-knee two-point discrimination distance is normal between 65 to 75 mm, diminished between 80 and 100 mm, and absent above 100 mm (Omer, 1971, 1984). Abnormal skin texture, such as heavy scales or calluses, has an influence on the test results (Fig. 3–9). Callus usually affects the light touch levels, but diminished protective sensibility can be measured. Testing can be performed in the presence of edema or infection, but the result demonstrates the sensibility present, which may not be the true status of the nerve (Omer, 1981a, 1981b, 1984).

A disc instrument designed by Moberg (1990), and the DISC-Criminator introduced by Dellon (1990) offer advantages over the former instruments such as the paper clip, eye caliper, Boley gauge, or Ridge sensitometer (Renfrew, 1969). The distance between the prongs is already determined and

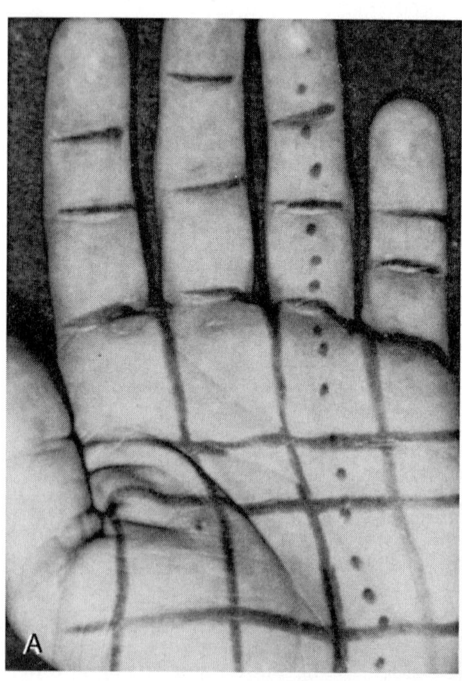
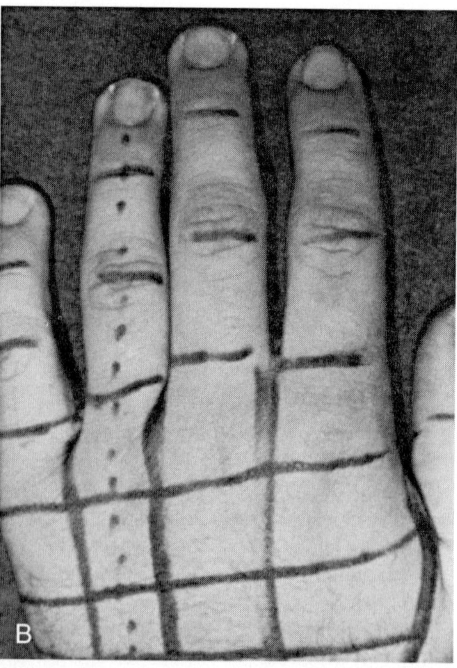

FIGURE 3–6. The hand is divided into seven theoretical zones of sensibility for testing: The seven palmar zones correspond to the flexion creases. Sensibility for two-point discrimination varies according to the zone being tested. Testing is begun at the more sensitive volar pulp tip. *A*, Volar; *B*, dorsal.

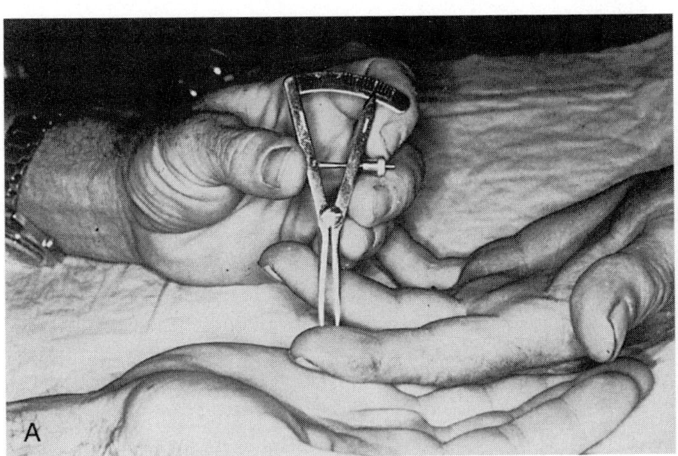
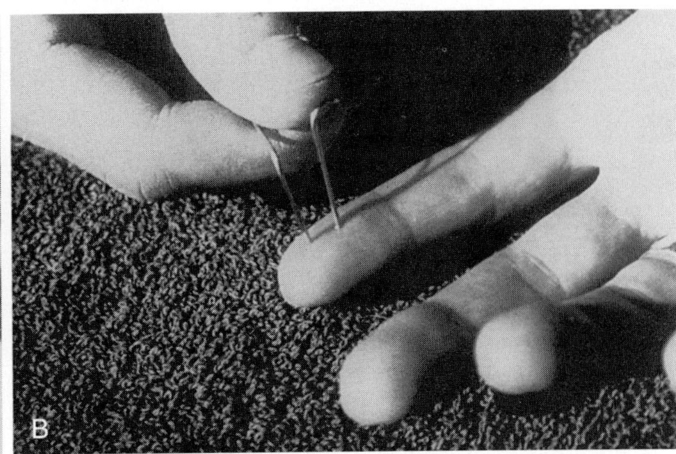

FIGURE 3–7. Technique for testing two-point discrimination distance with a blunt eye caliper. The line of application is in the longitudinal axis of the finger. The pressure from the instrument should not produce an ischemic area on the skin. (Omer GE Jr: Methods of assessment of injury and recovery of peripheral nerves. Surg Clin North Am *61*:310, 1981.) *B,* A paper clip may be used as a testing instrument for static two-point discrimination distance. The line of application is in the longitudinal axis of the finger. (Omer GE Jr: Physical diagnosis of peripheral nerve injuries. Orthop Clin North Am *12*:220, 1981.)

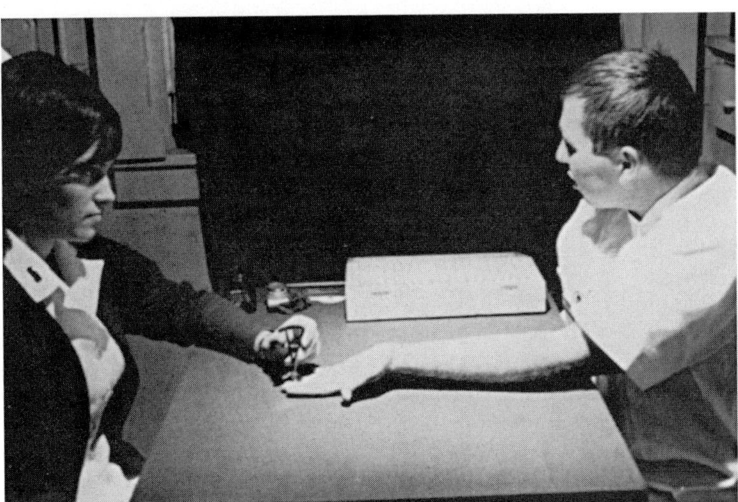
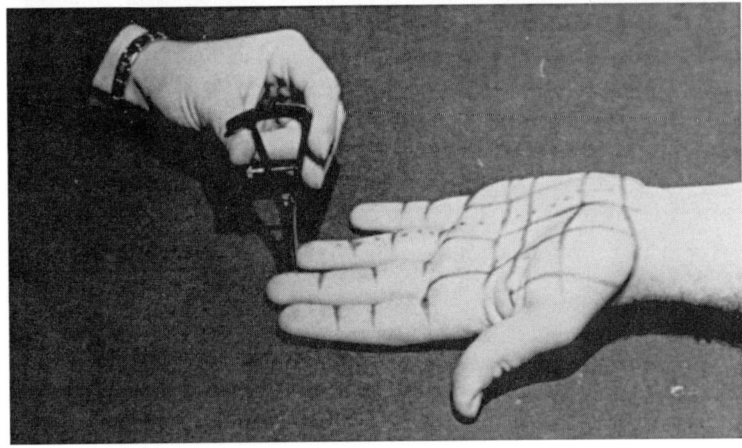

FIGURE 3–8. Weber two-point discrimination distance. Testing is begun distally and proceeds proximally. Both the examiner and patient should be comfortable.

▼ **TABLE 3–5**
Two-Point Discrimination Distance Volar Surface of Hand

	Hand Zone	Distance in Millimeters		
		Normal	*Diminished*	*Absent*
Between fingertip and D-I-P joint	7	3–5	6–10	10+
Between D-I-P joint and P-I-P joint	6	3–6	7–10	10+
Between P-I-P joint and finger web	5	4–7	8–10	10+
Between web and distal palmar crease	4	5–8	9–20	20+
Between distal crease and central palm	3	6–9	10–20	20+
Base of palm and wrist	1–2	7–10	11–20	20+

fixed, the prongs are not sharp but smooth, and these instruments are not as heavy as the Boley gauge. Testing by the DISC-Criminator instrument is most repeatable if the weight of the instrument is used as it rests against the hand rather than the examiner's applying variable force on application (Louis et al, 1984). The weight of the instrument alone is not enough to consider the stimulus force controlled. Even when held constant against the skin, the vibration of the examiner's hand greatly exceeds the resolution of normal touch by several orders of magnitude.

PROCEDURE FOR THE MOVING TWO-POINT DISCRIMINATION TEST

In the moving two-point discrimination test, the test is performed with an ordinary paper clip bent into two points in the same manner as the static two-point discrimination test. The finger is supported, and the paper clip is moved along the volar surface of the finger from a proximal to a distal direction (Fig. 3–10). The paper clip is moved parallel to the long axis of the finger. The ends of the paper clip are separated by 5 to 8 mm and closed in stages as the patient quickly indicates whether one point or two points are felt. The testing stimulus is alternated at random from one to two points until the patient begins to hesitate with the answer. Seven of 10 responses are then required to be correct before

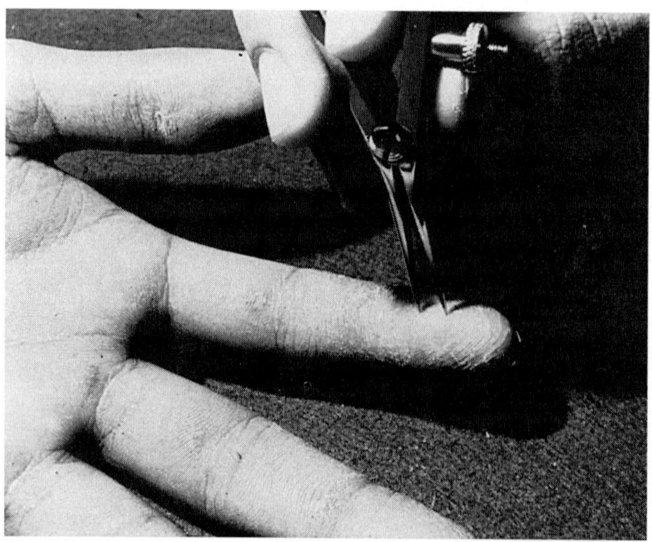

FIGURE 3–9. Abnormal skin texture can result in unstable test results. (Omer GE Jr: Physical diagnosis of peripheral nerve injuries. Orthop Clin North Am *12*:218, 1981.)

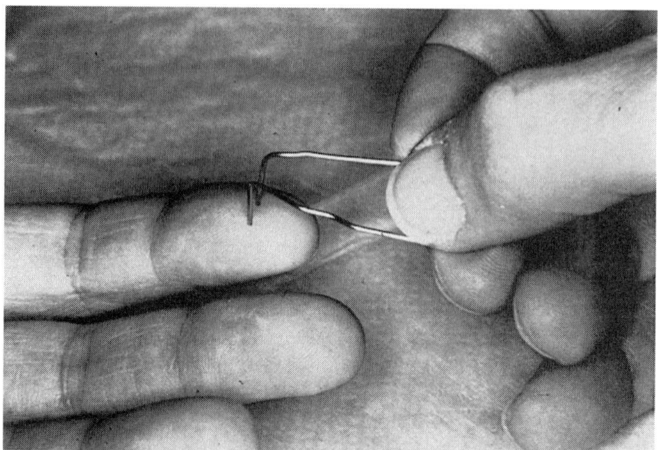

FIGURE 3–10. Dellon's technique for testing moving two-point discrimination. Pressure from the instrument should not produce an ischemic trail on the skin. (Omer GE Jr: Evaluation of the extremity with peripheral nerve injury and timing for nerve suture. Instr Course Lect Am Acad Orthop Surg *33*:475, 1984.)

proceeding to the next lower value (closer points). The normal moving two-point discrimination distance is 2 mm in the distal phalangeal pad, which is the only area tested. The test evokes a positive response from a recovering nerve before a response to a static two-point discrimination stimulus is detected.

Control of force of application may be the single most important factor in sensibility testing, as shown by the variable mapping of detection force possible with the Semmes-Weinstein pressure esthesiometer (Bell-Krotoski and Buford, 1988). Moberg supported the need for force control in two-point discrimination test instruments. Until controlled instruments become available, he suggested applying 5 and 10 g in testing and made a prototype design for a controlled instrument that would produce these two weights (Fig. 3–11*A* and *B*).

Other factors are important in stimulus control. The ends of the instrument used for testing should be equal in length and blunted to avoid eliciting pain. The tip geometry should be identical on the two prongs. The same type of instrument should be used in following a series of patients, because different instruments produce different stimuli (Omer and Spinner, 1975).

New computerized test instruments allow the two-point test to be applied with more specific force of application and throughout a range of sensitivities for the first time (Dellon, 1990; Horch et al, 1992a, 1992b). Testing with computerized stimuli could allow optimal test sensitivity and applications yet to be determined.

Within the limits of current instruments, two-point discrimination test results have been normal, whereas both the Semmes-Weinstein pressure esthesiometer and nerve conduction tests have been abnormal in both clinical and induced neuropathies (Bell, 1978; Szabo et al, 1984; Werner and Omer, 1970). Therefore, the two-point discrimination is not recommended as a single test for patients with nerve compression at this time. The test has widest application in patients with lacerations, in whom the presence of two-point discrimination usually indicates a significant return of peripheral nerve function.

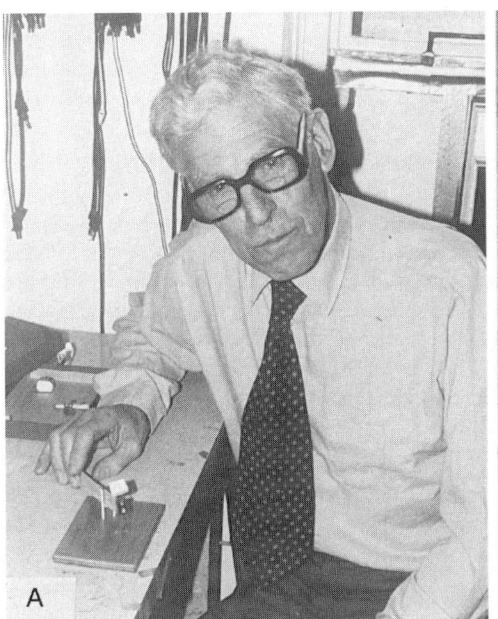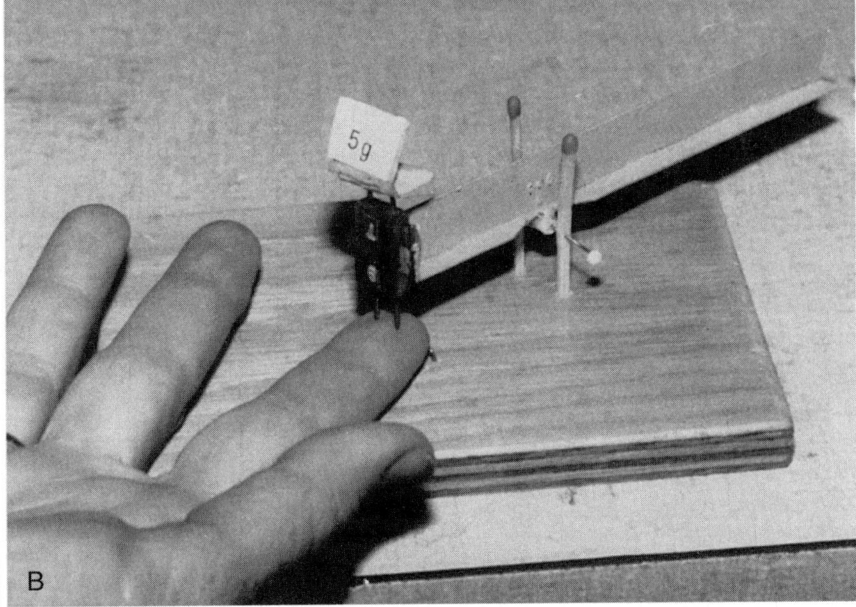

FIGURE 3–11. *A,* Photograph of Eric Moberg using matchsticks to develop a prototype design for a pressure-controlled instrument to measure two-point discrimination distance. *B,* Close-up of prototype instrument.

Picking-Up Test

Moberg (1965) emphasized measurement of what the hand can do, and coined the term tactile gnosis for normal cutaneous sensation, providing normal quality sensibility is present. Although two-point discrimination distance correlates with constant touch, such as various pinch or grip positions, it does not assess tactile gnosis, which requires movement (Wynn-Parry and Salter, 1976). In 1958, Moberg developed the picking-up test as a technique for determining the functional value of sensibility in the hand:

> *. . . pick up a number of small objects on a table and put them as quickly as he can into a small box, first with one hand and then with the other. After he has done this a few times he is asked to do the same thing blindfolded. It is then studied how rapidly and efficiently he picks up the objects; comparison is made between his right and left hands. The test with the patient blindfolded can be made harder by asking him to identify the objects as he picks them up.*

Moberg demonstrated the abnormal functional pattern in a hand with median cutaneous sensibility loss. The picking-up test is used only in patients with median or combined median and ulnar nerve injuries.

PROCEDURE

Omer quantitated the picking-up test by choosing nine objects of different size and shape (Omer, 1968, 1980) (Fig. 3–12). A normal result is considered to be five to eight seconds for young adult males, but a better normal measure-

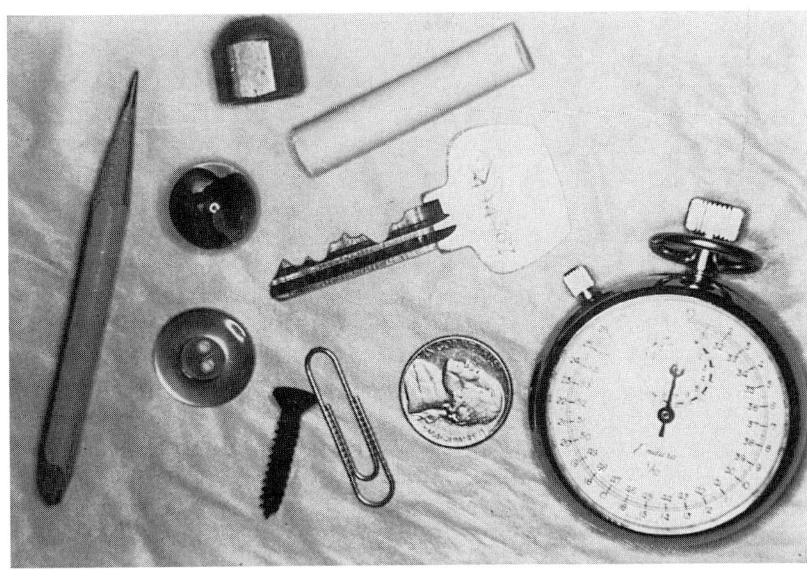

FIGURE 3–12. Items for a picking-up test. (Omer GE Jr: Methods of assessment of injury and recovery of peripheral nerves. Surg Clin North Am *61:*316, 1981.)

ment is the time required to complete the task with the uninvolved hand. The objects can include such things as a key, marble, small square piece of wood, nut and bolt, paper clip, short pencil, or safety pin.

The picking-up test is performed with the uninvolved hand and then with the injured hand, first with the eyes open and then with the eyes closed. The patient should attempt to identify the objects when the eyes are closed. The functional aptitude of the patient for picking up the objects is noted by the examiner. Sometimes a piece of chalk is substituted for one of the objects so that a trail of functional surfaces will remain on the hand (Omer, 1980, 1981a, 1981b, 1984) (Fig. 3–13). The patient is timed with a stopwatch each time the test is performed, and comparison of periodic tests indicates the changing status of function. Normal tactile gnosis requires motion and power as well as cutaneous sensibility.

The test is not static and will change with the level of homeostasis of the tissues and motor function capability as well as with sensibility recovery. Patients can improve results with experience doing the test (Omer, 1974) (Fig. 3–14).

Seddon stated that the precursor of the picking-up test was the coin test, as described by Riddoch in 1940 (Seddon, 1975). The patient, whose eyes must be closed, is given a coin and asked to identify it.

Localization

Resolution in point localization after nerve laceration repair begins wide and narrows with time. A filament or probe is used as a stimulus and is applied to the hand with the patient's vision occluded. The patient is asked to point to the area touched. Distance is recorded in centimeters, and direction is drawn as an arrow between the point touched and the point of response (see Fig. 3–6).

Normal sensibility localizes pressure between 2.44 and 2.83 at the distal end of the extremities, but normal pressure is between 4.08 and 4.17 at the proximal portion of the extremities.

Point localization is a useful test in demonstrating problems with referred touch following nerve repair, but is highly dependent on the cognitive spatial ability of the patient. Some normal subjects are unable to localize closer than 2 cm at sites on their palm. Like other hand-held tests, the results may vary because of changes in application force.

Body Position and Movement

The precision of sensibility for body position or movement is the reverse of that of cutaneous sensibility for the proximal and distal portion of the extremity. The patient can identify the position and directional change in a finger or toe when passive movements of the interphalangeal joints are performed. An interphalangeal joint requires 5 to 10 degrees of passive movement for recognition, but in the shoulder joint, less than 1 degree of passive movement can be recognized and a given position can be reproduced within 2 degrees.

Vibration

Vibration has had a resurgence in interest as a test for sensibility. Differential testing can be made at low and high frequencies, and compared with a physiological normal value. Testing requires a response by the patient that can easily be made a forced choice and will provide quantifiable data. Lundborg has used controlled computerized instruments to differentiate responses at various frequencies (Lundborg et al, 1986).

The application force produced by the examiner can be uncontrolled, and the patient may not be limited in ability to add additional force. Many instruments are set at one frequency and vary only in the intensity of that frequency.

Vibration as a separate sense may not exist, and the test has yet to be shown to correlate with patient function. It does not correlate with how much a patient can or cannot feel. The test is the subject of research in the identification of early carpal tunnel syndrome. Few studies compare the results of vibrometry with the other tests for sensation or sensibility.

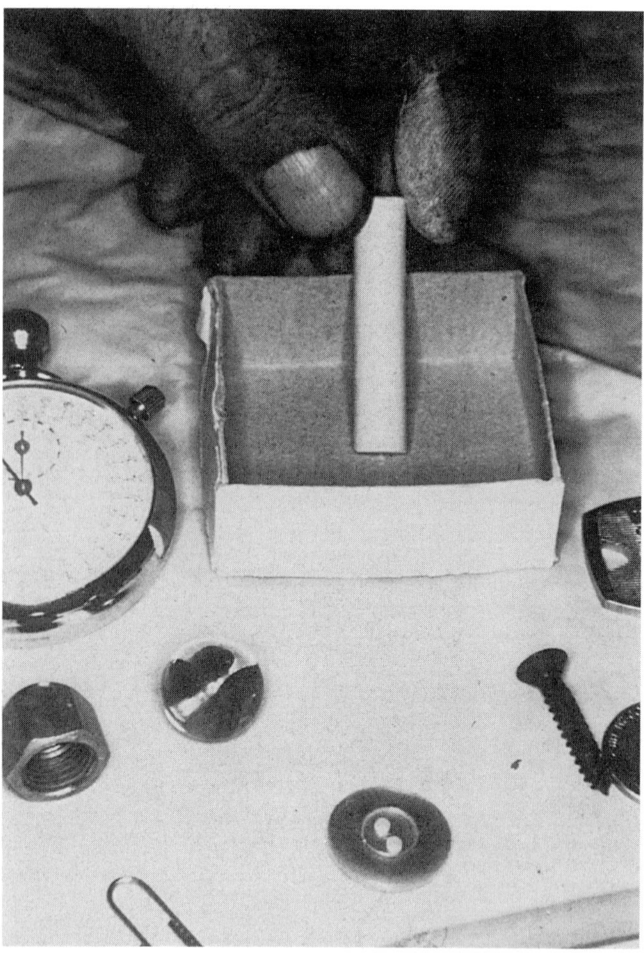

FIGURE 3–13. A piece of chalk, as one of the objects in the picking-up test, will demonstrate functional surfaces of digits. (Omer GE Jr: Methods of assessment of injury and recovery of peripheral nerve injuries. Surg Clin North Am *61*:317, 1981; and Omer GE Jr: Physical diagnosis of peripheral nerve injuries. Orthop Clin North Am *12*:225, 1981.)

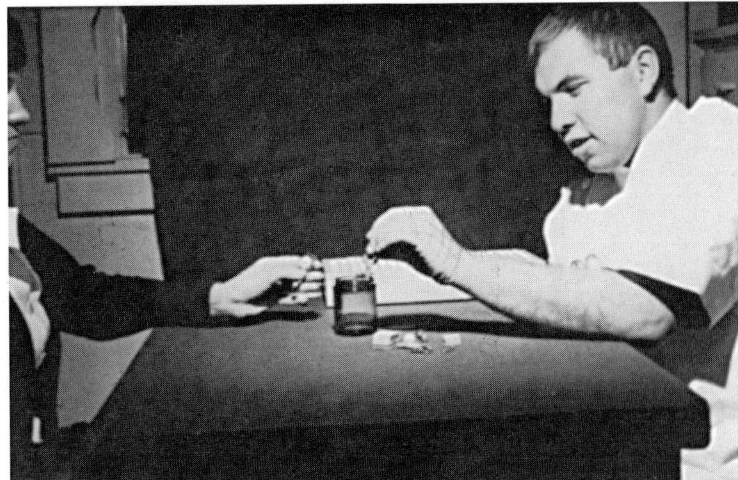

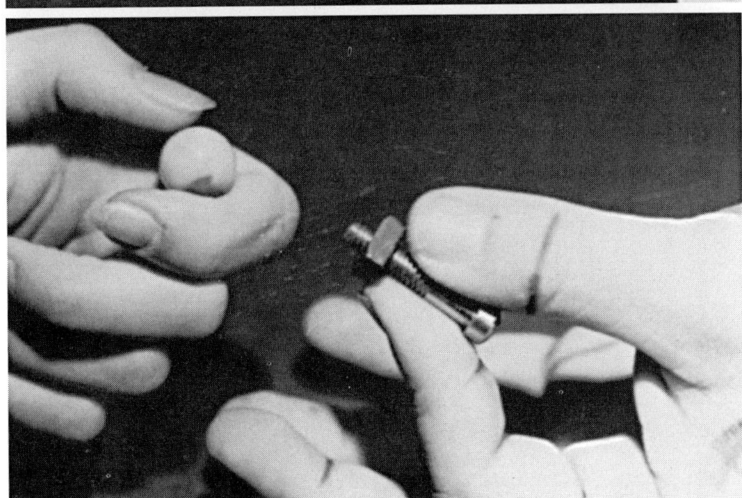

FIGURE 3–14. Timed picking-up test. The patient should attempt to identify each object, then is timed while transferring all objects from the table to the jar.

SENSATION TESTS

Temperature

Because of the summation of temperature and difficulty in obtaining objective data, temperature recognition is difficult to measure precisely. Normal resolution of temperature is in the order of plus or minus 5°C. Warm and cold test tubes are too gross for sensitive testing. Instruments that can measure exacting temperature responses have been designed, but these instruments are expensive and not yet generally available.

Tinel's Sign

Tinel (1918) described a so-called formication sign that indicates the presence of axons in the process of regeneration:

. . . when percussion is lightly applied to the injured nerve trunk, we find in the cutaneous region of the nerve a creeping sensation usually compared by the patient to that caused by electricity.

Tinel stated that sensibility in the distal cutaneous distribution could appear by the fourth to sixth week after the injury. He distinguished the abnormal sensibility in the cutaneous distribution from the pain sensation, which is perceived at the site of percussion.

PROCEDURE

The percussion should be performed with a tuning fork (30 cps) over the trunk of the involved nerve (Fig. 3–15). Percussion should begin at the distal portion of the extremity to delay the patient's discomfort until the final point of the test. The point of maximal response is measured from bony prominences. The reaction to percussion usually appears 6 weeks after injury or surgery (Henderson, 1948).

A nerve response that remains fixed at one level for several months probably indicates frustrated nerve regeneration, but an advancing level of response does not ensure a sufficient quantity of fibers for clinical function. In addition, there is no measurement of quality, so that the response may indicate paresthesia rather than useful sensibility.

Wrinkled Finger Test

O'Riain (1973) recorded a common but unappreciated observation: The skin of denervated fingers and toes does not wrinkle or shrivel as normal skin does when immersed in warm water. This objective test can be performed without

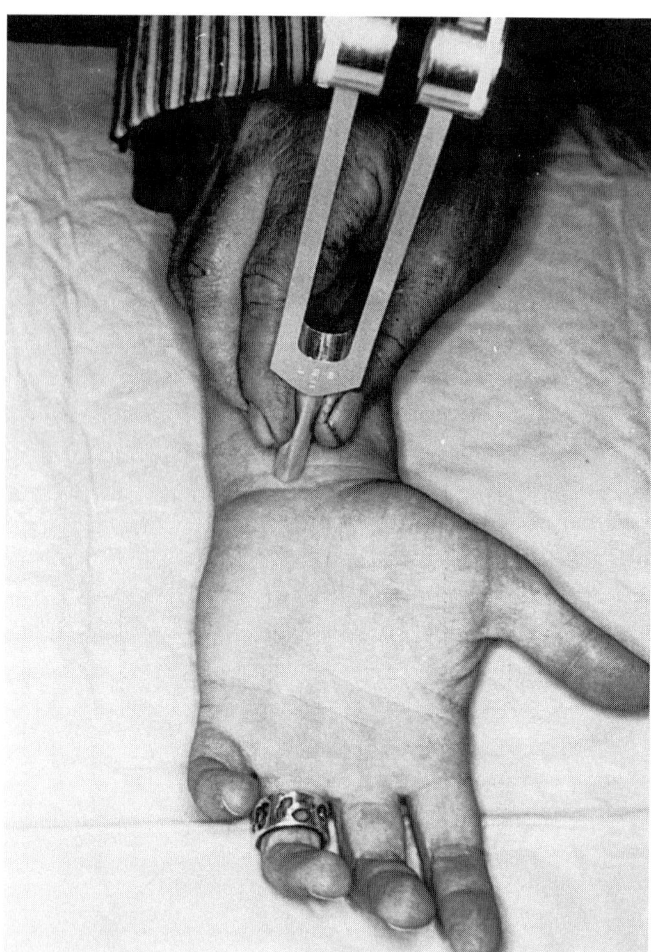

FIGURE 3–15. Technique of percussion with tuning fork (30 cps) over peripheral nerve to elicit Tinel's sign. The base of the tuning fork provides a vibration. (Instrument studies show that the stimulus of the instrument is controlled better when applied with its base than on its side. [Bell-Krotoski and Buford, 1988].) (Omer GE Jr: Evaluation of the extremity with peripheral nerve injury and timing for nerve suture. Instr Course Lect Am Acad Orthop Surg 33:470, 1984.)

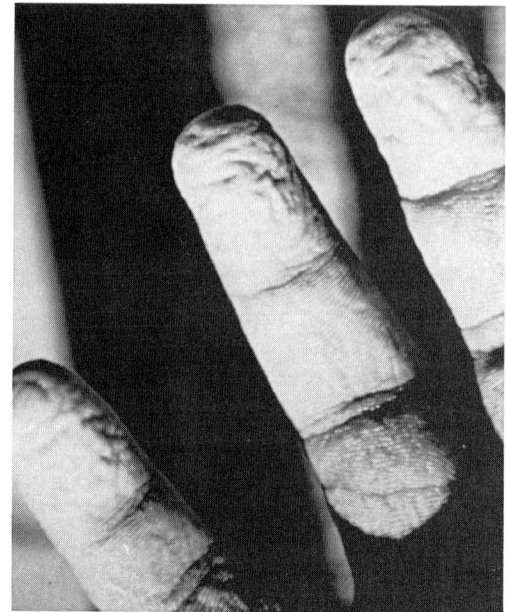

FIGURE 3–16. Normal fingertip wrinkling after immersion in warm water.

the patient's concentration or cooperation, and is indicated particularly for small children (Fig. 3–16). Shriveling of the skin returns progressively with recovery of nerve function. O'Riain recommends immersion in water at approximately 40°C for a period of 30 minutes. Smooth skin indicates loss of sensation. However, this is really a test of sympathetic nervous system activity and is not a test for sensibility (Omer and Spinner, 1984). In time, some patients will recover wrinkling without recovery of sensation.

GRADING RESULTS

Sensibility is more difficult to evaluate than motor strength and amplitude. Voluntary movement is an essential component of precise sensibility, and the moving finger with normal sensibility can identify textured fabrics, different grades of sandpaper, geometric shapes, and letters (Omer, 1984). In the hand, Moberg (1962) believed that a two-point discrimination distance of more than 12 mm provides only protective sensibility because the patient must use visual control of precise activity. Moberg (1978) believed that the

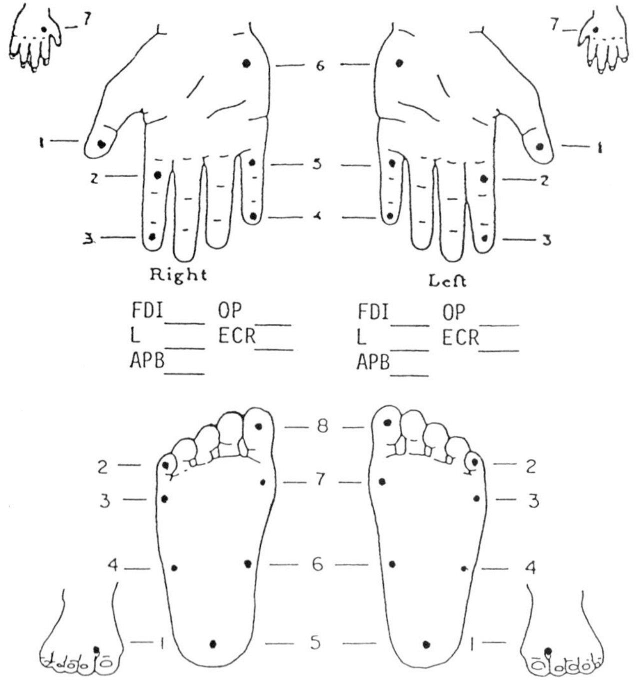

FIGURE 3–17. Hand and foot screen forms. Consistent sites allow monitoring and correlation with treatment. Dots are for sites tested for sensibility. Initials are for muscles tested, that is, first dorsal interosseous, opponens pollicis, lumbrical to the little finger, extensor carpi radialis (longus and brevis), and abductor pollicis brevis (graded 5 to 1). (Note: Semmes-Weinstein minikit monofilaments can be graded 5 to 1 at each site [5 = normal], and point-totaled for each nerve. Increasing or decreasing numbers then reflect the direction of change in status.) APB = abductor pollicis brevis; ECR = extensor carpi radialis (longus and brevis); FDI = first dorsal interosseous; L = lumbrical to the little finger; OP = opponens pollicis.

sensibility system adopted by the British Medical Research Council (1954) is inadequate to rate functional loss. However, this is the system generally used for evaluation.

MINIMAL ESSENTIAL TESTS

Patient history and physical examination of the nerve may be the most important, followed by monofilament, or two-point discrimination, and nerve conduction testing. An observational test such as the Moberg picking-up test is helpful in demonstrating how a patient uses the hand.

Once an appropriate initial examination has been made, it is not always necessary to repeat the entire testing sequence, but only those elements that are most significant. For example, once a nerve has been mapped in threshold response to the Semmes-Weinstein pressure esthesiometer, retesting can be concentrated on areas expected to change.

Hand and foot screens are being used as minimal critical measures with increasing frequency (Fig. 3–17). These screens provide consistent testing of only a few sites for each nerve, along with a few muscles from each nerve. The data can be numerically coded for response at these sites and totaled for each nerve. In this way, data from several patients can be compared (Bell-Krotoski, 1991).

By understanding the requirements for controlled stimuli, examiners can assess the objectivity of any current and future test instrument. Sensitive and controlled tests allow direct correlation of peripheral nerve status with treatment and help define the patient's treatment needs. In the future, it may be possible to determine whether or not a fascicular repair is superior to an epineural repair, or whether or not different chemical treatments of the nerve can affect sensibility.

References

Almquist E, Eeg-Olofsson O: Sensory-nerve-conduction velocity and two-point discrimination in sutured nerves. J Bone Joint Surg 52A:791–796, 1970.

Bell JA: Sensibility evaluation. In Hunter JM, Schneider LH, Mackin EJ, Bell JA (eds): Rehabilitation of the Hand. Philadelphia, C.V. Mosby Company, 1978, pp 269–291.

Bell-Krotoski JA: Pocket filaments and specifications of the Semmes-Weinstein monofilaments. J Hand Ther 3:26–29, 1990.

Bell-Krotoski JA: Advances in sensibility evaluation. Hand Clin 7:527–546, 1991.

Bell-Krotoski JA: Sensibility testing: Current concepts. In Hunter JM, Mackin EJ, Callahan AD (eds): Rehabilitation of the Hand, 4th ed. Philadelphia, C. V. Mosby Company, 1995, pp 109–128.

Bell-Krotoski JA, Buford WL: The force/time relationship of clinically used sensory testing instruments. J Hand Ther 1:76–85, 1988.

Bell-Krotoski JA, Fess EE, Hiltz D, Figarola J: Threshold detection and Semmes-Weinstein monofilaments: A comparative study. In Special Issue on Biomechanics of the Hand. J Hand Ther 8:155–162, 1995.

Bell-Krotoski JA, Tomancik E: The repeatability of the Semmes-Weinstein monofilaments. J Hand Surg 12A:155–161, 1987.

Bell-Krotoski JA, Weinstein S, Weinstein C: Testing sensibility, including touch-pressure, two-point discrimination, point localization, and vibration. J Hand Ther 6:114–123, 1993.

Brand PW, Ebner JD: Pressure sensitive devices for denervated hands and feet. J Bone Joint Surg 51A:109–116, 1969.

Breger DE: Correlating Weinstein-Semmes monofilament mapping with sensory nerve conduction parameters in Hansen's disease patients: An update. J Hand Ther 1:33–37, 1987.

Buford WL: Clinical assessment, objectivity, and ubiquitous laws of instrumentation. J Hand Ther 8:167–174, 1995.

Cohen LA: Analysis of position sense in human shoulder. J Neurophysiol 21:550–562, 1958.

Dellon AL: The moving two point discrimination test: Clinical evaluation of the quickly adapting fiber receptor system. J Hand Surg 3:474–481, 1978.

Dellon AL: The sensational contributions of Eric Moberg. J Hand Surg 15B:14–24, 1990.

Dellon AL, Curtis RM, Edgerton MT: Evaluating recovery of sensation in the hand following nerve injury. Johns Hopkins Med J 130:235–243, 1972.

Dellon AL, Curtis RM, Edgerton MT: Reeducation of sensation in the hand after nerve injury and repair. Plast Reconstr Surg 53:297–305, 1974.

Dyck PJ, Obrien PC, Bushek W, Oviatt KF, Schilling K, Stevens JC: Clinical versus quantitative evaluation of cutaneous sensation. Arch Neurol 33:651–656, 1979.

Fess E: The need for reliability and validity in hand assessment instruments. J Hand Surg 11A:621–623, 1986.

Greco RJ, Hunter JM, Schneider LH: The use of Semmes-Weinstein sensory evaluation in LTS. Presented at the Annual Meeting of the American Society of Plastic and Reconstructive Surgery, San Francisco, California, 1989.

Griffey RH, Eaton RP, Sibbitt RR, Sibbitt WL Jr, Bicknell JM: Diabetic Neuropathy: Structural analysis of nerve hydration by magnetic resonance spectroscopy. JAMA 260:2872–2878, 1988.

Henderson WR: Clinical assessment of peripheral nerve injuries: Tinel's test. Lancet 2:801–805, 1948.

Holewski JJ, Sress RM, Graf PM, Grunfield C: Aesthesiometry: Quantification of cutaneous pressure sensation in diabetic peripheral neuropathy. J Rehabil Res Dev 25:1–10, 1988.

Horch K, Hardy M, Jimenez S, Jabaley M: An automated tactile tester for evaluation of cutaneous sensibility. J Hand Surg 17A:829–837, 1992a.

Horch K, Hardy M, Jimenez S, Jabaley M: Evaluation of nerve compression with the automated tactile tester. J Hand Surg 17A:838–842, 1992b.

Hunter JM: Recurrent carpal tunnel syndrome, epineural fibrous fixation, and traction neuropathy. Hand Clin 7:491–504, 1991.

Juul-Jensen P, Mayer RF: Threshold stimulation for nerve conduction studies in man. Arch Neurol 15:410–419, 1966.

Kimura J: Principles and pitfalls of nerve conduction studies. Ann Neurol 16:415–427, 1984.

Levin S, Pearsall G, Ruderman RJ: von Frey's method of measuring pressure sensibility in the hand; an engineering analysis of the Semmes-Weinstein pressure aesthesiometer. J Hand Surg 3:211–216, 1978.

Lister G: The Hand: Diagnosis and indications. Edinburgh, Churchill Livingstone, 1977, pp 70–72.

Louis DS, Green TL, Jacobson KE, et al: Evaluation of normal values for stationary and moving two-point discrimination in the hand. J Hand Surg 9A:552–555, 1984.

Lundborg G, Lie-Strenstrom AK, Sollerman C, Stromberg T, Pyykko I: Digital vibrogram, a new diagnostic tool for sensory testing in compression neuropathy. J Hand Surg 11A:693–699, 1986.

Medical Research Council: Peripheral nerve injuries, Special Series No. 282. London, Her Majesty's Stationery Office, 1954.

Moberg E: Objective methods for determining the functional value of sensibility in the hand. J Bone Joint Surg 40B:454–476, 1958.

Moberg E: Criticism and study of methods for examining sensibility of the hand. Neurology 12:8–19, 1962.

Moberg E: Evaluation and management of nerve injuries in the hand. Surg Clin North Am 44:1019–1029, 1964.

Moberg E: Relation of touch and deep sensation to hand reconstruction. Am J Surg 109:353–355, 1965.

Moberg E: Sensibility in reconstructive limb surgery. In Fredericks S, Brody GS (eds): Symposium on the Neurologic Aspects of Plastic Surgery. St. Louis, C.V. Mosby Company, 1978, pp 30–35.

Moberg E: Two-point discrimination test. Scand J Rehabil Med 22:127–134, 1990.

Mountcastle VB: Medical Physiology, 14th ed. St. Louis, C.V. Mosby Company, 1980, pp 348–390.

Omer GE Jr: Evaluation and reconstruction of the forearm and hand after acute traumatic peripheral nerve injuries. J Bone Joint Surg 50A:1454–1478, 1968.

Omer GE Jr: The assessment of peripheral nerve injuries. In Cramer LM, Chase RA (eds): Symposium on the Hand. St. Louis, C. V. Mosby Company, 1971, pp 1–13.

Omer GE Jr: Sensation and sensibility in the upper extremity. Clin Orthop 104:30–36, 1974.

Omer GE Jr: Sensory evaluation by the pickup test. *In* Jewett DL, McCarroll HR Jr (eds): Nerve Repair and Regeneration: Its Clinical and Experimental Basis. St. Louis, C.V. Mosby Company, 1980, pp 250–252.

Omer GE Jr: Methods of assessment of injury and recovery of peripheral nerves. Surg Clin North Am *61:*303–319, 1981a.

Omer GE Jr: Physical diagnosis of peripheral nerve injuries. Orthop Clin North Am *12:*207–228, 1981b.

Omer GE Jr: Evaluation of the extremity with peripheral nerve injury and timing for nerve suture. Instr Course Lect Am Acad Orthop Surg *33:*463–486, 1984.

Omer GE Jr, Day DJ, Ratliff H, Lambert P: The neurovascular cutaneous island pedicles for deficient median nerve sensibility. New technique and results of serial functional tests. J Bone Joint Surg *52A:*1181–1192, 1970.

Omer GE Jr, Eversmann WW Jr: Peripheral nerve problems. *In* Burkhalter WE (ed): Orthopaedic Surgery in Vietnam. Washington, D.C., Medical Department of the U.S. Army in Vietnam, U.S. Government Printing Office, 1994, pp 155–188.

Omer GE Jr, Spinner M: Peripheral nerve testing and suture techniques. Instr Course Lect Am Acad Orthop Surg *24:*122–143, 1975.

Omer GE Jr, Spinner M: Management of peripheral nerve problems. Instr Course Lect Am Acad Orthop Surg *15:*461–530, 1984.

Omer GE Jr, Vogel JA: Determination of physiological length of a reconstructed muscle-tendon unit through muscle stimulation. J Bone Joint Surg *47A:*304–312, 1965.

O'Riain S: New and simple test of nerve function in the hand. BMJ *3:*615–616, 1973.

Renfrew S: Fingertip sensation: A routine neurological test. Lancet *1:*393, 1969.

Seddon H: Surgical Disorders of the Peripheral Nerves, 2nd ed. New York, Churchill Livingstone, 1975, pp 32–56.

Semmes J, Weinstein S, Ghent L, Tuber H: Somatosensory changes after penetrating brain wounds in man. Cambridge, MA, Harvard University Press, 1960.

Sillerud LO, Kirsch CF, Pennino RP, Miller G, Cappon JP, Kornfeld M, Kirsch W, Omer G: Monitoring of early wallerian degeneration in rat sciatic nerve using high-field proton NMR spectroscopy. Am Coll Surg *38:*555–558, 1987.

Stopford JSB: The nerve supply of the interphalangeal and metacarpophalangeal joints. J Anat *56:*1–11, 1921/1922.

Szabo RM, Gelberman RH: The pathophysiology of nerve entrapment syndromes, Part 2. J Hand Surg *12A:*880–884, 1987.

Szabo RM, Gelberman RH, Williamson RV, Dellon AL, Yaru NC, Dimick MP: Vibratory testing in acute peripheral nerve compression. J Hand Surg *9(A):*104–109, 1984.

Tinel J: Nerve Wounds: Symptomatology of Peripheral Nerve Lesions Caused by War Wounds. (Translated by F. Rothwell, edited by C.A. Joll.) New York, William Wood and Company, 1918.

Vallbo AB, Johansson RS: Properties of cutaneous mechanoreceptors in the human hand related to touch sensation. Hum Neurobiol *3:*313–314, 1984.

von Frey M: Zur physiologic der juckempfindung. Arch Neerl Physiol *7:*142–145, 1922.

von Prince K, Butler B: Measuring sensory function of the hand in peripheral nerve injuries. Am J Occup Ther *21:*385–396, 1967.

Weber EH: Ueber den tastsinn. Arch Anat Physiol Wissensch Med 152–160, 1835.

Weinstein S: Tactile sensitivity of the phalanges. Percept Mot Skills *14:*351–354, 1962.

Weinstein S: Intensive and extensive aspects of tactile sensitivity as a function of body part, sex, and laterality. *In* Kenshalo DR (ed): The Skin Senses. Springfield, IL, Charles C Thomas, 1968, pp 193–218.

Weinstein S: Fifty years of somatosensory research: From the Semmes-Weinstein monofilaments to the Weinstein Enhanced Sensory Test. J Hand Ther *6:*11–22, 1991.

Werner JL, Omer GE Jr: Evaluating cutaneous pressure sensation of the hand. Am J Occup Ther *24:*347–356, 1970.

Wynn-Parry CB, Salter M: Sensory re-education after median nerve lesions. Hand *8:*250–257, 1976.

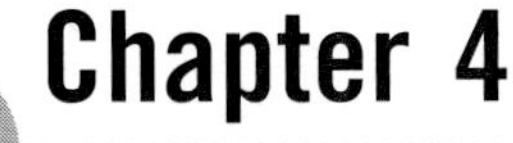

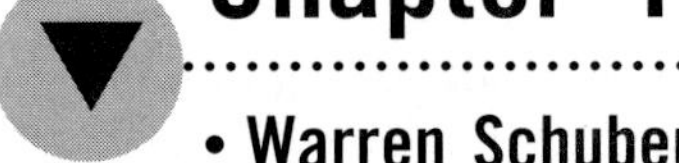

• Warren Schubert

Chapter 4

Trauma Involving the Key Motor and Sensory Nerves of the Face

This chapter reviews the anatomy, clinical findings, and indications for repair of the facial nerve and key sensory nerves to the face. The clinician is reminded that one of the most frequent mistakes made in treating patients, particularly following maxillofacial trauma, is the failure to document a complete neurological examination before the initiation of treatment. In many cases, patients are injected with a local anesthetic, and the lacerations are sutured, or the patient is taken to the operating room for an open reduction and internal fixation of facial fractures without a clear preoperative examination of motor or sensory function. It is hoped that this chapter will provide a better understanding of anatomy and emphasize the importance of a complete examination.

TRAUMA INVOLVING THE FACIAL NERVE

The facial nerve is the key motor nerve for facial expression. It controls all of the mimetic muscles but is not involved in oculomotor function or the muscles of mastication. Bell's palsy is one of the most common forms of facial nerve paralysis. Despite the fact that Bell performed some of the original work of sectioning the seventh nerve to study facial paralysis (Bell, 1821), the term is now used to refer to the idiopathic form of facial palsy. Although some clinicians associate the findings of a patient with Bell's palsy as representing a classic seventh nerve palsy, patients with Bell's palsy commonly have decreased corneal sensation; pain or numbness of the side of their head, ear, face, neck, and shoulder; and numbness of their tongue. These findings also suggest involvement of cranial nerves five, nine, and ten (May, 1979).

Clinical Findings

Despite the multiplicity of mimetic facial muscles, for the purposes of determining the degree of paralysis, determining the extent of recovery, or attempting reanimation, the muscle actions that are considered the most significant are the following: the frontalis, orbicularis oculi, zygomaticus major, and orbicularis oris muscles, and the lip depressors (depressor anguli oris, depressor labii inferioris, and to some extent, the platysma) (Anderson, 1994).

The clinical findings following injury to the facial nerve depend on the branches that are injured and the duration of the injury. Facial nerve injury results in the loss of facial wrinkles on the involved side. Symptoms of the upper face include loss of symmetrical facial expression, brow ptosis, lagophthalmos (due to unopposed action of the levator palpebrae superioris, following paralysis of the orbicularis oculi muscle), atonic lower lid, disturbance of lacrimal drainage due to ectropion of the puncta, compromise of the lacrimal sac pumping mechanism, corneal irritation, keratoconjunctivitis sicca, and possible corneal ulceration (Jelks et al, 1979; Seiff and Chang, 1992; Wells and Manktelow, 1990).

Disturbances of the lower face include loss of the nasolabial sulcus, droop of the anguli oris (following injury to the zygomatic branch), and inability to draw the lower lip downward or laterally evert the vermilion border with loss of the mandibular branch. Findings also include decreased ability to purse the lips; distortion of the oral sphincter, leading to problems with speech and drooling on the affected side; and with time, deviation of the mouth to the nonparalyzed side due to the unopposed pull of the facial muscles from the normal side (Conley et al, 1982; Miehlke et al, 1979; Moffat and Ramsden, 1977; Pollack, 1954).

Injury of the cervical branch of the facial nerve, such as may occur from neck exploration or a platysmal face lift operation, may also cause some weakness in depression of the lower lip. This has been referred to as a pseudoparalysis of the mandibular branch of the facial nerve (Ellenbogen, 1979).

Location of the Lesion

When evaluating facial paralysis, it is important to determine if the location of the lesion is supranuclear, nuclear, infranuclear-cerebellopontine angle, intratemporal, or extratemporal. In some cases of a simple deep laceration to the face, it may be obvious. In many cases, patients may have sustained multiple trauma, as in a motor vehicle accident, and present comatose or with marked facial edema and with multiple facial lacerations. These complex polytrauma patients are the ones in whom the surgeon is most likely to miss a significant lesion of the facial nerve.

Supranuclear lesions refer to lesions above the facial nucleus (which is located deep within the pons). Supranuclear lesions may involve the cerebral cortex or the upper motor neurons between the cortex and the pons. Causes include both traumatic and nontraumatic modalities, such as cerebrovascular accidents and neoplasm. Traumatic causes can be further divided into mass and nonmass lesions. Mass lesions include epidural, subdural, and intracerebral hematomas.

Nonmass lesions include contusions or sheer injury with diffuse axonal injury. Of all of these causes, cerebrovascular accidents are the most common. Clinical findings include preservation of function of the frontalis and orbicularis muscles (frontal branch of the facial nerve) due to the bilateral innervation of the upper motor neurons from the cortex, with contralateral paralysis of the lower facial muscles.

Lesions occurring at the level of the facial nucleus or below the nucleus (referred to as lower motor neuron lesions) result in ipsilateral weakness of all of the facial muscles, including the forehead. This includes injuries of the intratemporal and extratemporal course of the facial nerve (Baker, 1990; Wilson-Pauwels et al, 1988).

If the sixth and seventh cranial nerves are not functioning, this suggests a lesion in the pons. If the seventh and eighth cranial nerves are not functioning, it suggests a lesion near the internal acoustic meatus or in the intratemporal region, such as from an acoustic neuroma (Carpenter, 1978; Wilson-Pauwels et al, 1988).

Determination of the level of injury of the facial nerve within the intratemporal course depends on the evaluation of three key branches within the temporal bone (Adkins and Osguthorpe, 1991; Baker, 1990; May, 1979). The first branch is the greater petrosal nerve. This branch exits the petrous portion of the temporal bone through the greater petrosal foramen. It enters the middle cranial fossa, exits through the foramen lacerum, and then passes into the pterygoid canal. It then enters the pterygopalatine fossa, where it synapses with the parasympathetic pterygopalatine ganglion. It contin-

ues a rather circuitous route and finally supplies postganglionic fibers to the lacrimal gland to stimulate secretory function. The secretory function of the lacrimal gland can be tested with the Schirmer test.

The second key branch is the nerve to the stapedius muscle, which is responsible for the dampening of loud sounds. Paralysis of the stapedius results in hyperacusia (abnormal acuteness of hearing) due to the uninhibited movement of the stapes.

The third important branch is the chorda tympani, which passes through the petrotympanic fissure to join the lingual nerve, and supplies taste to the anterior two thirds of the tongue (Fig. 4–1). Tactile sensation to the tongue is supplied by the lingual nerve (a branch of the mandibular branch of the trigeminal nerve).

Various authors have discussed the anatomical detail of the intratemporal course of the facial nerve (May, 1973; Sunderland and Cossar, 1953); the various tearing, audiometric, taste, and radiological studies that are performed as part of the evaluation for intratemporal lesions (Anderson et al, 1982; Steenerson, 1986; Williams et al, 1992); as well as the indications and techniques for intratemporal nerve repair (Coker et al, 1987; Fisch, 1974; Glasscock et al, 1979; House and Crabtree, 1965; Jongkees, 1965; Kanzaki et al, 1991). Interpretation of the tests that study these three key intratemporal branches can be challenging and often of questionable merit (Adkins and Osguthorpe, 1991; Coker et al, 1987). The topic of intratemporal injury is further discussed in Chapter 39.

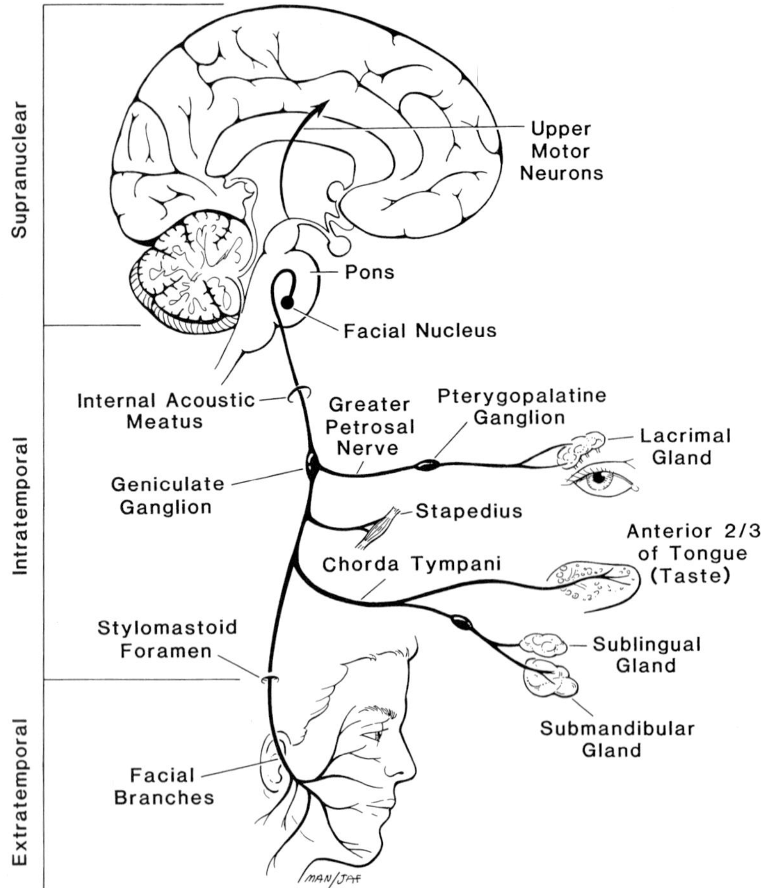

FIGURE 4–1. The course of the facial nerve, emphasizing the three key branches in the intratemporal course that are commonly tested. Note that this represents a simplified drawing of the facial nerve and does not include all of its branches or functions.

Anatomical Considerations for the Extratemporal Portion of the Facial Nerve

The facial nerve exits the stylomastoid foramen posterolateral to the styloid process, and anteromedial to the mastoid process. This is 20 mm deep to the skin (Rudolph, 1990), 10 mm deep and slightly inferior to the tragal pointer, and 6 to 8 mm deep to the inferior end of the tympanomastoid suture (Johns and Kaplan, 1987). The first minor extratemporal branch of the facial nerve is the posterior auricular, which supplies the occipitalis, and the posterior and superior auricular muscles (Hollinshead, 1982; Moore, 1985).

The main trunk of the facial nerve passes anteriorly and inferiorly, superficial to the styloid process and the posterior belly of the digastric muscle. It gives off additional minor branches to the posterior belly of the digastric and the stylohyoid muscle. Although many authors view the styloid process as a good landmark in identifying the proximal trunk of the facial nerve, one series (Davis et al, 1956) found it absent in over one third of cases, and "shielded completely or nonpalpable in many others" (p 410). As the nerve passes into the parotid, there is a great deal of variability in the relationship between the parotid and the facial nerve (McKenzie, 1948).

The facial nerve passes superficial to the external carotid artery and the posterior facial vein. The first major division of the facial nerve is generally into an upper and lower division known as the temporofacial and cervicofacial branches. This bifurcation generally "lies posterior and slightly medial to the ramus of the mandible and superiorly two-thirds of the distance between the external angle of the mandible" (p 624) and the temporomandibular joint (McCormack et al, 1945). The diameter of the temporofacial division is often two to three times larger than the cervicofacial division.

These two divisions then further divide to form the five main branches of the facial nerve; the temporal (frontal), zygomatic, buccal, mandibular (or marginal mandibular), and cervical branches. Some texts have suggested that the temporal and zygomatic branches are derived from the temporofacial, and the buccal, mandibular, and cervical are derived from the cervicofacial division (Hollinshead, 1982). Baker and Conley (1979c) usually found a bifurcation of the main trunk but sometimes found a trifurcation with the addition of the buccal branch, and occasionally found a quadrification, and rarely a plexiform pattern. They suggest that both the temporofacial and cervicofacial divisions contribute to the buccal area, with the temporofacial generally contributing two branches and the cervicofacial contributing one branch to the buccal area. These various divisions form the ill-defined boundary between the superficial and deep lobes of the parotid gland (McWhorter, 1917).

Along the course from the stylohyoid foramen and through the parotid, the facial nerve is relatively deep and well protected in adults. It is not likely to be injured from superficial lacerations but is more likely to be damaged due to a parotid malignancy, iatrogenic injury during a parotidectomy, and major traumatic injuries, such as from a gunshot wound. Numerous authors have discussed in detail landmarks for the antegrade dissection of the facial nerve and for the identification of the main trunk (Beahrs and Adson,

1958; Johns and Kaplan, 1987; Woods and Beahrs, 1976). Caution should be used in the evaluation of infants because the main trunk of the facial nerve is very superficial as it exits the stylomastoid foramen.

The five main branches of the facial nerve emerge from the superior, anterior, and inferior margins of the parotid gland (Moore, 1985). Rudolph (1990) studied the mean depth of the temporal, zygomatic, buccal, and mandibular branches along the parotid edge, and found that the depth was between 9.1 and 10.6 mm, with a gradual increase in depth while moving in the craniocaudal sequence. The motor branches lie deep to the superficial musculoaponeurotic system (SMAS; Mitz and Peyronie, 1976). It is in the anterior and more superficial areas in which damage to the nerve due to traumatic lacerations or rhytidectomy is more likely to occur. These branches innervate the 18 paired and one unpaired (orbicularis oris) muscles of facial expression (Anderson, 1994). The nerve supply to the most clinically important muscle groups is as follows (Fig. 4–2):

Frontalis—temporal branch
Orbicularis oculi—temporal and zygomatic branch
Zygomaticus major—zygomatic branch
Orbicularis oris—buccal and mandibular branch
Lip depressors—mandibular branch (in some patients, some component of lip depression may also be contributed by the platysma, which is innervated by the cervical branch)

Freilinger and colleagues (1987) studied the surgical anatomy of the mimic muscles. They divided the facial muscles into four layers and emphasized that most of the muscles receive their respective innervation of the facial nerve branches from the deep muscle surface. Notable exceptions included the muscles innervated by the temporal branches and the muscles in the fourth (deepest) layer, which included the levator anguli oris, buccinator, and mentalis muscles.

Baker and Conley (1979c) found that all of the five major branches of the facial nerve usually have multiple smaller branches to their respective areas distally, with the exception of the frontal area, which is supplied by just one branch of the frontal nerve. Authors have found multiple interconnections among the five major divisions of the facial nerve occurring in 70% to 90% of patients (Baker and Conley, 1979c; Davis et al, 1956; McCormack et al, 1945). Many others have also studied the variability of the anastomotic branches of the facial nerve (Bernstein and Nelson, 1984; Katz and Catalano, 1987).

The temporal and mandibular branches have interconnections in just 10% to 15% of cases (Baker and Conley, 1979c). This makes injury to these two main branches the least forgiving.

Pitanguy and Ramos (1966) described the course of the frontal branch of the facial nerve as starting from a point 0.5 cm below the tragus and passing in a line 1.5 cm above the lateral portion of the eyebrow (Fig. 4–3A). Stuzin and associates (1989) found that although there may be variations in the branching pattern of the frontal branch of the facial nerve, the nerve always travels in a "predictable and constant" plane (p 269). As it crosses the zygomatic arch, it travels within the temporoparietal fascia. As the frontal branch passes superiorly into the temporal region, it then travels deeper along the undersurface of this fascia. The frontal branch of the superficial temporal artery lies directly

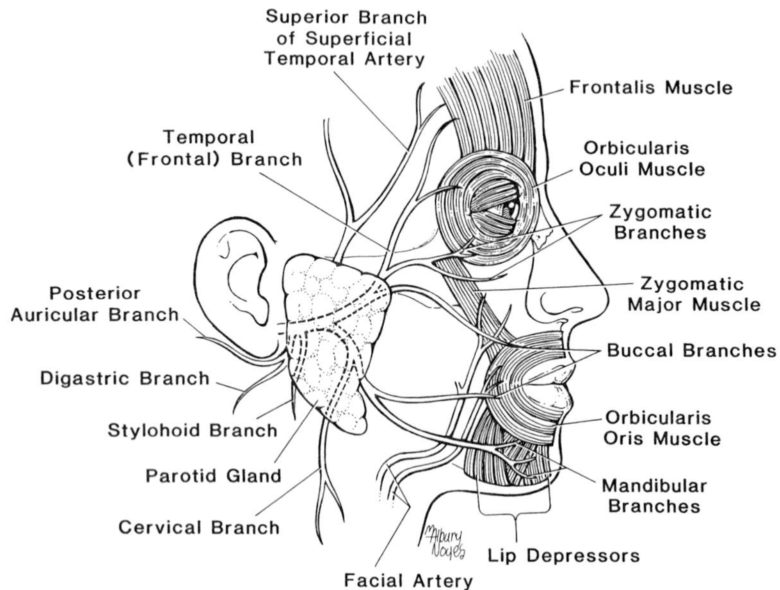

FIGURE 4–2. The five key motor branches of the facial nerve and the key muscle groups that are affected. Note the relative position of the superior branch of the superficial temporal artery to the temporal branch of the facial nerve. Note also the position of the facial artery and vein that pass deep to the mandibular branch of the facial nerve. Please refer to the text and Figure 4–5 regarding the numerous important controversies of the position of the mandibular nerve relative to the inferior border of the mandible.

cephalad and parallel to the frontal branch of the facial nerve. Stuzin described the danger of injury of the frontal branch as it passes over the zygomatic arch and described the safe dissection to the arch through the coronal approach (Fig. 4–4). This is through a dissection deep to the temporoparietal fascia and at a point 2 cm cephalad to the zygomatic arch, passing through and then remaining deep to the superficial layer of the deep temporal fascia. One is then in the layer of the superficial temporal fat pad. Stuzin emphasized the distinction between a superficial and deep layers of the deep temporal fascia.

Bernstein and Nelson (1984) described the anatomy of the frontal branches as they cross the zygomatic arch (Fig. 4–3B). The anteriormost ramus of the nerve averaged a distance of 2 cm posterior to the anterior origin of the zygomatic arch. On the average, the posteriormost ramus was found 1.8 cm anterior to a vertical line drawn from the anterior superior portion of the auricle. Ishikawa (1990) described the facial danger point as a gently curved line linking a point 7 cm posterior to the bony lateral canthus to a point 4 cm superior to the lateral canthus (Fig. 4–3C). Examination of the diagrams by Bernstein and Ishikawa is recommended. These studies suggest that contrary to Baker's findings, a multiplicity of rami of the frontal branch is a common occurrence.

In cadaveric studies of the mandibular branch of the facial nerve, Dingman and Grabb (1962) found that posterior to the facial artery, the nerve passed cephalad to the inferior

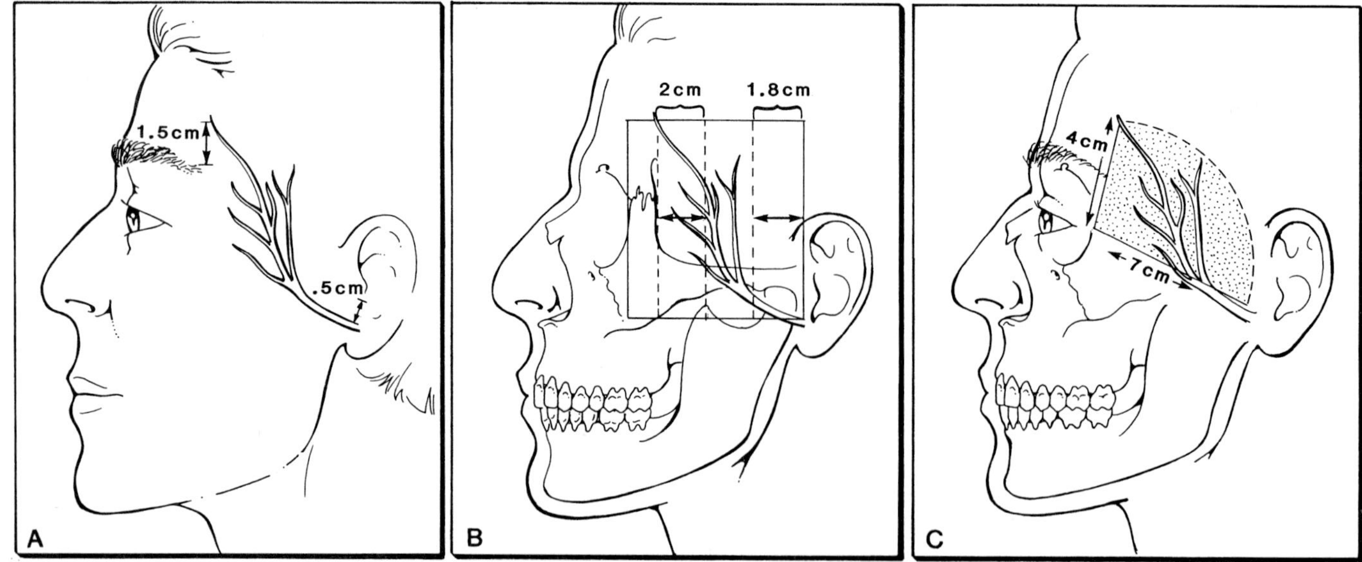

FIGURE 4–3. All three diagrams define the course of the frontal branch of the facial nerve as determined by different authors. A, Pitanguy and Ramos described the course as starting from a point 0.5 cm below the tragus, and passing in a line 1.5 cm above the lateral portion of the eyebrow. B, Bernstein and Nelson described the anatomy as the nerve crossed the zygomatic arch. C, Ishikawa described the potential path as lying within a gently curved line linking a point 7 cm posterior to the bony lateral canthus to a point 4 cm superior to the lateral canthus.

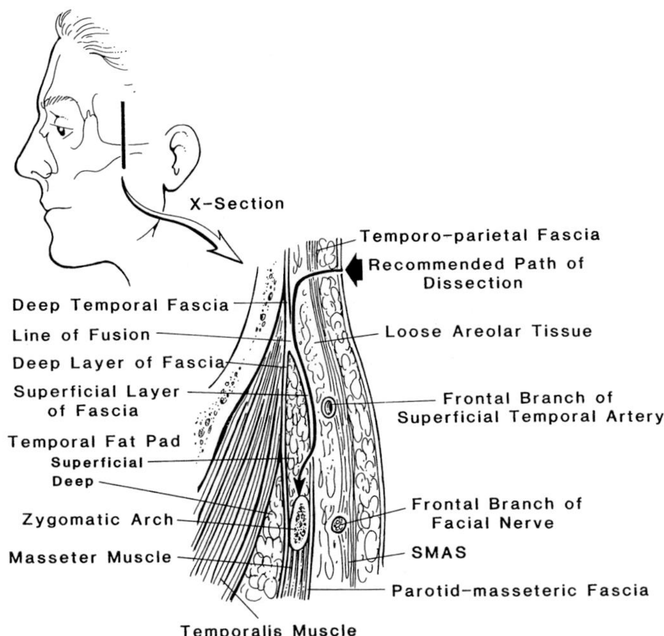

FIGURE 4–4. The cross-sectional view (coronal view) of the path of the frontal branch of the facial nerve, as described by Stuzin.

border of the mandible in 81% of patients, and caudad to the inferior border in 19% of dissections (Fig. 4–5A). In those patients in whom it passed inferiorly, the mandibular branch passed in an arch within 1 cm from the inferior border. Anterior to the facial artery, the mandibular nerve remained cephalad to the inferior border of the mandible in 100% of dissections.

Baker and Conley (1979c) pointed out that the cadavers in Dingman's study represented fixed specimens. They found that based on their clinical experience, the mandibular branch of the facial nerve was 1 to 2 cm caudad to the lower border of the mandible in almost every instance. In some individuals, the nerve was as low as 3 to 4 cm below the border of the mandible (Fig. 4–5B). They pointed out that extension of the neck in the operating room could lower the nerve farther. Both Dingman and Baker agreed that the mandibular branch or the facial nerve is the most common branch injured.

Nelson and Gingrass (1979) performed a detailed study of the various smaller and distal branches of the mandibular nerve while using a nerve stimulator. They concluded that they were able to study the branching of the nerve in greater detail and far more anteriorly than in the study by Dingman and Grabb. The nerve was always found deep to the platysma muscle. At the angle of the mandible, Nelson and Gingrass' recommendation was to make the incision through the platysma at least several centimeters (2 fingerbreadths) below the mandible. As Nelson and Gingrass dissected anteriorly, they continued to find significant branches of the mandibular nerve inferior to the mandible, even anterior to the facial vessels (Fig. 4–5C). When in the area of the submandibular triangle, they described the thin fascia over the submandibular gland as including the nerve. They emphasized the need to use the nerve stimulator and elevate the fascia as a flap with the nerve. Finally, Nelson was able to distinguish three separate branches of the mandibular nerve going to the mentalis, the depressor labii inferioris, and the depressor anguli oris muscles. Each branch could consistently be found at a different level, with the nerve to the mentalis lying the most inferior, followed by the nerve to the depressor labii inferioris in between, and the nerve to the depressor anguli oris the most superior. Perhaps the most important finding was that Nelson and Gingrass were able to identify certain branches below the inferior border of the mandible in all patients.

Liebman and co-workers (1988) studied the relative depth of the mandibular nerve during gross dissection and following serial histological sectioning. They found that at a distance of 4 and 3 cm from the corner of the mouth, the nerve was deep to the platysma. At a distance 2 cm from the corner of the mouth, the mandibular nerve interdigitates with and runs superficial to the platysma. Liebman and colleagues

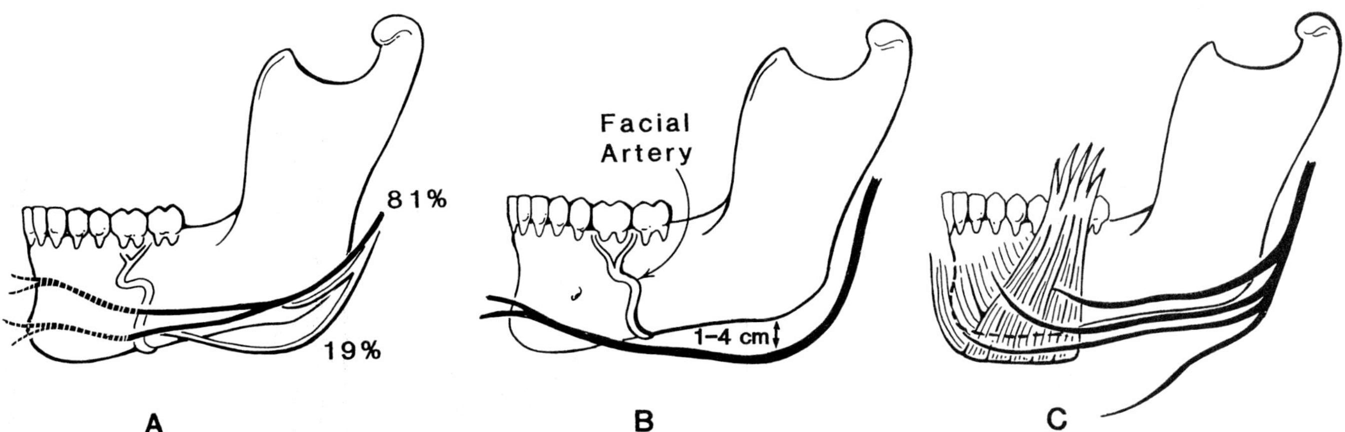

FIGURE 4–5. All three diagrams define the course of the mandibular branch of the facial nerve as determined by different authors. *A,* Dingman and Grabb found that posterior to the facial artery, the nerve passed cephalad to the inferior border of the mandible in 81% of cases and caudad to the inferior border in 19% of dissections (cadaveric study). *B,* Baker and Conley found that posterior to the facial artery the mandibular branch was 1 to 2 cm caudad to the lower border of the mandible in almost every instance, and in some individuals, it was as low as 3 to 4 cm caudad. *C,* Nelson was able to distinguish three separate branches of the mandibular nerve going to the mentalis, depressor labii inferioris, and depressor anguli oris muscles. Nelson studied the course of these branches anterior to the facial artery. The nerve to the mentalis was the most inferior, followed by the depressor labii inferioris in between, and the depressor anguli oris was the most superior. Some of these branches remained below the inferior border of the mandible in all patients. The exact level of branching is somewhat unclear and is probably more anterior than is suggested in diagram *C.*

also found that at this level, there is increased tissue adhesiveness and less subcutaneous fat, making the dissection in this area much more difficult. On the bases of these findings, they recommend that the surgeon not go medial to this point while performing face lift procedures.

Seckel (1994) has published a monogram with diagrams on avoiding injury to the facial nerve in the various danger zones.

Electrophysiological Evaluation

Various authors have summarized the electrophysiological testing measures that are available (Anderson, 1994; Kartush and Prass, 1988). One of the problems with many of the series that compare different techniques of testing is that most of the testing was performed on patients with Bell's palsy and not on patients with traumatic injuries to the major facial branches.

The nerve excitability test uses the minimum electrical current to elicit a facial twitch and compares this threshold to the contralateral side. The test does not reflect denervation at the moment it is occurring. Nevertheless, because it is inexpensive and because of its ease, it is one of the most common tests performed (Kartush and Prass, 1988; Hilger, 1964).

The maximal stimulation test uses higher milliamps than the nerve excitability test and ideally achieves supramaximal stimulation. May and colleagues (1971) reported that in patients with Bell's palsy, the maximal stimulation test becomes abnormal sooner than the nerve excitability test and is a more reliable guide to prognosis.

Electroneurography measures the electrically evoked muscle compound action potential using bipolar surface electrodes. The compound action potential amplitude is measured peak to peak on each side of the face. It is compared with the normal side and expressed as a percentage of the normal response (Hughes, 1982). Hughes found that quantitative results using electroneurography were more objective and more precise than those obtained using nerve excitability testing. The response on the abnormal side of the face was studied by Hardy and associates (1989) 1 week following acoustic neuroma surgery. They found that electroneurography was a good indicator of the likelihood of recovery in facial nerves that were known to be anatomically intact but demonstrated no evidence of function.

Electromyography uses intramuscular needles to study muscle that is voluntarily contracting (detection method) or in recording the muscle response to an electrical stimulus (stimulo-detection method) (Raimbault, 1984). A problem with electromyography is that evidence of degeneration may not appear for 14 to 21 days after a nerve injury (Kartush and Prass, 1988), and therefore, electromyography may be the least useful tool in the diagnosis of an acute paralysis. It may be useful for monitoring reinnervation, especially when using the stimulo-detection method.

Conservative Therapy

The decision to explore or not to explore for a facial nerve injury is based, in part, on the mechanism of injury and the anatomical location. Baker and Conley (1979c) found that injury to the facial nerve occurred in less than 1% in their series. More than 80% of these injuries had spontaneous return within 6 months.

Because of the interconnections between the main branches of the facial nerve, one may choose to be more conservative with a perceived weakness of the facial muscles in the zygomatic and buccal distribution than in the temporal and mandibular distribution. It is often difficult to know whether a delayed return of function is due to a resolution of a neuropraxia, a regeneration following axonotmesis, compensation due to the various neurointerconnections, or hypertrophy of other facial muscles that provide a similar function.

Most authors do not recommend exploration of the branches of the facial nerve for lacerations that are medial to a line drawn from the lateral canthus to the corner of the mouth (Mackinnon and Dellon, 1988). This seems to be the accepted standard of care, and it is unclear whether this is based purely on the small size and the multiplicity of branches distally, or whether there is a chance of random reinnervation of muscle this far distally. We have found that the branches of the mandibular nerve can often be followed medial to the commissure in an adult.

A case has been reported with strong electromyographical and clinical evidence for the return of the function of the depressor muscles in a 12-year-old boy who had suffered from a traumatic avulsion of his lower lip and chin from commissure to commissure. The lip and chin were replanted using the inferior labial artery; however, a microneural repair was not performed (Schubert et al, 1988). This suggests that for distal injuries, random nerve ingrowth or reinnervation may occur in children.

Operative Repair of the Facial Nerve

Before embarking on the exploration and repair of the facial nerve, an understanding of the anatomy of the nerve and its branches is essential. The surgeon should be comfortable with both the antegrade and retrograde dissection of the nerve.

Several authors have reviewed the use of primary nerve repair and interpositional nerve grafting (Anderson, 1994; Duel and Tickle, 1936; Fisch, 1974b; Kitamura et al, 1972; Lee and Terzis, 1984; Miehlke and Stennert, 1981; Miehlke, 1965; Millesi, 1979; Sade, 1975; Tucker, 1978; Wells and Manktelow, 1990). Primary repair offers the best possible outcome in wounds that are clean and without evidence of a crush injury, where there is not a significant segmental defect to result in coaptation under tension.

Proper technique includes the use of magnification and fine nylon suture on the order of 10-0 or 11-0. Whether to use the epineural, fascicular, or fascicular bundle technique and the total number of sutures needed for the repair remains controversial and, in part, may be related to the cross-sectional size of the nerve defect. Early exploration and repair are encouraged in order to take advantage of the fact that the facial muscles will continue to move for 72 hours after injury with the use of a nerve stimulator. This may be invaluable in identifying the various branches. In the event of a delayed final repair due to contamination or crush injury, early exploration for tagging of the nerve endings may still be beneficial.

Early exploration also makes the anatomical identification of the nerve branches as well as the various fascicles within the branches easier. Following a delay in the repair, fibrosis occurs, and the dissection and identification of the branches is more difficult. Fascicular mismatch is more likely, and an additional resection of the nerve ends will be required before the repair. Animal studies of the optimal timing for facial nerve repair have confirmed that the best results are found with early repair (Barrs, 1991).

Interpositional nerve grafting is required if coaptation of the nerves cannot be achieved without tension. Nerves to consider for nerve grafts include the greater auricular, medial antebrachial cutaneous, lateral antebrachial cutaneous, and sural nerves (Fisch, 1974a and b; Mackinnon and Dellon, 1988). Although nerve grafting requires the axonal sprouts from the proximal stump to cross two separate levels of nerve coaptation before reinnervation, the results have been highly preferable when compared with the results following primary repair under tension.

Spector and associates (1991) compared the results of patients with facial nerve regeneration with end-to-end coaptation with patients with interpositional nerve grafts. They found that tone and symmetry at rest, and electrophysiological tests were similar between the two groups. Voluntary motion was decreased and synkinesis was increased in patients with interpositional nerve grafts.

Various techniques have been described for mastoid and extratemporal rerouting of the facial nerve to gain extra length for coaptation without nerve grafting. In a cadaveric study by Yarbrough and colleagues (1993), as much as 17.6 ± 1.7 mm of facial nerve length could be gained using these techniques.

Reconstructive Alternatives

Various alternatives to reconstruction exist, and they include the following methods to achieve some degree of static support or reanimation:

1. Cross-facial nerve grafting (Anderl, 1979; Baker and Conley, 1979b; Burgess and Goode, 1994; Delbeke and Thauvoy, 1982; Freilinger, 1975; Miehlke and Stennert, 1981; Scaramella, 1979; Sobol et al, 1990).

2. Free muscle transfer with ipsilateral or cross-facial nerve grafting (Aviv and Urken, 1992; Hakelius, 1979; Hamilton and Terzis, 1984; Harii et al, 1976; Harii, 1979; Harrison, 1985, 1990; Manktelow, 1984a, 1984b; O'Brien et al, 1980, 1990; Sanger et al, 1991; Sassoon et al, 1991; Thompson, 1971; Tolhurst and Bos, 1982; Whitney et al, 1990).

3. Cranial nerve transfer (Alexander et al, 1954; Balance and Duel, 1932; Burgess and Goode, 1994; Coleman, 1940; Conley and Baker, 1979; Evans, 1974; Falbe-Hansen and Hermann, 1967; Gagnon and Molina-Negro, 1989; Gavron and Clemis, 1984; Hitselberger, 1974; Iansek et al, 1986; Kessler et al, 1959; Kunihiro et al, 1991; May et al, 1991; Pensak et al, 1986; Poe et al, 1989; Stennert, 1979).

4. The use of fascial strips or regional muscle transfer (Adams, 1946; Baker and Conley, 1979a; Burgess and Goode, 1994; Correia and Zani, 1973; Freeman, 1979; Gil-

lies, 1934; Hastings, 1920; Owens, 1947; Rubin, 1974; Sheehan, 1935; Tucker, 1979).

5. Gold weight or eye spring lid reanimation (Burgess and Goode, 1994; Jelks et al, 1979; Seiff and Chang, 1992; Sobol et al, 1990).

These methods of reanimation are discussed in Chapter 70. The plethora of means of reconstructions suggests limitations with each form of reconstruction. These alternatives should not be used as an excuse for the surgeon not to be maximally aggressive in attempting primary repair or interpositional nerve grafting when possible.

Marino (1953) reported a series of seven patients with paralysis due to injury of the mandibular branch of the facial nerve. Interestingly, the most common cause was due to incision and drainage of an abscess of the angle of the mandible, especially in children. In order to achieve symmetry, the patients were treated with neurectomy of the contralateral side. Blepharospasm and several other disorders have been successfully treated with botulinum toxin injection (Jankovic and Brin, 1991; Scott et al, 1985). A case has been reported of the use of botulinum toxin injection on the contralateral side of the frontal branch to achieve temporary symmetry for a frontal branch weakness following a rhytidectomy (Clark and Berris, 1989). The long-term role of contralateral paralysis to achieve symmetry has yet to be determined. The development of botulinum toxin allows for an interesting long-term and yet reversible trial for the patient.

TRAUMA INVOLVING THE SENSORY NERVES

The key sensory nerves of the face are represented by the three branches of the trigeminal nerve, and include the supraorbital (a branch of the ophthalmic division, V1), the infraorbital (a branch of the maxillary division, V2), and the mental nerve (a branch of the mandibular division, V3).

The frontal nerve (V1) passes through the superior orbital fissure superior to the annulus of Zinn. It passes along the orbital roof and branches to form the supraorbital and supratrochlear nerves (Zide and Jelks, 1985). The supraorbital and supratrochlear nerves supply sensation to the forehead and the anterior scalp. In a study of 80 skulls, we found that 92.5% of the time, the supraorbital nerve exited the roof of the orbit through a supraorbital notch. In the remaining 7.5%, it exited through a true foramen. Of the nine skulls in which the superior orbital foramen was a true foramen, in six it represented a unilateral finding and in three a bilateral finding (Schubert et al, 1992). In our experience, the departure of the supraorbital nerve from the orbit through the notch or foramen is easier to identify during a coronal incision by performing the entire dissection in the subpericranial (subperiosteal) layer. This nerve is most commonly damaged as a result of forehead lacerations and by iatrogenic means during coronal approaches for the repair of frontal sinus fractures and during brow lift procedures.

The maxillary division (V2) of the trigeminal nerve passes through the foramen rotundum. Divisions include the zygomatic nerve (with branches that include the zygomaticotemporal and zygomaticofacial nerves), the posterior superior alveolar nerve, the middle superior alveolar nerve, the anterior superior alveolar nerve, and the infraorbital nerve (Malamed, 1980; Zide and Jelks, 1985). Part of the nerve passes through the inferior orbital fissure and in the infraorbital groove in the posterior portion of the orbit and then into the infraorbital canal. This posterior portion of the nerve in the infraorbital groove may be injured during a periorbital dissection. The infraorbital nerve supplies sensation to the lower eyelid, cheek, lateral ala, and upper lip. The infraorbital nerve is most commonly injured following maxillary, zygomatic, and orbital floor fractures. The fractures commonly pass through the foramen of the infraorbital nerve, with bony fragments compressing the nerve. Small fragments suspicious for compression should be removed. The infraorbital foramen lies 6 to 7 mm below the infraorbital rim in adults, and care must be used in this area while degloving the mid-face to expose facial fractures, while performing a dissection as part of a subperiosteal face lift, or for the exposure and placement of malar implants.

The mandibular branch of the trigeminal nerve (V3) passes through the foramen ovale, with branches including the inferior alveolar nerve, which enters the posterior portion of the mandible medially at the mandibular foramen, passes through the mandible in the inferior alveolar canal, and exits at the mental foramen as the mental nerve. It then divides into three branches to supply sensation to the chin and mucosa of the lower lip and gingiva.

In our study of 80 mandibles, the position of the mental foramen was variable and ranged from the apex of the root of the first premolar to the apex of the root of the first molar. The mean position was near the second premolar (Schubert et al, 1992).

The mental nerve is commonly injured during mandibular fractures when they occur between the mental and mandibular foramen. As with maxillary fractures, mandibular fractures commonly occur through the mental foramen. The nerve may also be damaged with injury to the inferior alveolar nerve as part of a dental extraction (Buckley and Zuniga, 1993; Pogrel, 1990) or during the placement of osseo-integrated dental implants (Beirne and Worthington, 1991; Shulman and Shepherd, 1990). The mental nerve is also commonly injured as part of an open reduction and internal fixation of a mandible fracture due to traction on the inferior nerve while reducing the fracture or traction on the mental nerve while exposing the mandible, or resulting from drill holes or screws placed in the inferior alveolar canal (Block et al, 1990). The management of a nerve injury and the decision whether or not to remove hardware following anesthesia to the nerve branch remains controversial. Finally, the mental nerve may be injured due to traction following exposure for a chin implant or while performing a sliding genioplasty (Spear and Kassan, 1989).

Some authors have stated that reconstruction of sensory nerves is not worthwhile (Banks et al, 1985). Theoretically, any key sensory nerve that is cut and can be repaired should be, both to try to restore sensation and to diminish the chances of forming a painful neuroma. Unfortunately, most of the serious injuries to the infraorbital and mental nerve often occur precisely at the foramen as an avulsion injury. Several reports have documented the repair of the inferior alveolar nerve, but the indications remain undefined (Donoff and Colin, 1990; LaBanc and Van Boven, 1992; Meyer,

1992). Some authors have claimed to have been able to repair the infraorbital nerve as well (Epker and Gregg, 1992).

The great auricular nerve is the sensory nerve that is injured most often during a rhytidectomy, and the nerve is commonly damaged during the neck dissection for other procedures. The anatomy of the great auricular nerve and guidelines for avoidance were described by McKinney and Katrana (1980). The great auricular nerve is derived from the second and third cervical roots, and provides sensation to the lower two thirds of the ear and the preauricular and postauricular skin. The nerve comes from behind the posterior border of the sternocleidomastoid muscle and crosses the mid-belly of the muscle 6.5 cm caudal to the bony external auditory canal (and 0.5 cm posterior to the jugular vein at this point). From this point, the nerve runs superiorly toward the ear. McKinney believed that a platysmal flap could be safely elevated anteriorly, starting at a point 6.5 cm caudad to the ear and at the anterior border of the sternocleidomastoid muscle, without risk of injury to the great auricular nerve.

Acknowledgments

I would like to thank Dr. James Hoffman and LuAnn LaShomb from the Division of Plastic Surgery, and Dr. William Ganz from the Department of Neurosurgery of St. Paul-Ramsey Medical Center and the University of Minnesota, for their generous help and advice with this chapter.

References

Adams WM: The use of the masseter, temporalis and frontalis muscles in the correction of facial paralysis. Plast Reconstr Surg 1:216, 1946.

Adkins WY, Osguthorpe DJ: Management of trauma of the facial nerve. Otolaryngol Clin North Am 24:587, 1991.

Alexander E, Davis CH: Correction of peripheral paralysis of the facial nerve by hypoglossal-facial anastomosis. South Med J 47:299, 1954.

Anderl H: Cross-face nerve transplant. Clin Plast Surg 6:433, 1979.

Anderson R, Olson J, Merkle M, Dowart R, Schaefer S: CT air-contrast scanning of the internal auditory canal. Ann Otol Rhinol Laryngol 91:501, 1982.

Anderson RG: Facial Nerve Disorders and Surgery. Selected Readings in Plastic Surgery, Vol. 7. Dallas, Baylor University Medical Center, 1994, pp 1–36.

Aviv JE, Urken ML: Management of the paralyzed face with microneurovascular free muscle transfer. Arch Otolaryngol Head Neck Surg 118:909, 1992.

Baker DC: Facial paralysis. In McCarthy JG (ed): Plastic Surgery, Vol 3. Philadelphia, W. B. Saunders Company, 1990, pp 2237–2319.

Baker DC, Conley J: Regional muscle transposition for rehabilitation of the paralyzed face. Clin Plast Surg 6:317, 1979a.

Baker DC, Conley J: Facial nerve grafting: A thirty year retrospective review. Clin Plast Surg 6:343, 1979b.

Baker DC, Conley J: Avoiding facial nerve injuries in rhytidectomy: Anatomical variations and pitfalls. Plast Reconstr Surg 64:781, 1979c.

Balance C, Duel AB: The operative treatment of facial palsy. Arch Otolaryngol 15:1, 1932.

Banks P, Wilson JSP, Sanders R, Terry B, Whitlock TR, Chapman CW, Williams JL: Gunshot wounds. In Rowe NL, Williams JL (eds): Maxillofacial Injuries. Edinburgh, Churchill Livingstone, 1985, pp 561–694.

Barrs DM: Facial nerve trauma: Optimal timing for repair. Laryngoscope 101:835, 1991.

Beahrs OH, Adson MA: The surgical anatomy and technic of parotidectomy. Am J Surg 95:885, 1958.

Beirne OR, Worthington P: Problems and complications in implant surgery:

The surgeon's perspective. Oral Maxillofac Surg Clin North Am *3*:993, 1991.

Bell C: On the nerves, giving an account of some experiments on their structure and function, which leads to a new arrangement of the system. Trans R Soc Lond *3*:398, 1821.

Bernstein L, Nelson RH: Surgical anatomy of the extraparotid distribution of the facial nerve. Arch Otolaryngol *110*:177, 1984.

Block MS, Provenzano J, Neary JP: Complications of mandibular fractures. Oral Maxillofac Surg Clin North Am *2*:525, 1990.

Buckley MJ, Zuniga JR: Nerve dysfunction. Oral Maxillofac Surg Clin North Am *5*:137, 1993.

Burgess LPA, Goode RL: Reanimation of the Paralyzed Face. New York, Thieme Medical Publishers Inc., 1994.

Carpenter MB: Core Text of Neuroanatomy, 2nd ed. Baltimore, Williams & Wilkins, 1978.

Clark RP, Berris CE: Botulinum toxin: A treatment for facial asymmetry caused by facial nerve paralysis. Plast Reconstr Surg *84*:353, 1989.

Coker NJ, Kendall KA, Jenkins HA, Alford BR.: Traumatic intratemporal facial nerve injury: Management rationale for preservation of function. Otolaryngol Head Neck Surg *97*:262, 1987.

Coleman CC: Results of facio-hypoglossal anastomosis in the treatment of facial paralysis. Ann Surg *111*:958, 1940.

Conley J, Baker DC: Hypoglossal-facial nerve anastomosis for reinnervation of the paralyzed face. Plast Reconstr Surg *63*:63, 1979.

Conley J, Baker DC, Selfe RW: Paralysis of the mandibular branch of the facial nerve. Plast Reconstr Surg *70*:569, 1982.

Correia PC, Zani R: Masseter muscle rotation in the treatment of inferior facial paralysis. Plast Reconstr Surg *52*:370, 1973.

Davis RA, Anson BJ, Budinger JM, Kurth LE: Surgical anatomy of the facial nerve and parotid gland based upon a study of 350 cervicofacial halves. Surg Gynecol Obstet *102*:385, 1956.

Delbeke J, Thauvoy C: Electrophysiologic evaluation of cross-face nerve graft and treatment of facial palsy. Acta Neurochir *65*:111, 1982.

Dingman RO, Grabb WC: Surgical anatomy of the mandibular ramus of the facial nerve based on the dissection of 100 facial halves. Plast Reconstr Surg *29*:266, 1962.

Donoff RB, Colin W: Neurologic complications of oral and maxillofacial surgery. Oral Maxillofac Surg Clin North Am *2*:453, 1990.

Duel AB, Tickle TG: The surgical repair of facial nerve paralysis: A clinical presentation. Ann Otol Rhinol Laryngol *45*:3, 1936.

Ellenbogen R: Pseudo-paralysis of the mandibular branch of the facial nerve after platysmal face-lift operation. Plast Reconstr Surg *63*:364, 1979.

Epker BN, Gregg JM: Surgical management of maxillary nerve injuries. Oral Maxillofac Surg Clin North Am *4*:439, 1992.

Evans DM: Hypoglosso-facial anastomosis in the treatment of facial palsy. Br J Plast Surg *27*:251, 1974.

Falbe-Hansen J, Hermann S: Hypoglosso-facial anastomosis. Acta Neurol Scand *43*:472, 1967.

Fisch U: Facial paralysis and fracture of the petrous bone. Laryngoscope *84*:2141, 1974a.

Fisch U: Facial nerve grafting. Otolaryngol Clin North Am *7*:517, 1974b.

Freeman BS: Review of long-term results in supportive treatment of facial paralysis. Plast Reconstr Surg *63*:214, 1979.

Freilinger G: A new technique to correct facial paralysis. Plast Reconstr Surg *56*:44, 1975.

Freilinger G, Gruber H, Happak W, Pechmann U: Surgical anatomy of the mimic muscle system and the facial nerve: Importance for reconstructive and aesthetic surgery. Plast Reconstr Surg *80*:686, 1987.

Gagnon NB, Molina-Negro P: Facial reinnervation after facial paralysis: Is it ever too late? Arch Otorhinolaryngol *246*:303, 1989.

Gavron JP, Clemis JD: Hypoglossal-facial nerve anastomosis: A review of forty cases caused by facial nerve injuries in the posterior fossa. Laryngoscope *94*:1447, 1984.

Gillies H: Experience with fascia latae grafts in the operative treatment of facial paralysis. Proc R Soc Med *27*:1372, 1934.

Glasscock ME, Wiet RJ, Jackson CG, Dickins JRE: Rehabilitation of the face following traumatic injury to the facial nerve. Laryngoscope *89*:1389, 1979.

Hakelius L: Free muscle grafting. Clin Plast Surg *6*:301, 1979.

Hamilton SGL, Terzis JK: Surgical anatomy of donor sites for free muscle transplantation to the paralyzed face. Clin Plast Surg *11*:197, 1984.

Hardy DG, MacFarlane R, Baguley DM, Moffat DA: Facial nerve recovery following acoustic neuroma surgery. Br J Neurosurg *3*:675, 1989.

Harii K: Microneurovascular free muscle transplantation for reanimation of facial paralysis. Clin Plast Surg *6*:361, 1979.

Harii K, Ohmori K, Torii S: Free gracilis muscle transplantation with microneurovascular anastomoses for the treatment of facial paralysis. Plast Reconstr Surg *57*:133, 1976.

Harrison DH: The pectoralis minor vascularized muscle graft for the treatment of unilateral facial palsy. Plast Reconstr Surg *75*:206, 1985.

Harrison DH: Current trends in the treatment of established unilateral palsy. Ann R Coll Surg Engl *72*:94, 1990.

Hastings S: Transplantation of anterior half of masseter muscle for facial paralysis. Proc R Soc Med *13*:64, 1920.

Hilger JA: Facial nerve stimulator. Trans Am Acad Ophthalmol Otolaryngol *68*:74, 1964.

Hitselberger WE: Hypoglossal-facial anastomosis. Otolaryngol Clin North Am *7*:545, 1974.

Hollinshead WH: Anatomy for Surgeons: Volume 1, The Head and Neck, 3rd ed. Philadelphia, J. B. Lippincott Company, 1982, pp 291–323.

House WF, Crabtree JA: Surgical exposure of the petrous portion of the seventh nerve. Arch Otolaryngol *81*:506, 1965.

Hughes GB: Electroneurography: Objective prognostic assessment of facial paralysis. Am J Otol *4*:73, 1982.

Iansek R, Harrison MJG, Andrew J: Hypoglossal-facial nerve anastomosis: A clinical and electrophysiological follow-up. J Neurol Neurosurg Psychiatry 49:588, 1986.

Ishikawa Y: An anatomical study on the distribution of the temporal branch of the facial nerve. J Craniomaxillofac Surg *18*:287, 1990.

Jankovic J, Brin MF: Therapeutic uses of botulinum toxin. N Engl J Med *324*:1186, 1991.

Jelks GW, Smith B, Bosniak S: The evaluation and management of the eye in facial palsy. Clin Plast Surg *6*:397, 1979.

Johns ME, Kaplan MJ: Surgical Therapy of Tumors of the Salivary Glands. *In* Thawley SE, Panje WR, Batsakis JG, Lindberg RD (eds): Comprehensive Management of Head and Neck Tumors. Philadelphia, W. B. Saunders Company, 1987, pp 1104–1138.

Jongkees LBW: Facial paralysis complicating skull trauma. Arch Otolaryngol *81*:518, 1965.

Kanzaki J, Kunihiro T, O-uchi T, Ogawa K, Shiobara R, Toya S: Intracranial reconstruction of the facial nerve. Acta Otolaryngol 487(Suppl): 85, 1991.

Kartush JM, Prass RL: Facial Nerve Testing: Electroneurography and Intraoperative Monitoring. *In* Thomas JT, et al (eds): Instructional Courses of the American Academy of Otolaryngology, Head & Neck Surgery. St. Louis, CV Mosby, 1988, pp 231–247.

Katz AD, Catalano P: The clinical significance of the various anastomotic branches of the facial nerve. Arch Otolaryngol Head Neck Surg *113*:959, 1987.

Kessler LA, Moldaver J, Pool JL: Hypoglossal-facial anastomosis for treatment of facial paralysis. Neurology 9:118, 1959.

Kitamura T, Togawa K, Tsukamoto K, Naito J: Extratemporal facial nerve surgery. Arch Otolaryngol *95*:369, 1972.

Kunihiro T, Kanzaki J, O-Uchi T: Hypoglossal-facial nerve anastomosis. Clinical observation. Acta Otolaryngol *487*(Suppl):80, 1991.

LaBanc JP, Van Boven RW: Surgical management of inferior alveolar nerve injuries. Oral Maxillofac Surg Clin North Am *4*:425, 1992.

Lee KK, Terzis JK: Management of acute extratemporal facial nerve palsy. Clin Plast Surg *11*:203, 1984.

Liebman EP, Webster RC, Gaul JR, Griffin T: The marginal mandibular nerve in rhytidectomy and liposuction surgery. Arch Otolaryngol Head Neck Surg *114*:179, 1988.

MacKinnon SA, Dellon AL: Surgery of the Peripheral Nerve. New York, Thieme Medical Publishers Inc., 1988, pp 89–129, 393–321.

Malamed SF: Handbook of Local Anesthesia. St. Louis, C.V. Mosby Company, 1980, pp 112–129.

Manktelow RT: Free muscle transplantation for facial paralysis. Clin Plast Surg *11*:215, 1984a.

Manktelow RT: Muscle transplantation by fascicular territory. Plast Reconstr Surg *73*:751, 1984b.

Marino H: Paralysis of the muscles of the chin. Surgical treatment. Surg Gynecol Obstet *96*:433, 1953.

May M: Anatomy of the facial nerve (spatial orientation of fibers in the temporal bone). Laryngoscope *82*:1311, 1973.

May M: Facial paralysis: Differential diagnosis and indications for surgical therapy. Clin Plast Surg *6*:275, 1979.

May M, Harvey JE, Marovitz WF, Stroud M: The prognostic accuracy of the maximal stimulation test compared with that of the nerve excitability test in Bell's palsy. Laryngoscope 81:931, 1971.

May M, Sobol SM, Mester SJ: Hypoglossal-facial nerve interpositional-jump graft for facial reanimation without tongue atrophy. Otolaryngol Head Neck Surg *104*:818, 1991.

McCormack LJ, Cauldwell EW, Anson BJ: The surgical anatomy of the facial nerve with special reference to the parotid gland. Surg Gynecol Obstet *80*:620, 1945.

McKenzie J: The parotid gland in relation to the facial nerve. J Anat *82*:183, 1948.

McKinney P, Katrana DJ: Prevention of injury to the great auricular nerve during rhytidectomy. Plast Reconstr Surg *66*:675, 1980.

McWhorter GL: The relations of the superficial and deep lobes of the parotid gland to the ducts to the facial nerve. Anat Rec *12*:149, 1917.

Meyer RA: Applications of microneurosurgery to the repair of trigeminal nerve injuries. Oral Maxillofac Surg Clin North Am *4*:405, 1992.

Miehlke A: Extratemporal repair of the facial nerve. Arch Otolaryngol *81*:534, 1965.

Miehlke A, Stennert E: New techniques for optimum reconstruction of the facial nerve in its extemporal course. Acta Otolaryngol *91*:497, 1981.

Miehlke A, Stennert E, Chilla R: New aspects in facial nerve surgery. Clin Plast Surg *6*:451, 1979.

Millesi H: Nerve suture and grafting to restore the extratemporal facial nerve. Clin Plast Surg *6*: 33. 1979.

Mitz V, Peyronie M: The superficial musculo-aponeurotic system (SMAS) in the parotid and cheek area. Plast Reconstr Surg *58*:80, 1976.

Moffat DA, Ramsden RT: The deformity produced by a palsy of the marginal mandibular branch of the facial nerve. J Laryngol Otol *91*:401, 1977.

Moore KL: Clinically Oriented Anatomy, 2nd ed. Baltimore, Williams & Wilkins, 1985, pp 829–832.

Nelson DW, Gingrass RP: Anatomy of the mandibular branches of the facial nerve. Plast Reconstr Surg *64*:479, 1979.

O'Brien BM, Franklin JD, Morrison WA: Cross-facial nerve grafts and microneurovascular free muscle transfer for long established facial palsy. Br J Plast Surg *33*:202, 1980.

O'Brien BM, Pederson WC, Khazanchi RK, Morrison WA, MacLeod AM, Kumar V: Results of management of facial palsy with microvascular free-muscle transfer. Plast Reconstr Surg *86*: 12, 1990.

Owens N: Implantation of fascial strips through the masseter muscle for surgical correction of facial paralysis. Plast Reconstr Surg *2*:25, 1947.

Pensak ML, Jackson CG, Glasscock ME, Gulya AJ: Facial reanimation with the VII–XII anastomosis: Analysis of the functional and psychologic results. Otolaryngol Head Neck Surg *94*:305, 1986.

Pitanguy I, Ramos AS: The frontal branch of the facial nerve: The importance of its variations in face lifting. Plast Reconstr Surg *38*:352, 1966.

Poe DS, Scher N, Panje WR: Facial reanimation by XI–VII anastomosis without shoulder paralysis. Laryngoscope *99*:1040, 1989.

Pogrel MA: Complications of third molar surgery. Oral Maxillofac Surg Clin North Am *2*:441, 1990.

Pollack RS: Surgical significance of the marginal mandibular branch of the facial nerve. Arch Surg *68*:81, 1954.

Raimbault J: Electrical assessment of muscle denervation. Clin Plast Surg *11*:53, 1984.

Rubin LR: The anatomy of a smile: Its importance in the treatment of facial paralysis. Plast Reconstr Surg *53*:384, 1974.

Rudolph, R.: Depth of the facial nerve in face lift dissections. Plast Reconstr Surg *85*:537, 1990.

Sade J: Facial nerve reconstruction and its prognosis. Ann Otol Rhinol Laryngol *84*:695, 1975.

Sanger JR, Riley DA, Yousif NJ, Matloub HS, Bain JLW: Histochemical staining of nerve endings as an aid to free muscle transplantation. Microsurgery *12*:361, 1991.

Sassoon EM, Poole MD, Rushworth G: Reanimation for facial palsy using gracilis muscle grafts. Br J Plast Surg *44*:195, 1991.

Scaramella LF: On the repair of the injured facial nerve. Ear Nose Throat J *58*:45, 1979.

Schubert W, Kimberley B, Guzman-Stein G, Cunningham BL: Use of the labial artery for replantation of the lip and chin. Ann Plast Surg *20*:256, 1988.

Schubert W, Quillopa N, Shons AR: An analysis of the key sensory foramina of craniofacial surgery. Presented at the 49th annual meeting of the American Cleft Palate—Craniofacial Association, Portland, Oregon, May 12–15, 1992.

Scott AB, Kennedy RA, Stubbs HA: Botulinum A toxin injection as a treatment for blepharospasm. Arch Ophthalmol *103*:347, 1985.

Seckel BR: Facial Danger Zones. Avoiding Nerve Injury in Facial Plastic Surgery. St. Louis, Quality Med Publishers, 1994.

Seiff SR, Chang J: Management of ophthalmic complications of facial nerve palsy. Otolaryngol Clin North Am *25*:669, 1992.

Sheehan JE: The muscle-nerve graft. Surg Clin North Am *15*:471, 1935.

Shulman LB, Shepherd NJ: Complications of dental implants. Oral Maxillofac Surg Clin North Am *2*:499, 1990.

Sobol SM, May M, Mester S: Early facial reanimation following radical parotid and temporal bone tumor resections. Am J Surg *160*:382, 1990.

Spear SL, Kassan M: Genioplasty. Clin Plast Surg *16*:695, 1989.

Spector JG, Lee P, Peterein J, Roufa D: Facial nerve regeneration through autologous nerve grafts: A clinical and experimental study. Laryngoscope *101*:537, 1991.

Steenerson RL: Bilateral facial paralysis. Am J Otol *7*:99, 1986.

Stennert E: I. Hypoglossal facial anastomosis: Its significance for modern facial surgery. II. Combined approach in extratemporal facial nerve reconstruction. Clin Plast Surg *6*:471, 1979.

Stuzin JM, Wagstrom L, Kawamoto HK, Wolfe SA: Anatomy of the frontal branch of the facial nerve: The significance of the temporal fat pad. Plast Reconstr Surg *83*:265, 1989.

Sunderland S, Cossar DF: The structure of the facial nerve. Anat Rec *116*:147, 1953.

Thompson N: Autogenous free grafts of skeletal muscle. A preliminary experimental and clinical study. Plast Reconstr Surg *48*:11, 1971.

Tolhurst DE, Bos KE: Free revascularized muscle graft and facial palsy. Plast Reconstr Surg *69*:760, 1982.

Tucker HM: The management of facial paralysis due to extracranial injuries. Laryngoscope *88*:348, 1978.

Tucker HM: Restoration of selective facial nerve function by the nerve-muscle pedicle technique. Clin Plast Surg *6*:293, 1979.

Wells MD, Manktelow, RT: Surgical management of facial palsy. Clin Plast Surg *17*:645, 1990.

Whitney TM, Buncke HJ, Alpert BS, Buncke GM, Lineaweaver WC: The serratus anterior free-muscle flap: Experience with 100 consecutive cases. Plast Reconstr Surg *86*:481, 1990.

Williams WT, Ghorayeb BY, Yeakley JW: Pediatric temporal bone fractures. Laryngoscope *102*:600, 1992.

Wilson-Pauwels L, Akesson EJ, Stewart PA: Cranial Nerves: Anatomy and Clinical Comments. Toronto, B. C. Decker Inc., 1988, pp 82–95.

Woods JE, Beahrs OH: A technique for the rapid performance of parotidectomy with minimal risk. Surg Gynecol Obstet *142*:87, 1976.

Yarbrough WG, Brownlee RE, Pillsbury HC: Primary anastomosis of extensive facial nerve defects: An anatomic study. Am J Otol *14*:238, 1993.

Zide BM, Jelks GW: Surgical Anatomy of the Orbit. Hong Kong, Raven Press, 1985.

Chapter 5

• Robert C. Russell
• Jurgen Hussmann
• Mary Burns

Clinical Motor Function Testing—Upper Extremity

Clinical examination of upper extremity motor function is based on a sound comprehension of anatomical relationships. The major peripheral nerves of the upper extremity contain both sensory and motor axons, which activate the individual muscles of the limb and relay sensibility from the periphery to the brain. There are also anatomical variations such as the Martin-Gruber or Riche-Cannieu anastomoses, as well as peripheral sensory nerve overlap, which must be considered to prevent misinterpretation of clinical findings. A general evaluation of the patient is crucial to detect underlying causes of neuromuscular dysfunction that may mimic specific regional defects even in cases of acute and apparently obvious lacerations. These causes include diabetes mellitus, chronic alcohol abuse, systemic neurological disorders, rheumatoid arthritis, hypothyroidism, acromegaly, pregnancy, chronic hemodialysis with amyloid formation, hemophilia, tumor, neurofibromatosis, and others. Patients with such conditions may have abnormal motor and sensory nerve function before injury that can alter the physical findings, leading to erroneous conclusions regarding the site or degree of nerve injury.

Nerve or muscle damage in the upper extremity following trauma, surgery, or disease can be precisely located using straightforward clinical examination when the physician has mastered the anatomy of the upper extremity. Physical findings depend on the onset and duration of the pathological process, and may range from discrete paresthesias or faint weakness to progressive muscle wasting and complete loss of all sensory and motor nerve function. The widely accepted grading classification of muscle function (Table 5–1) has been suggested by the Medical Research Council (1976) and is a useful way to clinically document muscle strength.

ANATOMICAL CONSIDERATIONS

The motor axons to the upper extremity originate in the ventral horn of the spinal cord and the spinal nerves exit the spinal column through the intervertebral foramina. They merge with dorsal sensory ganglion axons to form the roots

▼ TABLE 5–1
Grading Classification of Muscle Function

0	No contraction
1	Flicker or trace of contraction
2	Active movement, gravity eliminated
3	Active movement against gravity
4	Active movement against gravity and some resistance
5	Normal power

of the cervicobrachial plexus, which contains fibers from cervical roots C5(4) to T1(2) (Fig. 5–1). Several functions of the upper extremity can be confined to specific roots. This aids in determining the level of a root or trunk lesion. The functions of corresponding cervical roots are listed in Table 5–2. Some muscles display a dual or variable pattern of nerve supply and require special consideration. Patients with long-standing nerve injury or those who have lost the function of individual muscles, for example, after a free flap transfer, usually recruit adjacent muscles to replace the extremity functions that are lost (Russell et al, 1986). Such movements may lead to false interpretation of standard muscle function tests.

The shoulder musculature is supplied by nerves that originate in the brachial plexus (see Fig. 5–1) and include the dorsal scapular, suprascapular, medial and lateral pectoral, subscapular, and thoracodorsal nerves. The five major nerves to the upper extremity, the axillary, brachial, median, radial, and ulnar, all carry both sensory and motor fibers to provide muscle function and sensibility to the upper extremity (Figs. 5–2*A* and *B* and 5–3*A* and *B*). Systemic diseases or nerve injury results in specific motor or sensory nerve loss, which can be tested by physical examination (Kendall, 1983).

Dorsal Scapular Nerve

The dorsal scapular nerve originates from the upper trunk of the brachial plexus with contributions from C4 and 5 roots. The nerve traverses the posterior triangle of the neck to innervate the rhomboids major and minor and part of the levator scapulae muscle. It can be injured from trauma usually associated with traction injuries to the brachial plexus occurring in high-velocity motor vehicle accidents or with penetrating injuries such as gunshot wounds. All of the muscles supplied by the dorsal scapular nerve attach the medial boarder of the scapula to the cervical or thoracic spine and act to adduct, elevate, and rotate the scapula. Function of these muscles can be tested with the patient in the prone position by attempting to pull the flexed elbow away from the body while pushing against the shoulder with the other hand (Fig. 5–4). This produces a downward and externally rotating force on the scapula, which, if the muscles are weak or absent, will abduct the scapula away from the spine and rotate the angle laterally. Paralysis or weakness of the serratus anterior muscle can cause unopposed action of the rhomboids resulting in adduction and elevation of the scapula into a contracted position. When paralyzed with brachial plexus avulsion, C5 supraganglionic injury is present. This unique finding makes examination of the rhomboid crucial.

▼ TABLE 5–2
Functional Anatomy by Region

Anatomical Region	Function	Root	Nerve	Key Muscles	Test	Muscles with Similar Function but Different or Dual Innervation
Shoulder	Abduction	C5	Suprascapular	Supraspinatus	Abduction of humerus against resistance, palpation through relaxed trapezius	Biceps, lat. head deltoid
			Axillary	Deltoid	Abduction against resistance without rotation	Supraspinatus
	Adduction	C7	Thoracodorsal	Latissimus dorsi	Adduction of internally rotated and extended arm against resistance	Biceps, short head pectoralis major, teres major, teres minor, and coracobrachialis triceps, lat. head
		C6–C8	Lateral and medial pectoral	Pectoralis major and minor	Horizontal adduction of flexed and abducted arm	See earlier
	External rotation	C5	Suprascapular	Infraspinatus, supraspinatus	See under individual muscle	Teres minor, deltoid, post. portion
	Internal rotation	C5	Subscapular	Subscapularis, teres minor	See under individual muscle	Deltoid, ant. portion, pectoralis major, latissimus dorsi
	Extension	C5–C8	Multiple	Multiple	Extension with different degrees of rotation	Posterior deltoid, latissimus dorsi, teres major, triceps, long head
	Flexion	C5–C7	Multiple	Multiple	Flexion with different degrees of rotation	Anterior deltoid, pectoralis major, biceps brachii, coracobrachialis
Elbow	Extension	C7	Radial	Triceps	Forearm extension at elbow with arm held horizontally in 90 degrees of flexion	Anconeus
	Flexion in neutral position	C5(6)	Radial	Brachioradialis	Elbow flexion against resistance	Biceps brachii, brachialis, pronator teres
	Flexion in supination	C5(6)	Musculocutaneous	Biceps brachialis	Elbow flexion against resistance with forearm in supination	Brachioradialis, pronator teres
	Supination of extended forearm	C6	Posterior interosseous (radial)	Supinator	Supination of extended forearm against resistance	Brachioradialis, biceps
	Pronation	C6	Median anterior interosseous (median)	Pronator teres, pronator quadratus	Pronation of forearm against resistance	Flexor carpi radialis, brachioradialis, palmaris longus
Wrist	Extension	C(6)7	Radial	All extensors, brachioradialis	Dorsal and radial wrist extension with forearm in supination	None
	Flexion	C7–C8	Median ulnar	All forearm flexors, flexor carpi ulnaris	Palmar wrist flexion	
Fingers	Abduction	T1	Ulnar	Interossei, abductor digitorum minimi		
	Adduction					
	Extension	C8	Radial	All extensors		
	Flexion	C8	Median ulnar	Flexor digitorum profundus II–III, flexor digitorum profundus IV–V		
Thumb	Abduction	T1	Median	Abductor pollicis brevis		
	Adduction	C8–T1	Ulnar	Adductor pollicis	Froment's sign	Extensor pollicis longus (weak)
	Pinch	C8	Median	Long flexor of thumb and index		

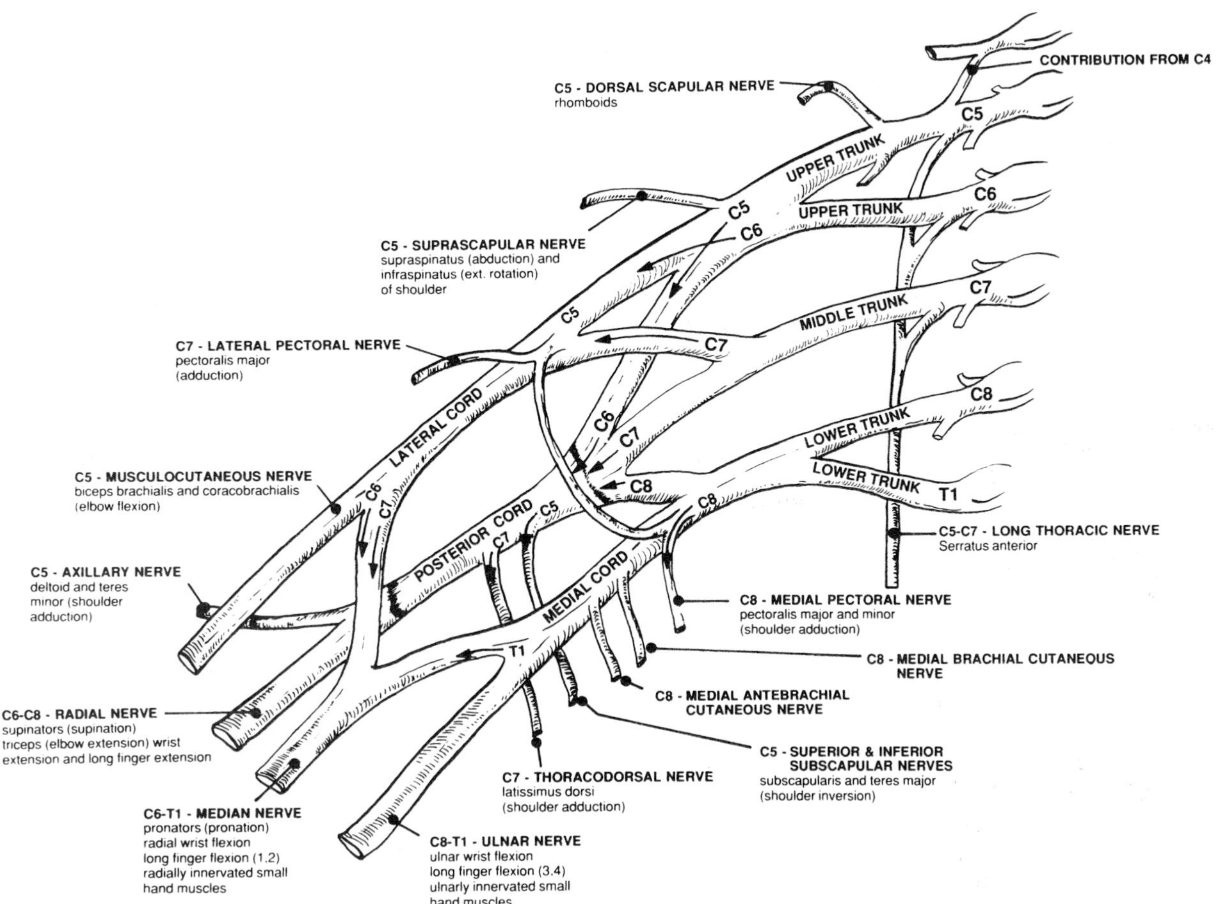

FIGURE 5–1. The cervicobrachial plexus is formed by dorsal sensory and ventral motor axons from the cervical roots of C5–T1. There are occasional contributions from C4 and T2.

Suprascapular Nerve

The suprascapular nerve originates from the upper trunk of the brachial plexus with contributions from C4, 5, and 6 and innervates the supraspinatus muscle. The nerve can be compressed as it courses under the superior or inferior transverse ligaments, or both, of the scapula. The muscle originates from the supraspinatus fossa of the scapular and inserts on the greater tuberosity of the humerus and the joint capsule of the shoulder. The muscle acts to abduct the shoulder and stabilizes the humerus in the glenoid fossa. The muscle can be tested with the patient standing with the arm at the side and the neck flexed to the same side while the head is rotated to the opposite side to relax the overlying trapezius muscle (Fig. 5–5). The muscle can then be palpated as the patient abducts the shoulder while the examiner holds pressure against the forearm in adduction.

Medial and Lateral Pectoral Nerves

The medial and lateral pectoral nerves arise from the medial and lateral cords of the brachial plexus in the axilla below the level of the clavicle, and innervate the pectoralis major and minor muscles. The pectoralis minor muscle originates from the third, fourth, and fifth ribs anteriorly, and inserts into the coracoid process of the scapula. Flexion of the muscle pulls the coracoid process forward and down, rotating the scapula forward and causing the angle to move posteriorly and medially. Shortness or contracture of the pectoralis minor holds the shoulder forward off the table when the patient is at rest in a supine position. Muscle function is tested by asking the patient to move the shoulder forward with the arm extended off the examining table against manual resistance of the examiners hand (Fig. 5–6).

The upper fibers of the pectoralis major muscle originate from the inferior portion of the medial clavicle while the lower fibers originate from the sternum and the first six or seven rib cartilages and fascia of external oblique muscle. The muscle acts to adduct and medially rotate the humerus toward the opposite side. The upper fibers innervated primarily by the lateral pectoral nerve are tested with the patient supine by holding the opposite shoulder on the table with the elbow extended and the shoulder at 90 degrees of flexion. The patient adducts the arm toward the opposite shoulder against resistance (Fig. 5–7). The lower fibers are tested in a similar fashion by asking the patient to adduct the extended arm toward the opposite hip, which is held on the table by the examiner's opposite hand (Fig. 5–8).

Subscapular Nerve

The superior and inferior subscapular nerves originate from the medial cord of the brachial plexus with contributions from C5, 6, and 7 and innervate the subscapularis

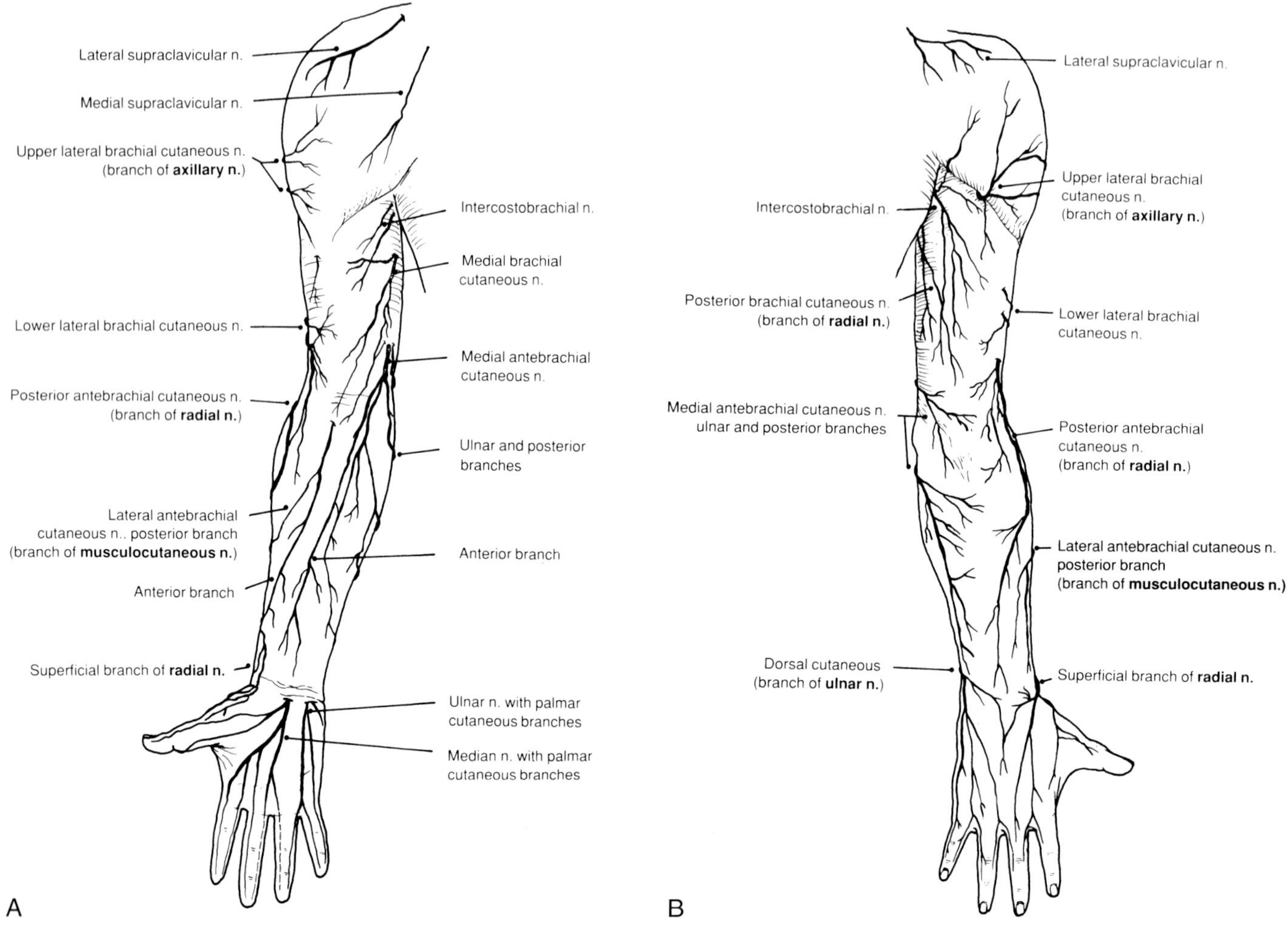

FIGURE 5–2. The sensory nerve distribution to the upper extremity: anterior *(A)* and posterior *(B)*.

muscle. The muscle originates in the subscapular fossa of the scapula and inserts into the lesser tubercle of the humerus and the joint capsule of the shoulder. It acts to rotate the shoulder medially and to stabilize the humeral head in the glenoid fossa. The subscapularis muscle cannot be tested independently but is tested as a group with the other muscles contributing to medial shoulder rotation. These muscles are the latissimus dorsi, pectoralis major, teres major, and subscapularis. The patient is asked to medially rotate the humerus with the elbow held at a right angle. The examiner stabilizes the humerus while applying pressure to the forearm in the direction of lateral or external rotation (Fig. 5–9).

Thoracodorsal Nerve

The thoracodorsal nerve carries fibers from C6, 7, and 8 and originates from the posterior cord at the level of the clavicle. The nerve carries motor axons to the latissimus dorsi muscle, which it enters with the thoracodorsal vascular pedicle in the distal third on the undersurface of the muscle. The muscle functions to adduct, internally rotate, and extend the shoulder joint. Injury to the nerve most commonly occurs as a complication of mastectomy surgery, when the axillary lymph nodes are removed, or with fracture dislocations of

the proximal humerus. Latissimus dorsi muscle function is tested in the prone position by forced abduction of the extended, medially rotated arm away from the patient's body (Fig. 5–10). The muscle contraction can also be palpated in the posterior axillary wall when the patient is asked to adduct the shoulder against resistance from a position of 90 degrees of abduction.

Axillary Nerve

The axillary nerve carries fibers from C5–C6 and originates from the posterior cord (see Fig. 5–1). It curves laterally and dorsally around the humerus, and together with the posterior humeral circumflex artery and vena comitans, it composes a neurovascular bundle. The nerve transverses the quadrangular space formed by the teres major and minor, the long head of the triceps, and the humerus, where avulsion transection and compression syndrome can occur. The axillary nerve supplies the deltoid, teres minor, and infraspinatus muscles. The deltoid is composed of anterior, middle, and posterior fibers. The anterior and posterior fibers stabilize shoulder abduction, and act as weak shoulder flexors and rotators. In the supine position, anterior fibers internally rotate the arm, and in the prone position, posterior fibers

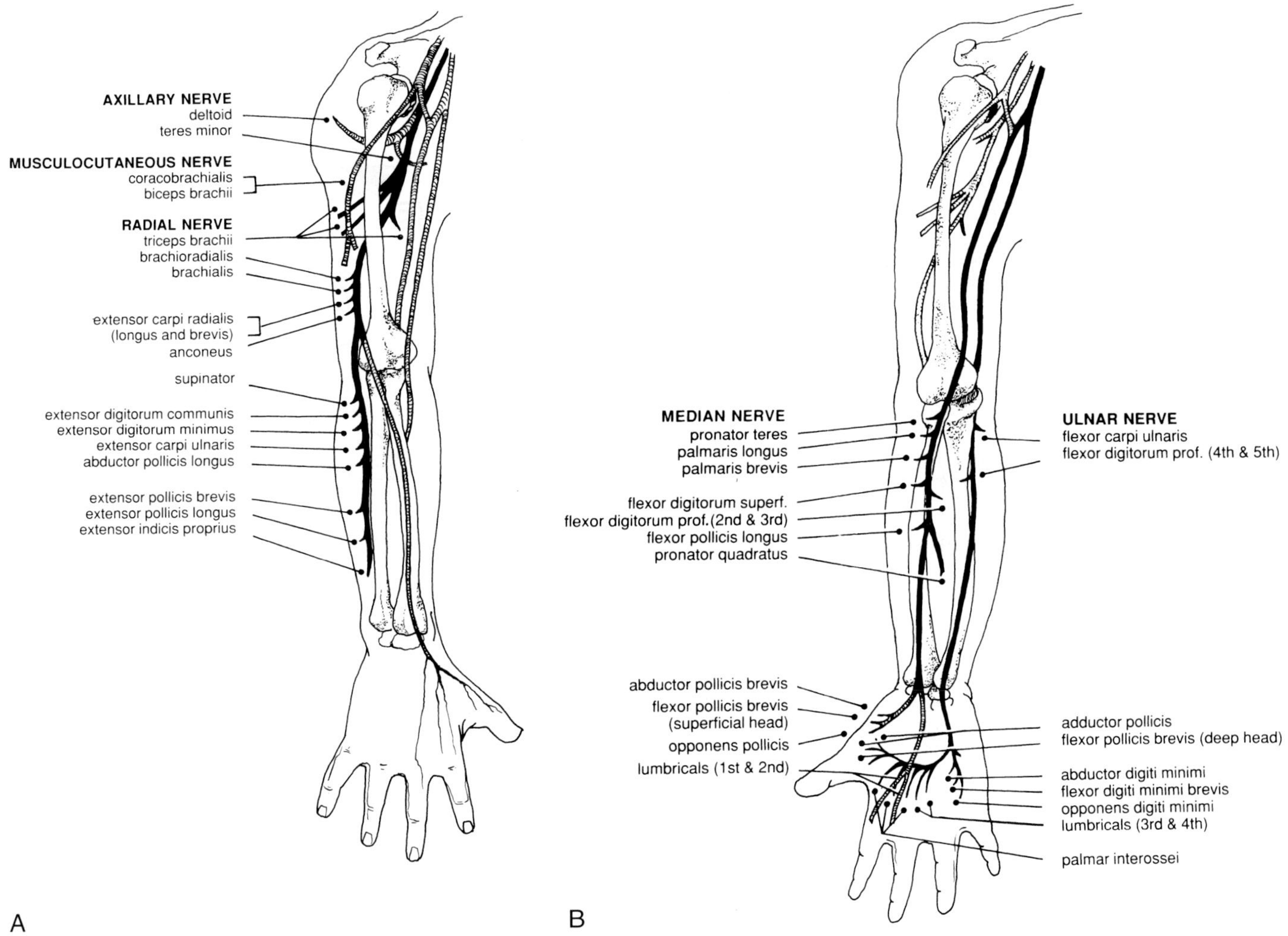

FIGURE 5–3. *A,* The course of the axillary, musculocutaneous, and radial nerves in the arm. *B,* The course of the median and ulnar nerves in the arm.

FIGURE 5–4. The dorsal scapular nerve from the upper trunk innervates the rhomboid major and minor and the levator scapulae muscles. These muscles are tested with the patient in prone position by attempting to pull the flexed elbow away from the body while pushing the shoulder down with the examiner's other hand. E = Examiner; P = patient.

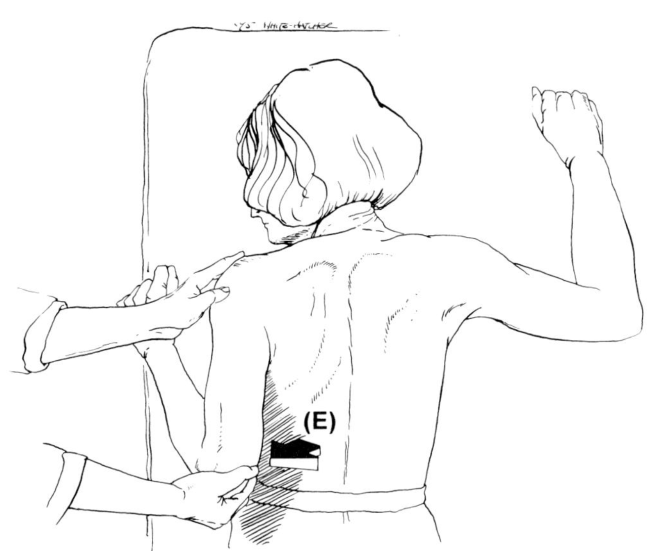

▼ TABLE 5–3
Upper Extremity: Motor and Sensory Nerve Contribution to Peripheral Nerves

Nerve	Branch	Muscle Innervation	Sensory Distribution
Dorsal scapular, C4–5		Rhomboid major, rhomboid minor, levator scapulae	None
Suprascapular, C4–6		Supraspinatus, infraspinatus	None
Nerve to subclavius, C5		Subclavius	None
Subscapular, C5–7		Teres major	None
Long thoracic, C5–7		Serratus anterior	None
Thoracodorsal, C6–8		Latissimus dorsi	None
Lateral pectoral, C6		Pectoralis major, pectoralis minor	None
Medial pectoral, C7–8		Pectoralis major, pectoralis minor	None
Axillary, C5–6	Lateral, brachial, cutaneous	Deltoid, teres minor	Over deltoid, lateral aspect of upper arm, lateral portion of shoulder joint
Musculocutaneous, C5–7	Lateral antebrachial cutaneous	Biceps brachii, brachialis, coracobrachialis (together with radial nerve), pronator teres	Volar radial forearm to wrist, may extend to thenar eminence
Medial brachial cutaneous (medial cord) C8–T1		None	Medial aspect of upper arm
Radial, C5–8	Posterior interosseous Posterior, brachial, cutaneous, posterior, antebrachial, cutaneous, superficial, radial	*Triceps brachii, brachioradialis,* anconeus, *extensor carpi radialis (brevis and longus), extensor digitorum communis II–V,* brachialis, supinator, *extensor carpi ulnaris, extensor digiti minimi, extensor pollicis longus, extensor pollicis brevis, extensor indicis proprius*	Dorsal distal upper arm Dorsal radial forearm Dorsal *first web space* Radial dorsum of hand, wrist joint
Medial antebrachial cutaneous, C8–T1 (medial cord)	Anterior ulnar	None	Ulnar forearm
Median, C5–T1	Anterior interosseous Recurrent motor branch Palmar cutaneous	Pronator teres, pronator quadratus, *flexor carpi radialis,* palmaris longus, flexor digitorum superficialis, flexor digitorum profundus (second and third), *flexor pollicis longus, abductor pollicis brevis,* flexor pollicis brevis (superficial head), opponens pollicis, lumbricales (first and second)	*Pulp of thumb and index, proximal palm and thenar eminence,* radial palm and radial fingers
Ulnar, C8–T1	Superficial palmar	*Flexor carpi ulnaris,* flexor pollicis brevis (deep head), flexor digitorum profundus (fourth and fifth), *flexor digiti minimi brevis, opponens digiti minimi,* palmaris brevis, adductor pollicis, flexor pollicis brevis, abductor digiti, lumbricales (third and fourth), interossei	*Pulp of little finger, dorsal ulnar surface of hand,* ulnar palm and ulnar fingers

Italics: key muscles, most reliable sensory distribution.

to the ulnar wrist and digital extensor muscles, and the superficial radial nerve sensory fibers to the dorsal first web space and proximal dorsal aspect of the thumb and index finger. The posterior interosseous nerve supplies the supinator, extensor digitorum communis, extensor digiti quinti,

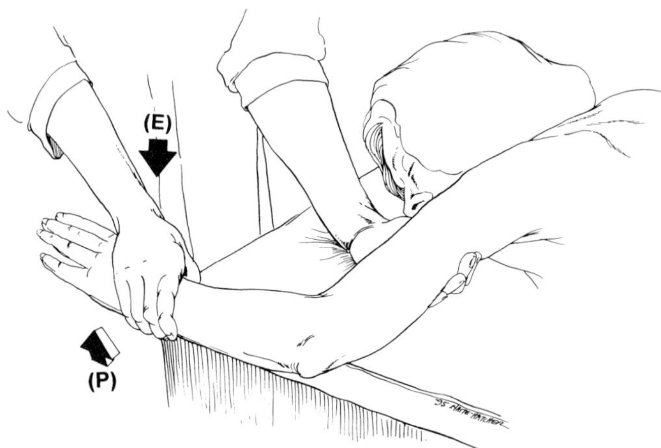

FIGURE 5–12. Teres minor and infraspinatus muscle function is tested by asking the patient to rotate the humerus laterally with the elbow held at 90 degrees as the examiner applies pressure to medially rotate the humerus.

extensor carpi ulnaris, extensor pollicis longus and brevis, extensor indicis proprius, and abductor pollicis longus. Posterior interosseus nerve palsy secondary to nerve transection is an important clinical entity and may be caused by penetrating lacerations, gunshot wounds, or fractures of the proximal third of the radius. Occupational overuse of the supinator, such as unaccustomed use of a screwdriver or arm wrestling, may produce compression of the posterior interosseous nerve and symptoms of proximal forearm pain and eventual weakness of digital and ulnar wrist extension and supination. Posterior interosseous nerve injury spares the brachioradialis and extensor carpi radialis longus muscles, allowing the patient weak wrist extension with radial deviation.

Proximal radial nerve lesions are diagnosed by testing triceps and anconeus function. The patient is asked to actively extend the elbow against resistance (Fig. 5–14). Radial nerve lesions at the middle third of the humerus usually leave the triceps intact. The brachioradialis may be affected and is tested by active elbow flexion against resistance when biceps and brachialis contraction are excluded by pronation of the forearm (Fig. 5–15). The extrinsic wrist or digital extensors are tested by active extension of the wrist or digital metacarpophalangeal joints with the proximal interphalangeal (PIP) and distal interphalangeal (DIP) joints flexed and the elbow in 90 degrees of flexion. Supinator function is

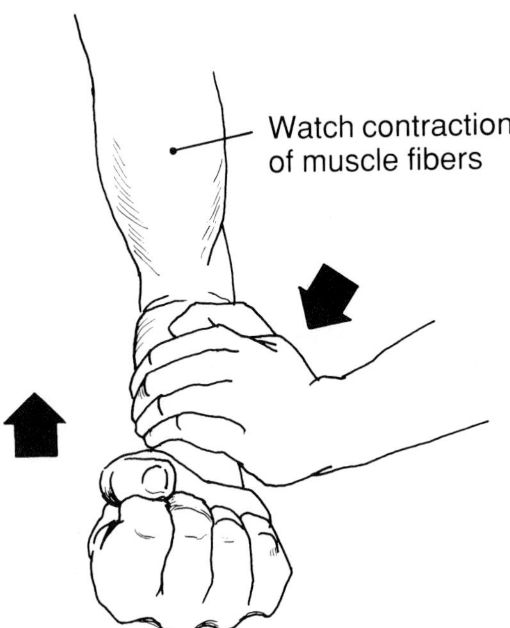

MUSCULOCUTANEOUS NERVE
elbow flexion in supination (biceps)
(brachioradialis is innervated by
radial nerve and is an elbow flexor
with forearm in pronation)

FIGURE 5–13. The musculocutaneous nerve innervates the biceps and brachialis muscles, which are tested by active flexion of the elbow against resistance with the forearm in supination.

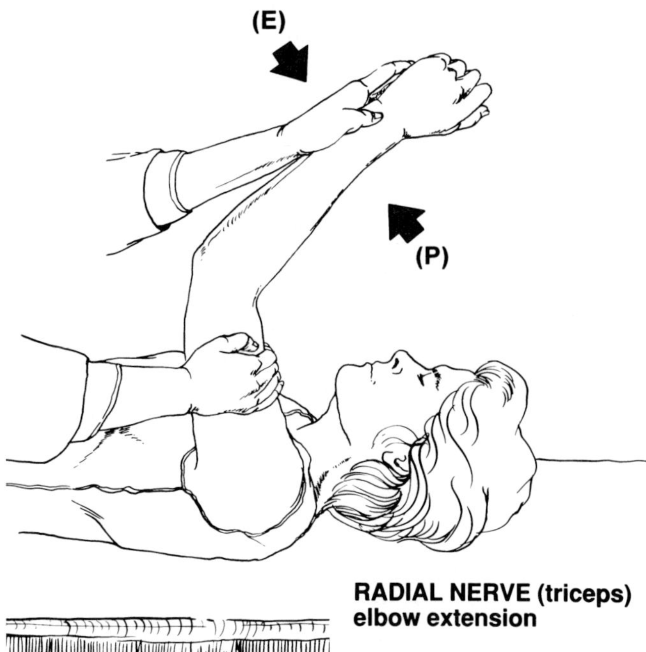

FIGURE 5–14. The triceps muscle is innervated by the radial nerve and is tested by asking the patient to extend the elbow against resistance.

tested by active supination of the forearm from a pronated position, with the elbow in 90 degrees of flexion (Fig. 5–16). Extensor digitorum communis function is tested by active extension of the metacarpophalangeal joints of the second to the fifth fingers, with the interphalangeal joints relaxed. Extensor indicis proprius and extensor digitorum quinti function are tested individually by active extension of the metacarpophalangeal joint of the index or little finger alone. Lumbrical and interosseous muscles combine with extrinsic extensor tendons to extend the PIP joints, whereas the DIP joints are extended by intrinsic muscles. The extensor pollicis brevis extends the thumb metacarpophalangeal joint, and the extensor pollicis longus extends the thumb interphalangeal joint. The abductor pollicis longus abducts and slightly extends the first metacarpal.

Median Nerve

The median nerve originates from cervical roots C5–T1, and is formed by a fusion of branches from the medial and lateral cords in front of the brachial artery (see Fig. 5–1). The median nerve and brachial artery travel distally in a neurovascular bundle located medial to the coracobrachialis and biceps muscles and tendons (see Fig. 5–3A). The median nerve at the elbow gives a branch to the pronator teres and travels through the two heads of this muscle, where it can sometimes be compressed. It runs under a fibrous arch, through the flexor digitorum superficialis muscle, and

courses throughout the forearm in the posterior fascia of this muscle. Distal to the elbow, the nerve gives off motor branches to palmaris longus, flexor digitorum superficialis, abductor pollicis brevis, superficial head of flexor pollicis brevis, opponens pollicis, and first and second lumbricals. The median nerve supplies sensation to the volar surface of the palm including the thumb, index, long, and half of the ring fingers (see Fig. 5–2A and B).

The anterior interosseous nerve is a branch of the median nerve, which arises in the midforearm and innervates the flexor pollicis longus, flexor digitorum profundus to the index and long fingers, and the pronator quadratus muscles.

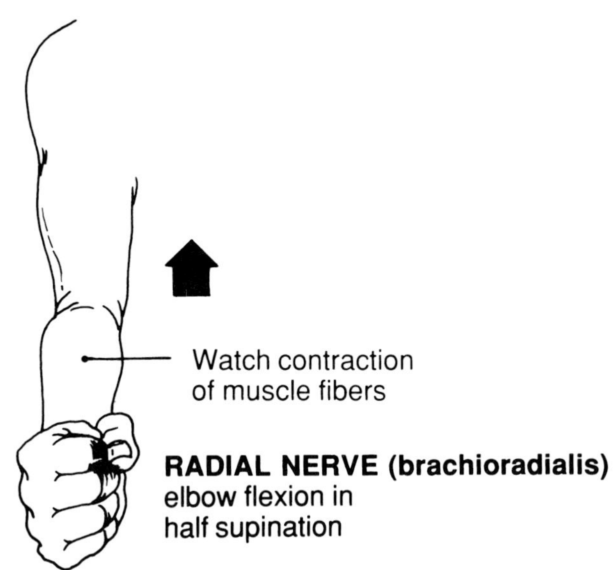

FIGURE 5–15. The brachioradialis is tested by active elbow flexion against resistance with the forearm in neutral to exclude the biceps and brachialis muscles.

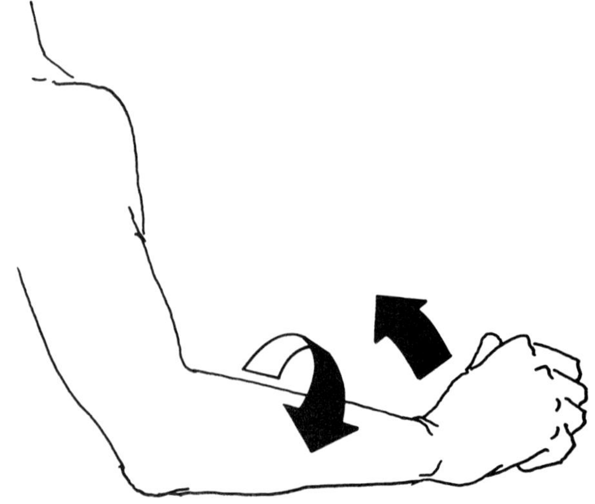

FIGURE 5–16. Wrist extension and supination can be tested with the elbow in 90 degrees of flexion when the patient attempts to extend the wrist and supinate the forearm against resistance.

Pronator teres function is tested by palpation of the muscle during pronation of the forearm with the elbow flexed at 30 degrees. The flexor carpi radialis is tested by active radial flexion of the wrist against resistance. The individual flexor digitorum superficialis muscle slips to each digit can be tested by flexing the proximal interphalangeal joints of the index, long, ring, and little fingers successively while the distal interphalangeal joints on adjacent fingers are held in extension. The flexor digitorum superficialis also assists in wrist and metacarpophalangeal joint flexion. The flexor digitorum profundus muscle slips to the index and long fingers are usually supplied by the median nerve, while those to the ring and little fingers are usually supplied by the ulnar nerve. Profundus muscle function should be tested by digital DIP joint flexion against resistance with the metacarpophalangeal and the PIP joints held in extension (Fig. 5–17). The flexor pollicis longus is tested by active thumb interphalangeal

joint flexion against resistance. The pronator quadratus pronates the forearm when the elbow is completely flexed, eliminating the pronator teres. The abductor pollicis brevis is tested by active abduction of the thumb away from the palm against resistance while the examiner stabilizes the hand and forearm. The opponens pollicis is tested by active opposition of the thumb against resistance.

Ulnar Nerve

The ulnar nerve is the terminal branch of the medial cord and contains fibers of C8–T1 (see Fig. 5–1). It runs together with the median and medial antebrachial cutaneous nerves in the upper arm and then pierces the medial intermuscular septum to lie anterior to the medial head of the triceps muscle (see Fig. 5–3A). It continues distally behind the medial epicondyle and then between the humeral and ulnar heads of the flexor carpi ulnaris muscle. The nerve travels behind the medial epicondyle of the elbow in the cubital tunnel, which is the most common site of ulnar nerve compression. It sends branches to the flexor carpi ulnaris and flexor digitorum profundus to the ring and little fingers. The nerve travels beneath the flexor carpi ulnaris muscle and at the wrist passes radial to the pisiform bone, across the pisohamate ligament, through the canal of Guyon, where it gives off branches to the palmaris brevis muscle. Exiting the canal, the nerve divides into superficial and deep ulnar nerve branches. The superficial branch provides sensation for the ulnar border of the hand, including the volar surface of the little and half of the ring fingers. The deep branch carries motor fibers across the palm of the hand together with the deep palmar arch of the ulnar artery. It branches to all four hypothenar muscles, the two ulnar lumbricals, and all interosseous muscles, and terminates in the adductor pollicis muscle.

Lesions of the ulnar nerve may occur on the medial side of the upper arm from superficial wounds, tourniquets, or improper positioning on the operating table but most commonly are located behind the medial epicondyle of the humerus in the cubital tunnel due to repeated minor trauma. At this level, all motor and sensory branches of the nerve are affected. Lesions at the heel of the hand compromise the interossei, the two ulnar lumbricals, the hypothenar musculature, and the volar sensory distribution (see Fig. 5–2A and

FIGURE 5–17. Profundus muscle function for each finger is tested by flexion of the DIP joint while the MP and PIP joints are held in extension.

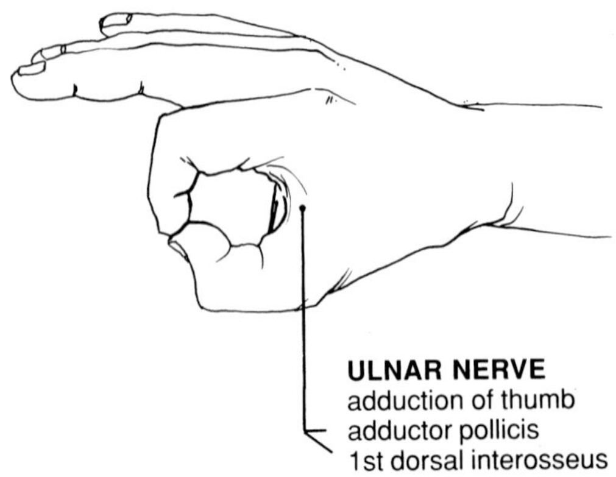

FIGURE 5–18. The first dorsal interosseous and adductor pollicis muscles can be palpated in the web space during pinch.

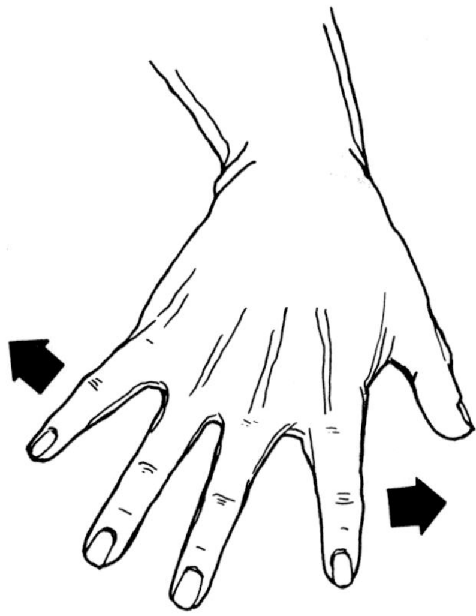

FIGURE 5–19. The intrinsic muscles of the hand are innervated by the ulnar nerve and can be tested by palpation of the first dorsal interosseous and hypothenar muscles during active abduction of the small and index fingers away from the hand against resistance.

B). The deep branch of the ulnar nerve may be affected by ganglia, fracture of carpal bones, or hemorrhage.

Muscles for lateral key pinch and for grip strength are primarily supplied by the ulnar nerve, but a complex clinical evaluation is required to determine the exact site of a lesion owing to considerable anatomical variations. The examiner palpates the first dorsal interosseous muscle contraction during pinch (Fig. 5–18). Reliable tests for extrinsic ulnar innervated muscle function include active flexion of the ulnar wrist and the distal phalanx of the little and ring fingers against resistance with the hand and forearm stabilized. Intrinsic muscle innervation of the first dorsal interosseus muscle is tested by palpating the muscles during active abduction of the little and index fingers against resistance (Fig. 5–19).

IMPORTANT ANATOMICAL VARIATIONS

These variations may camouflage peripheral nerve injury or mimic rapid healing after nerve repair. The most common upper extremity anatomical variations are the Martin-Gruber anastomosis in the forearm and the Riche-Cannieu anastomosis in the hand. The Martin-Gruber anastomosis (Gruber, 1870; Leibovic and Hastings, 1992; Martin, 1763) is a communication between the median nerve or its anterior interosseous branch and the ulnar nerve in the forearm. The anastomosis may be further subdivided according to pattern of course and distal innervation. Ulnar-to-median nerve anastomosis occurs as well. The Riche-Cannieu anastomosis (Cannieu, 1897; Riche, 1897) is a communication between the recurrent motor branch of the median nerve and the deep branch of the ulnar nerve. It may affect the innervation of the superficial head of the flexor pollicis brevis, the opponens pollicis, the first to third lumbricals, or the abductor pollicis brevis.

The two classic plexus paralyses of the upper extremities are

1. Upper plexus paralysis (C5–C6, Erb-Duchenne); classic clinical sign: arm hangs in adduction, internal rotation, elbow extension, and forearm pronation; paralysis of supraspinatus, infraspinatus, rhomboids, deltoid, biceps, brachialis; weakness of pectoralis major, triceps, and extensor carpi radialis if C6 is involved

2. Lower plexus paralysis (C8–T1, Déjerine-Klumpke): paralysis of all intrinsic hand muscles, weakness of flexor carpi ulnaris and flexor digitorum profundus to little finger if C8 is involved; additional Horner's syndrome indicates avulsion of T1 from spinal cord

References

Cannieu JMA: Recherches sur une anastomose entre la branche profonde du cubital et le median. Bull Soc Anat Physiol Bordeau *18*:339–340, 1897.

Gruber W: Uber die Verbindung des Nervus medianus mit dem Nervus ulnaris am Unterarme des Menschen und der Saugethiere. Arch Anat u Physiol *37*:501–522, 1870.

Kendall FP, McCreavy EK: Muscles: Testing and Function, 3rd ed. Baltimore, Williams & Wilkins, 1983, pp 59–128.

Leibovic SJ, Hastings H II: Martin-Gruber revisited. J Hand Surg *17A*:47–53, 1992.

Martin R: Tal om Nervus allamanna Egenskaper i Mannsikans Kropp. Stockholm, Lars Savius, 1763.

Medical Research Council: Aids to the examination of the peripheral nervous system. Memorandum No. 45. London, Her Majesty's Stationery Office, 1976.

Riche P: Le nerf cubital et les muscles de l'eminence thenar. Bul Mem Soc Anat *5*:251–252, 1897.

Russell RC, Pribaz JP, Zook EG, Leighton WD, Eriksson E, Smith CJ: Functional evaluation of latissimus dorsi donor site. Plast Reconstr Surg *78*:336, 1986.

Chapter 6

• William F. Blair
• John J. Callaghan

Clinical Motor Function Testing—Lower Extremity

GENERAL CONSIDERATIONS

Motor testing is used to determine whether specific muscles or muscle groups are capable of contraction and to assess the magnitude of that contraction. Muscle contraction depends on the integrity of the muscle and its tendons, normal passive motion in the joints across which the muscle acts, and the quality of innervation of the muscle. For the peripheral nerve surgeon, the question of the quality of innervation is paramount.

Motor testing is used clinically to assess the extent of injury or disease. It must be performed efficiently and systematically (Evarts, 1983). After trauma, the results of motor testing define the magnitude of the primary injury. In neuromuscular disease, motor testing defines the severity of involvement. These observations form the basis of the patient's prognosis. The results of initial motor testing are the baseline against which natural recovery or the results of treatment are assessed. The initial, baseline motor testing evaluation must be thorough and accurate. Motor testing is especially important after peripheral nerve injury and reconstruction, when the results are used to assess the quality and extent of reinnervation.

Muscle contraction can be assessed qualitatively, semiquantitatively, and quantitatively (Blair, 1991). Qualitative assessment is completed by having the patient describe muscle performance, by inspecting the muscle mass and contour, and by observing voluntary motion. Semiquantitative assessment, which is used most widely, is essentially manual motor strength testing. It is based on a grading system that requires thorough knowledge of muscle and peripheral nerve anatomy and muscle function (Hoppenfeld, 1976). Manual motor testing has the distinct advantage of providing information about either major nerves or specific branches of the nerves. It is fundamental to the assessment of peripheral nerve injury and treatment. This form of testing is convenient, inexpensive, and readily repeatable in the clinic setting, so it is appropriately the primary focus of this chapter. The quantitative assessment of muscle function in the lower extremity requires the use of one of a variety of machines. Many new computer-interfaced machines measure strength, power, and endurance. However, they do not isolate muscles well; therefore, they are not as specific as manual motor testing in the assessment of specific nerve deficits.

The clinical task of testing a specific muscle can be performed in two basic ways. In the first technique, the joints across which the muscle in question acts are placed in the position from which the muscle moves the joint, and the patient is asked to produce the desired motion or to contract the tested muscle. The patient's ability to produce the desired motion is assessed. For example, the knee is placed in flexion and the patient is asked to extend the knee to test the quadriceps muscle. In the second technique, the body part is placed in the position into which the tested muscle would normally move that part. The patient's ability to maintain that position against the examiner's resistance is assessed. For example, the patient's knee is placed in full extension and the patient is asked to maintain knee extension while the examiner offers a flexion force, thus testing the quadriceps. Practically, either or both of these test methods are used.

SPECIFIC TESTING STRATEGIES

The motor examination should begin first with an inspection of the lower extremity for muscle atrophy or deformity secondary to muscle imbalance. The inspection should then focus on gait. Gait testing may also be supplemented by functional testing. For example, the patient may be asked to walk on the toes or heels to elicit variations in complete motions that are characteristic of specific deficits. After inspection, motors are tested first about the hip, then the knee, and finally in the foot and ankle. In the presence of a lumbosacral plexus injury or injury to a specific peripheral nerve, the motor examination is performed along the course of each nerve, sequentially from proximal to distal. The grading scale for muscle strength in the lower extremity is normal (complete range of motion against gravity with full resistance), good (complete range of motion against gravity with some resistance), fair (complete range of motion against gravity), poor (complete range of motion without gravity), or absent (Table 6–1).

Abnormal Hip Gaits

A Trendelenburg gait is a classic finding, caused by a weak hip abductor. When the patient has a weak hip abductor

▼ TABLE 6–1
Muscle Power Grading

Grade	Description
0-None	No palpable muscle contraction
1-Trace	Palpable muscle contraction, detectable by examiner
2-Poor	Active joint motion present with gravity eliminated
3-Fair	Muscle can move joint through full range of motion against gravity
4-Good	Full range of motion against gravity and some resistance
5-Normal	Full range of motion with a maximal force that is normal for that muscle

muscle (primarily the gluteus medius), the weakness can best be detected when the patient is walking away from the examiner. The contralateral pelvis drops during the stance phase of gait.

The Trendelenburg gait must be differentiated from an abductor lurch, caused by hip pain. A patient with a painful hip but not gluteus medius weakness, in attempting to lower the forces on the joint, brings the torso over the involved hip joint during stance phase and produces an abductor lurch gait pattern.

When the patient has a weak hip extensor (primarily the gluteus maximus), a characteristic gait also results. This gait is best seen by evaluating the patient from the side. The patient will exhibit increased lumbar lordosis during the stance phase to counteract the anterior hip forces. This will decrease the workload required by the weakened hip extensors.

Other atypical gaits may also be detected. When the patient walks toward and away from the examiner, if the patient has a short leg for any reason, the head of the patient will be lowered when in stance phase on the involved side. This is called a short leg gait. When a patient is viewed from the side, if the hip is stiff, the pelvis will translate during gait rather than the femur. This is called a stiff hip gait. Unless the examiner watches the patient's pelvis closely, this abnormality can go unrecognized, even in a patient who has a completely fused hip. The patient's gait should be evaluated by having the patient walk toward, away from, to the left of, and to the right of the examiner.

The Hip

Motor testing about the hip sequentially tests the flexors, extensors, abductors, and adductors (Callaghan, 1994). Hip flexor strength can be assessed with the patient sitting with legs flexed 90 degrees at the knee. The examiner pushes against the distal, anterior aspect of the thigh as the patient flexes the hip (Fig. 6–1). This primarily tests the iliopsoas supplied by L1, L2, and L3 (the femoral nerve). Hip extensor

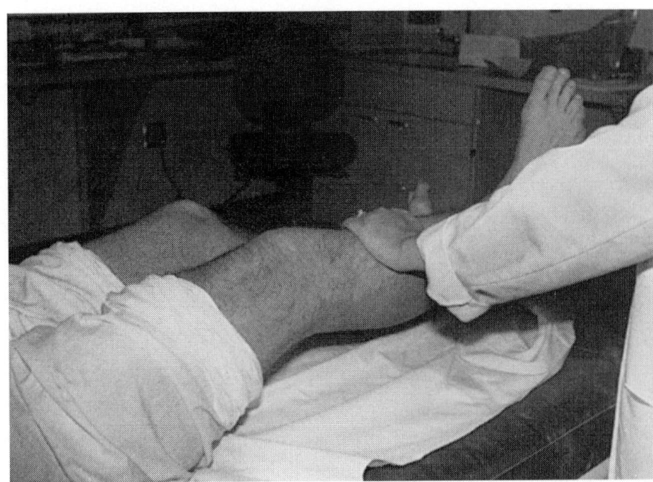

FIGURE 6–2. Resistance to active extension of the knee and flexion of the hip is used to evaluate quadriceps strength. The quadriceps muscle is innervated by the femoral nerve (L2, L3, L4).

strength is checked with the patient prone and by having the patient elevate the femur off the table with the examiner pressing over the distal, posterior thigh. The gluteus maximus, which is innervated by the inferior gluteal nerve (S1), is primarily responsible for hip extension. Hip abduction is evaluated with the patient lying on each side in turn and having him or her elevate the leg with the examiner pressing laterally on the knee. This test evaluates the strength of the gluteus medius and minimus muscles, the major abductors of the hip, which are supplied by the superior gluteal nerve (L5). Hip adductor strength is checked with the patient pushing the leg toward the midline while the examiner applies resistance to the medial aspect of the thigh. The major adductor muscles are the adductors longus, brevis, and magnus and the gracilis and pectineus muscles supplied by L2, L3, and L4 (the obturator nerve).

The Knee

The examination of the knee focuses primarily on extension and flexion (Tearse, 1994). Extension testing for the knee is performed with the patient in the sitting position. The knee is passively placed in maximal extension, and the patient is asked to maintain that position. The examiner then gently but firmly attempts to force the knee into flexion, grading the strength of resistance. Knee extension strength can also be tested by placing the knee in maximal flexion and then asking the patient to actively extend the leg, again while the examiner offers extension resistance. Quadriceps muscle function can also be assessed by examining combined knee extension and hip flexion (Fig. 6–2).

Examination of knee flexion strength is best performed with the patient in the prone position. With the knee in maximal flexion, the examiner attempts to gently but firmly extend the knee against resistance, again grading the strength of resistance (Fig. 6–3). Knee flexion strength can also be examined by placing the knee in maximal extension and asking the patient to flex the knee against manual resistance offered by the examiner.

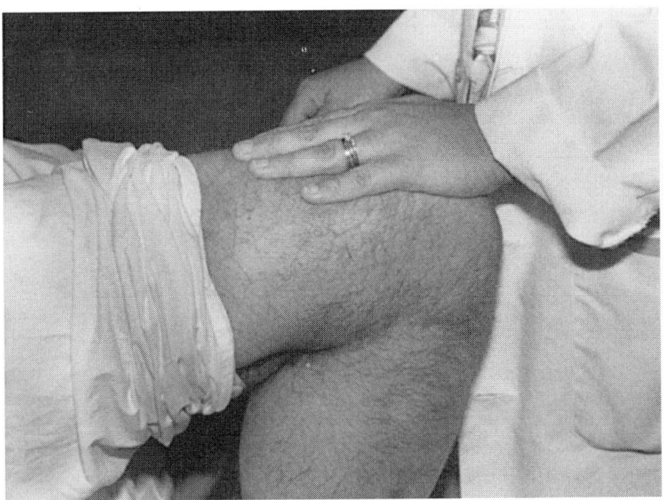

FIGURE 6–1. Resistance to active hip flexion with the patient seated is used to evaluate iliopsoas strength. The iliopsoas muscle group is innervated by L2, L3, and L4.

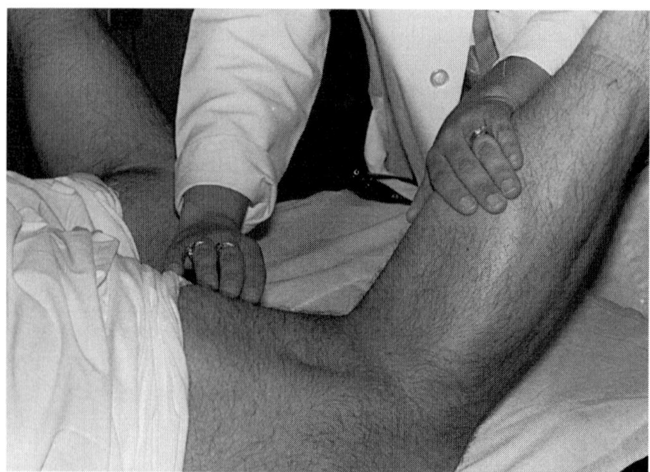

FIGURE 6–3. Palpation of the medial hamstrings, when knee flexion is resisted, is used to evaluate semimembranosus and semitendinosus motor function (innervation by tibial portion of sciatic nerve, L5). The biceps femoris (the lateral hamstring) is innervated by S1.

The Ankle and Foot

Dynamic testing of motor function may be helpful in identifying strength deficits. Because the muscles of the leg are usually much stronger than those of the examiner's forearm, subtle motor weaknesses may not be detected. However, this information may be gathered by observing the patient walk and exercise. A gait characterized by foot slapping indicates weakness of the ankle dorsiflexors and suggests a possible deep peroneal nerve problem. It may be helpful to ask the patient to stand on the toes or heels. An inability to stand on tiptoes suggests weakness of the ankle plantarflexors and signifies a potential underlying posterior tibial nerve problem. Selective weakness can also be secondary to problems with a muscle or its tendon. To differentiate weakness from the neurological versus musculotendinous origin, a careful sensory examination should complement the motor examination (Saltzman and Cooper, 1994).

The muscles that power the foot and ankle are all innervated by terminal branches of the sciatic nerve. The sciatic nerve bifurcates into the peroneal and posterior tibial nerves. The posterior tibial nerve continues down the posterior aspect of the leg into the plantar aspect of the foot. The common peroneal nerve winds around the neck of the fibula, dividing into the superficial and deep peroneal nerves, which continue onto the dorsum of the foot. These three nerves completely control the motor function of the foot and ankle.

The posterior tibial nerve innervates muscles originating both in the leg (extrinsics) and in the foot (intrinsics). To test the function of the extrinsic muscles, the examiner checks the power of ankle plantarflexion (gastrocsoleus complex), foot inversion and adduction (tibialis posterior muscle), flexion of the great toe (flexor hallucis longus), and flexion of the lateral four toes (flexor digitorum longus).

Above the ankle joint, the posterior tibial nerve bifurcates into medial and lateral plantar branches. The respective distributions of these two nerves closely parallel those of the median and ulnar nerves in the hand. The medial plantar nerve's motor function is to abduct and flex the great toe (abductor hallucis and flexor hallucis brevis), to flex the

proximal interphalangeal joint of the lesser four toes (flexor digitorum brevis), and to flex the second metatarsophalangeal (MTP) joint (first lumbrical). The lateral plantar nerve innervates the remainder of the muscles of the sole of the foot. Its function involves flexion of the lateral three MTP joints (lumbricals of the lateral three toes), flexion of the proximal phalanx of the little toe (flexor digiti minimi), adduction of the great toe (adductor hallucis), adduction of the lateral three toes (plantar interossei), and abduction of the second through the fifth toes (dorsal interossei and abductor digiti minimi).

As in the hand, the interossei and, to some extent, the lumbricals are responsible for flexion of the MTP joints and extension of the proximal and distal interphalangeal joints. Selective functional loss of the lateral plantar nerve results in a so-called intrinsic minus foot. This is characterized by hyperextension at the MTP joints and flexion at the proximal and distal interphalangeal joints.

The deep peroneal nerve is responsible for extension of the foot and ankle. The extrinsic muscles are tested by checking the power of inversion and dorsiflexion of the foot (tibialis anterior muscle) (Fig. 6–4), extension of the great toe (extensor hallucis longus) (Fig. 6–5), and extension of the lesser toes (extensor digitorum longus). The intrinsic muscles are tested by checking the power of extension at the MTP joints (extensor hallucis brevis and extensor digitorum brevis).

The superficial peroneal nerve innervates the extrinsic muscles on the lateral aspect of the leg. It is evaluated by assessing the power of the foot eversion (peroneus brevis) (Fig. 6–6) and plantar flexion of the medial border of the foot (peroneus longus).

The Lumbosacral Plexus

Rather than being functionally or anatomically based, the motor examination can be performed relative to the lumbosacral plexus and, thus, the neuroanatomy of the lower extremity (Mannerfelt, 1980). This strategy is most helpful when a focal nerve lesion is suspected or motor nerve recovery is

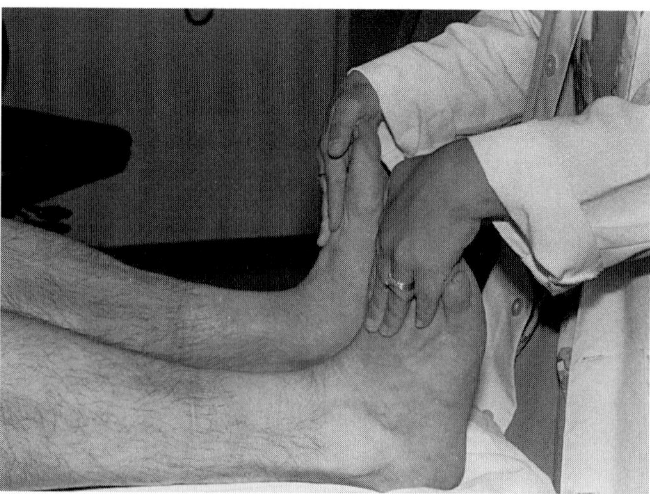

FIGURE 6–4. Anterior tibial muscle function is tested by applying resistance to active ankle dorsiflexion. The muscle is innervated by the deep peroneal nerve, L4.

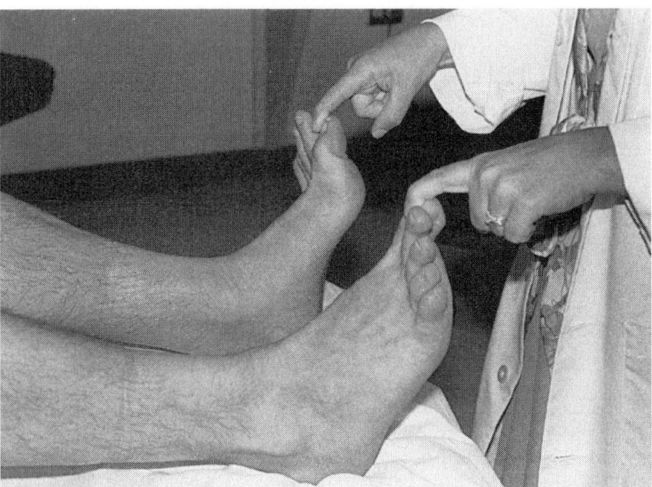

FIGURE 6–5. Extensor hallucis longus muscle function is tested by applying resistance to active dorsiflexion of the great toe. The muscle is innervated by the deep peroneal nerve, L5.

being followed after peripheral nerve repair or reconstruction.

The lumbosacral plexus is formed by contributions from roots T12 to S5. Anatomically the lumbar plexus emerges from behind the psoas muscle. The major nerves that exit the lumbar plexus innervate the thigh. The lumbar plexus can be considered as having anterior and posterior components. The anterior component, the obturator nerve, innervates the medial aspect of the thigh, and the posterior component, the femoral nerve, innervates the anterior thigh. The sacral plexus lies on the anterior surface of the piriformis muscle and exits through the greater sciatic foramen to enter the buttock. The sacral plexus, too, can be considered as having anterior and posterior components. The anterior parts of the plexus form the tibial nerve and additional small branches to the hip rotators. The posterior parts form the common peroneal nerve and branches of the buttock.

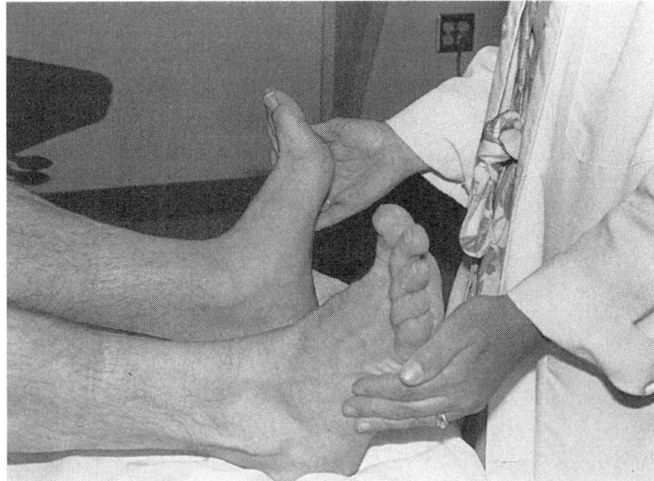

FIGURE 6–6. Resistance to active eversion of the foot is used to test peroneus longus and brevis function. These muscles are innervated by the superficial peroneal nerve, S1.

PERIPHERAL NERVES

Obturator Nerve (Fig. 6–7)

1. Adductor longus (L2, L3). The patient may be either sitting or supine, with the legs abducted. The patient is instructed to adduct the legs while resistance is applied on the medial aspect of the knees. Strong adduction indicates obturator integrity.

2. Adductor brevis (L3, L4) and magnus (L3–5). The test for these muscles is the same as that used for the adductor longus. These three muscles cannot be readily differentiated on clinical examination.

3. Gracilis (L3, L4). This muscle adducts the thigh and internally rotates the knee. It is tested in the same manner as the adductor group, muscles from which it cannot be isolated.

Femoral Nerve

1. Quadriceps (L2–4). This muscle group is best tested with the patient in the sitting position. The knee is allowed to flex fully over the edge of the examining table. The patient is instructed to actively extend the knee against

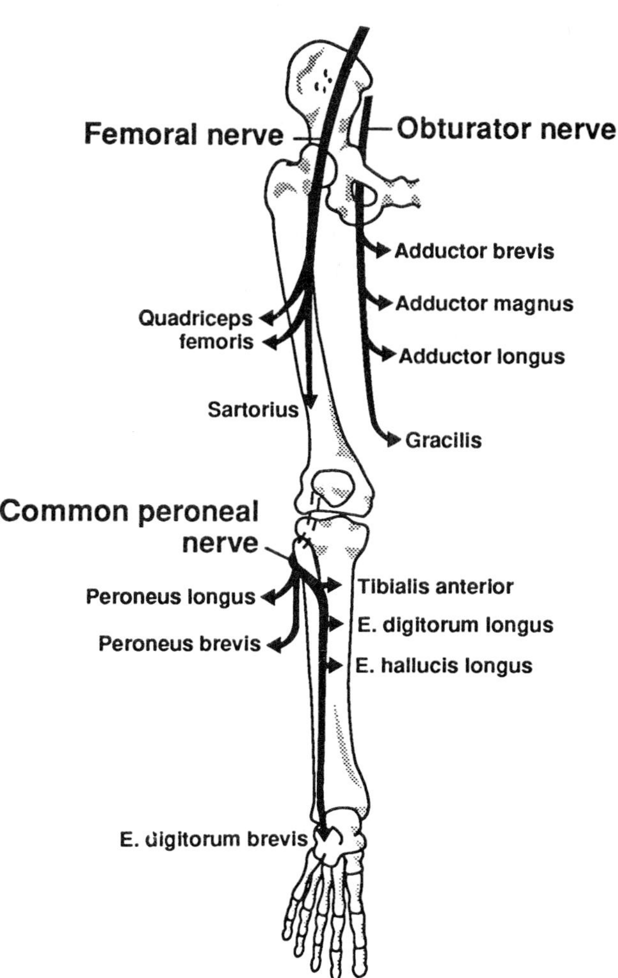

FIGURE 6–7. Muscle innervated by the femoral, obturator, and common peroneal nerves, as viewed from the anterior aspect of the lower extremity. E, extensor.

resistance, which is applied through the examiner's grasp at the ankle. Active knee extension indicates quadriceps muscle and obturator nerve function.

2. Sartorius (L2, L3). This muscle's actions are very similar to the quadriceps femoris. It is activated during active knee extension, and it cannot be readily differentiated from the quadriceps.

Sciatic Nerve in the Thigh (Fig. 6–8)

1. Semimembranosus (L5–S2). This muscle is one component of the hamstring group. To test it, the patient is positioned prone on the table and the knee is fully extended. The patient is instructed to flex the knee against resistance, which is applied through the examiner's grasp at the ankle. Strong knee flexion indicates intact motor branches from the sciatic nerve. To better isolate the medial hamstrings from the lateral hamstrings, the leg is internally rotated while the test is repeated.

2. Semitendinosus (L5–S2). This is the second of the two medial hamstring muscles. It is tested in the same manner as the semimembranosus. It cannot be differentiated from that muscle on clinical examination.

3. Biceps femoris (L5–S2). This muscle is the lateral

component of the hamstring group. It is tested in the same manner as the semimembranosus and semitendinosus muscles, except that it is better isolated by externally rotating the leg while performing the test.

In the posterior thigh, the sciatic nerve divides into the tibial and peroneal nerves. The tibial nerve continues down the posterior aspect of the upper extremity to innervate muscles in the posterior aspect of the leg. The peroneal nerve passes through the interval between the fibula and tibia to enter the anterior aspect of the leg. As it takes this course, it supplies the muscles of both the lateral and anterior compartments of the leg.

Tibial Nerve

1. Gastrocnemius, medial and lateral heads (S1, S2). The patient is easily examined in the sitting position with the knees flexed and the feet over the edge of the examining table. The feet are positioned plantigrade, and the examiner's hand is placed under the ball of the foot. The patient is instructed to flex the foot downward. Because this muscle is strong, it is difficult to grade strength using this maneuver. The patient should also be asked to walk on the toes.

2. Soleus (S1, S2). Because its anatomical location and function are very similar to those of the gastrocnemius, this muscle is tested in the same manner. The two muscles cannot be readily differentiated clinically. Changing the knee position to include or exclude gastrocnemius activity is not reliable.

3. Tibialis posterior (L5, S1). The tendon is palpable as it comes around the medial malleolus and inserts into the tarsal navicular. It is tested with the patient in the sitting position. The examiner stabilizes the distal tibia with one hand and instructs the patient to flex and invert the foot against resistance. Simultaneous ankle flexion and foot inversion confirm tibialis posterior function.

4. Flexor digitorum longus (L5, S1). This muscle to the lateral four toes is tested by stabilizing the calcaneus with the ankle in a neutral position. The patient is then instructed to bend or curl the toes downward. The examiner assesses strength by attempting to straighten the toes with the opposite hand. Sustained toe flexion indicates good innervation.

5. Flexor hallucis longus (L5, S2). This muscle to the great toe is tested by stabilizing the calcaneus with the ankle in a neutral position. The patient is then instructed to bend or curl the great toe downward. The examiner assesses the muscle's strength by attempting to straighten the great toe with the opposite hand.

6. Intrinsics on the plantar aspect of the foot (L5, S2). These muscles provide flexion of the toes through the MTP joint without simultaneous flexion of the other joints and contribute to abduction and adduction of the toes. Testing does not isolate them well. The patient can be instructed to alternate spreading the toes apart and then squeezing them together.

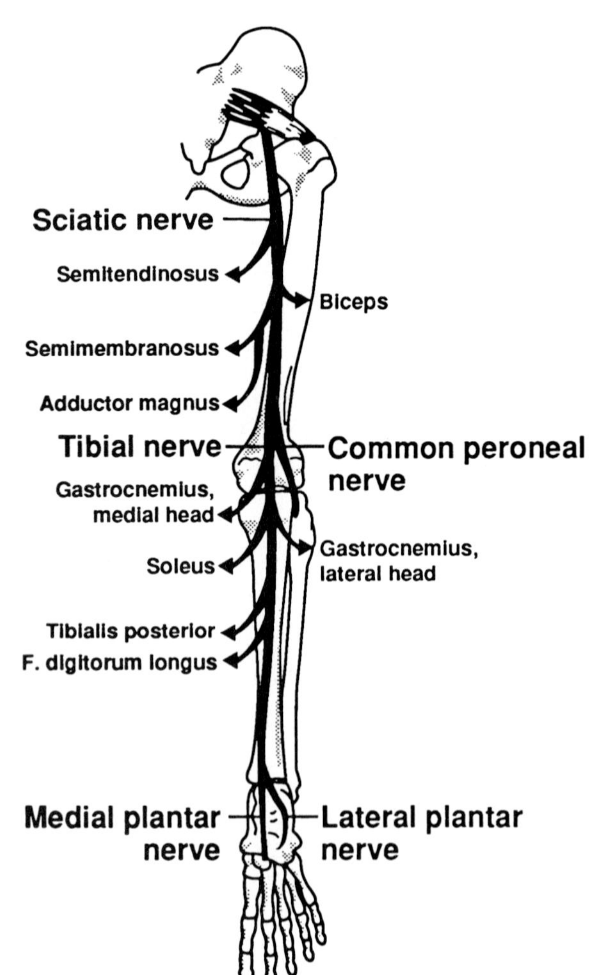

FIGURE 6–8. Muscles innervated by the sciatic nerve and its major tibial nerve branch, as viewed from the posterior aspect of the lower extremity. F, flexor.

Peroneal Nerve

The common peroneal nerve divides into superficial and deep nerves as it passes around the neck of the fibula. The superficial nerve continues down the leg to innervate the lateral compartment. The deep nerve travels distally and medially to enter and innervate the muscles of the anterior compartment of the leg.

1. Peroneus longus and brevis (L4–S1). These two tendons are just posterior to the lateral malleolus. They cannot be differentiated on clinical examination. The patient sits on the examining table with the knees bent 90 degrees. The examiner stabilizes the distal tibia with one hand. The foot is placed in flexion and eversion. The patient is asked to maintain that position while the examiner applies resistance to the lateral border of the fifth metatarsal. A sustained position of flexion and eversion indicates good innervation of the peronei.

2. Tibialis anterior (L4–S1). This muscle is the primary extensor or dorsiflexor of the foot; it is also an invertor. During contraction, it is visibly and palpably present on the anterior aspect of the ankle. To test it, the patient sits on the examining table with the knees flexed. The foot is placed in inversion and extension. The examiner stabilizes the distal tibia with one hand and grasps the patient's foot with the other. The examiner attempts to invert and flex the foot against the patient's resistance. Strong resistance confirms tibialis anterior integrity.

3. Extensor digitorum longus (L4–S1). This muscle is the primary extensor of the lateral four toes. To test it, the patient assumes the sitting position with the knees flexed. The patient is instructed to extend or pull the toes upward. The examiner's index finger is placed transversely across the toes and attempts to flex the toes downward. Peroneal nerve function allows the patient's toes to resist the flexion force.

4. Extensor hallucis longus (L4–S1). This muscle is the primary extensor of the great toe. It is tested in the same manner as the extensor digitorum longus, except that the great toe is actively extended and the examiner attempts to flex it downward with only the tip of the index finger.

5. Extensor digitorum and extensor hallucis brevis (L5–S1). These muscles are secondary toe extensors. They are tested in the same manner as for their long counterparts. They cannot be isolated for muscle testing.

Motor testing is easy to describe and comprehend, but it requires considerable retention of information and experience to translate these descriptions effectively into clinical practice. Optimal motor testing is not easily accomplished in every case. Associated muscle and tendon injury or decreased passive motion in joints across which each muscle acts confounds the interpretation of observations. Also, motor testing is predicated on the assumption that the patient is providing optimal effort. This may not always be the case, either because the patient does not understand the instructions, because the patient may be impaired from providing an optimal effort by systemic or psychological factors, or because the patient may have some interest in providing a suboptimal performance. These factors must be considered when interpreting the performance of each muscle test.

Despite these limitations, motor testing remains an invaluable method of systematically assessing the integrity of the peripheral nervous system.

References

Blair WF: Motor testing. *In* Gelberman RH (ed): Operative Nerve Repair and Reconstruction. Philadelphia, J.B. Lippincott Company, 1991, pp 159–170.

Callaghan JJ: Examination of the hip. *In* Clark CR, Bonfiglio M (eds): Orthopaedics. Essentials of Diagnosis and Treatment. New York, Churchill Livingstone, 1994, pp 65–74.

Evarts CM: Examination of the musculoskeletal patient. *In* Evarts CM (ed): Surgery of the Musculoskeletal System. New York, Churchill Livingstone, 1983, pp 9–17.

Hoppenfeld S: Physical Examination of the Spine and Extremities. New York, Appleton-Century-Crofts, 1976, pp 2–104, 153–235.

Mannerfelt L: Motor function testing. *In* Omer GE Jr, Spinner M (eds): Management of Peripheral Nerve Problems. Philadelphia, W.B. Saunders, 1980, pp 16–29.

Saltzman CL, Cooper RR: Examination of the ankle and foot. *In* Clark CR, Bonfiglio M (eds): Orthopaedics. Essentials of Diagnosis and Treatment. New York, Churchill Livingstone, 1994, pp 81–96.

Tearse DS: Examination of the knee. *In* Clark CR, Bonfiglio M (eds): Orthopaedics. Essentials of Diagnosis and Treatment. New York, Churchill Livingstone, 1994, pp 75–80.

PERIPHERAL NERVE INJURIES OF THE LOWER EXTREMITY

Lower extremity nerve injuries are less common than injuries of the upper extremity. The literature is replete with reports regarding upper extremity nerve injuries but there are few series of cases reporting significant numbers of cases regarding the management of lower extremity nerve injuries (Aldea and Shaw, 1986a, 1986b; Dolene, 1977; Hattrup and Wood, 1986; Hudson, 1984; Kline, 1972; Omer, 1981; Sedel, 1985; Sedel and Nizard, 1993; Trumble and Vanderhooft, 1994; Wood, 1991). The loss of digit dexterity, position and sensibility, combined with muscle paralysis, has immediate and long-term effects. These effects are minimized by effective management of nerve injuries (Gelberman, 1991). This chapter delineates the management of acute and delayed nerve repairs.

ANATOMY

The anatomy of the lower extremities peripheral nerves is crucial information for the surgeon (Grant, 1962; Pernkopf, 1980; Sunderland, 1968). Detection of the site of injury and surgical exploration hinge on the anatomy and examination (Halpern, 1989).

The femoral sciatic plexus has its origins at the level of first lumbar vertebrae and also has components from the fourth sacral level. The L1–L4 of the plexus give origin to the femoral nerve, the lateral cutaneous nerve of the thigh, the obturator nerve, and the genitofemoral nerve. L4 also contributes to the femoral nerve and genitofemoral nerve but begins the split between upper and lower components of the lumbosacral plexus. The lower half of the plexus starts at level L4 and extends to S4; it contributes to the sciatic nerve, the common peroneal nerve, the posterior cutaneous nerves of the thigh, the pudendal nerve, and the smaller motor nerve responsible for muscle function in the thigh or buttock areas. The proximal origins of the these nerves is difficult to access surgically, and injuries to the nerves at that level are rare (Fig. 7–1).

MECHANISM OF INJURY

Injuries to the lumbosacral plexus are rare and are associated with avulsive trauma, penetrating injuries, or traction injuries to the pelvis and lower spine (Edwards et al, 1987; Fassler et al, 1993; Hall et al, 1995; Hirasawa and Sakakida, 1983; Seddon, 1975; Sedel, 1985). Iatrogenic injury usually associated with tumor excision and other pelvic procedures has been reported by Edwards and associates (1987), Hall

and colleagues (1995), Kroll et al, 1990; Simmons and associates (1991), and Vrahas and co-workers (1992). During preoperative assessment, a careful clinical examination delineates the injury level. Imaging of the lumbar and sacral spine elements of the plexus may help with establishing the diagnosis and level of injury if fractures or disc problems are present. The potential of supraganglionic injury must be excluded and, in the presence of the cauda equina, makes the determination of supraganglionic injury difficult. Vertical fractures of the sacrum, dislocation of the sacral iliac joint, and disruption of the lumbosacral spine are associated with avulsion or disruption of the plexus.

SURGICAL EXPLORATION OF THE LUMBOSACRAL PLEXUS

Surgical exploration of the lumbar or sacral plexus is formidable. There is extremely limited experience reported in the literature regarding repair of the lumbosacral plexus or sciatic nerve (Sunderland et al, 1993).

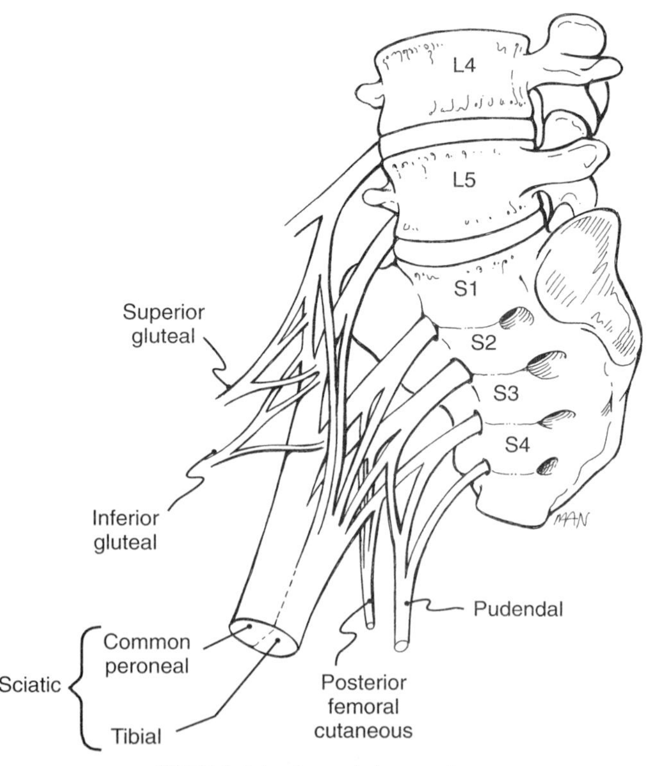

FIGURE 7–1. Lumbosacral plexus anatomy.

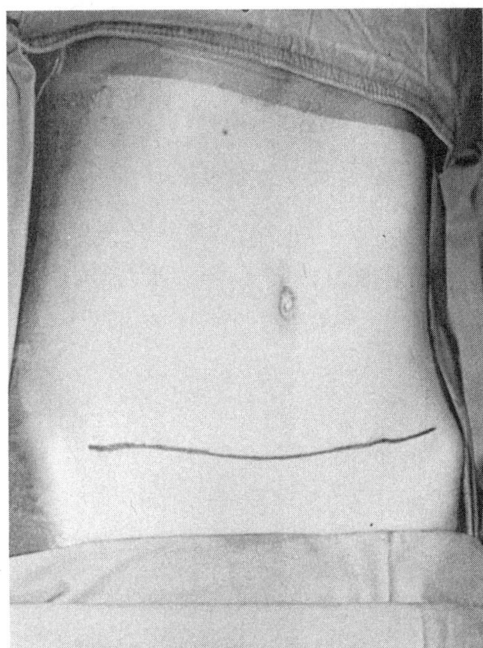

FIGURE 7–2. Abdominal exploration.

This author prefers a transabdominal exploration of the plexus (Fig. 7–2.) The ability to stent ureters, control major vessels, and improved visibility make this approach safer but still difficult. Retroperitoneal approaches or excision of the posterior sacral elements has not been tried by the author but have been reported. Unfortunately only a few cases of lumbar or sacral plexus repairs have been reported. The lumbar components are easier to access than are the sacral components. The sacrum tilts away vertically from the surgical access, which makes this exploration very difficult.

The delay in treatment and mechanism of injury accompanying these injuries results in significant nerve gaps, and the problem of obtaining appropriate numbers and lengths of nerve grafts poses a major challenge. Personal clinical experience and experience reported in the literature report repairs of either the femoral or sacral portions of the plexus but not both areas simultaneously.

During the exploration, it may be necessary to visualize the sciatic nerve outside the pelvis or within the sciatic notch. To accomplish this, it will be necessary to temporarily close the abdomen and rotate the patient to the supine position. The sciatic nerve is readily visualized and the sciatic foramen along with the sciatic nerve can be explored to its intrapelvic beginning (Figs. 7–3 and 7–4). From this position, the sural nerves are harvested, and if large amounts of nerve graft are required, it may be necessary to use the common peroneal from the injured side as a nerve graft (Fig. 7–5). The prone position during surgery facilitates harvesting both sural nerves and the ipsilateral common peroneal nerve for grafts if needed for nerve grafting. This decision is based on the greater need for function in the posterior tibial and femoral nerve. Sensibility to the bottom of the foot, establishing push off with the posterior calf compartment muscles, and knee extension have priority over ankle and digit extension. Repair of the sciatic or femoral plexus usually produces hip flexion, knee extension, knee flexion, and ankle plantar flexion. More distal function may not return.

Combined femoral and sciatic plexus reconstruction in cases in which the plexus is excised because of tumor excision is one of the areas in which reconstruction of the plexus may best be accomplished using heterografts and immunosuppression. The author has been unable to find a report of combined complete reconstruction of the sciatic and femoral plexus using autologous nerve grafts or heterografts in the literature.

The author's experience with two lumbosacral plexus explorations resulted in one instance of neurolysis with the removal of bone fragments from the plexus and one instance

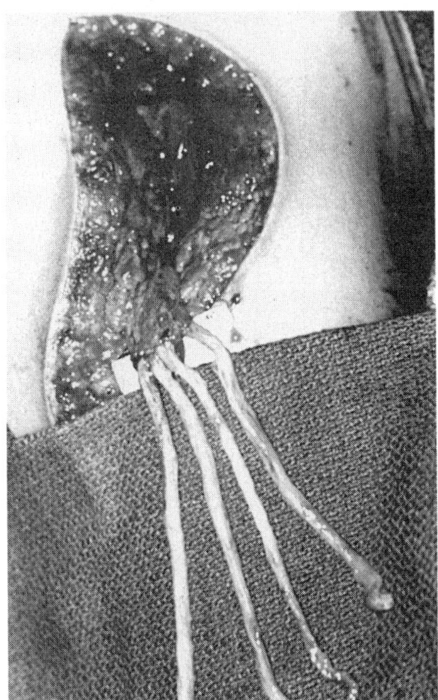

FIGURE 7–3. Post thigh: Grafts attached to distal sciatic nerve before being placed into pelvis.

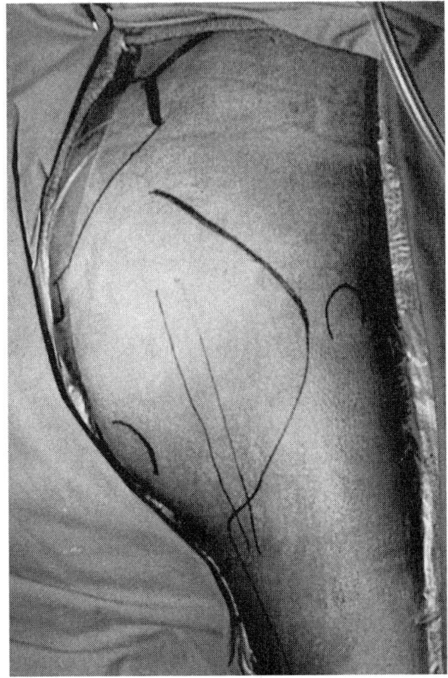

FIGURE 7–4. Posterior hip and thigh exposure.

of sacral plexus reconstruction with autologous grafts. The patient who was treated with neurolysis has had useful femoral nerve function recovery, and the author suspects that the seemingly intact nerves of the sacral components of the plexus were actually cauda equina components and that the patient sustained a supraganglionic injury of the sacral plexus. This patient has been followed for 6 years and ambulates with the help of orthotic devices, does not have plantar sensibility, and has not experienced return of function in the posterior tibial or common peroneal nerves. The second patient had graft reconstruction of the sacral plexus. The patient was referred for 18 months following a pelvic schwannoma resection that resulted in resection of the sacral plexus with the tumor. The lumbar components of the plexus S1, S2, and S3 were repaired using 22-cm nerve grafts from the sacral nerve stumps through the sciatic foramen to the sciatic nerve. In this patient, the sural nerves and the common peroneal portion of the ipsilateral sciatic nerve were used as nerve grafts. The patient has regained function of biceps femoris (M5), gastrocnemius (M4), soleus (M3), and tibialis posterior (M4), but had diminished protective sensibility to the plantar foot. During the follow-up of 9 years, the patient has not developed evidence of Charcot joint and has not had any foot ulcerations.

FEMORAL NERVE

The femoral nerve originates from the posterior divisions of the lumbar plexus arising from L2–L5 (Pernkopf, 1980; Sunderland, 1968). The nerve exits the lumbar origin, and its proximal course is covered anteriorly by the psoas muscle. Posterior to the nerve, the iliacus muscle forms the nerve's bed. As it courses further from its origin, the nerve is located in the retroperitoneal space and travels along the outline of the ilium (Fig. 7–6). The nerve then remains on the anterior muscle surface of the muscles within the groove between

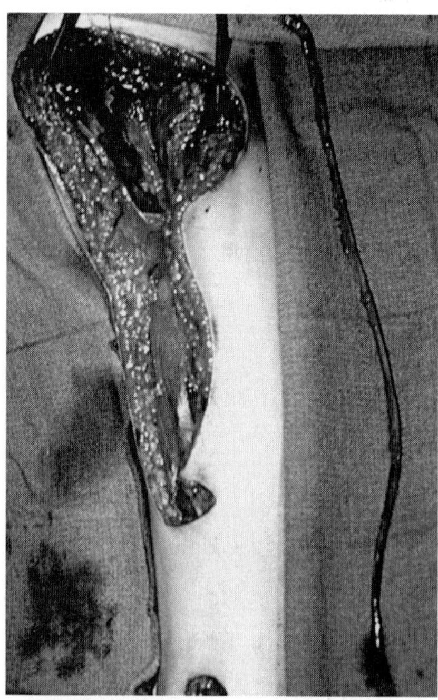

FIGURE 7–5. Harvested common peroneal nerve.

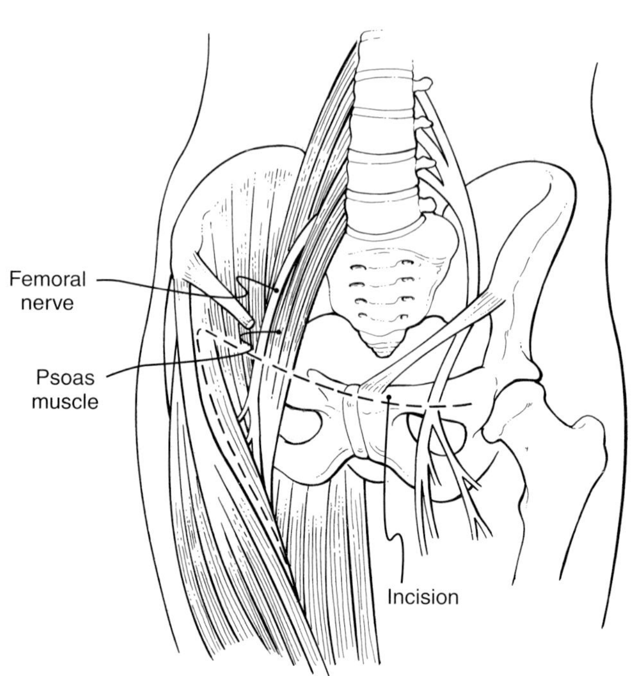

FIGURE 7–6. Femoral nerve access groin and thigh.

the psoas and iliacus muscle. It joins the external iliac vessels, and the vein, artery, and nerve then exits the pelvis through the femoral canal, under the inguinal ligament. Because of its location in the pelvis, it is readily identified unless fibrosis obscures dissection. During the proximal dissection, the hypogastric vessels can impair visibility and exposure. In the distal half of its intrapelvic course, the dissection is complicated by the external iliac vessels. Distal to the inguinal ligament, as the nerve enters the upper thigh, it lies lateral to the femoral vessels. The mnemonic "van" for vein, artery, and nerve describing the anatomical orientation of the femoral neurovascular structures in the groin from medial to lateral is particularly easy for the author to remember. The nerve begins to arborize 3 to 5 cm distal to the ligament (Fig. 7–6).

The femoral nerve provides innervation to the pectineus, sartorius, rectus femoris, vastas medialis, vastas intermedius, and vastas lateralis muscles. These muscles are responsible for extension of the knee.

Stabbing, gunshot, saw, stretch, compression, hemorrhage, retractor, and tourniquets have all been reported as causing femoral nerve injury (Aldea and Shaw, 1986a; D'Amelio et al, 1990; Kline, 1972; Mackinnon, 1993; Sammarco and Stephens, 1991; Seddon, 1975; Sunderland, 1993; Williams and Trzil, 1991). Iatrogenic injury during appendectomy, pelvic tumor excision, inguinal or femoral herniorraphy, vascular bypass surgery, and saphenous vein harvesting have all been recorded (Belsh, 1991; Birch et al, 1991; Hall et al, 1995; Infantino et al, 1994; Kroll et al, 1990; Simmons et al, 1991). Repair of the femoral nerve and when necessary nerve grafting following these events produced satisfactory outcomes.

When confronted with a femoral nerve injury, the surgeon's assessment must be directed at detecting where the nerve is injured, what functional deficits are present for both sensibility and motor function, and whether there are pain factors that need to be resolved. The surgeon must then decide what approach to use, and if nerve grafting is likely, what donor nerves will be used. Once it is determined where the nerve is injured, the surgical approach will be known. The mechanism of injury and site of injury indicate whether autologous grafts are necessary. The choice of donors may be predicated by the extent of nerve injury or associated injury.

For injuries to the femoral nerve near the origin of the nerve, a midline abdominal incision is preferred by the author. This permits vascular control, access, and evaluation of entire femoral plexus as well as the obturator nerve. When the injury is in the distal half of pelvic course of the nerve, the author prefers a direct approach. This includes division of the inguinal ligament with a step cut technique when the injury is near the ligament. Access for evaluation and subsequent repair make visualization of the injury essential to accurate repair.

Following division of the inguinal ligament, accurate repair and closure of the femoral canal is mandatory to prevent subsequent herniation through either the femoral or inguinal canals.

If necessary, the direct inguinal approach and midline abdominal approach can be combined. This provides easy access to the entire course of the nerve.

When the injuries are combined in the upper thigh area, exploration is below the inguinal ligament but starts directly over the femoral triangle, where the proximal nerve is identified lateral to the femoral artery. Distally, the dominant sensory portion of the femoral nerve continues as the saphenous nerve and lies lateral to the superficial femoral artery as it courses through the adductor canal. At the distal end of the canal, the saphenous nerve moves to a more superficial position behind the sartorius muscle, descends to the knee, and then becomes subcutaneous in location.

Injury to the femoral nerve results in loss of the quadriceps mechanism of the knee. Knee extension may still be possible because the gracilis muscle is innervated by the obturator nerve and the semitendinosus and semimembranosus muscles are innervated by the sciatic nerve. Extension, strength, and dexterity will be greatly impaired. The sensory loss that occurs following femoral nerve injury is not located in an area where sensibility is critical. However, neuroma sensitivity and hyperesthesia can occur following injury, and nerve repair may be required to alleviate those symptoms, even if the motor components of the nerve are functioning. Saphenous nerve neuromas have a propensity for producing painful sequelae following injury.

Following direct femoral nerve repair, the hip may be flexed 20 to 30 degrees to help close a gap between the ends of the nerve. However excessive tension across the repair must be avoided. A gap of over 4 cm usually requires nerve grafts. If a direct repair is accomplished, it is important to protect the nerve repair following surgery with a body cast that keeps the hip flexed for 3 weeks. Following a nerve graft, protected mobility and ambulation can resume 5 days following surgery.

SCIATIC NERVE

The largest peripheral nerve is the sciatic nerve. Injury to this nerve has devastating consequences with both immediate and long-term problems in the lower leg and foot (Clawson

and Seddon, 1960; Gelberman, 1991; Kline, 1972; Omer, 1980; Sunderland, 1968). The etiology of nerve problems is similar to that reported with plexus injuries, but childhood compression (Venna et al, 1991) and injection injuries of this nerve (Hudson, 1984; Villarejo et al, 1993), serve as reminders to consider all etiologies of nerve injury when confronted with peripheral nerve pathology.

In the gluteal area, the sciatic nerve is covered by the gluteus maximus, and gluteus medius muscles, and exits the sciatic foramen from under the inferior edge of the piriformis muscle. The inferior gluteal nerve is adjacent to the sciatic nerve within the sciatic foramen but is not a branch of the sciatic nerve. Exiting the sciatic foramen above the piriformis muscle and on the surface of the gluteus minimus, the superior gluteal nerve can be located. Both the inferior and superior gluteal nerves are direct branches of the sacral plexus. The superior gluteal nerve provides innervation of the tensor fascia lata.

In the upper thigh area and just after exiting the sciatic foramen, the sciatic nerve supplies motor branches to the adductor magnus, semitendinosus, semimembranosus, and to the long and short heads of the biceps femoris. The inferior gluteal artery, a branch of the internal iliac artery, accompanies the sciatic nerve as it exits from under the inferior edge of the gluteus maximus. At the junction of the upper and middle thirds of the thigh, the common peroneal and posterior tibial nerves have formed individual structures and can be easily separated into their components though they are loosely held together until approximately mid-thigh. When the posterior tibial nerve and common peroneal nerves reach the distal third of the thigh, they begin to enter the area of the popliteal fossa. In this area, the posterior tibial nerve is found between the medial and lateral heads of the gastrocnemius muscle, lying lateral to the popliteal artery and vein. The common peroneal nerve is found lying between the tendon of the biceps femoris and the lateral head of the gastrocnemius. It is located immediately under the investing fascia of the leg adjacent to the knee and also courses just inferior to the fibular head.

Surgical exposure of the proximal sciatic nerve requires prone positioning of the patient. In the prone position, exposure is accomplished by reflecting the gluteus maximus from lateral to medial by separating its insertion into the iliotibial band and the greater trochanter (see Fig. 7–4). The muscle is easily reflected medially, and the nerve visualized. Usually, the gluteus medius muscle can be retracted, allowing access to the proximal sciatic nerve. Great care must be taken to avoid injury to the superior and inferior gluteal nerves when the sciatic nerve has been injured because they serve as valuable innervators of the hip flexors and course through the foramen adjacent to the sciatic nerve.

The sciatic nerve has a massive cross-sectional area, and reconstruction of gaps in the nerve require large amounts of nerve graft. This is a key factor in the decision of how to repair a gap in the sciatic nerve. It should be planned that the sciatic nerve in its proximal one third would required 8 to 10 sural nerve cables to cover the cross-sectional area of the cut nerve. Therefore, a 10-cm nerve gap would require a donor nerve length totaling at least 100 cm. A second problem that seems apparent when repairing this large nerve is the circumstance of graft inosculation. Will the large amount of graft material prevent adequate revascularization of all of the grafts? The surgeon can attempt to splay the grafts to prevent inadequate revascularization of the grafts but even that may not be adequate. Mackinnon has reported the use of heterograft transplantation as a solution to large gaps. The use of vascularized nerve grafts for extremity reconstruction has been reported by Taylor (1976) and Briedenbach (1986), but sufficient amount of vascularized grafts for the sciatic nerve would be difficult to attain.

It is not advisable to harvest any branches of the femoral nerve in an extremity that has sciatic nerve compromise because the femoral nerve provides some sensory input from the dorsal foot and the obturator nerve provides for some flexion of the knee through function of the adductors and gracilis muscles.

There is little reported in the literature on the outcome of sciatic nerve grafting or even on direct repair of the sciatic nerve. The clinical data that are available, as well as the author's experience with sciatic nerve repair, indicates that return of motor and sensory function can be expected to levels below the knee with appropriate nerve repair. The actual microsurgical techniques of nerve repair is covered in other chapters.

POSTERIOR TIBIAL NERVE

The posterior tibial nerve is responsible for flexion of the toes and ankle, and assists with knee flexion. It provides the crucial sensory pathways for the plantar aspect of the foot. Injury to this nerve is not common and has many etiologies (Brunner and Spencer, 1990; Dellon and Mackinnon, 1991; Dendooven et al, 1990; Galardi et al, 1990; Gartsman et al, 1988; Kline, 1972; Pace et al, 1991; Satku et al, 1992; Seddon, 1975).

The posterior tibial nerve is easily identified in the popliteal fossa as it crosses the fossa along with the vessels. In the fossa, it gives rise to several motor and sensory branches, as outlined in the illustration. Of particular note for the surgeon are the branches to medial and lateral gastrocnemius, soleus motor branch, and medial sural nerve. These specific motor nerves originate in the fossa. Just below, the fossa branches arborize to the tibialis posterior, the flexor digitorum longus, and the flexor hallucis longus.

Surgical exposure of the posterior tibial nerve is easiest when the patient is prone (Figs. 7–7 to 7–9). As the vertically directed incision is crossing the popliteal fossa, the incision should parallel the popliteal fossa flexion crease. Below the crease, the incision should extend from the mid popliteal area on a direct line toward the medial malleolus. This incision also provides access to the sural nerve if it needs to be harvested. The lesser saphenous vein is also immediately in the vicinity of this incision. The sural nerve and lesser saphenous vein should not be injured because they are potential resources for future use. During exposure in the mid-calf area, the two heads of the gastrocnemius are easily separated, but the fibers of the soleus muscle are more difficult and the nerve is easiest to access by splitting the muscle fibers of the soleus. In the author's experience, trying to repair the nerve using a lateral approach between the tibialis posterior and the flexor digitorum longus is even more difficult and impedes microscopic visualization of the nerve. Even in emergent circumstances when the popliteal

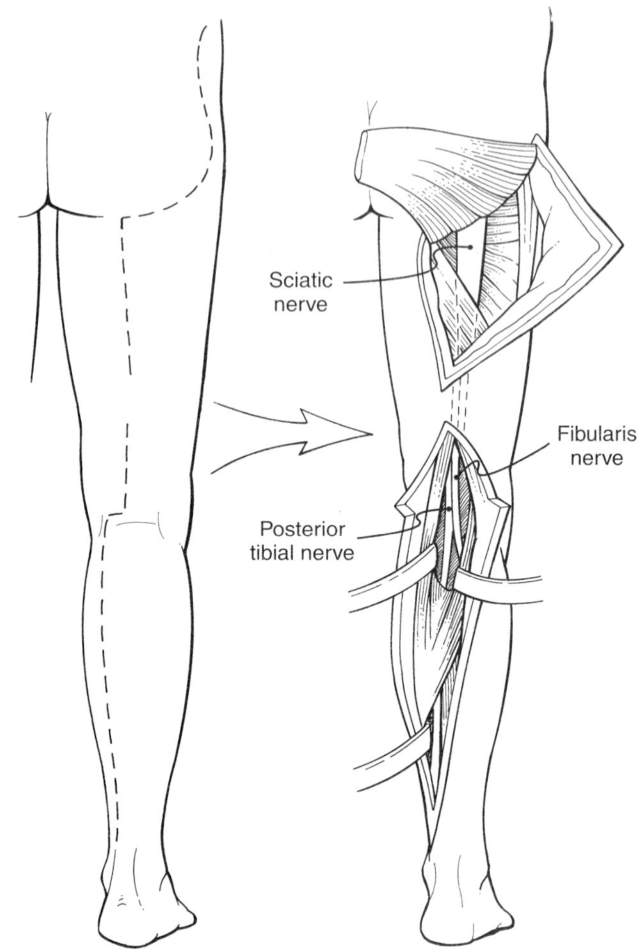

FIGURE 7–7. Posterior tibial nerve exposure prone.

artery or its branches are injured, the prone approach is very applicable (Visser et al, 1980).

When the nerve is observed during surgical repair, it is essential that viable and healthy fascicles are visualized. Repaired neuromas do not provide effective regeneration. Unless fascicle topography is clearly delineated, the apparent nerve that is observed may be a linear neuroma extending down the avulsed segment of nerve. The posterior tibial nerve is a polyfascicular nerve with at least 10 well-circumscribed fascicles. What appears to be a single large fascicle is not healthy nerve, and additional proximal removal of the neuroma is required. In avulsion injuries, the nerve can be injured for distances up to 20 cm proximal to the popliteal fossa. One reason lower extremity nerve repairs have not been as successful as the counterpart in the upper extremity may be because the entire injured segment of nerve has been underestimated.

The posterior tibial nerve usually requires at least five cables of sural nerve to cover the surface area of a transected nerve. In patients in whom the sural nerve origin is above the level of injury, the author prefers to use the contralateral sural nerve as the donor nerve. Because sensibility to the foot is already compromised, it seems important to avoid additional sensory compromise. If the injury is above the origin of the medial sural contribution to the sural nerve, the surgeon should still try to preserve the sural nerve because

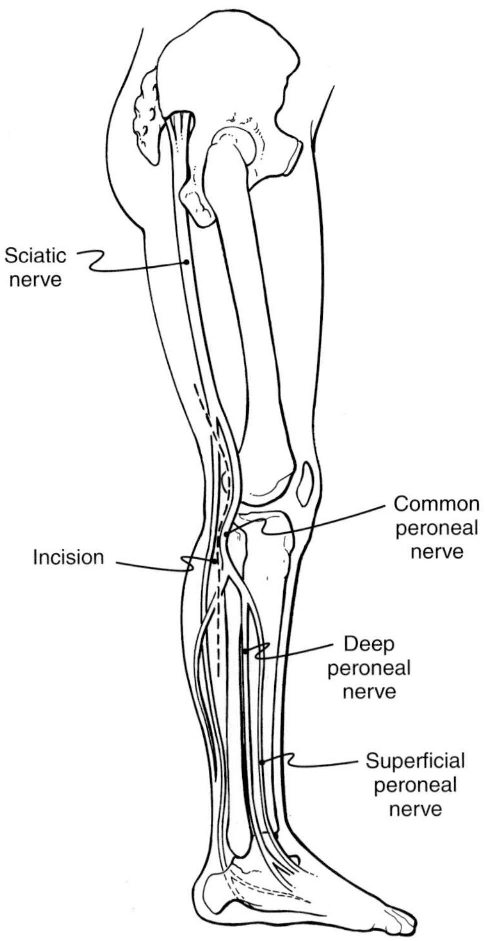

FIGURE 7–8. Exposure posterior tibial nerve mid–lower leg.

injured nerve in the lower extremity (Demuynck and Zuker, 1987; Hirasawa and Sakakida, 1983; Kline, 1972; Shevell and Stewart, 1988; Wood, 1991). Severe injuries disrupting the ligaments of the knee or dislocation following motorized vehicle accidents or athletic injuries make this nerve particularly vulnerable to stretch and disruption (McMahon and Craig, 1994; Terranova et al, 1986). Also because of its location, iatrogenic injury to this nerve may occur (Esselman et al, 1993; Herrara-Ornelas et al, 1986; Kirgis and Albrecht, 1992; Phillips et al, 1993). This nerve is also vulnerable to compression and neuritis (Chaise and Roger, 1985; Leach et al, 1989; Seddon, 1975; Sunderland, 1968).

After the common peroneal nerve branches from the sciatic nerve, it follows the biceps tendon and begins a lateral course away from the posterior tibial nerve. It is smaller than the posterior tibial nerve and is polyfascicular. In the popliteal fossa, it supplies the peroneal communicating branch that may join the medial sural nerve to form the sural nerve in the distal two thirds of the lower leg. It also supplies the lateral cutaneous nerve of the calf. Just after crossing under the biceps tendon and proximal to the fibular head, the nerve supplies a recurrent motor branch to the tibialis anterior. The nerve then divides into the superficial (musculocutaneous) and deep peroneal nerve (anterior tibial) branches. The superficial branch supplies the peroneous longus and brevis muscles and then continues to the dorsum of the foot, where it provides sensation as the dorsal cutaneous nerves of the foot.

The deep peroneal branch provides innervation to the tibialis anterior, extensor hallucis longus, extensor digitorum longus, and peroneus tertius muscles. The nerve then continues in a deep plane to the dorsum of the foot mimicking the posterior interosseous nerve's distal course in the forearm. On the dorsum of the foot, the nerve supplies the extensor digitorum brevis and extensor hallucis brevis muscles.

Exposure of the upper two thirds of the common peroneal nerve is easiest using a prone position. The incision should parallel but remain medial to the biceps femoris tendon by 2 cm. The incision should stay behind and below the fibular head.

If only the distal one third of the nerve is to be explored, surgical positioning in the lateral decubitus position permits access to the common peroneal's division into superficial and deep components and also repair at that level. Because the investing fascia of the peroneal muscles covers the nerve, injury during dissection must be avoided during exposure around the fibula's neck.

In severe trauma to the knee in which complete disruption of the supporting ligaments for the knee has occurred, the common peroneal nerve is particularly vulnerable to injury. Stretch injury and disruption can result in injury to the nerve for distance as great as 20 to 25 cm proximal to the knee. It is not known why avulsion most commonly occurs on the proximal side of the knee joint and is less common distal to the knee joint. The surgeon must beware of linear neuromas that can develop following stretch or avulsion injuries to this nerve. Repairing a linear neuroma does not provide innervation. This nerve has multiple fascicles, not a single or bifascicular topography. That may seem to be the circumstance when exploring this nerve following severe knee derangement, when injury to the common peroneal nerve may cause linear neuroma formation for distances as great as 20 cm above the knee following knee dislocation. Resec-

of the contribution from the common peroneal nerve via the lateral sural nerve. If larger donor nerves are used as grafts, the surgeon should plan accordingly because fewer cables would be necessary. In some circumstances, the motor branches are avulsed from the muscles they supply, leaving the surgeon with limited options. If that circumstance occurs, direct neurotization using grafts has been reported by Mackinnon and co-workers (1993).

Following a direct repair of the posterior tibial nerve, the nerve repair is protected for 3 weeks with the use of an anterior splint that permits flexion but precludes complete extension of the knee. If a nerve graft is used and the repair completed with the knee extended, the repairs are protected for 10 days and then motion started. Hematoma formation in the wound or around nerve graft cables can lead to unrecognized loss of nerve grafts and failure of the nerve to regenerate. Meticulous hemostasis after tourniquet deflation and appropriately used drains will help minimize the risk of hematoma formation.

COMMON PERONEAL NERVE

It is likely that the superficial location and its course directly over the lateral knee and adjacent to the head of the fibula make the common peroneal nerve the most commonly

tion of the nerve until suitable fascicular patterns are noted is essential if reinnervation is expected. The gap that follows must be grafted, and the author prefers to use the contralateral sural nerve and if necessary because of a long gap the ipsilateral nerve also. The technical steps involved with nerve grafting are reviewed in this book.

Direct repair of the common peroneal nerve must be protected from disruption by movement, similar to that used to protect the posterior tibial nerve. Nerve grafts must also be protected from mechanical disruption for 2 weeks.

RESULTS FOLLOW LOWER EXTREMITY NERVE REPAIRS

Following repair of any of the major nerves of the leg, the time to recovery of muscle reinnervation will precede recovery of distal sensory innervation.

When the sciatic nerve or posterior tibial nerve is injured and sensory reinnervation does not occur, long-term complications of recurrent plantar skin ulcers, paralytic clawing of the toes, Charcot joints, and gait changes will occur. All of these factors make reconstruction of the lower extremity peripheral nerves essential when possible and when other mechanical factors do not preclude repair. Support for repair of the lower extremities peripheral nerves is documented in the reports of Demuynck and Zuker, 1987; Dolene, 1977; Hattrup and Wood, 1986; Kline, 1972; Sedel, 1993; Truble and Vanderhooft, 1994; Visser et al, 1980; Wood, 1991. The recovery of function is usually commensurate with age, level of injury, nerve graft length, and time of delay between injury and repair. Nerve reconstruction of the femoral or sciatic nerve reliably produces some reinnervation of muscles above the knee. It can also be expected that large muscles such as the gastrocnemius, tibialis posterior, and tibialis anterior may reinnervate, especially if the injury is in the lower two thirds of the thigh.

The insensate foot can be retained in very compliant patients with meticulous care of the foot. However, in some circumstances, when sensibility cannot be restored and there are mechanical problems with the involved foot or ankle, the best treatment plan may be prosthetic reconstruction.

If the foot has sensibility but motor loss cannot be reconstructed, tendon transfers or bone stabilization is often required to enhance function of the extremity.

References

Aldea PA, Shaw WW: Lower extremity nerve injuries. Clin Plast Surg *13*:691–699, 1986a.

Aldea PA, Shaw WW: Management of acute lower extremity nerve injuries. Foot Ankle *7*:82–94, 1986b.

Belsh JM: Anterior femoral cutaneous nerve injury following femoral artery reconstructive surgery. Arch Neurol *48*:230–232, 1991.

Birch R, Bonney G, Dowell J, Hollingdale J: Iatrogenic injuries of peripheral nerves. J Bone Joint Surg [Br] *73*:280–282, 1991.

Breidenbach WC, Terzis JK: The blood supply of vascularized nerve grafts. J Reconstr Microsurg *3*:43–56, 1986.

Brunner WG, Spencer RF: Posterior tibial nerve neurotmesis complicating a closed fibial fracture. S Afr Med J *78*:607–608, 1990.

Chaise F, Roger B: Neurolysis of the common peroneal nerve in leprosy. A report on 22 patients. J Bone Joint Surg [Br] *67*:426–429, 1985.

Clawson DK, Seddon HJ: The results of repair of the sciatic nerve. J Bone Joint Surg *42B*:205, 1960.

D'Amelio LF, Musser DJ, Rhodes M: Bilateral femoral nerve neuropathy following blunt trauma. Case report. J Neurosurg *73*:630–632, 1990.

Dellon AL, Mackinnon SE: Results of posterior tibial nerve grafting at the ankle. J Reconstr Microsurg *7*:81–83, 1991.

Demuynck M, Zuker RM: The peroneal nerve: Is repair worthwhile? J Reconstr Microsurg *3*:193–197, 199, 1987.

Dendooven AM, Lissens M, Bruyninckx F, Vanhecke J: Electrical injuries to peripheral nerves. Acta Belg Med Phys *13*:161–165, 1990.

Dolene V: Microsurgical treatment of peripheral nerve injuries. Zentralbl Neurochir *38*:185–190, 1977.

Edwards BN, Tullos HS, Noble PC: Contributory factors and etiology of sciatic nerve palsy in total hip arthroplasty. Clin Orthop *218*:136–141, 1987.

Esselman PD, Tomski MA, Robinson LR, Zisfein J, Marks SJ: Selective deep peroneal nerve injury associated with arthroscopic knee surgery. Muscle Nerve *16*:1189–1192, 1993.

Fassler PR, Swiontkowski MF, Kilroy AW, Routt ML Jr: Injury of the sciatic nerve associated with acetabular fracture. J Bone Joint Surg [Am] *75*:1157–1166, 1993.

Galardi G, Comi G, Lozza L, Marchettini P, Novarina M, Facchini R, Paronzini A: Peripheral nerve damage during limb lengthening. Neurophysiology in five cases of bilateral tibial lengthening. J Bone Joint Surg [Br] *72*:121–124, 1990.

Gartsman GM, Bennett JB, Cain TE: Surgical correction of severe knee pterygium. Microsurgery *9*:246–248, 1988.

Gelberman RH: Operative Nerve Repair and Reconstruction. Philadelphia, J. B. Lippincott Company, 1991.

Grant JCB: Grant's Atlas of Anatomy, 5th ed. Baltimore, Williams & Wilkins, 1962.

Hall MC, Koch MO, Smith JA Jr: Femoral neuropathy complicating urologic abdominopelvic procedures. Urology *45*:146–149, 1995.

Halpern JS: Lower extremity peripheral nerve assessment. J Emerg Nurs *15*:333–337, 1989.

Harris WR: Avulsion of lumbar roots complicating fracture of the pelvis. J Bone Joint Surg *55A*:1436, 1973.

Hattrup SJ, Wood MB: Delayed neural reconstruction in the lower extremity: Results of interfascicular nerve grafting. Foot Ankle *7*:105–109, 1986.

Herrera-Ornelas L, Tolls RM, Petrelli NJ, Piver S, Mittleman A: Common peroneal nerve palsy associated with pelvic surgery for cancer. An analysis of 11 cases. Dis Colon Rectum *29*:392–397, 1986.

Hirasawa Y, Sakakida K: Sports and peripheral nerve injury. Am J Sports Med *11*:420–426, 1983.

Hudson AR: Nerve injection injuries. Clin Plast Surg *11*:27–30, 1984.

Infantino A, Fardin P, Pirone E, Masin A, Melega E, Cacciavillani M, Lise M: Femoral damage after abdominal rectopexy. Int J Colorectal Dis *9*:32–34, 1994.

Kirgis A, Albrecht S: Palsy of the deep peroneal nerve after proximal tibial osteotomy. An anatomical study [see comments]. J Bone Joint Surg [Am] *74*:1180–1185, 1992.

Kline DG: Operative management of major lesions of the lower extremity. Surg Clin North Am *52*:1247–1265, 1972.

Kroll DA, Caplan RA, Posner K, Ward RJ, Cheney FW: Nerve injury associated with anesthesia (see comments). Anesthesiology *73*:202–207, 1990.

Leach RE, Purnell MB, Saito A: Peroneal nerve entrapment in runners. Am J Sports Med *17*:287–291, 1989.

Mackinnon SE, Hudson AR: Clinical application of peripheral nerve transplantation. Plast Reconstr Surg *90*:695–699, 1992.

Mackinnon SE, McLean JS, Hunter GA: Direct muscle neurotization recovers gastrocnemius muscle function. J Reconstr Microsurg *9*:77–80, 1993.

McMahon MS, Craig SM: Interfascicular reconstruction of the peroneal nerve after knee ligament injury. Ann Plast Surg *32*:642–644, 1994.

Ninkovic M, Sucur D, Starovic B, Markovic S: A new approach to persistent traumatic peroneal nerve palsy. Br J Plast Surg *47*:185–189, 1994.

Omer GE Jr: Physical diagnosis of peripheral nerve injuries. Orthop Clin North Am *12*:207–228, 1981.

Omer GE, Spinner M: Management of Peripheral Nerve Problems. Philadelphia, W.B. Saunders Company, 1980.

Pace N, Serafini P, Lo Iacono E, Castricini R, Zanoli S: The tarsal and calcaneal tunnel syndromes. Ital J Orthop Traumatol *17*:247–252, 1991.

Pernkopf E: Atlas of Topographical and Applied Human Anatomy. Philadelphia, W. B. Saunders Company, 1980.

Phillips LH 2nd, Morgan RF: Anomalous origin of the sural nerve in a patient with tibial-common peroneal nerve anastomosis. Muscle Nerve *16*:414–417, 1993.

Salisbury RE, Dingeldein GP: Peripheral nerve complications following burn injury. Clin Orthop *163*:92–97, 1982.

Sammarco GJ, Stephens MM: Neurapraxia of the femoral nerve in a modern dancer. Am J Sports Med *19*:413–414, 1991.

Satku K, Wee JT, Kumar VP, Ong B, Pho RW: The dropped big toe. Ann Acad Med Singapore *21*:222–225, 1992.

Seddon HJ: Surgical Disorders of the Peripheral Nerves. Edinburgh, Churchill Livingstone, 1975.

Sedel L: The surgical management of nerve lesions in the lower limbs. Clinical evaluation, surgical technique and results. Int Orthop *9*:159–170, 1985.

Sedel L, Nizard RS: Nerve grafting for traction injuries of the common peroneal nerve. A report of 17 cases. J Bone Joint Surg [Br] *75*:772–774, 1993.

Shevell MI, Stewart JD: Laceration of the common peroneal nerve by a skate blade. Can Med Assoc J *139*:311–312, 1988.

Simmons C Jr, Izant TH, Rothman RH, Booth RE Jr, Balderston RA: Femoral neuropathy following total hip arthroplasty. Anatomic study, case reports, and literature review. J Arthroplasty *6*(Suppl):S57–66, 1991.

Sunderland S: Nerves and Nerve Injuries, Baltimore, Williams & Wilkins, 1968.

Sunderland S, McArthur RA, Nam DA: Repair of a transected sciatic nerve. A study of nerve regeneration and functional recovery: Report of a case. J Bone Joint Surg [Am] *75*:911–914, 1993.

Taylor EG, Hau FJ: The free vascularized nerve graft. Plast Reconstr Surg *57*:413, 1976.

Terranova WA, McLaughlin RE, Morgan RF: An algorithm for the management of ligamentous injuries of the knee associated with common peroneal nerve palsy. Orthopedics *9*:1135–1140, 1986.

Trumble T, Vanderhooft E: Nerve grafting for lower-extremity injuries. J Pediatr Orthop *14*:161–165, 1994.

Venna N, Bielawski M, Spatz EM: Sciatic nerve entrapment in a child. Case report. J Neurosurg *75*:652–654, 1991.

Villarejo FJ, Pascual AM: Injection injury of the sciatic nerve (370 cases). Childs Nerv Syst *9*:229–232, 1993.

Visser PA, Hermreck AS, Pierce GE, Thomas JH, Hardin CA: Prognosis of nerve injuries incurred during acute trauma to peripheral arteries. Am J Surg *140*:596–599, 1980.

Vrahas M, Gordon RG, Mears DC, Krieger D, Sclabassi RJ: Intraoperative somatosensory evoked potential monitoring of pelvic and acetabular fracture. J Orthop Trauma *6*:50–58, 1992.

Williams PH, Trzil KP: Management of meralgia paresthetica (see comments). J Neurosurg *74*:76–80, 1991.

Wood MB: Peroneal nerve repair. Surgical results. Clin Orthop *267*:206–210, 1991.

Diagnostic nerve blocks are useful procedures in the evaluation and localization of pain. They can also serve to predict the outcome of permanent denervation by section of a neuropathway in a given patient. In any discussion on the role of diagnostic and prognostic nerve blocks, an understanding of the types of pain and their causative mechanisms is essential for proper selection and application.

Pain may be either acute or chronic. Acute pain is usually caused by noxious stimuli traveling along neuropathways to the brain, where they are perceived as nociception. Noxious stimuli trigger specialized pain receptors known as nociceptors (Bonica and Albe-Fessard, 1976, 1990; Burgess, 1974); these are located in skin, subcutaneous tissue, viscera, muscle, and deep structures, and are characterized by high threshold (Bonica and Albe-Fessard, 1976, 1990; Burgess, 1974; Perl, 1971). They transmit a persistent discharge in response to a suprathreshold stimulus along small A-delta and C fibers (Bonica and Albe-Fessard, 1976; Burgess, 1974; Hallin and Torebiork, 1974; Iggo, 1972). Impulses travel along these fibers to the dorsal horn cells, where they are modulated by a highly developed process of selection, integration, and abstraction (Melzack and Wall, 1965; Wall, 1967; Wall and Melzack, 1994). Further modulation and selection also occurs in the ascending tracts of the spinal cord and in the mid-brain (Bonica, 1977). The stimulus finally reaches the primary somato-sensory cortex. The somato-cortex, through its discriminative function, and probably by regulating subcortical activity, will further modulate nociception (Bonica, 1977). However, the brain, through the descending neural systems, can influence transmission in the thalamus, reticular formation, and dorsal column of the spinal cord (Fetz, 1968; Taub, 1964; Wall, 1967; Winnie, 1983) and trigeminal system (Sessle and Greenwood, 1976).

Because pain is an emotional experience, psychological factors play a great role in the patient's total pain experience (Chapman, 1977; Merskey and Spear, 1967; Sternbach, 1968). Neocortical processes modulate cognitive and psychological factors such as anxiety, prior conditioning, experience, and emotional and cultural background (Melzack and Casey, 1968; Melzack and Wall, 1965; Wall and Melzack, 1994). Causes of pain are generally accepted as (1) nociception, (2) central pain states, (3) psychological factors, and (4) behavioral phenomena (Murphy, 1977; Cousins and Bridenbaugh, 1987).

Singly or in combination, the causes listed earlier can be responsible for pain. Certainly, nociception may play the primary role in acute pain. However, when pain is chronic, psychological factors become more important (Chapman, 1977; Melzack, 1974) and still persist after the cessation of nociception.

Central pain states (Noordenbos, 1974; Pagni, 1974) may be secondary to a lesion within the central nervous system (CNS); for example, tumor, herpes virus, trauma, or other CNS disease states (Bonica, 1990). However, in a great number of cases, no specific causative lesion is identifiable.

ROLE OF DIAGNOSTIC AND PROGNOSTIC NERVE BLOCKS

1. To localize the area where noxious stimuli are produced.

2. To define neuropathways where noxious stimuli may be transmitted.

3. To determine if transection of the nerve or root could be successful in eliminating pain. In this particular role, diagnostic nerve blocks play a definite role in subsequent patient management.

4. To evaluate patients' acceptance of prolonged denervation. Many patients find anesthesia more objectionable than the original pain.

5. To assess long-term nerve blocks with alcohol or phenol to determine the possible occurrence of permanent dysesthesia. To avoid permanent nerve damage, low concentrations of phenol are recommended, because denervation is not always reversible when high concentrations of phenol are used.

PREPARATION OF A PATIENT FOR NERVE BLOCK

In acute pain, simple interruption of the appropriate neural pathway will provide relief. At this point, patients are not usually addicted to any medication, and psychological factors do not usually play a major role. After a complete physical and neurological examination, one or more provisional diagnoses are usually arrived at. One of two approaches can be chosen at this point.

1. If the etiology of the pain is relatively clear, the block is expected to confirm the provisional diagnosis. There is no need for screening blocks; for example, spinal, epidural, or caudal. It is far less traumatic and disruptive to the patient to proceed with the least invasive technique. For instance, if a myofascial syndrome is suspected, simple local infiltration of the involved muscle or fascial plane will be the block of choice. More extensive blocks will be resorted to only if local infiltration fails. This would probably indicate that the causative mechanism may not be a simple myofascial syndrome limited to the particular area of infiltration.

2. If the nature of the pain is very indefinite and poorly localized, screening blocks can be helpful. For example, if a lumbar epidural with complete anesthesia below T12–L1 spinal dermatomes fails to alleviate leg pain, it is rather obvious that the pain will not be interrupted by blocking any neural pathway in the lower limbs. A different mechanism

for nociception in that leg should be searched for. If, however, the screening block is successful in eliminating the pain, then more distal blocks will be necessary to further localize the neural pathway involved.

In chronic pain states, patients often present for treatment at such a late stage that most of them have already been subjected to large amounts of narcotics, sedatives, and tranquilizers. These patients have become drug dependent, and it is impossible to differentiate whether most of their pain symptoms are actually indirect requests for medication or demonstrate true nociception. Sudden cessation of addictive drugs may produce severe withdrawal symptoms and even worse pain; therefore, gradual withdrawal of the drugs, with the help of qualified psychiatric assistance, is the most expedient approach. In the meantime, other methods for alleviating pain, such as continuous epidural block or percutaneous nerve stimulation, as well as any appropriate physical therapy during the period of drug withdrawal, should be employed. Only when the patient is no longer drug dependent can one proceed with diagnostic blocks.

Psychiatric evaluation prior to blocks should be required in all chronic pain problems even if the patient presents with valid reasons for chronic pain. Screening tests, such as the Minnesota Multiphasic Personality Inventory (MMPI), and many other psychological tests are helpful in defining the psychological component.

Weaning patients off narcotics, psychiatric evaluation, and supportive therapy is tedious and time consuming. However, unless ample time as well as effort is allocated, arriving at a correct diagnosis and initiation of therapy may be impossible. When a nerve block is finally selected, the patient is asked to abstain from analgesics for a few hours, after which the pain should be reassessed as to its degree, nature, duration, and triggering mechanisms. When the pain is paroxysmal or intermittent, it is very difficult to assess the value of the block, if, at the time of the block, the patient has been free of pain. Blocks of long duration with an indwelling catheter may be necessary. If pain does not recur within a few days it is safe to assume that the involved neural pathway has been interrupted.

KEY POINTS FOR EFFECTIVE DIAGNOSTIC BLOCKS

1. Success of a block should not be in doubt. It is imperative to be absolutely sure that the block is fully in effect by evaluating sensory deficits, signs of sympathetic blockade (e.g., Horner syndrome in head or neck), increases in skin temperature, and loss of motor power. Monitoring limb temperature by a sensitive thermocouple before and after a block would detect any change in temperature secondary to vasodilation of skin vessels when sympathetic hyperactivity is interrupted.
2. Blocks should be performed with minimal paresthesia and nerve damage. Repeated puncture of nerves may produce iatrogenic pain.
3. Several drugs of varying duration and placebos should be used to evaluate chronic pain. It may be wise not to inform the patient of the normal therapeutic duration of the drug utilized. During assessment of the block the patient should report on the duration and degree of relief.

ASSESSMENT OF BLOCK

Degrees of Pain Relief. The patient is asked to evaluate the degree of relief in percentages; if no or poor relief of pain is experienced, the patient should be asked to stimulate trigger points, if any, or to perform any movement or activity that is known to elicit pain, and then the amount of relief should be reassessed. Many patients will be surprised to find that they can perform many activities or movements that they were unable to perform prior to the block without eliciting a degree of pain sufficient to interrupt the activity.

Duration of Relief. This is important in assessing the value of the block. The usual responses from patients when asked about the duration of relief are as follows:

1. Duration of relief exceeds anesthetic duration of the drug. This is a common occurrence, the reasons for which are not understood at the moment; probably the relief is extended by prolonging the refractory period of the nerve (Condouris, 1966), thereby modulating neuro-information. This is typical also of causalgic pain, wherein patients sometimes report relief for 24 hours or longer. However, if the same effect is also obtained after a placebo, psychogenic factors should be suspected to be the actual causative mechanism; true central pain is rarely relieved consistently by placebos. Several blocks with agents of different anesthetic duration may be necessary to differentiate between pain of psychogenic nature and true nociception.
2. Duration of anesthesia produced by nerve block far exceeds relief. The amount of relief obtained is adequate, but only for a very short period and far less than the duration of sensory block; in such cases, the psychological component of pain may be the predominant factor. In some patients, drug addiction may play a role, especially if the patient demands the usual dose of narcotics to which he or she has been accustomed.
3. Duration of relief equals the anesthetic duration of the drug. This is typical of nociception, and these patients are proper candidates for permanent denervation if the permanent anesthesia that will develop is acceptable.
4. No relief at all is obtained. This can be attributed to an unsuccessful block, to nociception transmitted through a different neuropathway, to central pain states, or to pain of psychological origin. Screening blocks that would anesthetize large segments of the body are of value in this situation. If these screening blocks are unsuccessful in interrupting pain, further search of the true pathways should be made.

TYPES OF NERVE BLOCKS

Sympathetic

These blocks are primarily designed to interrupt sympathetic innervation to regions where sympathetic hyperactivity may be the causative mechanism of pain. Sympathetic hyperactivity (sympathetic reflex dystrophy) usually presents with burning pain, coldness, pallor, trophic changes of the skin, and excessive sweating (hyperhydrosis) (Doupe et al, 1944). Stellate and lumbar sympathetic blocks can provide pure sympathetic block, while spinal, epidural, caudal, or plexus blocks with low concentration of local anesthetics can produce a differential sympathetic block, owing to the fact that sympathetic fibers are very small and unmyelinated, and the minimum concentration (CM) required to block these fibers will hardly affect the larger sensory and motor fibers. For this reason, 0.25% lidocaine, 0.5% procaine or chloroprocaine, and 0.125% bupivacaine may be successful in producing a true sympathetic differential block. Continuous blocks with an indwelling catheter assess results of sympathetic blockade for up to 4 days. If the patient has complete relief for a few days with an indwelling catheter placed at the stellate or lumbar sympathetic chain, relief with a permanent chemical or surgical sympathectomy should be expected.

Sensory

1. Trigger point injections—local infiltration of trigger points in myofascial syndromes with the usual concentrations of anesthetics used for local infiltration is sufficient to provide pain relief. Long-acting anesthetics are preferable, although short-acting anesthetics or, at times, even placebos can be of value. These injections are used to determine if pain is due to a reflex mechanism triggered by local pathology.

2. Somatic nerve blocks are some of the most useful diagnostic tools available for pain syndromes. They range from large screening blocks (spinal, epidural, caudal, or plexus) to blocks involving individual small nerves.

3. Differential sensory nerve blocks are of value in achieving anesthesia without any major interruption of motor activity.

4. Placebo blocks are particularly helpful in assessing pain that appears to be psychosomatic in nature.

5. Motor nerve blocks are used if pain results from spasm of a muscle or group of muscles. These are usually prognostic and are done prior to surgery to determine if spasm in involved muscles can be relieved by interruption of the motor nerve supply.

LOCAL ANESTHETIC DRUGS

For the safe use of local anesthetics, the following rules should be observed:

1. Use the minimum dose and concentration necessary to produce adequate anesthesia. Increasing the concentration of the local anesthetic is not an efficient way of prolonging the block. Anesthetic solutions containing epinephrine should be used instead.

2. Aspirate carefully. Avoid intravascular injection; most toxic reactions occur when this simple precaution is neglected.

3. If a larger dose for a large area is needed, it is preferable to inject the drugs in divided doses.

4. For nerve blocks, place the needle carefully; with accurate placement of the anesthetic, smaller doses can be used.

5. Use nerve blocks instead of local infiltration when large areas are to be anesthetized.

6. Avoid injecting the anesthetic into any infected area.

7. Deposit anesthetic solution around the nerve. Do not puncture the nerve unnecessarily.

8. Allow sufficient time for the anesthetic agent to work.

A comprehensive description of these drugs is beyond the scope of this chapter, and the reader is advised to refer to the appropriate texts (Concepcion and Covino, 1989; Collins, 1976; Covino and Vassallo, 1976). A brief description of the most commonly used drugs will be included.

Local anesthetic drugs can be divided into two major groups; namely, amides and esters. The pertinent differences in their pharmacological properties are as follows:

1. Ester groups are generally of shorter duration of action, except tetracaine, which is the only compound of considerable duration.

2. Allergic reactions are more common in the esters group. Most complications with the amide group are due to either toxicity from overdosage or intravascular injection.

3. Onset of action is usually shorter in the ester compounds.

4. Esters are detoxified in the bloodstream by pseudocholinesterases, and therefore, the duration of action is considerably shorter if mixed with blood. Amides are detoxified mainly in the liver, and the effect of blood will not alter the duration of these compounds.

The most commonly used ester compounds are procaine (Novacaine) and 2-3-chloroprocaine (Nesacaine), and their pharmacological characteristics are listed in the previous list. Concentrations commonly used are 0.5% to 2 % for procaine and 1% to 3% for chloroprocaine. They may be mixed with 1/100,000 to 1/200,000 epinephrine solution to increase duration and reduce systemic absorption. Duration with no epinephrine added is approximately 30 minutes for 2-chloroprocaine and up to 45 minutes for procaine. If epinephrine is added, the duration can be increased by 50% to 100%, depending on the vascularity of the area being infiltrated. Maximum dose of chloroprocaine should not exceed 15 mg/kg for single injection.

In the amide group, lidocaine (Xylocaine), mepivacaine (Carbocaine), bupivacaine (Marcaine), and etidocaine (Duranest) are commonly used.

Lidocaine and mepivacaine are clinically similar and can be used in these concentrations:

1. For infiltration anesthesia, sympathetic differential nerve block 0.25% to 0.5%.

2. For block of small nerves and sensory differential nerve block: 1.0%.

3. For block of large nerves: 1.5%.

4. For spinal (Lidocaine): 2.0%.

5. For epidural (Lidocaine): 1.5% to 2.0%.

Their duration of action ranges from 45 to 90 minutes. Addition of 1/100,000 to 1/200,000 epinephrine solution may increase the duration 50% to 100%.

Bupivacaine is similar in structure to mepivacaine but is three to four times more potent; it owes its long duration of anesthesia to its binding property to tissue proteins. The duration of anesthesia is 3 to 4 hours, depending on the vascularity of the region. The concentrations used are:

1. For sympathetic blocks: 0.12% to 0.25%.

2. For small sensory nerve and sensory differential nerve blocks: 0.25%.

3. For large nerve blocks: 0.5%.

4. For spinal and epidural blocks: 0.25% to 0.75%.

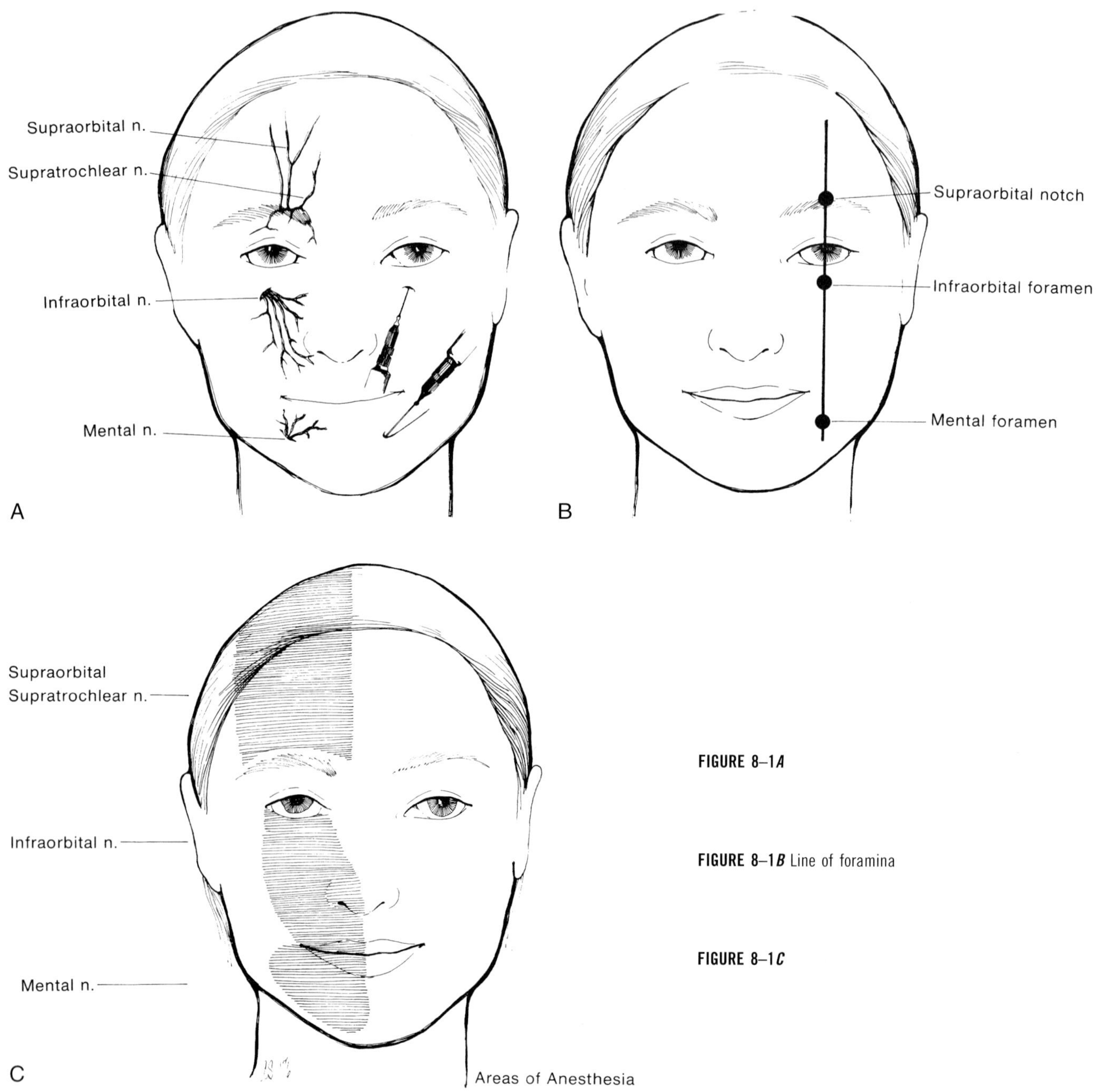

FIGURE 8–1*A*

FIGURE 8–1*B* Line of foramina

FIGURE 8–1*C*

Bupivacaine produces excellent differential blocks in smaller concentrations, because it has a particular affinity for sensory fibers. The onset of action is rather slow, and addition of epinephrine does not increase the duration of the drug to any appreciable degree. The maximum dose for a single injection is approximately 250 mg, although 400 mg has been used extensively and without any undesirable effects (Moore, 1975).

Etidocaine and ropivacaine are new drugs similar in properties to bupivacaine. Etidocaine concentration used is about twice that of bupivacaine. It affects the motor fibers more than bupivacaine (Moore et al, 1975) and would not be suitable for differential blocks. Ropivacaine is similar to mepivacaine, and it is a long-acting local anesthetic agent. Its major advantage is to produce profound analgesia without motor blockade. Adding clonidine to mepivacaine also prolongs the duration of anesthesia and analgesia (Singelyn et al, 1992). Bicarbonation and carbonation of local anesthetic, although shown to be clinically beneficial, remain controversial and are not widely used.

TECHNIQUES OF MOST FREQUENTLY USED DIAGNOSTIC BLOCKS

Head and Neck Region

INFRAORBITAL NERVE BLOCK

The infraorbital nerve supplies the lower eyelid, the lower third of the lateral surface of the nose, the upper lip (includ-

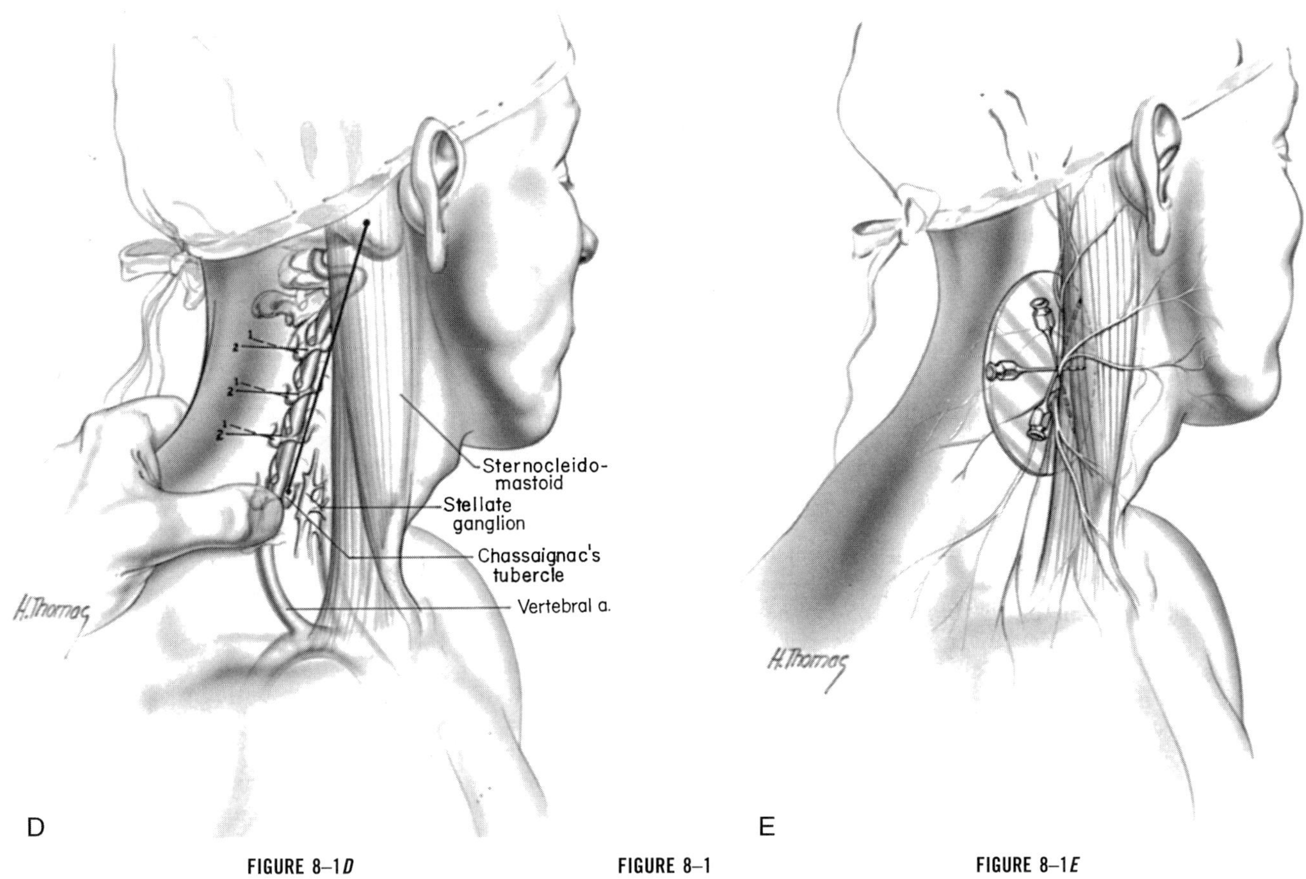

D

E

FIGURE 8–1*D*   **FIGURE 8–1**   **FIGURE 8–1***E*

ing mucous membrane), the columella, and the upper two incisors (Fig. 8–1*A* and *C*).

The infraorbital foramen can be very easily palpated below the infraorbital ridge, which is on the same line as the pupil when the eyes are looking straight forward (Fig. 8–1*B*). Three or four milliliters of a low concentration local anesthetic injected into or around the infraorbital foramen provides immediate anesthesia. Paresthesia is usually elicited as the needle is advanced along the infraorbital canal, which runs posteriorly, superiorly, and outward.

MENTAL NERVE BLOCK

The mental nerve supplies the chin and lower lip, including the mucous membrane and the lower cheek. It can be blocked at the mental canal or as it emerges from the mental foramen (see Fig. 8–1*A* and *C*).

The mental foramen lies below the second bicuspid tooth about midway between the upper and lower borders of the lower mandible. With age, in the edentulous patient, and with the progressive atrophy of the alveolar ridge, the foramen comes closer to the upper border of the mandible until it lies close to the very upper margin. The alveolar foramen can be entered with the needle pointing downward medially and forward. Paresthesia should be elicited to ensure a good block.

SUPRAORBITAL NERVE BLOCK

The supraorbital nerves can be blocked at the supraorbital notch, which is located 1 inch lateral to the midline at the inferior edge of the supraorbital ridge (see Fig. 8–1*A* and *C*). The supraorbital notch can be easily palpated with the finger; 3 ml of a local anesthetic agent deposited at the notch inferior to the supraorbital ridge render complete anesthesia for the corresponding half of the forehead.

SUPRATROCHLEAR NERVE BLOCK

The supratrochlear nerve exists from the orbit halfway between the supraorbital notch and the pulley of the superior oblique muscle. It emerges lateral to the medial border of the orbit to curve upward. It supplies the lower part of the forehead and the bridge of the nose. Paresthesia should be elicited if alcohol or phenol is used (Fig. 8–1*A* and *C*).

For blocks of maxillary nerves or their branches, readers should refer to the excellent descriptions by Kramer Jr. and Schmidt, 1977, and by Moore, 1965, and for overall information on head and neck anesthesia, readers should consult the publication by Abadir and Humayun (1991).

CERVICAL PLEXUS BLOCK

The patient is in the dorsal supine position, without a pillow, arms at sides, and head turned to the side opposite the side being blocked. One half inch posterior to a line connecting the tip of the mastoid process and Chassaignac's tubercle, palpate the second, third, and fourth transverse processes (see Fig. 8–1*D*). Landmarks can be easily checked by locating Chassaignac's tubercle and counting the transverse processes in the cephalad direction. Skin wheals are

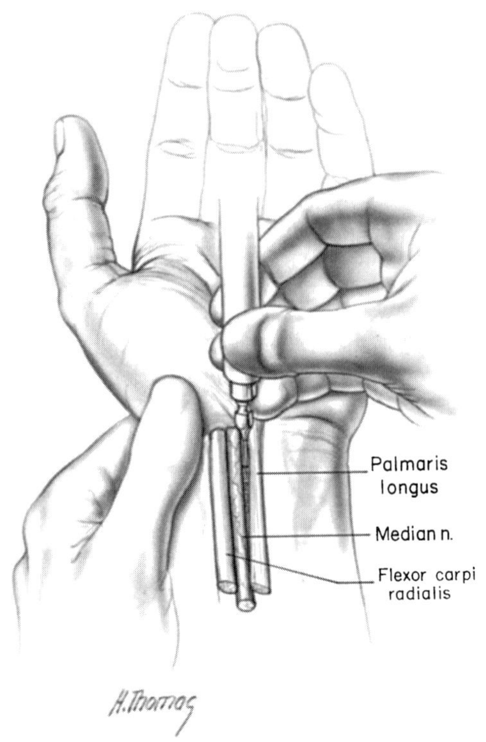

FIGURE 8–5

Lower Extremity

The three most frequently blocked nerves are the femoral, the sciatic, and the lateral femoral cutaneous.

FEMORAL NERVE BLOCK

The femoral artery is palpated. The femoral nerve is located immediately lateral to it. Through a skin wheal, a 22-gauge, 2-inch needle is inserted 1/2 inch lateral to the artery, 1/2 to 1 1/2 inches deep, depending on the amount of fat. At this point, 5 to 10 ml of a suitable anesthetic agent is injected.

SCIATIC NERVE BLOCK

A line is drawn between the posterior superior iliac spine and the greater trochanter, then at the midpoint of this line, a perpendicular line is dropped 3 to 3 1/2 inches long; at the end of this line, a skin wheal is raised, and a needle is inserted perpendicular to the skin (Fig. 8–6). The nerve is usually 2 to 3 inches deep, depending on the thickness of the buttocks. Paresthesia is then elicited but avoid injecting the nerve. Inject 10 to 20 ml of 2% lidocaine or a comparable strength of another local anesthetic. If epinephrine is used, anesthesia is usually complete within 15 or 20 minutes.

Lateral Femoral Cutaneous Nerve Block

One inch medial to and one inch inferior to the anterior superior iliac spine, the needle is inserted perpendicularly until it penetrates the fascia lata; 5 to 10 ml of 1% lidocaine, or a comparable dose of some other local anesthetic, are injected in a fanlike fashion cephalad and caudad (Fig. 8–7). The procedure is repeated, and another 5 ml is injected in a similar fashion.

OBTURATOR NERVE BLOCK

A wheal is made over the skin 1/2 inch below and 1/2 inch lateral to the pubic tubercle. A 22-gauge, 2-inch needle is advanced perpendicular to the skin through the wheal until it contacts the inferior ramus of the pubic bone. The needle is withdrawn and redirected and readvanced to a depth of 1/2 inch, at an angle of 60 degrees to the transverse axis, pointing laterally and cephalad (Fig. 8–8). When the needle point is no longer in contact with bone, it is again slightly withdrawn and redirected at an angle of 30 degrees to the transverse axis, pointing more laterally, and then advanced 1 1/2 inches. Paresthesia usually occurs at this point. The usual technique for aspiration is followed, and if blood is obtained, the needle should be withdrawn for a few millimeters and readvanced to elicit paresthesia. A volume of 15 ml of local anesthetic solution is deposited. The needle is withdrawn slowly and another 10 ml is injected.

INTERCOSTAL NERVE BLOCK

The intercostal nerves can be blocked at any point along their course 3 to 4 inches from the vertebral spine to the cartilaginous portion of the rib. They run in a neurovascular bundle located in a groove running along the lower border of each rib.

A wheal is raised along the lower border of the rib where the block should be performed. The needle is advanced carefully until the lowermost border of the rib is contacted, then the needle is walked along the lower border of the rib, then readvanced slowly for about one eighth inch (Fig. 8–9). Paresthesia may or may not be elicited at this stage. Careful aspiration for blood or air is made. The needle tip should be always under control and always in contact with the lower

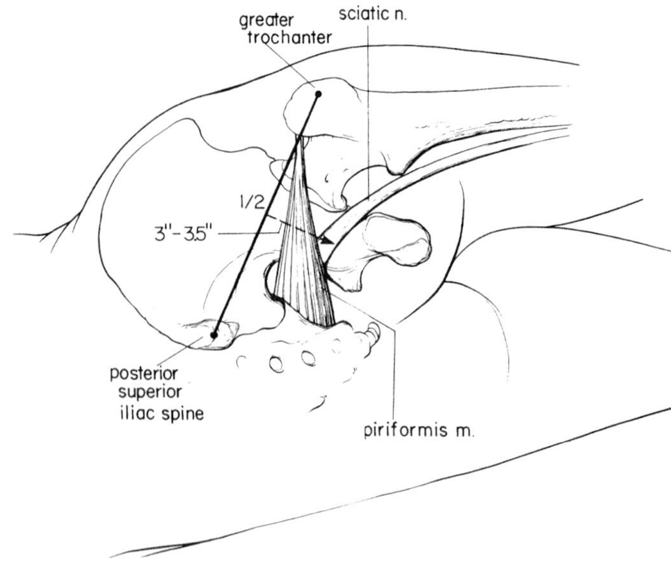

FIGURE 8–6

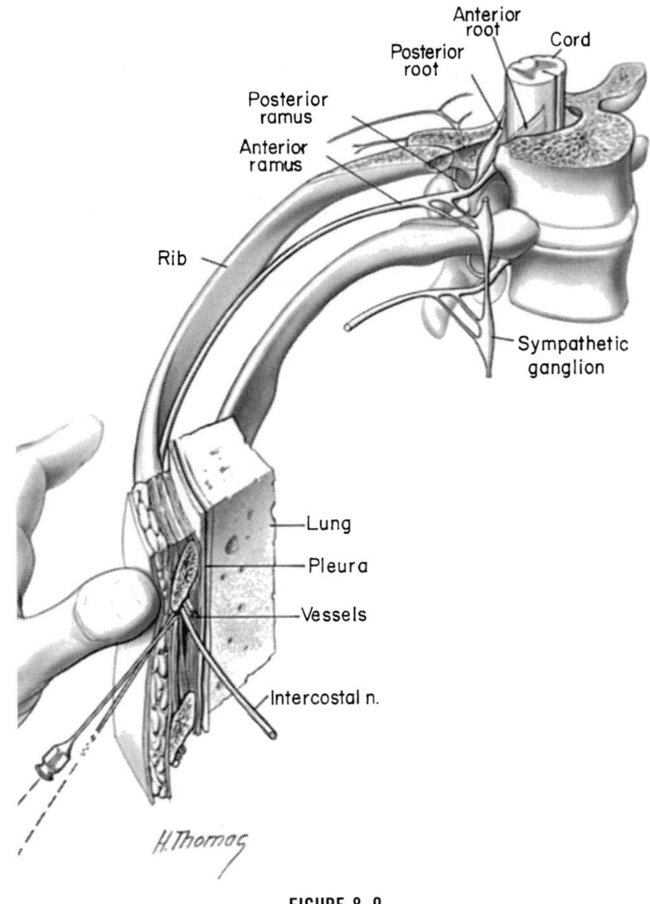

FIGURE 8–9

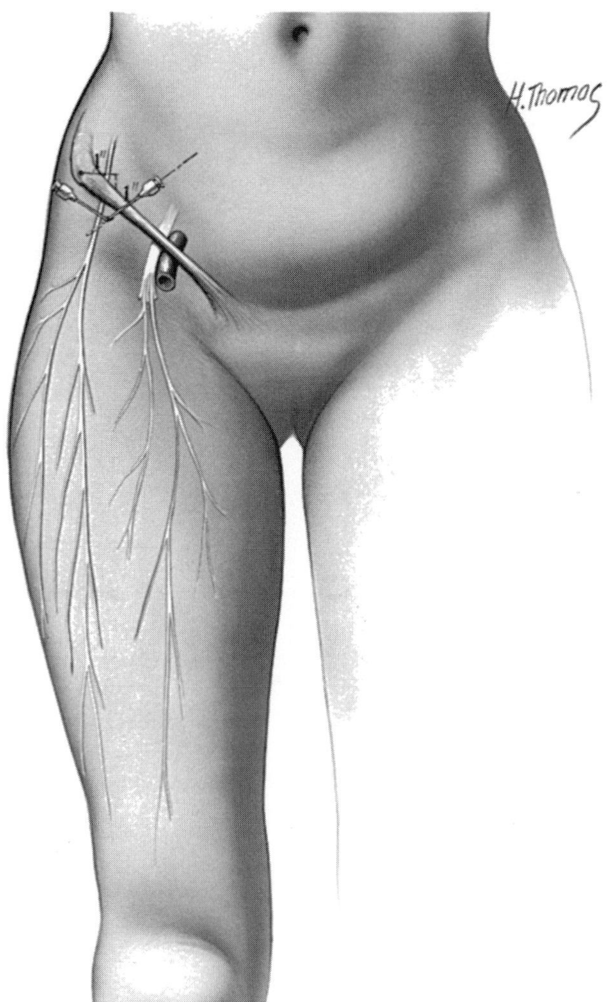

FIGURE 8–7

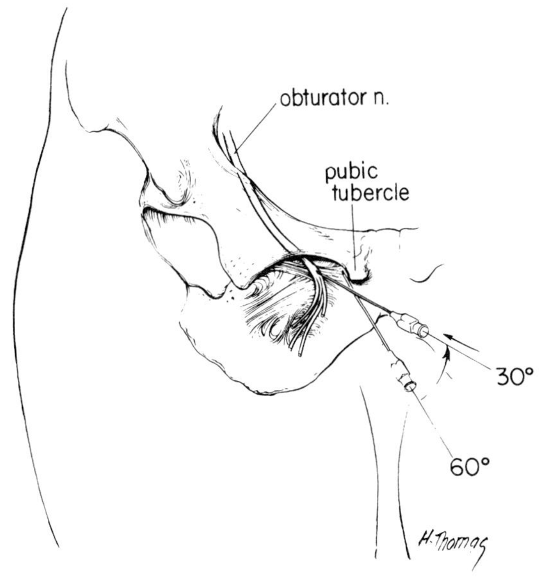

FIGURE 8–8

border of the rib. A few milliliters of a weak concentration of the chosen local anesthetic are then injected. Pneumothorax is the most common complication of this procedure. As many ribs as needed can be blocked to effect complete relief of pain. Bilateral blocks are necessary for lesions overlying the sternum or midline. Onset of anesthesia is immediate. High systemic blood levels of the drugs are common in intercostal blocks.

PARAVERTEBRAL SYMPATHETIC CHAIN BLOCK

The spine of the second or third lumbar vertebra is palpated and a skin wheal is raised at 2 1/2 to 3 inches lateral to the tip of the spine (Figs. 8–10 and 8–11). A 4-inch, 22-gauge needle is inserted through the skin wheal at an angle of 40 to 45 degrees to the perpendicular. The needle is withdrawn a few millimeters and walked off the tip. It is then readvanced at an angle of 40 to 50 degrees so it contacts the ventrolateral aspect of the lumbar vertebral body. It is then withdrawn and redirected until it slides off the lateral surface of the vertebral body. Advancement is carefully controlled to avoid puncturing any major vessels. The needle is withdrawn 1/2 cm, and a 5- to 10-ml dose of local anesthetic agent is deposited at this point. An image intensifier capable of two-plane visualization and televised x-ray screening can demonstrate the exact location of the tip of the needle in relation to the ventrolateral aspect of the vertebral body (Boas, 1976).

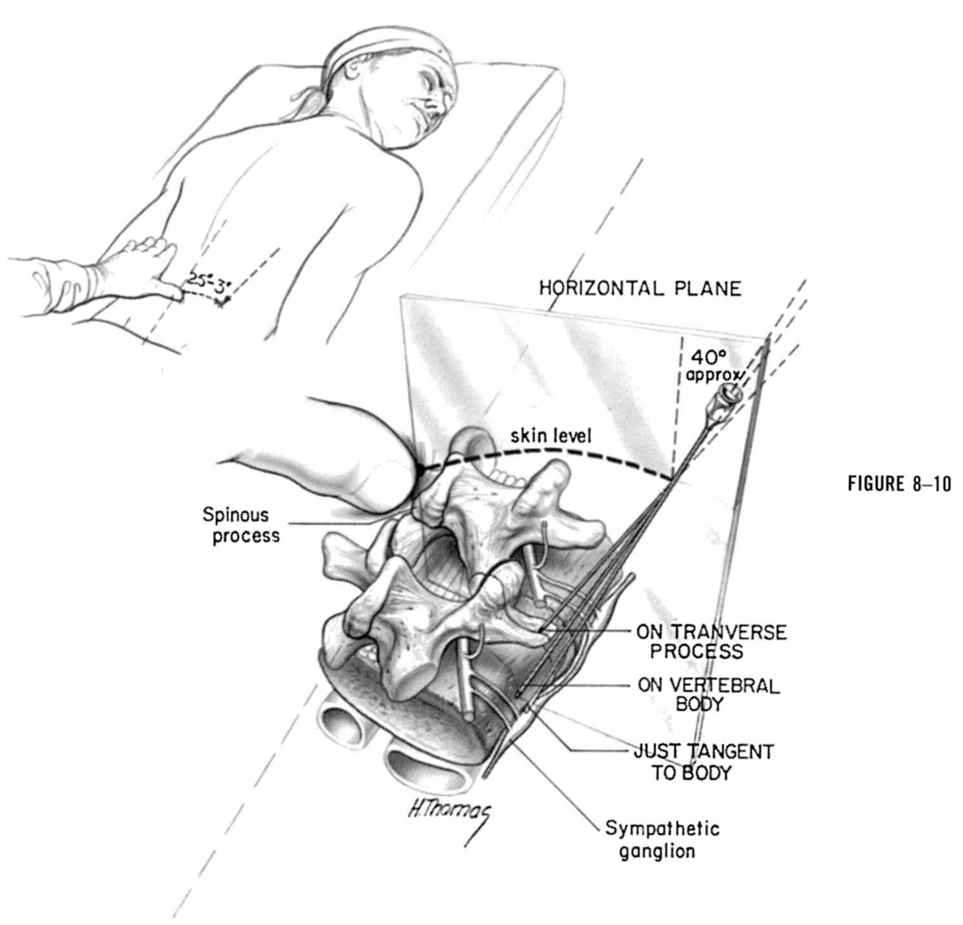

FIGURE 8–10

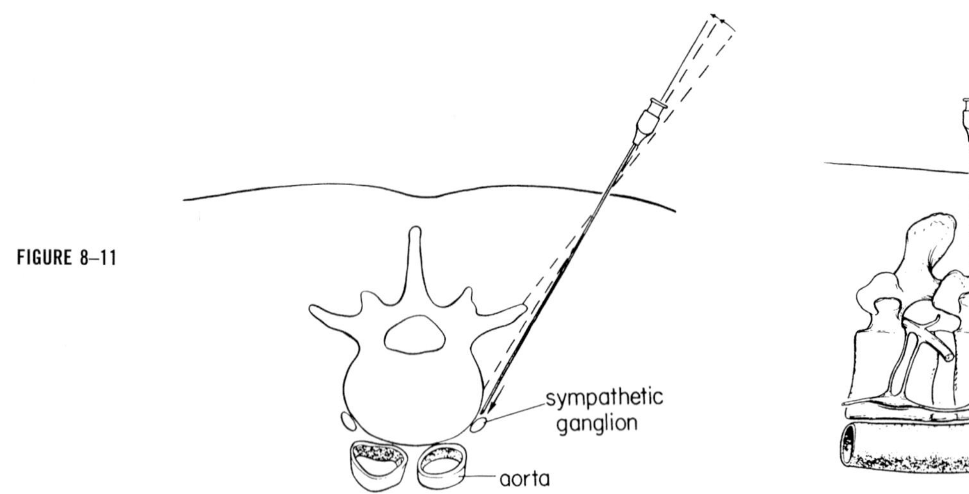

FIGURE 8–11

PARAVERTEBRAL SOMATIC NERVE BLOCK

In the thoracic region, this block is helpful in identifying intercostal neuralgia and cardiac pain, whereas in the lumbar region, it is helpful in localizing the pain in the inguinal region, legs, and lower back.

The same technique is used in both the lumbar and thoracic regions. However, one should note the difference in the anatomical landmarks. The tip of the thoracic vertebral spine corresponds to the body of the vertebra below. In the lumbar region, it corresponds to the same vertebral body. Skin wheals are raised over the selected transverse processes. The needle is inserted and advanced perpendicular to the skin until it contacts the transverse process. Then the needle is withdrawn a few millimeters and redirected, while advanced a few degrees caudad, until it slides off the lower border of the transverse process. Depending on the individual physique, a depth of 1¾ to 2¾ cm is required to contact the appropriate root. Paresthesia should be elicited with utmost care. After careful aspiration for blood and cerebrospinal fluid, a dose of 5 ml of suitable local anesthetic agent is deposited.

LUMBAR PLEXUS BLOCK

The lumbar plexus is sandwiched between the quadratus lumborum and the psoas muscles; hence it is enclosed in fascial envelopes. This block can be accomplished by a single injection using an anterior inguinal paravascular approach (Winnie, 1975). The technique is a simple modification of the femoral nerve block.

The femoral artery is palpated and retracted medially. Just lateral to the femoral artery, a skin wheal is raised. The needle is inserted into the fascial sheath and advanced until paresthesia of the femoral nerve is elicited. Digital pressure is applied firmly just distal to the needle while a suitable local anesthetic agent is injected. A volume of 30 to 35 ml is necessary. Following the injection, the needle is removed but digital pressure should be maintained for another few minutes. We have developed a curved-needle technique for celiac plexus and lumbar sympathetic block (Abadir et al, 1990). A 12.5-cm, 20-gauge spinal needle or a 12.5-cm Tuohy needle bent into a 100-degree arch provides significant advantage in placement of medication near the celiac plexus or lumbar sympathetic ganglion. Under contrast radiography, using a C-arm linkage, intensifies this technique, maintains close proximity to the vertebral body, and lessens the possibility of injuring a solid organ.

Classic regional anesthesia texts such as Moore, 1965, Bonica, 1990, Collins, 1976, Datta, 1992, and Winnie, 1983 should be referred to for further details regarding techniques for other blocks, particularly the commonly used screening blocks; for example epidural, caudal, and spinal (Inberg et al, 1993).

References

Aantaa R, Kirvelä O, Lahdenperä A, Nieminen S: Transarterial brachial plexus anesthesia for hand surgery: retrospective analysis of 346 cases. J Clin Anesth 6:189–192, 1994.

Abadir AR, Humayun SG: Anesthesia for Plastic and Reconstructive Surgery. St. Louis, Mosby–Year Book, 1991.

Abadir AR, Silverstein JH: A curved needle technique for celiac plexus and lumbar sympathetic block. Anesth Analg 70:1, 1990.

Baronowski AP, Pither CE: A comparison of three methods of axillary brachial plexus anesthesia. Anesthesia 45:632–635, 1990.

Bietar R: Comparison of local anesthetics. J Pharmacol 56:221, 1936.

Boas RA: Lumbar sympathectomy—a percutaneous chemical technique. In Bonica JJ, Albe-Fessard D: Advances in Pain Research and Therapy, Vol 1. New York, Raven Press, 1976, pp 685–690.

Bonica JJ: The Management of Pain, Philadelphia, Lea and Febiger, 2nd ed, 1990.

Bonica JJ: Current role of nerve blocks in diagnosis and therapy of pain. In Bonica JJ: Advances in Neurology, Vol 4. New York, Raven Press, 1974.

Bonica JJ: Neurophysiologic and pathologic aspects of acute and chronic pain. Arch Surg 112:750, 1977.

Bonica JJ, Albe-Fessard D: Proceedings of the first world congress on pain. In Bonica JJ, Albe-Fessard D: Advances in Pain Research and Therapy, Vol. 1. New York, Raven Press, 1976.

Burgess PR: Patterns of discharge evoked in cutaneous nerves and their significance for sensation. In Bonica JJ: Advances in Neurology, Vol 4. New York, Raven Press, 1974.

Chapman CR: Psychological aspects of pain patient treatment. Arch Surg 112:767, 1977.

Collins VJ: Principles of Anesthesiology. Philadelphia, Lea and Febiger, 1976.

Concepcion M, Covino BG: Criteria for selecting the best local anesthetic agent. Boston, Tutorial, Department of Anesthesia, Harvard Medical School, Brigham and Women's Hospital, 1989.

Condouris GA: Effects of local anesthetics on the refractory periods of peripheral nerves. Pharmacologist 8:187, 1966.

Condouris GA: Local anesthetics as modulators of neural information. In Bonica JJ, Albe-Fessard D: Advances in Pain Research and Therapy, Vol 1. New York, Raven Press 1976.

Cousins MJ, Bridenbaugh PO (eds): Neural Blockade in Clinical Anesthesia and Management of Pain. Philadelphia, J.B. Lippincott, 1987.

Covino BG: Pharmacology of local anesthetic agents. Br J Anesth 58:701, 1986.

Covino BG, Vassallo HG: Local anesthetics: Mechanism of action and clinical use. New York, Grune & Stratton, 1976.

Datta S: Pharmacology of Local Anesthetics. Annual Refresher Course Lectures, ASA, New Orleans, 1992.

Doupe J, et al: Post traumatic pain and causalgesic syndrome. J Neurosurg Psychiatry 7:33, 1944.

Fetz ED: Pyramidal tract effects on interneurons in the cat lumbar dorsal horn. J Neurophysiol 31:69, 1968.

Iggo A: The case for pain receptors. In Payne JP, Burt RAP (ed): Pain: Basic Principles, Pharmacology Training. London, Churchill Livingston, 1972.

Inberg P, Tarkilla PJ, Neuvonen PJ, Vilkkiss: Regional anesthesia for microvascular surgery: A combination of brahcial plexus, spinal and epidural blocks. Reg Anesth 18:98–102, 1993.

Kapral S, Kraft GP, Eibenberger K, Fitzgerald R, Gosch J, Weinstable C: Ultrasound-guided supraclavicular approach for regional brachial plexus. Anesth Analg. 78:507–513, 1994.

Koscielniak-Nielson ZJ, Horn A: Radial or brachial artery injections for intraarterial regional anesthesia for hand surgery? Reg Anesth 19:402–407, 1994.

Kramer HS, Schmidt WH: Regional Anesthesia of the Maxillofacial Region in Facial Pain, 2nd ed. Philadelphia, Lea and Febiger, 1977.

Melzack R: Psychological concepts and methods for the control of pain. In Bonica JJ: Advances in Neurology, Vol 4. New York, Raven Press, 1974.

Melzack R, Wall PD: Pain mechanism: A new theory. Science 150:971, 1965.

Merskey H, Spear FG: Pain: Psychological and Psychiatric Aspects. London, Baillière Tindall and Cassell Ltd, 1967.

Moore DC: Regional Anesthesia. Springfield, Charles C Thomas, 1965.

Murphy T: Current status of diagnostic and therapeutic nerve blocks. In 28th Annual Refresher Course Lectures. American Society of Anesthesiologists, 1977.

Noordenbos W: Pathologic aspects of central pain states. In Bonica JJ: Advances in Neurology, Vol 4. New York, Raven Press, 1974.

Pagni CA: Pain due to central nervous system lesions: physiopathological considerations and therapeutical implications. In Bonica JJ: Advances in Neurology, Vol 4. New York, Raven Press, 1974.

Perl ER: Is pain a specific sensation? J Psychiatr Res 8:272, 1971.

Rucci FS, Pippa P, Boccaccini A, Barbaglir: Effects of injection speed on anesthetic spread during axillary block using the orthogonal two needle technique. Europ J Anesth 12:4505–4511, 1995.

Sessle BJ, Greenwood LF: Role of trigeminal nucleus caudalis in the modulation of trigeminal sensory and motor neuronal activities. *In* Bonica JJ, Albe-Fessard D: Advances in Pain Research and Therapy, Vol 4. New York, Raven Press, 1976.

Singelyn FJ, Dangoisse M, Bartholomee S, Goiuverneur JM: Adding clonidine to mepivacaine prolongs the duration of anesthesia and analgesia after axillary brachial plexus block. Reg Anesth *17:*148–150, 1992.

Sternback RA: Pain: A Psychophysiologic Analysis. New York, Academic Press, 1968.

Taub A: Local, segmental supraspinal interaction with a dorsolateral spinal cutaneous afferent system. Exper Neurol *10:*357, 1964.

Wall PD: The Laminar organization of dorsal horn and effects of descending impulses. J Physiol *188:*403, 1967.

Wall PD, Melzack R: Textbook of Pain, 3rd ed. New York, Churchill Livingstone, 1994.

Winnie AP: Regional anesthesia. Surg Clin North Am *55*(4):861–892, 1975.

Winnie AP: Plexus Anesthesia: Perivascular Techniques of Brachial Plexus Block. Philadelphia, W. B. Saunders Company, 1983.

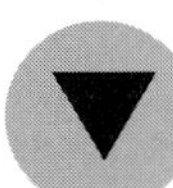

Chapter 9

• E. F. Shaw Wilgis

Special Diagnostic Studies

Diagnostic studies can be used in the search for an answer to peripheral nerve problems in addition to the standard tests, including physical examination and electrodiagnostic evaluation of the peripheral nerves. Most of these tests require the examining surgeon along with the aid of ancillary personnel. No one study is, in itself, diagnostic but should be used as an aid in the complete assessment of any given problem.

MAGNETIC RESONANCE IMAGING

High-resolution imaging of the upper extremity requires the use of surface coils and preferably mid- and high-field scanners with adequate gradient strength. Although they are less confining to the obese or claustrophobic patient, some low- and mid-field scanners may not have a large enough signal-to-noise ratio to produce state-of-the-art diagnostic quality imaging of the anatomy in the upper extremity.

The examination is tailored to the clinical problem. Routine examination of the upper extremity includes T1-weighted spin echo axial and coronal images, spin density and T2-weighted fast spin echo axial images, gradient echo coronal and axial images with repetition time (TR) 400–500 ms, an echo time (TE) 10 ms with a 20-degree flip angle, and a sagittal T1-weighted sequence. Magnetic resonance imaging (MRI) of the soft tissue, and particularly nerves, is useful in determining the location and involvement of tumors, particularly primary nerve tumors (Figs. 9–1 to 9–3). MRI can also be used to demonstrate nerve compression such as carpal tunnel syndrome as described by Mesgarzadeh and associates (1989).

MRI is also useful in evaluation of the cervical spine, and compression of the spinal cord and the roots by osteophyte formation in the foramina and is used extensively in the neurosurgical arena.

When evaluating lesions about the brachial plexus, especially metastatic disease causing brachial plexus symptoms,

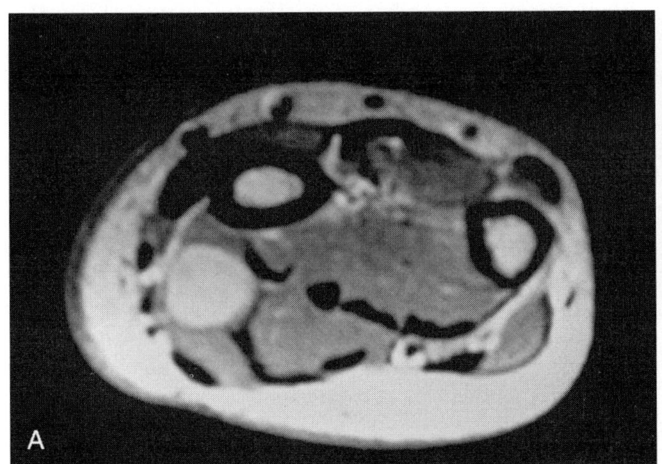

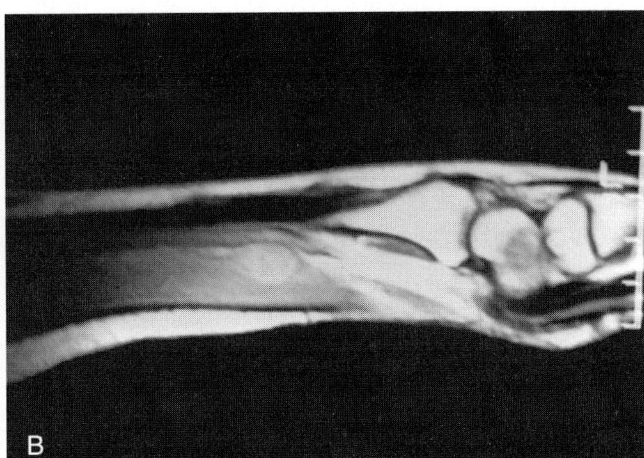

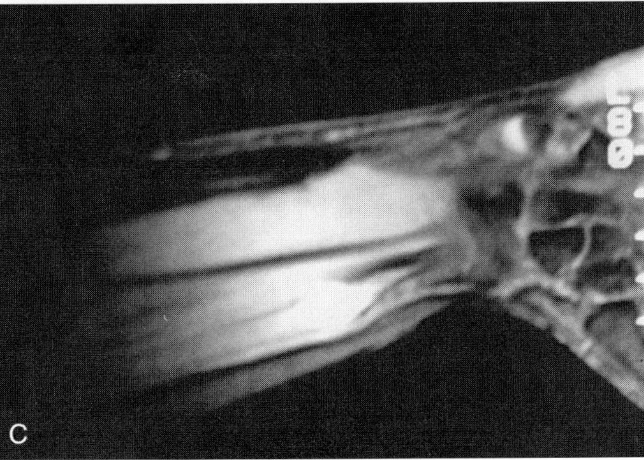

FIGURE 9–1. MRI of forearm showing median nerve tumor in cross section *(A)* and in lateral *(B)* and oblique *(C)* planes.

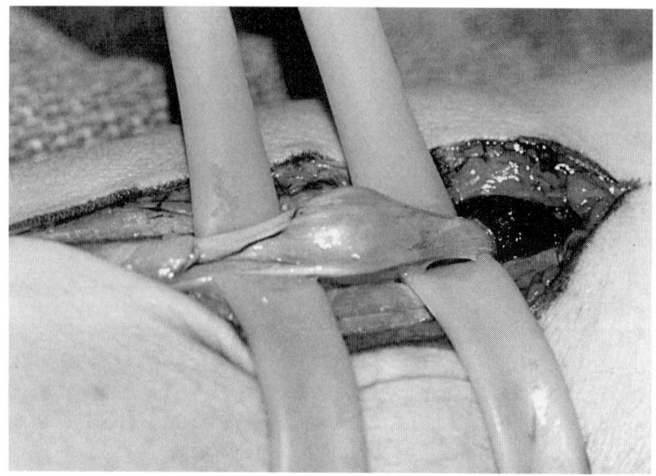

FIGURE 9–2. Median nerve exposed with intraneural tumor.

MRI is extremely useful because it gives the most complete picture of the anatomy and of lesions that can potentially cause brachial plexus nerve symptoms.

VASCULAR TESTS

The function of the peripheral nerves and extremity can be directly related to the quality of the circulation in the extremity. Studies by this author as well as others have shown that nerves respond quickly to ischemia, and if that ischemia is prolonged, they show a prolonged recovery (Wilgis et al, 1974). In 1917, Tinel described the consequences of ischemia from severing a main artery, and this was reconfirmed by Sedden in 1972.

Ischemia can be produced in several different ways. First, as a result of injury, there is occlusion of a major vessel that includes division, thrombosis, or embolism. Second, ischemia can be produced by a compressive force such as hematoma, subfascial edema, or a tumor growing in a closed space. These two methods of producing ischemia have two separate effects. First, there is a local effect on the adjacent nerve. This local effect is an ischemic neuritis or compression defect within a segmental area of that given nerve. Second, and just as important, is the distal effect of an ischemic event. This effect can involve the entire physiologic function of the nerve, including the sensory and motor end organs. We see this distal effect more often in the vascular lesions of diabetes, collagen vascular diseases, and severe peripheral arteriosclerosis, in which the entire circulatory input into the extremity is diminished.

For all of these reasons, it is most important to include a thorough vascular examination in any patient with a peripheral nerve lesion. The normal physical examination including blood pressure recordings, the palpation of pulses, and measurement of skin temperature should be performed. Specific maneuvers such as the Adson test and hyperabduction, which examines the shoulder, can be helpful in pinpointing local compressive forces. Several special diagnostic studies of varying degrees of complexity are also discussed.

The Allen Test

The Allen test is a useful clinical test to determine the patency of one of the arteries in a double arterial supply system. This is particularly useful in the hand, which is supplied by both the radial and ulnar arteries. The Allen test consists of compressing both the radial and ulnar arteries and then emptying the hand of all blood by flexion and extension of the digits. The pressure is then removed from the radial artery, and the hand is allowed to fill. The test is repeated by releasing pressure to the ulnar artery, and again the hand is allowed to fill. If one of the two arteries is occluded or if the palmar arch is incomplete, the compromised circulation will then become evident. In a study of 70 healthy subjects, Mozersky and colleagues (1973) reported that 1.6% had an incomplete radial dominant palmar arch with no antegrade circulation and that 8.4% had poor antegrade and retrograde collateral circulation, indicating the importance of detecting the adequacy of the entire arterial tree. A variant of this test can also be used in the digit by selectively compressing either digital artery and testing the capillary filling of that particular digit.

NONINVASIVE VASCULAR TESTING

Ultrasound

Sound is a longitudinal wave prorogated through a medium by mechanical stimulation. It can be categorized by frequency or the number of cycles per second (hertz [Hz]). Audible sound is generally described as ranging from 20 to 20,000 Hz. Ultrasound is defined as sound above the audible range and is measured in millions of cycles per second (megahertz). Ultrasound can be further subdivided into to basic types: (1) Doppler ultrasound and (2) pulse echo ultrasound.

DOPPLER ULTRASOUND

Doppler ultrasound uses the Doppler effect to evaluate the change in the sound wave reflected from the moving red blood cells. It studies the speed of the object or red blood

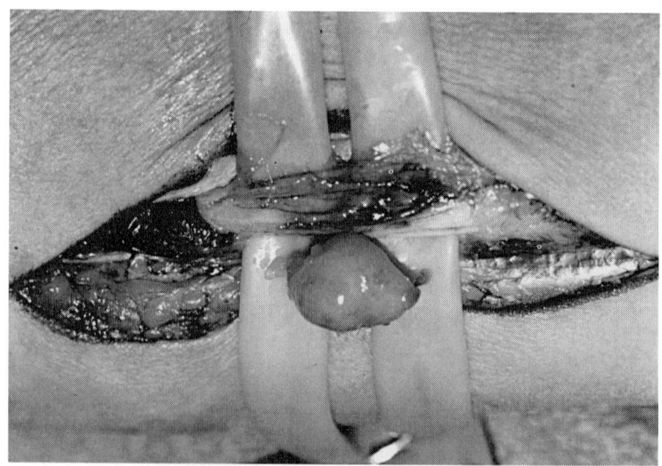

FIGURE 9–3. Median nerve tumor excised.

cells, the direction of their motion, or even more simply, the presence of motion itself. The gathered information is thus hemodynamic.

The heart of the Doppler ultrasound unit is a piezoelectric crystal. This crystal produces electrical energy when its physical state is altered. It is capable of transforming electrical energy into mechanical energy and vice versa. In practice, an oscillator in the unit vibrates at a set frequency and applies electrical energy to the crystal. This energy is then transformed into mechanical energy or sound and is transmitted to the body through an acoustic gel. The sound is reflected back to the crystal after deflection off the moving red blood cells. The sound waves are then transformed back into electrical energy by a second piezoelectric crystal, amplified, and displayed as a needle deflection cathode ray tracing, recorded analog tracing, or audio output. The full range of reflected frequencies in this signal can be studied in greater detail if processed by a spectrum analyzer.

Continuous Wave Doppler Unit. A continuous wave Doppler unit contains two crystals: (1) one to send signals and (2) the other to receive signals. This gives a steady stream of emitted ultrasound. It indiscriminately samples blood flow velocity, mixing all the various velocities found across the vessel. A further refinement will allow it to separate flow by its direction and is particularly helpful in upper extremity vascular examinations. These units are often found outside of the vascular laboratory and increasingly are a major component of the clinical examination.

Pulsed Wave Doppler Unit. A second type of Doppler unit is the pulsed wave Doppler unit, which contains just one crystal that sends and receives short bursts of sound. This method results in a more discrete sampling of the blood flow and can be very effective in localizing small areas of disturbed or turbulent flow. These units are most commonly found in vascular laboratories.

Velocity. The reflected sound from both continuous and pulsed Doppler units is dependent on multiple factors summarized in the Doppler Equation.

$$F = \frac{2 \mathrm{feV}(\cos 0)}{C}$$

In this equation, F = frequency shift (i.e., pitch), fe = frequency of transmitted sound, V = velocity of object (blood cells), 0 = incident angle, and C = velocity of sound in the medium. Because it is assumed that the Doppler unit probe frequency is constant throughout the examination, that the incident angle is a prescribed constant, and that the velocity of sound in the body is a constant, the listener is essentially hearing a frequency shift. This shift or pitch difference is directly dependent on the velocity of the object or red blood cells.

A common misconception is that pressure or force of flow is heard. Remembering that velocity equals pressure divided by resistance clarifies this falsehood. Another misconception is that the louder the signal, the better the blood flow. Signal loudness is a function of sound beam placement in relation to mainstream flow. It may also be a function of the selection of the appropriate Doppler transmitting frequency for the depth of the vessel.

When listening to a Doppler signal, it is important to be able to distinguish arterial from venous flow. Abnormal arterial signals can often resemble those of normal veins. The reverse may also be true. Remembering basic vessel hemodynamics will help. Normal arterial signals are pulsatile with a clear biphasic or triphasic sound resembling that of a heartbeat. The signals normally become more monophasic as the vessels become more distal. This phenomenon is a reflection of the decreasing peripheral resistance in the capillary beds. Normal venous signals are phasic against respiration with the sound ebbing and flowing in response to inhalation and exhalation, respectively. Venous signals are said to resemble the sounds of a wind tunnel (Strandness et al, 1966). Following replantation, venous return through repaired veins may pulsate and sound similar to arterial flow.

PULSE ECHO ULTRASOUND

The second type of ultrasound is pulse echo ultrasound. Sound is transmitted into the body in short bursts, and the time until the echo is returned is measured. A two-dimensional image is produced as differing proportions of sound are reflected by the interfaces between the different tissue layers. Although several types of pulse echo ultrasound are available, the most commonly used is brightness mode or B mode. The resulting image is an anatomic or structural representation of the vessel's contour and diameter. When B-mode images are rapidly viewed and erased many times per second, the vessels appear to be moving. This technique is called *real-time imaging.* Arteries can be seen pulsing, and veins can be collapsed with compression.

DUPLEX ULTRASOUND UNIT

A duplex ultrasound unit combines information from a pulsed Doppler and a real-time pulse echo unit simultaneously. It provides both functional and structural information. A further refinement displays the Doppler information in a color-coded visual format, producing dramatic pictures of vessel dynamics and the corresponding anatomic structures. This type of imaging is most commonly used to study the carotid arteries and the major arteries and veins of the lower extremities. It can be used, however, in examining the arteries at the wrist, in the palm, and in the digits themselves. Masses can be examined for vascularity. Flow through dialysis shunts or arterial bypass grafts can be studied.

Segmental Systolic Pressures

The second vascular testing tool is segmental systolic blood pressures. By combining an occlusive cuff and a Doppler unit, systolic blood pressures can be easily obtained at any level. Pressure patterns can be used to diagnose major or small vessel disease. They can be valuable when differentiating ischemia from other causes of rest pain. Pressures can be measured before and after exercise to detect work claudication (Darling et al, 1972).

Plethysmography

The third vascular testing tool is plethysmography. This method is probably the oldest technique to measure blood flow. It uses limb or digit volume changes to indirectly measure flow. Air-filled cuffs or photo sensors are usually used. Less commonly used techniques are mercury strain gauges or impedance sensors.

Air or pneumoplethysmography measures dimensional changes in a limb or digit in response to a change in blood content. These minute changes occur as a result of net blood flow into the limb or digit through pulsatile heart beats or an interruption in venous return during respiration. The Pulse Volume Recorder (Life Sciences, Greenwich, Connecticut) is one such plethysmograph that measures the limb volume changes through pressure transducers connected to air-filled cuffs (Raines et al, 1973). Specific pressure within the cuff is obtained by injecting a specific volume of air. This specificity ensures calibration and reliability of the resulting analog tracings. It also allows for comparison of results from digit to digit or test to test.

Photoplethysmography uses a photopulse transducer to emit near infrared light into the superficial tissue layers. A phototransistor creates a voltage output in proportion to the amount of back-scattered light from the capillary bed. Although not a true plethysmograph in the strictest interpretation, arterial pulsations or venous return can be recorded as an analog tracing identical to that of the pneumoplethysmographs. It cannot be easily calibrated and thus has more limited applications.

Volume pulse tracings from all types of plethysmographs can be used to demonstrate arterial contractility and perfusion. Normal arteries show a sharp upstroke with good amplitude and a second dicrotic notch. The volume tracings from diseased or stenotic vessels show a rounding of the upstroke and decreased amplitude. The dicrotic notch often disappears. Occluded arteries progress toward a straight-line tracing.

Segmental systolic pressures and volume tracings provide complementary information. Segmental pressures supply information from a specific artery or a specific section of an artery. Plethysmographic volume tracings present information on total limb or digit flow. An extremity or digit may have an arterial occlusion and still have a small volume tracing. This finding would reflect collateral flow, an important diagnostic finding.

BASIC NONINVASIVE EXAMINATION

One of the most important parts of an upper extremity examination is taking a thorough and detailed vascular-related history. The significance of this history is often overlooked. The wider the technologist's knowledge in the fields of internal medicine, vascular surgery, rheumatology, orthopedics, and the extremities, the more complete the history and testing will be. Subtle nuances can alter the testing procedures and subsequent therapy. Medical and surgical history, occupational activities, and physical limitations are all areas that require detailed review. Careful attention should also be paid to smoking patterns, intolerance to cold, and changes in skin color (Buehner and Koontz, 1993).

This step is followed by a basic clinical vascular examination, including both manual pulse palpations and Doppler signals. By using a standardized legend and hand mapping chart, this subjective information becomes a more objective testing reference.

Next, segmental systolic blood pressures and volume pulse tracings are taken at the upper arm, forearm, and digital levels. Both radial and ulnar forearm pressures are taken. Custom-designed digital cuffs allow for a very sensitive volume tracing. A modified Allen's test using plethysmography can provide information about artery dominance or occlusion. A similar procedure on a specific digit could provide information on isolated digital artery occlusion. When interpreting segmental pressures, a 20-mm Hg difference at different extremity locations is generally considered indicative of disease. The pattern of the segmental pressures can be used to localize stenosis or occlusion. These absolute segmental pressures can be valuable in differentiating ischemia from other causes of reported pain. The probability of claudication limiting activity or ischemia inhibiting wound healing can also be suggested. The total functional effect from multiple areas of stenosis can be accurately measured.

An index is then calculated for each level by dividing the systolic pressure for that area by the higher brachial pressure. This index indicates the amount of potential blood flow actually reaching that area. It allows for comparison of pressures over time when brachial pressures have changed. It also allows for comparison against standardized criteria. A normal index is 1.00 or higher. An index of 0.75 is generally associated with work-induced claudication. An index of 0.50 or lower usually indicates ischemic rest pain.

Formal protocols are established for specific vascular conditions and are thus requested by the referring physician. During the actual testing, however, the technologist must integrate the presenting symptoms, the patient history, and the preliminary findings to individualize each examination.

SUMMARY

In conclusion, the vascular system cannot be separated from the nervous system. When patients present with pain, paresthesias, and paralysis, they may well have a vascular lesion alone or a lesion that derives from both the nervous and the vascular systems. Complete evaluation of the vascular system, including the physical examination and the noninvasive testing, yields important information in the diagnosis of peripheral nerve problems.

References

Buehner JW, Koontz CL: The examination in the vascular laboratory. Hand Clin 9:5–11, 1993.

Darling RD, Raines JK, Brener BJ, Austen WG: Quantitative segmental pulse volume recorded: A clinical tool. Surgery 72:873, 1972.

Mesgarzadeh M, Schneck CD, Bonakdarpour A: Carpal tunnel: MR imaging. Part I. Normal Anatomy. Radiology 171:743–748, 1989.

Mesgarzadeh M, Schneck CK, Bonakdarpour A, et al: Carpal tunnel: MR imaging. Part II. Carpal tunnel syndrome. Radiology 171:749–754, 1989.

Mozersky DJ, Buckley CJ, Hagood CO Jr, Capps WF Jr, Dannemiller FJ Jr: Ultrasonic evaluation of the palmar circulation—a useful adjunct to radial artery cannulation. Am J Surg 126:810, 1973.

Raines JK, Jaffrin MY, Rao S: A noninvasive pressure pulse recorder development and rationale. Med Instrum 7:245, 1973.

Seddon H: Surgical Disorders of the Peripheral Nerves. Baltimore, Williams & Wilkins, 1972.

Strandness DE Jr, McCutcheon EF, Rushmer RF. Application of a transcutaneous Doppler flowmeter in evaluation of occlusive arterial disease. Surg Gynecol Obstet 122:1039, 1966.

Tinel J: Nerve Wounds. London, England, Bailliere, Tindall, and Cox, 1917.

Wilgis EFSW, Jezic D, Stonesifer GL Jr, Classen JN, Sekercan K: The evaluation of small vessel flow. J Bone Joint Surg 56A:1199, 1974.

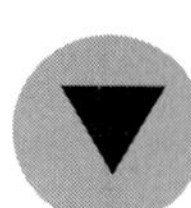

Chapter 10

- James D. Collins
- Marla L. Shaver
- Anthony C. Disher
- Theodore Q. Miller

Bilateral Magnetic Resonance Imaging of the Brachial Plexus and Peripheral Nerve Imaging: Technique and Three-Dimensional Color

Computed tomography (CT) and magnetic resonance imaging (MRI) are special radiographic modalities used to image the thorax, shoulder girdle, soft tissues (Collins et al, 1986). Vascular structures, surface anatomy, and the soft tissues are incompletely imaged by conventional x-ray techniques. CT extends the capabilities of x-ray imaging to obtain detailed transverse (axial) anatomic sections, but CT does not definitively distinguish tumors from vascular or neurovascular structures, or both. CT myelography allows imaging of spinal nerves; however, CT does not allow satisfactory images of the soft tissues. CT three-dimensional imaging of soft tissue anatomy is not satisfactory, and detailed peripheral nerve imaging is not possible. Multi-planer MRI displays the anatomy of the brachial plexus and peripheral nerves for investigation by sequential imaging of landmark anatomy according to proton density distribution (Collins et al, 1993).

The anatomy of the brachial plexus and peripheral nerves are graphically displayed in classic textbooks (Fig. 10–1) (Clemente, 1985, 1987). Anatomic and clinicopathologic nerve models allowed investigative radiological studies using MRI to correlate textbook descriptions (Fig. 10–2). Bilateral brachial plexus and peripheral nerve MRI three-dimensional reconstruction imaging makes possible demonstration of the relationship of nerves to their surrounding landmark anatomy. The knowledge of peripheral nerve and brachial plexus anatomical imaging offers new avenues in the teaching of medical students, residents, and other health professionals (Collins et al, 1991a; 1993). Understanding MRI of soft tissue landmark anatomy requires review of the brachial plexus anatomy.

The brachial plexus lies within the fascial planes of the neck and axilla, but it is routinely displayed on MRI of the thorax and shoulder girdle (Collins et al, 1986). Multiplane MRI in the supine position allows bilateral sequential imaging of the neck, thorax, and the brachial plexus. Mutiplanar sequential imaging gave us the idea to image a gross section of the brachial plexus from a fresh cadaver (Collins et al, 1989). As a result of our findings, we began to perform bilateral MRI of the brachial plexus and peripheral nerves. The anatomy and compromising abnormalities of the bra-

chial plexus and three-dimensional color images were displayed with MRI (Collins 1991a; 1993).

Disorders of the cervicothoracic vertebral column, first rib, vasculature supply, and soft tissues are compromising abnormalities of the brachial plexus and/or brachial plexopathies (Lord and Rosati, 1971; Lord, 1989). The anterior and middle scalene muscles, through which the brachial plexus nerve roots pass and adhere to the subclavian artery, arise from the cervicothoracic levels of the vertebral column. The muscles insert and, in part, support the first ribs. The first ribs are curved and flat, and slope obliquely to form most of the thoracic inlet. The slope that gives an antero-superiorly directed upper surface, changes with respiration, cervicothoracic spine scoliosis, pectus deformities, and affects structures crossing the rib. The anterior scalene muscle and the posterior insertion of the middle scalene muscle and the first ribs from the scalene (uneven) triangle. The change in the slope of the first rib affects the interscalene triangle contents (Collins et al, 1993; Sunderland, 1968). The scalene muscles and their effacement of the surrounding structures are important anatomical landmarks in the understanding of brachial plexopathy displayed by MRI.

The upper nerve roots of the brachial plexus descend along the margin of the middle scalene muscle and join the lower nerve roots to envelope the subclavian artery. The nerve roots bind to the artery within the scalene triangle to form a neurovascular bundle (Sunderland, 1945). This bundle passes with sympathetic fibers unprotected over the apex of the lung and first rib through the scalene triangle, beneath the clavicle and subclavius muscle, inferior to the coracoid process, and posterior to the tendon of the pectoralis minor muscle into the axilla. The imaging of these landmarks is an essential requirement to understand how effacement of the neurovascular bundle may result in clinical complaints related by patients with peripheral neurophaties.

The subclavian artery, similar to the artery within the femoral triangle, is unprotected (Clemente, 1987; Lord and Rosati, 1971), although it is not routinely cannulated for vascular studies. Different from the femoral artery, a muscle (the anterior scalene muscle) separates the subclavian vein from the subclavian artery. This makes the anterior scalene

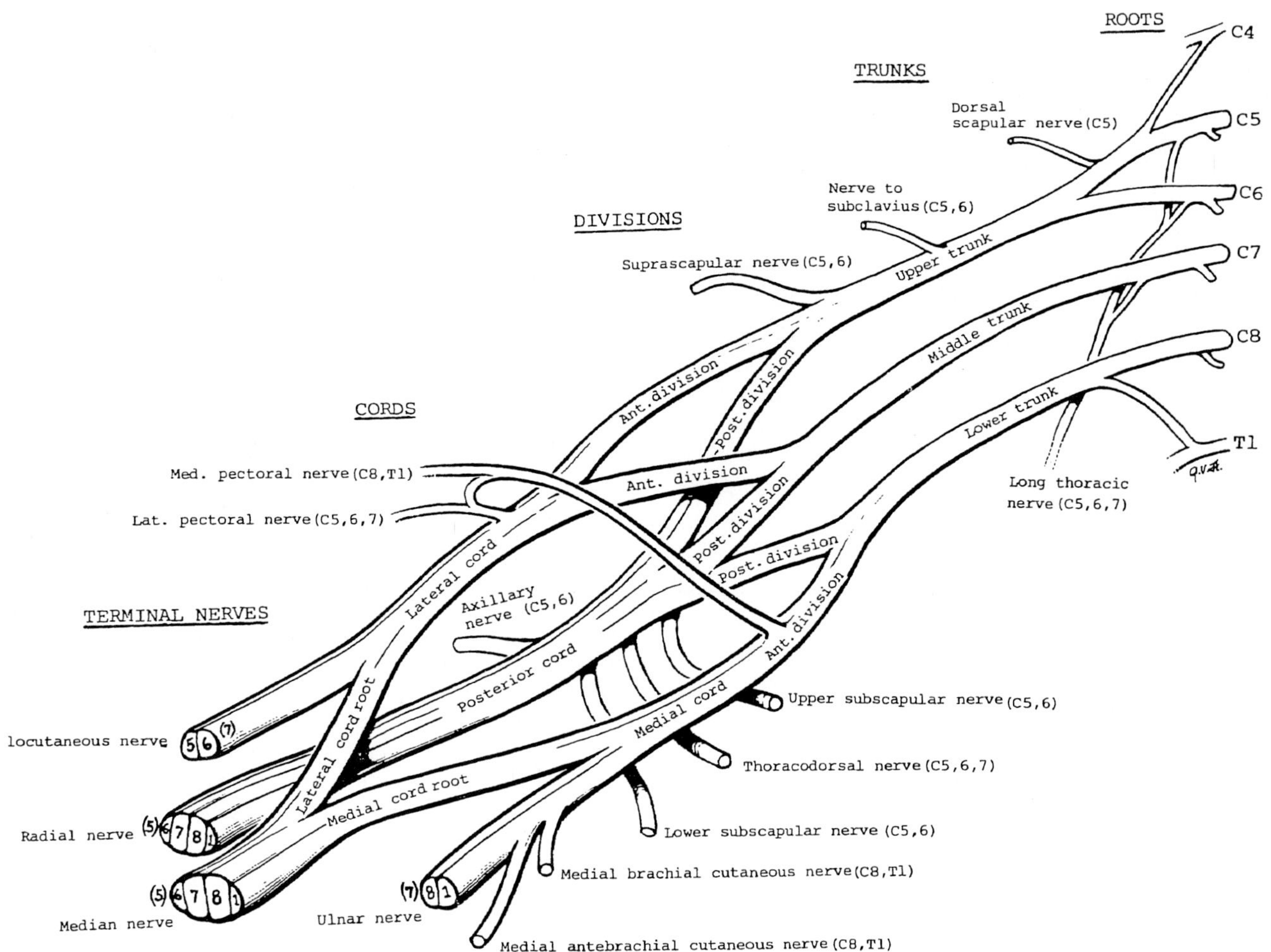

FIGURE 10–1. Diagram of the brachial plexus. (From Collins JD, Shaver ML, Disher AC, Miller TQ: Compromising abnormalities of the brachial plexus as displayed by magnetic resonance imaging. Clinical Anatomy 8:1–16, 1995. Copyright © 1995, Wiley-Liss, Inc. Reprinted by permission of Wiley-Liss, Inc., a subsidiary of John Wiley and Sons, Inc.)

muscle an important anatomical landmark in determining compression (effacement) of the contents of the scalene triangle. Enlargement of the anterior scalene muscle or atrophy of the anterior scalene muscle, or both increases or decreases the distance between the subclavian artery and the subclavian vein, as demonstrated on transverse MRI sequences (Collins et al, 1993). This distance may be measured on the first image or raw data of magnetic resonance angiography (MRA) two-dimensional Time Of Flight (TOF) of the brachial plexus (Collins et al, 1994). Abnormalities of the middle scalene muscle may also contribute changes on the MRA.

A thin layer of deep fascia envelopes the neurovascular bundle of the upper limb. Four spaces are formed from the root of the neck to the lower part of the axilla. The spaces that may have clinical problems that compromise the brachial plexus (Lord and Rosati, 1971) include the intervertebral foramina, scalene triangle, costoclavicular space, costocoracoid space, and the axilla. In most individuals, the fascial plane spacing between soft tissues and osseous structures is adequate to perform routine functions without compromising the nerves or the artery that combine to form the neurovascular bundle. Pathology involving peripheral nerves alters fascial planes. The acute or permanent changes may alter the adjacent tissues, thereby compromising the vascular supply

that nourishes the peripheral nerves (Collins et al, 1993; Dyck, 1984; Sunderland, 1968). This results in patients presenting with clinical symptoms. They may also occur from articular motion of the shoulder girdle, autoimmune disease, hypertrophic enlargement of the scalene triangle muscles, congenital rib anomalies, pressure by ligaments, instances of abnormal insertion of the scalene (anomalous) muscles, fractures (acute and chronic), primary and secondary lymphedema and tumors, crushing injuries of the thorax, and arteriosclerotic disease that results in nerve evulsions, vascular thrombosis, and ruptured silicone breast implants (Collins et al, 1993; Dyck, 1984; Lord, 1971; Sunderland 1968). Patients may complain of degenerative changes resulting in a shift in their osseous structures. Aging and laxity of their muscular structures may result in complaints originating from congenital abnormalities that were not obvious problems at a younger age (Collins et al, 1993; Lord and Rosati, 1971; Sunderland 1968).

MRI demonstrates soft tissue detail by proton distribution and provides high-resolution imaging of nerves, vascular structures, and lymphatics (Collins et al, 1986, 1991b, 1991c, 1993). The phospholipids found in the myelin of nerves (fascicles) may have intermediate- to high-intensity signals when visualized in in vitro studies and intermediate- to high-intensity signals when demonstrated in vivo. Positive-

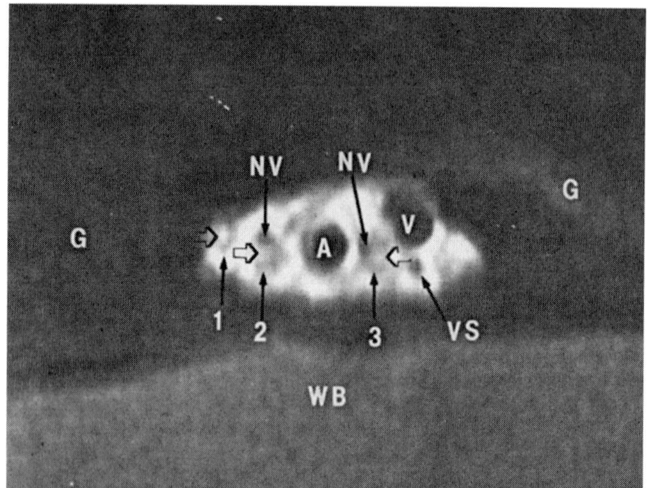

FIGURE 10–2. Transverse *magnetic resonance imaging* (MRI) scan of the gross specimen (A, artery; V, vein; and 1, 2, 3, nerve fascicles within the perineurium). The nerve fascicles *(transparent arrow)* are marginated by the intermediate low signal intensity of the perineurium. Nutrient artery (NV) superior to the nerves. The saline soaked gauze (G) and the saline water bag (WB) enhanced the imaging. (From Collins JD, Shaver ML, Batra P, Brown K: Nerves on magnetic resonance imaging. J Natl Med Assoc 81:129–134, 1989.)

mode T1-weighted images show blood flow as low signal intensities (black) and subcutaneous fat as high signal intensities (white). Diminished blood flow may appear as an intermediate signal intensity (Collins, 1989). The T1-weighted sequence displays the deep fascial layer of tissue containing the neurovascular compartments. Fast spin echo (FSE with nonfat and nonwater suppression technique) displays the long axis of peripheral nerves with high signal intensities (Collins et al, 1993). The signal-to-noise ratio decreases with FSE imaging, causing decreased contrast and resolution of the images. The low signal intensities of flowing blood and the high signal intensities of myelin combine to vary the high signal intensity of nerves. The signal intensity of nerves may then depend on the imaging axis of that nerve (Collins et al, 1986). The combination of a rich blood supply to the spinal cord and cerebrospinal fluid results in the intermediate signal intensity of the spinal cord. Nerve roots may have high signal intensities after they exit from the subarachnoid space. The low signal intensity vertical bands of nutrient vessels interrupt the high signal intensity of nerves (Collins et al, 1986, 1989, 1991c; Sunderland, 1945). Compression injuries of nerves involve an ischemic component and alter blood supply. Ischemia initiates inflammatory changes causing edema and fibrosis. Inflammation or edema, or both, diminishes the signal intensity of nerves and alters their architecture when compromised in autoimmune disease (Collins et al, 1991c).

Bilateral imaging of the brachial plexus is based on the fact that the brachial plexus envelopes and adheres to a major artery forming a neurovascular bundle, and that displaying the artery ensures imaging the nerves (Collins et al, 1995; Sunderland 1945, 1968). Bilateral imaging of the thorax is accomplished, and asymmetry of the neck and thorax may be identified. Sunderland's 1945 anatomical nerve model demonstrated the blood supply (microcirculation) of nerves (Fig. 10–3; see also color plate), and Collins and associates' (1989) gross anatomical nerve model demon-

strated with MRI the vascular supply (low signal intensity marginating the nerves), that is used to distinguish nerves from surrounding tissues (Collins et al, 1991c, Sunderland, 1945). Demonstrating effacement of the low signal surrounding a nerve has been correlated with MRIS of the brachial plexus (Collins et al, 1986; 1993; 1995). The objective of this presentation is to demonstrate a new technique that uses the knowledge of anatomy to correlate the various etiologies of thoracic outlet syndrome and to demonstrate effacement (compression) or compromising abnormalities of nerves correlated with the patients' clinical complaints, or both. Asymmetrical muscle building (seen in body builders); degenerative changes of cervical spine in a patient with bilateral cervical ribs; application of our technique to peripheral nerve (neurolemmoma) imaging of the upper extremity; an old fracture injury of the right first, second, and third ribs compromising the neurovascular bundle are the cases that have selected for presentation later in this chapter. A brief history and results are presented.

We are unable to display chest radiographs for each patient as well as the entire sequential images for the plane imaged. The images selected support each other as a group (Collins 1993, 1995; Lord and Rosati, 1971). Each image cannot be studied without considering the other images. The grainy nature of the figures (noise) results because of (1) the high magnification used, (2) the diminished signal intensity due to the small amount of fat and increased muscle mass, as is seen in body builders (Collins et al, 1993, 1995), and

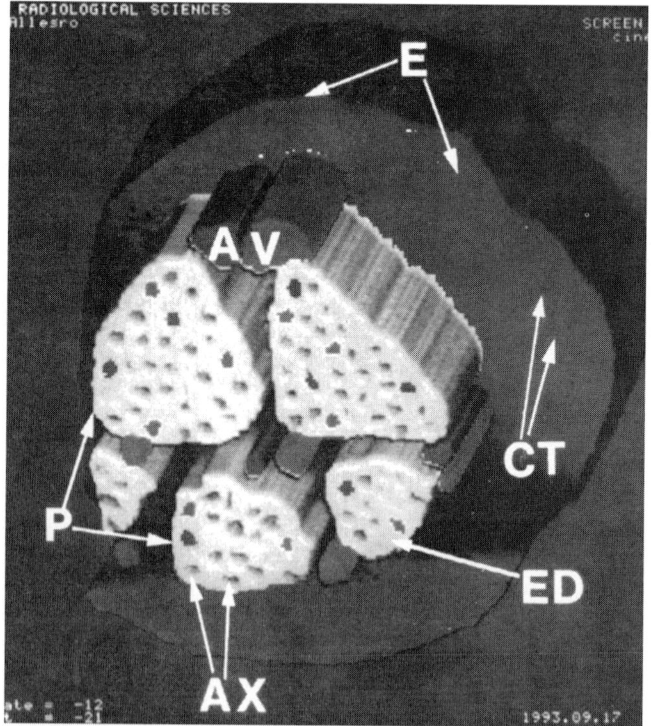

FIGURE 10–3. This is a three-dimensional, computer-generated transverse section of a peripheral nerve demonstrating the rich nutrient blood supply that Sunderland described in 1945. The collateral blood vessels have been omitted. Epineurium (E), small dark capillaries *(arrows)* in the red connective tissue (CT), rich nutrient supply to nerves. A, Arteries; V, veins; P, perineurium; ED, endoneurium; and AX, axons. (See also color plate.) (From Collins JD, Shaver ML, Disher AC, Miller TQ: Compromising abnormalities of the brachial plexus as displayed by magnetic resonance imaging. Clinical Anatomy 8:1–16, 1995. Copyright © 1995, Wiley-Liss, Inc. Reprinted by permission of Wiley-Liss, Inc., a subsidiary of John Wiley and Sons, Inc.)

(3) the 512 × 256 matrix 2 NEX increases the resolution but decreases contrast, resulting in a grainy appearance. The enlarged and windowed images demonstrate the anatomy of the brachial plexus by gray scale MRI. The three dimensional color reconstruction images simplify landmark anatomy and display compromising abnormalities of the neurovascular bundles.

METHODS AND MATERIALS

Magnetic Resonance Imaging Technique

The clinical history, physical examination, available neurological studies, and any outside radiographic studies are reviewed prior to the MRI examination. A posteroanterior and lateral radiograph is obtained and reviewed prior to the bilateral brachial plexus or peripheral nerve MRI, or both. The chest radiograph is obtained to detect osseous abnormalities or the possibility of unsuspected metallic objects. The procedure is discussed and the patient examined. Respiratory gating is applied throughout the procedure to minimize motion artifact and maximize the contrast of the soft tissue signal intensities. The patient is positioned supine in the body coil, arms down to the side, and imaging is monitored at the MRI station.

A body coil is used because it offers optimal full field of view for bilateral imaging of the brachial plexus and provides uniform signal-to-noise ratio across the imaging field that is necessary for three-dimensional reconstruction. Surface coils are limited to depth and field of view, and are not adequate for bilateral imaging of the brachial plexus. Intravenous contrast agents are not administered. A water bag (500 ml of normal saline) is placed on the right and the left sides of the neck above the shoulder girdle to increase the signal-to-noise ratio for higher resolution imaging. A full field of view (40–48 cm) of the neck and the thorax is used to image both supraclavicular fossae. Contiguous (4–5 mm) coronal, transverse (axial), oblique transverse, and sagittal T1-weighted images are obtained. If there is clinical evidence of scarring, tumor, or lymphatic obstruction, T2-weighted images or fast spin echo (FSE) pulse sequences are obtained. A minimal of four imaging sequences are acquired—coronal, transverse, oblique transverse, and sagittal. A coronal abduction and external rotation of the upper extremities may be obtained to determine if the change in arm position mimics the clinical complaint.

The coronal sequence is the first series to be imaged. The brachial plexus envelopes the artery (forming a neurovascular bundle), and the nerves are best imaged when the cursors are aligned to the arterial blood supply. The axillary artery margins vary in each patient, and the cursors must be adjusted for each bilateral MRI brachial plexus examination. The cursors are positioned from the skin surface of the posterior chest wall to the skin surface of the anterior chest wall for symmetry and three-dimensional reconstruction, and to detect abnormalities that may mimic brachial plexopathies. The superior landmark is set at the base of the skull, and the inferior landmark is set at the level of the kidneys. The image that best demonstrates the arterial blood flow to the upper extremities is selected as the baseline image for the remaining sequences. The transverse sequence is set from the baseline coronal image at the superior aspect of the

third cervical vertebral body to the carina. The lateral margins of the shoulder girdle are imaged to ensure bilateral, simultaneous display of the brachial plexus. The oblique transverse sequence is set by aligning the cursors to the arterial blood supply of each upper extremity using the baseline coronal sequence. The cursors are centered to the plane of the axillary artery 2 cm below the inferior cord of the brachial plexus to the superior margin of the coracoid process. This sequence is necessary to detect signal intensity, architecture, and effacement of the long axis of the nerves, arteries, and veins.

The sagittal sequence is obtained by aligning the cursors lateral to the coracoid process, medially to include the insertion of the anterior scalene muscle on the first rib and the middle third of the first thoracic vertebral body. It is necessary to use the sagittal plane to detect effacement of the neurovascular bundle by the coracoid process, pectoralis minor muscle, clavicle or subclavius muscle, axillary masses, and abnormalities of the scalene triangle. When an image sequence is completed, it is immediately transferred to another screen at an independent work station for review and three-dimensional reformat display. The software for this type of three-dimensional reconstruction is already prepared in the 1.5 Tesla General Electric Signa MRI scanner (General Electric Medical Systems, Milwaukee, Wisconsin). The images are stored on CT tape (GE 9800) format and on optical disks for three-dimensional color reconstruction on the ISG workstation (ISG Technologies Inc, Mississauga, Ontario, Canada). The entire study is monitored by the radiologist and requires 1½ hours. Selected Kodak color and black and white laser prints and transparencies are obtained for lectures and poster presentations, and annotated images are preserved on VHS, archived digital tapes, or optical discs.

Equipment

MRIs are obtained on the 1.5 Tesla General Electric Signa MRI scanner. The three-dimensional reformatted images are videotaped on a separate work console at the monitoring station, and computerized color is applied to the images using a ISG console (ISG Technologies Inc, Mississauga, Ontario, Canada). A 512 × 256 matrix format is used. The saline water bags are those supplied for intravenous use. There is no need for special prepared saline containers.

CASE REPORTS

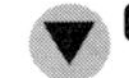 **CASE 1:**

BODY BUILDER: The patient is a 37-year-old, 87.0-kg asymmetrically built man with a 6- to 8-year history of excessive daily body building. He describes a 3-year history of bilateral equal pain in the upper extremities, and tingling and numbness of all fingers in the neutral and stress position (glovelike distribution); he describes an insensitivity to temperature for periods of 1 to 3 days with painful numbness that was relieved by weight lifting. Nerve conduction studies that were performed at another institution indicate a mild slowing of conduction velocity along the ulnar nerve measured at the elbow and a bilateral

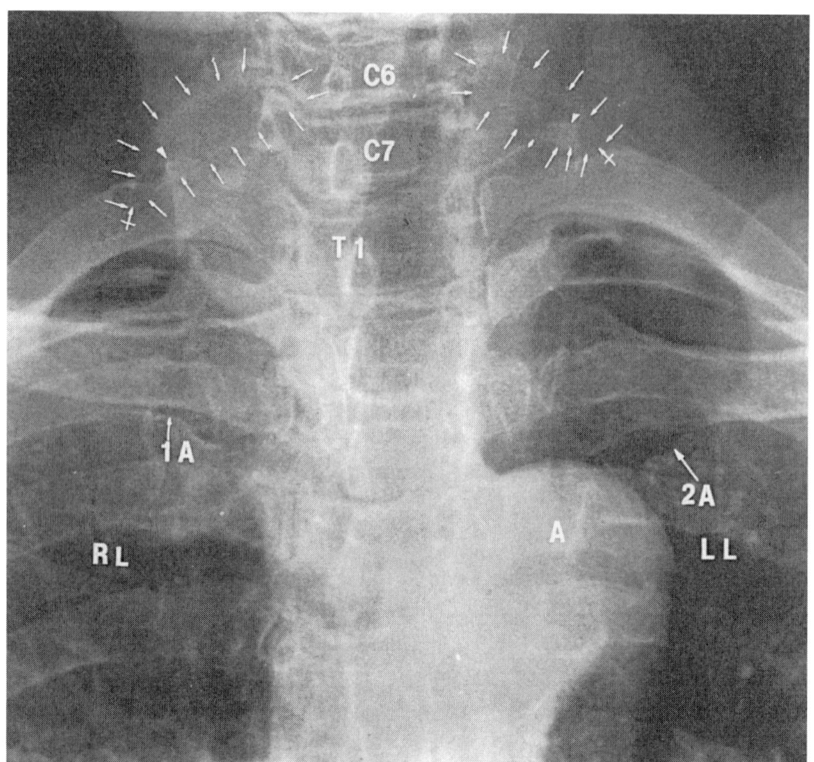

FIGURE 10–7. This is a posteroanterior (PA) chest radiograph demonstrating an apparent rotated appearance secondary to scoliosis. The larger right and left ribs are marginated by small arrows. Aorta (A), superior margin right first (1A) and left first ribs (2A), cervical vertebral bodies (C6, C7) transverse process of the right and left T1 vertebra *(arrowheads),* right lung (RL), left lung (LL), and ends of cervical ribs *(single bar arrow).* (From Collins JD, Batra P, Brown K, Shaver ML: Anatomy of the thorax and shoulder girdle as displayed by magnetic resonance imaging. J Natl Med Assoc *83:*46–52, 1991a.)

ribs at the sternum were present. The cervical ribs were small, asymmetrical, posterior, and faintly displayed. The right cervical rib was larger and angled anteromedially to its lower insertion on the first rib.

The bilateral brachial plexus MRI examination demonstrated asymmetrical cervical vertebral spine pillars, cervicothoracic spine scoliosis, degenerative compression of the cervicothoracic vertebra, and bilateral cervical ribs. The right cervical rib compressed the C8 and T1 nerve root proximal to the formation of the displaced inferior trunk (Fig. 10–8). The left cervical rib caused minimal superior effacement of the left eighth cervical nerve root and the adjacent sympathetic nerves.

The coronal images were the best sequence of the series to demonstrate the asymmetrical degenerative changes of the cervical spine pillars (higher on the right than left) and compression of the cervical vertebral bodies (C4–C6). The nerve roots followed the asymmetry of the cervical spine. Degenerative changes of the acromioclavicular joint accentuated the inferior angulation of the right clavicle and subclavius muscle. The subclavian arteries formed high loops over the first ribs, with the right subclavian artery higher than the left. The right cervical rib effaced the subclavian artery, the eighth cervical nerve and the first thoracic nerve, proximal to formation of the inferior nerve trunk (IT), which was displaced anteriorly by the descending loop of the right subclavian artery (see Fig. 10–8). The left cervical rib did not appear to cause significant effacement of the nerve roots.

The transverse sequence demonstrated the enlarged head of the right clavicle, which bowed anteriorly as compared with the left clavicle; the asymmetrical cervicothoracic spine; and atrophy of the right scalene muscles. The right nerve roots, divisions, and terminal branches appeared smaller. The cervical rib effaced the right C8–T1 nerve roots, sympathetic nerves, and the subclavian artery as the nerve roots crossed the apex of the right lung (Fig. 10–9), and the spinal cord was tethered to the right.

Blood flow decreased in the left internal jugular vein. The bilateral oblique transverse imaging sequence confirmed the above-mentioned findings and displayed mild effacement of the C8 nerve root by the smaller left cervical rib.

The right sagittal sequence demonstrated the cervical rib effacing the C8–T1 nerve roots complementing the coronal and transverse sequences. The small recurrent laryngeal nerve parallels its origin from the vagus nerve and the adjacent superior cardiac nerves were well displayed. The left sagittal sequence was normal.

The three-dimensional computer-generated images were cross referenced to the gray scale sequential images to demonstrate the in vivo anatomical relationship between the neurovascular bundles, osseous structures, and adjacent landmark anatomy. The three-dimensional image of the cervico-thoracic spine was rotated into a posterior oblique display to accentuate the degenerative compression of C4–C6 cervical vertebral bodies, the asymmetrical cervicothoracic spine scoliosis, and the bilateral cervical ribs. The thoracic spine was convexed to the right at the T5–T6 level. The nerve roots, nerve divisions, and terminal branches of the brachial plexus were imaged separately in the three-dimensional mode, which is not demonstrated here. The right cervical rib crossed the first rib. The lateral position of the radial nerve and the medial position of the right median and the ulnar nerves reflected the internal rotation adduction of the arms with the hands on the chest wall. The left brachial plexus appeared smaller.

The nervous, osseous, and vascular structures were combined into one image (Fig. 10–10; see also color plate). The image displayed asymmetry and the loops of the subclavian arteries. The left cervical nerve root joined the sympathetic chain. The right inferior nerve trunk and the median nerve roots (lateral to the inferior trunk) arched anteriorly and over the right subclavian artery. The right subclavian artery arched high over the first rib, and the cervical rib (CR) effaced the C8–T1 nerve

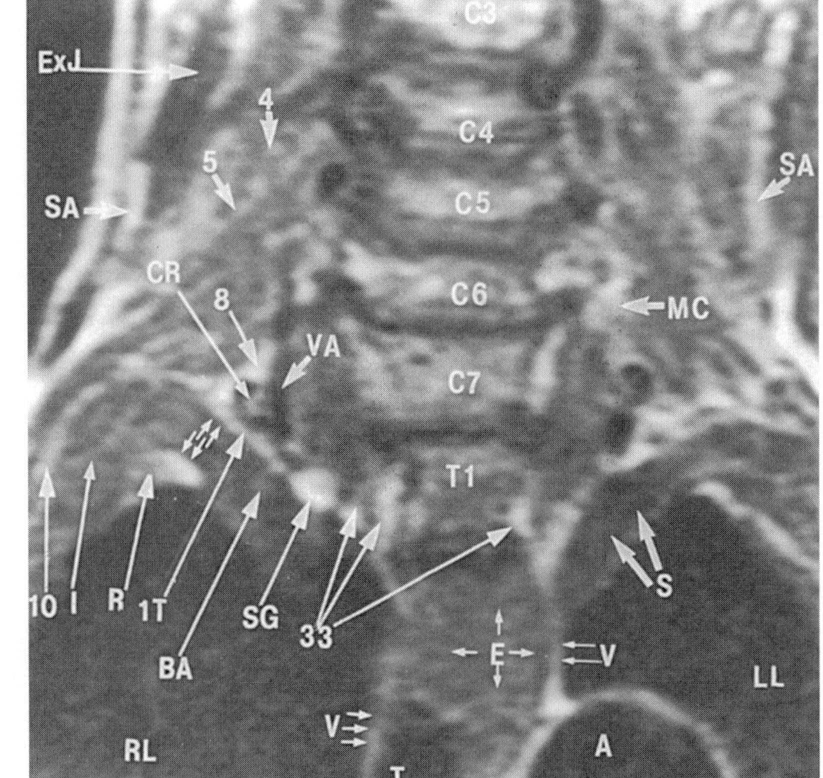

FIGURE 10–8. Image 27 of the coronal series demonstrates slight narrowing of the right subclavian artery *(four small arrows)* and compressed (C4–6) cervical vertebral bodies (C3–7). Right cervical rib (CR), C8 spinal nerve root (8), vertebral artery (VA), C4–5 spinal nerve roots (4, 5), external jugular vein (ExJ), spinal accessories nerves (SA), brachiocephalic artery (BA), first rib (R), stellate ganglia (SG), and inferior (I) and middle nerve trunks (10), sympathetic nerves and right first rib *(small arrows),* first thoracic nerve root (1T), right and left vagus nerves (V), first thoracic vertebra (T1), right (RL) and left (LL) lungs, recurrent laryngeal nerves (33), left subclavian artery (S), trachea (T), esophagus (E), and aorta (A). (From Collins JD, Batra P, Brown K, Shaver ML: Anatomy of the thorax and shoulder girdle as displayed by magnetic resonance imaging. J Natl Med Assoc *83*:46–52, 1991a.)

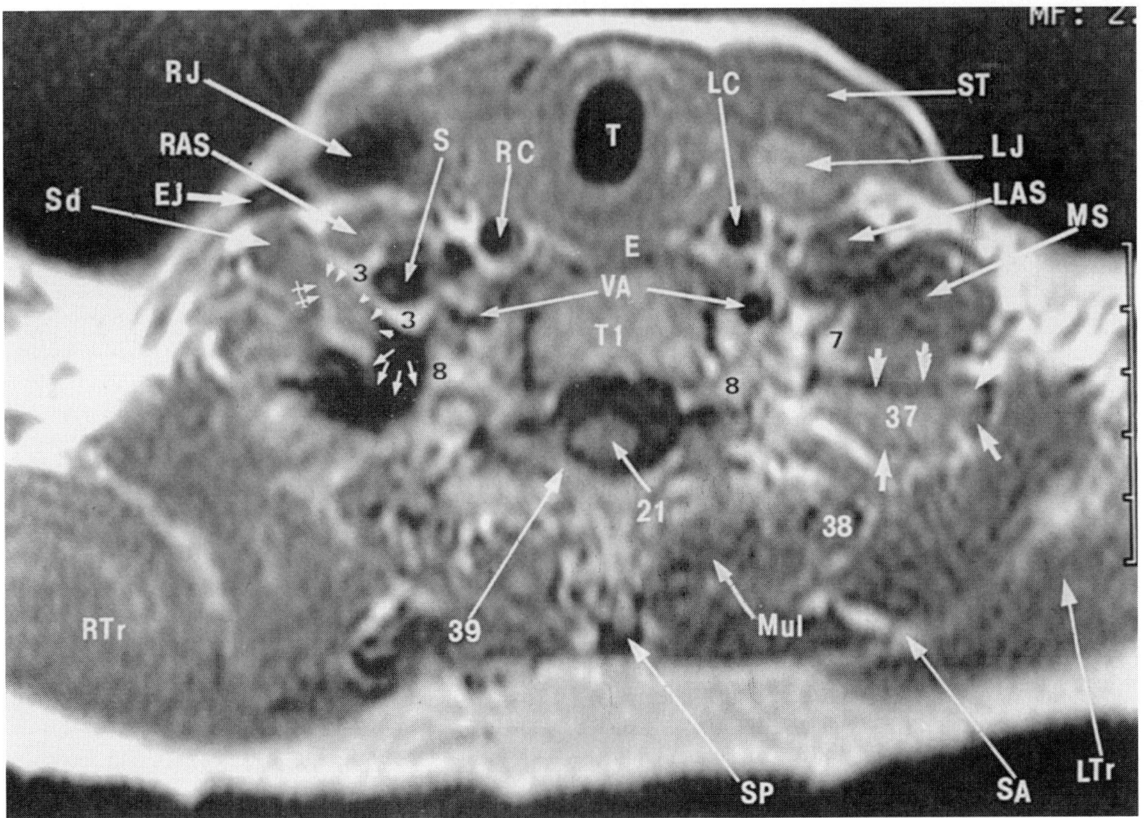

FIGURE 10–9. Transverse image 18 demonstrates effacement of nerves by the right cervical rib. Ansa subclavia (3), left normal C8 and right effaced C8 nerve roots (8), effaced first thoracic nerve root *(four small arrows)* joining T1 nerve root *(four arrowheads),* ascending (S) and descending (Sd) loops of subclavian artery, external (EJ) and internal jugular (RJ, LJ) veins, anterior scalene muscles (RAS, LAS), common carotid arteries (RC, LC), trachea (T), esophagus (E), vertebral arteries (VA), dorsal spine (Sp) and spinal cord (21), multifidus muscle (Mul), spinal accessories nerve (SA), trapezius muscles (RTr, LTr), left transverse process (38), C7 nerve root (7), middle scalene muscle (MS), left first rib (37 and *four large arrows*), vertebral arteries (VA), and sternocleidomastoid muscle (ST). (From Collins JD, Batra P, Brown K, Shaver ML: Anatomy of the thorax and shoulder girdle as displayed by magnetic resonance imaging. J Natl Med Assoc *83*:46–52, 1991a.)

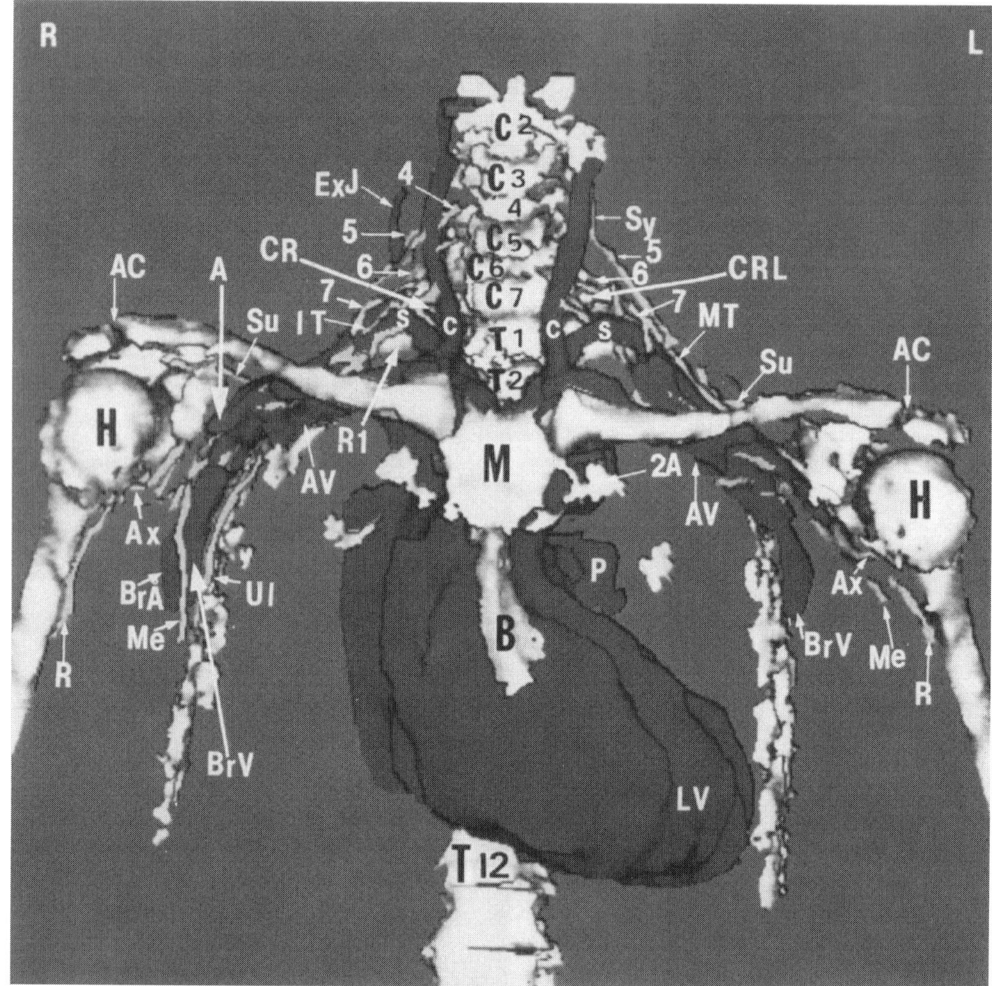

FIGURE 10–10. Three-dimensional image of osseous, neurovascular bundles, heart and great vessels demonstrating the mild right convexed cervicothoracic scoliosis. Right (R) 1st Rib (R1); cervical rib (CR); C4–7 nerve roots; small left (L) cervical rib (CRL); manubrium sterni (M); anterior rib (2A); acromioclavicular joints (AC); humerus (H); 1st, 2nd, and 12th thoracic (T1,T2,T12) and cervical (C2–7) vertebral bodies; body of the manubrium sternum (B); and middle (MT) and inferior (IT) trunks. Axillary (Ax), suprascapular (Su), radial (R), median (Me), ulnar (Ul), and long thoracic (LT) nerves. Pulmonary artery (P), and left ventricle (LV). Axillary (A), subclavian (S), common carotid (C) and brachial (BrA) arteries. Brachial (BrV), axillary (AV), and external jugular (ExJ) veins. Sympathetic nerve (Sy). (See also color plate.) (From Collins JD, Batra P, Brown K, Shaver ML: Anatomy of the thorax and shoulder girdle as displayed by magnetic resonance imaging. J Natl Med Assoc *83*:46–52, 1991a.)

roots. The smaller left cervical rib effaced the superior margin of the C8 nerve root (yellow) and sympathetic nerve branches. The manubrium sterni asymmetrical articulation with the clavicles complemented the posteroanterior chest radiograph (see Fig. 10–7).

The three-dimensional images confirmed the gray scale imaging series and displayed the compression changes of the cervical vertebral spine. The cervical rib compression and effacement was displayed. The patient was informed of our findings. Because of her age, surgery was not recommended. Her physician elected to continue observation and physical therapy as tolerated.

▼ CASE 3:

NEUROLEMMOMA OF THE MEDIAN NERVE: A 28-year-old man presented with a painful palpable mass on the medial aspect of the right upper arm. The neurological examination determined that the mass involved the median nerve. A bilateral brachial plexus MRI was requested to rule out possible multiple tumors prior to surgery. Bilateral brachial plexus imaging was performed with coronal and transverse sequences to ensure the proximal bilateral brachial plexus was normal. The coronal and transverse sequences were within normal limits, except for a mass involving the median nerve of the right upper arm. Oblique sagittal T1 (Fig. 10–11*A*) and oblique sagittal FSE (Fig. 10–11*B*) sequences were obtained of the right upper arm. The

tumor was demonstrated and surgically proved to be a neurolemmoma. The patient tolerated the surgery without sequelae.

▼ CASE 4:

OLD RIB FRACTURES (CALLUS FORMATION) COMPRESSING THE NEUROVASCULAR BUNDLE. This study focuses on a 22-year-old right-handed man who injured his right upper rib cage as a teenager playing football in high school. He did not remember the treatment, and old records were not available. He gave a history of numbness of the right upper extremity in various positions without specific tingling or pain in the right hand. The bilateral MRI of the brachial plexus was obtained to evaluate compromise of the right brachial plexus. A preliminary posteroanterior chest radiograph demonstrated an old fracture of the first, second, and third right ribs with fusion of the second and third ribs and medial deviation of the first rib (Fig. 10–12). The coronal sequence demonstrated the asymmetrical insertion of the clavicles, bowed right clavicle, and fractured fusion (fibrotic changes) of the first and second ribs lateral to the scalene triangle. The first rib compressed the upper right lung medially. The callus formation caused superior and anterior effacement of the neurovascular bundle at the axillary level (Fig. 10–13*A*). The right anterior scalene muscle was larger than the left scalene muscle and proximal in position to the left anterior scalene muscle on the transverse sequence. The margins of the right first and second ribs were inseparable and

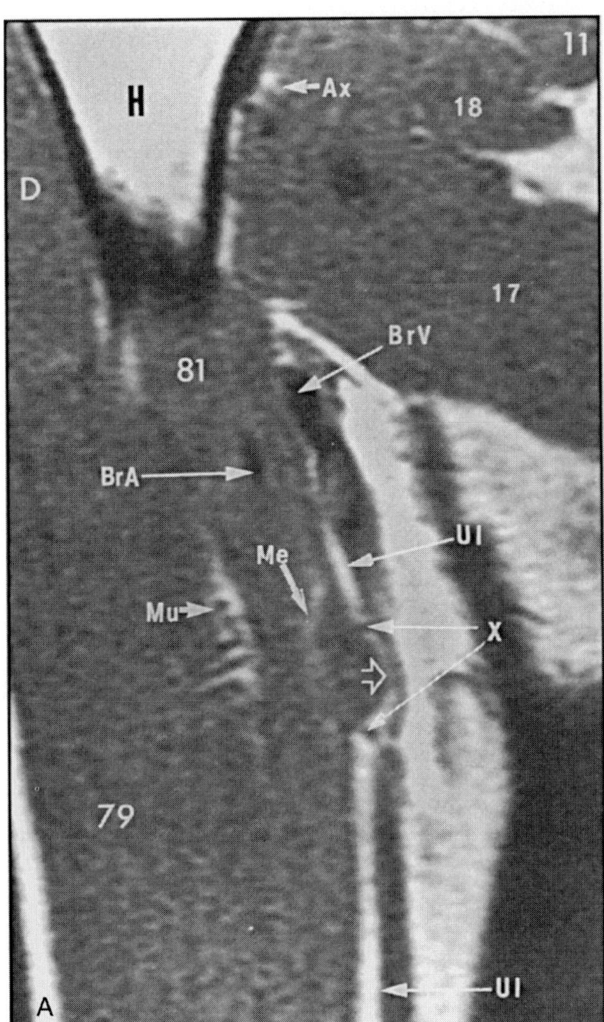
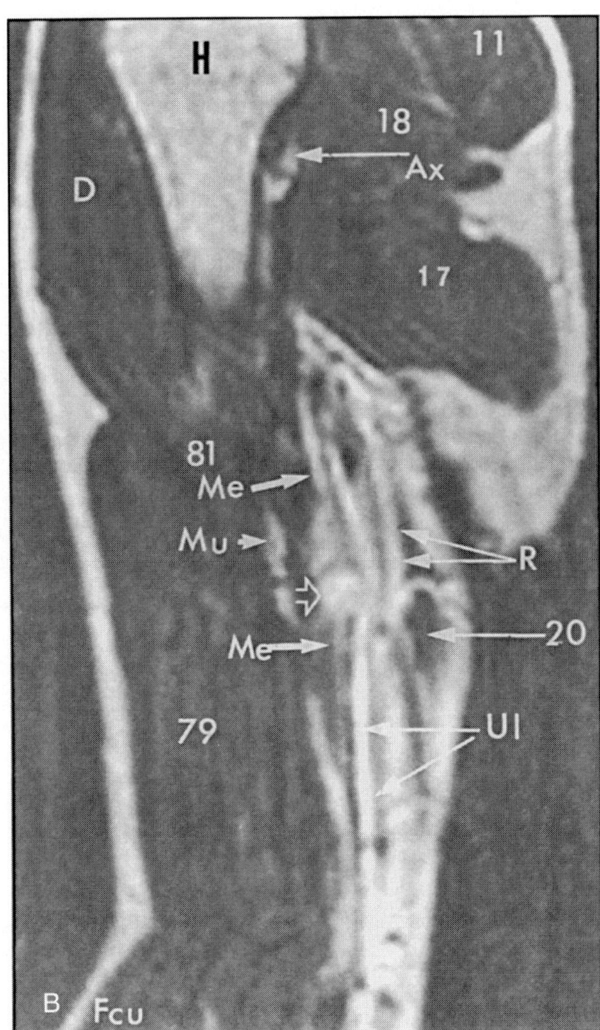

FIGURE 10–11. *A,* This is a T1-weighted sagittal oblique image of the right upper arm. The ulnar (Ul) nerve is effaced *(clear arrow)* by the neurolemmoma. Humerus (H), axillary (Ax), median (Me), and ulnar (Ul) nerves. Brachial (BrA) artery, brachial (BrV). Anterior deltoid (D) and posterior deltoid (11), short head of the biceps (79), teres major (17) and teres minor (18) and coracobrachialis (81) muscles. Musculocutaneous (Mu) nerve. Nutrient blood supply to the ulnar nerve (X). *B* This the fast spin echo (FSE) of *A* demonstrating decreased contrast, motion artifact, and tumor *(clear arrow)*. Humerus (H), axillary (Ax), radial (R), median (Me) and ulnar (Ul) nerves. Brachial (BrA) artery, brachial vein (BrV). Anterior (D) and posterior (11) deltoid, short head of the biceps (79), teres major (17) and minor (18), coracobrachialis (81), flexor carpi ulnaris (Fcu) and long head of the triceps (20) muscles. Musculocutaneus (Mu) nerve. (From Collins JD, Batra P, Brown K, Shaver ML: Anatomy of the thorax and shoulder girdle as displayed by magnetic resonance imaging. J Natl Med Assoc *83*:46–52, 1991a.)

the subclavian artery was narrowed with poststenotic dilatation of the axillary artery lateral to the scalene triangle. The left transverse oblique sequence (Fig. 10–13*C*). demonstrated callus effacement of the inferior nerve trunk (transparent arrow) and right axillary vein. The left sagittal sequence was unremarkable. The right sagittal sequence demonstrated the callus union of the 1st and 2nd rib and compression of the neurovascular bundle (Fig. 10-13*D*). The MRA confirmed the above-mentioned images. Surgery confirmed fibrosis and fusion of the first and second rib by callus formation, as demonstrated on the MRI. The right first rib, callus formation, and anterior scalene muscle were resected. The patient tolerated the surgery and returned to play football. He had no sequalae.

DISCUSSION

In Case 1 (the bodybuilder), compromise of the brachial plexus was caused by several problems: (1) scalene triangle compression by the scalene muscles as the neurovascular bundle is formed, (2) the sternocleidomastoid muscle, and (3) the clavicle and subclavius muscle at the thoracic outlet. The cervicothoracic scoliosis may be secondary to the shorter insertion of the anterior scalene muscle on the first rib, and the asymmetrical muscular development of the shoulder girdle muscles (see Figs. 10–4 to 10–6). In this case, surgery may be complicated by problems caused by the hypertrophy of the muscles.

In Case 2 (cervical ribs), the patient was 79 years of age before her complaints were presented to a physician. The cervical ribs were not identified. The consulting neurologist suggested a bilateral brachial plexus MRI examination because he was aware of our procedure. The MRI confirmed the clinical neurological examination. The bilateral cervical ribs, muscle laxity, and degenerative changes of the osseous structures all seem to have contributed to the diagnosis of a right thoracic outlet syndrome (Collins et al, 1995; Lord and Rosati, 1971; Sunderland, 1968). They may be present in patients and may not cause clinical complaints until an injury of some sort occurs (Lord and Rosati, 1971; Sunderland, 1968). Often, they go undetected and do not present a problem. Chest radiographs

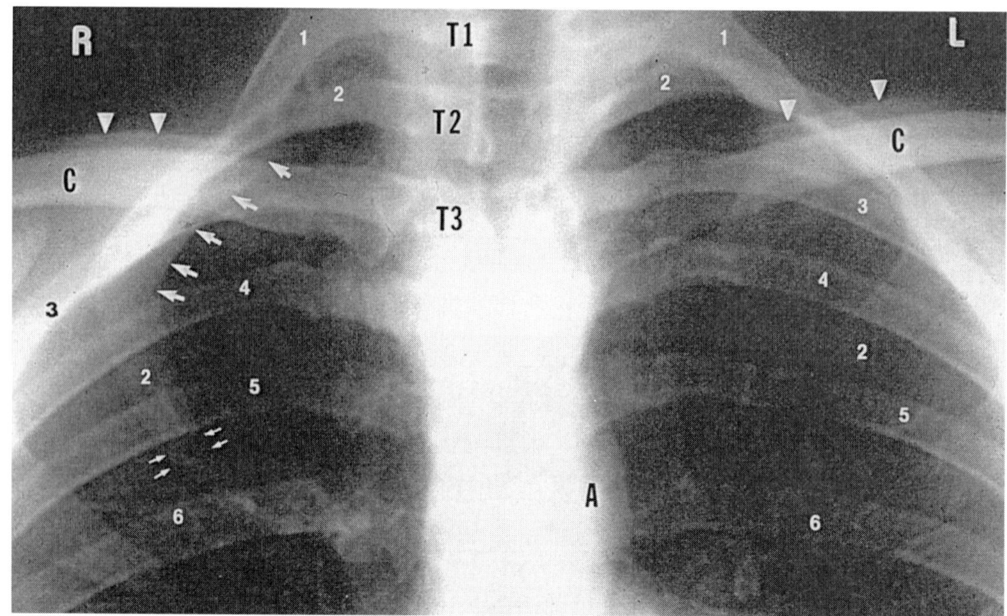

FIGURE 10–12. This is an enlarged PA upper chest radiograph at the time of the bilateral MRI of the brachial plexus. Observe the callus formation *(small arrows)* obscuring the second (2) and third (3) right ribs and medial displacement of the right first rib (1). Right lung (RL); clavicle (C); first, second, and third thoracic vertebral bodies (T1, T2, T3); aorta (A); fourth, fifth, and sixth ribs (4,5,6); and right (R) and left (L).

are reviewed, and the cervical ribs are routinely listed as an incidental finding. Seldom does the radiologist receive a follow-up communication of their detection.

The authors stress enlarging selected images to demonstrate the nerve effacement that we demonstrated in our cervical rib presentation (see Figs. 10–7 to 10–10). Cervical ribs are congenital abnormalities of the cervicothoracic spine.

The authors are aware of alternative diagnoses that may have caused her complaints. We are also aware that our narrative presentation included statements without all of the

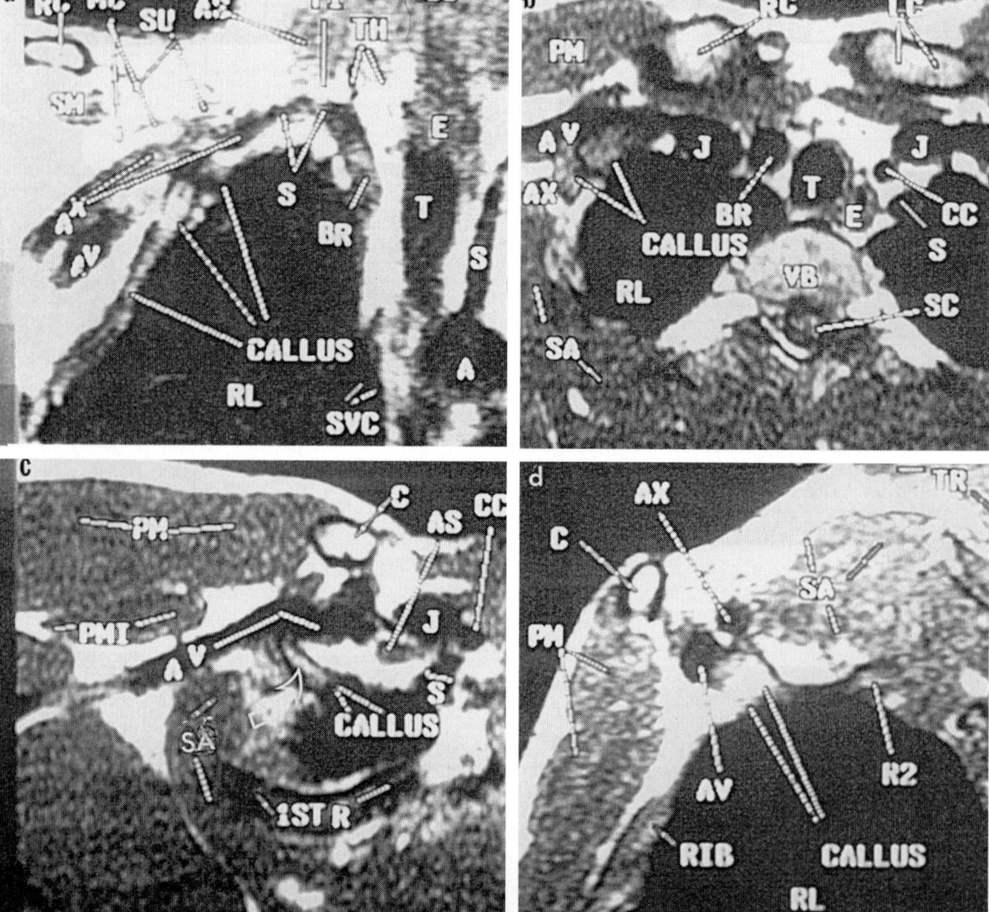

FIGURE 10–13. (*a* to *d*) This is the multiple imaging display of the patient in Figure 12. Coronal (*a*), transverse (*b*), right transverse oblique (*c*), and right sagittal (*d*). The callus formation effaces the neurovascular bundle superiorly (*a*), anteriorly in (*b* and *c*), and anterosuperiorly (*d*). RC, Right clavicle; LC, left clavicle; AX, axillary artery; AV, axillary vein; RL, right lung C, clavicle; 1st R, first rib, SA, first fascicle of the serratus anterior muscle; S, subclavian artery; BR, brachiocephalic artery; RIB, rib; R2, right 2nd rib; A, aorta, T, trachea; SVC, superior vena cava; CC, left common carotid; J, jugular vein; E, esophagus; PM, pectoralis major muscle; PMI, pectoralis minor muscle; TR, trapezius muscle; C6, cervical vertebral body; VB, first thoracic vertebral body; SC, spinal cord; AS, anterior scalene muscle; TH, thyrocervical artery; T1, first thoracic nerve; MC, medial cord; SM, subclavius muscle; SU, suprascapular nerve; C8-T1 nerve trunk *(clear arrow)*, C7 nerve trunk *(bar arrow)*.

images displayed. We did present a more extensive report for the patient's file supported by these selected images. Unlike x-ray images, a diagnosis is not made from a single plain film (Risler, 1931, 1976). Multiple images are provided in an MRI sequence, from which a selected group may best demonstrate the abnormality. Because it is not possible to present all of the images, those selected best demonstrated the pathology.

Radiology strives to increase the quality of imaging by eliminating the background or increasing the signal-to-noise ratio, or both. The simple placement of saline water bags next to the neck and next to the long axis of the extremities in Case 3 (neurolemmoma) provides increased on signal-to-noise ratio and increased definition of peripheral nerve and soft tissue imaging (Collins et al, 1989, 1990). Respiratory compensation (gating) diminishes artifacts caused by the uncontrolled movements of breathing (see Fig. 10–11*A*) and increases artifacts in FSE pulse sequence imaging (see Fig. 10–11*B*). Cursor lines indicate the position of each image and are required for cross referencing between sequences. The absence of the numbered cursor lines impedes interpretation. Surface coils are used exclusively by some institutions. Their studies are designed to include surface coils to image the brachial plexus. Although our institution has surface coils and the phased-array torso coils, these elements are not routinely used. Furthermore, the phased-array torso coils cost $250,000 or more. The surface penetration does not provide uniform imaging that the body coil provides. We have been using saline water bags to enhance MRI studies at our institution for more than 10 years. Most hospitals who might use this technique would not be able to afford the phased-array torso coils and the contiguous anatomic structures important in these cases would not be imaged.

The authors believe three-dimensional reconstruction is a useful tool to confirm gray scale MRI examinations. A tailored anatomical bilateral MRI imaging of the brachial plexus, correlated with the clinical history, does allow the study of brachial plexopathies (Collins et al, 1995). In 1985, we reviewed 80 patients who had chest radiographs correlated with surgery for thoracic outlet syndrome. The posteroanterior chest film findings correlated with the surgical findings: (1) smaller thoracic inlet on the concave side of the cervicothoracic spine scoliosis; (2) a shorter distance between the dorsal spine of the second or third thoracic vertebral body to the concavity of the first ribs, or both; (3) asymmetrical first ribs, clavicles, and coracoid processes; (4) synchondrosis of the first and second ribs; and (5) muscle atrophy on the side of the clinical complaints. Our 22-year-old patient in Case 4 (old rib fractures) did not seem to have complaints from his chest wall injury in his early teens. The chest wall injury and increased body size and musculature since participating in high school football seemed to compromise the right brachial plexus. The review of old chest films may have directed attention to the rib fractures as the etiology for his right upper extremity numbness. The diagnosis was suggested on the plain chest radiographs.

Anatomists, neurologists, vascular surgeons, and neurosurgeons have been made aware that bilateral MRI examination of the brachial plexus and peripheral nerve imaging were possible and patients' clinical complaints correlated with MRI. Since 1985, over 275 patients were imaged. One hundred and ninety-five of these patients were imaged with a 1.5 Tesla unit and three-dimensional reconstruction MRI. An important abnor-

mal anatomical landmark may appear on the plain radiograph. Most first-year medical school students participate in gross anatomy laboratory dissections of the human body. When the clinical history is presented, the students should imagine a three-dimensional image of the anatomy. The interpretation of MRI and CT examinations provides the experienced radiologist with a chance to superimpose a three-dimensional image of the anatomy while interpreting the plain radiograph. The radiologist masters the use of imaging equipment to acquire images that best display normal and abnormal anatomy. The full field of view MRI of the neck, thorax, and shoulder girdle provides detailed study of the brachial plexus and landmark anatomy. Although clinical presentations may change with different categories of disease and the diagnosis may vary, the knowledge of anatomy remains the most important feature in the use of MRI to detect nerve disorders.

References

Clemente CD: Gray's Anatomy, 31st ed. Philadelphia, Lea and Febiger, 1985.

Clemente CD: Anatomy: A Regional Atlas of The Human Body, 4th ed. Baltimore, Urban and Schwarzenberg, 1995.

Collins JD, Batra P, Brown K, Shaver ML: Anatomy of the thorax and shoulder girdle as displayed by magnetic resonance imaging. Anat Rec *214:*24A, 1986.

Collins JD, Shaver ML, Batra P, Brown K: Nerves on magnetic resonance imaging. J Natl Med Assoc *81:*129–134, 1989.

Collins JD, Batra P, Brown K, Shaver ML: Anatomy of the thorax and shoulder girdle as displayed by magnetic resonance imaging. J Natl Med Assoc *83:*46–52, 1991a.

Collins JD, Batra P, Brown K, Shaver ML: Imaging the thoracic lymphatics: Experimental studies of swine. Clinical Anatomy *4:*1–14, 1991b.

Collins JD, Batra P, Brown K, Shaver ML: Magnetic resonance imaging of chest wall lesions. J Nat Med Assoc *83:*352–360, 1991c.

Collins JD, Kovacs BJ, Shaver M, Hall T, Brown K, Batra P, Sinha S: Enhancement of magnetic resonance images using water bags. J Natl Med Assoc *82:*197–199, 1990.

Collins JD, Shaver ML, Disher A, Miller TQ: Compromising abnormalities of the brachial plexus as displayed by magnetic resonance imaging. Anat Rec (Suppl 1)*235:*44A, 1993.

Collins JD, Shaver ML, Disher A, Miller TQ: The vascular supply of the brachial plexus as displayed by magnetic resonance imaging: Magnetic resonance angiography (MRA). Presented at the Eleventh Annual Scientific Program of the American Association of Clinical Anatomists. University of Texas Medical Center, Galveston, Texas, June 16, 1994.

Collins JD, Shaver ML, Disher AC, Miller TQ: Compromising abnormalities of the brachial plexus as displayed by magnetic resonance imaging. Clinical Anatomy 8:1–16, 1995.

Dyck PK, Karnes J, Lais L Lofgren EP, Stevens JC: Pathologic alterations of the peripheral nervous system of humans. *In* Dyck PJ, Thomas PK, Lambert EH, Bunge R (eds): Peripheral Neuropathy, 2nd ed. Philadelphia, W.B. Saunders Company 1984; pp 760–870.

Lord JW, Rosati LM: Thoracic-outlet syndromes. Clinical Geigy *23:*1–32, 1971.

Lord JW: Critical reappraisal of diagnostic and therapeutic modalities for thoracic outlet syndromes. Surg Gynecol Obstet *168:*337–340, 1989.

Rigler LG: Roentgen diagnosis of small pleural effusions. JAMA *96:*104–108, 1931.

Rigler LG: A half century of radiology. Semin Roentgenol *11:*1–11, 1976.

Sunderland S: Blood supply of the nerves to the upper limb in man. Arch Neurol Psychol 53:91–115, 1945.

Sunderland S: Nerves and Nerve Injuries. Baltimore, Williams & Wilkins Company, 1968.

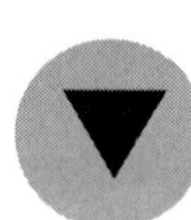

• Karen H. Prendergast Lauckhardt

Chapter 11

Decision Pathways for the Therapist's Management of Peripheral Nerve Injury

Critical to the future of quality medical therapy is the balance between diagnostic accuracy, treatment efficacy, and improved cost efficiency. Increased patient participation and responsibility will be necessary; passive attendance at therapy visits will no longer be possible. Likewise, costly professional time will be carefully delegated. Time-consuming tasks will be divided among less highly paid individuals on the caregiver pyramid.

As a uniform topic approach, I will present the so-called *think pathway* for preparation before and during a treatment session. First is the evaluation or *assessment* of the patient's condition. This assessment is derived from the objective and subjective information gathered at the start of the treatment session.

Assessment leads to goal setting. Short-term *treatment strategy* is the approach for one or two treatment sessions and the methodology to achieve the immediate goals.

The actual mechanics of the session are recorded in the therapist's chart note. Repeated upgrading of goals and strategy advances the patient through the rehabilitative process.

THERAPIST'S ASSESSMENT TOOLS FOR NEUROLOGICAL PROBLEMS

Objective measurements are the foundation of the therapist's assessment bank. As part of my treatment philosophy for the patient with a neurological problem, I emphasize frequent objective measures to assess treatment efficacy. One such objective measure is the *pain diagram* (Margoles, 1983). This tool has been shown to be a valid and reliable tool as a representation of the patient's perception of his or her current discomfort. Also valuable are *visual analog scales* (VASs) for measurement of the intensity and annoyance level of the pain, as described by Revill and co-workers (1976). Use of these parameters during successive treatment sessions is a powerful tool in confirming agreement on the nature and extent of the pain.

The most objective and reliable measure therapists have for sensory status is the *Semmes-Weinstein monofilaments*, which Omer and Bell-Krotoski describe in Chapter 4. When studied in a mapping series, nerve progression and regression are clearly seen.

If a monofilament test is impossible or results are improbable, sweating patterns are objective representations of pseudomotor activity. The triketohydrindene hydrate (Ninhydrin) sweat test is particularly effective for young patients. Ninhydrin spray and filter paper now make this test relatively easy

to perform. The skin is washed before mild heating for approximately 10 minutes. One presses the hand against the filter paper for 30 seconds. A small application of the Ninhydrin spray will turn the paper purple as it dries in the areas that sweat. If the paper is dried with a heat gun, the procedure must be performed in a well-ventilated area because the spray is noxious.

Other important assessment tools are provocative tests that, when they are repeated in a series, add valuable input:

- *Tinel mapping,* showing major and minor sites of nerve responsiveness.

- *Phalen's test* (flexed wrist held for 30 seconds)—reported symptoms should disappear on release of wrist flexion.

- *Symptom reproduction*—therapists can reproduce the pain pattern on deep palpation, making the developing diagnosis more credible.

The provocative test results can be included on the monofilament map or, better yet, be placed on the *pain diagram.* An example of the pain diagram is seen in Figure 11–1. The patient is able to represent his or her own perspective clearly and becomes an active member of the recovery team. The diagram not only aids in communicating with the patient but facilitates communication with the physician team, bypassing long verbal explanations that are less objective.

The pain diagram is most valid when the patient relates to the current condition of the pain, not last night or when it was particularly intolerable (Price et al, 1983). After the patient is given time to draw the description, the therapist then asks the patient to be even more specific. The example shows that the patient has drawn the pain as a shaded area. The therapist then guides the patient by asking specific questions regarding the pain. For instance, the therapist may ask about the time of day the pain occurs, activities that precipitate the pain, and the length of time for the pain to dissipate. The pain experienced after activity may be in a different location than the stiffness experienced on awakening. The therapist's examination points out trigger points and paresthesias that, when added to the diagram, provide a more complete picture. Further use of the pain diagram is included in the discussion on compression neuropathy.

The VASs (Joyce et al, 1975) seen alongside the pain diagram should be performed in conjunction with the diagram. Like the pain diagram, the VAS is most valid if it represents present pain rather than remembered pain. The left VAS is a 10-cm line representing pain intensity or pain

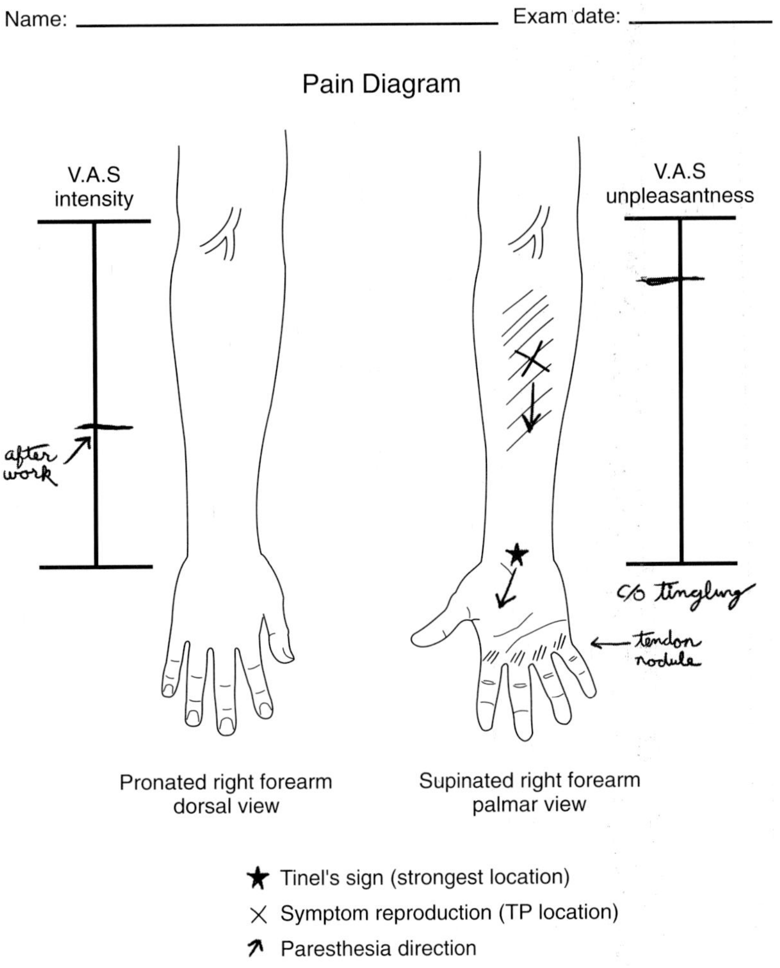

Name: _________________________________   Exam date: __________

Pain Diagram

FIGURE 11–1. The hatch markings on the pain diagram are the representation of the patient's concept of the pain. Superimposed on the diagram are symbols designating the provocative findings the therapist found on palpation of the extremity, which is the guided portion of the diagram. Alongside the diagram is the set of visual analog scales (VASs), quantifying the intensity as well as the frustration level of the pain. On this 10-cm line, the patient indicates the level of the pain from his or her own perspective. The comparison of the pain diagram against the dual levels of pain provides key information for therapist and physician alike.

loudness. The right VAS is more abstract because it represents the negative effect of pain on daily living and function. This annoyance and frustration scale reveals information about the patient's quality of life and personal coping.

The two scales are interpreted together. The numerical value can be expressed either in centimeters or as a ratio of intensity to annoyance. If the treatment strategy is effective, the annoyance scale value should reduce dramatically following the first few treatment sessions as coping improves. The intensity level reduces as the primary nerve lesion recovers. The pain area typically focuses at the primary lesion site as secondary pains are eliminated. The two tools used together enable the therapist to document the changing rather than static condition. The tools distinguish areas of secondary pain due to muscle spasm and fluid distention from the primary injury. They also document the patient's report of his or her ability to cope with daily function.

ACUTE NERVE TRAUMA: PERIPHERAL NEURORRHAPHY

Gathering baseline information is the therapist's first assignment. As regeneration progresses, ongoing assessment and the prevention of deterioration in the status of the extremity follow.

Assessment

MUSCLE TESTING

A formal manual muscle test takes skill and time and requires detailed knowledge of anatomy; however, for the information gained, it is well worth the trouble. Before the formal test, informally examine the patient for several minutes while he or she attempts several functional tasks. The denervated or weakened muscle will become apparent through the substitution maneuvers. This can be more revealing than the formal manual muscle grading system. I like to complete both types of examinations for my assessments. In addition, neuromuscular electrical stimulation (NMES) identifies which motor fibers are presently innervated and contractile versus which muscle units lack sufficient innervation to respond to the short-duration current. This examination does not rule out the possibility of tendon rupture as a reason for lack of voluntary motion.

SENSIBILITY TESTING

On the first visit, a baseline *Semmes-Weinstein mapping* is performed. This type of mapping documents any anatomical innervation anomalies or cross-over innervations that existed before the injury.

Mapping of *Tinel's sign* and paresthesias, in combination

with a *manual muscle test,* will detail the baseline status of the extremity before regeneration begins. Static and moving two-point discrimination tests on vibration assessment are also useful modalities.

Strategy

With the pain and sensory status clearly defined, the therapist can act on a strategy for early desensitization methods or electrical stimulation of nerve or muscle.

Motor nerve repairs can benefit from splinting to prevent capsular contractures, deformity, and overstretched, elongated muscle-tendon units. Beware of splinting that interferes with needed substitution patterns. The patient must remain functional during the daytime.

Insensate areas from sensory nerve injury need protection from abrasion and temperature extremes. This may be best accomplished with a thermoplastic splint cap or cloth covering over vulnerable areas. Proper clothing, mittens, and protective gloves are especially important for ulnar nerve insensate areas. Brand discusses management of the sensory-deprived extremity in Chapter 72. These principles are the same as those employed in splinting:

- Eliminate friction and shear stresses.

- Distribute pressures and forces over the widest area possible.

- Lubricate the skin or scar.

- Educate the patient.

Nerve Gliding

Nerves glide longitudinally in their bed as the extremity moves. Several authors have documented that nerves change in length as much as 20% (McLellan and Swash, 1976; Millesi, 1986) as the extremity flexes and extends. Just as tendons adhere to any surgical or trauma site, so does a repaired nerve. If the nerve is allowed to become "spot welded" to the surgical wound, gliding is prevented. Joint movement will cause pain from traction on the nerve within the wound. Therefore, massage and gliding techniques are incorporated into the postoperative program (Hunter and Totten, 1991). Gentle gliding is started early, avoiding traction so radical that a lasting paresthesia is elicited. When extremity range of motion (ROM) is completed without producing a paresthesia, then gliding has been effective.

Extremity use exhibiting good motor and sensory return in the form of functional patterns is the end goal of neurorrhaphy. Regenerated axons, motor and nerve end-organs, joint capsules, and muscle tissue must be in top shape to deliver optimal extremity function. The art is to have all structures ready as the nerve axons meet their terminal end points. Training must be appropriate to the amount of reinnervation: too much exercise training will fatigue newly innervated motor fibers; too little training perpetuates substitution patterns.

Exercise

A partially reinnervated extremity suffers greatly from balance problems. Team partnerships among muscle pairs have been lost. If satisfactory reinnervation has occurred, we attempt to re-establish pairing and balance by working in functional patterns. Isolated exercises of specific muscles are not recommended until gross patterns are re-established.

If optimal reinnervation does not occur and function is impaired, the next consideration may be surgical intervention with tendon transfer.

WHEN THERE IS NO REGENERATION: TENDON TRANSFER REBALANCING

The goal of reconstructive tendon transfer in the upper extremity is to restore the three functional patterns that are controlled by the peripheral nerves.

- *Median* innervated pattern—power pinch and pull, and precision pinch actions.

- *Ulnar* innervated patterns—digital power grasp, fist closure, refined intrinsic actions.

- *Radial* innervated patterns—wrist stabilization and tenodesis control to allow power and digital flexion sweep.

It is hoped that the patient considering tendon transfer procedures has sought the care of a highly experienced hand surgeon with access to a skilled, experienced hand therapy team. Above all, this surgery requires the utmost in judgment and experience. Planning the operative procedure should be a team effort. The physician team evaluation should be followed by the therapist's evaluation of

- Meticulous grading of a formal manual muscle test of all muscles of the extremity.

- Assessment of availability of donor tendons for transfer.

- A detailed understanding of the candidate's vocational and avocational interests.

- Joint ROM assessment, including reasons for any restrictions or laxities.

- The candidate's ability to isolate muscle function following high nerve injury.

This composite information is critical in deciding if the proposed donor transfer tendons are of sufficient power to be useful after the transfer procedure. Also important is preoperative assessment of joint mobility. Joint restrictions will block the desired line of pull of the transfer. Too much joint play with too many articulations will dilute the force of the transfer. The surgical transfer should be timed such that all innervated muscles are in top condition and all joint capsules have appropriate freedom of motion or appropriate stability. Surgical procedures are completed in stages. Operative procedures to stabilize and fuse excessively mobile joints are completed during a procedure separate from those that mobilize tendons. Patients are often anxious to move from stage to stage. Operative stages should not be rushed; the therapy team should spend 1 to 2 months before each operation to prepare the muscles and joints properly. The delay to gain optimal conditions preoperatively is well worth the wait (see Chapter 67).

THERAPIST'S TREATMENT AFTER TENDON TRANSFER

Assessment

Observation of the patient's attempt at motion after cast removal will quickly reveal weaknesses in the new muscle system. Typically, either the new transfer works immediately or problems have to be worked out through training. A gradual rise to perfection does not occur as in some other procedures.

Common postoperative problems with tendon transfer procedures include the following:

- Adhesions can restrict the gliding tendon.

- Inaccurate pulley angles and adhesions around the pulley may be present.

- Multiple articulations dilute forces to the target joint action.

- Substitution patterns hinder training of the transferred tendon.

- Mass muscle activity or co-contraction may occur in proximal nerve lesions.

Strategy for Therapy

The treatment of tendon transfer procedures centers on four concepts:

1. Protect the transferred tendon from overstretching and rupture until healing is complete.
2. Use the new pattern only; block all substitution patterns.
3. Develop a practice pattern that is compatible with both the old and the new action of the donor muscle.
4. Stabilize lax joints that impair the desired pattern of action until learning is complete.

Satisfactory transfer function depends on anticipating the common problems and using intervention strategies to avoid pitfalls. The therapist guides the patient by repeating functional use patterns until learning is accomplished. If all length relationships are correct, the pattern will be automatic without much deviation. If there is any adherence, abnormal line of pull, or joint instability, substitutions will corrupt the pattern. The action pattern may be unstable if too many joint articulations provide excessive mobility. Custom thermoplastic joint blocks and collars solve the problem by shunting forces to the desired joint and assisting proper tendon gliding. Repetition of the correct pattern elongates adhesions and strengthens the donor muscle. In time, the splints may be eliminated as the system becomes stronger and more balanced.

Surgical revisions are sometimes needed to fine tune the pattern. Tenolysis for adhesions, length tension balancing, and joint arthrodesis for stabilizations are not uncommon.

With more proximal injury and therefore more loss of functional use, surgery is planned in stages. Two or three procedures are often required to stabilize certain areas and to transfer groups of tendons. The most happy circumstances occur when all members of the medical team agree on the goals and expectations of each stage. It can be an exciting and rewarding challenge.

PERIPHERAL NERVE STRETCH INJURY

Assessment

Surgical intervention is postponed when there is hope that the stretched nerve will recover spontaneously. The therapist is in the best position to evaluate nerve progress continuously. These repeated examinations sway the decision toward or away from surgery. A typical example is the radial nerve stretch injury that occurs with a humeral fracture. Manual muscle testing, NMES, and mapping of Tinel's sign are recorded biweekly during regular therapy sessions. The muscle test may not pick up a subtle strength increase, but electrical stimulation may show firing of newly innervated motor fiber. A twitch is seen or palpated over the muscle long before strength is great enough to cause an increased ROM. The pain diagram may change, showing the recovering nerve moving distally. Change seen in these tests reflects the status of the nerve perhaps with more sensitivity than the electromyelographic findings. When no change is documented, it is a poor sign and will be confirmed by repeat electromyelography.

Strategy

Stretch injury treatment proceeds in the same manner as already described for neurorrhaphy, including nerve gliding and extremity protection. Unfortunately, the probability of dysesthesia problems with stretch injury is high. In my experience, the probability is far higher than for the surgically repaired nerve. I routinely prepare for dysesthesia pain and use programs that I use to prevent reflex sympathetic dystrophy (RSD).

SEVERE MULTILEVEL INJURIES AND GUNSHOT WOUNDS

Injuries of a severe nature are characterized by massive amounts of adhesive scarring. If it is immobilized, the extremity becomes cemented in scar and is rendered nonfunctional. This is perhaps the one situation when fracture immobilization takes a back seat to tissue mobilization. Loss of tissue elasticity results in more permanent damage to the extremity than a malunited fracture. Close coordination between the physician and the therapist is critical as they try to serve the goals of both bone stability and gliding tissue.

Assessment

Assessment of multilevel wounds includes the following factors:

- Joint contracture—developed or developing.

- Tenodesis restrictions caused by tendon scarring.

- Muscle fiber adhesions resulting in loss of muscle power and excursion.

- Functional motor imbalances caused by muscle fiber loss and nerve loss.

- Spasm of traumatized muscle.

Strategy

Following assessment of the above-mentioned factors, form a potential problem list. Early wound care coincides with edema control, tendon gliding (Wehbé, 1987) and nerve gliding, joint capsule motion, and muscle conditioning. Prioritize treatment according to which structures are in the most immediate jeopardy. Fibrous adhesions form within the first week, so there is no time for delay. The greater the magnitude of the injury, the more immediate the need for early therapy intervention.

While working around pins, plates, and grafts, the therapist protects unstable structures and actively exercises the stable ones. The emphasis must be on active muscular work and active joint compression. Passive range of motion (ROM) is not an effective substitute to salvage muscle fiber whether it is innervated or not. NMES is an excellent method to use to achieve active muscular pumping with all of its beneficial effects. The electrical intensity applied dictates how much motion and tendon glide will occur, and therefore, it can be adjusted to the amount of movement allowed. Open wounds and external fixators are not contraindications to this valuable modality. The physician can advise whether to allow moderate, minimal, or no tendon gliding and the same for the joint motion. There must be a patch of sensate normal skin in order to apply the electrode pads unless one uses the underwater method possible with dual pulsed high-voltage stimulators. If it is possible to use a personal NMES unit, the patient can keep the muscle fiber pumping and the tissues exercising for a prescribed time period, several times daily, every day of the week. This method results in a higher level of compliance than that seen with the most cooperative patient in a regular exercise regimen.

The key to treatment of traumatic injuries of complex severity is similar to that of burn treatment. Active motion must begin early and the soft tissues must keep gliding to prevent the adhesive gluing effect of the inevitable massive quantities of scar.

COLD INTOLERANCE

A residual of multiple trauma injuries can be extreme sensitivity to cold. Replantation injuries, revascularization, and crushing injuries seem to compromise the local blood flow and sympathetic nerves so severely that tolerance of cold temperatures takes years to normalize. These patients have difficulty with weather changes, in cool weather, and in locations such as the grocer's freezer compartment. The treatment is similar to that for Raynaud's disease.

Assessment

Documentation of cold sensitivity is sometimes needed when a change of occupation is being considered. If documentation of symptoms is necessary, the only test I have used is cold stress recovery time (Thulesius et al, 1981). This is a nonstandard examination and therefore is untested for validity and reliability. The test is based on the premise that skin temperature is a direct reflection of digital blood flow (Phelps et al, 1979). Because the test intentionally provokes a reaction, it is best to clear the test with the physician. One should probably not perform this test until the circulatory system is well established and at least 6 months after the injury.

Begin the test by establishing the baseline surface skin temperature of the digit and then provoke a cold stress reaction. I have used either an ice water bath or circumferential cold packs. Apply the cold stress for 30 seconds. After removing the cold application, one measures the same surface skin temperature immediately and charts it on a graph at 1-minute intervals. Watch the reaction as the body part attempts to re-establish baseline temperature. A steady rise to baseline is seen in normal digits. A delayed flat response indicates an abnormal reaction to cold. Further interpretation of the flow chart can be made by the physician. If the part does not re-establish baseline skin temperature within 20 minutes, Raynaud's phenomenon or chronic flow problem is confirmed. The test should be completed bilaterally, because Raynaud's phenomenon produces the same result on both sides. In the case of trauma, the two sides should be dramatically different.

The associated discomfort can be graded with a VAS for intensity. The intensity scale should be recorded before and immediately after the application of cold stress. The annoyance scale can record the patient's frustration with this problem.

Strategy

Aside from medications and biofeedback to increase blood flow (Hayduk, 1980) and decrease sympathetic influences, behavior modification is the treatment of choice. Patients should learn to anticipate cold stresses. Wearing of gloves with glove liners in all seasons should become second nature. Patients insulate hands against cold soda cans and glasses using a napkin or adapt by switching to plastic containers. They use a potholder to remove items from the freezer and cold storage areas. For some patients, these simple changes allow them to cope; for others, more radical lifestyle changes may be necessary. Certain occupations are not compatible with severe cold sensitivity. Outdoor jobs, meat and fish handling jobs, and severely air-conditioned areas may be out of the question.

Another aspect of behavior modification is reducing the fear associated with the condition. Patient education can give the patient a sense of power over the problem (locus of control) and reduce the fears that make the blood flow even more constricted. In biofeedback training, the patient actively intervenes at the onset of cold stress and he or she learns to place a positive effect on the sympathetic nerve response. As the patient relaxes, the sympathetic nerves relax, adding possibly 15% to 20% of vessel lumen diameter. To supplement this biofeedback training program, I prescribe soft putty or a squeeze ball to grasp and release whenever the patient is walking or standing outdoors. In cool weather, this action stimulates local blood flow before the cold stress reaction begins. The fewer incidents of stress reaction, the more confident the patient becomes. For the majority of patients, cold sensitivity will last one to two winters. The unfortunate few with severe trauma reactions and those with severe Raynaud's phenomenon will need to follow these methods for a lifetime.

COMPRESSION NEUROPATHY

In my experience, adult-onset compression neuropathy seldom exists by itself. A myofascial problem is the cause or another disease entity or trauma instigates the nerve compression (see Chapters 51, 53, and 56). In the upper extremity, the most discussed neuropathy is carpal tunnel syndrome. This is as exacting as saying the patient has a "headache." It does not identify the cause. I find that many instances of median nerve compression in the mature adult wrist are caused by thickening of the flexor tendons from tenosynovitis. As the digits flex into grasp, the thickened tendon is pulled proximally into the carpal canal. The canal space is now occupied by the thickened tendons, increasing the inner canal pressure. Over time, chronic inflammation of the tenosynovium produces long-term increased pressures. The patient experiences median nerve compression symptoms during digital flexion as well as the typical night-awakening scenario. Both the tenosynovitis and the nerve compression need to be addressed.

Another reason for compression is more proximal problems. Extrinsic forearm muscles encase the median, ulnar, and radial nerves as they course distally to the hand. If inflammation or spasm exists in one of these muscles, nerve compression symptoms may appear. In this scenario, the symptoms mimic more distal entrapments, depending on the mix of sensory or motor fibers at the level of compression.

Because there are underlying causes for nerve entrapment, it is imperative that treatment be directed not only at the nerve compartment but also at the inflamed structures creating the pressure within the compartment.

Some of the basic principles that hold true for most neuropathic compression conditions include assessment, reading the pain diagram, and strategy.

Assessment

Evaluate for the probable cause of the compression. A guided pain diagram (see Fig. 11–1) provides the best information about pain and sensory patterns. After the patient has drawn the initial diagram, the therapist guides the patient by querying for more information. Data are recorded about the pain when the extremity is at rest, on awakening, and after activity. Location of Tinel's signs and direction of paresthesias are drawn on the diagram. Markings locating tendon nodules, muscle trigger points, and areas of palpable muscle soreness are superimposed on the diagram.

READING THE PAIN DIAGRAM

The perception of tingling and numbness should follow a predictable pattern for each sensory nerve and each type of compression. Proper utilization of the pain diagram along with objective provocative testing gives valuable input to develop an effective treatment strategy. In the example of carpal tunnel syndrome, fluid builds in the carpal canal during sleep, and night awakening is characteristic of nerve compression. Work activity exacerbates tingling and inflammation when the causative factor is tenosynovitis; these patients are at their best on awakening. A complaint of joint stiffness on awakening is common when the inflammation is caused by degenerative disease. These indicators are clearly seen with the guided pain diagram and will assist the therapist greatly in forming a strategy that treats the underlying cause of the nerve compression pain.

Strategy

The treatment strategy for compression neuropathy and repetitive strain injury includes the following measures:

- Correct postural problems and neck positioning, and provide brachial plexus stretches.

- Construct a splint to rest inflamed tendons in an elongated position for healing.

- Stretch shortened muscle-tendon units.

- Relieve muscular trigger points through myofascial techniques.

- Rebalance muscle partners through a graded conditioning program combined with a stretch program.

- Educate patients in methods to reduce strain on muscles and tendons with activities of daily living adaptations.

The surgical decompression procedure relieves only the pressure on the nerve. It does not cure the underlying cause of the pressure or inflammation. The surgical procedure actually stresses the recuperation of inflamed tendons or muscles. With or without surgery to relieve the nerve, treatment and monitoring are the key to reducing the inflammation of the muscle, tendon, or joint. Once formal therapy is complete, self-monitoring and self-intervention is the management technique that allows the patient to return to and maintain full function.

PAIN PROBLEMS

Pain is a difficult term to define. I will try to sort pain problems into classes depending on the timing from onset, how much it has dispersed from its origin, and contributing factors. Once pain has been classified, a strategy for a therapy program can be developed. The first section to be discussed is assessment and strategy for acute pain symptoms. The second section addresses chronic pain problems. The third section focuses on problems that have a sympathetic component, classified as RSD.

Acute Pain

ASSESSMENT

In the first discussion about pain, assume that pain is directly attributed to a wound or inflammatory condition. The discomfort originates from a normal cellular response to wounding. If the diagnosis is acute inflammation, the subjective physical signs correlate with the objective measures: increased local skin temperature, increased fluid volume, and increased pain. A high VAS intensity scale value is the norm. The pain diagram should highlight the primary location; the area of spread can be more extensive than the diagnosis indicates. Complete extremity assessment identifies potential adjuncts to the pain. Prompt edema control, reduction of secondary muscle spasm, and proper position for rest and sleep all help make the acute pain more tolerable. Teaching of healing expectations can reduce fears and anxiety reflected on the level of the VAS frustration scale. Coping skills are invaluable in preventing acute pain problems from becoming chronic pain syndromes or having a sympathetic component.

STRATEGY

The completed examinations will highlight factors that can cause additional pain. Areas that are tender on palpation can be cushioned with splints and supported with soft wraps. Modalities like icing can produce short-term anesthesia; heat can relax painful muscles. Transcutaneous electrical nerve stimulation (TENS) is believed to be most effective in directly addressing acute pain. It is far less effective with chronic pain.

When Pain Becomes Chronic: Chronic Pain Versus Chronic Inflammation

Continued pain may be normal for a regenerating nerve. To remain within normal limits, it is important that the pain change. The pain diagram will illustrate this change. The regenerating nerve and its associated bizarre feelings require a program of sensory desensitization and techniques for coping. We do not classify this as chronic pain.

When pain has lingered longer than 6 months and is unchanged, it is considered chronic and is not considered normal as in the above-mentioned example. We are reluctant to label a problem "chronic pain syndrome." It is a defeat, a failure admitting that medical therapies have been exhausted; the condition is incurable. Likewise, chronic inflammation is an unpopular diagnosis because its very duration implies we have not been effective. The latter condition is more hopeful and should be thoroughly examined before settling on the diagnosis of chronic pain syndrome.

To begin the differential diagnosis among types of chronic pain problems, carefully review the type and duration of each therapy course already tried. Confirm that there has been full compliance with each form of medical therapy. Study the pain diagram to determine if the pain pattern follows a dermatome, a myotome, or the course of a nerve or tendon. Palpate specific structures for possible soreness. I

often find that patients are not aware that the muscle belly is sore or the tendon sheaths at the A1 pulley are tender.

Distinguish between the two diagnoses, and take a fresh approach. Unfortunately, many think all occupational and physical therapists deliver the same heat and ultrasound as treatment. In the upper extremity, a certified hand therapist will approach pain or chronic inflammatory problems very differently.

When the patient has suffered for months with continual pain, assessment is more difficult. After this length of time, muscle spasm, imbalance, and contracture become part of the pain syndrome. Multiple trigger points in the cervical and shoulder girdle muscles are typical. Additional radicular pain is not uncommon. Distorted functional patterns and muscle imbalances lend themselves to flare ups of myofascial pain and tendonitis. Patients report that they believe their condition is analogous to a cancer that spreads and grows. Patients report that their VAS frustration and anxiety level is extremely high, even though the VAS pain intensity level may be low. When the diagnosis is chronic pain, not pain from inflammation and not from nerve growth, the best therapy we can offer is comfort through modalities and improved coping skills.

STRATEGY FOR CHRONIC PAIN SYNDROMES

There are two treatment strategies: (1) to relieve the primary pain, and (2) to manage the secondary complications.

It takes a few visits with the therapist before patient rapport is developed. I begin by eliminating the easiest *secondary complications* first. By avoiding pain at the primary site, trust is established. In the upper extremity, begin proximally with neck and shoulder exercises and gradually work toward the primary pain area. This principle should hold true with the lower extremity as well. Make the patient aware of negative guarding posturing or abnormal gait patterns that create havoc with muscle balance and cause secondary pain. Ensure that medications are effective and are used as directed and that the patient is getting a quiet night's sleep. These basic techniques will go a long way toward making the patient's frustration with pain diminish.

Once headway has been made on the adjunct pain, the patient may be more confident in both himself or herself and the therapist. Optimism and home program compliance usually follow because the patient feels empowered by recent successes.

Patients can be so upset, frustrated, and angry that any compliance is impossible. One may have to block the pain response at the *primary pain site* so that exercise can begin at the secondary pain areas. Show care for the primary pain by cushioning or supporting the part during exercises. Give the patient some type of cushion or wrap to wear when out in public. This treatment may be controversial because some believe it encourages a sickness behavior. I find that those patients who need the pain or injury for other emotional reasons need someone to respect the fact that they are in pain. When that respect is shown, they may begin to resolve the issue or at least comply with a program that shrinks the pain site. Mutual trust can give the patient the courage to accept the steps necessary to gain control over the pain. A doubting, pessimistic patient will resist all methods to self-intervene. Faith in just one medical professional may propel the patient in a forward progression. With luck, the patient crosses the emotional bridge that leads from passivity to more responsible behavior.

I try to remain realistic that these most difficult patients stretch the limits of my knowledge and experience. Unconventional approaches and structures can work; your own flexibility is key.

INTERVENTION AND COPING SKILLS

The focus of therapy is to regain control by changing behavioral responses to the pain. The patient with long-standing pain feels a loss of control. Patients should learn to control the pain intensity by intervening with a behavior. If the patient can learn to apply intervention techniques at the appropriate time, much can be accomplished in coping with the situation.

Therapeutic modalities of benefit for chronic pain sites include

- Heat for relaxation and cold for anesthesia.

- Vibration desensitization.

- NMES to relax painful muscles in spasm.

- Myofascial massage techniques.

I routinely use heat, cold, and vibration desensitization to block or reduce primary pain. Modalities to relieve pain may also include TENS and contrast baths. Myofascial massage is used not only for current soreness but as a means to prevent increased muscle spasm. Pain from muscle guarding is particularly responsive to NMES—electrical stimulation at a tetanic level to force fiber relaxation. A home modality unit enables the patient to intervene at will. Patients are instructed to use the units both for muscular comfort and when the pain level rises above VAS intensity level 3. As with pain medications, it is believed that waiting until pain is overwhelming is harmful. A steady tolerable pain level is preferred. The NMES treatment both reduces painful spasm and tends to divert the focus away from the primary pain.

There are home stimulation units available that offer broad-frequency output permitting both a TENS-type and NMES treatments. The therapist can program one set of electrodes in an NMES mode to address the muscle fiber spasm and a second pair of electrodes over the primary pain area for a TENS-type sensory response.

Chronic Inflammation and Repetitive Strain Problems

Pain assessment may uncover a chronic inflammatory process that has resisted standard treatment. The diagnosis of chronic inflammation as in tendonitis or neuritis demands not a coping technique as mentioned earlier but inflammation management.

Job-related inflammation problems are becoming pervasive and are particularly disturbing. Patients seek help from their physician when the pain has recurred enough to disrupt their work capability. During the visit with the physician, they are advised to rest and are granted sick leave. Nothing is accomplished at home except a break from the job task that created the inflammation. When the vacation is over, they return to work. It is not surprising to me that the problem returns—again and again. A competitive athlete cannot perform without preparation and practice, and neither can working tissue; the time spent at home is not productive. The patient is not learning how to manage sore tissues for the present or the future. In addition to acute care, a regimen of preparation before an activity and stretch after activity is needed. Without therapy training, it is predictable that the inflammation will return and become a chronic problem.

ASSESSMENT

Volumetrics documents the level of edema in the extremity. This should always be performed bilaterally for comparison. It is important to rule out an inflammatory process like tenosynovitis and confirm that the edema is noninflammatory fluid pooling.

Skin temperature mapping satisfies both the therapist and the patient that the fluid accumulation is or is not inflammatory in nature. Home exercise programs and exercise levels are based on this differentiation.

Inflammatory Edema Versus Stasis Edema

Therapists may be unclear about the difference between inflammatory edema and pooling stasis edema. An inflammatory cellular response in a tissue produces edema in conjunction with vasodilation, heat, and pain. The tissue needs rest to proceed through the healing cycle. With this type of inflammation, we avoid exercise of the inflamed muscle or tendon, limiting the muscle pumping exercise to squeezing with the intrinsic muscles. The pooling type of noninflammatory stasis edema contains nonproteinaceous fluid, occupies space, and impedes joint movement but is not accompanied by vasodilation and pain. The long-term residual of injury to the lymphovenous return mechanism has been compared to poor plumbing. Joint motion, intrinsic muscle pumping, and tendon glide are the cure for this type of fluid accumulation; elevation and rest *retard* progress.

STRATEGY FOR EDEMA

When the edema is the result of poor plumbing, it takes *active* exercise to reduce it by assisting the impaired system with muscle pumping and joint compression. It is easy to become sidetracked with passive measures such as elevating, compressing, wrapping, and massaging. The fluid becomes the enemy and receives the focus of attention rather than active exercises.

I have trained students for years not to focus undue attention on relieving noninflammatory pooling edema as a treatment goal; focus on muscular contraction as the means to pump fluids. If there is any question about whether the exercise is producing acute inflammation, graph the skin temperature and volume studies as a guide. If there are no signs of inflammation, continue the active program.

The chronically inflamed structure should be supported during exercise or work and rest in between exercise or work bouts. Neoprene wraps and light thermoplastic supports are particularly helpful in assisting the patient in functioning actively while protecting the pain site.

NEURITIS

Chronic nerve irritation is a diagnosis of last resort. Because pain and weakness are the symptoms, the consequences of this diagnosis are devastating functionally. We try every therapy to cure the irritability of the nerve. However, sometimes the symptoms worsen. As reluctant as we are to label the problem as chronic nerve irritation, it is important to establish the diagnosis. Acceptance of this diagnosis then allows the patient to begin the process of re-establishing his or her life and function in a new modified form. Very often, job modifications and perhaps retraining are required. The patient's life must be reorganized to allow for function only when and for how long the nerve will perform. Sometimes this period is an hour, and sometimes it is minutes. For neuritis, as for chronic pain syndromes, the patient should have his or her own intervention program:

- Cushion and secure the nerve from excess mobility.

- Reduce demands on muscles within the nerve distribution.

- Reorganize life and work patterns, and reduce workload through tool modifications.

DYSESTHESIA AND NEUROMA PAIN

In the early stages following nerve injury, pain of some sort is characteristic. Discriminating between the types of discomfort can be difficult. By definition, *dysesthesia* means abnormal sensibility. It is the abnormal interpretation of the sensory input on a skin surface affected by local nerve injury. Like RSD, it tends to spread beyond the site of local injury and its pain is more disturbing than the injury itself. Unlike RSD, it does not carry a sympathetic component. It is responsive to therapy and can be reversed without residual impairment.

Neuroma pain is also an anticipated side effect of nerve injury—either direct laceration or stretch injury. Incomplete axon regeneration into the distal segment of the nerve forms a ball of axons that is highly sensitive to touch or stretch. There is not necessarily pain when the neuroma is undisturbed, but added dysesthesia pain may be present. Neuromas can be responsive to sensory desensitization therapy, although only surgical repair or displacement can truly make the pain disappear.

Assessment

A guided pain diagram illustrates the perceived sensations. This information allows discrimination between expected reinnervation pains, localized neuroma pain, spreading dysesthesia, and lastly, RSD. The dysesthesia diagram shows pain spreading in a pattern radiating away from the local injury site. This area of sensory disturbance is painful with any contact and is interpreted as intense beyond the known level of pressure applied. It is frightening to the patient in its intensity and is functionally disabling. Avoidance of use patterns derails the patient's compliance with therapy programs.

The neuroma pain diagram will show local pain on percussion that the patient reports as electricity shooting down the course of the nerve distribution. This is much like Tinel's sign but more painful. The degree of severity depends on the size and location of the neuroma. It may be mixed with dysesthesia pain.

OBJECTIVE MEASURES

Measures that aid in the assessment include the following:

- Sweat mapping with Ninhydrin can document sympathetic function.

- Skin temperature mapping can confirm or rule out sympathetic vascular instability.

- VASs quantify degrees of pain intensity or frustration levels.

Strategy

Through objective testing, try to determine the type and extent of the painful area. The therapist should begin much as one would with RSD but reinforce that the learning pathways need stimulus to progress toward normalization of sensory perception. A hierarchy of contact stimuli is applied—gradually producing desensitization and progress toward normal sensory interpretation and perception of the part.

In the case of the painful neuroma, the surrounding area will desensitize and the acute pain will localize, giving the patient the option to undergo surgical revision or to learn coping techniques.

When the above-mentioned strategies have been followed and the pain is persistent, referral to a pain clinic may be in order. Entrance into the pain clinic system should not mean discontinuation of active physical programs. In the flurry of activity to institute new passive interventions, exercise regimens are often suspended. Pain postures reign and joints become stiffened while the new intervention program gets under way. The active program should be used in conjunction with passive programs.

REFLEX SYMPATHETIC DYSTROPHY

Characterized by extremely painful sensory and sympathetic disturbance, RSD is a frustrating condition to deal with for even the most experienced clinicians. Many variations are seen, and predictor threads are inconsistent. Once the diagnosis of RSD is made, the treatment emphasis shifts from the causative injury to the pain itself. Certain methods appear effective in converting pain from intolerable to functional. Once pain is under the patient's control, more assertive therapy can address goals like ROM and functional strength.

Assessment

The pain diagram allows the patient to express discomforts graphically. It is important to illustrate the worst of times as well as during activity, during inactivity, and after sleep. Patients who are trapped in RSD or a chronic pain syndrome may not be accurate at first. Repeated comparison diagrams are helpful, along with use of the VAS scales. As the patient begins to take control, a steady decrease in VAS annoyance pain is seen regardless of the VAS intensity level.

OBJECTIVE MEASURES

Objective assessment measures include the following:

- VASs quantify degrees of pain intensity or frustration levels.

- Trace sweat patterns of hyperhydrosis-Ninhydrin can be used for objectivity.

- Skin temperature mapping documents sympathetic vascular vasodilation.

Skin temperature mapping can document vascular changes at the surface due to sympathetic disturbance. It is not easy to distinguish a sympathetic disturbance from underlying inflammation. I use the pain diagram, and palpation of the tendon sheaths and muscle bellies to differentiate the two. On the basis of this information, I establish a treatment strategy.

Strategy

At the first meeting between the patient and the therapist, rapport begins with a mutual understanding of the patient's pain perception. Strategy for RSD in the short term is to encourage patient participation through a gentle form of intrinsic muscle fluid flushing and bone loading. Both can be performed with a minimum of discomfort using putty; one cannot take a "bite the bullet approach" to the treatment of RSD. The therapist coaxes and urges the patient to perform beneficial exercises that do not cause pain. I choose simple bimanual activities or crafts that can be done without effort. The patient's mental concentration is placed on the task and not on the pain.

DO NOT BECOME DIVERTED BY EDEMA

RSD spreads into the tissues filled with edema. Patients strongly relate the edema to the pain. They become convinced that there is an undiscovered cause for the fluid; the fluid is the pain source, and when the swelling leaves, so will the pain. Unfortunately, they also believe that the edema will exit by resting and that it is better to leave it alone. This approach ensures the continuation of this cycle of edema, pain, and immobility, and consequently, ensures the continuation of the RSD.

As noted under the heading entitled Chronic Inflammation and Repetitive Strain Problems, the pooling type of noninflammatory edema contains nonproteinaceous fluid, occupies space, and impedes joint movement. With RSD, the injury and immobility have produced poor plumbing. Intrinsic pumping, gentle joint movements, and tendon glides are the cure for this type of fluid accumulation. The duration of the therapy both in minutes per session and in number of visits is extended. The motions are small and pain is always respected.

THE PATIENT CONTROLS THE CURE

Teach the patient that he or she owns the pain and controls the process. A minimum of passive therapy modalities should be incorporated into the program. Self-application of hot and cold packs, self-massage, and self-administered bone-loading exercises that are structured and self-monitored clearly re-enforce that it is the patient who controls the cure, not the pain. Day splinting is used only to promote function. A support or cushioned wrap that does not immobilize but that enhances use of the extremity can be very beneficial; it affirms the problem but validates use of the extremity. Neoprene soft wraps are especially good for this use.

The patient is the most important participant—a chart of compliance is an excellent way to show a cause and effect relationship between the patient's intervention and a tissue reaction or change. Change is the desired goal; pain relief may not be the first reaction encountered. With luck, the patient who truly desires to recover will accept change as a sign of progress and not quit when tight muscles react to stretch. The patient is taught that "motion is lotion" to blood flow, edema control, synovial fluid exchange, and soft tissue elasticity—the key to resolving the pain and restoring function.

MODALITIES OF BENEFIT

Several modalities of benefit for RSD include

- Nonpainful muscle contraction to reduce edema levels and initiate muscular work—intrinsic exercises with soft putty are excellent.

- Self-controlled bone loading—begin with soft putty rolling that includes all joints of the extremity in a relaxed pattern.

- Self-massage of muscles and desensitization massage of most painful areas; vibration is effective in diverting the pain.

- Bimanual tasks—relatively simple; minimal resistance; steady-paced repetitive tasks such as weight well rolling and pedaling exercises help posture and trunk patterning.

MODALITIES IN USE THAT ARE OF LIMITED BENEFIT

Contrast Baths. As yet, there are no objective controlled studies with data to confirm the efficacy of contrast baths. Many therapists are convinced of their value in the treatment of RSD. This treatment might be useful in the clinical setting if it is supervised by an aide and not billed as therapist time. When the patient completes the contrast baths on his or her own, it fulfills the criteria for patient control over pain and patient recovery.

TENS. The goal of TENS treatment for RSD must be carefully considered. Its use to mask pain and gain compliance is foreseeable, but it should not be used alone. At its best, it should encourage movement and function much like a splint.

CONCLUSION

I have illustrated what I consider the proper relationship between the therapist's assessment and the formulation of a treatment strategy.

I have chosen assessments that I use for neurological conditions that yield valuable data on which strategy decisions are made. The therapist uses this information in differential decison-making about exercise levels and home programs. It is only through complete objective examination that therapists can accurately choose exercise levels from the broad range that exists within the definitions of active, passive, and resistive exercise.

Much like an operative report, this therapist's data base is a form of communication that assists the team of patient, therapist, and physician. All members of the team are better served when there is a trail of objective information indicating the thought pattern that led to modifications in the treatment program throughout the course of patient recovery.

References

Hayduk A: Increasing hand efficiency at cold temperatures by training hand vasodilation with a classical conditioning—biofeedback overlap design. Biofeedback Self Regul 5:307–326, 1980.

Hunter JM, Totten PA: Therapeutic techniques to enhance nerve gliding in thoracic outlet syndrome and carpal tunnel syndrome. Hand Clin 7:505–520, 1991.

Joyce C, Zutshi D, Hrubes Y, Mason R: Comparison of fixed interval and visual analogue scales for rating chronic pain. Eur J Clin Pharmacol 8:415–420, 1975.

Margoles MS: The pain chart: Spatial properties of pain. *In* Melzack R (ed): Pain Measurement and Assessment. New York, Raven Press, 1983, pp 215–225.

McLellan DL, Swash M: Longitudinal sliding of the median nerve during movements of the upper limb. J Neurol Neurosurg Psychiatry 39:566–570, 1976.

Millesi H: The nerve gap: Theory and clinical practise. Hand Clin 4:651–663, 1986.

Phelps D, Rutherford R, Boswick J: Control of vasospasm following trauma and microvascular surgery. J Hand Surg 4:109–117, 1979.

Price DD, McGrath PA, Rafii A, Buckingham B: The validation of visual analog scales as ratio scale measure for chronic and experimental pain. Pain 17:45–56, 1983.

Revill S, Robinson J, Rosen M, Hogg M: Anaesthesia 31:1191–1198, 1976.

Thulesius O, Burbakk A, Berlin E: Response of digital blood pressure to cold provocation in cases with Raynaud's phenomenon. Angiology 32:113–118, 1981.

Travell JG, Simons DG: Myofascial Pain and Dysfunction: The Trigger Point Manual. Baltimore, Williams & Wilkins, 1983.

Wehbé M: Tendon gliding exercises. Am J Occup Ther 41:164–167, 1987.

Part III

PAIN

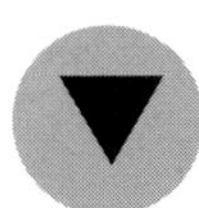

Chapter 12

- L. Andrew Koman
- J. Leonard Goldner
- Thomas L. Smith

The Effect of Extremity Blood Flow on Pain and Cold Tolerance

Abnormalities in upper extremity blood flow may cause pain, cold intolerance, or both. Alterations in activities of daily living and decreased work productivity secondary to these symptoms are a significant societal burden. Aberrant microvascular flow and cold intolerance are seen after vascular compromise (occlusive, vasospastic, or vaso-occlusive) or trauma (autonomic dysfunction or reflex sympathetic dystrophy) and have a negative impact on millions of people. Pain and cold intolerance secondary to abnormal blood flow are estimated to affect over 10% of the general population (Cleophas and Niemeyer, 1993).

Symptoms result from congenital or acquired abnormalities in the integrity of vascular structure, function, or both. Structural abnormalities in the vasculature or vascular control mechanisms may be either congenital or acquired; even when abnormalities of neurovascular control occur in the presence of structurally adequate vasculature, they can result in abnormal perfusion. Regardless of etiology, blood flow that adversely affects cellular perfusion and causes cell damage results in symptoms that range from mild discomfort to severe disability. The purpose of this chapter is to define the anatomy and physiology of normal and abnormal vascular and microvascular flow and to present an approach to evaluating and understanding the pain and cold intolerance related to abnormalities of vascular flow.

EXTREMITY PERFUSION: ANATOMIC AND PATHOLOGIC CONSIDERATIONS

Extremity vascular competency requires that the vascular system be capable of fulfilling metabolic needs of the extremity under both stressed and unstressed conditions. Vascular perfusion depends on arterial inflow, venous outflow, lymphatic drainage, local factors, autonomic microvascular control mechanisms, and central nervous system responses (Figs. 12–1 and 12–2) (Koman, 1983). Pain associated with inadequate extremity blood flow is the result of cellular damage. The perception of pain depends on the initiating event, afferent input, efferent modulation, and central interpretation (Fig. 12–3) (Dray et al, 1994). Therefore, vascular incompetency induces or enhances extremity pain when the microcirculation is not sufficient to provide for cellular metabolic needs. To prevent the activation of polymodal (or primary) afferent neurons (pain receptors), it is necessary to have both adequate arterial *structure* and appropriate physiologic *function*. Damage to the vascular system (e.g., occlusion of the brachial artery and major collateral arteries due to trauma) or inappropriate microvascular regulation and control (e.g., vasospasm and inappropriate arteriovenous

shunting secondary to collagen vascular disease) causes pain, tissue necrosis, or both. The pain accompanying major arterial occlusion is relatively easy to diagnose and understand; however, the discomfort secondary to inappropriate microvascular perfusion and relative segmental ischemia in a normal-appearing extremity with good pulses may be a perplexing clinical problem.

Thermoregulatory and Nutritional Flow

Thermoregulatory flow and nutritional flow constitute total peripheral flow (Burton, 1939; Coffman, 1972). Thermo-

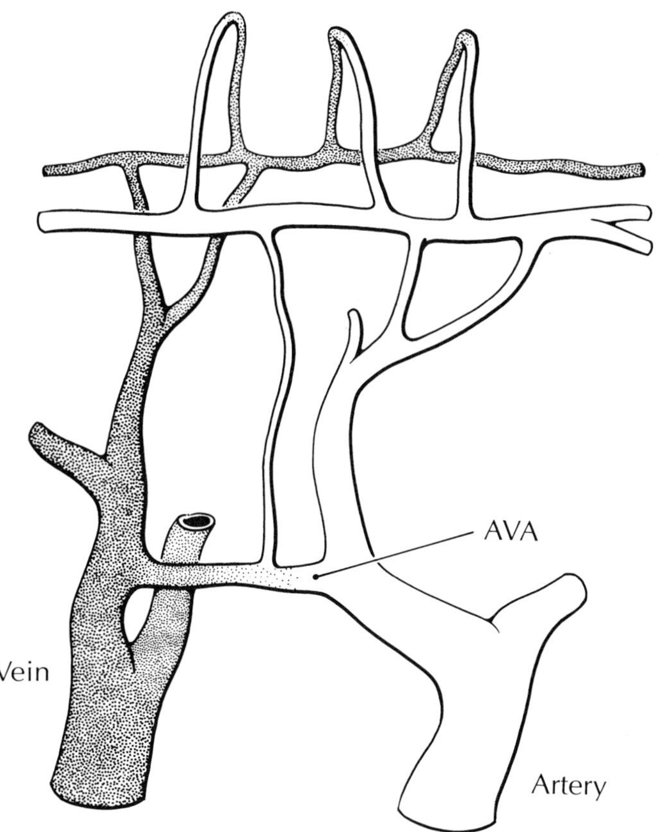

FIGURE 12–1. Cutaneous papillary capillaries of the digits with supplying arterioles and venules. Note the presence of the arteriovenous anastomosis (AVA), which can bypass the nutritive capillaries, permitting thermoregulatory cutaneous blood flow. Included in this representation is a nutritive arteriole that branches off the AVA, a feature noted by direct observations. (Reproduced with permission of the Extremity Laboratory, Department of Orthopaedic Surgery, Bowman Gray School of Medicine, Wake Forest University.)

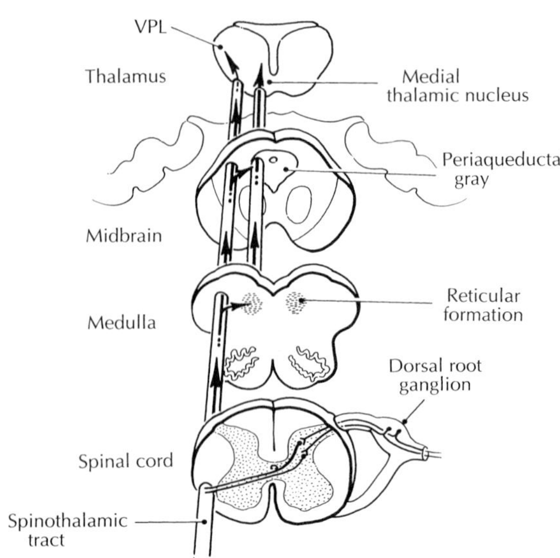

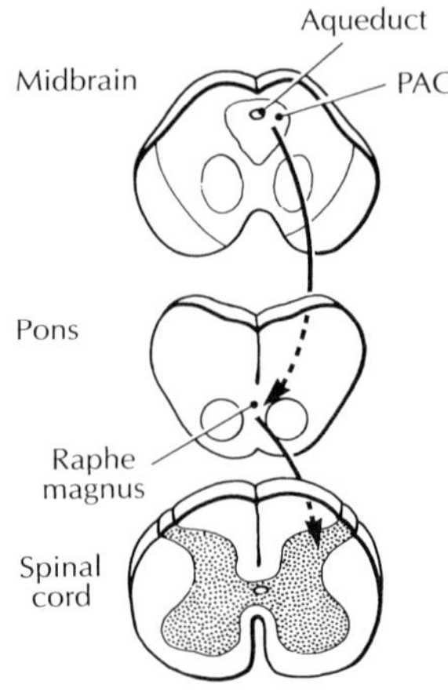

FIGURE 12–2. Ascending nociceptive pathways to the thalamus *(left panel)* and descending modulatory pathways from cortex and brainstem *(right panel)*. (From Koman LA: Painful upper extremity. ASSH Hand Surgery Update *1*:24–2, 1994. Reproduced by permission of American Society for Surgery of the Hand. New York, Churchill Livingstone, 1994.)

regulatory flow (80% to 90% of total flow) passes through arteriovenous anastomoses, and it is these shunts that help regulate core body temperature. Nutritional flow (10% to 20% of total flow) provides the cellular metabolic needs of the extremity and requires (1) *adequate blood volume and pressure within the macrocirculation* to perfuse the microvasculature and papillary or nutritional capillary beds during stressed and unstressed conditions (see Fig. 12–1), and (2) *appropriate distribution* of microvascular perfusion. When nutritional flow is inadequate, a nociceptive cellular insult results in the activation of polymodal afferent pain receptors, which provide input through ascending pathways (see Fig. 12–3). This information is modified by descending pathways (see Fig. 12–2) and then subjected to cortical interpretation of the magnitude and intensity of pain. An extremity is considered to be vascularly competent when arterial inflow

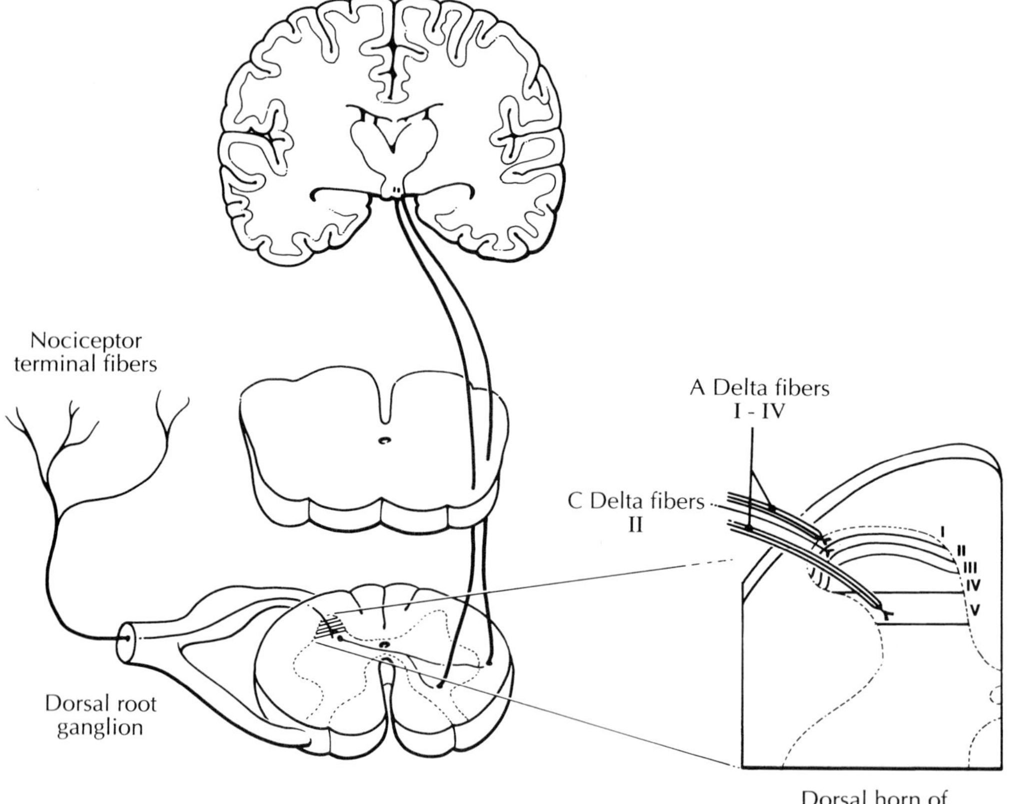

FIGURE 12–3. Primary afferent nociceptor fibers (polymodal afferent neurons) impinge on the dorsal horn of the spinal cord. Information is then relayed to the thalamus and cortex. (From Koman LA: Painful upper extremity. ASSH Hand Surgery Update *1*:24–1, 1994. Reproduced with permission of American Society for Surgery of the Hand. New York, Churchill Livingstone, 1994.)

can reach nutritional capillary beds in sufficient quantity to meet stressed and unstressed metabolic demands and prevent symptoms of pain, cold intolerance, and claudication.

The thermoregulatory component of extremity blood flow may be 20 to 30 times the nutritional component and is characterized by large fluctuations. Absolute requirements for nutritive perfusion are low (1 to 2 ml/min/100 g tissue), and there is little fluctuation in an unstressed state. In pathologic conditions, small increases in the nutritional flow component can play a dramatic role in decreasing ischemic symptoms.

Macrocirculation/Microcirculation

The macrocirculation is composed of vessels greater than 100 micrometers in diameter; it functions by delivering nutrients to smaller microcirculatory vessels and providing thermoregulatory capacity to arteriovenous connections. In contrast, the 100-micrometer and smaller vessels that make up the microcirculation deliver nutrients at a cellular level without large fluctuations in volume (see Fig. 12–1), and they help to control temperature through arteriovenous anastomoses. The macrocirculation is vital, and its injury or compromise may result in arterial insufficiency and tissue necrosis. The extent of symptoms following injury to large vessels is directly related to the adequacy of the collateral circulation, existing vasomotor tone, local control mechanisms, and neuroendocrine factors (Koman, 1983). Distal to the elbow and knee, parallel arteries with multiple interconnections exist in the majority of extremities (Coleman and Anson, 1961) (Fig. 12–4). Large vessel flow with sufficient pulse pressure to provide pulsatile digital flow is necessary for painless, normal function. Redundancy within the microcirculation allows significant injury to occur without microvascular compromise. In the upper extremity, a mid-forearm

laceration of the radial or ulnar artery is compensated over time by an increase in flow through the remaining vessel, and symptoms are minimal despite a drop in digital blood pressure (Gelberman et al, 1982).

Control Mechanisms

Assuming normal, adequate large-vessel blood delivery is present, distribution of flow to thermoregulatory or nutrient microvascular beds depends on (1) local control mechanisms, (2) the sympathetic nervous system, (3) myogenic autoregulation, (4) humoral and blood-borne agents, and (5) environmental conditions. In normal hands, feet, and digits, local control mechanisms tend to be overridden by the central (sympathetic) nervous system (Coffman and Cohen, 1988; Fig. 12–5). Myogenic autoregulatory control provides a basal level of microvascular tone (Hwa and Bevan, 1986), with major cutaneous circulatory control being provided by vasoconstrictor, α-adrenergic tone, which is further modified by humoral agents and environmental temperature (Abramson, 1972; Egloff et al, 1982; Flatt, 1980; Flavahan et al, 1987).

EVALUATION TECHNIQUES

Pathologic States and the Importance of Stress

Pathologic alterations in extremity blood flow that may produce symptoms include congenital deformities, trauma, and acquired diseases. Symptoms may be precipitated by events within the macrocirculation, the microcirculation, or both. If either large or small vessels sustain structural damage or if function is compromised by abnormal control mechanisms, compromised perfusion of the nutritional capil-

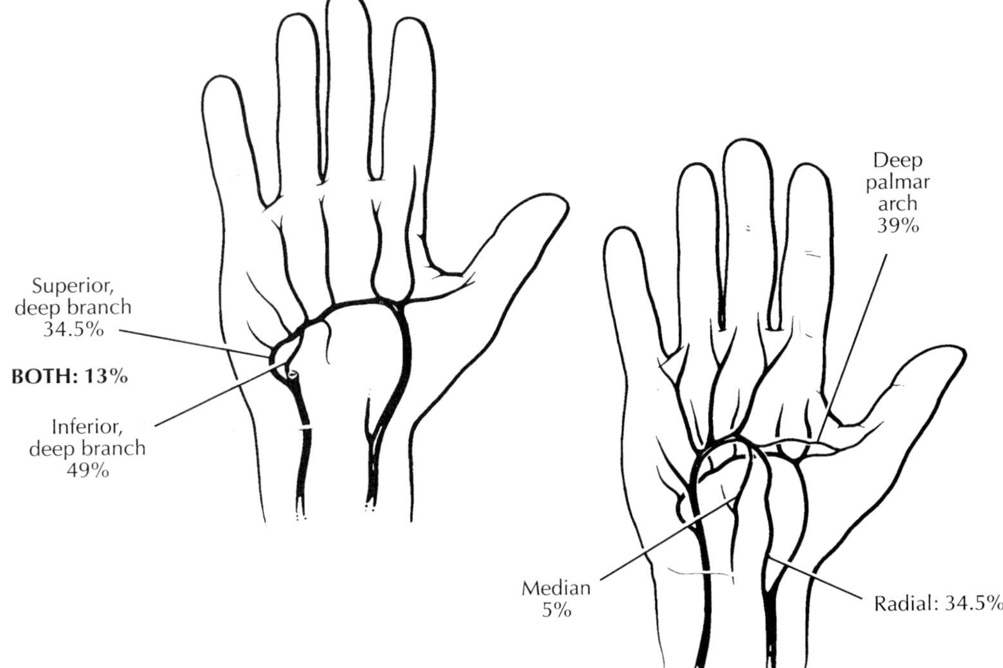

FIGURE 12–4. Vascular supply of the hands demonstrating superficial and deep aspects of the circulation of the upper extremities. Common variations of the vascular anatomy are noted. Modified from Koman LA, Smith BP, Smith TL: Stress testing in the evaluation of upper-extremity perfusion. Hand Clin 9(1):60, 1994.

Causes of Pain Associated with Extremity Blood Flow

Congenital	Primary Abnormal System
Absence of arterial development	Macrocirculation
Arteriovenous malformation	Macrocirculation
Traumatic	
Transection	Macrocirculation
Occlusive disease	Macrocirculation
Embolic disease	Macrocirculation and microcirculation
Dystrophic response	Microcirculation
Acquired	
Systemic Disease	
• Diabetes mellitus	Macrocirculation and microcirculation
• Collagen vascular disease	Macrocirculation and microcirculation
• Erythromelalgia	Macrocirculation and microcirculation
• Atherosclerosis	Macrocirculation and microcirculation
Genetic Disease	
• Sickle cell	Macrocirculation and microcirculation

laries induces cellular damage and pain (Table 12–1). Evaluation of pain secondary to altered perfusion requires an analysis of structure and function with and without stress (Koman et al, 1993a, 1993b; Wilgis, 1981). *In order to appreciate causal relationships between pain and blood flow, it is crucial to use testing that provides a comprehensive analysis of both static and dynamic vascular perfusion at a macrocirculatory and a microcirculatory level, and to be able to differentiate thermoregulatory flow from nutritional flow.*

Techniques Available for Evaluating Upper Extremity Blood Flow

The physical examination of the extremity can reveal a great deal about the underlying disease. Proper evaluation requires a thorough history and detailed clinical examination, including evaluation of pulses, wrist and digital Allen tests, timed Allen test, and segmental blood pressure determinations (Koman, 1985; Koman et al, 1993a, 1993b). In addition, specialized testing may be necessary to delineate the level, magnitude, and complexity of the abnormality. Testing must be capable of evaluating both large and small vessels under controlled conditions.

Laboratory Evaluation

NONINVASIVE VASCULAR LABORATORY EVALUATION

The three basic techniques employed in a noninvasive vascular laboratory evaluation are *Doppler ultrasound, segmental systolic pressures, and plethysmography* (Berger and Kleinert, 1993; Koman, 1983; Koman et al, 1993b). Use of these techniques allows the diagnosis of large or small vessel disease.

Doppler ultrasound provides hemodynamic information based on the Doppler effect of moving cells on sound wave frequency as received by a piezoelectric crystal. Continuous wave and pulsed wave Doppler units may be employed to provide subjective information regarding primarily macrovascular flow. Pulse echo ultrasound provides real-time B-mode imaging of vessels (Fig. 12–6*A* and *B*) (Koman et al, 1985) and can be combined with a pulsed wave Doppler ultrasound to provide functional and structural information for the accurate assessment of stenoses, occlusions, and aneurysms (Fig. 12–7).

Segmental systolic pressures can be used to differentiate large and small (macrovascular) lesions, and an objective estimation of static extremity perfusion is possible with the use of an index calculated by dividing the systolic pressure of the distal extremity by that of the proximal extremity. A

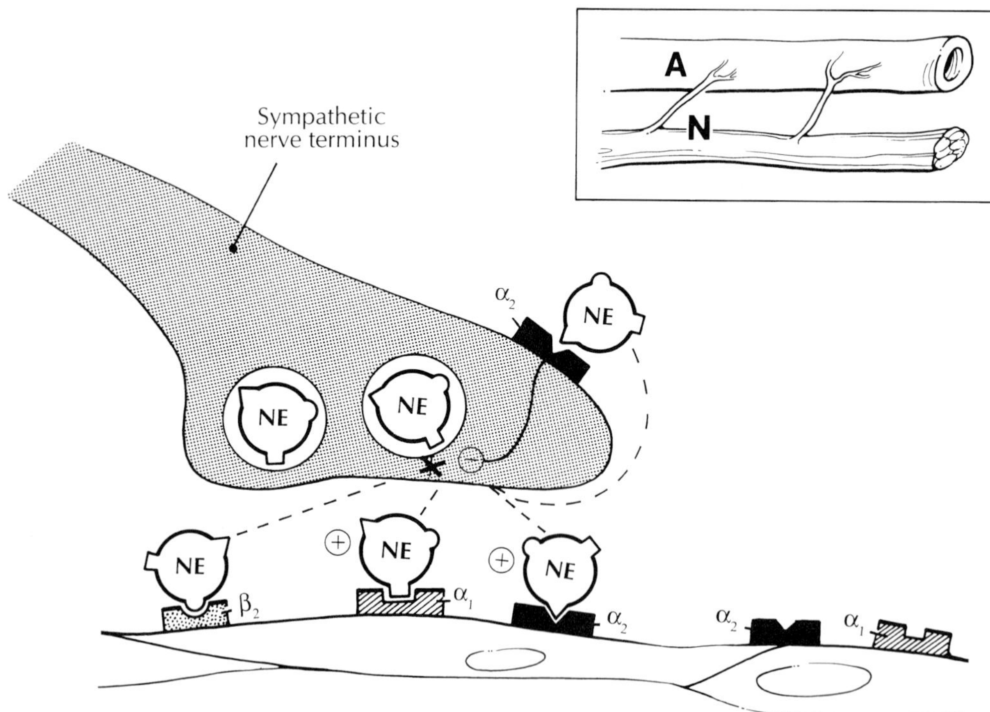

FIGURE 12–5. Sympathetic innervation of the digital vasculature *(upper right)* with the neurovascular junction on the vascular smooth muscle cells *(lower left)*. Norepinephrine (NE) is the primary adrenergic neurotransmitter at these sites. Note that the primary postsynaptic receptors present are α_1 and α_2 (vasconstrictive) and β_2 (vasodilatory) receptors. The presynaptic α_2-receptor on the nerve terminus inhibits further release of NE from the neuron when the α_2 receptor is stimulated. (Reproduced with permission by Extremity Laboratory, Department of Orthopaedic Surgery, Bowman Gray School of Medicine, Wake Forest University.)

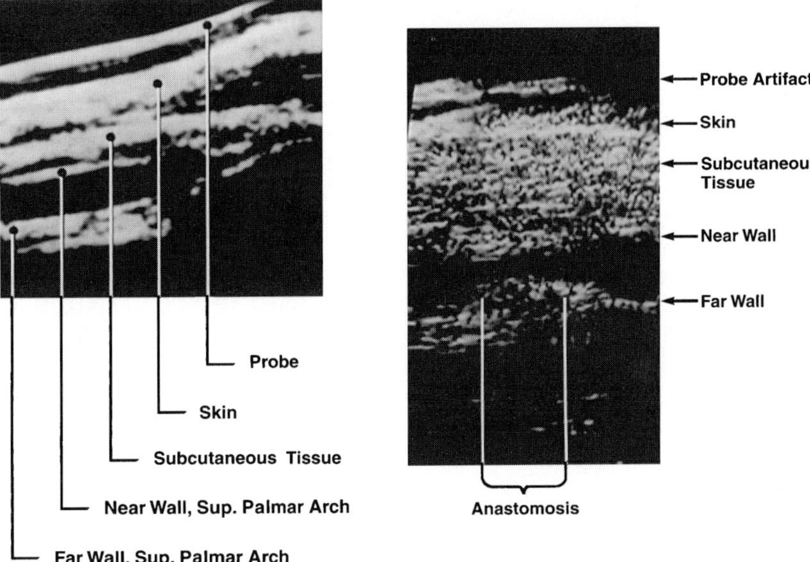

FIGURE 12–6. High-resolution (10 MHz) ultrasound of the superficial palmar arch *(on right)* and a stenosis at an end-to-end anastomosis of the ulnar artery. (Reproduced with permission by Extremity Laboratory, Department of Orthopaedic Surgery, Bowman Gray School of Medicine, Wake Forest University).

20-mmHg difference indicates the presence of disease, and the patterns of segmental pressure can be used to localize stenosis or occlusion.

Digital plethysmography can be performed by air-filled cuffs, mercury-in-rubber strain gauges, photosensors, or occlusion techniques (Jones, 1991; Kleinert and Gupta, 1993; Koman, 1983). Plethysmographic techniques are noninvasive and may be used to evaluate forearm, calf, hand, foot, or digital blood flow (see Fig. 12–7). Occlusion plethysmography provides an objective, accurate measurement of volume change following occlusion, that is, a measure of total flow. The other techniques measure changes in diameter or skin motion and provide linear assessments of relative total flow (Jones, 1991). Plethysmographic techniques cannot discriminate between cutaneous and skeletal muscle blood flow or differentiate between nutritional and thermoregulatory perfusion (Koman et al, 1993b). Digital plethysmography provides qualitative information regarding total digital flow and complements segmental pressure data, which evaluate specific arteries (structural data) (Koman, 1985).

MICROVASCULAR ANGIOLOGY LABORATORY EVALUATION

The clinically applicable techniques that evaluate digital microcirculatory performance include temperature, laser Doppler digital fluxmetry and vital capillaroscopy. When coupled with stress techniques, these methods provide significant objective determinations of total digital flow and allow the differentiation of thermoregulatory flow from nutritional flow (Koman et al, 1993a).

Skin surface temperature provides an estimate of total flow (Felder et al, 1954). At temperatures below 30°C, skin surface temperature is linearly proportional to flow (Conrad and Green, 1963). At higher temperatures, large increases in flow may accompany relatively small temperature alterations, because skin temperature measurements are insensitive to rapid changes in cutaneous flow, and further may be affected by core temperature, blood flow in adjacent structures, muscle activity, and sweating. Therefore, skin temperature is best used to evaluate trends in total digital flow (Koman et al, 1993). For example, skin temperature is excellent for monitoring flow following digital replantation (Stirrat et al, 1978). However, skin temperature cannot differentiate nutritional flow from thermoregulatory flow, and thus it is relatively nonspecific. Thermography is a method of measuring temperature, but in spite of providing a large amount of data, it is subject to the same limitations as surface temperature probes.

Laser Doppler fluxmetry, a noninvasive technique, allows the rapidly repeatable evaluation of perfusion by low-power

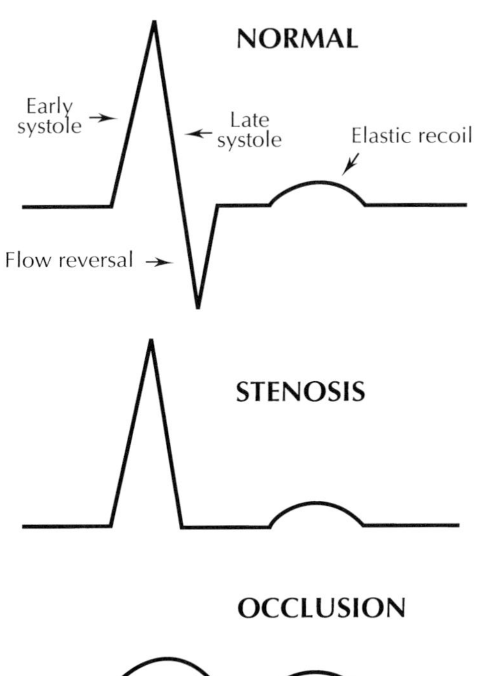

FIGURE 12–7. Plethysmographic pulse contours. Normal patterns *(top)* are compared with recordings obtained beyond a stenosis *(middle)* and an occlusion *(bottom)*. (Reproduced with permission by Extremity Laboratory, Department of Orthopaedic Surgery, Bowman Gray School of Medicine, Wake Forest University.)

helium-neon light transmitted through a quartz glass fiberoptic connection (Öberg et al, 1984). It relies on the Doppler effect and produces a signal proportional to the movement of the red blood cells. The technique allows the measurement of relative blood flow without invading microvascular beds. Conventional probes provide 0.1-second frequency response data from a single area. Laser Doppler perfusion imaging provides two-dimensional mapping of tissue perfusion over a 12 × 12-cm area at 4- to 5-minute intervals and permits the evaluation of spatial and (to some extent) temporal variations in skin perfusion (Fig. 12–8) (Wärdell, 1994; Wärdell et al, 1994).

Vital capillaroscopy, a noninvasive technique, is the only practical method for assessing nutritional blood flow and microvascular structure (Fig. 12–9) (Bollinger et al, 1974; Houtman et al, 1987; Koman et al, 1993b). The nutritional or papillary capillary bed can be visualized directly through an appropriately designed epi-illumination microscope. Although portions of capillary loops can be seen in all skin areas, the capillary loops at the digital nailfold of the hand and feet are oriented parallel to the skin surface and thus are the easiest to observe (Fagrell, 1973, 1974). These papillary capillary loops consist of an arterial limb (7 to 12 μm) and a venous limb (10 to 20 μm) and may be evaluated structur-

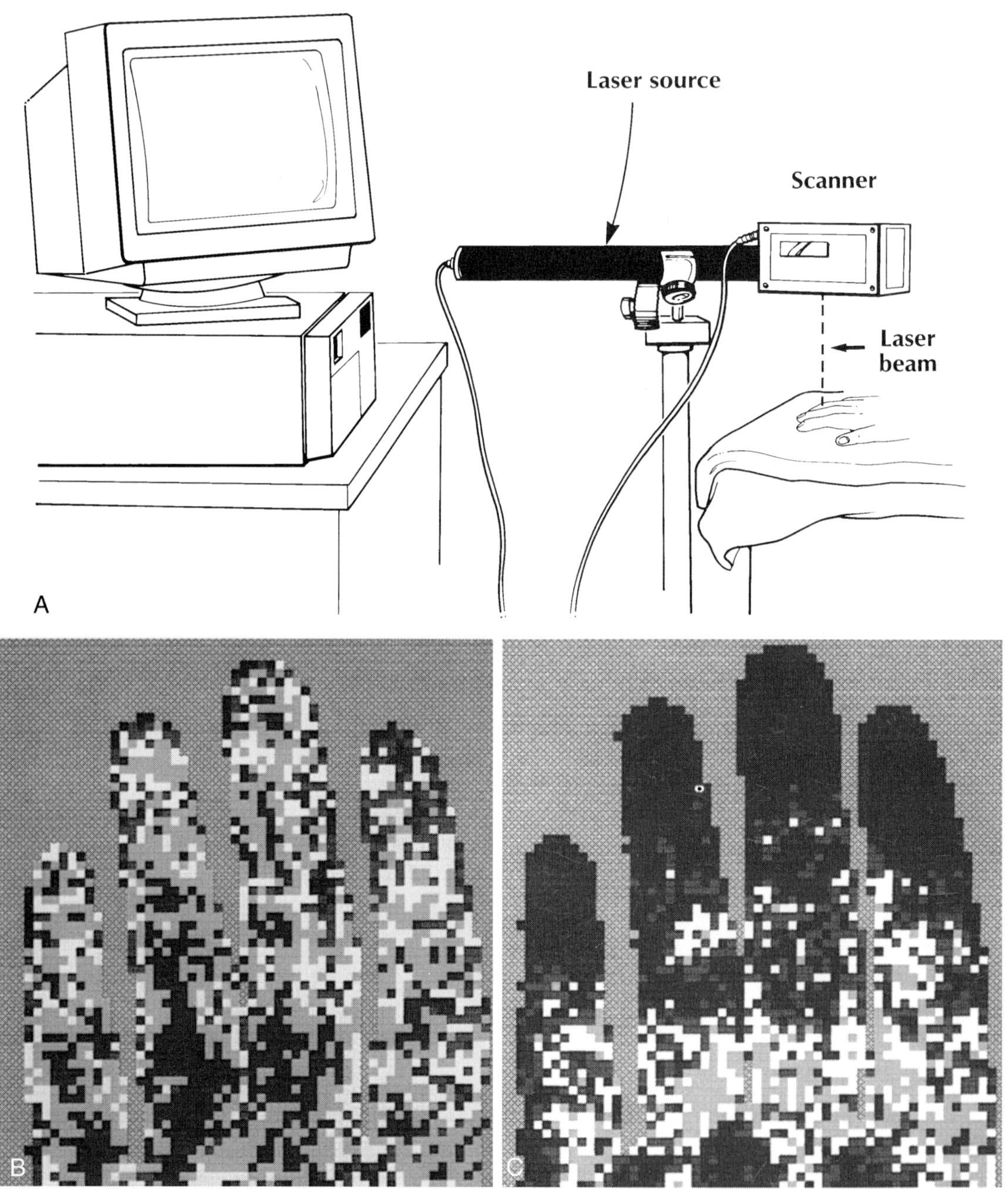

FIGURE 12–8. *A,* Laser Doppler perfusion imaging monitor with helium-neon laser source, scanner head, controller (microcomputer) and subject extremity. (Reproduced with permission by Extremity Laboratory, Department of Orthopaedic Surgery, Bowman Gray School of Medicine, Wake Forest University.) *B* and *C,* Spatial distribution of cutaneous perfusion of a volunteer's hand at room temperature (23°C) *(B)* and after cooling (14.2°C) *(C).* Note the dramatic heterogeneous decrease in cutaneous perfusion following 3 minutes' exposure to cool air. (Reproduced with permission by Extremity Laboratory, Department of Orthopaedic Surgery, Bowman Gray School of Medicine, Wake Forest University.)

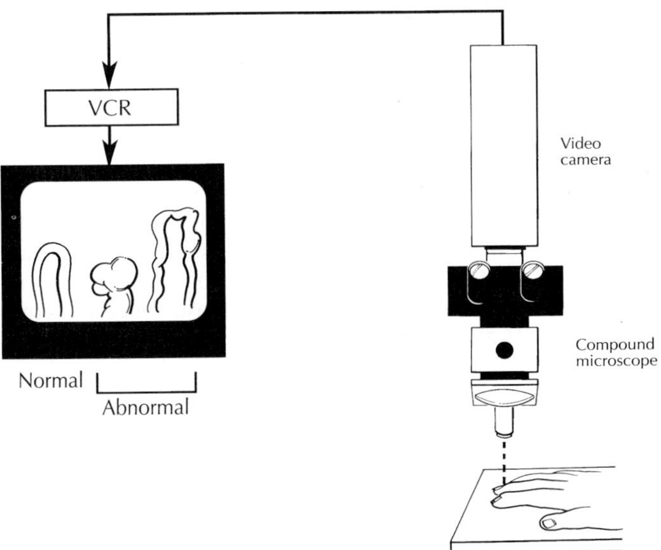

FIGURE 12–9. Nailfold capillaroscopy performed using a compound microscope with epi-illumination, video camera and video cassette recorder (VCR), and television monitor image. Note the differing normal and pathologic anatomy of the nailfold capillaries. (Reproduced with permission by Extremity Laboratory, Department of Orthopaedic Surgery, Bowman Gray School of Medicine, Wake Forest University.)

ally by photomicrography or dynamically by using dynamic videomicrography (Rosén et al, 1988). Structural analysis includes an assessment of density, shape, and diameter; dynamic data include measurements of velocity and volume, which allow calculations of nutritional flow in microliters per second.

Isolated Cold Stress Testing. In order to determine the effect of blood flow on pain and cold intolerance, the microcirculation must be evaluated under stressed and non-stressed conditions (Pollock et al, 1989, 1993). Stress may be induced by high or low temperature, a transient ischemia, or psychological manipulation. Cold stress may be achieved by ice water immersion (Nielson, 1976), application of cold to the nape of the neck (Jamieson et al, 1971a, 1971b), total body cooling (Nielson, 1976), or temporary hand or foot enclosure in a refrigeration unit (Koman et al, 1984; Koman and Nunley, 1986). Isolated cold stress testing is a nonimmersion technique that is performed under physiologic temperatures and provides insight into microcirculatory responses (Koman, 1994). By combining temperature with laser Doppler fluxmetry and vital capillaroscopy, qualitative and quantitative data reflecting flow during stressed and unstressed conditions can be obtained. Isolated cold stress testing evaluates the ability of a given vascular bed to respond to a moderately cold local stress and then to recover in a thermoneutral environment. Skin surface temperature is used as an index of total blood flow; skin microvascular perfusion is measured and analyzed by laser Doppler fluxmetry. In addition, vital capillaroscopy data may be incorporated. Normal response patterns of laser Doppler, temperature, and capillaroscopy have been established, and abnormal responses can be correlated with clinical signs and symptoms (Koman et al, 1993a).

PATHOLOGIC CONDITIONS

Pathologic changes leading to microvascular compromise and digital pain include large vessel and small vessel occlusion, trauma, and abnormalities of neurovascular control (Cardelli and Kleinsmith, 1989; Maricq, 1982; Wilgis, 1981, 1985). Events that lead to arterial flow abnormalities and resultant pain may be associated with vascular insults at the macrovascular or microvascular level (e.g., thrombosis of the ulnar artery at the wrist), with trauma to nonvascular structures (e.g., reflex sympathetic dystrophy) (Christensen and Henriksen, 1983; Kleinert et al, 1973), with combined vascular and neural injury, with abnormal sympathetic control (e.g., vasospastic disease), or with congenital abnormalities (e.g., hemangiomas).

Vascular Injury/Compromise

Occlusion of large vessels above the elbow or knee from atherosclerotic disease or trauma and the subsequent ischemic pain at rest of claudication is easy to understand and diagnose. In the presence of adequate collateral circulation, however, symptoms may be minimal or nonexistent without significant provocation. Below the elbow or knee, isolated disruption of a single vessel with an intact parallel vessel results in increased flow in the remaining vessel or vessels, decreased digital blood pressure, and minimal symptoms (Gelberman and Blasingame, 1981; Gelberman et al, 1979, 1982) unless the damage occurs distal to collateral inflow or involves a significant end artery (Koman and Urbaniak, 1981; Koman et al, 1983) as with a distal injury from emboli. For example, symptoms following thrombosis of the ulnar artery at the wrist depend on (1) the adequacy of the collateral circulation after thrombosis and (2) the effect of the event on sympathetic tone. A short-segment thrombosis with completion of the superficial arch by a large collateral from the radial artery may present with a wide spectrum of symptoms—from trivial to incapacitating. Because the macrocirculation is adequate structurally, symptoms are based on inappropriate functional control with vasospasm, abnormal shunting, and relative ischemia, or neuropathic symptoms from segmental ischemic neuropathy. Conversely, thrombosis that occurs in the absence of adequate collateral circulation or distal to collateral inflow that involves end arteries, or that is accompanied by embolism, may produce ischemia with subsequent cellular injury and pain. Noninvasive vascular testing allows the diagnosis of occlusion or stenosis (see Fig. 12–7). Testing in the microvascular angiology laboratory can determine the degree of arteriovenous shunting and sympathetic tone (see Fig. 12–8).

Occlusive Disease

Thrombosis of the ulnar artery at the wrist (so-called hypothenar hammer syndrome) is a frequent complication in patients whose occupations encourage using the palm of the hand as a tool (Koman and Urbaniak, 1981). Many patients with ulnar artery thrombosis never consult a physician and are able to compensate due to adequate collateral circulation and appropriate sympathetic tone. Symptomatic patients ex-

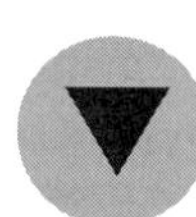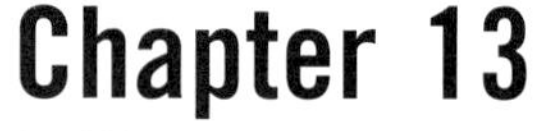

Chapter 13

• George E. Omer, Jr

Continuous Peripheral Epineural Infusion for the Treatment of Acute Pain

Pain is an unpleasant sensory and emotional experience associated with actual or potential tissue damage and is described in terms of such damage (Mersky, 1979). The U. S. Commission on the Evaluation of Pain (1987) notes that pain is a "complex experience, embracing physical, mental, social, and behavioral processes, which compromises the quality of life of many individuals." The recognition of pain is subjective and depends on the intensity of the peripheral stimulus, central summation, and the personality of the patient (Omer, 1978a, 1978b, 1984c; Omer and Pirela-Cruz, 1994). Individually, pain is an intensely personal reaction, and Aristotle and Plato considered it to be a "passion of the soul" (Geldard, 1972).

PREVENTION OF PAIN

Pain can be totally incapacitating after iatrogenic procedures on the peripheral nerves. For elective surgical procedures, the prevention of pain is an important aspect of treatment (Omer, 1979, 1984b). If a cutaneous nerve is partially cut, such as the superficial radial nerve, the laceration should be sutured promptly. In extensive injuries of extremities, venous repair is important for the prevention of edema. Surgical release of fascial sheaths is performed as indicated. During the early postoperative period (24–72 hours), attempts should be made to halt the development of edema. Early motion should be initiated, such as active shoulder exercises when the fingers should not move after elective surgery. Medications to consider during the early postoperative period include aspirin and a mild tranquilizer. Aspirin blocks the metabolic pathway from injured cells to the formation of prostaglandins and thromboxanes (Halpern, 1977). A mild tranquilizer promotes the inhibition of anxiety and reduces the incidence of analgesic side effects, including nausea and vomiting (Mayer and Hayes, 1975). Postoperative pain should be evaluated promptly; a pain syndrome never should be allowed to develop fully before aggressive treatment is initiated. For example, the osteoporosis of Sudek's atrophy is not evident by plain radiography for 5 to 8 weeks after injury, but the patient has pain from the time of initial injury.

The attending physicians and therapists must learn to identify the unstable emotional personality. Psychological factors include not only the patient's personality but also the social circumstances surrounding the injury and the potential for primary or secondary gain from continued disability. In these patients, the pain state becomes a permanent memory bank, and the total personality may become focused on the pain problem (Omer, 1978a, 1978b; Zancolli and Zancolli, 1991). These patients require much more time and explanation preoperatively in order to cope with their potential postoperative pain problem.

Sympathetic nervous system dysfunction is the secondary component of pain dysfunction (Amadio, 1988). Lankford (1980, 1991, 1993) has emphasized that reflex sympathetic dystrophy is not present unless three conditions are present at the same time: (1) a persistent, painful lesion (traumatic or acquired); (2) dysesthesia (predisposition, body characteristic, susceptibility); and (3) an abnormal sympathetic reflex.

SUBJECTIVE RELIEF OF PAIN

There are two principles in a treatment program for extremity pain: (1) relieve the pain, and (2) institute active physical use of the involved extremity (Omer, 1978a, 1978b, 1984a, 1984b, 1984c, 1987a). A local trigger point is the immediate physical event that usually initiates the pain.

In those patients with an established pain pattern, it is useful to differentiate localized pain along the course of major peripheral nerves, such as a painful neuroma, from generalized pain that may be stocking-level in distribution or that may follow the watershed, delta-shaped area of major blood vessels. The extremity should be palpated and tapped very gently with a finger from distal to proximal to demonstrate any trigger points of extreme irritation. If a trigger point is obvious, it is marked with a sterile marking pen, and the area is surgically prepared and draped.

After local cutaneous anesthesia, a 16-gauge needle is inserted into the area of irritation (Fig. 13–1A). The needle is aspirated to prevent blood vessel penetration, and a flexible 18-gauge polyethylene intravenous catheter is inserted through the 16-gauge needle (Fig. 13–1B). If performed in this manner, the intravenous catheter should not penetrate a nerve or blood vessel (Omer and Eversmann, 1994). The large-bore, 16-gauge needle is then removed, leaving the 18-gauge intravenous catheter in place (Fig. 13–1C). One-half milliliter of 0.5% lidocaine hydrochloride (Xylocaine) is then injected through the intravenous catheter for local anesthetic effect (Fig. 13–2A and B). If the trigger-point pain is relieved, the intravenous catheter is capped and taped in place (Fig. 13–3A and B). The anesthetic block usually is insufficient for complete motor and sensory paralysis, and the pain-free patient is asked to exercise the extremity, to walk, and to perform assigned physical therapy activities

116

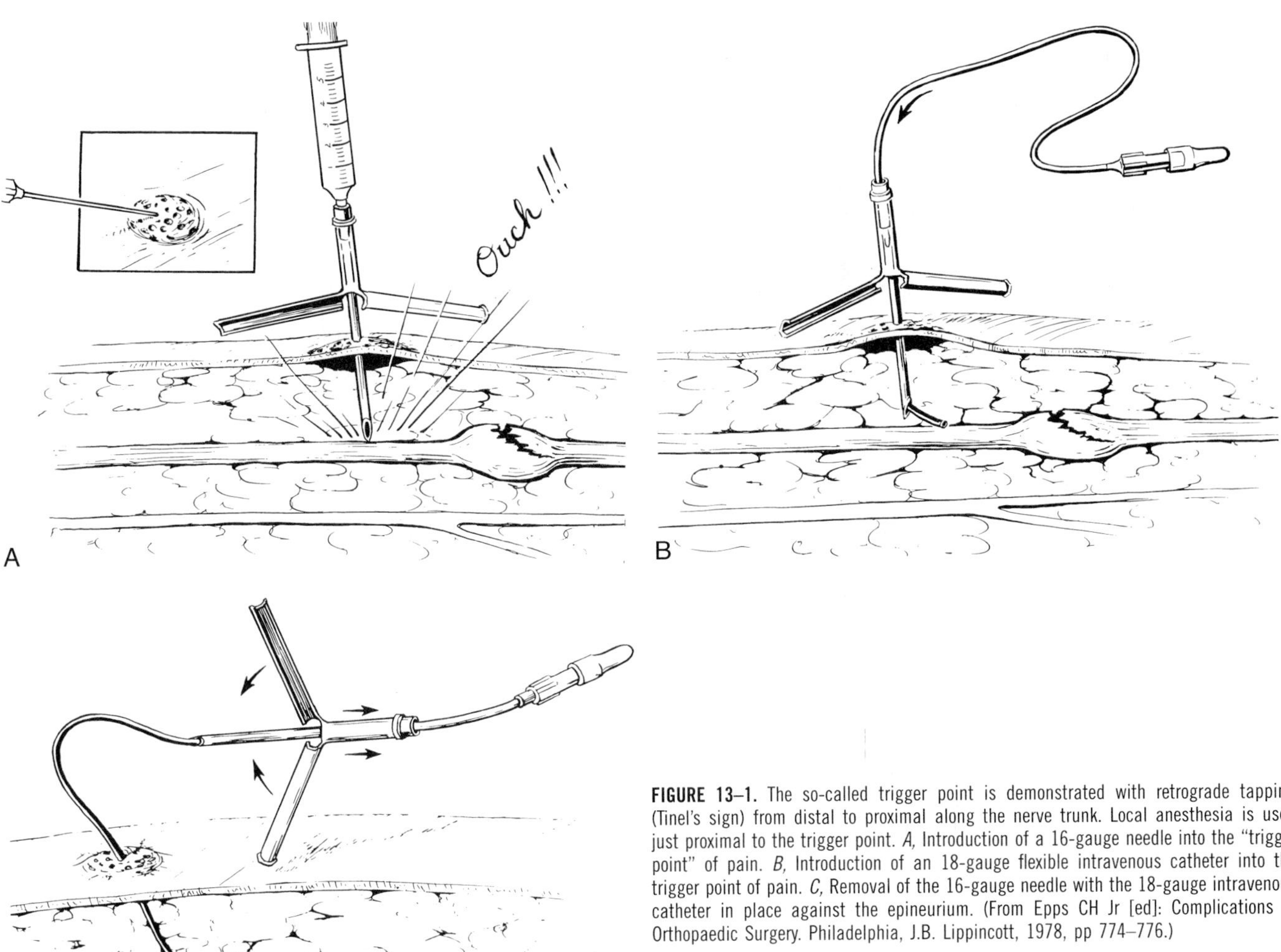

FIGURE 13–1. The so-called trigger point is demonstrated with retrograde tapping (Tinel's sign) from distal to proximal along the nerve trunk. Local anesthesia is used just proximal to the trigger point. *A,* Introduction of a 16-gauge needle into the "trigger point" of pain. *B,* Introduction of an 18-gauge flexible intravenous catheter into the trigger point of pain. *C,* Removal of the 16-gauge needle with the 18-gauge intravenous catheter in place against the epineurium. (From Epps CH Jr [ed]: Complications of Orthopaedic Surgery. Philadelphia, J.B. Lippincott, 1978, pp 774–776.)

FIGURE 13–2. *A,* Injection of local anesthetic agent to obtain a peripheral perineural infusion block. (From Epps CH Jr [ed]: Complications of Orthopaedic Surgery. Philadelphia, J.B. Lippincott, 1978, p 776.) *B,* Anesthetic agent is given on the ward. Additional injections may be given to provide pain-free activity. (From Omer GE Jr, Pirela-Cruz M: Complications in peripheral nerve injuries. *In* Epps CH Jr [ed]: Complications of Orthopaedic Surgery, 3rd ed. Philadelphia, J.B. Lippincott, 1994, p 834.)

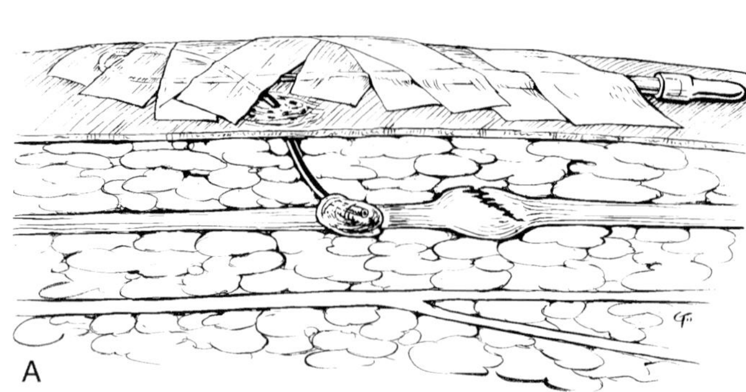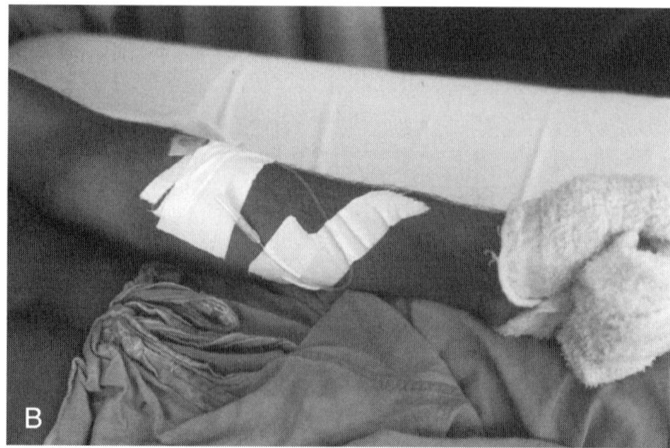

FIGURE 13–3. *A,* If pain is relieved, the intravenous catheter is capped and taped in place for continuous (periodic) peripheral perineural infusion blocks. (From Epps CH Jr [ed]: Complications of Orthopaedic Surgery. Philadelphia, J.B. Lippincott, 1978, p 777.) *B,* The extremity is free to perform physical therapy. If the block cannot sustain relief after 2 or 3 days, the catheter is replaced to obtain an effective block. (From Omer GE Jr, Pirela-Cruz M: Complications in peripheral nerve injuries. *In* Epps CH Jr [ed]: Complications of Orthopaedic Surgery, 3rd ed. Philadelphia, J.B. Lippincott, 1994, p 834.)

(Omer, 1978a, 1978b, 1979, 1984a, 1984b, 1984c, 1984d, 1986, 1987a, 1987b; Omer and Thomas, 1971, 1974).

If the anesthetic block is not effective to relieve the trigger-point pain, an additional milliliter of lidocaine hydrochloride is injected. If the additional amount also is not effective after a few minutes, the intravenous catheter is withdrawn. The peripheral epineural infusion block may be repeated at least once if the first attempt is unsuccessful.

If the peripheral epineural infusion block is effective, it should be used for treatment. Additional periodic injections of anesthetic solutions such as lidocaine hydrochloride (Xylocaine), mepivacaine hydrochloride (Carbocaine), bupivacaine hydrochloride (Marcaine), or prilocaine hydrochloride (Citanest) may be used. The patient decides the frequency of injection, depending on the time of pain-free activity. Our usual regimen has been one-half millimeter of 2% lidocaine hydrochloride (Xylocaine) solution with 1/100,000 epinephrine or mepivacaine hydrochloride (Carbocaine) every 4 hours. The volume for each injection has ranged from 0.5 to 1 ml, and the time range between injections has been 1 to 10 hours. The average time between injections was 2.2 hours during the acute stage, lengthening to 3.4 hours as the cumulative effect of the periodic peripheral epineural infusion and enforced extremity activity decreased pain and improved circulation and muscle function (Omer and Thomas, 1971). The periodic infusion is injected through the intravenous catheter without need for further skin puncture, and has been continued for 2 weeks in only a few cases (Omer and Thomas, 1974).

If there is more than one area of localized irritation, separate intravenous catheters should be used for each trigger point. In contrast to a central chemical stellate block, the peripheral perineural infusion is a ward procedure that can be performed simultaneously with other modes of treatment. The peripheral perineural infusion should block the local formation of neurokinin more effectively than the central chemical stellate block (Omer, 1987c; Omer and Eversmann, 1994).

If a peripheral trigger point of pain cannot be identified, then early treatment includes chemical central interruption of an abnormal sympathetic reflex and a cervical sympathetic block should be performed as a diagnostic test as well as a

therapeutic procedure (Omer, 1987c). Leffert and colleagues (1978) at the Massachusetts General Hospital have developed a technique for continuous sympathetic blockade that uses an indwelling catheter for injection about the stellate ganglion. The initial technique for periodic chemical sympathetic blocks involved the lumbar area (Thomason and Moritz, 1949).

FUNCTIONAL ACTIVITY AS TREATMENT

The second principle in all treatment for established pain syndromes is functional activity (Omer, 1978a, 1978b, 1979, 1984a, 1984b, 1984c, 1984d, 1986, 1987a, 1987b).

Passive treatment modalities improve circulation, decrease edema, and prepare the patient for voluntary participation in active treatment modalities, such as athletics. Passive modalities include massage to relieve discomfort, vibrators, stump wrapping, faradic muscle stimulation, ice packs, hot packs, paraffin packs, microwaves, ultrasound, and inflatable splints with positive-negative pressure. It is important that these passive modalities do not initiate pain with their use. In an apprehensive patient, use of these modalities may have to be preceded by such delicate techniques as stroking the skin with a feather. Our methods of desensitization include handling foam rubber chips, jelly beans, navy beans, and rice to provide progressively greater contact pressure. Some passive modalities may be contraindicated, such as the whirlpool bath when its dependent heat results in increased edema. The passive program should maintain joint motion, prevent contracture, and desensitize hyperesthetic areas. It also increases the patient's confidence in the treating team.

The more important phase is voluntary functional activity. Special care should be directed toward warming up key areas of circulation, such as the rotator cuff muscles in a patient with a shoulder-arm-hand syndrome. Total body conditioning is important, and the patient should be ambulatory, if possible. Function can be developed with diversionary games, athletics, assigned physical work, and activities of daily living. It is important that the health care team be compassionate yet obtain maximum effort from the patient. The best functional activity occurs when the patient returns to his or her usual work. With the continued use of functional activity, patients ultimately cure themselves.

LIMITATIONS OF TREATMENT

The indications for the periodic peripheral epineural infusion include a trigger point of pain, and when it is to be used in combination with a central chemical sympathetic block (stellate ganglion) when the central block had an initial effective duration but subsequent central blocks have given progressively shorter pain-free periods and there is an associated peripheral trigger point of pain. The contraindications for the periodic peripheral epineural infusion include established pain syndromes that have been unrelieved for 3 months or longer, and brachial plexus or lumbar plexus level pain in which the pain has occurred in the unaffected contralateral extremity. In addition, there is potential for necrosis at the injection site in a severely injured extremity with marginal vascularity. One should expect the periodic peripheral infusion to relieve painful symptoms for a variable period of time, but the technique will not produce permanent relief of pain without associated active use of the extremity by the patient.

Periodic peripheral epineural infusion is much less effective in those cases in which the pain has been untreated and unrelieved for 3 or more months. Interviews with patients who were not improved by peripheral chemical blocks or surgical sympathectomy indicated a trend toward gradual tolerance to the pain after 3 years or more (Omer, 1986; Omer and Eversmann, 1994). In time, almost all patients used their involved extremities. Under emotional stress, the pain seemed as severe as it was during active treatment but no longer dominated the patient's life, and most activities of daily living could be performed. Experience has also demonstrated that if the chemical peripheral or central sympathetic blockade is not effective, permanent improvement by surgical sympathectomy should not be expected.

References

Amadio PC: Pain dysfunction syndromes. J Bone Joint Surg *70A*:944–949, 1988.

Commission on the Evaluation of Pain, U.S. Department of Health and Human Services, Social Security Administration Office of Disability, SSA Pub. No. 64-031. Washington, D.C., March, 1987.

Geldard FA: The Human Senses, 2nd ed. New York, John Wiley and Sons, 1972.

Halpern LM: Analgesic drugs in the management of pain. Arch Surg *112*:861–869, 1977.

Lankford LL: Reflex sympathetic dystrophy. *In* Omer GE Jr, Spinner M (eds): Management of Peripheral Nerve Problems. Philadelphia, W.B. Saunders Company, 1980, pp 216–244.

Lankford LL: Reflex sympathetic dystrophy of the upper extremity. *In* Jupiter JB (ed): Flynn's Hand Surgery, 4th ed. Baltimore, Williams & Wilkins, 1991, pp 656–670.

Lankford LL: Reflex sympathetic dystrophy. *In* Green DP (ed): Operative Hand Surgery, 3rd ed. New York, Churchill Livingstone, 1993, pp 627–660.

Leffert RD, Lenson MA, Todd DP: The use of continuous sympathetic blockade in the treatment of reflex dystrophy. Personal communication, 19 June 1978.

Mayer DJ, Hayes R: Stimulation-produced analgesia: Development of tolerance and cross-tolerance to morphine. Science *188*:941–943, 1975.

Mersky H: Pain terms: A list with definitions and notes on usage. International Association for the Study of Pain (IASP) Subcommittee on Taxonomy. Pain *6*:249–252, 1979.

Omer GE Jr: Management of pain syndromes in the upper extremity. *In* Hunter JM, Schneider LH, Mackin EH, Bell JA (eds): Rehabilitation of the Hand. St. Louis, C.V. Mosby, 1978a, pp 341–349.

Omer GE Jr: The reflex sympathetic dystrophies and other pain syndromes. *In* Fredricks S, Brody GS (eds): Symposium on the Neurologic Aspects of Plastic Surgery, vol 17. Educational Foundation of the American Society of Plastic and Reconstructive Surgery. St. Louis, C.V. Mosby, 1978b, pp 100–107.

Omer GE Jr: Management of the painful extremity. *In* Ahstrom JP (ed): Current Practice in Orthopaedic Surgery, vol 8. St. Louis, C.V. Mosby, 1979, pp 86–98.

Omer GE Jr: Present thoughts on the management of pain in the upper extremity, Clin Plastic Surg *11*:85–94, 1984a.

Omer GE Jr: Management techniques for chronic pain of the upper extremity. Bull Hosp J Dis *44*:381–405, 1984b.

Omer GE Jr: Management techniques for the painful upper extremity, Part V. *In* Omer GE Jr, Spinner M: Management of Peripheral Nerve Problems, American Academy of Orthopaedic Surgeons, Instructional Course Lectures, vol 33. St. Louis, C.V. Mosby, 1984c.

Omer GE Jr: Management of pain syndromes in the upper extremity. *In* Hunter JM, Schneider LH, Mackin EJ, Callahan AD (eds): Rehabilitation of the Hand, 2nd ed. St. Louis, C.V. Mosby, 1984d, pp 503–508.

Omer GE Jr: Posttraumatic dystrophy. *In* Boswick JA (ed): Complications in Hand Surgery. Philadelphia, W.B. Saunders, 1986, pp 87–93.

Omer GE Jr: Nerves. *In* McFarlane RM (ed): Unsatisfactory Results in Hand Surgery. Edinburgh, Churchill Livingstone, 1987a, pp 209–212.

Omer GE Jr: The management of pain. *In* Lamb DW (ed): The Paralyzed Hand. Edinburgh, Churchill Livingstone, 1987b, pp 216–231.

Omer GE Jr: Management techniques for the painful upper extremity. *In* Terzis JK (ed): Microreconstruction of Nerve Injuries. Philadelphia, W.B. Saunders, 1987c, pp 145–159.

Omer GE Jr, Eversmann WW Jr: Peripheral Nerve Problems. *In* Burkhalter WE (ed): Orthopaedic Surgery in Vietnam. Washington, D.C., Office of the Surgeon General and Center of Military History, U.S. Army, 1994, pp 155–188.

Omer GE Jr, Pirela-Cruz M: Complications of peripheral nerve injuries. *In* Epps CH Jr (ed): Complications in Orthopaedic Surgery, 3rd ed. Philadelphia, J.B. Lippincott, 1994, pp 811–856.

Omer GE Jr, Thomas SR: Treatment of causalgia: Review of cases at Brooke General Hospital. Tex Med *67*:93–96, 1971.

Omer GE Jr, Thomas SR: The management of chronic pain syndromes in the upper extremity. Clin Orthop *104*:37–45, 1971.

Thomason JR, Moritz WH: Continuous lumbar paravertebral sympathetic block maintained by fractional installation of procaine. Surg Gynecol Obstet *89*:447–453, 1949.

Zancolli EA, Zancolli ER Jr: The Painful Hand, Problems and Solutions. *In* Wynn Parry CB (ed): Management of Pain in the Hand and Wrist. Edinburgh, Churchill Livingstone, 1991, pp 114–138.

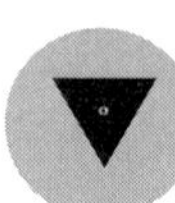

Chapter 14

• David Schultz

Indications for Utilization of a Pain Clinic

Knowledge and understanding of pain have grown considerably in recent years, and there is increasing national awareness that effective pain management is important (Carr et al, 1992). The medical practice of pain management is evolving from a field dominated by an assortment of practitioners into a sophisticated medical subspecialty recognized by the American Board of Medical Specialties, with its own qualification examination and board certification process.* A basic knowledge of current pain theories, treatment options, and referral alternatives will help the surgeon to deal more effectively with patients experiencing persistent pain. In this chapter, we will explore why pain sometimes persists beyond normal healing, discuss how abnormal pain is best diagnosed and treated, and identify criteria to use for appropriate referral to the chronic pain specialist.

HISTORICAL PERSPECTIVES

In times past, pain was thought to be transmitted in a simple, straightforward fashion from peripheral tissue to central nervous system by telephone-wire–like neural connections first postulated by Descartes in 1664 (Fig. 14–1). The concept of wirelike pain transmission led to the liberal use of neurosurgical destruction. Surgeons of an earlier era often believed that persistent pain states could be effectively treated by resecting the involved sensory nerves. It seemed logical that if a nerve was transmitting unnecessary and troublesome pain messages, then it should be clipped and removed. Experience has shown, however, that the nervous system often responds adversely to neurodestruction and seems to find clever ways to reroute neuropathic pain messages to consciousness despite repeated attempts to destroy what is viewed as the offending pathway. Simple destruction of pain pathways at points along their course has often led to functional loss combined with recurrent, amplified, and even more refractory pain (Loeser, 1972, 1990; Superville et al, 1975).

Pain pathways are not simple telephone-wire–like connections from peripheral tissue to central nervous system; they are extremely complex systems of neural connections capable of intense modulation and adaptation at various sites within the peripheral nerve, spinal cord, and brain. Basic

science research into pain mechanisms and clinical research into the efficacy of pain treatments have led away from the simplistic approach of neurodestruction and toward the use of medications, nondestructive nerve blocks, stimulating devices, and multidisciplinary approaches to chronic pain management. We are slowly gaining insight into the complex workings of the nervous system and the many complexities of pain (Bonica JJ, 1990a; Yaksh, 1993b).

DEFINITION OF TERMS

Pain. The International Association for the Study of Pain defines pain as ''an unpleasant sensory and emotional experience associated with actual or potential tissue damage, or described in terms of such damage.'' Inherent in this elegant and widely accepted definition of pain are the following points:

- Pain has both sensory and emotional components.

- Pain may exist without tissue damage and, conversely, tissue damage may exist without pain.

- Pain is a purely subjective phenomenon and therefore cannot be measured objectively.

The experience of pain is uniquely personal, and pain behavior is shaped by personality, culture, and past experience. It follows that there is great individual variation in the

---

*Available for board-certified anesthesiologists through the American Board of Anesthesiology, 100 Constitution Plaza, Hartford, Connecticut 06103, and for nonanesthesiologist board-certified physicians through the American College of Pain Medicine, 5700 Old Orchard Road, Skokie, Illinois 60077-1057.

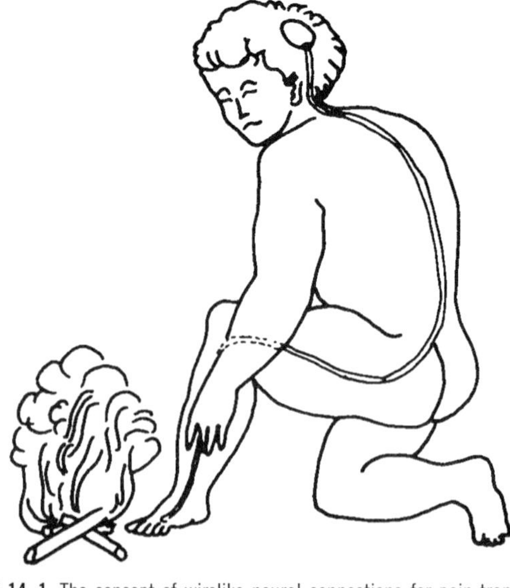

FIGURE 14–1. The concept of wirelike neural connections for pain transmission.

human response to similar noxious physical processes and that the medical management of pain can sometimes be confusing and frustrating. Furthermore, pain is always subjective and is variable from one individual to another. It is, therefore, difficult to study pain in a controlled, scientific fashion.

Nociception. Nociception is the biological transmission of pain impulses through the nervous system, resulting in certain reflex processes and in the conscious perception of pain (Bonica, 1990d).

Acute Pain. Acute pain can be considered to be the physical and emotional experience of nociception. It functions as a physiological warning system for the body. Acute pain usually has a readily identifiable source and a predictable course and resolves as healing progresses (Bonica, 1990d).

Chronic Pain. Chronic pain is a process that differs fundamentally from nociception and acute pain. Chronic pain can be considered to be a destructive force without biological purpose. It persists long after healing has occurred and often bears little relationship to any underlying physical pathology. Causes of chronic pain are often obscure; its course is prolonged and its treatment difficult and involved. It is a process that involves the entire person and not simply a bodily structure, and has aptly been described as a complex "biopsychosocial phenomenon" (Lippe, 1993).

Ongoing Acute Pain. These terms can be used to describe the persistent nociception that accompanies certain chronic conditions, including arthritis, neuropathy, and migraine headache. It is important to distinguish between ongoing acute pain and chronic pain because causes and treatments are often very different (Bonica, 1990d).

In times past, acute pain was considered to be short-lived, and chronic pain was thought to persist for a period of at least 6 months (Bonica, 1990d). However, in certain situations acute pain can persist, and, conversely, chronic pain behavior can become apparent early in the course of disease. Therefore, criteria other than duration are sometimes used to distinguish between acute and chronic pain states. These criteria include the presence or absence of an identifiable underlying nociceptive focus, the psychosocial impact of the pain on the individual, the specific behavioral reaction of the individual toward the pain, and the premorbid personality of the patient (Bonica, 1990d, 1990e; Lippe, 1993). We now accept that chronic pain can begin weeks after injury and acute pain can sometimes persist for a lifetime.

PATHOPHYSIOLOGY OF ACUTE PAIN

Anatomically, pain pathways have been clearly identified (Fig. 14–2). Typically, nociception begins when a peripheral noxious stimulus activates receptors on sensory afferent A delta and C polymodal nociceptive nerve fibers. A delta fibers are small, myelinated, and relatively fast conducting, whereas C fibers have small, unmyelinated axons that conduct more slowly. These primary afferent pain fibers have a unipolar or pseudounipolar cell body contained within the dorsal root ganglion from which extends both a central and a peripheral process. The peripheral process of the pain

afferent neuron typically travels outward from the spinal cord within a peripheral somatic nerve to innervate body tissues. Pain impulses are carried from the peripherally arborized terminals of these afferent fibers toward the spinal cord and enter the cord through the central process of the dorsal root ganglion cell. This central process, in turn, terminates within various lamina of the spinal cord dorsal horn and synapses with interneurons capable of activating powerful spinal reflexes. Nociceptive spinal reflexes include flexion muscle spasm (splinting) mediated by the alpha motor neuron pool in the anterior horn and sympathoadrenal responses such as vasoconstriction, tachycardia, and hypertension mediated by sympathetic preganglionic neurons that lie within the intermediolateral cell column of the spinal cord (Fig. 14–3). From the dorsal horn, afferent impulses ascend to higher brain centers within the contralateral *anterolateral fasciculus* of the spinal cord, which consists of the spinothalamic, spinoreticular, and spinomesencephalic tracts. Ultimately, pain impulses act on sites within the brain, initiating hormonal responses and triggering neural activity within powerful, inhibitory descending fiber tracts that project back down to the spinal cord dorsal horn and modulate further nociception (Bonica, 1990b).

As an illustrative example, when a finger touches a hot stove there is an immediate sharp, well-localized pain associated with a withdrawal reaction. This *first pain* is mediated by the fast conducting A delta fibers, has an immediate protective effect for the organism, and constitutes what is known as the sensory-discriminative component of pain. The second component of the pain is slower in onset and less well localized, but more prolonged and agonizing. This *second pain* has a profound emotional and psychological impact on the organism and is responsible for the learned avoidance behavior and unpleasant memory associated with the painful experience. This so-called affective-motivational component of pain is mediated by the slower conducting C fibers. Ultimately, the behavioral response of the individual to the pain will be a function of the amount and type of modulation that is occurring within the central components of the pain pathway.

C fibers are unique in that they contain a number of inflammatory mediators within their axons that are released on repeated stimulation. These compounds include such substances as bradykinin, prostaglandins, histamine, serotonin, and other vasoactive and neuroactive peptides that serve to create a localized inflammatory reaction in peripheral tissue (Bonica, 1990a, 1990b; Dubner, 1991; Yaksh, 1993b). This process is called *neurogenic inflammation* and is the basis for the wheal, flare, and hyperalgesia of the axon reflex, first described as the *triple response* by Lewis in 1942.

Many of these inflammatory neuropeptides have the capacity to sensitize pain afferent fibers, and in the presence of neurogenic inflammation, C fiber peripheral terminals develop lower firing thresholds and depolarize more readily throughout the region of injury. Furthermore, because nociceptive impulses are normally conducted orthodromically toward the spinal cord as well as antidromically out to the arborized, peripheral terminals of the particular nerve, the mediators of inflammation contained within the nerve are released over a relatively wide peripheral area (see Fig. 14–3). As this peripheral sensitization occurs, a clinical state termed *primary hyperalgesia* develops in which further

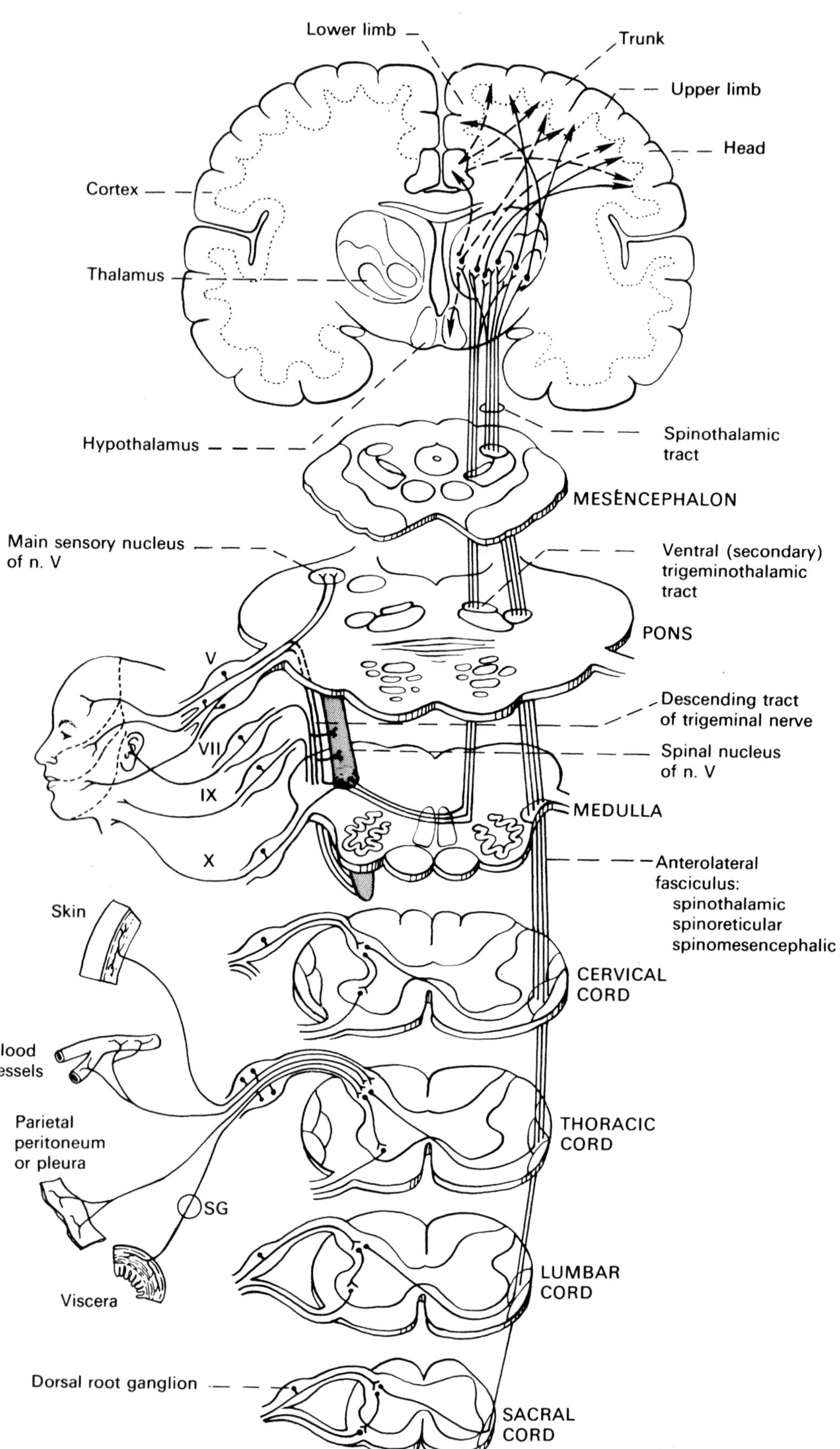

FIGURE 14–2. Anatomical pain pathways. (Bonica JJ: The Management of Pain. Baltimore, Williams & Wilkins, 1990. © Lea & Febiger, 1990.)

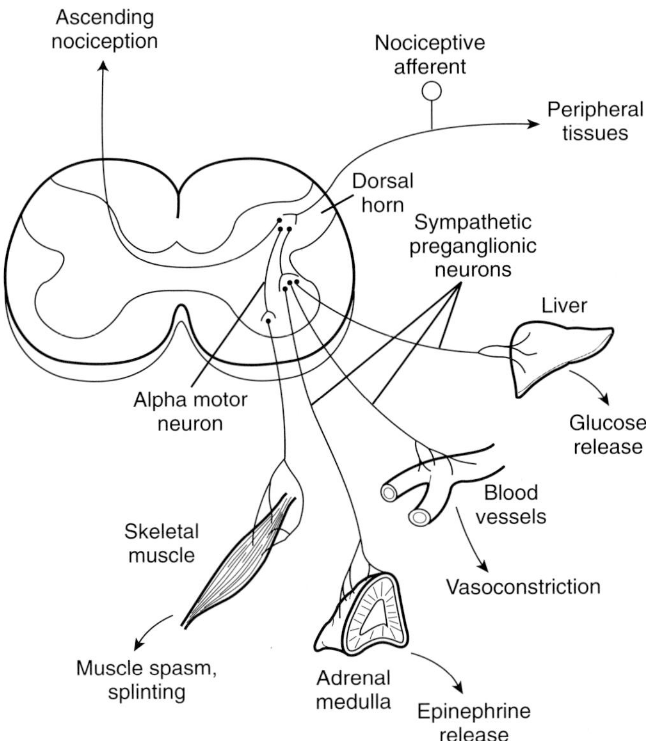

FIGURE 14–3. Nociceptive spinal reflexes.

noxious stimulation is sensed more intensely (Sinatra, 1992; Yaksh and Aimone, 1989). As nociceptive impulses course centrally toward the dorsal root ganglion cell body and then through the cell's central axon process to the spinal cord, the same set of inflammatory neuropeptides is released from central C fiber terminals into the spinal cord dorsal horn. The release of inflammatory mediators into the spinal cord results in central neurogenic inflammation and what has been termed *secondary hyperalgesia* (Sinatra, 1992; Yaksh and Aimone, 1989). Specifically, central pain afferent fibers make connections with a population of dorsal horn interneurons in lamina V of the dorsal horn called *wide dynamic range neurons*. These neurons are involved in transmitting nociceptive input to higher brain centers and have been shown to become sensitized by repeated nociceptive input, increasing their peripheral receptive fields and lowering their firing thresholds. This results in marked facilitation of spinal cord pain processing and the clinical phenomenon known as spinal cord windup (Yaksh, 1993b). Current recommendations regarding preemptive analgesia for the management of postoperative pain are aimed at reducing this spinal cord windup phenomenon* (Dahl and Kehlet, 1994).

The inherent ability of certain neurons to change their

---

*Preemptive analgesia is the term used to describe the clinical administration of opioids and/or local anesthetics before a painful stimulation such as surgical incision. Local anesthetics block afferent pain impulses from reaching the dorsal horn, and opioids prevent afferent pain neurotransmitters from acting on dorsal horn neurons. Theoretically, either of these classes of drugs, if administered before skin incision, should prevent the spinal cord windup phenomenon that accompanies surgery. Clinical studies have supported this concept. Interestingly, inhalational anesthetics do not prevent windup even at high concentrations.

firing thresholds, the size of their receptive fields, and even the types of stimulation to which they respond is now well documented, and the term *neuroplasticity* has been coined to describe it (Dubner, 1991). There is evidence at present that neuroplastic changes within the nervous system can be profound and long lasting, and it is likely that these changes play a significant role in the perpetuation of pain. Nitric oxide, a newly discovered class of neurotransmitter, may play a pivotal role in the neuroplastic up regulation of pain processing and may eventually spawn the development of a new class of analgesic (Malmberg and Yaksh, 1993).

The end result of persistent nociceptive input is a peripheral and central neurogenic inflammatory response, profound neuroplastic changes within the nervous system, the sensitization of pain pathways in the peripheral tissue and within the central nervous system, and the facilitation of pain processing. There are muscular as well as hemodynamic and hormonal consequences to this persistent pain.

WHY DOES PAIN PERSIST?

There are a variety of reasons that pain might persist beyond the period of normal healing. Some of these reasons are relatively simple and straightforward, but others are more complex and multifaceted. Following are some possible explanations for persistent pain.

Ongoing Nociception. The most readily understood source for ongoing pain is ongoing nociception. Many acute, subacute, and chronic physical processes can result in the continued activation of pain pathways. Because nociception is the normal physiological response to tissue damage, ongoing nociception may indicate ongoing physical pathology. Examples include persistent inflammation, ischemia, neural compression, and fracture nonunion. The first step in any evaluation for persistent pain is a thorough workup to rule out any readily identifiable physical cause.

Sometimes, even an extensive and detailed workup will fail to reveal an underlying physical cause for the patient's pain complaints. In other cases, pain will persist despite identification and treatment of a potential source for ongoing tissue damage.

Neuropathic Pain. Whereas nociception represents pain transmitted from injured tissue through normal nerves, neuropathy is the condition in which pain impulses are generated and perpetuated by injured, malfunctioning nervous tissue itself (Cimino, 1992; Devor, 1983; Myers, 1995). Abnormal and persistent pain may result from neural injury at any point within the peripheral or central nervous system. Examples include pain associated with diabetic neuropathy, nerve compression, painful neuroma, and nerve root avulsion. Neuropathic pain is characterized by the following attributes (Cimino, 1992):

- Burning quality

- Numbness or paresthesia in the distribution of pain

- Allodynia and/or hyperalgesia of skin in the area of pain

- Lack of identifiable physical source

Reflex Sympathetic Dystrophy and Causalgia. These conditions represent a subcategory of neuropathic pain in which an abnormal interaction seems to occur between the sympathetic and somatic nervous systems, resulting in persistent pain, trophic changes, and autonomic instability in the affected part. Sympathetic pain syndromes have been identified with a variety of names, including reflex sympathetic dystrophy (RSD), causalgia, Sudeck's atrophy, and shoulder-arm-hand syndrome. Causalgia is defined today as "a syndrome of sustained burning pain, allodynia, and hyperpathia after a traumatic nerve lesion, often combined with vasomotor and sudomotor dysfunction and later, trophic changes" (Bonica, 1990d). Causalgia, first described in detail by the Civil War battlefield surgeon Weir Mitchell, is most often precipitated by gunshot wound and usually involves direct injury to the brachial plexus, median nerve, or sciatic nerve (Bonica, 1990c).

Reflex sympathetic dystrophy is the term currently used to identify the identical syndrome when no macroscopic nerve injury is apparent. There is a paucity of controlled scientific research on the topic of sympathetic pain for a variety of reasons, including the lack of consensus regarding specific diagnostic criteria, the variability in clinical presentation, and the difficulties inherent in studying a diverse population of patients with chronic pain (Bonica, 1990c). Nonetheless, it is believed that RSD and causalgia represent a variety of disorders in which persistent pain is associated with sympathetic dysfunction. The hallmarks of sympathetically maintained pain include the following signs and symptoms, usually occurring in an extremity (Bonica, 1990c).

- Persistent burning pain

- Allodynia (pain resulting from a stimulus that does not ordinarily produce pain)

- Skin temperature and/or color changes

- Edema

- Atrophic changes in skin, nails, bone

- Reversal of pain with sympathetic block

Exact mechanisms underlying sympathetically maintained pain are not well understood, although recent advances in knowledge regarding pain transmission have shed some light on the process. It is believed that nerve injury, or at least nerve dysfunction, is the initial precipitating event. With causalgia, this injury is obvious and identifiable, but with RSD the injury may be undetectable or is discernable only at the microscopic or submicroscopic level. As previously noted, pain in the normal nervous system is transmitted via A delta and C-type nerve fibers from peripheral tissues to spinal cord. The sympathetic nervous system is, on the other hand, an exclusively efferent system. First-order sympathetic neurons reside within the intermediolateral spinal cord, and second-order neurons lie within thoracolumbar sympathetic chain ganglia. These second-order sympathetic neurons then send their peripheral postganglionic fibers through gray rami communicans into the peripheral somatic nervous system.

The efferent sympathetic fibers then course through somatic peripheral nerves on their way to innervate blood vessels and skin structures. Because sympathetic efferent fibers and pain afferent fibers are in close proximity within

certain peripheral nerves (Fig. 14–4), it is possible that injury at the macroscopic or microscopic level causes afferent pain fibers to interact inappropriately with efferent sympathetic fibers. Although no anatomical ephapses have been demonstrated, there is evidence that abnormal "cross-talk" between the afferent C fiber and the adjacent sympathetic efferent

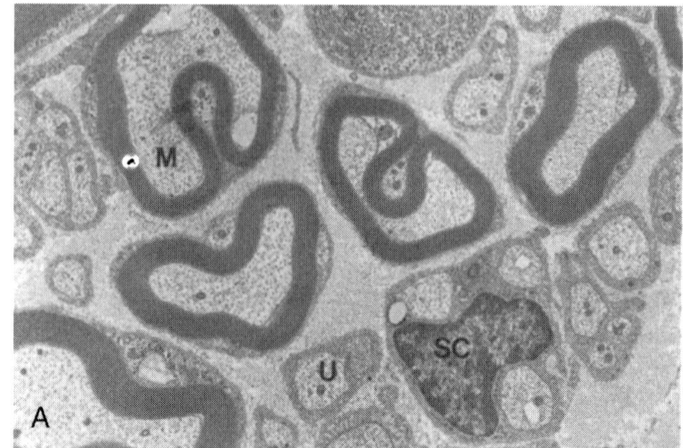

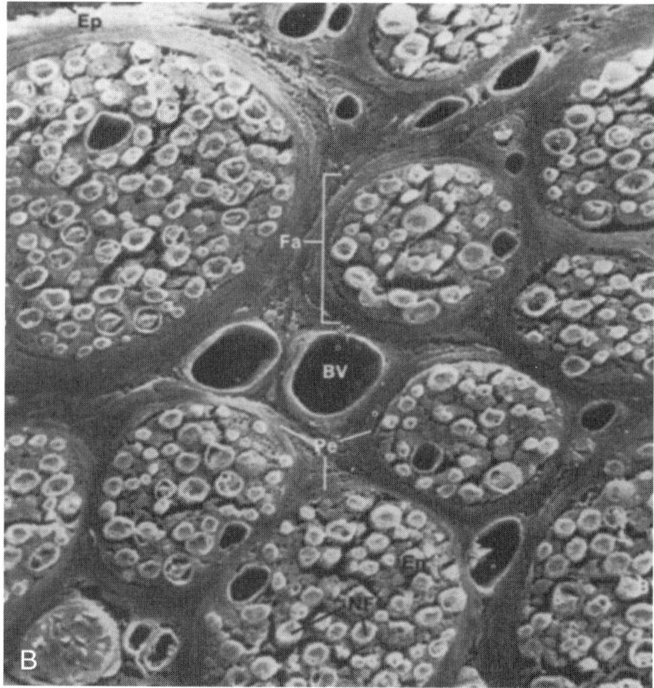

FIGURE 14–4. *A,* Electron micrograph of normal human peripheral nerve illustrating coexistence of myelinated (with dark-staining myelin sheaths) (M) and unmyelinated (U) fibers. A Schwann cell nucleus (SC) is seen in the lower right associated with a group of three unmyelinated fibers. Mitochondria and smaller organelles can be seen in the axoplasm of both myelinated and unmyelinated fibers. (Uranyl acetate and lead citrate) (From Cousins MJ, Bridenbaugh PO: Neural Blockade in Clinical Anesthesia and Management of Pain, Philadelphia, JB Lippincott Company, 1980; courtesy of Dr. Henry C. Powell, University of California, San Diego, California.) *B,* Scanning electron micrograph of a peripheral nerve in cross section. Nerve fibers (NF) are organized in bundles called fascicles (Fa), each of which is surrounded by a collagen-rich sheath, the perineurium (Pe). Loose connective tissue forms the epineurium (Ep), which encircles groups of fascicles. The endoneurium (En) is a division of the perineurium that forms thin layers of connective tissue surrounding nerve fibers. In practice, the entire space bounded by the perineurium is referred to as endoneurial space. Blood vessels (BV) with fenestrated endothelial cells are numerous in the epineurial space. Somewhat smaller vessels within the endoneurium form the vasa nervorum with tight endothelial cell junctions. These two circulations communicate via vessels that pass obliquely through the perineurium. (Kessel RG, Kardon RH. Tissue and Organs. New York, W.H. Freeman, 1979, p 79.)

fibers does occur (Bonica JJ, 1990c). This cross-talk could theoretically result in a situation where C-fiber afferent discharge could trigger inappropriate sympathetic efferent depolarization. The inappropriate sympathetic efferent impulses are propagated along the sympathetic axon and, on arrival at the nerve terminal endings, cause norepinephrine to be discharged into tissue. Afferent C-fiber axons have been shown to become sensitized when exposed to norepinephrine and will fire at lower thresholds (Cline et al, 1989). Vasomotor instability results from the effects of norepinephrine on local vasculature. Furthermore, because afferent C-fiber nerves contain a large number of vasoactive and neuroactive peptides, which are mediators of inflammation and which are released into tissue on the stimulation of C-fiber terminals, neurogenic inflammation with localized edema will occur. This neurogenic inflammation serves to further sensitize C fibers, which, in turn, tend to fire spontaneously, further stimulating efferent sympathetic discharge. A vicious cycle is thereby created, resulting in persistent pain, persistent sympathetic discharge, and the clinical syndrome of RSD.

Central Pain. It is becoming clear that RSD and other neuropathic pain states have a central as well as a peripheral basis. Furthermore, certain pain syndromes such as phantom limb pain, "thalamic pain," and post-stroke pain seem to have a central basis without any peripheral component. As previously noted, sensitization and facilitation of spinal cord neurons have been shown to occur when repetitive barrages of nociceptive impulses travel to the dorsal horn along intact C fibers. Similarly, it has been observed that peripheral nerve transection can result in central nervous system sensitization and persistent pain with neuropathic characteristics (Cimino, 1992; Tasker, 1980). The term *deafferentation pain* has been used to describe the pain that sometimes occurs after peripheral sensory afferent fiber input into the central nervous system is disrupted. Specifically, when a peripheral C fiber is destroyed, the cell body within the dorsal root ganglion dies, and input from its central process into the dorsal horn ceases. This causes certain dorsal horn neurons to increase their peripheral receptive fields, lower their firing thresholds, and exhibit spontaneous activity independent of any further peripheral input. Because these central nervous system nociceptive neurons are spontaneously firing despite the lack of peripheral nociceptive input, the perception of pain persists without any identifiable physical cause and without evidence of ongoing tissue damage (Myers, 1995).

It is likely that pain processing within the brain can similarly be altered by peripheral deafferentation as well as by direct brain injury. Little is known, however, about nociceptive physiology within the brain, and conclusions about brain contributions to central pain states must await further study.

Psychosocial Dysfunction. The diverse patient population treated for peripheral nerve injury will include some patients with significant psychosocial and emotional components contributing to the perpetuation of their pain behaviors. The anatomical and physiological basis for the association of pain with behavior and emotion is inherent in the organism and has a firm anatomical and physiological basis that lies in the extensive projections of pain afferent fiber tracts into the limbic system of the brain (Bonica, 1990a). The limbic system, composed of the hippocampus, amygdala, cingulate gyrus, and hypothalamus, comprises the paleocortex and is responsible for affect, mood, motivation, and emotional behavior. This is in contrast to the neocortex, or cerebral cortex, which is responsible for sensory processing and integration and formal intellectual activity. Given the extent of the neural connections between pain afferent fibers and emotional centers in the brain, it is not surprising that many patients with persistent pain exhibit significant emotional behavior. The extent and expression of this emotional behavior will depend on the personality, temperament, and cultural background of the individual involved and is not necessarily predictive of any underlying psychopathology. Nonetheless, persistent pain does occur in individuals with underlying psychopathology, and this increases the likelihood that a maladaptive reaction to the pain will occur and that the subsequent persistence of pain behaviors will be linked more to psychosocial processes than to ongoing nociception (Lippe, 1993). Clinical depression is also commonly associated with chronic pain, although depressive behavior may be masked and not readily apparent to the examining physician. An important task for the chronic pain specialist is to identify the depressed patient and the individual in whom pain behavior is influenced by an underlying psychiatric condition, issues of secondary gain, maladaptive personality factors, and, although rare, malingering (Lippe, 1993). In this way, the diverse population of patients with persistent pain can be separated into those who might benefit from invasive procedures, those who are candidates for surgery, those who will likely respond to medications, and those for whom behavioral therapy and psychological counseling are more appropriate. Of course, many patients with complex chronic pain problems respond best when treated with combinations of invasive and noninvasive interventions, including medications, physical therapies, psychological therapies, and invasive procedures when appropriate, in a coordinated and multidisciplinary fashion (Bonica JJ, 1990e; Lippe, 1993). Consequently, the single modality pain clinic has often been less successful at treating chronic pain than the multidisciplinary center (Bonica JJ, 1990e; Lippe, 1993; Turk and Chapman, 1982).

There are a number of psychiatric diagnoses associated with persistent pain and, in some patients, these psychological conditions are largely responsible for the ongoing pain behavior. *The Diagnostic and Statistical Manual of Mental Disorders* (DSM-IV) (1994) classifies these conditions as follows.

Somatoform Pain Disorder. This condition is synonymous with psychogenic pain and tends to occur in individuals with evidence of premorbid neurotic functioning. Inherent in the diagnosis is a history of preoccupation with pain for which there is no demonstrable etiology but that is associated with evidence of psychological dysfunction. If pain becomes the central focus of a neurotic obsession, then the term *pain neurosis* may be used to describe the condition, whereas preoccupation with financial compensation is termed *compensation neurosis*. DSM-IV diagnostic criteria are listed as follows.

1. Pain in one or more anatomical sites is the predominant focus of the clinical presentation and is of sufficient severity to warrant clinical attention.

2. The pain causes clinically significant distress or impairment in social, occupational, or other important areas of functioning.

3. Psychological factors are judged to have an important role in the onset, severity, exacerbation, or maintenance of the pain.

4. The symptom or deficit is not intentionally produced or feined (as in factitious disorder or malingering).

5. The pain is not better accounted for by a mood, anxiety, or psychotic disorder and does not meet criteria for dyspareunia.

Hypochondriasis. Patients with hypochondriasis are abnormally fixated on their physical symptoms and fail to be reassured by the absence of pathology on extensive workup. They often feel compelled to undergo further diagnostic evaluation and believe that an underlying physical abnormality is responsible for their pain. DMS-IV diagnostic criteria are as follows.

1. Preoccupation with fears of having or the idea that one has a serious disease, based on the person's misinterpretation of bodily symptoms.

2. The preoccupation persists despite appropriate medical evaluation and reassurance.

3. The belief in 1 is not of delusional intensity (as in delusional disorder, somatic type) and is not restricted to a circumscribed concern about appearance (as in body dismorphic disorder).

4. The preoccupation causes clinically significant distress or impairment in social, occupational, or other important areas of functioning.

5. The duration of the symptoms is at least 6 months.

6. The preoccupation is not better accounted for by generalized anxiety disorder, obsessive-compulsive disorder, panic disorder, a major depressive episode, separation anxiety, or another somatoform disorder.

Malingering. Malingering is the voluntary, deliberate, and intentional feigning of signs or symptoms of physical or psychological conditions for personal gain. This fraudulent practice is rare in the pain clinic setting (Lippe, 1993), and usually involves individuals with significant psychopathology. Malingering may be driven by issues of financial, familial, or social gain or may occur with drug-seeking behavior. According to DMS-IV diagnostic criteria, malingering should be considered in the presence of one or more of the following criteria.

1. There is a medicolegal context of presentation (e.g., the person is referred by his or her attorney to the physician for examination).

2. There is a marked discrepancy between the person's claimed distress or disability and the objective findings.

3. There is a lack of cooperation with the diagnostic evaluation and prescribed treatment regimen.

4. There is the presence of an antisocial personality disorder.

Schizophrenia. Patients with schizophrenia live with a distorted reality and may misinterpret the meaning of bodily sensations. Pain complaints may be voiced as part of a bizarre constellation of symptoms that do not make medical sense. These patients are usually easily identifiable and are not commonly referred to pain centers, although physical pain syndromes can certainly occur coincident with schizophrenia. The rather lengthy DMS-IV diagnostic criteria can be summarized as follows.

1. Some of the following symptoms of psychosis are present.
   a. Delusions
   b. Hallucinations
   c. Loose association
   d. Grossly disorganized or catatonic behavior
   e. Flat affect
2. There is marked disruption in social, vocational, and/or familial functioning.
3. Self-care is inadequate.
4. An underlying toxic metabolic etiology to the aberrant behavior has been ruled out.

Depression. Although depression is quite common in patients with chronic pain, there is not always a causal relationship between pain and depression. In some cases, depression is a reaction to chronic pain, but in other cases, depression precedes the onset of pain and may be a factor in the perpetuation of the chronic pain behavior. Furthermore, some patients with chronic pain are not depressed, although signs and symptoms of depression should always be actively sought during the initial evaluation phase of pain center treatment. DSM-IV diagnostic criteria for depression include the following.

1. Poor appetite or significant weight loss (when not dieting) or increased appetite or significant weight gain.
2. Insomnia or hypersomnia.
3. Psychomotor agitation or retardation.
4. Loss of interest in or enjoyment of sex.
5. Social withdrawal.
6. Feelings of worthlessness, self-reproach, or excessive inappropriate guilt.
7. Recurrent thoughts of death, wishes to be dead, suicidal ideation or suicide attempt.
8. Fearfulness or crying.

The broad continuum of patients with persistent pain includes those with predominantly physical ongoing nociception and those with predominantly psychological etiologies to their pain behaviors. Most patients with chronic pain have elements of physical pathology as well as psychological dysfunction, and when pain persists, there are psychological, social, and familial ramifications for even the most well-adjusted individual. A considerable amount of expertise and experience is required to separate the physical from the psychological and social aspects of persistent pain and, for this reason, effective management of patients with complex chronic pain is beyond the scope of most office medical practices. Appropriate referral to the chronic pain specialist is in the best interests of the patient and the referring physician.

DIAGNOSIS

Adequate efforts at identifying the etiology for persistent pain often involve the use of radiologic imaging studies, including magnetic resonance imaging and computed tomography; electrodiagnostic investigations, including nerve conduction studies and electromyography; and nuclear medicine examinations, such as the three-phase bone scan (Kosin et al, 1981). These diagnostic techniques are covered in detail elsewhere in this text and will not be discussed here except to say that there is no substitute for the appropriate use of these powerful modalities to rule out occult malignancy, infection, hematoma, nerve damage, and structural anatomical defects as possible causes for persistent pain.

There are a number of other diagnostic interventions that can be used by the pain specialist in an attempt to determine the source for ongoing pain. Specifically, it may be possible to determine whether pain emanates from somatic as opposed to visceral structures; whether it is mediated by the peripheral, central, or sympathetic nervous system; and to what extent psychological factors are involved in the perpetuation of pain behaviors. Although it is often not possible to determine the exact etiology of chronic pain, useful information can often be gained by using one or more of the following diagnostic techniques.

Diagnostic Nerve Blocks

Selective Somatic Neural Blockade. Reversible, local anesthetic nerve blocks may be helpful for identification of abnormal sensory nerves, localization of tissue pathology, and determining the anatomical site of pain generation. Theoretically, if pain is relieved by neural blockade of a specific branch of a peripheral nerve, then pain is originating either from the somatic bodily structure innervated by that nerve or from the neuropathic firing of the nerve itself. Furthermore, pain is probably originating at, or peripheral to, the site of the block. Through the use of careful and selective somatic nerve block, pain originating in body wall structures can sometimes be distinguished from visceral pain, and pain of peripheral neuropathy can sometimes be distinguished from pain of more central origin. Peripheral nerves that lend themselves to isolated neural blockade are listed in Table 14–1.

Although useful information can sometimes be gained by selective neural blockade, there are a number of problems with this approach. First, it is often difficult, and sometimes impossible, to selectively block peripheral nerves, especially in areas such as the proximal brachial plexus, without affecting other nerves in the area. Second, there is some question as to whether pain relief obtained from selective blockade of a specific nerve truly identifies that nerve as responsible for propagation of the clinical pain. For instance, it has been shown that peripheral blockade of the sciatic nerve in the leg can relieve lumbar radicular pain for prolonged periods even when this pain has been proved to be related to acute disc herniation in the lumbar spine (Abram, 1988). There is also a placebo response that is significant in more than 30% of patients (Orne, 1992; Turk and Melzack, 1992). Nevertheless, many chronic pain specialists today believe that valuable information about the anatomical location of pain generators can be obtained in certain circumstances from selective, diagnostic nerve block.

▼ **TABLE 14–1**
Peripheral Nerves Used for Neural Blockade

Peripheral Nerve	Site of Blockade
Ilioinguinal and iliohypogastric nerves	Medial to the anterior-superior iliac spine
Genitofemoral nerve	Pubic tubercle
Supraorbital nerve	Superior orbit
Supratrochlear nerve	Superior orbit
Infraorbital nerve	Inferior orbit
Auriculotemporal nerve	Anterior to the ear
Mental nerve	Mental foramen of the mandible
Facial nerve	Mastoid process
Greater occipital nerve	Occipital skull at the superior nuchal line
Lesser occipital nerve	Posterior to the mastoid process
Greater auricular nerve	Posterior to the sternocleidomastoid muscle
Musculocutaneous nerve	Proximal humerus
Suprascapular nerve	Suprascapular notch
Intercostobrachial and medial cutaneous nerve of the arm	Subcutaneous tissue of the proximal arm
Radial nerve	Midshaft humerus, elbow or wrist
Median nerve	Elbow or wrist
Ulnar nerve	Elbow or wrist
Digital nerves	Medial and lateral digit
Intercostal nerves	Beneath the rib
Sciatic nerve	Greater sciatic notch
Lateral femoral cutaneous nerve	Inferomedial to the anterior-superior iliac spine
Obturator nerve	Obturator foramen
Common peroneal nerve	Head of the fibula
Saphenous nerve	Medial condyle of the femur or the medial malleolus
Deep peroneal nerve	Medial to the extensor hallucis longus tendon
Superficial peroneal nerve	Subcutaneous tissue of the anterior ankle
Tibial nerve	Medial to the Achilles tendon
Sural nerve	Lateral to the Achilles tendon

Selective Sympathetic Blockade. Because the sympathetic nervous system is functionally and anatomically separate from the somatic nervous system, it is theoretically possible to selectively block the sympathetic nervous innervation to an affected part without blocking somatic nervous innervation. Selective sympathetic blockade is commonly used to diagnose sympathetically maintained pain. If pain resolves after selective sympathetic blockade, it is inferred that the sympathetic nervous system is responsible for the continuation of pain. The sympathetic nervous system is commonly blocked at the following points.

Stellate Ganglion Block. The cervicothoracic (stellate) ganglion is the confluence of the inferior cervical and the first thoracic sympathetic ganglion located ventral to the transverse process of the seventh cervical vertebra. The stellate ganglion contains synapses between sympathetic preganglionic axons and the cell bodies of the postganglionic axons that supply sympathetic innervation to the head, neck, and upper extremity on the ipsilateral side. The technical aspects of this block are described elsewhere in this text. Because the neck contains many important structures within a confined space, complications from stellate ganglion block can be severe. Specifically, injection of local anesthetic into a dural cuff deep to the transverse process may result in total spinal anesthesia with resultant hypotension and inability to spontaneously ventilate. Also, injection of local anesthetic into a vertebral artery may cause seizures and loss of consciousness.

Signs of a successful sympathetic block include increase in temperature to the upper extremity as well as a Horner's syndrome (ptosis, miosis, and anhydrosis) of the ipsilateral face. The presence of intact sensation and strength in the upper extremity denotes the absence of somatic blockade. Pain relieved by stellate block is assumed to be perpetuated by sympathetic nervous system dysfunction. The block has a role in both diagnosis and therapy for persistent pain in the head, neck, and upper extremity.

Lumbar Sympathetic Block. Most of the sympathetic outflow to the lower extremities passes through the ipsilateral L2, L3, and L4 lumbar paravertebral ganglia. These sympathetic ganglia lie at the anterolateral aspect of the lumbar vertebral bodies, medial to the body of the psoas muscle, and can be blocked with needles placed into the posterolateral flank and then directed to the anterolateral surface of the vertebral body as described elsewhere in this text. Sympathetic blockade is documented by noting temperature and blood flow changes in the ipsilateral foot. The absence of somatic block can be inferred if sensation and strength are intact in the lower extremity. As with the stellate ganglion block, pain relief may denote sympathetically maintained pain. The block has both diagnostic and therapeutic value.

Sympathetic innervation to the thorax and abdomen can similarly be interrupted by thoracic sympathetic block and celiac plexus block, respectively.

Successful selective sympathetic blockade should be accompanied by an identifiable increase in blood flow to the affected part as well as an increase in skin temperature approaching core body temperature. If sensory changes are noted in the extremity after sympathetic blockade, then somatic fibers have also been blocked and, by definition, the sympathetic blockade is not selective. No conclusions regarding the mechanism of pain can be drawn from such a combined block, although the therapeutic efficacy of the block for treating sympathetically maintained pain is unchanged. It is often difficult to block sympathetic fibers without also blocking somatic fibers to some degree; therefore, a careful check for sensory deficit should be made.

Differential Spinal Blockade. Within the spinal cord, fibers of differing diameters serve differing physiological functions. As described in greater detail elsewhere in this text, the smallest diameter axons consist of sympathetic preganglionic fibers, followed by larger A delta and C fibers transmitting somatic pain. The largest fibers are A alpha and A beta axons responsible for motor and tactile sensation, respectively. Theoretically, it should be possible to differentially block sympathetic fibers independently of A delta and C pain afferent fibers by subjecting them to gradually increasing concentrations of local anesthetic within the epidural or intrathecal space. In the past, differential epidural and differential subarachnoid neural blockades have been used for the purpose of differentiating among sympathetically maintained pain, somatically mediated pain, and central pain syndromes. With this technique, gradually increasing concentrations of local anesthetic are applied to the spinal

neuraxis. In theory, dilute concentrations of local anesthetic will selectively block sympathetic fibers, whereas higher concentrations will progressively block somatosensory and somatomotor axons.

There is currently significant doubt as to the reliability of differential spinal block in determining the origin of pain. It has been shown that the concentration of local anesthetic required to block nerves is not solely a function of fiber diameter (Heavner and deJong, 1974). Experiments have shown that A delta and B fibers can be blocked at concentrations of local anesthetic below those required to block the smaller C fibers. It is also doubtful whether it is possible to produce a pure block of sympathetic or a pure block of somatic nerve fibers within the epidural or subarachnoid space. Furthermore, there are questions regarding the reliability and reproducibility of subjective patient response in the setting of spinal anesthesia (Strichartz, 1988; Wurm, 1992).

Spinal local anesthetic blockade does, however, have a role in pain diagnosis. First, if complete somatosensory spinal blockade fails to produce pain relief, it may be reasonable to conclude that pain originates from higher sites within the central nervous system (central pain), that pain is psychogenic, or that the patient is malingering. Second, valuable information regarding the segmental somatic level of nociceptive input may be obtained by blocking increasingly higher spinal segments.

Pharmacological Blockade of the Nervous System. There are two pharmacological interventions that are sometimes helpful in the diagnosis of persistent pain. The lidocaine challenge test involves the intravenous administration of lidocaine at a dose of 1.2 to 2 mg/kg titrated until the patient reports tingling or lightheadedness. There is some evidence that patients with central pain states will obtain analgesia with systemic lidocaine infusion, whereas patients with peripheral tissue etiology for ongoing pain will not obtain analgesia (Backonja, 1994). Analgesia with intravenous lidocaine may also be predictive of favorable response to oral local anesthetics such as mexiletine. These drugs may be reasonable alternatives for the long-term treatment of persistent pain.

Psychometric Testing

Because psychometric testing yields imprecise data, the psychological assessment of the patient with chronic pain requires a thorough psychological interview by an experienced and qualified behavioral pain specialist (Kinney and Brin, 1992; Turk and Chapman, 1982). Many multidisciplinary pain centers have psychiatrists or psychologists on staff to complete this aspect of patient evaluation. The psychological interview concentrates on revealing the patient's attitude toward pain; the impact that pain has on employment, family relations, and feelings of self-worth; and uncovering any signs or symptoms of clinical depression. Concurrently, there are a number of psychological tests that help to shed light on the personality and mental state of the patient with chronic pain. Three commonly used psychological screening tests are listed below along with a brief description of the information they can provide.

MMPI. The Minnesota Multiphasic Personality Inventory is perhaps the best known and the most widely used psychological screening test today (Hathaway et al, 1989). There is a significant amount of data supporting its validity and reliability. The MMPI can give insight into the personality characteristics of the patient with pain and provide clues as to the presence or absence of depression and psychosis. The test has more than 500 questions and may take 2 hours for completion.

Mcgill Pain Questionnaire. This commonly used test offers some insight into how the patient perceives the pain experience (Melzack, 1975). The test is relatively simple and asks the patient to describe the pain by selecting a number of adjectives such as "agonizing," "stabbing," "suffocating," and "killing." There is a pain drawing that allows the patient to mark the anatomical distribution of pain onto a figure of the human body (see Fig. 14–3). This test helps to define the quality, location, and meaning of the patient's pain. The test is probably less reliable than the MMPI, but it is easier to administer and score and allows the pain specialist to follow changing patterns of pain perception over time.

Beck Depression Inventory. This quick and easy test has been used successfully to identify depression in patients with persistent pain (Beck and Ward, 1961). The test consists of 21 questions regarding the patient's thoughts and feelings and can be administered and scored in 15 minutes or less.

TREATMENT

Many patients who are referred to a chronic pain center have already been evaluated and treated by a number of physicians. Most patients are convinced that there is a physical source for their pain and if only this source could be eradicated, everything would be fine. Physicians, on the other hand, are trained to take definitive action against disease and suffering and sometimes feel compelled to offer aggressive therapies with a chance for cure even if that chance is slim. Therefore, patients often undergo multiple invasive procedures and surgeries for obscure chronic pain conditions, with no lasting benefit. The patient initially has great hope but, when invasive therapy is ineffective, loses faith in the initial physician and seeks care from another physician who provides a different invasive therapy. This cycle repeats itself again and again as the patient continues to believe that the magic cure waits behind the next physician's office door, and each successive physician believes that his or her invasive intervention will work better than the last one. Although many patients benefit greatly from surgery and other invasive procedures aimed at pain control, the successful practice of chronic pain management requires the practitioner to accept the fact that certain patients have incurable pain conditions and will not benefit from invasive attempts to eradicate physical pathology. A major objective of the multidisciplinary pain center is to help patients avoid unnecessary surgeries and invasive procedures and to learn to live productive and fulfilling lives despite chronic pain. This is no easy undertaking and, to be effective, it requires a motivated patient as well as a coordi-

nated, multidisciplinary effort on the part of health care professionals.

There are a large number of treatments available for recurrent acute and chronic pain. In general, these treatments can be divided into invasive and noninvasive techniques. Invasive techniques include nerve blocks, neuroablative procedures, and implantable devices. Noninvasive therapies include medications, physical therapies, and behavioral pain management. A brief discussion of various therapies in use today follows.

Invasive Interventions

Reversible Neural Blockade. Therapeutic nerve blocks have been used to alleviate a number of different types of persistent pain. Some patients receiving local anesthetic nerve blocks for diagnostic or therapeutic reasons obtain pain relief that far outlasts the pharmacological duration of effect of the local anesthetic in tissue (Bonica, 1990f). This prolonged analgesia is sometimes enhanced if steroid medication is added to the local anesthetic mixture (Devor, 1985) or if the nerve blocks are carried out in series (Bonica, 1990f). There are a number of theories as to why repeated neural blockade, with or without added steroid, might result in prolonged analgesia (Bonica, 1990f). Certainly, local anesthetics can inhibit the afferent limb of pain reflexes, alter regional blood flow, reverse muscle spasm mediated by somatomotor nerves, and block sympathetic input to an affected part. Local anesthetics may also prevent the self-sustaining, inappropriate depolarization of abnormal neurons in dorsal root ganglia or spinal cord. Whatever the mechanism, there is good evidence that neural blockade can be helpful as adjunctive therapy, and sometimes curative, in many conditions, including the following (Bonica, 1990; Devor et al, 1985; Strichartz, 1988; Wurm, 1992).

- Herpes zoster and postherpetic neuralgia
- Reflex sympathetic dystrophy and causalgia
- Peripheral neuritis and neuralgia
- Radiculopathy
- Entrapment neuropathy
- Malignant invasion of a nerve or plexus
- Myofascial pain syndrome

Neuroablative Procedures. There is currently a movement away from neuroablative procedures for chronic noncancer pain. After many years of experience with neurodestruction, there is little in the way of documented long-term success for procedures that have previously been widely recommended (Loeser, 1972, 1990). Problems with neuroablation have included functional loss, recurrent pain, and creation of neuropathic pain states that are more bothersome than the original pain. Neuroablation for sympathetically maintained pain has not been consistently effective for a number of reasons. First, not all sympathetic fibers follow the usual course from their origins in the intermediolateral cell column of the spinal cord through ventral root and white rami communicans into the adjacent paravertebral sympathetic ganglion (Loeser,

1990). Some preganglionic fibers travel a variable distance within the sympathetic chain before synapsing with postganglionic fibers in a ganglion several segments higher or lower. Other preganglionic fibers follow an aberrant course through dorsal root or gray rami communicans on their way to a ganglionic synapse. This variability in the sympathetic pathway is in part responsible for the disappointing results with surgical sympathectomy.

Problems have also arisen when the decision to proceed with neurodestruction has been based on the results of antecedent reversible neural blockade. There is ample evidence in the literature that favorable response to local anesthetic nerve block does not predict the effect of surgical or chemical neuroablation (Loeser, 1972, 1990). This is especially true when results of local anesthetic sympathetic blocks are used to predict the effect of surgical sympathectomy. Pain relief from the local anesthetic block may result in part from unintentional somatic block, whereas surgical sympathectomy will not affect somatic nerves.

Nonetheless, neurodestruction has proved to be efficacious in a variety of cancer pain syndromes as well as in certain types of chronic benign pain, including brachial plexus avulsion (Friedberg, 1992; Loeser, 1990), trigeminal neuralgia (Sweet et al, 1981), and sometimes sympathetically maintained pain (Cousins, 1979).

Localized Injections. Local infiltration of soft tissue with local anesthetic and/or steroid has been advocated for the treatment of a number of conditions, including myofascial pain syndrome (Simons, 1988), painful scar (Defalque, 1982), and painful neuroma (Cimino, 1992; Devor et al, 1985). In myofascial pain syndrome, it is believed that a pathological reflex arc develops as injured areas of muscle send nociceptive impulses into the spinal cord. Spinal reflexes are then initiated that result in alpha motor neuron and sympathetic output to the site of injury, leading to the clinical syndrome of chronically painful, tender areas in skeletal muscle. Injection of local anesthetic into the muscular trigger point allows relaxation of muscle fibers, increased blood flow, decreased nociceptive input into the central nervous system, and improvement in pain (Simons, 1988; Simons and Travell, 1983; Sola and Bonica, 1990). When done in series and coordinated with physical therapy, trigger point injections have been successful at permanently reversing chronic and sometimes debilitating myofascial pain (Sola and Bonica, 1990). With painful scar and neuroma, there is evidence that repeated injection of local anesthetic and steroid solution may permanently relieve pain by stabilizing neuronal membranes and reducing spontaneous ectopic discharge from injured nerve (Defalque, 1982; Devor et al, 1985). As persistent nociceptive input into the spinal cord is decreased, central nervous system sensitization resolves, thus contributing to the resolution of the chronic pain state.

Implantable Devices. The implantation of devices to control chronic pain has gained wider acceptance in recent years as technology has improved and patient selection has become more stringent. Currently, two different implantable therapies are being used with good results: spinal cord stimulation and spinal drug delivery.

Spinal Cord Stimulation. This technique was developed about 25 years ago and after initial uncontrolled use, fell into disfavor because of poor success rates. Recently, outcome has improved as patients have been more carefully selected and as the original monopolar lead systems have been replaced by multipolar systems capable of creating a number of different stimulation patterns and amenable to external reprogramming (North et al, 1993; Urban and Nashold, 1978). Currently, a number of pain syndromes have been identified as amenable to spinal cord stimulation therapy. The following is a list of indications ranked in order of decreasing efficacy (North et al, 1993). Spinal cord stimulation is discussed in detail elsewhere in this text.

1. "Failed back syndrome" with chronic radiculopathy.
2. Peripheral vascular disease with chronic ischemic pain.
3. Sympathetically maintained pain (RSD and causalgia).
4. Phantom limb pain.

Implantable Drug Delivery Systems. The two fundamentally different types of implantable drug delivery systems currently available are subcutaneous injection ports attached to subcutaneously tunneled intraspinal catheters and subcutaneous infusion pumps attached to subcutaneously tunneled intraspinal catheters.

Subcutaneous injection ports can be used for patients who require a prolonged course of intermittent injections to treat such conditions as refractory RSD. Most commonly, these systems are placed to deliver epidural medication on a regular basis over a period of weeks or months so that repeated epidural instrumentation can be avoided.

The drug infusion systems commonly consist of a tunneled intrathecal or epidural catheter attached to an infusion pump. The catheter can be externalized and attached to a continuous infusion pump, or the infusion pump can be implanted into a subcutaneous tissue pocket and filled percutaneously. Implanted drug infusion systems are commonly used for patients with terminal cancer pain, but they are also increasingly being used to treat selected patients with chronic benign pain as an alternative to oral opioid therapy (Onofrio and Yaksh, 1990). Advantages of spinally administered over orally administered opioids include less somnolence and a more powerful, segmental analgesia (Cousins and Mather, 1984).

Noninvasive Therapies

There are certain chronic pain conditions that are, for all practical purposes, incurable by medical or surgical means. This is not to say, however, that the patient must live in misery. Suffering and nociception are distinct and independent entities, and suffering can often be improved even when nociception persists. Suffering constitutes the emotional component of pain and is dependent, in part, on the presumed consequences of pain, expectations for the future, and the specific meaning of the pain to the individual. Cassell (1982) describes suffering as occurring when "an impending destruction of the person is perceived . . . suffering can be defined as the state of severe distress associated with events that threaten the intactness of the person." By this definition, suffering from chronic pain that is not associated with ongoing injury to the organism may be in part alleviated through patient education and reassurance. Furthermore, there is certainly a connection between the psychological state of a person and his or her perception of, and reaction to, nociception. For these reasons, noninvasive, nonmedicinal approaches to chronic pain designed to improve patient's coping skills, decrease anxiety, change beliefs and attitudes toward pain, improve family dynamics, and minimize pain behavior can improve quality of life more effectively than any medical or surgical approach and with less risk of iatrogenic injury. There are a significant number of noninvasive interventions that may be efficacious for the treatment of chronic pain, including transcutaneous electrical nerve stimulation (TENS), biofeedback, hypnosis, relaxation, and cognitive-behavioral therapy. Such treatments can be used alone or in combination and can be incorporated into a comprehensive approach to pain relief that includes invasive, medicinal, and behavioral treatments simultaneously. A brief discussion of several noninvasive pain therapies follows.

Transcutaneous Electrical Nerve Stimulation. This has been used to treat pain for more than two decades and represents a therapy with a theoretical basis in the gate control theory of pain. Gate control theory postulates that intense modulation of afferent nociceptive input occurs at the level of the dorsal horn of the spinal cord (Melzack and Wall, 1965). Pain impulses traveling through A delta and C-fiber nociceptive afferent nerve fibers cause the gate to open, and these impulses pass through the dorsal horn to the brain, where pain is consciously perceived. Conversely, the gate is closed by the activity of large A beta fibers carrying pressure and touch sensation to the cord. This is perhaps why we shake our hand after burning our finger. With TENS, an external generator creates an electrical current that is delivered to the painful segment via skin electrode or acupuncture needle, thus closing the gate by selectively stimulating large fiber axons. The mechanism of gate closure is unclear, but it is thought to involve the presynaptic inhibition of nociceptive dorsal horn neurons by large fiber axons. Routine high-frequency TENS delivered through skin electrode is not naloxone-reversible and does not involve opioid receptors. Interestingly, TENS delivered via acupuncture needles is more powerful and is reversed by naloxone, indicating an endorphin-dependent mechanism (Lorenz et al, 1992).

Biofeedback. With biofeedback, patients learn to alter certain physiological parameters such as heart rate, skin temperature, electroencephalogram waveforms, and electromyographic recordings from skeletal muscle through the voluntary use of mental processes. This technique has been popularized in the lay press in recent years, and numerous claims have been made regarding its usefulness in the treatment of chronic pain (Urban and Nashold, 1978). Although results of controlled studies have been variable, there currently is some evidence for the efficacy of biofeedback in pain management (Turk and Chapman, 1982). Because the treatment is harmless and patient acceptance is high, biofeedback is widely used in the treatment of a number of pain problems, including muscle contraction headache, Raynaud's syndrome, arthritis, and lower back pain.

Hypnosis and Relaxation Therapy. Profound relaxation has been shown to have a significant effect on a number of physiological parameters, including respiratory rate, heart rate, blood pressure, oxygen consumption, and brain wave patterns (Benson, 1975; Turk and Chapman, 1982). Changes in these parameters are consistent with a reduction in the output of the sympathetic nervous system and have been collectively defined as the *relaxation response* (Benson, 1975). Considered to be the opposite of the sympathetically mediated *fight or flight response,* the relaxation response has been shown to be elicited by a large number of different activities associated with relaxation, including meditation, prayer, yoga, and hypnosis. Relaxation training, in one form or another, is a common theme in most multidisciplinary pain centers today, and there is evidence that benefits demonstrable during the relaxation period carry over into the post-relaxation period (Benson, 1975; Orne, 1992; Turk and Chapman, 1982). Because persistent pain is often associated with psychological stress, the ability to relax at will is certainly a valuable skill for this group of patients.

Medicinal Approach to Pain Management

There are a number of medications that have proved helpful in the management of persistent pain. Presently, these medications fall into five broad categories:

- Opioids
- Nonsteroidal anti-inflammatory drugs
- Tricyclic antidepressants
- Anti-seizure medications
- Oral local anesthetics

These different classes of drugs tend to alleviate pain by separate and independent mechanisms and, when used in logical combinations, may act synergistically.

Opioids. The analgesic properties of opium and its derivatives have been known for hundreds of years. Recent research has determined that these powerful analgesics exert their effects by binding to a number of different receptor subtypes within brain and spinal cord. Receptor binding prevents the presynaptic release and modifies the postsynaptic effects of nociceptive neurotransmitters (Benson, 1975; Yaksh, 1986, 1992). Opioids may also have a peripheral site of action because receptors have been discovered in joint synovium, and morphine instilled into joints after arthroscopy has shown to be analgesic. The appropriate use of opioid analgesics is now mandated by federal guidelines for the control of severe acute pain and for the pain of terminal cancer (Carr et al, 1992). The long-term treatment of chronic benign pain with opioid analgesics is, however, more controversial. Recently, the use of long-term opioids in selected individuals with chronic benign pain has been advocated. A subset of chronic pain patients can obtain analgesia, improve function, and become more productive with opioid therapy (Portenoy, 1990). Fear of addiction has been a major factor in the long-standing reticence of physicians to prescribe opiate analgesics for persistent pain. On objective analysis, however, drug addiction, defined as psychological dependence on a drug associated with nonmedicinal use of the drug and pervasive, drug-seeking behavior, has been shown to be rare in patients who are using opioids to control pain. Drug addiction, in contrast to physical dependence on and tolerance to opioids, has been identified to be a psychosocial phenomenon driven by underlying personality traits and not simply the result of opioid intake (Portenoy, 1990). Physical dependence and tolerance, on the other hand, are biophysiological consequences of opioid use and will occur in any person taking opioid drugs over time. Patients being treated with chronic opioids may therefore require increasing amounts of drug to obtain similar analgesia over time (tolerance) and will manifest a withdrawal syndrome if the drug is abruptly withdrawn (physical dependence) without being drug addicted in the psychosocial sense. Nevertheless, the use of opioid medications to treat chronic benign pain is controversial. If this method of therapy is to be used effectively, opioids must be administered in a controlled and methodical way following published guidelines and recommendations. This type of therapy has proved to be labor intensive and requires a long-term commitment by involved health professionals. The practice is perhaps best accomplished through a centralized community program rather than through a private physician office practice.

Antidepressants. Tricyclic antidepressants such as amitriptyline have long been used in the management of persistent pain. Studies have consistently demonstrated pain relief greater than placebo at doses below those usually required for the treatment of depression (Spiegel et al, 1983; Watson et al, 1982). It is thought that these agents provide analgesia by enhancing the effects of serotonin within the central nervous system. These drugs are sometimes effective for pain relief at low blood levels. At higher doses, however, tricyclic antidepressants are often poorly tolerated, with side effects including sedation, dry mouth, constipation, and confusion. The newer central nervous system serotonin-uptake blockers such as fluoxetine (Prozac), paroxetine (Paxil), and sertraline (Zoloft) are well tolerated and efficacious at treating the depression that often accompanies chronic pain, but these compounds have not been shown to possess intrinsic analgesic properties.

Nonsteroidal Anti-inflammatory Drugs (NSAIDs). This class of drugs acts by inhibiting cyclooxygenase, decreasing the production of prostaglandins, and diminishing the inflammatory response accompanying nociception. The NSAIDs have traditionally been considered to act peripherally, but recent attention has been focused on their effects within the central nervous system. The anti-inflammatory potency of the various NSAIDS has little correlation to their analgesic potency, and this has led to the discovery that these drugs also inhibit prostaglandins within the spinal cord (Yaksh, 1993a). It is thought that spinal cord prostaglandins interfere with endogenous descending pathways responsible for blocking pain transmission.

Antiepileptic Drugs. Medications such as carbamazepine (Tegretol) and phenytoin (Dilantin) have been used as analgesics for persistent pain. These drugs suppress spontaneous and inappropriate neuronal firing and are most commonly used in neuropathic pain states in which neurons are thought to be firing spontaneously. Pain responsive to antiepileptic medication often has a paroxysmal, lancinating quality related to the pathological depolarization of neuron pools within the central nervous system. Conditions responsive to this type of therapy include trigeminal neuralgia, postherpetic neuralgia, diabetic neuropathy, and phantom limb pain. Although efficacious in some patients, these drugs are often poorly tolerated. Side effects include dizziness, dysphoria, confusion, and gastrointestinal distress.

Systemic Local Anesthetics. The systemic infusion of lidocaine has been used in the treatment of persistent pain since shortly after its synthesis 50 years ago. Most commonly, this form of therapy has been advocated for the treatment of neuropathic pain, and there is evidence that at least some patients obtain long-term benefit from infusions done in series (Backonja, 1994). Systemic local anesthetics seem to have effects that outlast the pharmacological activity of the drug in tissue, similar to the phenomenon seen with local anesthetic nerve blocks. The recent development of orally administered local anesthetics such as mexiletine has made it possible to use these drugs long-term in the outpatient setting.

SUMMARY

Persistent pain can be extremely frustrating for the patient and the physician. Many uncomplicated pain problems can be effectively treated in the physician's office or by the physician pain specialist. In contrast, the effective management of complex, enigmatic pain syndromes associated with significant psychosocial disruption often requires the resources of a multidisciplinary pain center able to draw on the expertise of specialized physicians and other health professionals from a number of different disciplines.

In some cases, even the most sophisticated and thorough workup will fail to uncover the etiology for chronic pain, and the best efforts at treatment will fail to prevent its disabling consequences. More often, when persistent nociception cannot be completely eradicated, patients can live fuller, more productive, and less painful lives if cared for in an organized, coordinated, and comprehensive manner. The surgeon familiar with current trends in pain management will be better able to care for patients with persistent pain and to identify those patients who require specialized pain management.

References

Abram SE: Pain mechanisms in lumbar radiculopathy. Anesth Analg 67:1135–1137, 1988.

Backonja MM: Local anesthetics as adjuvant analgesics. J Pain Symptom Manage 9:491–499, 1994.

Beck AT, Ward CH: An inventory for measuring depression. Arch Gen Psychiatry 4:561–571, 1961.

Benson H: The Relaxation Response. New York, Academic Press, 1975.

Bonica JJ: Anatomic and physiologic basis of pain. *In* Bonica JJ (ed): The Management of Pain, ed 2. Philadelphia, Lea & Febiger, 1990, p 88.

Bonica JJ: Biochemistry and modulation of nociception and pain, *In* Bonica JJ (ed): The Management of Pain, ed 2. Philadelphia, Lea & Febiger, 1990c, pp 220–221, 238.

Bonica JJ: Definitions and taxonomy of pain. *In* Bonica JJ (ed): The

Management of Pain, ed 2. Philadelphia, Lea & Febiger, 1990d, pp 19–21.

Bonica JJ: General considerations of chronic pain. *In* Bonica JJ (ed): The Management of Pain, ed 2. Philadelphia, Lea & Febiger, 1990e, p 187.

Bonica JJ: Regional anesthesia with local anesthetics. *In* Bonica JJ (ed): The Management of Pain, ed 2. Philadelphia, Lea & Febiger, 1990f, pp 1883–1996.

Carr DB, Jacox AK, Chapman CR, et al: Acute Pain Management: Operative or Medical Procedures and Trauma. Clinical Practice Guideline/ AHCPR publication no. 92-0032. Agency for Health Care Policy and Research, Rockville, MD, 1992.

Cassell EJ: The nature of suffering and the goals of medicine. N Engl J Med 306:639, 1982.

Cimino C: Painful neurological syndromes. *In* Aronoff G (ed): Evaluation and Treatment of Chronic Pain. Baltimore, Williams & Wilkins, 1992.

Cline MA, Ochoa J, Torebjork HE: Chronic hyperalgesia and skin warming caused by sensitized C nociceptors. Brain 112:621–647, 1989.

Cousins MJ: Neurolytic lumbar sympathetic blockade: Duration of denervation and relief of rest pain. Anaesth Intensive Care 7:21, 1979.

Cousins MJ, Mather LE: Intrathecal and epidural administration of opioids. Anesthesiology 61:276–310, 1984.

Dahl JB, Kehlet H: Preemptive analgesia: Is it effective in postoperative pain? Pain Digest 4:106–109, 1994.

Defalque RJ: Painful trigger points in surgical scars. Anesth Analg 61:518, 1982.

Devor M: Nerve pathophysiology and mechanisms of pain in causalgia. J Auton Nerv Syst 7:371, 1983.

Devor M, Govrin-Lippman R, Raber P: Corticosteroids suppress ectopic neuronal discharge originating in experimental neuromas. Pain 22:127, 1985.

Diagnostic and Statistical Manual of Mental Disorders, ed 4. American Psychiatric Association, Washington, DC, 1994.

Dubner R: Neuronal plasticity in the spinal and medullary dorsal horns: A possible role in central pain mechanisms. *In* Casey KL (ed): Pain and Central Nervous System Disease. New York, Raven, 1991, pp 77–83.

Friedberg SR: The neurosurgeon's approach to pain. *In* Aronoff GM (ed): Evaluation and Treatment of Chronic Pain. Baltimore, Williams & Wilkins, 1992, pp 229–237.

Hathaway SR, McKinley JC, Butcher JN: Minnesota Multiphasic Personality Inventory 2: Manual for Administration. Minneapolis, University of Minnesota Press, 1989.

Heavner JE, deJong RH: Lidocaine blocking concentrations for B- and C-nerve fibers. Anesthesiology 40:228–233, 1974.

Kinney WW, Brin EN: Diagnostic evaluation and management of the patient with chronic pain. *In* Aronoff G (ed): Evaluation and Treatment of Chronic Pain. Baltimore, Williams & Wilkins, 1992.

Kosin F, Soin JS, Ryan LM, Carrera GF, Wortmann RL: Bone scintigraphy in reflex sympathetic dystrophy syndrome. Radiology 13:4437–4438, 1981.

Lewis T: Pain. New York, Macmillan, 1942, pp 57–84.

Lippe PM: Pain. *In* American Medical Association Guides to the Evaluation and Treatment of Permanent Impairment, ed 4. Chicago, American Medical Association, 1993, p 305.

Loeser JD: Dorsal rhizotomy for the relief of chronic pain. J Neurosurgery 36:745, 1972.

Loeser JD: Ablative neurosurgical procedures—Introduction. *In* Bonica JJ (ed): The Management of Pain, ed 2. Philadelphia, Lea & Febiger, 1990, p 88.

Lorenz KI, Jefferson JK, Mathew HM: Acupuncture: A neuromodulation technique for pain control. *In* Aronoff GM (ed): Evaluation and Treatment of Chronic Pain. Baltimore, Williams & Wilkins, 1992, pp 291–298.

Malmberg MB, Yaksh TL: Spinal nitric oxide synthesis blocks NMDA induced thermal hyperalgesia and produces antinociception in the formalin test in rats. Pain 54:291–300, 1993.

Melzack R: The Mcgill Pain Questionnaire: Major properties and scoring methods. Pain 1:277–299, 1975.

Melzack R, Wall P: Pain mechanisms: A new theory. Science 150:971, 1965.

Myers RR: The pathogenesis of neuropathic pain. Reg Anesth 20:173–184, 1995.

Nehme AM, Warfield C: Diagnostic measures. *In* Warfield C (ed): Principles and Practice of Pain Management. New York, McGraw-Hill, 1993, pp 58–59.

North R, Kidd M, Zuharak M, James P, Long D: Spinal cord stimulation for chronic intractable pain: Experience over two decades. Neurosurgery 32:384–395, 1993.

Onofrio B, Yaksh TL: Long term pain relief produced by intrathecal morphine infusion in 53 patients. J Neurosurg 72:200–209, 1990.

Orne M: Nonpharmacological approaches to pain relief: Hypnosis, biofeedback, placebo effects. *In* Aronoff G (ed): Evaluation and Treatment of Chronic Pain, ed 2. Baltimore, Williams & Wilkins, 1992, p 435.

Pagni CA, Canavero S: Pain, muscle spasms and twitching following brachial plexus avulsion. J Neurol 240:468–470, 1993.

Portenoy R: Chronic opioid therapy in nonmalignant pain. J Pain Symptom Manage 5(Suppl):46–61, 1990.

Simons DG: Myofascial pain syndromes of head, neck and low back. *In* Dubner R, Gephart GF, Bond MR (eds): Pain Research and Clinical Management, vol 3. Proceedings of the 5th World Congress on Pain. New York, Elsevier, 1988, pp 186–200.

Simons DG, Travell JG: Myofascial origins of low back pain: Part I, II, and III. Postgrad Med 73:66, 1983.

Sinatra RS: Pathophysiology of acute pain. *In* Sinatra RS, Hord AH: Acute Pain: Mechanisms and Management. St. Louis, Mosby, 1992.

Sola AE, Bonica JJ: Myofascial pain syndromes. *In* Bonica JJ (ed): The Management of Pain, ed 2. Philadelphia, Lea & Febiger, 1990, pp 363–365.

Spiegel K, Kalb R, Pasternak GW: Analgesic activity of tricyclic antidepressants. Ann Neurol 13:462, 1983.

Strichartz GR: Neural physiology and local anesthetic action. *In* Cousins M, Bridenbaugh P (eds): Neural Blockade, ed 2. Philadelphia, Lippincott, 1988, pp 36–37.

Superville B, Rasminsky M, Finlayson MM: Complications of phenol neurolysis. Arch Neurol 32:226, 1975.

Sweet WH, Poletti CE, Macon JB: Treatment of trigeminal neuralgia and other facial pain by retro gasserian injection of glycerol. Neurosurgery 9:647, 1981.

Tasker R: Deafferentation and causalgia. *In* Bonica JJ (ed): Advances in Pain Research and Treatment. New York, Raven, 1980, pp 305–329.

Turk DC, Chapman CR: Psychological intervention for chronic pain: A critical review. I. Relaxation training and biofeedback. Pain 12:1, 1982.

Turk DC, Melzack R: The measurement of pain and the assessment of people experiencing pain. *In* Turk DC, Melzack R (eds): Handbook of Pain Assessment. London, Guilford, 1992, pp 3–12.

Urban BJ, Nashold BS: Percutaneous stimulation of the spinal cord for relief of pain. J Neurosurg 48:323, 1978.

Wall PD, Melzack R: Introduction. *In* Wall PD, Melzack R (eds): Textbook of Pain. New York, Churchill Livingstone, 1984, pp 13–14.

Watson CP, Evans RJ, Reed K, Merskey H, Goldsmith L, Warch J: Amitriptyline vs. placebo in postherpetic neuralgia. Neurology 32:671–673, 1982.

Wurm HW: Role of diagnostic and therapeutic nerve blocks in the management of pain. *In* Aronoff G (ed): The Evaluation and Treatment of Chronic Pain. Baltimore, Williams & Wilkins, 1992, pp 118–219.

Yaksh TL: The central pharmacology of primary afferents with emphasis on the disposition and role of primary afferent substance P. *In* Yaksh TL (ed): Spinal Afferent Processing. New York, Plenum, 1986, pp 165–195.

Yaksh TL: The spinal pharmacology of acutely and chronically administered opioids. J Pain Symptom Manage 7:356–361, 1992.

Yaksh TL: Spinal actions of NSAIDS in blocking spinally mediated hyperalgesia: The role of cyclooxygenase products. Agents Actions Suppl 41:89–100, 1993a.

Yaksh TL: The spinal pharmacology of facilitation of afferent processing evoked by high threshold afferent input of the postinjury state. Curr Opin Neurol Neurosurg 6:250–256, 1993b.

Yaksh TL, Aimone LD: The central pharmacology of pain transmission. *In* Wall PD, Melzack R (eds): Textbook of Pain. New York, Churchill Livingstone, 1989.

Recommended Reading

Aronoff G: The Evaluation and Treatment of Chronic Pain, ed 2. Baltimore, Williams & Wilkins, 1992.

Bonica JJ: The Management of Pain, ed 2. Philadelphia, Lea & Febiger, 1990.

Cousins M, Bridenbaugh P: Neural Blockade. Philadelphia, Lippincott, 1988.

Sinatra R: Acute Pain: Mechanisms and Management. St. Louis, Mosby, 1992.

Warfield C: Principles and Practice of Pain Management. New York, McGraw-Hill, 1993.

Spinal Cord and Peripheral Nerve Stimulation for Management of Peripheral Pain

Fascination with the therapeutic uses of electricity dates to ancient times. In the first century A.D., electric fish were used to numb aches and pains associated with headache and gout (Ray, 1975a). In more recent times, Benjamin Franklin used electrostatic generators to treat a variety of medical maladies, especially pain. Numerous stimulating or shocking devices were touted as panaceas in the early 1800s, but their use declined with the development of drugs and the abhorrence of device quackery.

The now classic gate control theory of Melzack and Wall (1965) reintroduced the use of electrical stimulation for pain control by providing a rationale for its effects. The first practical implanted stimulation device for pain control was devised by Shealy and co-workers in 1967. Stimulation of the dorsal column of the spinal cord proved to be a successful method for addressing certain cases of severe, chronic pain of the lower extremities. By the early 1970s, the method was being adopted widely and uncritically. After the initial wave of poor results that inevitably followed—due to improper patient selection criteria and fragile equipment—the therapy fell into disfavor. Nevertheless, some investigators deeply involved in the clinical application of electrical stimulation continued to experience good to excellent results in patients considered unsalvageable by other therapeutic means (Burton, 1975; Campbell and Long, 1976; Nielson et al, 1975; North et al, 1978; Ray, 1975a, 1975b).

By the latter part of the 1970s, it had become apparent that about half of the patients treated by stimulator implants would receive lasting relief of approximately 50% of their prestimulation pain, regardless of the intensity or duration of the pain (Burton, 1975; Burton et al, 1977). Since then, development of specific patient selection criteria and improvements in neurostimulation devices and techniques have contributed to enhanced safety and efficacy of neurostimulation for the treatment of chronic, intractable pain.

This chapter addresses two types of neurostimulation for chronic, intractable pain: spinal cord stimulation and peripheral nerve stimulation. Both therapies use implantable electrodes to superimpose a pattern of paresthesia within the painful area to block pain signals. In the case of spinal cord stimulation, electrodes are implanted along the dorsal column of the spinal cord at a position corresponding to the painful area. Peripheral nerve stimulation is helpful for very localized pain involving no more than two nerve roots. The electrodes are placed on the involved nerve distribution

branch to achieve very targeted relief. For each type of neurostimulation therapy, the electrode-bearing leads are connected to a stimulus-pulse source, which provides the power for stimulation.

Each of these therapies, when properly applied to the appropriate patient, is safe and effective. They offer alternatives differing from all other therapeutic modes and should be considered before destructive and irreversible procedures or more costly regimens are chosen (Fig. 15–1).

SPINAL CORD STIMULATION

Neuroanatomy of the Two Pain Systems

Activation of normally present inhibitory circuits is probably the principal mode of operation for neurostimulation control of pain (and other stimulation-treatable disorders). There are two pain systems of humans, each of which passes through the substantia gelatinosa of the dorsal spinal cord, the site of the inhibitory spinal gate in the gate control theory. The first pain system is a rapid, direct skin and lining structure or surface-activated, somatotopically specific system. Its constituents include primary afferent small A-delta and C fiber (pain, itching, thermal) input into the marginal cells and substantia gelatinosa of the dorsal spinal cord.

Integrative and filtering effects take place in the dorsal spinal cord that exercise considerable control over what is transmitted upstream. The next-order neurons in this system for conveying localizing pain information cross and ascend in the lateral neospinothalamic tract, passing through the medial lemniscus to terminate in the ventrobasal thalamus. Higher order neurons ascend to the postcentral gyrus of the cortex. Some of the descending system connects principally through the dorsolateral corticospinal system to the spinal segment of pain origin. The overall effect of the oligosynaptic somatotopic lateral pain system is localization, fast withdrawal, and protection against injury.

Stimulating peripheral nerves, dorsal columns, and the contralateral posterolateral sensory-specific thalamus produce localized tingling that can inhibit the experience of pain in the same somatotopic area. This paresthesia effect has been shown to be mediated by an organization involving gate control at the segmental level (Kerr, 1980; Krainick et al, 1980). There is further evidence that this tingling pain-

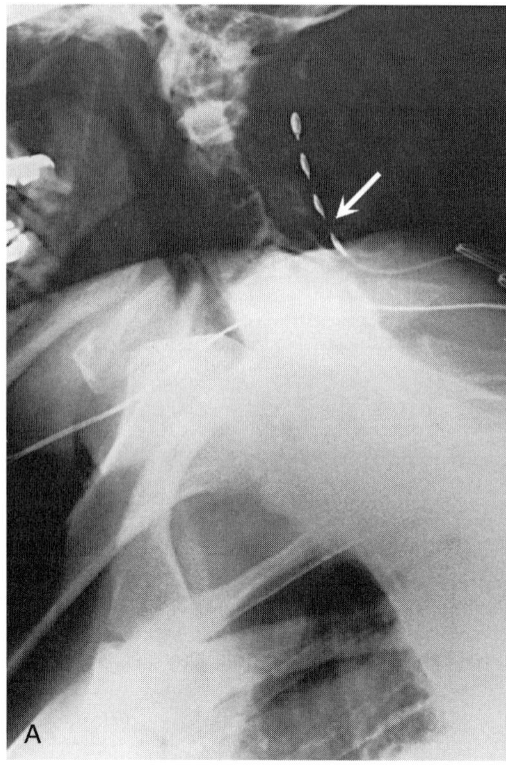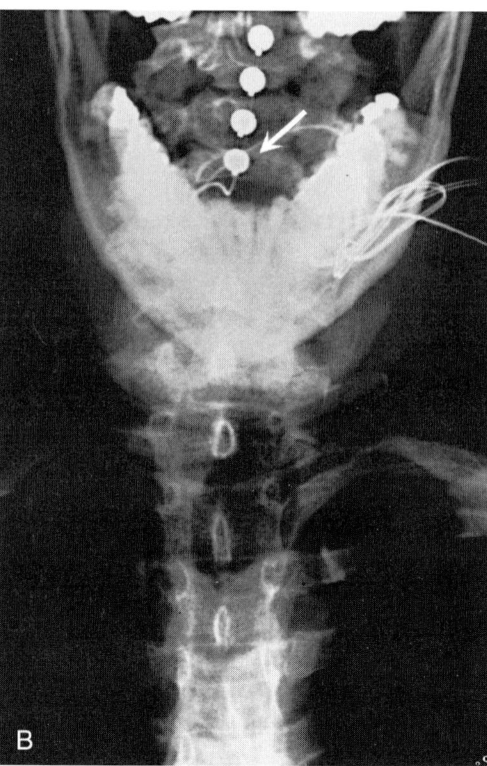

FIGURE 15–1. Anteroposterior *(A)* and lateral *(B)* views of Resume SCS lead (Medtronic, Inc.) in the cervical spine.

suppression effect arises in part from a signal modification (so-called jamming) and is not mediated by the endogenous opioids. For example, the effect is not modified by injection of the narcotic antagonist naloxone (Freeman et al, 1983; Horowitz et al, 1976; Liebeskind et al, 1982; Ranck, 1975).

The second pain system is a slow, indirect, deep structure–activated nonsomatotopic system. Its pathway is one of primary afferent small fiber input, similar to the first system, and local polysynapses to neurons that cross to ascend in the ventral paleospinothalamic tract. Fibers pass upward through the mesencephalic reticular system with its connections to the hypothalamus and limbic system. Bulbar reticular neurons also connect to the periaqueductal gray and the medial and intralaminar thalamus. Further rostral to these structures are connections to the hypothalamus, limbic system, and cortex. This complex system is involved in nondiscriminative aspects of pain as well as motivational and affective states. The system is enkephalin and opiate activated and, when disturbed, is likely the major source of chronic pain in humans (Ray et al, 1981).

Stimulation in the medial, intralaminar, nonspecific thalamic and periaqueductal gray system in humans leads to a reduction in chronic, agonizing pain; there is also an accompanying rise in the intraventricular endorphin content (Akil, 1978). Naloxone reverses these effects. Unlike stimulation of the first system, no somatotopic (tingling) sensations are produced. Thus, the second of the two pain inhibitory systems may be loosely characterized as primarily a chemical-like or opioid system, whereas the other is primarily signal like in function.

Possible Mechanisms of Pain Relief

It is unclear precisely what mechanisms are responsible for the pain relief afforded by electrical stimulation of the spinal cord. In many patients, pain relief begins about 15 minutes after the stimulation is initiated and persists for a half-hour to 2 hours or more after the stimulation is turned off (North, 1991). The prolonged pain relief following cessation of stimulation implies the activation of some neurochemical processes, but the specific processes have not yet been identified. Spinal cord stimulation is known to produce an increase in cerebrospinal fluid levels of substance P and to be associated with serotonin release in the dorsal horn (Linderoth et al, 1992). The extracellular concentration of gamma-aminobutyric acid in the lumbar dorsal horns has been found to increase significantly after 30 minutes of spinal cord stimulation (SCS) in rats (Linderoth et al, 1994, 1993). This finding is particularly notable given the known role of gamma-aminobutyric as an inhibitory neurotransmitter in the central nervous system.

Another possible inhibitory mechanism for SCS is frequency-related conduction block occurring at branch points of primary afferents, with collaterals to the dorsal horn (Campbell et al, 1990). Abram (1993) has postulated that the analgesia resulting from spinal stimulation is associated with both stimulation of large fiber ascending tracts and blockade of spinothalamic pathways. Detailed studies of neural excitation patterns in anesthetized monkeys by Chandler and associates (1993) suggest that spinal cord stimulation reduces pain by inhibiting the firing of spinothalamic tract cells that are activated by small-fiber afferents, while the paresthesias associated with the stimulation result from activation of spinothalamic tract cells that are excited by large-fiber afferents.

In any case, there is little evidence that electrical stimulation applied anywhere in the central nervous system directly produces more than transient inhibition. Thus, whether electrical stimulation for pain control functions either by signal inhibition or by neurochemically mediated pain inhibition processes, or both, *it is a reversible method.* In addition, it is a nondrug, nondestructive method with relatively few side effects. When side effects do occur, they are usually eliminated or greatly minimized by reducing the stimulus parameters. The majority of selected patients with implanted stimulators continue to enjoy good to excellent results for several years (De La Port et al, 1983, 1993; Krainick et al, 1980; Kumar et al, 1991; Lazorthes et al, 1983; Lifson et al, 1985; Long et al, 1981; North et al, 1993; Ray et al, 1982; Siegfried and Lazorthes, 1982). With recent improvements in the major components of SCS systems, the major reasons for failures, when they occur, are faulty patient selection, incorrect lead placement, inappropriate use of the devices, or misinterpretation of results.

Recent Experience with Spinal Cord Stimulation

North and associates (1993) have reviewed their experience over two decades with 320 patients who underwent implantation of temporary or permanent spinal cord stimulators, or both. Of the 205 patients available for follow-up interview by a disinterested third party (mean follow-up time of 7.1 ±4.5 years), 171 had received permanent implants. Of these, 52% reported at least 50% continued pain relief. Sixty percent reported that they would be willing (knowing what they know now) to repeat the implantation procedure. Additionally, the majority of patients reported improvements in lifestyle and reduced use of analgesics.

In an earlier study, North and colleagues (1991) reported on a series of 62 patients followed for an average of 2.14 years after implantation to treat failed back syndrome, lumbar arachnoid fibrosis, spinal cord injuries, and peripheral pathology or stump pain. A majority of patients reported at least 50% sustained relief of pain, and indicated to a disinterested third party that they would go through the procedure again for the same result. Superposition of stimulation paresthesias upon a patient's topography of pain was found to be a statistically significant predictor of successful relief of pain (Fig. 15–2).

De La Porte and Van de Kelft (1993) have reviewed their experience with SCS for 78 failed back syndrome patients, of whom 64 underwent permanent implantation following a 1-week period of trial stimulation. At a mean follow-up period of 4 years, 55% continued to experience at least 50% pain relief, and 90% were able to reduce their medication. LeDoux and Langford (1993) reported on a series of 32 failed back syndrome patients, of whom 26 received permanent implants. At least 50% pain reduction was reported by 74% of their patients at the 2-year follow-up. Electrode migration was the most common complication in this series.

Kumar and co-workers (1991) reported on their experience with 121 patients over 10 years, with pain of widely varied benign organic etiology. Patients were followed for from 6 months to 10 years, with a mean follow-up of 40 months. Lower extremity pain secondary to arachnoiditis or perineural fibrosis seemed to respond favorably. Good results were also obtained with lower extremity pain due to multiple sclerosis and advanced peripheral vascular disease. Paraplegic pain, phantom-limb pain, midline back pain without radiculopathy, pain due to cauda equina injury, and pain due

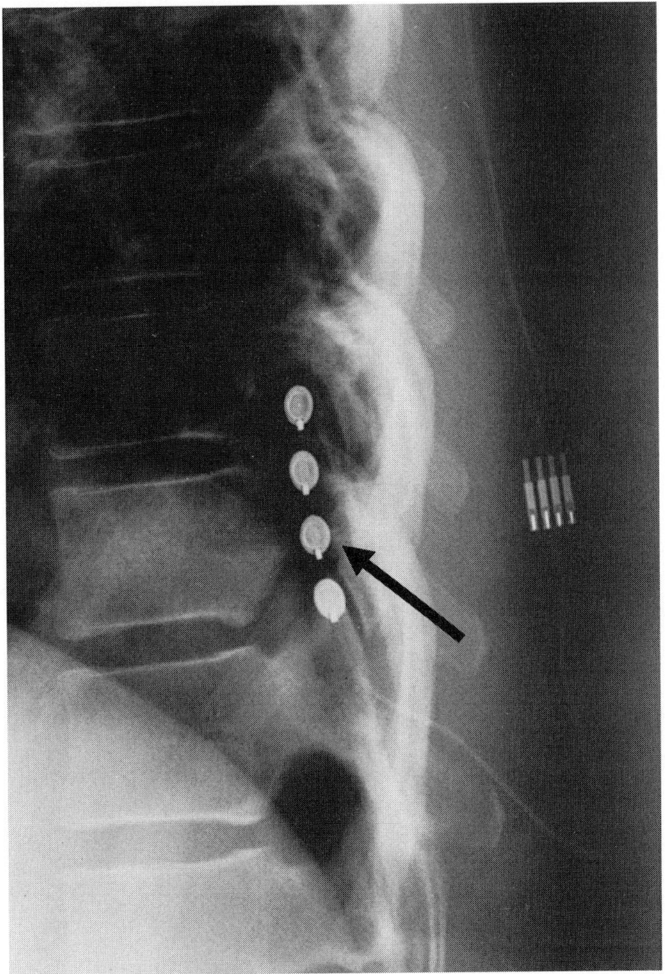

FIGURE 15–2. Resume lead in the epidural space about T9.

to primary bone or joint disease seemed to respond less well. Overall, 40% of patients were able to control their pain by SCS alone.

Reports of smaller patient series have shown SCS to be a procedure of potential benefit for pain relief in postherpetic neuralgia (Meglio et al, 1989a, 1989b), traumatic paraplegia (Buchhass et al, 1989), idiopathic Raynaud's disease and reflex sympathetic dystrophy of the upper limbs (Robaina et al, 1989), and deafferentation pain (Sanchez-Ledesma et al, 1989). Overall, more than 50 articles are now in the literature reporting on the use of SCS for syndromes ranging from multiple sclerosis to reflex sympathetic dystrophy with results fairly consistently showing that approximately half of the patients receiving permanent stimulator implants experience at least 50% pain relief over the long term.

Patient Selection

In selecting patients for neurostimulation, one must first ascertain that the problem cannot be appropriately treated by, or has not responded to, other standard means. Next, in overall importance for good results, the following must be determined:

A. Psychosocial criteria (Daniel et al, 1985; Long, 1979; Ray, 1981)
   1. Assurance that the pain is not a manifestation of disordered thinking—there is an objective basis for the complaint (e.g., myelographically documented lumbar arachnoid fibrosis).
   2. Motivation and cooperation by the patient.
   3. Freedom from drug habituation or drug-seeking behavior.
   4. Absence of impending legal actions, unsettled compensation disputes, or other sources of secondary gain.
   5. Absence of major marital, familial, social, or occupational conflict.
B. Clinical criteria
   1. Location and distribution of pain: The topography of the pain must be amenable to overlap by stimulation paresthesias. Trial placement of a temporary electrode to demonstrate relief addresses this issue.
   2. Provokability of the pain: Some mechanical maneuver (e.g., joint movement or direct pressure over the painful area) should reliably provoke or augment the pain, and some other mechanical state (rest, positioning, exercise) should reliably relieve it.
C. Technical criteria
   1. Location of the stimulus site: The technical detail of greatest importance is electrode location. Uncertain or random placement of an electrode almost invariably produces useless results.
   2. Stimulus parameters: The most important parameter is the amplitude or strength of the pulses. Pulse frequency and pulse width may also affect the results and patient comfort.
D. Less important considerations for lasting results
   1. The cause of pain (distribution being considerably more important). North (1993) lists the following specific indications in decreasing order of frequency of application and reported success rates:
      a. Lumbar arachnoid fibrosis (arachnoiditis) or failed back syndrome with radiculopathic pain, ideally predominating over axial low back pain, in particular mechanical pain (North et al, 1991).
      b. Peripheral vascular disease, with ischemic pain (Broseta et al, 1986).
      c. Peripheral nerve injury, neuralgia, or causalgia (including reflex sympathetic dystrophy).
      d. Phantom limb or stump pain (Krainick et al, 1980).
      e. Spinal cord lesions, with well-circumscribed segmental pain (North et al, 1993).
   2. The duration of pain (months or years).
   3. The extent of disability caused by the pain.

Types of Leads

Leads can be categorized according to whether they are for temporary use only or implanted for long-term use. Among leads for definitive implant, models with either percutaneously inserted wire-type or surgically implantable plate-type electrodes exist. Finally, among plate-type electrodes arrayed on a paddle, models with either in-line or a mix of in-line and lateral electrodes are available (Fig. 15–3).

A temporary screening lead can provide a cost-effective

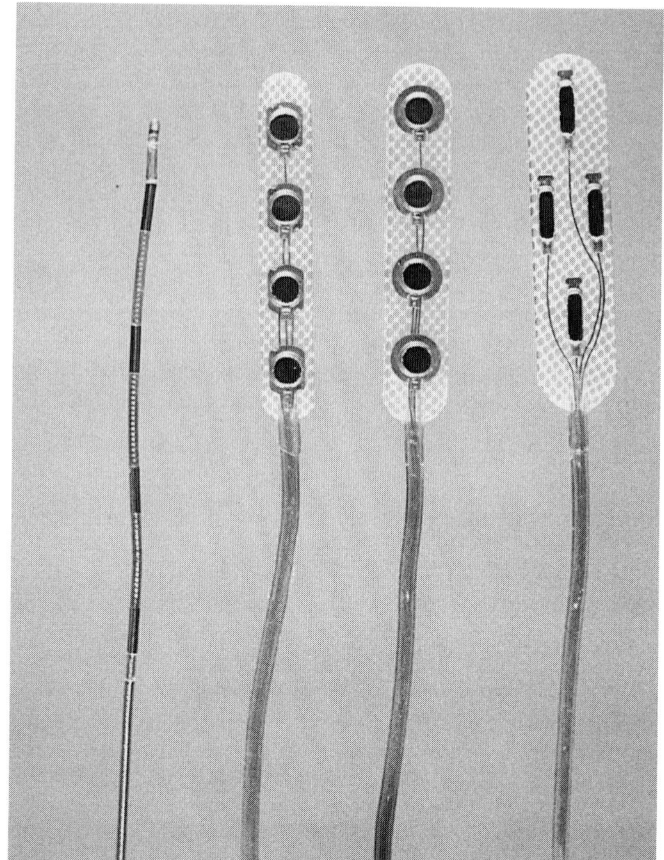

FIGURE 15–3. Types of leads from left to right: percutaneously inserted lead with wire-type electrodes and three surgically implantable leads (Medtronic, Inc.).

way to conduct a stimulation trial with a patient to determine whether SCS therapy may be successful. During trial screening, the physician and patient can determine what configuration of electrodes and settings of stimulation parameters are effective in "covering" the painful area, and can determine appropriate lead positioning. These factors are among the most crucial in obtaining a successful outcome.

Temporary screening leads are typically of the wire type, with several electrodes arranged linearly along the distal end of the electrode. The lead is inserted percutaneously using a Touhy needle, as described later. Temporary screening leads are available that replicate the capabilities of definitive-implant percutaneous leads (such as the Verify screening lead, which replicates the capabilities of the Pisces-Quad, both from Medtronic Neurological, Minneapolis, Minnesota). The screening lead can be left in place for up to 10 days, which is usually sufficient for evaluation of the SCS therapy. If desired, most leads used for definitive implant can be used for the trial stimulation period as well, by means of adapters available from the manufacturer. North (1993) reports that it has been the practice of his group to conduct a minimum 3-day trial with a temporary percutaneous electrode, after which time the electrode is discarded to minimize the risk of infection.

Leads with plate-type electrodes are placed epidurally by a laminotomy procedure, which is described later. The distal end of these electrodes consists of a flat paddle containing several electrodes placed either in a linear or diamond pattern. The paddle-shaped end has the advantage of providing greater stability in the epidural space, reducing the likelihood of treatment failure due to lead migration. In the event that previous epidural scarring, spinal stenosis, or an abnormally small epidural space is encountered, the same electrode configuration and surface area as a standard paddle-shaped lead can be obtained in a smaller size. Models with widths as small as 6.6 mm and with a thickness of 1.37 mm are available (Resume TL, Medtronic Neurological, Minneapolis, Minnesota). For patients with bilateral or a broad area of pain, leads with a diamond pattern of oval-shaped electrodes on the paddle (e.g., SymMix, Medtronic Neurological, Minneapolis, Minnesota) produce stimulation across the patient's midline to optimize broad or bilateral coverage of painful areas.

Stimulation Systems

There are two types of stimulation systems: fully implantable pulse generators, and radiofrequency systems (sometimes called external systems) involving an implanted receiver and an external power source. Fully implanted pulse generators, containing long-lasting (3 to 10 years) lithium batteries, have the advantages of improved patient acceptance and compliance. These systems are turned on and off by an external magnet; parameters are reprogrammed using an external, physician-operated control unit. Radiofrequency systems have the advantage of not requiring surgery when the battery has reached the end of life. Patients requiring high-amplitude stimulation (as determined during the clinical trial) would benefit most from a radiofrequency system. Most leads can be adapted to attach to either type of stimulator system, using connectors supplied by the manufacturers (Fig. 15–4).

Although most SCS systems are designed to power quadripolar leads, systems accommodating eight electrodes are also available to provide broad or bilateral coverage (e.g., Neuromed's Dual Quattrode system and Medtronic's Mattrix system). The Mattrix system uses a fully selectable dual-channel system powered by an external radiofrequency transmitter configured to function either as a single channel (1 × 8) or a true dual channel (2 × 4) system. Changes in electrode combinations and polarities of electrodes may be made externally, as desired. This selectability not only may shorten the duration of the trial period but also may prevent long-term loss of effectiveness in some cases.

Surgical Procedures

Before undertaking the procedure, the surgeon and the nurse or technician who will follow the patient should be familiar with the manufacturer's literature and audiovisual materials. It is worthwhile to visit a clinical center where implants are being performed on a regular basis.

Before the insertion of any of the electrodes discussed here, the patient should completely understand the potential risks and benefits of the procedure. It is helpful to require that the patient and closest relatives view an audiovisual education program covering these matters (Ray, 1980). Because pain is a subjective sensory experience, patients must

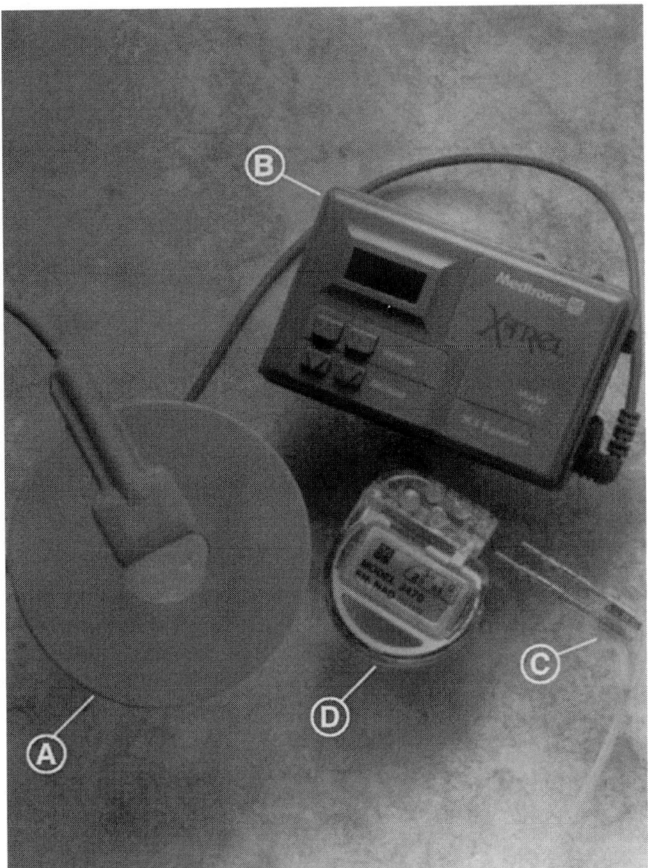

FIGURE 15–4. Components of the X-Trel system (Medtronic, Inc). A—Antenna, B—External Control Unit, C—Extension Lead, D—Receiver.

have their electrode inserted using local (and vocal, or verbal, reassurance) anesthesia. Patients must be convinced that the procedure will be almost painless and that they will be informed of everything before it happens, that is, there will be no surprises.

CHOICE OF LEAD TYPE

The percutaneous type of lead has the advantage of being inserted through a Touhy needle passed via a small incision. On the other hand, it is sometimes easily or spontaneously dislodged, with a loss of stimulation. Also, the smallness of the electrode surface can make this type of lead less beneficial for permanent implant.

The author has found that the results using larger surface electrodes (plate-type leads) have more than compensated for the apparent increased complexity of implantation. However, because percutaneous electrodes are appropriate for temporary screening purposes (North, 1993), the practitioner will do well to become proficient at both of the insertion procedures described here.

With either type of lead, the technical detail of greatest importance in successful use of SCS is electrode location. If this is not correct, all else fails to compensate.

LEAD INSERTION TECHNIQUE: PERCUTANEOUS TYPE

Whether a percutaneous lead is inserted for the stimulation trial or following the decision to do a definitive implant, the insertion technique is the same.

Oral diazepam, 10 mg, is given when the patient is called to the operating room, and a single-dose, broad-spectrum antibiotic is administered while the patient is in the preanesthetic holding area. Intravenous diazepam and fentanyl is used in conjunction with the local anesthetic, as needed. Moderate analgesia and mild sedation will not interfere with the patient's ability to cooperate; control of the pain is not the objective of this phase of the technique. Percutaneous electrode insertion requires an image-amplifying fluoroscope. The patient lies prone on the fluoroscopic table, with a pillow under the abdomen to promote slight forward flexion. Technical details described here were developed for use with the Neurological Pisces system (Medtronic Neurological, Minneapolis, Minnesota) but are basically applicable to other similar epidural wire-type implant systems (Ray, 1981a, 1981b).

A short (3 cm) axial incision is made, passing over the dorsal processes of the T12 and L1 vertebral levels (or about T6 for cervical electrode placement). A Touhy needle introduces the lead through the interlaminar ligament, entering the epidural space beneath the fluoroscopic shadow of the spinous process of the T11 vertebral level. A careful two-handed technique is used to push the needle into the space. If the ligament is slightly calcified, the hub of the needle is tapped with an instrument (scissors or large hemostat) to drive it gently into the epidural space. Entry into this space is detected by a slight decrease in insertion pressure. An arterial guide wire is then passed into the posterior epidural space. Some wire-type electrodes, such as the Pisces, may be bent about 20 degrees, 1 cm below the tip, to permit guiding the electrode through the epidural space (somewhat as one would guide a cardiac catheter) by rotating the external portion of the stylet during insertion. This is carefully followed on the fluoroscopic image.

The midline of the spinal cord may be significantly displaced from the apparent anatomical midline; one must follow the patient's reports of the location of the tingling to determine appropriate electrode positioning. Intraoperative test stimulation is begun. If possible, the patient should be given the stimulator unit so that he or she may alter the stimulus energy, keeping it comfortable as the testing progresses. Because the negative electrode is about four times more effective than the positive electrode in depolarizing nerves, one usually connects the superior of the bipolar pair of electrodes to the negative terminal of the stimulator.

The physician moves epidural electrode(s) until a good pattern of tingling is obtained, beginning with the rate setting high (above 100 pulses per second). The pulse width is set fairly wide (0.5 msec). Changes in pulse width often produce a change in the distribution of stimulation. Amplitude changes are gradual, preferably under the control of the patient. One searches for an effect (location) of the tingling and absence of radicular stimulation or tingling in an uninvolved area. Having achieved good location, the lead is anchored in the deep tissue using a device provided by the manufacturer or a Hemoclip that is carefully applied so that it does not damage the insulation.

If the physician is conducting a trial of stimulation with the percutaneous lead, extension wires are brought out through a stab wound made far enough away from the posterior wound so that these wires, and not the lead, pass through the skin. The wounds are closed. Over the next several days (usually 1 week or less) trial stimulation is then carried out, searching for the pain-masking effect and optimal setting of the stimulus parameters.

If the trial is completed and the percutaneous lead is being placed for definitive implant, the physician will then proceed to subcutaneous tunneling of the extension and the implantation of the power source.

LEAD INSERTION TECHNIQUE: PADDLE-TYPE

Paddle-type leads have plate electrodes with significantly larger effective surface areas than the percutaneously inserted wire-type electrodes. Furthermore, the paddle-type spinal cord stimulation electrodes are insulated on the side away from the dura, bringing more stimulus energy to their ventral surface. This description is based on extensive personal experience, and the unit described here is the Resume electrode system of Medtronic Neurological, Minneapolis, Minnesota. Other plate electrode systems use similar implantation techniques.

The procedure is performed under a combination of epidural and local anesthesia, and preoperative diazepam and antibiotics are administered (as discussed earlier). The patient is placed prone using lateral chest rolls. The spinous process of the T10 vertebral level is identified by counting down the spine from the C7 level. A linear wheal is raised in the midline skin overlying the spinous processes of T9–T10 or T10–T11 using bacteriostatic saline (0.9% benzyl alcohol preservative is an excellent nonburning preanesthetic) to prevent the pain from subsequent injection of the local 1% procaine or lidocaine. The deeper fascia is injected with either of the latter two local anesthetics. An 8-cm, 22-gauge needle then is used to strike the lamina, where about 10 ml of anesthetic is injected; the anesthetic diffuses along muscle/fascial planes to block most of the posterior sensory branches. Some caution is required so as not to puncture the lung or the dura. The region around the costovertebral joint capsule is also infiltrated to accommodate the placement of a retractor. The paraspinous deep fascia on the opposite side is also injected. A total of about 60 ml is used and will be refreshed as needed.

In a personal communication, Krainick of Mainz, Germany has described the use of an epidural catheter inserted in the upper lumbar level and then maneuvered upward to the level of the incision (T9–T10 vertebral body) under fluoroscopic control. Small volumes of dilute bupivacaine can be administered through this catheter. Krainick reports that the local epidural block provides adequate anesthesia for that level and some degree of analgesia below, but the patient can clearly feel tingling paresthesias in the legs while remaining pain free at the incision wound (Krainick, 1986). The author routinely uses 10 to 15 ml of 0.5% bupivacaine, injected into the epidural space just cephalad to the planned incision site, via a Husted needle. No epidural catheter is required.

The insertion technique for plate electrode units requires a hemilaminotomy at the T9 or T10 vertebral level on the painful side. The electrode assembly (four plates) is simply slipped into the epidural space (Fig. 15–5).

A small laminotomy 8 to 10 mm wide and 8 to 12 mm long is performed very close to the lateral base of the T9 or T10 spinous process. The ligamentum flavum is usually

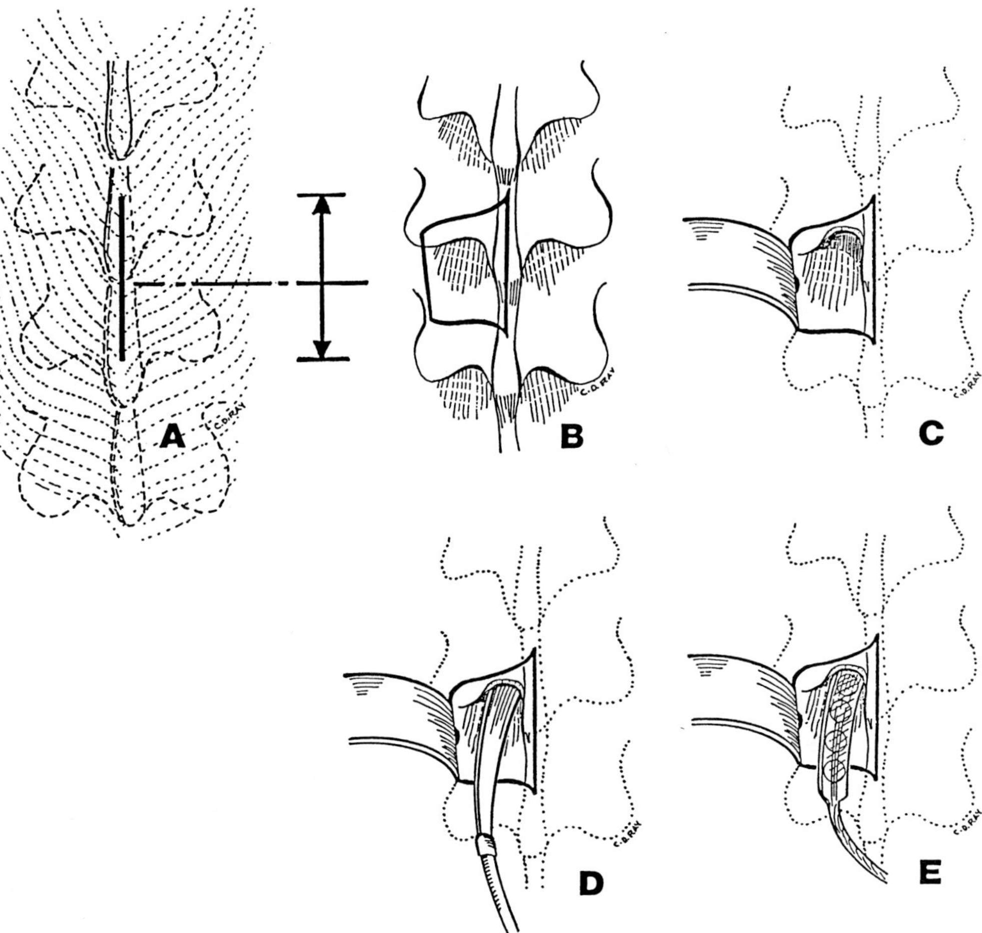

FIGURE 15–5. Diagrams showing technique for implantation of plate-type SCS electrode. *A,* Exposure under local anesthesia for left-sided pain. Area outlined is to be exposed during the procedure. *B,* Laminotomy. The skin, muscle, and other tissues are retracted, prying against the pars and costovertebral joint capsule. *C,* Curved dissector passed to provide tract for the electrode. *D,* Electrode passed into the epidural space, angulated slightly to cross the midline. *E,* The platinum electrode surfaces face the dura.

removed (unless the space is large). The patient is warned that the ensuing manipulations in the epidural space might be uncomfortable. A Penfield No. 3 dissector is passed cephalad in the epidural space, followed by a curved plastic dissector. These clear a path through possible epidural adhesions. The laminotomy must be wide enough to permit some medial and lateral movement of the electrode as it is slipped into place. The electrode passes from the painful side toward the midline and may even cross it slightly. The location is determined by test stimulation, and the electrode is moved about as needed. The patient should operate the amplitude control of the stimulator unit as the electrode is repositioned. Close interaction between the surgeon and patient is essential. The sole task at that moment is to find a position where the tingling covers all of the painful areas with no unwanted stimulation, (e.g., radicular burning or stimulation) into uninvolved areas. The testing is not performed to determine if the stimulation has any effect on the old pain problem (Fig. 15–6).

In some cases, the painful area cannot be covered well, especially in the deep midline low back. Sometimes, it may be necessary to extend the laminotomy into the lower lamina and slip the electrode into the epidural space in the caudal direction. At times, the search for the best placement may be frustrating, especially if this takes a long time and the patient begins to suffer from increasing pain. In any case, a poor location of stimulation paresthesias during on-table testing will *not* improve later; it must be correct the first time. The trial period and methods used are essentially identical with those for the percutaneously inserted systems.

Trial Period

It is usually advisable to wait at least a day after the insertion of the electrodes before beginning trial stimulation; the sensitivity of the fresh wound often causes a distortion of the perceived paresthesias. Over the next 3 to 7 days, the patient tries the device while keeping a diary of electrode combinations (with polarities and electrode configurations used), stimulus parameters, sensations produced, latency and persistence of effectiveness, degree of pain relief, and physical activity level. Nurses' notes are checked for consistency with the patient's observations and for medications required. The patient should once again review audiovisual or other teaching materials (Ray, 1980). Time must also be spent answering questions. Patients must be taught when, how, and why to alter the parameters of stimulation and the effect of these on outcome. If need be, the patient can be sent out of the hospital for several days before deciding whether or not the system should be internalized. Appropriate skin care must be carefully maintained.

When the results show subjective and objective improvement in pain behavior, reported pain level, physical activity, and reduced need for medication, the system will be internalized. Several authors believe that unless the improvement is

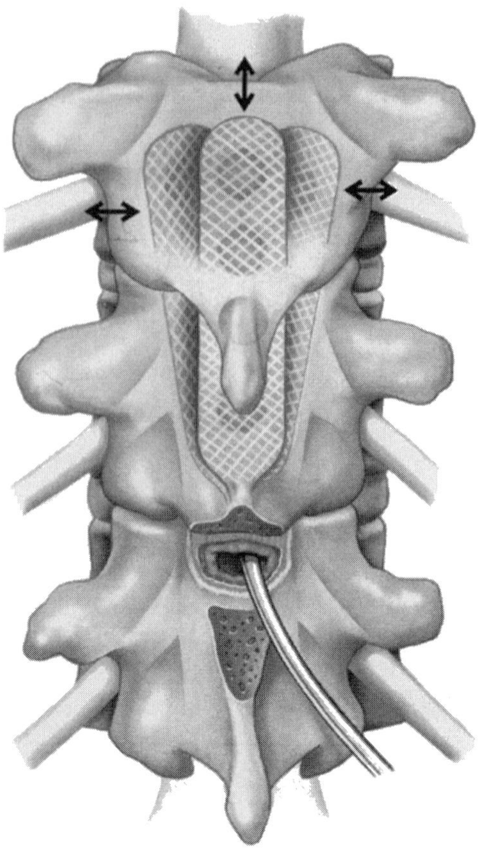

FIGURE 15–6. Laminotomy for placement of surgically implanted SCS lead. The laminotomy should be wide enough to permit some medial and lateral movement of the lead within the epidural space.

at least 50% better than the preimplant state, the results are, or will become, poor and the system should not be implanted (Burton, 1975; Burton et al, 1977; Long, 1979; Nielson et al, 1975; Ray et al, 1982; Siegfried and Lazorthes, 1982).

Internalization of Implanted Stimulators

If a percutaneous lead has been inserted, the negative electrode (as selected between the two electrodes during the trial period) is marked by tying a knot in the percutaneous extension or by placing a Hemoclip on it. This should be done about 1 cm beyond the point of emergence from the skin. Of course, multielectrode units are coded and need not be marked. In all cases, final selection of the combination should be written in the daily clinical record before internalization. In implantable stimulators with the capability of having electrode combinations changed after implantation, there is less need for such notation.

The location of the subcutaneous pocket for the receiver or implantable pulse generator is selected after ascertaining the patient's wishes. The author typically places the pocket on the anteroinferior chest wall or in the subclavicular space. In these protected locations, the receiver is supported against the ribs and cannot rotate or migrate into deeper fat. Abdominal area placements are also common. The pocket should have between 5 and 10 mm of overlying fat.

The technique of internalization has been well described

elsewhere (Ray, 1981a, 1981b); the manufacturer's surgical procedure manual should also be reviewed. Internalization of the receiver is almost always performed under general anesthesia. A one-dose preoperative antibiotic is again given. The passage of interconnecting lead wire must be planned with some care. A small intermediate or passing incision may be required for long lead wires. Pockets adequate to accommodate the connector and redundant lead wires must also be planned. Percutaneous extensions are cut off (after being previously marked, if necessary.) Routine preparation is followed by draping the patient with a self-adherent plastic sheet. The midline incision is reopened, and the cut ends of the extensions are brought through. The receiver or pulse generator is implanted in its pocket; its leads are then passed, being careful not to traverse muscle, and are also brought out through the posterior midline wound. The leads are connected and sealed as specified in the manufacturer's instructions. Throughout this procedure, one must be careful not to injure the insulation, leads, or connectors.

Postoperative instructions are given to the patient (or responsible relatives) so that all important details are well understood. With percutaneously inserted spinal cord stimulation implants, patients should be reminded not to bend excessively, especially to the side away from the pocket location, for the first 2 months after implantation. This allows the tissues to heal in position around the electrodes and lead, reducing the likelihood of displacement. This admonition is rarely needed for patients implanted with paddle-type leads. Before leaving the hospital, the patient must completely understand techniques of care of the skin overlying the implant and care of any external components of the system. Good descriptive material is available from the manufacturers.

The proper and continuous use of such life-modifying implanted devices is not to be taken lightly by the physician in charge of the case. Personal visits are required at least twice within the first year, yearly thereafter, and by correspondence as often as needed. Most device adjustments for optimization of parameters can be performed by well-trained nurses or technicians at follow-up.

Complications

The most common complication is loss of effectiveness because of mechanical failure (of the lead or insulation) or because of some undetermined physiological change. Other complications rarely occur in experienced hands (Bishop, 1980; Lazorthes and Verdie, 1983). In nearly 700 implants performed by the author's group for 15 years, a system has had to be removed on only four occasions for infection, and never for spinal cord compression or cerebrospinal fluid leakage. The effective lifetime for a spinal implant is about 3 to 7 years, at which time the most likely failure is mechanical breakage of the lead or insulation around the wire or battery depletion. The recently developed totally implantable pulse generators may continue to function for 5 to 10 years.

Effectiveness and Outlook

It is the author's conclusion that the techniques presented here are valid and serve a definite role in the management of selected patients with severe chronic pain. Others (such as Kallgren, 1994) agree that spinal cord stimulation is one of the safest and most effective procedures available for the management of chronic pain. Alternative surgical procedures, such as dorsal root entry zone (DREZ) lesioning, can be effective for relief of chronic pain (e.g., pain secondary to brachial plexus avulsion [Thomas and Kitchen, 1994] and differentiation pain [Ianoco et al, 1992]), and can be applied in situations in which SCS is not applicable, such as the treatment of trigeminal neuralgia (Chen, 1993). However, because DREZ lesioning is a destructive procedure, it is irreversible. Complications of DREZ lesioning, including sensory loss, motor weakness, and new pain, have been reported in substantial percentages in some series of patients (Kumagai et al, 1992). In contrast, SCS is a nondestructive procedure that can be performed on a trial basis, as described. The applications of SCS should continue to expand with the development of more widespread understanding and acceptance of the methods.

PERIPHERAL NERVE STIMULATION FOR FOCUSED PAIN AREAS

When pain is highly focused, involving not more than two nerve roots, peripheral nerve stimulation may be an appropriate intervention. This neuroaugmentation technique is used less commonly than SCS, but the principles involved are the same. Gybels and Van Calenbergh (1990) report an 81% success rate in a carefully selected group of patients at follow-up (mean 4.3 years, range 1.1 to 7.6 years). Patients with intractable pain secondary to peripheral nerve damage or reflex sympathetic dystrophy are the best candidates for this therapy. Indications include direct or indirect nerve trauma, reflex sympathetic dystrophy, causalgia, repetitive stress, and postherpetic neuritis. Other patient selection criteria for peripheral nerve stimulation are the same as for spinal cord stimulation.

The most common peripheral nerves to be treated with peripheral nerve stimulation are ulnar, median, radial, tibial, and common peroneal nerves. In the 1960s, surgical technique for peripheral nerve stimulation involved the placement of cuffs proximal to the injury on the nerve. Direct contact between the electrodes lowered the long-term success rates. Today, both percutaneous and plate-type leads are used in peripheral nerve stimulation. The injured nerve is separated from the lead by using intramuscular septum or split fascia. A special-purpose peripheral nerve stimulation lead has been developed (On-Point, Medtronic Neurological, Minneapolis, Minnesota) to provide greater lead stability and facilitate implantation and anchoring. This paddle-type lead, designed to fit in small spaces, has a skirt of mesh polyester for suturing to the fascia (Fig. 15–7).

As with spinal cord stimulation, patients being considered for peripheral nerve stimulation must meet the standard selection criteria and undergo preoperative evaluation to determine the exact location and extent of the nerve damage. Implantation of a peripheral nerve stimulation system involves lead placement, trial screening, and system implantation. Some clinicians use transcutaneous electrical nerve stimulation (TENS) devices for trial screening (Gybels and Van Calenbergh, 1990).

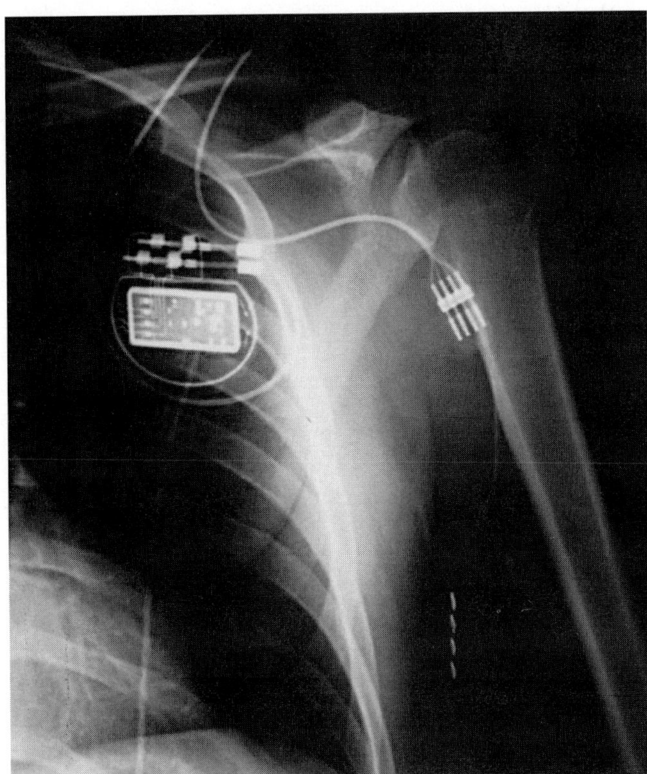

FIGURE 15–7. Peripheral nerve electrode on the ulnar nerve. Transmitter and receiver in the left upper anterior chest wall. (Resume TL lead and Itrel spinal cord stimulation system, by Medtronic, Inc.)

Unlike SCS lead placement, peripheral lead placement is performed under general anesthesia. The lead is placed beneath the involved nerve proximal to the nerve damage and anchored with sutures. Techniques specific to the nerve involved may vary. For example, a consideration in a lead implant involving the ulnar or median nerve is that the elbow should be flexed and extended several times to ensure that there is no undue stress on the lead. Manufacturers' surgical technique manuals provide details pertinent to each implant location (Lewis and Racz, 1992).

Once optimal positioning is achieved, a harvested fascial flap is sewn between the nerve and electrode plate to prevent direct contact. Care should be taken to ensure that the lead body does not rub against the nerve. Percutaneous wires are tunneled subcutaneously and connected to an external temporary power source for a trial of stimulation that may last one or more days. The goal of the trial screening is to determine that the area of pain is covered by the paresthesia and that an acceptable level of pain relief is obtained.

If the patient experiences at least 50% pain relief during the screening trial, the system can be implanted under general anesthesia. The site where the power source will be implanted is identified, and a pocket is formed. Chest or abdominal wall locations are common sites, with the selection dependent on the lead location. An extension is tunneled subcutaneously from the pocket to the lead incision site, and then connected to both the lead and the power source. Incisions are closed and dressed.

The power source should be programmed in the recovery room when the patient is responsive. Because parameter settings are a function of the resistance between the lead and stimulated nerve, movement of the extremity may cause positional sensitivity. Patients can compensate by adjusting the amplitude. Early and aggressive physical therapy is recommended. Return of function and strength is proportional to the patient's use of the limb. Following removal of the sutures, activities are unrestricted.

CONCLUSIONS

Both spinal cord stimulation and peripheral nerve stimulation are neuroaugmentation techniques that contribute significantly to the clinician's armamentarium against chronic, intractable pain. It is the author's conclusion that the techniques presented here are valid and serve a definite role in the management of selected patients with severe chronic pain. Others (e.g., Kallgren, 1994) agree that spinal cord stimulation is one of the safest and most effective procedures available for the management of chronic pain.

Alternative surgical procedures, such as DREZ lesioning, can be effective for relief of chronic pain (e.g., pain secondary to brachial plexus avulsion [Thomas and Kitchen, 1994] and differentiation pain [Ianoco et al, 1992]), and can be applied in situations in which SCS and peripheral nerve stimulation are not applicable, such as the treatment of trigeminal neuralgia (Chen, 1993). However, because DREZ lesioning is a destructive procedure, it is irreversible. Complications of DREZ lesioning including sensory loss, motor weakness, and new pain have been reported in substantial percentages in some series of patients (Kumagai et al, 1992). In contrast, SCS and peripheral nerve stimulation are nondestructive procedures that can be performed on a trial basis, as described. The applications of SCS and peripheral nerve stimulation should continue to expand with the development of more widespread understanding and acceptance of these methods.

References

Abram SE: 1992 Bonica Lecture. Advances in chronic pain management since gate control. Reg Anesth *18(2)*: 66–81, 1993.

Akil H, Richardson DE, Hughes J, Barchas JD: Enkephalin-like material elevated in ventricular cerebrospinal fluid of pain patients after analgesic focal stimulation. Science *201*:463–465, 1978.

Bishop B: Pain: Its physiology and rationale for management. Physical Ther *60*:13–37, 1980.

Broseta J, Barbera J, DeVera J, et al: Spinal cord stimulation in peripheral arterial disease. J Neurosurg *64*:71–80, 1986.

Buchhaas U, Koulousakis A, Nittner K: Experience with spinal cord stimulation (SCS) in the management of chronic pain in a traumatic transverse lesion syndrome. Neurosurg Rev *12*(Suppl 1):582–587, 1989.

Burton CV: Dorsal column stimulation: Optimization of application. Surg Neurol *4*:171–176, 1975.

Burton CV, Ray D, Nashold BS (eds): Symposium on the safety and clinical efficacy of implanted neuroaugmentive devices. Neurosurgery *1*:185–232, 1977.

Campbell JN, Long DM: Peripheral nerve stimulation in the treatment of intractable pain. J Neurosurg *45*:692–699, 1976.

Campbell JN, Davis KD, Meyer RA, North RB: The mechanism by which dorsal column stimulation affects pain: Evidence for a new hypothesis. Pain 5:S228, 1990.

Chandler MJ, Brennan TJ, Garrison DW, Kim KS, Schwartz PJ, Foreman RD: A mechanism of cardiac pain suppression by spinal cord stimulation: Implications for patients with angina pectoris. Eur Heart J *14*:96–105, 1993.

Chen HJ: Facial pain relieved by dorsal root entry zone lesions in the trigeminal nucleus caudalis: Report of two cases. J Formos Med Assoc *92*:583–585, 1993.

Daniel MS, Long C, Hutcherson WL, Hunter S: Psychological factors and outcome of electrode implantation for chronic pain. Neurosurgery *17*:773–777, 1985.

De La Porte C, Siegfried J: Lumbosacral spinal fibrosis (spinal arachnoiditis): Its diagnosis and treatment by spinal cord stimulation. Spine 8:593–603, 1983.

De La Porte C, Van de Kelft E: Spinal cord stimulation in failed back surgery syndrome. Pain *52*:55–61, 1993.

Freeman TB, Campbell JN, Long DM: Naloxone does not affect pain relief induced by electrical stimulation in man. Pain *17*:189–195, 1983.

Gybels J, Van Calenbergh F: The treatment of pain due to peripheral nerve injury by electrical stimulation of the injured nerve. Advances in Pain Research and Therapy *13*:217–222, 1990.

Horowitz P, Grodzins L, Ladd W, Ryan J, Merriam G, Lechene C: Vertebrate central nervous system: Same neurons mediate both electrical and chemical inhibitions. Science *194*:1166–1170, 1976.

Ianoco RP, Guthkelch AN, Boswell MV: Dorsal root entry zone stimulation for differentiation pain. Stereotact Funct Neurosurg *59*:56–61, 1992.

Kallgren MA: Comment on: North RB, et al: Spinal cord stimulation for chronic, intractable pain: experience over two decades. Survey of Anesthesiology *38(3)*:162–163, 1994.

Kerr FWL: The structural basis of pain: Circuitry and pathways. *In* Bonica JJ (ed): Pain. New York, Raven Press, 1980, pp 49–60.

Krainick J-U, Thoden U, Riechert T: Pain reduction in amputees by long-term spinal cord stimulation (five year study). J Neurosurg *52*:346–350, 1980.

Krainick J-U: Personal communication. July, 1986.

Kumagai Y, Shimoji K, Honma T, Uchiyama S, Ishijima B, Hokari T, Fujioka H, Fukuda S, Ohama, E: Problems related to dorsal root entry zone lesions. Acta Neurochir *115*:71–78, 1992.

Kumar K, Nath, R, Wyant GM: Treatment of chronic pain by epidural spinal cord stimulation: A 10-year experience. J Neurosurg *75*:402–407, 1991.

Lazorthes U, Verdie J-C: Technical evolution and long-term results of chronic spinal cord stimulation. *In* Lazorthes U, Upton ARM (eds): Neurostimulation: An overview. Mt. Kisko, NY, Futura Publishing Company, Inc., 1983, pp 61–86.

LeDoux MS, Langford KH: Spinal cord stimulation for the failed back syndrome. Spine *18*:191–194, 1993.

Lewis R, Racz G: Peripheral Nerve Stimulation Surgical Technique Notebook. Minneapolis, Medtronic, Inc., 1992.

Liebeskind JC, Sherman JE, Cannon T: Neural and neurochemical mechanisms of pain inhibition. Anaesth Intensive Care *10*:139–143, 1982.

Lifson A, Burton CV, Ray CD, Gracie KW: Spinal cord stimulation with multiple contact epidural electrode for intractable pain control. 8th International Congress in Neurologic Surgery, Toronto, Poster #8:17, July, 1985.

Linderoth B, Bazelius B, Franck J, Brodin E: Dorsal column stimulation induces release of serotonin and substance P in the cat dorsal horn. Neurosurgery *31*:289–297, 1992.

Linderoth B, Stiller CO, O'Connor WT, Hammarstrom G, Understedt U, Brodin E: An animal model for the study of brain transmitter release in response to spinal cord stimulation in the awake, freely moving rat: Preliminary results from the periaqueductal grey matter. Acta Neurochir Suppl *58*:156–160, 1993.

Linderoth B, Stiller CO, Gunasekera L, O'Connor WT, Ungerstedt U, Brodin E: Gamma-aminobutyric acid is released in the dorsal horn by electrical spinal cord stimulation: An in vivo microdialysis study in the rat. Neurosurgery *34*:484–488, 1994.

Long DM: Current status of neuroaugmentation procedures for chronic pain. *In* Beers RF, Bassett EG (eds): Mechanisms of Pain and Analgesic Compounds. New York, Raven Press, 1979, pp 51–69.

Long DM, Erickson D, Campbell J, North R: Electrical stimulation of the spinal cord and peripheral nerves for pain control. A 10-year experience. Appl Neurophysiol *44*:207–217, 1981.

Meglio M, Cioni B, Prezioso A, Talamonti G: Spinal cord stimulation (SCS) in the treatment of postherpetic pain. Acta Neurochir Suppl *46*:65–66, 1989a.

Meglio M, Cioni B, Prezioso A, Talamonti G: Spinal cord stimulation (SCS) in deafferentiation pain. Pacing Clin Electrophysiol *12*:709–712, 1989b.

Melzack R, Wall P: Pain mechanisms: A new theory. Science *150*:971–979, 1965.

Nielson KD, Adams JE, Hosobuchi Y: Experience with dorsal column stimulation for relief of chronic intractable pain: 1968–1973. Surg Neurol 3:148–152, 1975.

North RB: The role of spinal cord stimulation in contemporary pain management. APS Journal 2:91–99, 1993.

North RB, Ewend MG, Lawton MT, Piantadosi S: Spinal cord stimulation for chronic, intractable pain: Superiority of "multi-channel" devices. Pain 44:119–130, 1991.

North RB, Fischell TA, Long DM: Chronic dorsal column stimulation via percutaneously inserted epidural electrodes: Preliminary results in 31 patients. Appl Neurophysiol 40:184–191, 1978.

North RB, Kidd DH, Zahurak M, James CS, Long DM: Spinal cord stimulation for chronic, intractable pain: Experience over two decades. Neurosurgery 32:384–394, 1993.

Ranck JB Jr: Which elements are excited in electrical stimulation of mammalian central nervous system: A review. Brain Res 98:417–440, 1975.

Ray CD (ed): Pain Symposium. Electrical stimulation of the human nervous system for the control of pain. Surg Neurol 4:61–204, 1975a.

Ray CD: Control of pain by electrical stimulation: A clinical follow-up review. In Penzholz, H, Brock M, Hamer J, et al (eds): Advances in Neurosurgery, Vol 3. Heidelberg, Springer-Verlag, 1975b, pp 216–224.

Ray CD: Neuroaugmentation—Neurostimulation Training Series (audiovisuals): IES-1 Introduction of electrical stimulation. PDBS-1 Relieving your pain with deep brain stimulation. PSCS-1 Relieving your pain with spinal cord stimulation. Sister Kenny Institute (2727 Chicago Ave., Minneapolis, MN 55407), Educational Materials Listing. Spring, 1980, pp 2–3.

Ray CD: Percutaneous spinal cord stimulation: Technique. In Hosobuchi Y, Corbin T (eds): Indications for Spinal Cord Stimulation. Amsterdam, Exerpta Medica, 1981a, pp 17–33.

Ray CD: Spinal epidural electrical stimulation for pain control: Practical details and results. Appl Neurophysiol 44:194–206, 1981b.

Ray CD: Electrical and chemical stimulation of the CNS by direct means for pain control: Present and future. Clin Neurosurg 28:564–588, 1981.

Ray CD, Burton CV, Lifson A: Neurostimulation as used in a large clinical practice. Appl Neurophysiol 45:160–166, 1982.

Robaina FJ, Dominguez M, Diaz M, Rodriguez JL, de Vera JA: Spinal cord stimulation for relief of chronic pain in vasospastic disorders of the upper limbs. Neurosurgery 24:63–67, 1989.

Sanchez-Ledesma MJ, Garcia-March G, Diaz-Cascajo P, Gomez-Moreta J, Broseta J: Spinal cord stimulation in deafferentiation pain. Stereotact Funct Neurosurg 53:40–45, 1989.

Shealy CN, Mortimer JT, Reswick JB: Electrical inhibition of pain by stimulation of the dorsal columns: Preliminary clinical report. Anesth Analg 46:489–491, 1967.

Siegfried J, Lazorthes Y: Long-term follow-up of dorsal column stimulation in the treatment of causalgic pain. Appl Neurophysiol 45:201–204, 1982.

Thomas DG, Kitchen ND: Long-term follow-up of dorsal root entry zone lesions in brachial plexus avulsion. J Neurol Neurosurg Psychiatry 57:737–738, 1994.

Herndon, JH: Neuromas. *In* Green DP (ed): Operative Hand Surgery Vol 2. New York, Churchill Livingstone, 1993, p 1389.

Herndon JH, Eaton RG, Littler JW: Management of painful neuromas in the hand. J Bone Joint Surg *58A*:369–373, 1976.

Kanaya F, Jevans AW: Rapid histochemical identification of motor and sensory fascicles: Preparation of solutions. Plast Reconstr Surg *90*:514–515, 1991.

Laborde KJ, Kalisman M, Tsai T: Results of surgical treatment of painful neuromas of the hand. J Hand Surg *7*:190–193, 1982.

Mackinnon SE: Surgical management of the peripheral nerve gap. Clin Plast Surg *16*(3):587, 1989.

Mackinnon SE, Glickman LT, Dagum A: A technique for the treatment of neuroma in continuity. J Reconstr Microsurg *8*:379–383, 1992.

Melzak R, Wall PD: Pain mechanisms—a new theory. Science *150*:971, 1965.

Millesi H: The nerve gap—theory and clinical practice. Hand Clin *2*(4):651, 1986.

Mitchell SW: Traumatic neuralgia: Section of the median nerve. Am J Med Sci *67*:2–16, 1874.

Moldaver J: Brief note: Tinel's sign. J Bone Joint Surg *60A*:412–414, 1978.

Omer GE Jr: Nerve, neuroma, and pain problems related to upper limb amputations. Orthop Clin North Am *12*:751–762, 1981.

Poth EJ, Bravo-Fernandez E: Prevention of neuroma formation by encasement of the severed nerve end in rigid tubes. Proc Soc Exp Biol Med *56*:7, 1944.

Seddon HI: Three types of nerve injury. Brain *66*:237, 1943.

Smith JR, Gomez NH: Local injection therapy of neuromata of the hand with triamcinolone acetonide. A preliminary study of twenty-two patients. J Bone Joint Surg *52A*:71–83, 1970.

Snyder CC, Knowles RP: Traumatic neuromas. J Bone Joint Surg *47A*:641, 1965.

Stedman TL: Stedman's Medical Dictionary, 24th Edition, Baltimore, Williams and Wilkins, 1982, p 947.

Sunderland S: Nerves and Nerve Injuries, 2nd ed. Edinburgh, Churchill Livingstone, 1978.

Swanson AB, Boeve NR, Lumsden RM: The prevention and treatment of amputation neuromata by silicone capping. J Hand Surg *2*:70–78, 1977.

Terzis J, Faibisoff B, Williams HB: The nerve gap: Suture under tension vs graft. Plast Reconstr Surg *56*:166, 1975.

Tupper JW, Booth DM: Treatment of painful neuromas of sensory nerves in the hand: A comparison of traditional and newer methods. J Hand Surg *1*:144–151, 1976.

Wall PD, Gutnick M: Properties of afferent nerve impulses orginating from a neuroma. Nature *248*:740–742, 1974.

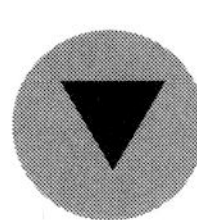

Chapter 17

• Victoria R. Masear
• Ekkehard Bonatz

Painful Neuromas of the Lower Extremity and Postneurectomy Pain

Painful neuromas, whether end neuromas or neuromas in continuity, can have devastating effects. The pain can lead to addictive, drug-seeking behavior; disruption of interpersonal and family relationships; and loss of employment. Sunderland (1978) classified neuromas into three types: bulb neuromas form on the ends of transected nerves, spindle neuromas (e.g., Morton's neuroma) are neuromas in continuity with an intact perineurium, and lateral neuromas occur when the perineurium has been interrupted. All neuromas have the potential to become painful.

Painful neuromas may lead to a reflex sympathetic dystrophy (RSD; Sudek's dystrophy). Weir Mitchell (1872) coined the term causalgia in gunshot wounds to mean intractable burning pain. Leriche described causalgia as caused by vasospasm resulting from abnormal vasomotor reflexes (Homans, 1960). RSD is now described as a common form of causalgia and is called minor causalgia (Girgis and Parry, 1988). Major causalgia is from nerve injuries, while minor causalgia may result from a trivial injury. The differentiation of causalgia pain from painful neuroma may be difficult. If the neuroma symptoms can be relieved, the RSD will usually subside (Kenzora, 1986). For a pain to be defined as causalgic, Sunderland (1978) outlined various criteria: (1) the pain is severe, spontaneous, and persistent; (2) the nature of the pain is burning, tingling, crushing, or tearing; (3) it must occur following injury to a nerve; (4) it must be present for 5 weeks; and (5) it may be exacerbated by emotional or environmental factors.

As a normal abortive attempt at repair, all lacerated nerves form neuromas (Spencer, 1974). Not all neuromas become painful. Multiple factors may play a role in the development of a painful peripheral nerve lesion. Nerve injuries in certain anatomical locations are predisposed to becoming painful. In the lower extremity, the development of painful neuromas is most likely on the dorsum of the foot. These are usually secondary to a crushing injury or to a surgical incision or laceration. Painful foot neuromas have been described in the sural, deep peroneal, medial plantar, and common digital nerves to the lesser toes (Kenzora, 1986). The most highly symptomatic neuromas were on the dorsal medial foot (Kenzora, 1984). The dorsal medial proper digital nerve to the hallux may be injured in as many as 30% of bunionectomies (Meier and Kenzora, 1985). Although usually not as severe as the dorsal foot neuroma, the sural nerve is often painful following harvest or biopsy (Staniforth and Fisher, 1978). The infrapatellar branch of the saphenous nerve is frequently injured with surgical incisions or arthroscopy portals about the knee.

Fibrosis or a scarred bed will make neuromas more painful. Intraneural fibrosis secondary to a crush injury or external scar causing nerve constriction and decreased vascularity can lead to painful nerve lesions (Wilson, 1981). External nerve adhesions resulting from fractures, infections, or surgery can cause loss of nerve gliding, with pain caused by nearby joint or tendon movement (Fig. 17–1). End neuromas in amputation stumps have the greatest propensity for being painful when they reside in a scarred bed.

There may be a genetic predisposition to developing pain following injury to a peripheral nerve (Girgis and Parry, 1988). Personality also seems to play a role in the development of painful nerve lesions (Williams, 1987).

Most peripheral nerve lesions cause little or no pain, but 5% to 10% will develop devastating symptoms of causalgia (Girgis and Parry, 1988). Pain usually develops after a few days or weeks and will progress in severity for several months. Other symptoms include numbness, dysesthesias, burning, tingling, aching and paresthesias. Pain is often worse at night and is unrelieved by medication. Pain is most pronounced with local contact to the area (such as a shoe, clothing, or touch).

Sunderland (1978) described the trophic changes of the skin as cold, clammy, thin, glistening, and sweaty. The skin may also be red and mottled, dry, or warmer than normal. A scar over the area of nerve lesion will be painful. Hypersensitivity and dysesthesias to light tapping or rubbing are classic. A painful tingling sensation is present over the neuroma. There is decreased sensation distal to the injury. Either guarding and lack of use or prolonged pain may cause

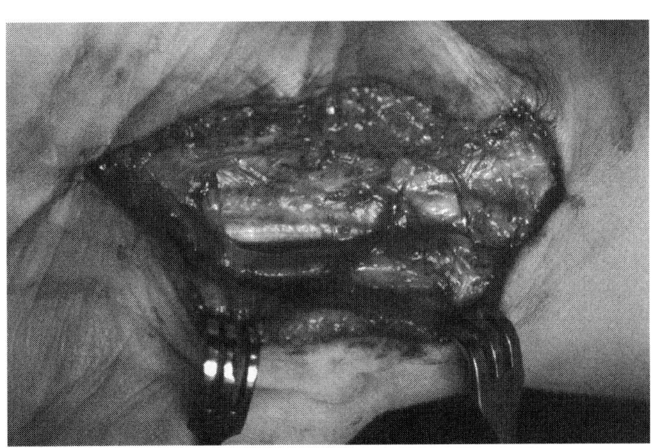

FIGURE 17–1. Severe extraneural fibrosis.

joint stiffness and fibrosis. Radiographs often demonstrate osteopenia of the involved limb.

Electrodiagnostic studies may reveal a complete or incomplete nerve lesion. Computed tomography (CT) (Singson et al, 1987) and magnetic resonance imaging (MRI) (Donnal et al, 1990; Singson et al, 1990) scans have been used for identifying neuromas in amputation stumps. Some promise was shown in distinguishing neuromas from other causes of stump pain, but whether or not these tests are more helpful than a good clinical examination remains to be seen. They obviously can not distinguish between a painful versus a nonpainful neuroma.

TREATMENT

Desensitization by repeated nerve stimulation should be the first line of treatment for painful neuromas (Granville, 1838). Light massage, percussion, and tapping are used. Initially, smooth textures are rubbed over the dysesthetic area, followed later by increasingly coarse textures (Wilson, 1981). Normal activities and active use are encouraged. Static splinting may be used to help pain, but active and active assistive exercises to regain movement in stiff joints is imperative. Dynamic splinting should be used with caution because it may increase pain and thus stiffness. Scar tenderness is aided with scar massage (usually with vitamin E or cocoa butter) and elastomer molds applied to the scar. Edema needs to be controlled with range of motion exercises, elevation, and compression wraps.

High-frequency, low-amplitude nerve stimulation with a transcutaneous electrical nerve stimulator (TENS) may help spontaneous pain. One electrode is placed over the neuroma and the other more proximally over the same nerve. The TENS unit may give pain relief only while in place or for several hours after removal. Long (1977) obtained improvement in 33% of patients.

Narcotics should be used only in the acute injury period. After that, only nonnarcotic pain medications or nonsteroidal anti-inflammatory drugs should be given. Amitriptyline hydrochloride (a tricyclic antidepressant), 50 to 75 mg just before bed may aid in sleep and reduce nerve irritability. Phenoxybenzamine, a sympatholytic alpha blocker, is sometimes helpful (Wilson, 1981). Carbamazepine (Tegretol) might help but is more beneficial for diabetic neuropathy.

Sympathetic nerve blocks are helpful in the treatment of dystrophy and causalgia, and may be of some benefit in the treatment of painful neuromas. An indwelling catheter to give a continuous Marcaine block for several days will sometimes give lasting relief (Omer, 1978; Girgis and Parry, 1988). Stellate ganglion blocks have been most commonly used, but they are unpleasant and many patients will refuse repeat blocks. A series of three to six blocks is usually given on successive or alternate days. An increase in skin temperature is indicative of sympathetic blockade. Therapy for range of motion is then given while the block is still effective.

A longer-acting sympathetic block can be achieved by an intravenous regional block. Guanethidine binds to norepinephrine storage vesicles, thus releasing norepinephrine from the sympathetic nerve endings (Hanninton-Kiff, 1974). A continuous sympathetic blockade is produced and lasts for up to 3 weeks. Girgis and Parry (1988) recommend a series of guanethidine blocks given on alternate days until pain and hyperpathia are reduced. If there is no effect by the sixth block, they are discontinued. Initially the pain may only be relieved for 2 to 3 days. Serial blocks may steadily increase the length of relief. In his series of 78 patients, Girgis had 23 excellent results, but in 18, the pain recurred later and required more blocks. Crush injuries were helped the least. Bretylium tosylate has been introduced as an intravenous regional sympatholytic blocking agent with effects comparable to guanethidine (Ford et al, 1988).

Chemical injections of painful neuromas can give long-lasting improvement. Multiple local steroid injections gave relief in 70% of patients (Smith and Gomez, 1970). For end neuromas or pure sensory nerves, alcohol or phenol injections may be used and can stop pain for up to 6 months. At times, there will be some toxic effect to the other local tissues.

It is beneficial to all chronic pain patients, and often their families, to enter a good, supportive counseling program. Coping measures, biofeedback, and hypnosis will benefit some patients.

Patients responding to sympathetic blocks may be able to obtain longer-lasting relief with surgical sympathectomy. Horner's syndrome, which is commonly seen following cervical sympathectomy, can be avoided with a thoracic sympathectomy. This normally required the removal of one or two ribs, but good success with less morbidity has been achieved endoscopically. The main remaining problem with surgical sympathectomy is that although early results may show dramatic relief, the lasting results are unpredictable and regeneration of the sympathetic nervous system will cause pain to recur (Girgis and Parry, 1988).

Nerve stimulators have met with some success in the treatment of painful neuromas. Dorsal column stimulation will give relief in about 50% of patients but the relief often lessens with time (Wilson, 1981). Implanted peripheral nerve stimulators placed proximal to the neuroma may give relief in approximately 30% to 62% of patients (Law et al, 1980; Long, 1980; Nashold and Goldner, 1975). They should be used only in those patients who have responded to TENS. Again, pain may recur with time.

Resection of painful neuromas is probably the most common surgical treatment. Resection should be recommended only if the involved nerve can be sacrificed without a serious functional loss (e.g., bulb neuromas, pure sensory nerves not supplying a significant tactile area, and nerves with no chance of recovery). The nerve should be resected away from the area of scar and joint so it is not tethered and susceptible to traction with joint motion. Because of shoe contact, neuromas of the foot are usually best treated with a resection proximal to the ankle. Excisional neurectomy has been successful in approximately 65% to 83% of patients (Tupper, 1976; Kenzora, 1984, 1986).

Neurectomy may be combined with several other procedures: (1) burying of the resected nerve, (2) transposition to a healthier bed, (3) nerve capping or sleeves, or (4) nerve repair or grafting.

The resected nerve end may be buried in bone (Snyder, 1961; Gluck, 1880) but is most commonly placed beneath a healthy muscle (Dellon and Mackinnon, 1986; Dellon et al, 1984; Petropoulos and Stefanko, 1961). It is probably best to leave some redundancy in the resected nerve buried beneath the muscle so contraction of the muscle will not place traction on the nerve. For neuromas in continuity that cannot be sacrificed, a local muscle flap transferred over the neuroma may decrease local sensitivity.

Transposition of the involved nerve can be performed with or without neuroma resection. Herndon and colleagues (1976) recommended keeping the encapsulating scar and neuroma intact but transposing it to an area less exposed to trauma and free of scar. Amputation neuromas are often treated with transposition away from the end of the stump and scar, with or without neurectomy.

Nerve capping has been performed with both artificial materials and with local tissues. Millipore (Campbell et al, 1963), Micropore (Freeman, 1965), gold foil (Freeman et al, 1969), tantalum (Swanson et al, 1977), and silicone (Tauras and Frackelton, 1967) have all been used. Silicone has been the most common capping material. The neuroma is first freed from the surrounding scar, and the epineurium is pulled over the end of the neuroma. Two sutures are placed into the silicone cap, which, in turn, is tethered to an area free of scar. Williams (1987) reported a 70% success rate, but in a series of 348 painful neuromas, Tupper (1976) reported a 65% success rate with excisional neurectomy whether or not the nerve was also capped. Epineurial sleeves are a form of capping with local tissue. The fascicles are cut shorter than the epineurium, which is then double or triple ligated over the end of the nerve stump (Chapple, 1917). Silicone capping combined with an epineurial sleeve may improve results (Williams, 1987).

Probably the best prevention of, or treatment for, painful neuromas is direct nerve repair. Unfortunately, the freshened nerve ends will often not approximate following excision of the neuroma. Autografting of the nerve gap has been recommended for pain control (Lusskin et al, 1986). Conduits other than nerve autografts (such as freeze-thawed muscle grafts) have been used to restore the continuity of nerves following resection of the painful neuroma (Thomas et al, 1994). They are, however, not effective when the nerve gaps are large. Centrocentral anastomosis involves an end-to-end anastomosis of interposed nerve grafts between fascicular groups of the proximal nerve stump. In a series of 20 patients, the neuroma pain was relieved in all, but there

was no improvement of the phantom pain (Barbera and Albert-Pamplo, 1993).

Neurolysis alone gives little relief from the pain associated with neuromas. However, if the neurolysis allows the neuroma to retract into a bed of healthy tissue, approximately 60% of patients will obtain pain relief (Williams, 1987). Neurolysis with vein wrapping to prevent the recurrence of adhesions to the surrounding tissues will help that pain associated with traction secondary to nearby joint or tendon motion (Masear et al, 1989; (Figs. 17–2*A* and *B*, and 17–3 *A* and B). It also improves but does not totally relieve the pain associated with direct contact to the area of the neuroma. It also does not relieve the phantom pain. We reserve vein wrapping with either autograft or gluteraldehyde-preserved human umbilical vein for nerves with adherent surrounding scar and/or for neuromas in continuity that cannot be resected because the sacrifice of function would be unacceptable (Fig. 17–4). In the latter case, the added transfer of a local muscle flap over the area of the nerve/vein complex may further improve the result.

Although the success rate with most of the procedures described here is 60% or more, the chance of improvement with repeated surgeries is significantly diminished. Other methods of treatment for painful neuromas such as chemical fixatives, sclerosis, freezing, coagulation, diathermy, and crushing have been relatively unsuccessful (Snyder, 1961; Williams, 1987).

INTERDIGITAL PLANTAR NEUROMA (MORTON'S NEUROMA)

The affliction of plantar digital neuromas was first described by Durlacker (1845) and then by Morton (1876). It is most commonly seen in women, particularly those wearing high-heeled shoes. Also, aerobic exercises involving weight bearing on tip toes are a common cause. The pain is usually described as sharp or burning, often with radiation to one or two toes. The pain is exacerbated by walking. There is pain with compression between the metatarsal heads of the involved interspace, and sometimes the mass is palpable. There may be a reproduction of pain with complete dorsiflexion of the metatarsophalangeal and interphalangeal joints of the toes (Gauthier, 1979). Usually, pain is elicited

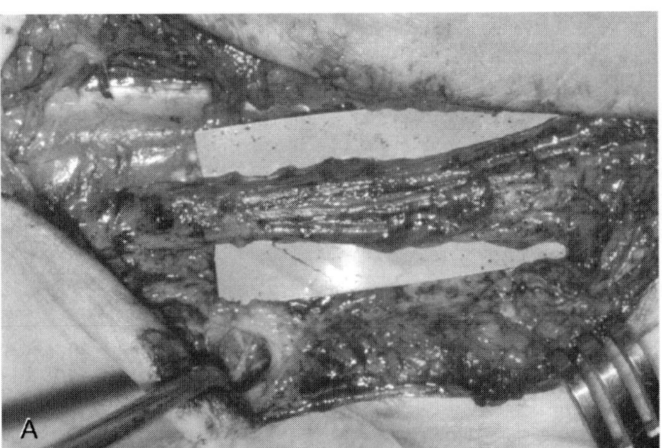
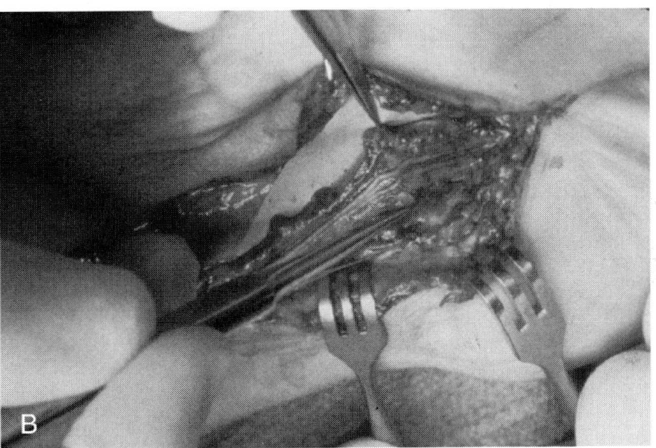

FIGURE 17–2. *A,* Extraneural fibrosis prior to neurolysis. *B,* Nerve following neurolysis.

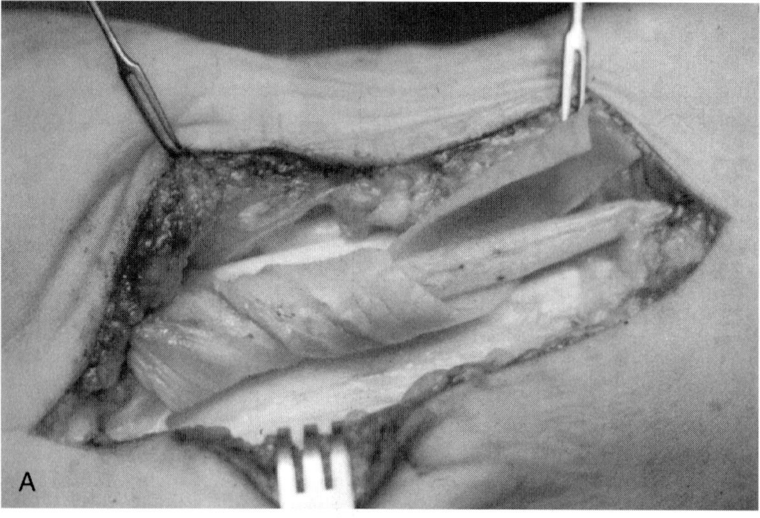

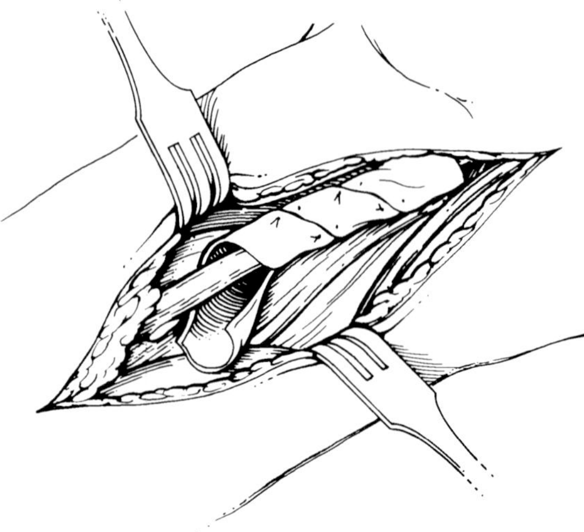

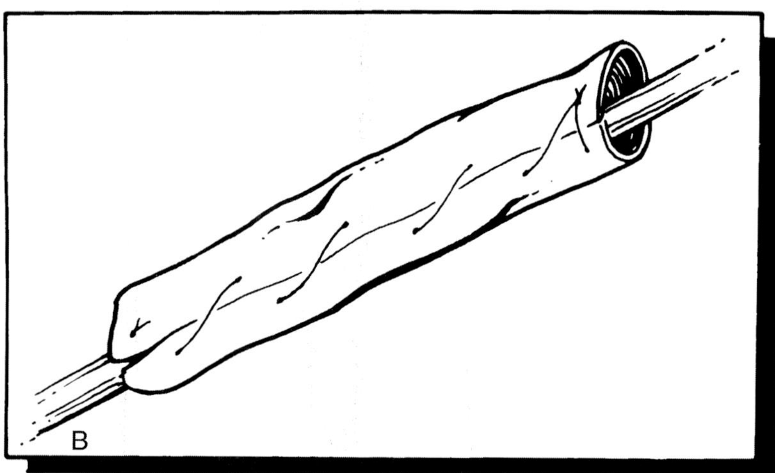

FIGURE 17–3. *A*, The intima of the vein is placed adjacent to the nerve, and the vein spiraled loosely around the involved nerve. The vein junctures are sutured to one another with 6-0 nylon. *B*, When a smaller nerve is involved, the vein may be slit and wrapped around the nerve and then closed with a running 6-0 nylon suture. Care must be taken not to make the vein wrap too tight.

with medial to lateral compression of all metatarsal heads (Mulder, 1951).

The common digital nerves of the second and third web spaces are the most commonly involved (Levitsky et al, 1993). Normally, only one web space is involved. A second plantar interdigital neuroma of the same foot is rare (Thompson and Deland, 1993). It has been proposed that the neuroma is secondary to tethering of the common digital nerve by its contributions from medial and lateral plantar nerves with dorsiflexion of the toes (Betts, 1940). The communicating branch between third and fourth webs is present in 27% of feet, but it does not increase the risk of neuroma formation (Levitsky, 1993). Other theories as to the cause of Morton's neuromas include an entrapment (Gauthier, 1979; Guiloff, 1984; and Lassman et al, 1976) or a nerve ischemia (Nissen, 1948). There is a smaller distance between the metatarsal heads in the second and third webs when compared with the first and fourth webs. Calluses on the plantar aspect of the second and third metatarsal heads are common. This is indicative of an increased weightbearing on those metatarsal heads. This increased weightbearing and the decreased intermetatarsal head distance in the second and third webs may cause a form of entrapment neuropathy or ischemia.

Routine, standing x-ray studies should be performed for a suspected Morton's neuroma. They often reveal other causes of metatarsalgia such as stress fractures, arthritis, and avascular necrosis of the metatarsal head. An MRI or CT scan, or sonography may be helpful in diagnosing a Morton's neuroma, but we have found a good clinical examination and relief of pain following a steroid injection of the involved interspace to be more predictive and much less expensive.

A Morton's neuroma is not an actual neuroma. The epi-

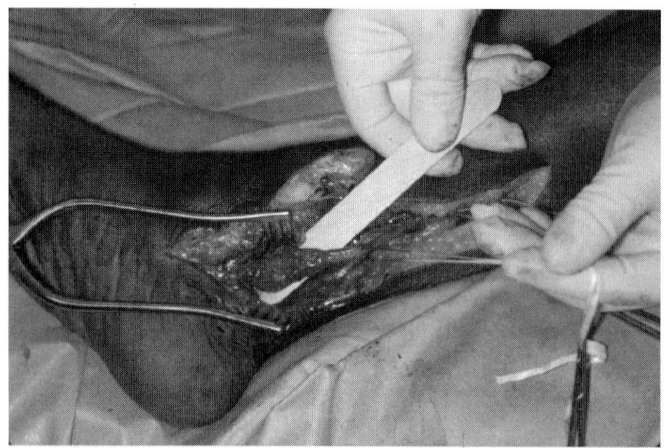

FIGURE 17–4. A tibial neuroma following a tarsal tunnel release and postoperative extraneural scar constriction.

neurium and perineurium are thickened and pathologically show fibrosis, and there may be wallerian degeneration (King, 1946; Lassman et al, 1976). There may also be vascular and perivascular proliferation.

Nonoperative therapy should be the first line of treatment for Morton's neuromas. Most patients will improve with shoe modifications or steroid injections. The shoes should have a wider toe box, low or no heel, and a well-cushioned sole. A pad placed proximal to the metatarsal heads may effect spreading of the metatarsal heads, thus relieving pressure on the nerve (Milgram, 1991). Repeated steroid injections, possibly as often as once per month, may afford relief in as many as 80% of patients (Greenfield et al, 1984).

Surgical intervention is recommended for those who are unresponsive to nonoperative treatment, or for those unwilling to change foot wear. Good results have been achieved following division of the intermetatarsal ligament (Gauthier, 1979), but most recommend resection of the involved nerve. Typically, it is assumed that resection of the nerve will allow the nerve to retract proximally (Amis et al, 1992; Mann and Reynolds, 1983). However, plantar nerve branches or scar may prevent retraction. Because the resected digital nerve will form a new neuroma, we recommend that this new neuroma be placed proximal to the weightbearing area. This is accomplished by transecting the nerve proximal to the level of the metatarsal neck.

A dorsal longitudinal approach is made over the involved web. The transverse metatarsal ligament is transected longitudinally and the neuroma is found either just beneath or just proximal to the ligament (Fig. 17–5). A blunt instrument such as a hemostat is introduced through the dorsal wound and is felt on the plantar aspect of the foot to identify the level of nerve resection and place it proximal to the weightbearing area (Fig. 17–6). We believe that this is safer than relying on the cut nerve to retract. With this technique, 87 consecutive patients have experienced relief of the neuroma pain associated with weightbearing. The new neuroma

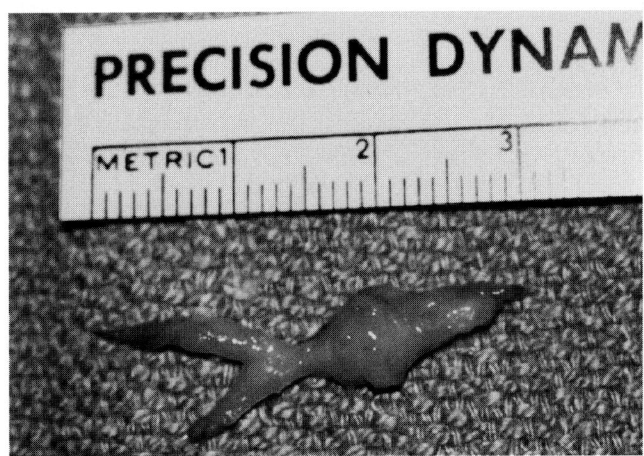

FIGURE 17–6. Morton's neuroma after resection proximal to the weight-bearing area.

is tender when palpated on the plantar arch but it is not symptomatic.

More distal resections of the involved nerve have not met with such good success (Greenfield et al, 1984). In our experience, the most common cause of pain following resection of an interdigital neuroma is a new neuroma located on the weightbearing surface. The next most common cause is failure to actually resect the neuroma or common digital nerve. Our approach to reoperation for Morton's neuroma is through a dorsal incision. Over 90% can be resected through this approach. Occasionally, the resected nerve neuroma is adherent to the plantar aspect of an MP joint or flexor tendon and cannot be located from the dorsal approach. If this is the case, a longitudinal plantar incision is made proximal to the weightbearing area of the metatarsal heads, and the neuroma is resected. If either an unresected neuroma or a new neuroma in the weightbearing area is found and is resected proximally, the success following reoperation for Morton's neuromas should be as good as that of a primary resection.

References

Amis JA, Siverhus SW, Liwnicz BH: An anatomic basis for recurrence after Morton's neuroma excision. Foot Ankle *13*(3):153–156, 1992.

Barbera J, Albert-Pamplo R: Centrocentral anastomosis of the proximal nerve stump in the treatment of painful amputation neuromas of major nerves. J Neurosurg *79*:331–334, 1993.

Betts LO: Morton's metatarsalgia: Neuritis of the fourth digital nerve. Med J Aust *1*:514–515, 1940.

Campbell JG, Bassett CAL, Bohler J: Frozen irradiated homografts shielded with microfilter sheaths in peripheral nerve surgery. J Trauma *3*:303, 1963.

Chapple WA: Re-amputation. BMJ *2*:242, 1917.

Dellon AL, Mackinnon SE: Treatment of the painful neuroma by neuroma resection and muscle implantation. Plast Reconstr Surg *77*:427–436, 1986.

Dellon AL, Mackinnon SE, Restron KA: Implantation of sensory nerve into muscle: Preliminary, clinical, and experimental observations of neuroma formation. Ann Plast Surg *12*:30–40, 1984.

Donnal JF, Blinder RA, Coblentz DL, Moylan JA, Fitzpatrick KP: MR imaging of stump neuroma. J Comput Assist Tomogr *14*(4):656–657, 1990.

Durlacker L: Treatise on corns, bunions, the disease of nails and the general management of feet. London, Simpkin, Marshal & Co., 1845, p 52.

Fisher GT, Boswich JA Jr: Neuroma formation following digital amputations. J Trauma *23*:136–142, 1983.

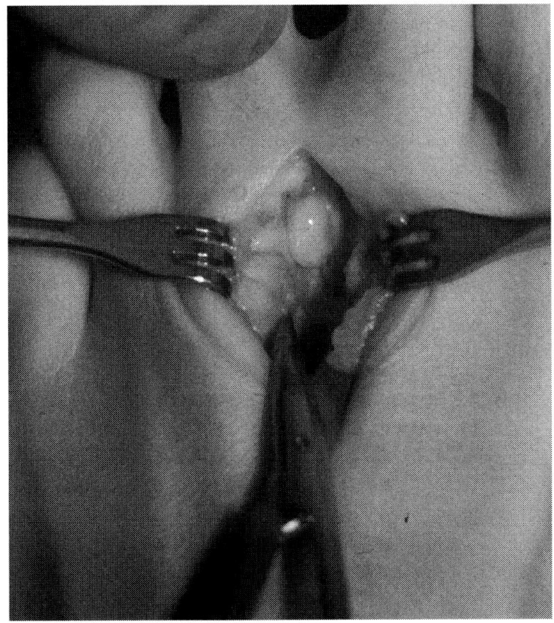

FIGURE 17–5. Dorsal approach to a Morton's neuroma. The neuroma is visible just proximal to the deep transverse metatarsal ligament.

Ford SR, Forrest WH Jr, Eltherington L: The treatment of reflex sympathetic dystrophy with intravenous regional bretylium. Anesthesiology *68*:137–140, 1988.

Freeman BS: Adhesive neural anatomses. Plast Reconstr Surg *35*:167, 1965.

Freeman BS, Perry J, Brown D: Experimental study of adhesive surgical tape for nerve anastomoses. Plast Reconstr Surg *43*:174, 1969.

Gauthier G: Thomas Morton's disease: A nerve entrapment syndrome. Clin Orthop *142*:90-92, 1979.

Girgis FL, Parry CB: Management of causalgia after peripheral nerve injury. Int Disabil Studies *11*:15–20, 1988.

Gluck T: Ueber Neuroplastik auf dem wege der transplantation. Arch Klin Chir 25:606, 1880.

Graham CE, Graham DM: Morton's neuroma: A microscopic evaluation. Foot Ankle *5*(2):150–153, 1984.

Granville AB: Counter irritation: Its principles and practice. Philadelphia, A Waldie, 1838.

Greenfield J, Rea J, Ilfeld FW: Morton's interdigital neuroma. Indications for treatment by local injections versus surgery. Clin Orthop Rel Res *185*:142–144, 1984.

Guiloff RJ, Scadding JW, Klenerman L: Morton's metatarsalgia. J Bone Joint Surg *66B*(4):586–591, 1984.

Hanninton-Kiff JG: Intravenous regional sympathetic block with guanethidine. Lancet *1*:1019–1020, 1974.

Herndon JH, Eaton RG, Littler JW: Management of painful neuromas in the hand. J Bone Joint Surg *58A*:369, 1976.

Homans J: Minor causalgia: A hyperesthetic neurovascular syndrome N Engl J Med *222*:870–874, 1960.

Kenzora JE: Sensory nerve neuromas -Leading to failed foot surgery. Foot Ankle *7*(2):110–117, 1986.

Kenzora JE: Symptomatic incisional neuromas on the dorsum of the foot. Foot Ankle *5*(1):2–15, 1984.

King LSL: Note on the pathology of Morton's metatarsalgia. Am J Clin Pathol *16*:124–128, 1946.

Lassman G, Lassman H, Stockinger L: Morton's metatarsalgia: Light and electron microscopic observations and their relation to entrapment neuropathies. Virchows Arch *370*:307–321, 1976.

Law JD, Swett J, Kirsch WM: Retrospective analysis of 22 patients with chronic pain treated by peripheral nerve stimulation. J Neurosurg 52:482–485, 1980.

Levitsky KA, Alman BA, Jeusevar DS, Morehead J: Digital nerves of the foot: Anatomic variations and implications regarding the pathogenesis of interdigital neuroma. Foot Ankle *14*(4):208–214, 1993.

Long DM: Electrical stimulation for the control of pain. Arch Surg *112*:884–888, 1977.

Long DM: Surgical therapy of chronic pain. Neurosurgery 6:317–328, 1980.

Lusskin R, Battista A, Lenzo S, Price A: Surgical management of late post-traumatic and ischemic neuropathies involving the lower extremities: Classification and results of therapy. Foot Ankle *7*(2):95–104, 1986.

Mann RA, Reynolds JD: Interdigital neuroma—a critical clinical analysis, Foot Ankle *3*(4):238–243, 1983.

Masear VR, Tulloss J, St. Mary E, Meyer RD: Venous Wrapping of Nerves to Prevent Scarring. American Society for Surgery of the Hand, 44th Annual Meeting, Seattle, WA, September 15, 1989.

Meier PJ, Kenzora JE: The risks and benefits of distal first metatarsal osteotomies. Foot Ankle *6*:7–17, 1985.

Milgram JE: Padding and devices to relieve painful feet. *In* Jahss MH (ed): Disorders of the Foot and Ankle. Medical and Surgical Management, 2nd ed. Philadelphia, W.B. Saunders Company, 1991, pp 2838–2840.

Morton TG: A peculiar and painful affection of the fourth metatarsophalangeal articulation. Am J Med Sci *71*:37–45, 1876.

Mulder JD: The causative mechanism in Morton's metatarsalgia. J Bone Joint Surg *33B*:94–95, 1951.

Nashold BS, Goldner JL: Electrical stimulation of peripheral nerves for relief of intractable chronic pain. Med Instrum 9:224–225, 1975.

Nissen KI: Plantar digital neuritis: Morton's metatarsalgia. J Bone Joint Surg *30B*:84–94, 1948.

Omer GE: Management of pain syndromes in the upper extremity. *In* Hunter JM, Schneider LH (eds): Rehabilitation of the Hand. St. Louis, C.V. Mosby Company, 1978, pp 341–349.

Petropoulos PC, Stefanko S: Experimental observations on the prevention of neuroma formation. J Surg Res *1*:241, 1961.

Singson RD, Feldman F, Slipman CW, Gonzalez E, Rosenberg ZS, Kiernan H: Postamputation neuromas and other symptomatic stump abnormalities: detection with CT. Radiol *162*(3):743–745, 1987.

Singson RD, Feldman F, Staron R, Fechtner D, Gonzalez E, Stein J: MRI of postamputation neuromas. Skeletal Radiol *19*:259–262, 1990.

Smith JR, Gomez NH: Local injection therapy of neuromata of the hand with triamcinalone acetonide: a preliminary study of 22 patients. J Bone Joint Surg *52A*:71–83, 1970.

Snyder CC: The surgical handling of tissue. Fort Worth, TX, Proceedings of the Seventh Annual Convention. American Association of Equine Practice, 1961.

Spencer PS: The traumatic neuroma and proximal stump. Bull Hosp Joint Dis 35:85, 1974.

Staniforth P, Fisher TR: The effects of sural nerve excision in autogenous nerve grafting. Hand *10*:187, 1978.

Sunderland S: Nerve and Nerve Injuries. 2nd ed. New York, Churchill, Livingstone, 1978.

Swanson AB, Boeve NR, Lumsden RM: The prevention and treatment of amputation neuromata by silicone capping. J Hand Surg 2:70, 1977.

Tauras AP, Frackelton WH: Silicone capping of nerve stumps in the problem of painful neuromas. Surg Forum *18*:504, 1967.

Thomas M, Stirrat A, Birch R: Freeze-thawed muscle grafting for painful cutaneous neuromas. J Bone Joint Surg *76B*(3):474–476, 1994.

Thompson FM, Deland JT: Occurrence of two interdigital neuromas in one foot. Foot Ankle *14*(1):15–17, 1993.

Tupper JW: Treatment of painful neuromas of sensory nerves in the hand: A comparison of traditional and newer methods. J Hand Surg *1*:144, 1976.

Weir Mitchell S: Injuries of Nerves and Their Consequences. 1872. Reprinted 1965. Dover Publications, New York.

Williams HB: The painful stump neuroma and its treatment. *In* Terzis JK (ed): Microreconstruction of Nerve Injuries. Philadelphia, W.B. Saunders Company, 1987, pp 161–172.

Wilson RL: Management of pain following peripheral nerve injuries. Orthop Clin North Am *12*(2):343–359, 1981.

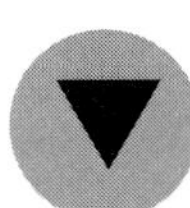

Chapter 18

• Erdoğan Atasoy
• Harold E. Kleinert

Surgical Sympathectomy and Sympathetic Blocks for the Upper and Lower Extremities, and Local and Plexus Levels

OVERVIEW AND HISTORY

In 1852, French physiologist Claude Bernard reported his classic work regarding the effects of sympathetic nerves in maintaining normal constrictor tone in the blood vessels of the skin. In 1858, he demonstrated that sectioning of the cervical sympathetic nerve caused papillary constriction and blushing of the conjunctiva and ear. Horner, a Swiss ophthalmologist, in 1869 reported the complete description of full eye and skin changes following sympathetic disturbance in the neck; the syndrome now bears his name (Firkin and Whitworth, 1987). In Europe, the condition is called Bernard-Horner syndrome. The French surgeons Leriche (1913) and Jabouley (1899) first applied and tested the concepts of sympathetic denervation as a treatment of peripheral vascular diseases. This sympathetic denervation was used and advocated by Leriche (1916) in the form of periarterial sympathectomy for the great variety of painful and circulatory disorders of the extremities.

The first successful cervicothoracic sympathectomy was performed and reported in 1920 by Jonnesco, a French surgeon, for the relief of angina pectoris. In 1924, Royle of Australia used sympathetic ramus sectioning for the treatment of lower extremity spastic paralysis, and he observed improved circulation in the legs of the patients. During the same year, Julio Diez of Argentina, who was dissatisfied with the results of periarterial sympathectomy, first performed and reported the lumbar sympathectomy for the treatment of occlusive arterial disease of the lower extremities (Diez, 1926; Moore, 1991).

These observations led Adson and Brown to use cervical and lumbar sympathectomies in 1925, 1929, and 1935 for the treatment of Raynaud's disease and hyperhidrosis. In 1930, Glen Spurling reported the first dorsal sympathectomy for the treatment of causalgia. In 1955, Palumbo reported that the upper extremity sympathectomy could be performed without any residual Horner's syndrome. Before this, during the sympathectomy, total removal of the stellate ganglion and T2 to T3 thoracic ganglion was performed. The total stellate ganglionectomy usually leaves the patient with unsightly, undesirable, permanent Horner's syndrome. Palumbo first performed and advocated removal of only the lower third of the stellate ganglion in order to prevent permanent Horner's syndrome.

Smithwick (1940) and Gibbon (1962) proposed the removal of the second and third intercostal nerves, including the intraspinal portions of both anterior and posterior roots, to eliminate the possibility of residual vasomotor symptoms, because in 15% of patients, there is the presence of an intermediate ganglion (Skoog, 1947; Wrete, 1935). This ganglion, if present, usually is found in the upper thoracic region and is located very close to the second and third intercostal nerves.

In 1980, Adrian Flatt introduced digital sympathectomy for the treatment of cold injuries and several vasospastic disorders of the digits. It has gained increasing popularity for the treatment of these conditions, and even the success rate has been stated as being better than that with the thoracic sympathectomy for predominant digital symptoms in patients with vasospastic disorders and cold injuries.

As to sympathetic blocks, the first classic anterior approach to stellate ganglion blocks was initiated by Leriche (1933, 1934). Mandl first described the technique of the lumbar sympathetic block in 1926.

ANATOMY AND PHYSIOLOGY

The autonomic nervous system, which controls smooth muscles, cardiac muscle, glands, and blood vessels, functions independently. However, it has been demonstrated that some visceral mechanisms can be brought under partial voluntary influence.

The autonomic nervous system has two major divisions: the sympathetic or thoracolumbar division, and the parasympathetic or craniosacral division (Fig. 18–1).

The preganglionic (central) neurons of the sympathetic division are located in the gray matter of the spinal cord intermediolateral position. They extend from the first thoracic segment to the third lumbar segment.

The axons of sympathetic preganglionic neurons emerge from the spinal cord through the ventral root as white fibers because they are myelinated. These preganglionic fibers enter the sympathetic ganglions and usually synapse with the postganglionic neurons of the same level, or after traveling

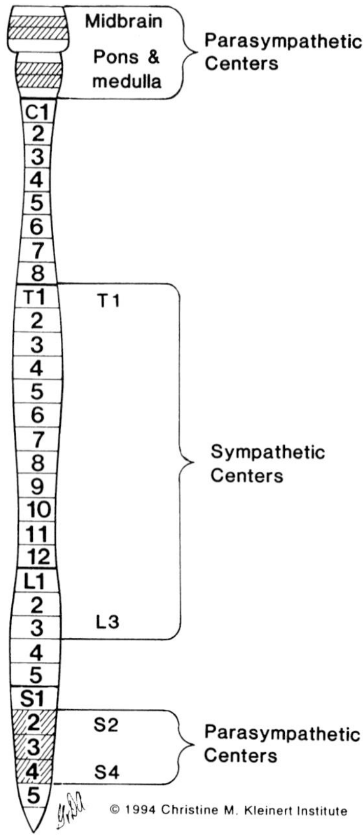

FIGURE 18–1. Anatomical locations of sympathetic and parasympathetic centers in the central nervous system. (© 1994 Christine M. Kleinert Institute.)

a distance they may synapse in the ganglions above or below (Fig. 18–2). Some preganglionic fibers pass without any relay through the sympathetic chain, and they synapse in the collateral ganglions, such as the celiac and the superior and inferior mesenteric ganglions. The inconstant relay and synapse in the chain may be partially responsible for a number of disappointing results from an apparently technically successful block.

The postganglionic axons are almost all myelinated and widely distributed; some join peripheral nerves by gray communicants to their autonomic targets, and some join to vessels to their target organs (see Fig. 18–2).

There are three cervical ganglions. Thoracic sympathetic ganglions are segmentally located in the chest from T1 to T11 and sometimes T12. There are four to five lumbar, four sacral, and one coccygeal ganglion. The superior cervical ganglion is the largest cervical ganglion and is located close to the base of the skull on the anterior aspect of the transverse process of C1 and C2. The middle cervical ganglion is the smallest and is located at the anterior lateral aspect of the C6 vertebral body. Postganglionic fibers supply blood vessels; glands; smooth muscles of the head and neck, thyroid, and parathyroid; and send superior and middle cardiac nerves to the heart. The inferior cervical ganglion is usually fused with the T1 ganglion, occasionally T2, forming a long stellate ganglion. It is located at the anterolateral aspect of the C7 vertebral body, extending caudally to the neck of the first rib (Fig. 18–3). It sends fibers in the distribution of the C7–C8 cervical nerves and the first and second thoracic nerves, and the lower cardiac nerve takes its origin from it.

Some postganglionic fibers form a plexus on the subclavian artery and its branches, supplying sympathetic innervation along these vessels. These vascular nerves, after arriving in the vessels, unite and form an extensive perivascular adventitial plexus and then ramify into the plexus between the adventitia and the media, and between the media and the intima. Some of the terminal branches extend to the ciliary muscle for its dilatory function (Williams et al, 1989).

The preganglionic fibers to the upper limb usually arise from T2–T7 thoracic cord segments and reach the corresponding ganglion by the way of white rami, and pass up and down the chain (see Fig. 18–2). After a series of synapses, they leave the ganglion through gray fibers from the T1, T2, T3, and sometimes T4 ganglions, and finally enter the limb through the C7, C8, and T1 branches of the brachial plexus. The preganglion fibers to the lower limb arise from the T10–L3 spinal cord segment, then usually synapse in the T1–T4 lumbar ganglions and enter the roots of the lumbar and sacral plexus to innervate the lower extremity (Kandel et al, 1991).

Sympathetic commands enable the organism to mobilize and expand energy and perform well during emergencies; cardiac acceleration is accompanied by relaxation of the coronary artery wall, contraction of peripheral arteries, elevation of blood perfusion pressure, increased ventilation by relaxing bronchial muscles, increased blood volume by contracting splanchnic veins to the skeletal muscle for use, and widening of the pupils for more light.

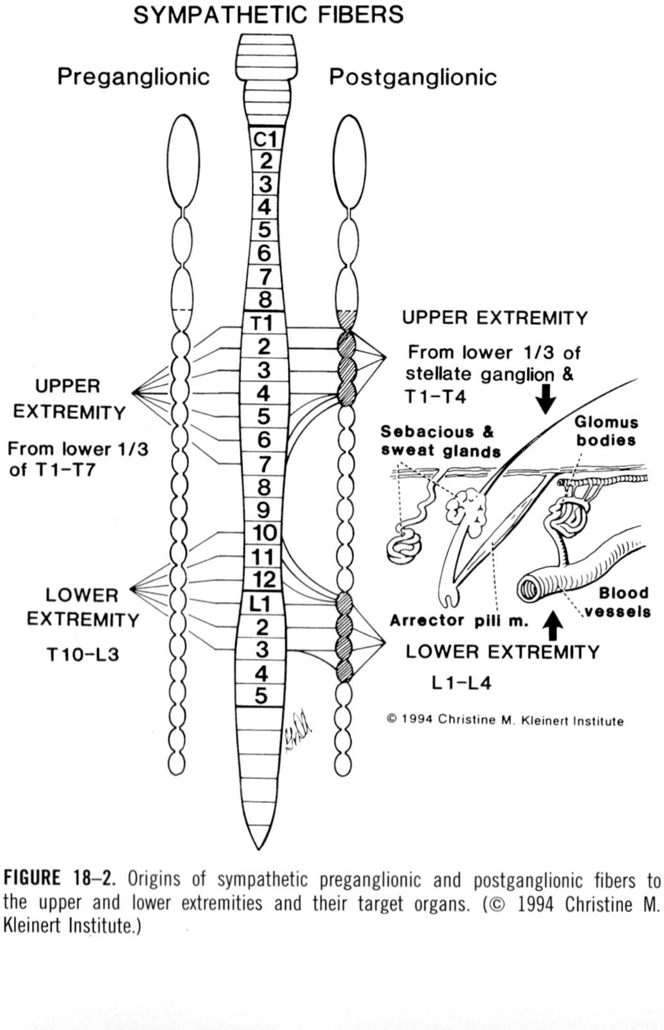

SYMPATHETIC FIBERS

FIGURE 18–2. Origins of sympathetic preganglionic and postganglionic fibers to the upper and lower extremities and their target organs. (© 1994 Christine M. Kleinert Institute.)

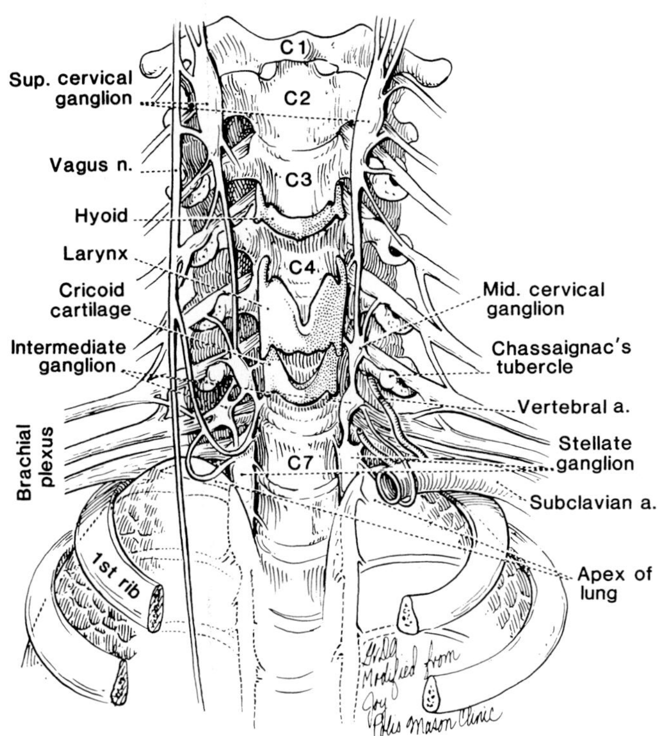

FIGURE 18–3. Anterior view of the cervicothoracic portion of the sympathetic nervous system.

In the sympathetic system, preganglionic fibers spread over to several sympathetic ganglions. Postganglionic fibers often extend to more than one visceral organ.

The predominant neurotransmitter in sympathetic systems is norepinephrine, which has a prolonged, generalized effect following stimulation of sympathetic nervous systems. This effect results in the release of a mixture of epinephrine and norepinephrine from the adrenal medulla, causing an increase in vascular tone, blood sugar, metabolic rate, and stronger contracture of the skeletal muscles (Best and Taylor, 1991).

Function

The sympathetic nervous system has a wide range of effects on several organs, such as vasoconstriction on peripheral and splanchnic arteries and veins through alpha receptors; increased heart rate and contractility; increased cardiac output with coronary vessel relaxation by beta 1 receptor stimulation; bronchial tree relaxation through β_2 receptor stimulation; a minor vasodilation effect on the muscular vessel wall; and a wide variety of metabolic, smooth muscle relaxation, and sphincter contraction effects in the bladder and bowel by β_2 receptor stimulation. We will discuss primarily here the sympathetic effect on pain and peripheral blood flow.

Pain. Recent evidence suggests that sympathetic efferents may influence pain perception in the extremities. Release of neurotransmitters from the sympathetic nerve endings increases the sensitivity of peripheral nociceptors.

Sympathetic Effect on Peripheral Blood Flow. In a normal person, a sympathetic block will cause vasodilation of arteries and veins, and increased capillary flow in the extremities. This blood flow increase is largely restricted to the skin and produces increased skin temperature and a marked feeling of warmth.

Because muscle blood flow is automatically regulated by muscle metabolism, a sympathetic block will not affect muscle blood flow during rest, work, and ischemia. Thus, reduced blood flow (e.g., claudication) may not be helped by a sympathetic block. But it seems logical to use a sympathetic block to improve blood flow and relieve rest pain in a patient with insufficient peripheral skin blood circulation because of vasospasm or obstructive arterial disease.

However, it is not possible to predict the effect of a sympathetic block in a patient with peripheral arterial disease. An increase in skin temperature is not always related to an increase in blood flow through the skin; it could merely reflect venous pooling and local inflammatory change.

In patients with severe occlusive vascular disease who have low ankle blood pressure because of proximal stealing, which occurs often, a distally decreasing blood flow is followed by vasodilation in vessels located proximally. Although rare, there are some reports of worsening of pain and gangrene after sympathectomy.

Sympathetic activity can be blocked pharmacologically by an α receptor blocker (phentolamine, dibenzyline), by a β receptor blocker (propranolol [β_1 and β_2 receptors] or practolol [mainly β_1 receptor]), or by a depletor of norepinephrine activity in the sympathetic nerve endings (guanethidine or reserpine).

Sympathetic nerve fiber block can be performed intradurally or extradurally (blocking preganglionic fibers by subarachnoid or epidural block), at the sympathetic chain by sympathetic block, at the peripheral nerves by a nerve block, or at the vessel by perivascular infiltration (Cousins and Bridenbaugh, 1988).

STELLATE GANGLION BLOCK AND CERVICOTHORACIC SYMPATHECTOMY

Anatomy. The stellate ganglion is formed by the fusion of the inferior and first thoracic ganglions and, occasionally, the second thoracic ganglion. Because of several efferent and afferent fibers entering and leaving the ganglion, it may appear in the shape of a star or dumbbell, depending on the amount of fusion. It is about 2.5 mm long, 1 cm wide, and 0.5 mm thick. The ganglion lies over the neck of the first rib and extends up to the transverse process of C7, with the longus colli muscle just medial to it (Fig. 18–4A). The dome of the pleura covers the lower third. The vertebral artery is on its anterolateral aspect. It has a close relationship with the subclavian artery (anterior and lower), the inferior thyroid artery (lateral), the first intercostal nerve, and the recurrent laryngeal nerve (posterior and medial locations, respectively). At the level of C6, the vertebral artery dives posteriorly and goes through the foramen of the transverse process of C6. Because of this passage, the transverse process is prominent anteriorly and is called Chassaignac's tubercle; it is an important landmark when the stellate ganglion block is performed (Fig. 18–4B).

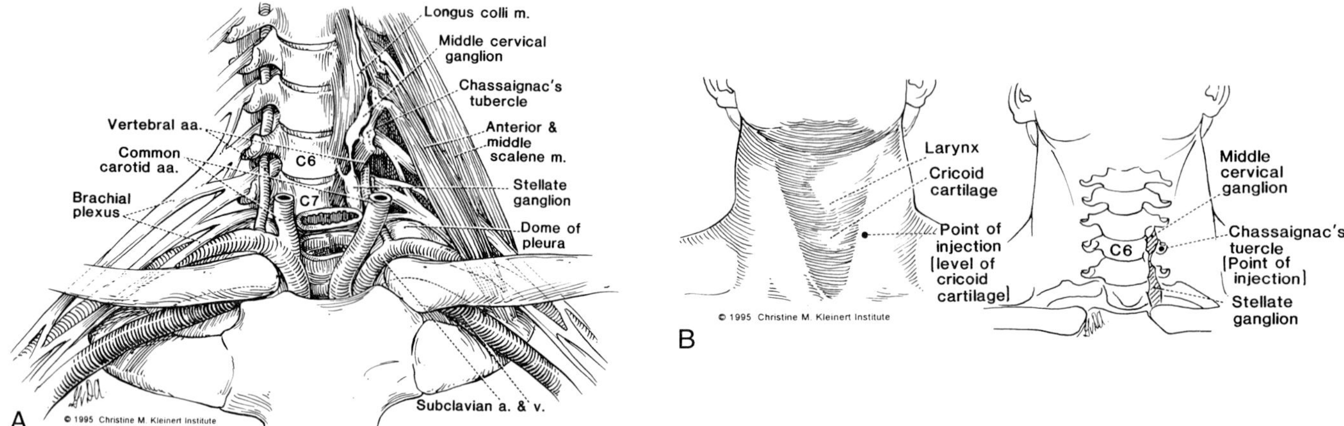

FIGURE 18–4. *A* and *B*, Regional anatomy of middle cervical and stellate ganglion and their relationship to neurovascular, osseous, and muscular structures. Note the points of injections (skin and bone levels; see text). (© 1995 Christine M. Kleinert Institute.)

The sympathetic preganglionic fibers for the head, neck, and upper limb leave the spinal cord from T1 down to T7 (see Fig. 18–2). They converge and pass upward anteriorly to the neck of the first rib and usually pass through the stellate ganglion, but sometimes they may bypass the stellate ganglion completely on their way into the head, neck, and upper extremity. For the best result, the local anesthetic solution should fill the prevertebral space from C6 down to the T3–T4 level. This can be done by injecting 15 to 20 ml of local anesthetic material in front of the transverse process of C6. This injection should not be given below C6 because of the greater risk of a pneumothorax and the danger of intra-arterial injection inside the vertebral artery.

Indications. Indications for the stellate ganglion block include pain relief for such conditions as reflex sympathetic dystrophy (RSD), phantom pain, central pain, and postfrostbite syndrome; to improve circulation in the arm in some vasospastic and vascular conditions, including scleroderma, Raynaud's disease, and acrocyanosis; following embolectomy, traumatic or embolic, and occlusive vascular conditions (e.g., Buerger's disease); and finally, to remedy conditions such as axillary or upper extremity hyperhidrosis.

The stellate ganglion block is most commonly used for RSD and related conditions. Before considering this type of block for this condition, several weeks of conservative treatment, including physical therapy modalities and medications (anti-inflammatory, neurologic blocking, and psychotropic drugs), should be tried. Because of improved conservative treatment programs, the necessity for the stellate ganglion block has been reduced in our institution.

A failure rate of 30% to 35% has been reported with the stellate ganglion block. This could be due to some diagnostic and anatomical abnormalities such as the presence of intermediate ganglion (Skoog, 1947), presence of Kuntz' nerve (Flatt, 1980) (this is a direct nerve fiber from the T2 ganglion to the brachial plexus), and direct sympathetic connection from the spinal cord to the brachial plexus from the same and opposite sides through the ventral roots (presence of 27% unmyelinated fiber has been demonstrated under the electronic microscope, and significant numbers of these fibers are sensory and sympathetic).

The most commonly used and easily performed anterior approach is described. The patient is placed in the supine position with a pillow under the shoulder and the neck slightly hyperextended. The mouth is slightly opened to relax the anterior neck muscles.

Following routine preoperative preparation and with sterile gloves on the hands, the trachea, cricoid cartilage, and carotid pulse are felt with two fingers; then Chassaignac's tubercle, which is between the trachea and the sternocleidomastoid muscle, is palpated at the level of the cricoid cartilage. Thus, the cricoid cartilage, Chassaignac's tubercle, and the middle cervical ganglion are all at the same level (Fig. 18–5A). The left index and middle fingers are kept apart slightly and used to retract the carotid sheath and sternocleidomastoid muscle laterally, and a 30-gauge needle is used to raise a skin wheal a little lateral to the cricoid cartilage or on the palpated Chassaignac's tubercle. The deeper tissues are then anesthetized (usually with a long-lasting local anesthetic material such as bupivacaine (Marcaine) (0.5% is used). By using a two-needle technique and first anesthetizing the patient's skin and deeper structures, the patient's apprehension is relieved and confidence in the doctor will increase. A 25-gauge, 1½ inch long needle with a 20-ml controlled syringe is inserted slowly through the anesthetized area down to the transverse process of C6. When bony resistance is felt, the needle is withdrawn 2 to 4 mm (see Fig. 18–5B). While doing this, the left index and middle fingers maintain the position, and an aspiration test is performed. If no blood is seen in the syringe, a test dose of 1 or 2 ml Marcaine 0.5% is given, then gradually the rest of the solution is slowly injected (usually 15–20 ml). A high level of resistance indicates a periosteal injection, so the needle should be withdrawn 2 to 3 mm. During the injection, the proximal one of the two fingers retracting the sternocleidomastoid muscle and carotid sheath should firmly press the area. The distal finger should ease off its pressure to facilitate the spread of the solution distally toward the stellate ganglion. At the completion of the injection, the patient's head and chest are elevated at least 45 degrees and the injection site is gently milked caudally to push the anesthetic solution distally toward the stellate ganglion and below. The patient should be warned that the injection of local anesthetic could cause some discomfort, such as feeling a lump in the throat, temporary hoarseness, or some difficulty swallowing. Also,

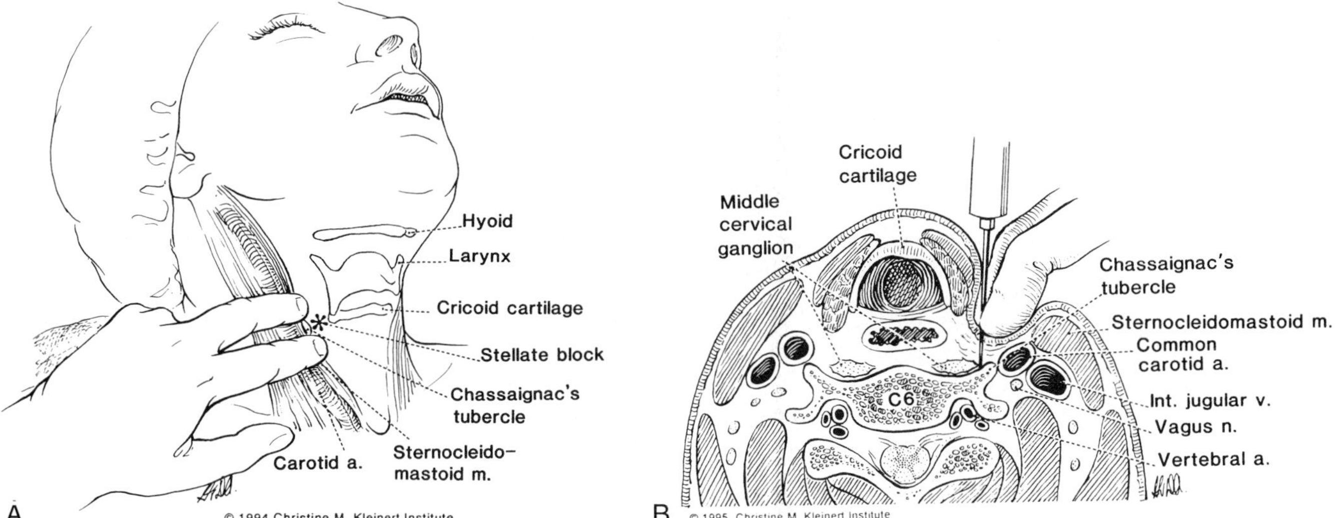

FIGURE 18–5. *A* and *B,* Anterior approach for stellate ganglion block. The carotid sheath and sternocleidomastoid muscle are retracted with two fingers. By using a two-needle technique, the transverse process of C6 is approached. (© 1995 Christine M. Kleinert Institute.)

the possibility of Horner's syndrome should be explained to the patient (Green, 1993; Kleinert et al, 1973; Moore, 1965).

The signs of Horner's syndrome (ptosis, myosis, and enophthalmus) are usually accepted as an indication of a satisfactory block (Fig. 18–6). Also, sometimes stuffiness of the nasal passages and flushing of the conjunctiva on the injected side are observed. Although generally the occurrence of Horner's syndrome is accepted as the sign of a successful stellate ganglion block, the best and the most reliable signs are the occurrence of a warm, dry extremity with dilated and distended veins in the hand on the injected side. A continuous block can be performed by inserting a thin intravenous plastic cannula with a stylet. It should be kept in mind that the catheter could move near the dura or vertebral artery and other structures.

Complications. The most serious complications result from intra-arterial or intradural injections. Because a negative aspiration test does not exclude the chance of an intradural or intra-arterial injection, it is very important that the inserted needle be on the bone and a resistance felt before the injection. If the needle passes through the ligament between transverse processes, the tip may be near or in the vertebral artery or dural sac, and if the injection proceeds, immediate seizure or spinal anesthesia may occur. Bilateral injection should not be done because of the danger of airway problems resulting from blocking both recurrent laryngeal nerves. Also, brachycardia and hypotension may occur owing to loss of cardiac accelerator activity. A low-level injection could cause pneumothorax, especially if it is conducted at the level of C7. Other complications are brachial plexus block, hematoma formation, and rarely, osteitis of the transverse process caused by the needle traversing the esophagus before reaching the transverse process (Cousins and Bridenbaugh, 1988).

Cervicothoracic Sympathectomy, and Thoracoscopic and Digital Sympathectomy

Stellate and T1 ganglions make only a 15% to 30% sympathetic nerve contribution to the upper extremity, but both these ganglions make considerable contributions to the eye. Most of the upper extremity sympathetic supply comes from the T2 and T3 ganglions, but there is an additional sympathetic supply to the upper extremity through anomalous intermediate ganglions and connections, which could be one of the reasons for failure of a sympathectomy.

Usually, a satisfactory result is obtained by removing the lower third of the stellate ganglion and the T2 and T3 ganglions. Avoiding the upper two thirds of the stellate

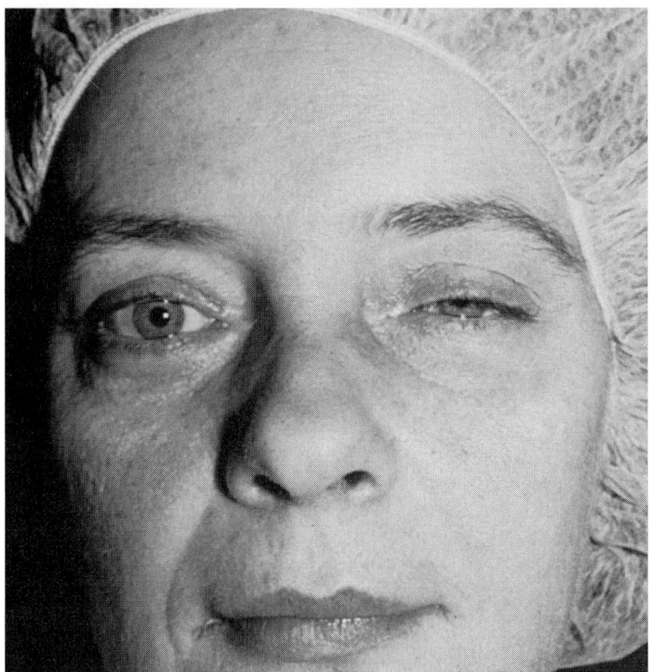

FIGURE 18–6. The stellate ganglion block and appearance of Horner's syndrome in left eye.

ganglion eliminates the risk of Horner's syndrome because the preganglionic sympathetic fibers supplying the pupils, after arising from the lateral horn of the spinal cord, emerge with the anterior roots of C8 and T1 and traverse the upper part of the stellate ganglion.

After complete sympathetic denervation, a 40% to 100% increase in total resting blood flow in the acutely ischemic extremity has been reported, usually by opening the arteriovenous shunts with little change in muscle blood flow. Maximum peripheral vasodilatation is usually seen immediately after sympathectomy, and progressive declination is usually observed in most patients, starting 1 to 2 weeks after the procedure.

This gradual recovery has been explained on the bases of incomplete sympathectomy, regeneration of fibers, and increased sensitivity of α_2 vascular smooth muscle receptor to circulatory catecholamines.

It is generally believed that the sympathectomy will have a temporary effect on the resting blood flow of the extremity, but its effects on sweating and vasoconstrictor responses to cold are more persistent if it is complete. It is also difficult to make a good assessment about the effect of sympathectomy on neurogenic and ischemic pain, but it has been shown that pain tolerance is usually increased in the extremities after sympathectomy.

Generally, sympathectomy increases the blood flow to the ischemic skin in the limb and promotes healing of small superficial skin ulcers. Also, ischemic and neurogenic pain tolerance is increased. It has been reported that 47% to 70% of patients claim that their pain was relieved.

Best results are obtained in reflex dystrophy, hyperhidrosis, and vasospastic disorders, even with some skin ulceration.

Patient selection is critical when considering surgical sympathectomy. An adequate response with relief of symptoms must occur with the stellate ganglion block. At least four or five stellate ganglion blocks should be administered, and if they result in temporary relief, especially with reflex dystrophy, then the surgical sympathectomy is considered.

Indications for surgical sympathectomy include RSD in its various forms; vasospastic disorders such as primary Raynaud's disease, Raynaud's phenomenon secondary to scleroderma, and other collagen diseases such as lupus; periarterial nodosa; severe hyperhidrosis; acrocyanosis, which is painless, persistent coldness and cyanosis of the hands and feet, especially with exposure to cold, without ulcerations; Buerger's disease; vascular insufficiency secondary to trauma; arteriosclerosis with ischemic lesions; and vasomotor changes.

Thoracic outlet compression with marked symptoms of sympathetic overactivity in the extremity and subclavian or axillary artery involvement with peripheral emboli can be managed with a transaxillary first rib resection and thoracic sympathectomy combined with a transcervical scalenectomy (Fig. 18–7).

Contraindications to sympathectomy are poor pulmonary

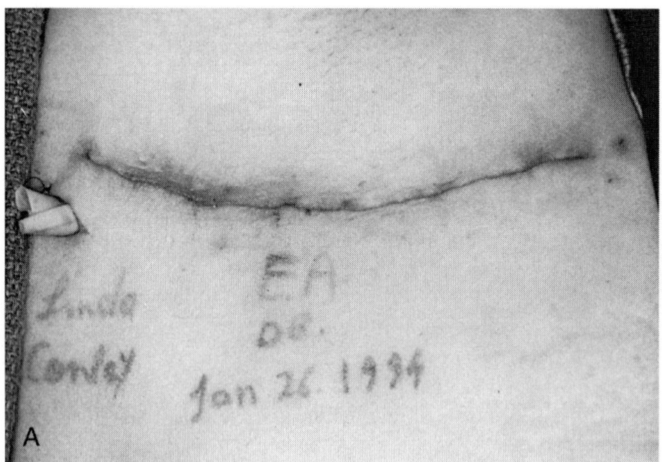

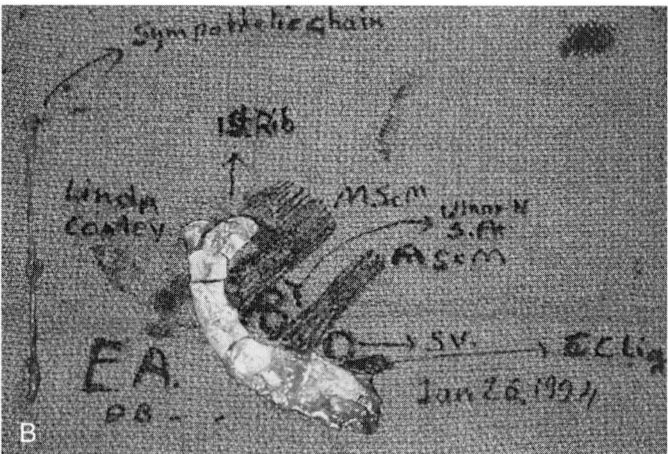

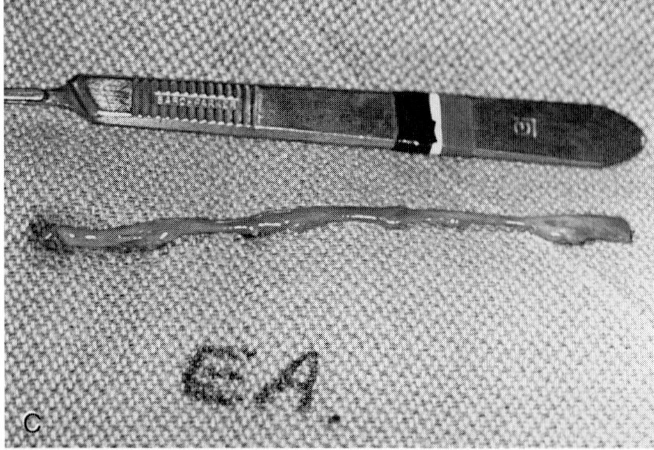

FIGURE 18–7. Transaxillary sympathectomy combined with first rib resection. Incision *(A)* removed first rib and related structures *(B)* and sympathetic chain *(C)*.

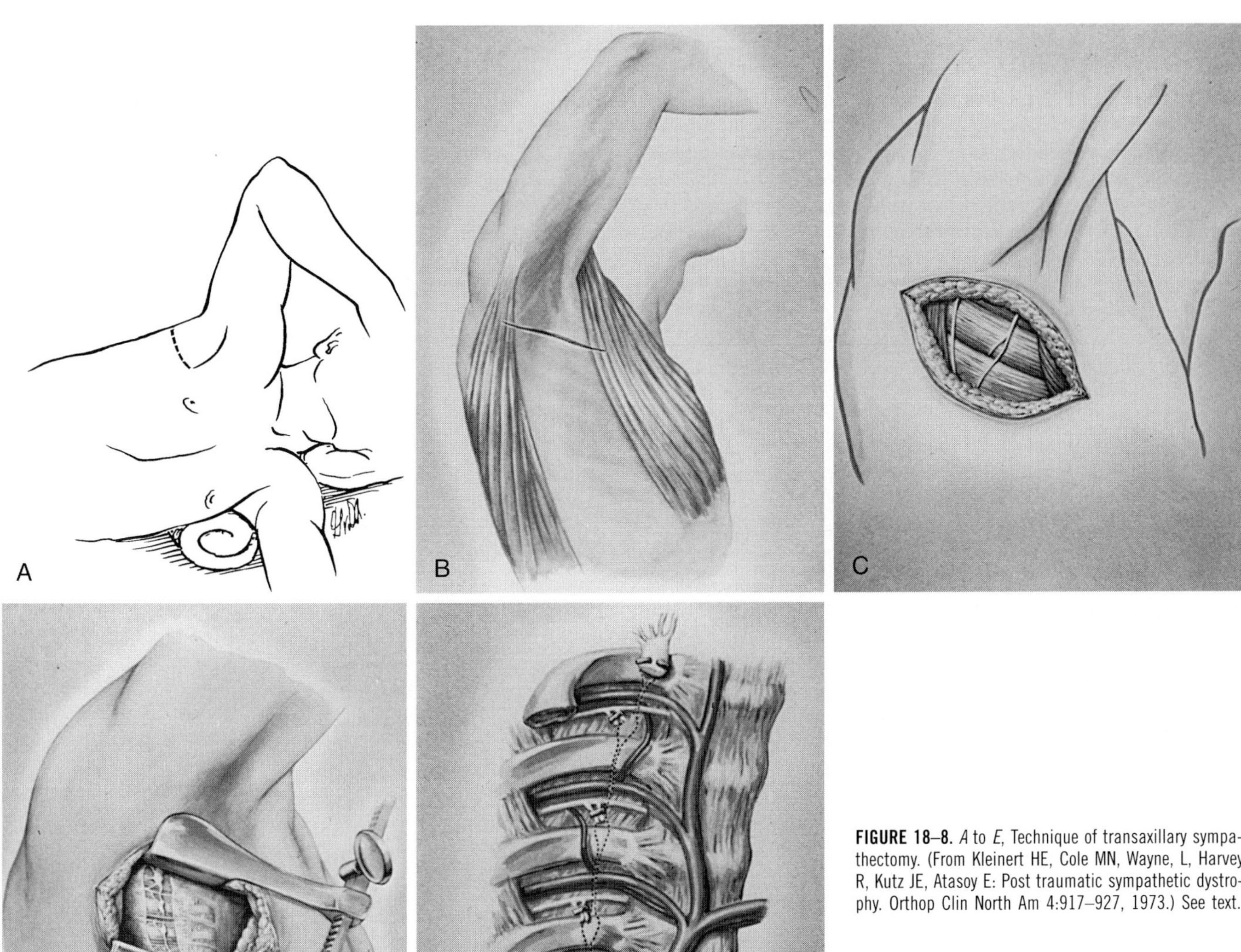

FIGURE 18–8. *A* to *E*, Technique of transaxillary sympathectomy. (From Kleinert HE, Cole MN, Wayne, L, Harvey R, Kutz JE, Atasoy E: Post traumatic sympathetic dystrophy. Orthop Clin North Am 4:917–927, 1973.) See text.

reserve, advanced cardiovascular disease, Pancoast's tumor, and factitious lymphedema. Erythromelalgia, which is defined as a warm, hyperemic, painful extremity with an obscure etiology, is not an indication for sympathectomy.

Operative Technique. The four approaches described in the literature include the supraclavicular, posterior transthoracic (Adson and Brown, 1929), anterior transthoracic (Palumbo, 1955), and transaxillary transthoracic. The latter is the most commonly used and produces excellent exposure of the stellate ganglion as well as the upper four thoracic ganglions. This exposure was originally used by Shutze and Goets (Kleinert et al, 1965). In 1949, Atkins first reported his experience with this approach in eight cases (Kleinert et al, 1965). Kleinert and colleagues (1965) popularized this approach with their experience in 51 operative cases.

The procedure is carried out with the patient under general anesthesia. The patient is placed in the lateral position, and a towel covered with 4 inches of thick foam roll is placed under the opposite axilla. One pillow is placed under the leg laying on the table, and another between the flexed legs. Adhesive tape and a padded chest brace are used to maintain this position. The arm may be supported on a padded arm rest or Mayo stand, or it may be held by an assistant in 90 to 100 degrees of abduction with gentle, controlled intermittent traction. Abduction should not exceed 120 degrees to avoid any stretch injury to the brachial plexus. The skin incision is made over the third rib level from the lateral border of the pectoralis major to the border of the latissimus dorsi, just below the axillary hair line. The incision is deepened through the distal part of the axillary fat pad, just below the lymph nodes down to the chest wall, exposing the digitation of the serratus anterior and the third rib. During the dissection, care is taken to preserve the second and third intercostal brachial cutaneous nerves that innervate the skin of the medial and lateral portions of the upper arm down to the elbow (Fig. 18–8*A* to *E*). The most important nerve in this area is the long thoracic nerve. It is identified along the anterior border of the latissimus dorsi on the digitation of the serratus anterior. The thoracodorsal nerve is located more posteriorly under the latissimus dorsi with the subscapular artery. The serratus anterior is split posteriorly until the long thoracic nerve is reached. It is carefully preserved, and the second and third digitation of this muscle is dissected off the second and third rib with care. The pleural cavity is entered through either the third space or the bed of the third rib after freeing it from the surrounding periosteum. The pleural opening is extended anteriorly and posteriorly, then by using either a small laminectomy or small Finochietto rib spreader, the space is slowly opened to prevent or minimize any rib fracture. Adhesions, if present, are sharply dissected, then the lung is pulled down and packed with folded laboratory pads and gently retracted with a wide malleable retractor.

The sympathetic chain is readily visualized beneath the parietal pleura in the posterior mediastinum lying on the head of the ribs; it can be rolled under the tip of a long pickup. The intercostal vessels are usually located under the chain, but sometimes the first intercostal vein may cross it. On the right side, the sympathetic chain runs lateral to the azygos vein and vagus. On the left side, it is lateral to the vagus and phrenic nerves and the origin of the subclavian artery (Fig. 18–9).

The stellate ganglion, which is usually formed by fusion of the inferior cervical and T1 ganglions, may not be fully seen from this approach, but at least its lower half is usually identified. Occasionally, the second thoracic ganglion may be incorporated with the stellate ganglion.

The posterior pleura overlying the sympathetic chain is incised down to the level of the T5 ganglion, and the chain is exposed by gently pushing the pleura on both sides of the chain (Fig. 18–10). The chain is elevated with a nerve hook at the middle portion, rami are clipped around the fourth thoracic ganglion, and it is divided below this ganglion. Following mobilization of the distal half of the chain, a long right angle clamp is applied to the middle of the chain. Gentle traction helps the rami stand out, and they are clipped with ease proximal to the lower part of the stellate ganglion. Only the distal third of the exposed stellate ganglion is resected together with the rest of the chain. The bleeding vessel can be controlled with a long tip bovie or hemoclip (Kleinert et al, 1980).

A No. 24 or 28 Fr chest tube is passed through either the fifth or sixth intercostal space into a stab wound at about the midaxillary line, placed to the apical part of the chest cavity, and sutured to the skin. The chest cavity is irrigated with lactated Ringer's and bacitracin solution (50,000 units in 1000 ml of Ringer's solution). Usually, three No. 2 Vicryl pericostal sutures are inserted over the upper rib and through holes drilled in the lower rib to avoid injury to the intercostal nerve and artery. The intercostal muscles are sutured with either interrupted or running 5-0 or 4-0 Vicryl sutures. During closure, the chest tube is connected to a Pleur-Evac–type drainage system. The axillary fascia is closed with interrupted 5-0 Vicryl sutures, and the skin is closed with continuous subcuticular 5-0 Vicryl sutures and a Steri-Strip is applied to the skin.

Early postoperative pain may be decreased by an intercostal nerve block, which can be given through the chest cavity before closure by injecting 0.5% Marcaine with epinephrine 5 ml to each intercostal space, two spaces above and below the incision site. Complete lung expansion is verified by

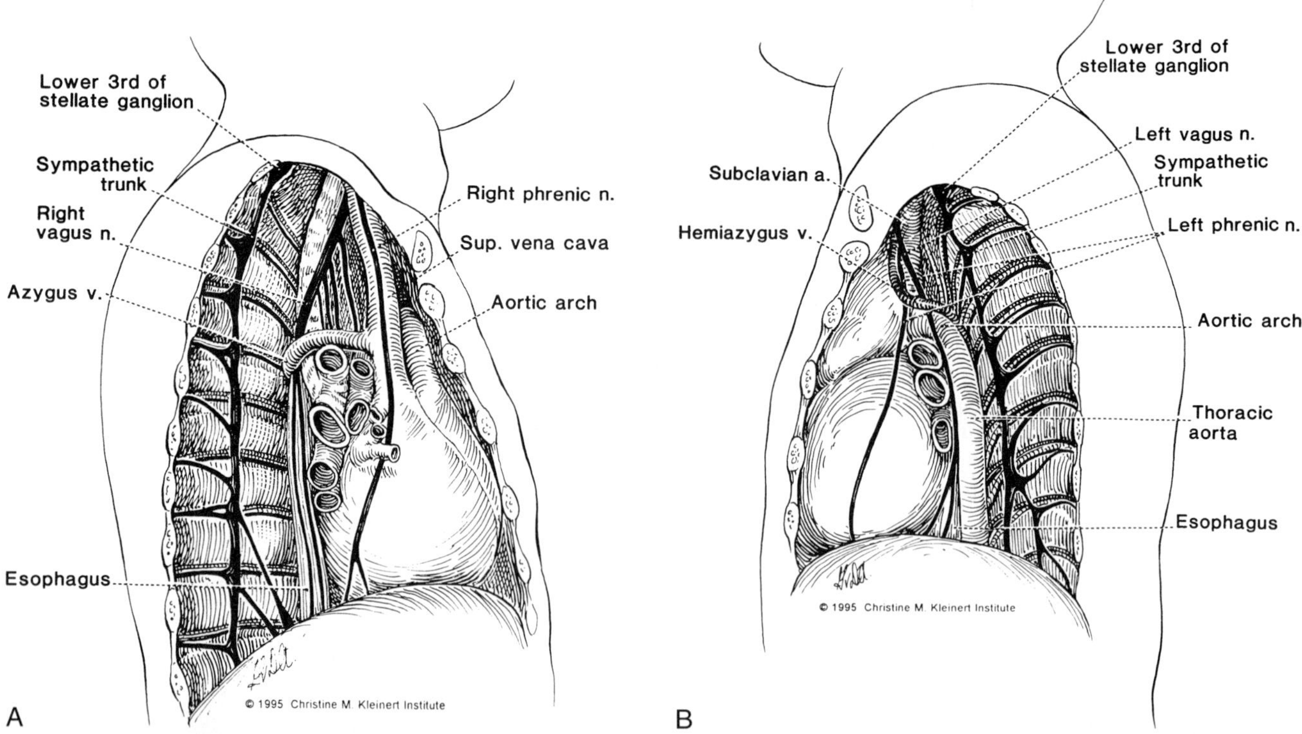

FIGURE 18–9. *A* and *B*, Anatomy of the right and left thoracic sympathetic chain. (© 1995 Christine M. Kleinert Institute.)

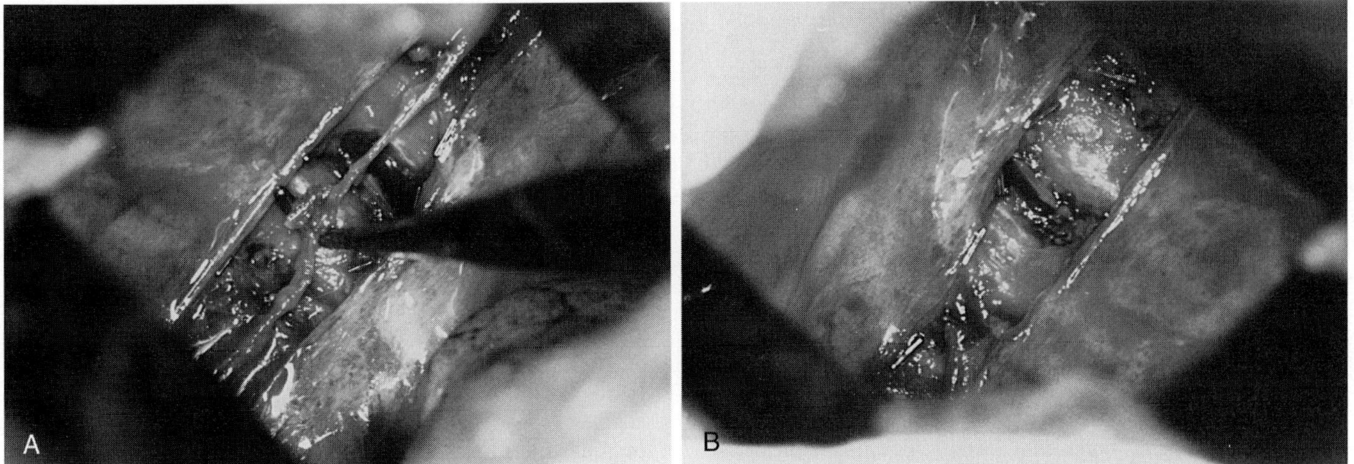

FIGURE 18–10. *A* and *B*, Dissection and removal of upper thoracic sympathetic chain during right transaxillary, transthoracic sympathectomy. (© 1994 Christine M. Kleinert Institute.)

chest x-ray study. Vigorous deep breathing and coughing exercises and intermittent positive breathing are begun the same day. Intravenous antibiotics (Kefzol 1g q6h for 2–3 days) followed by oral cephalosporin are continued for about 1 week. The chest tube is milked every hour to keep it open.

Early mobilization is started on the evening of surgery. The chest tube is usually removed on the second day, and full lung expansion is verified by follow-up chest x-ray study. Most patients go home by the fourth or fifth postoperative day.

The most common complication is intercostal neuritis, which can last weeks or months. This is usually treated with analgesics, repeat intercostal nerve blocks, and application of transcutaneous electrical nerve stimulation (TENS) units.

Recurrent upper extremity pain could be a problem for patients and surgeons if it is caused by residual reflex sympathetic dystrophy or regeneration of the sympathetic nerves. If the third and fourth thoracic ganglions are not removed, the sympathectomy will be incomplete. In some patients, residual sympathetic innervation is from the contralateral side. Wrete (1935) and Skoog (1947) have described an accessory or intermediate ganglion, which usually can be found in the second spinal nerve. This accessory ganglion could be responsible for the recurrent symptoms.

Although the thoracoscopic sympathectomy has not gained uniform popularity, since the early 1970s in this country, it has been successfully used, especially for treatment of bilateral palmar hyperhidrosis and RSD. Recent advances in optics, lighting, and better equipment could increase its popularity because of lower morbidity, shortened hospital stay, less postoperative discomfort, and a quick return to normal lifestyle and work. It is usually performed under general anesthesia with a double-lumen endobronchial tube with full-lung ventilation at the contralateral side and lung collapse on the surgical side for better visualization. For a single-sided sympathectomy, the patient is placed in a lateral position; for bilateral sympathectomy, the patient is placed in the supine position. During the procedure usually three ports are used (Fig. 18–11). Sometimes the fourth port may be necessary for an expandable lung retractor with multiple prongs. The first port is on the fourth space at the midaxillary line. Following collapse of the ipsilateral lung,

a 10- to 12-mm trocar is inserted in the first port, and a thoracoscope is introduced through the trocar. Second and third ports are placed at the third space, one on the anterior and the other on the posterior axillary line for grasper and scissors, respectively. These are also introduced through trocars. With the endoscopic scissors and grasping instruments, the pleura over the sympathetic chain is incised longitudinally. The veins crossing the chain are clipped and cut. The chain is elevated with a blunt nerve hook and resected, including T4, T3, T2, and the lower third of the stellate ganglion. Some authors do not recommend using hemoclips on the chain because it has been postulated that they may contribute to postoperative neuralgia. At completion, the trocar sides are closed, and for safety, a No. 24 or 28 Fr chest tube with a Pleur-Evac–type drainage system can be used and removed the next day (Kaiser and Daniel, 1993). In an alternative technique that can be simpler and easier, only two ports are used: one for the thoracoscope, the other for the grasper. First, the ipsilateral lung is collapsed by a double-lumen endobronchial tube. If desired, a maximum collapse can be achieved by insufflation of 600 to 1000 ml of carbon dioxide to the pleural cavity through a Verres

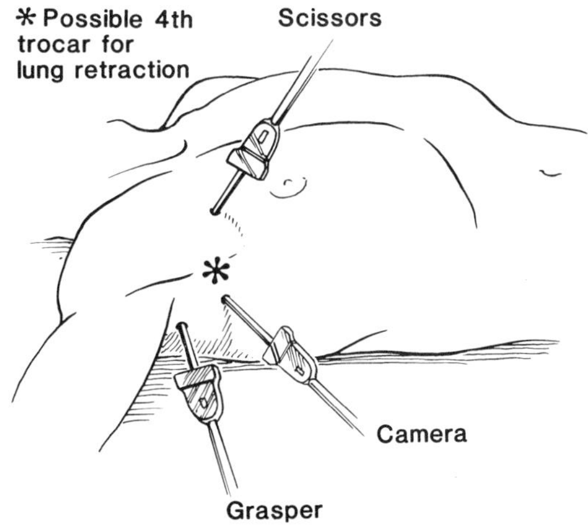

FIGURE 18–11. Position of the patient and location of the trocars during the thoracoscopic sympathectomy.

insufflation needle. After the removal of the needle, two trocars are inserted through the 3rd and 4th intercostal spaces. The thoracoscope and the grasper are then introduced through the trocars. Following visualization of the sympathetic chain, the ganglia to be resected are grasped and lifted together with the parietal pleura (mainly T2–T3 and sometimes T4 and the lower third of the stellate ganglion); they are cauterized without opening the parietal pleura. At the end of the procedure, the lung is inflated while the trocar is kept open. A small amount of pneumothorax can be ignored. Occasionally, a chest tube may be inserted. A bilateral procedure can be performed in one setting for hyperhidrosis.

Wilkinson (1984) reported on radio frequency percutaneous upper thoracic sympathectomy by using probes under local anesthesia in an outpatient setting. The probe produced tissue necrosis at the side of the thoracic ganglion. He reported 18 good results in 19 patients, but this approach has not gained much popularity.

Digital artery sympathectomy was first introduced by Flatt in 1980. This is a periarterial sympathectomy. The concept was first used by Leriche around 1913 in the form of periarterial sympathectomy on the proximal femoral artery on a patient who was suffering a peripheral vascular insufficiency.

The cervicothoracic sympathectomy has been tried for patients with chronic peripheral vascular insufficiency because of the central role of the sympathetic nervous system on blood vessel tone. Disappointing long-term results from this type of sympathectomy on improvement of ulcer healing and pain relief have been explained on the basis of inadequacy of this procedure. Flatt explained these failures by the fact that the brachial plexus did not receive its sympathetic fibers exclusively from the upper thoracic and stellate ganglions. Additional sympathetic branches may reach the extremity through the carotid plexus, sinuvertebral nerve, or the nerve of Kuntz, which is a direct nerve fiber from the T2 ganglion to the brachial plexus (Flatt, 1980).

There are some other reported direct sympathetic connections between the spinal cord and the brachial plexus. Sometimes the sympathetic fibers bypass the sympathetic chain by going through the intermediate ganglion (Skoog, 1947), which is closely located to the T2 spinal nerve. These aberrant pathways, especially the Skoog ganglion, usually remain intact during sympathectomy and later play an important role in residual or recurrent symptoms. Because of these aberrant pathways, a complete upper extremity sympathectomy is nearly impossible, and there is about a 30% to 35% failure rate with the stellate ganglion block. These failures led Flatt (1980) to perform more digital sympathectomies in the palms of patients suffering from digital vascular insufficiency by stripping the adventitial layer of the common and proper digital arteries about 3 to 4 mm in length at the level of their junction. He has reported 1.5° to 2.5°F increases in skin temperature on frostbite patients following digital sympathectomy, and he also reported healing of ulcers and improvement of preexisting symptoms. Morgan and Wilgis (1986) have reported a 1.2°C temperature increase in rabbit ears following sympathectomy on the central artery.

Preoperative pulse volume recording and especially cold stress testing have been recommended by Wilgis (1985) and others. To evaluate the patient with chronic digital ischemia, pulse volume recordings are obtained in the resting state and after cold stress testing, which involves immersing the hand in water (12° to 14°C) for 3 minutes and measuring the pulse volume at 1 and 5 minutes following immersion. In the normal hand, a significant change can be observed by cold stress with markedly decreased pulse volume amplitude at 1 minute. At 5 minutes the pulse volume rebounds to normal or even higher than normal level, which is a normal response. Next, the sympathetic nerve blocks are performed at the distal palm by blocking digital nerves with Marcaine, and pulse volume recordings are obtained at rest and at 1 and 5 minutes following 3 minutes of cold stress. If the cold stress and past cold stress recordings demonstrate good improvement, the digital sympathectomy is considered. Some people use the elevation of digital temperatures in response to peripheral block with Marcaine as a criterion for digital sympathectomy for patients with digital vascular insufficiency. The best responses can be expected in patients with postfrostbite and crush syndromes of the digits. The other vasospastic disorders such as scleroderma, Raynaud's disease, Raynaud's phenomenon, and other arterial insufficiencies associated with vasospasm in diabetes and arteriosclerotic ischemic disease usually respond less favorably.

Wilgis (Morgan et al, 1983; Wilgis, 1985) modified the original technique and removed longer adventitia about 2 cm in length from the common and digital arteries after separating connections between digital nerves and arteries, including the four sympathetic branches traveling from digital nerve to the vessel (Figs. 18–12 to 18–14). The procedure can be performed under high loop magnification or preferably under an operative microscope so as not to damage the media and intima (Egloff et al, 1982). A crease or zigzag incision can be used (Fig. 18–15).

In 1991, Jones reported a more extensive technique of digital sympathectomy, especially in patients who had connective tissue disease with vascular insufficiency. After observing significant fibrosis in the palms and proliferative fibrosis around the common and proper digital arteries in these patients, he did extensive stripping of the superficial arch and common digital arteries. In some cases, the sympathectomy extended to the digital arteries. For this extensive sympathectomy, the incision along the course of the superficial arch can be extended to the fingers in a zigzag manner. If a segment occlusion is present, it can be bypassed with

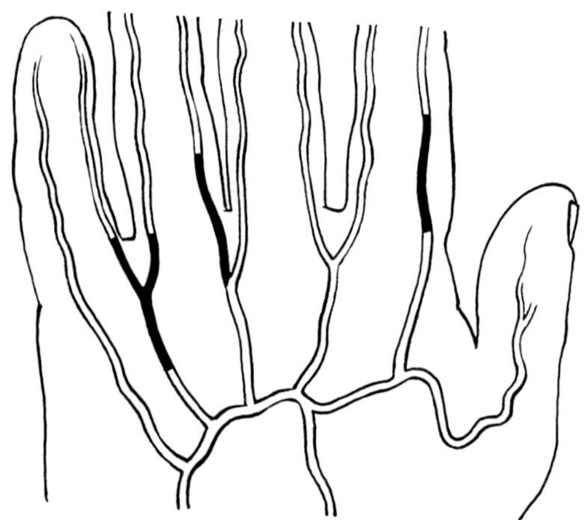

FIGURE 18–12. Levels of digital sympathectomy.

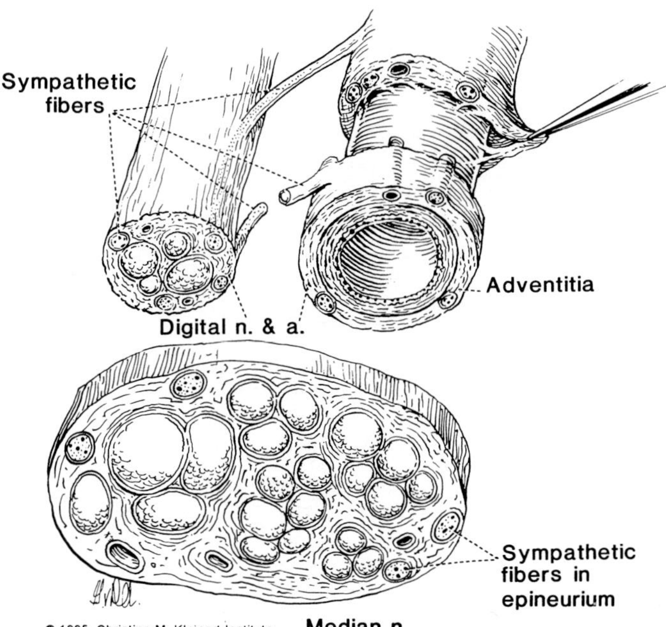

FIGURE 18–13. Location of the sympathetic fibers in epineurium of median nerve and sympathetic innervation of a digital artery. (© 1995 Christine M. Kleinert Institute.)

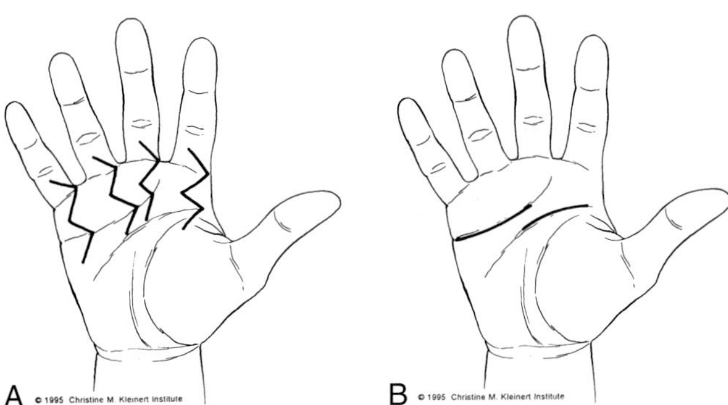

FIGURE 18–15. *A,* Zigzag incision for digital sympathectomy. *B,* Crease incision of digital sympathectomy. (© 1995 Christine M. Kleinert Institute.)

periarterial sympathectomy. The areas distal to it maintain their adrenergic innervation. He postulated that the beneficial effect of periarterial sympathectomy could be due to loss of support around the artery, and he called the procedure an *adventitiectomy* rather than a sympathectomy.

Although Jones (1987) reported decreased pain, decreased cold intolerance, and improved healing of digital ulcers with extended sympathectomy, this remains to be seen after long-term follow up (El-Gammal and Blair, 1991).

PARAVERTEBRAL LUMBAR SYMPATHETIC BLOCK AND LUMBAR SYMPATHECTOMY

Anatomy. The preganglionic sympathetic center for the lower extremity is located in the T10–L3 spinal cord segments (see Fig. 18–2). Fibers originating from these centers usually make synapses in the L1–L4 lumbar ganglions. The postganglionic gray fibers enter the roots of the lower lumbar and sacral plexus to innervate the lower extremity. Similar to cervicothoracic sympathetic systems, usually a small percentage of preganglion fibers (about 15%) either cross over to innervate the opposite side through conventional pathways or synapse in the more peripherally located intermediate ganglion. Most of the sympathetic supply of the lower limbs, especially below the knee, comes through the L2–L3 ganglions; L1–L4 has little contribution.

The lumbar part of the sympathetic ganglionic chain is separated from the somatic nerves by the psoas muscle and its fascia, and lies along the anterolateral side of the vertebral bodies. Usually about four or five ganglions are present in the lumbar region (Fig. 18–16).

Theoretically, one injection to the L2–L3 level should produce enough sympathetic block. Clinically, to obtain a complete block, injections are given at the L2–L3 levels.

Indications. Indications for lumbar sympathetic block include pain relief in RSD, phantom pain, central pain, and postfrostbite syndrome; to improve circulation in some vasospastic and vascular conditions, such as scleroderma, Raynaud's disease, and acrocyanosis; and in Buerger's disease and some embolic, traumatic, and other occlusive vascular diseases.

An accurate diagnosis is important in RSD because it may be confused with such neurovascular disorders as Raynaud's disease, Raynaud's phenomenon, scleroderma, acrocyanoses,

an interpositional vein graft if the patient has satisfactory distal run off on arteriogram. After this extensive sympathectomy, Jones (1987) observed that there were three components that contributed to ischemia in the fingers of the patients with connective tissue disease: vasoconstrictive response, periarterial fibrosis producing external compression on the digital vessels, and intimal proliferation.

Thus, the sympathectomy may produce improved blood flow in the arteries not only by relieving the sympathetic vasoconstrictive effect on the vessel but also by removing the vasoconstrictive layer of adventitial fibrosis around the arteries. This type of decompression of the digital arteries is called decompression arteriolysis.

Kaarela (Junila et al, 1991; Kaarela, 1991; Kaarela et al, 1991) has shown in animal models that adrenergic innervation of the blood vessels will disappear only at the site of

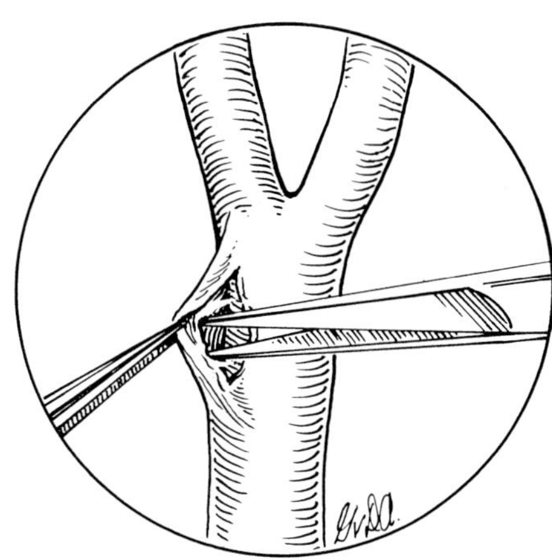

FIGURE 18–14. Technique of digital periarterial sympathectomy; elevation and dissection of adventitia approximately 2 cm in length from common and proper digital arteries.

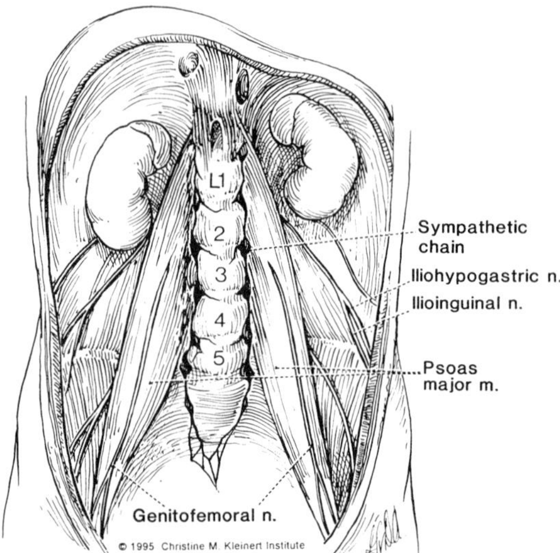

FIGURE 18–16. Posterior abdominal wall including lumbar sympathetic chain with its relationship to lumbar vertebral column, iliopsoas muscle and genitofemoral nerve.

and erythromelalgia, all of which should be considered in the differential diagnosis. Lack of response or a marginal response to adequate conservative treatment in sympathetic dystrophy is an indication for a trial of paravertebral lumbar sympathetic block (Kleinert et al, 1980).

Technique of Paravertebral Lumbar Sympathetic Block. The lumbar sympathetic block is technically more difficult to perform than a stellate ganglion block. Although a one-needle technique has been described, the most complete and best possible result is obtained by using the three-needle technique to block the L2, L3, and L4 ganglions. Not only is the block more difficult to perform, but its success is also more difficult to evaluate. For this reason, the block has been discredited as a predictor of the success of sympathectomy. The most important objective finding is vasodilation of peripheral veins and a feeling of warmth. Vasodilation and relief of symptoms are the best indicators of a satisfactory block. If relief of symptoms is good but only temporary after an L3–L4 lumbar sympathetic block, lumbar sympathectomy may be indicated (Kleinert et al, 1980).

The patient is placed in the prone position, and a pillow is placed under the abdomen to flatten the lumbar curvature. The midline is marked, and three transverse lines are drawn through the 2nd, 3rd, and 4th spinal processes, which correspond to the 2nd, 3rd, and 4th lumbar ganglions to be blocked. A second line is drawn approximately four fingerbreadths (8 to 10 cm) lateral and parallel to the midline. The intersections of this lateral line and transverse lines mark the sites of injections (Fig. 18–17). First, skin wheals are raised at the intersections by using a 30-gauge needle; then 10-cm long, 22-gauge spinal needles are inserted through these three sites at approximately a 45-degree angle to the midline, inclining toward the lumbar vertebra until the needle touches the vertebral body about 4 to 5 cm in. If it does not strike the vertebral body, the needle should be reangled. After the needle touches the vertebral body, it is slid off 2 to 3 mm, and 10 ml of 0.5% plain Marcaine is injected after one is certain that no blood can be aspirated (Fig. 18–18). The

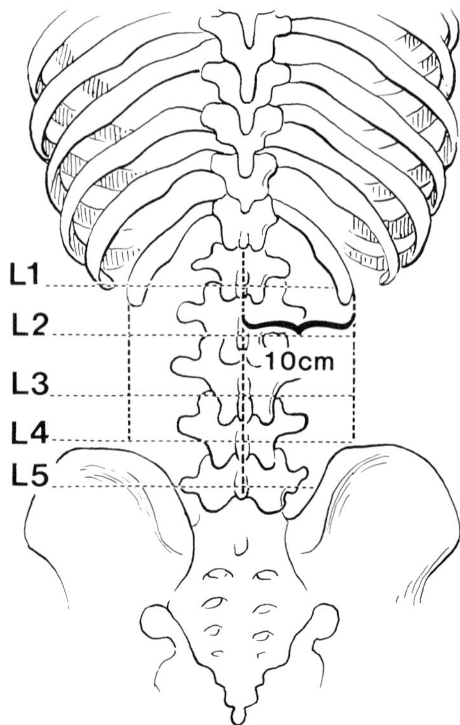

© 1995 Christine M. Kleinert Institute

FIGURE 18–17. Lumbar sympathetic block. Topographical anatomy. Location of two or three injection sites at the junction of three horizontal lines with perpendicular line (see text). (© 1995 Christine M. Kleinert Institute.)

injection is repeated at the L2, L3, and L4 levels (Cousins and Bridenbaugh, 1988; Kleinert et al, 1980).

Lumbar Sympathectomy

The first lumbar sympathectomy was performed by Diez in 1924 for arterial occlusion disease of the lower extremity. Today, controversy still exists concerning its indications, physiological effects, and long-term results on ischemia and neurovascular disorders of the lower extremity.

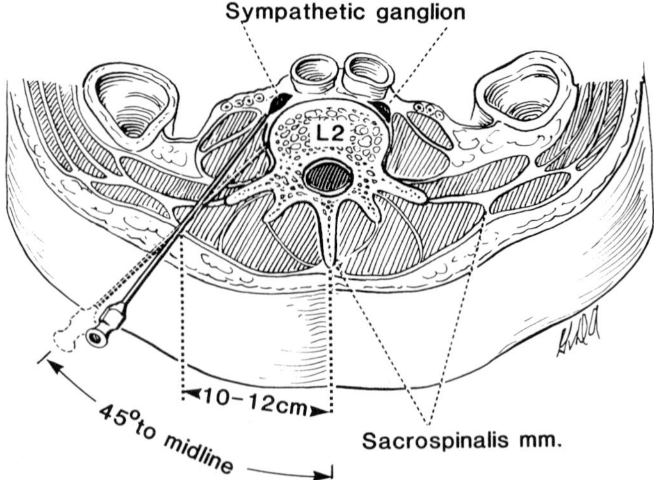

FIGURE 18–18. Technique of the lumbar sympathetic block (see text).

Although four to five lumbar ganglions have been described, their numbers sometimes vary from two to eight. They usually are located on the anterolateral aspect of the corresponding lumbar vertebrae and are separated from the somatic nerves by psoas muscle and fascia.

Cross communication usually is present between both sides of the sympathetic chain, and the intermediate ganglions are present on the rami communicantes in about 15% of cases. For this reason, it is important to divide all of the rami during the sympathectomy. Usually, removal of L2–L3 will give satisfactory sympathetic denervation of the lower limb, but to achieve a more complete denervation the L4 is also included. Indications for lumbar sympathectomy are similar to those for upper extremity sympathectomy and include RSD; phantom pain; central pain; postfrostbite syndrome; hyperhidrosis; insufficient circulation in some vasospastic and vascular problems, such as scleredema, Raynaud's disease and phenomenon, and acrocyanosis; and Buerger's disease and other occlusive ischemic arterial diseases. The most common indication is RSD. Before considering a lumbar sympathectomy for this condition, the patient should have a series of successful lumbar sympathetic blocks resulting in transient relief of pain and other symptoms.

In the 1940s and 1950s, lumbar sympathectomy was an important procedure in the management of occlusive arterial disease of the lower extremity. Now its role is limited to certain conditions. Its physiological effect on the arterial vessel wall of the lower extremity is not well defined. It has been shown that following sympathectomies, arteriovenous shunts open and increased blood flow is usually restricted to the skin, with increased skin temperature and a feeling of warmth. This usually occurs through vasodilation of veins and arteries with increased capillary flow. The muscle blood flow, which is automatically regulated according to muscle metabolism, is not affected by lumbar sympathectomy (Cronenwett and Lindenauer, 1977; Walker and Johnson, 1980).

Clinical series have demonstrated that the major benefits of lumbar sympathectomy are improvement of pain at rest, healing of some superficial skin ulcers, and an increase in the circulation of the skin without helping claudication (Moore and Hall, 1973).

If sympathectomy is used as an adjunct to arterial reconstruction, it may increase total blood flow to the extremity, decrease vascular resistance, and reduce the early graft thrombosis, but long-term follow-up has not shown much difference (Terry et al, 1970). It has also been tried as an alternative to amputation in cases in which the arterial reconstruction is practically impossible. During the early postoperative period, it is very important for the patient to stop smoking, to care for any foot lesions, and to avoid other factors leading to vasoconstriction. These all may be helpful for the effectiveness of the lumbar sympathectomy (Collins and Rich, 1981; Walker and Johnson, 1980).

Contraindications to lumbar sympathectomy are poor general condition of the patient and advanced cardiovascular disease.

Operative Technique. Access to the lumbar sympathetic chain is best achieved with an oblique midabdominal or umbilical level transverse abdominal muscle splitting incision using the extraperitoneal approach (Fig. 18–19). General anesthesia is used, and the patient is placed in the lateral

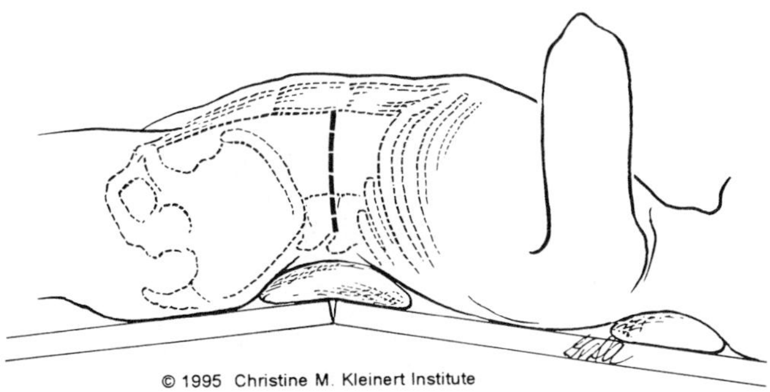

© 1995 Christine M. Kleinert Institute

FIGURE 18–19. Patient's position for left lumbar sympathectomy. Patient's lower back slightly hyperextended, and a lumbar support is used. Also patient is slightly rotated to opposite side. (© 1995 Christine M. Kleinert Institute.)

jack-knife position with adequate padding between the knees and in the axilla. If an oblique incision is used, it is carried in the flank, starting near the anterior superior iliac crest and extending proximally superior and lateral to the tip of the twelfth rib. The incision is carried to the muscle layer. The external and internal oblique muscles are split with the rectus sheath. The transversalis muscle and fascia are opened in the direction of its fibers. The peritoneum is gently separated by blunt and finger dissection from the lateral abdominal wall and retracted medially from the lumbar adipose tissue. Further retraction and dissection brings the psoas major muscle into view. It is located more anteriorly, and the quadratus lumborum muscle is located laterally and posteriorly. Dissection between these muscles should be avoided. The ilioinguinal and genitofemoral nerves are on the medial aspect of the psoas muscle and follow a downward and lateral course. The genitofemoral nerve, which is more medial, can be mistaken for the lumbar sympathetic chain. When the correct plane is entered, the dissection will elevate the kidney, ureter, and genital vessels, which are reflected medially with the peritoneum. The ureter and genital vessels should be identified under the peritoneum so as to avoid any injury.

By further retraction and dissection, the lateral aspect of the vena cava on the right and the aorta on the left are exposed. On the right, the chain is located posterior to the vena cava on the anterior lateral aspect of the vertebral column at the junction of the vertebrae and the medial aspect of the psoas muscle. It may be necessary to divide several lumbar veins to visualize it. On the left, the chain lies in the groove between the psoas muscle and the vertebral body. The aorta is usually located anterior medial to it, making dissection somewhat easier. The chain is usually palpable as a bow string on the vertebral body.

After adequate dissection and exposure, the chain is lifted with a blunt nerve hook (Fig. 18–20). Usually two or three ganglions, including T2, T3, and T4, are removed by clipping and dividing all rami between the silver clips. When the L3 ganglion is not found in its usual location, exposure to a higher level may be necessary. Sometimes, fused L2–L3 or L3 alone can be found deeper posteriorly after separation of the medial fibers of the psoas muscle. In males, the T1 ganglion should be left intact, especially in bilateral lumbar sympathectomy, to avoid impotence.

Following satisfactory hemostasis, any rent in the peritoneum is repaired, and following operative field irrigation, it

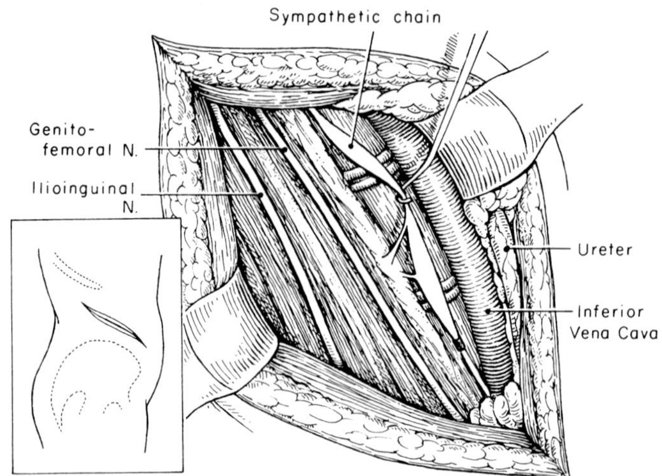

FIGURE 18–20. Alternative incision for right lumbar sympathectomy and technique of lumbar sympathectomy.

is allowed to fall back into position. The muscle layers are sequentially closed with interrupted Vicryl sutures, and the skin is closed with continuous subcuticular 5-0 Vicryl suture. The nasogastric tube usually is removed on the first or second postoperative day, and early ambulation is encouraged (Effeney and Stoney, 1993; Haimovici, 1989; Kleinert et al, 1973, 1980).

Complications. Major complications are hemorrhage from lumbar veins and injury to major vessels, such as the vena cava, aorta, and ureter. The somatic nerves can also be mistakenly removed as the sympathetic chain.

As a late complication, postsympathectomy neuralgia can occur fairly frequently about 2 weeks after surgery. The pain is fairly severe, of a burning-aching type, and occurs mainly at night over the cutaneous distribution of L1–L3, and occasionally T12. The distribution, often with hyperesthesia, is usually along the anterior and lateral femoral cutaneous, genitofemoral, and ilioinguinal nerves. Its etiology is not clear but is usually attributed to neuroma formation in the chain, ischemia, or traumatic neuritis of the sensory nerves adjacent to the sympathetic chain. It is usually self-limiting and treated conservatively (Haimovici, 1989).

The lumbar sympathectomy may not be effective because of an incomplete removal of the sympathetic chain, presence of intermediate ganglions, cross over from the contralateral side, variations and distribution of the sympathetic ganglions and rami, (rarely) regeneration of the chain, and an increased sensitivity of the blood vessels. This is usually explained by the exaggerated response of the smooth muscles of the vessel walls to the circulating catecholamines.

References

Adson AW, Brown GE: Treatment of Raynaud's disease by lumbar ramisection and ganglionectomy and perivascular sympathetic neurectomy of the common iliacs. JAMA *84*:1908, 1925.

Adson AW, Brown GE: The treatment of Raynaud's disease by resection of the upper thoracic and lumbar sympathetic ganglia and trunks. Surg Gynecol Obstet *48*:577, 1929.

Adson AW, Graig WM, Brown GE: Essential hyperhidrosis cured by sympathetic ganglionectomy and trunk resection. Arch Surg *31*:794, 1935.

Best CH, Taylor NB: Best and Taylor's Physiological Basis of Medical Practice, 21st ed. Baltimore, William & Wilkins, 1991.

Collins GJ Jr, Rich NM: Clinical results of lumbar sympathectomy. Am Surg 47:31–35, 1981.

Cousins, MJ, Bridenbaugh PO (eds): Neural Blockade in Clinical Anesthesia and Management of Pain, 2nd ed. Philadelphia, J.B. Lippincott Company, 1988.

Cronenwett JL, Lindenauer SM: Direct measurements of arteriovenous anastomotic blood flow after lumbar sympathectomy. Surgery *82*(1):82–89, 1977.

Diez J: Le traitement des affections trophiques et gangrenenses des memebres inferieurs par la resection du sympathique lombo-sacre'. Reo Neurol *33*:184–192, 1926.

Effeney DJ, Stoney RS (eds): Wylie's Atlas of Vascular Surgery—Disorders of the Extremities. Philadelphia, J.B. Lippincott Company, 1993.

Egloff DV, Mifsud RP, Verdan CL: Superselective digital sympathectomy in Raynaud's phenomenon. Hand; *12*:110–114, 1982.

El-Gammal TA, Blair WF: Digital periarterial sympathectomy for ischemic digital pain and ulcers. J Hand Surg: *16B*(4):382–385, 1991.

Firkin BG, Whitworth JA: Dictionary of Medical Eponyms. Carnforth, Lancs, UK, The Parthenon Publishing Group, 1987.

Flatt, A: Digital artery sympathectomy. J Hand Surg *5A*(6):550–556, 1980.

Gibbon JH: Surgery of the Chest. Philadelphia, W.B. Saunders Company, 1962.

Green DP (ed): Operative Hand Surgery, 3rd ed. New York, Churchill Livingstone, 1993.

Haimovici H (ed): Haimovici's Vascular Surgery—Principles and Techniques. Norwalk, Appleton & Lange, 1989.

Jabouley M: Le traitment de quelgues troubles trophiques de le pied et de la jambe par la denudation de L'artere et la distension des nerfs vasculaires. Med Lyon *91*:457, 1899.

Jones FN, Imbriglia JE, Steen VD, Medsger TA: Surgery for scleroderma of the hand. J Hand Surg *12A*(3):391–400, 1987.

Jones FN: Acute and chronic ischemia of the hand pathophysiology, treatment, and prognosis. J Hand Surg *16A*(6):1074–1083, 1991.

Jonnesco T: Angine de poitrine querie par la resection du sympathique cervicothoracique. Bull Acart Med Paris *84*:93, 1920.

Junila J, Kaarela IO, Waris T: Failure of perivascular sympathectomy to remove adrenergic nerves from peripheral vessels of the rabbit ear skin. Scand J Plast Reconstr Hand Surg 25(3):199–202, 1991.

Kaarela IO: Perivascular sympathectomy of the metacarpal artery of the rabbit paw fails to remove distal adrenergic innervation. Scand J Plast Reconstr Hand Surg *25*:121–124, 1991.

Kaarela O, Raatikainen CS, Huopaniemi T, Waris T: Effect of perivascular sympathectomy on distal adrenergic innervation in the hands of monkeys. J Hand Surg *16B*(4):386–388, 1991.

Kaiser LR, Daniel TM: Thoracoscopic surgery. Boston, Little Brown & Company, 1993.

Kandel E, Schwartz JH, Jessell TM (eds). Principles of Neural Science, 3rd ed. New York, Elsevier, 1991.

Kleinert HE, Cole MN, Wayne L, Harvey R, Kutz JE, Atasoy E: Post traumatic sympathetic dystrophy. Orthop Clin North Am *4*:917–927, 1973.

Kleinert HE, Cook FW, Kutz JE: Neuro-vascular disorders of the upper extremities treated by transaxillary sympathectomy. Arch Surg *90*:612–616, 1965.

Kleinert HE, Norberg H, McDonough JJ: Surgical sympathectomy upper and lower extremity. *In* Omer GE, Spinner M (eds): Management of Peripheral Nerve Problems, 1st ed. Philadelphia, W. B. Saunders Company, 1980, pp 285–302.

Leriche R: De L'elongation et de la section des nerfs perivasculaires dans certaines syndromes douloureux d'origine arteriele at dans quelques troubles trophiques. Lyon Chirc *10*:378, 1913.

Leriche R, Fontaine R: L'anesthesie isolee du ganglion étoile: sa technique, ses indications, ses resultatas. Press Medicale *42*:849, 1934.

Leriche R, Fontaine R: Technique de l'ablatian du ganglion étoile. J Chir *41*:353, 1933.

Leriche R: De la causalgie enuisagée commeune neurite sympathetique et de son traitement par la denudation et L'excision de plexus nerveux periarteriels. Presse Med 25: 178–180, 1916.

Mandl F: Die paravertebrale Injektion. Vienna, Springer-Verlag, 1926.

Miller LM, Morgan RF: Vasospastic disorders etiology recognition, and treatment. Hand Clin 9(1)171–187, 1993.

Moore DC: Regional Block, 4th ed. Springfield, IL, Charles C Thomas, 1965.

Moore WS (ed): Vascular Surgery: A Comprehensive Review. Philadelphia, W.B. Saunders Company, 1991.

Moore WS, Hall AD: Effects of lumbar sympathectomy in skin capillary blood flow in arterial occlusion disease. J Surg Res *14*:151, 1973.

Morgan FR, Reisman NR, Wilgis EFS: Anatomic localization of sympathetic nerves in the hand. J Hand Surg *8*(3)283–288, 1983.

Morgan FR, Wilgis EFS: Thermal changes in a rabbit ear model after sympathectomy. J Hand Surg *11A*(1)120–124, 1986.

Palumbo LT: Upper dorsal sympathectomy without Horner's syndrome. Arch Surg *71*:743–751, 1955.

Royle ND: A new operative procedure in the treatment of spastic paralysis and its experimental basis. Med J Aust 1:77, 1924.

Skoog T: Ganglia in the communicating rami of the cervical sympathetic trunk. Lancet 253:457, 1947.

Smithwick RH: The rationale and technique of sympathectomy for relief of vascular spasm of the extremities. N Engl J Med 222:699–703, 1940.

Spurling RG: Causalgia of the upper extremities. Treatment by dorsal sympathetic ganglionectomy. Arch Neurol Psychiatr *23*:784, 1930.

Terry HJ, Allen JS, Taylor GW: The effect of adding lumbar sympathectomy to reconstructive arterial surgery in the lower limb. Br J Surg *57*(1):51–55, 1970.

Walker PM, Johnson KW: Predicting the success of a sympathectomy: A prospective study using discriminant function and multiple regression analysis. Surg. 97:216, 1980.

Wilgis EFS: Digital sympathectomy for vascular insufficiency. Hand Clin *1*(2)361–367, 1985.

Wilkinson HA: Radio frequency percutaneous upper thoracic sympathectomy. N Engl J Med *311*:34–38, 1984.

Williams PL, et al (eds): Gray's Anatomy, 37th ed. New York, Churchill Livingstone, 1989.

Wrete M: Entwicklung der intermediaren Ganglien beim Menschen. Gegenbaurers Morphol Jahrb *75*:229, 1935.

Part IV

ANATOMICAL OVERVIEW

Chapter 19

• Miguel A. Pirela-Cruz

Surgical Exposures of the Peripheral Nerves in the Extremities

OVERVIEW

The primary objective of this chapter is to provide a basic review of surgical anatomy and common surgical approaches to the exposure of peripheral nerves of the extremities. Clinical correlation is presented. For practical reasons, extensile approaches have been described, which can be modified to suit the clinical demands of a given case.

NERVES OF THE UPPER EXTREMITY

Brachial Plexus

ANATOMY

The brachial plexus is formed by the anterior rami of C5 to T1. It provides innervation to the muscles and skin of the upper extremity (with the exception of the trapezius muscle) that originate from the back and chest wall. At times, it may receive contributions from C4 (prefix) and T2 (postfix). In addition to the sensory and muscle innervation, the brachial plexus also provides a conduit for sympathetic nerves to the upper extremity. As memorized in medical school, the mnemonic *Robert Taylor Drinks Cold Beer* comes to mind. This is an easy way to recall the segments of the plexus. The brachial plexus is composed of five *r*oots, three *t*runks, six *d*ivisions, three *c*ords, and fifteen peripheral *b*ranches.

The roots of C5 and C6 form the upper trunk. The C7 root continues to become the middle trunk and the C8 and T1 roots form the lower trunk of the plexus. Each trunk divides into an anterior and posterior division that continue as medial lateral and posterior cords. The nomenclature is derived from the position of the cord with respect to the axillary artery. The medial cord is a continuation of the anterior division of the lower trunk. The lateral cord is formed by the confluence of the anterior division of the upper and middle divisions. The posterior cord is composed of all three posterior divisions combined.

The long thoracic (C5, C6, and C7) and the dorsal scapular (C5) nerves branch off at the root segment. The long thoracic with branches innervates the serratus anterior muscle. The dorsal scapular nerve supplies the levator scapulae and the rhomboid muscles.

Two additional nerves come off at the trunk level—the nerve to the subclavius (C5 and C6) and the suprascapular nerve (C5 and C6) to innervate the supraspinatus and infraspinatus muscles.

From the lateral cord, two additional nerves originate. The lateral pectoral (C5, C6, and C7) supplies the pectoralis major and the musculocutaneous nerve (MCN) (C5, C6, and C7) to the muscles of the anterior compartment of the arm. After innervating the anterior compartment muscles, the MCN then surfaces and continues as the lateral antebrachial cutaneous nerve and provides sensation to the radial forearm. The median nerve (C6, C7, and C8) is formed by nerve contributions from the medial and lateral cords. The median nerve, usually, supplies all the muscles of the forearm except the flexor carpi ulnaris (FCU) and the ulnar two profundi of the flexor digitorum profundus (FDP) tendon. Within the hand, the median nerve supplies all the intrinsic muscles of the thumb except for adductor pollicis, the deep head of the flexor pollicis brevis, and the ulnar two lumbricals which are innervated by the ulnar nerve. The median nerve also provides volar sensibility for the radial 3 1/2 digits and radial side of the hand.

The medial pectoral nerve (C8 and T1) originates from the medial cord of the plexus and supplies the pectoralis minor and pectoralis major muscles. The important ulnar nerve (C8 and T1) arises from the medial cord of the brachial plexus includes and supplies the FCU muscle and the two ulnar profundi in the forearm. The ulnar nerve also innervates the adductor pollicis, deep head of the flexor pollicis brevis of the thumb, and all of the intrinsics of the hand except for the radial two lumbrical muscles. The ulnar nerve's most common skin innervation pattern is sensibility to the ulnar half of the ring finger, the entire surface of the small finger, and both the volar and dorsal surfaces of the ulnar side of the hand. Two large sensory branches originate from the medial cord, the medial brachial cutaneous (C8 and T1) and the antebrachial cutaneous nerves (C8 and T1). These nerves supply the ulnar aspect of the arm and forearm, respectively.

The posterior cord of the plexus is the largest cord and gives origin to several nerves. The upper subscapular nerve (C5 and C6) innervates the subscapular muscle. The lower subscapular nerve (C5 and C6) innervates part of the subscapularis and the teres major muscles. The thoracodorsal nerve (C5, C6, and C7) also originates from the posterior cord to innervate the latissimus dorsi muscle. The axillary nerve (C5 and C6) is the next nerve to originate from the posterior cord. It passes through the quadrangular space enroute to innervate the teres minor and deltoid muscles, and then provides sensibility to the skin over the lateral shoulder. The largest nerve to come off the posterior cord is the radial nerve (C5, C6, C7, C8, and T1). The radial nerve

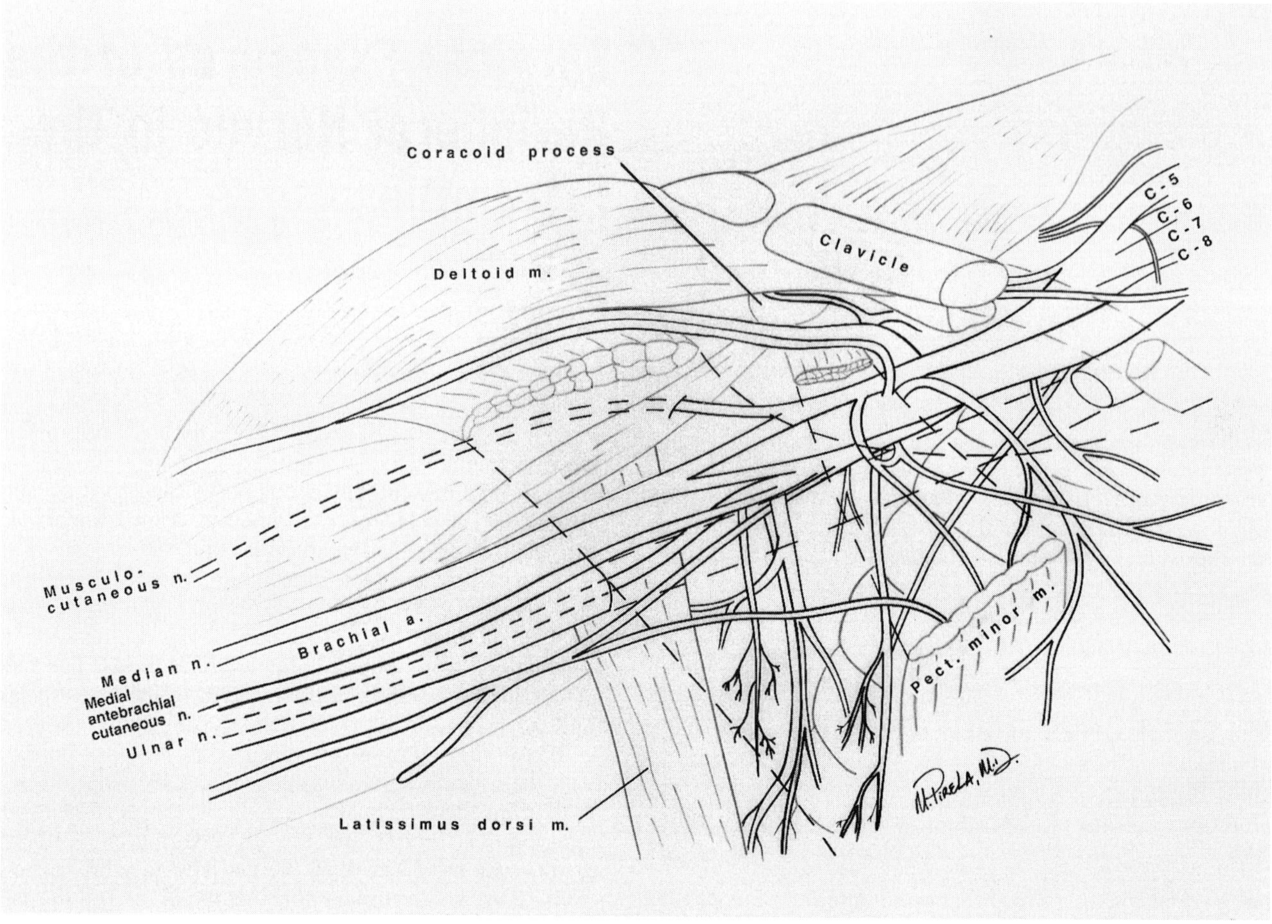

FIGURE 19–1. The brachial plexus.

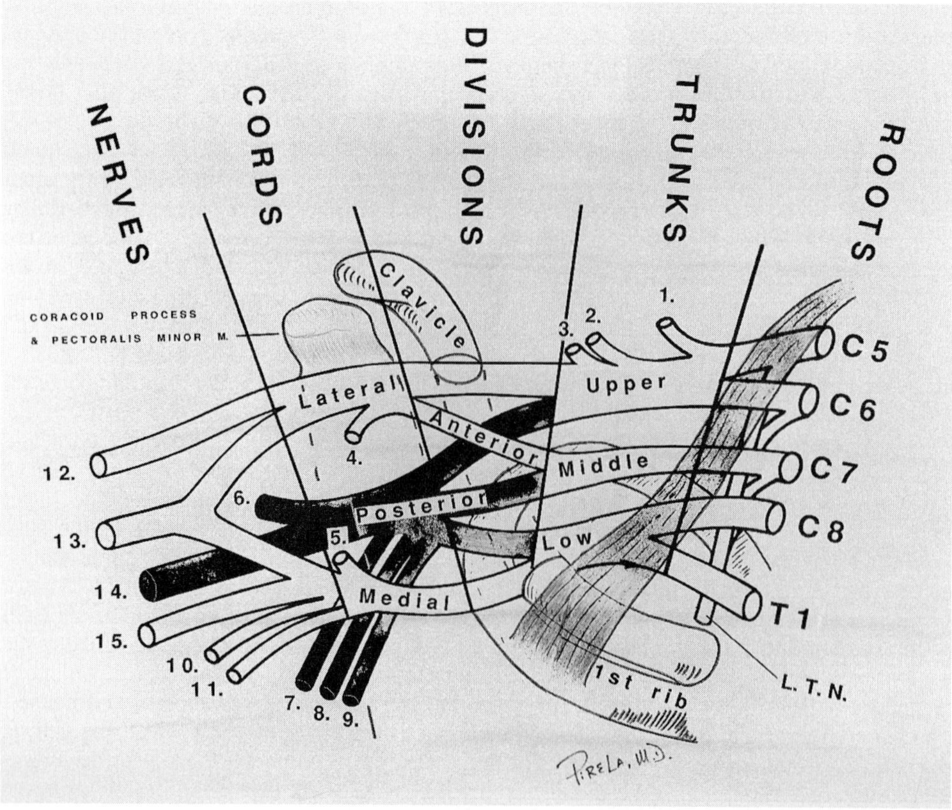

FIGURE 19–2. The brachial plexus of the right upper extremity. 1, Dorsal scapular nerve. 2, Suprascapular nerve. 3, Subclavian nerve. 4, Lateral pectoral nerve. 5, Medial pectoral nerve. 6, Axillary nerve. 7, Lower subscapular nerve. 8, Thoracodorsal nerve. 9, Upper subscapular nerve. 10, Medial antebrachial cutaneous nerve. 11, Medial brachial nerve. 12, Musculocutaneous nerve. 13, Median nerve. 14, Radial nerve. 15, Ulnar nerve. As a review exercise, cover the legend and identify the branches and segments of the plexus. LTN, Long thoracic nerve.

provides innervation to all of the extensors of the arm and forearm. It also supplies sensibility to the extensor surface of the arm, forearm, radial side of the hand to approximately the 4th metacarpal, and lastly, the dorsal skin of the radial 3 1/2 digits distally to about the distal interphalangeal joint level.

The anatomical description of the brachial plexus given is a simple overview of the most common presenting pattern. The operating surgeon should be familiar with the anatomical variations that may exist. The goals of surgery should be very clear to the patient and surgeon. The surgeon should also be equipped to handle all aspects of the reconstruction including, but not limited to, neurological repair, muscle and tendon transfers, and arthrodesis of joints, depending on the clinical circumstances.

Patient Position. Supine.

Surgical Equipment. Hand table, small bolster under the upper back and shoulder, nerve stimulator, and somatosensory evoked potentials.

General Comments. The extensile anterior approach to the brachial plexus is the exposure that is most commonly used when surgically addressing the brachial plexus (Kerr, 1918; Walsh, 1877). However, it can be modified to address specific problems above or below the clavicle, or involving the middle portion of the plexus. An osteotomy of the clavicle should be avoided because the development of a nonunion is possible and the clavicle does provide support to the upper extremity. However, if an osteotomy is performed, stable internal fixation and bone grafting of the clavicle is beneficial to obtain union. Additionally, segmented removal of the midportion of the clavicle offers excellent exposure of the plexus in difficult cases. Lastly, when exposing the inferior segment of the plexus, an attempt should be made to avoid the anterior axillary fold because this region is notorious for developing a thick scar and causing an adduction contracture of arm. The anatomy of the brachial plexus can be reviewed (Figs. 19–1 and 19–2).

EXPOSURE OF THE BRACHIAL PLEXUS

Anterior Extensile Exposure

With the arm abducted, begin just anterior to the anterior border of the deltoid muscle following the orientation of the deltoid distally (Fig. 19–3). Lateral and inferior to the anterior axillary fold, the incision is curved posteriorly (avoiding the skin fold entirely) and then curved along the medial border of the arm, following the course of the neurovascular bundle (ulnar nerve and brachial artery). If so desired, the length of the incision can be extended further distally.

Superiorly, the approach can be extended toward and across the clavicle, crossing the clavicle approximately at the junction of the middle and distal thirds and then curved medially 3 to 4 cm toward the anterior border of the sternocleidomastoid muscle. As the incision approaches the base of the sternocleidomastoid muscle, it is then curved in a cephalad direction toward the inferior angle of the mandible.

Medially, the dissection is carried out through the superficial fascia and platysma muscle, exposing the external jugular vein and omohyoid muscle. If required, the external

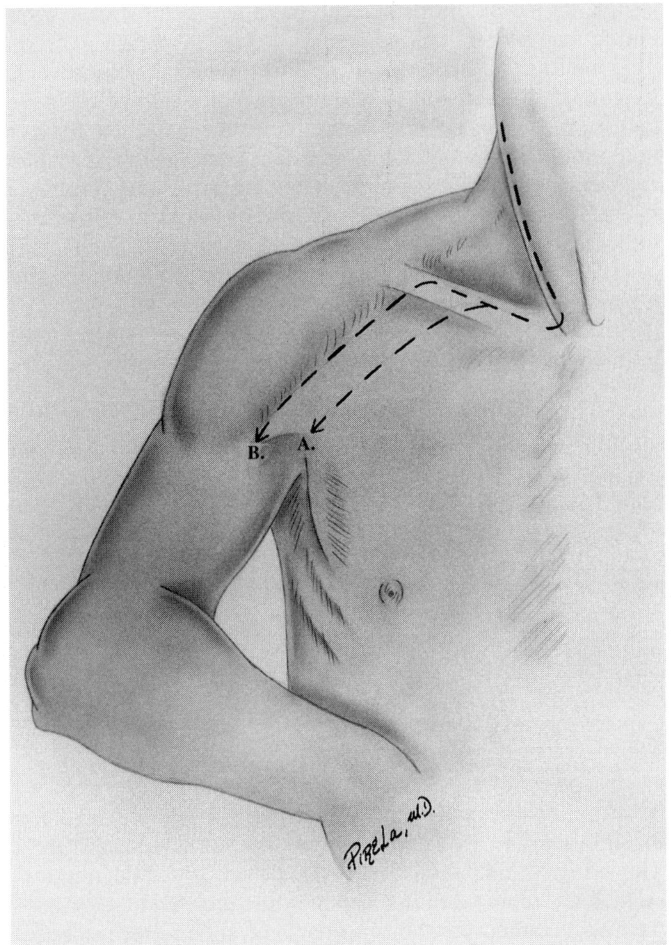

FIGURE 19–3. Incisions used for the extensile exposure of the brachial plexus. Incision A offers a more direct approach. Incision B can be used if simultaneous exposure of the shoulder joint is required.

jugular may be ligated and transected for additional exposure. The inferior belly of the omohyoid muscle is divided and tagged for later repair and is reflected inferiorly. The dissection is continued to the deep fascia. If additional medial exposure is required, the clavicular insertion of the sternocleidomastoid muscle may be released to visualize the roots of the plexus. At this point, identify the anterior scalenus muscle, the phrenic nerve lying superficial to the muscle, and the deep transverse cervical artery. Ligate and transect the deep transverse cervical artery. With extreme care, mobilize the phrenic nerve and retract it medially. A word of caution is warranted—overzealous retraction can cause injury to this nerve, causing paralysis of the diaphragm.

The lateral (transected) segment of the deep transverse (superficial) cervical artery can be used to help identify the C7 nerve root that usually lies just inferior to it on the posterior border of the scalenus anterior muscle. If the dissection is extended superiorly, the ascending cervical artery can be seen also lying on the scalenus anterior muscle. The suprascapular nerve and nerve to the subclavius help identify the junction of the C5 and C6 roots or upper trunk of the plexus. If the C5 root is followed laterally, the dorsal scapular nerve is seen. Inferior to the C7 root, the suprascapular artery can be found, and inferior to this artery, the C8 root can be located. After identifying these nerve roots, dissection along the plexus is performed proximally and distally. Labeling of the various branches can facilitate identification later during surgery.

Sometimes, only a distal or inferior plexus exposure is required. This decision should be made clinically. To expose the distal inferior portion of the brachial plexus, the dissection should be continued in the deltopectoral interval. The cephalic vein is a key landmark for the exposure. Once this interval is adequately developed, the insertion of the pectoralis muscle on the humerus is released, leaving a small cuff of tissue to facilitate closure. The pectoralis minor muscle origin on the coracoid is tagged, released, and reflected inferiorly. Medially, the clavipectoral fascia is opened parallel to the neurovascular structures. Identify the axillary artery and vein, as well as the medial and lateral cords of the plexus. A useful method of confirming the identification of the lateral cord is by finding the coracobrachialis muscle and tracing it toward its origin and following the MCN to the lateral cord. The posterior cord can be located behind the axillary artery. If additional exposure is needed, a segment of clavicle can be removed using a small oscillating saw. Most of the time, osteotomizing the clavicle is not required. If an osteotomy of the clavicle is performed, good internal fixation needs to be obtained during closure to avoid iatrogenic complications such as delayed union or nonunion.

Transaxillary Approach

The indications for exposure of the brachial plexus using the transaxillary exposure are very limited (Breslau, 1983). The primary indication for this approach is for decompression of the thoracic outlet region when indicated (see Chapter 52). It offers the ability to perform an anterior scalenectomy and first rib resection. Women and thin men are the prime candidates for this approach, whereas obese and muscular individuals are not good candidates owing to the limited exposure. The transaxillary approach is not a good choice for brachial plexus exploration because of the limited exposure and inability to convert easily to an extensile ap-

proach. Moreover, the potential for vascular complications also limits the usefulness of the transaxillary approach.

Place the patient in the lateral decubitus position, and prep the chest wall, axilla, and shoulder region, with the extremity free. A surgical scrub nurse should assist by holding the extremity in the correct position. Place a transverse incision at the base of the axilla just distal to the hair line. Continue the dissection toward the chest wall with minimal undermining of the soft tissues to prevent postoperative problems resulting from dead space. Divide the pectoris major muscle close to the humerus, leaving a small cuff of tissue for reattachment later. Identify the rather large intercostobrachial nerve that supplies some sensibility to the upper arm and a small area of the prepectoral skin. This nerve should be handled carefully in an attempt to prevent a painful neuroma. It can also serve as a donor nerve for neurorrhaphy procedures if needed. If the intercostobrachial nerve is to be transected, it should be cut as proximal as possible to allow for adequate padding of the proximal stump. Palpate the axillary artery, and continue the dissection toward the neurovascular bundle. Open the neurovascular bundle. Identify the lateral cord of the brachial plexus, axillary artery, and vein. The medial cord of the plexus is the cord most commonly involved in iatrogenic injury during rib resection; therefore, identification and protection of this cord before resection is advisable.

Musculocutaneous Nerve

The MCN originates from the lateral cord of the brachial plexus, with fibers coming from C5 and C6 levels. About the level of the subscapularis muscle, it is located in a superolateral position relative to the axillary artery and vein. As the MCN proceeds distally, it pierces the coracobrachialis muscle, which, at times, may be very proximal and near to the coracoid process. Laterally on the arm, the nerve travels between the biceps and brachialis muscles (Fig. 19–4). After innervating these muscles, the MCN surfaces just lateral to

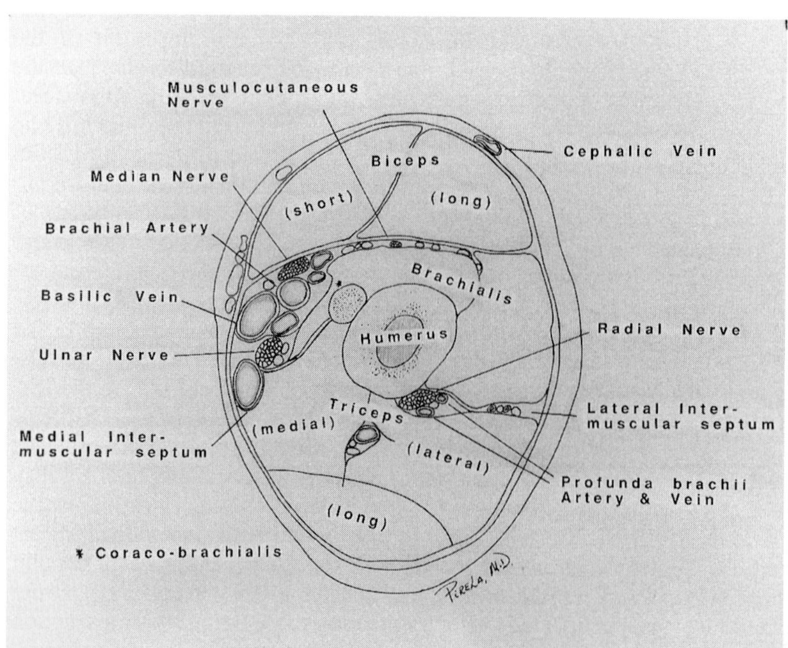

FIGURE 19–4. Cross-sectional view of the mid-arm. Note the relationship of the musculocutaneous nerve in the anterior compartment of the arm as well as the other neurovascular structures.

the laceratus fibrosa and continues as the lateral antebrachial cutaneous nerve (LACN), supplying sensation to the lateral forearm.

Should the need to explore the MCN arise, the exposure is similar to that used for the infraclavicular approach to the brachial plexus (see the description given earlier). First, the exposure should be from its origin on the lateral cord of the plexus to as far distal as needed. Second, detachment of the insertion of the pectoralis major muscle from the humerus facilitates exposure, allowing good visualization of the plexus including the MCN. Occasionally, there is a high take-off of the MCN from the brachial plexus. Specific branches to the coracobrachialis, biceps, and brachialis muscles can be traced. To expose (or decompress) the lateral antebrachial cutaneous nerve, refer to the following section.

Medial Antebrachial Nerve

ANATOMY

The medial antebrachial cutaneous nerve (MACN) is of particular interest in peripheral nerve surgery because of its value as a potential donor in reconstruction (Nunley et al, 1989). On occasion, the MACN may develop symptomatic neuromas from iatrogenic causes, such as venopuncture, surgery related to the ulnar nerve, and medial approaches to the elbow joint (Dellon and MacKinnon, 1985; Horowitz, 1994). Neuromas can also form as a result of direct trauma.

The MACN commonly originates from the medial cord of the brachial plexus with contributions from C8 and T1. As described by Masear and colleagues (1989), there can be some variation in the origin and distribution of this nerve. It may arise from the medial brachial or medial anterior thoracic nerve, or both. The MACN can arise from the lower trunk of the plexus. Internervous communication between the brachial and ulnar nerve has also been described.

In the distal arm (7 to 22 cm above the medial humeral condyle), the MACN divides into anterior and posterior branches, with variations in their cutaneous distribution. The most common distribution pattern is shown in Figure 19–5. The posterior division can cross in a posterior direction within a span of 12 cm above and below the medial condyle. Ninety percent of the time, the posterior division crosses at or above the medial condyle. The anterior division follows the course of the basilic vein running within the subcutaneous tissue. Its innervation may extend as far distal as the level of the wrist.

EXPOSURE OF THE LATERAL ANTEBRACHIAL CUTANEOUS NERVE

The LACN can be involved in entrapment neuropathies (Bassett and Nunley, 1982; Felsenthal et al, 1984). Symptomatic neuromas can develop from trauma (Yuan and Cohen, 1985). The LACN may also serve as donor nerve graft for neurorrhaphy procedures. The anatomical location of the LACN has been studied by Bourne and associates (1987). They found a consistent location of the LACN in the cadaveric specimens they dissected. The location of the LACN was clinically confirmed in 10 volunteers using a lidocaine blockade. Specifically, the LACN was found on the radial

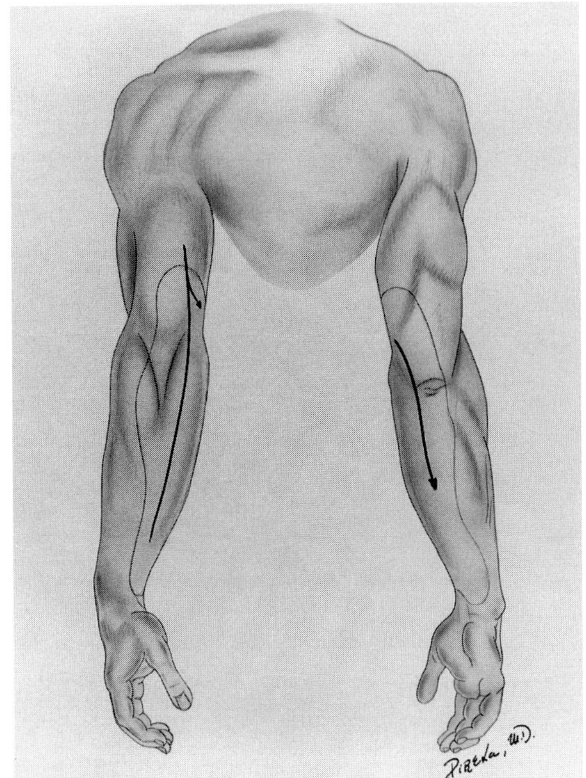

FIGURE 19–5. The anterior and posterior distribution of the medial antebrachial cutaneous nerve.

side of the biceps tendon at the level of the interepicondylar line (Heuter's line). Mackinnon and Dellon (1985) found some degree of overlap in the cutaneous territory of the LACN and the superficial branch of the radial nerve (Fig. 19–6).

Median Nerve

ANATOMY

The median nerve is derived from the medial and lateral cords of the brachial plexus. In the upper arm, it is initially located in an anterolateral position with respect to the brachial artery. It then proceeds distally, crossing the brachial artery in the mid-arm, where it ultimately lies medial to the artery in the region of the elbow joint. Just distal to the elbow joint, the anterior interosseous nerve or branch originates from the median nerve.

As the median nerve leaves the cubital region, it passes between the two heads of the pronator teres. It then proceeds distally in an interval between the flexor digitorum superficialis and the FDP.

In the forearm, the median nerve supplies all flexor muscle except the FCU and the ulnar half of the FDP, which are supplied by the ulnar nerve. The anterior interosseous branch of the median nerve is given off in the proximal forearm. This branch supplies the flexor pollicis longus, the radially located FDP, most commonly the FDP to the index finger but rarely the middle finger. The pronator quadratus is the last muscle to be innervated by the anterior interosseus branch of the median nerve.

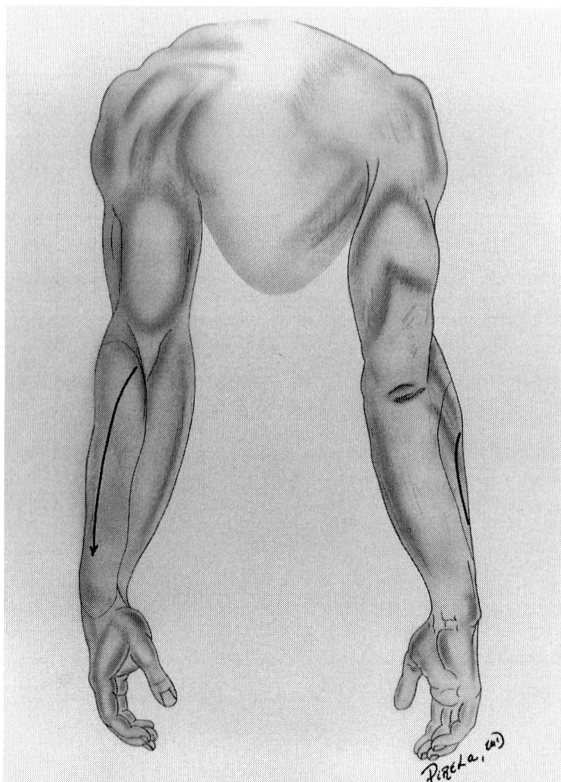

FIGURE 19–6. The anterior and posterior distribution of the lateral antebrachial cutaneous nerve.

At approximately 6 to 10 cm proximal to the flexor crease of the wrist, the palmar cutaneous branch of the median nerve is given off. The nerve then proceeds radially at the subcutaneous level to supply sensibility to the thenar eminence. At the level of the wrist, the median nerve surfaces to be found just radial and posterior to the palmaris longus tendon, where it is very susceptible to laceration injuries.

The median nerve, along with the flexor tendons to the fingers and thumb, travels through the carpal tunnel to innervate all the thenar muscles except the adductor pollicis and the deep head of the FPB. Moreover, the recurrent motor branch of the median nerve, which commonly follows an extraligamentous course, passes distal to the transverse carpal ligament and then returns back (proximal) to gain access to the thenar muscles. The reader is referred to the anatomical work of Lanz and colleagues, who have categorized the various patterns of the recurrent branch of the median nerve (Lanz, 1977; Pirela-Cruz et al, 1992). Flaconer and Spinner (1985) have also observed variations in the motor (and sensory) supply to the thumb, including the Riche-Cannieu variant. Specifically, the motor recurrent branch innervates the opponens pollicis, the superficial head of the FPB, and the abductor pollicis brevis. The radial two lumbricals are also supplied by the median nerve. However, these muscles are supplied by motor branches that travel with the digital sensory nerves to the index and middle fingers.

Once the median nerve is distal to the carpal tunnel, it provides sensibility to the palmar surface of the thumb, index, middle, and radial half of the ring finger. The median nerve also provides sensibility to the central area of the palm

and thenar eminence through its palmar cutaneous branch. The sensory distribution pattern does vary to some degree.

Entrapment of the median nerve may occur at several points along its course (Spinner, 1984):

1. The thoracic outlet.
2. At the ligament of Struthers in patients with a supracondylar process in the distal arm.
3. The lacertus fibrosis.
2. Between the heads of the pronator teres.
4. At the fibrous arcade between the heads of the flexor digitorum superficialis in the proximal forearm.
5. By Gantzer's muscle (Kaplan, 1942; Mangini, 1960) (an anomalous muscle) in the proximal forearm.
6. Within the carpal tunnel in the hand.

EXPOSURE OF MEDIAN NERVE IN THE ARM AND ELBOW

To expose the median nerve in the distal arm, elbow, and proximal forearm, make a so-called lazy S curvilinear incision on the antecubital region on the medial side (Fig. 19–7). The dissection proceeds just medial to the biceps tendon in the arm and just lateral to the flexor-pronator muscle group in the forearm. The median nerve (and brachial artery) can be located between the two heads of the pronator teres muscle (Fig. 19–8A and B). Do not confuse the biceps tendon with the median nerve because, at first glance, these two structures may have a strikingly similar appearance.

Exposure of the median nerve in the hand (see later).

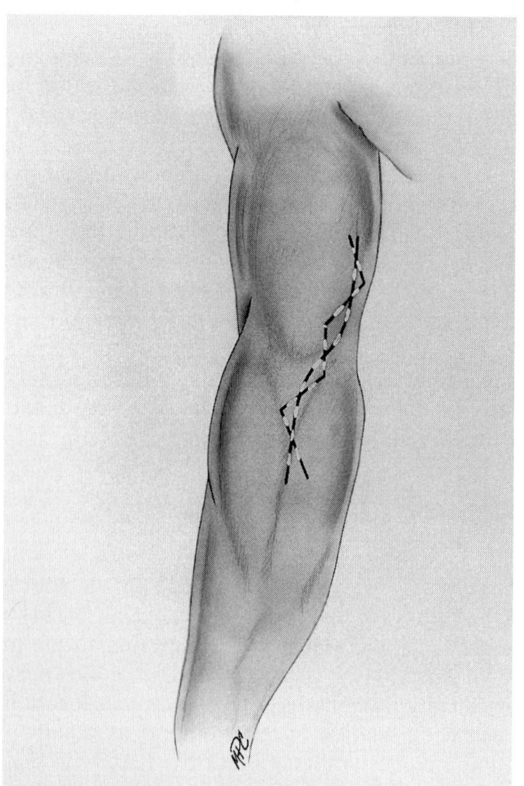

FIGURE 19–7. The so-called "lazy S incision" for exposing the median nerve in the proximal forearm and distal arm.

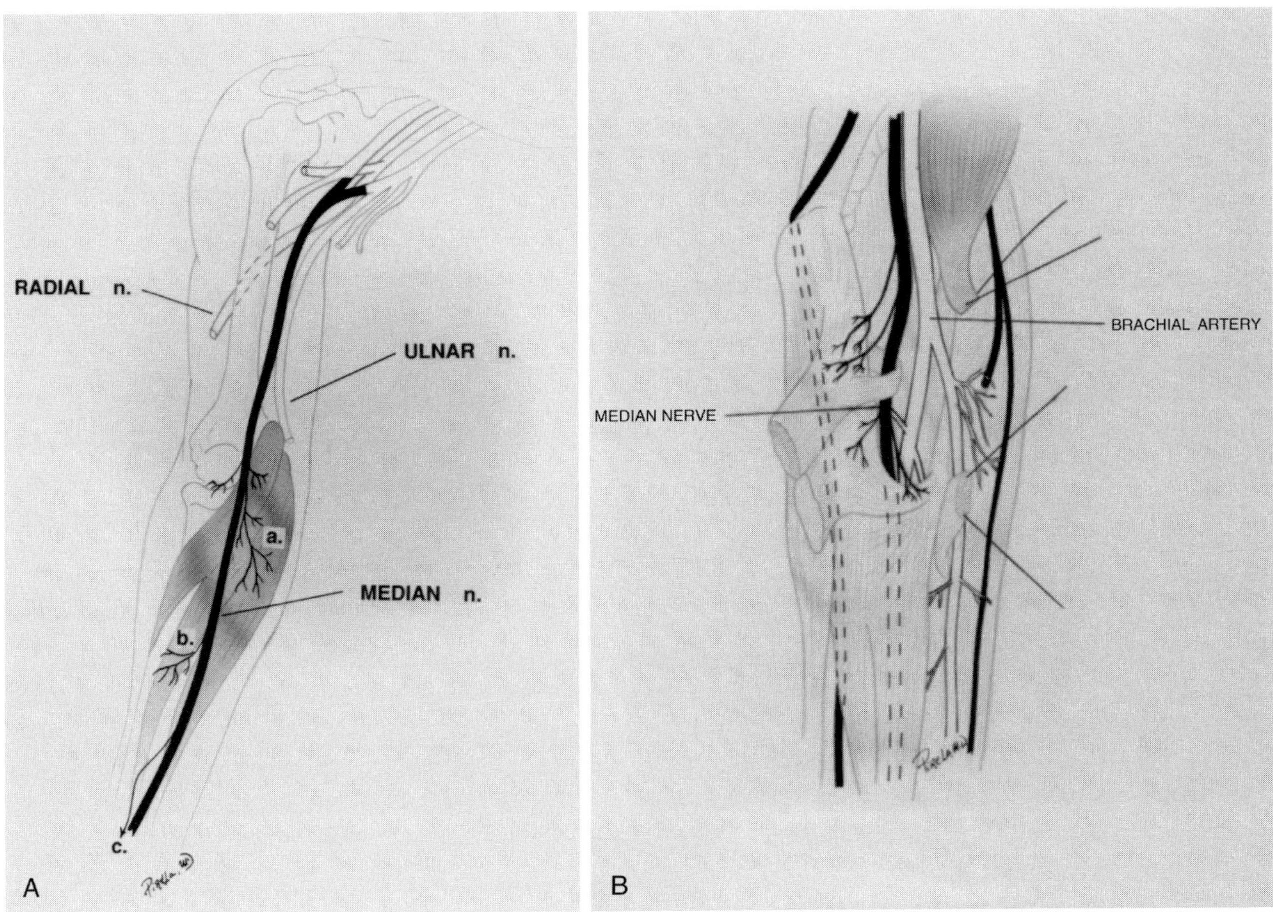

FIGURE 19–8. *A,* The course of the median nerve as it comes off the brachial plexus and proceeds distally. The median nerve gives off multiple branches to the finger flexors and pronator muscle group, (a). The anterior interosseous nerve, (b), comes off farther distal. The palmar cutaneous nerve (c) can be seen as a distinct branch in the distal forearm. *B,* The relationship of the median nerve to surrounding structures at the elbow.

Axillary Nerve

Patient Position. Lateral decubitus, arm on support, or prone (distal portion), and supine (proximal segment).

Surgical Equipment. Airplane splint, abduction pillow, or shoulder spica cast that may be required postoperatively.

ANATOMY

The pertinent surgical anatomy of the axillary nerve has been described by many authors (Alnot and Valenti, 1991; Artico et al, 1991; Flatow and Bigliani, 1992) (Fig. 19–9*A* and *B*). The axillary nerve is a continuation of the posterior cord of the brachial plexus. The nerve comes off the posterior cord at about the level of inferior border of the subscapularis muscle and then passes through the quadrangular space posteriorly. The axillary nerve is accompanied by the posterior humeral circumflex artery as it passes through the quadrangular space. The nerve then gives off a branch to the teres minor as it is leaving the quadrangular space and continues in a posterolateral direction toward the deltoid muscle. This portion of the axillary nerve divides into two major segments, the smaller branch supplying the posterior third of the deltoid and the larger branch continuing around to supply the middle and anterior thirds of the deltoid. Also

traveling with the anterior division of the axillary nerve are cutaneous fibers that form the lateral cutaneous nerve about the axillary line to supply sensation to the skin overlying the shoulder.

EXPOSURE

Surgical exposure of the axillary nerve is difficult. Careful preoperative evaluation is useful to decide if only an anterior exposure or a combination of an anterior and posterior exposure is needed. If an extensile exposure is required (anterior and posterior), then consideration to starting the exposure with the patient in the supine position and then either placing the patient into the prone or lateral decubitus position should be given. Although it is somewhat difficult to operate in the shoulder region with the patient in the lateral position, the position does offer some degree of latitude for simultaneous anterior and posterior approaches. The benefit of operating intially in the supine position and then prone position is the ability to use the operating microscope. However, critical decisions such as the location (e.g., the quadrilateral space) of the injured nerve segment, and length and amount of cable grafts to be used do pose many practical problems. These are just some of the dilemmas that must be considered when preparing to operate on the axillary nerve.

To expose the distal half of the axillary nerve, the patient

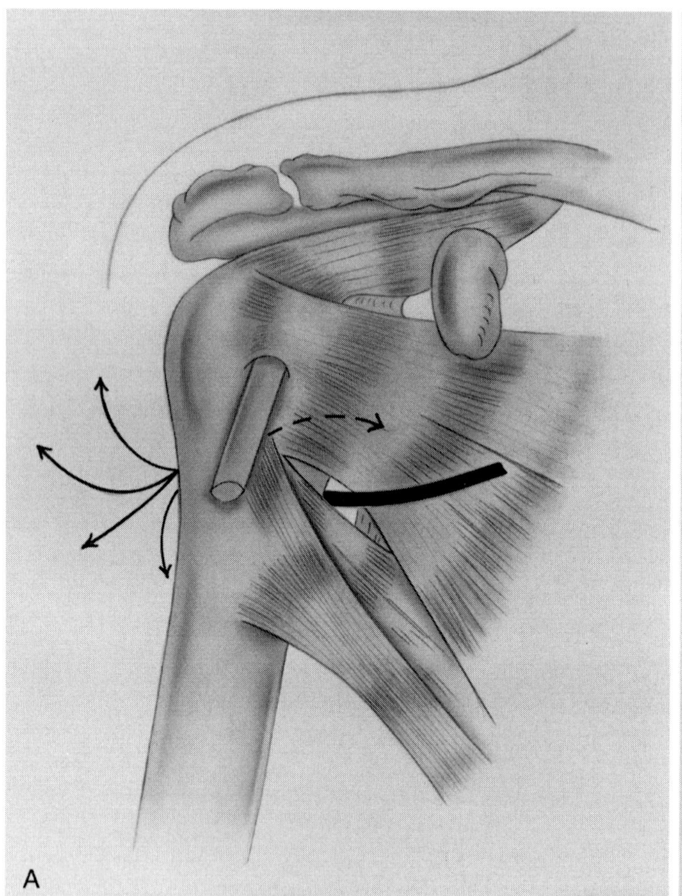

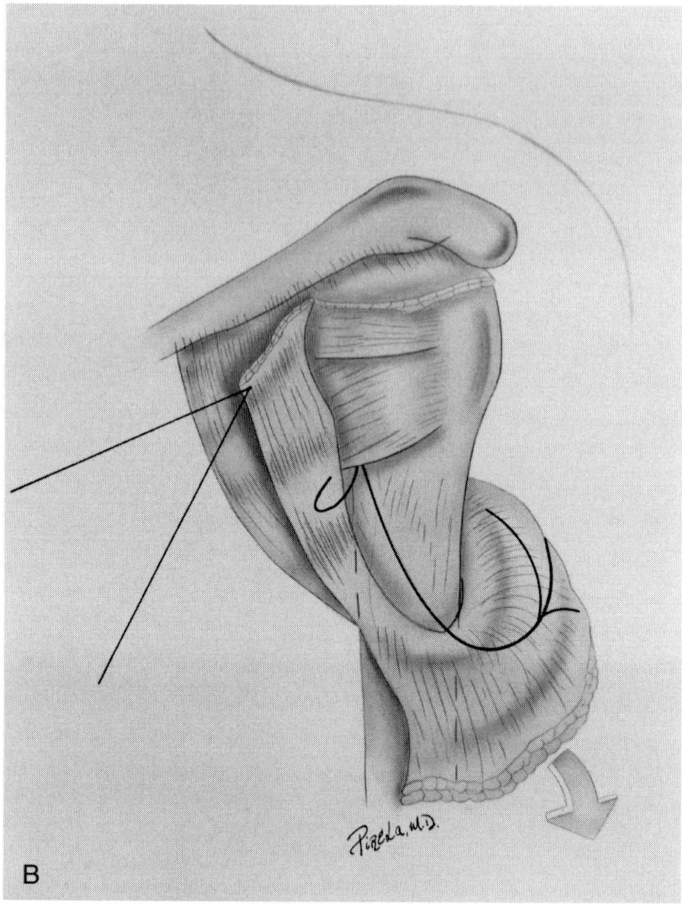

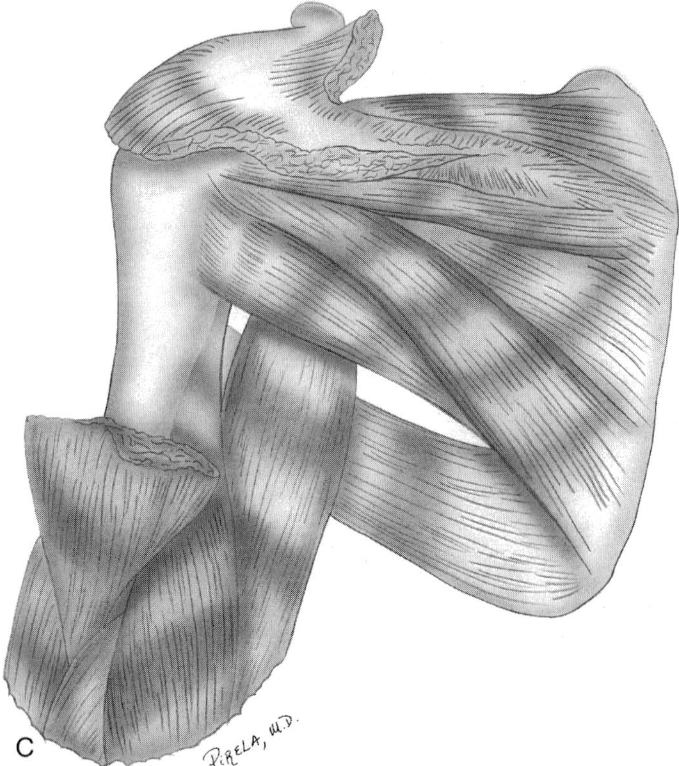

FIGURE 19–9. The course of the axillary nerve about the shoulder. *A,* Posteriorly, the axillary nerve passes through the quadrangular space with the posterior humeral circumflex artery. The quadrangular space is formed by the teres minor, the teres major, the humerus, and the long head of the triceps muscle. *B,* Laterally, adjacent to the quadrangular space, the triangular space can be seen. The hiatus is based laterally and bounded by the long head of the triceps. The teres major and teres minor make up the superior and inferior borders. *C,* Posterior view of the left shoulder with the deltoid removed. The quadrangular and triangular spaces are noted.

should be placed in either the lateral decubitus or prone position. The extremity should be draped free for intraoperative placement. The deltoid muscle needs to be considered in order to perform an adequate exposure. The deltoid muscle consists of three major muscle groups, with the interval between the middle and posterior third being better defined than the interval between the anterior and middle muscle groups. The dissection uses the interval between the middle and posterior portions of the deltoid because this internervous plane is relatively avascular.

Begin the incision posteriorly over the spine of the scapula, extending laterally to about the angle of the acromion, then proceed distally over the arm to the level of the posterior axillary fold. Once hemostasis is established, the lateral half of the posterior (third) of the deltoid and the medial half of the middle deltoid is detached from its origin in the spine and acromion of the scapula and is opened like a book superiorly. The dissection is then continued inferiorly in the interval between the middle posterior third of the deltoid. By identifying the teres minor muscle with its obliquely oriented fibers, then the quadrangular space, axillary nerve, and posterior humeral circumflex artery can be identified. This exposure allows visualization of the terminal portion of the nerve. If a more proximal approach is required, a separate anterior exposure needs to be performed. (The reader should refer to the section on exposure of the infraclavicular portion of the brachial plexus.) Reattachment of the deltoid to the acromion and clavicle should be performed with small drill holes to ensure secure closure. It is advisable to support the extremity in an abduction pillow postoperatively to allow the deltoid to heal at its normal myofascial resting tension.

Suprascapular Nerve

Patient Position. Prone or lateral decubitus position.

Surgical Equipment. Bean bag or peg board, extremity holder, fiber optic light, and nerve stimulator.

EXPOSURE

The suprascapular nerve can be involved in entrapment syndromes (Bateman, 1980; Garcia and McQueen, 1981; Murray, 1974; Rengachary et al, 1979; Sarno, 1983). This nerve is also susceptible to injury by arthroscopic surgical procedures. Surgical exploration may be required for decompression or neurorrhaphy procedures

To expose the distal two-thirds of the suprascapular nerve, place the patient in either the lateral decubitus or prone position. If the patient is placed into the lateral position, an extremity holder or well-padded Mayo stand is required. The extremity can be draped free or covered. If the patient is placed in the prone position, turn the head opposite the operated side with a small bolster under the head and ipsilateral shoulder. An approximately 8- to 10-cm transverse incision is made over the spinous process of the scapula (Fig. 19–10). Care should be exercised to keep a relatively dry field because this region can be very vascular and impede visibility and dissection. Subperiosteal dissection is used to elevate the trapezius and supraspinatus muscles above the spine and the infraspinatus below. Above the spine, the

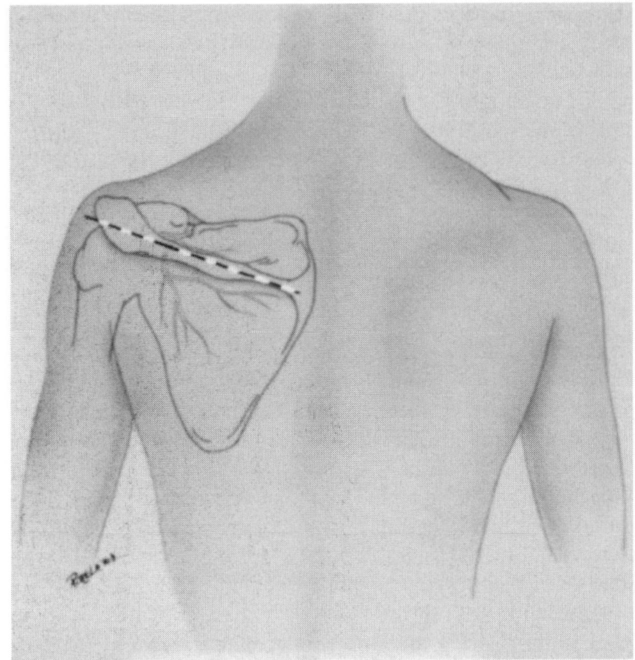

FIGURE 19–10. Incision used for exposure and decompression of the suprascapular nerve as it exits from the suprascapular notch.

dissection is continued to the suprascapular notch, which is a considerable distance anteriorly. The use of a small fiberoptic light, a nerve stimulator, and a scapula bone model facilitates the dissection. The surgeon removes the transverse scapular ligament with a Kerrison rongeur, taking care to protect the nerve. Once the nerve is located, it can be traced distally (inferiorly) below the spine (Fig. 19–11). If more proximal

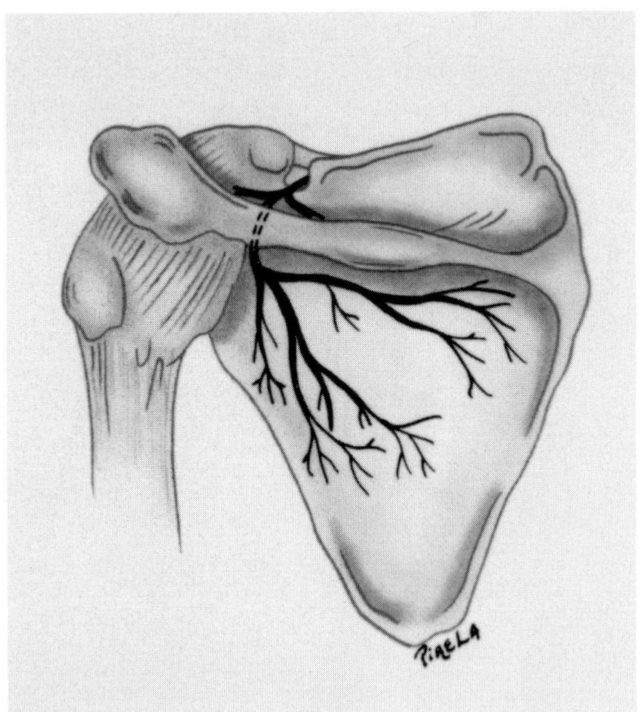

FIGURE 19–11. The course of the suprascapular nerve about the shoulder. Note the proximity of the nerve to the glenohumeral joint.

exposure is required, the reader is referred to the article by Bateman (1980), who states that the patient should be placed in a semi-seated position and an oblique incision (direct approach) should be used from the mid-posterior cervical triangle, which allows visualization of the C5 and C6 nerve roots. This exposure can also be performed in the prone position.

Radial Nerve

ANATOMY

The posterior cord of the brachial plexus is the largest cord of the plexus, and the radial nerve is the largest branch. It is a continuation of the posterior cord of the brachial plexus made up of fibers from C6, C7, and C8. At its take-off from the brachial plexus, it is located posterior to the axillary artery and then proceeds posteriorly between the long head of the triceps and the teres major muscle. The radial nerve continues posteriorly and laterally around the humeral neck, giving off branches to the medial and lateral heads of the triceps and proceeds distally within the spiral groove of the humerus. In this upper region of the arm, the radial nerve is joined by the profunda brachii artery (Fig. 19–12). At about the distal third of the arm, the nerve surfaces, piercing the lateral intermuscular septum to proceed between the brachialis and brachioradialis (BR). At the level of the lateral condyle of the elbow, the radial nerve gives off branches to the brachialis, BR, and extensor carpi radialis longus. Distally about the elbow joint, branches to the extensor carpi radialis brevis and the anconeus muscle are given.

There are numerous sites along the course of the radial nerve that are of clinical significance:

1. The lateral intermuscular septum (proximal to the radial tunnel).

2. At the junction of the middle and distal thirds of the humerus in patients with the Holstein-Lewis fracture (1963).

3. Fibrous bands anterior to the radial head.

4. At the arcade of Frohse (Frohse and Frankel, 1908) (proximal border of the supinator).

5. Extensor carpi radialis brevis origin.

6. The radial neck (the so-called bare area [Spinner, 1978]).

7. Radial recurrent vessels (leash of Henry) to BR and extensor carpi radialis longus.

8. At the wrist (cheiralgia paraesthetica, Wartenberg's disease).

Radial Nerve (Proximal)

Patient Position. Supine or lateral decubitus position.

Surgical Equipment. Bolster under the shoulder (supine), nerve stimulator, arm table (supine), and sturdy (well-padded) Mayo stand (lateral decubitus position).

EXPOSURE OF THE RADIAL NERVE IN THE ARM

As with the axillary nerve approach, a critical decision needs to be made when surgically exposing the proximal radial nerve. The most important factor is where the lesion is. Is it proximal or distal to the triceps innervation? Does the exposure require access to the posterior shoulder region? If the answer is proximal (i.e., triceps is not functioning), then a standard anterior exposure to the brachial plexus with exploration of the posterior cord with the patient in the supine position is indicated. If it is possible that a posterior arm exposure is needed, then placing the patient into the lateral decubitus position should be considered in order to have access to the posterior arm region, anterior chest, and shoulder. If on the other hand, the exploration that is required is distal to the origin of the triceps, then the patient can be placed into either a lateral decubitus or supine position, with the extremity resting on an arm table. As a practical note, if the patient is placed into the lateral decubitus position, the extremity can be rested on a sturdy, well-padded Mayo stand or small table for support. The use of a sterile tourniquet, which can be used for exposure of the radial nerve in the distal arm during the initial part of the dissection, can aid tremendously.

The incision that offers the best approach for the radial nerve follows its course. Draw the incision on the skin beginning on the posterolateral aspect of the arm if the exposure is to be carried out in this region (Fig. 19–13). Progress distally until just distal to the mid-arm and then curve the incision anteriorly, moving anteriorly toward the antecubital fossa. The sterile tourniquet can now be used to help locate the nerve in its more superficial location between

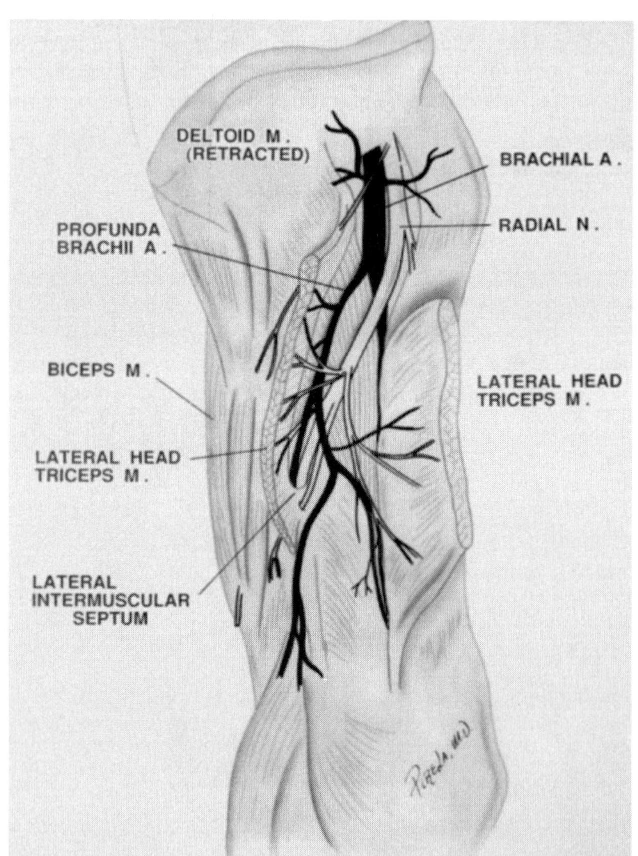

FIGURE 19–12. The course of the radial nerve in the arm. Note its relationship to the surrounding anatomical structures.

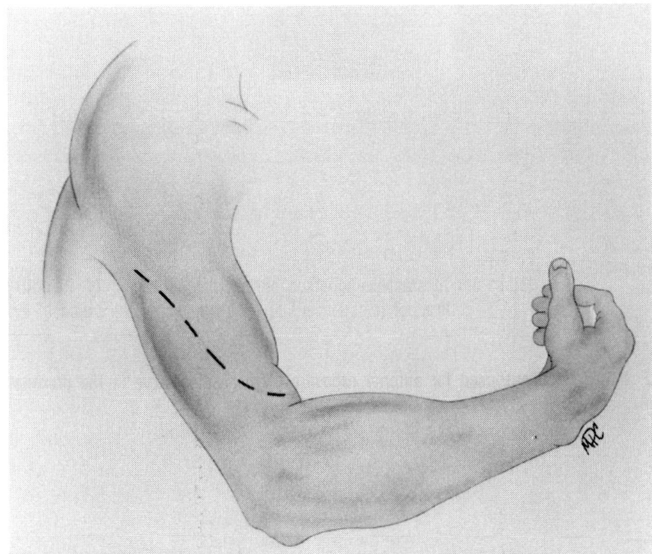

FIGURE 19–13. Incision used for exposing the radial nerve in the mid-arm. This incision can be used for limited or extensile exposures.

the brachialis and brachioradialis muscles in the middle and distal third of the arm. From this location, the nerve can be traced either proximally or distally, depending on the clinical situation. If the dissection is carried out proximally, remove the tourniquet and continue the dissection proximally. The lateral head of the triceps muscle is encountered. Do not divide this muscle but rather develop the interval between the lateral head and long head of the triceps (see Fig. 19–13).

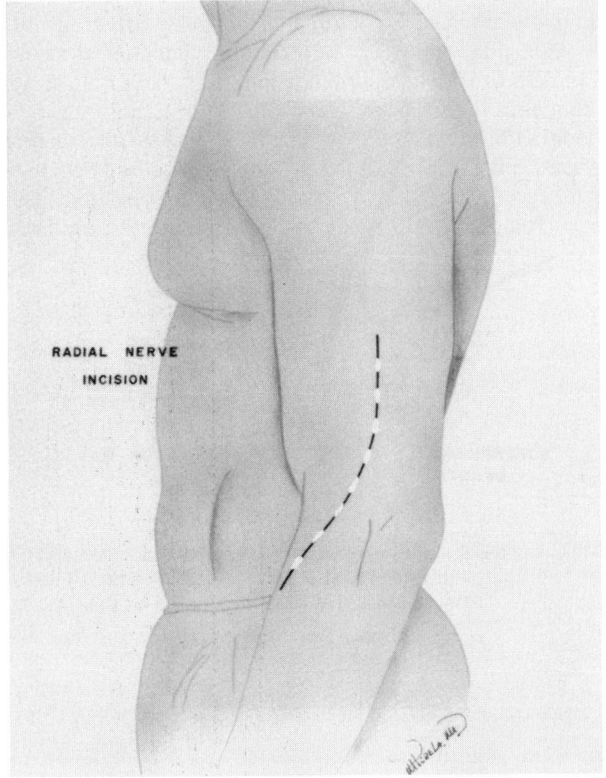

FIGURE 19–14. Incision used for exposure of the radial nerve in the distal arm and anterior proximal forearm.

Access to the nerve can be obtained by working around the lateral head of the triceps.

EXPOSURE OF THE RADIAL NERVE AT THE ELBOW AND PROXIMAL FOREARM

The radial nerve in the distal third of the arm can be consistently located between the BR and brachialis muscles. If an anterior exposure is required, begin the incision on the lateral aspect of the elbow and then carry the incision anteriorly toward the antecubital fossa. On the proximal forearm, follow along the ulnar border of the mobile wad (Fig. 19–14). Like other exposures, this incision can be modified to accommodate the clinical demands. If the dissection is carried out in a proximal to distal direction, the radial nerve should be located between the brachialis and BR because the dissection is easier in this region. On the other hand, if a distal to proximal approach is desired, locating the superficial branch of the radial nerve under the BR muscle and tracing it proximally is a relatively simple method of locating the radial nerve in the proximal forearm and distal arm. A nerve stimulator is useful to help locate the posterior interosseous nerve (PIN).

Posterior Interosseous Nerve

Patient Position. Supine position.

Surgical Equipment. Arm table, nerve stimulator, and arm tourniquet.

ANATOMY

The indications for exploring the PIN in the proximal forearm primarily include traumatic injuries such as laceration or avulsion and entrapment neuropathy by an anatomical structure or a tumor. Distally, the PIN can be a donor nerve graft tissue for segmental defects such as digital nerve lacerations. Although the PIN is considered a motor nerve, occasionally it is the culprit in an obscure extra-articular pain syndrome of the wrist due to its capsular innervation (Dellon, 1985).

In the proximal forearm, the PIN can be explored from either an anterior or posterior approach. Each approach has its advantages and disadvantages. To perform the anterior approach, begin by identifying the mobile wad of Henry (BR, extensor carpi radialis longus, and extensor carpi radialis brevis) and drawing the incision from just proximal to Hueter's line (interepicondylar line) to approximately third of the length of the forearm distally (Fig. 19–15). Open the antebrachial fascia, and continue the dissection between the BR and the flexor carpi radialis muscles (Fig. 19–16). Do not mistake the LACN, which is located in the subcutaneous fascia, for the superficial branch of the radial nerve, which runs underneath the BR muscle. The simplest method of locating the PIN is by initially finding the superficial branch of the radial nerve and tracing it proximally from its origin (radial nerve). Next, locate the proximal edge of the supinator muscle (arcade of Frohse; Frohse and Frankel, 1908). According to Fuss and Wurzl (1991), the arcade of Frohse is located 3 to 5 cm below Hueter's line. If further exposure

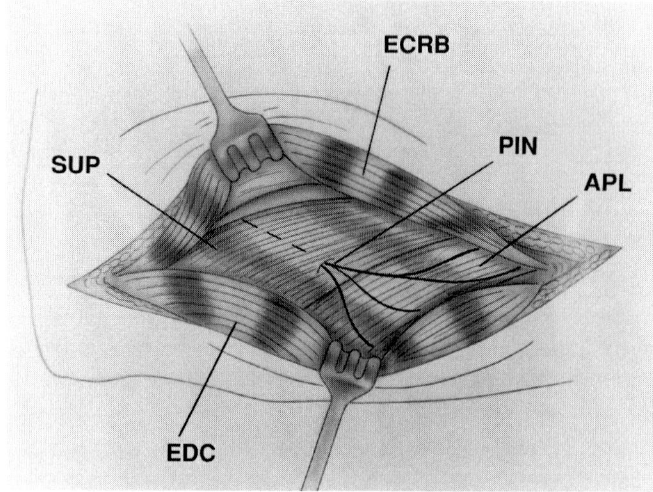

FIGURE 19–19. The posterior interosseous nerve (PIN) as it exits the supinator muscle. Note the orientation of the supinator muscle fibers. For adequate exposure of the PIN, this muscle must be cut. (APL, Abductor pollicis longus; ECRB, extensor carpi radialis brevis; EDC, extensor digitorum communis; SUP, supinator muscle.)

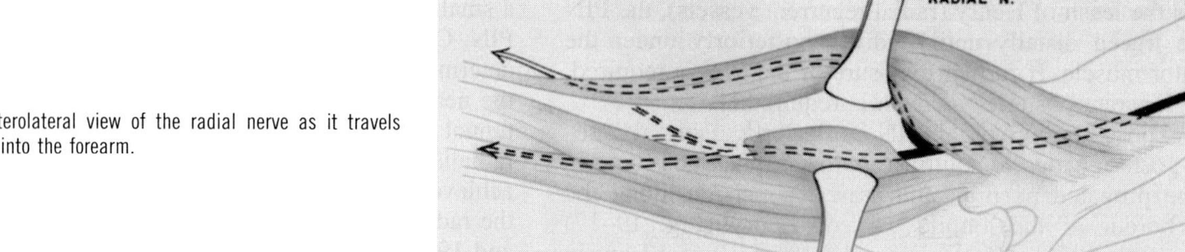

FIGURE 19–20. Posterolateral view of the radial nerve as it travels from the distal arm into the forearm.

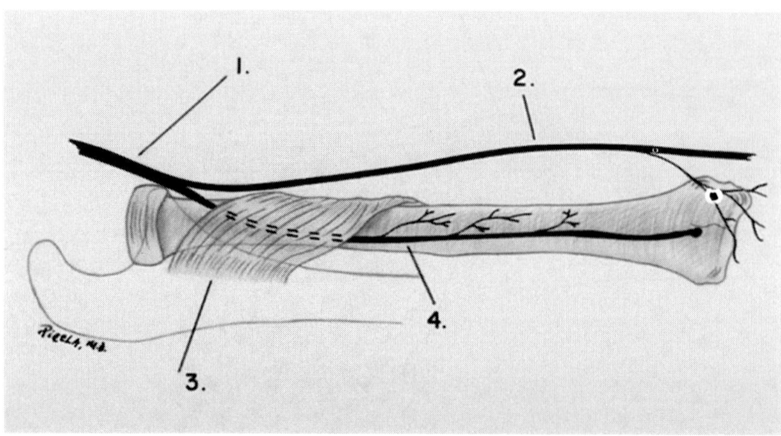

FIGURE 19–21. The course of the radial nerve in the forearm. The radial nerve (1) gives off the superficial branch (2), which travels under the cover of the brachioradialis muscle. The posterior interosseous nerve (PIN) (4) penetrates the substance of the supinator (3) as it gains entrance to the posterior forearm.

consistent location of the terminal PIN deep within a separate fascicle sheath of the fourth extensor compartment. The diameter of the nerve ranged from 1 to 5 mm with 1 to 5 fascicles. he length of available donor graft ranging from 5 to 10 cm could be harvested. They found the distal PIN to be ideal for digital nerve grafting with no donor site morbidity. Make a straight dorsal incision mid-line over the distal forearm at the level of the radial styloid process and extend proximally. Locate the fourth extensor compartment, and open it longitudinally, preserving the distal half of the extensor retinaculum. Care should be exercised when opening the extensor retinaculum completely in a longitudinal fashion, and a special effort should made to repair it in order to prevent bowstringing problems of the extensor tendons postoperatively. Retract the extensor digitorum communis (EDC) and extensor indicis proprius (EIP) tendons laterally. Locate the PIN on the radial side of the compartment adherent to the periosteum of the radius. The PIN can now be traced proximally to obtain the desired length.

EXPOSURE OF THE SUPERFICIAL BRANCH OF THE RADIAL NERVE AT THE WRIST AND DISTAL FOREARM

The superficial branch of the radial nerve at the wrist and distal forearm can be easily exposed through a longitudinal zigzag or transverse incisions. The longitudinal and zigzag incisions can be developed into an extensile approach and are more versatile. The transverse incision, on the other hand, gives a more cosmetically appealing scar, but the exposure is limited.

The SBRN gains access to the distal forearm and wrist by traveling under the cover of the BR. At about the junction of distal and middle thirds of the forearm it exits. Distally about the wrist, the SBRN sends off multiple small branches to provide sensibility to the dorsoradial aspect of the hand and radial three fingers.

Ulnar Nerve

ANATOMY

The ulnar nerve arises from the medial cord of the brachial plexus. It receives contributions from C7, C8, and T1 nerve roots. At its take-off, it is the most medially positioned major nerve of the plexus. It is medially related to the median nerve and axillary artery throughout its course on the extremity. The ulnar nerve passes through the mid-brachium, and it pierces the medial intermuscular septum as it moves from the posterior compartment anteriorly. As it progresses distally, the nerve surfaces just before its entry into the cubital tunnel, where it is frequently traumatized. The ulnar nerve passes posterior to the medial epicondyle and gains access to the forearm by passing between the two (humeral and ulnar) heads of the FCU. Within the forearm, it descends under the cover of the FCU in an anteromedial location. Within the distal third of the forearm, two cutaneous branches originate—the dorsal and palmar cutaneous branches—to provide cutaneous innervation. Distally, at the junction of the wrist and forearm, the nerve is again in a precarious superficial (palmar) position. The nerve has an intimate relationship to the ulnar artery as it travels into

Guyon's canal (1861). Just past the hook of the hamate, the ulnar nerve divides into sensory and motor branches. The sensory branch continues medially to gain access to the ulnar two fingers. The motor branch curves sharply in a radial direction around the hamulus to gain access to the radial side on the hand.

The ulnar nerve innervates the FCU and the two ulnar heads of the FDP in the proximal forearm. At approximately 6 to 10 cm from the wrist flexor crease, a dorsal cutaneous nerve that supplies the dorsal medial aspect of the hand and fingers is given off. The palmar continuation of the ulnar nerve innervates all of the hypothenar muscles, the ulnar two lumbricals, all of the interossei (dorsal and palmar), the adductor pollicis and the deep head of the flexor pollicis brevis through its motor branch. The sensory portion of the ulnar nerve usually supplies the ulnar one and one-half digits (little finger and the ulnar half of the ring finger). There can be considerable variation in the innervation pattern.

Neural interconnections between the median and ulnar nerve occur in the forearm (Gruber, 1870; Martin, 1763) and palm (Cannieu, 1897; Riche, 1897). These interconnections can at times present a confusing clinical picture.

Clinically important sites in the course of the ulnar nerve include (Eversmann, 1993)

1. The thoracic outlet (i.e., first rib and scalene muscles).
2. The arcade of Struthers and the medial intermuscular septum in the arm (Spinner, 1984).
3. The cubital tunnel (Osborne's fibrous arcade [Osborne, 1970]).
4. The septum within the FCU in the forearm—Spinner's ligament (Inserra and Spinner, 1986; Plancher et al, 1996).
5. Guyon's tunnel at the wrist (e.g., pisohamate ligament) (Guyon, 1861).
6. Adductor origin in the hand (Ruder and Wood, 1993).

EXPOSURE OF THE ULNAR NERVE IN THE ARM, ELBOW, AND PROXIMAL FOREARM

In the region of the proximal forearm or distal arm, the ulnar nerve can be exposed directly through a medial approach using either a curvilinear or zigzag incision (Fig. 19–22). Surgery should be under tourniquet control. A sterile tourniquet can aid greatly. If mid-arm exposure of the nerve is required, a sterile tourniquet should be used for the initial part of the dissection and then removed. After the incision is made, the dissection is carried down to the antebrachial fascia with extreme caution to prevent any injury to branches of the brachial and antebrachial cutaneous nerves that can develop into significant painful neuromas. Palpate the medial epicondyle, and continue the dissection just above this region, where the nerve can be easily located. From this region, the nerve can be traced either proximally or distally. In the upper arm, the ulnar nerve can be located just posterior to the brachial artery and anterior to the long head of the triceps muscle. In the distal arm, the nerve is located posterior to the medial intermuscular septum and anterior to the medial (deep) head of the triceps (Fig. 19–23).

EXPOSURE OF THE ULNAR NERVE IN THE HAND AND DISTAL FOREARM

After obtaining tourniquet control, a curvilinear incision can be made to gain access to the ulnar nerve in the hand

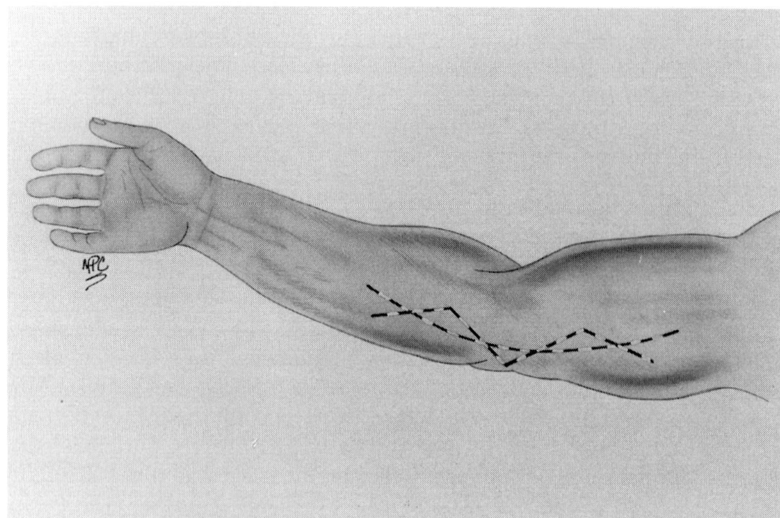

FIGURE 19–22. Incisions used for exposure of the ulnar nerve in the forearm and distal arm. The incision can be modified depending on the clinical demands.

and distal forearm. The incision can be modified depending on the clinical demands. In the proximal forearm, the ulnar nerve runs between FCU and FDP tendons (Fig. 19–24). Within the distal forearm, the ulnar nerve can be located just radial to the FCU tendon and traced proximally or distally. In the hand, the classic incision parallels the thenar eminence and is in line with the fourth ray. This incision is similar to the one used for the median nerve except that it is placed a little more ulnarly (medially). It can be developed into an extensile exposure for access to the ulnar (and median) nerve in the forearm. If only the ulnar nerve is to be exposed, the dissection requires a little more strategy because there are few anatomical landmarks to guide the dissection. Guyon's tunnel is located palmar (anterior) and ulnar to the carpal tunnel. Moreover, the roof of the carpal tunnel is the transverse carpal ligament (TCL), which is the floor of Guyon's tunnel (Fig. 19–25). The volar carpal ligament (VCL) is the roof of Guyon's tunnel. Therefore, the dissection is carried just medial to the line of Taleisnik, deep to the palmar aponeurosis. Incising the volar carpal ligament (VCL) opens Guyon's tunnel.

The simplest method to gain entry into Guyon's tunnel is by identifying the superficial palmar arterial arch distally and tracing it proximally (backwards) toward the volar carpal ligament. This approach takes you into Guyon's tunnel through the back door. The ulnar nerve can be located just medial (ulnar) to the artery within the tunnel (Fig. 19–26). As the ulnar nerve exits from the tunnel, the nerve divides into its sensory and motor branches (Fig. 9–27).

Median and Ulnar Nerves (Wrist and Palm)

Patient Position. Supine position.

Surgical Equipment. Arm table and tourniquet.

OVERVIEW

Numerous surgical incisions have been described for the exposure of the median nerve at the palm and distal forearm. Recently, because of the development of the endoscopic

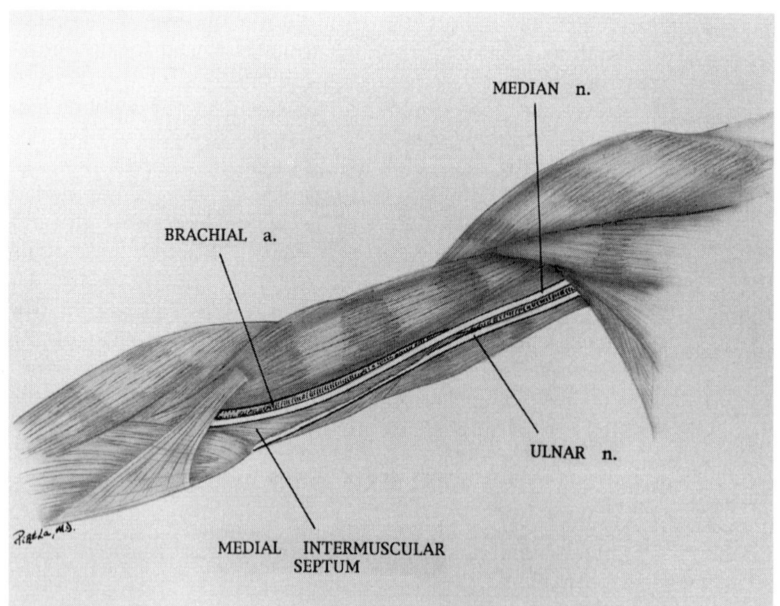

FIGURE 19–23. The ulnar nerve in the arm. The use of a sterile tourniquet (which can be removed) can facilitate the dissection.

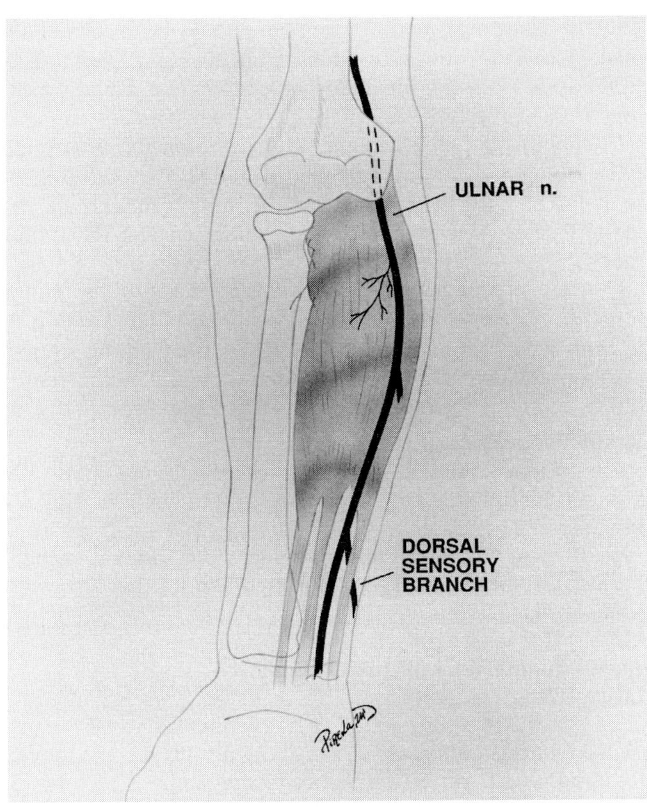

FIGURE 19–24. The course of the ulnar nerve in the forearm.

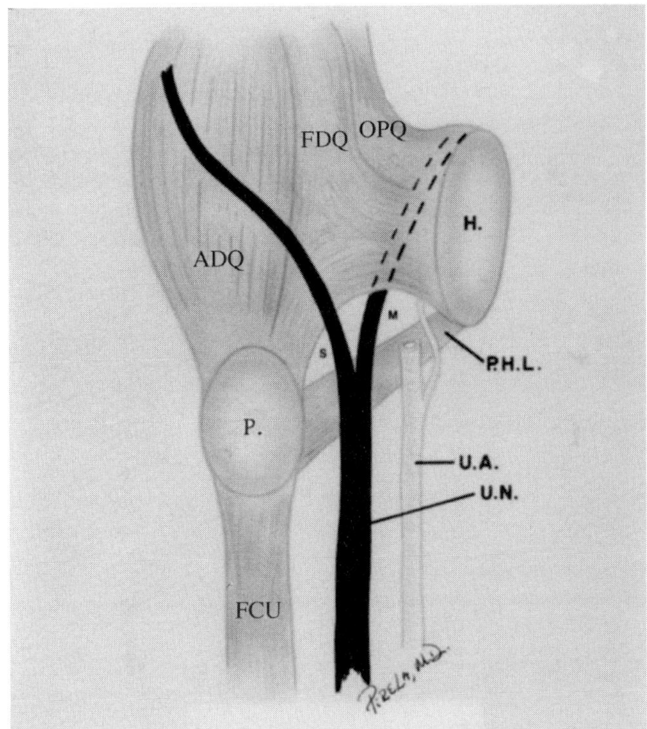

FIGURE 19–26. The course of the ulnar nerve in the palm. As the nerve exits from Guyon's tunnel, it divides into sensory (S) and motor (M) branches. The relationship of the ulnar nerve to the pisohamate ligament (PHL) and hypothenar muscles is shown.

carpal tunnel release procedures that use small surgical portals, the length of the incision for the conventional open carpal tunnel decompression has been reduced (Poitevin, 1994). New terms such as limited and mini-exposure are commonly being used. An incision that compromises between the classic extensile exposure and the very limited incision can be used for most cases (Fig. 19–28). With this in mind, it is even more important that the hand surgeon be familiar with the anatomical variations that may exist with respect to the median and ulnar nerves in the palm in order to avoid iatrogenic complications, which may be more disabling than the initial presenting problem (Conolly, 1987; Murphy et al, 1994; Taleisnik, 1973).

GENERAL PRINCIPLES

Some general surgical principles that are of particular concern to the surgeon operating on peripheral nerves in the hand, wrist and distal forearm include the following:

FIGURE 19–25. An axial view of Guyon's and the carpal tunnel. Note relationship of the transverse carpal ligament (TCL) forming the roof of the carpal tunnel but forming the floor of Guyon's tunnel. The volar carpal ligament (VCL) makes up the roof of Guyon's tunnel. Also, note how the fibers of the VCL meet the fibers of the TCL over the carpal tunnel. The relationship of the ulnar nerve and ulnar artery can be seen entering Guyon's tunnel as these structures travel distally. (C, Capitate; H, hamate; L, lunate; P, pisiform; S, scaphoid; Tq, triquetrum; Tr, trapezium.)

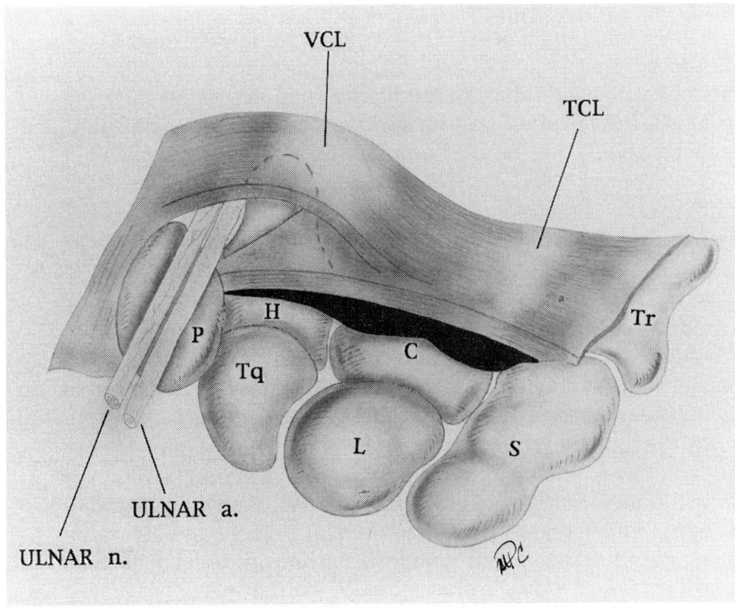

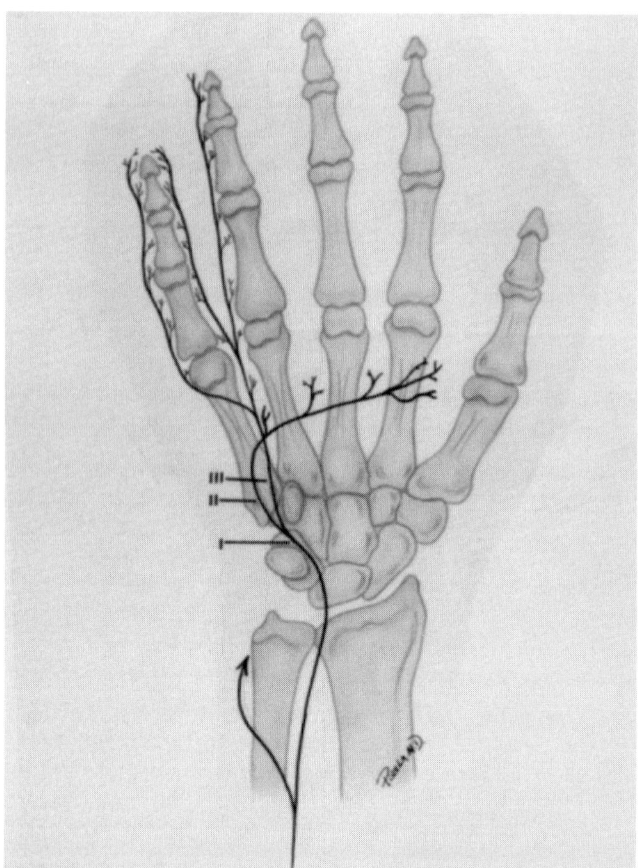

FIGURE 19–27. The course of the ulnar nerve in the distal forearm, palm, and fingers. The ulnar nerve (I) in Guyon's tunnel can be appreciated. The motor branch (II) takes a direct posterior (dorsal) course immediately as the ulnar nerve comes out of the tunnel to innervate the intrinsic muscles of the hand. The sensory branch (III) as it travels distally to supply the ulnar 1 and 1/2 digits. Note the sensory branches as they come off the proper and common portions of the ulnar nerve.

1. Straight incision across joints on the palm should be avoided. Violating this basic principle may cause severe scarring, chronic ulceration with the development of a flexion contracture, and restricted range of motion of the wrist.

2. A longitudinal incision and not a transverse incision should be used to reduce risk of injury to palmar cutaneous branches, or even injury to the median and ulnar nerves.

3. At the level of the flexor crease of the wrist, the incision should not be on the radial side of the axis of the ring finger. As noted by Taleisnik, an incision on the radial side of the axis places the palmar cutaneous branch at increased risk of injury (Murray, 1994).

4. The surgical exposure should be performed under exsanguination and tourniquet control whenever possible to minimize bleeding and difficulty with visualization. There are some occasions when the use of a tourniquet is contraindicated and meticulous hemostasis is essential, such as a patient with chronic renal failure and a carpal tunnel entrapment neuropathy requiring surgical decompression and having an arteriovenous access shunt on the symptomatic side.

5. Surgery can be facilitated by the use of magnification to help visualize and identify peripheral branches, which at times may be very small. Loupe magnification of 3.5 × is usually adequate. Procedures such as internal neurolysis, if indicated, are best performed with the operating microscope.

6. The transverse carpal ligament should be incised only when visualized—directly when using the open method or indirectly when using the endoscopic technique. Blind procedures invite problems.

7. Opening the carpal tunnel should be on the ulnar side of the transverse carpal ligament just radial to the hook of the hamulus to avoid injury to the motor branch of the median nerve (see the section on variations of the motor branch).

8. After opening the carpal tunnel, identify the motor branch of the median nerve and determine its relationship to the transverse carpal ligament. If a transligamentous course is present, consider a Chevon decompression of the motor branch. (Surgical prophylaxis for a traction neuropathy of the motor branch).

9. Inspect the contents of the carpal tunnel, and check the floor for pathology. Rarely, a tumor or ganglion may be discovered.

10. In general, incisions used should be flexible enough to allow proximal or distal exposure if the need arises.

SURFACE TOPOGRAPHY OF THE HAND AND EXAMINATION

Understanding the palmar anatomical surface landmarks of the hand can be of assistance in assessing structures at risk. Moreover, these landmarks are of particular importance in performing closed or relatively closed procedures, such as endoscopic carpal tunnel release, percutaneous A-1 pulley

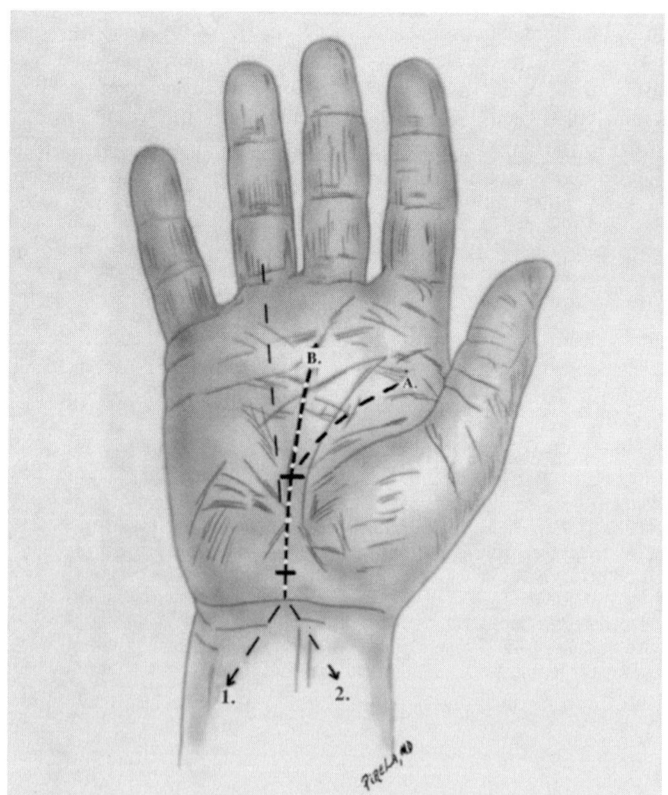

FIGURE 19–28. Incisions used for exposure or decompression of the median and ulnar nerves in the palm and distal forearm. If more proximal exposure is required, the incision can be extended in an ulnar (1) or radial (2) direction, depending on the clinical demands.

release, or needle insertion into the palm for diagnostic or therapeutic procedures. Actual or imaginary topographical lines of the hand can be drawn. These lines are built around Kaplan's cardinal line—the primary line (Fig. 19–29).

EXPOSURE OF ULNAR NERVE (VOLAR APPROACH)

Patient Position. Supine.

Surgical Equipment. Arm table and tourniquet.

There are three volar methods of exposing the ulnar nerve at the wrist and hand—the retrograde palmar approach (back door approach) to Guyon's tunnel and the antegrade ap-proach, which involves following the ulnar nerve and artery distally. The third, medial (ulnar) approach involves mobiliz-ing the abductor digiti quinti and piriform. The more com-mon (volar) exposure is described first.

Make an incision on the palm similar to the incision used for the a carpal tunnel release, but the incision should be slightly longer and placed a little more toward the ulnar side of the palm (please refer to Fig. 19–28). Opening the carpal tunnel facilitates the exposure of the ulnar nerve and artery (i.e., not the median nerve). However, when only the ulnar nerve is of interest, incising the transverse carpal ligament is not essential. The simplest method of locating the ulnar neurovascular bundle is by tracing the superficial palmar arch proximally into Guyon's tunnel. As discussed earlier, using a blunt instrument such as a small hemostat, the distal end of the tunnel can be located and opened, thereby exposing the ulnar artery. Using careful dissection, the ulnar nerve can be located just medial (ulnar) to the artery. If the ulnar nerve is traced further proximal, the motor branch can be identified at about the pisiform or approximately 1 cm proximal to the hook of the hamate as it comes off the ulnar nerve.

The antegrade approach to Guyon's tunnel is described. Begin the incision in the distal forearm on the ulnar side just radial to the FCU tendon. Distally, cross the flexor crease of the wrist obliquely. Locate the ulnar artery and nerve, and trace the neurovascular bundle distally into Guyon's tunnel.

EXPOSURE OF ULNAR NERVE (MEDIAL APPROACH)

The medial approach to the ulnar nerve can accomplished by initially making an incision along the ulnar border of the 5th metacarpal, curving into the volar surface of the hand at the base of the hypothenar region, and following the FCU tendon proximally. The abductor digiti quinti is reflected palmarly. Within the plane of the abductor digiti quinti and opponens digiti quinti, the sensory portion of the ulnar nerve, the ulnar artery, and the branch to the abductor can be found. In order to gain adequate exposure, the pisiform needs to be mobilized volarly. This is accomplished by releasing the retinacular restraining fibers from the FCU tendon. The ulnar nerve at the base of the palm is now visible, and with careful dissection, the motor branch can be identified. To trace the motor branch distally, the opponens digiti quinti needs to be mobilized and retracted volarly. Now the motor division of the ulnar can be followed until it curves radially toward the 4th metacarpal.

EXPOSURE OF THE DIGITAL NERVES

Two surgical approaches are commonly used for exposing the digital nerves in the fingers—the mid-axial and the volar. The mid-axial exposure described by Bunnell and the volar incision described by Bruner both are useful in reducing the amount of postoperative scar formation in the digits, which can be a significant problem (Bruner, 1951; Bunnell, 1948). These approaches have stood the test of time in reducing postoperative scar-related problems.

The mid-axial or mid-lateral incision is performed by locating an imaginary plane located between the dorsal and palmar aspect of the finger. If the surgeon is given a choice, he or she should place the incision on the nondominant side

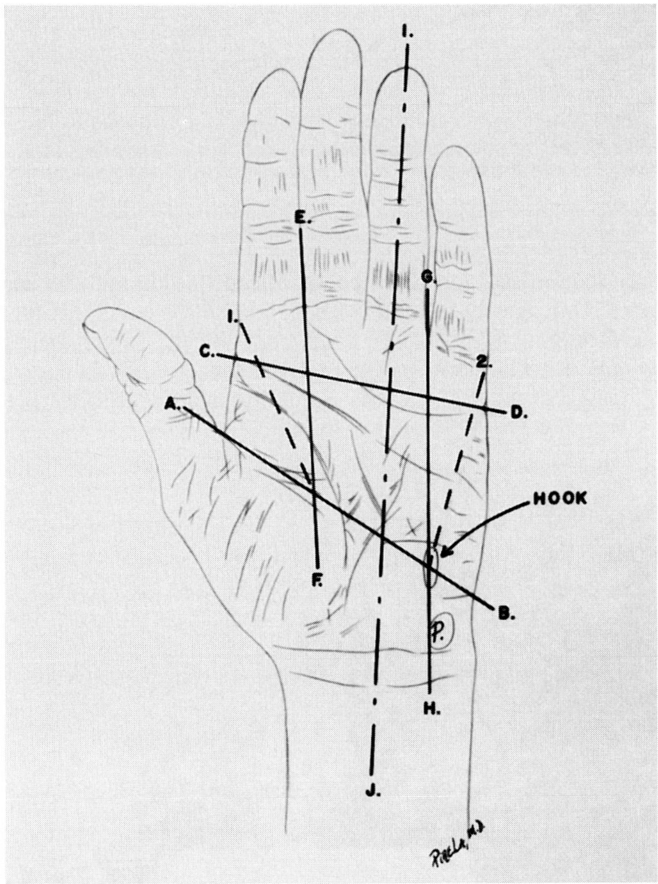

FIGURE 19–29. The topographical lines of the hand that are of clinical importance. As a review exercise, cover the legend and name the anatomical structure associated with the given line. Line A to B is Kaplan's cardinal line. It is projected from the first web space (with the thumb in extension) to the hook of the hamate. This line is somewhat parallel to the transverse palmar crease. The deep palmar arch is found in the mid-portion of this line (between lines E to F and G to H). Line C to D is drawn across the distal transverse palmar crease. The superficial palmar arch is located between lines E to F and G to H at this level. Line E to F is projected along the radial border of the long finger, where it intersects Kaplan's line ((line A to B), the motor branch of the median nerve can be located as it enters the thenar muscles. Line G to H is drawn along the ulnar border of the ring finger. Between lines A to B and C to D, the common digital nerve to the ring and little fingers can be located. Line number 1 begins at the intersection of A to B and E to F and extends distally to the base (metacarpophalangeal joint flexion crease) of the index on the radial side of the digit. The proper radial digital nerve can be found in this region. Line number 2 is drawn from the intersect of line A to B and G to H to the base of the little finger on the ulnar side (metacarpophalangeal joint flexion crease). The proper ulnar digital nerve is located here. Line I to J is the line of Taleisnik. If this line is projected to the flexion crease of the wrist, 90% of the time the palmar cutaneous branch of the median nerve is on the radial side of this line.

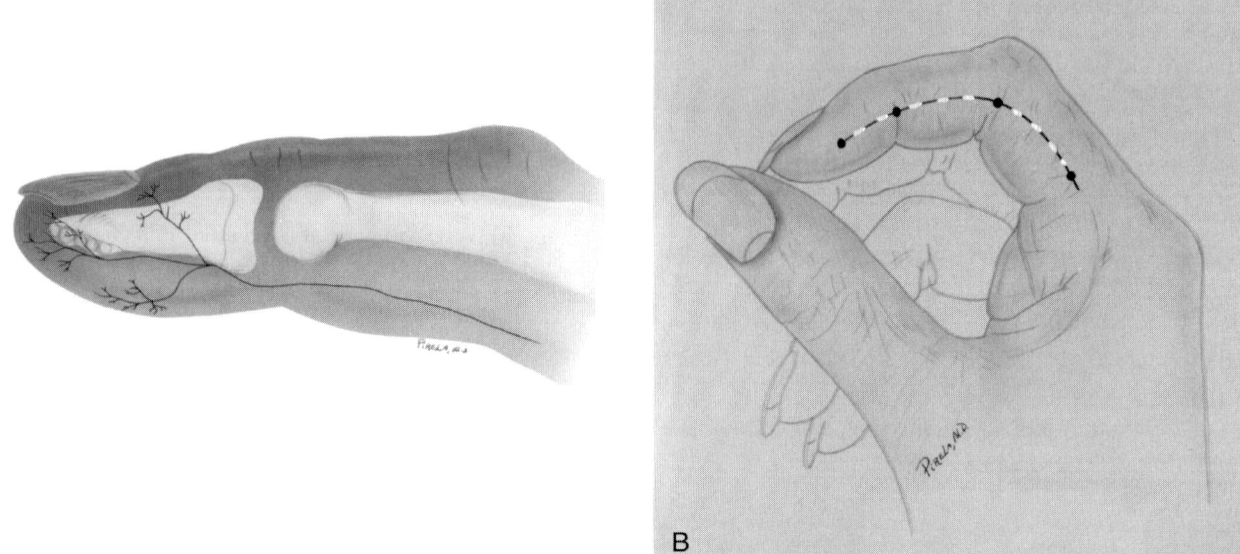

FIGURE 19–30. *A,* The course of a typical digital nerve to its trification distally. *B,* The mid-lateral (mid-axial) incision. Ideally, the incision should be placed on the nondominant side of the digit.

of the digit (radial side of the small, ulnar side of the index, and radial side of the thumb). The incision is performed between the palmar and dorsal branches of the palmar digital nerve (Fig. 19–30*A* and *B*). Care must be observed when extending the incision proximally in order to avoid injury to the dorsal digital branch.

The volar approach is the preferred route to the digital nerves because it offers great flexibility in accommodating various clinical situations (Fig. 19–31). The Bruner incision is performed by connecting a point just to the axilla of the base of the finger (proximal digital flexor crease) to almost the axilla of the opposite side of the finger distally on the middle digital flexor crease (proximal interphalangeal crease). The incision can be extended distally to the distal digital flexor crease (distal interphalangeal crease) or proximally into the palm, as needed.

Spinal Accessory Nerve

Injuries to the spinal accessory nerve (SAN) can occur from iatrogenic and noniatrogenic causes. Causes include sharp transections due to knife injuries, as seen in civilian altercations or during routine lymph node biopsy procedures (Donner and Kline, 1993). Moreover, rare surgical complications of carotid endarterectomy, rhytidectomy, and coronary bypass surgery with injury to the SAN as been documented (Blackwell et al, 1994; Marini et al, 1991; Sweeney et al, 1992). Stretch and blunt trauma are some other unusual causes of injury (Aziz and Shakespeare, 1989; Dellon et al, 1990). Tumors originating from within the nerve, such as a neurofibroma or a neurilemmoma, or extrinsic tumors with contiguous invasion can also cause paralysis of the SAN (Chang et al, 1990; Fabrizi et al, 1992; Lanotte et al, 1994; McShane et al, 1986; Noyek et al, 1992; Ortiz and Reed, 1995). Surgical reconstructive procedures such as neurotization for brachial plexus injuries, restoration of the blink reflex, and motor function through facial nerve reinnervation

may require that the SAN be sacrificed (Allieu and Cenac, 1988; Danziger et al, 1995; Ebersold and Quast, 1992; Samardzic et al, 1989, 1990). Lastly, oncological surgery, such as radical neck dissection may require sacrifice of this nerve, although, at present, there is a trend to spare or reconstruct

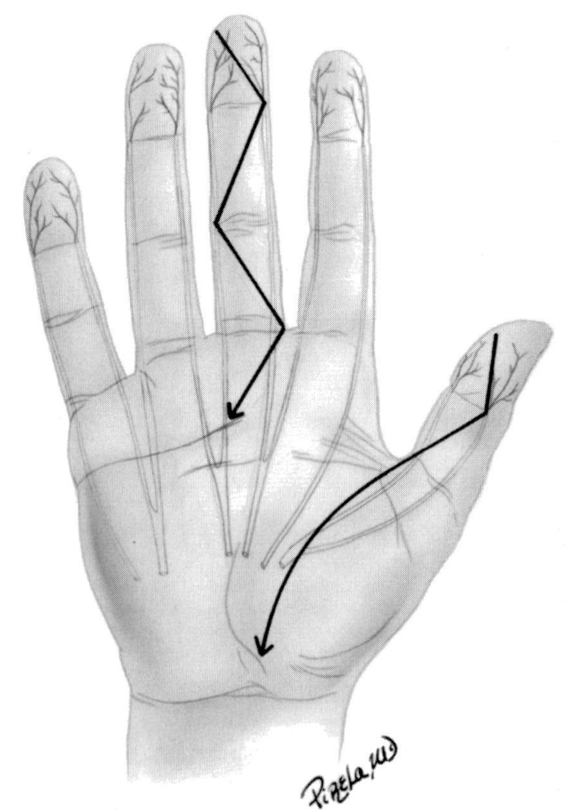

FIGURE 19–31. Bruner's incisions for exploration of the digital nerves using the palmar approach.

the SAN whenever possible (Beck et al, 1991; Eisele et al, 1991; Jori et al, 1992; Lederman and Wilbourn, 1991; Weisberger and Lingeman, 1987). However, some investigators have found no significant difference in survival of patients or improved neck control between the classic radical neck dissections and modified radical neck dissections sparing the SAN (Andersen, 1994; Saunders et al, 1985).

ANATOMY

The SAN is cranial nerve XI, and it is composed of two portions—cranial and spinal. The cranial segment originates in the brainstem and quickly joins the spinal contribution after formation. The entire nerve proceeds through the jugular foramen and then separates into the cranial and spinal divisions. The cranial segment joins the vagus nerve to innervate the musculus uvulae, the levator veli palatini, the pharyngeal constrictor muscles, and lastly, the muscles of larynx esophagus.

The spinal division of the SAN originates in the motor cells of the ventral horns of spinal levels C1 through C5. After formation, the nerve proceeds superiorly, entering the foramen magnum, where it joins its cranial division. The entire nerve then proceeds inferiorly to exit the jugular foramen (as described earlier) and separates. The spinal division continues into the posterior triangle of the neck, passing medial (deep) to the jugular vein and upper portion of the sternocleidomastoid muscle and supplying innervation to this muscle. As the SAN travels through the posterior triangle of the neck, it picks up communicating twigs from the cervical plexus (C2 and C3). Within the posterior triangle of the neck, the SAN lies on the levator scapulae, dividing this muscle essentially in half along its longitudinal axis, and then proceeds to innervate the trapezius muscle.

SURGICAL EXPOSURE OF THE SPINAL ACCESSORY NERVE

The posterior triangle of the neck is bounded by the posterior margin of the sternocleidomastoid muscle anteriorly, the anterior margin of the trapezius muscle posteriorly, and the middle third of the clavicle inferiorly (Fig. 19–32). The posterior triangle of the neck is further subdivided into the occipital and subclavian triangle by the inferior belly of the omohyoid muscle. Initially, it is best to locate the SAN within the occipital triangle and then work from this region.

Make a vertical incision approximately 1 cm anterior to the trapezius muscle parallel to its margin. Begin the incision in the middle third of the occipital triangle and extend it proximally and distally, if needed. Meticulous hemostasis is required for good visualization. Once the dissection is carried deep to the dermal layer, identify the posterior border of the sternocleidomastoid muscle. If the dissection is carried out superiorly, within the upper half of the border, the lesser occipital and the great auricular nerves can be identified, with the lesser occipital nerve being located a few centimeters above the great auricular nerve. Cutaneous twigs from the cervical plexus may also be encountered. Next, the trapezius and the levator scapulae muscles should be identified. The SAN can be found lying on the levator, running in a somewhat parallel course to the muscle fibers. Cervical branches to the accessory nerve also can be identified. The

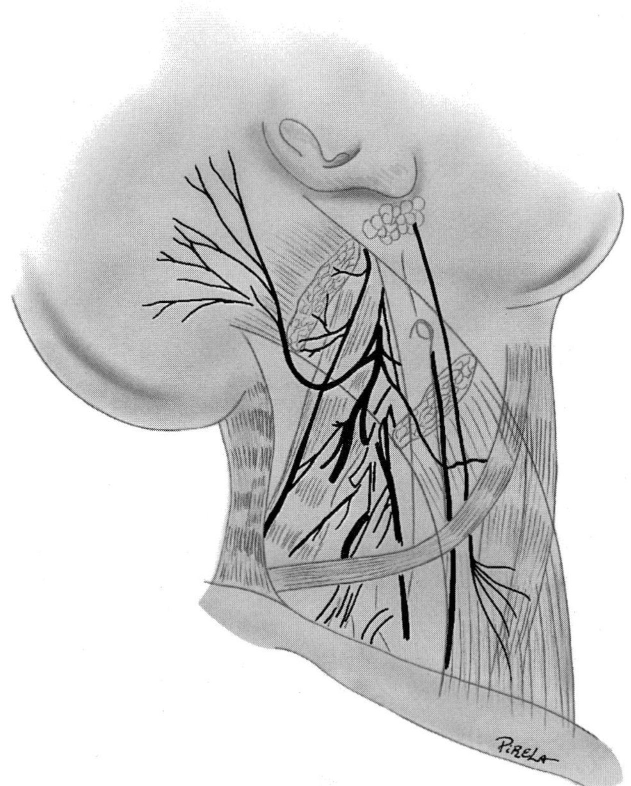

FIGURE 19–32. The spinal accessory nerve in the posterior triangle of the neck.

nerve can now be traced proximally into the sternocleidomastoid muscle and distally toward the trapezium.

NERVES OF THE LOWER EXTREMITY

Lumbosacralcoccygeal Plexus

Peripheral nerves to the pelvis, buttock, perineum, and lower extremity originate from the lumbosacral and coccygeal plexus. The spinal terminology in this region can be somewhat confusing. The lumbosacral plexus consists of spinal levels L1 through the coccygeal nerve (Cn). The lumbar plexus includes levels L1 to L4. The sacral plexus is made up of spinal levels L5 to S3, and lastly, the coccygeal plexus refers to levels S4, S5, and the Cn. The pudendal plexus is made from nerve segments originating from S2, S3, and S4.

The lumbar plexus is composed of mainly L2, L3, and L4 (Fig. 19–33A). It also receives a small cutaneous contribution from L1 root, which ultimately terminates as the ilioinguinal nerve. The major peripheral nerves that arise from the lumbar plexus include the genitofemoral nerve (GFN, L1, L2), the obturator nerve (ON, L2–L4), the lateral femoral cutaneous nerve (L2, L3), and the femoral nerve (FN, L2–L4).

The sacral plexus is predominately made up of L5, S1, S2, and S3 (Fig. 19–33B). It also receives some contribution from L4 via the lumbosacral trunk. The major peripheral nerves that originate from the sacral plexus include the superior gluteal nerve (L4–S1), the inferior gluteal nerve (L5–S2), and the two divisions of the sciatic nerve—the

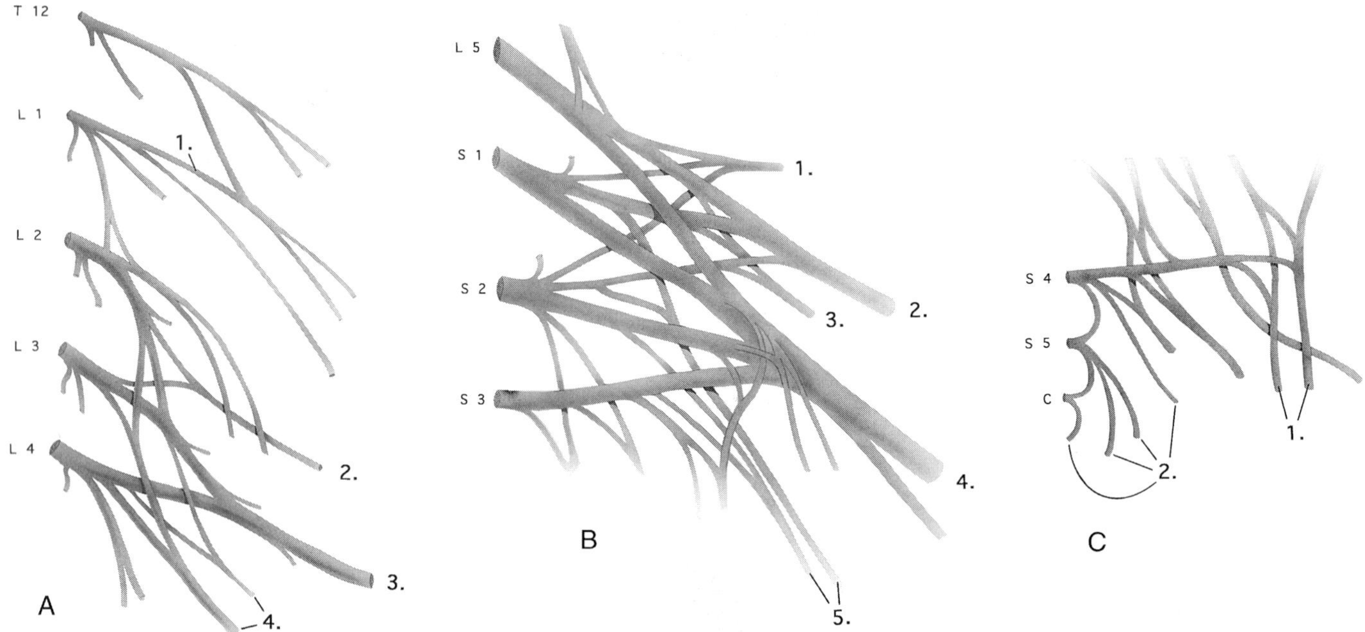

FIGURE 19–33. *A,* The lumbar plexus. 1, Genitofemoral nerve. 2, Lateral femoral cutaneous nerve. 3, Femoral nerve. 4, Obturator nerve. *B,* The sacral plexus. 1, Superior gluteal nerve. 2, Common peroneal nerve. 3, Inferior gluteal nerve. 4, Tibial nerve. 5, Posterior femoral cutaneous nerve. *C,* Coccygeal plexus. 1, Inferior cluneal nerve. 2, Pudendal branches. 3, Anococcygeal nerves.

common peroneal nerve (CPN; L4–S2) and the tibial nerve (TN; S1–S3). The last major nerve to originate from the sacral plexus is the posterior femoral cutaneous nerve, which supplies sensation to the posterior thigh.

The pudendal plexus is composed of fibers from levels S2 to S4. It is the main sensory and motor nervous supply to the perineum. Sacral levels S4, S5, and the Cn are the predominate contributors to the coccygeal plexus (Fig. 19–33C). These nerves form fine filaments that provide cutaneous sensation to the skin of the anococcygeal region. Major nerves to the lower extremity of interest to the peripheral nerve surgeon are discussed in the following sections.

Sciatic Nerve

Patient Position. Prone or lateral decubitus position.

Surgical Equipment. Bean bag or peg board, nerve stimulator, and somatosensory evoked potentials.

ANATOMY

The sciatic nerve is the largest nerve in the body. It is part of the lumbosacral plexus and receives contributions from L4, L5, S1, S2, and S3. The sciatic nerve enters the gluteal region through the lower part of the greater sciatic foramen underneath the piriformis muscle. The sciatic nerve is formed by the joining of the CPN and the tibial nerve. The contributions from each of the respective nerves may be identified as a distinct bundle as high as the sciatic notch, which is a valuable practical note for the peripheral nerve surgeon. As the sciatic nerve leaves the pelvis, it travels under the gluteus maximus muscle. If an imaginary line is drawn between the greater trochanter and ischial tuberosity

and is bisected, the nerve is usually located within the medial half of this region. It then proceeds inferiorly to enter the posterior compartment of the thigh in the interval between the adductor magnus muscle anteriorly and the long head of the biceps muscle posteriorly. As the nerve enters the lower part of the thigh, it divides into the tibial and CPNs.

The innervation to the muscles of the thigh is relatively consistent. Branches from the common peroneal division supply the short head of the biceps muscle. The tibial portion of the sciatic nerve supplies the long head of the biceps, the semimembranosus, the semitendinosus, and the adductor magnus muscles.

EXPOSURE OF THE SCIATIC NERVE

Exposure of the sciatic nerve can be performed through the classic question mark incision, or a modification thereof, depending on the extent of exposure required (Henry, 1973) (Fig. 19–34). For exposure in the proximal (buttock) region of the extremity, reflection of the gluteus maximus is required (Fig. 19–35). Exposure inferior to the gluteal fold may be achieved through a direct linear incision (Fig. 19–36). Preoperatively, using the simple percussion test over the course of the sciatic nerve may elicit a Tinel's sign and aid in the localization of the level of the lesion.

The extensile approach, which allows visualization of the nerve from the sciatic notch to as far distally as the popliteal region, is described. Make an incision parallel to the posterior iliac crest at about 3 to 5 cm inferior to the superior border of the crest. Begin at the posterosuperior spine and work laterally toward the greater trochanter. The incision is then directed inferiorly for approximately 4 to 5 cm, curving slightly medially. At a level just inferior to the gluteal fold, the incision is brought back medially to almost the midline of the thigh and then is curved inferiorly over the sciatic

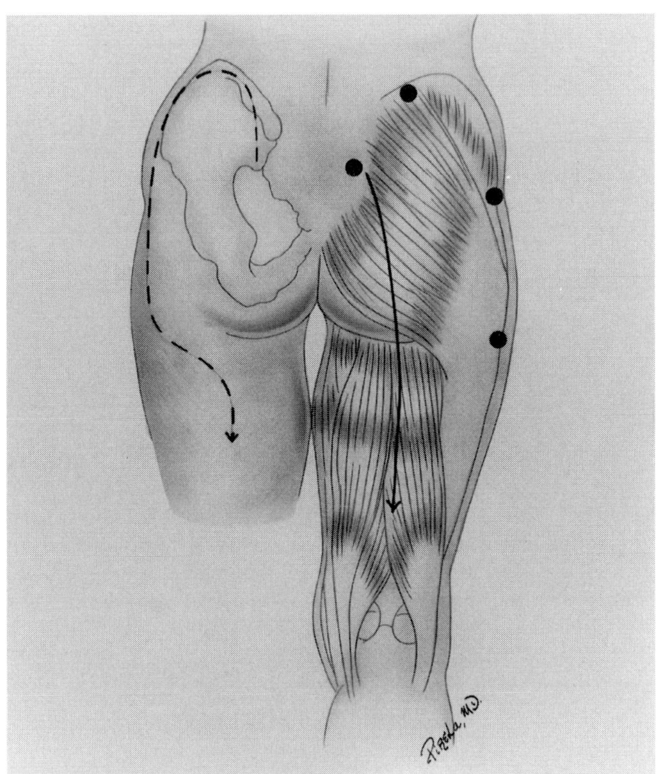

FIGURE 19–34. The classic question mark incision of Henry for the surgical exploration of the sciatic nerve in the gluteal region. To achieve adequate exposure, all four corners of the gluteus maximus must be elevated and reflected. The exposure then proceeds in an interval between the biceps femoris and semitendinosus muscles. In the proximal and mid-levels of the posterior thigh, good mobilization of the biceps muscle is required in order to work around the muscle without detaching it from its origin.

nerve. The incision can be extended distally in a linear fashion until about 10 cm proximal to the popliteal fold. If only exposure inferior to the gluteal fold is required, a direct linear incision may be used (see Fig. 19–36). At 10 to 20 cm from the knee flexion crease, the incision can be extended further distally on either the medial or lateral side of the knee, depending on the clinical situation.

Deeper in the proximal buttock, the interval between the gluteus maximus and medius needs to be carefully identified and developed after the iliotibial band and fascia lata are opened in order to allow for adequate reflection of the gluteus maximus muscle medially. After all corners have been released, the gluteal maximus is retracted medially, the piriformis muscle is identified, and the dissection is continued medially. Once adequate dissection is obtained, the inferior gluteal nerve (and artery), the sciatic nerve (greater sciatic nerve), and posterior femoral cutaneous nerve (lesser sciatic nerve) can be visualized. If further proximal exposure is required, the piriformis muscle can be incised to carry the dissection to the sciatic notch. The sciatic notch can be expanded with a rongeur for additional exposure. In the proximal thigh, dissect, isolate, and protect the biceps muscle with a large Penrose drain. The muscle belly can be mobilized superiorly and inferiorly for exposure as needed. The sciatic nerve can now be traced as far distally as necessary and curved in either a medial or lateral direction (Fig. 19–37). On occasion, there are clinical situations that may war-

rant a direct (linear) approach within the popliteal region; under these circumstances, a Z-plasty of the incision is recommended to prevent a flexion contracture of the knee (Figs. 19–38A and B, and 19–39).

Femoral Nerve

The FN receives contributions from the posterior divisions of the L2, L3 and L4 nerve roots, and it is the largest branch of the lumbar plexus. It emerges from the lateral border of the psoas muscle at the level of the iliac crest and descends between the iliacus and psoas to pass inferior to the inguinal ligament to gain access to the femoral triangle. Just distal to the inguinal ligament, the FN branches into anterior and posterior divisions. The anterior motor segment innervates the pectineus and sartorius muscles. The sensory portion of the anterior division further divides to provide sensibility for the anterior and medial aspect of the thigh. The posterior division of the FN gives rise to the saphenous nerve, which supplies sensibility to the anteromedial aspect of the leg, medial ankle region, and the arch of the foot. The motor portion of the posterior division provides innervation to the rectus femoris and the three vastus muscles (lateralis, intermedius, and medialis).

Isolated complete FN paralysis is relatively rare because of the early ramifications that are given off shortly after the nerve exits from the pelvis. These ramifications are given off in a corda equina–like fashion, and because of the compensatory actions of the adjacent muscles, clinically it is difficult to detect paralysis of only one or two muscles. But FN paralysis can be associated with coagulopathies secondary to anticoagulation therapy (Giuliani et al, 1990; Jamjoom et al, 1993; Lanz, 1977; Merrick et al, 1991; Probst et al, 1982). Although immediate, formal, open surgical decompression may be contraindicated in abnormal coagulopathy states, Merrick and colleagues (1991) suggest that percutaneous decompression may be a practical alternative. Traumatic iliac hematoma from other causes also can be the underlying cause of an isolated femoral neuropathy (Kumar et al, 1992).

EXPOSURE OF THE FEMORAL NERVE

Patient Position. Supine position.

Surgical Equipment. Nerve stimulator.

In preparation for exposure of the FN, palpate and mark the anterosuperior iliac spine (ASIS), the symphysis pubis, and the femoral artery. Draw a line between ASIS and the pubis (line A–B, Fig. 19–40). Draw a second vertical line along the femoral artery intersecting the superior oblique line (line C–D, Fig. 19–40). The skin incision follows these lines somewhat depending on the body habitus. Begin the incision midway between the vertical line and the ASIS, and just inferior (distal) to the oblique line. The incision continues medially to approximately 2.0 cm lateral to the vertical line and is then curved inferiorly. A Z-plasty of the skin may be required to avoid a contracture across the flexion crease if a perpendicular vertical incision is used. The incision is extended as far distally as required. Beware and protect the ilioinguinal nerve. Proximally, carry the dissec-

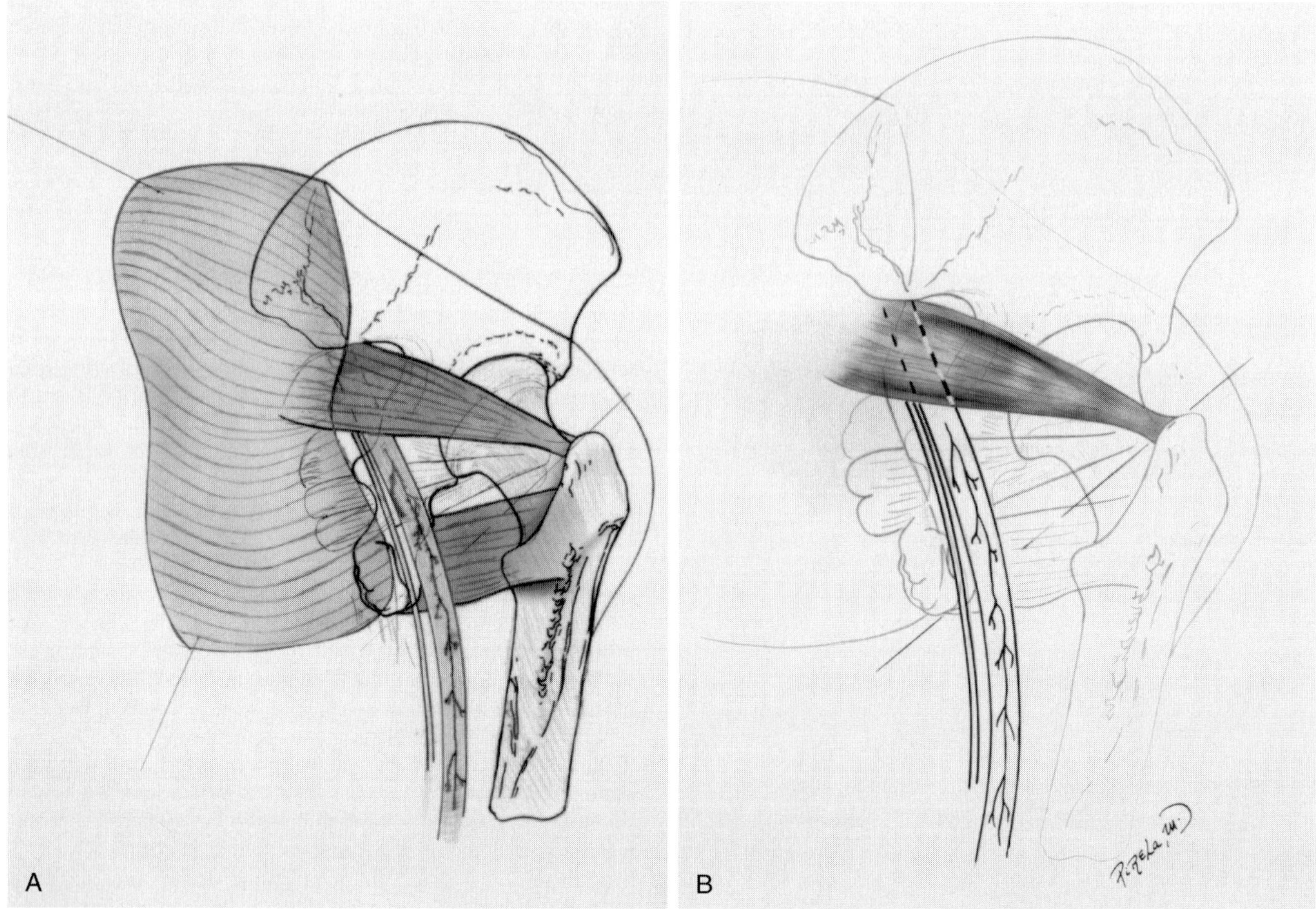

FIGURE 19–35. *A* and *B*, With the gluteus maximus muscle reflected medially, the sciatic nerve can now be visualized exiting from the greater sciatic foramen. Note the relationship of the piriformis to the nerve.

tion through the deep fascia and open the fascia of the external abdominal oblique muscle. The dissection on the anterior thigh is carried to the inguinal ligament (Fig. 19–41). If exposure is difficult, divide the ligament and tag the ends for later closure. Retract the peritoneum superior and medially, exposing the iliac fascia. Identify the psoas muscle, and open the fascia. The FN can be identified along the lateral border of the muscle from which it emerges. The use of a nerve stimulator also can facilitate the identification of motor branches.

EXPOSURE OF THE SAPHENOUS NERVE

The saphenous nerve is the largest branch of the FN. It provides sensibility to the medial thigh and knee. On occasion, it can serve as a source of nerve graft for neurorrhaphy procedures when other donor nerves are not available. In the proximal thigh, the exposure for the saphenous branch is the same as for the FN. The saphenous nerve (branch) can be identified by its medial location and its relatively large size. As mentioned earlier, the use of a nerve stimulator can also facilitate in the identification of motor branches.

Obturator Nerve

ANATOMY

The ON is formed by the anterior divisions of the L2, L3, and L4 nerve roots in the substance of the psoas major muscle. It emerges from the medial side of the psoas. In the pelvis, it descends posterior to the common iliac vessels to pass along the lateral wall to exit through the obturator foramen as it gains entry into the thigh. Cutaneous branches from the ON supply the medial thigh and may extend as far distally as the knee. The motor segment of the nerve divides into an anterior and posterior divisions shortly after entering the thigh. The divisions pass on either side of the adductor brevis muscle. The anterior division innervates the adductor longus, adductor brevis, gracilis, and pectineus muscles. This anterior division can be located between the adductor brevis and longus muscles. Articular branches to the hip joint are also given off the anterior division. The posterior division occasionally innervates the adductor brevis, adductor magnus, and obturator externus. The posterior division can be found between the adductor brevis and adductor magnus muscles. The pectineus and adductor magnus muscles have duel innervation. The pectineus receiving additional supply from the FN and the adductor magnus receiving contributions from the tibial division of the sciatic nerve.

EXPOSURE

Patient Position. Supine position.

The ON may be injured during genitourinary surgical procedures, resulting in weak adduction. Formal exploration

Text continued on page 203

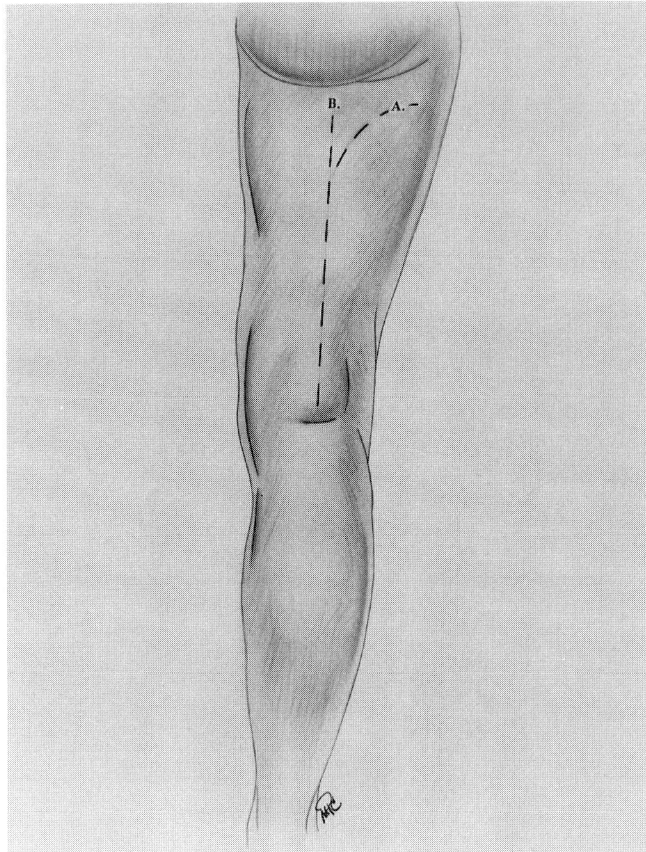

FIGURE 19–36. Incisions used for exposure of the sciatic nerve inferior to the gluteal fold.

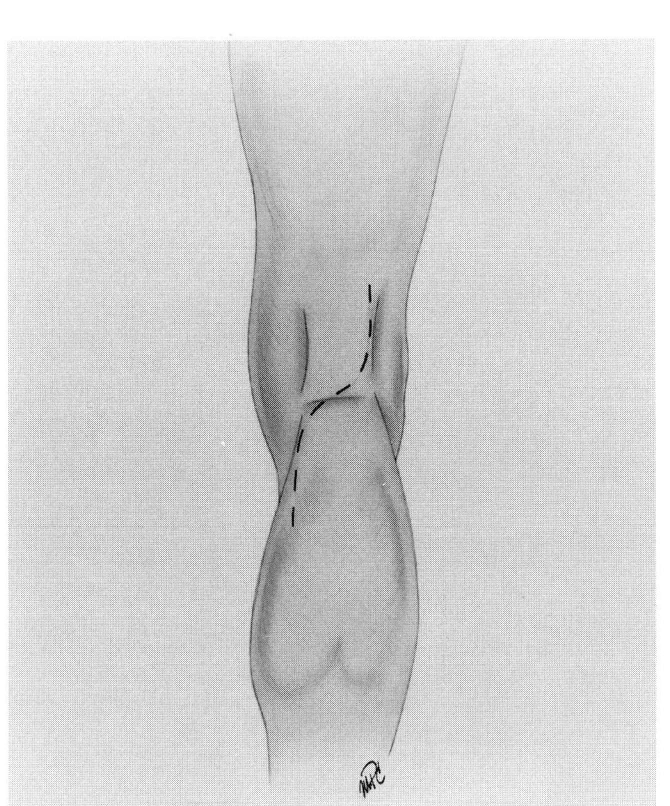

FIGURE 19–37. Incision used for the exposure of the tibial nerve in the popliteal region of the knee.

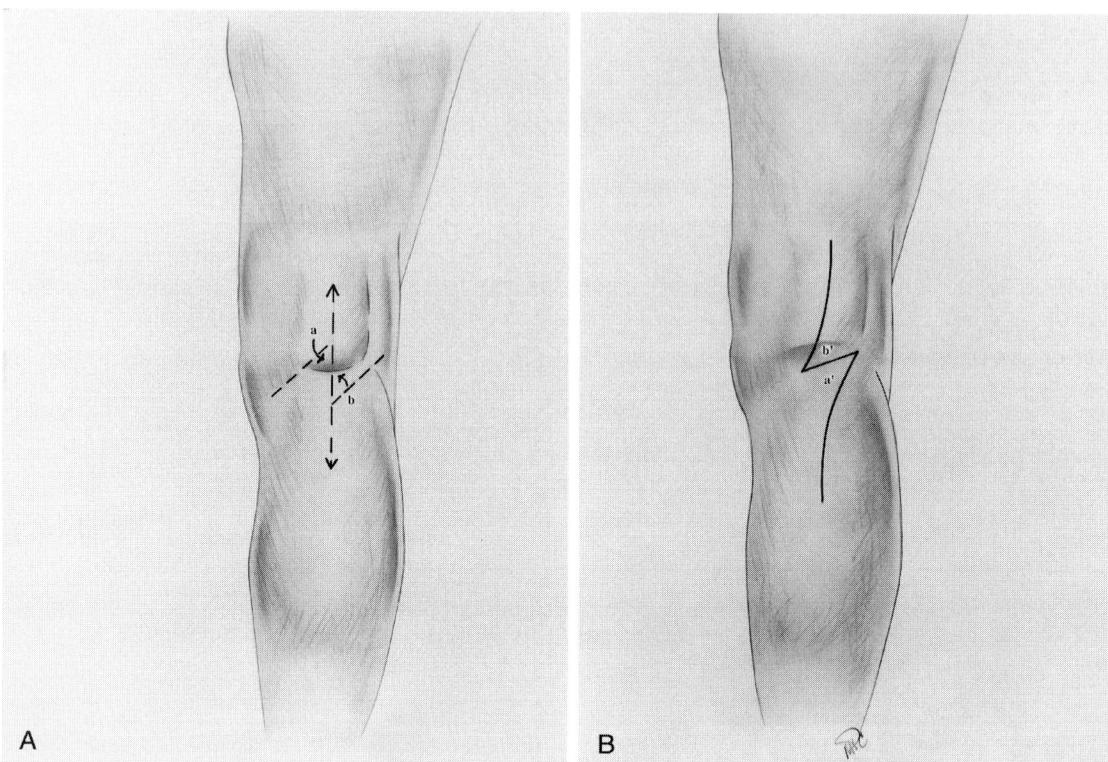

FIGURE 19–38. *A,* An alternative incision for exposure of the neurovascular structures in the popliteal region of the knee. *B,* The linear incision is converted to a Z-plasty to help prevent scar tissue with the development of the knee flexion contracture. The Z-plasty can also be used as the primary incision, avoiding flap transposition.

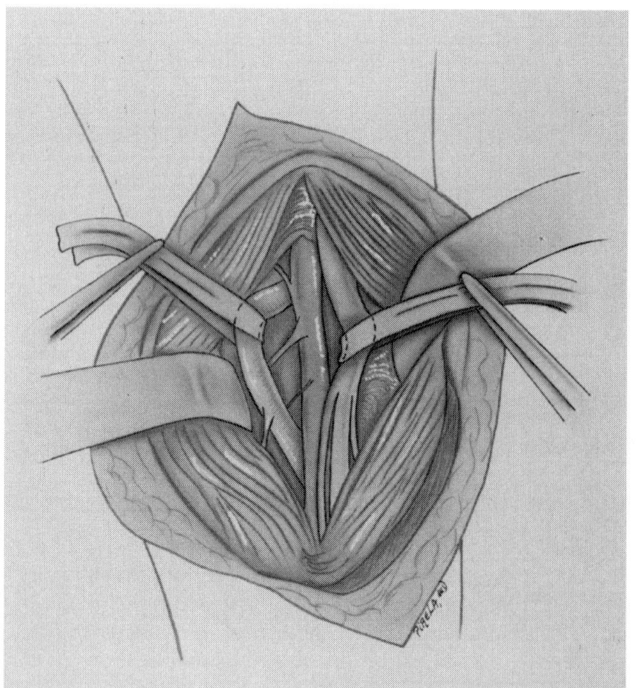

FIGURE 19–39. The popliteal region of the knee with exposure of the tibial nerve, popliteal artery, and vein.

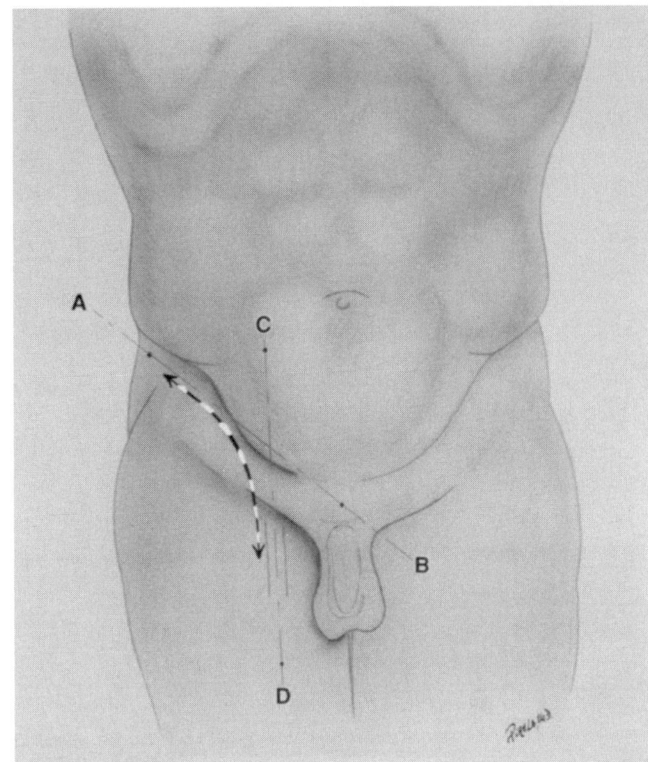

FIGURE 19–40. Incision used for the exposure of the femoral nerve. Useful landmarks include the inguinal line drawn by connecting the anterosuperior iliac spine, *A,* to the symphysis pubis, *B.* A second vertical line, C-D, is drawn over the femoral artery. The incision should be placed inferior to line A-B and just lateral to line C-D.

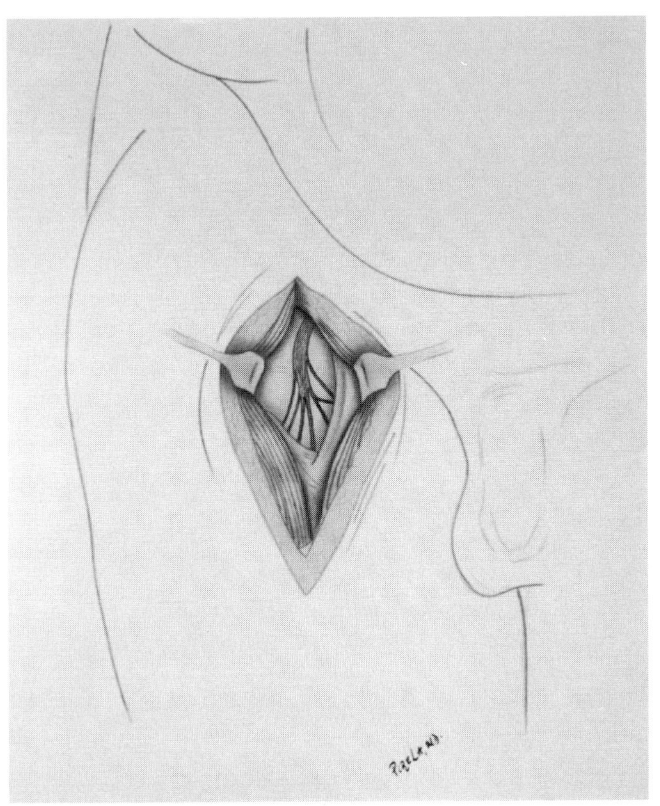

FIGURE 19–41. The femoral nerve with its ramifications. Note the largest (and medial) branch is the saphenous nerve. The mnemonic NAVEL (N, nerve; A, artery; V, vein; E, empty space; and L, lacuna ligament) helps us recall the anatomical structures in this region as we travel in a lateral to medial direction.

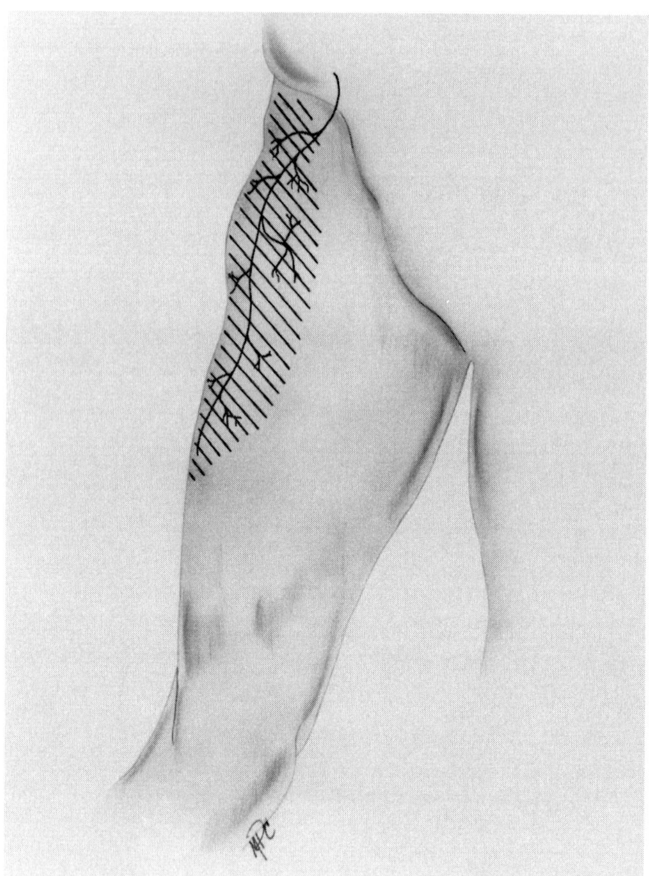

FIGURE 19–42. The cutaneous distribution of the lateral femoral cutaneous nerve.

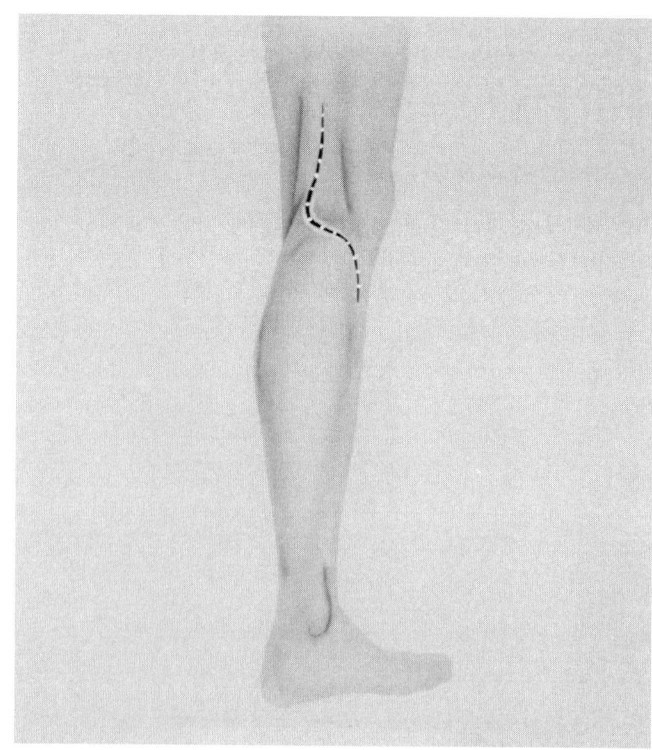

FIGURE 19–43. Incision used for the extensile surgical exposure of the common peroneal nerve.

and simple epineurial repair may be indicated (Vasilev, 1994).

Exposure of the extrapelvic segment of the ON in the upper thigh can be performed through a direct medial approach. Make an incision along the upper medial aspect of the thigh beginning at the pubis symphysis and extending distally for 20 to 25 cm. Identify the adductor magnus laterally and the adductor longus medially. Separate these muscles, and develop this interval. The obliquely oriented muscles fibers of the adductor brevis can now be identified. The anterior branch of the ON can be located on the anterior surface of the adductor brevis muscle. If exposure of the posterior branch of the ON is also necessary, incise the adductor brevis muscle carefully and locate the nerve on the posterior surface.

Lateral Femoral Cutaneous Nerve

Patient Position. Supine with a bolster under the ipsilateral buttock.

The lateral femoral cutaneous nerve is composed of the L2 and L3 nerve roots. On its path to the lateral region of the thigh, it courses just medial to the anterosuperior iliac spine (Fig. 19–42). At about 10 cm inferior to the inguinal ligament, the nerve perforates the fascia lata as it surfaces to the subcutaneous level.

The indications for surgical decompression of the lateral femoral cutaneous nerve are very rare, although this nerve may be involved in entrapment neuropathies (e.g., meralgia paraesthetica, Roth-Bernhardt's syndrome).

Common Peroneal Nerve

Patient Position. Supine with a bolster under the leg or buttock, lateral or prone.

Surgical Equipment. Pneumatic tourniquet, nerve stimulator.

The CPN can be identified as a discrete branch within the sciatic nerve anywhere from its origin in the pelvis to the popliteal region. It is composed of spinal segments L4, L5, S1, and S2. The anatomy of the peroneal nerve about the proximal fibula is of particular interest to the surgeon performing arthroscopy of the knee (Esselman et al, 1993) or osteotomies of the fibula (and tibia), to correct malalignment problems of the leg, or harvesting the fibular as a vascularized or nonvascularized bone graft (Rodeo et al, 1993; Satku and Kumar, 1992; Slawski et al, 1994; Soejima et al, 1994). The incision for exposing the CPN is shown (Fig. 19–43). Although the extensile incision is shown, a limited approach may be all that is required (Fig. 19–44). In a study by Soejima and colleagues (1994), the anatomical considerations of the peroneal nerve for division of the fibula were analyzed. Soejima and coworkers found a relatively safe area located 20.5 mm from the tip of the fibula head distally where osteotomies can be safely performed. They further described a safe angle of 64.1 degrees to perform the osteotomy to avoid injury to the proximal branch to the extensor hallucis longus muscle.

Two sensory branches come off the common peroneal: the lateral sural cutaneous branch and the peroneal anastomotic branch. The lateral sural nerve provides sensibility to the lateral knee region and extends distally to the proximal calf. The peroneal anastomotic branch combines with the tibial anastomotic nerve to form the sural nerve, which supplies the posterolateral calf and lateral malleolus. The CPN spirals around the fibular neck and shortly divides into a superficial and a deep branch. The superficial branch of the peroneal nerve passes between the extensor digitorum longus, the peroneal longus muscles, and the intermuscular septum, giving off branches to these muscles and the peroneal brevis as it travels distally. In the distal third of the leg, the superficial branch of the peroneal nerve divides into two cutaneous nerves to supply the anterolateral aspect of the leg and dorsal and lateral aspect of the foot.

The deep peroneal nerve exits the CPN just distal to the neck of the fibula in the proximal leg. The DPN continues medially, passing posterior to the extensor digitorum longus to lie between the tibia and fibula anterior to the interosseous membrane (Figs. 19–45 and 19–46). Once in this region, the nerve continues distally to supply the tibialis anterior, extensor digitorum longus, extensor hallucis longus, peroneus tertius, extensor digitorum brevis, and the first dorsal interosseous muscles. After the first dorsal interosseous branch is given off, the DPN surfaces to supply cutaneous innervation to the dorsal web space, ultimately terminating as two dorsal digital nerves to supply the skin to the dorsolateral great toe and dorsomedial second toe. This region is the autonomous zone of the DPN. The anatomy about the first web space is of particular interest to the reconstructive hand surgeon who uses anatomical parts based on the arterial distribution of the first metatarsal artery (Fig. 19–47).

Posterior Tibial Nerve

Patient Position. Supine with a bolster under the contralateral buttock.

Surgical Equipment. Pneumatic tourniquet.

In the proximal leg, access to the tibial (posterior tibial) nerve can be approached through a direct medial approach just anterior to the muscles of the posterior compartment (Fig. 19–48). This approach can be modified to accommodate limited or extensile exposure, depending on the clinical situation. After incising the deep fascia, the interval between the soleus and the flexor digitorum longus is developed. Deep retraction is required for adequate exposure. The tibial nerve can be located buried within the flexor digitorum longus and soleus muscles (Fig. 19–49). Distally, the posterior tibial nerve can be easily located posterior to the medial malleolus along with the tibialis posterior tendon, the flexor digitorum longus, the flexor hallucis longus (which can be remembered by the mnemonic Tom, Dick, and Harry), and the posterior tibial artery (Figs. 19–50 and 19–51). If distal exposure of the posterior tibial nerve is required, more often than not, it is advisable to initially locate the nerve just above the medial malleolus and then trace it proximally because the nerve quickly dives at approximately 3 to 4 cm above the malleolus and searching for the nerve at this level (or higher) may be a little more difficult.

Sural Nerve (Lateral Sural)

Patient Position. Prone or lateral decubitus position, or supine (with some difficulty).

Text continued on page 208

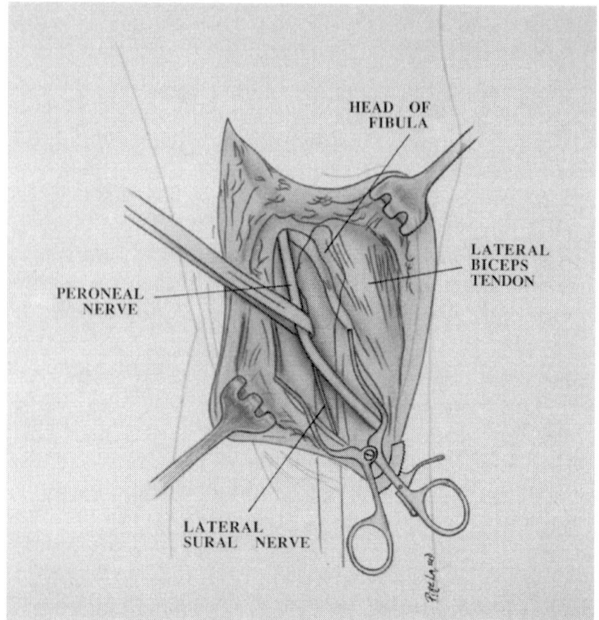

FIGURE 19–44. The common peroneal nerve in the lateral knee region.

FIGURE 19–45. The deep peroneal nerve in the mid-leg. Note the interval between the anterior tibialis and toe extensors muscles where the neurovascular bundle can be found. EDC, Extensor digitorum communis; EHL, extensor hallucis longus.

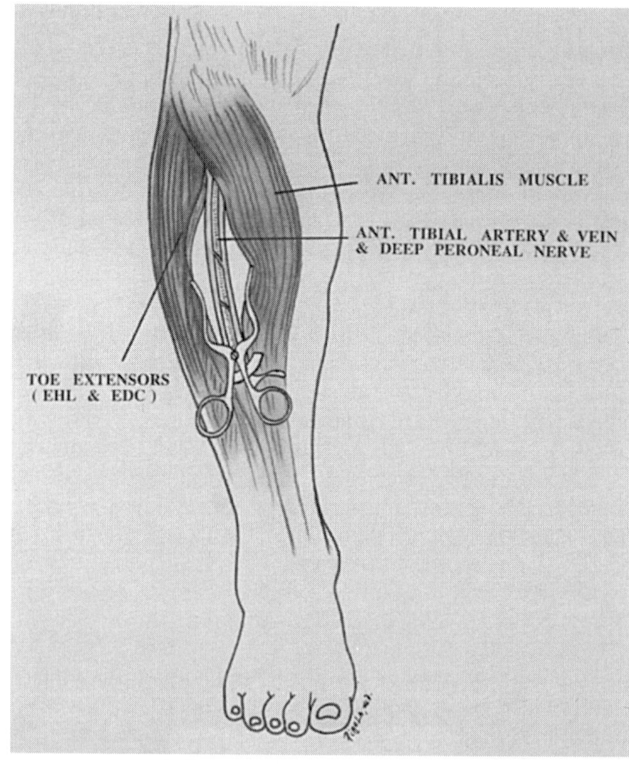

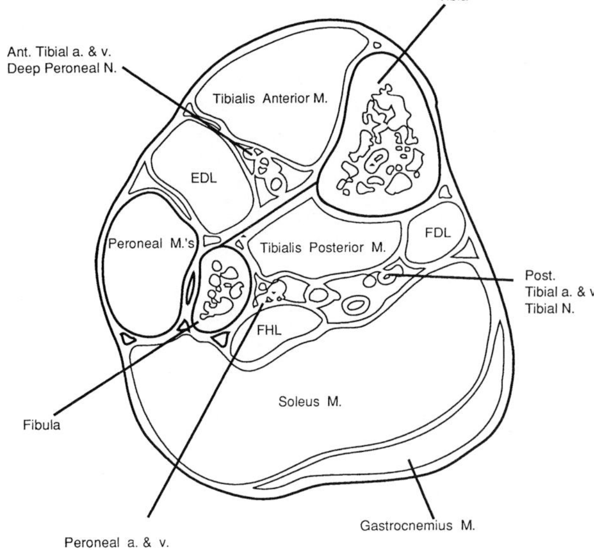

FIGURE 19–46. Cross-sectional view of the leg at the midlevel. The muscles of the extensor digitorum longus (EDL), flexor digitorum longus (FDL), and the flexor hallucis longus (FHL) can be seen.

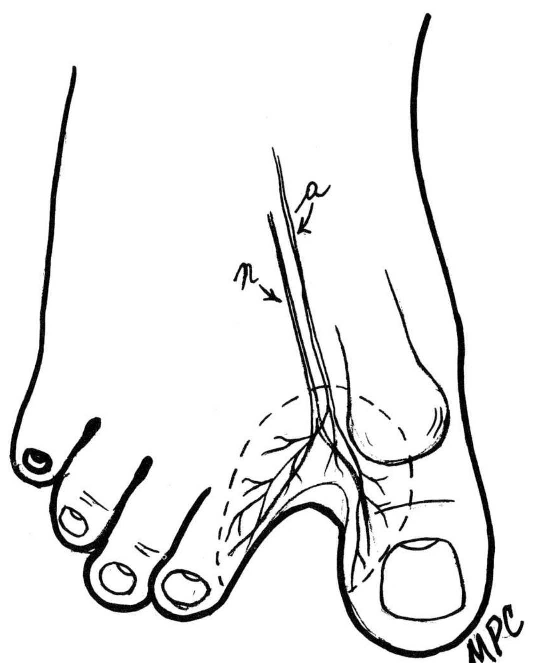

FIGURE 19–47. The first toe web space with its associated metatarsal artery and nerve.

Surgical Equipment. Pneumatic tourniquet.

The sural nerve is commonly used as a donor nerve graft for neurorrhaphy procedures because of the relatively low morbidity associated with harvesting this nerve. Moreover, because of its relatively low morbidity, it is the donor nerve of choice for major nerve reconstructive procedures. A neural interconnection between the tibial nerve and CPN has been described by Phillips and Morgan (1993) in a patient. They also found the sural nerve to be arising entirely from the CPN.

Harvesting of this sural nerve should be performed under pneumatic tourniquet control to minimize bleeding. The exposure should be performed through one long incision to reduce the surgical trauma on the nerve. The initial incision to locate the nerve should be performed just above and posterior to the lateral malleolus because the nerve is relatively superficial here. If there is difficulty locating the nerve at this level, the foot should be placed into the equinus position and the incision extended distally. Eastwood and coworkers (1992) found the main trunk to be located in this region with a 95% confidence limit. If only a small segment of nerve is required, it is advisable that the actual nerve graft be obtain well above the ankle region because symptomatic neuroma formation is possible and may interfere with shoe wear. Once the sural nerve is located distally, it can easily be traced proximally to the popliteal region.

References

Allieu Y, Cenac P: Neurotization via the spinal accessory nerve in complete paralysis due to multiple avulsion injuries of the brachial plexus. Clin Orthop 237:67–74, 1988.

Alnot JY, Valenti P: Surgical repair of the axillary nerve. Apropos of 37 cases. Int Orthop 15:7–11, 1991.

Andersen PE, Shah JP, Cambronero E, Spiro RH: The role of comprehensive neck dissection with preservation of the spinal accessory nerve in the clinically positive neck. Am J Surg 168:499–502, 1994.

Artico M, Salvati M, D'Andrea V, Ramundo EO, Nucci F: Isolated lesion of the axillary nerve: Surgical treatment and outcome in 12 cases. Neurosurgery 29:697–700, 1991.

Aziz NH, Shakespeare DT: Blunt injury to the spinal accessory nerve. Injury 20:381–382, 1989.

Bassett FH 3rd, Nunley JA: Compression of the musculocutaneous nerve at the elbow. J Bone Joint Surg (Am) 64:1050–1052, 1982.

Bateman JE: Nerve lesions about the shoulder. Orthop Clin North Am 11:319–321, 1980.

Beck DL, Maves MD, Stith JA: Spinal accessory nerve preservation. Laryngoscope 101(Pt 1):1386, 1991.

Blackwell KE, Landman MD, Calcaterra TC: Spinal accessory nerve: An unusual complication of rhytidectomy. Head Neck 16:181–185, 1994.

Bourne MH, Wood MB, Carmichael SW: Locating the lateral antebrachial cutaneous nerve. J Hand Surg (Am) 12(Pt 1):697–699, 1987.

Breslau RC: Transaxillary approach to the upper dorsal spine. In Watkins RG (ed): Surgical Approaches to the Spine. New York, Springer-Verlag, 1983, pp 58–68.

Bruner JM: Incisions for plastic and reconstructive (non-septic) surgery of the hand. Br J Plast Surg 4:448–455, 1951.

Bunnell S: Surgery of the Hand, 2nd ed. Philadelphia, J. B. Lippincott, 1948.

Cannieu JMA: Recherches sur une anastomose entre la branche profonde du cubital et le mé dian. Bull Soc Anat Physiol Bordeaux 18:339–340, 1897.

Chang KC, Huang JS, Liu KN, Tsai CS, Chen TY: Neurinoma of the spinal accessory nerve: Report of a case. Taiwan I Hsueh Hui Tsa Chih 89:593–597, 1990.

Conolly WB: Minor surgical procedures and infections. In McFarlane RM (ed): Unsatisfactory Results in Hand Surgery. New York, Churchill Livingstone, 1987, pp 41–64.

Danziger N, Chassande B, Lamas G, Fligny I, Soudant J, Willer JC: Partial

restoration of blink reflex function after spinal accessory–facial nerve anastomosis. J Neurol Neurosurg Psychiatry 58:222–226, 1995.

Dellon AL: Partial dorsal wrist denervation: Resection of the distal posterior interosseous nerve. J Hand Surg (Am) 10:527–533, 1985.

Dellon AL, Campbell JN, Cornblath D: Stretch palsy of the spinal accessory nerve. Case report. J Neurosurg 72:500–502, 1990.

Dellon AL, MacKinnon SE: Injury to the medial antebrachial cutaneous nerve during cubital tunnel surgery. J Hand Surg 10B:33–36, 1985.

Donner TR, Kline DG: Extracranial spinal accessory nerve injury. Neurosurgery 32:907–910, 1993.

Eastwood DM, Irgau I, Atkins RM: The distal course of the sural nerve and its significance for incisions around the lateral hindfoot. Foot Ankle 13:199–202, 1992.

Ebersold MJ, Quast LM: Long-term results of spinal accessory nerve–facial nerve anastomosis. J Neurosurg 77:51–54, 1992.

Eisele DW, Weymuller EA, Price JC: Spinal accessory nerve preservation during neck dissection. Laryngoscope 101(Pt 1):433–435, 1991.

Esselman PC, Tomski MA, Robinson LR, et al: Selective deep peroneal nerve injury associated with arthroscopic knee surgery. Muscle Nerve 16:1188–1192, 1993.

Eversmann WW Jr: Entrapment and compression neuropathies. In Green DP (ed): Operative Hand Surgery, 3rd ed. New York, Churchill Livingstone, 1993, p 1341.

Fabrizi AP, Poppi M, Giuliani G, Gambari PL, Gaist G: Benign solitary nerve sheath tumors of the spinal accessory nerve in the posterior triangle of the neck. J Neurosurg Sci 36:247–250, 1992.

Falconer D, Spinner M: Anatomic variations in the motor and sensory supply of the thumb. Clin Orthop 195:83–96, 1985.

Felsenthal G, Mondell DL, Reischer MA, Mack RH: Forearm pain secondary to compression syndrome of the lateral cutaneous nerve of the forearm. Arch Phys Med Rehabil 65:139–141, 1984.

Flatow EL, Bigliani LU: Tips of the trade. Locating and protecting the axillary nerve in shoulder surgery: The tug test. Orthop Rev 21:503–505, 1992.

Frohse F, Frankel M: Die Muskeln des Menschlichen Armes. Bardeleben's Handbuch der Anatomie des Menschlichen. Jena, Fisher, 1908.

Fuss FK, Wurzl GH: Radial nerve entrapment at the elbow: Surgical anatomy. J Hand Surg (Am) 16:742–7, 1991.

Garcia G, McQueen D: Bilateral suprascapular-nerve entrapment syndrome. J Bone Joint Surg (Am) 63:491–492, 1981.

Giuliani G; Poppi M; Acciarri N; Forti A: CT scan and surgical treatment of traumatic iliacus hematoma with femoral neuropathy: case report. J Trauma 30:229–231, 1990.

Gruber W: Ueber die Verbindung des Nervus medianus mit dem Nervus ulnaris am Unterarme des Menschen und der Sängethiete. Arch Anat Physiol 37:501–522, 1870.

Guyon F: Note sur une disposition anatomique propre à la face antérieure de la région du poignet et non encore décrite. Bull Soc Anat Paris 6:184–186, 1861.

Henry AK: Exposures in the lower limb. Sec. IV. In Henry AK (ed): Extensile Exposure, 2nd ed. New York, Churchill Livingstone, 1973, pp 180–307.

Holstein A, Lewis GB: Fractures of the humerus with radial nerve paralysis. J Bone Joint Surg (Am) 45A:1382, 1963.

Horowitz SH: Peripheral nerve injury and causalgia secondary to routine venipuncture. Neurology 44:962–964, 1994.

Inserra S, Spinner M: An anatomic factor in transposition of the ulnar nerve. J Hand Surg (Am) 11:80–82, 1986.

Jamjoom ZA, al-Bakry A, al-Momen A, Malabary T, Tahan AR, Yacub B: Bilateral femoral nerve compression by iliacus hematomas complicating anticoagulant therapy. Surg Today 23:535–540, 1993.

Jori J, Savay L Cziger J: Recontruction of the spinal accessory nerve after radial neck dissection. Acta Chir Hung 33:79–86, 1992–1993.

Kaplan EB: Correction of a disabling flexion contracture of the thumb. Bull Hosp Joint Dis 3:51–54, 1942.

Kerr AT: The brachial plexus of nerves in man, the variations in its formation and branches. Am J Anat 23:285, 1918.

Kumar S, Anantham J, Wan Z: Posttraumatic hematoma of iliacus muscle with paralysis of the femoral nerve. J Orthop Trauma 6:110–112, 1992.

Lanotte M, Massaro F, Scienza R, Faccani G: Intracisternal schwannoma of the spinal accessory nerve presenting as a normal pressure hydrocephalus syndrome. Case report and review of the literature. Neurosurg Rev 17:225–227, 1994.

Lanz U: Anatomical variations of the median nerve in the carpal tunnel. J Hand Surg 2:44–53, 1977.

Lederman RJ, Wilbourn AJ: Spinal accessory nerve palsy. Arch Phys Med Rehabil 72:604–605, 1991.

Lister GD, Belsole RV, Kleinert HE: The radial tunnel syndrome. J Hand Surg 4:52–59, 1976.

MacKinnon SE, Dellon AL: The overlap pattern of the lateral antebrachial cutaneous nerve and the superficial branch of the radial nerve. J Hand Surg (Am) 10:522–526, 1985.

Mangini U: Flexor pollicis longus muscle. Its morphology and clinical significance. J Bone Joint Surg (Am) 42A:467–470, 1960.

Marini SG, Rook JL, Green RF, Nagler W: Spinal accessory nerve palsy: An unusual complication of coronary artery bypass. Arch Phys Med Rehabil Mar 72:247–249, 1991.

Martin R: Tal om Nervus allmanna Egenskaper i Mannsikans Kropp. Stockholm, Lars Salvius, 1763.

Masear VR, Meyer RD, Pichora DR: Surgical anatomy of the medial antebrachial nerve. J Hand Surg 14A:267–271, 1989.

McShane D, Noyek AM, Chapnik JS, Steinhardt MI, Cooter N: Schwannoma of the intersternomastoid portion of the spinal accessory nerve: Sophisticated preoperative CT diagnosis and appropriate surgical management. J Otolaryngol 15:282–285, 1986.

Merrick HW, Zeiss J, Woldenberg LS: Percutaneous decompression for femoral neuropathy secondary to heparin-induced retroperitoneal hematoma: Case report and review of the literature. Am Surg 57:706–711, 1991.

Murphy RX Jr, Jennings JF, Wukich DK: Major neurovascular complications of endoscopic carpal tunnel release. J Hand Surg (Am) 19:114–118, 1994.

Murray JWG: A surgical approach for entrapment neuropathy of the suprascapular nerve. Orthop Rev 3:33–35, 1974.

Noyek AM, Chapnik JS, Wortzman G, Kandel R: Schwannoma of the intrasternomastoid portion of the spinal accessory nerve: Sophisticated pre-operative MRI diagnosis and appropriate surgical management. J Otolaryngol 21:286–289, 1992.

Nunley JA, Ugino MR, Goldner RD, Regan N, Urbaniak JR: Use of the anterior branch of the medial antebrachial cutaneous nerve as a graft for the repair of defects of the digital nerve. J Bone Joint Surg (Am) 71:563–567, 1989.

Ortiz O, Reed L: Spinal accessory nerve schwannoma involving the jugular foramen. Am J Neuroradiol 16(Suppl):986–989, 1995.

Osborne G: Compression neuritis of the ulnar nerve at the elbow. Hand 2:10–13, 1970.

Phillips LH 2nd, Morgan RF: Anomalous origin of the sural nerve in a patient with tibial–common peroneal nerve anastomosis. Muscle Nerve 16:414–417, 1993.

Pirela-Cruz MA, Omer GE, Benzel EC: Surgical exposure of the peripheral nerves of the upper extremity. *In* Benzel EC (ed): Practical Approaches to the Peripheral Nerve Surgery. Park Ridge, Illinois, American Association of Neurological Surgeons, 1992, pp 131–151.

Plancher KD, McGillicuddy JO, Kleinman WB: Anterior intramuscular transposition of the ulnar nerve. Hand Clin 12:435–444, 1996.

Poitevin LA: Carpal tunnel syndrome—limited open release. ASSH Correspondence Newsletter 33:194, 1994.

Probst A, Harder F, Hofer H, Thiel G: Femoral nerve lesion subsequent to renal transplantation. Eur Urol 8:314–316, 1982.

Rengachary SS, Neff JP, Singer PA, et al: Suprascapular entrapment neuropathy: A clinical, anatomical, and comparative study. Part 2: Anatomical study. Neurosurgery 5:441–446, 1979.

Riche P: Le nerf cubital et les muscles de l'é minence thenar. Bull Mem Soc Anat Paris 5:251–252, 1897.

Rodeo SA, Sobel M, Weiland AJ: Deep peroneal nerve injury as a result of arthroscopic meniscetomy. A case report and review of the literature. J Bone Joint Surg (Am) 75:1221–1224, 1993.

Ruder JR, Wood VE: Ulnar nerve compression at the arch of the origin of the adductor pollicis muscle. J Hand Surg (Am) 18:893–895, 1993.

Samardzic M, Grujicic D, Antunovic V, Joksimovic M: Reinnervation of avulsed brachial plexus using the spinal accessory nerve. Surg Neurol 33:7–11, 1990.

Samardzic M, Joksimovic M, Antunovic V, Grujicic D: Regional donor nerves in the reinnervation of brachial plexus palsy due to upper spinal roots avulsion. Neurol Res 11:181–185, 1989

Sarno JB: Suprascapular nerve entrapment. Surg Neurol 20:493–497, 1983.

Satku K, Kumar VP: Palsy of the deep peroneal nerve after proximal tibial osteotomy. An anatomical study (letter; comment). J Bone Joint Surg (Am) 74:1180–1185, 1992.

Saunders JR Jr, Hirata RM, Jaques DA: Considering the spinal accessory nerve in head and neck surgery. Am J Surg 150:491–494, 1985.

Slawski DP, Schoenecker PL, Rich MM: Peroneal nerve injury as a complication of pediatric tibial osteotomies: A review of 255 osteotomies. J Pediatr Orthop 14:166–172, 1994.

Soejima O, Ogata K, Fukahori Y, et al: Anatomic consideration of the peroneal nerve for division of the fibula during high tibial osteotomy. Orthop Rev 23:244–247, 1994.

Spinner M: Injuries to the Major Branches of the Peripheral Nerves of the Forearm, 2nd ed. Philadelphia, W.B. Saunders, 1978.

Sweeney PJ, Wilbourn AJ: Spinal accessory (11th) nerve palsy following carotid endarterectomy. Neurology Mar 42(Pt 1):674–675, 1992.

Spinner M: Management of nerve compression lesions. Instr Course Lect 33:498–512, 1984.

Taleisnik J: The palmar cutaneous branch of the median nerve and the approach to the carpal tunnel. J Bone Joint Surg (Am) 55A:1212–1217, 1973.

Walsh JF: The anatomy of the brachial plexus. Am J Med Sci 74:387, 1877.

Wartenburg RA: Sign of Ulnar Palsy. JAMA 112:1688, 1939.

Waters PM, Schwartz JT: Posterior interosseus nerve: An anatomic study of potential nerve grafts. J Hand Surg (Am) 18:743–745, 1993.

Weisberger EC, Lingeman RE: Cable grafting of the spinal accessory nerve for rehabilitation of shoulder function after radial neck dissection. Laryngoscope 97(Pt 1):915–918, 1987.

Yuan RT, Cohen MJ: Lateral antebrachial cutaneous nerve injury as a complication of phlebotomy. Plast Reconstr Surg 76:299–300, 1985.

Vasilev SA: Obturator nerve injury: A review of management options. Gynecol Oncol 53:152–155, 1994.

Zinberg EM: Surgical approaches for decompression of the posterior interosseous nerve in the radial tunnel syndrome. Am Soc Surg Hand Correspondence Newsletter 120, 1994.

Chapter 20

• Greg P. Watchmaker
• Michael E. Jabaley

Pertinent Internal Topography of Peripheral Nerves

HISTORICAL OVERVIEW

Early Studies of Topography

Early accounts of human anatomy failed to distinguish between peripheral nerves and blood from vessels. In ancient Greece in 200 AD, Galen wrote, "Some persons are convinced that the nerves originate in the heart because they are unable to distinguish a sinew from a nerve" (Siegel, 1976). Galen himself accurately described "voluntary impulses" that originated in the brain and propagated to the nerves and muscles. Although detailed and accurate accounts of the gross peripheral nerve anatomy followed, the intraneural plexuses were first described in 1779 by Prochaska in his treatise "De structure nervorum; tractatus anatomicus" (Fig. 20–1).

Interest in nerve injuries intensified during World War I, when physicians on both sides recognized their disappointing results following repair of nerve lesions. In 1913, Stoffel described his larger-than-life models of the internal topography of the sciatic nerve at various levels. Following 110 operations and 50 cadaveric dissections, he concluded that the intraneural arrangement was relatively constant between individuals. Three years later, Heinemann presented his investigations of the inner and gross anatomy of the upper extremity nerves (Heinemann, 1916). In contrast to Stoffel, he described irregular internal plexuses, which were illustrated through longitudinal dissections.

Langley and Hashimoto (1917) are credited with the first comprehensive investigation of nerve plexuses and their clinical relevance. Their investigation included dissections of the sciatic nerves of cats, dogs, and humans. They pointed out that several factors delay or prevent complete nerve recovery: (1) Fibers of the central (proximal) end, as they grow out, pass into connective tissue instead of the nerve fibers of the distal (peripheral) end; (2) some fibers, although they grow, are unable to make functional endings, as when efferent fibers grow into afferents and visa versa; and (3) some fibers make functional nerve endings but the central connection is different from that existing before the nerve lesion. Their rationale for the existence of fascicular bundles is interesting: "The advantage of the formation of bundles is that the arteries and veins can be kept outside the perineurium and thus pressure on the nerve fibres is avoided . . ." Regarding the role of intraneural plexuses, "The internal plexus obviously serves to collect together the afferent and efferent fibres of different nerve roots for the areas supplied by the peripheral nerves." They noted that certain fascicles run for a considerable distance without interconnection and they also commented that connections were more frequent *within* groups of fascicles than *between* groups of fascicles. Finally, they correctly recognized that connective tissue growth at the repair site could be an important impediment to regeneration, and they felt individual fascicular suture could hinder regeneration by causing increased scarring. Thus, almost 80 years ago, Langley and Hashimoto de-

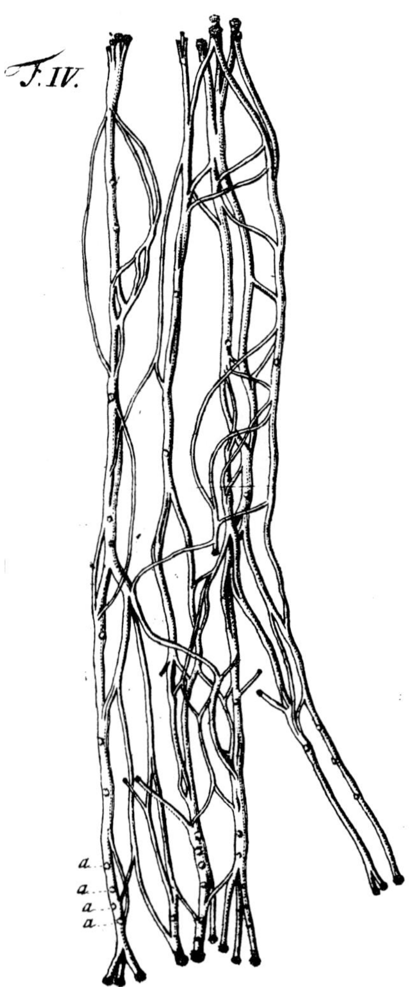

FIGURE 20–1. An early drawing by Georg Prochaska, 1779. Prochaska clearly recognized that fascicles could be separated from one another and that interconnections produced a plexus of bundles. (From Prochaska G: De Structura Nervosum; Tractus Anatomicus. Vindobonae, Apud Rudolophum Graeffer, 1779. OCLC: 11273305.)

scribed most of the principles of intraneural anatomy and fascicular suture.

During the same period, other investigators were examining internal topography. Compton (1917) described the "twisting" orientation of fascicles within a nerve, whereby the fascicles maintained constant internal anatomy but twisted about the axis of the nerve. He ascribed this phenomena to the rotation of the extremities during fetal development, as they assumed their final orientation. In 1918, Dustin performed both longitudinal and cross-sectional examinations of the median nerve and, to a lesser extent, the radial and ulnar nerves. In 1921, McKinley studied the entire adult sciatic nerve through cross sections at 3-mm intervals. He illustrated the extensive divisions and interconnections between fascicles, describing them as a "continuous exchange of fibers." He thus refuted the theory of Dustin, which described a quadrantic relationship of fibers within the nerve. McKinley further disproved the idea of quadrantic relationship by performing partial transections of the proximal sciatic nerve of dogs then studying the distribution of wallerian degeneration distally. He found degeneration to be widely distributed and not confined to certain quadrants.

The matter of mixing of individual nerve fibers within a plexus remained unclear. Kraus reported on electrical stimulation studies in human upper extremity nerves and found that motor fasciculi took a straight course from brachial plexus to distal motor branches (Krause, 1920). In contrast, Goldberg (1924) dissected human cadaver nerves and concluded that, "No two sciatic nerves present exactly the same internal topography; in fact, there is a considerable variation in internal structure."

The variation in these studies was due partly to the choice of nerve studied (sciatic nerve versus peroneal or tibial and lower versus upper extremity) and the dissection technique (cross-sectional versus longitudinal). Longitudinal dissections tend to disrupt small plexus connections and thus underestimate the complexity of the architecture. Cross-sectional studies typically suffer from small sample size due to the intensive labor involved. Table 20–1 summarizes the early and more recent studies which have been performed.

The Midcentury

Following the investigations of 1910 to 1920, little reference was made to intraneural topography for the next 25 years. Surgical technique was based on whole nerve suture, with little attention paid to internal alignments.

With World War II came a huge number of nerve-injured patients and renewed interest in nerve suture. Shortly after the war, Sunderland published his examination of the intraneural topography of the radial, median, and ulnar nerves (Sunderland, 1953). The accompanying plates gave detailed accounts of the fascicular arrangement (or funiculi as he preferred to call them) and their course within the nerves. Sunderland was able to provide this level of detail by tracing each fascicle's course and branching patterns in 0.25-mm increments along the nerves (our own investigations have confirmed that this small interval is necessary if the study is to correctly account for all changes in topography along the nerve).

Sunderland studied a small number of nerves by cross section: one radial nerve, one median nerve, and two ulnar nerves. Based on these four specimens, along with additional longitudinal dissections, he concluded that "there was no constant or characteristic funicular pattern for any nerve. Variations occurred at different levels along the same nerve, at the same level on the two sides of the body, and from nerve to nerve and subject to subject at any given level." He added that the average distance over which the pattern remained constant varied between 0.25 and 0.5mm (Fig. 20–2).

▼ **TABLE 20–1**
Internal Topography Studies

Year	Author	Dissection Technique	n	Nerve(s)	Magnification	Interval
1913	Stoffel	Cross section	50	Sciatic		?
1918	Dustin	Cross section		Median, radial, ulnar		
1921	McKinley	Cross section	1	Sciatic		3 mm
1945	Sunderland	Cross section	4	Radial (1), median (1), ulnar (2)		25 mm
1959	Sunderland	Cross section	15	Axillary (5), musculocutaneous (5), obturator (5)		?
1980	Jabaley	Cross section	3	Median (1 total, 2 partial)		0.1–1 mm
1986	Chow	Cross section	10	Median and ulnar		5 mm
1991	Watchmaker	Cross section	16	Median (distal)		.25–1 mm
1994	Watchmaker	Cross section	5	Ulnar (elbow)		.33–1 mm
1916	Heinemann	Longitudinal		Median, radial, ulnar	?	
1917	Compton	Longitudinal	12	Sciatic	lens	
1917	Langley	Longitudinal	3	Sciatic	?	
1924	Goldberg	Longitudinal	10	Sciatic/obturator	none	
1945	Sunderland	Longitudinal	20	Median, radial, ulnar	?	
1980	Jabaley	Longitudinal	10	Median (4), ulnar (4), radial (2)	4.5–25×	
1986	Chow	Longitudinal	17	Median and ulnar	?	
1992	MacKinnon	Longitudinal	23	Median (distal 2nd/3rd web)	3.5 loupe	
1968	Hakstian	Intraoperative stimulation	13	Ulnar (8), median (5)		
1983	Schady	Percutaneous stimulation	4	Median		
1990	Hallin	Percutaneous stimulation	15	Median		
1990	Marchettini	Percutaneous stimulation	27	Ulnar		

n, Number

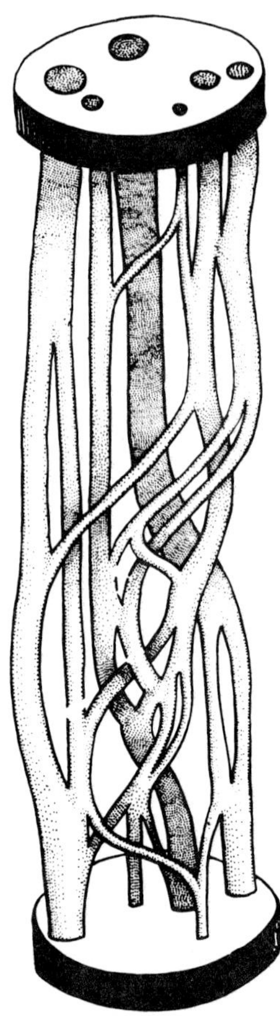

FIGURE 20–2. Reconstruction of the musculocutaneous nerve, produced from serial sections by the late Sir Sidney Sunderland, who recognized interconnections between bundles of fibers. (From Sunderland S: Nerves and Nerve Injuries. New York, Churchill Livingstone, 1968.)

Despite his views of topographic complexity, Sunderland found specific areas where fascicular anatomy could be used to the surgeon's benefit. In 1953, he noted the principles of funicular suture and funicular exclusion. When repairing a nerve such as the radial nerve in the arm, he recommended separating the motor and sensory components so that selective repair or grafting could be performed (Sunderland, 1953). Sunderland later performed similar investigations into the circumflex, musculocutaneous, and obturator nerves (Sunderland, 1959). These findings are summarized in his text Nerve and Nerve Injuries (Sunderland, 1968).

The Modern Era

It must be recalled that the majority of early studies were by anatomists and tended to emphasize the internal complexity of nerves. Beginning in the 1960s, however, improvements in magnification and instrumentation led surgeons to examine nerve repair in more detail. With these examinations came an appreciation of the practical anatomy of nerves. It became apparent that, when necessary, epineurium could be incised or excised and that fascicles could be separated and identified over distances greater than the fractions of a millimeter that Sunderland had proposed.

To confirm these clinical impressions, surgeons repeated the classic studies of topography, performing serial histologic sections and longitudinal dissections (Jabaley et al, 1980). These investigations led to the following conclusions: (1) The musculocutaneous nerve, as depicted by Sunderland, is not typical of the major nerves of forearm and wrist. Instead, fascicles can be easily separated for greater distances without apparent injury. (2) Even when interconnections occur, fibers still travel in fairly uniform fashion in specific quadrants, and (3) functional components can be identified, even when they are several centimeters apart and joined, if necessary, by grafts.

Overall, these findings were more encouraging to surgeons, who were trying to improve clinical results and have been subsequently corroborated by several other investigators (Chow et al, 1986; Watchmaker et al, 1991; Williams and Jabaley, 1986).

CLINICALLY RELEVANT TOPOGRAPHY

Median Nerve in the Forearm and Wrist

In cases in which a nerve is cleanly transected or has a limited zone of injury, knowledge of the general topography may assist in accurate alignment of fascicles. Jabaley, Wallace, and Heckler comment on their results from microdissections and serial sections: "In the median nerve in the upper third of the forearm, the motor branches to the extrinsic muscles lie about the periphery, primarily on the radial and ulnar sides" (Jabaley et al, 1980). The remainder occupy the central core and dorsal quadrant. In the middle third of the forearm, there are very few branches and no major quadrant changes. In the distal third, the components are well separated and can be isolated for repair. They were able to identify the motor branch to the thenar muscles on the volar-radial aspect of the median nerve and trace it for distances of up to 30 mm proximal to the radial styloid.

From these investigations, Jabaley and co-workers proposed a much more organized anatomy in the distal aspect of peripheral nerves (Fig. 20–3). They suggest that axons themselves may maintain definite quadrantic positions over long distances and that it is the varying arrangement of internal epineurium that is responsible for much of the change observed in cross-sectional analysis.

As noted above, this view of axonal organization (despite plexus interconnection) has been independently substantiated by several investigators using a variety of techniques. Brushart (1991) studied the axonal organization in primates. Using retrograde transport of horseradish peroxidase, he demonstrated that axons to a single digital nerve remained well localized even at the level of the brachial plexus. In the upper arm, individual digital nerve axons occupied only one third to one sixth of the nerve cross section with only moderate intermingling. This view is also supported by Perotto and Delagi (1979), who found sharp demarcation of sensory loss in persons with partial median nerve lacerations. Direct electrical studies of the median nerve on four human volunteers by Schady and colleagues (1983) reached a similar conclusion. Stimulation of sensory fascicles in the arm projected to no more than 20% of the median nerve sensory territory, suggesting that most of the rearrangements of spinal root fibers occurs at the brachial plexus level. Based on

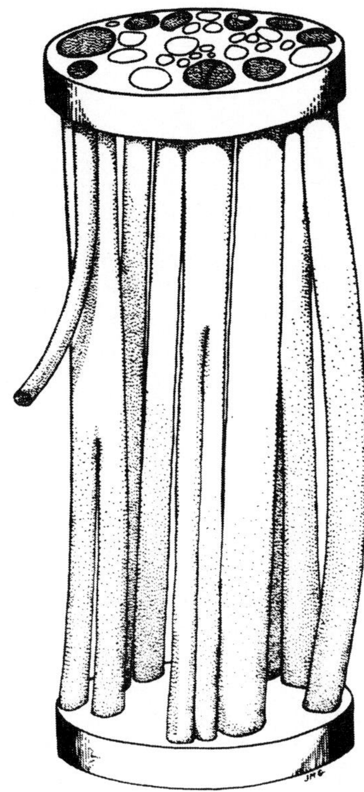

FIGURE 20–3. The more distal portions of the median nerve. In contrast to Figure 20–2, the fascicular arrangement is more orderly, with individual bundles travelling for several centimeters and with relatively few connections between them.

intrafascicular recordings using very fine concentric electrodes, Hallin (1990) has suggested the concept of intrafascicular micro-bundles. Fibers within these micro-bundles remain well localized within the nerve despite fascicular rearrangements. These studies all argue strongly in favor of proper axial alignment during nerve repair, whether or not fascicular topography is conserved.

Watchmaker and associates (1991) studied the topography of the median nerve in the distal forearm and wrist in a large number of specimens and found that the sensory fibers to the second and third web space remained well localized well into the forearm with few intergroup connections. The sensory and motor fascicles to the thumb communicated more freely along the volar-radial aspect of the nerve at this level. Ross (1992) confirmed these findings and suggested a technique using the third web space fascicles as a donor nerve by proximal dissection to provide graft material for 3- to 6-cm median nerve gaps. MacKinnon (1988) has previously confirmed the safety of this intraneural dissection in the primate model.

From a practical standpoint, the significance of such studies is twofold: (1) When a nerve is transected, individual bundles or fascicles can be separated from one another for purposes of identification and suture. If one knows the dissection distances (Fig. 20–4), it is immediately apparent how far separation can be accomplished. Such information is especially helpful in partial transections where a loop suture is indicated, in grafting situations, or when a specific branch, such as the motor branch of the median nerve, must be identified. (2) When epineurotomy and fascicular separation (internal neurolysis) is indicated. The most com-

mon example is the median nerve in previously operated carpal tunnel syndrome, in which a simple external decompression might be considered inadequate.

Ulnar Nerve in Forearm and Wrist

The fascicular anatomy of the distal ulnar nerve is relatively straightforward and should be familiar to the peripheral nerve surgeon. Three discrete fascicular groups arise from the ulnar nerve in the distal forearm: (1) the dorsal sensory group, (2) the volar sensory group to ring and small finger, and the (3) intrinsic motor group. Sunderland (1945) identified the deep motor branch along the dorsal-ulnar aspect of the distal nerve. More proximally, the dorsal cutaneous sensory fascicles enter on the medial aspect of the nerve, moving the motor branches to a more central location. Chow and colleagues (1985, 1986) have confirmed this dorsal-ulnar location of the motor fascicular group of the ulnar nerve. The ulnar motor bundles may be identified as a separate group up to 50 mm proximal to the level of the radial styloid (Williams and Jabaley, 1986).

The stable anatomic relationship of fascicles in the distal ulnar nerve underscores the importance of proper alignment during repair. To confirm the functional role of bundles, intraoperative nerve stimulation in the awake patient can aid the surgeon. Hakstian (1968), Gaul (1986), and Jabaley and co-workers (1984) have all described the use of intraoperative nerve stimulation to assist in repair, and Kline and Hudson have encouraged stimulation and recording of individual nerves (Gaul, 1986). Lastly, histochemical techniques have also been advocated as a means of assigning specific function to specific fascicles.

Ulnar Nerve at the Elbow

Clinically, knowledge of the fascicular anatomy of the ulnar nerve is more commonly used for decompression at the elbow than for repair. In anterior transposition, Learmonth originally recommended proximal dissection of the posterior

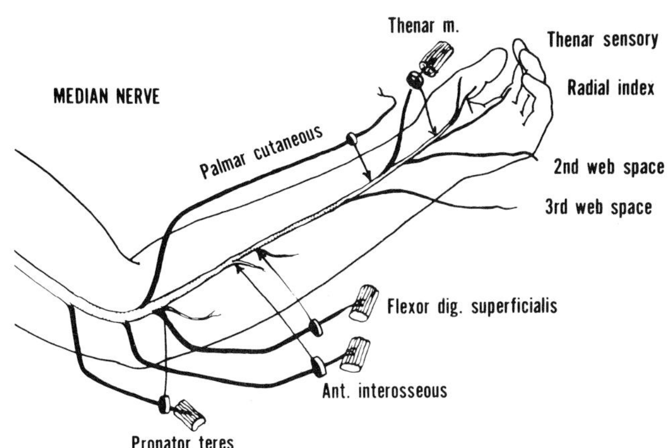

FIGURE 20–4. A partially dissected median nerve (not to scale). Four branches are shown, illustrating their dissection distances. The ring and arrow indicated the original branch point. Proximal to this, the dark line indicates the distance that the branch can be separated without damaging interconnections. (Jabaley ME. Wallace WH, Heckler FR: Internal tomography of major nerves of the forearm and hand: A current view. J Hand Surg 5:1–18, 1980.)

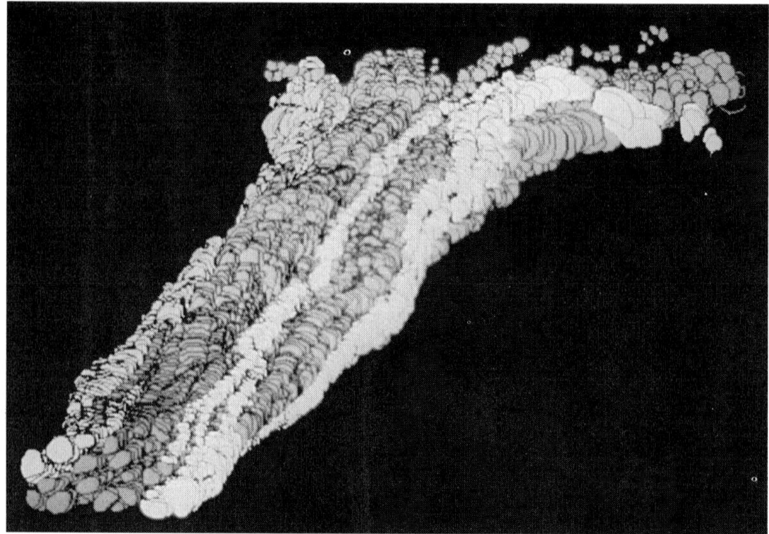

FIGURE 20–5. Longitudinal reconstruction of a right median nerve, seen from the proximal end (left lower corner to distal end [right upper corner]). The original nerve was sectioned serially, and each section was digitized; the image was generated by computer. Thenar motor fibers are shown initially as two fascicles, which become confluent just before exiting from main trunk.

branches to the flexor carpi ulnaris and flexor digitorum profundus to prevent tethering of the nerve close to the epicondyle, and this has remained the standard technique. Recently, Watchmaker and associates (1994) has investigated the plexus anatomy in this region and confirmed that no fascicular interconnections occur over a distance of 6.0 cm (Fig. 20–5). Therefore, proximal dissection of ulnar motor branches may be safely performed above the elbow without injury to the intraneural plexus.

RADIAL NERVE

The major area of interest in radial nerve anatomy is one joint proximal to those of the median and ulnar nerves—at the elbow.

Beginning at the dorsal hand at the superficial radial nerve, sensory fibers travel proximally to join motor and sensory axons of the posterior interosseous nerve and form the radial nerve proper. This union occurs in the proximal forearm at the supinator level, but the two components remain separate and distinct for a distance of 7 to 9 cm before any interconnections are noted (Jabaley et al, 1980; Sunderland, 1945). As one proceeds further proximally, the specific fascicles still maintain a fairly constant quadrantic relationship, well up to the area of the spiral groove of the humerus.

The significance of these findings is obvious. Correct alignment in terminal radial injuries is usually apparent and relatively simple to obtain. This, coupled with the relatively few fascicles in the radial nerve and short distance to target muscles, is largely responsible for the favorable prognosis in radial nerve injuries, compared with median and ulnar transections at the same level.

SUMMARY

Fascicular topography has been investigated in detail for the nerves of the upper extremity, and the peripheral nerve surgeon may use knowledge of this anatomy to her or his benefit. Whatever suture technique is selected, correct fascic-

ular alignment is the basic goal of repair. This may be especially true in the more commonly involved distal injuries.

Many unresolved questions remain regarding fascicular topography and fascicular repair in humans. Although laboratory studies suggest no advantage to fascicular versus external epineurial repair, no series in humans has addressed the clinical results in a controlled manner. Brushart and associates (1983) have shown more appropriate innervation following fascicular suture in the rat. Wall and co-workers (1986) demonstrated major topographic changes in the primate cortex following median nerve transection and repair that was not found after nerve crush and regeneration. These studies support again the importance of fascicular alignment.

Today, the greatest unanswered question facing investigators is the primary role of the fascicular plexus. Whether it serves as a sorting mechanism or is simply an artifact of development is not known. No investigator has successfully mapped the course of individual axons in human peripheral nerves to determine the degree of mixing within the plexus. Cortical mappings in the primate have shown much less axonal mixing than the fascicular plexus would suggest, providing a more optimistic view toward correct regeneration and reinnervation in major mixed nerves.

Whatever the nature of intraneural plexuses within nerves, this much can be said with certainty: The surgeon who understands the general nature of nerve makeup and the specifics of such areas as the terminal portions of the three major nerves in the upper limb will be better able to make correct anatomic alignment of transected nerves. By recognizing the functional significance of specific fascicles or fascicular bundles and connecting them correctly, one is assured that regenerating axons are given the best chance of reaching their proper end organs and restoring function.

References

Brushart TM, Edward CT, Mesulan M: Specificity of muscle reinnervation after epineurial and individual fascicular suture of the rat sciatic nerve. J Hand Surg 8:248–253, 1983.

Brushart TM: Central course of digital axons within the median nerve of Macaca Mulatta. J Comp Neurol *311*:197–209, 1991.

Chow JA, Van Beek AL, Meyer DL, et al: Surgical significance of the motor fascicular group of the ulnar nerve in the forearm. J Hand Surg *10A*:867–872, 1985.

Chow JA, Van Beek AL, Bilos ZJ, et al: Anatomical basis for repair of ulnar and median nerves in the distal part of the forearm by group fascicular suture and nerve-grafting. J Bone Joint Surg *68A*(2):273–280, 1986.

Compton AT: The intrinsic anatomy of the large nerve trunks of limbs. J Anat *51*:103–117, 1917.

Dustin AP: La fasciculation des nerfs. Ambulance de l'Ocean *2*:135–154, 1918.

Gaul JS: Electrical fascicle identification as an adjunct to nerve repair. Hand Clinic *2*(4):709–722, 1986.

Goldberg I: The internal architecture of the tibial, peroneal and obturator nerves. Am J Anat *32*:447, 1924.

Hakstian RW: Funicular orientation by direct stimulation. J Bone Joint Surg *50A*:1178–1186, 1968.

Hallin RG: Microneurography in relation to intraneural topography: Somatotopic organization of median nerve fascicles in humans. J Neurology Neurosurg Psych *53*:736–744, 1990.

Heinemann O: Ueber Schussverletzungen der peripheren Nerven. Nebst anatomischen Untersuchungen uber den inneren Bau der grossen Nervenstamme. Arch F Klin Chir 108:107–150, 1916.

Jabaley ME, Wallace WH, Heckler FR: Internal topography of major nerves of the forearm and hand: A current view. J Hand Surg *5*:1–18, 1980.

Jabaley ME: Electrical nerve stimulation in the awake patient. Bull Hosp Jt Dis *44*:248–259, 1984.

Kraus WM, Ingham SD: Peripheral nerve topography. Arch Neurol Psych *4*:259–296, 1920.

Kraus WM, Ingham SD: Electrical stimulation of peripheral nerves exposed at operation. JAMA *74*:586–589, 1920.

Langley JN, Hashimoto M: On the suture of separate nerve bundles in a nerve trunk and on internal nerve plexuses. J Physiol *51*:318–346, 1917.

Learmonth JR: Technique for transplanting the ulnar nerve. Surg Gynecol Obstet *75*:792, 1942.

MacKinnon SE, Dellon AL: Evaluation of microsurgical internal neurolysis in a primate median nerve model of chronic nerve compression. J Hand Surg *13*:345–351, 1988.

McKinley JC: The intraneural plexus of fasciculi and fibers in the sciatic nerve. Arch Neurol Psych *6*:377–399, 1921.

Perotto AI, Delagi EF: Funicular localization in partial median nerve injury at the wrists. Arch Phys Med Rehabil *60*:165–169, 1979.

Prochaska G: De structura nervorum; tractatus anatomicus. Vindobonae, Apud Rudolphum Graeffer, 1779. OCLC: 11273305.

Ross D, Mackinnon SE, Chang YL: Interneural anatomy of the median nerve provides "third web space" donor nerve graft. J Reconstr Microsurg *8*(3):225–232, 1992.

Schady W, Ochoa JL, Torebjork HE, et al: Peripheral projection of fascicles in the human median nerve. Brain *106*:745–760, 1983.

Segal RE: Galen on the Affected Parts: Translation from the Greek Text with Explanatory Footnotes. New York, S. Karger, 1976.

Sunderland S: The intraneural topography of the radial, median and ulnar nerves. Brain *68*(4):243–299, 1945.

Sunderland S: Funicular suture and funicular exclusion in the repair of severed nerves. Br J Surg *40*:580–587, 1953.

Sunderland S, Marshall RD, Swaney WE: The intraneural topography of the circumflex, musculocutaneous and obturator nerves. Brain *82*:116–129, 1959.

Sunderland S: Nerves and Nerve Injuries. New York, Churchill Livingstone, 1968.

Wall JT, Kaas JH, Sur M, et al: Functional reorganization in somatosensory cortical areas 3b and 1 of adult monkeys after median nerve repair: Possible relationships to sensory recovery in humans. J Neurosci *6*(1):218–233, 1986.

Watchmaker GP, Gumucio CA, Crandall RE, et al: Fascicular topography of the median nerve: A computer based study to identify branching patterns. J Hand Surg *16A*:53–59, 1991.

Watchmaker GP, Lee G, Mackinnon SE: Intraneural topography of the ulnar nerve in the cubital tunnel facilitates anterior transposition. J Hand Surg *19A*:915–922, 1994.

Williams HB, Jabaley ME: The importance of internal anatomy of the peripheral nerves to nerve repair in the forearm and hand. Hand Clin *2*(2):689–707, 1986.

Lower Extremity Nerve Topography (Sciatic and Femoral Nerve)

SCIATIC NERVE: ANATOMY AND FASCICULAR ARRANGEMENT

The internal arrangement of the sciatic nerve with regard to the location of fascicles with different functions is less known than that of the nerves of the upper limb (Goldberg, 1924; Infante and Kennedy, 1970; Libassi and Vigasio, 1988; McKinley, 1921; Sunderland and Bradley, 1949; Sunderland and Ray, 1948). That is due to less frequent traumatic involvement, less investigation, and less frequent surgery of the nerve.

The sciatic nerve originates from the ventral branches of the spinal nerves L4, L5, S1, S2, S3, that is, from the sacral plexus, which is made up of the lumbosacral trunk (L5 plus part of L4) and by spinal nerves S1, S2, and S3.

Anterior to the plexus are the pelvic colon on the left and the rectum in the mid-line, the lymph nodes of the sacral hollow, and the internal iliac vessels with the ureter. The lateral sacral arteries run medially on the plexus, the ilio-lumbar artery ascends to pass anterior to the lumbosacral trunk, the superior gluteal artery runs posteriorly between the lumbosacral trunk and the first sacral nerve, and the inferior gluteal courses between the second and the third sacral nerve.

Before forming the sciatic nerve, the sacral plexus gives off the common nerve for the tensor fasciae latae and smaller and middle gluteus as well as the single branches to pyramidal, superior and inferior gemellus, and quadratus femoris muscles.

After the confluence of its roots, the sciatic trunk emerges as a somewhat flattened band, 20 mm in width, which leaves the pelvis through the greater sciatic foramen below the lower margin of the piriformis and above the superior gemellus, and passes in the gluteal region. It proceeds in a caudad and lateral direction in a deep groove formed medially by the ischium and laterally by the greater trochanter. It lies beneath the gluteus maximus. The superior gluteal nerve leaves the foramen a little proximally, just distal to the (superior) gluteal artery. Even if anatomy books, like Testut's, say that at this level the fibers going to peroneal nerve are anterior and those of the tibial nerve are posterior, in our dissections, the authors found that the fibers for the common peroneal nerve are lateral and those for the tibial nerve are medial.

The gross internal arrangement from medial to lateral is as follows: the fibers to the hamstring muscle, those for the tibial and common peroneal nerve, and those for the nerve to the short head of biceps.

In the gluteal region, the nerve runs downward beneath the gluteus maximus, passing laterally to the ischial tuberosity and medially to the greater trochanter before descending vertically to the thigh. Anteriorly, the obturator-gemelli group and the quadratus femoris are interposed between the nerve and the capsule of the hip joint. The nerve is accompanied by the arteria comitans (a continuation of the inferior gluteal artery). The nerve continues down the mid-line of the thigh on the adductor magnus and is closely related to the shaft of the femur. It gives branches to the hamstrings, the adductor magnus (ischial fibers), and the hip joint. Just below the ischial tuberosity, it is crossed obliquely by the long head of biceps and below this again is overlapped by the contiguous margins of the semimembranosus and biceps muscles. In the thigh, the sciatic trunk gives off branches first to the semitendinous muscle, second to the long head of the biceps, third to the adductor magnus and semimembranosus, and fourth to the short head of the biceps. Toward the apex of the popliteal fossa, it divides into its two terminal branches: the common peroneal and the tibialis nerves. Less commonly, it divides above this level and, more rarely, below.

After the separation, the common peroneal nerve divides into the lateral cutaneous nerve of the leg and the superficial and the deep peroneal nerves.

The superficial peroneal nerve (lateral compartment), in turn, divides into the nerves to the muscles peroneus longus and peroneus brevis, and a sensory nerve that supplies the first seven dorsal digital nerves.

The deep peroneal nerve (anterior compartment) gives off four branches: the nerves to the muscles tibialis anterior, extensor digitorum longus, extensor hallucis longus and third peroneus, and sensory branches for the first web.

The tibial nerve descends in the plane between the gastrocnemius and soleus muscles posteriorly and the tibialis posterior anteriorly, sharing a common neurovascular sheath with the posterior tibial vessels, then it descends directly toward the internal retro malleolar zone.

The tibial nerve divides into several motor branches (one or even two for each posterior muscle of the leg and plantar muscles of the foot) and several sensory branches: the cutaneous medialis of the calf, the sural nerve, the internal calcaneus nerve, and the plantar cutaneous nerve.

INTRANEURAL TOPOGRAPHY OF THE SCIATIC NERVE

In order to know the internal arrangement of the fascicles having different destiny and function, we have dissected

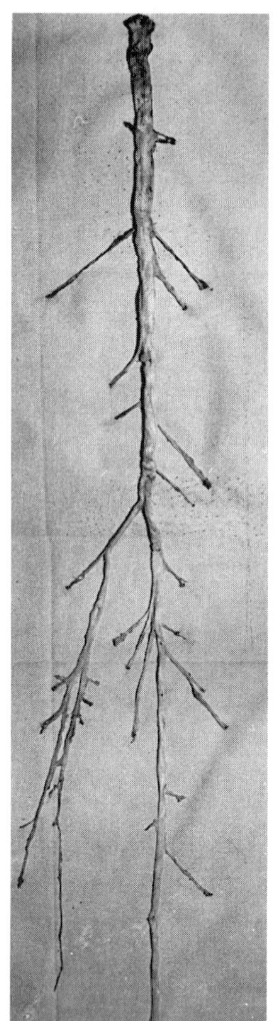

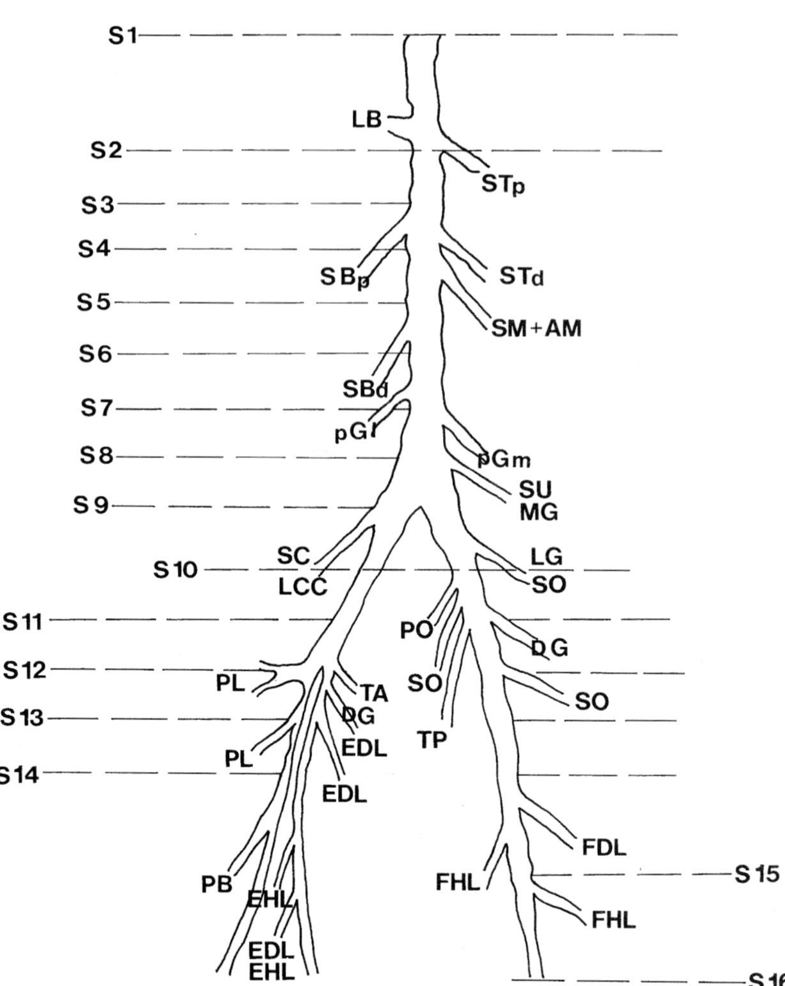

FIGURE 21–1. Intraneural topography of the sciatic nerve. (From Brunelli G [ed]: Textbook of Microsurgery. Milano, Italy, Masson Publishing Company, 1988.)

three cadavers (Fig. 21–1). The terminal and collateral branches of the sciatic nerve were identified distally, and their fascicles were isolated and followed proximally as far as possible (depending on the exchanges of fibers, which are more frequent in proximity of the sacral plexus).

Dissection was performed under loupe and operating microscope magnification. Cross sections were taken from the contralateral sciatic nerve, and the specular quadrantic location of the fascicles was identified and photographed by light microscopy. Instead of giving distances in centimeters from osseous reference points, which vary with the size of the subject, the nerves of the lower limb have been divided into two halves (the thigh and the leg) and divided, in turn, into eighths, so that the sections correspond to the same level in subjects of different size.

Cross sections were taken as follows (Fig. 21–2):

Section 1: at the sciatic notch
Section 2: at the gluteal crease
Section 3: between the 1st and 2nd eighth of the thigh
Section 4: between the 2nd and 3rd eighth
Section 5: between the 3rd and 4th eighth
Section 6: between the 4th and 5th eighth
Section 7: between the 5th and 6th eighth
Section 8: between the 6th and 7th eighth
Section 9: between the 7th and 8th eighth

Section 10: knee joint
Section 11: between the 1st and 2nd eighth of the leg
Section 12: between the 2nd and 3rd eighth
Section 13: between the 3rd and 4th eighth
Section 14: between the 4th and 5th eighth
Section 15: tibial nerve between the 6th and 7th eighth
Section 16: tibial nerve to the tibialis malleolus.

The tibial and the common peroneal nerves below the sciatic notch are described separately because although they are both contained in the common sciatic nerve, they are well defined.

Constitution of the Collateral and Terminal Branches of the Sciatic Nerve and Location of Their Constituents (According to Our Research)

Long Head of Biceps and Semitendinous Muscles. At the sciatic notch, they are found on the medial quadrant, together with the fascicles for the adductor magnus, semitendinosus, plantar, and flexor hallucis longus muscles. They descend in this position until they reach the gluteal crease, where they detach from the principal trunk.

Adductor Magnus and Semimembranosus Muscles. At the sciatic notch, they are found in the anterior half, together with other fascicles of the plantar nerves, flexor hallucis longus, semitendinosus and lateral head of biceps. They descend in the same position until the first eighth of the thigh, where they move laterally and remain in this position until the fourth eighth where they detach with a common trunk.

THE TIBIAL NERVE FROM THE SCIATIC NOTCH TO THE TIBIAL MALLEOLUS (MEDIAL CONTINGENT OF THE SCIATIC NERVE)

In the passage from the middle third of the thigh to the popliteal fossa, the tibial nerve changes its cross-sectional pattern and its shape from oval to round. This change is due to a redistribution of all the fascicles in the quadrantic location corresponding to the direction of the branches.

Genicular Branches

Proximal Branch. At the level of the sciatic notch, some fascicles are joined to those of the tibialis posterior, plantar, and flexor hallucis longus muscles, forming a group situated in a lateral position until the detachment of the proximal branch (sixth eighth of the thigh). The other fascicles in the fifth eighth of the thigh are in medial position, then they move anteriorly and laterally until their detachment.

Distal Branch. The fascicles in the eighth section of the thigh take a medial position until the first eighth of the leg, where they detach from the nerve.

Soleus Muscle

It is innervated by the proximal, middle, and distal branches.

The Proximal Branch. This branch in the third eighth is mixed with the fascicles to the medial head of the gastrocnemius and to the sural nerve. The fascicles in the sixth eighth of the thigh are in a posterior position. They frequently originate with a single branch at the eighth section of the thigh.

Distal and Middle Branches. The fascicles at the seventh eighth of the thigh are in central position, mixed with other fascicles of the plantar nerves and of the tibialis posterior; toward the knee, they move laterally and descend in this position below the knee. At the level of the second eighth of the leg, the proximal and the distal branches originate.

Popliteus and Lateral Head of the Gastrocnemius Muscle

The course and location of these fascicles are similar. Their fibers group starting from the sixth eighth of the thigh in a posterior position. On descending toward the knee, they move into a lateral position. The branch for the lateral head of the gastrocnemius originates at the eighth section of the thigh, while that of the popliteus is at the first eighth of the leg.

Tibialis Posterior Muscle

The fascicle is in a lateral position at the level of the sciatic notch, joined to that of the soleus, flexor hallucis longus, plantar, and genicular nerves. It descends in this position until its origin (second eighth of the leg).

Flexor Digitorum Longus Muscle

The fascicles are found at the level of the seventh eighth of the thigh in the central position, joined to the fascicles of the tibialis posterior, soleus, flexor hallucis longus, and plantar nerves.

This group descends toward the knee and the leg, moving into an anterior position and dividing itself so that, at the level of the first eighth of the leg, the fascicles of the flexor digitorum longus can be isolated in the anterior position, where it remains until its origin (fourth eighth of the leg).

Flexor Hallucis Longus Muscle

This muscle is innervated by two branches: proximal and distal.

Proximal Branch. The proximal branch can be recognized starting from the eighth section of the thigh in a superficial anterior position. It remains in this position until the second eighth of the leg. At the level of the third eighth, it moves laterally, and at the fourth eighth, it detaches from the nerve trunk.

Distal Branch. At the level of the sciatic notch, it is made up of two groups of fascicles. One in a lateral position tied to fascicles for the tibialis posterior, genicular, soleus, and plantar nerves, and the other in a medial position, together with the plantar ones.

The fascicles of the first group maintain their lateral position until the knee. Below the knee, they separate: Those to the flexor hallucis longus remain with the medial plantar fascicles situated on the medial part of the nerve until the fifth eighth of the leg, where the distal branch originates. The other group descends in a medial position and, at the level of the sixth eighth of the thigh, moves anteriorly until the knee. Then they separate from the plantar fascicles and join the fascicles of the flexor hallucis longus of the previous group.

Plantar Nerves

Their fascicles from the sciatic notch until the knee are mixed with the fascicles of all the branches, with the exception of those for the posterior muscles of the thigh. Below the knee, at the first eighth of the leg, the fascicles of both the plantar nerves are located in the posterior part. At the level of the second eighth, they stay in the central part. At the third eighth, the two fascicles groups part, becoming located in the lateral and medial zone of the nerve, respectively, until the medial malleolus.

THE COMMON PERONEAL NERVE FROM THE SCIATIC NOTCH TO THE INTERNAL MALLEOLUS (LATERAL CONTINGENT OF THE SCIATIC NERVE)

Branches of the Common Peroneal Nerve

Lateral Cutaneous of the Calf and Communicating Sural Branch. The fibers of the lateral cutaneous of the calf and the communicating sural branch group at the second eighth of the thigh in central position. In the descent toward the knee, they move first laterally and then, at the fifth eighth, posteriorly, and finally, at the sixth eighth, they go to the medial quadrant until their origin from the trunk.

Proximal Genicular and Distal Short Head of the Biceps Branches. They appear at the level of the gluteal crease in anterolateral position, then descend toward the knee, moving anteriorly, and detach from the trunk.

Proximal Branch of the Short Head of the Biceps. The fascicle appears at the first eighth of the thigh in lateral position. On descending toward the knee, it moves posteriorly and detaches at the third eighth of the thigh.

Superficial Peroneal Nerve

Sensitive Branches (Medial and Intermediate Cutaneous-Dorsal Nerves). The fibers of the medial and intermediate cutaneous-dorsal nerves group in fascicles at the eighth eighth of the thigh in central position. At the sixth eighth, they detach from the trunk.

Peroneus Brevis and Longus. The fascicles appear at the seventh eighth of the thigh in centrolateral position. On descending toward the knee, they move toward the medial half of the common peroneal nerve until the neck of the fibula. At the second eighth of the leg, the nerve undergoes torsion and the fascicles move laterally. The branch of the peroneus longus detaches in the second eighth.

Deep Peroneal Nerve

The Distal Branches. The sensitive distal branches assemble at the second eighth of the leg in central position, until the sixth eighth where they move medially.

Branches for the Extensor Hallucis Longus Muscle. The fascicles gather in the leg in a lateral position and remain in the same position until the detachment of their branches: the proximal at the fourth and the distal at the fifth eighth.

The Extensor Digitorum Longus Muscle. This muscle is innervated by three branches: proximal, middle, and distal. The fascicles of the proximal branch appear at the second eighth of the leg in the lateral position until their detachment (third eighth). The fascicles for the middle and distal branches assemble in the third eighth of the leg in the lateral quadrant. They detach from the nerve at the fifth eighth (intermediate branch) and seventh eighth (distal branch).

The Tibialis Anterior Muscle. This muscle is usually innervated by three branches: The first rises from the deep peroneal nerve or from the common peroneal nerve in the point of its division at the level of the first eighth of the leg, the second at the second eighth, and the third at the third or fourth eighth. Their fibers gather to form fascicles at the second eighth of the leg in the medial position until their detachment.

TOPOGRAPHICAL ARRANGEMENT OF THE FASCICLES

Section 1 (Sciatic Notch). It is not possible to recognize all the single fascicles and their destinations (see Figs. 21–2, 21–3, and 21–4). Two fascicles, destined to the short head of the biceps, are situated at the extreme of the medial quadrant. The fascicles for the branches of the tibialis posterior, soleus, flexor hallucis longus, plantars, genicular, and semimembranosus are in the anterolateral quadrant; the fascicles for the adductor magnus, semitendinosus, long head of biceps, plantars, and flexor hallucis longus are anteromedially located.

Section 2 (Gluteal Crease). The fascicle arrangement changes very slightly. The two fascicles of the short head of the biceps merge and move in the posterior zone.

Thigh

Section 3 (Between the First and the Second Eighth). The fascicle of the short head of the biceps moves to a lateral zone.

Section 4 (Between the Second and Third Eighth). The fascicle of the short head of the biceps divides into two: one for the proximal and the other for the distal branch, situated in the lateral part. The central zone is occupied by the fascicles of the sural communicating nerve, lateral cutaneous nerve of the calf, and proximal genicular nerve. The fascicles for the long head of biceps and semitendinosus disappear.

Section 5 (Between the Third and Fourth Eighth). The anteromedial zone is occupied by fascicles of the genicular and short head of biceps (distal branch), the lateral part by the sural communicating and the lateral cutaneous of the calf, and the posterior zone by the short head of biceps (proximal branch). The other fascicles cannot be recognized.

Section 6 (Between the Fourth and Fifth Eighth). The fascicles for the sural communicating and lateral cutaneous of the calf are in the posterolateral quadrant, and the fascicle for the short head of biceps (distal branch) is in the anterior quadrant. The fascicles for the tibial nerve do not undergo important modifications in their positions. The fascicles for the adductor magnus and semimembranosus disappear.

Section 7 (Between the Fifth and Sixth Eighth). There are few changes in the fascicle arrangement. The fascicles for the flexor hallucis longus and genicular are found in medial position.

Section 8 (Between the Sixth and Seventh Eighth). The fascicles of the sural communicating and lateral cutaneous of the calf occupy the medial zone.

The fascicles for the genicular and flexor hallucis longus travel a little anteriorly; the other fascicles are separated in numerous small groups of fascicles, the function of which is still unclear.

Section 9 (Between the Seventh and Eighth). The fascicles of the sural communicating and lateral cutaneous nerves of the calf are in medial position, whereas those of the deep peroneal nerve are centrally located. The fascicles of the various distal branches start to be recognizable. The fascicles to the flexor hallucis longus are in the anteromedial quadrant, and those to the flexor digitorum longus are in the anterolateral quadrant. Those of the popliteus, the lateral head of the gastrocnemius, and the sural are found in the posterolateral quadrant, and those to the medial head of the gastrocnemius are found in the posteromedial quadrant.

The fascicles to the plantar nerves and to the soleus muscle are spread in the anterolateral, posterolateral, and posteromedial quadrants, whereas those to the tibialis posterior are located both in the anterolateral and posterolateral positions.

Section 10 (Knee Joint). The fascicles of the deep peroneal nerve are in lateral position, and those of the peroneus longus and brevis are medially located. The central zone is occupied by the fascicles destined to travel to the sensory branch. In the anterolateral quadrant are fascicles to flexor hallucis longus, plantars, and flexor digitorum longus. In the anterolateral position are fascicles to the soleus, tibialis posterior, popliteus, and flexor hallucis longus muscles. In the posteromedial quadrant stay fascicles for plantar muscles and the sensory genicular branch. In the posterolateral quadrant, again are fascicles to flexor hallucis longus and soleus.

Leg (Peroneal Nerve)

Section 11 (Between the First and Second Eighth). There is little change in the arrangement of the fascicles.

Section 12 (Between the Second and Third Eighth). When the common peroneal nerve turns around the neck of the fibula in order to enter the anterolateral compartment, the anterior surface becomes posterior and the medial one become lateral. The lateral quadrant is occupied by the fascicles of the superficialis peroneal nerve and the medial quadrant by the deep peroneal nerve.

Section 13 (Between the Third and Fourth Eighth). The division of the two branches has already occurred. The sensitive fascicles of the superficial peroneal nerve are arranged medially, and those for the peroneus brevis nerve are arranged laterally. The fascicles of the deep peroneal, and genicular and tibialis anterior nerves are situated medially; those for the extensor digitorum longus nerve, extensor hallucis longus nerve, and the sensitive branches are laterally located.

Section 14 (Between the Fourth and Fifth Eighth). The fascicular arrangement of the superficial peroneal nerve does not change. As regards the deep peroneal nerve, the fascicles to the extensor digitorum longus are medially located, whereas those to the extensor hallucis longus and the sensitive branches are centrally located.

Leg (Tibial Nerve)

Section 11 (Between the First and Second Eighth). The anteromedial quadrant is occupied by the plantar, genicular, and flexor hallucis longus nerves. The anterolateral quadrant is occupied by the tibialis posterior, popliteus, flexor digitorum longus, and flexor hallucis longus; more fascicles to the plantars are contained in the posteromedial and in the posterolateral quadrant. Fascicles to the soleus are also posteriorly and laterally located.

Section 12 (Between the Second and Third Eighth). The tibialis posterior, soleus, and flexor hallucis longus are in the lateral part; the flexor hallucis longus fascicles and the flexor digitorum longus are medially located. The fascicles for the plantar group are in the central zone.

Section 13 (Between the Third and Fourth Eighth). The arrangement does not change much except for the gathering of the fascicles in groups with the same functional meaning.

Section 14 (Between the Fourth and Fifth Eighth). There are no changes.

Section 15 (Between the Sixth and Seventh Eighth). The fascicles for the flexor hallucis longus and flexor digitorum longus are in the medial part, and the rest of the nerve is occupied by the fascicles for the plantar nerves.

Section 16 (at the Level of the Internal Malleolus). The fascicles for the lateral plantars are in the lateral, and those for the medial plantars in the medial quadrant.

We hope that our study may be useful to the reader and that it can enable correct connection of the fascicles both in suturing and in grafting the sciatic nerve.

FEMORAL NERVE

The knowledge of the internal map of the femoral nerve (Bartolaminelli, 1988; Hepburn, 1887; Lanz and Wachsmuth, 1935; Omer and Spinner, 1980; Sunderland, 1978; Testut, 1908) may appear of less interest than that of the other nerves of the human body because below the inguinal liga-

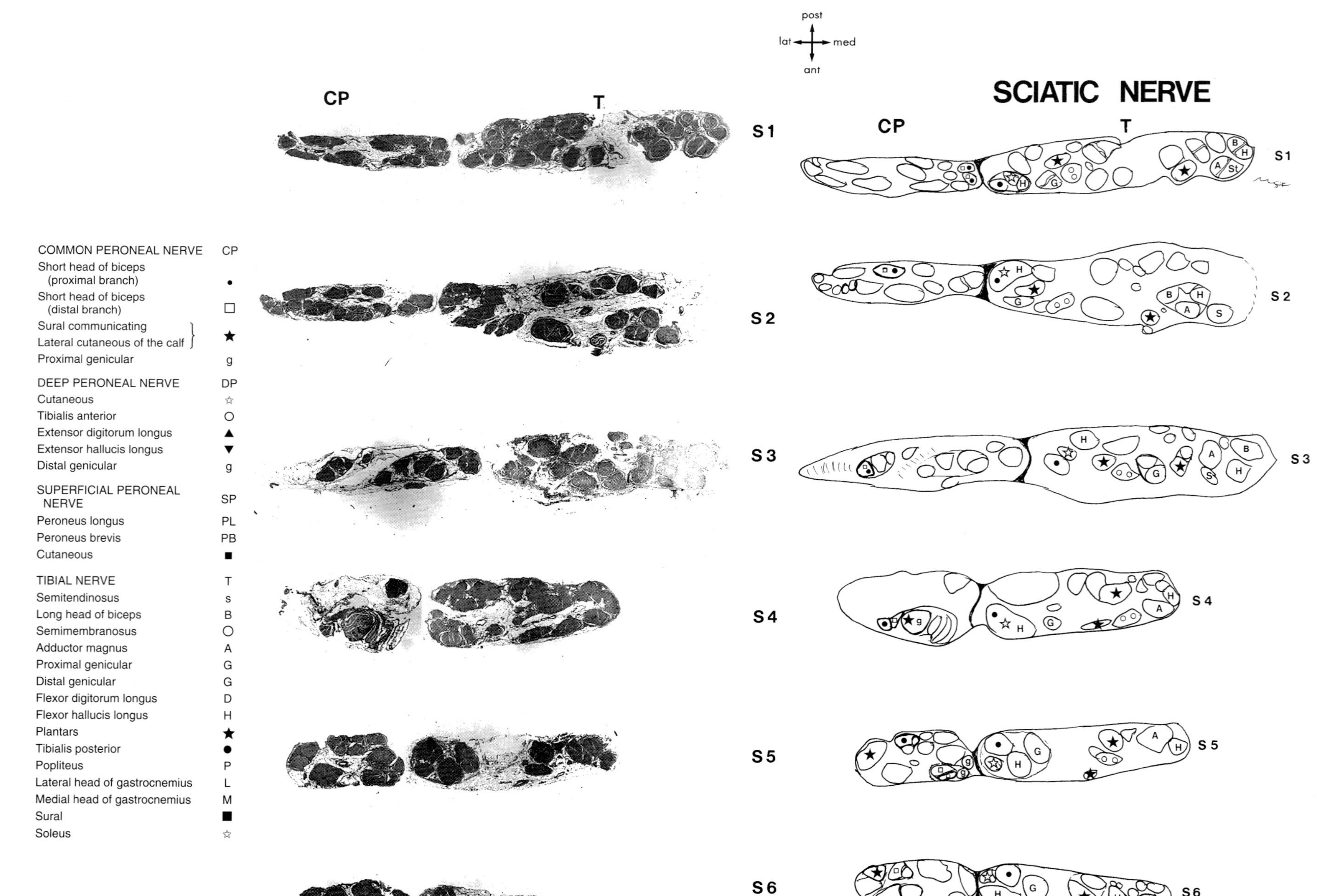

FIGURE 21–2. The sciatic nerve, sections 2 through 6. (From Brunelli G [ed]: Textbook of Microsurgery. Milano, Italy, Masson Publishing Company, 1988.)

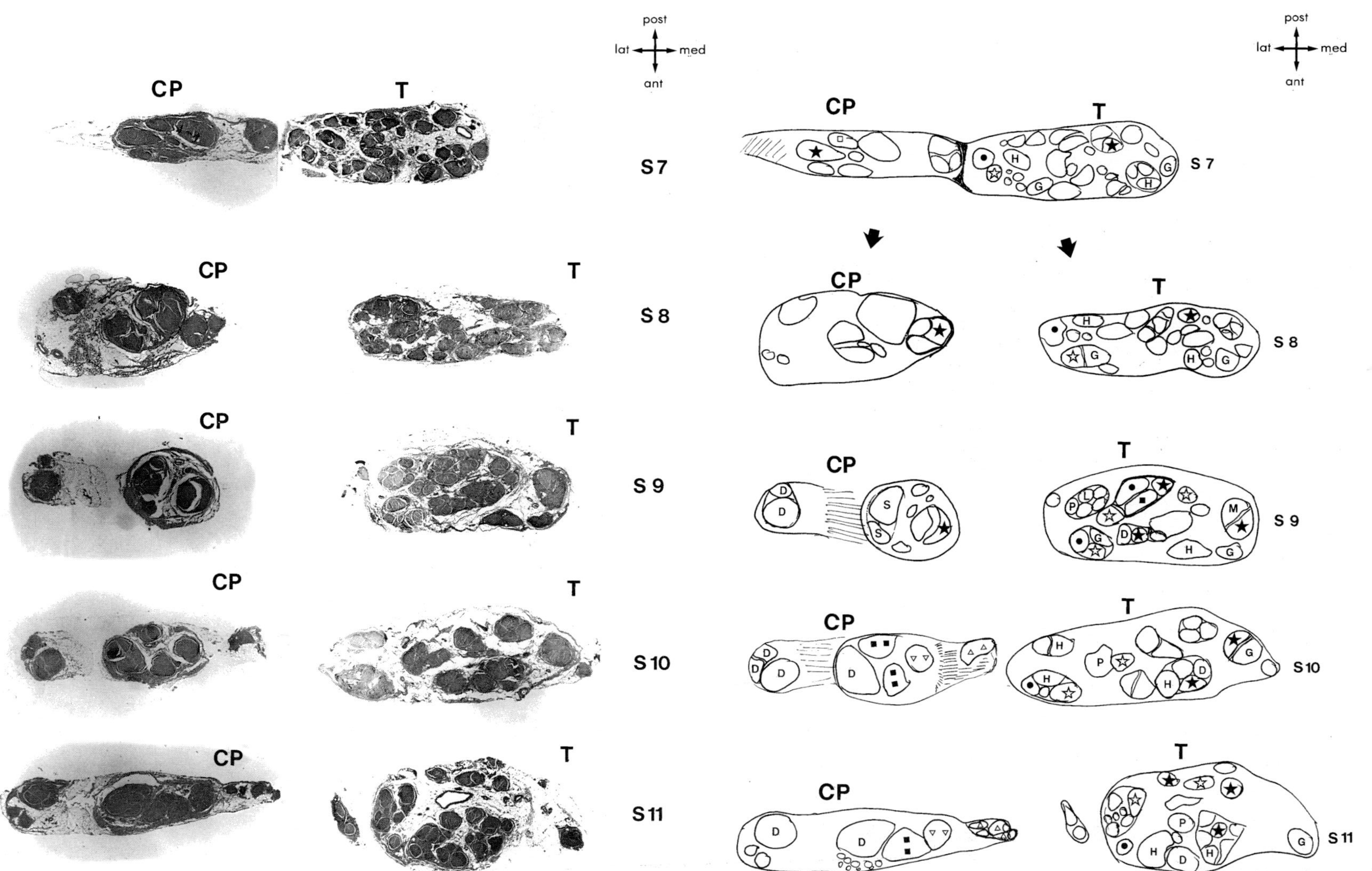

FIGURE 21–3. The sciatic nerve, sections 7 through 11. (From Brunelli G [ed]: Textbook of Microsurgery. Milano, Italy, Masson Publishing Company, 1988.)

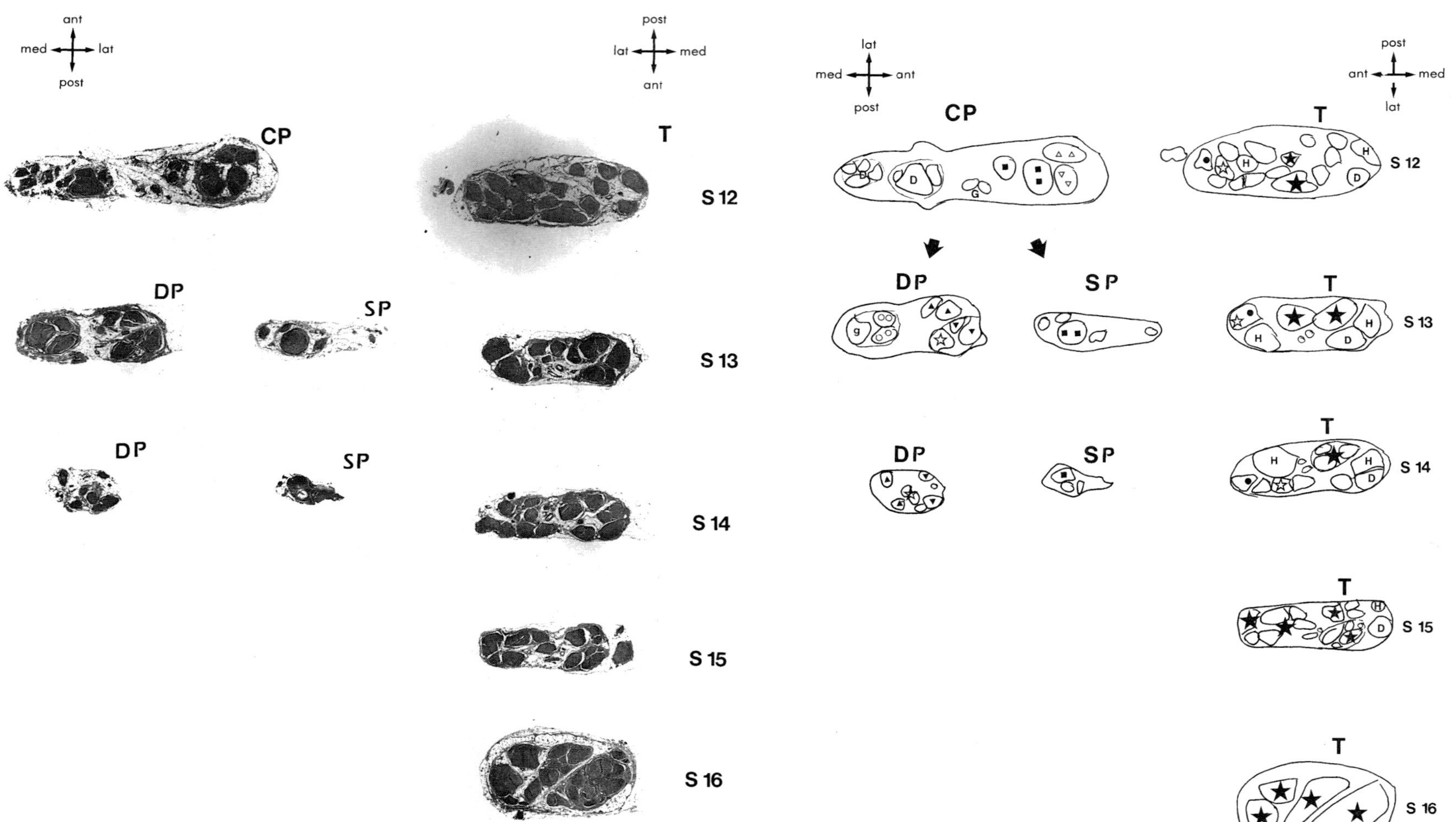

FIGURE 21–4. The sciatic nerve, sections 12 through 16. (From Brunelli G [ed]: Textbook of Microsurgery. Milano, Italy, Masson Publishing Company, 1988.)

ment, the only motor function is the extension of the knee with minor participation in the flexion of the hip.

The nerve has many different sensory functions. Therefore, it is very important, from the surgical point of view, to know which are the motor and sensory fascicles and which cutaneous area is supplied by each of these types of fascicles. The trunk of the nerve lies inside the abdomen (extraperitoneal) and would seem of minor surgical interest. However, we had to operate inside the abdomen on several patients due to lesions such as professional accidental knife cut in two butchers, knife cut resulting from an assault, stab wounds resulting from an altercation, some gunshot wounds, removal of very large neurinomas (two patients: one in a 3-year-old child, and one in an adult man), section by screwed hip prosthesis cup (one patient) and other, traumatic lesions due to penetrating fragments of glass or metal. More patients were not operated on, such as those with severe long-lasting palsies due to irradiation.

The femoral nerve is the largest (terminal) branch of the lumbar plexus, which is composed by the ventral branches of the first three lumbar nerves and of the upper part of the ventral branch of the fourth lumbar nerve. Various patterns are possible.

The femoral nerve is the longest branch and derives its fibers from L2, L3, and L4. Other branches of the lumbar plexus are the iliohypogastric, the ilioinguinals, the lateral femoral cutaneous, and the obturatorius nerves and the lumbosacral trunk, which travels to the sacral plexus. The roots of the femoral nerve converge inside the psoas muscle to form the trunk of the nerve, which emerges from the lateral aspect of the psoas muscle and runs distally in the groove formed by the psoas and the iliacus muscle along the lateral aspect of the psoas. Beneath the inguinal ligament, the femoral nerve is crossed by the circumflex iliac artery and is separated from the femoral artery by the iliopectineus fascia. In one third of patients, some fibers may arise separately from the lumbar plexus and course independently anterior to the femoral nerve to terminate in the saphenous or one or more of the femoral cutaneous branches. This is the accessory femoral nerve. During its pelvic course, the nerve gives off branches for the iliac and psoas muscles as well as roots and branches for pectineus muscles and the branch for the femoral artery. Beneath the inguinal ligament, it divides into its terminal branches as follows:

1. The lateral musculocutaneous nerves: It is a mixed nerve, supplying both the sartorius muscle and the skin of the anterior and medial aspect of the thigh.

2. The medical musculocutaneous nerve: It supplies the middle adductor and pectineus muscle as well as the internal superior skin of the thigh.

3. The saphenous nerve: It is a pure sensory nerve and is the deepest and most medial branch of the femoral nerve. It begins laterally to the femoral artery from which it is separated by the ileopettineal band. It penetrates the femoral vessel sheath at the middle of the thigh, running in front of the artery. In the adductor canal it is placed medially to it for 5 cm, then pierces the Hunter's canal while traveling toward the medial condyle of the femur, running first between the adductor magnus and the vastus medialis muscles and then between the gracilis and the sartorius muscles. Then it becomes superficial, perforating the superficial fascia

of the leg at the level of the internal tuberosity of the tibia, where it gives off small branches to the medial skin of the thigh, the knee, and the proximal part of the sura. The two terminal branches are

- the infrapatellar nerve, arising at the medial epicondyle of the femur and piercing back the sartorius muscle and then the fascia. It bends under the patella, traveling laterally and innervating the anteromedial skin of the knee.

- the tibial branch, arising at the level of the articular crease of the knee. It runs between the sartorius muscle and the insertion tendon of the gracilis muscle at the level of the medial condyle of the tibia. It then perforates the fascia, getting close to the long saphenous vein and running along with it to the medial malleolus. It then runs posterior to the malleolus and breaks up into cutaneous filaments that extend to the root of the big toe. At the level of the medial third of the leg, it gives origin to a posterior branch going to the skin of the malleolar region. Along the leg, the tibial branch gives off small branches traveling to the skin of the medial part of the leg.

4. The nerve of the quadriceps: It is the deepest and most lateral branch of the femoral nerve. It divides in four branches for four muscles of the quadriceps. Their patterns are variable. The *classic* arrangement is as follows:

- The *branch to the anterior rectus muscle,* which penetrates the muscle through its posterior part and divides into three branches, the superior of which gives off a branch to the hip joint;

- The *branch to the vastus lateral muscle,* which initially runs beneath the sartorius muscle, then divides into three or four branches to the vastus lateralis muscle. A branch to the hip may arise from the superior branch;

- The *branch to the vastus medialis muscle,* which may start with a common trunk with the saphenous nerve. It runs along with the artery to the Hunter's canal, dividing into small branches that supply the vastus medialis from the anterior part. It also gives off articular branches to the knee and to the patellar branches;

- The *nerve of the vastus intermedius muscle,* which reaches the anterior aspect of the muscle with two or three small filaments.

INTRANEURAL MAP OF THE FEMORAL NERVE

Careful dissection of three cadavers under magnification was carried out in an attempt to localize the different fascicles inside the trunk of the femoral nerve (Fig. 21–5).

Dissection was carried out by isolating the terminal and collateral branches of the nerve distally and by following them proximally inside the trunk. Magnification was obtained by means of loupes ($\times$ 4) and by operating microscope when exchanges of fibers from one fascicle to another occurred. Assuming that, except for some rare cases, in one person the arrangement of fibers is the same on both sides, the cross sections were taken from the contralateral nerve to show the fascicular maps. Cross sections were taken from the roots before their fusion in the common trunk (Sections

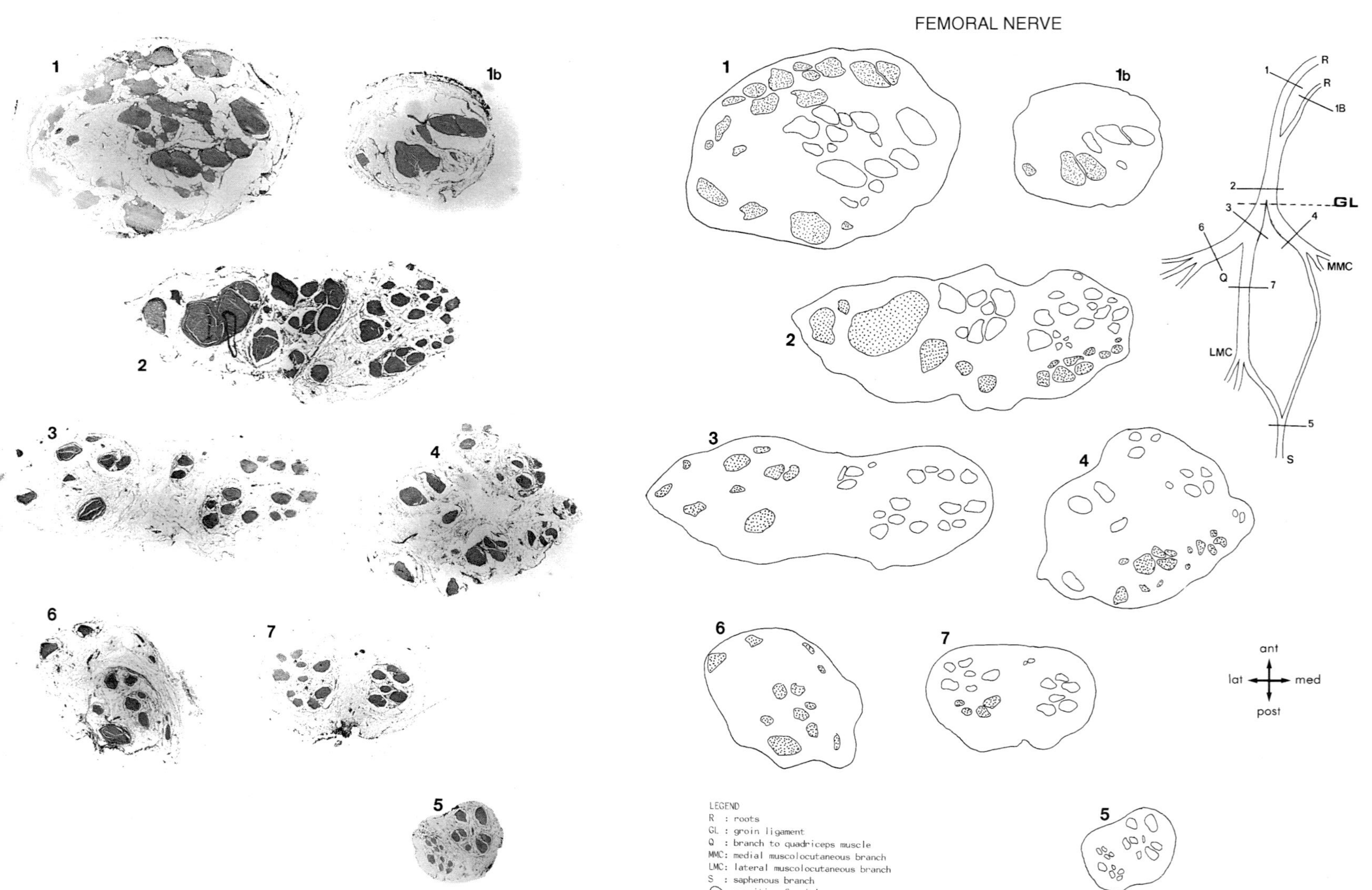

FIGURE 21–5. The femoral nerve. (From Brunelli G [ed]: Textbook of Microsurgery. Milano, Italy, Masson Publishing Company, 1988.)

1 and 1B) at the middle part of the common trunk (Section 2). Immediately after the first division (Sections 3 and 4) and at the saphenous (Section 6) and quadriceps and lateral musculocutaneous (Section 7) nerves are found (see Fig. 21–1). The internal arrangement of fascicles at the origin depends on the spatial location of the branches constituting the nerve and distally on the quadrantic position of the fibers that group before constituting the collateral or terminal branches.

In the proximal part of the femoral nerve, it was very difficult to discern the individual fascicles that are well distinguished in the second half of the nerve. This is due to the shortness of the segment of the nerve, inside which the fibers coming from the spinal nerves mingle before assuming their quadrantic location. In fact, roots of the nerve unite at the upper third of the iliac muscle and start to divide before the inguinal ligament. In the second half of the nerve, the fascicles that make up the lateral musculocutaneous nerve run toward the anteroexternal side of the femoral nerve trunk. However, some bundles of fibers of this contingent cross the anterior part of the trunk and join the bundles of fibers of the medial musculocutaneous nerve. The main fascicles of the medial musculocutaneous nerve lie in the medial portion of the anterior part of the nervous trunk.

The fascicles to the quadriceps muscle have the following locations:

- The fibers to the rectus anterior muscle lie in the dorsal or external dorsal portion;

- Also, the fibers to the vastus lateralis muscle lie in the dorsal portion, medially to the bundles to the rectus anterior;

- The fibers to the vastus medialis muscle occupy the most medial part of the femoral nerve trunk.

The bundles making up the saphenous nerve lie in the central portion of the nerve under the fascicles of the medial musculocutaneous and medially to the fascicles to the vastus medialis. A branch to the hip branches off from the superior branch.

References

Bartolaminelli P: Femoral nerve: Anatomy and fascicular arrangement. *In* Brunelli G (ed): Textbook of Microsurgery. Milano, Italy, Masson, 1988, pp 591–593,

Goldberg I: The internal architecture of the tibial peroneal and obturator nerves. Am J Anat *32*:447, 1924.

Hepburn D: Some variations in the arrangement of the nerves of the human body. J Anat *21*:511, 1887.

Infante E, Kennedy WR: Anomalous branch of the peroneal nerve detected by electromyography. Arch Neurol *22*:162, 1970.

Lanz T, Wachsmuth W: Pratkische Anatomie. Part 1, Vol. 3, Berlin, Arm-Springer, 1935.

Libassi G, Vigasio A: Sciatic nerve: Anatomy and fascicular arrangement. In Brunelli G (ed): Textbook of Microsurgery. Milano, Masson, 1988, pp 583–590.

McKinley JC: Intraneural plexus of fasciculi and fibers in sciatic nerve. Arch Neurol Psychiatr *6*:377, 1921.

Omer G, Spinner M: Management of Peripheral Nerve Problems. Philadelphia, W. B. Saunders Company, 1980.

Sunderland S: Nerves and Nerve Injuries. London, Churchill Livingstone, 1978.

Sunderland S, Ray LJ: The intraneural topography of the sciatic nerve and its popliteal divisions in man. Brain *71*:242, 1948.

Sunderland S, Bradley KC: The cross-sectional area of peripheral nerve trunks devoted to nerve fibers. Brain *72*:428, 1949.

Testut L: Trattato di anatomia topografica, Vol II. Torino, Un Tip Torinese, 1908.

Normal and Anomalous Innervation Patterns of the Face and Neck

The anatomy of the major cervicofacial sensory and motor nerves has been exhaustively studied and carefully detailed. Anatomical descriptions of location, depth, and relationship to surface landmarks aid the head and neck surgeon in finding and avoiding these various nerves. Other than parotid gland surgery, and repair of the injured facial nerve or cutaneous sensory nerves, the usual goal is to avoid these nerves while operating on the surface and deeper structures of the cervicofacial region.

Clearly, it is impossible to know the exact anatomy of a given nerve in a given individual without carefully dissecting the nerve and visually inspecting its course, branching pattern, and variations from normal. Because this is not a reasonable option in the majority of cases, how then does one safely perform surgery and avoid injury to these nerves? Although nothing in anatomy is 100%, knowledge of the normal anatomy of a nerve and its usual location relative to fixed surface landmarks is essential if nerve injury is to be avoided. The purpose of this chapter is to provide the reader with the above-mentioned information for the facial nerve, the cutaneous sensory branches of the trigeminal nerve, and the cervical plexus.

FACIAL NERVE

The branches of the facial nerve most commonly injured during surgery include the marginal mandibular and frontal branches. Not surprisingly, the majority of facial nerve anatomical studies are directed to these two major branches, in addition to identification of the facial nerve trunk as it exits the skull base and enters the parotid gland.

Basic Anatomy and Branching Patterns

There are two major divisions of the facial nerve: the temporofacial and the cervicofacial. Davis and colleagues described the basic branching (anastomotic) patterns of the facial nerve in a large anatomical study of 350 specimens (Fig. 22–1). Greater than 30% of facial nerves have no anastomoses between the cervicofacial and temporofacial divisions, and 13% have no anastomoses between any branches of the two major divisions. The significance of the absence of anastomoses between major divisions and between branches of major divisions is that it is not possible to rely on anastomoses to maintain facial nerve function in

lieu of meticulous dissection and preservation not only of the larger but also of the smaller branches.

Identification of the Facial Nerve at Surgery

Facial Nerve Trunk. Numerous landmarks and techniques have been described to help locate the trunk of the facial nerve (see Chapter 4). Many of these are based on surface sites that are too variable for routine use. Safe and consistent localization of the trunk of the facial nerve has perhaps best been described by Furnas (1965) (Fig. 22–2). The angle formed by the tympanic ring (bony external auditory canal) and the mastoid process continues medially to the vaginal-mastoid angle. The styloid process, when present, protrudes from the vaginal process of the tympanic portion of the temporal bone. By following the deepest extension of the cartilaginous portion of the external auditory canal medially and posteriorly in the groove between the tympanic ring and the mastoid process, the vaginal process comes into view. On entering the loose areolar tissue between the parotid gland and the above bony landmarks, gentle spreading with a small hemostat in the direction of the facial nerve (anterior to posterior) exposes the facial nerve. Confirmation of identification of the facial nerve with the adjustable nerve stimulator set on the lowest setting is appropriate. "Squeezing or pinching" the suspected nerve with forceps or hemostats is to be avoided. The styloid process is not a reliable landmark, because it has been reported to be absent or excessively short to preclude its use as a landmark in up to 50% of cases (Davis et al, 1990, 1994). When present and palpable, the styloid process is always medial to the facial nerve.

Bifurcation of the trunk of the facial nerve into its two major divisions is usually posteromedial to the mandibular ramus, approximately at the junction of the middle and upper third of the mandibular ramus, measuring from the angle of the mandible to the temporomandibular joint. This is not a specific landmark, and the location of the bifurcation has considerable variation in anteroposterior and inferosuperior locations. The trunk can actually bifurcate before its exit from the stylomastoid foramen, and one should always be aware of the possibility of multiple branches of the facial nerve trunk when approaching it between the parotid gland and skull base.

Frontal Branch. In addition to the brief description by Pitanguy and Ramos of the location of the frontal branch of the facial nerve in 1961, which stated that the nerve followed

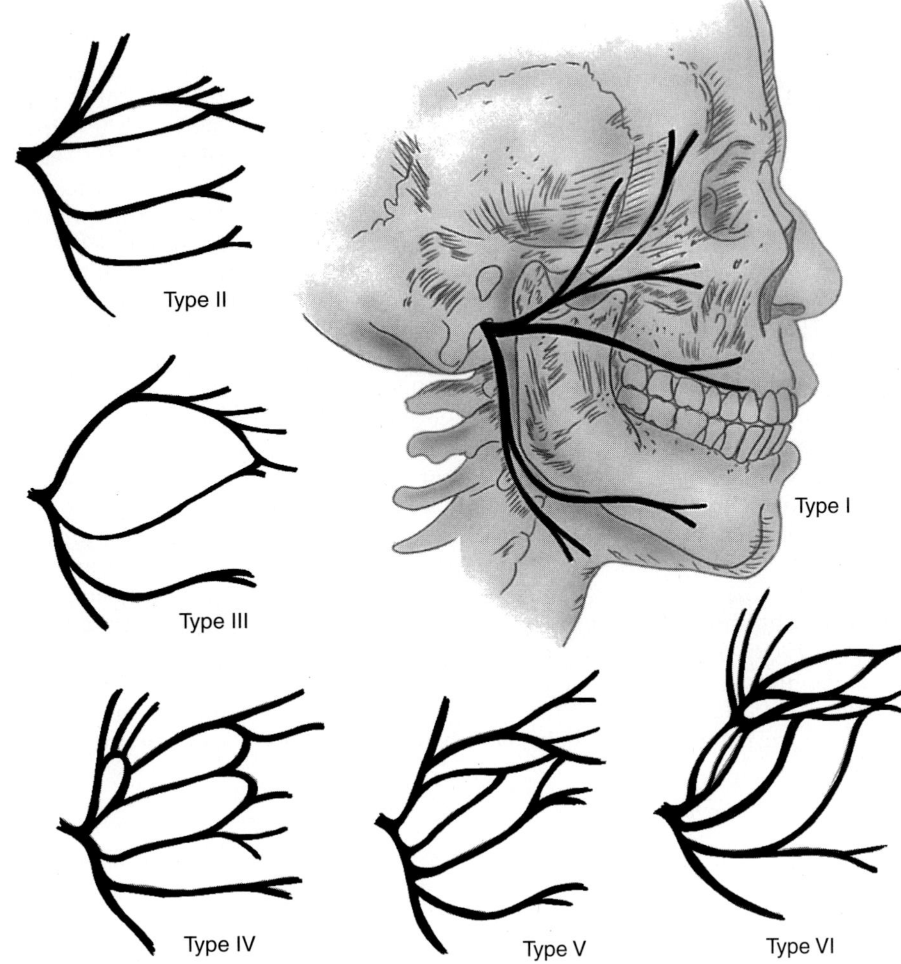

FIGURE 22–1. Basic branching patterns of the facial nerve. (Modified from Davis RA, Anson BJ, Budinger JM, Kurth LE: Surgical anatomy of the facial nerve and parotid gland based upon a study of 350 cervicofacial halves. Surg Gynecol Obstet *102*:385, 1986.) By permission of Surgery, Gynecology & Obstetrics, now known as the Journal of the American College of surgeons.

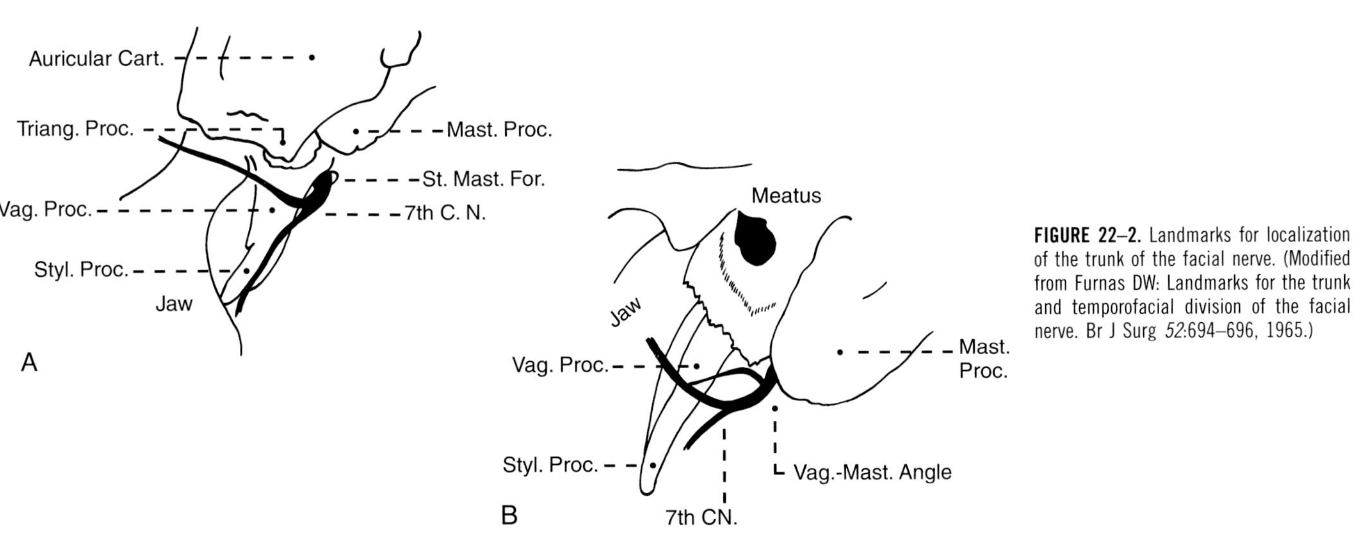

FIGURE 22–2. Landmarks for localization of the trunk of the facial nerve. (Modified from Furnas DW: Landmarks for the trunk and temporofacial division of the facial nerve. Br J Surg *52*:694–696, 1965.)

a course starting 1/2 inch below the tragus, passing in the direction of the eyebrow, other authors have further elaborated on relevant surface anatomy (Furnas, 1965; Peterson and Johnston, 1987). To localize the frontal branch on the skin surface, draw a line starting 0.5 cm below the tragus (i.e., the intertragal notch) to a point 1.5 cm above the lateral extent of the eyebrow. This line should overlie or be slightly superior to the frontal branch. A method of confirming the location of the frontal branch as it crosses the zygomatic arch is to draw a line from the lateral canthus of the eyelids to the auricle. Halfway along this line is approximately where the frontal branch crosses the zygoma. Seckel (1994) defined danger zones of the face where the nerves are at greatest risk from surgical trauma. Seckel's danger zone for the frontal branch of the facial nerve is described as a "triangle circumscribed by lines drawn from 0.5 cm below the tragus to a point 2 cm above the lateral eyebrow, along the zygoma to the lateral orbital rim and from the point above the eyebrow, through the lateral end of the eyebrow to the zygoma." It is in this area, especially inferiorly, over the zygomatic arch, that the frontal branch lies just deep to the SMAS layer and is more easily injured (Fig. 22–3).

Marginal Mandibular Branch. Dingman and Grabb's classic study (1962) on the surgical anatomy of the marginal mandibular branch of the facial nerve was based on the dissection of 100 facial specimens. They described the relationship of the marginal mandibular branch to the inferior border of the mandible anterior and posterior to the facial artery. Posterior to the facial artery the nerve dropped no more than 1.0 cm below the inferior border of the mandible in approximately 20% of cases. In the remainder, the nerve stayed above the inferior mandibular border. Anterior to the facial artery, the marginal mandibular branch remained above the inferior border of the mandible in 100% of cases (Fig. 22–4). The nerve was found to be superficial to the posterior facial vein in 98% and superficial to the anterior facial vein in 100% of cases. In 50 patients, Peterson and Johnston (1987) quickly and easily identified the marginal mandibular branch inferior to the angle of the mandible, measuring 4.0 to 4.5 cm from the earlobe sulcus (Fig. 22–5). Seckel's danger zone for the marginal mandibular nerve describes an area more anteriorly, where the nerve overlies the body of the mandible, before innervating the lip depressors and inferior orbicularis muscles. The danger zone is defined as a 4-cm diameter circle with its center overlying the mandibular body, 2.0 cm posterior to the oral commissure (Fig. 22–6). In this area, the platysma-SMAS layer may be thinner, providing less protection. In addition, troublesome bleeding from the facial artery or vein may require electrocautery, resulting in injury to the marginal mandibular branch of the facial nerve.

Zygomatic and Buccal Branches. The main zygomatic branch may be found just inferior to the zygoma and superior to the parotid duct. The buccal branches have a

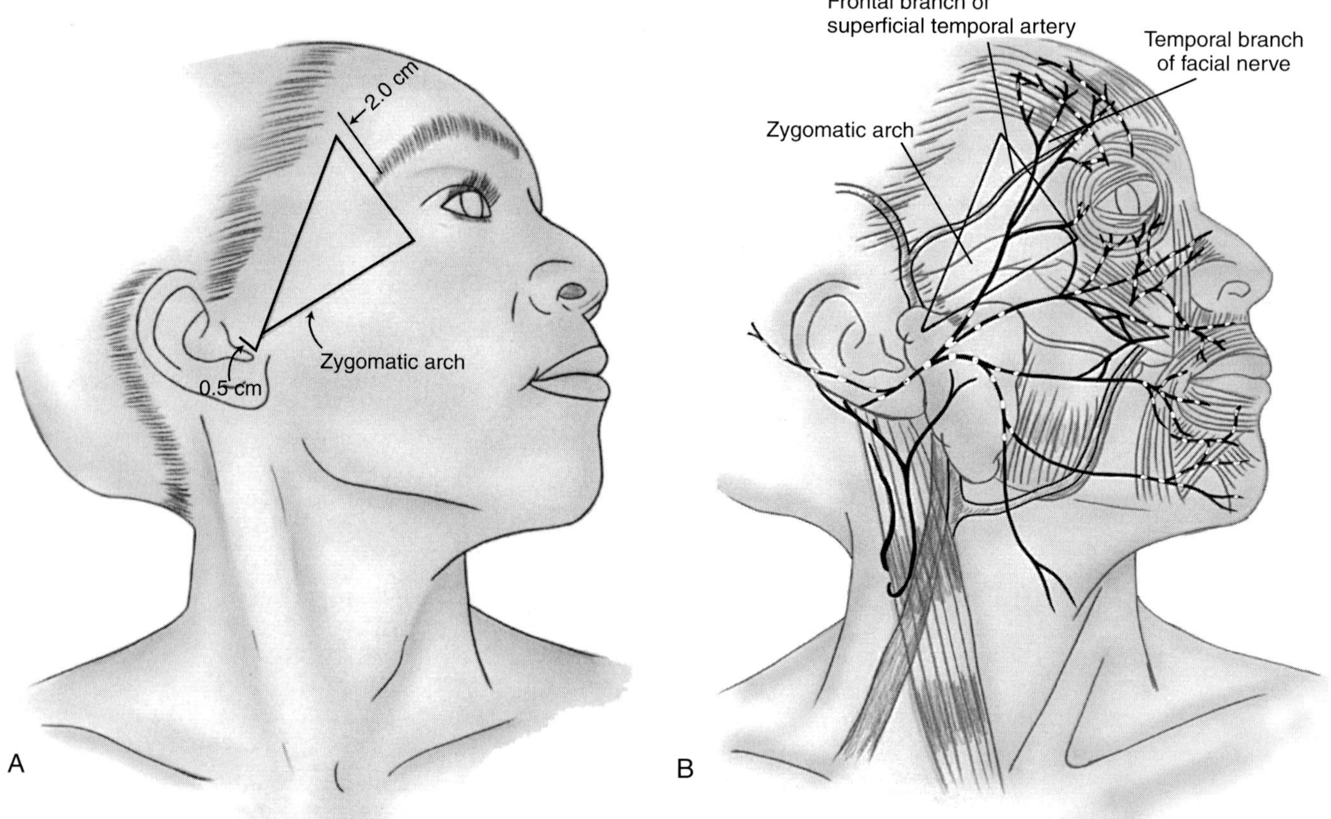

FIGURE 22–3. Danger zone in which the frontal branch of the facial nerve is more easily injured. *A,* Surface landmarks. *B,* Detail of nerve distribution. (Modified from Seckel BR: Facial Danger Zones: Avoiding Nerve Injury in Facial Plastic Surgery. St. Louis, Missouri, Quality Medical Publishing, Inc., 1994.)

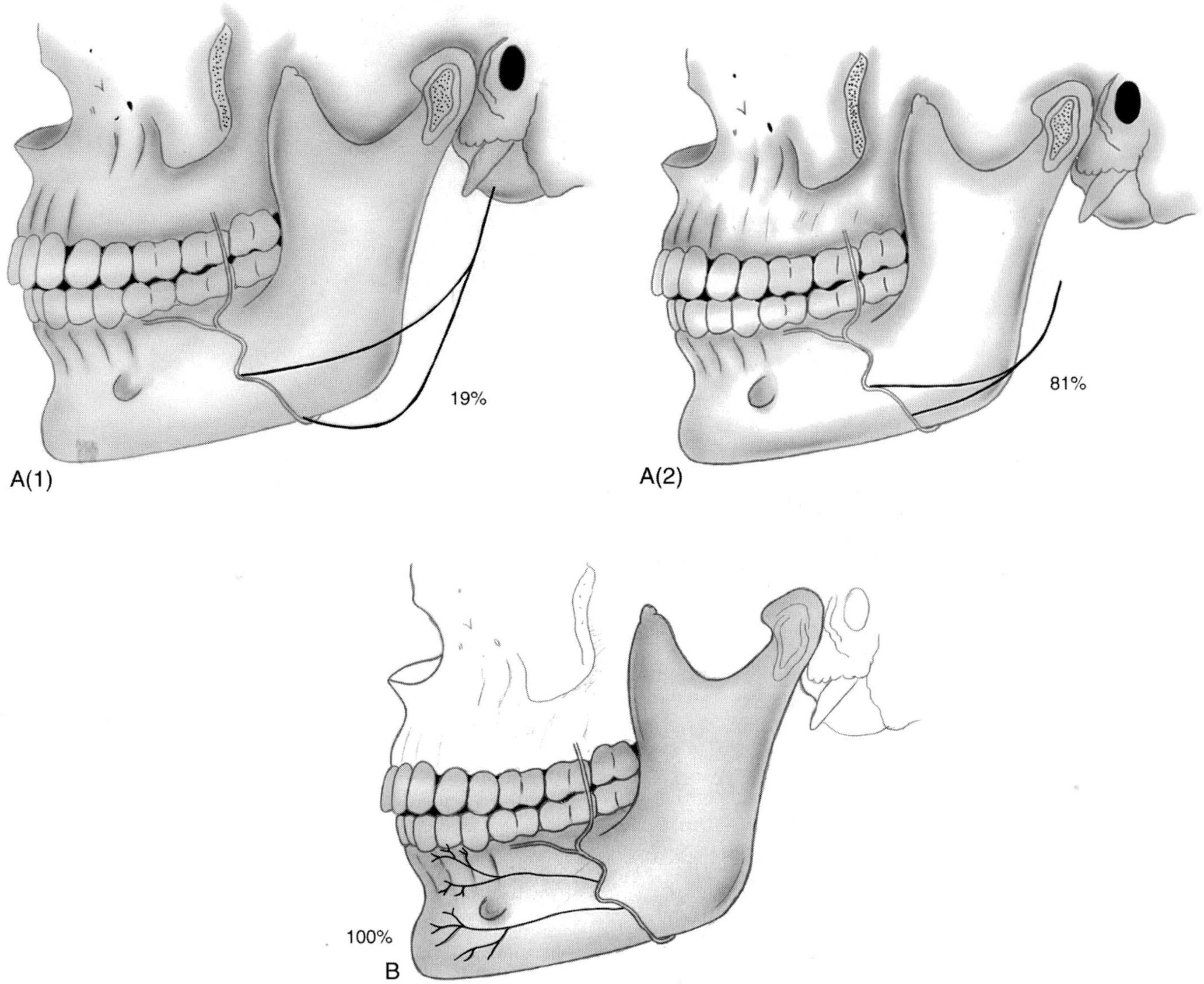

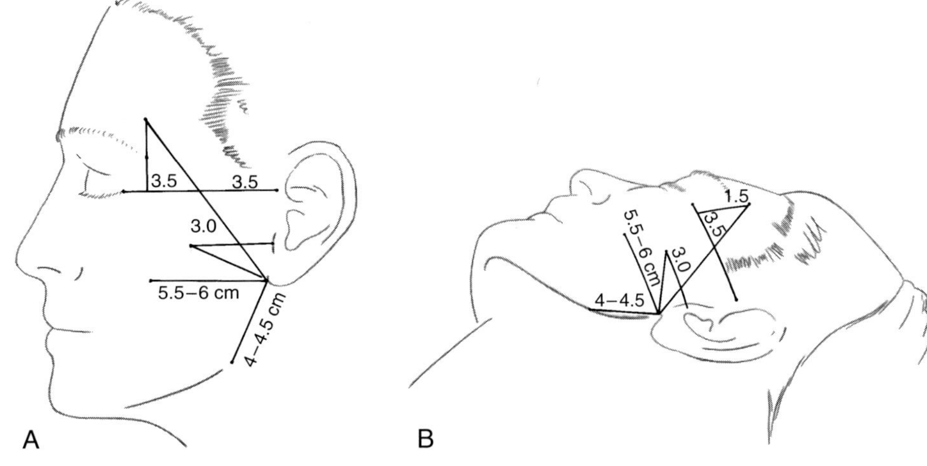

FIGURE 22–4. *A,* Posterior to the facial artery, the marginal mandibular branch drops below the inferior border of the mandible in about 20% of cases (1) and stays above the border in about 80% of cases (2). *B,* Anterior to the facial artery, the marginal mandibular branch remains above the inferior border of the mandible in virtually all cases. (Modified from Dingman RO, Grabb WC: Surgical anatomy of the mandibular ramus of the facial nerve based on dissection of 100 facial halves. Plast Reconstr Surg *29*:266–272, 1962. © Williams & Wilkins, 1962.)

FIGURE 22–5. Landmarks for localization of the marginal mandibular branch of the facial nerve. (Modified from Peterson RA, Johnston DL: Facile identification of the facial nerve branches. Clin Plast Surg *14*:785–788, 1987.)

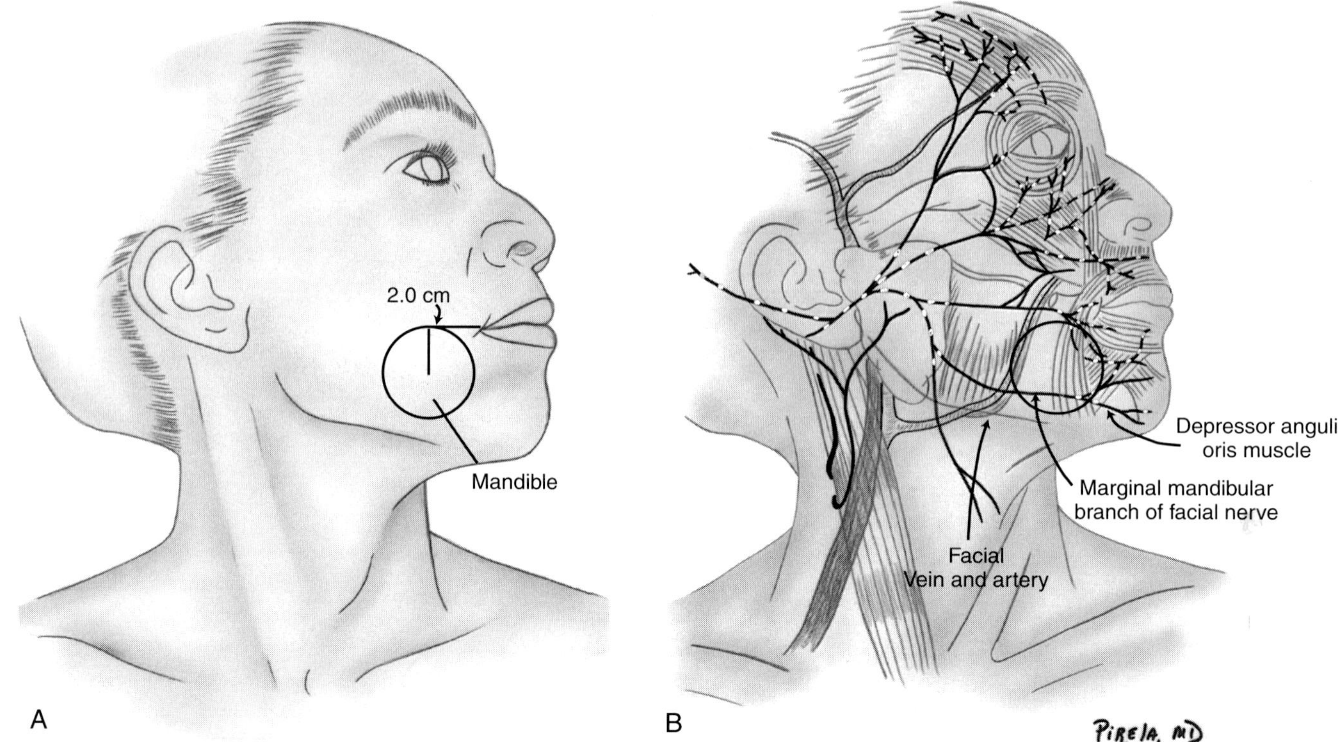

FIGURE 22–6. Danger zone in which the marginal mandibular branch of the facial nerve is more easily injured. *A,* Surface landmarks. *B,* Detail of nerve distribution. (Modified from Seckel BR: Facial Danger Zones: Avoiding Nerve Injury in Facial Plastic Surgery. St. Louis, Missouri, Quality Medical Publishing, Inc., 1994.)

varied anastomotic pattern anterior to the parotid gland, overlying the anterior masseter muscle and the buccal fat pad. Careful dissection in the direction of the facial nerve branches generally allows rapid identification of one or more nerve branches in this area.

TRIGEMINAL NERVE

The trigeminal nerve has three major cutaneous nerve branches: the supraorbital, infraorbital, and mental nerves. The supraorbital and infraorbital nerves are not infrequently injured during cutaneous reconstructive facial surgery and maxillofacial trauma, respectively. These injuries may be unavoidable and unrepairable and are usually well tolerated by the patient. Mental nerve injuries, on the other hand, are poorly tolerated because of associated problems with drooling and biting the lip.

Supraorbital Nerve

The sensory nerve supply to the forehead and anterior scalp is from the frontal nerve, a branch of the first division (ophthalmic) of the trigeminal nerve. The frontal branch divides into a lateral (supraorbital nerve) and medial branch (supratrochlear nerve) usually within, but occasionally following its exit from the superior orbit (Fatah, 1991). The most medial nerve branch (supratrochlear) exits the orbit 1.5 to 2.5 cm from the mid-line. The supraorbital nerve emerges in a periosteal condensation through a notch or groove in the supraorbital rim and less frequently through a foramen. The supraorbital notch can usually be palpated along the

supraorbital rim just superior to the mid-pupil. On exiting the orbit, these nerves lie deep to the overlying muscles. The most medial nerve branch rapidly penetrates the muscle, changing to a subcutaneous position. The other, more lateral branches subsequently penetrate the muscle at successively higher levels, with the most lateral branch continuing deep to the frontalis muscle, almost to the hairline (Fig. 22–7). The pattern of branching of these nerves to the forehead is quite variable.

Infraorbital Nerve

The infraorbital nerve is a branch of the second division (maxillary) of the trigeminal nerve and exits the skull

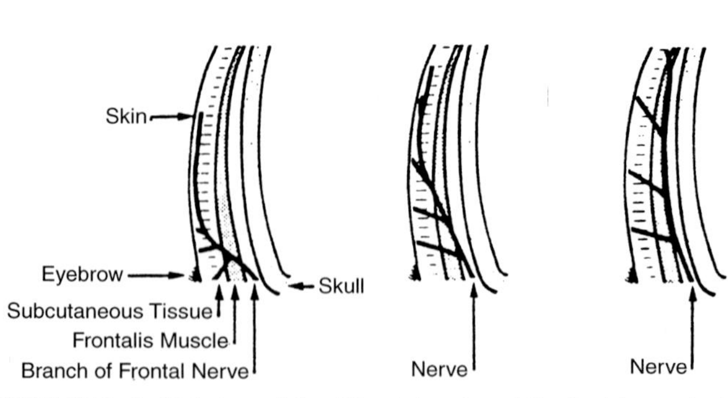

FIGURE 22–7. Sagittal views of the different branches of the frontal nerve in the forehead. Note that each subsequent nerve changes plane from submuscular to subcutaneous, starting from medial (at left) to lateral (at right). (From Fatah MF: Innervation and functional reconstruction of the forehead. Br J Plast Surg *44*:351–358, 1991.)

through the infraorbital foramen approximately 1.0 cm below the infraorbital rim. The infraorbital foramen can usually be palpated through the skin, but it can also be located 1.0 cm inferior to the infraorbital rim along a line drawn from the supraorbital notch or foramen through the mid-pupil inferiorly to the second mandibular premolar (Seckel, 1994). Damage to this nerve during facial surgery is infrequent, and injury can usually be avoided with careful dissection in the area of the infraorbital foramen.

Mental Nerve

The mental nerve is a branch of the third division (mandibular) of the trigeminal nerve. The mental foramen lies below the second mandibular premolar approximately midway between the superior and inferior borders of the mandible. In the long-standing edentulous patient, the foramen is relatively more superior on the mandibular body as a result of the loss of alveolar bone. Injury to the mental nerve occurs most commonly with mandibular trauma or surgery and chin implantation, and it is of major significance because of problems with drooling and lip biting. Repair of the nerve, within the mandible or after its exit from the mental foramen, should be considered whenever possible.

CERVICAL PLEXUS

Branches of the cervical plexus to the skin include the great auricular, lesser occipital, anterior cutaneous, and the supraclavicular trunk (Paff, 1973). The cutaneous nerves of the cervical plexus radiate to the skin from a point along the posterior margin of the sternocleidomastoid muscle midway between the mastoid tip and clavicle (Fig. 22–8A and B).

Great Auricular

The great auricular nerve is formed by the dorsal sensory roots of the spinal cord segments C2 and C3 and provides nerve supply to the lower two thirds of the ear and the preauricular and postauricular skin (McKinney and Katrana, 1980). Temporary numbness is not infrequent after face-lift surgery; however, significant injury to the main trunk may result in permanent sensory loss and a painful neuroma. With the head turned away from the surgeon, as in parotid gland or face-lift surgery, the nerve crosses the mid-portion of the sternocleidomastoid muscle 6.5 cm below the inferior margin of the external auditory canal (Fig. 22–9). At this point, the external jugular vein may be found 0.5 cm anterior to the nerve.

Lesser Occipital

The lesser occipital nerve (C2) supplies the postauricular scalp and occipital region after traveling superiorly along the posterior border of the sternocleidomastoid muscle.

Anterior Cutaneous

The anterior cutaneous nerve (C2, C3) crosses anteriorly over the sternocleidomastoid muscle to supply the skin of the anterior neck.

Supraclavicular Trunk

The medial, intermediate, and lateral supraclavicular nerves (C3, C4) supply the skin over the lower lateral neck, supraclavicular, and upper pectoral regions.

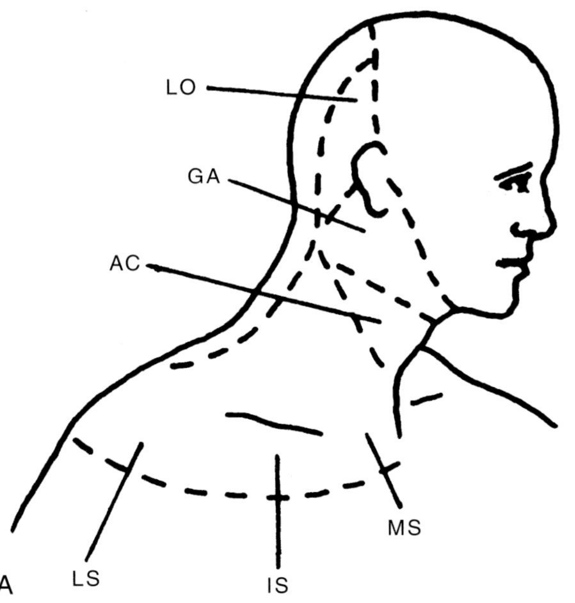

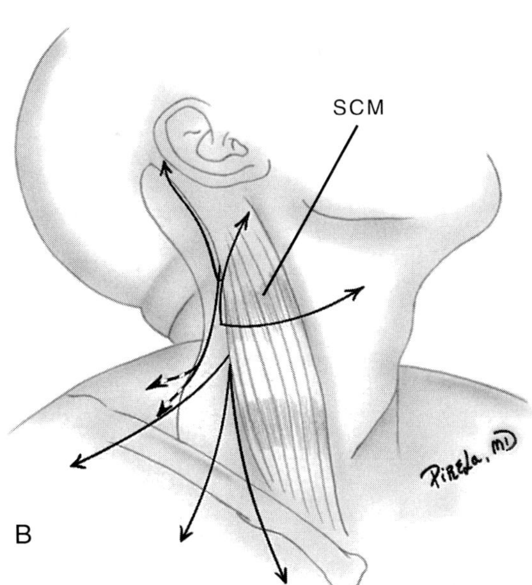

FIGURE 22–8. *A*, Areas of skin supplied by the peripheral cutaneous branches of the cervical plexus. GA, great auricular; LO, lesser occipital; AC, anterior cutaneous; LS, IS, MS, supraclavicular nerves. *B*, Radiation of the cutaneous nerves of the cervical plexus. SCM, sternocleidomastoid. (Modified from Paff GE: Anatomy of the Head and Neck. Philadelphia, W. B. Saunders Company, 1973.)

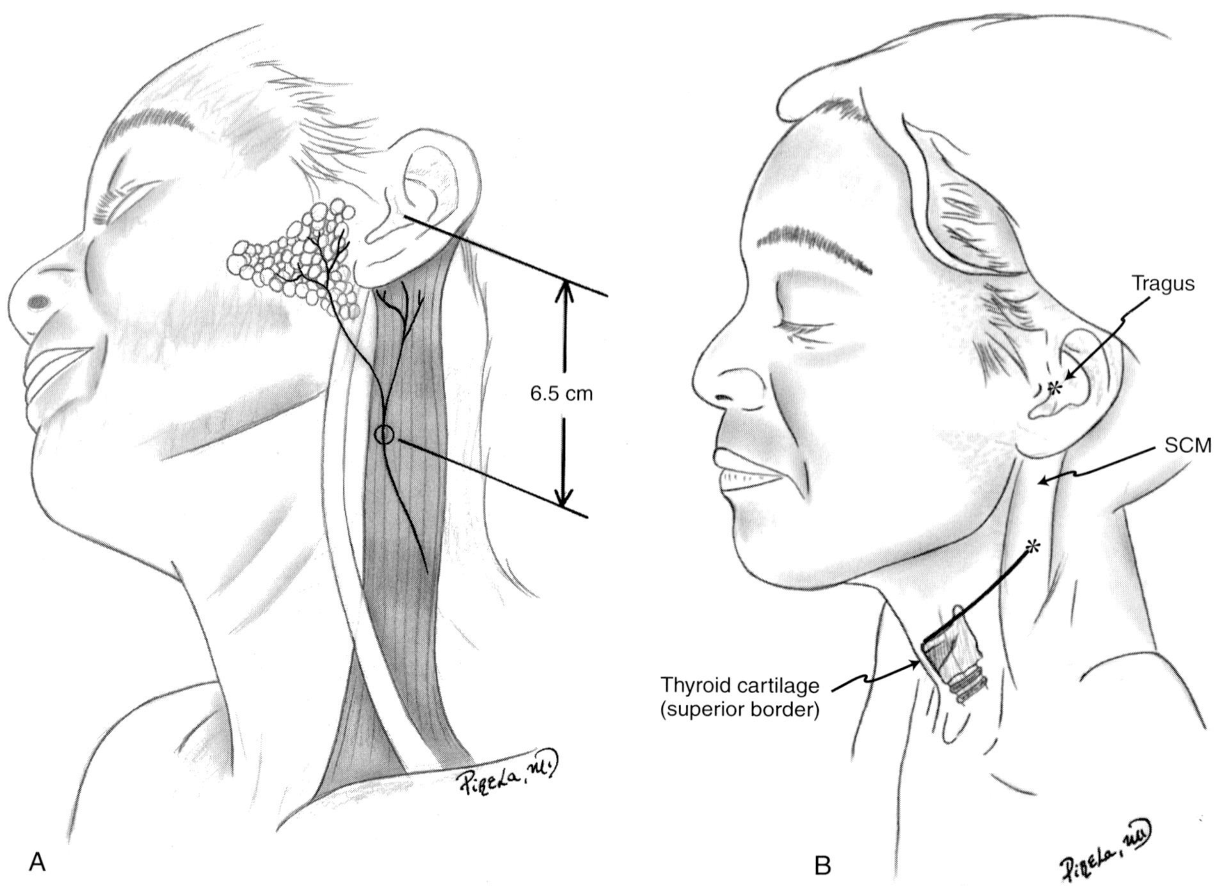

FIGURE 22–9. *A,* The course of the great auricular nerve. *B,* An incision in the platysma muscle that lies a safe distance from the marginal branch of the great auricular nerve; this is a useful approach in face-lift surgery. SCM, sternocleidomastoid. (Modified from McKinney P, Katrana DJ: Prevention of injury to the great auricular nerve during rhytidectomy. Plast Reconstr Surg *66*:675–679, 1980. © Williams & Wilkins, 1980.)

SUMMARY

Knowledge of the anatomy of the major sensory cutaneous and motor nerves of the face and neck is essential for safe surgery in these regions. Although nerve injury may be unavoidable, ignorance of normal anatomy is inexcusable.

References

Davis RA, Anson BJ, Budinger JM, Kurth LE: Surgical anatomy of the facial nerve and parotid gland based upon a study of 350 cervicofacial halves. Surg Gynecol Obstet *102*:385, 1986.

Dingman RO, Grabb WC: Surgical anatomy of the mandibular ramus of the facial nerve based on the dissection of 100 facial halves. Plast Reconstr Surg *29*:266–272, 1962.

Fatah MF: Innervation and functional reconstruction of the forehead. Br J Plast Surg *44*:351–358, 1991.

Furnas DW: Landmarks for the trunk and the temporofacial division of the facial nerve. Br J Surg *52*:694–696, 1965.

McKinney P, Katrana DJ: Prevention of injury to the great auricular nerve during rhytidectomy. Plast Reconstr Surg *66*:675–679, 1980.

Paff GH: Anatomy of the Head and Neck. Philadelphia, W. B. Saunders, 1973.

Peterson RA, Johnston DL: Facile identification of the facial nerve branches. Clin Plast Surg *14*:785–788, 1987.

Pitanguy I, Ramos AS: The frontal branch of the facial nerve: The importance of its variations in face lifting. Plast Reconstr Surg *38*:352–356, 1964.

Seckel BR: Facial Danger Zones: Avoiding Nerve Injury in Facial Plastic Surgery. St. Louis, Quality Medical Publishing, 1994.

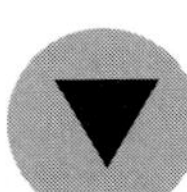

Chapter 23

• Thomas Marshall Brushart

Trophic and Tropic Influences on Peripheral Nerve Regeneration

The term neurotrophism is derived from the Greek *tro-phikos*, or nursing. It was originally coined to describe an interaction between developing neurons and their targets, in which a substance produced by the target is taken up by innervating axons and transported back to the neuron, preventing its death. This definition has been broadened to include positive effects on events of neuronal differentiation, such as axonal growth and transmitter production. The so-called neurotrophic hypothesis relates primarily to development, and it is in this context that neurotrophic interactions have been most completely studied. During vertebrate development, many neurons die during the process of forming connections with the periphery (Oppenheim et al, 1991). Neuronal survival is promoted by access to a limited supply of trophic factors provided by the target tissue. This competition serves to match axonal and target populations, eliminating inappropriate connections. The neurotrophic hypothesis predicts that neuronal survival may be increased by any maneuver that increases the supply of trophic factor, such as increasing the target field or providing exogenous factors, and may be diminished by any manipulation that decreases trophic factor supply, such as decreasing target size or blocking the transport or activity of the factor itself. It has also been recognized that neurotrophic interactions in the periphery may involve ensheathing glial cells in addition to target tissues, and in the central nervous system may include influences from afferent neurons, or even the neuron itself (Korsching, 1993). The neurotrophic concept is introduced by examination of the actions of nerve growth factor (NGF), the first neurotrophic factor to be isolated. The best defined of the growth factors acting in the peripheral nervous system is then described in the context of injury and regeneration. Although some general patterns may be derived, the recent explosion of growth factor research has complicated, rather than unified, the overall picture. Future directions in neurotrophism research and clinical application also are discussed.

Neurotropism is derived from the Greek *trope*, a turning. It is used in neurobiology to describe regeneration of an axon up a concentration gradient of a diffusible substance to reinnervate a specific target. Neurotropism, sometimes referred to as chemotropism, has been studied since the time of Ramon y Cajal to draw regenerating axons en mass to a distal nerve stump, generating specificity at the tissue level (Brushart, 1991). Current debate centers on the action of neurotropism in the generation of higher levels of specificity, such as at the level of the nerve trunk or even end-organ. A critical review of this literature indicates only a limited role for neurotropism in generating higher levels of regeneration specificity.

NERVE GROWTH FACTOR AND NEUROTROPHISM

NGF was first isolated in small quantities from mouse sarcoma tissue (Levi-Montalcini and Hamburger, 1951). It was later found in abundance in the mouse submandibular gland, which produces enough NGF to allow determination of its structure. The NGF molecule is assembled from three pairs of subunits, termed alpha, beta, and gamma. The beta subunit, the seat of growth-promoting activity, is a 118 amino acid chain, joined to its beta counterpart by noncovalent bonds to form a strongly associated dimer (Angeletti et al, 1971). This general structure is shared by a family of molecules, the neurotrophins: brain-derived neurotrophic factor and neurotrophins 3 (NT-3), 4 (NT-4), and 5 (NT-5). NGF is produced by peripheral tissues, which serve as the target for developing sensory and sympathetic neurons. For instance, during development of the skin, NGF is made by cells of both the dermis and the epidermis (Davies et al, 1987). This synthesis is timed to coincide with the arrival of developing axons but is regulated independently by an endogenous clock, which is not under axonal control (Thoenen et al, 1988). When the developing axon arrives, NGF from the target binds a specific receptor on the axonal membrane. Two receptor types are found: a rapidly binding, low-affinity NGF receptor (Johnson et al, 1986) and a slowly binding, high-affinity receptor. The slowly binding, high-affinity receptor has recently been found to be a member of the trk family of tyrosine kinases (Cordon-Cardo et al, 1991). The high-affinity receptor was initially thought to be exclusively responsible for the initiation of neurotrophic activity within the neuron. However, the possibility has been raised that the two receptors may sandwich the NGF molecule in a complex that then initiates neurotrophic activity (Bothwell, 1991). Once NGF is bound to its receptor or receptors on the membrane, the NGF-receptor complex is internalized, and it sets off a cascade of reactions (summarized in Altin and Bradshaw, 1993) that convey the signal to the cell nucleus. One pathway includes tyrosine phosphorylation and activation of phospholipase C, whereas another occurs through tyrosine phosphorylation of the GTPase-activating protein. Once the signal is received within the nucleus, it results in synthesis of tubulin, neurofilament and calcium-binding proteins, and neurotransmitters.

The neurotrophic hypothesis has found strong confirmation in the results of experiments that purposefully alter specific components of the above-mentioned process. When mice are genetically altered so that their skin produces an excess of NGF, sensory and sympathetic nerves serving these areas hypertrophy, confirming that NGF produced by the cutaneous target controls neuronal survival and thus the level of innervation (Albers et al, 1994). Proximal transport of NGF is suggested by experiments in which pharmacological disruption of transport leads to buildup of NGF within the distal target tissue but not within the dorsal root ganglion (Korsching and Thoenen, 1985). At the neuronal level, experimentally induced neuronal death can be reduced by administration of exogenous NGF (Hamburger and Yip, 1984), whereas exposure in utero to antibodies to NGF, which block the molecule's bioactivity, results in increased neuronal loss (Johnson et al, 1980).

NEUROTROPHIC FACTORS IN PERIPHERAL NERVE INJURY AND REGENERATION

Nerve Growth Factor

Axon transection is rapidly followed by a marked reduction in the amount of NGF and NGF receptor transported to the neuronal cell body from the periphery (Raivich et al, 1991). This reduction in peripheral message results in a secondary decrease in the production of NGF receptor within the neuron (Raivich et al, 1990). When continuity with the periphery is restored through axonal regeneration, the concentrations of NGF and NGF receptor within the neuronal nucleus return to normal (Raivich et al, 1991). The peripheral pathway responds to transection with a biphasic increase in NGF synthesis by non-neuronal cells. The first increase is seen in the injured areas of both proximal and distal stumps within 6 hours of transection (Heumann et al, 1987). After an additional 2 to 3 days, blood-borne macrophages enter the degenerating distal stump and produce interleukin-1, a potent stimulator of NGF production (Lindholm et al, 1987). Beginning 3 to 4 days after axotomy, low-affinity NGF receptor is also produced by Schwann cells in massive quantities (Taniuchi et al, 1988). The receptor is displayed on all denervated Schwann cells, regardless of whether or not their previous axonal partners were sensitive to NGF, and its production is down regulated when axonal contact is re-established. These receptors bind NGF and display it on the Schwann cell surface. The Schwann cell may thus provide trophic support, and perhaps even tropic guidance, for regenerating axons (Taniuchi et al, 1988). This observation mandates refinement of the original neurotrophic hypothesis, because the pathway is clearly providing what was originally thought of as the reward for successful end-organ contact.

The effects of exogenous NGF on peripheral nerve regeneration have been studied extensively in the silicon chamber model. After nerve transection, proximal and distal nerve stumps are introduced within opposite ends of a silicon tube, creating an enclosed neural gap that may be filled with a solution of NGF. In the rabbit facial nerve, the addition of NGF to the chamber fluid resulted in a larger nerve cable at 5 weeks when axons successfully crossed the gap but did not increase the frequency of successful regeneration (Chen

et al, 1989). Studies of the rat sciatic nerve are consistent with a transient stimulation of regeneration through NGF effects on supporting cells rather than on axons themselves (Derby et al, 1993; Hollowell et al, 1990; Rich et al, 1989). In 10-mm and 15-mm gap experiments, NGF administration resulted in enhanced initial outgrowth of both non-neuronal cells and axons (Derby et al, 1993). After 3 weeks, three times as many myelinated axons were regenerating through NGF-containing tubes as through controls. However, by 4 weeks, the NGF effect was lost at mid-tube, where equal numbers of myelinated and unmyelinated axons were present in treated and untreated groups. At 10 weeks, in an 8-mm gap model, there was complete regeneration of both NGF-treated and control groups (Hollowell et al, 1990). The addition of NGF to the chamber fluid thus appears to give regeneration a head start but does not appear to alter the final outcome (Derby et al, 1993). These findings are consistent with the results of experiments in which regeneration of crushed axons was not impaired by the addition of antibodies to NGF (Diamond et al, 1992), and recent work specifically addresses the positive effect of NGF on Schwann cell migration (Anton et al, 1994).

Ciliary Neurotrophic Factor

Ciliary neurotrophic factor (CNTF) is a 200 amino acid protein, derived originally from the chick eye, which was found to promote survival of ciliary ganglion neurons (Barbin et al, 1984). In subsequent tissue culture experiments, CNTF has been shown to support the survival of a variety of other neuronal types, including sensory neurons of the dorsal root ganglion and motoneurons (Raivich and Kreutzberg, 1993). CNTF support of cultured motoneurons is enhanced by basic fibroblast growth factor (bFGF), demonstrating a synergistic effect of these two growth factors in the tissue culture environment (Arakawa et al, 1990). However, in the living animal, CNTF fails to rescue ciliary, sympathetic, or sensory neurons from programmed cell death, demonstrating a positive effect only on motoneurons (Oppenheim et al, 1991). A possible role for CNTF as a motoneuron growth factor is further supported by experiments in which application of CNTF to transected neonatal motor axons prevents motoneuronal cell death that would normally result (Sendtner et al, 1990), and local application of CNTF to muscle results in motoneuron sprouting (Gurney et al, 1992). Mutant mice lacking CNTF undergo normal development but then develop progressive motoneuron atrophy and degeneration (Masu et al, 1993).

Adult peripheral nerve is the richest source of CNTF, which is localized predominantly to the cytoplasm of myelinating Schwann cells (Friedman et al, 1992). Through the use of sensitive antibody techniques, CNTF has also been found within myelinated neuronal axoplasm (Rende et al, 1992). However, the absence of a hydrophobic leader sequence on the CNTF molecule, a prerequisite for secretion, and its presence within Schwann cell cytoplasm rather than on basement membrane suggest that CNTF may not be secreted from the Schwann cell under physiological conditions (Sendtner et al, 1992). After nerve injury, mRNA coding for CNTF in Schwann cells decreases to 5% of normal levels, and CNTF production declines rapidly (Rabinovsky et al, 1992; Seniuk et al, 1992; Smith et al, 1993). This presents a paradox: Why do levels of a potential trophic factor decrease at a time when the factor is presumably needed most? The answer may lie in the observation that, while CNTF production drops precipitously, CNTF bioactivity is maintained at one third of normal levels (Sendtner et al, 1992). This persisting activity reflects CNTF that is present in extracellular locations, where it may be available to regenerating axons as a so-called injury factor rather than as a target-derived trophic factor. The inability to demonstrate CNTF within skin or muscle, which are normal sources of trophic factor, is consistent with this interpretation (Dobrea et al, 1992).

The finding of low CNTF levels in a peripheral nerve after axotomy suggests that the addition of exogenous CNTF may improve the course of axon regeneration. Accordingly, both systemic and local applications of CNTF have been found to increase the number of myelinated axons distal to a nerve repair after 4 to 6 weeks (Badalamente et al, 1993; Sahenk et al, 1994). CNTF thus appears to be a glial-derived factor, and the role of this factor in normal nerves remains obscure. Sufficient CNTF may be released into the extracellular space after injury to provide some support to regenerating axons. Although exogenous CNTF may function as a motor nerve growth factor, it does not appear to be a target-derived trophic factor in the classic sense. The complexity and potential contradictions of the CNTF story to date point out several of the pitfalls inherent in the study of trophic factors: (1) activity in vitro does not accurately predict activity in vivo; (2) a trophic factor may be present in a given location, but if it lacks a mechanism for secretion, it may not be biologically active; (3) trophic factors may be present in incredibly small quantities, so that newer genetic techniques of biological amplification may demonstrate their presence in areas previously thought to be barren.

Insulin-like Growth Factors

The two insulin-like growth factors (IGF-I, originally termed somatomedin-C, and IGF-II) are proteins that structurally resemble proinsulin. In tissue culture, IGF-I or IGF-II can stimulate outgrowth of motor (Caroni and Grandes, 1990), sensory (Bothwell, 1982), and sympathetic (Recio-Pinto et al, 1986) neurites in physiological concentrations. In adult animals, both motor and sensory neurons produce IGF-I, which is transported anterogradely to the periphery (Hansson et al, 1987). Small amounts may also be transported in retrograde fashion from the periphery to the central neuron (Hansson, 1993). However, IGF-I and IGF-II do not appear to be peripherally derived, centrally transported neurotrophic factors in the usual sense. Binding of IGFs to their receptors occurs on the extracellular surface of cells and activates kinases within the cell (Ishii et al, 1993). If the subsequent activity of these kinases is the event necessary for neurotrophic activity, then the IGF molecules themselves may not need to cross the membrane, a possibility borne out by experiments in which the receptors are successfully tricked into producing a central effect by non–insulin-like molecules (summarized in Ishii et al, 1993).

IGF-I activity has been detected in small amounts within the Schwann cells of the normal rat sciatic nerve (Hansson

et al, 1986). After nerve transection, IGF-I levels increase within reactive Schwann cells, especially when the nerve ends are enclosed within a silicon tube. Application of exogenous IGF-I to the site of sciatic nerve freeze injury increases the speed of axon regeneration in a concentration-dependent manner (Sjoberg and Kanje, 1989), and this effect may be augmented by simultaneous application of platelet-derived growth factor (Hansson, 1993). In separate experiments, exogenous IGF-II was found to stimulate regeneration of motor nerves (Near et al, 1992). The importance of IGFs for axon regeneration is also suggested by experiments in which antibodies to IGFs inhibited regeneration of both sensory and motor axons in vivo (Ishii et al, 1993).

The IGFs also play a crucial role in neuromuscular development and regeneration. The IGF-II gene is vigorously expressed in developing rat limb during polyneuronal innervation but is down regulated when extra synapses are eliminated (Ishii, 1989). Application of even low concentrations of IGF-I or IGF-II to adult muscle results in intramuscular nerve sprouting (Caroni and Grandes, 1990). Recent work has begun to define separate roles for IGF-I and IGF-II in the neuromuscular system (Glazner et al, 1993). After nerve injury, levels of mRNA for IGF-II were increased much more in muscle than in nerve; IGF-I mRNA was more abundant in nerve than in muscle, both innervated and denervated. IGF-I thus appears to be primarily involved in the stimulation of axon regeneration, and IGF-II mediates the establishment of neuromuscular synapses.

Fibroblast Growth Factors

The fibroblast growth factors (FGFs) are polypeptides whose growth-promoting and mitogenic activities are strongly dependent on the co-factor heparin. The most well-characterized are bFGF and acidic fibroblast growth factor (aFGF), which share more than half of their amino acid sequence identities (Sensenbrenner, 1993). In tissue culture, both bFGF and aFGF promote the development of sensory and sympathetic neurites (Eckenstein et al, 1990), bFGF enhances the level of choline acetyltransferase in rat spinal cord (motoneuron) cultures (McManaman et al, 1989), and both are potent mitogens for Schwann cells (Davis and Stroobant, 1990). In vivo, application of bFGF to the cut rat sciatic nerve prevents the dorsal root ganglion neuron death that would normally follow this lesion (Otto et al, 1987). Similarly, bFGF rescues motor neurons after hypoglossal nerve injury in neonatal rats (Grothe and Unsicker, 1992). Although these findings support a role for FGFs as target-derived neurotrophic factors, evidence for their retrograde transport is incomplete (Hassan et al, 1994), and bFGF fails to rescue embryonic chick neurons from programmed cell death (Oppenheim et al, 1992). In normal sciatic nerve, aFGF is present in high levels, rapidly decreasing after nerve transection. It has been suggested, on the basis of the above-mentioned observations, that aFGF is released from peripheral nerve soon after injury, activating Schwann cells and promoting neural regeneration (Eckenstein et al, 1991). Attempts to stimulate regeneration by the addition of exogenous FGFs to enclosed neural gaps are consistent with this hypothesis. In qualitative studies, both aFGF and bFGF were found to promote rat sciatic nerve regeneration across a 15-

mm gap, a distance that is not normally bridged by regenerating axons in this model (Aebischer et al, 1989; Walter et al, 1993). The addition of aFGF to a 5-mm gap resulted in peripheral reinnervation by higher numbers of motoneurons (Cordeiro et al, 1989), and bFGF was found to promote migration of both neural and non-neural elements across a gap at early time periods. The FGFs are thus potent stimulators of peripheral nerve regeneration and are likely to find clinical application in the near future.

Neurotrophism—The Future

Trophic factors will soon be used to improve the outcome of peripheral nerve repair in humans. However, several aspects of trophic factor biology must be understood and manipulated before this can occur. First, we must learn which trophic factors normally participate in peripheral nerve regeneration. New factors still burst on the trophic scene with alarming frequency. A recent addition is glial cell line–derived neurotrophic factor (GDNF) (Henderson et al, 1994), which promotes the survival of developing motoneurons at much lower concentrations than members of the NGF family of neurotrophins. Fortunately, techniques for analyzing trophic factor production and activity have improved significantly in the last decade. Early research on NGF relied on standard biochemical techniques of molecular analysis and required vast quantities of neural tissue to isolate minute quantities of NGF. More recently, the revolution in molecular biology has shifted the focus from the molecule under study to the DNA and RNA sequences that code for it in the cell nucleus. One of the most powerful of these techniques is polymerase chain reaction, which allows amplification (replication) of individual DNA sequences and is so sensitive that it can detect a single copy of DNA at the genomic level. The DNA under study is denatured, then replicated in a chain reaction catalyzed by heat-resistant DNA polymerase from bacteria, such as *Thermus aquaticus* cultured from hot springs in Yellowstone National Park. This technique has been used to detect differences in brain-derived neurotrophic factor concentrations in muscle and cutaneous nerve (Rapoza et al, 1994), in contrast to previous techniques that could barely detect brain-derived neurotrophic factor in peripheral nerve at all. Another neurogenetic technique brought to bear on trophic interactions involves the production of transgenic mice in which a given trophic factor is either absent or produced in excess. Resulting changes in neuroanatomy or regeneration biology help pinpoint the role of the manipulated factor in the development and regeneration of the normal animal. For instance, mice that overproduce NGF in the skin develop novel sympathetic projections to sensory neurons (Davis et al, 1994). This observation provides support for the hypothesis that increased NGF expression is a crucial link in the development of sympathetic hyperalgesia. Conversely, lack of CNTF production leads to a mouse model of human motoneuron disease, with normal development but progressive deterioration in adulthood (Davis et al, 1994).

When trophic factor participation in neural regeneration has been defined, we must then decide which factors to manipulate in our efforts to improve clinical outcome. One approach is to add factors that seem to play a vital role but that decrease after nerve injury (vide supra, CNTF). Another strategy would be to analyze separately neural regeneration in juveniles, in whom regeneration proceeds successfully, and in adults, in whom it is substantially flawed. Restoration of the adult trophic factor mix to that seen in juveniles would then be expected to improve adult outcome. Such manipulations would doubtless be complicated by the interdependency of trophic factor production in the living organism. For instance, addition of exogenous NGF has been found to increase brain-derived neurotrophic factor production in dorsal root ganglia (Apfel et al, 1994).

Once an optimal trophic factor mix is identified, an appropriate delivery system must be designed and tested. One approach has been to enclose a nerve repair within a bioresorbable tube that releases trophic factors as it dissolves (Aebischer et al, 1989). Beta FGF delivered with this system stimulated rat sciatic axons to cross a 15-mm gap, one that could not be crossed in controls without bFGF. An even more sophisticated potential approach would be to alter the genetic material within the parent neuron, so that it could make the appropriate trophic factors itself. Viral particles can be altered to contain the genetic material for production of specific trophic factors. In initial experiments, virus containing the DNA for NGF was introduced into superior cervical ganglion cells. The gene was transcribed, and NGF was produced (Federoff et al, 1992). Furthermore, the infected cells gained the ability to survive interruption of NGF transport from the periphery. It might thus be possible to add genetic material to injured neurons at the time of nerve repair; this material would then be transported proximally to the neuron, where it could stimulate production of trophic factors needed to optimize axon regeneration.

NEUROTROPISM

Neurotropism involves guidance of regenerating axons to a specific target, and it is thus usually discussed in the context of regeneration specificity. Peripheral axon regeneration may exhibit specificity at many levels and is most easily understood when arranged in a hierarchical framework (Brushart, 1991). The term *tissue* specificity refers to the guidance of regenerating axons as a group to the distal nerve stump rather than to other tissues such as tendon or muscle. *Fascicular* or *nerve trunk* specificity describes guidance of axons to their fascicle of origin, for instance reinnervation of the distal peroneal stump by peroneal axons after sciatic nerve repair. *Sensory* versus *motor* specificity separates efferent motor axons from afferent sensory axons and plays a crucial role in determining the population of axons reinnervating tributary nerves. Within both sensory and motor systems, *topographic* specificity refers to the return of axons to the topographic area they previously served, such as index finger axons to the index finger after median nerve repair, and *end-organ* specificity describes reinnervation of each type of end-organ by axons that previously served and are centrally wired to serve that specific end-organ. Neurotropism has been directly implicated in the generation of both tissue and fascicular specificity. The relevant experimental evidence will be reviewed to ascertain the validity of these claims.

Chemotropism, guidance of regenerating axons by chemical influences emanating from the distal nerve stump, was first proposed by Forssman (1898; reviewed in Ramon y Cajal, 1928). Ramon y Cajal then subjected regenerating axons to a variety of influences, concluding that "the action exerted by the peripheral stump—the cells of Schwann, etc.—on the growth of the young fibers is not individual and specific, that is, from tube to tube, but is general and collective, similarly directing the new axons towards the periphery" (Ramon y Cajal, 1928). He coined the term neurotropism to describe this activity. The next major investigation of neurotropism was performed by Weiss and Taylor (1944) in the course of a broad survey of regeneration specificity. On the basis of critically flawed experiments (Ochi et al, 1994), Weiss and Taylor dismissed neurotropism, discouraging further work for several decades. Interest in the topic was then revived by Lundborg in the 1970s. Working at Lund University, the site of Forssman's earlier experiments, he showed that axons will regenerate obliquely across a tissue chamber to reinnervate a distal stump placed in the opposite corner (Lundborg et al, 1982). Work on tissue specificity soon followed in this and other laboratories (Lundborg et al, 1986; Mackinnon et al, 1986). In these experiments, regenerating axons were given a choice of distal targets by introducing them into the base of a silicon Y chamber. The two targets were then introduced into the limbs of the Y, so that axons would have equal access to both targets and the inert silicon environment would not interfere with the action of target-generated substances. Axons uniformly reinnervated distal nerve as opposed to tendon, muscle, or granulation tissue (Lundborg et al, 1986; Mackinnon et al, 1986). It is important to note that these findings are consistent with the action of neurotropism but do not specifically prove its effect. Neurotropism can be proved only by observing axons regenerating selectively toward a target that they have not yet reached. In these experiments, analyzed after several weeks of regeneration, axons that reached correct targets could already be receiving neurotrophic support not available to axons reaching incorrect targets, resulting in their selective survival. It is also unclear whether the distal stump influences regenerating axons directly or indirectly through an attractive action on migrating Schwann cells. Although it does not rule out neurotropic axon guidance, attraction of Schwann cells to the distal stump in the absence of regenerating axons has been demonstrated (Abernethy et al, 1994). The elegant experiments of Kuffler (1989) have successfully answered the question of early axon trajectory. Axons regenerating from the proximal stump of the transected frog cutaneous pectoris nerve wander randomly when no distal stump is present. However, these axons exhibit marked directionality in their growth toward a distal nerve target, even before this target is reached. This work firmly establishes the action of neurotropism in guiding axons or Schwann cells, or both, to the distal nerve stump in the generation of tissue specificity.

Specificity at the nerve trunk level was first examined by Weiss and Hoag (1946), who concluded that "the concept that there is any selectivity, absolute or relative, in the establishment of regenerative connections between motoneurons and muscle fibers is . . . contradicted by the facts." Interest in the topic was later revived by Politis, who believed that nerve trunk specificity could be generated through the action of neurotropism (Politis, 1985). He provided re-

generating rat peroneal or tibial axons with a choice of peroneal or tibial nerve grafts across a 5-mm gap in a silicon Y chamber (vide supra). These experiments demonstrated nearly absolute selectivity in the growth of peroneal axons to the peroneal graft, and tibial axons to the tibial graft. However, results were evaluated at 3.5 weeks, after distal stump reinnervation, and therefore cannot be used as evidence for neurotropism. To overcome this objection in discussing similar experiments, Politis and colleagues (1982) argued that neurotropism, rather than neurotrophism, was the likely mechanism because (1) preferential *survival* of axons reaching the correct target was unlikely, because no axonal degeneration was observed in the incorrect target; and (2) preferential *maturation* was also unlikely, because there was no difference in the size of the largest axons projecting correctly or incorrectly.

Attempts to reproduce these findings in the rat Y-tube model, using intact distal nerve instead of graft and assessing regeneration with myelinated axon counts, have met with variable results. Seckel and co-workers (1986) examined growth of peroneal axons across an 8-mm gap and found a 2:1 preference for the distal peroneal nerve after 6 weeks. Davey and colleagues (1992) used a 10-mm gap and demonstrated greater than 2:1 preference of both tibial and peroneal axons for the distal peroneal nerve after 8 to 12 weeks. Abernethy and associates (1992) examined regeneration across a 6-mm gap and found no preference of either tibial or peroneal axons to selectively reinnervate the appropriate distal stump after 4 to 6 weeks. Zhao and co-workers (1992) returned to the original Politis model and compared the outcome with either a nerve graft or an intact distal nerve stump. Specificity was generated at 1 month when axons could reinnervate muscle through intact distal pathways but not when the only peripheral pathway was present in the form of nerve graft. In aggregate, these experiments suggest that some type of fascicular specificity may be unmasked under the appropriate experimental conditions and that it may be based on the ease with which muscle is reinnervated rather than on a particular characteristic of the peripheral nerve pathway. However, as mentioned previously, rigid criteria must be satisfied before regeneration specificity can be attributed to the action of neurotropism. Appropriately directed axonal growth must be visualized before the target is reached; directed regeneration in the presence of target contact might result from initially random reinnervation, followed by selective maintenance of correctly projecting axons at the expense of those projecting to inappropriate targets. The Y-tube experiments on fascicular and nerve trunk specificity thus provide no evidence for the action of neurotropism. Reliance on neurotropism to direct axons across a gap properly (Dellon and Mackinnon, 1988) thus appears unwarranted.

References

Abernethy DA, Rud A, Thomas PK: Neurotropic influence of the distal stump of transected peripheral nerve on axonal regeneration: Absence of topographic specificity in adult nerve. J Anat *180*:395, 1992.

Abernethy DA, Thomas PK, Rud A, King RHM: Mutual attraction between emigrant cells from transected denervated nerve. J Anat *184*:239, 1994.

Aebischer P, Salessiotis AN, Winn SR: Basic fibroblast growth factor released from synthetic guidance channels facilitates peripheral nerve regeneration across long nerve gaps. J Neurosci Res *23*:282, 1989.

Albers K, Wright D, Davis B: Overexpression of nerve growth factor in epidermis of transgenic mice causes hypertrophy of the peripheral nervous system. J Neurosci *14:*1422, 1994.

Altin J, Bradshaw R: Nerve growth factor and related substances: Structure and mechanism of action. *In* Loughlin S, Fallon J (eds): Neurotrophic Factors. New York, Academic Press, 1993, p 129.

Angeletti R, Bradshaw R, Wade R: Subunit structure and amino acid composition of mouse submaxillary gland nerve growth factor. Biochemistry *10:*463, 1971.

Anton E, Weskamp G, Reichardt L, Matthew W: Nerve growth factor and its low-affinity receptor promote Schwann cell migration. Proc Natl Acad Sci USA *91:*2795, 1994.

Apfel SC, Dormia C, Newell ME, Kessler JA: Nerve growth factor administration alters the expression of other neurotrophins in adult sensory ganglia. (Abstract.) Soc Neurosci Abstr *20:*1302, 1994.

Arakawa Y, Sendtner M, Thoenen H: Survival effect of ciliary neurotrophic factor (CNTF) on chick embryonic motoneurons in culture: Comparison with other neurotrophic factors and cytokines. J Neurosci *10:*3507, 1990.

Badalamente MA, Hurst LC, Pecoraro M: Ciliary neuronotrophic factor (CNTF) as an *in vivo* adjunct to peripheral nerve repair. (Abstract.) ORS Abst *39:*91, 1993.

Barbin G, Manthorpe M, Varon S: Purification of the chick eye ciliary neuronotrophic factor. J Neurochem *43:*1468, 1984.

Bothwell M: Insulin and somatomedin MSA promote nerve growth factor—independent neurite formation by cultured chick dorsal root ganglionic sensory neurons. J Neurosci Res 8: 225, 1982.

Bothwell M: Keeping track of neurotrophin receptors. Cell *65:*915, 1991.

Brushart TME: The mechanical and humoral control of specificity in nerve repair. *In* Gelberman RH (ed): Operative Nerve Repair and Reconstruction. Philadelphia, J. B. Lippincott Company, 1991, p 215.

Caroni P, Grandes P: Nerve sprouting in innervated adult skeletal muscle induced by exposure to elevated levels of insulin-like growth factors. J Cell Biol *110:*1307, 1990.

Chen Y-S, Wang-Bennett L, Coker N: Facial nerve regeneration in the silicon chamber: The influence of nerve growth factor. Exp Neurol *103:*52, 1989.

Cordeiro PG, Seckel BR, Lipton S, D'Amore P, Wagner J, Madison R: Acidic fibroblast growth factor enhances peripheral nerve regeneration in vivo. Plast Reconstr Surg *83:*1013, 1989.

Cordon-Cardo C, Tapley P, Jing S, Nanduri V, O'Rourke E, Lamballe F, Korvary K, Klein R, Jones K, Reichardt L, Barbacid M: The TRK tyrosine protein kinase mediates the mitogenic properties of nerve growth factor and neurotrophin-3. Cell *66:*173, 1991.

Davey DF, Brown CS, Ansselin AD: Pathway selection by regenerating peripheral nerve axons growing through a Y-shaped tube is related to distal stump size. Soc Neurosci Abstr *18:*609, 1992.

Davies A, Bandtlow C, Heumann R, Korsching S, Rohrer H, Thoenen H: Timing and site of nerve growth factor synthesis in developing skin in relation to its innervation and expression of the receptor. Nature *326:*353, 1987.

Davis BM, Katz DM, Seroogy KB, Albers KM: Overexpression of NGF in transgenic mice induces novel sympathetic projections to primary sensory neurons. Soc Neurosci Abstr *20:*1090, 1994.

Davis JB, Stroobant P: Platelet-derived growth factors and fibroblast growth factors are mitogens for rat Schwann cells. J Cell Biol *110:*1353, 1990.

Dellon L, Mackinnon S: An alternative to the classical nerve graft for the management of the short nerve gap. Plast Reconstr Surg *82:*849, 1988.

Derby A, Engleman W, Frierdich G, Neises G, Rapp S, Roufa D: Nerve growth factor facilitates regeneration across nerve gaps: Morphological and behavioral studies in rat sciatic nerve. Exp Neurol *119:*176, 1993.

Diamond J, Foerster A, Holmes M, Coughlin M: Sensory nerves in adult rats regenerate and restore sensory function to the skin independently of endogenous NGF. J Neurosci *12:*1467, 1992.

Dobrea G, Unnerstall J, Rao MS: The expression of CNTF message and immunoreactivity in the central and peripheral nervous system of the rat. Dev Brain Res *66:*209, 1992.

Eckenstein FP, Esch F, Holbert T, Blacher RW, Nishi R: Purification and characterization of a trophic factor for embryonic peripheral neurons: A comparison with fibroblast growth factors. Neuron *4:*623, 1990.

Eckenstein FP, Shipley GD, Nishi R: Acidic and basic fibroblast growth factors in the nervous system: Distribution and differential alteration of levels after injury of central versus peripheral nerve. J Neurosci *11:*412, 1991.

Federoff HJ, Geschwind MD, Gellers AI, Kessler JA: Expression of nerve growth factor in vivo from a defective herpes simplex virus 1 vector prevents effects of axotomy on sympathetic ganglia. Proc Natl Acad Sci USA *89:*1636, 1992.

Forssman J: Ueber die Ursachen, welche die Wachstumsrichtung der peripheren Nervenfasern bei der Regeneration bestimmen. Beitr Z Pathol Anat 24:56, 1898.

Friedman B, Scherer SS, Rudge JS, Helgren M, Morrisey D, McClain J, Wang D, Wiegand S, Furth M, Lindsay RM, Ip NY: Regulation of ciliary neurotrophic factor expression in myelin-related Schwann cells in vivo. Neuron 9:295, 1992.

Glazner GW, Wright WG, Ishii DN: Kinetics of insulin-like growth factor (IGF) mRNA changes in rat nerve and muscle during IGF-dependent nerve regeneration. Soc Neurosci Abstr (Abstract.) *19:*253, 1993.

Grothe C, Unsicker K: Basic fibroblast growth factor in the hypoglossal system: Specific retrograde transport, trophic, and lesion-related responses. J Neurosci *32:*317, 1992.

Gurney M, Yamamoto H, Kwon Y: Induction of motor neuron sprouting in vivo by ciliary neurotrophic factor and basic fibroblast growth factor. J Neurosci *12:*3241, 1992.

Hamburger V, Yip H: Reduction of experimentally induced neural death in spinal ganglia of the chick embryo by nerve growth factor. J Neurosci *4:*767, 1984.

Hansson H-A: Insulin-like growth factors and nerve regeneration. Ann NY Acad Sci *692:*161, 1993.

Hansson HA, Dahlin LB, Danielsen N, Fryklund L, Nachemson AK, Polleryd P, Rozell B, Skottner A, Stemme S, Lundborg G: Evidence indicating trophic importance of IGF-I in regenerating peripheral nerves. Acta Physiol Scand *126:*609, 1986.

Hansson H-A, Rozell B, Skottner A: Rapid axoplasmic transport of insulin-like growth factor I in the sciatic nerve of adult rats. Cell Tissue Res *247:*241, 1987.

Hassan S, Kerkhoff H, Troost D, Veldman H, Jennekens F: Basic fibroblast growth factor immunoreactivity in the peripheral motor system of the rat. Acta Neuropathol (Berl) *87:*405, 1994.

Henderson CE, Pollock RA, Armanin M, Phillps HS, Rosenthal A: Glial cell line–derived neurotrophic factor (GDNF), a potent survival factor for spinal motoneurons, is present in developing limb. (Abstract.) Soc Neurosci Abstr *20:*1095, 1994.

Heumann R, Korsching S, Bandtlow C, Thoenen H: Changes of nerve growth factor synthesis in nonneuronal cells in response to sciatic nerve transection. J Cell Biol *104:*1623, 1987.

Hollowell J, Villadiego A, Rich K: Sciatic nerve regeneration across gaps within silicon chambers: Long-term effects of NGF and consideration of axonal branching. Exp Neurol 110:45, 1990.

Ishii DN: Relationship of insulin-like growth factor ii gene expression in muscle to synaptogenesis. Proc Natl Acad Sci USA *86:*2898, 1989.

Ishii DN, Glazner GW, Whalen R: Regulation of peripheral nerve regeneration by insulin-like growth factors. Ann NY Acad Sci *692:*172, 1993.

Ishii DN, Loughlin SE, Fallon JH (eds): Neurotrophic Factors. San Diego, Academic Press, 1993, p 415.

Johnson D, Lanahan A, Buck C, Sehgal A, Morgan E, Mercer E, Bothwell M, Chao M: Expression and structure of human NGF receptor. Cell *47:*545, 1986.

Johnson E, Gorin P, Brandeis L, Pearson J: Dorsal root ganglion neurons are destroyed by exposure in utero to maternal antibody to nerve growth factor. Science *210:*916, 1980.

Korsching S: The neurotrophic factor concept: A reexamination. J Neurosci *13:*2739, 1993.

Korsching S, Thoenen H: Treatment with 6-hydroxydopamine and colchicine decreases nerve growth factor levels in sympathetic ganglia and increases them in the corresponding target tissues. J Neurosci *5:*1058, 1985.

Kuffler DP: Regeneration of muscle axons in the frog is directed by diffusible factors from denervated muscle and nerve tubes. J Exp Neurol *281:*416, 1989.

Levi-Montalcini R, Hamburger V: Selective growth stimulating effects of mouse sarcoma on the sensory and sympathetic nervous system of the chick embryo. J Exp Zool *116:*321, 1951.

Lindholm D, Heumann R, Meyer M, Thoenen H: Interleukin-1 regulates synthesis of nerve growth factor in non-neuronal cells of rat sciatic nerve. Nature *330:*658, 1987.

Lundborg G, Dahlin LB, Danielsen N, Johannesson A, Hansson H-A: *In* Lee AJC, Albrektsson T, Branemark PI (eds): Clinical Applications of Biomaterials. Chichester, UK, John Wiley & Sons, Ltd., 1982, p 323.

Lundborg GL, Dahlin N, Danielsen N, Nachemson AK: Tissue specificity in nerve regeneration. Scand J Plast Reconstr Surg *20:*279, 1986.

Lundborg G, Hansson H-H: Regeneration of peripheral nerve through a preformed tissue space. Preliminary observations on the reorganization of regenerating nerve fibers and perineurium. Brain Res *178*:573, 1979.

Mackinnon SE, Dellon AL, Lundborg G, Hudson AR, Hunter DA: A study of neurotrophism in a primate model. J Hand Surg *11A*:888, 1986.

Masu Y, Wolf B, Holtmann B, Sendtner M, Brem G, Thoenen H: Disruption of the CNTF gene results in progressive motoneuropathy. Nature *365*:27, 1993.

McManaman JL, Crawford FG, Clark R, Richker J, Fuller F: Multiple neurotrophic factors from skeletal muscle: Demonstration of effects of basic fibroblast growth factor and comparisons with the 22 kDa choline acetyltransferase development factor. J Neurochem *53*:1763, 1989.

Near SL, Whalen R, Miller JA, Ishii DN: Insulin-like growth factor II stimulates motor nerve regeneration. Proc Natl Acad Sci USA *89*:11716, 1992.

Ochi M, Matsuda T, Ikuta Y, Yonehara S: Further experimental evidence of selective nerve regeneration in aortic Y-chambers. Scand J Plast Reconstr Hand Surg *28*:137, 1994.

Oppenheim RW: Cell death during development of the nervous system. Annu Rev Neurosci *14*:453, 1991.

Oppenheim RW, Prevette D, Fuller F: The lack of effect of basic fibroblast growth factors on the naturally occurring death of motoneurons in the chick embryo. J Neurosci *12*:2726, 1992.

Oppenheim RW, Prevette D, Qin-Wei Y, Collins F, MacDonald J: Control of embryonic motoneuron survival in vivo by ciliary neurotrophic factor. Science *251*:1616, 1991.

Otto D, Unsicker K, Grothe C: Pharmacological effects of nerve growth factor and fibroblast growth factor applied to the transected sciatic nerve on neuron death in adult rat dorsal root ganglia. Neurosci Lett *83*:156, 1987.

Politis MJ: Specificity in mammalian peripheral nerve regeneration at the level of the nerve trunk. Brain Res *328*:271, 1985.

Politis MJ, Ederle K, Spencer PS: Tropism in nerve regeneration in vivo. Attraction of regenerating axons by diffusable factors derived from cells in distal nerve stumps of transected peripheral nerves. Brain Res *253*:1, 1982.

Rabinovsky ED, Smith GM, Browder DP, Shine HD, McManaman JL: Peripheral nerve injury down-regulates CNTF expression in adult rat sciatic nerves. J Neurosci Res *31*:188, 1992.

Raivich G, Hellweg R, Kreutzberg G: The expression of growth factor receptors during nerve regeneration. Restorative Neurol Neurosci *1*:217, 1990.

Raivich G, Hellweg R, Kreutzberg G: NGF receptor–mediated decrease in axonal uptake and retrograde transport of endogenous NGF following sciatic nerve injury and during regeneration. Neuron *7*:151, 1991.

Raivich G, Kreutzberg GW: Peripheral nerve regeneration: Role of growth factors and their receptors. Int J Dev Neurosci *11*:311, 1993.

Ramon y Cajal S: Degeneration and Regeneration of the Nervous System. London, Oxford University Press, 1928.

Rapoza MP, Aldous MD, Archibald SJ, Rohwer RJ, Madison RD: BDNF levels increase in the terminal motor branch following lesions of the parent femoral nerve: A competitive PCR study. (Abstract.) Soc Neurosci Abstr *20*:1500, 1994.

Recio-Pinto E, Rechler MM, Ishii DN: Effects of insulin, insulin-like growth factor-II, and nerve growth factor on neurite formation and survival in cultured sympathetic and sensory neurons. J Neurosci *6*:1211, 1986.

Rende M, Muir D, Ruoslahti E, Hagg T, Varon S, Manthorpe M: Immunolocalization of ciliary neuronotrophic factor in adult rat sciatic nerve. Glia *5*:25, 1992.

Rich K, Alexander T, Pryor J, Hollowell J: Nerve growth factor enhances regeneration through silicon chambers. Exp Neurol *105*:162, 1989.

Sahenk Z, Seharaseyon J, Mendell JR: CNTF potentiates peripheral nerve regeneration. Brain Res *655*:246, 1994.

Seckel BR, Ryan SE, Gagne RG, Ho-Chiu T, Watkins E: Target-specific nerve regeneration through a nerve guide in the rat. Plast Reconstr Surg *78*:793, 1986.

Sendtner M, Kreutzberg GW, Thoenen H: Ciliary neurotrophic factor prevents the degeneration of motor neurons after axotomy. Nature *345*:440, 1990.

Sendtner M, Stockli KA, Thoenen H: Synthesis and localization of ciliary neurotrophic factor in the sciatic nerve of the adult rat after lesion and during regeneration. J Cell Biol *118*:139, 1992.

Seniuk N, Altares M, Dunn R, Richardson PM: Decreased synthesis of ciliary neurotrophic factor in degenerating peripheral nerves. Brain Res *572*:300, 1992.

Sensenbrenner M: The neurotrophic activity of fibroblast growth factors. Prog Neurobiol *41*:683, 1993.

Sjoberg J, Kanje M: Insulin-like growth factor (IGF-I) as a stimulator of regeneration in the freeze-injured rat sciatic nerve. Brain Res *485*:102, 1989.

Smith GM, Rabinovsky ED, McManaman, JL, Shine HD: Temporal and spatial expression of ciliary neurotrophic factor after peripheral nerve injury. Exp Neurol *121*:239, 1993.

Taniuchi M, Clark H, Schweitzer J, Johnson E: Expression of nerve growth factor receptors by Schwann cells of axotomized peripheral nerves: Ultrastructural location, suppression by axonal contact, and binding properties. J Neurosci *8*:664, 1988.

Thoenen H, Bandtlow C, Heumann R, Lindholm D, Meyer M, Rohrer H: Nerve growth factor: Cellular localization and regulation of synthesis. Cell Mol Biol *8*:35, 1988.

Walter MA, Kurouglu R, Caulfield JB, Vasconez LO, Thompson JA: Enhanced peripheral nerve regeneration by acidic fibroblast growth factor. Lymphokine Cytokine Res *12*:135, 1993.

Weiss P, Hoag A: Competitive reinnervation of rat muscles by their own and foreign nerves. J Neurophysiol *9*:413, 1946.

Weiss P, Taylor AC: Further experimental evidence against neurotropism in nerve regeneration. J Exp Zool *95*:233, 1944.

Zhao Q, Dahlin LB, Kanje M, Lundborg G, Lu S-B: Axonal projections and functional recovery following fascicular repair of the rat sciatic nerve with Y-tunnelled silicon chambers. Restorative Neurol Neurosci *4*:13, 1992.

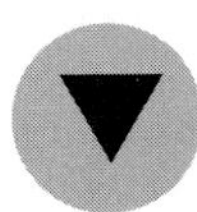

Chapter 24

• Lawrence C. Hurst
• Marie A. Badalamente

Histochemical Aids to Control Specificity in Peripheral Nerve Repair

When mixed peripheral nerves are severed, the selective reanastomosis of motor and sensory fascicles is a factor that may lead to more optimal functional recovery. The internal topography of sensory and motor axons within a peripheral nerve is complex and cannot be differentiated using conventional histology or electron microscopy (Figs. 24–1 and 24–2). It has been reported that in proximal segments of peripheral nerve, there is little organization of motor and sensory axons (Sunderland, 1980). However, distally axons may be organized into distinct fascicles or fascicular groups that can innervate specific motor and sensory targets (Sunderland, 1980). As Jabaley has reported,

". . . although the cross-sectional appearances of major nerves varies with the level, the path of functional units is less changeable and can be predicted over a reasonably long length of nerve. In an attempt to increase the specificity of target reinnervation, the focus of nerve repair has shifted to the accurate alignment of functional fascicles. Current repair techniques require the surgeon to understand the internal topography of nerves and to be capable of internal dissection of nerves where necessary" *(Jabaley, 1991).*

Several histochemical and biochemical techniques have been developed over the past three decades that aid in differentiating between motor and sensory components of mixed peripheral nerves. Using these histochemical or bio-

chemical techniques, the surgeon may accurately map the location of motor or sensory fascicles or fascicular groups before nerve repair. The basis by which motor and sensory axons may be differentiated relates to components within their cytoplasmic structure. These components are synthesized within anterior horn cell bodies of the spinal cord for motor axons or within dorsal root ganglia cell bodies for sensory axons. Axoplasmic transport is the mechanism that moves the cellular components to their functional sites and is critical to neuron survival (Sheetz et al, 1989). The classic works on axoplasmic transport defined two broad categories based on speed: fast and slow axoplasmic transport (Atwood and MacKay, 1989; Bradford, 1986; Hammerschlag and Brady, 1989; Hammerschlag and Stone, 1986; Lasek et al, 1984; Noback and Demerest, 1981; Ochs, 1987). Fast axoplasmic transport can move cellular components at a rate of up to 410 mm per day and is bidirectional. Slow axoplasmic transport has been divided into three types: slow component A, with a transport rate of 1 mm per day; slow component B, with a transport rate of 2 to 4 mm per day; and intermediate slow transport, with a rate of 4 to 8 mm per day. Slow axoplasmic transport is unidirectional in the antegrade direction.

The components that allow differentiation between sensory and motor axons are enzymes that are produced within

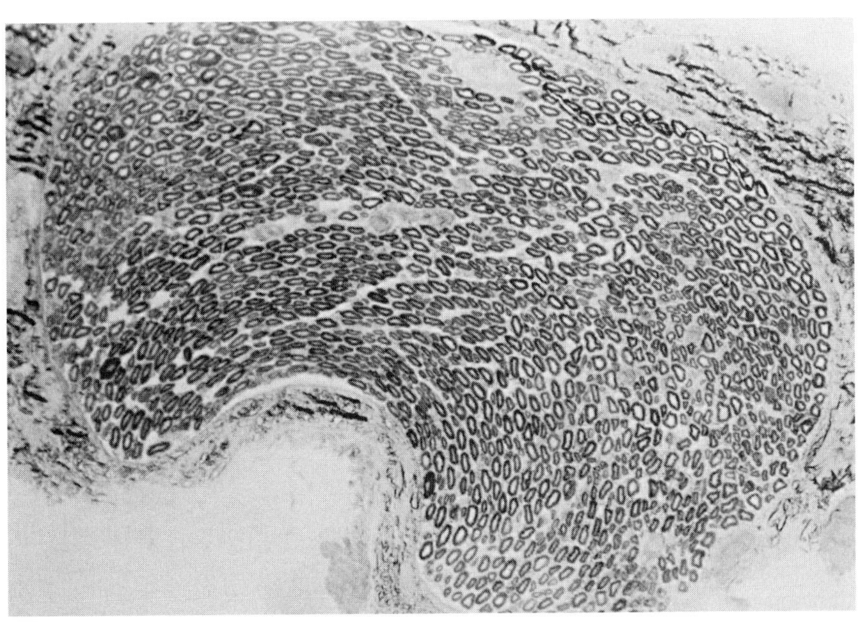

243

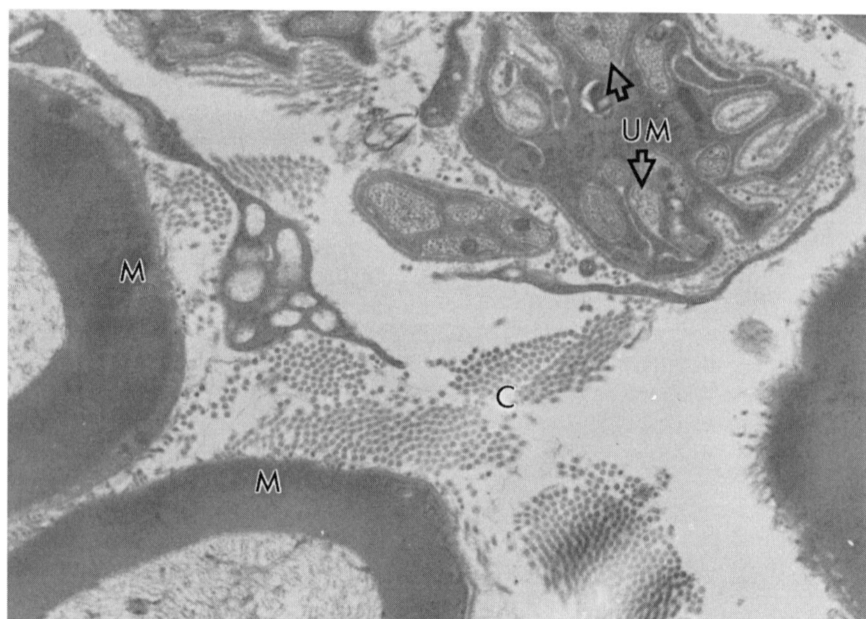

FIGURE 24–2. Electron micrograph of a rat peroneal nerve showing myelinated (M) and unmyelinated (UM) axons within endoneurial collagen (C). It is not possible to distinguish motor or sensory axons. × 15,000.

cell bodies and moved by axoplasmic transport distally. Acetylcholinesterase and choline acetyltransferase are enzymes contained within motor axons. Carbonic anhydrase is an enzyme contained predominantly within sensory axons.

ACETYLCHOLINESTERASE HISTOCHEMISTRY FOR DIFFERENTIATION OF MOTOR AXONS

Many histochemical techniques have been used to stain cholinesterases in animal models (Adams et al, 1967; Baljet and Drukker, 1975; Hebb, 1963; Kasa and Rakonczay, 1982; Koelle and Freidenweld, 1949; Lubinska et al, 1963). Karnovsky and Roots (1964) were the first to demonstrate that when sectioned nerve tissue is incubated in a solution containing acetylthiocoline, copper sulfate, and potassium ferricyanide, cytoplasmic acetylcholinesterase hydrolyzes the acetylthiocoline ester to thiocholine. Thiocholine further reduces ferricyanide to ferrocyanide and then combines with copper irons to form a very dark brown precipitate—copper ferrocyanide, which is visible in the light microscope. In 1973, Gruber and Zenker (1973) further expanded on the use of acetylcholinesterase histochemistry to differentiate between motor and sensory axons in a rat model. These authors showed that the Karnovsky and Roots' histochemical method stained approximately 80% of motor and less than 10% of sensory fibers in this rat model. In 1976, Gruber and colleagues (1976) applied the acetylcholinesterase technique to human peripheral nerves in a clinical situation of nerve repair. Further clinical and experimental studies were reported by Freilinger and associates (1975), and since 1979, these authors have applied the method in humans for nerve injuries at the wrist (Deutinger et al, 1993).

One of the major disadvantages that Gruber and co-workers (1973, 1976) identified in the 1970s was that the use of acetylcholinesterase histochemistry for clinical nerve repair required laboratory processing that took 24 to 36 hours. This led to a two-stage approach to the nerve repair. Yunshao and Shizhen (1988) have reported that histochemical acetylcho-

linesterase identification in human peripheral nerves during operative nerve repair can take as little as 1 hour. However, in another report, Deutinger and associates (1993) have stressed that it takes 4 hours of incubation of sectioned nerve tissue to accurately stain motor fascicles and fascicular groups.

Surgical Technique

Most investigators using histochemistry as an aid to nerve repair obtain cross-sectional proximal and distal debridement trimmings 2 to 4 mm in thickness as a biopsy (Lang et al, 1991). In order to avoid scar, these biopsies must be obtained after excision of the proximal neuroma and distal glioma. It is also important to recognize that, in both the proximal and distal segments before the debridement samples are resected, marking sutures should be placed epineurally for orientation. The sample is then taken to the laboratory and the histochemical staining performed. After motor fascicles or fascicular groups are identified by deposits of acetylcholinesterase, a photomicrograph is obtained and the motor portions identified (Fig. 24–3). This photomicrograph is essentially a map of the internal topography of the proximal and distal stump, which is reviewed by the microsurgeon in the operating room before realignment.

An extremely serious problem with the histochemical use of acetylcholinesterase is that the staining in the distal portion of the nerve decreases with time. This is due to the fact that the distal stump undergoes wallerian degeneration. Therefore, the reliability of this technique is probably limited to the first 7 to 10 days after injury (Lang et al, 1991). In contrast, it has been reported (Lang et al, 1991) that the proximal nerve stump staining persists and may actually increase with time, probably due to the axoplasmic transport of the enzyme from the cell body.

CHOLINE ACETYLTRANSFERASE ASSAY

Ganel and colleagues (1980, 1982) have also reported on the use of choline acetyltransferase nerve identification in

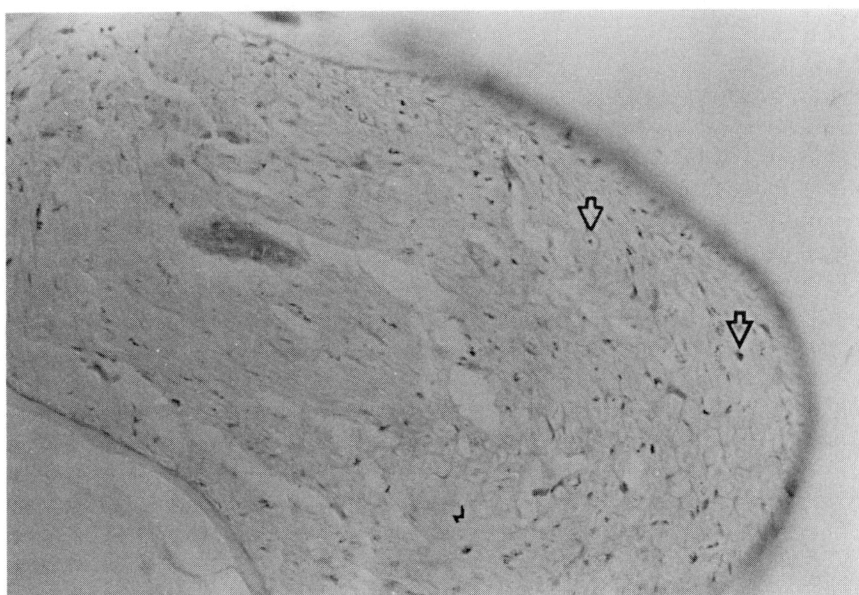

FIGURE 24–3. Photomicrograph of a rat peroneal nerve 5 mm distal to a nerve repair site, 28 days after repair, acetylcholinesterase histochemistry. The black deposits *(arrows)* represent intra-axonal acetylcholinesterase staining within myelinated motor axons. × 315.

early and late nerve repair. Choline acetyltransferase is an additional enzyme that has an activity that is greater in motor axons than in sensory axons. This enzyme was described in the early 1940s by Nachmansohn and Machado (1943) and is found in all cholinergic axons. The use of radiochemical assays was developed by Engel and co-workers (1980), who demonstrated fairly rapid nerve fascicle identification of homogenized fresh cadaver nerve samples. It has been reported that the assay must be performed within 96 hours of injury due to the fairly rapid decrease with time of this enzyme activity in the distal nerve stumps (Lang et al, 1991). The time to perform the assay is between 2 to 4 hours. According to Engel and associates (1970) and Lang and colleagues (1991), debridement trimmings from the proximal and distal nerve trunks are transferred to separate wells of a microtiter plate and kept moist with Ringer's buffer. Fascicles are dried and cut into 3.5- to 5-mg slices. Weights are recorded, the tissue is buffered, and the radioactive substrate reagent is added (tritiated acetylcholine). After the reaction is terminated, an average count per minute of the samples is recorded and corrected for fascicle weight. This data, consisting of each sample's identification number, counts per minute, corrected counts per minute, fascicle slice weight, and corrected counts per milligram nerve, is then provided to the surgeon. Using this technique, Lang et al (1991), reported that motor nerve fascicle choline acetyltransferase activity is usually greater than 350 counts per minute per milligram of nerve, whereas the sensory nerve fascicle activity was usually less than 80 counts per minute per milligram of nerve.

CARBONIC ANHYDRASE HISTOCHEMISTRY FOR DIFFERENTIATION OF SENSORY AXONS

Carbonic anhydrase is a ubiquitous enzyme that occurs in three forms (Holmes, 1977; Jeffrey and Carter, 1980; Register et al, 1978; Tashian et al, 1980). This enzyme has been purported to be useful in differentiating sensory axons of peripheral nerves. As Carson and Terzis (1985) have stated, carbonic anhydrase occurs in bacteria, plant, and animal tissue. The enzyme catalyzes the hydration of carbon dioxide and the dehydration of bicarbonate ions, and in general is found at sites of gas exchange and ion transport across membranes. In a review article, these authors have further reported that in mammals, significant carbonic anhydrase activity has been found in many tissues including the colon, erythrocytes, salivary glands, gastric mucosa, pancreas, liver, intestine, kidney, sweat glands, endometrium, and nervous system. The exact role for carbonic anhydrase has been suggested to be in the metabolism of acid-secreting cells, bicarbonate transport, sodium and chloride transport, carbon dioxide metabolism, and potassium transport.

In tissues, histochemical staining for carbonic anhydrase depends on the loss of carbon dioxide from the surface of frozen sections. Riley and associates (1981) showed that carbonic anhydrase histochemistry could be used to differentiate between large myelinated dorsal root and ventral root axons in the rat model. Their results demonstrated the complex distribution of carbonic anhydrase isoenzymes in the neuromuscular system and pointed out that carbonic anhydrase isoenzyme content depended on both the type of tissue as well as age and sex in the rat model. Subsequently, Riley and Lang (1984), as well as Carson and Terzis (1985), proposed that carbonic anhydrase histochemistry could be used clinically as an aid to nerve repair in humans. The surgical technique used to mark proximal and distal debridement trimmings with subsequent laboratory procedures for carbonic anhydrase and a resultant photomicrograph (Fig. 24–4) is similar to that already described for acetylcholinesterase histochemistry.

A disadvantage to the use of carbonic anhydrase histochemistry in nerve repair is the fact that some motor ventral root axons may also be stained using this technique. Also, as in acetylcholinesterase histochemistry, time after nerve injury is a factor for the use of carbonic anhydrase. For example, it has been reported in a human ulnar nerve that carbonic anhydrase activity persisted for only 24 hours in

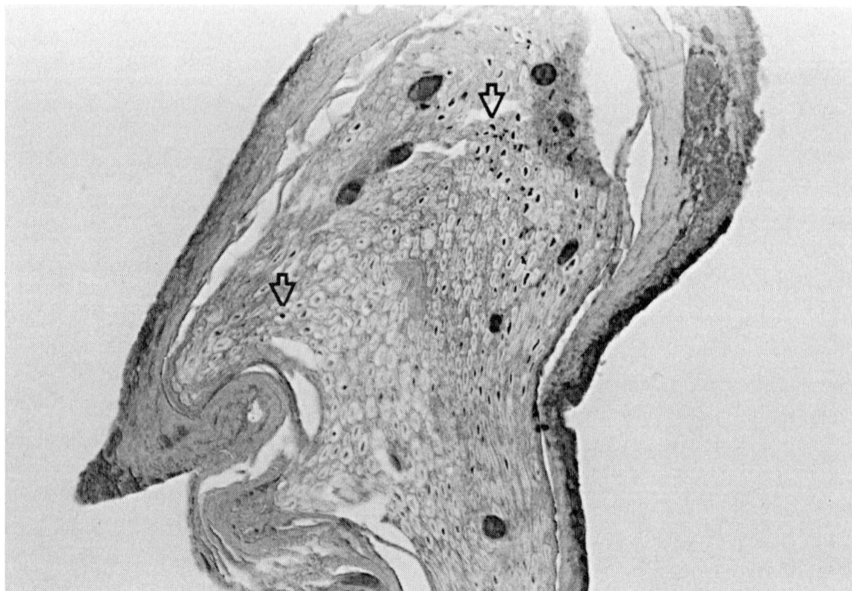

FIGURE 24–4. Photomicrograph of a rat peroneal nerve 5 mm distal to a nerve repair site, 28 days after repair, carbonic anhydrase histochemistry. The black desposits *(arrows)* represent intra-axonal carbonic anhydrase staining within myelinated sensory axons. × 315.

the distal stump, whereas activities were increased in the proximal nerve stumps (Riley and Lang, 1984).

Although numerous authors have reported on the potential use of carbonic anhydrase as a histochemical aid to peripheral nerve repair in humans, none has published a definitive article or series using this method. A very recent report by Deutinger and colleagues (1993) used acetylcholinesterase histochemistry only as an intraoperative aid to median and ulnar nerve repair in humans.

Additional techniques for the identification of sensory and motor axons have been reported in a rabbit animal model using immunohistochemical methods (Xiao-Song, 1990). A monoclonal antibody was prepared by fusing SP2/0 myeloma cells with splenic cells from mice. This antibody is purportedly specific for sensory axons only, with the entire course of the immunostaining requiring 50 minutes. However, to date, this technique has not been applied to nerve repair in humans. Although it is only speculation, the localization of nitric oxide synthase, an enzyme involved in synthesis of nitric oxide, may conceivably be applied to the differentiation of motor and sensory axons for nerve repair. There have been no studies published on the clinical use of nitric oxide synthase in nerve repair. However, it has been reported by Yu (1994) that after transection of peripheral nerve in an animal model, nitric oxide synthase expression was significantly up regulated in sensory ganglion cells, whereas in motor neurons, nitric oxide synthase was not present unless axon regeneration was prevented and cell death became massive.

In summary, many authors have shown that use of histochemical staining to differentiate motor and sensory fascicles and fascicular groups as an intraoperative aid in human peripheral nerve repair is technically feasible. However, the use of these histochemical techniques has not been used routinely because they increase intraoperative time and may require specialized training for accurate interpretation of laboratory results for selective reanastomosis. Future studies are required in large numbers of patients in whom histochemical aids are used to determine whether the added

intraoperative time is justified on the basis of improved return of motor and sensory function.

References

Adams CW, Grant RT, Bayliss B: Cholinesterases in nervous system. I. Mixed, motor and sensory trunks. Brain Res 5:366–376, 1967.

Atwood H, MacKay W: Essentials of neurophysiology. Philadelphia, BC Decker 1989, pp 1–64.

Baljet B, Drukker J: An acetylcholinesterase method for in toto staining of peripheral nerves. Stain Technol 50:1, 1975.

Bradford H: Chemical neurobiology: An introduction to neurochemistry. New York, WH Freeman, 1986, pp 1–495.

Carson KA, Terzis JK: Carbonic anhydrase histochemistry: A potential diagnostic method for peripheral nerve repair. Clin Plast Surg 12(2):227–232, 1985.

Deutinger M, Girsch W, Burggasser G, et al: Clinical and electroneurographic evaluation of sensory/motor-differentiated nerve repair in the hand. J Neurosurg 78:709–713, 1993.

Engel J, Ganel A, Melamed S, et al: Choline acetyltransferase for differentiation between human motor and sensory nerve fibers. Ann Plast Surg 4:5, 1980.

Freilinger G, Gruber H, Holle J, et al: Zur methodik der "sensomotorisch" differenzierten faszikel-naht peripherer nerven. Handchirurgie 7:133–137, 1975.

Ganel A, Engel J, Luboshitz S, et al: Choline acetyltransferase nerve identification method in early and late nerve repair. Ann Plast Surg 4:228–230, 1980.

Ganel A, Farine I, Aharonson Z, et al: Intraoperative nerve fascicle identification using choline acetyltransferase: A preliminary report. Clin Orthop 165:228–232, 1982.

Gruber H, Freilinger G, Holle J, et al: Identification of motor and sensory funiculi in cut nerves and their selective reunion. Br J Plast Surg 29:70, 1976.

Gruber H, Zenker W: Acetylcholinesterase: Histochemical differentiation between motor and sensory fibers. Brain Res 51:207–214, 1973.

Hammerschlag R, Brady S: Axonal transport and the neuronal cytoskeleton. In Siegel G, Agranoff B, Albers R, Molinoff P (eds): Basic Neurochemistry. New York, Raven Press, 1989, pp 457–478.

Hammerschlag R, Stone G: Prelude to fast axonal transport: Sequence of events in the cell body. In Iqbal Z (ed): Axoplasmic transport. Boca Raton, FL, CRC Press, 1986, pp 21–34.

Hebb C: Formation, storage and liberation of acetylcholine. In Handbuch der Experimentellen Pharmakoligie. Berlin, Springer, 1963, pp 56–88.

Holmes RS: Purification, molecular properties and ontogeny of carbonic anhydrase isozymes. Evidence for A, B and C isozymes in avian and mammalian tissues. Eur J Biochem 78:511, 1977.

Jabaley ME: Internal topography of peripheral nerves as related to repair. *In* Gelberman RH (ed): Operative Nerve Repair and Reconstruction. Philadelphia, J.B. Lippincott Company, 1991, pp 231–240.

Jeffrey S, Carter N: A comparison of carbonic anhydrase III isozymes from human, baboon, pig and sheep muscle. Comp Biochem Physiol (B) 66:439, 1980.

Karnovsky MJ, Roots CA: A "direct coloring" thiocholine method for cholinesterases. J Histochem Cytochem 12:219–221, 1964.

Kasa P, Rakonczay Z: Histochemical and biochemical demonstration of the molecular forms of acetylcholinesterase in peripheral nerve of rat. Acta Histochem 70:244–257, 1982.

Koelle GB, Freidenweld JS: A histochemical method for localizing cholinesterase activity. Proc Soc Exp Biol Med 70:617–622, 1949.

Lang DH, Lister GD, Jevans AW: Histochemical and biochemical aids to nerve repair. *In* Gelberman RH (ed): Operative nerve repair and reconstruction. Philadelphia, J.B. Lippincott Company, 1991, pp 259–270.

Lasek R, Garner J, Brady S: Axonal transport of the cytoplasmic matrix. J Cell Biol 99:212–221, 1984.

Lubinska L, Niemierko S, Oderfeld B, et al: The distribution of cholinesterase in peripheral nerves. J Neurochem 10:25–41, 1963.

Nachmansohn D, Machado AL: The formation of acetylcholine. A new enzyme "choline acetylase" J Neurophysiol 6:397–404, 1943.

Noback C, Demarest R: The Human Nervous System: Basic Principles of Neurobiology, 3rd ed. New York, McGraw-Hill, 1981, pp 49–123.

Ochs S: A brief history on present status of transport mechanism models. *In* Smith R, Bisby M (eds): Axonal Transport. New York, Alan R Liss, 1987, pp 1–14.

Register AM, Koester MK, Noltmann EA: Discovery of carbonic anhydrase in rabbit skeletal muscle and evidence for its identity with basic muscle protein. J Biol Chem 253:4143, 1978.

Riley DA, Ellis S, Bain J: Carbonic anhydrase histochemistry reveals subpopulations of myelinated axons in the dorsal and ventral roots of rat spinal nerves. Soc Neurosci Abst, 7:257, 1981.

Riley DA, Lang DH: Carbonic anhydrase activity of human peripheral nerves: A possible histochemical aid to nerve repair. J Hand Surg 9A(1):112–120, 1984.

Sheetz M, Steuer E, Schroer T: The mechanism and regulation of fast axonal transport. Trends Neurosci 12:474–478, 1989.

Sunderland S: The anatomic basis of nerve repair. *In* Jewett DL, McCarroll HR (eds): Nerve Repair and Regeneration. St. Louis, CV Mosby, 1980, pp 35–50.

Tashian RE, Hewett-Emmett D, Stroup SK, et al: Evolution of structure and function in the carbonic anhydrase isozymes of mammals. *In* Bauer C, Gross G, Bartels H (eds): Biophysics and Physiology of Carbon Dioxide. Berlin, Springer-Verlag, 1980, pp 176–176.

Xiao-Song G: The identification of sensory and motor nerve fibers by an immunohistochemical method. Am Soc Reconstr Microsurg 6th Annual Meeting, Toronto, 1990; p 74.

Yu WH: Nitric oxide synthase in motor neurons after axotomy. J Histochem and Cyotochem 42(4):451–457, 1994.

Yunshao H, Shizhen Z: Acetylcholinesterase: A histochemical identification of motor and sensory fascicles in human peripheral nerves and its use during operation. Plast Reconstr Surg 82:125–132, 1988.

Part V

SUTURE TECHNIQUES

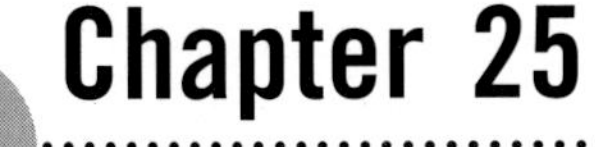

Chapter 25

• Allen L. Van Beek

Intraoperative Nerve Stimulation and Recording Techniques

There is a long, well-documented history associated with evaluating the nature, level, and severity of peripheral nerve injuries. The history of civilian nerve injuries is punctuated by the great wars and the casualties that inevitably followed. World War II, the Korean War, and the Viet Nam War all produced large numbers of peripheral nerve injuries. Both civilian and military injuries resulted in techniques that permitted systematic clinical evaluation and documentation of injuries preoperatively and postoperatively (Bristow, 1947; Gelberman, 1991; MacKinnon and Dellon, 1988; Omer, 1974; Posch and Cruz-Saddul, 1980; Sakellarides, 1962; Seddon, 1975; Sunderland, 1951). The time-tested systems for the clinical evaluation of peripheral nerve injuries must be thorough, chronological, and documented. However, the advent of electrical recording of nerve action potential (Dimitrijevic et al, 1978; Gaul 1986; Hakstain, 1968; Jones, 1979; Kline, 1968; Kline and Hackett, 1970; Lehman and Calloway, 1979; Terzis et al, 1976; Williams and Terzis, 1976) and the use of computer chip technology (Aminoff, 1980; Giblin, 1964; Hallin et al, 1981; Morrison and Morrison, 1961; Van Beek et al, 1983) have changed the systems of evaluation and will change the grading of nerve injuries in the future. Since their development in the 1980s, computer-assisted nerve conduction studies, computer-assisted physical evaluations of strength and dexterity, computer-assisted assessment of sensibility, central nervous system–evoked electrical potential studies, electronic scanning techniques, magnetic scanning techniques, and spectrographic scanning techniques (Fahr, 1988) are going to dramatically change our systems of evaluation and understanding of peripheral nerve problems, including pain. It is astonishing to think that the clinical methods for nerve repair have not changed dramatically during this period of time.

This chapter discusses the techniques associated with using nerve stimulating and recording techniques in the operating room. These techniques are becoming necessary for elaborate methods of reconstruction after nerve injuries and in some circumstances are essential for accurate assessment of some nerve injuries.

ELECTROPHYSIOLOGIC ASSESSMENTS

Hakstain in 1968 used a nerve stimulator to evaluate the fascicular topography of the proximal end of peripheral nerves. He then found the corresponding distal innervation by direct dissection. Kline (1982) popularized the technique of assessing nerve-evoked responses by directly recording evoked responses from the surface of the nerve. Terzis (1976) confirmed the ability to use intraoperative nerve stimulation and recording techniques for the evaluation of nerves intraoperatively. In 1974, Matthews and associates demonstrated that cervical somatosensory responses could be recorded. In 1980, Yamada and colleagues demonstrated that evoked responses could be reliably recorded from the median nerve. Van Beek in 1983 and 1986 reported on the clinical use of intraoperative nerve conduction studies using the signal-averaging computer to eliminate some of the technical problems associated with nerve conduction studies on peripheral nerves in the operating room. Intraoperative use of recording evoked responses from the brain stem, spinal cord, brachial plexus, or brain is now a routine part of many surgical procedures (Baines et al, 1985; Calder et al, 1994; Jones, 1979; Nelson, 1988; Sloan and Koht, 1985; Stone et al, 1985; Sugioka, 1984; Yiannikas, 1983).

It must be emphasized that the information obtained from the intraoperative evaluation of nerves must be preceded by an accurate clinical assessment of the nerve. The cognitive ability of the brain to interpret incoming data varies remarkably between individuals, and this ability can be assessed only with the patient awake and the physician carefully examining the status of the nerve and the patient connected to the nerve injury.

PRINCIPLES

The details of nerve physiology are discussed in Chapter 37. However, some of the principles (Sumner, 1980; Starr, 1976) associated with intraoperative conduction studies are particularly important and should be emphasized.

Nerve conduction velocity is directly related to body temperature, myelin thickness, and internode distance (Alberts, 1989; Berne, 1983; Dorfman et al, 1981). Aging slows nerve conduction velocity, but this is related to internode and myelin changes (Aminoff, 1980). If during general anesthesia the patient's core temperature decreases or because of surgical exposure the extremity temperature decreases, the nerve conduction velocity will decrease. Because of these factors, the surgeon using intraoperative conduction studies must have a built-in control to eliminate some of these variables. The best control, when possible, is the nerve proximal to the nerve lesion being explored. Using direct recording from the surface of a nerve is difficult because of electrical interference from other equipment in the operating room. The stimulator stimulus artifact wave may further complicate the recording by obscuring the initial phase of the nerve's evoked response curve and the changes in neurophysiology induced by nerve dissection. Use of the tourniquet may alter the normal waveform.

The magnitude of an evoked response being conducted along a peripheral nerve is directly related to the number of fibers and the diameter of the fibers that are transmitting the pulse. When testing a nerve intraoperatively, a sufficient stimulus is given to the nerve to assume all the nerves are transmitting the information along the nerve. To create this circumstance, a supramaximal electrical stimulus is used to elicit the evoked response (Fig. 25–1). The evoked response is transmitted simultaneously along nerve fibers toward the central nervous system and toward the digits. When recorded from the surface of the nerve, magnitudes of evoked responses in the millivolt range are detected. Amplification of the recorded responses makes display and analysis possible on cathode ray tubes or recording devices.

When recording a nerve's evoked response with a signal-averaging computer to assist recording, the evoked response is recorded from the surface of the skin directly over the nerve being studied (Fig. 25–2). Because of the distance between the recording electrode on the skin and the underlying nerve, impedance in the structures and tissues makes the evoked response amplitude very small. The recorded response is in the range of 0.5 to 10 μv, which could not be seen or recorded using the usual recording techniques (Cracco, 1973). The signal-averaging computer improves the recording process and permits the signal to be visualized and recorded. Using this technique, hundreds of evoked responses are recorded along with the accompanying electrical noise and then summed by the computer. This technique accentuates repeated events, and random electrical noise that would otherwise mask this response is removed in the process of summing the responses (Fig. 25–3). The signal-averaging equipment used for nerve action potential from the skin surface is widely available and is usually found in neurology or electroenceophalography laboratories.

EQUIPMENT AND PREPARATION

The equipment used for direct nerve stimulation consists of a nerve stimulator, stimulus isolation unit, and stimulation electrodes (Fig. 25–4). The stimulation electrodes can be unipolar or bipolar. When using unipolar electrodes, the electrons flow from the tip of the anode to the grounding cathode. The field of electron flow induced using monopolar electrodes may stimulate adjacent nerve tissue to a greater

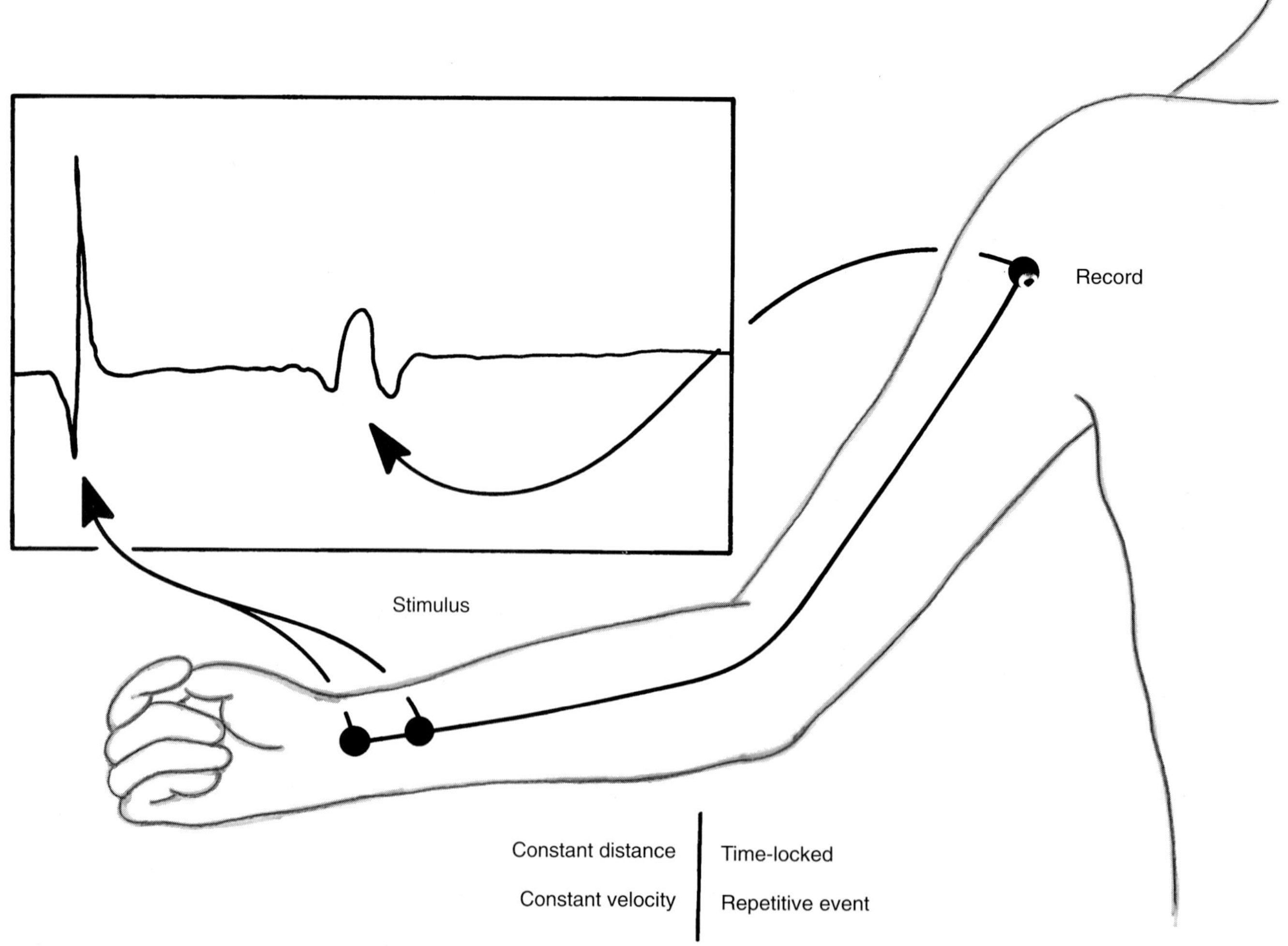

FIGURE 25–1. Stimulation of the nerve fiber with evoked depolarization.

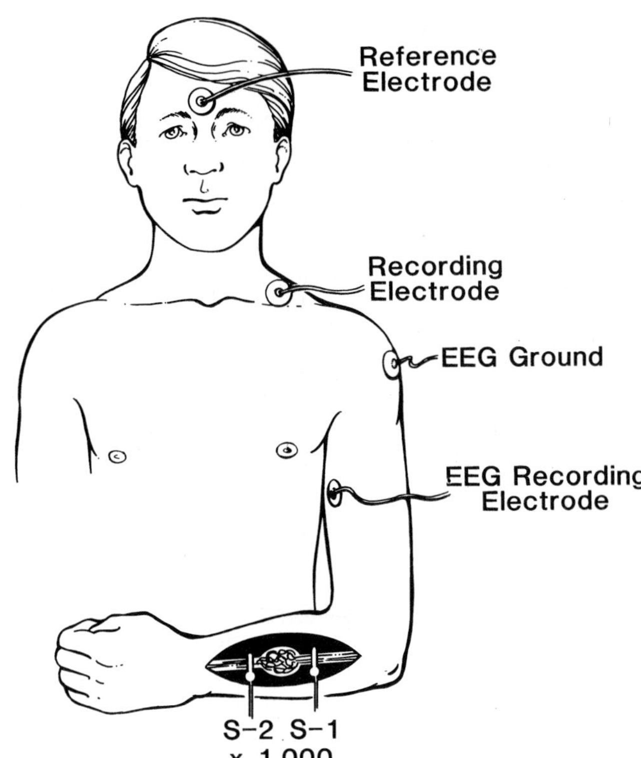

FIGURE 25–2. Peripheral nerve–evoked responses can be obtained using cutaneous electrodes at a remote site along the nerve course.

degree than bipolar electrodes. Bipolar electrodes have a more defined field of electron flow between the closely positioned anode and cathode. The size of the bipolar electrodes can be very small and the distance between them only a millimeter. This permits stimulation of even single fascicles of a nerve. In practice, because of availability and disposability, the monopolar disposable electrode is the most widely used nerve stimulator.

When stimulating the nerve and then recording an evoked response, the complexity of technology increases. To record the evoked response either from the surface of the nerve or at a remote site requires amplification of the evoked response by thousands or hundreds of thousands. The recording electrodes detect the passing of the potential difference associated with the nerve fibers' depolarization wave underneath the electrode. The response is then amplified by the preamplifier of the recording device. The display device will then again amplify the signal to permit visualization on a cathode ray tube or recording device. The preamplifier also has to process the signal to eliminate electrical noise. The preamplifier will have a low-filter and high-filter system. Filtering permits electrical noise waveforms with lower or

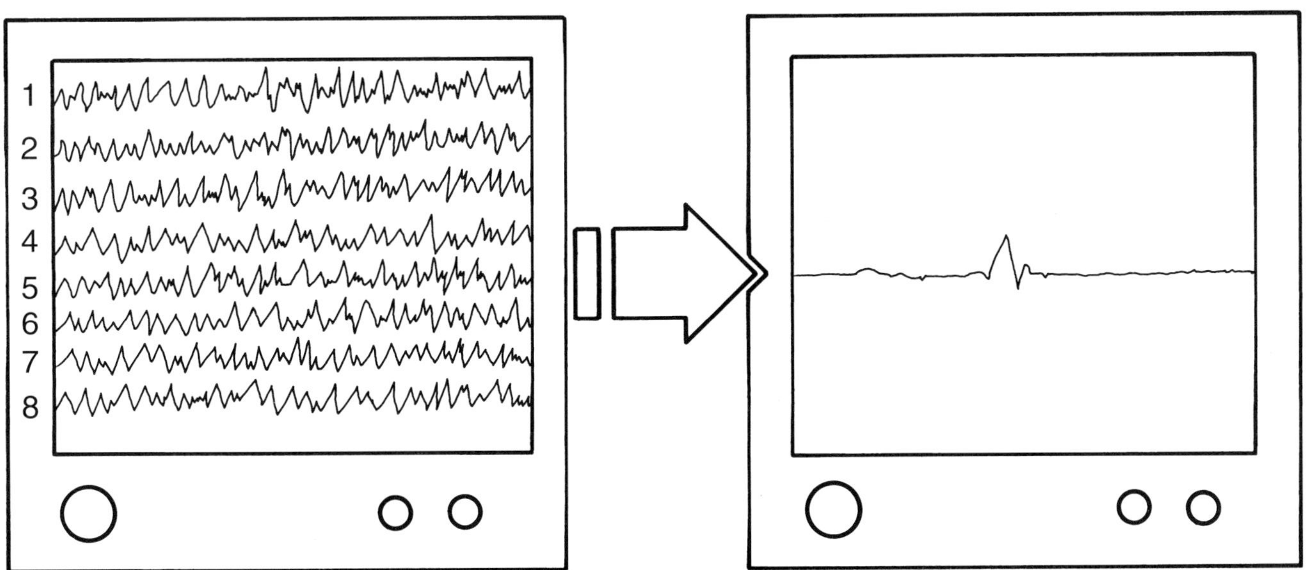

FIGURE 25–3. The computer microprocessor sums the repetitive response, but summation of noise cancels those random electrical activities.

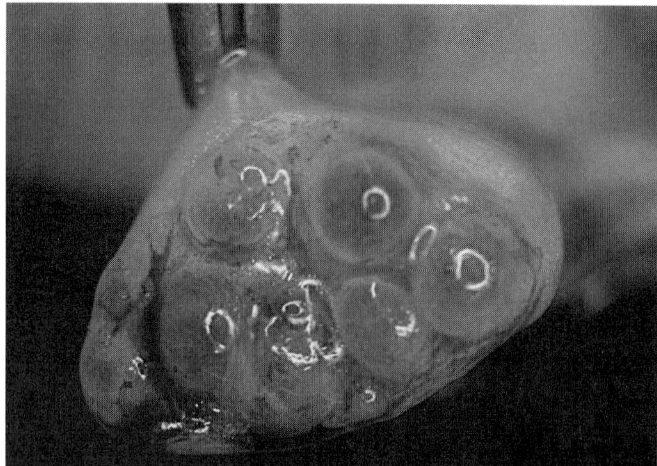

FIGURE 25–7. Proximal nerve stump stimulation for topographical mapping. Distal alignment is possible by dissection only after wallerian degeneration is complete.

distance from the stimulation to the recording electrode is more than 25 cm.

CLINICAL TECHNIQUES

Nerve Stimulation

Nerve stimulation is the most widely used and easiest of electrical techniques for analyzing nerve function. Nerve stimulators can be disposable or fixed hardware. They are used for nerve localization in the nonparalyzed patient, for motor fascicle identification during free muscle transfers (Harii, 1979; Manktelow and McKee, 1978; Van Beek et al, 1986), and, to a lesser extent, for sensory fascicle identification when aligning nerve repairs during secondary nerve reconstruction (Gaul, 1986; Hakstain, 1968; Jabaley et al, 1980; Van Beek, 1986; VanDePut et al, 1969).

Sensory Fascicle Stimulation

Sensory fascicle stimulation is an important adjunct for the surgeon when the topography of the nerve has been altered by previous surgery or is difficult because of a long segmental loss of nerve structure. The location of the injury is extremely important. When attempting to accurately restore nerve alignment, unless the surgeon reliably knows the distal orientation of the fascicles by dissection or nerve appearance, it will be of little help to understand the proximal topography. Assuming the distal topography can be determined by dissection or topography maps (Chow et al, 1986; Jabaley et al, 1980; Sunderland, 1978), the proximal topography can be determined by awake stimulation of the fascicles of the proximal nerve stump. Using this technique, the patient tells the surgeon where sensation is perceived when stimulating various fascicles. This can then guide the alignment with the distal fascicles. The patient's nerve problem can usually be exposed using intravenous regional anesthesia. Once the nerve is exposed and determination made that the injured segment needs to be resected, the area is resected, local anesthetic is injected into only skin, and the block is reversed. Approximately 20 minutes after reversing the block, reliable stimulation of the proximal nerve stump can begin. To obtain the patient's trust and cooperation, start with low stimulation intensity and increase slowly as tolerated by the patient. Use only an intensity needed to obtain a repeatable response. A stimulation rate of 3 Hz will be perceived as a tapping sensation in a very specific location if bipolar electrodes are used. If a fascicle does not elicit a definite strong response, it is probably a motor fascicle. For these types of stimulation techniques, disposable stimulators are disadvantageous because they are too rapid, lack sufficient stimulus variability, and the monopolar configuration may not be specific enough for small fascicles. There are many available nerve stimulators available for the surgeon. Unfortunately, the availability of electrodes of suitable size is still a problem. An easy solution to this problem is to use two needle electroencephalogram (EEG) electrodes to create a very small bipolar stimulating electrode. The sharpened, very small needles make excellent electrodes for single fascicle stimulations (Fig. 25–8).

Once the fascicle pattern is determined, the patient is provided a general anesthetic and the nerve repairs are completed. Remember: It is necessary to determine the distal topography by direct dissection of the nerve or by using well established patterns of topography.

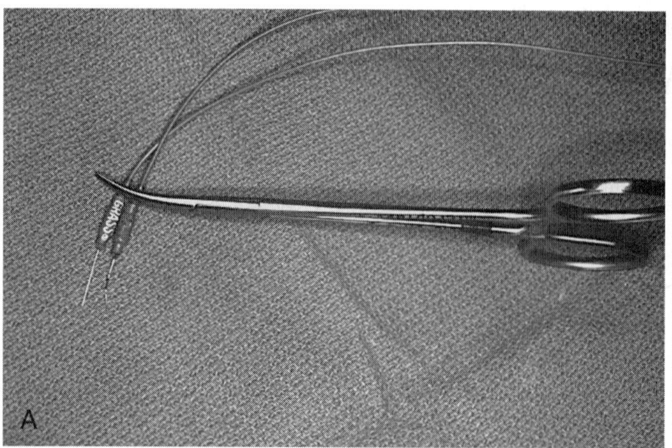
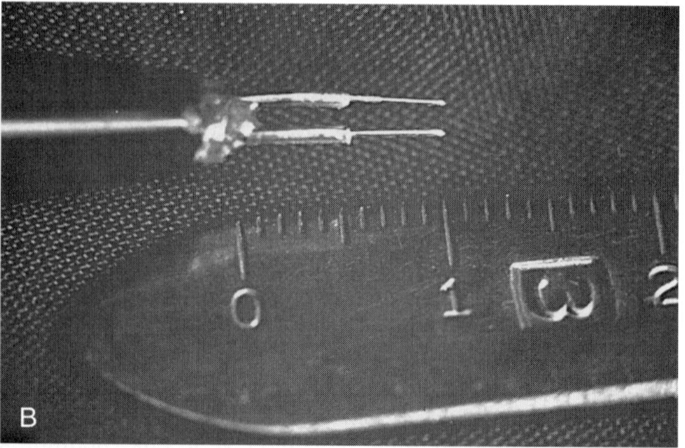

FIGURE 25–8. Small stimulating electrodes are essential for fascicle studies. Custom electrodes *(A)* or EEG electrodes *(B)* are options available when very small electrodes are required for single fascicle stimulation.

MOTOR FASCICLE TERRITORIES

Motor fascicles have distinct areas of innervation within muscles (Van Beek, 1983). This information is important when harvesting portions of muscle for reanimation procedures for the face or when splitting a single free muscle transfer when it may be advantageous to have two functions provided by the muscle.

Motor fascicle stimulation can occur when the muscles are not paralyzed. Single fascicles, or in some circumstances, groups of fascicles, are stimulated and the area of the muscle that is dominantly contracting, which is the major area of distribution of the fascicle, is noted. Small bipolar stimulating electrodes are used for stimulating the nerves (see Fig. 25–8).

The gracilis and latissimus dorsi muscles can be divided into segments of innervated muscle. The gracilis muscle can be split into two separate linear segments of contracting muscle (Fig. 25–9). If differentially innervated by two different motor nerve branches, these two segments of muscle can provide separate function. Motor fascicle stimulation is accomplished while both origin and insertion of the muscle are still intact. The initial stimulation using a twitch-inducing stimulus must be of sufficient strength to induce a strong response. The twitch response is not an effective way to determine the territory of a fascicle, but it does establish the stimulus parameter that will induce a motor response. Once the parameters are set, a tetanus-inducing frequency is used.

This can be accomplished by 30 to 60 Hz stimulations. By adjusting the frequency, it is possible to see the cleavage planes of different fascicles' motor distributions within a muscle (see Fig. 25–9). If supra-maximal stimulation or large stimulating electrodes are used, it will not be possible to reliably stimulate small fascicles. If the origin or insertion is taken down, the mechanical contraction of the muscle will interfere with continuous contact between the electrodes and the nerve; it may also obscure the area of muscle most dominantly contracting. Linear separation of fascicle groups will also help to separate function. Two keys to successful stimulation of motor fascicles are using the minimal twitch-inducing stimulus and then increasing to a tetanus-producing stimulus frequency. The stimulus duration should be kept at 0.1 msec, and the tetanus-inducing frequency should be altered to give the most indicative muscle contraction.

STIMULATION AND RECORDING STUDIES

Stimulation and recording studies for abnormal segments of peripheral nerves are most applicable when a nerve injury is being explored early and distal innervation could not have occurred (Kline, 1968; Van Beek, 1986). This makes reliable clinical assessment of recovery by reinnervation difficult. Exploration of a nerve and discovery of a neuroma incontinuity complicate judgment, and if there is some nerve function across the neuroma, decision-making becomes even

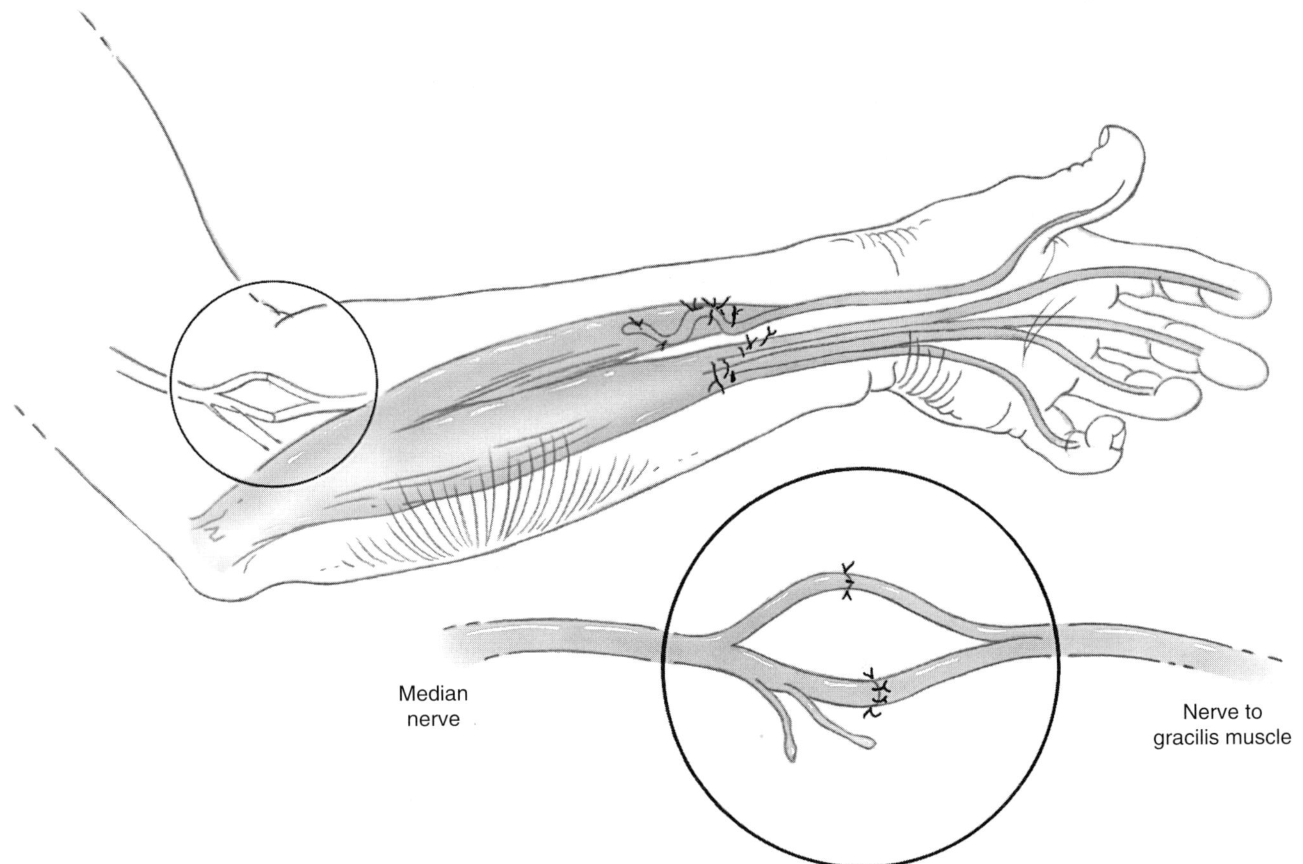

FIGURE 25–9. Motor fascicle territory determination by differential fascicle stimulation with twitch- or tetany-producing stimuli is helpful in some skeletal muscle animation procedures.

more difficult. The observed clinical or electrical function could be through uninjured areas of the nerve or possibly even from early regeneration across the injured areas of the nerve. Partially transected nerves can sometimes be detected and, by careful microscopic dissection, separated from injured nerve, but partial reinnervation across a repair site often makes the decision between neurolysis and resection and grafting difficult to make. In these circumstances, the availability of additional data may be essential and certainly reassuring to the surgeon. When stimulating and recording across a neuroma incontinuity, the previous principles must be applied, and additional clinical factors will make the task of electrical recording easier. While surgical preparations are being made, insert EEG electrodes to Erb's point or the apex of the axilla and the midline of the forehead. Secure the electrodes with tape. Explore the nerve with the tourniquet elevated, but after dissection and release of the tourniquet, wait 20 minutes before beginning recordings. Record the nerves' evoked response by stimulating proximal to the injury and recording at Erb's point or the axilla (see Fig. 25–3). Once the normal evoked response is seen and recorded, repeat the study a second time. If the waves are congruent, a reliable study has been completed. Repeat the studies by stimulating on the distal side of the neuroma. The evoked response may not be present. It may have a smaller amplitude or demonstrate a marked slowing in conduction velocity across the injury site. In circumstances in which the velocity is not slowed and the amplitude is diminished, be suspicious of a partial injury to the cross section of the nerve. Ensure that there is at least 2 cm of nerve exposed proximally and distally to the neuroma to improve the quality of the study. Ensure that accurate marking of sites of stimulation on each side of the neuroma occurs and that the distance between the two stimulating sites is known. This information will permit accurate calculation of the conduction velocity across the neuroma. If the previously listed parameters are not met and the clinical assessment supports the decision, the nerve segment being studied should be removed and the nerve repaired directly or by using grafts.

In some institutions, neurologists or technicians are available to assist the surgeon in the operating room. However, if one is working with complex nerve problems, understanding how to set up and run the equipment will be most helpful to everyone. Performing somatosensory-evoked response testing on oneself and spending time in the neurology laboratory to gain confidence with how the equipment is set up and used are recommended.

The surgeon today must use today's technology to help solve some of the difficult peripheral nerve problems encountered in the operating theater.* Without the use of technology, one is like a pilot with a compass but without an altimeter, radio, and radar.

References

Alberts B, Bray D, Lewis J, Raff M, Roberts K, Watson JD: Molecular Biology of the Cell. New York, Garland, Inc., 1989.

---

*Some companies that provide the equipment for performing these studies include Grass Electronics (nerve stimulator, stimulus isolation unit, EEG needle electrodes, NER equipment), Nicolet (NER equipment, electrodes), TECA (NER equipment, electrodes).

Aminoff MJ: Electrodiagnosis in Clinical Neurology. New York, Churchill Livingstone, 1980.

Baines DB, Whittle IR, Chaseling RW, et al: Effect of halothane on spinal somatosensory evoked potentials in sheep. Br J Anaesth 57:896–899, 1985.

Berne RM, Levy MN: Physiology. St. Louis, Mosby, 1983.

Bristow WR: Injuries of peripheral nerves in two World Wars. Br J Surg 34:333, 1947.

Calder HB, Mast J, Johnstone C: Intraoperative evoked potential monitoring in acetabular surgery. Clin Orthop 305:160–167, 1994.

Chow JA, Van Beek AL, Bilos ZJ, Meyer DL, Johnson MC: Anatomical basis for repair of ulnar and median nerves in the distal part of the forearm by group fascicular suture and nerve grafting. J Bone Joint Surg 68A:273–280, 1986.

Cracco RQ: Spinal evoked response: Peripheral nerve stimulation in man. Electroencephalogr Clin Neurophysiol 35:379, 1973.

Dimitrijevic MR, Larsson LE, Lehmkuhl D, Sherwood A: Evoked spinal cord and nerve root potentials in humans using a non-invasive recording technique. Electroencephalogr Clin Neurophysiol 45:331, 1978.

Dorfman LJ, Cummins KL, Leifer LJ: Conduction velocity distributions: A population approach to electrophysiology of nerve. New York, Alan R. Liss, 1981.

Emerson RG, Seyal M, Pedney TA: Somatosensory evoked potentials following median nerve stimulation: The cervical components. Brain 107:169–182, 1984.

Gaul JS Jr: Electrical fascicle identification as an adjunct to nerve repair. 2:709–722, 1986.

Gelberman RH: Operative Nerve Repair and Reconstruction. Philadelphia, JB Lippincott, 1991.

Giblin DR: Somatosensory evoked potentials in healthy subjects and in patients with lesions of the nervous system. Ann NY Acad Sci 112:93–142, 1964.

Hallin RG, Wiesenfield Z, Lungnegard H: Neurophysiological studies of peripheral nerve functions after neural regeneration following nerve suture in man. Int Rehabil Med 3:187–192, 1981.

Harii K: Microneurovascular free muscle transplantation for reanimation of facial paralysis. Clin Plast Surg 6:361, 1979.

Jabaley ME, Wallace WH, Heckler FR: Internal topography of major nerves of the forearm and hand: A current view. J Hand Surg 5:1, 1980.

Jones SJ: Investigation of brachial plexus traction lesions by peripheral and spinal somatosensory evoked potentials. J Neurol Neurosurg Psychiatry 42:107, 1979.

Kline DG: Early evaluation of peripheral nerve lesions in continuity with a note on nerve recording. Am Surg 34:77, 1968.

Kline DG: Operative management of major nerve lesions of the lower extremity. Surg Clin North Am 52:1247, 1972.

Kline DG: Timing for exploration of nerve lesions and evaluation of the neuroma-in-continuity. Clin Orthop 163:42–49, 1982.

Kline DG, Hackett ER: Value of electrophysiologic tests for peripheral nerve neuromas. J Surg Oncol 2:299–310, 1970.

Lehman D, Calloway E: Human evoked potentials. In Desmedt JE (ed): Somatosensory Evoked Responses: Maturation, Cognitive Parameters, and Clinical Uses in Neurological Disorders. New York, Plenum, 1979.

MacKinnon SE, Dellon AL: Surgery of the Peripheral Nerve. New York, Thieme Medical Publishers, 1988.

Manktelow RT, McKee NH: Free muscle transplantation to provide active finger flexion. J Hand Surg 3:416, 1978.

Matthews WB, Blanchamp M, Small DG: Cervical somatosensory evoked responses in man. Nature 252:230, 1974.

Morrison P, Morrison E: Charles Babbage and His Calculating Engines. New York, Dover Publications, 1961.

Nelson KR: Use of peripheral nerve action potentials for intraoperative monitoring. Neurol Clin 6:917–933, 1988.

Omer GE: Injuries to nerves of the upper extremity. J Bone Joint Surg 56A:1615, 1974.

Omer GE, Spinner M: Management of Peripheral Nerve Problems. Philadelphia, WB Saunders, 1980.

Posch J, Cruz-Saddul F: Nerve repair in trauma surgery: A ten year study of 231 peripheral injuries. Orthop Rev 9:35–45, 1980.

Sakellarides H: A follow-up study of 172 peripheral nerve injuries in the upper extremity in civilians. J Bone Joint Surg 44A:140, 1962.

Seddon H: Surgical Disorders of the Peripheral Nerve. Edinburgh, Churchill Livingstone, 1975.

Sloan TB, Koht A: Depression of cortical somatosensory evoked potentials by nitrous oxide. Br J Anaesth *57*:849–852, 1985.

Starr A: Auditory brain-stem responses in brain death. Brain *99*:543, 1976.

Stone RG, Weeks LE, Hajdu M, Stinchfield FE: Evaluation of sciatic nerve compromise during total hip arthroplasty. *201*:26–31, 1985.

Sugioka H: Evoked potentials in the investigation of traumatic lesions of peripheral nerve and the brachial plexus. Clin Orthop *184*:85–92, 1984.

Sumner AJ: The Physiology of Peripheral Nerve Disease. Philadelphia, WB Saunders, 1980.

Sunderland S: A classification of peripheral nerve injuries producing loss of function. Brain *74*:491–515, 1951.

Sunderland S: Nerves and Nerve Injuries. Edinburgh, Churchill Livingstone, 1978.

Terzis JK, Dykes RW, Hakstain RW: Electrophysiologic recordings in peripheral nerve surgery: A review. J Hand Surg *1*:52–66, 1976.

Van Beek AL: Electrodiagnostic evaluation of peripheral nerve injuries. Hand Clin *2*:747–760, 1986.

Van Beek A, Hubble B, Kinkead L, et al: Clinical use of nerve stimulations and recording techniques. Plast Reconstr Surg *71*:225–238, 1983.

Van Beek AL, Massac E, Smith DO: The use of the signal averaging computer for evaluation of peripheral nerve problems. Clin Plast Surg *13*:407–419, 1986.

VanDePut J, Tanner JC, Huypens L: Electrophysiological orientation of the cut ends in primary peripheral nerve repair. Plast Reconstr Surg *44*:378, 1969.

Williams HB, Terzis JK: Single fascicular recordings: An intra-operative diagnostic tool for the management of peripheral nerve lesions. Plast Reconstr Surg *57*:562, 1976.

Yamada T, Kimura J, Nitz DM: Short latency somatosensory evoked potentials following median nerve stimulation in man. Electroencephalogr Clin Neurophysiol *48*:367, 1980.

Yiannikas C, Walsh JD: Somatosensory evoked responses in the diagnosis of thoracic outlet syndrome. J Neurol Neurosurg Psychiatry *46*:234–240, 1983.

• Allen L. Van Beek
• Miguel A. Pirela-Cruz

Chapter 26

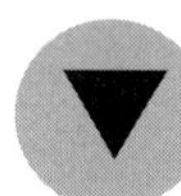

Microsurgical Nerve Repairs

The introduction of the surgical binocular microscope for ear and eye surgery in the 1920s by Nylen (1954) and Holmgren (1923) initiated an era when advances in surgical technique would parallel advances in technology. As technology improved, so did the surgeon's ability to manage difficult problems.

The history of nerve repairs is interesting and reflects the understanding regarding the nature of the peripheral nerve regeneration through various historic periods of time (Bunnell, 1928; Ramon y Cajal, 1959; Sanders, 1942; Seddon, 1947; Sunderland, 1968; Young and Medaware, 1940). Smith (1964) is credited for popularizing the use of the operating microscope for nerve repairs.

This chapter will illustrate the surgical techniques associated with the microscopic assessment, manipulation, and repair of peripheral nerves.

SETUP

The microscope is an invaluable asset for the surgical evaluation and repair of peripheral nerves. The enhanced visualization of the nerve permits accurate assessment of the injury, nerve anatomy and topography, vascularity, function, and ultimately suture placement (Fig. 26–1). Without microscopic visualization, these key features may not be perceived or may even be misjudged.

When setting up the microscope for a nerve repair, several factors are essential. The following guidelines will make the task of microneurorrhaphy easier (O'Brien et al, 1990). When repairing facial or lower extremity nerve injuries, a microscope body objective with a focal length of 200 to 300 mm permits the surgeon to create a comfortable working position and provides appropriate magnification. When working in a cavity or deep plane, a focal length of 250 to 300 mm should be used, depending on the depth of the structures. Remember to have long instruments available. If working closer to the skin surface, the 200-mm objective is used. Occasionally, it is necessary to repair single fascicles, and higher magnification may be required. This can be achieved by using a shorter focal length on the microscopic body, usually a 150- to 175-mm focal distance. Using this setup will give excellent resolution and high magnification, but the depth of field is difficult to work within. Unfortunately, as the magnification increases, the depth of field decreases. The most commonly used objective is the 200-mm objective in conjunction with 10 to 12.5× ocular objectives. Higher powered ocular objectives (15–20×) may also be used to produce higher magnifications, but they can distort visual resolution. When available and conditions

permit, changing the microscope body objective to increase magnification is preferred.

If the microscope base stand is placed behind the surgeon, it permits the surgical assistant and the surgical technician easy access to the surgical field for assisting (Fig. 26–2).

When repairing nerves in the face or neck, it is very helpful to place the head of the patient at the foot of the surgical table. This will allow the surgeon more comfortable access to the patient during microscopic repairs. The surgeon will be able to get his or her knees under the surgical table, making foot pedal control and access easier (Fig. 26–3).

When repairing nerves in the lower fourth of the lower extremity, access is made easier by using the position shown in Figure 26–4.

In addition to visual enhancement by magnification, nerve approximators, background material, methylene blue staining, suction irrigation devices, and proper microsurgical instruments (Fig. 26–5) are essential to a meticulous and efficient repair (Van Beek, 1980).

The availability of a gas-sterilized extremity tourniquet for use on the arm or lower extremity when nerve injuries are more proximal may be helpful in preventing blood loss and in providing safer dissection in a bloodless field.

If nerve grafts might be required, placing tourniquets before skin preparation, draping, and beginning the operation will be helpful and save considerable time when it is time to harvest the nerve grafts.

SURGICAL TECHNIQUE

Using tourniquet hemostasis during exploration of nerves is advisable, and using the incisions discussed in Chapter 19, which discusses extensile exposure of the nerves, will aid surgical exposure of the nerves. Initial dissection of the nerve is performed with 3 to 4× loupes with exposure of the normal nerve proximal and distal to the site of injury and neuroma formation. The nerve is then traced into the zone of injury using the microscope. When the nerve stumps are identified, final dissection and nerve end preparation is completed using the microscope. The ability to magnify the nerve's structure permits identification of intact fascicles and fascicle crossovers before they are injured. Crossovers in the distal forearm are few and permit group fascicular dissection (Chow et al, 1980; Jabaley et al, 1980; Sunderland, 1968). These structures are not readily visualized with loupes. When dissection of the nerve and its injury is completed, the microscope is used to determine where and how the nerve is to be repaired (Buncke, 1972; Chabaud et al, 1976; Edsage, 1964; Grabb, 1968; Hakstain, 1973; Larsen, 1958;

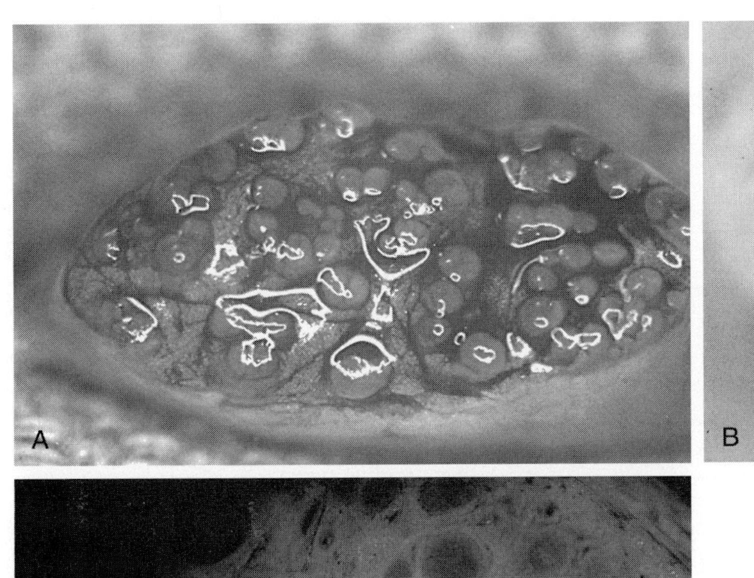
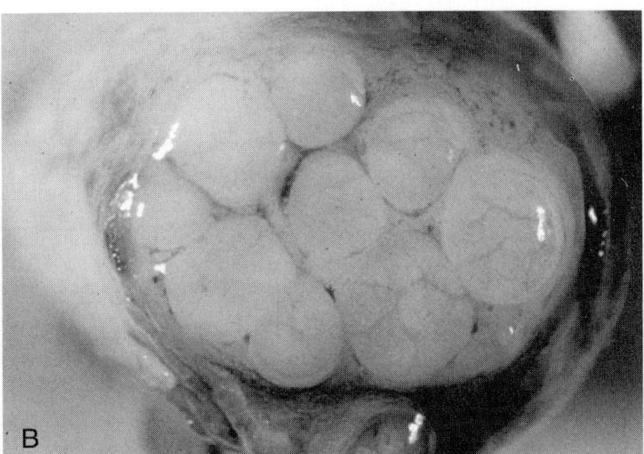
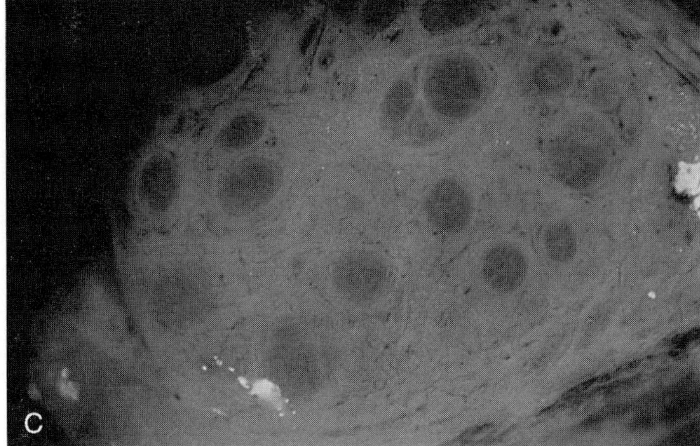

FIGURE 26–1. Operating microscopic visualization of *(A)* a normal sciatic nerve, *(B)* a median nerve, and *(C)* a median nerve with intraneural fibrosis.

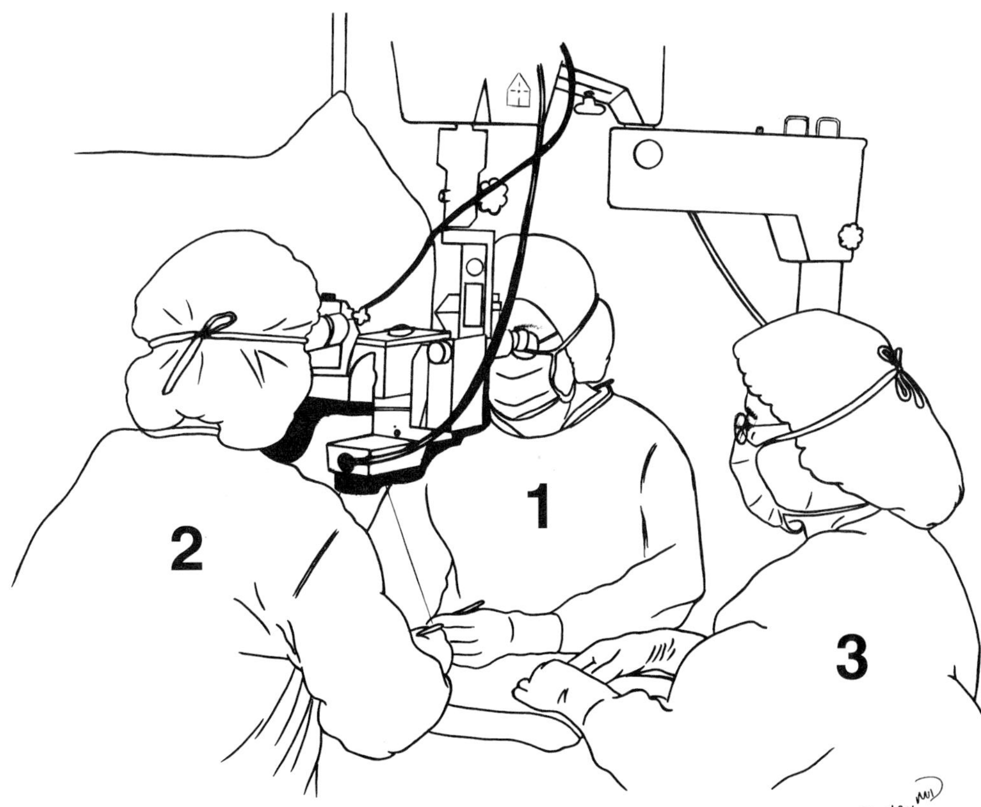

FIGURE 26–2. With the microscope stand located behind the surgeon, assistants have easy access to the operative field.

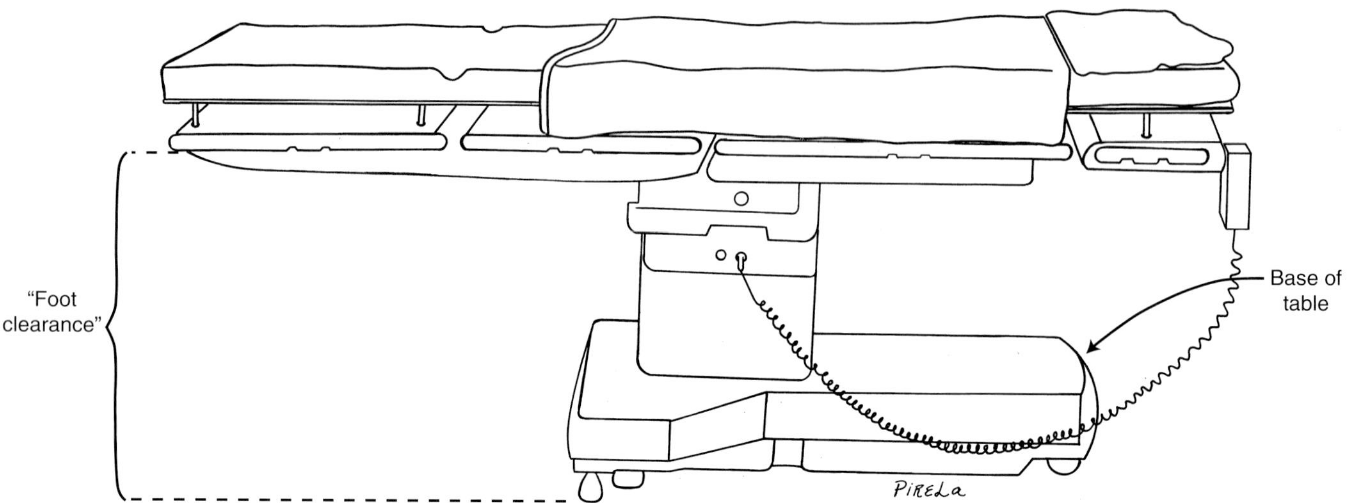

FIGURE 26–3. When repairing facial nerves, it is useful to place the patient's head at the foot of the operative table. This will permit the surgeon to position his legs under the table while using the microscope.

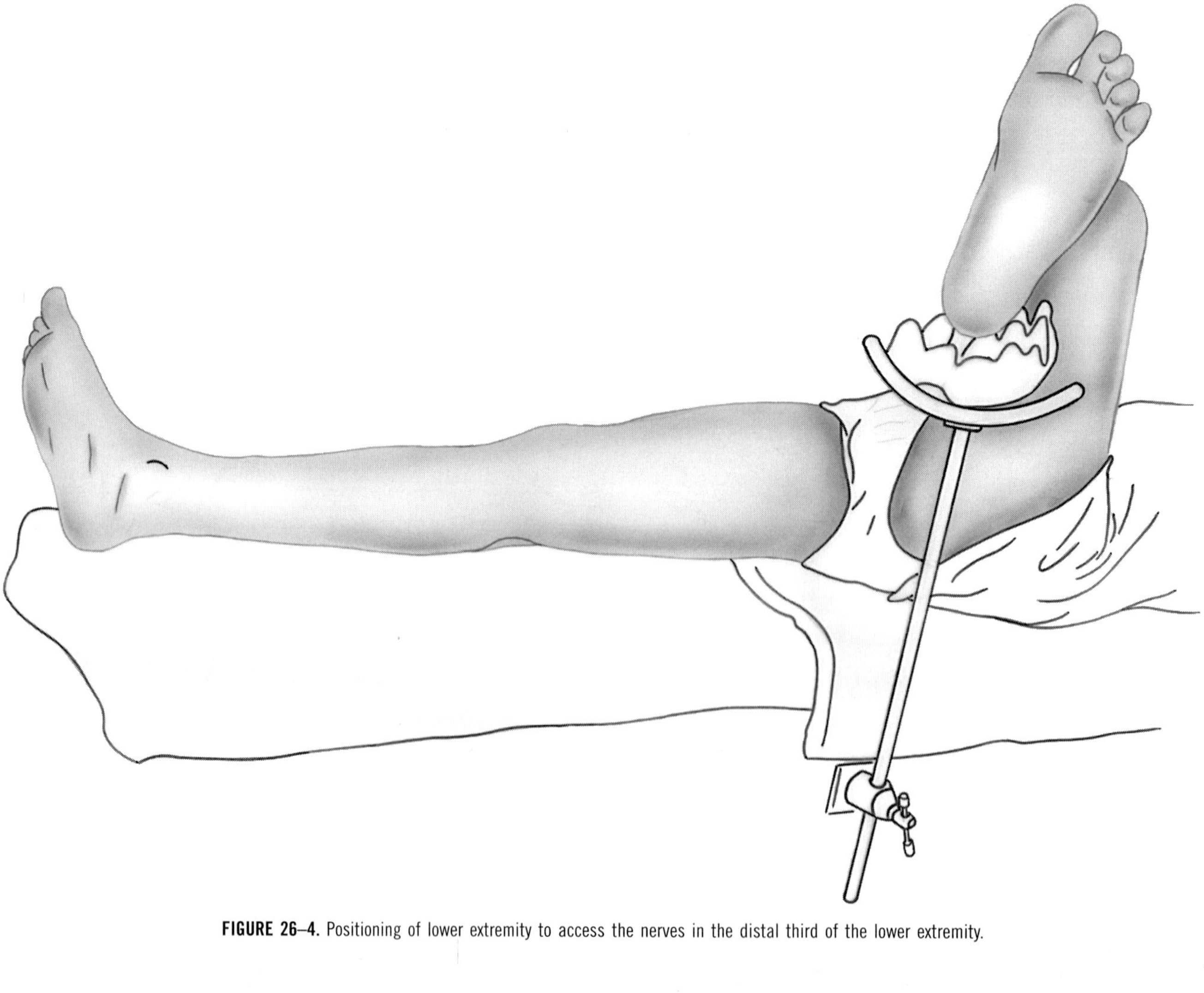

FIGURE 26–4. Positioning of lower extremity to access the nerves in the distal third of the lower extremity.

Technical Tips

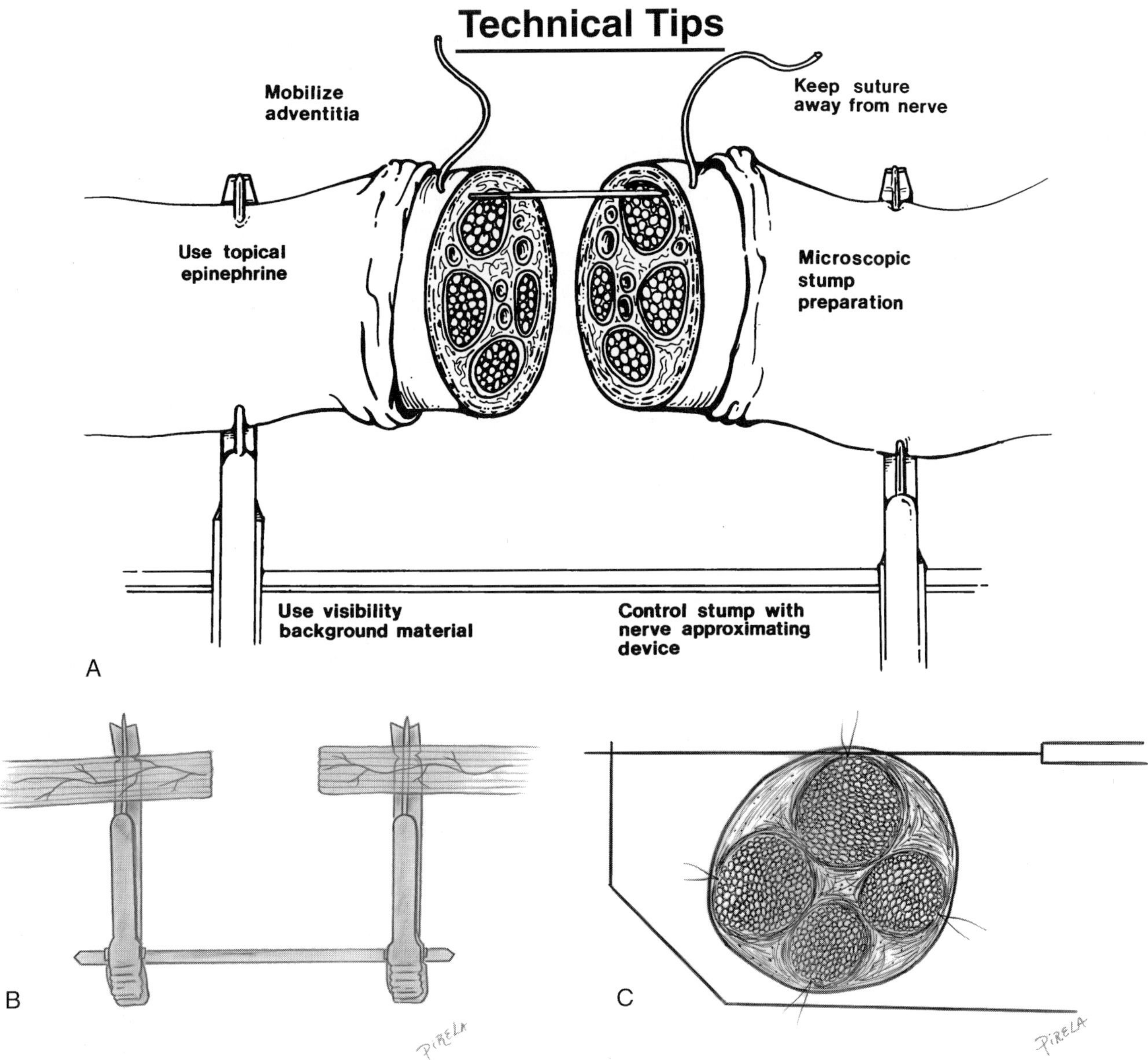

FIGURE 26–5. *(A)* The nerve repair set up should include background sheeting, nerve approximator, and a dry surgical field. *(B)* The nerve-approximating device relieves stress across the repair site and allows rotation of the repair site for easy access. *(C)* The retention needles for the nerve-approximating device penetrate only the external epineurium.

Lilla et al, 1979; Merle et al, 1986; Millesi, 1973; Orgel and Terzis, 1977). In acute injuries, the topography of the nerve is readily discernible, and alignment of the nerve's fascicles is more accurate if the microscope is used for enhanced visualization.

Nerve Dissection

When a delay in exploration of a nerve injury has occurred, the nerve is identified near the injury and then surgically exposed toward the injury or neuroma. In acute injury exploration, the nerve is found immediately adjacent to the injury and inspected along with other injured structures. Because of the nature of injuries that are associated with nerve damage, the nerve is often the last structure repaired before skin closure. For this reason, the repairs are often done with the tourniquet deflated. Bleeding from the cut

ends of a nerve during a repair is annoying and should be controlled. Bleeding can be stopped after direct microscopic visualization of the bleeding point and control by bipolar coagulation or topical application of dilute epinephrine solution.

Anatomy and Terminology

The peripheral nervous system (PNS) comprises all nervous tissue outside of the brain and spinal cord (central nervous system [CNS]). Its primary function is to serve as a conduit for communication with the CNS. The PNS can be further subdivided into afferent and efferent systems. The afferent nerve fibers carry information or stimuli toward the CNS, and efferent fibers conduct impulses away from the CNS. A typical peripheral nerve has mixed elements of both afferent and efferent fibers. For example, the ulnar nerve

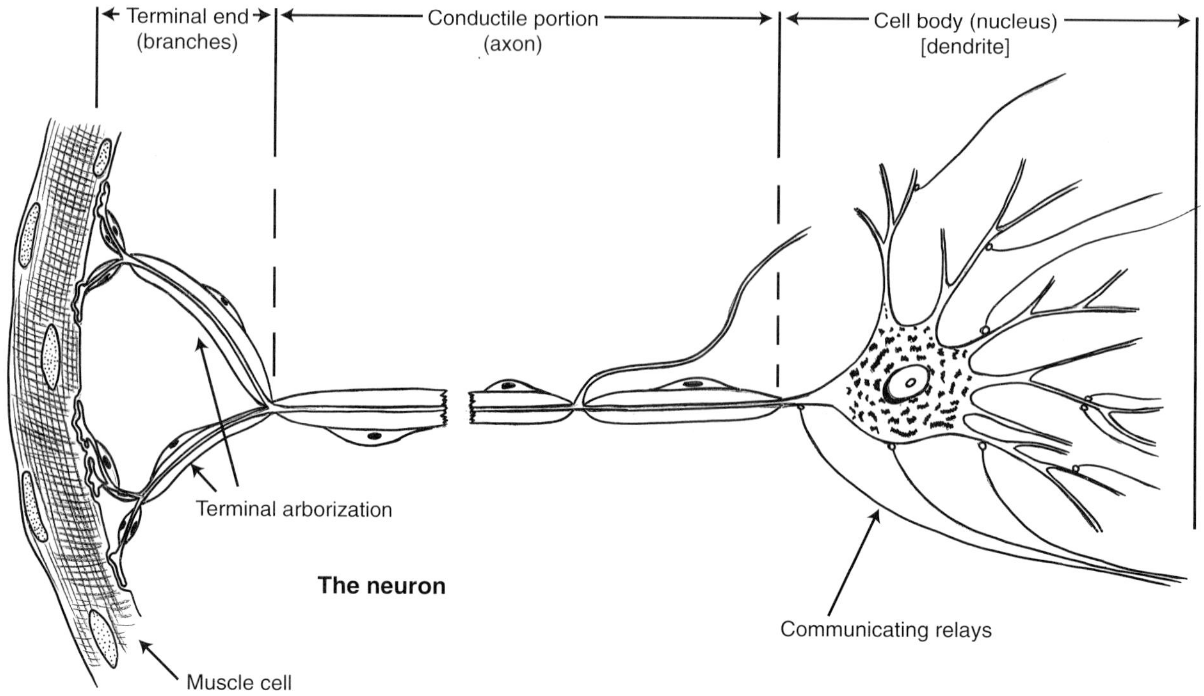

FIGURE 26–6. The cellular component of a nerve fiber has three dominant components—the central cell body, the nerve fiber, and the terminal end-organ complex.

typically provides sensibility to the ulnar side of the hand, which is an afferent function. The sensory input is ultimately sent to the brain for analysis. The ulnar nerve also innervates the flexor carpi ulnaris, which is an efferent function. Nerves that are thought to be "pure motor nerves" also have afferent fibers. For example, the posterior interosseous nerve provides proprioceptive and sensory feedback to the CNS via its afferent fibers.

A peripheral nerve is composed of three sections (Fig. 26–6): a central portion (the cell body), a conductile portion (the nerve fiber), and a terminal end portion. The cell bodies are located within the spinal cord. The nerve fibers connect the cell body with its terminal end.

Microsurgical repair of a peripheral nerve is really the attempted repair of damaged nerve fibers (axotomy); therefore, understanding the cross-sectional anatomy and the nomenclature of nerve fibers components is essential (Fig. 26–7).

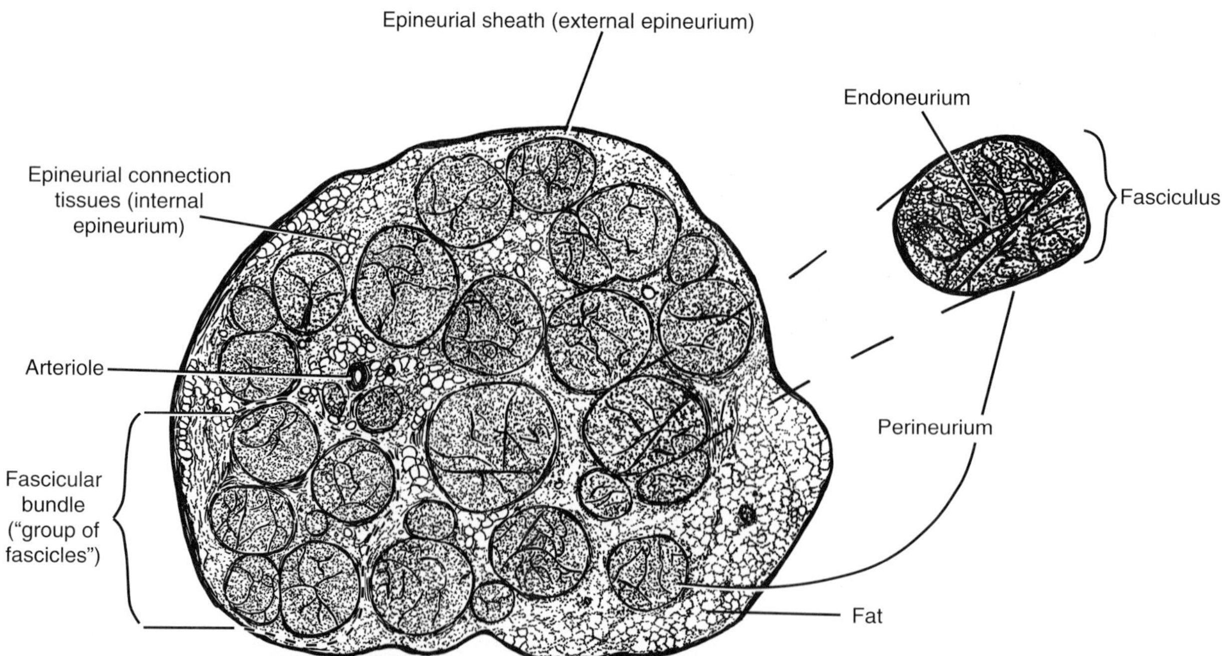

FIGURE 26–7. Surgical nomenclature for a nerve cross section.

With the operating microscope, on cross-sectional analysis the external epineurium of the peripheral nerve is noted to have a dense connective tissue that encapsulates the nerve. The epineurium is invested by a loose adventitial layer. The primary function of the external epineurium seems to be bundling of fascicles and supporting their position. In response to injury or irritation, the epineurium can become very thick and constrictive; removing thickened epineurium is an important part of nerve repair. Fat, blood vessels, and lymphatics are normal components located within the structure of nerves.

The internal epineurium is a loose array of connective tissue bridging the external epineurium and surrounding all the nerve fascicles in continuous envelope of supportive tissue.

Like the external epineurium, the perineurium is composed of a lamellar, dense connective tissue and cellular stroma. On electron microscopy, a prominent basement membrane and tight junctures are noted. The perineurium serves as a blood nerve barrier and constrains nerve fibers.

The endoneurium is the interstitial tissue encompassing the nerve fibers within the perineurium. It also provides support to the Schwann cell. Each nerve fiber, myelinated or unmyelinated, is surrounded by a Schwann cell and its accompanying Schwann cell sheath.

Fascicles are nerve subcomponents. They vary in size and number within the nerve. Each fascicle is surrounded by a perineurial sheath and epineurium. The fascicle is the smallest nerve component that can be surgically repaired.

ACUTE DIRECT NERVE REPAIR

The most common type of nerve repair is the direct microscopic nerve repair. After complete or partial transection of a nerve, the best repair is a meticulous direct coaptation of the nerve without tension. Microscopic visualization during a repair aids visualization of the topography, helps with debridement of extruded fascicle content, minimizes traumatic handling of the nerve, and ensures appropriate placement of sutures (Buncke, 1972; Kutz et al, 1981; Posch and delaCruz-Saddul, 1980; Snyder et al, 1968; Wise et al, 1969; Young et al, 1981). To minimize suture foreign body reaction within the nerve repair, the suture material used should be 10-0 or smaller for digital nerve repairs and 9-0 or smaller for larger nerve repairs (Van Beek et al, 1985). The minimum number of sutures needed to accurately coapt the nerve is preferred to excessive numbers of sutures.

External epineurial (Fig. 26–8) and group fascicular nerve repairs (Fig. 26–9) are the most commonly used repair techniques for direct nerve repair (Buncke, 1972; Merle et al, 1986; Millesi et al, 1972; Sakellarides, 1962). In general, single fascicle repairs (Fig. 26–10) are not advocated for repairing transected nerves, but they may be the technique of choice under special circumstances (Kutz et al, 1981).

External epineural repair is used for the repair of digital nerves and larger nerves such as the median or ulnar nerve. Group fascicular repair is used for larger nerves of the arm, forearm, and lower extremity and in anatomical locations where the nerve has definable groups of fascicles. The improved internal alignment of nerves with larger cross-sectional areas may produce improvement in the specificity of nerve regeneration and decrease stump interface fibrosis. Each fascicle around the perimeter of the nerve should have at least a single suture placed as shown in Figure 26–9. Additional sutures may aid in nerve alignment and constraint of fascicle content. After coaptation of the nerve, excess fascicle content often extrudes from between the sutures. This excess material is removed to permit the fascicles to be coapted by the existing sutures without buckling or misalignment.

When larger cross-sectional areas need to be coapted, a group fascicle repair is preferred. This repair will permit more accurate coaptation of the nerve ends and improve spatial alignment.

Groups of fascicles are readily identified with the microscope, and in the preterminal areas of the nerve, the groups

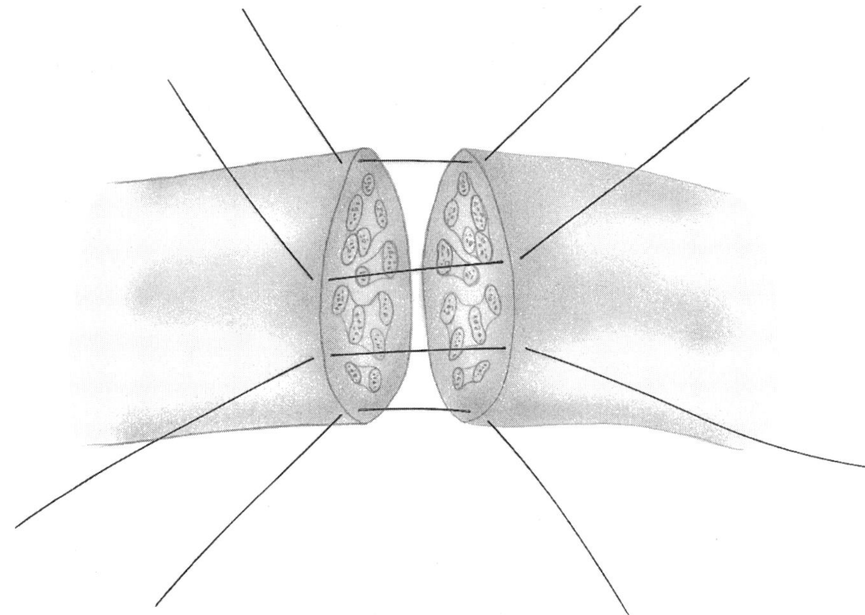

FIGURE 26–8. During external epineurial repair, microsutures are placed in the epineurium adjacent to fascicles.

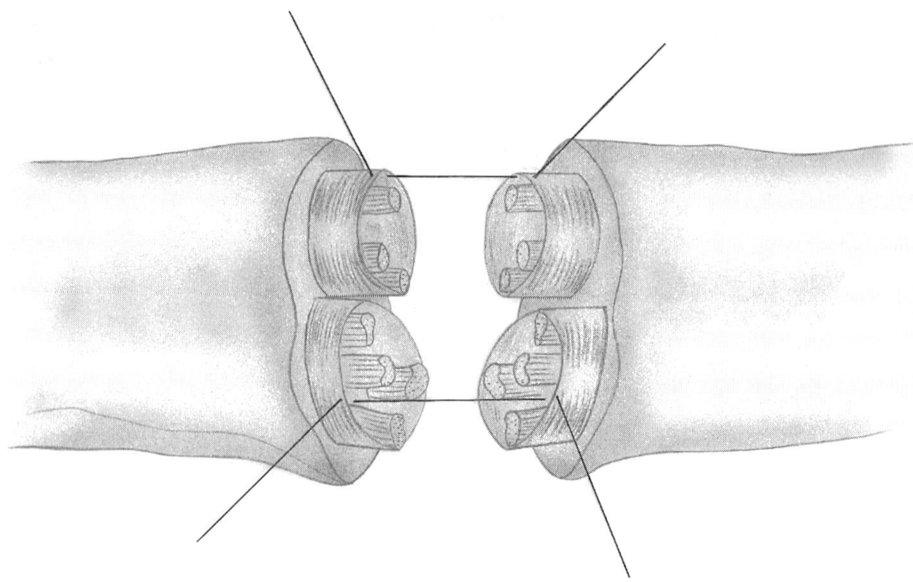

FIGURE 26–9. During group fascicular repair, dominant groups of fascicles are separated and the perimeter of the groups sutured. Sutures are used to align the fascicles in each group.

can be separated for distances of 1 to 2 cm. This separation of the groups from each other makes alignment and suturing of the groups easier. After coapting the groups of fascicles, some fascicles may extrude between the sutures. The extruding fascicles should be shortened to permit better coapting of the nerve ends between the sutured areas of the epineurium. This is similar to excising extruding fascicle content, except the entire fascicle component is shortened.

A word about suture placement seems appropriate. When placing sutures through the nerve substance, the needle should stay out of the fascicle content and should only be placed through external, internal, or the outer lamella of the perineurium (Van Beek, 1975). Avoid including nerve fibers within the repair suture's loop (Fig. 26–8).

Nerve Grafts

The decision to provide coaptation of the stumps of an injured nerve with a nerve graft is important. As emphasized by Millesi (1973, 1987), when the gap between the stumps of an injured nerve cannot be approximated without excessive tension, a nerve graft is indicated. The measurement of excessive tension is elusive. Our rule of thumb is that if a suture larger than 7-0 is required to bring the ends of the nerve together, then a nerve graft should be considered. Many conditions must be present for a nerve graft to be successful (Briedenbach and Terzis, 1986; Kline and Nulsen, 1972; MacKinnon, 1988; Millesi, 1972; Seddon, 1975). A suitable proximal and distal nerve stump must be present.

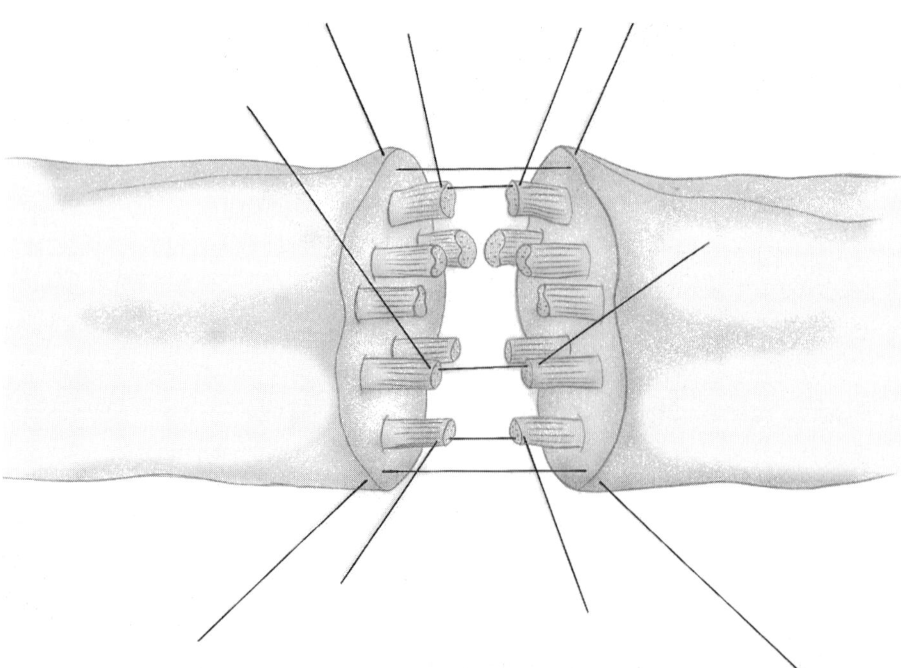

FIGURE 26–10. During single fascicle repairs, two or three sutures are placed within the epineurium and the outer lamella of the perineurium to align each fascicle. This repair is very technically demanding and is reserved for special circumstances.

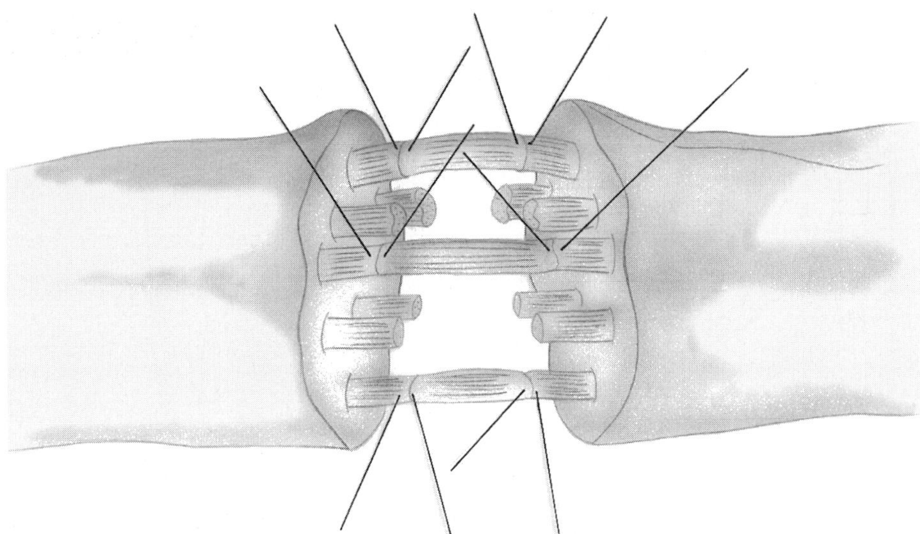

FIGURE 26–11. Alignment of nerve grafts is difficult because of dissimilar patterns of fascicle topography between nerve stumps and nerve graft.

The tissue bed where grafts will be placed must be pliable and well vascularized. An acceptable donor nerve site and careful preoperative informed consent are essential.

Commonly used donor sites for nerve grafts are lateral antebrachial cutaneous nerve, medial antebrachial cutaneous nerve, sural nerve, sensory component posterior interosseous nerve, and nerves retrieved from amputated parts. The morbidity of the donor sites should not be overlooked and must be explained to the patient.

Once the injured nerve is prepared for nerve grafting by trimming to acceptable fascicle appearance, the nerve graft can be prepared for placement. Excessive adventitia and external epineurium should be removed. The graft is reversed to preserve all fibers entering the graft. Without reversal, some fibers may be lost to small branches along the course of the nerve. Estimate the number of cables that will be required and make sure that ample nerve grafts are available. If the tissue conditions are not favorable, the nerve graft should be delayed, provisions should be made to improve those conditions, or a vascularized nerve graft should be provided.

Nerve graft fascicle topography is essential to alignment of nerves (Chow et al, 1985; Jabaley et al, 1980; Sunderland, 1968). The injured nerve will have topography that will be completely dissimilar to the topography of the nerve graft being used for the repair. Therefore, the surgeon must provide the best coaptation of dissimilar nerve facets between the graft and the injured nerve and try to align the proximal and distal fascicles of the proximal and distal nerve stumps (Gaul, 1986; Hakstian, 1968; Van Beek, 1985). Each strand of nerve graft is secured with 3 or 4 sutures around each graft, using the operating microscope to enhance alignment (Figs. 26–11 and 26–12). This provides for secure coaptation and improved alignment. Extruding fascicle content is removed with a sharp scissor to improve alignment and coaptation of the nerve ends. Fibrin glue to aid coaptation has been advocated by Young and Medaware (1940) and by Narakas (1990).

The assessment of nerve injuries is an integral part of caring for patients with nerve injuries. A systematic and chronological assessment is advocated. This permits the early recognition of recovery or failure to recovery. The timing of secondary intervention or reconstruction is determined by the clinical status after nerve repair. The form in Figure 26–13 is a useful tool to guide and record assessments.

After a direct nerve repair, the repair site should be protected from distracting forces for 3 weeks. Nerve graft repair sites should be protected for 2 weeks. This does not preclude movement-only motion that would distract the repair site. For example, a digital nerve repair in combination with a flexor tendon injury does not mean that passive motion exercises could not be used. Passive flexion can be started early, but only if the digit is blocked from being completely extended during active or passive extension by appropriate splinting techniques.

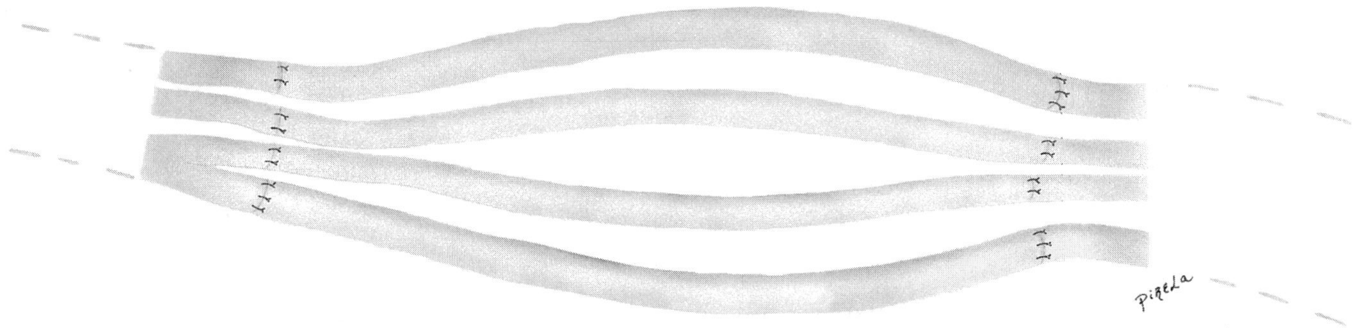

FIGURE 26–12. Enough sutures are placed on the nerve graft ends to ensure accurate coaptation. This usually requires four to six sutures for each end of the graft.

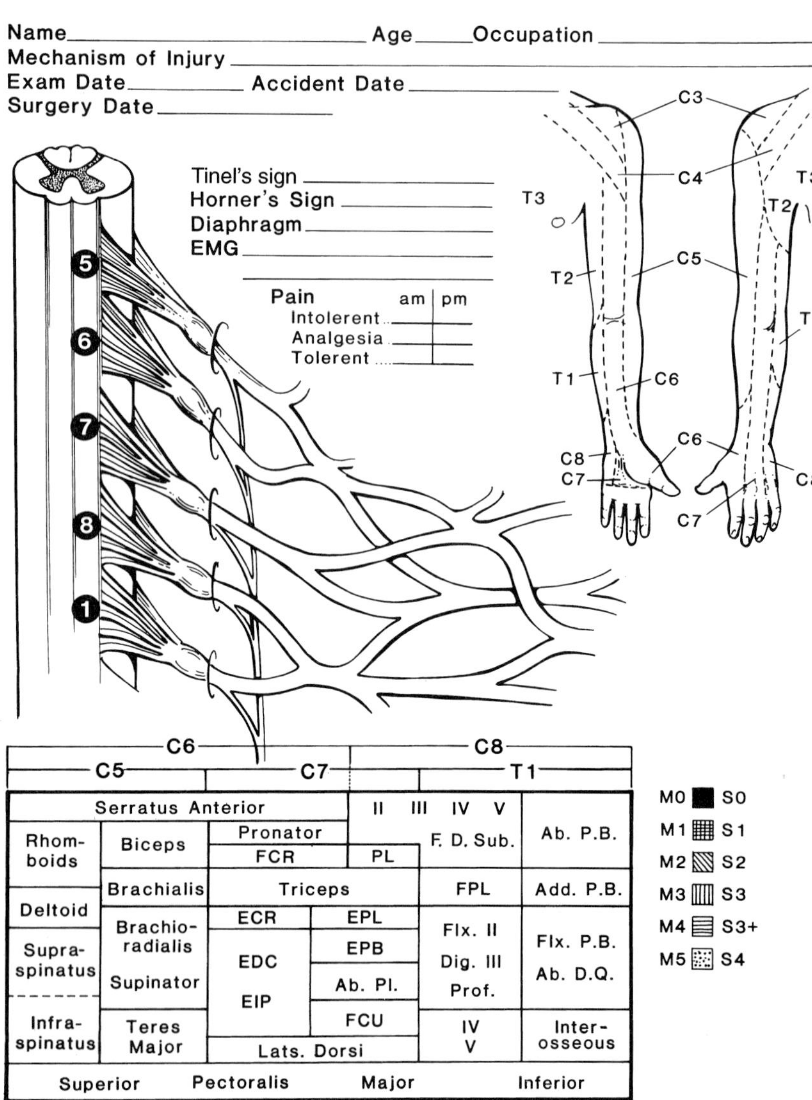

FIGURE 26–13. Accurate chronologic assessment of improvement is essential to determine the timing and necessity of additional reconstructive surgery. An assessment form is helpful for recording information and for patient education.

What size suture should be used during nerve repair? For digital nerve repairs, 10-0 is preferred. When repairing larger nerves, 9-0 or 10-0 is preferred. Single fascicle repairs are usually accomplished with 10-0 or 11-0 suture. Suture size recommendations must be tailored to match the circumstances of the repair, and the surgeon's role is to minimize foreign body reaction at the risk of repair site disruption because of insufficient strength at the site of nerve coaptation.

Is the microscope better than binocular loupe magnification? Improved lighting, higher magnification, surgical assistance, controlled meticulous technique, delicate tissue manipulation, and improved visualization make nerve repair easier when using the microscope as compared with loupe magnification. Because it is easier and more accurate, microscopic repair is the gold standard for neurorrhaphy.

References

Breidenbach WC, Terzis JK: The blood supply of vascularized nerve grafts. J Reconstr Microsurg 3:43–56, 1986.

Buncke HJ: Digital nerve repairs. Surg Clin North Am 52:1267–1285, 1972.

Bunnell S: Repair of nerves and tendons of the hand. J Bone Joint Surg 10:1–16, 1928.

Chabaud HE, Rodkey WG, McCarroll HR, et al: Epineural and perineurial fascicular nerve repairs: A critical comparison. J Hand Surg 1:131–137, 1976.

Chow JA, Sunderland S, Van Beek AL: Surgical significance of the motor fascicular group of the ulnar nerve in the forearm. J Hand Surg [Am] 9:605, 1985.

Clawson DK, Seddon HJ: The results of repair of the sciatic nerve. J Bone Joint Surg 42B:205, 1960.

Edsage S: Peripheral nerve suture: A technique for improved intraneural topography. Acta Chir Scand (Suppl) 331:1–104, 1964.

Gaul JS: Electrical fascicle identification as an adjunct to nerve repair. Hand Clin 2:709–722, 1986.

Grabb WC: Median and ulnar nerve suture. J Bone Joint Surg 50A:964–972, 1968.

Hakstian RW: Funicular orientation by direct stimulation: An aid to peripheral nerve repair. J Bone Joint Surg 50A:1178–1186, 1968.

Hakstian RW: Perineurial neurorrhaphy. Orthop Clin North Am 4:945–956, 1973.

Highet WB, Sanders FK: The effects of stretching nerves after sutures. Br J Surg 30:355, 1943.

Holmgren G: Some experiences in the surgery of otosclerosis. Acta Otolaryngol (Stockh) 5:460, 1923.

Jabaley ME, Wallace WH, Heckler FR: Internal topography of major nerves of the forearm and hand: A current view. J Hand Surg 5:1–8, 1980.

Kline DG, Nulsen FE: The neuroma incontinuity: Its preoperative and operative management. Surg Clin North Am 52:1189–1209, 1972.

Kutz JE, Shealy G, Lubbers I: Interfascicular nerve repair. Orthop Clin North Am 12:277–286, 1981.

Larsen RD, Posch JL: Nerve injuries in the upper extremity. Arch Surg 77:469–482, 1958.

Lilla JA, Phelps DB, Boswick JA: Microsurgical repair of peripheral nerve injuries in the upper extremity. Ann Plast Surg 2:24–31, 1979.

MacKinnon SE: Nerve Repair and Nerve Grafting. Surgery of the Peripheral Nerve. New York, Thieme Publishers, 1988, pp 89–130.

Merle M, Amend P, Cour C, Foucher G, Michon S: Microsurgical repair of peripheral nerve lesions: A study of 150 injuries of the median and ulnar nerves. Peripheral Nerve Repair Regeneration 2:17–26, 1986.

Millesi H: Microsurgery of peripheral nerves. Hand 5:157–160, 1973.

Millesi H: The nerve gap: Theory and clinical practice. Hand Clin 2:651–664, 1987.

Millesi H, Meissl G, Berger A: The interfascicular nerve-grafting of the median and ulnar nerves. J Bone Joint Surg 54A:727–750, 1972.

Millesi H, Meissl G, Berger A: Further experience with interfascicular grafting of the median, ulnar and radial nerves. J Bone Joint Surg 58A:29–118, 1976.

Narakas AO: Brachial plexus injuries. In McCarthy JG (ed): Plastic Surgery. Philadelphia, WB Saunders, 1990.

Nylen CO: The microscope in aural surgery: Its first use and later development. Acta Otolaryngol Suppl (Stockh) 116:226–240, 1954.

O'Brien BM, Morrison WA, Gumley GJ: Principles and techniques of microvascular surgery. In McCarthy JG (ed): Plastic Surgery. Philadelphia, WB Saunders, 1990.

Omer G: Injuries to nerves of the upper extremities. J Bone Joint Surg 56A:1615–1624, 1974.

Orgel MG, Terzis JK: Epineurial versus perineural repair: An ultrastructural and electrophysiological study of nerve regeneration. Plast Reconstr Surg 60:80–91, 1977.

Posch JL, delaCruz-Saddul F: Nerve repair in trauma surgery: A 10-year study of 231 peripheral injuries. Orthop Rev 9:35–45, 1980.

Ramon y Cajal S: Degeneration and Regeneration of the Nervous System (RM May, translator). Hafner Publishing, New York, 1959.

Russell RC: Transmission and scanning electron microscopy of peripheral nerves. Hand Clin 2:665–676, 1986.

Sakellarides H: A follow-up study of 173 peripheral nerve injuries of the upper extremity of civilians. J Bone Joint Surg 44A:140–148, 1962.

Sanders PK: The repair of large gaps in peripheral nerves. Brain 65:281–337, 1942.

Seddon HJ: The use of autogenous grafts for the repair of large gaps in peripheral nerves. Br J Surg 35:151–167, 1947.

Seddon HJ: Surgical Disorders of Peripheral Nerves. Baltimore, Williams & Wilkins, 1975.

Smith JW: Microsurgery of peripheral nerves. Plast Reconst Surg 33:317–329, 1964.

Snyder CC, Webster H, Pickens JE, et al: Intraneural neurorrhaphy: A preliminary clinical and histological evaluation. Ann Surg 167:691, 1968.

Sunderland S: Nerves and Nerve Injuries. Baltimore, Williams & Wilkins, 1968.

Thomas PK: The cellular response to nerve injury. J Anat 100:287–303, 1966.

Thomas PK, Jones DG: The cellular response to nerve injuries: Regeneration of the perineurium after nerve section. J Anat 101:45–55, 1967.

Van Beek AL, Glover JL, Zook E: Primary versus delayed primary neurorrhaphy in rat sciatic nerve. J Surg Res 18:335–339, 1975.

Van Beek AL, Kleiner HE: Peripheral nerve injuries and repair. In Rand RW (ed): Microneurosurgery. St. Louis, Mosby, 1985.

Van Beek AL, Zook EG: A nerve approximating device. Plast Reconst Surg 66:143–147, 1980.

Wise AJ Jr, Topuzlu C, Davis P, Kaye IS: A comparative analysis of macro- and microsurgical neurorrhaphy techniques. Am J Surg 117:566–572, 1969.

Woodall B, Beebe WG: Peripheral Nerve Regeneration. A Follow-Up Study of 3,656 World War II Injuries. Washington, DC, U.S. Government Printing Office, VA Medical Monograph, 1956.

Young JZ, Medaware PB: Fibrin suture of peripheral nerves. Lancet 2:126, 1940.

Young L, Wray RC, Weeks PM: A randomized prospective comparison of fascicular and epineural digital nerve repairs. Plast Reconstr Surg 68:89–92, 1981.

Zachery RB, Homes W: Primary suture of nerves. Surg Gynecol Obstet 82:632–651, 1946.

Chapter 27

• E. F. Shaw Wilgis

Epineurial Repair: Technique and Long-Term Results

The purpose of all nerve repair techniques is to restore continuity of the nerve trunk, including all of its elements, in order to achieve optimal and useful reinnervation of both sensory and motor end-organs. There are many accepted techniques for coaptation of the ends of a severed nerve. No single repair method is appropriate for every instance of nerve injury. The choice of repair technique depends on several overriding anatomical factors.

TYPES OF NERVES

Nerves are subdivided into three types (Millesi and Terzis, 1984). A **monofascicular** nerve is one containing one large fascicle with many axons. An example is one of the terminal branches of a digital nerve. Monofascicular nerves are usually either predominately sensory or predominately motor. An **oligofascicular** nerve is one in which the cross section consists of few fascicles. Examples are the digital nerves and the ulnar nerve at the elbow. The ulnar nerve at the elbow usually contains four fascicles. Oligofascicular nerves can be either single-purpose or mixed nerves with both sensory and motor components. **Polyfascicular** nerves are nerves in which the cross section consists of many small fascicles, such as the radial nerve in the upper arm.

In its course from the brachial plexus to the fingertips, the nerve may undergo changes (polyfascicular in the upper arm, oligofascicular in the elbow region, and monofascicular in the hand). The ulnar nerve, as it emerges from the brachial plexus, is classified as polyfascicular; at the elbow, as oligofascicular; and after the division to the motor branch in the hand, as monofascicular. One selects the type of nerve repair according to both nerve type and location.

EXCURSION

A second anatomical feature to be considered when treating a transected nerve is longitudinal neural excursion. During limb movement, peripheral nerve accommodates changes in the length of its bed. The longitudinal excursion of nerve during motion has been studied recently in several ways.

McLellan and Swash (1976) recorded action potentials in the median nerve before and during active and passive motion of limbs. They found that active and passive movement had equal effects. The greatest excursions were produced by extension of the wrist and fingers and by flexion of the elbow. Extension of the wrist and fingers caused a 7.4 mm excursion, and flexion of the elbow caused a 4.3-mm excursion. The authors estimated that hyperextension of the wrist caused the median nerve to glide 10 to 15 mm. They also found that displacement of the median nerve during flexion of the wrist and fingers was two to four times greater at the wrist than in the upper arm.

Dellon and co-workers (1984) postulated that the radial sensory nerve had a significant excursion on radial and ulnar deviation of the wrist. Wilgis and Murphy (1986), using 15 fresh intact adult cadaveric arms, dissected the entire peripheral nervous system, focusing on longitudinal nerve excursion. They noted that the brachial plexus had an average excursion of 15 mm when ranged from the frontal plane with the arm in full abduction to full adduction. The median and ulnar nerves at the elbow moved an average of 7.3 and 9.8 mm, respectively, with full motion. The greatest excursion of peripheral nerves occurred at the wrist, proximal to the carpal tunnel. Here, the median and ulnar nerves had 15.5 and 14.8 mm of longitudinal sliding, respectively, with the wrist ranged through a full arc of flexion and extension in the sagittal plane.

These studies are consistent with the studies of McLellan and Swash (1976). In the palm and digits, the excursion was considerably less. To summarize the amount of motion of the median nerve and the digital nerves at the wrist and fingers, the excursion of these components approaches 2 cm.

When planning repair of a divided peripheral nerve, the surgeon must consider not only the internal elastic tension of nerve but also the need for longitudinal excursion during limb movement. For example, the normal retraction of the median nerve at the level of the wrist is 1.5 cm after a clean division. By adding the 1.5 cm of longitudinal excursion needed when taking the wrist from full flexion to full extension, the immediate demand for appropriate length of the nerve becomes apparent.

Acutely, when the nerve can be approximated with minimal tension, one would expect normal longitudinal excursion to occur once local scarring factors have subsided. However, conditions are altered with the prolonged delays brought about by secondary nerve suture. Nerve loses elasticity as a result of the injury itself and subsequent scarring. Therefore, the stumps often cannot be approximated under normal tension with the anticipation of normal excursion, without acute flexion of an adjacent joint. In other words, nerve length is lost owing to both the injury and the elapsed time interval. If nerve is sutured under tension with the wrist in acute flexion, the nerve becomes unable to slide adequately when the adjacent joint is moved into the position opposite the one in which it was placed for the repair. The existing gap between the two ends is increased because of the excursion factor.

For example, in a secondary repair of the median nerve at the wrist, when the existing gap after resection of a neuroma is 2 cm, the surgeon should consider the additional 1.5 cm that must be provided in order to accommodate the nerve's requirement for longitudinal excursion. This creates a physiological gap of 3.5 cm—a gap sufficient to influence the surgeon to choose an alternative method of repair, such as nerve grafting.

At the elbow, the need for excursion can be satisfied by transposing the ulnar nerve anteriorly, thereby reducing its need for longitudinal excursion and bridging the gap. This aspect of nerve anatomy, in its dynamic state, is of particular importance to the surgeon undertaking primary and secondary repair of peripheral nerve.

PRINCIPLES OF REPAIR

The four overriding principles for coaptation of divided nerve were outlined by Millesi and Terzis in 1984:

1. Preparation of the stump, which often involves resection or interfascicular dissection with separation of individual fascicles or groups of fascicles. In this step, the zone of injury is removed as completely as possible by microscopic dissection.
2. Approximation with special reference to the length of the gap between the stumps, as well as the amount of tension present.
3. Coaptation of the nerve stumps. Coaptation connotes the apposition of corresponding nerve ends with special attention to bringing fascicles into original contact. A direct neurorrhaphy apposes stump to stump, fascicle to fascicle, or fascicle group to fascicle group, in the corresponding ends. An indirect coaptation is performed by interposing a nerve graft. In this section, we deal only with direct coaptation by epineural group or group fascicular repair.
4. Maintenance of coaptation involving the use of sutures.

In performing any of the repair techniques, proper fascicular identification is mandatory. Hakstian (1968), Jabaley (1984a, 1991), and Gaul (1983) have proposed using electrical stimulation to aid in the identification of the fascicular structure. Intraoperative nerve stimulation is also helpful in identifying specific motor and sensory bundles.

A second aid in the proper identification of fascicles is the use of histochemical reaction and staining techniques, as described by Lister. It is particularly helpful to use the histochemical techniques in situations of late repair when proximal fascicle identification is needed. In the acute phase, the cleanly transected and divided nerve can usually be matched without the use of staining techniques.

Epineurial Repair

Epineurial repair is enhanced with the use of magnification, either with magnifying loupes or the operating microscope.

In accomplishing the epineurial suture technique in the primary situation, the surgeon first divides the nerve ends proximal and distal to the injury site until all visible signs of damage have been debrided. Fascicles then mushroom from the neural stumps, and the epineurium retracts slightly. The goals of epineurial repair are to establish continuity without tension with proper alignment (Wilgis, 1991).

The nerve is inspected for longitudinal blood vessels that can be aligned in the epineurium. Also, fascicular arrangement is noted and fascicles from both stumps are matched. This method ensures appropriate rotational alignment.

The sutures are placed in the external epineurium using nonabsorbable sutures. We usually use 8-0 nylon for larger nerves and 10-0 nylon for smaller nerves, such as the digital nerves. The nylon is placed through the epineurium proximally and distally, and tied. The epineurium is not closed so tightly that the fascicular ends become mismatched and malaligned by bunching up. It is preferable to leave a small gap in the epineurium held together by a small suture with the fascicular ends in more appropriate alignment. Therefore, the suture, which is not tied tightly, acts as the guiding suture rather than a retention suture.

The second suture is placed opposite the first, and then the epineurium is closed by halving the distance on the anterior and posterior aspects of the nerve. The number of sutures to be used is the minimum number required to ensure coaptation of the nerve stumps. If the nerve cannot be approximated with 8-0 nylon suture, tension is considered excessive and further mobilization or nerve grafting should be performed.

At the end, no fascicles should protrude between the suture lines, and the fascicles should not be bunched up or mismatched within the epineurium.

One very helpful technique is to perform a combined partial epineurial and group fascicular repair, as described by Jabaley (1984b, 1991). In this technique, the same preparation occurs as that for the standard epineurial repair. After this preparation, a longitudinal incision is made through the external epineurium on the superficial surface of the nerve end. The anterior epineurium is then trimmed off, preserving the posterior or dorsal epineurium. The posterior epineurium is then used as a stent or a bridge, which then serves as a bed for the group fascicular repair. The posterior bridge is sutured using 8-0 nylon, and then the fascicular coaptation can be performed with smaller suture material.

POSTOPERATIVE CARE

Before closure of the wound, the repair site should be visually inspected. The joints should be moved through a range of motion to ensure that the repair site is under the appropriate tension. The surgeon should then select a position in which the tension is less than complete for the splinting position. That position should then be maintained for 2 weeks. The adjacent joints should be actively flexed and extended. This allows some very minimal motion at the repair site and minimizes the likelihood of adherence of the repaired site to the surrounding tissue, particularly tendons. At 3 weeks, the joints are allowed to extend to neutral, and there should be no forcible tension applied to the repair site. If necessary, a dorsal splint protecting the repair site should be placed on for another 6 weeks, at which time a full active range of motion is permitted.

The desired result is to have normal excursion of the nerve in the postoperative state. This is rarely possible because of the natural biological tendency of scarring and adherence of the nerve repair site to the surrounding tissue, but if it is minimized, the excursion will return to near normal and the potential of having a painful neuroma at the repair site is decreased.

RECOVERY

There are very few reports of long-term results following nerve repair suture available in the literature. Any study reporting nerve repair results before 2 years after nerve suture is inadequate.

There are several factors affecting nerve recovery. The patient's age is probably the most important factor. Younger patients respond better, and in fact, children under the age of 6 years have almost normal recovery following nerve suture. As the patient ages, normal recovery is impossible. The other significant factors affecting nerve recovery are the level of injury and the type of injury. It is logical to assume that a crushing or avulsive type of injury in the upper arm will have a poorer outcome than a sharp cut at the wrist. Therefore, when evaluating recovery, the site and type of injury are very important. Rarely are these differentiated in the reports.

The amount of nerve defect is also important in assessing the recovery. The nerve defect is important for two reasons: (1) it is more difficult to approximate accurately the nerve endings over a defect of several centimeters, and (2) the tension at the nerve site is increased once the defect reaches several centimeters. Increased tension has been associated with increased scarring.

Another factor affecting nerve recovery is the type of nerve. Nerves of predominantly a single type of fiber, either motor or sensory, appear to repair better than mixed nerves. For example, the radial nerve, largely a motor nerve, heals better than the median nerve, whereas digital nerves, which are primarily sensory, heal better than the mixed nerves. This is purely related to alignment of appropriate nerve fibers to their appropriate epineurial tubes. Other factors influencing the ultimate result are the delay from the time of injury to the time of suture and associated injuries. A nerve injury associated with an accompanying vascular injury or major crushing trauma, or both, to the region has a poorer chance of recovery than a sharp clean injury. The time of suture is important for proper alignment and for the proper coaptation of the nerve ends without tension.

Unfortunately, even with the aid of magnification, the operating microscope, interfascicular nerve grafting, and other techniques, the ultimate result of nerve repair, by any technique, has not improved significantly. The overriding important element is the patient's age. In patients under the age of 12, one could expect full motor and sensory recovery

with discrimination. As the age of the patient increases, sensory recovery diminishes, so that in patients over the age of 50 years, only protected sensibility can be promised with any technique. If one adds the component of a defect, then interpositional nerve grafting clearly yields superior results to a suture under tension. In an interesting study reported in 1982, Gaul showed that in adult patients after ulnar nerve repair, there was 7% intrinsic motor recovery at 14 months, which improved to an average of 82% after 26 to 51 months. In the author's opinion, this is the best long-term result of ulnar nerve repair using the epineurial technique.

SUMMARY

The epineurial technique of repairing nerves is a useful method and should be employed when differentiation of the motor and sensory branches is not clearcut. This is particularly true in the upper arm. When repairing a nerve with a clearcut motor and sensory difference at the wrist, the group fascicular technique with or without an epineurial stint yields better alignment (Sunderland, 1979). As a general rule, better alignment yields better results, but one should be cognizant of the fact that the patient's age is the most important factor in determining the ultimate long-term result.

References

Dellon AL, Mackinnon S, Pestronk A: Implantation of sensory nerve into muscle: Preliminary clinical and experimental observations on neuroma formation. Ann Plast Surg *12*:30–40, 1984.

Gaul S: Electrical fascicle identification as an adjunct to nerve repair. J Hand Surg *8*:289, 1983.

Gaul JS Jr: Intrinsic motor recovery: A long term study of ulnar nerve repair. J Hand Surg *7*:502–508, 1982.

Hakstian RW: Funicular orientation by direct stimulation. J Bone Joint Surg *50*:1178, 1968.

Jabaley ME: Electrical nerve stimulation in the awake patient. Bull Hosp Jt Dis *4*:248–259, 1984a.

Jabaley ME: Technical aspects of peripheral nerve repair. J Hand Surg *9*:14–19, 1984b.

Jabaley ME: Modified techniques of nerve repair: Epineural splint. *In* Gelberman R (ed): Operative Nerve Repair & Reconstruction. Philadelphia, J.B. Lippincott, 1991, pp 315–327.

Lister G: Histochemical and biochemical aids in nerve repair. *In* Gelberman R (ed): Operative Nerve Repair & Reconstruction. Philadelphia, J.B. Lippincott, 1991, pp 259–271.

McLellan DL, Swash M: Longitudinal sliding of the median nerve during movements of the upper limb. J Neurol Neurosurg Psychiatry *39*:566, 1976.

Millesi H, Terzis JK: Nomenclature in peripheral nerve surgery. Clin Plast Surg *11*:3, 1984.

Sunderland S: The intraneural topography of the radial, median and ulnar nerves. Brain *68*:243, 1945a.

Sunderland S: The adipose tissue of peripheral nerves. Brain *68*:118, 1945b.

Sunderland S: The pros and cons of funicular nerve repair. Founder's Lecture, the American Society for Surgery of the Hand. J Hand Surg *4*:201, 1979.

Wilgis EFSW, Murphy R: The significance of longitudinal excursion in peripheral nerves. Clin Hand Surg *2*:761–776, 1986.

Wilgis EFSW: Techniques of epineural and group fascicular repair. *In* Gelberman R (ed): Operative Nerve Repair & Reconstruction. Philadelphia, J.B. Lippincott, 1991, pp 287–295.

Chapter 28

• Jack W. Tupper

Fascicular Nerve Repair

Within a peripheral nerve, the nerve fiber (the axon and its sheath) is the smallest functional unit (Fig. 28–1). Bundles of these fibers contained in a specialized tubular membrane, the perineurium, form the smallest surgical unit, the fascicle (Figs. 28–2 and 28–3). (Note: In the older literature, funiculus equals fascicle.)

Fascicle size may vary from less than 0.1 mm to several millimeters in diameter. The fascicular contents are under axoplasmic pressure and are, therefore, always round in cross section. In contrast to the epineurium, the perineurium forms not only a physical but a physiological barrier, allowing preferential passage of some materials. Capillaries form the only true intrafascicular vessels. Breaching the perineurium of a fascicle in continuity causes at least local demyelinization. Therefore, lysis and repair of the contents within the perineurium is not only physically but physiologically impossible.

Fascicles may pass singly along the nerve, or in larger nerves, they may be arranged in groups (fascicular bundles). Surrounding fascicles and fascicular bundles, binding all together, is loose areolar tissue, the epineurial connective tissue. In this tissue are the blood and lymph vessels and sympathetic fibers to the arterioles. This areolar tissue surrounding the fascicle groups is condensed to form a suturable membrane. Surrounding all of these elements to form the outer layer of the peripheral nerve is a condensed membrane of the same material, the epineurial sheath (see Fig. 28–1).

It is the perineurium of the fascicle, the condensed epineurial connective tissue around the fascicular bundles, and the epineurial sheath that the peripheral nerve surgeon can identify and suture. From an anatomical standpoint, the nerve repairs may be of several types:

1. Epineurial: Sutures through the epineurial sheath only.
2. Epineurial plus a few sutures in the fascicles or fascicular bundles (in a large nerve).
3. Large bundle repair: Removal of epineurial sheath and suturing of the condensed epineurial connective tissue surrounding the fascicular bundles.
4. Perineurial: Both epineurial sheath and areolar epineurial connective tissue are discarded at the repair site. Fascicles are repaired with sutures in the perineurium only. Even in this type, groups of very small fascicles (less than 0.5 mm) are sutured as a unit.

There are approximately 25 fascicles in the median nerve at the wrist and 3 to 5 in a proper digital nerve (see Figs. 28–6 and 28–7). If an epineurial repair is done, there is gross orientation of the nerve ends but poor fascicular coaptation (Edshage, 1964). A tight closure inhibits escape of budding axons but may make an intraneurial hematoma more likely. Because a peripheral nerve is often 50% interfascicular tissue (Fig. 28–4), it would follow that regenerating axons would have a significant chance of not growing down a distal perineurial tube but rather into the tissue between the tubes. If motor and sensory fibers can be identified accurately, theoretically a larger number of functioning nerve fibers could regenerate to their proper end-organs. On the other hand, fascicular mismatch would preclude accurate return. Accurate fascicular matching can be done only in primary repair of sharply divided nerves by visual mapping. (Work

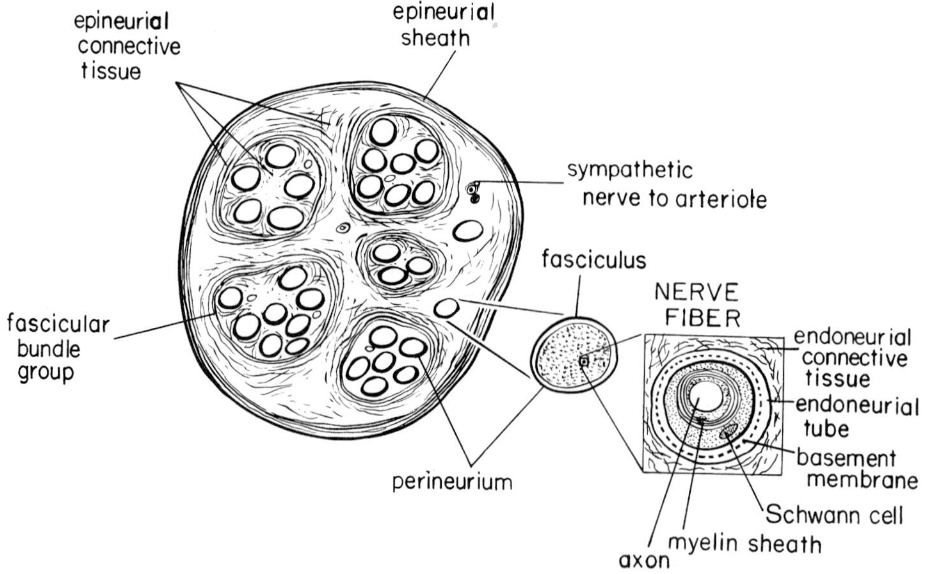

FIGURE 28–1. Composite peripheral nerve represented diagrammatically.

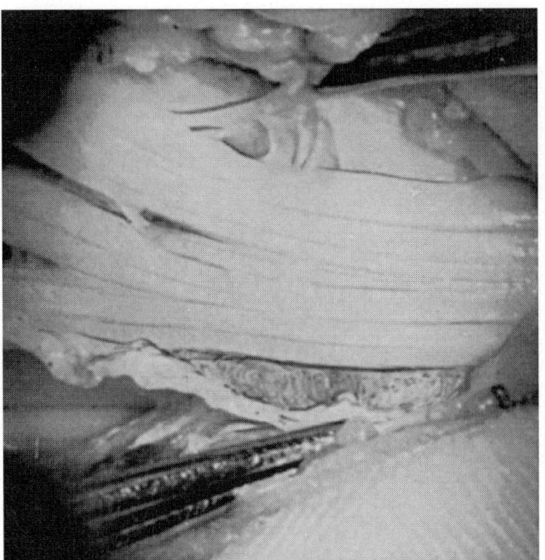

FIGURE 28–2. The two forceps hold the epineurial sheath. The median nerve at the wrist is seen trifurcating at the distal end of the carpal tunnel.

has been conducted on enzymatic identification, but it has not received widespread acceptance [Freilinger et al, 1975; Zhong et al, 1988].)

At the wrist level, the motor fasciculus of the median nerve is separate and can be identified distally by dissection from the known motor branch and proximally by visual mapping (Jabaley et al, 1980). Attempts have been made to do this by electrical stimulation at the time of surgery by Gaul (1983). The motor fascicle group of the ulnar nerve at the wrist is posteroulnar and readily identified (Chow et al, 1985; Jabaley et al, 1980). Proximal to 5 cm from the flexion crease of the wrist, there is motor-sensory mixing and specific identification is more difficult. Under these conditions epineurial repair may be the best approach rather than to chance a specific mismatch of motor to sensory nerves.

If a graft is to be used, the repair may be either epineurial or perineurial. The sural nerve is the usual donor. If a fascicular graft is to be used, the epineurium must be re-

moved and the fascicles dissected into a length determined by the distance between branching fascicles so that the length of a fascicular graft is one homogeneous strand. Not all fascicles within a nerve are useful; many are too small.

TECHNIQUE OF FASCICULAR REPAIR

An operating microscope is a necessity. A piece of ordinary light blue latex balloon serves nicely as a background. This is readily available, cheap, and nonreflective. A piece of long, narrow balloon yields a flatter surface than a spherical one. Frequent flushing, using a plastic balanced salt solution bottle* with a blunt needle, allows easier identifica-

---

*Alcon Company, P.O. Box 2664, Ft. Worth, TX 76161

FIGURE 28–3. This median nerve is seen with both a fascicle and a fascicular group dissected. A latex background is in place.

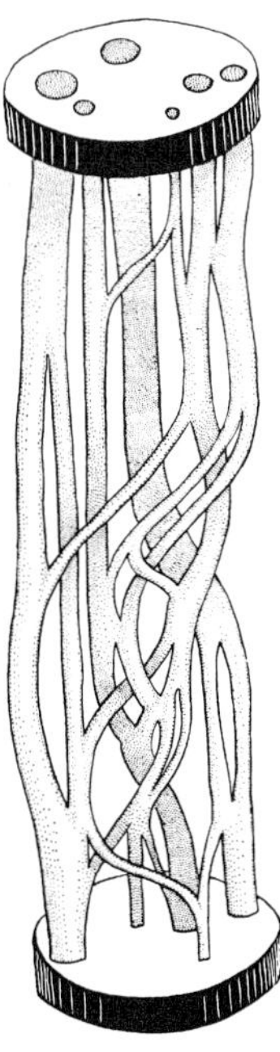

FIGURE 28–4. Fascicular pattern in peripheral nerves. (From Sunderland S: Nerves and Nerve Injuries. Baltimore, Williams & Wilkins, 1968.)

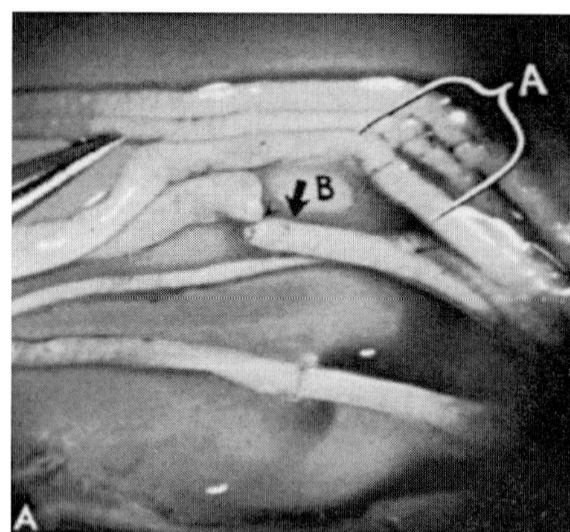
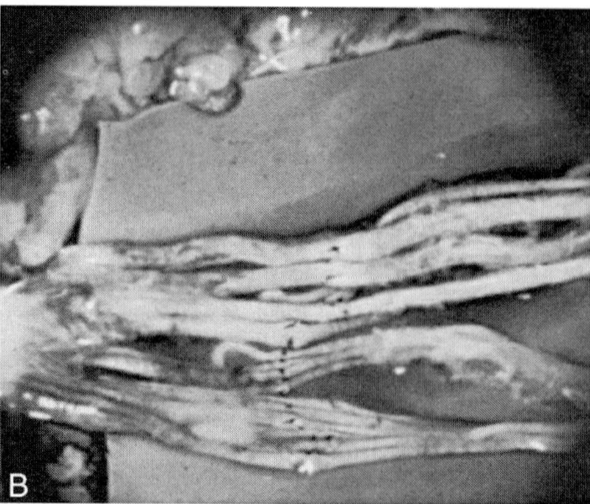

FIGURE 28–5. *A*, Fascicular graft. Graft segments (forceps) are sutured individually (A). Note one fascicle (B) with only one suture in place has poor approximation. *B*, Completed fascicular graft of ulnar nerve. Note the varying sizes of the fascicles.

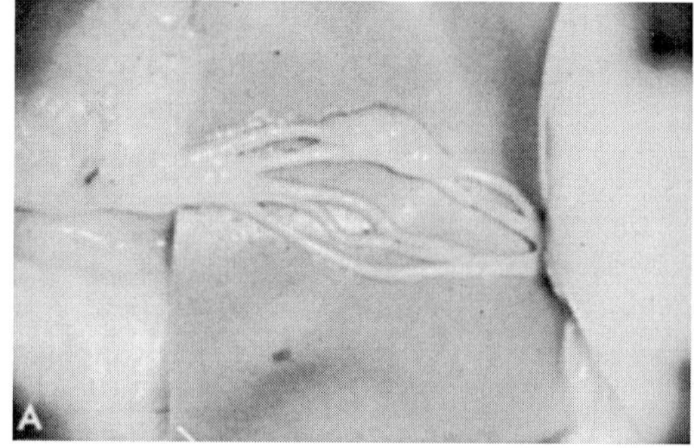
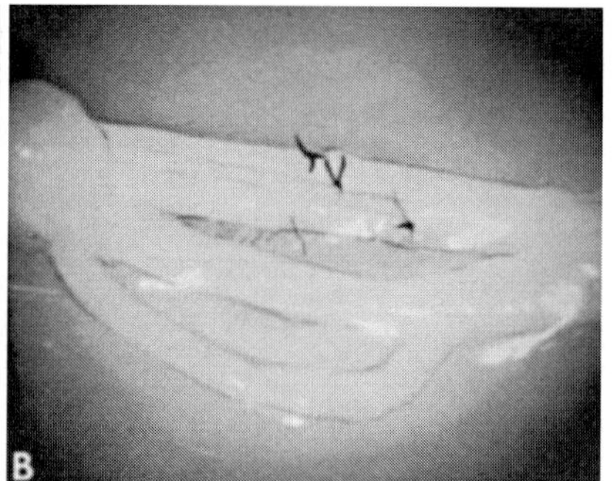

FIGURE 28–6. *A*, Partially divided digital nerve with some sensory loss and a painful neuroma. Two fascicles had been severed. *B*, Repair of the two severed fascicles resulted in improved sensation and loss of neuroma tenderness.

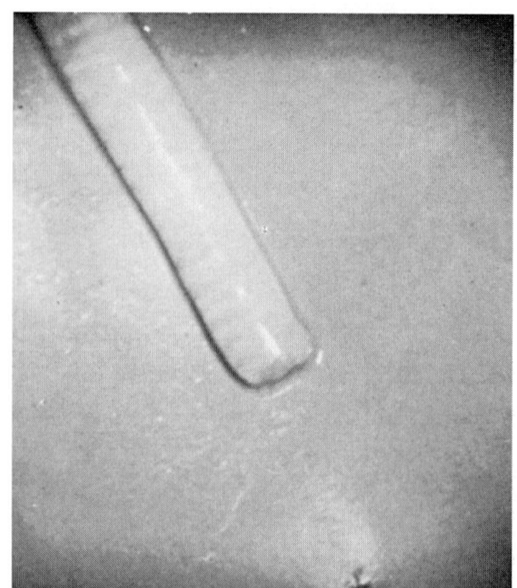

FIGURE 28–7. Single fascicle from a sural nerve. Note the spiral markings in the perineurium.

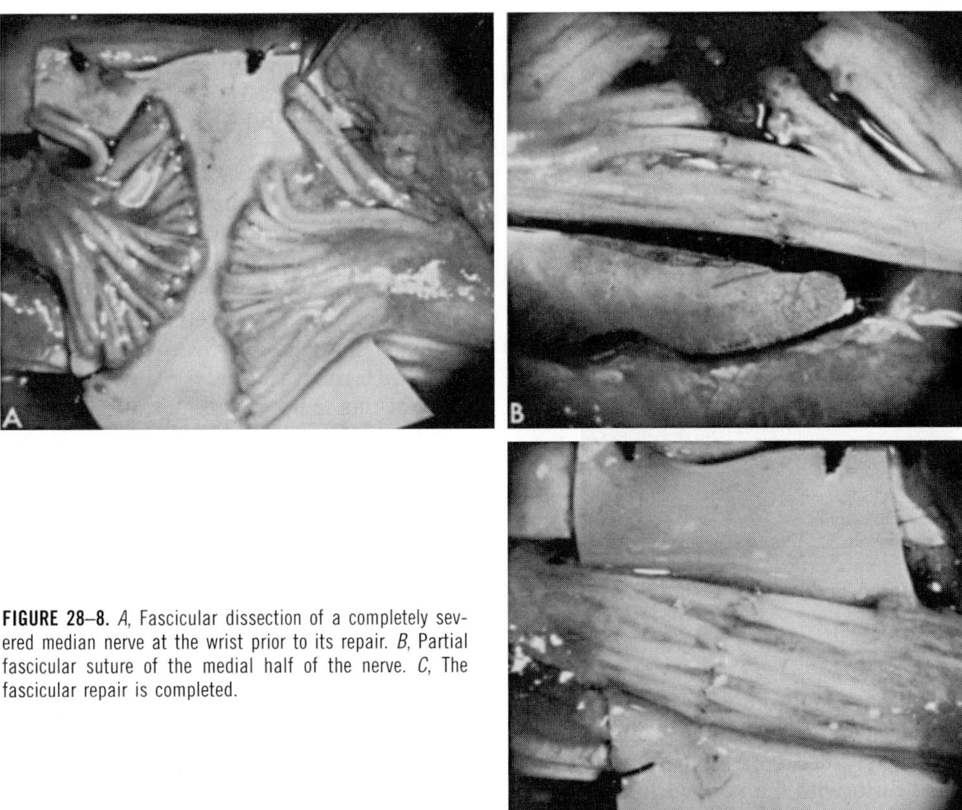

FIGURE 28–8. *A*, Fascicular dissection of a completely severed median nerve at the wrist prior to its repair. *B*, Partial fascicular suture of the medial half of the nerve. *C*, The fascicular repair is completed.

tion of tissue to be debrided. The irrigating solution is heparinized saline, which keeps the suture material from sticking to the wound surface and also tends to dissipate any static charge that may develop on the suture material. Depending on the situation, either the specific fascicles (recognizable motor) or, more commonly, fascicular groups can be isolated to accomplish repair at either the perineurial or the group fascicle level. Often the repair is a combination of the two. For perineurial suture, a 10–0 nylon on a 50-μm needle, either curved or 3 mm straight, is preferred (Figs. 28–5 and 28–6). It is difficult to do precise work with larger needles, and it is difficult to use a straight needle longer than 3 mm. (Stiffness increases by the cube as the length of the needle decreases.)

1. Dissect away the epineurial sheath from the end of the nerve for a distance approximately equal to the diameter of the nerve.

2. When dealing with a large nerve, very soon after injury, identify the fascicular bundles and dissect them initially as bundle groups, proximally and distally; match with what appear to be the corresponding units; and temporarily loosely suture. If dealing with the median or ulnar nerve at the wrist, identify the motor bundles and suture them first. If some bundles have had shredding of the enclosing epineurial connective tissue or have been cut on the bias, then dissect the fascicles from each other, removing the loose areolar tissue. Frequent flooding of the field will aid in cleanly repairing each fascicle. Each fascicle shows a spiral pattern in the perineurium (Fig. 28–7). These are the bands of fontana, pleats that disappear on axial stretch and reappear when tension is relaxed. The fascicles from two paired bundles

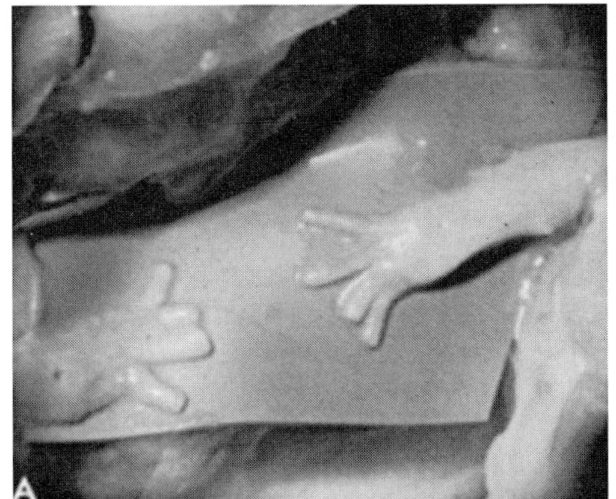

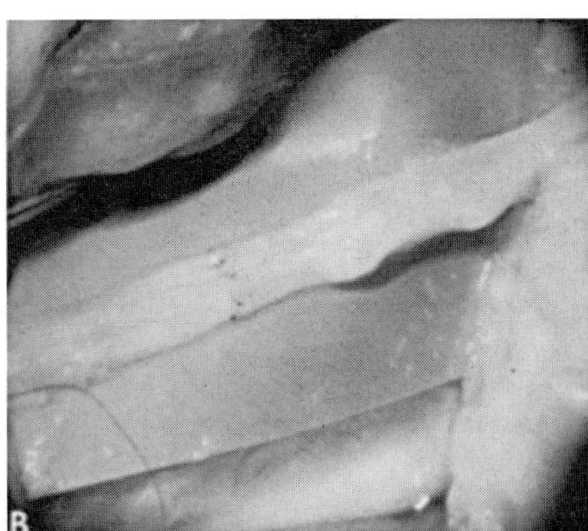

FIGURE 28–9. *A*, A digital nerve prepared for fascicular repair. *B*, The fascicular suture completed.

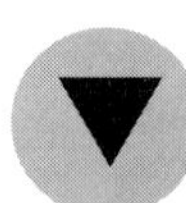

Chapter 29

• H. Millesi

Nerve Grafts:
Indications, Techniques, and Prognoses

BASIC CONSIDERATIONS

The logical technique for the repair of a transected peripheral nerve is end-to-end neurorrhaphy. In this procedure, there is only one gap and one site of coaptation that the regenerating axon sprouts must cross to reach the distal stump immediately. In an ideal situation, with no nerve defect, the fascicular structures of the proximal and the distal stumps are equal, and there is no jump in the fascicular pattern. If there is a defect caused by the changing fascicular pattern (Sunderland, 1951), a difference of the pattern exists that makes it more difficult for the axon sprouts to reach the proper peripheral destination. Having crossed the line of coaptation, into the endoneurium of the distal stump, the axons immediately find an optimal environment within the Büngner bands, which are columns, or tubes, of proliferated Schwann cells. These Büngner bands represent the end stage of wallerian degeneration caused by the nerve injury.

If the distance between the two nerve stumps is bridged by nerve graft, the regenerating axon must cross two lines of coaptation, one at the proximal and one at the distal end of the nerve graft. Thus, there are two jumps of the fascicular pattern. The environments that the axon sprouts meet within the nerve graft may be different, depending on the survival of the graft. If graft survival is optimal, the environmental conditions are identical in both nerve stumps. If graft survival is not optimal, fibrotic changes may impede the neurotization of the graft. The distal side of coaptation may be blocked by scar tissue when the axon sprouts arrive (Fig. 29–1).

There is general agreement that under optimal conditions, an end-to-end nerve repair offers the best chances of functional recovery. However, under less than optimal conditions, if end-to-end repair is impossible or unsuitable, nerve grafting offers excellent chances, provided that the unfavorable factors can be minimized. Because these unfavorable factors play different roles in different techniques, we cannot discuss nerve grafts in general but rather must consider the value of specific nerve grafting procedures. Among the many factors to be considered, the following are the most important:

1. Survival of the nerve graft
2. Optimal coaptation
3. Optimal imitation and restoration of the fascicular pattern of the nerve to be repaired by the nerve grafts
4. Minimal surgical trauma to reduce tissue damage

Survival of Nerve Grafts

As with other tissues, nerve tissue can be grafted as free or as vascularized nerve grafts. The free nerve graft remains after transplantation for a short period of time without blood supply. The restoration of circulation is achieved by vessels penetrating the surface of the graft. Optimum survival, therefore, depends on a soft tissue bed, which should contain many small vessels and no or minimal scar tissue, and on the relationship between the surface and the tissue mass of the graft. If a whole nerve trunk is grafted as a free graft, the time needed for spontaneous revascularization is too long to avoid anoxic damage to the central part of the graft. These parts develop fibrosis, and the Schwann cells may not survive.

Thin skin nerves, having a more favorable relationship between surface and mass, have a much better chance for complete survival if placed individually with circumferential contact to the wound bed. This advantage is lost if the skin nerves are packed together to form a cable of the size of the nerve to be repaired, as was done in the old cable graft technique (Seddon, 1947), because a great part of the surface is in contact with other grafts and not with the surrounding tissue.

It is important to note this difference and, therefore, cutaneous nerve grafts should be placed individually. We should stop talking about cable grafts if we mean cutaneous nerve grafting. If a nerve trunk is to be used as a free graft, such as the ulnar nerve in brachial plexus lesion with avulsion of C8 and T1, or if a limb was amputated and nerve trunks without function are available, we can split these nerve trunks by careful microscopic dissection according to their group pattern. By doing so, we can obtain long segments of fascicle groups without much crossing between the groups or of approximately the size of a cutaneous nerve. This procedure was called split nerve grafting (Eberhard and Millesi, 1996).

To avoid the problem of the initial ischemic periods of free nerve grafts, it was suggested already in the 1940s to transplant nerves like a pedicled flap, preserving their blood supply and using the complete grafting procedure (McCarty, 1951; Shelden, 1947; Strange, 1947; Strange, 1950). This technique can be used only if two nerve trunks running in parallel have been injured and then one is repaired at the expense of the other. The approach never became really popular and has become obsolete with the development of microsurgery.

The blood circulation within a nerve segment to be grafted can be preserved if a nerve trunk is transferred like an island flap on its vascular pedicle. The ischemic period can be minimized if a nerve trunk is transferred as a free flap and the blood supply is immediately restored by microvascular anastomosis (Taylor and Ham, 1976). It is obvious that the survival of a graft is optimal, even at an unfavorable recipi-

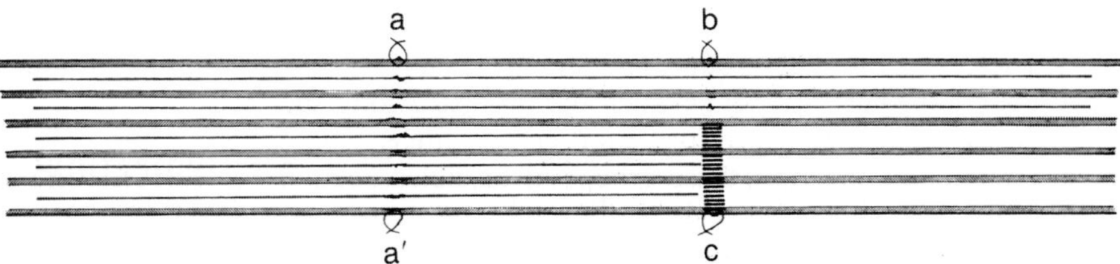

FIGURE 29–1. Nerve grafting. The proximal coaptation a–a' is crossed by axons. At the distal end, only a part of the axons reaches the distal nerve stump (b). At c, scar tissue blocks the further outgrowth of the axons. In this case, the distal site of coaptation is to be resected in a second stage with a new coaptation.

ent site, as long as the circulation is maintained. However, if an occlusion of the artery or the vein occurs, this nerve graft is completely lost. The relative merits of vascularized nerve grafts versus free nerve grafts are discussed later.

Optimal Coaptation

As long as the outgrowth of axons was believed to develop at random, according to the experiments of Weiss and Taylor (1944), optimal coaptation of the fascicular tissue was regarded as a basic requirement. Because long nonfascicular tissue represents between 40% and 60% of the cross-sectional area of polyfascicular nerve stump, a resection of the external epineurium and partially the interfascicular epineurium after interfascicular dissection of the stumps helps achieve optimal coaptation. Epineurial fibroblasts proliferate much faster than Schwann cells and tend to fill the gap between the two stumps. To reduce this proliferation and to give the slowly reproducing Schwann cells a better chance to fill the gap, a strip of epineurium is resected at the proximal and distal stumps.

Ideal healing is achieved if the two nerve stumps are coapted exactly under microsurgical vision, and tension at the site of coaptation is completely avoided (Millesi, 1977). If there is tension, the two cross sections of the two stumps tend to separate, and a zone of unstructured tissue develops between the two stumps that must be crossed by regenerating axon sprouts (Fig. 29–2).

Because the work of Lundborg and Hanson (1979) proved

in contrast to Weiss and Taylor (1944) that there is a tissue-specific outgrowth of axon sprouts, many studies have been focused on neurotropism.

The question can be raised whether a very exact coaptation might impede neurotropic effects and, therefore, a rather loose coaptation should be preferred. Consequently, Lundborg (1995) avoided close coaptation in end-to-end nerve repairs without defect and leaves the space between the two stumps protected from the outside by a silicone tube. However, a significant improvement was not achieved. In 1991 a symposium was organized to discuss this question (Millesi, 1990).

There is no question that neurotrophic effects exist—the question is rather the range of the effectivity. In nerve grafting procedures using cutaneous nerve grafts to connect fascicle groups of the proximal and the distal stump, a very exact coaptation of fascicular tissue is not possible owing to the different fascicular pattern. In spite of this fact, excellent recovery can be achieved (Millesi, 1981). This is most probably due to neurotropic and neurotrophic effects within fascicle groups. Brushart and colleagues (Brushart, 1993; Brushart and Seiler, 1987) demonstrated convincingly that in the first 2 weeks, the outgrowth of axons occurs at random, and only from the 3rd week onward, as an effect of neurotropism, the sprouts that are in the correct distal pathway survive and the ones having entered the wrong pathway degenerate. From this evidence, we may conclude that we still should try to obtain the best possible coaptation at the fascicular level, if we have to deal with large fascicles, or at the fascicle group level, if we have to deal with smaller fascicles of a polyfascicular pattern.

Restoration of Fascicular Pattern

Each nerve has an individual fascicular pattern. A trunk graft, even one from a corresponding donor nerve (e.g., median for a median nerve), has no identical fascicular pattern. The differences in the pattern are much more pronounced if another nerve, such as the ulnar nerve, is used to coapt with the median nerve in vascularized nerve grafting. Optimal restoration of the fascicular pattern cannot be achieved. However, a rough restoration of the pattern may be accomplished after preparing the two nerve stumps by interfascicular dissection into individual fascicles, or fascicle groups, respectively, as is discussed later.

Sunderland's (1945) description of the rapidly changing fascicular pattern and the plexiform arrangement of the fascicles within the nerve trunks seemed to make any attempts to restore the exact fascicular pattern impossible.

If intraneurial dissection of a peripheral nerve is performed, one will note that some fascicles are packed together more closely than others, forming groups. Between these

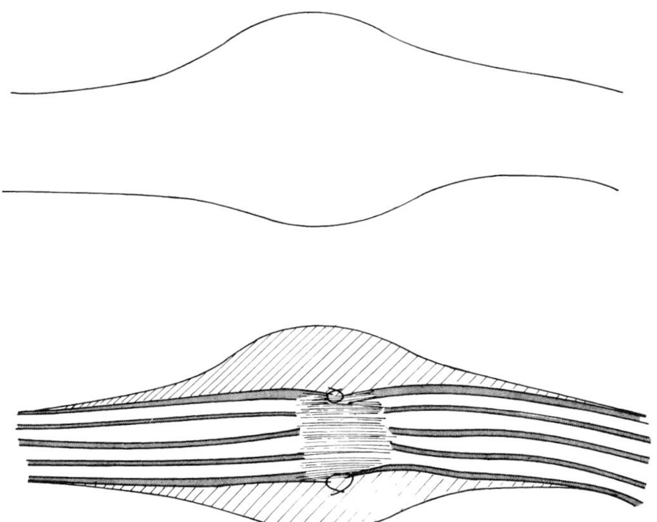

FIGURE 29–2. Scheme of a nerve repair showing the unstructured tissue between the stumps and the epineurial proliferation.

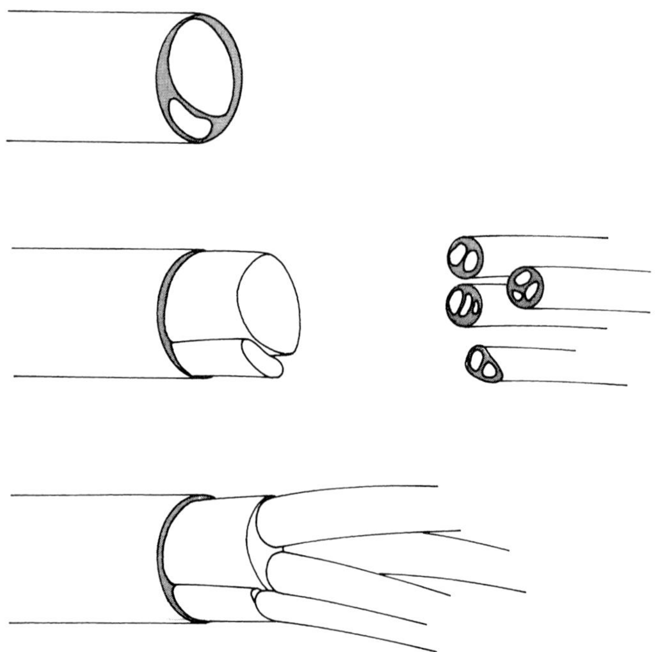

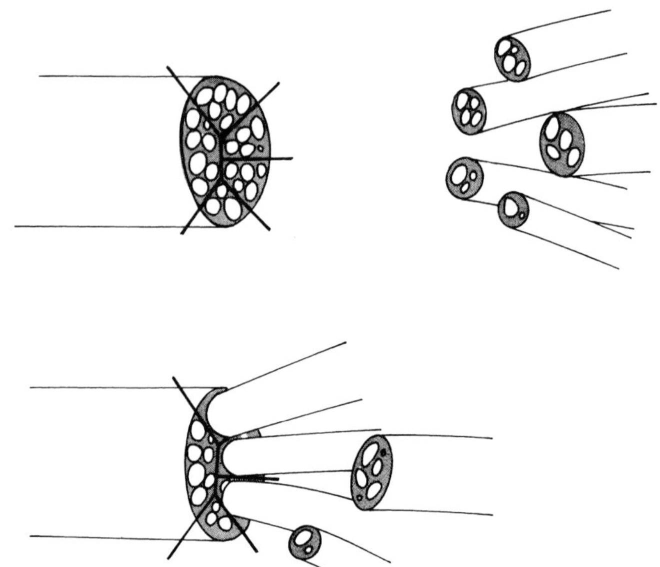

FIGURE 29–6. Coaptation (polyfascicular nerve without group arrangement). Each sector of the cross section is coapted with one graft (sectoral nerve grafting).

FIGURE 29–5. Coaptation (oligofascicular nerve). The cross section of the large fascicle is covered by three grafts (fascicular grafting 1:3) and the smaller one by one graft (fascicular grafting 1:1).

dissection in order to separate the fascicles and to perform a real fascicular nerve grafting, with each fascicle coapted to one graft. In this case, the preparation is done by interfascicular dissection and the epifascicular epineurium is resected.

POLYFASCICULAR NERVES WITH GROUP ARRANGEMENT

There are many, rather small fascicles of different sizes in the peripheral portion of the major nerve trunks. Proximal to the division of such a trunk, the fascicles destined for a specific branch are already arranged in a fascicle group. In many cases, this group arrangement is maintained proximally over varying distances. If this occurs, interfascicular dissection, as described above, can be performed. This internal arrangement is present in most of all peripheral nerves, in the distal portion, which is the most common site of nerve injuries. Under these circumstances the corresponding fascicle groups (see Fig. 24–5) are united by individual nerve grafts (interfascicular nerve grafting; (see Fig. 29–5).

The individual fascicle groups separated by interfascicular dissection are transected at different levels. After coapting the nerve grafts to these fascicle groups, an interdigitation between the fascicle groups and the nerve grafts can be achieved in a way that each graft has not only an end-to-end coaptation with the fascicle group but also has side-to-side contact with neighboring fascicle groups. This approach helps stabilize the coaptation, and it is, therefore, rarely necessary to use more than one stitch per each graft. Coaptation is maintained by normal fibrin coagulation, and the application of glues seems not to be necessary.

POLYFASCICULAR NERVES WITHOUT GROUP ARRANGEMENT

These are nerves consisting of many fascicles that are not arranged in fascicle groups but are distributed rather dif-

fusely over the cross section. These fascicular patterns can be met at very proximal levels such as at the root level of brachial plexus. These fascicular patterns are also present at particular levels of peripheral nerves where major exchange of fibers between the groups occurs.

In this case, no attempt for interfascicular resection is undertaken. Each section of the cross section is covered by a nerve graft (Fig. 29–6), until the whole cross section is satisfied.

An attempt to perform a fascicular nerve grafting procedure in a polyfascicular nerve with many small fascicles without group arrangement, as suggested by Tupper (1980), is not recommended. Too much surgical trauma is involved to isolate each fascicle. The identification of corresponding fascicles is impossible. Also, the grafts are to be split into individual fascicles, to achieve a proper size relationship (Fig. 29–7).

If a vascularized nerve graft is to be used, the preparation of the stumps has to be by segmental resection and a trunk-to-trunk coaptation has to be performed. This is actually due to the unpredictable intraneurial arrangement of the fascicles

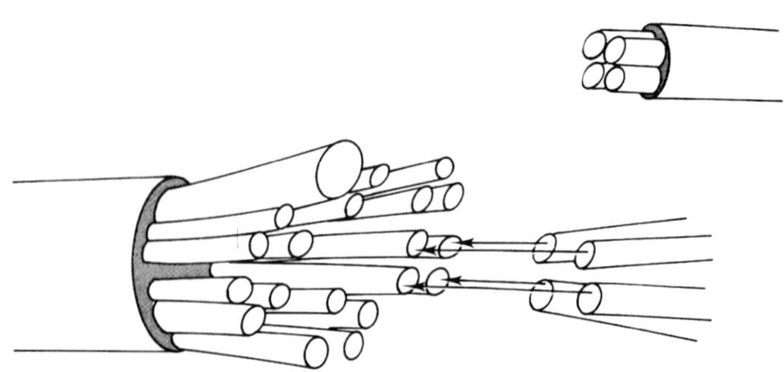

FIGURE 29–7. To achieve a fascicular coaptation in a polyfascicular nerve, each fascicle has to be isolated and the graft split into its individual fascicles. This involves too much surgical trauma. The identification of corresponding fascicles is impossible. Therefore, this procedure is not recommended.

in a nerve trunk over a long distance. It cannot be predicted whether the specific axons, entering the proximal end of the graft at a specific point, would leave a vascularized graft at the distal end.

Harvesting a Nerve Graft

After the stumps have been prepared and the tourniquet removed, precise hemostasis is performed using bipolar coagulation. The surgeon now must decide on several questions:

1. Should a free nerve graft or a vascularized nerve graft be used?
2. What is the proper length of the nerve graft?
3. Which nerve graft is to be used?

Whether to Use a Free Nerve Graft or a Vascularized Nerve Graft

After introduction of the vascularized nerve grafts, there were great expectations that these vascularized nerve grafts would be significantly superior to the free nerve grafts, as far as the results are concerned. In this case, vascularized nerve grafting should have become the treatment of choice. Because vascularized trunk grafts are not always available without creating a functional loss, an enormous amount of anatomical studies has focused on making expandable nerves, like the sural nerve and the saphenous nerve, available as vascularized nerve grafts (Townsend and Taylor, 1984). However, these expectations were not realized.

It could not be proved that vascularized nerve grafts are much superior to free nerve grafts, provided that conditions are equal. Of course, if the recipient site does not provide optimal conditions for free grafting, a vascularized nerve graft is the better choice, because it is independent of the recipient bed. The vascularized nerve graft is certainly not as sensitive to longitudinal traction as is the free nerve graft. The vascularized nerve graft also provides gliding tissue and does not form adhesions with the surrounding tissue as the free nerve graft has to do in order to survive.

The disadvantage of the vascularized nerve graft is the fact that, as already mentioned, it is not possible to connect elected points of the proximal stump with elected points of the distal stump. There is the possibility of the vascular complication with complete loss of the graft. Because we know well that Schwann cells do survive free grafting in spite of the ischemic period (Aguayo et al, 1977a, 1977b), the advantage of avoiding the ischemic period is not too important.

A personal series of brachial plexus cases, in which vascularized nerve grafts were used to neurotize one muscle and free nerve grafts were used to neurotize another muscle, did not show significant superiority of the vascularized nerve grafts. It was suggested (Doi et al, 1984) that vascularized nerve grafts are the only way to successfully bridge long defects. This might be true for very long defects (30 cm, or more) because they have to be bridged, such as in the C7 transfer from the same side to the contralateral avulsed brachial plexus. If a trunk graft should be used as a nerve

graft, it can be used only as a vascularized graft. Otherwise, if a trunk graft is a donor of free nerve grafting, it has to be split into minor units (Eberhard and Millesi, 1996).

In summary, the free nerve graft remains the workhorse of nerve grafting. Vascularized nerve grafts have their place in the treatment of nerve defects and offer relative advantages, especially if there are unfavorable conditions for free grafting as far as the recipient site is concerned.

What Is the Proper Length of the Nerve Graft?

Seddon (1975, p 194) recommended approximating the two ends of the nerve to be repaired as much as possible and to bridge the remaining defect by nerve grafts. This was certainly one of the reasons for the limited success of nerve grafts at this period. If one approximates the two nerve stumps as much as possible, such as by flexing the adjacent joints, a shorter nerve graft can be used. However, this procedure combines the disadvantages of a suture under tension with the disadvantage of having two sites of coaptation at the distal end of the nerve graft. As already mentioned, nerve grafts are very sensitive to longitudinal traction, because they have to form adhesions in order to survive and they are, therefore, not mobile. When the flexed joints are mobilized again, the proximal and the distal site of coaptation of the graft are exposed to traction and tension.

Instead of electing the length of the graft according to the *minimal* defect, it is much better to elect the length of the graft according to the *maximal* defect. This means to bring the joints in extended position first, then to measure the length of the distance between the two stumps in this situation, and then to elect the length of the graft by 20% longer than the length of the distance, in order to have a relaxed situation. If after grafting in this relaxed situation the limb is mobilized again, the nerve graft is rather relaxed and extended. This provides a big advantage, because after a nerve grafting procedure performed in this way, the time of immobilization is not longer than 8 days.

The advantage of this procedure can be offset, however, if the limb is immobilized in flexed position postoperatively. Even if the graft has been elected in proper length, the graft will form adhesions now in the flexed, relaxed position and will be fixed in this position. After the period of immobilization, when the limb will be mobilized again, the graft will not be able to adapt to the extended position and, therefore, a difficult situation will exist as if the graft had been elected too short from the beginning. Likewise, an excessively long graft will buckle and kink, producing untoward consequences.

The disadvantage of electing the graft in extended position would mean that a longer graft will have to be used. In the literature, one can find information that the result is relative to the length of the graft—and this would be a strong indication to use short nerve grafts! However, the conclusion is based on a misunderstanding of the problem.

The result deteriorates with the length of the nerve defect. It is obvious that the longer the nerve defect is, the greater is the difference in the fascicular pattern, and the more difficult it might be for the axons to find the proper destination. But the length of a nerve defect is not the same as the distance between the two stumps. If there is a given nerve defect, the distance can be arranged by flexing and extending the adjacent joints. With the same nerve defect in an extended position, a longer graft is needed. In this case, the length of the graft within certain limits does not play a significant role as far as the result is concerned, which is determined by the length of the nerve defect. It is, therefore, no real disadvantage if we elect longer grafts to bridge the same nerve defect in an extended position.

Which Nerve Is To Be Used?

SURAL NERVE

The sural nerve is ideal for grafting. One can obtain a piece of nerve 30 to 40 cm in length. This nerve divides distally behind the lateral maleolus. The sural nerve is a branch of the posterior tibial nerve arising behind the knee joints. It receives an additional communicating branch from the peroneus nerve, which unites at different levels with the fibers coming from the posterior tibial nerve. In the strict sense of anatomical nomenclature, the sural nerve would begin after the merging of these two sources. However, in clinical practice, we are using the term ''sural nerve'' for the total length of the nerve up to its origin from the posterior tibialis nerve.

The sural nerve can be exposed through a small transverse incision behind the lateral area of the ankle, following the lines of Langer. The proximal course of the nerve can be palpated by a gentle pull. A second incision is made 3 or 4 cm proximal, and the sural nerve, which can be bound with the short saphenous vein, can be lifted on a tape. After transection of the main trunk of the nerve at the level of the first incision, two or three additional branches can be palpated at this level by a gentle longitudinal tugging at the second incision. After these branches have been defined and transected, the nerve can easily be extracted through the second incision. Again, the course of the nerve is located by pulling longitudinally and palpating the calf more proximally. Usually, two more incisions, one at the lower border of the popliteal fossa and one in the middle of the calf, are sufficient to excise the whole nerve.

If a very long nerve graft is needed, the sural nerve can be followed in a proximal direction within the posterior tibial and sciatic nerve. It forms a distinct fascicle group in these nerves and can be excised up to the middle of the thigh without significant damage to other fascicle groups. If the nerve is followed by continuous palpation under gentle traction of the distal end, the communicating branch from the peroneus nerve can be located and harvested as well, using additional small transverse incisions. If a nerve stripper is used, the communicating peroneus branch might be destroyed, which is certainly a disadvantage outweighing the facility otherwise offered by the stripping technique.

In order to avoid traction, some surgeons prefer to use a long longitudinal excision with complete exposure of the sural nerve. Such long incisions are justified in babies for obstetric brachial plexus surgery, because the sural nerve is very thin and can be damaged easily. In adults, however, we think that the sequence of transverse incision is the better choice also from the cosmetic point of view. The traction during extraction of the nerve is not the real trauma, because the nerve will undergo wallerian degeneration anyway and what we need is the connective tissue framework with the Schwann cells, and not the endoneureal structures themselves. At the present time, harvesting the sural nerve with endoscopic techniques may become an alternative.

Attempts were made to use the sural nerve as a vascularized nerve graft. Fachinelli and colleagues (1981) and Gilbert (1982) developed a technique to transplant the sural nerve as a vascularized nerve graft with the arteria suralis superficialis, a branch of the arteria suralis medialis or lateralis, as a pedicle.

Doi and associates (1984) used a muscle branch of the peroneal artery with a skin island for observation of the circulation. Townsend and Taylor (1984) used the small saphenous vein for an anastomosis with an artery to arterialize the venous system. Gu and co-workers (1985) used the sural nerve including a skin flap as a free tissue transfer for covering a skin defect and repairing the nerve simultaneously.

MEDIAN CUTANEOUS NERVE OF THE FOREARM

This nerve is located at the lower border of the axillary grove. After incising the fascia, the nerve is found in close proximity to the brachial vein. Usually through two or more incisions, one in the mid-arm and the other at the elbow level, the medial cutaneous nerve of the forearm can be excised. One can obtain an about 20-cm graft.

LATERAL FEMORAL CUTANEOUS NERVE

This nerve is exposed through a transverse incision below the anterior superior iliac spine. By a gentle pull and distal palpation, the further course of the nerve is defined. The whole nerve is excised through several transverse incisions. About 20 cm of nerve tissue can be obtained. If more is needed, the nerve can be followed into the pelvic cavity and resected there.

SUPERFICIAL RADIAL NERVE

This nerve has been sacrificed on a few occasions to cover defects of the brachial plexus when an enormous amount of nerve grafts were needed. Otherwise the author would not use this nerve, especially if the median nerve or the ulnar nerve of the same extremity is involved, because of increased sensory loss due to overlapping of the cutaneous nerve territories. In addition, the superficial radial nerve tends to develop painful neuromas. The superficial radial nerve has been used occasionally as a vascularized nerve graft, either alone or in conjunction with a radialis forearm flap.

LATERAL ANTEBRACHIAL CUTANEOUS NERVE

This is the terminal branch of the musculocutaneous nerve, and it is identified at the lateral border of the biceps tendon. It has been used successfully by McFarlane and associates (1976).

SAPHENOUS NERVE

This nerve has been used in rare instances. It should not be excised if the sural nerve of the same extremity is to be harvested as well. The loss of sensibility incurred will be greater than the sum of the zone of hypesthesia after an isolated nerve graft excision. The saphenous nerve is a proper donor for a vascularized nerve graft.

THE DORSAL CUTANEOUS BRANCH OF THE ULNAR NERVE

This nerve yields only a rather small nerve graft and has not been used.

INTERCOSTAL NERVES

These nerves have the advantage that they contain both motor and sensory fibers, rather than sensory fibers only, as do the other donors. However, because they have many branches along their course, a great number of axons are lost. Intercostal nerves, therefore, are used mainly as axon donors in brachial plexus cases and not as nerve grafts.

CERVICAL PLEXUS

The sensory branches of the cervical plexus can be used to restore the facial nerve.

ULNAR NERVE

The ulnar nerve can be used as a nerve graft only if no functional loss is caused by harvesting the nerve. This is the case if there is an upper arm amputation or an avulsion of the roots C8 and T1 in brachial plexus lesions. Bonney and colleagues (1954) used the ulnar nerve as a vascularized nerve graft based on the brachial artery and vein. Breidenbach and Terzis (1983, 1984) studied the vascular anatomy of nerves in a very profound way. They realized that the whole ulnar nerve can depend on the superior collateral ulnar artery. This artery may serve as pedicle to transpose the nerve in proximal direction to bridge defects within the brachial plexus, but it is also suitable for vascularized anastomosis in free grafting. If transfer of the ulnar nerve as a vascularized graft is not possible or not suitable, the ulnar nerve can be split into minor units to be used as free nerve grafts.

PERONEUS NERVE

The superficial peroneus nerve was one of the nerves used early as vascularized nerve grafts (Taylor and Ham, 1976). Comtet* suggested using the peroneus nerve as a vascularized nerve graft to bridge defects of the sciatic nerve. This suggestion is based on the fact that in sciatic nerve lesions, the muscles innervated by the tibialis posterior nerve do recover well, but the muscles innervated by the peroneus nerve do not. It seemed, therefore, justified to concentrate on the tibialis posterior nerve in large sciatic nerve lesion and sacrifice the peroneus nerve. The peroneus nerve in such conditions can be used also as a split nerve graft.

---

*Personal communication, 1984.

Preparation of the Graft

The two ends of the graft have to be prepared carefully. In free nerve grafts, especially if the graft is already in place and has to be trimmed, we prefer to use special scissors with eradicated plates to avoid shifting the nerve tissue when cutting. The nerve is transected fascicle by fascicle, each time the epineurium is shifted slightly away from the cut end (Fig. 29–8). Overlapping of the cut surface by epineurium must be avoided. It is not necessary to resect the epineurium at both ends of the nerve graft. Because the grafts are free grafts, the epineurium will begin to proliferate after circulation of the graft is restored with a certain delay, depending on epineurial proliferation of the two nerve stumps. There is no danger that epineurial proliferation originating from the graft will interfere with the neurial regenerative process at the site of coaptation.

Vascularized nerve grafts are prepared by segmental resection in the usual manner.

DEFINITION OF CORRESPONDING FASCICLES AND FASCICLE GROUPS IN PROXIMAL AND DISTAL STUMPS

As we approach the division of a nerve, we find that more and more nerve fibers of a particular function are arranged in well-defined fascicle groups. This is in contrast to the more proximal sites, where the fibers are rather diffusely distributed over the cross-sectional area.

The end result depends on the recognition of corresponding fascicle groups. It is essential to unite motor fascicles of the proximal stump with motor fascicles of the peripheral stump. The staining technique of Gruber and Zenker (1973), which was applied by Freilinger and colleagues (1975), allows the surgeon to recognize the presence of motor fibers in a biopsy. Recent improvements in the technique have reduced the necessary time to get the result of this study based on the concentration of acetylcholine esterase within several hours, which means that the results will be available during a long operation.

One can also get an exact idea of the fascicular pattern of the peripheral stump by exposing the nerve until it branches, and then following the individual fascicles in a proximal direction. A sketch is made of the fascicular pattern of the distal stump. Another sketch is made of the fascicular pattern of the proximal stump. By matching the sketches, an approximate assumption is made of the corresponding fascicle groups in the proximal stump and the distal stump. The

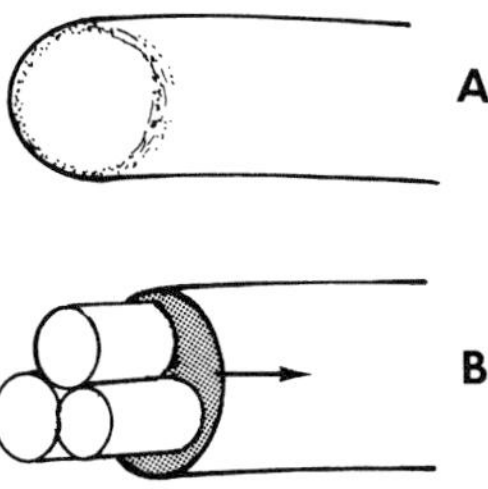

FIGURE 29–8. The epineurium may overlap the cut end of the graft *(A)*. It has to be shifted away before coaptation *(B)*.

functional result indicates that in the majority of cases, the guess has been correct. The well-defined points of the proximal and distal stumps are then united by individual segments of cutaneous nerve grafts. Of course, this selective technique cannot be applied if vascularized nerve grafts are used.

Approximation and Coaptation

The individual segments of free grafts are placed into the defect. A graft is selected for each fascicle group, the fascicular pattern of the sural nerve changes along its course. In a proximal level, it consists of one or a few fascicles, but the number of fascicles increases toward the periphery. Of course, one tries to select the best-fitting graft for each fascicle group. The graft is approximated to the cross-sectional area of the fascicle group using a 10.0 nylon stitch, which catches the epineurium of the graft. The suture is anchored in the remaining interfascicular connective tissue between the fascicles of the group (Fig. 29–9A) or in the perineurium of one of the fascicles of this group (Fig. 29–9B).

By manipulating the ends of the stitches, the graft is approximated to the cut end of the fascicle group, and without touching the nerve tissue. Now much attention is paid to achieve optimal coaptation of the fascicular tissue. If the extension is in a longitudinal direction, the approximation is close to the point where the suture is located, and because of the tension, the opposite perineurial and endoneurial tissue tend to separate (Fig. 29–10A and B). Thus, more stitches are needed to provide abutment of the cut ends. If tension is avoided completely, as it is a condition for this type of nerve grafting, good contact of the whole surface of each end can be achieved with one stitch, especially if the

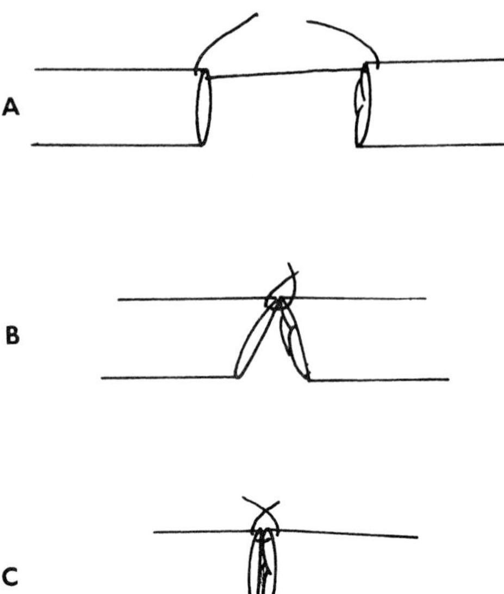

FIGURE 29–10. Coaptation by one stitch *(A)* under slight tension *(B)*. The site of the stitch is coapted but the remaining cross-sectional area is still spreading apart. If tension is avoided, one loose stitch is sufficient to achieve a broad contact of the whole cross section *(C)*.

stitch is placed in the correct point (Fig. 29–10C). If optimal contact is achieved between the whole surface of the two ends, no further attempt needs to be made to secure the coaptation. Natural fibrin clotting is sufficient to maintain the coaptation, if tension is completely avoided! This is especially the case if grafts and fascicle groups of a polyfascicular nerve with group arrangements are interdigitated. The tensile strength of such a neural juncture is minimal but sufficient if the graft is long enough and there is no separating force. In this way, grafting procedures can be performed with minimal surgical trauma or foreign body reaction. It cannot be stressed enough that the whole technique is based on coaptation without tension. A compromise in this regard will yield a poor result.

It has been suggested that the coaptation can be secured by the application of tissue glue. There is a vast literature on the advantages of application of tissue glue. In the early years, it was strictly recommended that tissue glue should not interfere with the cross-sectional area of the coaptation. Now this seems not to be important. All surgeons supporting the application of tissue glue are also using some stitches, especially for manipulation. The author believes that if tension is completely avoided, these stitches are enough to maintain the coaptation. An additional application of tissue glue may make the coaptation safer against longitudinal traction, but if the advice to keep longitudinal traction to zero is followed, it is not really necessary.

The coaptation vascularized nerve graft is performed as a trunk-to-trunk coaptation secured by epineurial stitches.

Wound Closure

After hemostasis has been achieved, the skin wound is closed very carefully to avoid shearing forces, which might dislocate the grafts. No suction drainage is used.

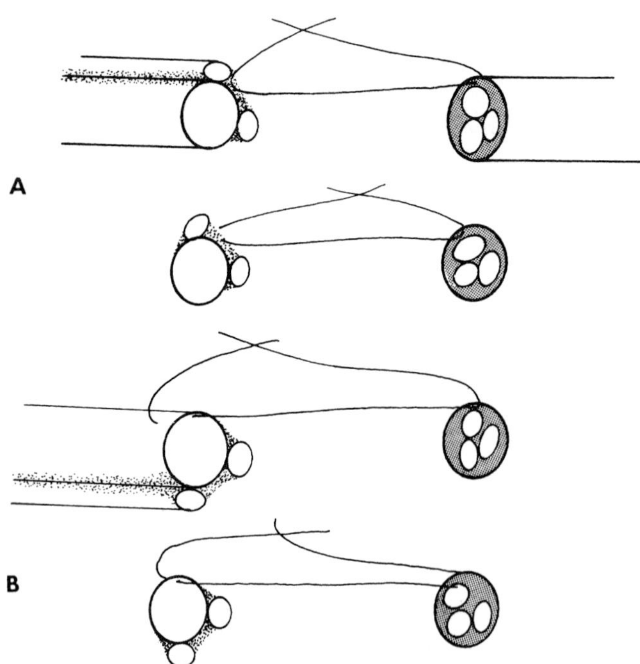

FIGURE 29–9. Approximation of the graft *(right)* to a fascicle group *(left)*. One stitch catches the epineurium of the graft and the interfascicular tissue *(A)* of the fascicle group or the perineurium of one fascicle of the graft and of the fascicle group *(B)*.

Immobilization

The extremity is immobilized in the exact position in which it was placed during the operation. An exact immobilization is extremely important, especially during the first 24 hours and the first postoperative days. Experiments have shown that the tensile strength after such a grafting operation, using a few stitches and natural fibrin coagulation, increases during the first days. After 6 days, tensile strength reaches a sufficiently high level to allow mobilization. Therefore, from a clinical viewpoint, active and passive mobilization can start 8 days after surgery.

PROGNOSIS

Resection of Distal Coaptation

It has already been mentioned that scar tissue formation at the peripheral end of the graft may cause an obstacle for further advancement of the axon sprouts. The frequency of this problem depends on the amount of connective tissue reaction at the distal end of the graft and on the time elapsed since the grafting procedure when the axons reach the distal neural junction. In our first 50 operations, the scar block at the distal coaptation was observed in seven patients (14%). One gets suspicious that a scar block may have formed if the Tinel-Hoffmann sign, after having advanced along the graft, then stops with its maximum at the distal end of the graft and does not proceed. If this situation remains unchanged for 2 or 3 months, surgical exploration is indicated. If thickening is detected at the distal suture site, it is resected and a new coaptation performed. In the majority of the cases, the Tinel-Hoffmann sign resumes its advancement and useful recovery occurs.

In later operations, the frequency of the scar block has decreased and is now between 1% and 2%. One must bear this possibility in mind. A lack of understanding is demonstrated by one who reports on failure of nerve grafts and does not even mention the possibility of a block at the distal suture site.

Reasons for Failure of Nerve Grafting

Many factors influence the quality of nerve regeneration, but in general, advanced age of the patient and a long interval following neural injury and treatment are unfavorable factors. In some cases, the results have been compromised by delayed wound healing and infection. Scars crossing the nerve graft may cause compression and impede regeneration. The plastic surgical procedure before or at the time of nerve grafting can prevent this outcome. In one case avulsion of the graft, including the proximal and distal coaptation sites, was observed. After new resection of the nerve stumps, the grafting procedure was repeated and satisfactory regeneration occurred. No reason for the occurrence of fibrosis could be detected. One might suspect that rupture of one of the suture sites may cause some failures, but the findings in the author's cases proved contrary. In the number of cases that the author re-explored for any reason, the author observed that in none of these cases, a rupture of the suture site had occurred.

References

Aguayo AJ, Attiwell M, Trecarten J, Perkins S, Bray GM: Abnormal myelination in transplanted Tremblar mouse Schwann cells. Nature *265*:73–75, 1977a.

Aguayo AJ, Kasarjian J, Skamene E, Kongshavn P, Bray GM: Myelination of mouse axons by Schwann cells transplanted from normal and abnormal human nerves. Nature *268*:753–755, 1977b.

Bonney G, Birch R, Jamieson AM, Eames R: Experience with vascularized nerve grafts. Clin Plast Surg *11*:137, 1954.

Breidenbach WB, Terzis JK: Vascularised nerve grafts. (Scholarship Contest) American Society for Plastic and Reconstructive Surgery, 1983.

Breidenbach WB, Terzis JK: The anatomy of free vascularised nerve grafts. Clin Plast Surg *11*:65–71, 1984.

Brushart TM: Motor axons preferentially reinnervated motor pathway. J Neurosci *13*:2730–2738, 1993.

Brushart TM, Seiler WA: Selective reinnervation of distal motor stumps by peripheral motor axons. Exp Neurol 97:290–300, 1987.

Doi K, Kuwata N, Kawakami F, Tamaru K, Kawai S: Free vascularized sural nerve graft. Microsurgery 5:175–184, 1984.

Eberhard D, Millesi H: Split nerve grafting. J Reconstr Microsurg *12*:71–76, 1996.

Fachinelli A, Masquelet A, Restrepo J, Gilbert A: The vascularized sural nerve. Anatomy and surgical approach. Int J Microsurg *3*:57, 1981.

Freilinger G, Gruber H, Holle J, Mandl H: Zur Methodik der sensomotorisch differentierten Faszikelnaht peripherer Nerven. Handchirurgie 7:133, 1975.

Gilbert A: Vascularized nerve grafts. Paper presented at Reconstructive Microsurgery. An indepth course in microsurgery. Oklahoma City, May 24–28, 1982.

Gruber H, Zenker W: Acetylcholinesterase: Histochemical differentiation between motor and sensory fibers. Brain Res *51*:207, 1973.

Gu YD, Wu MM, Zheng YH, Li HR, Xu YN: Arterialized venous free sural nerve grafting. Ann Plast Surg 15:332–339, 1985.

Lundborg G, Hansson HA: Regeneration of a peripheral nerve through a preformed tissue space. Brain Res *178*:573, 1979.

Lundborg G: Presentation at the Meeting of the American Society for Surgery of the Hand in San Francisco, September, 1995.

McCarty CS: Two-stage autograft for repair of extensive damage to sciatic nerve. J Neurosurg 8:319, 1951.

McFarlane RM, Mayer: Digital nerve grafts with the lateral cutaneous nerve. J Hand Surg *1*:169–173, 1976.

Meissl G: Die intraneurale Topographie des extrakraniellen Nervus facialis. Acta Chirurgica Austriaca (Suppl 28):1–17, 1979.

Millesi H: Healing of nerves. Clin Plast Surg 4:459–473, 1977.

Millesi H: How exact should coaptation be? *In* Gorio A, Millesi H, Mingrino S (eds): Posttraumatic Peripheral Nerve Regeneration (Experimental Basis and Clinical Implications). New York, Raven Press, 1981, pp 301–304.

Millesi H: Peripheral nerve surgery today: Turning point or continuous development? J Hand Surg *15B*:281–285, 1990.

Seddon HJ: The use of autogenous grafts for the repair of large gaps in peripheral nerves. Br J Surg *35*:151, 1947.

Seddon HJ: Surgical Disorders of the Peripheral Nerves, 2nd ed. Edinburgh, Churchill Livingstone, 1975, pp 194, 297.

Shelden CH, Pudenz C, McCarthy S: Two stage autograft for repair of extensive median and ulnar nerve defects. J Neurosurg 4:492–496, 1947.

Sunderland S: The intraneural topography of the radial, median and ulnar nerve. Brain 68:243, 1945.

Sunderland S: A classification of peripheral nerve injuries producing loss of function. Brain 74:491, 1951.

Strange FG St C: An operation for nerve pedicle grafting. Preliminary communication. Br J Surg 34:423, 1947.

Strange FG St C: Case report on pedicled nerve graft. J Surg 331, 1950.

Taylor GI, Ham FJ: The free vascularized nerve graft. Plast Reconstr Surg 57:413–426, 1976.

Townsend PLG, Taylor GI: Vascularised nerve grafts using composite arterialised neuro-venous systems. Br J Plast Surg *37*:1–17, 1984.

Tupper J: Fascicular nerve repair. *In* Jewett DL, McCarrol HR (eds): Nerve Repair and Regeneration: Its Clinical and Experimental Basis. St. Louis, CV Mosby, 1980, p 320.

Weiss P, Taylor AC: Further experimental evidence against "neurotropism" in nerve regeneration. J Exp Zool 95:233, 1944.

Nerve Lengthening Using Balloon Expansion

One of the most significant advances in peripheral nerve surgery has been the successful use of autologous nerve grafts to repair gaps in peripheral nerves following injury. The success of nerve grafts is well documented, and it remains the standard technique for the management of nerve gaps (Mackinnon, 1989; Millesi, 1986; Terzis, 1975). There are some circumstances in which nonvascularized nerve grafts are not an ideal choice for overcoming nerve gaps, and there are reports that regeneration following nerve grafting does not compare with direct nerve repairs when there is no tension across the direct repair site.

The ability for a peripheral nerve to slowly lengthen and maintain function is well established during limb-lengthening procedures (Galardi et al, 1990), tumor displacement of nerves, and accommodation of nerves to obesity, pregnancy, and other circumstances where normal body morphology is stretched to unusual disproportion over a long period of time. We observed that during skin expansion using an inflatable balloon, nerves that passed through the skin and over the expanders were stretched without loss of nerve function. This was first observed while expanding the skin of the posterior calf where the sural nerve was directly over the skin expansion balloon.

The concept of lengthening the nerve distal to a gap, proximal to a gap, or on both sides of a gap must be emphasized. When lengthening the proximal nerve, the intact nerve fibers, including associated supporting Schwann cells, are being lengthened. When lengthening the distal nerve, the nerve fiber has degenerated and the lengthening involves only the supporting Schwann cells filling the neural sheath (Figs. 30–1 and 30–2). The exact nature of this process is not completely understood. Expanding an intact nerve fiber is a slow process because of the potential for injury to the nerve fiber and patient discomfort. Distal expansion is easier because the nerve is not connected centrally. The risk here is to attempt a rapid expansion because of the warning signs are missed.

With this information, nerve lengthening using a silicone balloon device has become a useful way to manage some nerve gaps.

There are numerous reports of the successful lengthening of nerves using balloon expansion of the nerve in research models (Battison et al, 1992; Endo and Nakayama, 1993; Hall et al, 1993, Hall and Van Way, 1994; Milner, 1989; Milner and Wilkins, 1992; Orbay et al, 1993; Wood and McMahon, 1989; Wood et al, 1991). Manders and colleagues (1987) and the authors of this chapter have reported successful clinical cases of nerve expansion with good long-term results. This chapter describes the indications and potentials for using nerve expansion to overcome gaps in peripheral nerves.

At this time, the indications for using nerve lengthening rather than nerve grafting are fibrosis of the recipient bed that precludes nerve grafting, anticipated poor outcomes from nerve grafting, and inadequate autologous donor nerve supply.

The longest nerve gap that has been repaired directly using nerve lengthening is a 10-cm nerve gap in the proximal sciatic nerve (Van Beek and Hoffman, 1995) (Fig. 30–3). When nerve gaps are longer than 6 to 8 cm, one must consider using a proximal and distal balloon for lengthening the proximal and distal nerve stumps (Fig. 30–4). Nerve gaps less than 6 cm in length usually can be managed with a single balloon expander (Fig. 30–5). Each balloon usually provides approximately 5 to 8 cm of nerve lengthening, depending on the size of the expander that can be placed. In our series of nine patients, nerve lengthening has been used to repair gaps directly in the median nerve, upper trunk of the brachial plexus, posterior tibial nerve, sciatic nerve, and the common peroneal nerve. With the exception of one patient who did not achieve nerve repair, the outcome of these repairs is comparable to nerve grafting.

CASE SELECTION

Nerve lengthening is reserved for those cases in which it is believed that nerve grafting is not possible because of problems with the recipient bed or when nerve grafting does not consistently provide good results. Nerve lengthening

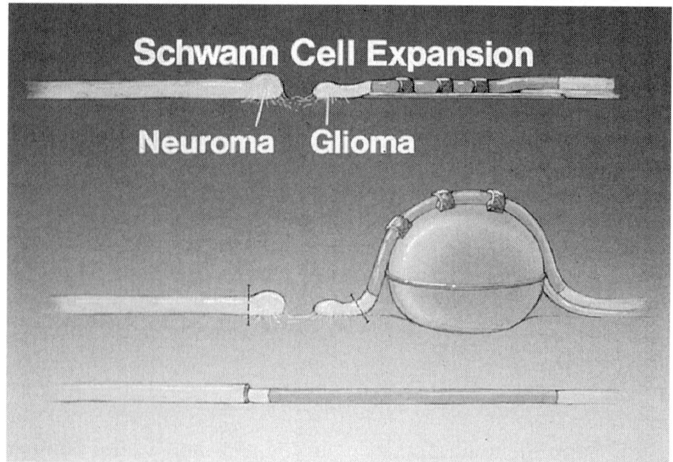

FIGURE 30–1. Lengthening the distal stump of a nerve results in lengthening only Schwann cell cords. The length gained by expansion must be sufficient to overcome the gap that results following identification of suitable nerve.

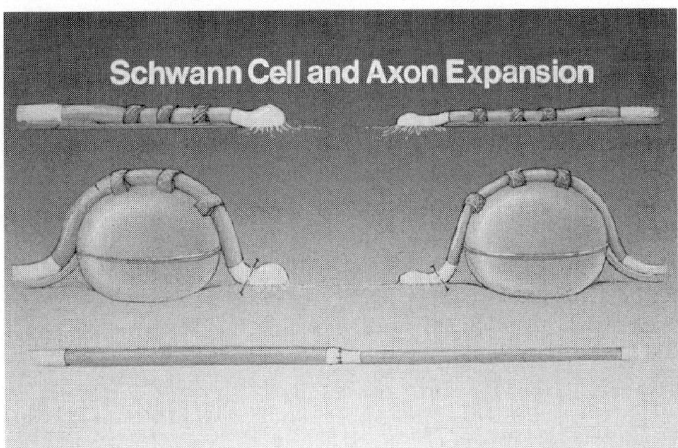

FIGURE 30–2. Simultaneous lengthening of proximal nerve fibers and distal Schwann cell cords can provide up to 12 cm of nerve length. Proximal nerve lengthening is a slower process than distal nerve lengthening.

is a two-stage procedure that is associated with all the complications of tissue expansion (Van Beek and Hoffman, 1995). Case selection is crucial to success, and the surgeon's experience with skin flap expansion is an important prerequisite in recommending this procedure.

TECHNIQUE

The injured nerve is exposed, and the length of the gap between the distal and proximal ends after neuroma resection is estimated. If the injury is located near major divisions of the nerve or other anatomical obstacles, it must be deter-

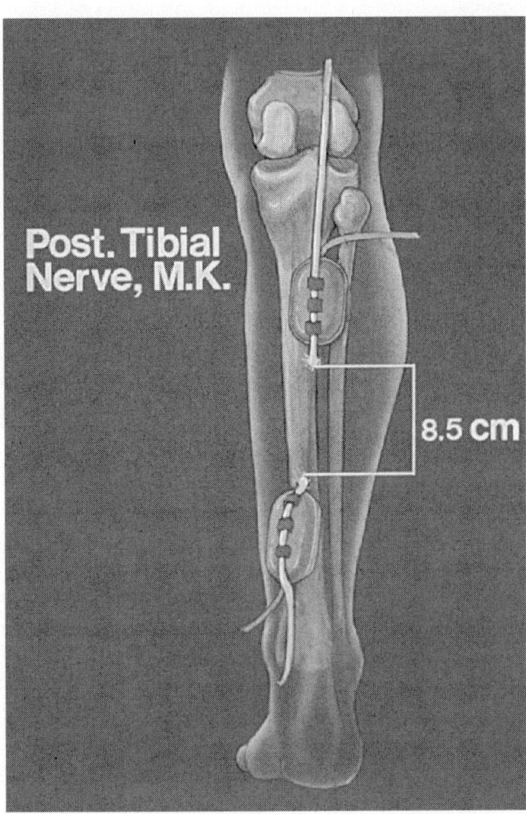

FIGURE 30–4. An example of expander placement for a mid-calf posterior tibial nerve injury.

mined what portions of the nerve can be expanded, because branching makes placing the expanders more difficult. If a short gap exists and nerve lengthening is necessary, the first choice would be to expand the distal nerve segment. If it is not possible to expand the distal segment of nerve, the proximal segment may need to be lengthened. In gaps that are over 6 cm in length, it will usually be necessary to lengthen both the proximal and distal nerve segments. Skin coverage over the nerve expansion sites must be pliable and usually without excessive scarring of the skin. This will permit balloon placement and subsequent expansion. When

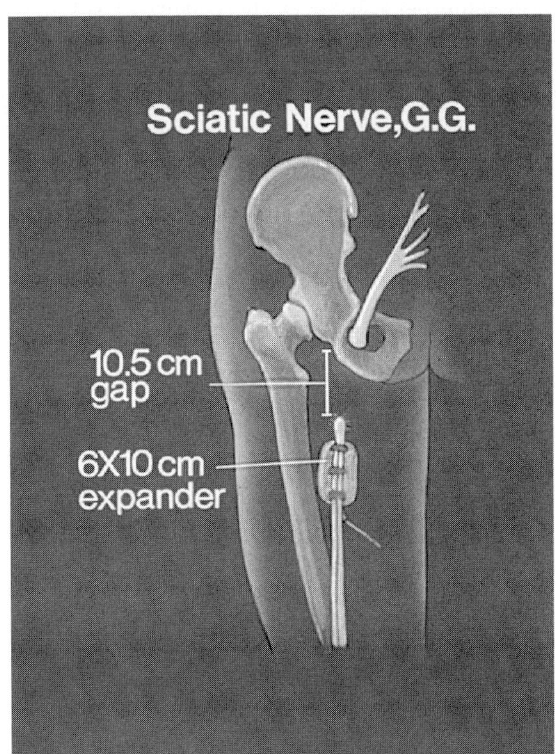

FIGURE 30–3. An example of expander placement for proximal sciatic nerve injury.

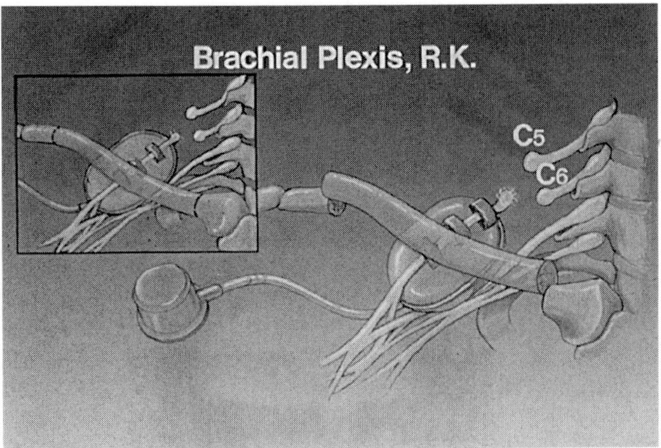

FIGURE 30–5. An example of expander placement and clavicle osteotomy to permit expansion of the upper trunk of the brachial plexus.

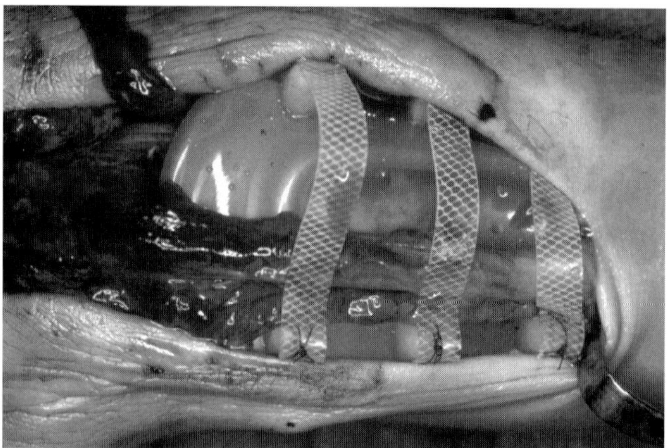

FIGURE 30–6. A median nerve restrained by the balloon's nerve retention straps.

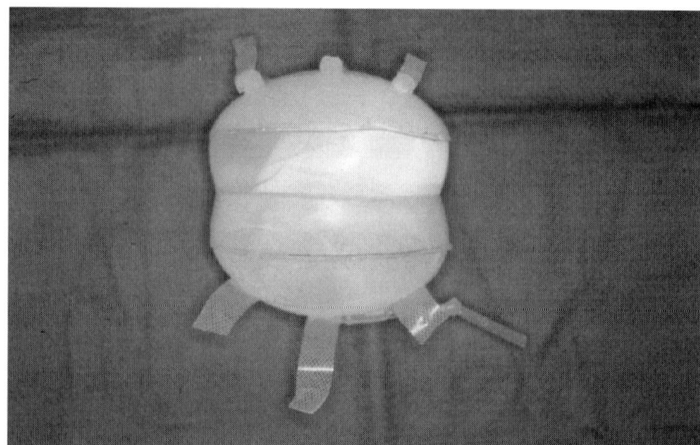

FIGURE 30–8. Dual chamber expansion devices elevate at least 5 cm if the overlying skin can tolerate the device.

possible, try to keep the incisions away from the area where the balloon will need to expand the skin. This is also sound advice for nerve grafts because an incision immediately over neuromas causes serious problems.

Expansion of the balloons positioned under a nerve so that it can be lengthened takes a longer amount of time than routine skin expansion. Nerve expansion requires at least 3 months, and in our experience, the balloons are inflated once every week. If proximal intact fibers are being lengthened, pain will occur if the balloon is expanded too rapidly. Unless the nerve is retained on the surface of the balloon, it will slip to the plane of least resistance and not be elongated

(Fig. 30–6). The expansion device must also be restrained, or it may shift to a position when being inflated. A shift in position could result in a loss of effective nerve lengthening (Figs. 30–7 to 30–9). Using a texture expander will help maintain fixation of the implant during expansion and also may prevent shifting of the balloon to a plane of less resistance (see Fig. 30–3). At the time of placement of the nerve expander, avoid detaching the proximal and distal stumps of the nerve from the surrounding area of fibrosis. Fibrous fixation allows secure fixation of the nerve stumps during expansion. If stump mobilization is essential, the mobilized stumps must be attached by sutures to adjacent tissue to ensure that they do not migrate over the nerve expander rather than expand their length. The nerve expander must be placed under normal nerve structure, not a neuroma. Because the nerve expander is designed for achieving maximum height, planning its placement and expansion is crucial (see Fig. 30–4).

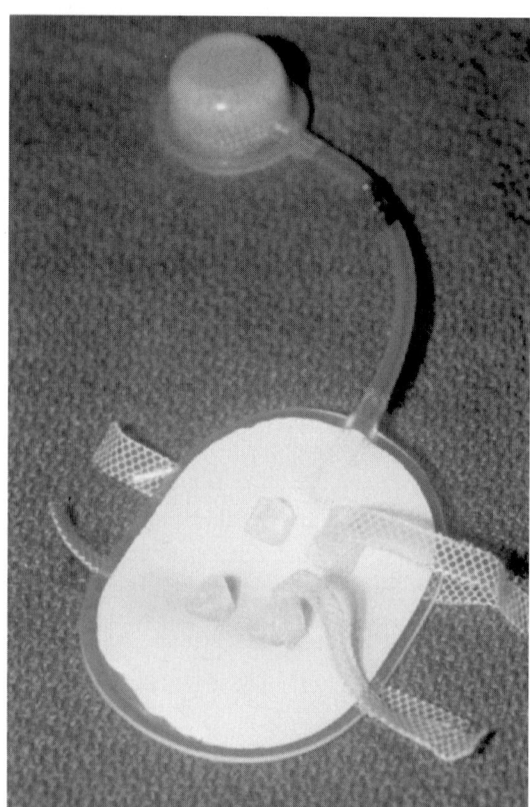

FIGURE 30–7. Deflated nerve expansion balloon with nerve retention straps and balloon retention straps.

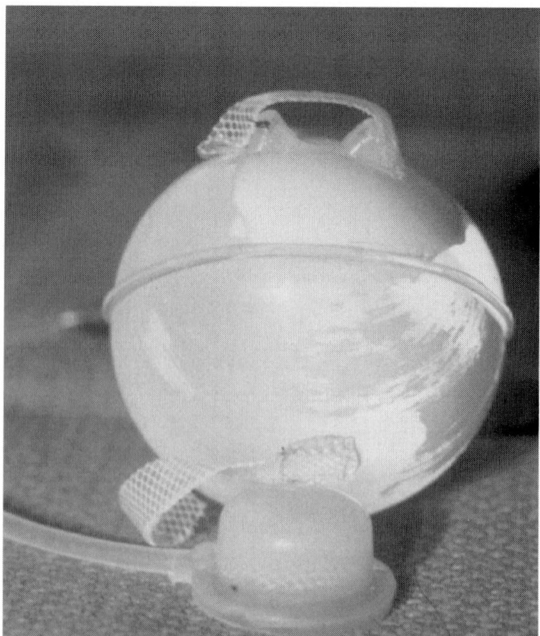

FIGURE 30–9. The nerve retention device is necessary to prevent the expanded nerve from migrating off the apex of the balloon.

Following expansion when the nerve is explored, find the nerve distal to the distal expander and proximal to the proximal expander. It is easier to trace the expanded nerve from those areas (see Fig. 30–6). The expander capsule must be released from surrounding tissue to permit nerve migration to close the gap between the nerve ends. Following mobilization from the expander's surface, the nerve will recoil to a small degree, but direct repair without excessive tension is possible if surgical planning has been appropriate. The expanded nerve is highly vascular and is readily identified as it passes over the balloon and under the expander retention straps. An external epineurial repair is performed using 8-0 to 10-0 sutures. Following nerve repair, the repair site is protected from disruption for 3 weeks by using splints and managing the nerve similar to a direct repair of a nerve following transection.

In our clinical series of eight carefully selected patients, the results of nerve lengthening to overcome nerve gaps has compared favorably with the results produced by nerve grafting. However, this is an evolving clinical technique and could be used in circumstances in which nerve grafting may not be successful for the reasons delineated earlier.

References

Battiston B, Buffoli P, Vigasio A, Brunelli G, Antonini L: The effects of lengthening on nerves. Ital J Orthop Traumatol *18(1)*:79–86, 1992.

Endo T, Nakayama Y: Histologic examination of peripheral nerves elongated by tissue expanders. Br J Plast Surg *46*:421, 1993.

Galardi G, Cami G, Lozza L, Marchettini P, Novarina M, Facchini R, Paronzini A: Peripheral nerve damage during limb lengthening: Neurophysiology in five cases of bilateral tibial lengthening. J Bone Joint Surg (Br) *72*:121–124, 1990.

Hall GD, Van Way CW: A comparison of nerve grafting and tissue expansion techniques in the rat. Microsurgery *15*:439–442, 1994.

Hall GD, Van Way CW, Kung FT, Campton-Allen M: Peripheral nerve elongation with tissue expansion techniques. J Trauma *34*:401–405, 1993.

MacKinnon SF: Surgical management of the peripheral nerve gap. Clin Plast Surg *16*:587, 1989.

Manders EK, Saggers GD, Diaz-Alonso P, Finn L, Sipio SC, Glumac T, Au VK, Wang RK, Mottaleb M: Elongation of peripheral nerve and viscera containing smooth muscle. Clin Plast Surg *14*:551–562, 1987.

Millesi H: The nerve gap: Theory and clinical practice. Hand Clin *2*:651, 1986.

Milner RH: The effect of tissue expansion of peripheral nerves. Br J Plast Surg *41*:414–421, 1989.

Milner RH, Wilkins PR: The recovery of peripheral nerves following tissue expansion. Br J Hand Surg *17b*:78–85, 1992.

Orbay J, Lin H, Kummer FJ: Repair of peripheral nerve defects by controlled distraction. A preliminary study. Bull Hosp Jt Dis *52(2)*:7–10, 1993.

Terzis J, Faibisoff BA, Williams HB: The nerve gap: Suture under tension vs. graft. Plast Reconst Surg *56*:166–170, 1975.

Van Beek AL, Hoffman JA: Peripheral nerve elongation by tissue expansion in eight patients. Scientific presentation at the Annual Meeting of the American Society for Peripheral Nerve, Montreal, 1995.

Wood FM, McMahon SB: The response of the peripheral nerve field to controlled soft tissue expansion. Br J Plast Surg *41*:682–686, 1989.

Wood RJ, Adson MH, Van Beek AL, Peltier GL, Zubkoff MM, Bubrick MP: Controlled expansion of peripheral nerves: Comparison of nerve grafting and nerve expansion and repair for canine sciatic nerve defects. J Trauma *31*:686–690, 1991.

Chapter 31

• Warren C. Breidenbach

Vascularized Nerve Grafts

Nerve grafting of peripheral nerve defects is an established technique with predictable, albeit less than perfect, results (Millesi et al, 1972, 1976). Because of the limited results, methods of improving nerve grafting have been sought. One technique proposed in 1976 by Taylor and Ham was to move a nerve graft with its blood supply: a vascularized nerve graft (VNG).

This chapter examines the technique of vascularized nerve grafting, explains how it is done, and examines its usefulness in peripheral nerve reconstruction. First, the theory of VNG is examined, then the different types of VNG are outlined. Experimental and clinical evidence for VNG are reviewed, and the indications for VNG are presented. Finally, the donor nerve anatomy and method of transfer are presented.

THEORY

A nerve graft functions not as a nonliving conduit but rather as a device for transferring living Schwann cells. Experiments have shown that freeze-dried or lyophilized nerve grafts do poorly (Best and Mackinnon, 1994; Sunderland, 1978; Trumble and Parvin, 1994). This is because the Schwann cells are killed. A nerve graft is a method of Schwann cell transfer, but it is exactly that—a graft. It is the transfer of a segment of nerve without its blood supply. Once in the recipient bed, the nerve graft must revascularize. Before completing the revascularization, a period of ischemia occurs that may damage Schwann cells (Lux et al, 1988).

The theory supporting the use of a VNG is that it allows transfer of a nerve with its blood supply, thereby avoiding damage to the Schwann cell population (Breidenbach and Terzis, 1986, 1987). This improved Schwann cell population, along with increased vascularity, may allow more rapid and complete axonal regeneration, which will enhance final nerve function outcome.

CLASSIFICATION OF NERVE GRAFTING

A nerve graft may be classified by its blood supply (Table 31–1). If a nerve is grafted without its blood supply, it is referred to as a nonvascularized nerve graft (NNG). If a nerve is moved with a blood supply, it is called a VNG. (Technically, because a VNG is moved with its blood supply, it is a true flap and not a graft; however, the term VNG is firmly established in the literature and is used throughout this chapter.)

Not all VNGs are transferred with the same blood flow characteristics. Normally, a VNG is a segment of nerve with an associated artery and vein, which are anastomosed to the recipient artery and vein. Blood flows from the recipient artery into the artery, capillaries, and vein of the VNG and exits out the recipient vein. This type of circulatory arrangement is referred to as a VNG. In addition, VNG is the generic term used for any nerve transferred with its blood supply, regardless of its circulatory characteristics.

A nerve may be transferred with only the artery attached (Rose et al, 1989). In this situation, blood flows from the proximal recipient artery into the artery associated with the nerve and then out into the distal recipient artery or vein. Venous outflow is not established. When the outflow recipient vessel is an artery, this graft is referred to as an arterialized nerve graft (ANG); if the outflow recipient vessel is a vein, it is called an arterialized fistula nerve graft (AFNG).

A nerve may be transferred with only an associated vein (Gu et al, 1985; Rose et al, 1989; Townsend and Taylor, 1984). Blood flows from the proximal recipient artery into the vein of the nerve graft and then out into the recipient artery or vein. When the outflow recipient vessel is an artery, the graft is referred to as an arterialized venous nerve graft (AVNG); if the outflow recipient vessel is a vein, it is called an arterialized venous fistula nerve graft (AVFNG).

Finally, venous blood may flow from the recipient vein into the vein associated with the nerve and then out into the distal recipient vein. This represents a vascularized venous nerve graft (VVNG) (Arakaki et al, 1994).

This chapter focuses primarily on VNG. The alternate forms of nerve grafting are referenced where appropriate, and the reader should be aware of these alternate forms

▼ TABLE 31–1
Definitions of Types of Vascularized Nerve Grafts

Abbreviations	Definitions
VNG	Vascularized nerve graft: A general term used for all types of vascularized nerve grafts (i. e., all of those listed in this table), or a reference specifically to a nerve transferred with its normal circulatory pattern.
ANG	Arterialized nerve graft: Artery only attached to the nerve, no vein. Arterial blood flows into the artery connected to the nerve, and drains into the recipient artery. No established venous outflow.
AFNG	Arterialized fistula nerve graft: the same as ANG, except outflow is into recipient vein.
AVNG	Arterialized venous nerve graft: Vein only attached to the nerve, no artery. Arterial blood flows into the reversed vein connected to the nerve, and then drains into the recipient artery. No established venous outflow.
AVFNG	Arterialized venous fistula nerve graft: Same as AVNG except outflow is into the recipient vein.
VVNG	Vascularized venous nerve graft: Venous blood flow into a vein associated with a nerve. There is no arterial blood. Outflow is into a vein.

when reviewing the literature. Obviously, it is incorrect to assume that all nerves transferred with their blood supply are equivalent when the methods of vascularization are different.

EXPERIMENTAL RESULTS

The purpose of performing a VNG rests on the premise that a VNG avoids a detrimental period of ischemia because it transfers a blood supply with the nerve. Therefore, to properly compare a VNG with an NNG, three questions should be addressed: (1) How does a nerve graft revascularize? (2) Does the graft undergo an ischemic period? (3) If an ischemic period exists, to what extent and severity?

A nerve graft revascularizes in two ways: (1) centripetal revascularization, which results from ingrowth of vessels from the surrounding tissue, and (2) inosculation, in which the vessels hook up from the ends of the graft. Different articles have reported the predominance of one type of revascularization over the other (Best and Mackinnon, 1994; Table 31–2).

The importance of the method in which a nerve graft revascularizes is more than an academic question. If inosculation predominates, then a nerve graft may receive adequate revascularization from each end, revascularization from the surrounding bed becomes less relevant, and a VNG would offer little advantage. If centripetal revascularization predominates, then the status of the recipient bed is important. In this situation, a VNG may provide an advantage over an NNG.

CLINICAL RESULTS

Several clinical studies have addressed the question regarding the superiority of VNG compared with NNG (Table 31–3). Unfortunately, most have problems in experimental design because of small numbers, no controls, and alternate circulatory characteristics.

The first report of a VNG and AVNG was presented by Taylor and associates (Taylor and Ham, 1976; Taylor, 1978; Townsend and Taylor, 1984). These studies are important because they show the feasibility of the concept. With the VNG study, the number of cases was small, the follow-up period was short, and there was no control. In place of the NNG control group, the authors used their clinical experience. They concluded that the VNG produced a superior result compared with their clinical experience with NNG. Likewise, a similar approach was taken with the AVNG study. Again their numbers were small, the follow-up period was short, and they used clinical experience as a control. They concluded that AVNG was superior.

Fachinelli and co-workers (1981) reported the first use of a vascularized sural nerve graft. Follow-up was not reported.

Merle and colleagues (1985) and Bonney and associates (1984) reported the use of ulnar nerves in brachial plexus reconstruction and arrived at different conclusions. Merle and colleagues found that with enough time, NNG results were equivalent to ulnar nerve VNG. Bonney and associates found ulnar nerve VNG was superior. Neither study used control groups.

Several authors have reported superior results with VNG using alternate circulatory patterns. Rose and co-workers (1985, 1989) reported superior results comparing an NNG to both AVNG and AVFNG (with control groups). These studies are intriguing because they are well designed and imply superior results with a VNG using altered circulatory patterns. Gu et al (1985) also studied AVNG and reported superior results to NNG, but there were no controls.

Many of the above-mentioned studies have inadequacies in experimental design, which preclude drawing firm conclusions that a VNG is superior to an NNG. This includes the studies on VNGs with altered circulatory characteristics, with the exception of the studies by Rose and co-workers (1985, 1989). The later studies show superior results with AVNG and ANG in digital nerve reconstruction. Although this represents an important contribution, it still begs the question regarding mixed peripheral nerves.

Studies by Doi and co-workers (1984, 1987, 1992) address the significant question of what type of grafting should be used with mixed peripheral nerves. The authors randomized peripheral nerve injuries that required grafting into two groups. Twenty-seven patients were reconstructed with a sural VNG and 22 with a sural NNG. The follow-up period was 24 to 40 months. The following parameters were clearly delineated in the study: age, skin defect, length of nerve gap, speed of axonal regeneration, time to S2 and electromyogram (EMG) return, and sensory and motor outcome. The results clearly show a statistically significant superior result for VNG compared with NNG in terms of the rate of axonal regeneration, rate of EMG return, and final sensory and motor outcome. This is an important study because it demonstrates this superior result in normal recipient beds and in relatively small defects. In other words, this study demonstrates better results in most peripheral nerve defects with VNG. It is not a technique isolated only to badly scarred beds or large nerve defects.

However, despite the results noted in this excellent paper, caution is indicated for the following reasons: First, this is only one study. Second, the randomization process the authors used is questionable because the numbers in each group were not equivalent. Third, the statistical analysis is questionable. The authors do not clearly state their methods of statistical analysis. In addition, the categorical variable

▼ **TABLE 31–2**
Summary of Experiments with Vascularized Nerve Grafts

Author	Animal	Nerve	Nerve Gap	Recipient Bed	Methods of Evaluation
Restrepo et al, 1985	Rabbit	Sciatic	4.5	Optimal	Morphometric
Pho et al, 1985	Rat	Femoral	2	Optimal	Morphometric
McCullough et al, 1984	Rat	Sciatic	2.5	Optimal	Morphometric, electrophysiological
Mani et al, 1992	Rabbit	Sciatic	3–4	Optimal and adverse	Morphometric, electrophysiological
Koshima and Harii, 1985a	Rat		1.5	Adverse	Morphometric, electrophysiological
Shibata et al, 1988	Rabbit	Median	3	Optimal	Morphometric, electrophysiological function
Kanaya et al, 1993	Rat	Sciatic	3	Optimal	Morphometric, electrophysiological function

▼ **TABLE 31–3**
Clinical Studies of Vascularized Nerve Grafts

Author	Indication for VNG	Donor Nerve	Type	No. of Cases	Control	Follow-up	Results
Taylor, 1976	Volkmann's contracture	Superficial radial	VNG	3	No	9 m–2 yr	VNG > NNG
Taylor, 1978	Burn trauma	Sural	AVNG	7	No	5 m–3 yr	AVNG > NNG
Fachinelli et al, 1981	Volkmann's contracture	Sural	VNG	6	No	None	Not stated
Bonney et al, 1984	Brachial plexus	Ulnar	VNG	12	No	5–28 m	VNG > NNG
Merle et al, 1985	Brachial plexus	Ulnar	VNG	8	No	?-2 yr	VNG = NNG
Rose and Kowalski, 1985	Previously failed digital nerve grafts	Deep peroneal	ANG	6	Yes	28 m	ANG > NNG
Rose et al, 1989	Complex digital injuries	Deep peroneal	AVFNG	12	Yes	6 m–2 yr	AVFNG > NNG

ANG, Arterialized nerve graft; AVNG, arterialized venous nerve graft; NNG, nonvascularized nerve graft; VNG, vascularized nerve graft.

used with the parameter's sensory and motor evaluation was analyzed as a continuous variable. This author has recalculated the results as a categorical variable and found that the results are significant but not with as many parameters. Finally, Doi and colleagues (1992) avoided stating that VNGs are superior in all situations, which their study seems to show. Rather they state that "our preliminary conclusion is that vascularized sural nerve grafting is indicated when nerve gap of more than 6 cm is associated with a large skin defect or amputation." This is a curious conclusion because only two patients in the whole study had a peripheral nerve defect greater than 6 cm with an associated skin defect or amputation. The average defect for the VNGs and NNGs were 6.5 and 6.6 cm, respectively. In other words, the defects were not large and often not associated with a large skin defect, yet the VNG demonstrated a superior result. It appears that the authors were trying to be conservative in their conclusions. The raw data, however, clearly challenge the conventional wisdom regarding the use of NNG. The data show that in relatively small defects and in a normal recipient bed, criteria that supposedly favor an NNG, the VNG produces a better result.

Mackinnon and associates (1988) published a unique case report that allowed a comparison between VNG and NNG. A median nerve defect was reconstructed with a vascularized superficial radial nerve graft and a nonvascularized sural nerve graft. This was done in two stages, with the proximal coaptation done first and the distal coaptation completed 7 months later. This allowed biopsies to be taken from both the VNG and NNG. Histological examination demonstrated superior regeneration in the VNG. Furthermore, the portion of the median nerve reconstructed with the VNG produced a superior sensory function.

INDICATIONS FOR A VASCULAR NERVE GRAFT

The indication for a VNG should be based on our understanding of the experimental and clinical evidence. As was pointed out in the previous sections, the results in both types of work are contradictory.

This author believes that the experimental and clinical studies should be interpreted in the following manner. Regardless of the method of revascularization (centripetal versus inosculation), there is evidence that an NNG undergoes approximately a 3-day period of ischemia in a normal bed. As the length of the nerve graft increases, placing greater requirements on inosculation, and as the scarring of the

bed increases, placing greater requirements on centripetal revascularization, it is likely that the ischemic period will increase. Ischemia is most likely detrimental to nerve graft outcome.

Therefore, the indication for a VNG is the clinical situation in which nerve graft ischemia is likely. Herein lies the debate. Some believe that the nerve is susceptible to ischemic damage in many situations, whereas others believe that it is not likely. Those who believe that the nerve is susceptible to ischemic damage, which include this author, recommend VNG as the deficit increases in size and the recipient bed becomes increasingly more scarred. In general, VNG should be considered for a deficit of greater than 6 cm and a recipient bed with extensive trauma. Finally, there may be a role for VNG in the repair of proximal lesions because VNG may allow more rapid axonal growth.

TRANSFER OF THE VASCULAR NERVE GRAFT

If one elects to proceed with a VNG transfer, four areas must be addressed: (1) donor nerve selection, (2) method of vascularization, (3) method of cable formation, and (4) monitoring. Each of these areas are addressed.

Donor nerve selection depends on an understanding of nerve vascular anatomy and the clinical situations in which its use is most beneficial. There are six potential types of VNGs (note that any nerve may be a VNG if vascular supply is present). Tables 31–3 to 31–6 list potential types of VNGs, their associated blood supply, and specifics about their anatomy (Breidenbach and Terzis, 1986). This author has used four of these types clinically, and they are reviewed.

The superficial radial nerve was the first proposed donor

▼ **TABLE 31–4**
Nerves and Vessels that May Be Used as Vascularized Nerve Grafts

Nerve	Blood Supply
Superficial radial	Radial
Ulnar	Superior ulnar collateral
Sural	Superficial sural
Anterior tibial	Anterior tibial
Superficial peroneal	Superficial peroneal
Saphenous	Saphenous

From Breidenbach WC, Terzis JK: The blood supply of vascularized nerve grafts. J Reconstr Microsurg 3:43,1986.

▼ **TABLE 31–5**
Cadaver Dissection Results of Donor Vascularized Nerve Grafts

Nerve	No. of Dissections	% Suitable as VNG	Artery (mm)		Artery Pedicle Length (cm)		Vein (mm)		Vein Pedicle (cm)	
			Average	*Range*	*Average*	*Range*	*Average*	*Range*	*Average*	*Range*
Superficial radial	20	100	3.6	2.5–5.5	6.4	3.5–13	2.5	1.0–5.0	6.4	3.5–13
Ulnar	25	96	1.8	0.8–2.5	4.9	3–9	1.9	1–3	4.0	1–8
Sural	20	30	1.2	1.1–1.4	5.0	3–7	1.3	0.8–1.9	4.8	3–7
Anterior tibial	20	95	4.4	3.1–5.5	4.2	3–7	3.4	1–5	4.2	3–7
Superficial peroneal	20	90	1.7	0.9–2.5	4.1	3–5	1.9	0.6–3.2	4.0	2–6
Saphenous	20	80	2.0	1.9–2.7	3.1	2.5–6	2.1	1.1–2.8	4.6	2.5–9
Lateral antebrachial cutaneous nerve of the forearm	20	30	1.81	0.8–2.9	3.17	1.5–5	1.8	1.1–3.0	3.2	1.5–5

From Breidenbach WC, Terzis JK: The blood supply of vascularized nerve grafts. J Reconstr Microsurg; *3*:43, 1986.

nerve as a VNG (Taylor and Ham, 1976). Its advantages include an easy dissection, an associated skin flap (forearm flap), a dominant artery (radial artery), and a high neural/connective tissue content. Disadvantages include the sacrifice of the radial artery and its short graft length.

The ulnar nerve may be used as a VNG based on either the ulnar artery (Bonney et al, 1984) or the superior ulnar collateral vessels (Breidenbach and Terzis, 1986). The latter is probably the preferable method to avoid ulnar artery sacrifice. In most cases, a limited skin flap may be attached (Breidenbach et al, 1987; Breidenbach and Terzis, 1986). The disadvantage of the ulnar VNG is that it is normally limited to brachial plexus injuries with preganglionic injuries of C8–T1.

The saphenous nerve has excellent length and an associated skin paddle (Breidenbach and Terzis, 1986). However, the anatomy is variable, making dissection of the associated skin paddle difficult and resulting in potential absence of the pedicle. Furthermore, the dissection is extensive, requiring exposure of Hunter's canal.

The sural nerve probably represents the best choice for a VNG for reconstruction of a peripheral nerve defect. There are two methods of transferring this nerve. The first bases the nerve on the blood supply coming from the popliteal fossa. The second is based on the peroneal system. The method using the blood supply from the popliteal fossa identifies the sural artery usually arising from the popliteal vessels. This is a relatively uncomplicated dissection. However, a significant number of cases (30% to 60%) may not have a pedicle (Breidenbach and Terzis, 1986; Fachinelli et al, 1981).

This led Doi and associates (1984) to develop an alternate method of carrying out a VNG. What is so interesting about the technique is that it is based on a dominant pedicle; the

▼ **TABLE 31–6**
Results of Measurements From Cadaver Dissections of Donor Vascularized Nerve Grafts

Nerve	Origin to Entry of Blood Supply (cm)		Length Pedicle Runs with the Nerve (cm)		Graft Length (cm)		Nerve Length Before First Branching		Nerve Length Before Last Motor Branch		Special Measurements (cm)
	Average	*Range*	*Average*	*Range*	*Average*	*Range*	*Average*	*Range*	*Average*	*Range*	
Superficial radial	9.0	4.5–14	11.8	9–17.5	23.8	20–28	21.3	18–24	NA	NA	Avg 26.3* Range 22–29
Ulnar	16.6	14–20	10.5	4–15	55.7	46–62	29.7	16–38	NA	NA	Avg 57.8* Range 48–64 Avg 17.8† Range 14–22
Sural	—	—	—	—	—	—	—	—	—	—	—
Anterior tibial	6.4	4–8	NA	NA	24.6	19–30	—	—	10.7	6–22	NA
Superficial peroneal	8.4	6–12	9.1	3–18	23.6	14–30	—	—	7.7	1–12	Avg 10.7‡ Range 7–15
Saphenous	27.4	17–42	13.2	17–23	40.4	31–49	23.2	6–39	NA	NA	NA
Lateral antebrachial cutaneous nerve of the forearm	—	—	4.1	1–9	34	19–41	—	—	NA	NA	NA

*, Length of extremity (cm).
†, Medical epicondyle to origin of blood supply in cm.
‡, Centimeters below head of fibula at which pedicle joins the nerve.
—, no measurement obtained.
NA, measurement not applicable.
From Breidenbach WC, Terzis JK: The blood supply of vascularized nerve grafts. J Reconstr Microsurg *3*:43, 1986.

peroneal or its perforators, which supply the fascia; and the blood supply of the fascia supports the nerve.

This author currently uses the vascularized sural nerve, as described by Doi, for peripheral reconstruction, and the vascularized ulnar nerve in appropriate brachial plexus lesions. The operative technique is outlined at the end of this chapter.

METHODS OF VASCULARIZING THE NERVE

As described earlier, alternate circulatory methods may be used to carry out a VNG. The literature reports three donor nerves: (1) the sural nerve with the associated vein transferred as an ANG (Gu et al, 1985), (2) the deep peroneal nerve with associated artery as an ANG (Rose and Kowalski, 1985), and (3) the deep peroneal nerve with associated vein as an AVNG (Rose et al, 1989).

These techniques are appealing because they simplify the procedures of harvesting and positioning a VNG. For example, with the sural nerve, it may be transferred with the associated saphenous vein. This nerve vein complex may then be reversed and anastomosed into an arterial deficit. In essence, a reverse vein graft is used in reconstructing the arterial deficit with the nerve attached to the vein. The advantage of this approach is that the dissection is simple, the anatomy is predictable, and it avoids sacrifice of a major artery.

Problems with these techniques include the following: First, attaching a flap for monitoring or coverage is problematic. Second, and most important, all of these techniques are based on the assumption that an alternate circulatory system will maintain nerve survival. For example, with the sural nerve–saphenous vein complex transferred as an AVNG, the arterialized blood must enter the vein, then pass in a retrograde fashion through the venous-nerve connections into the nerve. Clinical and experimental studies claim good results (Gu et al, 1985).

Experiments in our laboratory have evaluated the short-term effect on the nerve when it is transferred as an AVNG. The rabbit median nerve was the experimental model. Within the first 24 to 48 hours, extensive damage to the blood-nerve barrier occurred, followed by complete cessation of blood flow by 72 hours (Arakaki et al, 1994). Gu and co-workers (1985) used the same animal model of an AVNG and evaluated nerve conduction velocity, nerve density, and muscle weight at 3.5 months. The AVNG produced results similar to that of a VNG, and both were superior to an NNG (Gu et al, 1985). More work obviously needs to be done before one can definitively determine if there are benefits to these alternate methods of vascularizing a nerve graft.

METHOD OF CABLE FORMATION

A technical problem of VNG transfer is cable formation. Nerve cables need to be formed to overcome the size discrepancy between the recipient nerve and donor VNG. Forming cables may result in devascularization unless specific attention is given to maintaining blood supply. To understand how this is accomplished, a thorough understanding of nerve blood supply is necessary.

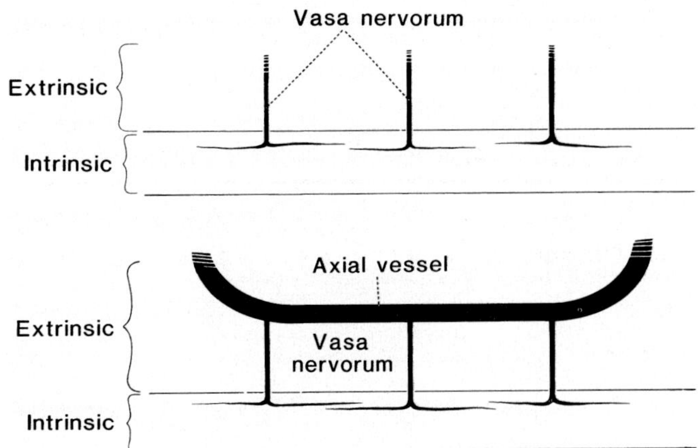

FIGURE 31–1. Blood is supplied to nerves by either extrinsic vessels, which lie outside the epineurium, or intrinsic vessels, which lie inside the epineurium. Extrinsic vessels may arise from fascial, musculocutaneous, and periosteal vessels *(upper diagram)* or from axial vessels *(lower diagram)*. This axial vessel is referred to as the dominant system. Vasa nervorum regress to any nutrient vessel of a nerve. (From Breidenbach WC, Terzis JK: The blood supply of vascularized nerve grafts. J Reconstr Microsurg 3:43, 1986, with permission.)

Nerve blood supply is either extrinsic or intrinsic. All vessels outside of the epineurium are extrinsic, while all those within the epineurium are intrinsic. Many small vessels, such as myocutaneous perforators and periosteal and fascial branches, provide extrinsic blood supply to nerves. These vessels are too small for microsurgical transfer. In a few cases, a large axial vessel runs with the nerve for a portion of its length and is suitable for transfer. Such vessels are called a dominant vessel (Fig. 31–1).

Nerves may be classified as having no, one, or multiple dominant systems (Breidenbach and Terzis, 1986). For example, the medial antebrachial cutaneous nerve of the forearm has no dominant vessel, the radial artery has one dominant vessel (radial), and the ulnar nerve has two dominant vessels (ulnar and ulnar collateral) (Fig. 31–2).

When the dominant system runs the whole length of the nerve, then cables may be easily formed. Fachinelli and associates (1981) introduced a technique of folding the nerve (Fig. 31–3), thereby maintaining blood supply to each segment.

The problem is that in most nerves, the dominant vessels

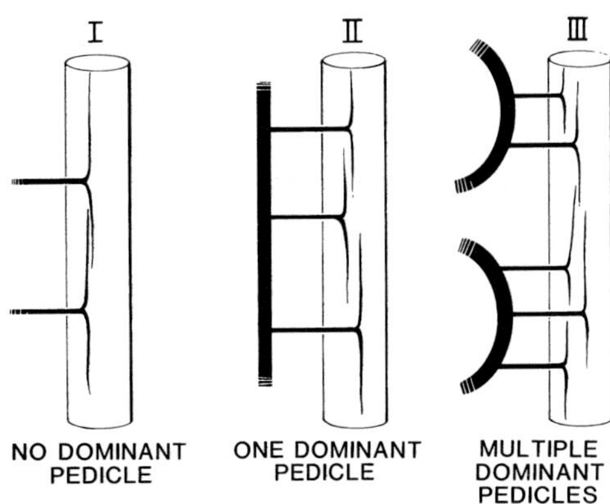

FIGURE 31–2. Classification of blood supply to nerves. (From Breidenbach WC, Terzis JK: The blood supply of vascularized nerve grafts. J Reconstr Microsurg 3:43, 1986, with permission.)

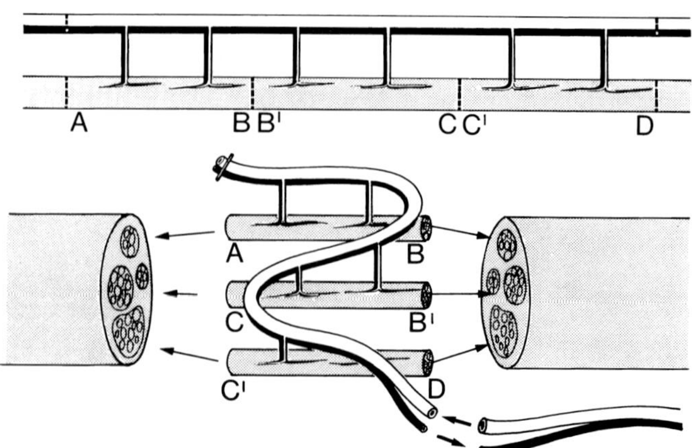

FIGURE 31–3. The method presented by Fachinelli and associates (1981) in which a nerve with a dominant blood supply may be cut and folded into cables and transferred as a vascularized nerve graft. (From Breidenbach WC, Terzis JK: The blood supply of vascularized nerve grafts. J Reconstr Microsurg 3:43, 1986, with permission.)

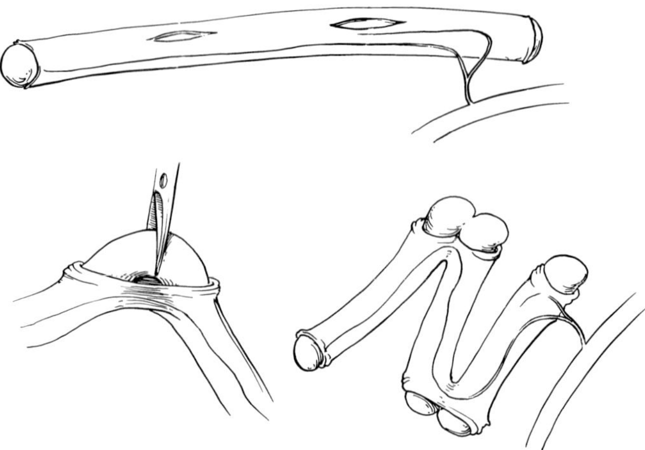

FIGURE 31–5. Vascularized cables are formed by transecting epineurium longitudinally and transecting the nerve transversely.

run with the nerve for less than its total length. The segment of nerve without a dominant vessel is supplied by small extrinsic vessels. This segment is referred to as a free segment. When such a nerve is elevated as a VNG, it has one segment supplied by the dominant vessel and a free segment (so named because it is free of a dominant system) supplied by the intrinsic system (Fig. 31–4). The portion of nerve supplied by a dominant vessel is easily separated into segments. However, the length of nerve without a dominant system, the free segment, is not easily divided into cables.

To fold the free segment into cables, the perineurium between each segment must be preserved. This is accomplished in the following manner. Under the microscope, the free segment is examined. Vessels can be seen coursing through the epineurium. A longitudinal incision is made in the epineurium, carefully preserving longitudinal vessels. The nerve itself is delivered out from the epineural incision and transected (Fig. 31–5). Each segment is prepared in a

similar fashion. Once prepared, each nerve is folded into cables, maintaining blood flow between each segment through the epineural vessels (Fig. 31–6).

The author has used this technique many times with the sural, saphenous, and ulnar nerves. Using this technique, free segments have been divided into a maximum of three cables, and bleeding has been observed in all segments. Furthermore, our laboratory investigated the blood flow in the median nerve of the rabbit folded into cables using this technique. Blood flow was maintained in each cable (Kanaya et al, 1993).

MONITORING A VASCULARIZED NERVE GRAFT

Ideally, a VNG should be monitored. Those who argue that monitoring is not necessary note that if a vessel thromboses, the VNG simply becomes an NNG. Beyond the academic argument that the outcome cannot be definitively associated with vascularity, there is a problem with vessel thrombosis. With a VNG, a venous failure may cause congestion, leading to nerve damage. With vascularized ulnar nerve transfer in brachial plexus reconstruction, thrombosis will probably lead to central necrosis. Ultimately, if it is worth carrying out a VNG, it is worth monitoring.

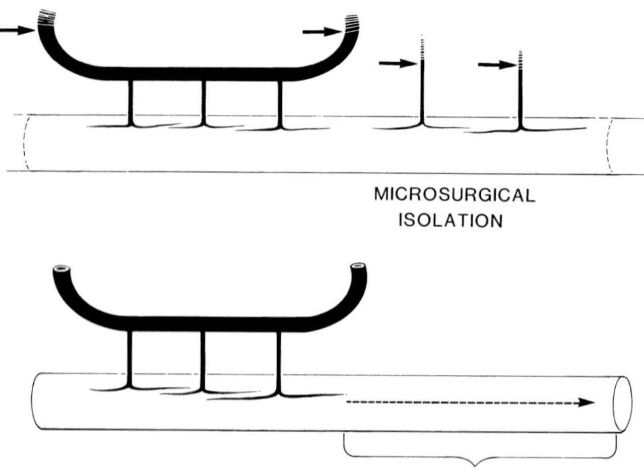

FIGURE 31–4. All extrinsic vessels must be transected (*arrows in upper diagram*) to transfer a nerve. Microsurgical anastomosis is carried out only on the dominant vessel. The free segment of the nerve (*lower diagram*), which was supplied by fascial, musculocutaneous, or periosteal vessels, must now be supplied by intrinsic vessels fed from the dominant pedicle. (From Breidenbach WC, Terzis JK: The blood supply of vascularized nerve grafts. J Reconstr Microsurg 3:43, 1986, with permission.)

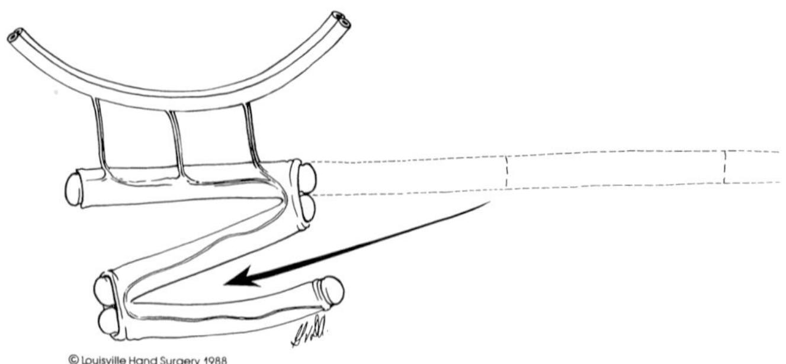

FIGURE 31–6. Dotted line represents the original position of the free segment. The epineurium is transected longitudinally and the nerve transversely, as in Figure 31–5. Blood supply is maintained through the folded epineurium. In this way, vascularized cables are formed when the dominant pedicle does not run the entire length of the nerve. (© Louisville Hand Surgery, 1988.)

For the sural nerve graft, as described by Doi and colleagues (1984), a skin paddle is easily attached. For the saphenous and ulnar nerves, an associated skin flap is based on the dominant artery. Unfortunately, the anatomy is variable, and the dissection is somewhat complex.

OPERATIVE TECHNIQUE

Vascularized Sural Nerve Graft

The sural nerve is harvested from the leg contralateral to the injured upper extremity. The patient is positioned supine, with the hips rotated to a lateral decubitus position. The donor leg is positioned upward and flexed to 90 degrees, with support. In this manner, two teams work, one harvesting the sural nerve while the other prepares the recipient site.

The vessels in the posterior crural septum are identified with Doppler imaging. Doi and associates (1984, 1987) note that the sural nerve has two dominant pedicles: The inferior pedicle arises from the peroneal artery, and the superior pedicle arises from the posterior tibial artery. The monitoring skin island is positioned over these perforators. A curvilinear incision begins at the distal leg posterior to the lateral malleolus over the sural nerve (Fig. 31–7). The incision is carried down through skin and subcutaneous tissue until identification of the sural nerve and short saphenous vein is made. Then the incision extends proximally toward the skin island, which it encompasses, and proceeds immediately to the popliteal fossa. A large subcutaneous flap is developed above the fascia from lateral to medial (Fig. 31–8). An incision is made on the medial side of the short saphenous vein and taken deep to the fascia. The short saphenous vein and sural nerve are identified proximally and distally, and then transected. (The sural nerve may dive deep to the gastrocnemius; if this is the case, it will need to be dissected from the muscle substance.)

Care is taken to visualize any pedicle as the proximal nerve is identified. A pedicle arises from the popliteal or

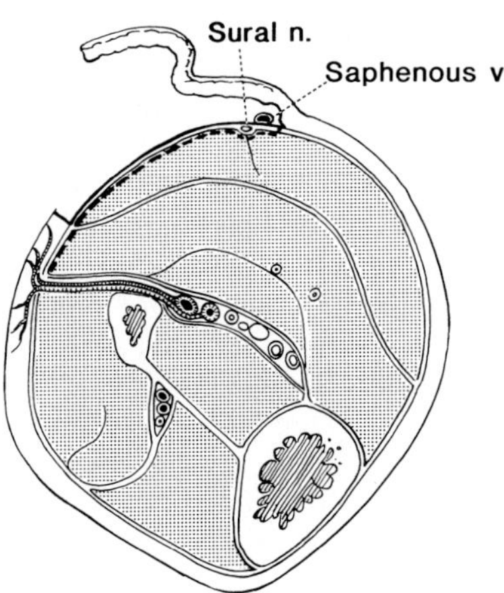

FIGURE 31–8. The subcutaneous skin flap is elevated. The dotted line indicates where the next dissection should proceed, below the fascia, starting medial to the short saphenous vein.

sural vessels in 30% to 60% of cases; this may be used as an alternative pedicle if the intermuscular septum's vessels are damaged (Breidenbach and Terzis, 1986; Fachinelli et al, 1981).

The posterior crural septum is approached next. Dissection is taken deep to the fascia toward the intermuscular septum (see dotted lines in Figs. 31–8 and 31–9) until the vessels are identified. It is often helpful to first identify the vessels; an incision is made anterior to the skin island and then pierces the fascia, dissecting posterior toward the intermuscular septum until the vessels are identified. The critical step is to identify the vessels within the intermuscular septum. These vessels will vary in origin, course, and size, and in some cases, will course directly through the muscle, not through the intermuscular septum (Wei et al, 1986). The dominant vessel may be superior, arising from the posterior tibial, or inferior, arising from the peroneal (Doi et al, 1984, 1987). This pedicle is followed down to the peroneal vessel. The peroneal vessel is a vessel of larger diameter than those in the intermuscular septum. The inferior or superior intermuscular septal vessel may be used to vascularize the nerve. If, however, the recipient artery is large, then a section of the peroneal vessel (from which the intermuscular septal

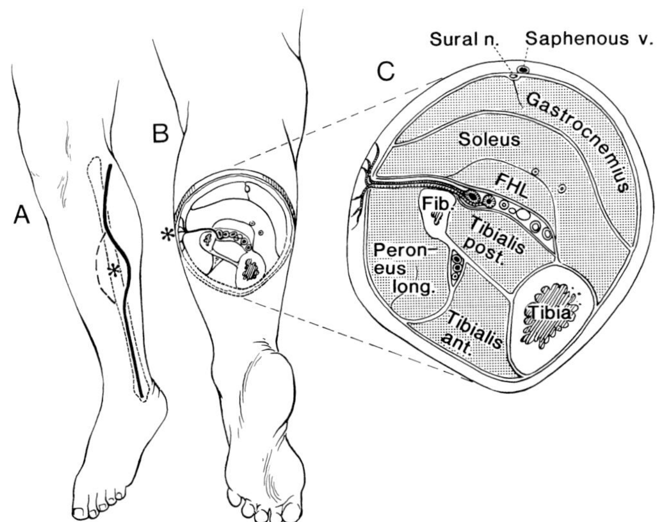

FIGURE 31–7. Lateral view of left leg *(A)* with solid line indicating the opening incision. Asterisk shows the skin island over the intermuscular septum. *B* and *C* illustrate cross section of same leg.

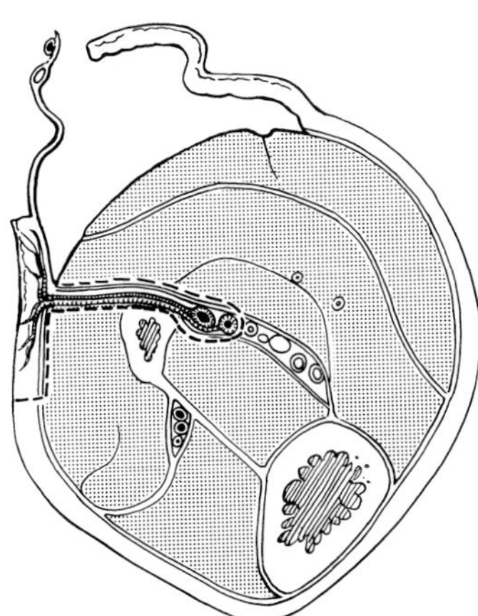

FIGURE 31–9. Fascia, including the sural nerve, is elevated to the posterior crural intermuscular septum. Dissection next proceeds along the dotted line.

vessel arises) may be used as the main pedicle. The vascularity of the leg is checked before sacrificing the peroneal vessels because it may be the dominant blood supply to the foot.

The fascia to the nerve is handled appropriately. Only some is preserved because it can make the flap too bulky. The fascia is preserved between the skin island and the nerve (Fig. 31–10). An edge of fascia 2 to 3 mm is left on both sides of the sural nerve as it extends both proximally and distally from this central segment.

After the nerve is elevated on the fascial segment and the appropriate pedicle isolated, it is transected. The vascularized nerve complex—consisting of skin island, fascia, and nerve (see Fig. 31–10)—is transferred to the recipient site.

Inserting the flap is the first priority. After the skin island has been inserted and stabilized, attention is turned to performing the microvascular anastomoses. After completion of the anastomoses, both the flap and the nerve are checked for bleeding. When it is firmly established that circulation is present, nerve reconstruction can be carried out. Great care is taken to maintain nerve blood flow to each cable segment of the sural nerve, which is divided into cables attached either to the epineurium of the nerve or to the fascial segment (Fig. 31–11). The appropriate length of cables is determined by measuring the nerve defect and calculating the requisite number of cables. Median and ulnar nerve reconstruction at the mid-forearm usually requires three or four cables. The length of each cable is measured, and the microscope is brought into the field. The nerve is teased out from the fascia, which is left attached to the central cable. The nerve will extend beyond the fascia proximally and distally. These segments are made into cables, as described earlier. A longitudinal incision is made in the epineurium, and the nerve is transected transversely. Epineural blood supply is thus maintained (see Fig. 31–11). Segments supplied by the only epineural vessels are then folded. The nerve segments are placed in the defect, and nerve repair is completed under the microscope. Bleeding is visualized from each segment.

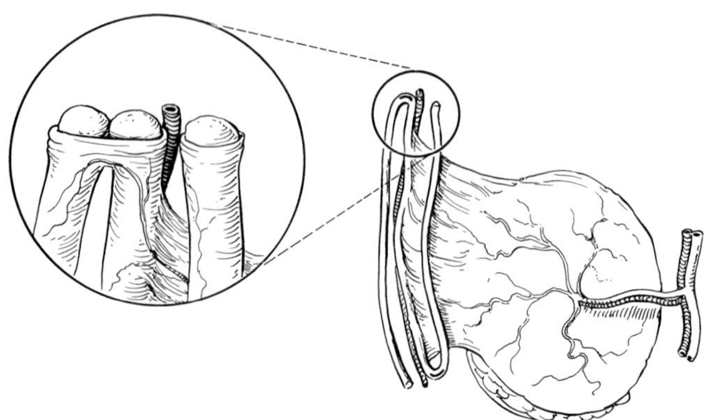

FIGURE 31–11. How blood supply is maintained to each of the segments. A middle cable is supplied by the fascia, while the two remaining cables are supplied through the epineurium. The large diagram shows the longitudinal transection in the epineurium prior to nerve transection. The blow-up view shows nerve after transection with epineurium intact.

When nerve repair is complete, the wound is closed and the flap is monitored constantly. All flaps are monitored with a photoplethysmograph at the time of closure and for 4 days thereafter. All nerve graft reconstructions are splinted postoperatively for 3 to 4 weeks.

Vascularized Ulnar Nerve Graft

The ulnar nerve may be used in brachial plexus reconstruction when there is a firmly established preganglionic lesion of C8 and T1.

To begin, the supraclavicular brachial plexus is explored thoroughly. This requires visualization of the C8 and T1 avulsed root or empty foramina to establish the presence of a preganglionic lesion. This author does not believe that myelography or somatosensory tests indicating avulsion of C8 and T1 are sufficient evidence to make a decision to sacrifice the ulnar nerve. The additional step of direct visualization of the brachial plexus is recommended. Along with this, obviously, some postganglionic lesions must be at C5, C6, or C7 to have sufficient proximal nerve for reconstruction.

Next, infraclavicular exploration is performed, and the most proximal portion of the normal nerves are identified. In this manner, the nerve graft that is present can be determined. A decision is made regarding use of the ulnar nerve as a VNG only after careful consideration of the size of the gap; the nature of the bed; the status of the proximal nerve roots at C5, C6, and C7; and the presence of a preganglionic lesion at C8 and T1. If one elects to proceed, the ulnar nerve is harvested.

The incision begins at the cubital tunnel and is carried proximally to expose the nerve in the same manner as in ulnar nerve subcutaneous transposition at the elbow. After the ulnar nerve is identified at the cubital tunnel, dissection is carried proximally. The superior ulnar collateral artery and vein will normally be visualized several centimeters proximal to the cubital tunnel. These vessels run on the inner aspect of the nerve (as viewed by the surgeon) and terminate by connecting with the branches of the ulnar recurrent vessels (Fig. 31–12). The ulnar nerve is elevated by transecting

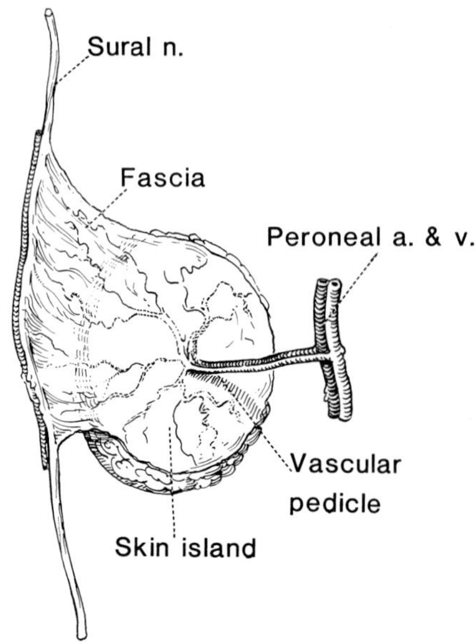

FIGURE 31–10. View from the bottom of the skin-fascia-nerve complex. Note that in this graft, a portion of the peroneal vessels was used.

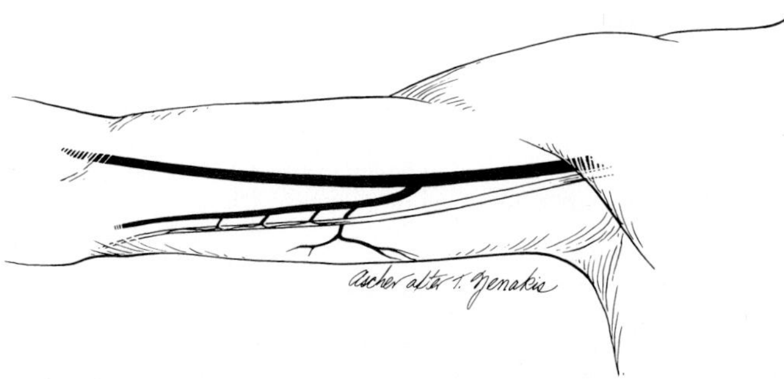

FIGURE 31–12. Right arm viewed from the medial aspect. Brachial artery is shown with superior ulnar collateral artery supplying the ulnar nerve and skin. (Grace Von Drake after T. Zenakis. Christian M. Kleinert Institute, Louisville, Kentucky.)

the branches holding it to the ulnar recurrent vessels. Dissection is then carried proximally, maintaining the superior ulnar collateral vessels on the nerve with a cuff of tissue around the whole neurovascular complex. Dissection may prove difficult because of the many branches to the surrounding muscle, which must be transected.

Two anatomical structures are carefully sought as the dissection proceeds from distal to proximal. First and most important, the origin of the superior ulnar collateral artery from the brachial artery is identified. This normally arises 14 to 22 cm above the medial epicondyle (Breidenbach and Terzis, 1986). Thus, it may originate as high as the axilla. The vein begins in the same region or slightly lower, coming from the plexus formed by the basilic and brachial veins. These vessels proceed in a medial direction to join the nerve, then course with the nerve on its inner deep side for 4 to 15 cm before turning away, always above the cubital tunnel.

The second important group of structures to visualize are the vessels running from the superior ulnar collateral vessel out to the medial skin. These are the vessels used to make a skin island monitor. In only 80% of the cases does a vessel run directly from the superior ulnar collateral vessels to the skin. In the remaining 20%, the vessel comes directly off the brachial vessels, making a skin island monitor impossible (Breidenbach et al, 1987).

After identifying the origin of the superior ulnar collateral artery from the brachial vessels, dissection proceeds rapidly in a more proximal direction until the ulnar nerve joins the brachial plexus. Here, the nerve is transected. Dissection then begins from the level of the cubital tunnel distally. The flexor carpi ulnaris fascia and muscle is split, and the nerve is harvested from the elbow to the wrist. Caution is used not to damage the ulnar artery, which is not harvested with the distal ulnar nerve. The distal ulnar nerve is transected at the wrist after it is elevated.

The entire length of the ulnar nerve may be harvested, obtaining a nerve graft length of 55.7 cm. The proximal and distal portions without extrinsic blood supply are dissected. The epineurium is left intact to protect the epineural vessels. If these vessels are damaged, the portion of the nerve without extrinsic blood supply may not survive. A decision is then made to use the nerve as a pedicle graft or as a free VNG. This decision will depend on the amount of nerve graft tissue needed to reconstruct the defect. If only one proximal root is intact, a pedicle nerve graft is sufficient.

The superior ulnar collateral vessels are left attached to the junction with the brachial vessels. The nerve graft is rotated so that the distal end, which is a free segment, is brought up into a position to reconstruct the defect. The epineurium is cut longitudinally, and the nerve is cut transversely to maintain epineural blood flow. Blood supply of the nerve graft is thus maintained, and the nerve defect is reconstructed.

When several proximal nerve roots are available for reconstruction and nerve gaps are large, 30 to 40 cm of a large-caliber nerve graft may be necessary. Here, the nerve would be transferred as a free VNG. As described earlier, the nerve is transferred based on the superior ulnar collateral vessels. Recipient vessels in the neck are identified; often, the transverse cervical is used as the artery. The external or internal jugular vein may serve as the recipient vein with an end-to-side anastomosis. After establishing blood flow, nerve graft reconstruction is done. The ulnar nerve is divided into cables corresponding to each of the defects to be reconstructed, using the techniques described earlier. After the nerve cables are constructed, nerve repairs are performed in standard fashion under the microscope.

If a vascular thrombosis is missed, the vascularized ulnar nerve is converted to a nonvascularized graft. Because the ulnar nerve has a large diameter, it becomes a trunk graft, which undergoes central necrosis. The results of trunk grafting are inferior compared with those of cable NNGs (Best and Mackinnon, 1994). Therefore, thrombosis in an ulnar VNG produces results that are inferior compared with those obtained with conventional nerve grafting. To avoid this problem, the ulnar VNG is monitored, when possible.

CONCLUSION

VNGs were introduced in 1976. Since then, experimental evidence from various animal models has suggested, but not decisively proved, that VNGs are superior to NNGs. The clinical evidence was also unclear, until the recent publication of Doi and colleagues (1992). This article seems to clearly demonstrate the superiority of VNG in mixed peripheral nerve reconstruction. Obviously, more clinical studies from other centers are indicated for confirmation of these findings. Doi's article also changes concepts of indications for VNGs. Previous indications were (1) scarred recipient bed, (2) proximal losses, and (3) large defects. Doi's work seems to imply that smaller defects in minimally scarred beds may also benefit from a VNG.

The sural nerve is the best choice for a VNG for peripheral nerve reconstruction when it is transferred on its peroneal system or perforators. In brachial plexus reconstructions with preganglionic losses of C8–T1, the vascular ulnar nerve is indicated.

When using a VNG, the surgeon should be familiar with the techniques necessary to form nerve cables while maintaining blood supply and attach a skin flap for monitoring.

References

Arakaki A, Tsai Tm, Firrell J, Breidenbach WC: Vascular filling and protein extravasation in three varieties of vascularized nerve grafts. J Reconstr Microsurg *10(3)*:166, 1994.

Best TJ, Mackinnon SE: Peripheral nerve revascularization: A current literature review. J Reconstr Microsurg *10*:193, 1994.

Bonney G, Birch R, Jamieson AM, Eames RA: Experience with vascularized nerve grafts. Clin Plast Surg *11*:137, 1984.

Breidenbach WC, Adamson W, Terzis JK: Median arm flap revisited. Ann Plast Surg *18*:150, 1987.

Breidenbach WC, Terzis JK: The blood supply of vascularized nerve grafts. J Reconstr Microsurg *3*:43, 1986.

Breidenbach WC, Terzis JK: Vascularized nerve grafts: An experimental and clinical review. Ann Plast Surg *18*:137, 1987.

Doi K, Kuwata N, Kawakami F, Tamaru K, Kay S: The free vascularized sural nerve graft. Microsurgery *5*:175, 1984.

Doi K, Kuwata N, Sakai K, Tamaru K, Kawai S: A reliable technique of free vascularized sural nerve grafting and preliminary results of clinical applications. J Hand Surg (Am) *12*:677, 1987.

Doi K, Tamaru K, Sakai K, Kuwata N, Kurafuji Y, Kawai S: A comparison of vascularized and conventional sural nerve grafts. J Hand Surg *17A*:670, 1992.

Fachinelli A, Masquelet A, Restrepo J, Gilbert A: The vascularized sural nerve. Int J Microsurg *3*:57, 1981.

Gu YD, Wu MM, Zheng YL, Li HR, Xu YN: Arterialized venous free sural nerve grafting. Ann Plast Surg *15*:332, 1985.

Kanaya F, Firrell J, Breidenbach WC: Blood flow of segmentally cut and folded vascularized rabbit sciatic nerve. J Reconstr Microsurg *9(6)*:429, 1993.

Koshima I, Harii K: Experimental study of vascularized nerve grafts: Morphometric study of axonal regeneration of nerves transplanted into silicone tubes. Ann Plast Surg *14*:235, 1985a.

Lux P, Breidenbach WC, Firrell J: Determination of temporal changes in blood flow in vascularized and nonvascularized nerve grafts in the dog. Plast Reconstr Surg *82*:133, 1988.

Mackinnon S, Kelly L, Hunter D: Comparison of regeneration across a vascularized versus conventional nerve graft: Case report. Microsurgery *9*:226, 1988.

Mani GV, Shurey C, Green CJ: Is early vascularization of nerve grafts necessary? J Hand Surg (Br) *17B*:536, 1992.

McCullough CJ, Grady O, Higginson DW, et al: Axon regeneration and vascularization of nerve grafts: An experimental study. J Hand Surg (Br) *9*:323; 1984.

Merle M, Lebreton E, Froucher G, et al: Vascularized nerve grafts: Preliminary results. Presented to the American Society for Reconstructive Microsurgery, Las Vegas, 1985.

Millesi H, Meissl G, Berger A: The interfascicular nerve grafting of the median and ulnar nerves. J Bone Joint Surg (Am) *54*:727, 1972.

Millesi H, Meissl G, Berger A: Further experience with interfascicular grafting of the median, ulnar and radial nerves. J Bone Joint Surg (Am) *58*:209, 1976.

Pho RWH, Lee YS, Rujiwetpongstorn V, Pang M: Histological studies of vascularized nerve graft and conventional nerve graft. J Hand Surg (Br) *10B*:45, 1985.

Restrepo Y, Merle M, Michon J, Folliguet B, Barrat E: Free vascularized nerve grafts: An experimental study in the rabbit. Microsurgery *6*:78, 1985.

Rose EH, Kowalski TA: Restoration of sensibility to anesthetic scarred digits with free vascularized nerve grafts from the dorsum of the foot. J Hand Surg (Am) *10*:514, 1985.

Rose EH, Kowalski TA, Norris MS: The reversed venous arterialized nerve graft in digital nerve reconstruction across scarred beds. Plast Reconstr Surg *83*:593, 1989.

Shibata M, Tsai TM, Firrell J, Breidenbach WC: Experimental comparison of vascularized and nonvascularized nerve grafting. J Hand Surg (Am) *13*:358, 1988.

Sunderland S: Nerve and Nerve Injuries, 2nd ed. Edinburgh, Churchill Livingstone, 1978, p 626.

Taylor IG: Nerve grafting with simultaneous microvascular reconstruction. Clin Orthop *133*:156, 1978.

Taylor IG, Ham FJ: The free vascularized nerve graft. Plast Reconstr Surg *57*:143, 1976.

Townsend PLG, Taylor GI: Vascularized nerve grafts using composite arterialized neuro-venous systems. Br J Plast Surg *37*:1, 1984.

Trumble TE, Parvin D: Physiology of peripheral nerve graft incorporation. J Hand Surg *19A*:420, 1994.

Wei FC, Chen HC, Chuang CC, Noordhoff MS: Fibular osteoseptocutaneous flap: Anatomic and clinical application. Plast Reconstr Surg *78*:191, 1986.

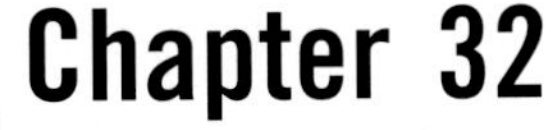

Chapter 32

• David T. W. Chiu

Autogenous and Synthetic Conduits for Nerve Repair

Essential to the success of repairing a peripheral nerve is to achieve a tensionless union between the proximal and distal stumps. When a gap exists between the proximal and distal stumps as a result of segmental destruction of the nerve, the most effective method of reconstruction is to bridge the gap with an autogenous nerve graft. However, the number of dispensable nerves suitable as donor nerves in the human body is limited. A search for alternatives for autogenous nerve grafts is more than warranted.

Indeed, since the beginning of the nineteenth century, numerous attempts have been made to identify a method of bridging a nerve gap by using either a biological or nonbiological tube. The evolution of the concept of tubulization, the early experimentation, the present development, and various types of conduits are presented in this chapter.

HISTORICAL REVIEW

The early conceptualization of using a tube to bridge a nerve gap was rather mechanical in nature. The earliest experimentation on utilizing a tube to bridge a nerve gap was the work of Gluck, who attempted to use a decalcified bone as a bridge graft for repair of a nerve gap in 1880. Eleven years later, Bungnar (1891) used a segment of brachial artery to repair the hypoglossal nerve of a dog and, reportedly, observed fasciculation of the reinnervated tongue muscle. In subsequent years, Foramitti (1904) and Nageotte (1921) independently used vein as bridge graft. However, none of these experiments was reportedly successful. Nageotte detailed his study and reported the dissolution of the vein graft with the extravasation of nerve fibers.

In the early twentieth century, the interest in peripheral nerve repair was heightened owing to the abundance of debilitating peripheral nerve injuries inflicted during the first World War. In 1919, Platt in England presented 26 cases of peripheral nerve repair using fascial tubes surrounding a nerve graft, the fascial tube surrounding strains of cat gut sutures, or a vein as a bridge graft. The space circumscribed by the fascial sheath was filled with sterile olive oil or petroleum jelly. The nerve that was bridged with a vein graft was a musculospiral nerve with a 6-inch defect. The vein lumen was filled with sterile olive oil. There was no success in any one of the cases reported in this series. Stopford (1920), a contemporary of Platt, also treated 12 patients with a fascial sheath in combination of autogenous or heterogenous nerve grafts. None of these cases proved to be successful with 2 years or more of observation. These two clinical trials not only cast a nearly irreparable blow to the concept of tubulization but also nearly doomed the development of autogenous nerve graft as well.

In fact, the interest in pursuing the development of the nerve conduit waned until near the end of World War II, when Paul Weiss' reports rekindled the interest of tubulization (Weiss, 1943, 1944a, 1944b; Weiss and Taylor, 1943, 1946) He designed a series of special instruments and developed the technique of sutureless splicing of nerve stumps with fragments of artery. He observed that, on the first postoperative day, the nerve stump was held together by blood clot. The erythrocytes lysed during the second postoperative day, leaving behind longitudinally oriented fiber meshwork filled with leukocytes. Further hemolysis was noted on the third day; however, the longitudinally oriented fibrils not only resisted proteolysis but appeared to have increased in diameter. He hypothesized that these fibrils provide a scaffolding for the advancing sheath cells to follow. At this stage, he also observed the presence of macrophages, even though he did not decipher the role of the macrophages during the process of nerve regeneration. He further observed that wallerian degeneration of the distal stump completed by the fourth day and connection of the proximal and distal stumps was achieved by the fifth day. Basically, this technique involved utilizing the arterial graft as a coupler rather than a bona fide bridge. In fact, he expressed doubt about the applicability of such a bridging technique in lesions larger than the diameter of the nerve. However, one should note that up to the time of Weiss, the concept of immunocompatibility and immunorejection was yet to be established. In many of his experiments, one could not determine whether the vessel grafts used were autogenous or homologous.

In 1970, Gibb described the use of a vein sleeve to protect the coapted nerve stump in a patient who had undergone facial nerve repair and reported success. However, in this instance, the vein graft was, in all likelihood, used as a coupler rather than as a bridge. In an anecdote cited as a cross reference, Gibb did remark on the success of Wilmot using a vein cylinder to bridge a 1-cm defect of a facial nerve in a patient with long-standing facial paralysis. The differentiation between a vein graft used as a coupler and a vein graft used as a bridge graft was not clear.

The experimentation on the nonbiological tubulization lagged behind the development of the biological bridge graft by a century. Payr (1900) reported the use of a magnesium tube; Auerbach (1915), casein treated with formalin; Lotheisen (1901), gelatin and agar tubes; and Steinthal (1917), rubber tubes. None of these methods proved to be successful. Interest subsided until Weiss (1944) reported his experimentation with tantalum foil to bridge nerve gaps. He developed a heat treatment technique to harden the tantalum foil and to fashion it into cylinders of various calibers that were used to bridge nerve gaps of a few millimeters in monkeys and rats. After 7 weeks of observation, he noted reconnection of the distal and proximal stumps. However, the excitement caused by this finding was short lived because the tantalum foil underwent fragmentation, and induced fibrosis and calcification, requiring its removal. In 1955, Garrity reported a clinical trial of using rubber, polyvinyl, and polytene tubes as a bridging device for nerve lesions. In one patient, he bridged a 12-cm nerve defect with a rubber tube. The bridging device was removed from the first, second, and third patient at 9 months, 7 weeks, and 13 days respectively. In no instance was continuity of the nerve restored, but neuroma formation was not observed either. Despite the lack of success in achieving restoration of nerve continuity, each patient experienced lessening of symptoms and required no further therapy. Such a less-than-discouraging result might have provided impetus for further search for different materials as a nerve bridging device. Campbell and Bassett (1957) conducted a series of studies using millipore, which is a cellulose-acetate plastic that is chemically inert and porous. The porosity was believed to be able to allow free exchange of nutrients while inhibiting the ingrowth of scar tissue. Initially, the millipore cylinder was made by wrapping the millipore around a glass rod saturated with water. However, such a cylinder was prone to rupture and led to subsequent neuroma formation. As a modification, the cellulose-acetate was applied over a cylinder made of steel mesh (Noback et al, 1958). Such a cellulose-acetate impregnated steel mesh nerve bridge was used to repair a nerve gap of 2.5 cm in the sciatic nerve of cats. Histological study at 3 to 4 weeks after repair revealed regeneration of axons in Schwann cell tubules. However, similar to the result with tantalum, the cellulose-acetate implemented steel mesh device was encapsulated and was found to undergo calcification and subsequent fragmentation (Bassett and Campbell, 1960). Despite this shortcoming, in 1961, Campbell and colleagues did report a trial of using cellulose to bridge an irreducible nerve gap in a major peripheral nerve in three healthy young men. The conduits were formed from reinforced matrix implemented with millipore and a nylon helix. All three repairs ended in failure. Re-exploration in one patient in whom the common peroneal nerve was repaired revealed collapse of the reinforced millipore bridging device presumably by the compression of the surrounding muscle. The clinical failure of this nonbiological bridging device indeed dampened the enthusiasm for tubulization for the next 2 decades. As of 1978, in the second edition of his monumental treatise "Nerve & Nerve Injury," the late Sir Sunderland facing the massive body of discouraging data was compelled to conclude that "the use of nonbiological materials is of no value in the bridging of gaps in nerves and may even introduce new complications in the form of infection or foreign body reaction and more extensive fibrosis. The method is now only of historical value."

AUTOGENOUS CONDUITS

The success of autogenous nerve grafts and the dawn of the understanding of the effect of tension on nerve repair propelled a new enthusiasm for the search for alternatives for autogenous nerve grafts. The latter part of the twentieth century has witnessed a renewal of the interest in the clarification of the concept of tubulization and refinement of the technique with encouraging success in clinical application.

Autogenous Venous Nerve Conduit

Through recognizing the unique regenerative potential of nerve fibers, understanding the contribution of Schwann cell as a supporting structure for the nerve regeneration, accepting the necessity of healthy vascularization as a physiological cushion for both Schwann cell proliferation and axonal regeneration, accepting the importance of banishing the invasion of scar tissue into the "vital space of regeneration" between the nerve gaps, Chiu and his colleagues at Columbia challenged the conventional dogma and re-examined the validity of autogenous vein graft as a nerve conduit (Campbell and Bassett, 1957; Campbell et al, 1961; Chiu et al, 1980, 1982, 1983). In 1980, at the surgical forum, Chiu presented histological and electrophysiological evidence of nerve regeneration through an autogenous vein graft in rodents and introduced the term autogenous venous nerve conduit (AVNC). In this study, a 1-cm segment of the sciatic nerve was removed bilaterally in Spraque Dawley rats. On one side, the nerve gap was bridged with interposition vein graft, while the other side was left unrepaired as a control. It was observed that plantar ulcers were uniformly present. However, the plantar ulcer was smaller on the vein graft side and eventually healed, whereas the ulcer on the control unrepaired side showed no signs of improvement. Muscle mass on both the control and the vein graft sides atrophied. However, the atrophy on the vein-grafted side plateaued at 3 to 5 months postoperatively, whereas the control side had persistent wasting. Three months after nerve reconstruction with the vein graft, direct electrical stimulation of the vein-grafted nerve resulted in distal muscle contraction. At 4 months, in vitro electrophysiological study on the vein-grafted limb revealed multiphasic muscle action potential, which is consistent with nerve regeneration and reinnervation of the previously denervated muscles. In vitro study with the vein-grafted nerve suspended in an isolated chamber demonstrated bona fide action potential. Histological examination revealed that, at 1 month, nerve fiber had passed the proximal venoneural junction. At 2 months, the regenerated nerve fiber had passed the distal venoneural junction and was invading the distal stump. At 5 months, the vein graft lumen was found to be filled with wavy nerve fibers that ran longitudinally from the proximal to distal border of the vein graft with no signs of obstruction. Histological examination of the control side only revealed neuroma formation. This study presented irrefutable data that autogenous venous nerve conduits could indeed serve as a protected passage for the regeneration of nerve fibers (Chiu et al, 1982). The amicable physiological environment that the vein graft provides allowed the nerve fiber to grow and mature. Having successfully passed through the vein graft, these regenerated nerve fibers are capable of recapturing the distal neuromuscular end-plate. This study was later supported by the findings of Rice and Berstein (1984) and Wang and co-workers (1993). In addition to confirming the previous finding, Wang and colleagues also noted the effect of the vessel diameter on regeneration.

To elucidate the relative efficacy of autogenous venous nerve conduit Chiu and associates then performed a quantitative study comparing the electrophysiological efficacy of autogenous venous nerve conduit compared with that of the autogenous nerve graft (Chiu et al, 1983). In this study, serial nerve conduction studies as well as terminal histological analysis were performed. This study provided quantitative electophysiological and microscopic data that supported the concept that AVNC is capable of supporting the regeneration of nerve fibers and their subsequent maturation. This study was subsequently confirmed by the study of Suematsu and associates (1988). The histological study revealed intact myelinated fiber growing through both grafts, with a remarkable absence of scar tissue within either the autogenous nerve graft (ANG) or the AVNC. This study represents the first report providing quantitative electrophysiological data comparing nerve conduit to nerve graft.

These findings were subsequently confirmed by Suematsu and associates (1988). The 50% less in nerve action potential most likely indicates that there are about half of the number of nerve fibers passing through the AVNC as compared with the ANG. Based on these findings, Chiu further hypothesized that this limited number of nerve fibers could successfully regenerate and pass through the bridge provided by the AVNC and could bring about the return of a critical level of functionality, such as protective sensation. To test this hypothesis, prospective clinical trials were conducted to compare the efficacy of AVNC with that of ANG and direct neurorrhaphy as treatment of distal sensory nerves. The criterion in determining the modality of treatment was the length of the nerve gap. If the nerve gap was small enough to allow direct repair without undue tension, the defect would be closed by direct neurorrhaphy. If the defect was not amenable by direct repair with minimum tension, but was larger than 3 cm, the defect was repaired with autogenous sural nerve graft. If the nerve gap was less than 3 cm, but not amenable to direct repair, it was then repaired by AVNC (Figs. 32–1 to 32–3). The result was evaluated by an independent and blinded evaluator. The data indicated that the parts innervated by the repair were uniformly functionally useful. There was no significant pain in the operative

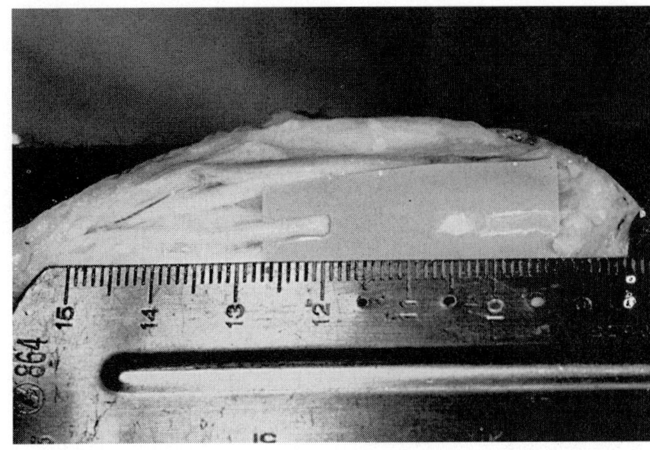

FIGURE 32–2. After resection of the neuroma, there was a nerve gap of 2.7 cm.

site in any of the patients, there was uniform satisfaction with the operation, and there was no request for a corrective operation. Examination revealed uniform return of pseudomotor activity and recovery of protective sensation. Two hundred and fifty-six and 30 cycles per second (CPS) vibration sensation are similar among all three treatment modalities. In the 12 palmar distal nerves treated with direct repair, static and moving two-point discrimination was found to be 7.4 ± 1.54 and 5.7 ± 1.7 mm, respectively. In the 10 palmar digital nerves treated with AVNC, the static and moving two-point discrimination was found to be 11.1 ± 3.4 and 6.5 ± 2.56 mm, respectively. In the four palmar digital nerves repaired with ANG, static and moving two-point discrimination were found to be 9.0 ± 1 and 5.78 ± 2.38 mm, respectively. Applying the sensory index, which registers a normal sensitivity with a value of 10 and total anesthesia with a value of 0, the result among direct repair, ANG, and AVNC were similar, with values of 7.7 ± 1, 7 ± 1, and 7.4 ± 0.15, respectively. These results not only confirm the validity of the author's hypothesis but also refute the dismal results reported by previous investigators. Although the superiority of the direct repair was readily apparent, this fact did not diminish the practicality of AVNC

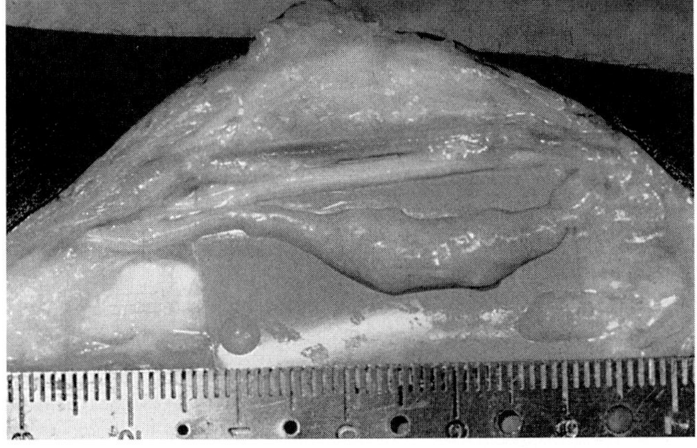

FIGURE 32–1. Neuroma of a branch of the superficial radial nerve of the distal forearm of a mail deliverer.

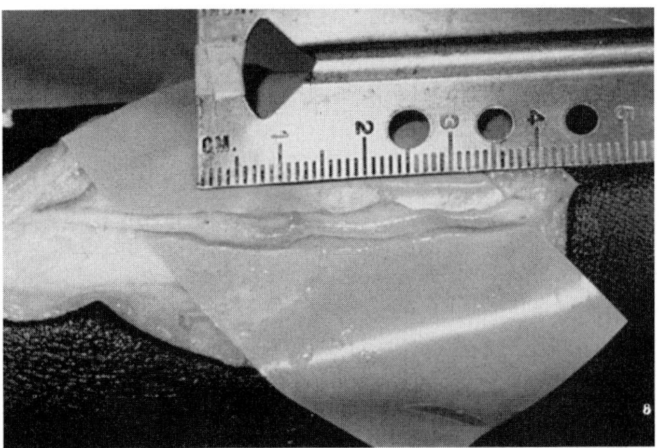

FIGURE 32–3. A segment of the adjacent basilic vein was used as AVNC. The nerve stumps were telescoped into the lumen and were secured with two 9-0 mattress sutures.

for treatment of short nerve gaps of 3 cm or less, particularly on nonessential cutaneous nerves. The preliminary data of this study were first reported at the Plastic Surgery Research Council Meeting in Boston in 1987, and the final result was published in 1990 (Chiu and Strauch, 1990). Walton and colleagues (1989) reported their findings on a retrospective study analyzing the results of 18 distal nerve repairs with interpositional vein grafts. This report indicated a recovery to S3+ level if nerve was repaired acutely and recovery of S3 level if the repair was delayed.

Empty Perineurial Tube

Restrepo and associates (1983) investigated the application of so-called empty perineurial tube grafts to bridge a 2.5-cm nerve defect using a rabbit sciatic nerve model and recorded more favorable electromyographic recovery and earlier revascularization compared with conventional autogenous nerve grafts. The myelinization, however, was less in the perineuronal tube-grafted group. The limited availability of the perineuronal tube renders the technique less attractive as an alternative to ANG.

Muscle as Conduit

In 1986, Glasby and co-workers presented the use of freeze-dried autogenous nerve muscle grafts as nerve conduits based on the assumption that the basement membrane of the skeletal muscle fiber could provide a suitable matrix for regenerating fibers. In this study, a gluteal maximus muscle in rats was dissected free, frozen with liquid nitrogen, and then thawed in distilled water to promote osmotic cellular membrane disruption. The treated muscle graft was then used to bridge a 1-cm nerve gap in the ipsilateral sciatic nerve. In another group of animals, a similar nerve gap was bridged with an untreated muscle graft serving as controls. A comparison was made between placing the muscle grafts perpendicular to the longitudinal axis of the nerve stumps and parallel to the longitudinal axis of the nerve. Histological study at 51 days revealed no regeneration in the control group. In the group with co-axially aligned muscle graft, axons were noted to course through the graft and to reach the distal stem. However, no axons were seen in the distal stump in the group with the muscle fibers aligned perpendicularly to the direction of growth of the axons. In a study on primates, marmosets had 3-cm ulnar or radial nerve lesion repairs with autogenous muscle graft. The graft was treated with the similar freezing technique described by Glasby and colleagues (1986). At 6 months, histological examination showed axons regenerating through the graft and reaching the distal stumps. Based on the qualitative evidence of nerve regeneration in rats and primates, Norris and colleagues (1988) performed a clinical trial on nine patients using the freeze-dried muscle autograft obtained from the patients' pectoralis major muscle. The ages of the patients ranged from 15 to 61. The nerve gap ranged from 15 to 25 cm. Follow-up at 3 to 11 months revealed S4 in one patient, S3+ in four patients and less than S3 in three patients. Some degree of two-point discrimination was noted in seven of eight patients. The freeze and thaw muscle graft conduit

has an interesting appeal; however, the experimental data are in need of objective confirmation and lack quantitative experimental data as compared with an autogenous sural nerve graft.

SYNTHETIC CONDUITS

Pseudosynovial Tube

Concurrent with the development of AVNC, Lundborg and co-workers (1982b) explored the technique of mesothelial tube as a means of providing a biological conduit to bridge a nerve gap. In their report in 1982, three groups of 10 rats had sciatic nerve gaps of 10 mm with a bridge of either a mesothelial tube or autogenous nerve graft; 10 rats had no repair and served as controls. The mesothelial tube was created by subcutaneously implanting a silicone rod surrounded by a thin metal spiral. The silicone rod was removed at 3 to 4 weeks, leaving behind a tubular mesothelial chamber held open by the metal spiral. This was then used to bridge the 10-mm gap in the sciatic nerve. Results in both show, at 1 month, fibers coursing through the longitudinal chamber and, at 3 months, fibers reaching the distal stumps. The control group showed only sparse ingrowth of nerve fibers into the distal stump at 3 months. Fluid removed from the mesothelial chamber at 3 days demonstrated neuronotrophic activities (Lundborg et al, 1982). This technique is clearly an advancement compared with the cellulose acetate steel mesh preparation. In 1985, Mackinnon and Dellon repeated Lundborg's study on five baboons with 3-cm ulnar nerve gaps bridged with pseudosynovial sheaths. Histological examination at 3, 5, 7, and 9 months demonstrated nerve regeneration across the gaps, supporting Lundborg's findings. In a subsequent study in 1988, Mackinnon and Dellon compared the efficacy of sural nerve grafts and pseudosynovial sheaths in bridging a 3-cm ulnar nerve gap on cynomolgus monkeys. In this study, 3-cm ulnar nerve gaps were created on both arms. On the left arm, the nerve gap was bridged with sural nerve graft and, on the right, pseudosynovial sheaths. After 1 year of follow-up, histological study revealed regeneration through both conduits. However, electrophysiological data for both conduits were significantly less than for the value obtained from normal ulnar nerves. More importantly, no statistical differences were noted between electrophysiological data of nerve graft in pseudosynovial sheaths. It was concluded that tubulization compared favorably with nerve grafting. Nonetheless, the need for multistage surgical intervention renders this technique less practical.

Polyglactin Mesh Tube

In 1982, Molander and co-workers presented their study using bioabsorbable polyglactin mesh tubes to bridge nerve lesions of 7 to 9 mm in the tibial nerve of 24 rabbits. Histological observation over a period of 8 weeks revealed gradual reabsorption of the mesh tubes, with the emergence of a new connective tissue tube containing fiber, blood vessels, and collagen, which were capable of guiding the outgrowing nerve fiber to the distal nerve stump. It was observed that the new connective tissue tube contained numerous fascicles, which displayed increased axonal regeneration and myelinization after 16 weeks. No scar tissue or neuroma formation was noted in the group treated with polyglactin, whereas the control group exhibited neuroma formation.

Polyglycolic Acid Tube

In view of the impracticality of the two-stage approach in using the pseudosynovial sheath procedure, Dellon and MacKinnon (1988) developed bioabsorbable polyglycolic acid tubes. With a similar ulnar nerve gap modeled on cynomolgus monkeys, they again demonstrated regeneration of nerve fibers through both autogenous nerve and bioabsorbable conduits. The conduction velocity and amplitude were also significantly less than normal, but no difference was found between the sural nerve graft and the bioabsorbable conduits.

The heightened interest in developing an off-the-shelf conduit for nerve reconstruction extended to a trial of using silicone tubes and polyethylene tubes. However, the concern of long-term complications of nonabsorbable, nonbiological conduits such as silicone and ethylene continued to have a dampening effect on the further developments (Merle et al, 1989). The application of bioabsorbable material appeared to be the more likely viable alternative. In 1990, MacKinnon and Dellon presented a clinical series of 15 patients, mean age 30.5 ± 7.6 years with a distal nerve gap ranging from 0.5 to 3.0 cm reconstructed with bioabsorbable polyglycolic acid tubes. Examination at a mean postoperative interval of 22.4 months (ranging from 11 to 32 months) showed that 53% (eight) of their patients had recovery of static two-point discrimination between 7 and 15 mm and moving two-point discrimination between 4 and 7 mm, 33% (five) of their patients had static two-point discrimination less than or equal to 6 mm and a moving two-point discrimination of less than or equal to 3 mm, and 14% (two) had poor results. MacKinnon and Dellon thus concluded that for reconstruction nerve gaps less than 3 cm, bioabsorbable polyglycolic tube gives at least clinical results comparable to that of autogenous nerve grafts yet is free of donor-site morbidity. These results are encouraging, future prospective studies with objective evaluation would likely enhance the advisability of its clinical application.

CONCLUSION

The concept of tubulization was revived toward the end of the last decade of the twentieth century. Both the autogenous biological conduit and the synthetic conduit has been tested extensively, both experimentally and, to a degree, clinically. At this juncture, by virtue of the consistency of both the qualitative and quantitative data, AVNC has emerged as an accepted surgical technique in bridging small nerve gaps of 3 cm or less. To expand the application potential of the autogenous venous conduit or other nonbiological conduits, one sees the future of potentiating such a conduit with neuronotrophic factors such as laminin or activated Schwann cells to serve as the source of neuronotrophic factors (Cor-

deiro et al, 1989; Danielson et al, 1988; DaSilva et al, 1985; DaSilva and Langone, 1989; Madison et al, 1985, 1987, 1988; Rich et al, 1989; Satou et al, 1986; Williams et al, 1987; Williams, 1987; Wooley et al, 1990). Such exciting possibilities certainly add a brilliant glow of optimism to the ever-evolving horizon of neuroscience and peripheral nerve surgery.

References

Auerbach S: Zur Frage der Nerveneinsheidung Mittelst Gulalith. Munch Med Wschr 63:1573.

Bassett CAL, Campbell JB: Calcification of millipore in vivo. Plast Reconstr Surg 26:132, 1960.

Bungnar OV: Die Gegenerations und Regenerations. Vorgange Am Nerven nack Verletzungen Beitr. Pathol Anat 10:321–393, 1891.

Campbell JB, Bassett CAL: The surgical application of monomolecular filters (millipore) to bridge gaps in peripheral nerves and to prevent neuroma formation. Surg Forum 7:570, 1957.

Campbell JB, Basset CA, Husby J, et al: Microfilter sheaths in peripheral nerve surgery: A laboratory report and preliminary clinical study. J Trauma 1:139–157, 1961.

Chiu DTW, Yui LT, Lovelace R, Wolff M, Stengel S, Middletown L, Ianecka I, Krizek T: Autogenous vein graft as a conduit for nerve regeneration. Surg Forum 31:550, 1980.

Chiu DTW, Janeka I, Krizek TJ, Wolffm, Lavelace RE: Autogenous vein graft as a conduit for nerve regeneration. Surgery 91:226–232, 1982.

Chiu DTW, Yui LT, Lovelace R, Wolff M, Stengel S, Middletown L, Ianecka I, Krizek T: A comparative electrophysiologic evaluation of nerve grafts and vein grafts as nerve conduits. Surg Forum 34:601–603, 1983.

Chiu DTW, Yui LT, Lovelace R, Wolff M, Stengel S, Middletown L, Ianecka I, Krizek T: Comparative electrophysiologic vein grafts as nerve conduits: An experimental study. J Reconstr Microsurg 4:303–310, 1988.

Chiu DTW, Strauch B: A prospective clinical evaluation of autogenous vein grafts used as a nerve conduit for distal sensory nerve defects of 3 cm or less. Plast Reconstr Surg 86:928–934, 1990.

Cordeiro PG, Seckel BR, Lipton SA, et al.: Acid fibroblast growth factor enhances peripheral nerve regeneration in vivo. Plast Reconstr Surg 83:1013–1019, 1989.

Danielson N, Pettmann B, Vahlsing HL, et al.: Fibroblast growth factor effects on peripheral nerve regeneration in a silicone chamber model. J Neurosci Res 20:320–330, 1988.

DaSilva CF, Madison R, Dikkes P, et al.: An in vivo model to quantify motor and sensory peripheral nerve regeneration using bioresorbable nerve guide tubes. Brain Res 342:307–315, 1985.

DaSilva CF, Langone F: Addition of nerve growth factor to the interior of a tubular prosthesis increases sensory neuron regeneration in vivo. Braz J Med Biol Res 22:691–694, 1989.

Dellon AL, MacKinnon SE: An alternative to the classical nerve graft for the management of the short nerve gap. Plast Reconstr Surg 82:849–856, 1988.

Dellon AL, MacKinnon SE: Selection of the appropriate parameter to measure neural regeneration. Ann Plast Surg 23:197, 1989.

Dellon AL: Discussion of autogenous vein graft repair of digital nerve defects in the finger: A retrospective clinical study. Plast Reconstr Surg 84:950–952, 1989.

Dellon AL: Wound healing in nerve. Clin Plast Surg 17:545–570, 1990.

Derby A, Engleman VW, Frierdich GE, et al: Nerve growth factor facilitates regeneration across nerve gaps: Morphological and behavioral studies in rat sciatic nerve. Exper Neurol 119:176–191, 1993.

Foramitti C: Zur Technik der Nervennaht. Arch Klin Chir 73:643, 1904.

Garrity RW: The use of plastic and rubber tubing in the management of irreparable nerve injuries. Surg Forum 6:517, 1955.

Gibb A: Facial nerve sleeve graft. J Laryngol Otol 84:577–582, 1970.

Glasby MA, Gschmeissner S, Hitchcock RFI, et al.: Regeneration of the sciatic nerve in rats: The effect of muscle basement membrane. J Bone Joint Surg Br 68:829–833, 1986a.

Glasby MA, Gschmeissner SE, Huang CLH, et al.: Degenerated muscle grafts used for peripheral nerve repair in primates. J Hand Surg Br 3:347, 1986b.

Gluck T: Ueber Neuroplastic Auf dem Wege de Transplantation. Arch Klin Chir 25:606, 1880.

Hollowell JP, Villadiego A, Rich KM: Sciatic nerve regeneration across gaps within silicone chambers: Long term effects of NGF and consideration of axonal branching. Exp Neurol *110*:45–51, 1991.

Khouri RK, Chiu DTW, Feinberg J, et al.: Effects of neurite-promoting factors on rat sciatic nerve regeneration. Microsurgery *10*:206–209, 1989.

Lotheisen G: Zur Technik der Nervenund Sehnennaht. Arch Klin Chir *64*:310, 1901.

Lundborg G, Dahlin LB, Danielsen N, et al.: Nerve regeneration in silicone chambers: Influence of gap length and of distal stump components. Exp Neurol *76*:361–375, 1982a.

Lundborg G, Dahlin LB, Danielsen N, et al.: Nerve regeneration across an extended gap: A neurobiological view of nerve repair and the possible involvement of neuronotrophic factors. J Hand Surg *7*:580–587, 1982b.

Mackinnon SE, Dellon AL, Hudson AR, et al.: Nerve regeneration through a pseudosynovial sheath in a primate model. Plast Reconstr Surg *6*:833, 1985.

Mackinnon SE, Dellon AL: A comparison of nerve regeneration across sural nerve graft and a vascularized pseudosheath. J Hand Surg *6*:935, 1988.

Mackinnon SE, Dellon AL: Clinical nerve reconstruction with a bioresorbable polyglycolic acid tube. Plast Reconstr Surg *85*:419–424, 1990.

Mackinnon SE, Dellon AL, O'Brien JP: Changes in nerve fiber numbers distal to a nerve repair in the rat sciatic nerve model. Muscle Nerve *14*:1116–1122, 1991.

Madison R, DaSilva CF, Dikkes P et al.: Increased rate of peripheral nerve regeneration using bioresorbable nerve guides and a laminin-containing gel. Experimental Neurology *88*:767–772, 1985.

Madison R, DaSilva CF, Dikkes P, et al.: Peripheral nerve regeneration with entubulation repair: Comparisons of biodegradable nerve guides versus polyethylene tubes and the effects of a laminin-containing gel. Exp Neurol *95*:378–390, 1987.

Madison R, Da Silva CF, Dikkes P: Entubulation repair with protein additives increases the maximum nerve gap distance successfully bridged with tubular prostheses. Brain Res *447*:325–334, 1988.

Merle M, Dellon AL, Campbell JN, Chang PS: Complications from silicon polymer intubulation of nerves. Microsurgery *10*:130–133, 1989.

Molander H, Olsson Y, Engkvist O, et al.: Regeneration of peripheral nerve through a polyglactin tube. Muscle Nerve *5*:54–57, 1982.

Nageotte J: de Processus de la Cicatrisation des Nerfs. CT Sea NC Soc Biol *78*:249, 1921.

Norris RW, Glasby MA, Gattuso JM: Peripheral nerve repair in humans using muscle autografts: A new technique. J Bone Joint Surg Br *70B*:530–533, 1988.

Noback CR, Hushy J, Girado JM, Basett CAL, Campbell JB: Neural regeneration across gaps in mammalian peripheral nerve: Early morphological findings. Anat Rec *131*:633, 1958.

Payr E: Beitrage Zur Technik der Blietgefass und Netvennacht nest Mitthei lungon uber die Verewentung resorbirbaren Metalles in der Chiruge. Arch Klin Chir :62–67, 1900.

Platt H: On the results of bridging gaps in injured nerve trunks by autogenous fascial tubulization and autogenous nerve grafts. Br J Surg *7*:384–389, 1919–1920.

Restrepo Y, Merle M, Michon J, Folliquet B, Petry D: Fascicular nerve graft using an empty perineurial tube: An experimental study in the rabbit. Microsurgery *4*:106–112, 1983.

Rice DH, Berstein FD: The use of autogenous vein for nerve grafting. Otolaryngol Head Neck Surg *92*:410, 1984.

Rich K, Alexander TD, Pryor JC, et al.: Nerve growth factor enhances regeneration through silicone chambers. Exp Neurol *105*:162–170, 1989.

Satou T, Nishida S, Hiruma S, et al.: A morphological study on the effects of collagen gell matrix on regeneration of severed rat sciatic nerve in silicone tubes. Acta Pathol Jpn *36*:199–208, 1986.

Steinthal C: Die Ueberdechung von Grossern Nervendef iekten Mittels Tabularnaht. Zenthl Chir *94*:646, 1917.

Stopford J: The treatment of large defects in peripheral nerve injuries. Lancet *2*:1296, 1920.

Suematsu N, Atsuta Y, Hirayama T: Vein graft for repair of peripheral nerve gap. J Reconstr Microsurg *4*:313–318, 1988.

Sunderland S: Nerve & Nerve Injuries, 2nd ed. New York, Churchill Livingstone, 1978, p 605.

Walton RL, Brown RE, Matory WE, et al.: Autogenous vein graft repair of digital nerve defects in the finger: A retrospective clinical study. Plast Reconstr Surg *84*:944–949, 1989.

Wang KK, Costas PD, Jones DS, et al.: Sleeve insertion and collagen coating improve nerve regeneration through vein conduits. J Reconstr Microsurg *9*:39–48, 1993.

Weiss P: The technology of nerve regeneration: A review. Sutureless tubulation and related methods of nerve repair. J Neurosurg *1*:400–448, 1944a.

Weiss P, Taylor AC: Histomechanical analysis of nerve reunion in the rat after tubular splicing. Arch Surg *47*:419–450, 1943.

Weiss P: Experiments on nerve repair. Trans Am Neurol Soc *69*:42–51, 1943.

Weiss P: Sutureless reunion of severed nerves with elastic cuffs of tantalum. J Neurosurg *1*:219, 1944b.

Weiss P, Taylor AC: Guides for nerve regeneration across gaps. J Neurosurg *3*:375–389, 1946.

Williams LR, Danielsen N, Muller H, et al.: Exogenous matrix precursors promote functional nerve regeneration across a 15-mm gap within a silicone chamber in the rat. J Comp Neurol *264*:284–290, 1987.

Williams LR: Exogenous fibrin matrix precursors stimulate the temporal process of nerve regeneration within a silicone chamber. Neurochem Res *12*:851–860, 1987.

Wooley AL, Hollowell JP, Rich KM: Fibronectin-laminin combination enhances peripheral nerve regeneration across long gaps. Otolaryngol Head Neck Surg *103*:509–518, 1990.

Chapter 33

• Edward Almquist

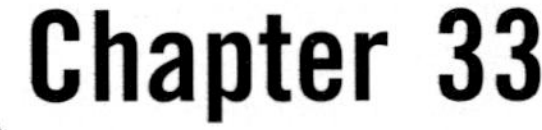
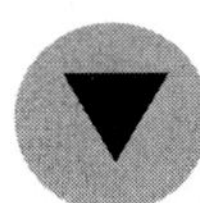

Adjuncts to Suture Repair of Peripheral Nerves: Laser, Glue, and Other Techniques

HISTORY OF ADJUNCTS TO NERVE REPAIR

Humans have used surgery to treat disease for at least 12,000 years. Skulls dating back to the late Ice Age clearly demonstrate that ancient practitioners performed trephination and that their subjects survived the procedure. Egyptian writings ca 2500 B.C. describe methods of approximating wounds of the flesh, dressing them, and applying grease and honey to promote healing. Egyptian practitioners did not treat open fractures, however, because they considered them untreatable and fatal. Hippocrates (460–377 B.C.) first described the instruments of surgery used in his time—knives, catheters, spatulas, forceps, curettes, rasps, and various needles. Surgeons of Hippocrates' time were able to excise hemorrhoids, drain empyemas, and ligate and excise aneurysms and varicose veins. Although these surgeons' understanding of general anatomy was fairly accurate, they directed little attention to nerves before Galen's time.

Galen (A.D. 130–200), whose works constituted the primary medical reference in Europe for 1700 years, practiced surgery in Alexandria before his career took him to Rome. There, he found that physicians such as himself were perceived as generalists, who were limited to diagnosis and medical treatments—only a specialized surgeon class performed surgery. Nonetheless, he wrote seven treatises on surgery, which at the time, focused mostly on treatment of combat wounds and the infections that resulted from those wounds.

Galen both identified and treated nerve injuries. He prescribed various medical treatments for a pricked nerve, a dreaded injury because of the severe pain it caused. There is evidence that Galen attempted to agglutinate wounds involving severed nerves with substances such as egg albumin. This technique suggests he understood the importance of rejoining the two severed nerve ends (Kuhn, 1965).

In the seventh century, Paul of Aegina (translated, 1844–1847) described nerve repairs. He stressed that nerve sutures should be "very superficial in order to avoid pinching or puncturing the nerve." He also suggested agglutination to approximate nerve ends. In the fourteenth century, Guy de Chauliac reported the restoration of nerve function after nerve suturing and commented that young patients seemed better able than adults to obtain renewed function (translated, 1923).

Even during the eighteenth century, after the microscope had come into wide use, nerve anatomy remained poorly understood. Research of that period had not yet ascertained whether axons come from the cell body or are part of a web closely associated to the nerve cell but not specifically part of it. Cruikshank, working in John Hunter's laboratory, began conducting experiments on nerve regeneration in 1776 and concluded that such regeneration, at least in large nerves, does occur, and that it occurs along a nerve element by axonal regeneration (Cruikshank, 1795). His view, however, was not widely accepted. The reunionist faction cited examples of nerves regaining function after severance within a few days to weeks following repair, and used this evidence to substantiate that nerve elements are two separate factions that can heal independently. This controversy continued even after Waller published his works on wallerian degeneration (Waller, 1852).

It was not until 1928 that the classic experiments of Ramon y Cajal settled the controversy regarding nerve regeneration and that surgical repair of nerves became generally encouraged (Cajal, 1928). By that time, tendon repairs and transplants had already been common for 30 years, and the advent of general surgery and anesthetic technique had made such procedures feasible. Surgeons recognized that suturing a nerve together was a difficult procedure and that the sutures themselves, even if they were restricted as much as possible to the epineurium, would likely produce disorganization of the fibers.

Young, Medawar, Holmes, and Saunders (1940) reported a new method by which nerve stumps could be held together. This technique involved approximating the cut nerve ends and pouring around them plasma mixed with a fibrinogen concentrate obtained from cockerel blood. Based on histological evaluation in experiments with rabbits, the researchers concluded that this method was superior to nerve sutures in rabbits and dogs (Fig. 33–1). Two years later, Seddon and Medawar (1942) used this method on humans and reported satisfactory functions as a result.

In the United States, Tarlov noted that conventional repair of severed nerves using silk sutures proved unsatisfactory because, he believed, the nerve fibers were unavoidably caught by the suture and strangulated, hence producing faulty longitudinal alignment when the stumps became pressed against each other in a tangle of fibers. He found the technique of Young and Medawar unsatisfactory as well because it produced excessive inflammation and fibrosis

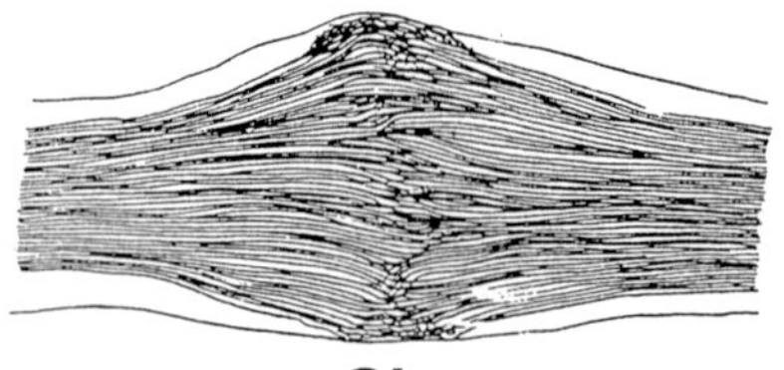

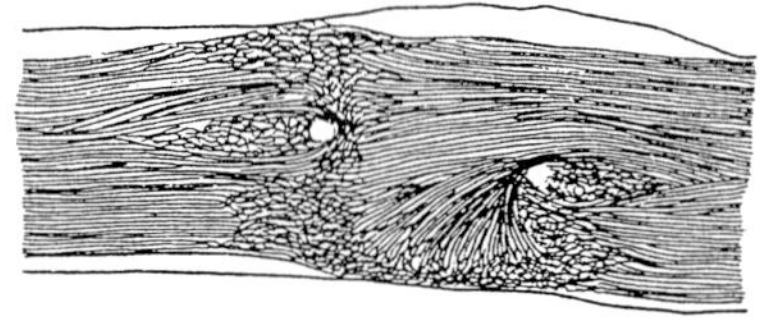

FIGURE 33–1. A drawing from the article by Young and Medawar, 1940, showing the superiority of glued nerve anastomosis. (From Young JZ, Medawar PB: Fibrin structure of peripheral nerves. Lancet *3*:126–127, 1940.)

around the repair site. He attributed this consequence to a foreign body reaction and suggested the use of fresh, unmodified autogenous plasma as an adherent. He designed a rubber mold to hold the nerve ends being glued and used a fine tantalum wire suture some distance from the repair site to reduce strain across the coaptation. Tarlov (1944) reported considerable success in 14 cases.

In the decade following Tarlov's work, several European studies described experiments using fibrinogen cryoprecipitates and the refinements of technique that resulted. Matras' study reported satisfactory clinical outcomes (Matras et al, 1975). Experiments and clinical trials in the use of adhesives ensued once human fibrinogen from pooled plasma, highly concentrated and rich with Factor VIII, began to be produced commercially in Vienna in the late 1970s.

Up to that point, the 1954 British Medical Research Council's special report on nerve injuries during World War II had been the most extensive evaluation of nerve injuries. It portrayed a pessimistic view of the return of adequate nerve function following repair. At that time, many believed that a biological limitation on the ability of adult axons to regenerate may exist, a limitation perhaps not surmountable by any type of repair. Researchers noted that much better function could be restored in young patients, and some suggested the probable reason for this outcome is a greater capacity in youth to regenerate the axon. Edshage and others, particularly in Sweden, countered this pessimistic view and asserted that the major factor in poor return of function in any age group is poor alignment and disruption at the repair site (Matras et al, 1975).

Experiments by Almquist and associates (1970, 1983) indicated that adult nerve regeneration can produce distal axon growth essentially equal to that among children and suggested that a major factor in the better return of function in children's nerves compared with those of adults is better central reorganization following misalignment of the nerve repair site. Such conclusions challenged the theory of an inherent inability of adult axons to regenerate and suggested that if axial alignment is improved, even an adult's ability to obtain function will also be improved. These optimistic views encouraged renewed attempts to improve techniques for peripheral nerve repair.

With the advent of very fine swedged-on needles, microsurgical repair techniques became possible. Microsutures caused less mechanical disruption of the nerve repair site and afforded finer detail in coaptation, resulting in less foreign body reaction. Nevertheless, the mechanical limitations of any form of suture repair in nerves inspired investigators to look elsewhere for additional improvements.

A small group of European researchers continued to experiment with adhesive repairs such as acrocyanate glues, which were found to be extremely toxic to tissues and, therefore, were soon abandoned. Human-derived fibrin glue

seemed to be an attractive alternative. Following the works of Matras and colleagues (1975, 1973), Duspiva (1978), and Kuderna (1976), others began using fibrin glues, both experimentally and clinically. By the mid-1980s, clinical results of several serial studies using fibrin glue had been published. These included reports by Eglof and Narakas (1983), Eglof and associates (1986), and Meyer and co-workers (1986). Since then, the popularity of fibrin glue adhesive nerve repair has grown. This form of repair has proved to be particularly useful in cases of multiple nerve grafting such as brachial plexus injuries.

The fibrinogen used is a derivative of pooled human plasma. Concentrated to 75 mg/ml, it is mixed with bovine aprotinin 300 IU and 5.88 mg of calcium chloride. A second, separate component is 500 IU/ml of lyophilized bovine thrombin. These two products are mixed together immediately before or during application, after which they coalesce to form an adhesive. This process is similar to a two-system epoxy glue. The fibrinogen components can be applied with a dual syringe spray set. Several manufacturers have developed kits for this type of application.

The pooled plasma derivative has not been approved for clinical use in the United States, although several groups in this country have used it experimentally. The possibility of transmissible disease from pooled plasma has been a concern with this protocol. In order to eliminate that possibility, Feldman and co-workers (1987) devised a method of autogenous fibrin collection—patients can have fibrinogen processed from their own donated blood. This process has not been reported for quantitative results in humans. Even in Europe, the use of commercially available fibrin adhesive has not gained universal acceptance (Herter, 1988). The primary clinical studies reported have focused on complex nerve injuries and are difficult to compare with other published results. Many well-known investigators are strong advocates of the use of fibrin glue, particularly in brachial plexus injuries and in grafts in which no tension is required (Narakas, 1988). These authors cite the speed of operating time and the ability to seal several cable grafts together at the repair site and then approximate them in the larger stump (Fig. 33–2). One author claimed a technical advantage to freezing the approximated ends, then trimming them accurately and applying the glue while the nerve ends are still frozen (Bertilli and Mira, 1993). The principal advantage reported in all clinical investigations using fibrin glue seems to be time saved in performing complex multiple nerve repairs or grafts.

Experimental studies comparing sutured nerve repair with fibrin clot repair do not demonstrate a clear advantage for using the glue repair; several authors even report a disadvantage. Of the 10 comparative experimental studies, six papers showed no difference in electrophysiological, histological, or functional results between fibrin glue and microsurgical

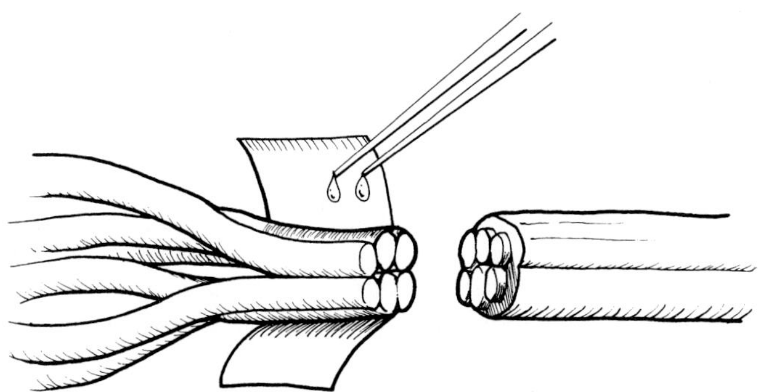

FIGURE 33–2. The two components for fibrin glue are applied to the multistrand cable graft near the anastomosis site. The contour is maintained by a sleeve until the glue is firm, hence allowing more accurate trimming and easing anastomosis to the nerve stump.

repair (Becker et al, 1985a; Becker et al, 1985b; Bertilli and Mira, 1993; Cruz et al, 1986; Faldini et al, 1984; Feldman et al, 1987; Herter, 1988; Moy et al, 1988; Narakas, 1988; Smahel et al, 1987). The study by Faldini and co-workers (1984) did report better results for glued nerves than for those sutured with nylon. These researchers repaired the rat peroneal nerve and recorded the isometric contraction of the extensor digitorum longus muscle using a strain gauge. In a rat sciatic nerve model, Cruz and colleagues (1986) noted an 80% dehiscence rate when using homogenous fibrin alone compared with no dehiscence when using suture alone. They also observed increased inflammation. Herter (1988) found that the fibrin glue dissolved prematurely; he also noted frequent fibrosis and gaping at the repair site. In a well-controlled study, Moy and associates (1988) determined that the fibrin seal did not produce equally good clinical function in electrophysiological evaluation or histological evaluation compared with 10-0 nylon sutured nerves, but the surgical time for repair was significantly faster. Narakas (1988) reported an approximately 25% increase in motor strength using glue when compared with his earlier cases using suture alone.

THE TECHNIQUE OF FIBRIN GLUE NERVE REPAIR

The technique of fibrin glue nerve repair shares the principles of sutured nerve repair. A clean, noncrushing cut is made back to definable fascicles. If an epineurial repair is required, most authors suggest a stay suture in the epineurium at some distance from the repair site. The proximal and distal corresponding fascicles should be identified using microscopic control, and the matched fascicular alignment should be controlled through the gluing process. The fibrin glue should be ready for application soon after the trimming of the nerve ends is done. Prolonged delay may allow protrusion of the axoplasms and a less technically satisfactory repair. A transparent sleeve is used to hold the glue in contact at the repair site; and the glue is applied circumferentially to afford, in essence, a minitubule. The fibrin glue should extend 2 to 5 mm to each side of the repair site. In group fascicular repairs a similar technique is used after appropriate dissection of each side of the nerve and removal of the epineurium. A distant suture is applied to relieve tension. The group fascicles are glued using the same technique, which can be technically demanding. The group fascicles are tiny, and many have to be adhered in a small area.

At present, the use of glue for nerve grafting is more popular. In the most commonly advocated technique, the nerve ends are cut appropriately to well-preserved fascicles on each side. The use of a cutting tool such as described by Meyer or Stenstrom is advised in order to avoid crushing the nerve during the trimming (Edshage, 1964; Narakas, 1988). The cable grafts are aligned with appropriately matched fascicles at the stump, and a mosaic of the cable fascicles is glued together to match the recipient site. This technique allows one large section of the graft to be approximated at the repair site, yet the adherent graft is only a few millimeters long. Thus, the desired revascularization of the thin cables is not compromised (see Fig. 33–2). A stay suture is placed in the epineurium at the recipient site and in the fibrin glue interface on the graft. The graft should be approximately 20% longer than the gap distance to ensure that there is no tension. The smallest effective amount of glue should be used in order to avoid getting glue between the anastomosis.

NERVE REPAIRS WITH LASERS

Microsurgical repairs with monofilament sutures (which produce relatively little tissue reaction) and swedged-on needles (the sutures placed primarily in the intrafascicular epineurium) has advanced the standard of surgical technique to the point where group fascicles, if not fascicle repairs, are possible. This technique is almost certainly approaching its limitations, which is unfortunate because the great deficiency of limb reconstruction still continues to be the inability to obtain excellent nerve regeneration.

The tubulation techniques initially employed by Paul Weiss and more recently evaluated by Lundborg and associates (1980, 1982), MacKinnon and co-workers (1985), and others have offered hope that by manipulating the biological system to provide a suitable environment, the nerve fibrils would seek their own appropriate reattachments. Lundborg's group has clearly shown that neurobiotaxis occurs, and a variety of agents that attract the regenerating axon* have been identified. Recent investigation by Brushart (1991a and b) may explain why this technique has provided less-than-optimal clinical results. Brushart clearly shows that chemotaxis takes place, that motor axons will reinnervate distal motor pathways, and that sensory axons will reinnervate into the sensory pathway.

Brushart showed that no specific attraction exists between the varying distal segments but that the axon will be pruned if it enters a nonhospitable host, that is, a motor axon will not pass through a sensory distal pathway. Brushart's later studies suggest there is no selectivity from one pathway to the other. There does not appear to be a biological system that selectively realigns the regenerated axons to their appropriate distal pathways. Maximizing realignment remains the ultimate task of the surgeon.

The unique properties of lasers can provide the surgeon

---

*Common terminology compels the use of the term *axon* for both motor and sensory anatomical situations, even though the true distal attachment to a sensory cell is in fact a dendrite.

with the ability to unite severed nerve ends with extreme precision. The word *laser* is an acronym for *l*ight *a*mplified by *s*timulation *e*missions of *r*adiation. Ordinary light consists of photons, with random wavelengths scattered in all directions, but laser light is almost exclusively one wavelength or color and is monodirectional. Photons are sources of electromagnetic energy in the form of light waves. In laser emissions, these wavelengths are sinusoidal, phased with one another, and parallel, and they produce an equal wave front—all of which allows the energy to be focused in a very small beam. Laser light can manifest a wide variety of lengths, from far infrared to extreme ultraviolet. At least 12 different laser systems are in medical use, and new uses continually evolve (Table 33–1).

The effect of a laser varies with its defining characteristics, which are wavelength, beam energy, diameter of the beam, pulse duration, and exposure time. Lasers affect tissue in one of three ways: photochemically, photothermally, or photomechanically. With the photochemical effect, light stimulates a chemical reaction such as that seen when light energy strikes melanin cells in the skin and results in tanning. There are a number of photothermal effects. An example of one is the heating of tissue to 60° to 70°C, which causes unraveling and cross-binding of the protein molecules and produces the glassy effect of coagulation seen in light microscopy.

Some evidence suggests that infrared lasers can split mitochondria selectively. Ultraviolet lasers seem to have more effect on proteins. Cell nuclei may respond differently to laser stimulation than do the organelles and the surrounding cytoplasm. In each case, a particular structure absorbs a laser energy differently than do neighboring structures, and, therefore, each is mechanically affected differently by that energy. The differential effect of each such structure to surrounding structures defines each as a chromophobe. Because of lasers' extreme focusing power and this differential effect on tissue, applications of this type offer the ability to micromanipulate tissue.

Lasers can also vaporize tissue. At present, lasers are most commonly used for tissue ablation in a medical setting. The water in the cell, when heated to 100°C, turns to steam and literally explodes. A rapid explosion may even cause a wave effect, an acoustical effect that further damages tissue. When heated to around 400°C, tissue will carbonize—this phenomenon is responsible for the effective cutting coagulation tool commonly used in medicine (Fig. 33–3).

The tissue welding technique in nerve repair uses laser energy to heat tissue to 65° to 70°C, thereby causing the protein to coagulate and thus create an adhesive glue that binds the nerve ends together. Tissue welding began in the 1960s with the use of the argon laser for coagulating detached retinas and retinal blood vessels. Since that time, a variety of laser systems have been developed for welding techniques, each with different properties and different uses. In nerve repair, lasers weld the tissue together, using either the nerve tissue itself or an additive such as hemoglobin to effect adherence.

Tissue Welding with the Argon Laser

The argon laser is used in conjunction with the chromophobe hemoglobin. A blue-green laser in the 0.488- to 0.518-mμ range, the argon laser is also visible as blue-green light.

▼ TABLE 33–1
A Selection of Current Medical Lasers

Laser Type	Predominant Wavelength(s) (μm)	Typical Power Energy	Form of Output	Delivery System(s)	Tissue Interaction
Excimer	0.19–0.35	0.5–50 W (effective)	Repet. Pulsed	Fiber	Thermal/ photochemical
Argon ion	0.49–0.51	3–20 W	C W	Fiber	Thermal/ photochemical
KTP	0.53	5–15 W	C W	Fiber	Thermal
Krypton ion	0.52 0.57–0.53 0.65	1 W	C W	Fiber	Thermal
Helium-neon	0.63	1–5 mW	C W	Fiber	Thermal
Gold vapor	0.63	2 W (av.)	Repet. Pulsed	Fiber	Thermal/ photochemical
Dye	0.4–0.9 (tunable)	1–5 W	C W/ Pulsed	Fiber	Thermal
GaAs	0.84	20 mW	Repet. Pulsed	Fiber	Thermal
Nd:YAG	1.06	1–100 W	C W/ Pulsed	Fiber	Thermal
Er:YAG	1.54	10 J	Pulsed	Fiber (development)	Thermal
Ho:YAG	2.15	10 W	C W/ Pulsed	Fiber	Thermal
CO_2	10.6	1–80 W	CW/Repet. Pulsed	Mirror/ hollow guide	Thermal

$(\mu_1=1/\text{attenuation coefficient})$

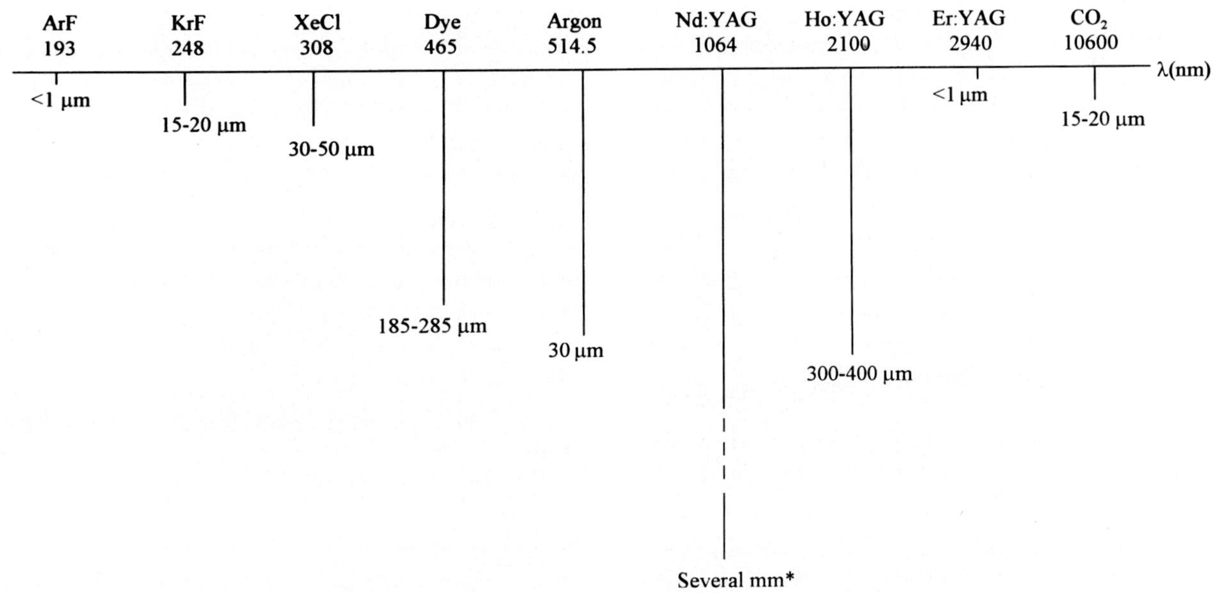

FIGURE 33–3. The differential penetrating depth in tissue of various lasers.

As reported by Almquist and colleagues (1988), the argon laser can pass through a fiberoptic system much as does regular light and, hence, can be delivered to a site relatively easily. The objective is to use red hemoglobin as an energy-absorbing chromophobe for the blue-green light of the laser. The blue-green light reflects from the white-surfaced nerve and, therefore, does not damage the nerve tissue. In experimental studies using the rat sciatic nerve model and the primate median nerve model, these researchers subjected a small portion of blood applied to the coaptated nerve segments to 75 mW of energy for 1/2 second in several areas around a group fascicular repair, thus turning the blood into an adherent coagulum (Fig. 33–4). Evaluation performed up to 1 year after repair in primates noted satisfactory electrophysiological and total axon counts. Neuroma formation was minimal, indicating that few axons escaped through the repair site. The control nerves, where similar amounts of laser energy were applied, showed no neuronal damage. These studies were thought to be qualitative, and the authors subsequently performed quantitative evaluation and clinical trials, evaluating argon laser secondary repairs 3 to 5 years after repair (Almquist, 1992). These repairs took place in median, ulnar, interdigital, and digital nerves. The clinical evaluation of 13 patients revealed outcomes that were at least comparable with standard microsurgical repairs if not better than what the authors had reported previously. The difference between the two types of repairs (laser and surgical) was not great. The technical difficulties with the laser nerve repairs and the awkwardness in using the argon system were significant enough for the authors to decide not to recommend this system in its present form as an alternative to standard microsurgical repair.

Carbon Dioxide Laser Nerve Repairs

Carbon dioxide lasers are of two general types. The standard high-energy, continuous-wave laser is generally in the 100-W range and is used medically as a cutting and coagulating tool. The second laser is the milliwatt pulse system. It produces energy in the 1500-mW range and has been used as a coagulating tool in nerve repairs. The carbon dioxide laser, which operates in the infrared range, cannot be passed through a fiberoptic system and is invisible—it must be accompanied by a directing visible light laser. For use in this technique, it must also be passed through a reflective system, such as a microscope. These constraints increase the awkwardness of its use. The principle behind carbon dioxide laser nerve repair is to apply sufficient energy to coagulate

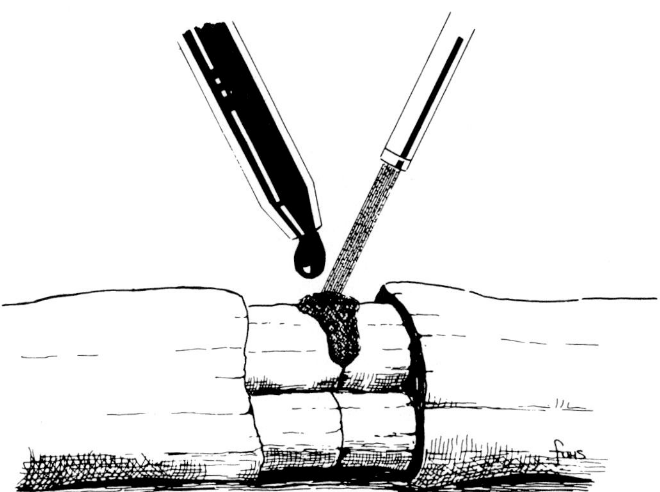

FIGURE 33–4. Argon laser nerve repair. The laser beam energy is absorbed by the chromophobe hemoglobin, turning the blood into an adherent coagulum.

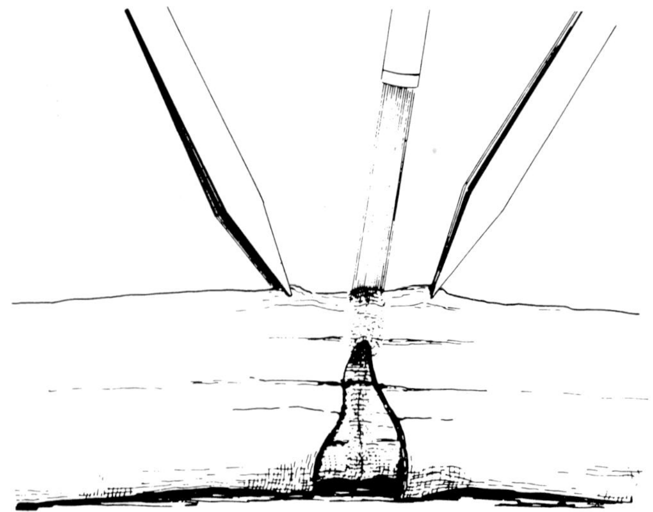

FIGURE 33–5. Carbon dioxide nerve repair. The laser beam energy is absorbed by adjacent tissue nonselectively forming a weld around and within the nerve.

the protein tissues within the nerve, sealing them in a layer. Carbon dioxide laser energy is absorbed by water, so essentially all tissues, excluding bone, are affected. It has no chromophobe and no specificity within the nerve tissue—it works by pulsing a small amount of energy to anneal the surface area at the repair site (Fig. 33–5). Its use requires a delicate balance in the amount of energy produced, a requirement that is met through a sensing device that terminates the laser energy when tissue in the beam reaches 60°C, that is, the temperature of coagulation. Despite this protection technique, however, some axoplasmic tissue is probably still affected by the laser system.

Works using experimental animal models with only a few clinical trials have been published by Fischer and co-workers (1985), Beggs and colleagues (1986), Neblett (1982), Schrober and co-workers (1985), and Huang and colleagues (1992). These reports have shown that densities of axonal fibers distal to the repair site are at least equal to the control of sutured nerves. Electrophysiological data have also shown clear evidence of nerve fibers transgressing the repair sites. Little, if any, quantitative data exist to underscore the superiority of carbon dioxide minipulse laser repairs to conventional repairs.

Neodymium:Yttrium-Aluminum-Garnet Laser

The neodymium:yttrium-aluminum-garnet (Nd:YAG) laser has also been used in peripheral nerve repairs. The acronym YAG is derived from the crystal. Two types of Nd:YAG lasers exist—one in the 106-μ wavelength, the other in the 132-μ wavelength. Both are in the near-infrared spectrum, so this laser's wavelength falls somewhere between that of the carbon dioxide laser and that of the argon laser. The more recently developed 132-mμ-wavelength laser seems to be more applicable to medical systems, in part because it can be passed through fiberoptics.

Schrober and colleagues (1985) have studied the effects of this laser on tissue. It has produced an adherent, amorphous coagulum when applied to collagen, and the collagen has

lost its periodicity. Schrober's work on nerve repair has shown axonal outgrowth across the anastomosis, myelin regeneration, and favorable growth overall compared with that resulting from the standard control sutures. There seemed to be no detrimental effects on the nerve from the laser energy.

Other Lasers

A variety of new lasers have been developed, among them excimer lasers, the krypton ion KTP laser, and even gold vapor lasers, although none has yet been reported in use for laser repairs (see Table 33–1).

Similar to the argon laser, the KTP laser is simpler to use and probably would be substituted for argon if it were sufficiently applicable. Whether these other laser systems have any value for nerve repair or regeneration awaits investigation.

The Future of Lasers in Nerve Repair

It is apparent that nerve regeneration research in the last 10 to 15 years strongly suggests that there is no major biological hindrance to adequate nerve regeneration. If we can adequately realign the nerve fascicles, regeneration will occur. The ideal, of course, would be to place each proximal axon to its appropriate distal recipient axon cylinder and allow that regenerating tissue to proceed down the tube, which is now lined with Schwann cells, to reach its end organ. Although in theory, precise realignment could produce extremely efficient nerve regeneration, this goal probably will never be completely realized. Misalignment appears to be the major factor contributing to poor clinical results in adults.

No suturing technique will ever produce the ideal repair. However, a technique of tissue welding in a variety of areas within and around the nerve could allow excellent approximation, alignment, and adherence with relatively little straying of sprouting axons. The ability of laser energy to be absorbed by intercellular and intracellular chromophobes could, in theory, make it possible to achieve the highest accuracy. Chromophobes could be placed at multiple matching points within and around the nerve repair site where laser energy could be targeted to create an adherent glue. The potential for exact approximation from such a technique is theoretically feasible, although the technique has certainly not been developed at this time.

Another possible technique might use stereoscopic radiation. Two beams of laser energy could be focused on a predetermined series of spots on and within a nerve. Focused minutely on these welding spots, the energy could then precisely adhere the nerve in a nearly exact approximation.

Low-Energy Laser Therapy on Nerve Regeneration

Mentioned here as an adjunct to nerve regeneration and not as a repair technique, low-energy laser therapy has been used for the last 25 years primarily in Eastern European countries that have had relatively little exposure to Western medicine until recently. This technique has been widely viewed with skepticism and controversy but is becoming more broadly accepted.

Low-energy laser therapy is defined as photon stimulation low enough to produce only biological effects without heating the tissue. By definition, the temperature cannot elevate more than 0.1° to 0.5°C, therefore, considerably limiting the power sources, probably to the 50-mW range. A number of laser systems can meet these requirements, among them the helium-neon (HeNe) laser, the GaAlAs laser, the GaAs laser, the ruby laser, the argon laser, and others. Many of the articles concerning these systems were published in large clinical reports with relatively little experimental data (Collins, 1989; Parrish and Wilson, 1991; Thomsen, 1991; Welch et al, 1991). The studies included treatments for osteoarthritis, neuralgia, diabetes, Peyronie's disease, rheumatoid arthritis, pain, dental disease, and tendinitis. There have been very few controlled clinical trials.

Work on the cellular response to laser therapy has been increasing. Although the approach is still controversial, sufficiently measurable responses have been observed in evaluations that are adequately scientific and specific for us to take laser therapy seriously (Parrish and Wilson, 1991). We have known cellular responses to light therapy for generations (tanning and the effect of vitamin D are two examples). The experimental work has included increased collagen and protein synthesis, increased RNA synthesis and cell proliferation, adenosine triphosphate synthesis, and prostaglandin synthesis.

In terms of nerve physiology, the findings are mixed. Some studies suggest that conduction velocities increase, axonal potentials become larger, and synaptic functions following radiation may improve. Others suggest that little difference can be detected (Basford, 1989). Radiation has been observed to improve migration of axons in in vitro tissue culture studies. Rochkind and Ouaknine (1992) have shown startling results in nerve regeneration of canine spinal cord injuries and peripheral nerve injuries following transplantation experiments with low-level laser radiation. These studies have not been confirmed by others. Although a variety of experimental works suggest some effect, the application of low-level laser energy to nerve regeneration is moving in no specific direction. Its efficacy appears to be remarkably dependent on wavelength and pulse duration. Although many clinical improvements have been asserted, all remain as yet unconfirmed, and the validity of any of them will be ascertained through detailed experimental work.

References

Almquist EE: Evaluation of argon laser nerve repair: Three to five year follow-up. Presented at Sunderland Society Peripheral Nerve Surgery Group, Malmö, Sweden, 1992.

Almquist EE: Nerve repair by laser. Orthop Clin North Am *19*:201–208, 1988.

Almquist EE, Eeg-Olofsson O: Sensory-nerve-conduction velocity and two-point discrimination in sutured nerves. J Bone Joint Surg *52*:791–796, 1970.

Almquist EE, Smith OA, Fry L: Nerve conduction velocity, microscopic, and electron microscopy studies comparing repaired adult and baby monkey median nerves. J Hand Surg *8*:406–410, 1983.

Almquist EE, Nachemson A, Auth D, Almquist B, Hall S: Evaluation of the use of the argon laser in repairing rat and primate nerves. J Hand Surg *9*:792–799, 1984.

Basford JR: Low-energy laser therapy: Controversies and new research findings. Editorial. Lasers Surg Med *9*:1–5, 1989.

Becker C, Gueuning C, Graff G: Peripheral nerve repair: Value of biological glues and epiperineural suture in late interventions. Experimental study in rats. Ann Chir Main Memb Super *4*:259–262, 1985a.

Becker CM, Gueuning CO, Graff GL: Sutures or fibrin glue for divided rat nerves: Schwann cell and muscle metabolism. Microsurgery *6*:1–10, 1985b.

Beggs JL, Fischer DW, Shetter AG: Comparative study of rat sciatic nerve microepineurial anastomoses made with carbon dioxide laser and suture techniques: Part 2. Neurosurgery *18*:266–269, 1986.

Bertilli JA, Mira JC: Nerve repair using freezing and fibrin glue: Immediate histologic improvement of axonal coaptation. Microsurgery *14*:135–140, 1993.

Brushart TM: Preferential molecular reenervation: A sequential double-labeling study. Restorative Neurobiology and Neuroscience *1*:218–287, 1991a.

Brushart TM: The mechanical and humoral control of specificity of nerve repair. *In* Gelberman R (ed): Operative Nerve Repair and Reconstruction. Philadelphia, J. B. Lippincott, 1991b, pp 215–230.

Cajal S: Degeneration and Regeneration of the Nervous System. (Translated by R. M. May, 1928.) Reprinted, New York, Hafner, 1968.

Collins L: Lasers in medicine—some current issues. Australas Phys Eng Sci Med *12*:215–227, 1989.

Cruikshank W: Experiments on the nerves, particularly on their reproduction; and on the spinal marrow of living animals. Philos Transactor Royal Society London 85:512, 1795.

Cruz NI, Debs N, Fiol RE: Evaluation of fibrin glue in rat sciatic nerve repairs. Plast Reconstr Surg *78*:369–373, 1986.

Duspiva W: Nerve Erkenntnisse zur Anastomosierung durchtrennter peripherer Nerven. Forster Med *96*:2214–2218, 1978.

Edshage S: Peripheral nerve suture. A technique for improved intraneural topography. Acta Chir Scand Suppl *331*:1–104, 1964.

Egloff DV, Narakas AO: Nerve anastomoses with human fibrin. Ann Chir Main Memb Super *2*:101, 1983.

Egloff DV, Narakas AO, Bonnard C: Results of nerve grafts with tissucol (tisseel) anastomosis. *In* Schlag G, Redl H (eds): Fibrin Sealant in Operative Medicine, Vol. 2, Ophthalmology, Neurosurgery. Berlin, Springer, 1986, pp 181–185.

Faldini A, Putoni P, Magherini PC, Lisanti M, Carlucci F, Risaliti R: Comparative neurophysiological assessments of nerve sutures performed by microsurgical methods and with fibrin glue: Experimental study. Ital J Orthop Traumatol *10*:527–532, 1984.

Feldman MD, Sataloff RT, Epstein G, et al: Autologous fibrin tissue adhesive for peripheral nerve anastomosis. Arch Otolaryngol Head Neck Surg *113*:963–967, 1987.

Fischer DW, Beggs JL, Kenshalo, Jr DL, et al: Comparative study of microepineurial anastomoses with the use of carbon dioxide laser and suture techniques in rat sciatic nerves: Part 1. Neurosurgery *17*:300–307, 1985.

Guy de Chauliac: On Wounds and Fractures. (Translated by W.A. Brennan.) Chicago: Published by translator, 1923.

Herter T: Problems of fibrin adhesion of the nerves. Neurosurg Rev *11*:249–258, 1988.

Huang TC, Blanks RH, Berns MW, Crumley RL: Lasers vs suture nerve anastomosis. Otolaryngol Head Neck Surg *107*:14–20, 1992.

Kuderna H: Klinische Anwendung der Klebung von nervenanastomosen mit Fibrinogen. Fortschr Kiefer Gesichtschir *21*:135, 1976.

Kuhn KG: Claudii Galeni Opera Omnia, Vol. XIII, De compositione medicamentorum secundum locus, libri X, decompositive medicamentorum per genera libri XII. Hildesheim, 1965 Olms.

Lundborg G, Dahlin LB, Danielsen N, Gelberman RH, Longo GM, Powell HC, Varon S: Nerve regeneration in a silicone chamber: Influence of gap length and of distal stump components. Exp Neurol *76*:361–375, 1982.

Lundborg G, Hansson H: Nerve regeneration through preformed pseudosynovial tubes. J Hand Surg *5*:35–38, 1980.

MacKinnon SE, Dellon AL, Hudson AR, Hunter DA: Nerve regeneration through a pseudosynovial sheath in a primate model. Plast Reconstr Surg *75*:833–839, 1985.

Matras H, Dinges HP, Mamoli B, et al: Nonsutured nerve transplantation. J Maxillofac Surg *1*:37, 1973.

Matras H, Mamoli B, Lassmann H: Zur Klebung von Nervenanastomosen mit Gerinnungssubstanzen. Fortschr Kiefer Gesichtschir *20*:112, 1975.

Meyer VE, Smahel J, Backem U: Reconstruction of peripheral nerves: Fibrin glue versus suture. An experimental study. Summary of the joint meeting of the European Society for Surgical Research and the Group for Advancement of Microsurgery: Peripheral Nerve Repair and Regeneration 3:82, 1986.

Moy OJ, Peimer CA, Koniuch MP, Howard C, Zielezny M, Katikaneni PR: Fibrin seal adhesive versus nonabsorbable microsuture in peripheral nerve repair. J Hand Surg *13*:273–278, 1988.

Narakas A: The use of fibrin glue in repair of peripheral nerves. Orthop Clin North Am *19*:187–199, 1988.

Neblett CR: Reconstructive vascular surgery with the use of carbon dioxide laser. Presented at the Congress on Laser Neurosurgery II, Chicago, Illinois, 1982.

Parrish JA, Wilson BC: Current and future trends in laser medicine. Overview. Photochem Photobiol *53*:731–738, 1991.

Paulus Aegenta (Paul of Aegina): Seven Books of Paulus Aegenta Commentar Embraced a Complete view of the Knowledge passed by the Greeks, Romans and Arabians on all subjects connected with Medicine and Surgery, vol II. (Translated by F. Adams.) London, Sydenham Society, 1844–1847.

Rochkind S, Ouaknine GE: New trend in neuroscience: Low-power laser effect on peripheral and central nervous system (basic science, preclinical and clinical studies). Review. Neurol Res 14:2–11, 1992.

Schrober R, Ulrich DW, Sander T, Dürselen H, Hessel S: Laser-induced alteration of collagen substructure allows microsurgical tissue welding. Science *232*:1421–1422, 1985.

Seddon HJ, Medawar PB: Fibrin suture of human nerves. Lancet 2:87–88, 1942.

Smahel J, Meyer VE, Bachem U: Gluing of peripheral nerves with fibrin: Experimental studies. J Reconstr Microsurg *3*:211–220, 1987.

Tarlov IM: Autologous plasma clot suture of nerves: Its use in clinical surgery. JAMA *126*:741–748, 1944.

Thomsen S: Review article. Pathologic analysis of photothermal and photochemical effects of laser-tissue interactions. Photochem Photobiol *53*:825–835, 1991.

Waller AV: Sept ième mémoire sur le système nerveux. C R Hebd Academic Sci Paris *35*:301, 1852.

Welch AJ, Motamedi M, Rastegar S, et al: Review article. Laser thermal ablation. Photochem Photobiol *53*:815–823, 1991.

Young JZ, Medawar PB: Fibrin structure of peripheral nerves. Lancet 2:126–127, 1940.

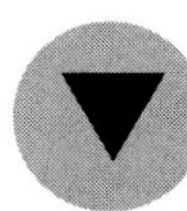

Chapter 34

- Rajiv Midha
- David G. Kline

Evaluation of the Neuroma in Continuity

The majority of nerve injuries associated with a significant functional deficit leave the nerve in gross continuity rather than transect it. Thus, lesions in continuity comprise between 60% and 70% of all peripheral nerve injuries (Kline and Hackett, 1975). Unfortunately, the majority of lesions in continuity represent an unknown quantity, especially during the early months following injury. On the one hand, based on clinical criteria, their course may take several months to unfold. On the other hand, a limiting factor to prolonged expectant observation is the irreversible changes that occur in denervated muscle over time that prevent full recovery despite the eventual reinnervation by axons (Gutmann and Young, 1944; Sunderland, 1991). Therefore, the surgeon is presented with a complex management problem because of the variable and unpredictable natural history of the neuroma in continuity. Specifically, the challenge is to develop and employ techniques that will accurately predict either recovery without resection and repair or the need for the same (Kline and Nulsen, 1972; Woodhall et al, 1957).

Our overall approach to the neuroma in continuity encompasses two stages: a preoperative assessment and, when necessary, an operative evaluation. The initial assessment relies on a thorough clinical analysis, aided by electrophysiological tests. Repeat and serial clinical follow-up examinations are critical to ascertain the possible natural history of the lesion. During these initial 3 to 4 months following injury, one may identify the potential for spontaneous recovery and also allow nerve regeneration to occur, which is electrically measurable at operation (Kline and Hackett, 1975). For those lesions in continuity that fail to demonstrate the ability of the nerve or nerve elements to successfully regenerate, operative exploration is indicated (Kline and Nulsen, 1972). At operation, the lesion is carefully exposed and inspected. However, mere inspection and palpation of the nerve may be misleading (Fig. 34–1), providing an unreliable indication of the pathology hidden by the surrounding epineurium (Kline and Nulsen, 1972). Over many years, therefore, the authors have relied greatly on the information provided by direct stimulation of the exposed nerve and the evoked compound nerve action potential across the neuroma in continuity in directing neurolysis versus resection and repair (Kline and Happel, 1993). In this chapter, the authors briefly discuss the neuropathology of the neuroma in continuity and then proceed to a more detailed presentation of our clinical and electrophysiological approach to its diagnosis and treatment.

NEUROPATHOLOGY

Any traumatic insult to a peripheral nerve may produce a neuroma in continuity. Injuries likely to do so include contusions, stretch or traction injuries, gunshot wounds, fractures adjacent to nerves, and even some sharply made lacerations (Sunderland, 1978). The most common mechanism of nerve injury involves stretch and contusive forces. In all of the above-mentioned settings, the entire cross section of the nerve is usually affected. In nerves that maintain continuity despite serious damage, a wide spectrum of internal derangement may exist. Sunderland's grading scale for in-continuity lesions ranges from mild, neuropraxic types that contain little or no apparent structural damage (Grade 1) to severe types that affect all components (Grade 4) of the internal nerve structure (Sunderland, 1978). Between these extremes are a variety of conditions that constitute partial or less severe nerve injuries. Moreover, a significant subset of lesions in continuity manifest more than one grade of injury across the cross section of the involved nerve element (Mackinnon and Dellon, 1988). This is critical because, to a great extent, return of function over time depends on the underlying neuropathology of the nerve, because those with a large neurotmetic component generally do not recover whereas those with neuropraxic and or axonotmetic pathology may recover (Seddon, 1972).

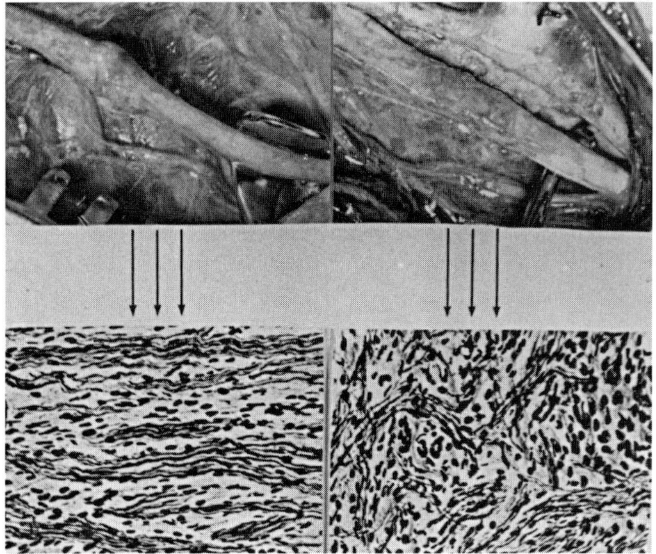

FIGURE 34–1. The external appearance of a neuron in continuity may have poor correlation with its internal structure, complicating surgical decision-making and management. The firm, irregular lesion *(upper left)* contained well-organized, regenerating nerve fibers *(lower left)*. On the other hand, the smooth and relatively well-modeled neuroma in continuity *(upper right)* was associated with extensive intrafascicular scar and a disordered axonal architecture *(lower right)*. (Modified from Kline DG, Nulsen FE: The neuroma in continuity: Its preoperative and operative management. Surg Clin North Am *52*:1189, 1972.)

In neuropraxia, the mildest form of injury, there is minimal or no discernible histopathological alteration in nerve structure. Rather, there is a reversible conduction block, manifested clinically as loss of function that persists for hours to days. In some neuropraxic injuries (Sunderland Grade 1), axons have localized thinning and mild segmental demyelination but are still characterized by excellent spontaneous recovery (Sunderland, 1978). Occasionally, neuropraxic lesions come to clinical attention because of slightly more severe damage to some axons, sufficient to lead to wallerian degeneration and attendant denervation changes in scattered distal motor fibers. Because the internal and endoneurial structure is maintained, effective regeneration and recovery ensues over a matter of months and electromyographic denervation changes gradually reverse.

There exists a small fraction of nerve injuries, usually secondary to mild stretch, prolonged compression, or the concussive effect of a bullet that traverses close to but does not impact the nerve, that present clinically with reduced motor function and little sensory loss in the nerve distribution (Happel and Kline, 1991). Across the cross section of the involved nerve are a mixture of neuropathological changes, including uninvolved nerve fibers, neuropraxic regions, and frankly axonotmetic areas. Return of complete or nearly full function is the rule in this situation. More frequently, a lesion in continuity is predominantly axonotmetic (Sunderland Grade 2), in which axon continuity is disrupted but with relative sparing of the connective tissue structure of the nerve (Sunderland, 1978). Importantly, fascicular integrity is maintained, as is the fine endoneurial network, with minimal endoneurial edema and fibrosis. Wallerian degeneration and Schwann cell proliferation is followed by regeneration of axons, whose elongating tips are guided toward the end-organ by the relatively intact endoneurial basement membrane. The rate of regeneration averages approximately 1 mm a day or an inch per month, parameters useful in serial clinical evaluation of the patient while awaiting possible return of function (Seddon et al, 1943; Sunderland, 1947a, 1947b). Patients with Grade 2 injuries usually recover effectively without the need for operative intervention, although the completeness of recovery is governed by additional factors such as the location of the injury and the specific nerve or nerve element involved.

The lesion in continuity all too frequently exhibits both loss of axonal continuity and a disruption in the connective tissue structures. When the damage is confined to the membranous structures within the fascicle, a Sunderland Grade 3 lesion is present, whereas additional involvement of extrafascicular connective tissue denotes a Grade 4 injury (Sunderland, 1978). In Grade 3 injuries, the intrafascicular endoneurial network is damaged, producing extensive edema and hemorrhage. Vascular compromise leading to frank necrosis is occasionally superimposed (Lundborg, 1975). A variable degree of intrafascicular fibrosis results, frustrating regenerating axons and leading to their aberrant regrowth, despite gross continuity of the nerve itself. Depending on the degree of internal disruption, spontaneous recovery may or may not occur. Therefore, a wide range of clinical outcomes is possible, from no function to return of full function. With the more severe Grade 4 injuries, the entire connective tissue framework of the nerve is damaged, setting in motion an exuberant fibroblastic response, associated with extensive and haphazard deposition of connective tissue. This presents a formidable barrier that obstructs successful nerve fiber regrowth. The resulting neuroma contains a meshwork of connective tissue entwined with fine-caliber, poorly myelinated axons. The Grade 4 injury represents the most severe pathology for a neuroma in continuity. Clinical recovery seldom occurs, unless operative resection and repair is undertaken.

Preoperative Assessment

CLINICAL

In the patient with nerve damage, a knowledge of the wounding agent may be useful in the assessment of the potential pathology and the likelihood of spontaneous recovery (Seddon, 1972). For example, lacerating injuries from a piece of glass or a knife are likely to lead to transections, although 20% of such cases associated with a complete deficit still leave the nerve in continuity, and some of these can heal without operative intervention (Kline and Hackett, 1975). Nerve injuries associated with closed fractures and dislocations heal spontaneously approximately 85% of the time, and in the vast majority, this recovery is evident within 4 months of the injury, obviating the need for surgical exploration (Siegel and Gelberman, 1991). Following gunshot wounds that result in a nerve or nerve element damage with total loss of function, spontaneous recovery can occur, varying from 40% to 50% of the time in civilian practice (Kline, 1989) to up to 69% in wartime experience (Omer, 1991). Those injuries not demonstrating recovery require not only operative exploration and intraoperative electrophysiological evaluation but also resection and repair in the majority of cases (Kline, 1989). Injuries from severe stretch, crush, and contusion are usually Grade 3 or 4 and, therefore, even more likely to require operative intervention if deficits fail to reverse in the early months (Kline and Hackett, 1975).

Careful, detailed and repetitive motor and sensory examinations are essential for adequate evaluation of any nerve injury. Initial clinical testing identifies those nerves and nerve elements that are associated with complete loss of function, a situation that frequently predicts the need for subsequent surgical exploration (Kline and Nulsen, 1972). In this context, the clinician should be aware that some complete median and ulnar nerve lesions may appear to be partial because of the anomalous innervation of hand muscles (Murphy et al, 1946) and the many variations of the Martin-Gruber anastomosis. Based on history and examination, the patient's function is documented and serves as a baseline for subsequent assessment. Therefore, recovery related to reversal of neuropraxic elements is easily detected when recovery occurs over days to weeks. On the other hand, early recovery secondary to regeneration of axonotmetic elements occurs at a rate of 1 mm per day and is thus clinically manifest over weeks to months (Seddon, 1972; Seddon et al, 1943). For example, in a suspected mid-humeral level injury to the radial nerve associated with complete loss, one would carefully test the next distal muscle supplied (i.e., the brachioradialis) at intervals to detect early evidence of recovery. However, in many nerve injuries, the wait for voluntary motor activity is long, especially if it does not occur when predicted by such calculations. This leads to a lengthy delay in repair, potentially compromising the eventual functional result (Sunderland, 1991). Therefore, other types of tests are important in assessing the nerve lesion.

Clinical tests other than motor examination include evaluation of autonomic and sensory function and the elicitation of Tinel's sign. Autonomic function, such as sweating, is subserved by fine fibers, which regenerate first. Therefore, it is tempting to use return of sweating as a sign of useful regeneration. However, the presence of fine fibers, even at such distal sites as the autonomous sensory zones for the median or ulnar nerve, may favor subsequent regeneration of large sensory and motor axons but do not reliably predict it (Nulsen and Kline, 1973). Similarly, return of sensation to an autonomous zone suggests the potential for useful motor fiber regeneration but does not guarantee it (Moberg, 1975). Moreover, recovery of motor function in the distribution of the nerve can precede return of function in a sensory territory, making serial sensory testing less valuable. Tinel's sign is present when paresthesias are evoked in the distribution of the nerve by tapping over it. Elicitation of Tinel's sign signifies the presence of fine, irritable, regenerated nerve fibers. Therefore, an advancing Tinel's sign over time along the distal anatomical course of the nerve signifies regeneration of nerve fibers (Henderson, 1948). However, this is again limited by not consistently presaging subsequent functional recovery (Henderson, 1948; Kline and Hackett, 1975). Indeed, many patients with an advancing Tinel's sign need resection and repair of the lesion in continuity (Nulsen and Kline, 1973; Woodhall et al, 1957). Alternatively, the absence of a Tinel's sign below the injury site is perhaps even more significant because it denotes the lack of regeneration of even small nerve fibers and suggests the need for surgical intervention (Henderson, 1948; Kline and Hackett, 1975; Nulsen and Kline, 1973).

ELECTRICAL

In addition to clinical testing, the patient with a neuroma in continuity undergoes preoperative electrophysiological assessment, which includes electomyographic (EMG) examination, electrical stimulation of the nerve in an attempt to evoke muscle contractions, and nerve conduction studies. Each of these tests provides supplemental information to the clinical examination that can aid the clinician in assessing the likelihood of spontaneous recovery. For instance, electrical studies for a Grade 1 lesion are characteristic and virtually diagnostic (Happel and Kline, 1991). Stimulation of the nerve proximal to the neuropraxic lesion produces little or no distal motor activity, indicating complete conduction block, yet axonal continuity is demonstrated by the ability to evoke muscle activity by applying the stimulus to the nerve distal to the injury site. Similarly, the nerve displays good compound nerve action potentials (NAPs) proximal and distal to the lesion but not across the lesion. Needle EMG examination shows only an occasional fibrillation or denervational potential. In most cases, each of these electrical abnormalities reverse over a relatively short time period, although they can persist for several weeks in the more severely neuropraxic lesion.

The electrophyiological findings of Grade 2 to 4 injuries are initially identical and not helpful in distinguishing one from the other. This is because all three of these grades of injury show unequivocal evidence of profound loss of motor axons (Kimura, 1983). In the first 72 hours following axonal injury, distal stimulation of the nerve may still produce muscle contraction because dissolution of the axon to the motor end-plate and the wallerian process of degeneration takes a finite length of time, and therefore electrical tests are not valid during this early period (Kline and Nulsen, 1972). After 2 to 4 weeks, depending on the distance between nerve injury and muscle examined, the EMG study shows signs of denervation, including fibrillation potentials, markedly reduced or absent electrical activity as the needle is inserted into the muscle, and inability to evoke muscle activity despite maximal voluntary effort by the patient (Kimura, 1983; Sumner, 1980). Additionally, electrical stimulation of the nerve either proximal or even distal to the injury no longer results in muscle contraction.

A particular value of serial electrical studies is in helping distinguish Grade 2 and some (mild) Grade 3 injuries from more severe insults. With successful regeneration and early re-input of axons into muscles and motor end-plate reconstruction, the electromyographer finds an increase in insertional activity, a decrease in the number of fibrillation potentials, and examples of nascent muscle action potentials (Bowden, 1954). At this earlier stage of reinnervation, stimulation of the regenerating nerves may evoke muscle contraction, which can antedate voluntary contraction by a period of several weeks (Grundfest et al, 1956; Nulsen and Lewey, 1947). If signs of reinnervation in the most proximal muscles are seen by the above-mentioned electrical criteria, the clinician is reassured that functional recovery is likely to follow. However, it is incumbent on the clinician to continue to observe the patient for clinical restoration in the apparently reinnervated muscle and also for further progression of electrical and clinical recovery in more distal muscles groups over time. Failure of progression of recovery or lack of clinical evidence of reinnervation of muscles beyond a suitable calculated interval for axons to reach and connect with the motor end-plate is a criterion for surgical exploration.

Because clinical (and EMG) examination relies on the reinnervation of muscle, a major limitation is imposed in the most common types of nerve injuries and nerve levels involved by them owing to the long distance from the site of the lesion to the nearest testable muscle. In most cases, many months may elapse before such reinnervation occurs, restricting the usefulness of EMG and electrically evoked muscle activity in documenting early regeneration. This becomes critical in more severe (Grade 3 or 4) neuromas in continuity, which usually require surgical repair and would be poorly served by a prolonged waiting period and unnecessarily delayed repair. Similarly, lesions in continuity involving plexus or proximal segments of major nerves may require relatively early repair if subsequent innervation is to be useful. Fortunately, the availability of another electrophysiological modality, the measurement of NAPs, provides evidence of a good quality of regeneration as early as 6 to 10 weeks after injury (Kline and Nulsen, 1972). This is well before reinnervation may occur. Also, the greater the distance between nerve injury and the first downstream muscle (as in brachial plexus or sciatic nerve injuries), the greater the value of the NAP.

The NAP can be obtained noninvasively and transcutaneously by stimulating and recording electrodes placed on the skin surface and yet over the anatomical course of the nerve, using computer summation techniques to amplify the response and reduce the level of noise and artifacts (Gilliatt and Sears, 1958; Seddon, 1972). In this fashion, NAP conduction evidence of relatively early (6 weeks or greater) nerve regeneration can sometimes be obtained. This technique works best for median, ulnar, and some radial nerve lesions at the elbow, forearm, and wrist levels. It is only of limited use in more proximal lesions by stimulating and recording from elements distal to a brachial plexus or sciatic nerve injury. Although these computer-averaging methods have greatly increased the sensitivity of noninvasive NAPs in ascertaining regeneration, the uncertainties of transcutaneous nerve stimulation and recordings undermine confidence in the information obtained. In the authors' experience, there is at least a 5% incidence of false-positive and false-negative results. The incidence of misleading results will fluctuate depending on the nerve being tested, the level of the lesion, the presence of complicating soft tissue wounds, the size of the limb and thus distance between nerve and electrode site, and how much potential regenerative time has elapsed between the occurrence of the injury and attempts at recording. For these reasons, this technique is not as accurate as the more direct operative assessment of NAPs discussed in the next section.

Operative Evaluation of a Neuroma in Continuity

SURGICAL TIMING, EXPOSURE, AND OBSERVATION

The measurement of NAPs provides evidence of good quality regeneration as early as 6 to 10 weeks after injury (Kline and Nulsen, 1972). However, the optimal *timing* for exploration and recording from a neuroma in continuity is influenced greatly by the mechanism of injury (Hudson and Hunter, 1977; Kline and Hackett, 1975). Injuries that are relatively more focal, such as those produced by gunshot wounds, iatrogenic causes, stab wounds, lacerations, and fracture associated contusions, are associated with significant (electrically measurable) regeneration much earlier than lengthier lesions resulting from severe contusion or stretch injuries. Therefore, the authors explore gunshot- and fracture-associated injuries at 2 to 3 months after wounding, whereas plexus stretch injuries are ideally tested 4 to 5 months after onset.

Careful proximal and distal exposure of a suspected lesion in continuity is performed first. Working in both directions toward the injury, using sharp dissection techniques, the lesion itself is then exposed. It is essential to obtain a generous exposure. Longitudinal blood supply to the nerve, which is subperineurial and deep, should be preserved, but most collaterals can be sacrificed to gain a 360-degree exposure of the nerve (Kline et al, 1972; Lundborg, 1975). The lesion in continuity is then inspected and palpated. Certain operative findings may predict internal pathology. For example, lateral neuromas suggest partial nerve transection, especially in the presence of partially spared function in the nerve distribution, known from preoperative clinical and or electrical examination. If the portion of spared clinical function relates to an unimportant distal structure, it can be

sacrificed to facilitate repair of the whole nerve. Also, if more than two thirds of the nerve is found to be clearly divided, complete resection and repair usually is advisable.

In the majority of cases, the neuroma is fusiform in shape. When the neuroma does have this fusiform shape, inspection and palpation provide only marginal information (see Fig. 34–1). The size of the neuroma is noted because a swelling of up to twice normal is compatible with either axonotmesis or neurotmesis, whereas swelling larger than that favors neurotmesis. A firm or hard consistency suggests heavy internal scar and favors neurotmesis. Exceptions to these simple guidelines make generalization somewhat hazardous (see Fig. 34–1). As a rule, the internal architecture of the neuroma is almost always worse than it appears on examination (Seddon, 1972). Various surgical maneuvers have been advocated to enhance the amount of information derived. These maneuvers include injection of saline into the neuroma in an attempt to delineate fascicular planes; microsurgical dissection of the fascicles proximal and distal to the lesion, followed by attempts to trace the pattern through the neuroma; and visualizing sequential sections through the epicenter of the neuroma until a fascicular pattern is visualized (Kline and Hackett, 1984). We do not recommend these methods because they give no information about intrafascicular pathology, where scarring may be severe in the face of milder extrafascicular changes. Additionally, despite the most meticulous dissection techniques, damage may result to a proportion of axons. In our opinion, an intraoperative electrophysiological approach to testing the neuroma in continuity is preferable.

ELECTROPHYSIOLOGICAL EVALUATION

After the lesion is exposed and examined, electrodes are used to stimulate the nerve proximal and then distal to the injury site in an attempt to evoke muscle contractions. Because both a retrograde and anterograde effect are possible, muscles that receive their innervation proximal and distal, respectively, to the injury site may be activated. Attention to positioning and draping the limb to allow the exact sites of muscle contraction to be felt and seen is helpful in analyzing the situation. Thus, proximal contracting elements are readily detected, preventing these elements from being confused with observations of contracting muscles in the distal distribution of the nerve. The contracting muscles are sought to provide evidence of successful regeneration. Another source of misleading information occurs with stimulus voltage that is either too excessive or prolonged. Impulse spread to adjacent, possibly intact, nerves with resulting contraction of their muscles then becomes a confounding factor. However, the major limitation of evoked muscle testing is the many months that must elapse before regeneration and reinnervation occur to allow a measurable response to be generated. Therefore, early regeneration will not be detected. Alternatively, the measurement of an NAP across the lesion provides early evidence of regeneration.

A detailed review of the background and our techniques for obtaining intraoperative NAPs has been published (Kline and Happel, 1993). The technique is essentially straightforward, requiring a basic set of electrophysiological equipment, mainly a set of appropriately designed electrodes, and an EMG machine (Figs. 34–2 and 34–3). As with all meth-

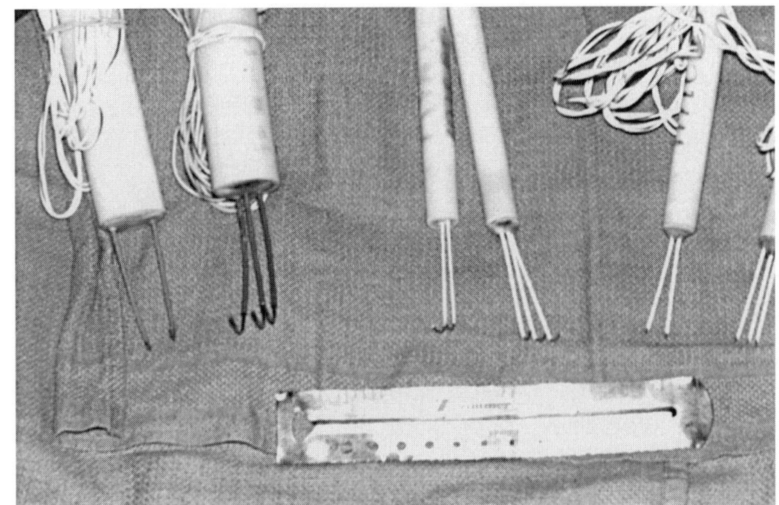

FIGURE 34–2. Electrodes used for NAP assessment. Three different-sized pairs of three-pronged stimulating *(on right of each pair)* and two pronged *(on left)* recording electrodes are illustrated. The different-sized electrodes are used selectively depending on nerve or nerve element diameter. (Modified from Kline DG, Happel LT: A quarter century's experience with intraoperative nerve action potential recording. Can J Neurol Sci *20*:3, 1993.)

ods, there is a learning curve that applies to learning the approach, and the best way to master the technique is to employ it as frequently as possible to develop experience and learn the nuances involved. For example, the senior author has used the technique in assessing all types of nerve injuries, including entrapment neuropathies, recording intraoperative NAPs in well over 2000 patients (Kline and Happel, 1993; Kline and Hudson, 1995). Practical considerations related to the successful use of the requisite equipment follows.

Electrode Design, Configuration, and Set-up. Our method of generating and recording NAPs employs electrodes constructed of stainless steel alloy. The electrode wire is insulated in Teflon, embedded within a plastic handle, with the bare tips bent into a shepherd's crook (see Fig. 34–2). The crook allows the nerve to be suspended in air, away from other tissue and tissue fluid during recording (Fig. 34–4). Stimulating electrodes are placed proximally and recording electrodes are placed distally in virtually all situations. *Stimulating electrodes* are separated by a distance of at least 3 mm to allow the current to spread sufficiently to excite all the axons in the nerve. If stimulating electrodes are placed too close to each other, current flow through the volume of the nerve is suboptimal, preventing many fibers from being stimulated. To accommodate a larger diameter nerve (e.g., the sciatic nerve), the area of separation between the electrodes is increased to 5 to 7 mm. We prefer to use a three-pronged electrode configuration for stimulation (see Fig. 34–2). The outer two tips of such an electrode are anodes, whereas the middle tip is a common cathode (Happel and Kline, 1991; Kline and Happel, 1993). This type of array decreases stimulus artifact and delivers a more precise point of stimulation, partially by reducing longitudinal spread of the stimulating current (Happel and Kline, 1991). The *recording electrodes* are of a bipolar configuration, with the tips placed far enough apart so that one contacts an active region of the nerve while the other is placed on an inactive zone. The amplitude of the NAP may be decreased if the electrodes are too close to each other. Under most circumstances, an optimal recording is achieved when the electrodes are separated by 3 to 5 mm. Even a greater gap between electrodes is needed for studying a long length (25 cm or greater) of nerve to compensate for the increased distance of nerve that is active from its constituent axons conducting at different velocities. A very important practical

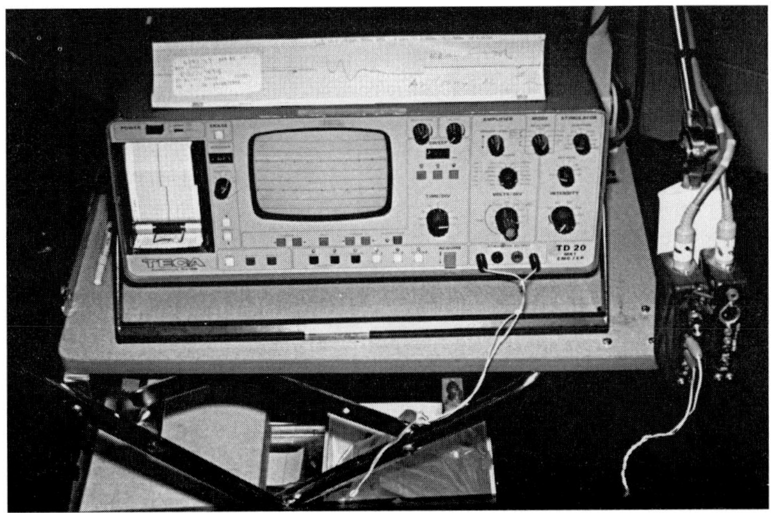

FIGURE 34–3. A self-contained electromyographic machine that is used at our institution for recording intraoperative NAPs. A strip from an actual recording is displayed across the top of the unit.

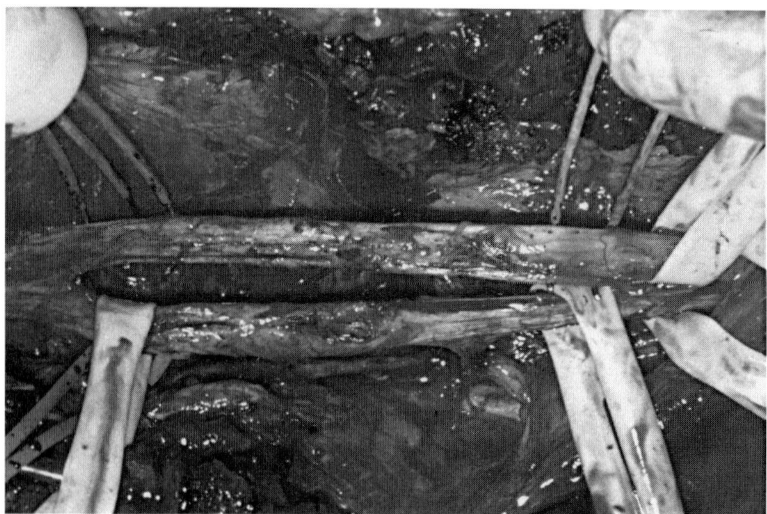

FIGURE 34–4. Intraoperative photo demonstrating the technique for electrophysiological evaluation of a neuroma in continuity. The sciatic nerve *(proximal to left)* and its tibial (shown undergoing electrophysiological testing) and peroneal division (suspended by Penrose drains) are shown. Note that the nerve undergoing recording is suspended away from surrounding tissue, cradled within the bent three prongs of the proximally placed stimulating and two prongs of the distally located recording electrodes.

consideration is the distance between the stimulating and recording electrodes. Placing the electrodes too close to one another not only magnifies the stimulus artifact, because of resistance and capacitance between the stimulating and recording electrode, but may also superimpose the NAP on the stimulus artifact, because of the short conduction time. The end result is a stimulus artifact that partially or totally obscures the NAP. In most cases, increasing distance to over 4 cm provides sufficient separation of the artifact from the evoked response to permit easy recognition and measurement of the NAP. Connecting cables from the stimulating and recording electrodes are separated by several inches to decrease capacitance between wires and to dampen electrical noise (Happel and Kline, 1991). The system is grounded by attaching the leads from the electrosurgical grounding pad, which are affixed to the patient's skin, to the grounding portion of the machine, after which the Bovie unit is turned off while recording. Sixty-cycle interference is further reduced, if necessary, by temporarily disabling battery-operated and motor-driven machines and turning off fluorescent lights.

Electromyographic Machine. Any modern single- or double-channel EMG machine has the capability of adequately stimulating and recording an NAP. A critical aspect of the component is that it must allow interfacing of single output from the stimulator with a resulting evoked response to be displayed as solitary traces on the oscilloscope. The goal of intraoperative NAP recording is to obtain single, not summated and averaged, responses because these responses most adequately sample the population of axons that are clinically significant (Kline and Happel, 1993; Van Beek et al, 1983). In the past, we had used a Grass stimulator and stimulus isolation unit, with recordings done by a differential amplifier and oscilloscope. At present, we are using a TECA (Pleasantville, New York), Model TD-20, EMG machine for intraoperative recordings (see Fig. 34–3). Self-contained units such as this one offer ease of mobility and simplicity but lack some flexibility with respect to stimulation parameters and filter settings. The authors' parameters for the stimulation parameters and filter settings are in the 5- to 10-Hz range for the low frequency filter and 2500 Hz or greater for the high-frequency filter setting. These settings most

optimally decrease stimulus artifact without filtering out the NAP response (Happel and Kline, 1991). Some machines have a 60-Hz notch filter built into the recorder. Because this filter device itself can generate a wave resembling an NAP, we recommend that it not be used.

Stimulation and Recording Parameters. Stimuli of brief duration and high intensity (voltage) are used. *Stimulation* needs to be brief in *duration* (0.05 to 0.1 milliseconds) because distances between stimulating and recording electrodes are often very short. Aside from reducing stimulus artifact, short-duration pulses also decrease activation of very small axons. These fibers may represent an unproductive degree of regeneration, not maturing further with time to result in useful function. The trade off to using brief pulses is the requirement to increase voltage for adequate stimulation. In contrast to healthy nerves, which require *voltage* between 3 to 15 V, regenerating nerves may need up to 50 V and occasionally more to be activated. To prevent damage with such a short-duration, high-intensity stimuli, the *frequency* should be kept below 2 per second. *Recording* parameters reflect the machine's ability to adequately display the evoked NAP. Because the amplitude of the NAP recorded can vary over a wide range between 20 μV and 2 mV, the oscilloscope settings must be able to encompass this range. The recorder is set between 50 μV and 5 mV per divison to display amplitude and the time base is set between 0.5 to 2.0 milliseconds per division to assess latency. Because the distance between stimulating and recording electrodes is often short, a time base of 1 millisecond (and sometimes 0.5 millisecond) per division is most frequently appropriate to discern the NAP that follows soon after the stimulus artifact. Starting with the recorder set at 100 μV per divison to display potentials (which are typically in the range of 200 to 500 μV in amplitude), the sensitivity of the machine is adjusted to suit the circumstances. In the situation in which no response is elicited even with the most sensitive setting (20 μV per division), the shock intensity is gradually raised until the upper limit of stimulation is reached.

Technique. Baseline NAPs are obtained first. These potentials usually require low levels of stimulation (3 to 5 V) and moderate sensitivity on the recorder (200 to 500 μV per division). It helps to expose 4 to 5 cm of the nerve above the lesion to assess the NAP proximally. A successfully recorded NAP here immediately confirms the integrity of the equipment. In those circumstances of very proximal stretch lesions or lengthy neuromas in continuity in which a proximal NAP cannot be assessed, a neighboring intact nerve is sought to obtain a baseline recording. The electrodes are then positioned above and below the lesion in continuity in an attempt to record across it (see Fig. 34–4). Starting with the parameters that evoke a baseline response, stimulation intensity is gradually increased (requiring up to 125 V at times) and amplification levels on the recorder are adjusted to progressively greater sensitivity until *single* consecutive NAP traces are viewed on the oscilloscope screen. A permanent record of either the single or an averaged trace is then made (Fig. 34–5). If a potential is recorded immediately distal to the neuroma in continuity, the recording electrode is moved even further down the distal nerve to ascertain how far the potential and, thus presumably regenerating axons of adequate number, caliber, and maturation have extended (Kline et al, 1969; Kline and Happel, 1993).

If an NAP is not elicited despite maximal stimulation and other appropriate adjustments of stimulating and recording parameters, it generally indicates the lack of sufficient regenerated axons across the electrode sites. Steps to exclude a false-negative result are important, however. The surgeon ensures that the nerve is elevated from surrounding tissue, blood, and fluid, and that excellent electrode contact, which is maximized by the nerve being cradled perpendicular to the electrode within its crook, with the nerve is present (see Fig. 34–4). The spacing of the electrodes is checked as per the previously mentioned guidelines. Low wound and nerve temperature are reversed with warm saline soaked sponges. Ischemia of tissue is precluded as a factor by waiting at least 20 minutes after letting down a tourniquet (which we do not use) before initiating recordings. The total lack of conduction across the neuroma, despite use of the above-mentioned maneuvers, mandates its resection and repair. Additionally, in those patients in whom NAPs are successfully recorded 6 months or more after injury but require maximal stimulation and very high amplification (10 μV per division), and conduct with velocities at less than 20 m/second, poor regeneration is likely present, and resection and repair are indicated.

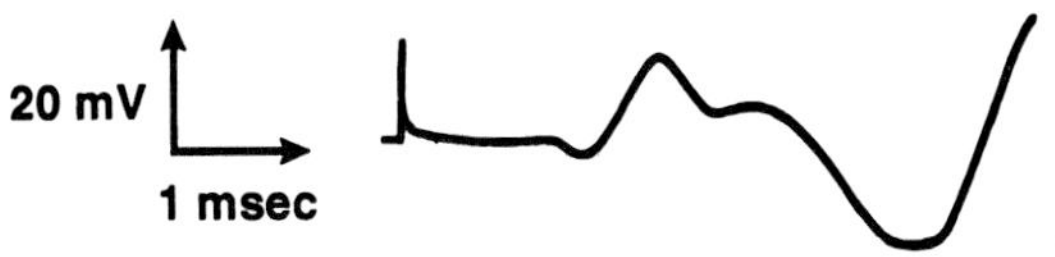

FIGURE 34–5. Example of an NAP recorded across a lesion in continuity involving the radial nerve at mid-humeral level. The patient had sustained a humeral fracture 9 weeks previously, resulting in complete radial palsy with no clinical or EMG evidence of recovery. The presence of an NAP across the lesion at operation indicated excellent regeneration, prompting the surgeon to perform an external neurolysis only. The patient went on to make a very good recovery (Grade 4) in all radial innervated muscle groups. C.D., complete denervation; S to R, distance between stimulating and recording electrodes. (Modified from Kline DG, Hudson AR: Nerve Injuries: Operative Results from Major Nerve Injuries, Entrapments, and Tumors. Philadelphia, W.B. Saunders Company, 1995.)

The surgeon should also be aware of generating false-positive recordings. For example, in proximal plexus lesions, in which the spinal nerves or roots are injured at a preganglionic level but are intact postganglionically, fast-conducting (60 to 80 m/second), high-amplitude NAPs are seen, reflecting activation of spared large-diameter sensory fibers. These responses are often even faster and larger than adjacent intact plexus elements and can be differentiated easily from the NAPs of regenerated nerves, which are much slower and of low amplitude. The absence of somatosensory evoked potentials from stimulating the proximal part of the spinal nerve confirms the preganglionic nature of these injuries. An evoked muscle action potential may also confuse the observer. These potentials can be distinguished from the NAP by their delayed latency (conduction velocity less than 20 m/second), increased amplitude, and polyphasic morphology. Use of a muscle-paralyzing agent will eliminate the motor response without affecting the NAP. Finally, 60-cycle interference can simulate an NAP, and steps to decrease this type of noise have already been addressed in an earlier section of this chapter.

Differential evaluation, including splitting, of the nerve or nerve element, is an important adjunct in interpreting NAPs and making intraoperative decisions. This factor is well illustrated by the sciatic nerve injury associated with severe distal clinical loss, which nevertheless conducts an NAP, implying that the observed response is only from one division whereas the other division needs resection and suture (Fig. 34–6). If the sciatic injury is close to its natural division into peroneal and tibial components, one can accomplish evaluation by stimulating the whole sciatic nerve and recording alternatively from each of the two components. A similar approach is useful in dealing with brachial plexus lesions. For example, lesions of the lateral and medial cord can be handled by stimulating the cord proximal to the neuroma in continuity and recording distally from the musculocutaneous nerve and lateral head of median nerve (for lateral cord injuries) or ulnar and median nerve (for medial cord injuries). Similarly, lesions to trunks of the plexus may require stimulation of roots and recording from either distal trunk, its divisions, or cords. At more distal levels, an injury to the radial nerve, for example, may be evaluated by stimulating the whole nerve while recording from both the superficial sensory and posterior interosseous branch. These techniques can result in a split repair of the neuroma in continuity, in which a portion of the cross section of the lesion that conducts an NAP is maintained, whereas the nonconducting portion is dissected away, resected, and grafted. At a finer level, particularly useful for very distal partial ulnar and median nerve injuries, the nerve may be split into fascicles or groups of fascicles, and recordings across the fascicles can be performed to direct resection and repair of nonconducting fascicles, as well as sparing of intact fascicles (Williams and Terzis, 1976).

RESULTS OF NERVE ACTION POTENTIAL RECORDINGS

The main objective of the intraoperative electrophysiological evaluation of a neuroma in continuity is to measure an NAP across and distal to the lesion. To a great extent, the ability of the lesion to transmit a single NAP determines the operative outcome. Moreover, in the initial months following

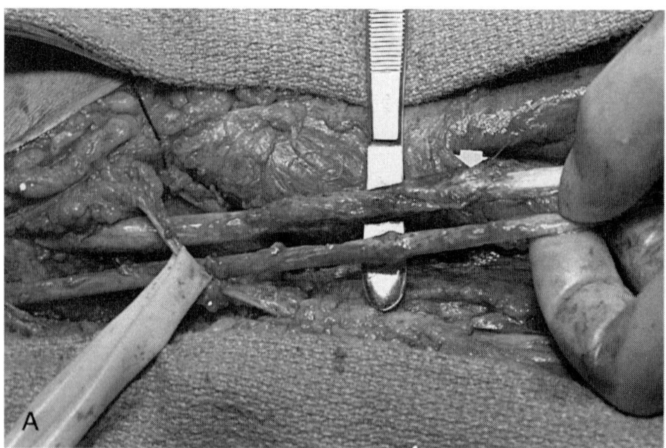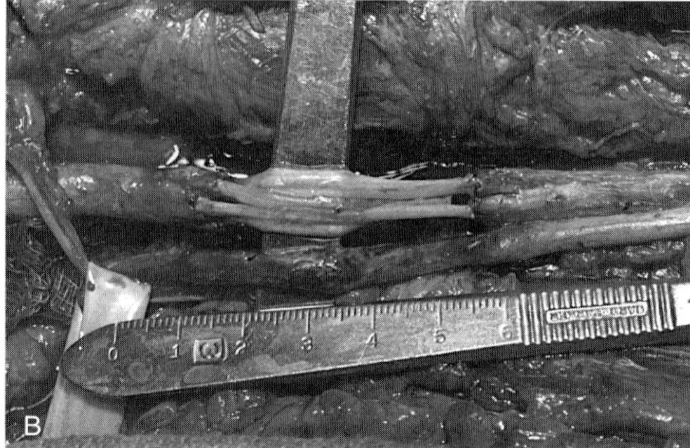

FIGURE 34–6. Intraoperative photos demonstrating differential evaluation of a neuroma in continuity involving the sciatic nerve divisions at proximal thigh level. *A*, The sciatic nerve is sharply dissected and split into its tibial *(white arrow)* and peroneal divisions, after which NAPs are elicited. *B*, This led to neurolysis of the conducting peroneal component, and resection and intrafascicular nerve grafting using five 4.5-cm long sural donor nerve for the nonconducting tibial component. (Modified from Kline DG, Hudson AR: Nerve Injuries: Operative Results from Major Nerve Injuries, Entrapments, and Tumors. Philadelphia, W.B. Saunders Company, 1995.)

injury, the simple presence or absence of an NAP is of much greater significance than the parameters of the trace, such as amplitude and conduction velocity. Again, it bears stressing that in all cases, the authors strive to record single, not averaged, NAPs. High amplification, summation, and integration techniques may allow a few hundred nerve fibers between the electrode sites to be discerned in an averaged NAP trace. Alternatively, single NAP recordings require several thousand moderately well-myelinated fibers as a substrate (Kline and Happel, 1993). The presence of an NAP reflects sufficient axons in at least some portion of the cross section of the sampled nerve to predict useful return of function (Kline and Happel, 1993). Therefore, when single evoked NAPs are obtained, external neurolysis is usually performed. Conversely, the absence of an NAP indicates that recovery will not occur without resection of the neuroma and repair of the nerve gap by either neurorrhaphy or grafting.

A review of the senior author's cases of lesions in continuity over a 25-year period (1965–1990) bears out the value of intraoperative electrophysiological evaluation (Kline and Happel, 1993). The information from NAP recording, procedures performed, and patient results from these cases are summarized in Table 34–1. Although varying slightly from nerve to nerve, the presence of a recordable NAP is consistently predictive of subsequent acceptable recovery, as shown in Table 34–1. These nerve and nerve elements underwent neurolysis alone, and 93.5% of the time, the patient obtained a useful (defined as Grade 3 or better) return of function in the distribution of the nerve. In 82% of cases, a Grade 4 (good) or 5 (excellent) outcome resulted (Kline and Happel, 1993). When NAPs are absent, our policy is to resect the neuroma in continuity. The pathological examination of the resected specimen in these cases invariably demonstrates a neurotmetic or Sunderland Grade 4 lesion. This pattern of pathology essentially precludes successful spontaneous regeneration leading to useful function, and such cases require resection of the lesion and repair by suture or grafting if there is any hope of functional return. The eventual recovery in these cases is somewhat unpredictable. In the Louisiana State University experience, the useful outcome results of such repairs have varied between 50% to 75%, depending on the nerve or nerve element involved (see Table 34–1).

To summarize, the evaluation of a patient with a suspected neuroma in continuity rests on a thorough knowledge of the possible underlying neuropathology. Serial clinical and electrophysiological assessment over the initial 2 to 4 months distinguishes those individuals who demonstrate spontaneous recovery from those who do not. A proactive decision to intervene operatively in the group of patients who do not demonstrate spontaneous recovery is indicated to optimize outcome. At surgery, the information derived from electrophysiological recording of NAPs is critical because it directs the surgeon: The lesions that conduct an NAP are left alone (neurolysed), whereas the lesions that fail to conduct an NAP are resected and repaired. Experimental studies in primates and clinical experience have validated this approach to the intraoperative evaluation of the neuroma in continuity.

▼ **TABLE 34–1**
Neuroma in Continuity Cases Studied

Nerve or Nerve Element	NAP Present: Neurolysis/Result*	NAP Absent: Repair/Result*
Median	72/70 (97%)†	49/37 (76%)
Radial	49/46 (94%)	84/61 (73%)
Ulnar	70/67 (96%)	38/22 (58%)
Combined upper extremity‡	55/48 (87%)	61/40 (66%)
Brachial plexus element	346/324 (94%)	562/289 (51%)
Lower extremity nerves§	193/175 (90%)	216/110 (51%)
Totals:	785/730 (94%)	1010/559 (55%)

*Number of patients operated on/number achieving useful, Grade 3 (proximal muscles contracting against gravity sund some resistance; distal muscles against gravity), or better outcome in follow-up.

†Percentage of patients (in parens) achieving Grade 3 or better results.

‡Combinations of median-ulnar, median-radial, or median-ulnar-radial nerves.

§Includes sciatic, tibial, peroneal, and femoral nerves.

Modified from Kline DG, Happel LT: A quarter century's experience with intraoperative nerve action potential recording. Can J Neurol Sci 20:3, 1993.

References

Bowden REM: Electromyography. *In* Seddon HJ (ed): Peripheral Nerve Injuries. Medical Research Council Special Report Series No. 282. London, Her Majesty's Stationery Office, 1954, p 263.

Gilliatt RW, Sears TA: Sensory nerve action potentials in patients with peripheral nerve lesions. J Neurol Neurosurg Psychiatr *21*:109, 1958.

Grundfest H, Oester YT, Beebe GW: Electrical evidence of regeneration. *In* Woodhall B, Beebe GW (ed): Peripheral Nerve Regeneration. Washington, DC, US Government Printing Office, 1956, p 203.

Gutmann E, Young JZ: Re-innervation of muscle after various periods of atrophy. J Anat *78*:15, 1944.

Happel LT, Kline DG: Nerve lesions in continuity. *In* Gelberman RH (ed): Operative Nerve Repair and Reconstruction. Philadelphia, J. B. Lippincott Company, 1991, p 601.

Henderson WR: Clinical assessment of peripheral nerve injuries. Tinel's test. Lancet *ii*:801, 1948.

Hudson AR, Hunter D: Timing of peripheral nerve repair: Important local neuropathologic factors. Clin Neurosurg *24*:392, 1977.

Kimura J: Electrodiagnosis in Diseases of Nerve and Muscles: Principles and Practice. Philadelphia, FA Davis, 1983.

Kline DG: Civilian gunshot wounds to the brachial plexus. J Neurosurg *70*:166, 1989.

Kline DG, Hackett ER: Reappraisal of timing for exploration of civilian peripheral nerve injuries. Surgery *78*:54, 1975.

Kline DG, Hackett ER: Management of the neuroma in continuity. *In* Wilkins RH, Rengachary SS (eds): Neurosurgery. New York, McGraw-Hill, 1984, p 1864.

Kline DG, Hackett ER, Davis GO, Myers MB: Effect of mobilization on the blood supply and regeneration of injured nerves. J Surg Res *12*:254, 1972.

Kline DG, Hackett ER, May P: Evaluation of nerve injuries by evoked potentials and electromyography. J Neurosurg *31*:128, 1969.

Kline DG, Happel LT: A quarter century's experience with intraoperative nerve action potential recording. Can J Neurol Sci. *20*:3, 1993.

Kline DG, Hudson AR: Nerve Injuries: Operative Results from Major Nerve Injuries, Entrapments, and Tumors. Philadelphia, W. B. Saunders Company, 1995.

Kline DG, Nulsen FE: The neuroma in continuity: Its preoperative and operative management. Surg Clin North Am *52*:1189, 1972.

Lundborg G: Structure and function of the intraneural microvessels as related to trauma, edema formation and nerve function. J Bone Joint Surg [Am] *57*:938, 1975.

Mackinnon SE, Dellon AL: Surgery of the Peripheral Nerve. New York, Thieme Medical Publishers Incorporated, 1988.

Moberg E: Methods for examining sensibility of the hand. *In* Flynn J (ed): Hand Surgery, 2nd ed. Baltimore, Williams & Wilkins, 1975, p 295.

Murphy F, Kirklin JW, Finlaysaon AI: Anomalous innervation of the intrinsic muscles of the hand. Surg Gynec Obstet *83*:15, 1946.

Nulsen FE, Kline DG: Acute injuries of peripheral nerves. *In* Youmans JR (ed): Neurological Surgery, 1st ed. Philadelphia, W. B. Saunders Company, 1973, p 1089.

Nulsen FE, Lewey FH: Intraneural bipolar stimulation: A new aid in the assessment of nerve injuries. Science *106*:301, 1947.

Omer GE: Nerve injuries associated with gunshot wounds of the extremities. *In* Gelberman RH (ed): Operative Nerve Repair and Reconstruction. Philadelphia, J. B. Lippincott Company, 1991, p 655.

Seddon HJ: Surgical Disorders of the Peripheral Nerves. Baltimore, Williams & Wilkins, 1972.

Seddon HJ, Medawar PB, Smith H: Rate of regeneration of peripheral nerves in man. J Physiol *102*:191, 1943.

Siegel DB, Gelberman RH: Peripheral nerve injuries associated with fractures and dislocations. *In* Gelberman RH (ed): Operative nerve repair and reconstruction. Philadelphia, J. B. Lippincott Company, 1991, p 619.

Sumner A: The Physiology of Peripheral Nerve Disease. Philadelphia, W. B. Saunders Company, 1980.

Sunderland S: Rate of regeneration in human peripheral nerves. Arch Neurol Psychiatr *58*:251, 1947a.

Sunderland S: Rate of regeneration in human peripheral nerves: Analysis of interval between injury and onset of recovery. Arch Neurol Psychiatr *58*:291, 1947b.

Sunderland S: Nerve and Nerve Injuries. Edinburgh, Churchill Livingstone, 1978.

Sunderland S: Nerve Injuries and Their Repair. A Critical Appraisal. Melbourne, Churchill Livingstone, 1991.

Van Beek A, Hubble B, Kinkead L: Clinical use of nerve stimulation and recording. Plast Reconstr Surg *71*:225, 1983.

Williams HB, Terzis JK: Single fascicular recordings: An intraoperative diagnostic tool for the management of peripheral nerve lesions. Plast Reconstr Surg *57*:562, 1976.

Woodhall B, Nulsen F, White J, Davis L: Neurosurgical Implications. *In* Woodhall B, Beebe GW (eds): Peripheral Nerve Regeneration. Washington, DC, Veterans Administration Monograph, 1957, p 569.

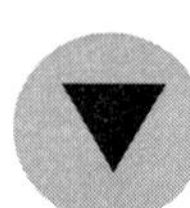

Chapter 35

• Susan E. Mackinnon

Evaluation of Nerve Gaps: Upper and Lower Extremities

Management of the peripheral nerve gap that precludes primary suture has been the focus of surgical research and debate for over a century and continues to be a current topic of interest and discussion. Several chapters in this textbook address related nerve repair and nerve grafting. In this chapter, I discuss my particular philosophy toward management of the nerve gap. The classic management of the nerve gap with either nerve repair or grafting is reviewed, as are the newer techniques using various conduits to bridge the short nerve gap. The concept of nerve transfer is reviewed as an option to obviate the need for a nerve graft or provide critical nerve function for extensive or very proximal nerve injuries. Finally, the role of nerve allografts for otherwise irreparable nerve injury is discussed (Fig. 35–1).

NERVE GAP VERSUS NERVE DEFICIT

The difference between the concept of nerve gap versus nerve deficit has been discussed (Mackinnon, 1989). The actual amount of nerve tissue lost refers to the nerve deficit. The nerve gap simply refers to the distance between the proximal and distal ends of the nerve. Thus, if a nerve has simply been divided and no nerve tissue is lost, the nerve deficit will be 0 cm. The nerve gap may also be 0 cm or it may be much greater if the two ends of the nerve are separated either mechanically by the surgeon or with scar retraction. If nerve tissue has been lost and a nerve deficit exists, then the nerve gap will be at least the same length as the nerve deficit and may, of course, be longer if the two ends of the nerve are separated further by the forces of wound healing (Fig. 35–2).

EXCURSION

Anatomical and mechanical factors affect longitudinal gliding of the nerve. The degree of longitudinal motion and the elasticity of the peripheral nerve varies between nerves and with the location of the nerves in the extremity. Excursion and gliding of a nerve is essential in order to distribute tension in both the normal and pathological state. Nerve compression and traction neuropathy may result when a nerve is tethered. The ulnar nerve is an example of a peripheral nerve that must glide to accommodate motion as it crosses behind the elbow joint. It has a longitudinal excursion of 7 to 11 mm proximal to the elbow. In the instance of a laceration of the ulnar nerve in the region of the cubital tunnel, the author performs an anterior submuscular transposition in order to decrease tension at the nerve repair site. Even greater excursion is noted at the wrist, where both median and ulnar nerves glide approximately 14 mm. Distally in the hand, the excursion decreases dramatically, with digital nerves gliding only 1 to 1.3 mm. Thus, although there may be some laxity gained by mobilization of the nerve and extremity positioning with more proximal injuries, little gain can be obtained in the digits. A very short defect in the digital nerve may be impossible to treat adequately with a simple nerve repair (Fig. 35–3).

Division of the radial nerve in the spiral groove may be associated with significant proximal and distal retraction of the nerve. By contrast, similar division of the radial sensory nerve in the forearm results in little retraction and minimal gap. In both situations, the nerve deficit will be 0 cm but the gap may vary significantly. Following injury, the formation of scar tends to tether the nerve and produce secondary

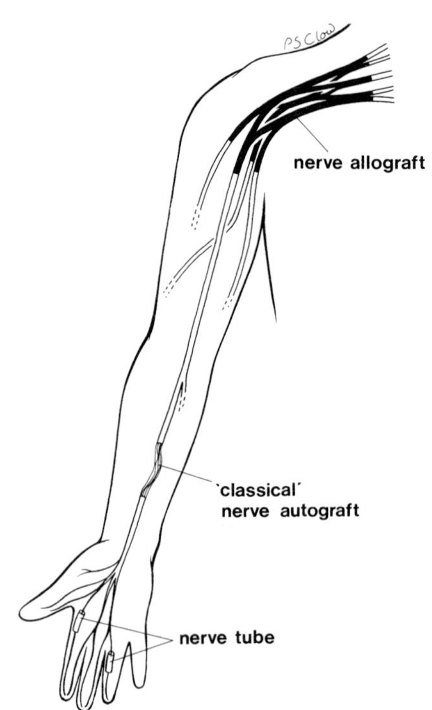

FIGURE 35–1. In general, the nerve gap is reconstructed with a classic nerve autograft. The extremely long gap requires the use of a nerve allograft. A nerve conduit can direct nerve regeneration over short distances. (From Mackinnon SE: Surgical management of the peripheral nerve gap. Clin Plast Surg *16*:587–603, 1989.)

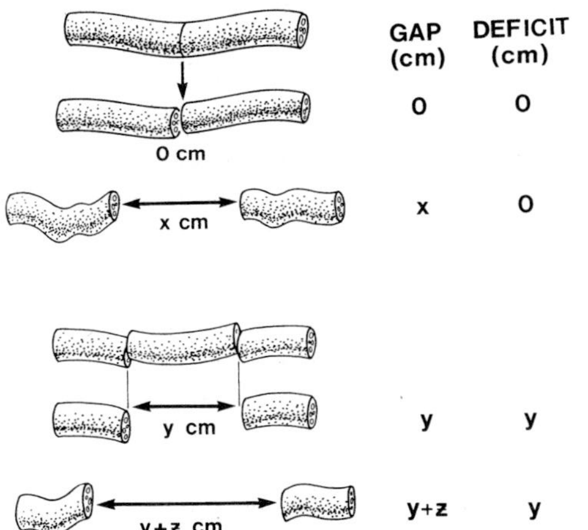

FIGURE 35–2. A schematic representation of the concept of nerve gap versus nerve deficit. The nerve deficit represents the amount of actual nerve tissue loss. The nerve gap is simply the distance between the proximal and distal nerve ends and may be the same distance as the nerve deficit or greater if the proximal and distal ends are pulled apart. Thus, although the nerve deficit will remain constant, the nerve gap can vary. (From Mackinnon SE: Surgical management of the peripheral nerve gap. Clin Plast Surg *16*:587–603, 1989).

traction neuropathy. Thus, early protected postoperative motion ensures that the adhesions that form will be long enough to accommodate full excursion of the nerve without traction from obligatory scar formation. The benefits of early protected motion following any peripheral nerve reconstruction can be emphasized and are underrecognized at present.

NERVE REPAIR

Basic Principles

We have modified our list of basic principles that form the basis of our current management of the nerve gap (Mackinnon and Dellon, 1988):

1. Quantitative assessment of motor and sensory function preoperatively and postoperatively, including assessment of strength (pinch/grip) and wasting, as well as the innervation threshold (vibration/pressure) and density (two-point discrimination).

2. Microsurgical repair with magnification and appropriate sutures and instrumentation.

3. Tension-free coaptation.

4. Interposition nerve grafting when otherwise a direct repair would require tension.

5. Avoidance of postural maneuvers to decrease tension.

6. Primary repair when the clinical and surgical conditions permit.

7. Secondary repair (at 3 weeks or when the wound permits) usually with a nerve graft technique if the proximal and distal extent of the nerve injury cannot be satisfactorily determined at the time of the injury.

8. Group fascicular repair when intraneural anatomy permits. Epineural repair when topography is indeterminate or mixed.

9. Early protected postoperative mobilization to encourage the formation of long scar adhesions that will not result in subsequent scar traction neuropathy.

10. Motor and sensory re-education to maximize the functional result.

Tension

Tension at the repair site encourages gaping, as well as scar and adhesion formation. It will also reduce blood flow and prevent early mobilization of the injured extremity due to concern over continuity at the nerve repair. Although, to some degree, the amount of tension that is accepted is subjective, the author uses a simple rule to gauge the amount of tension at the repair. If the first epineurial suture with an 8-0 monofilament nylon can bring the nerve into approximation without postural maneuvers, then it is appropriate to proceed with a direct primary repair. We rarely mobilize the nerve more than 1 to 2 cm to achieve repair. Novel techniques of tissue expansion to achieve increased length have

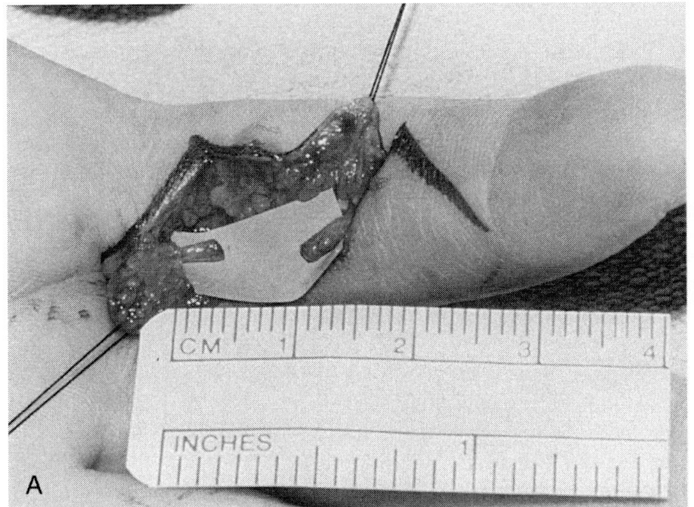

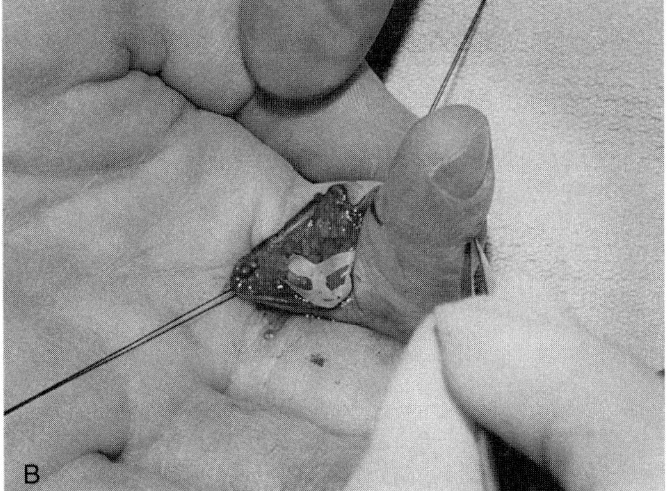

FIGURE 35–3. *A,* Even a short gap in the digital nerve is not easily overcome with direct repair. *B,* Even flexion of the proximal interphalangeal joint to 90 degrees does not allow a primary nerve repair. Note that the nerve deficit in both *A* and *B* are the same, but the nerve gap varies.

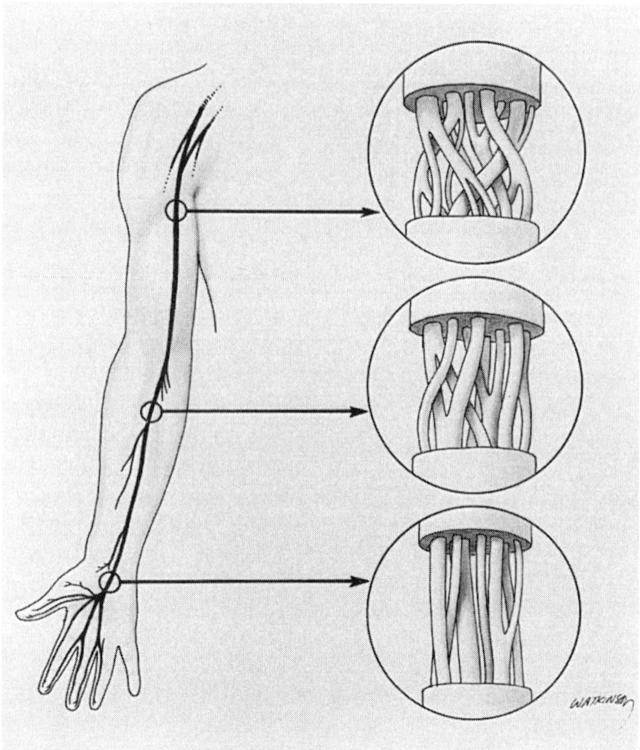

FIGURE 35–4. The internal topography of the median nerve. The degree of plexus formation that occurs between fascicles decreases in the distal portion of the extremity. (From Mackinnon SE, Dellon AL: Surgery of the Peripheral Nerve. New York, Thieme Medical Publishers, 1988.)

not met the expectations of the initial optimism. For example, in a case report after 3 months of expansion, only 2 cm of advancement was gained (Manders et al, 1987).

Fascicular Topography

Fascicular organization of the extremity nerves is not constant over the length of the nerve. Proximally in the extremity, there is an intricate pattern of intermingling between fascicles. In the distal extremity, there is less complex topography (Figs. 35–4 and 35–5).

Microneurography and horseradish peroxidase tracing studies have demonstrated that there is distinct somatotopic organization *within* the fibers of a fascicle. Thus, nerve territories remain localized even in the proximal portion of the extremity, suggesting the feasibility of awake stimulation to identify motor-sensory topography.

Certain relationships are clinically useful. The topographic organization of the distal ulnar nerve is relatively constant at the wrist and distal forearm. The motor fascicular group, is just slightly smaller than the sensory fascicular group and is located at the ulnar dorsal position. In the forearm, the motor group lies between the slightly larger fascicular group, giving sensation to the ulnar digits, and the small dorsal cutaneous group, giving sensation to the dorsum of the wrist and hand (Fig. 35–6).

At the wrist, the median nerve is divided into three main fascicular groups: sensory supply to the third web space, the

second web space, and the thumb index space, including motor supply to the thenar muscles (Fig. 35–7).

In the management of radial nerve injuries, proximal awake stimulation can be useful in identifying motor and sensory bundles. Distally, the radial sensory nerve is identified and followed proximally to the site of the nerve injury. The radial sensory nerve can be excluded from the distal nerve repair to ensure that the motor fascicles that have been identified by awake stimulation technique proximally are grafted into the motor component of the radial nerve and not lost in the sensory component. Special care is taken to reinnervate the extensor carpi radialis brevis, which will be the most proximal of the wrist extensors to be reinnervated. The radial sensory nerve can be used, if necessary, as nerve graft material (Fig. 35–8).

The intramuscular topography of the musculocutaneous nerve has been well worked out and is important in brachial plexus reconstruction for biceps function (Brandt and Mackinnon, 1993). The motor fibers to the biceps innervate the muscle in its mid-portion. Approximately 13 cm from the medial epicondyle, there are no more motor branches, and the cutaneous component (lateral antebrachial cutaneous [LABC] nerve) is easily separable from the motor component of the musculocutaneous nerve at this level (Fig. 35–9).

In the lower extremity, the fascicular group to the tibialis anterior muscle in the region of the fibular head and popliteal fossa is distinct. It is located in the medial aspect of the nerve, and recurs acutely around the fibular head to innervate the tibialis anterior muscle. In general, the principles for management of upper and lower extremity nerve gaps are the same. However, in the lower extremity, the surgeon may prioritize the requirements for reconstruction if there is a lack of donor graft material. For example, with respect to the peroneal nerve, recovery of tibialis anterior function is clearly the most critical in functional recovery. By contrast, with respect to the posterior tibial nerve, recovery of functional sensibility on the sole of the foot is more important than motor recovery. The surgeon uses awake stimulation proximally to identify sensory or motor fascicles and then specifically direct the most critical part of the reconstruction toward motor recovery for the peroneal nerve and sensory recovery for the posterior tibial nerve. The remainder of the reconstruction is completed with the remainder of potential available donor graft material. In the situation of posterior tibial nerve injury at the level of the popliteal fossa, we have recovered good protective sensibility on the sole of the foot with the transfer of a functioning sural nerve to the lateral plantar portion of the posterior tibial nerve, using a direct repair at the level of the ankle in an older patient in whom otherwise a nerve allograft or amputation would have been necessary (Mackinnon et al, 1993).

Mobilization and Primary Repair

Primary repair of an acutely and sharply transected nerve presents few problems. However, when the treatment is delayed or the nerve ends are slightly traumatized, a short nerve gap results. The dilemma then exists between performing a nerve repair under slight tension or using an interposition nerve graft. The author performs a limited mobilization of the nerve, and then an assessment is made

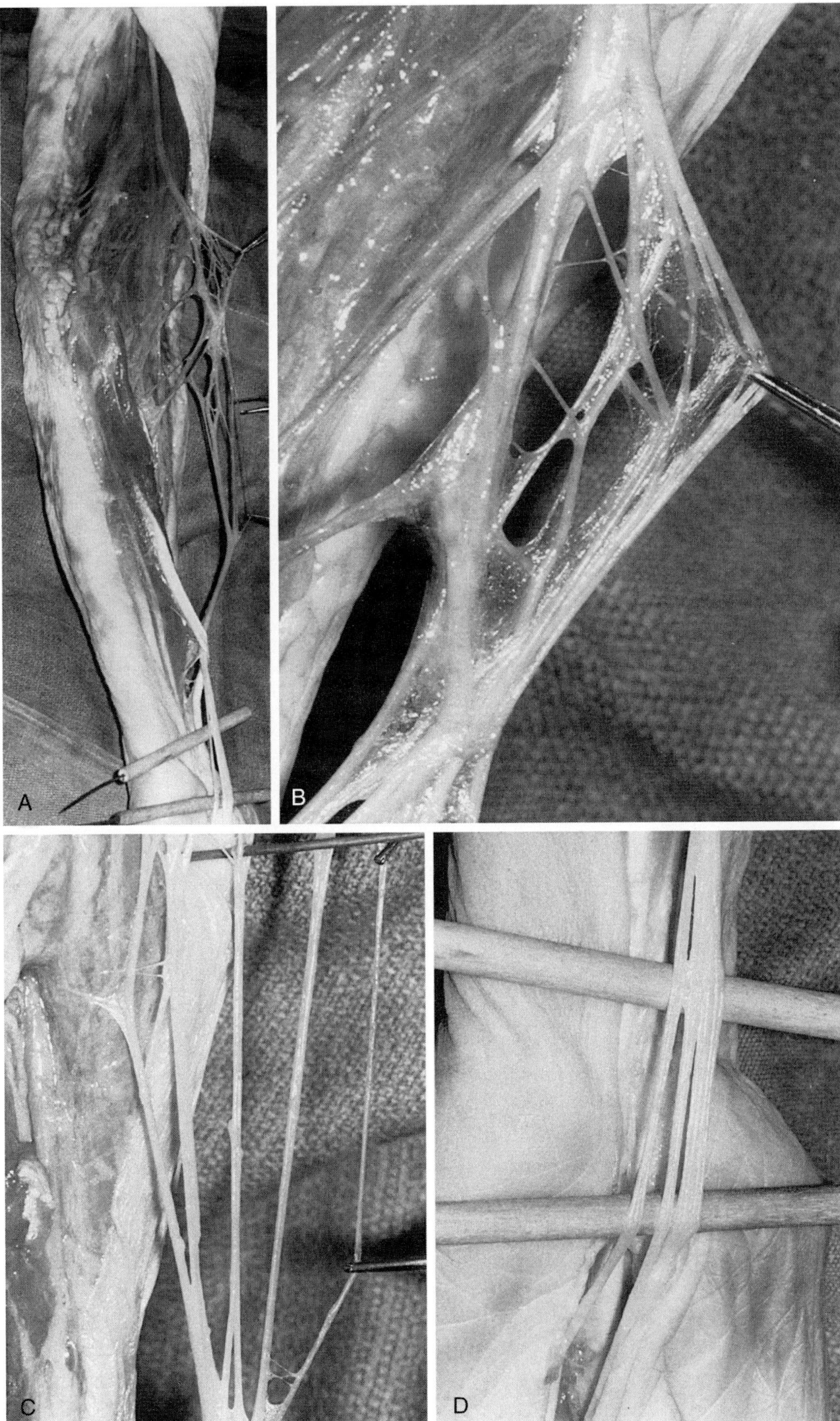

FIGURE 35–5. *A,* A cadaver dissection of the left median nerve, with the hand at the bottom of the photograph and the axilla at the top of the photograph. The fascicles of the median nerve have been dissected by means of a microneurolysis technique. *B,* Marked plexus formation is apparent in the region of the antecubital fossa. *C,* In the mid-forearm, less plexus formation is noted between fascicles. *D,* In the distal portion of the extremity at the level of the wrist, there is little plexus formation between fascicles.

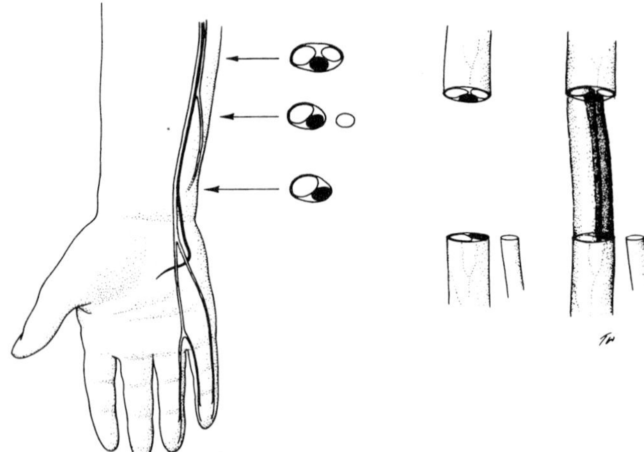

FIGURE 35–6. The internal topography of the ulnar nerve is such that the motor group is located between and just dorsal to the two sensory groups in the proximal part of the forearm. After the dorsal cutaneous branch of the ulnar nerve separates from the main ulnar nerve, the motor nerve is found medially and just dorsal to the sensory group. In Guyon's canal, the motor branch curves around the hook of the hamate bone dorsal to the sensory branches to the small and ring fingers. When a nerve graft is performed in the distal forearm and wrist area, awake stimulation can be used to identify motor and sensory groups in the proximal part of the nerve. In the distal portion of the nerve, dissection into Guyon's canal is performed so that the surgeon may clearly determine the sensory and motor components of the nerve (motor fascicles are black, and sensory fascicles white). (From Mackinnon SE: Nerve injuries: Primary repair and reconstruction. Cohen ML (ed), Mastery of Surgery—Plastic Surgery. Boston, Little, Brown, and Company, 1994, pp 1598–1624.)

FIGURE 35–7. The critical internal topography of the median nerve in the distal forearm and wrist is comparatively simple, because there are only one or two critical motor fascicles and they are usually located on the radial volar aspect of the nerve. The majority of the nerve is sensory. Thus, during nerve grafting procedures, there is little motor contamination of the distal nerve by proximal motor fibers. Awake stimulation can be used on the proximal nerve stump to exclude these contaminant fibers, although it is probably not necessary because there are so few. Anatomic dissection of the distal stump can be carried out to exclude the motor fibers to the thenar eminence if the time since injury is so long to preclude reinnervation of the thenar muscle and the surgeon is moving toward a tendon transfer for this function. (From Mackinnon SE: Nerve injuries: Primary repair and reconstruction. Cohen ML (ed): Mastery of Surgery—Plastic Surgery. Boston, Little, Brown, & Company, 1994, pp 1598–1624.)

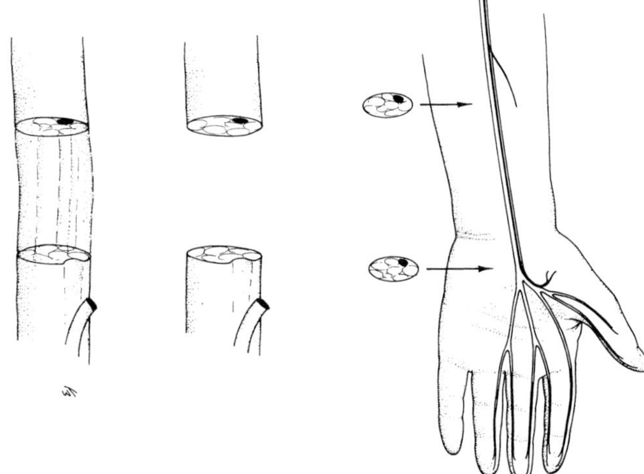

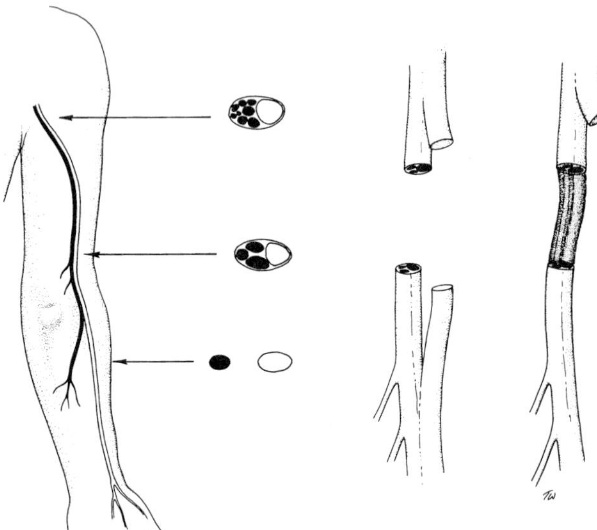

FIGURE 35–8. The fascicles of the radial nerve in the proximal arm are divided into discrete sensory and motor fascicles. Thus, awake stimulation can be used to determine the motor component of the nerve. Distally, just proximal to the elbow, the two motor branches to the extensor carpi radialis longus and brachial radialis tendon can be identified. It is important to innervate the branch to the extensor carpi radialis longus muscle. The radial sensory component can be identified and excluded from the nerve grafting procedure to ensure that no proximal motor fibers are directed to the cutaneous radial sensory nerve territory. Nerve grafts are directed from the proximal motor *(black)* fascicles to the distal motor *(black)* fascicles, excluding the sensory fascicles. (From Mackinnon SE: Nerve injuries: Primary repair and reconstruction. Cohen ML (ed): Mastery of Surgery—Plastic Surgery. Boston, Little, Brown, & Company, 1994, pp 1598–1624.)

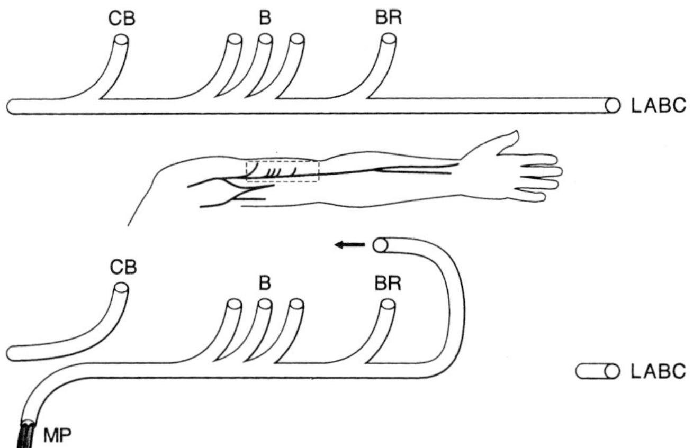

FIGURE 35–9. The technique of biceps reinnervation would involve exclusion of the branches to the coracobrachialis muscle (CB) and division of the lateral antebrachial cutaneous (LABC) nerve just distal to the last branch to the brachialis muscle (BR). This portion of the nerve would then be transposed into the biceps in a position near the motor end plates to the biceps (B) medial pectoral (MP) nerve. Rather than turning the LABC back into the biceps muscle, we have followed the advice of M. Wood, Mayo Clinic, and transferred this LABC to the radial nerve in effort to direct motor fibers to the wrist extensors rather than losing them into the cutaneous distribution of the LABC. (From Mackinnon SE: Technique for maximizing biceps recovery and brachial plexus reconstruction. J Hand Surg 726–733, 1993.)

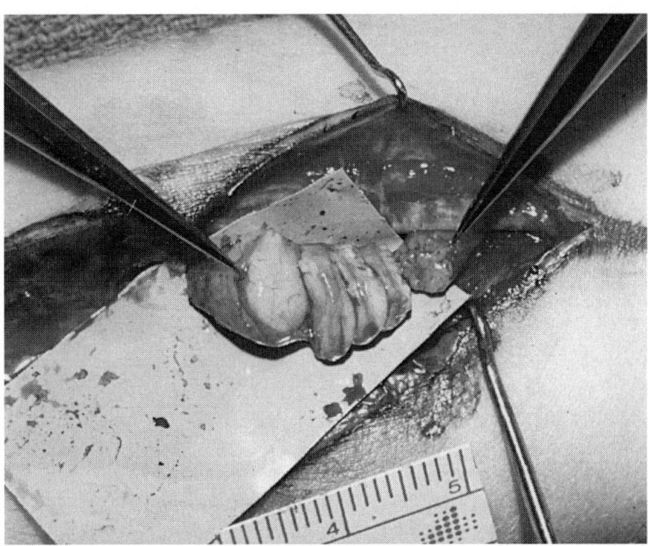

FIGURE 35–11. The bread-slicing technique is noted in this median nerve. Dense scarring is replaced with a nice fascicular pattern over a distance of several millimeters.

of the degree of injury to the proximal and distal sites of the transection. Minimal sharp trimming of the nerve ends may be done. If it is a clean injury, then a primary repair is performed. If there is marked contusion of the nerve ends, then the nerve is approximated using 6-0 nylon sutures. An attempt is made to align the nerve appropriately, taking advantage of the acute situation where fascicular patterns and vascular marking in the epineurium may assist in appropriate alignment of the nerve. At 3 weeks or when the wound permits, the nerve is re-explored and the nerve is sliced proximal and distal from the area of injury until a healthy fascicular pattern is noted (Figs. 35–10 and 35–11). A repair is performed, if possible. Otherwise, a short nerve graft is usually necessary.

There will be some injuries that are categorized as intermediate with respect to the degree of contusion. If the surgeon is somewhat concerned about the viability of the proximal and distal components of the transected nerve but is relatively confident that a definitive nerve repair is appropriate, a direct repair is performed. However, the patient will be told that if Tinel's sign does not advance at the appro-

priate rate of 1 inch a month, then within 2 to 3 months, a recommendation will be given to re-explore the area and evaluate the nerve for consideration of a nerve graft.

AUTOGENOUS NERVE GRAFTING

Donor Nerve Grafts

For reconstruction in the upper extremity, the available nerves include the medial antebrachial cutaneous (MABC), LABC, dorsal ulnar sensory, radial sensory, and sural (Fig. 35–12). It is also possible to scavenge neural tissue from regions distal to the site of transection. This approach eliminates creating additional morbidity from a new donor site. For example, noncritical components of a nerve may be used as donor nerve graft material (Fig. 35–13). In established median nerve injuries or following failed median nerve re-

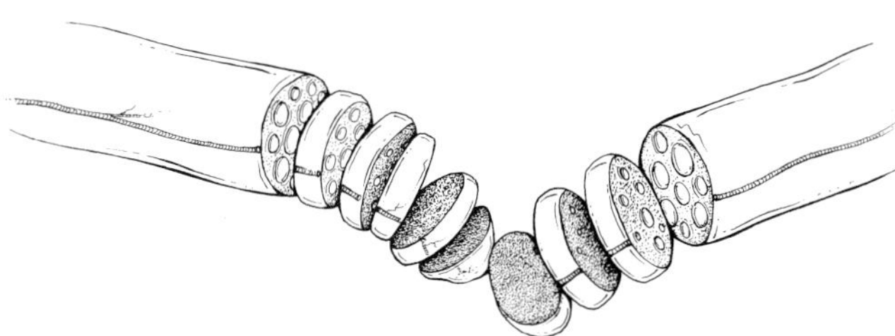

FIGURE 35–10. Serial section through a previously failed nerve repair demonstrates the technique of bread-slicing. The scarred ground-glass appearance through the center sections does not demonstrate any fascicular architecture. Eventually, normal, healthy nerve is noted both proximally and distally. (From Watchmaker GP, Mackinnon SE: Nerve repair and reconstruction. Peimer CA [ed]: Surgery of the Hand and Upper Extremity. New York, McGraw-Hill, 1996, 1251–1276.)

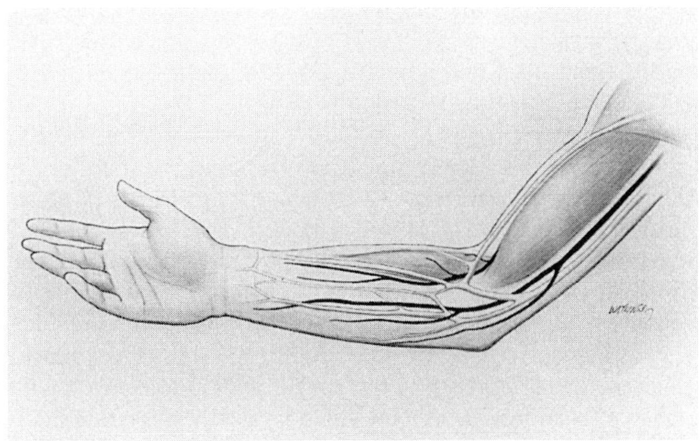

FIGURE 35–12. The anatomic relationships of the medial and lateral antebrachial cutaneous nerves (MABC and LABC). Note that the LABC maintains close relationship to the cephalic vein, aiding in its identification. Note the two branches of the MABC lying on either side of the basilic vein. (From Watchmaker GP, Mackinnon SE: Nerve repair and reconstruction. Peimer CA [ed]: Surgery of the Hand and Upper Extremity. New York, McGraw-Hill, 1996, pp 1251–1276.)

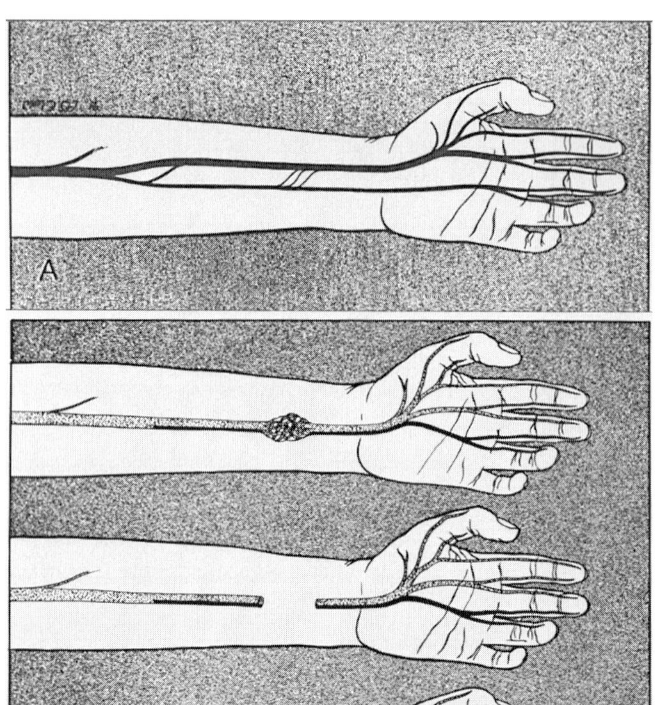

FIGURE 35–13. *A*, The internal topography of the median nerve allows fascicles dedicated to the third web space of the hand to be separated easily across a long distance before significant plexus formation occurs. *B*, The fascicles to the third web space can be harvested to the level of the first major plexus at approximately 14 cm proximal to the wrist crease and can be used as nerve graft material to reconstruct the remainder of the median nerve. (From Ross D, Mackinnon SE, Change Y: Intraneural anatomy of the median nerve provides "third web space" donor nerve graft. J Reconstr Microsurgery 8:225–232, 1992.)

pair, we will frequently harvest the fascicles to the third web space both proximal and distal to the area of injury as a donor source for nerve graft material (Ross et al, 1992). Similarly, the dorsal cutaneous branch of the ulnar nerve for ulnar nerve and radial sensory nerve repairs may be a source of graft material. In the lower extremity, the superficial sensory branch of the peroneal nerve is a satisfactory nerve donor besides the sural nerve. In general, the upper extremity nerves have a greater neural–to–connective tissue ratio than the lower extremity nerves. The patients are involved in discussion of the donor sites, because some patients prefer not to add additional sensory deficit to an already affected extremity. By contrast, others will want to keep all of their problems confined to one extremity. When faced with a short gap in an upper extremity nerve, the author uses the anterior branch of the MABC or the LABC. These nerves are ideal for digital nerve grafts. The author prefers the anterior branch of the MABC over the LABC, given that the medial arm scar is more readily concealed. Larger defects require the use of sural nerves.

Surgical Technique

Tourniquet technique is used whenever possible, and the injured nerve is approached through normal tissue both prox-

imally and distally. Intraoperative electrodiagnostic testing is performed either within the first 15 minutes of the tourniquet run or after the tourniquet has been released, unless there has been absolute confirmation preoperatively that a complete transection is present. If evidence of conduction is found, then the injury is treated like a neuroma in continuity (Mackinnon et al, 1992; Mackinnon, 1994; Watchmaker and Mackinnon, 1995). If no conduction is found, then the nerve is followed toward the area of injury. Starting in the obvious area of injury, the nerve is resected in both a proximal and distal direction until a healthy fascicular pattern is noted (see Fig. 35–10). Establishing the most distal level of healthy nerve tissue on the proximal stump is important because this sets the distance between the regenerating front of axons and the distal motor and sensory targets. Once the length of the nerve gap is identified and the ends have been prepared, a suitable donor nerve is harvested. The polarity of the nerve grafts is reversed, and all fascicles will be kept at the same level on the proximal and distal faces of the nerve trunk (Fig. 35–14). This maneuver increases the possibility that any fibers that escape from the repair site are more likely to be caught in an adjacent nerve graft. The extremity is then moved through the full range of motion to ensure that there is no tension on either end of the nerve grafts. The major nerves in both the upper and lower extremities typically require several interpositional grafts (five to seven), whereas the digital nerves require only one or two. Two or three 9-0 or 10-0 sutures are used to align each graft. Glickman has described the following technique: When multiple cables are being directed toward the face of a major nerve, use a single suture to pick up one area of each of the multiple grafts and to create a so-called rosebud effect (Glickman, 1995). This allows the multiple nerve grafts to be delivered toward the proximal or distal face of the main nerve as one bundle.

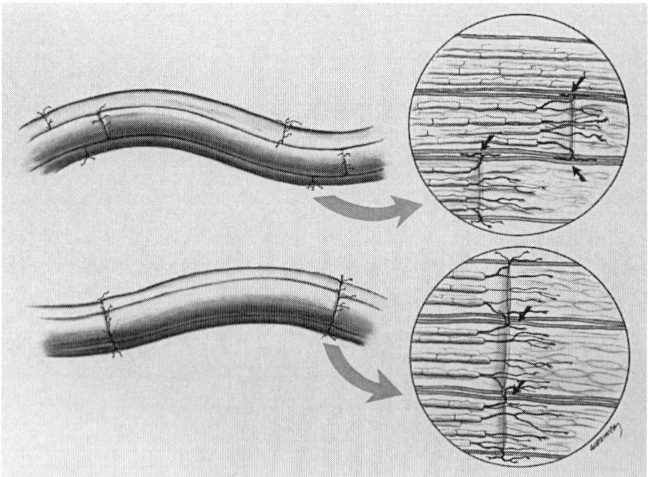

FIGURE 35–14. Nerve grafting technique: When the fascicles have been resected back to normal tissue and the suture lines for each of these grafts are slightly staggered, the nerve is divided in such a way that all nerve grafts are at the same level. Fibers that escape from the nerve repair sites may then be captured by adjacent nerve grafts. This technique maximizes the number of nerve fibers directed toward the distal nerve. However, if the surgeon does not want nerves from one fascicular group in the adjacent nerve grafts (for example, to avoid contamination of motor and sensory grafts), the staggered or step technique *(top)* is warranted. (From Mackinnon SE: Nerve injuries: Primary repair and reconstruction. Cohen ML (ed): Mastery of Surgery—Plastic Surgery. Boston, Little, Brown, & Company, 1994, pp 1598–1624.)

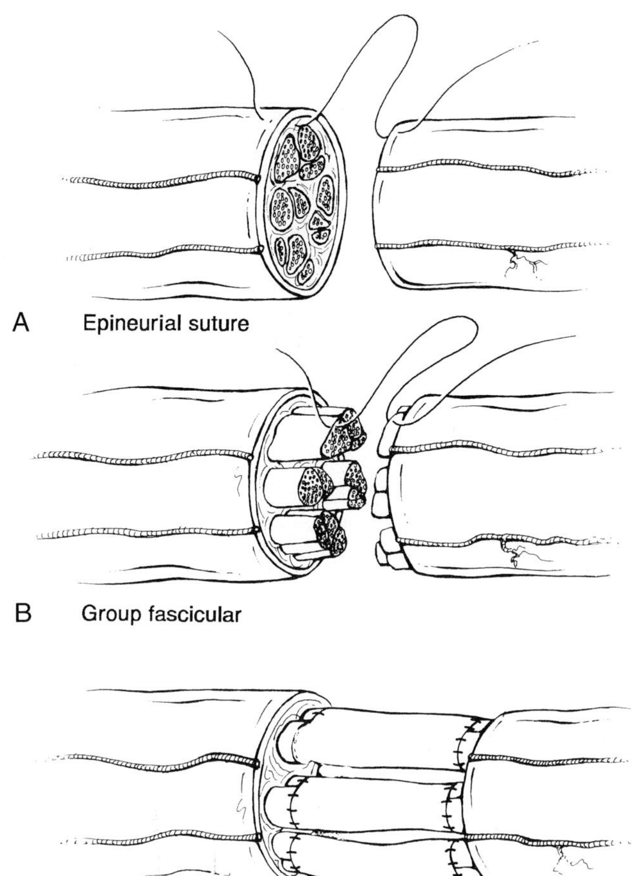

FIGURE 35–15. Techniques of nerve repair. *A,* A direct epineurial suture utilizing surface vessels for alignment. *B,* Group fascicular repair. *C,* Nerve grafting using multiple strands of donor nerve to bridge a gap. (From Watchmaker GP, Mackinnon SE: Nerve repair and reconstruction. Peimer CA (ed): Surgery of the Hand and Upper Extremity. New York, McGraw-Hill, 1996, pp 1251–1276.)

Group fascicular repair is performed when the motor or sensory topography is understood (Fig. 35–15). Once the repair has been completed, the repair site is re-examined to ensure that there is not excessive gaping at the repair sites and that no fascicles are protruding from the suture line. If there is gaping and fascicles do protrude, then microscissors are used to cut back the protruding axons and realign them so that proximal and distal fascicles directly face each other. Depending on the duration of denervation, the distal nerve stump may be smaller than the proximal nerve stump and there may be some maneuvering necessary in order to align the nerve grafts to facilitate this difference. Once the graft is completed, the extremity is once again put through a full range of motion to ensure that there is no tension on either repair site and that the graft tolerates complete range of motion of the extremity. The limb is immobilized in a fiberglass splint, and if the injury is located in the upper extremity, the splint fashioned to encourage early protective movement of the digits.

Vascularized Nerve Grafts

The initial enthusiasm for the vascularized nerve graft first described in 1976 by Taylor and Hamm has not been supported clinically, and conflicting experimental reports suggest that if any advantages do exist, they are likely to be marginal.

Awake Stimulation

Awake stimulation is a useful technique that requires cooperation from both the patient and the anesthesiologist. The initial surgical dissection is carried out with neuroleptanalgesia and regional or local anesthesia. A nerve injury is evaluated, and a short-acting anesthetic hypnotic agent is useful when the proximal portion of the nerve is sharply transected, because this maneuver is painful for the patient. Preoperatively, the patient will have been advised that the nerve will be stimulated and that he or she will be asked to respond to this stimulation. Motor fibers contain afferent sensory fibers, and the stimulation of motor groups is interpreted by the patient as a dull, nonspecific sensation. By contrast, stimulation of sensory fascicles is interpreted by the patient as a type of burning or electrical pain in a specific cutaneous distribution. This technique is extremely useful in the evaluation of the motor component of the peroneal and posterior tibial nerves and the deep motor branch of the ulnar nerve.

CONDUITS

Various types of conduits have been investigated, and this topic has recently been extensively reviewed (Doolabh et al, 1996). Silicone polymer tubulization is a recognized model for nerve compression, and if a silicone conduit is used, then the surgeon must eventually remove the silicone. Lundborg has demonstrated in a group of patients with mixed nerve injuries that regeneration across a short-nerve silicone conduit is similar to that seen across a primary nerve repair, although not any better.

Evans and associates (1994) have shown that selective reinnervation occurred across a 5-mm conduit equivalent to that achieved across an exact primary nerve repair, whether the nerve was correctly oriented in the conduit or rotated 180 degrees. Thus, this suggests that an incorrectly aligned nerve will reorient across a conduit and yield a result similar to that across a correctly aligned nerve repair.

Regeneration across vein grafts has been investigated clinically and experimentally, and can be used clinically for gaps less than 3 cm in noncritical sensory nerves.

The similarity between the basement membrane matrix of muscle and nerve has stimulated the use of treated muscle grafts for nerve repair. Glasby and his group have shown that regeneration will occur across short distances through pretreated muscle grafts. However, poor results were noted in major nerves and across long gaps.

The use of synthetic bioabsorbable conduits has been the focus of several studies. These conduits combine the benefits of ease of repair with bioabsorbability and lack of antigenicity. In our laboratory, we have demonstrated that the placement of a small (1–2 mm) slice of nerve material in the center of a conduit enhances regeneration (Francel et al, in press). Hypothetically, this sandwich of nerve graft materials acts as a source of Schwann cells and trophic factors, enhancing nerve regeneration and acting as a stepping stone between the proximal and distal nerve. Although the use of nerve conduits is still limited to controlled clinical trials, it is likely that this technique will soon be a standard tool for the reconstruction of short peripheral nerve gaps.

NERVE TRANSFERS

Tendon transfers are a standard method for reconstruction of neurological deficits. Similarly, direct nerve-to-nerve transfers (neurotization) can be very useful in providing functional recovery. With very proximal nerve injuries, the addition of a distal nerve transfer to compliment the more proximal reconstruction can be useful for the patient. For example, in a high upper brachial plexus injury, transfer of functioning, noncritical digital nerves to the digital nerves supplying the first web space provides rapid reinnervation in this critical area (Fig. 35–16). Similarly for high lower plexus or ulnar nerve injuries, the functioning median nerve–innervated third web space nerves can be transferred over to the sensory component of the ulnar nerve (Fig. 35–17). The author has also used transfers of the dorsal cutaneous branch of the ulnar nerve and the radial sensory nerve for recovery of more critical palmar sensation.

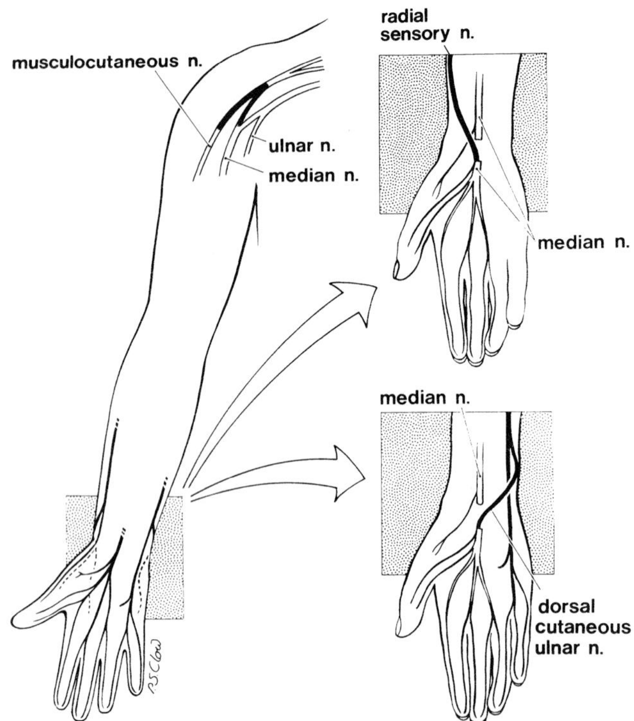

FIGURE 35–16. In the situation of a very high nerve injury, the proximal nerve will be reconstructed using standard autograft technique. Consideration may be given to distal neurotization procedures. In the situation diagrammed, the lateral cord has been injured, and nerve grafts are carried out proximally to reconstruct this injury. The lateral cord contributes the sensory component to the median nerve. Although sensory recovery can be expected across this proximal nerve graft, it will take 2 to 3 years for this to occur. Consideration can be given to distal neurotization procedures such as transfers of the dorsal cutaneous branch of the ulnar nerve or the radial sensory nerve to the radial side of the median nerve to provide protective sensibility to the median nerve distribution (note that the medial cord provides intrinsic median nerve muscle function, and this is maintained in this neurotization procedure by preserving the motor fascicles to the intrinsic median muscles). (From Mackinnon SE: Surgical management of the peripheral nerve gap. Clin Plast Surg *16*:587–603, 1989.)

Additional nerve transfers can be used in high ulnar nerve injuries. In several patients, the author has repaired the terminal branch of the anterior interosseus nerve, innervating the pronator quadratus muscle to the deep motor branch of the ulnar nerve. Neurolysis of the motor branch of the ulnar nerve from the main ulnar nerve facilitates a direct repair in the distal forearm between it and the anterior interosseus nerve.

It is in reconstruction of brachial plexus injuries that nerve transfer has the greatest role to play. For example, the author has successfully reinnervated the musculocutaneous nerve with medial pectoral, thoracodorsal, and long thoracic nerve transfers (see Fig. 35–9). The latter two transfers require a degree of motor re-education. Consideration of nerve transfers within the brachial plexus can obviate the need for long nerve grafts by using a proximal source of nearby motor nerve fibers. The variability and creativity seen with tendon transfer reconstruction can now be used in a similar fashion with nerve transfers.

Injury to the long thoracic nerve results in significant morbidity. In several patients, the author has transferred a branch of the thoracodorsal nerve to the distal portion of the long thoracic nerve in order to reinnervate the serratus anterior muscle and stabilize scapular movement (Fig. 35–18).

NEUROMA IN CONTINUITY

Management of the neuroma in continuity is a particularly challenging problem that requires an understanding of the degrees of nerve injury and their associated clinical and electrophysiological findings. In essence, the surgeon wishes to manage conservatively first-, second-, and third-degree injuries that show varying degrees of spontaneous recovery. By contrast, he or she will want to reconstruct the fourth- or fifth-degree component of the injury. The clinical examination and electrodiagnostic studies are critical in determining which component of the nerve is likely to recover and which component will require surgical intervention.

Detailed motor and sensory examination in all components of the injured nerve is necessary and has been discussed in previous chapters. Briefly, a Sunderland I–degree injury (neurapraxia) would be expected to show the most rapid recovery, and because there is no loss of axonal continuity, distal muscles do not show evidence of denervation, and Tinel's sign is not present because there are no regenerating nerve axons. A Sunderland II–degree (axonotmesis) would be expected to demonstrate the signs of axonal transection with an advancing Tinel's sign and muscle fibrillation. However, inasmuch as the endoneurial tubes are intact, the regeneration should be appropriate. A Sunderland III–degree injury has a potential for motor and sensory cross reinnervation because of disruption of the endoneurial tubes. This degree of injury displays the most variable extent of recovery, depending on the amount of scarring within the endoneurium. Electrodiagnostic studies demonstrate the presence of nascent units or motor unit potentials (MUPs) in Sunderland II– and Sunderland III–degree injuries. Sunderland IV– and Sunderland V–degree injuries are functionally equivalent, although the Sunderland IV–degree injury is physically in continuity. Neither injuries have potential for recovery. Surgical exploration of the neuroma in continuity is the

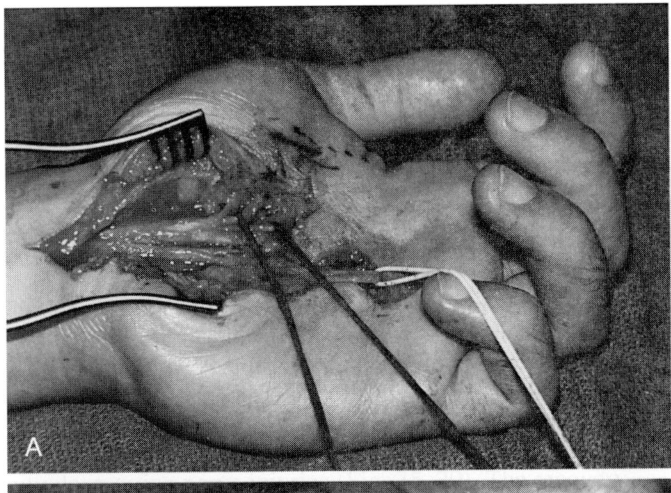

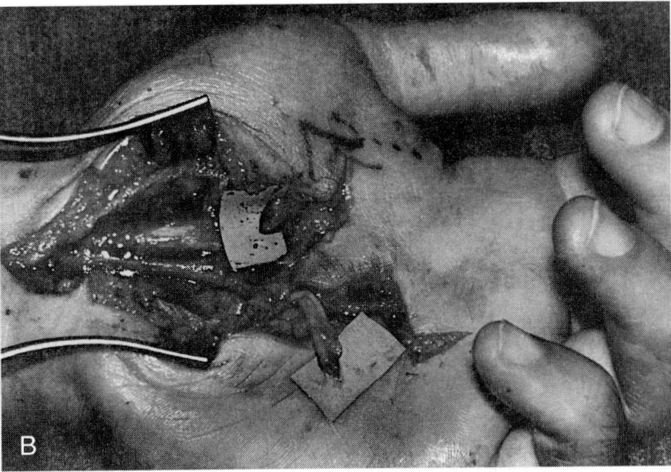

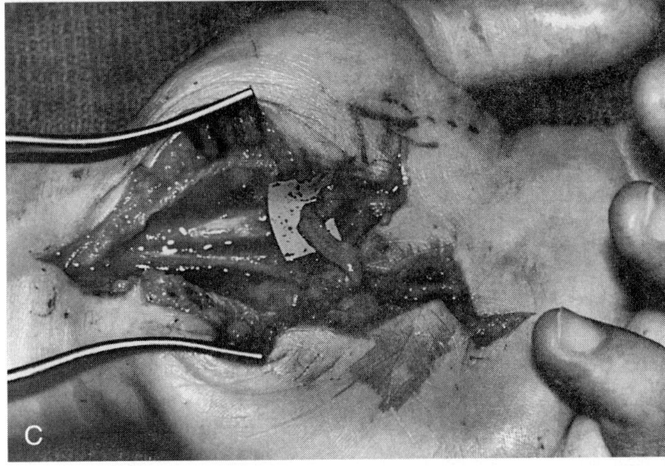

FIGURE 35–17. *A,* In a patient with a high upper plexus injury, sensation in the third web space was normal, but there was no sensibility in the first web space. The common digital nerve to the third web space is seen with a white vessel loop around it. The darker vessel loops are around the ulnar digital nerve to the thumb and the radial digital nerve to the index finger. *B,* These nerves are divided. *C,* A direct repair between the fascicles to the third web space is performed to the ulnar digital nerve to the thumb and the radial digital nerve to the index finger.

same as for a completely transected nerve, but because intraoperative nerve stimulation is frequently necessary, care must be taken to keep the ischemia time to a minimum (30 minutes or less).

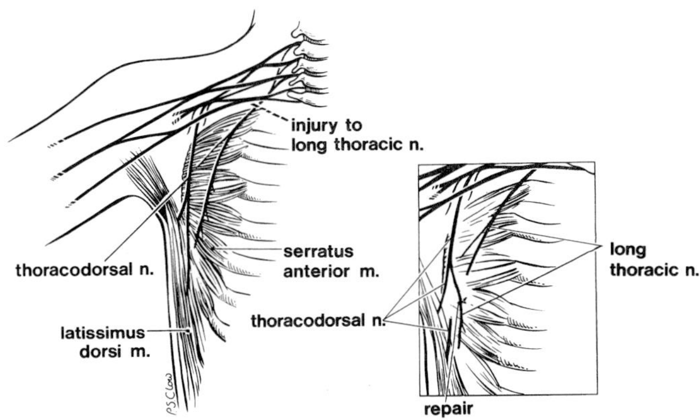

FIGURE 35–18. A rare instance is an isolated proximal lesion of the long thoracic nerve. Such a proximal injury in the long thoracic nerve would virtually preclude the possibility of recovery of serratus anterior muscle function. Consideration can be given to transferring the posterior or medial branch of the thoracodorsal nerve to the distal long thoracic nerve to provide rapid reinnervation of the serratus anterior muscle. Note the arrow marks through repair site between the thoracodorsal nerve and the long thoracic nerve. Note the proximal site of injury to the long thoracic nerve. (From Mackinnon SF: Surgical management of the peripheral nerve gap. Clin Plast Surg *16*:587–603, 1989.)

We have developed a surgical technique for the management of neuroma in continuity in which motor function is preserved and sensory function is reconstructed with nerve grafting (Mackinnon et al, 1992). A tedious and potentially damaging dissection within the neuroma in continuity can be avoided if the functioning motor fascicles are identified proximal and distal to the injury site with electrical stimulation, eliciting muscle contraction. These motor fascicles can then be preserved using a neurolysis technique, and the electrically silent and nonfunctioning sensory fascicles are divided proximal and distal to the neuroma and are reconstructed with nerve grafts. These nerve grafts essentially bypass the functioning motor component of the neuroma in continuity (Fig. 35–19). In the reverse situation, when the sensory fascicles are to be protected but motor fascicles are to be reconstructed, the surgeon may elect to proceed with tendon transfers. However, if the motor component is believed to be best reconstructed with the nerve grafting technique, then direct nerve-to-nerve stimulation is necessary through the neuroma in continuity in order to preserve the functioning sensory component and reconstruct the nonfunctioning or silent motor component.

A similar technique for primary nerve grafting for reconstruction of a nerve tumor extirpation, which necessitates resection of a critical nerve, can be used (Lee et al, 1993). Before removing the tumor, the various fascicular groups of the nerve proximal and distal to the tumor are stimulated so

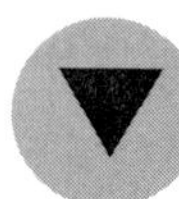

Chapter 36

• George E. Omer, Jr
• Judith Bell-Krotoski

The Evaluation of Clinical Results Following Peripheral Nerve Suture

Surgery to repair a peripheral nerve is successful only when there is subsequent pain-free useful function of the involved extremity. A major problem in the evaluation of nerve repair is the definition of a good clinical result. There are no worldwide accepted criteria for evaluation of a functional recovery after nerve suture. A minimal evaluation of functional recovery should include (1) motor strength and range of motion, (2) sensibility level and associated pain interference, and (3) biomechanical balance and coordination of the extremity.

MOTOR STRENGTH

Grading Systems

The British Medical Research Council introduced a system of grading in 1954 (Seddon, 1954) that attempted to assess the recovery of an entire peripheral nerve in relation to total extremity function. It is most useful in proximal (high) nerve lesions (Seddon, 1975) (Table 36–1). The peripheral nerve research study group of the United States Veterans Administration modified this scale into seven levels (Woodhall and Beebe, 1956) (Table 36–2).

Both the British and American reports attempted to evaluate and grade huge numbers of war injuries to determine management policy for treatment. They are confusing because they have different levels for grading. These grading levels have become entrenched in clinical practice but have come into question in recent years owing to lack of useful functional basis, inadequate picture of ultimate outcome, and lack of any attempt to ascertain if the code did in fact equate with the restoration of useful function (lecture by Sunderland [Kline and Hudson, 1993] [read after Sunderland's death by E. Almquist and G. Omer]).

Voluntary Muscle Testing

Techniques to examine muscle strength are based on the use of gravity and resistance. Robert W. Lovett, Professor of Orthopaedic Surgery at the Harvard Medical School, devised tests for function against gravity in 1912; and in collaboration with E.G. Martin, added a spring balance test for resistance in 1916 (Daniels et al, 1946). In Lovett's text on the treatment of infantile paralysis, published in 1917, he listed the combined gravity and resistance tests for good and normal ratings. In 1932, Arthur T. Legg and Janet B. Merrill listed further development of the tests given in Lovett's

book, including tests for a greater number of muscles and adding poor and fair ratings. A percentage system for recording the results of manual muscle grading was devised in 1936 by Henry O. Kendall and Florence P. Kendall, who were physical therapists at the Children's Hospital School in Baltimore. The common manual tests for muscle power in use today are based on the Lovett method (Table 36–3).

The manual grading of muscle strength demands precise anatomical knowledge and is based on the examiner's ability to grade both muscle power by palpation of the involved muscle-tendon unit and resisting movement of a bone-joint lever arm motored by the involved muscle (Omer, 1981a, 1981b, 1983, 1984). The relaxed muscle should be palpated for fibrosis or painful areas that could limit excursion. Trick movements must be detected (Omer, 1971). If there is questionable motor activity, a local anesthetic is indicated to block competing innervation, but this is used with the understanding that there are anastomotic variations among peripheral nerve branches. Pain always has an adverse effect on muscle testing, and use of a local anesthetic to block a pain point may assist the examiner in evaluating function. The test is voluntary and should be explained to the patient; it should be discontinued if the patient becomes tired or lacks concentration (Omer, 1971).

Voluntary muscle strength testing remains somewhat subjective until a precise way of measuring muscle contraction is generally available. The 5-to-0 grading system has become standard and is surprisingly repeatable among experienced examiners. When data reviewed from this grading are further reduced to normal, weak, and absent, they are even more repeatable and have higher confidence because some of the more subtle differences in the grades are eliminated. Electromyographic studies can help confirm motor

British Medical Research Council Grading System

Grade	Description
M5	Complete recovery
M4	All synergetic and independent movements are possible
M3	All important muscles act against resistance
M2	Return of perceptible contractions in both proximal and distal muscles
M1	Return of perceptible contractions in proximal muscles
M0	No contraction

From Seddon HJ: Surgical Disorders of the Peripheral Nerves, 2nd ed. Edinburgh, Churchill Livingstone, 1975.

▼ **TABLE 36–2**
United States Veterans Administration Grading System

Grade	Description
M6	Complete recovery
M5	Some synergetic and isolated movements possible
M4	All important muscles have sufficient power to act against resistance
M3	Proximal muscles act against gravity; perceptible contraction in intrinsic muscles
M2	Proximal muscles act against gravity; no return of power in intrinsic muscles
M1	Return of perceptible contraction in the proximal muscles
M0	No contraction

From Woodhall B, Beebe GW (eds): Peripheral Nerve Regeneration: A Follow-Up Study of 3,656 World War II Injuries. Veterans Administration Medical Monograph. Washington, D.C., U.S. Government Printing Office, 1956, pp 116, 257.

▼ **TABLE 36–3**
The Lovett Method

Percent of Function	Level			Description
	Numerical	Symbol	Evaluation	
100	5	N	Normal	Complete range of motion against gravity with full resistance
75	4	G	Good	Complete range of motion against gravity with some resistance
50	3	F	Fair	Complete range of motion against gravity
25	2	P	Poor	Complete range of motion with gravity eliminated
10	1	T	Trace	Evidence of slight contractility; no joint motion
0	0	0	Zero	No evidence of contractility

function of specific muscles or groups of muscles, particularly if these muscles are being considered for surgical transfers.

Omer (1981a, 1981b, 1983; Omer and Spinner, 1984) additionally quantitates the active range of motion with a goniometer across an appropriate joint and documents strength with resistance-measuring instruments such as a grip meter or pinch meter. The Jamar dynamometer is the preferred instrument for grip strength (Macey and Burke, 1995). A double-exposure photograph or serial photographs of specific repeatable positions often demonstrate the absence of function (Fig. 36–1A, and B). Amplitude and strength are not the only factors in muscle motor function. Other factors that should be considered and recorded are speed of endurance, speed of motion, and independence of action of individual muscles, especially those with associated function, such as the flexor digitorum superficialis and flexor digitorum profundus. Brand and Hollister (1993) use a metronome and document the number of times a patient can extend or contract a muscle or group of muscles against a known weight (e.g., 5 lbs).

SENSIBILITY LEVEL

Sensibility is the capacity for precise interpretation of sensation. For example, two-point discrimination is a judgment, not a primary sensation (Wynn-Parry, 1973). Normal cutaneous sensation provides normal quality sensibility that has been termed tactile gnosis by Moberg (1962). At present, all tests used to examine the degree of functional loss of sensibility are related to cutaneous touch-pressure sensation (Omer and Spinner, 1975).

Grading Systems

Sensibility testing often depends on the age and subjective response of the patient (March, 1990). The test is most objective if the instrument used for testing is itself repeatable and consistent. Objective findings of some tests may indicate paresthesia rather than useful function. W. B. Highet described an assessment of sensory recovery in 1954 (Wynn-Parry, 1973) (Table 36–4).

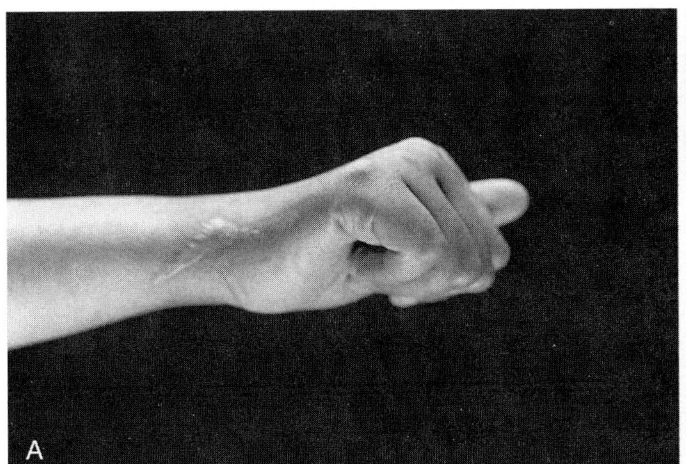

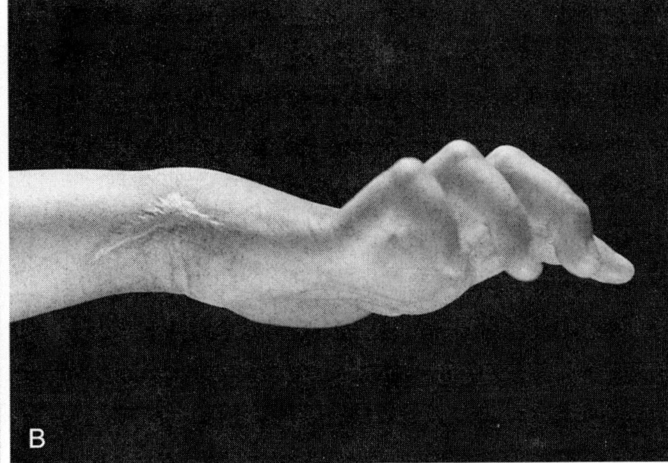

FIGURE 36–1. A double-exposure photograph or serial photographs of specific repeatable positions often demonstrate the absence of muscle function. *A,* A hand with ulnar nerve paralysis can assume a relatively normal fist. *B,* The same hand can be seen to be intrinsic minus on extension of the fingers.

▼ TABLE 36–4
Highet Scale of Sensory Recovery

Grade	Description
S5	Recovery of two-point discrimination within the autonomic zone
S4	Superficial pain and tactile sense in the autonomic zone, with disappearance of overresponse
S3	Superficial pain and tactile sense in the autonomic zone
S2	Deep cutaneous pain in the autonomic zone
S1	No sensation

From Wynn Perry CB: Rehabilitation of the Hand, 3rd ed. London, Butterworths, 1973.

The British Medical Research Council has six levels (Seddon, 1975) (Table 36–5).

Techniques for evaluating sensibility during World War II included pinprick, von Frey hairs, the Weber two-point discrimination test, and cotton wool for localization. However, most tests, other than pinprick and cotton wool localization, were not performed routinely, and the precise distance for some two-point discrimination was not defined.

A more precise rating of sensibility was presented by Moberg (1962) for the autonomous areas of the median and ulnar nerves (Table 36–6).

Moberg (1978) believed that a two-point discrimination distance greater than 12 mm provides only decreased functional sensibility because the patient must use visual control for hand activities.

The Semmes-Weinstein monofilament touch threshold test (modern version of the von Frey hairs) quantifies sensibility into levels (Table 36–7).

With the advent of computerized testing, vibration testing has been used more frequently. Vibration testing has yet to be associated with specific functional levels of sensibility.

These several tests address various aspects of sensibility and together provide a clearer picture of returning function than any one isolated test. They need extensive clinical comparison studies before one technique can be determined to be of greater value than another in measuring peripheral nerve recovery. At present, the two-point discrimination distance test is the most frequently used, followed by monofilament pressure threshold.

▼ TABLE 36–5
British Medical Research Council System of Assessment of Sensory Recovery

Grade	Description
S4	Complete recovery
S3+	Some recovery of two-point discrimination within the autonomous area
S3	Return of superficial cutaneous pain and tactile sensibility throughout the autonomous area with disappearance of any previous overreaction
S2	Return of some degree of superficial cutaneous pain and tactile sensibility within the autonomous area of the nerve
S1	Recovery of deep cutaneous pain sensibility within the autonomous area of the nerve
S0	Absence of sensibility in the autonomous area

From Seddon HJ: Surgical Disorders of the Peripheral Nerves, 2nd ed. Edinburgh, Churchill Livingstone, 1975.

▼ TABLE 36–6
Moberg's Rating Scale of Sensibility—Median and Ulnar Sensibility Two-Point Discrimination Distance

Grade	Distance
Good	< 12 mm
Fair	12–15 mm
Poor	15–20 mm
Bad	> 20 mm

From Moberg E: Criticism and study of methods for examining sensibility in the hand. Neurology 12:8–19, 1962.

The techniques for sensibility testing are discussed in Chapter 3.

PAIN

Because the neurophysiological aspects of pain cannot be divorced from the psychological, it is important that the patient realize that paresthesias and electrical sensations are normal in the course of recovery from injury. Unsuspected pain and unfamiliar sensations are alarming and usually associated with the protective mechanisms of the body. Patients who understand these unwanted signals tend to normalize over time with maturation of the nerve repair, and patients who view these signals as signs of recovery rather than as unwanted and potentially life-long changes are less likely to be concerned. Patients who are alerted to these complications before surgery seem more able to accept them as a necessary occurrence than patients who have not been informed.

Lesions that trigger pain, such as neuromas, are different problems. If these lesions can be protected or shielded during the course of recovery, then the extremity that may not otherwise be used is sometimes used to an extent sufficient to encourage discrimination of returning sensibility (Fig. 36–2).

Pain can complicate measurement of motor function as well as sensibility. Pain will limit the exploratory feedback system during use and can greatly restrict the discrimination of sensory input, particularly when referred touch is present secondary to neural fascicles growing into other fascicles during recovery. Guides to the Evaluation of Permanent Impairment (Omer, 1992; Dodge, 1993), published by the American Medical Association, lists the intensity of pain. Major points include

Minimal: The pain is annoying, but it has not resulted in diminution in an individual's capacity to carry out daily

▼ TABLE 36–7
The Semmes-Weinstein Touch and Pressure Threshold Test

Grade	Sensibility Level
1.65–2.83	Normal light touch
3.22–3.61	Diminished light touch
4.31–4.56	Diminished protective sensation
4.56–6.65	Loss of protective sensation
> 6.65	Untestable

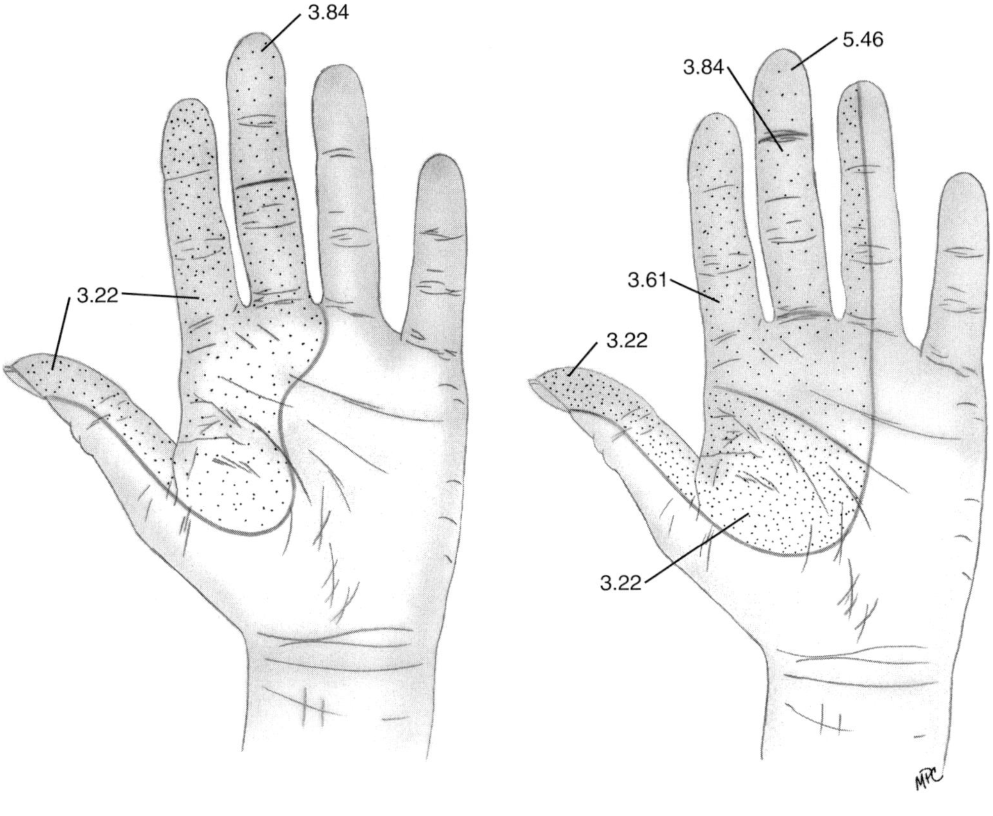

FIGURE 36–2. A woman who injured her left wrist with glass has previously had the median nerve explored and a compartment released in the forearm. She complains of a neuroma at the level of the wrist and difficulty in typing, although there is moderately functioning median nerve thenar musculature. *A,* A monofilament mapping of the median nerve shows a defined area of median nerve diminution with close to normal innervation except for the distal portion of the long finger. *B,* Shows a decrease in median nerve response following injection of lidocaine (Xylocaine) around the neuroma. Opponens function was lost as well. A decision was made against excision of the neuroma because of the potential for increased sensory loss and resultant impact on employment.

activities. The pain does not interfere with sleep, and it requires occasional use of non-narcotic medication.

Slight: The pain is tolerated but has been documented to cause diminution in an individual's capacity to carry out some specified daily activities. The pain may interfere with sleep. Non-narcotic medication may be consumed regularly, and occasional administration of narcotic medication may be required.

Moderate: The pain has been documented medically to result in extensive diminution in an individual's capacity to carry out specific activities of daily living. The pain interferes with sleep. It frequently requires use of narcotic medication, or it may require invasive procedures. Recreation and socialization are severely limited.

Marked: The pain precludes carrying out most activities of daily living. Sleep is disrupted. Recreation and socialization are impossible. Narcotic medication or invasive procedures are required and may not result in complete pain control.

A simple classification has been made according to how the pain interferes with the activities of daily living (Swanson et al, 1984) (Table 36–8).

EXTREMITY COORDINATION

Biomechanical Balance

Retention of some muscles in the absence of others causes mechanical imbalances within the extremity during activity. These mechanical imbalances go beyond incoordination. They affect the grasp and release patterns that are important in stabilizing the skeletal structures during function. This is most dramatic in peripheral nerve injuries with retention of extrinsic muscles and loss of intrinsic muscles. The extrinsic flexors must fully flex the digits before an object can be grasped, and the selective positioning of the digits with objects is lost, resulting in incoordination (Fig. 36–3).

Evaluation of the muscle strength alone can be misleading regarding coordination and balance for function. Other factors that should be considered are the speed of motion, endurance, and the independence of action of individual muscles (Omer and Spinner, 1975, 1984). Because the extremity is often loaded distally with objects held in a variety of positions, it also needs to be tested in various positions to evaluate function. A hand with intrinsic weakness or paralysis can sometimes look normal at the beginning of an evaluation, but after time, the digits can be shown to collapse structurally when they pick up a weighted object (Fig. 36–4).

▼ **TABLE 36–8**
Pain Severity Scale

Percent of Interference with Activity	Grade	Description
100	P4	Severe enough to prevent all activity and causes distress
75	P3	Prevents some activity
50	P2	Interferes with activity
25	P1	Annoying

From Swanson AB, Goran-Hagert C, Swanson G deG: Evaluation of impairment of hand function. *In* Hunter IM, et al (eds): Rehabilitation of the Hand. St Louis, CV Mosby Company, 1978.

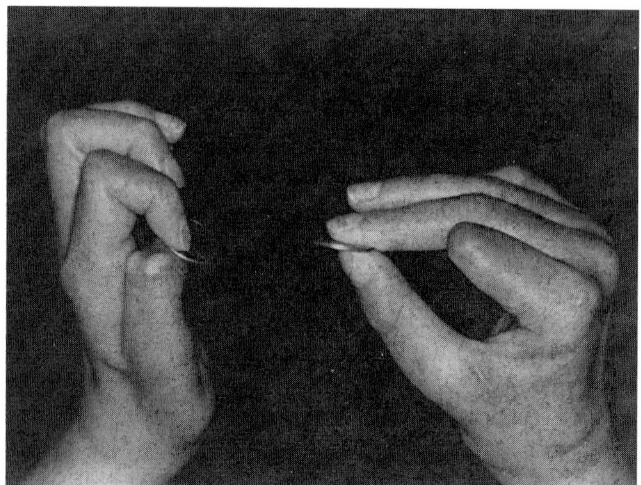

FIGURE 36–3. Positioning of digits in hands with bilateral ulnar and median nerve paralysis. The hand on the right has had intrinsic replacement procedures, and shows improved control and positioning of the digits with objects despite amputation of the distal index. The amputation was secondary to injury from insensitivity and previous biomechanical imbalance causing concentration of high stress at fingertips.

Following peripheral nerve repair the intrinsic muscles of the hand or foot are the least likely to return. The abnormal motor function that usually accompanies nerve palsy enhances the distorted sensibility patterns and contributes to dysesthesia. Motor reconstruction should be done before sensory reconstruction, because precise sensibility depends as much on muscle control as on sensory end-organs.

The amount of resistance a joint can sustain before collapse and the amount of joint stiffness a muscle or muscle group has to overcome to produce motion can now be measured on a commercial strain gauge (Brand and Hollister, 1993). Many possibilities exist for demonstrating hand, finger, and joint imbalance with common objects. These observational tests should be simple, consistent, and graded in progression. Graded weights are helpful in ascertaining the amount of pinch or grasp that can be sustained before col-

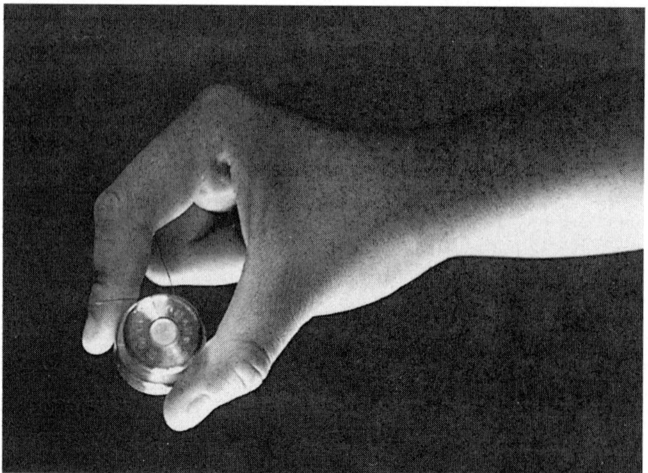

FIGURE 36–4. A hand with weakness or paralysis can sometimes look normal at the beginning of evaluation. Hands are required on use to function against weighted objects, and muscle imbalances are manifested as the hands are used. Progressive increases in weight demonstrate at what point there is structural collapse of the fingers and joints, and substitution from positioning and use of other muscles.

lapse of joints. Clear plastic cylinders can be used to demonstrate contact areas of the hand and fingers on grasp and pinch (Brand and Hollister, 1993).

Coordination

Coordination is the end product of the highly specialized motor and sensory systems, and evaluation of coordination should include both activities.

The picking-up test was introduced by Erik Moberg in 1958. The patient "should pick up a number of small objects on a table and put them as quickly as he can into a small box. After he has done this a few times, he is asked to do the same thing blindfolded. The test with blindfolding can be made more difficult by asking the patient to identify the objects as he picks them up" (Moberg, 1958, p 454). Omer (1968, 1980) quantitated the picking-up test by measuring the time required to pick up nine objects of different size and shape. The objects may include such items as a key, marble, nut, bolt, paper clip, coin, short pencil, or safety pin (Figs. 36–5 and 36–6). On occasion, a piece of chalk is used to demonstrate the functional surfaces of the hand (Omer, 1971, 1980, 1984). Normal time for completion of the test with nine objects is considered to be less than 10 seconds, but the results from a sequence of tests are more important than an individual test and indicate the changing status of coordination. Seddon (1975) states that the precursor of the picking-up test was the coin test. In the coin test, the patient, whose eyes must be closed, is given a coin and asked to identify it.

Greenseid and McCormack (1968) designed 12 functional tests requiring the use of pinch, grip, range of grasp, and finger manipulation. Tests are timed with a stopwatch, and the scored result is the fastest time of three performances on each test.

Tactile gnosis can be tested by writing numbers on the patient's digit (Bowden and Napier, 1961) or using Porter's letter test (Porter, 1966) in which the patient palpates type set in a block. A current term would be graphesthesia sensibility.

Standardized tests of hand coordination are now available. For medium-sized objects, the Minnesota Rate of Manipulation Test is useful. For objects of various sizes, the Jebsen Hand Function Test is useful. For fine dexterity, the Crawford Small Parts test can be used. For index finger-thumb manipulation in median or radial nerve injuries, the Purdue Pegboard test is useful (Fess, 1986, 1989). These tests meet criteria for instrument validity and reliability, as well as clinical validity. Other tests, such as an observational test, provide significant information when they are used properly.

Coordination tests are not static but will change with the level of homeostasis of the extremity or through experience with the test used for the evaluation. Re-education programs following nerve suture include repeated stimulation and motor-sensory activity to improve coordination through experience. Tests used for retraining should not also be used for evaluation.

CLINICAL CONSIDERATIONS

The length of time required to attain maximum clinical recovery depends on the level and severity of the nerve

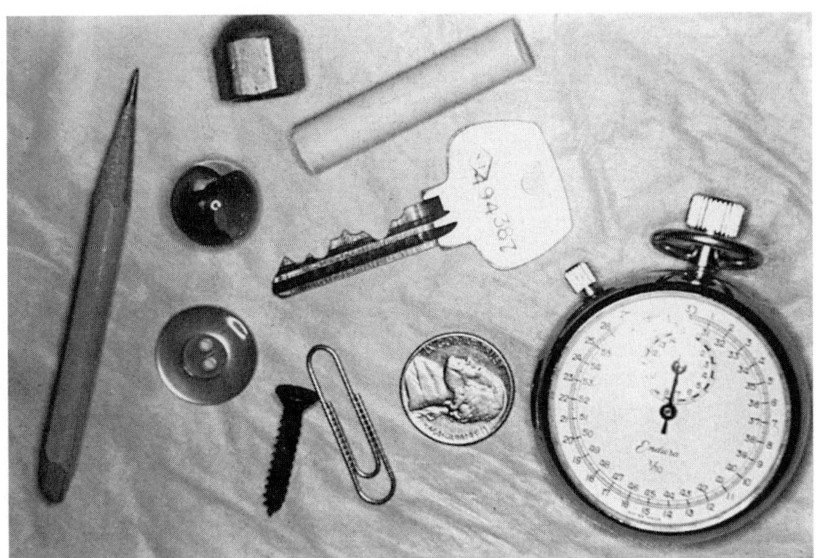

FIGURE 36–5. Items in a picking-up test for median and ulnar nerves. (From Omer GE Jr: Methods of assessment of injury and recovery of peripheral nerves. Surg Clin North Am *61*:316, 1981.)

lesion. Sunderland (1991) noted that improvement after nerve suture continues slowly and irregularly over several years but for exactly how long is not known. Zachary (Seddon, 1954) extended the period to 5 years in the casualties of World War II, and Stromberg and colleagues (1961) also concluded that maximum recovery requires 5 years in adults and 2 years in children. Sunderland (1991) states that the

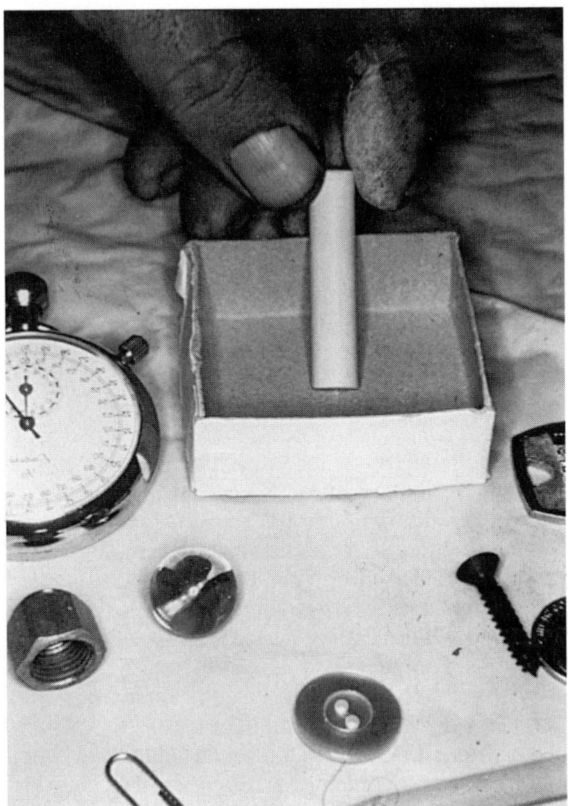

FIGURE 36–6. A piece of chalk, as one of the objects in the picking-up test, will demonstrate functional surfaces of digits. (From Omer GE Jr: Methods of assessment of injury and recovery of peripheral nerve injuries. Surg Clin North Am *61*:317, 1981; and Omer GE Jr: Physical diagnosis of peripheral nerve injuries. Orthop Clin North Am *12*:225, 1981.)

progress of recovery should be followed by regular clinical examinations that should be continued for 5 years; the timing of the examinations should be monthly in the first year, quarterly in the second year, and then biannually.

Sensory function usually returns before motor function. The earliest sign of recovery following nerve suture is paresthesia distal to the nerve suture when the nerve is percussed lightly. Early return of trace muscle activity usually improves with maturation of the repair. Any partial recovery of muscle function is a reasonable indication that more extensive recovery will follow. In general following injury, the earlier the return of function, the better the eventual result, if time has been allowed for the distance the regenerating nerve has to regrow.

In nerve lesions high above the elbow or knee, nerve repair is performed more to regain sensory function without pain than for motor recovery. Intrinsic muscle reinnervation is not always expected because of the time required for regeneration of the nerve to the periphery. In contrast to sensory end-organs, muscle fibers atrophy and lose most of their potential for reinnervation.

Appropriate range of motion exercises must be performed to ensure that the regenerating nerve is mobile and not adhered in scar tissue. Aggressive exercise and undue traction on the nerve repair should be avoided during the early phase of recovery. Overuse of the extremity with associated edema and pain can compromise the eventual result. Serial evaluations are pertinent to determine and document any change in nerve function (Bell-Krotowski, 1995), particularly in the first year following nerve repair.

One year following nerve repair is an accepted but probably inappropriate time for measurement of the extent of recovery with assessment of the functional level, because continued recovery with functional improvement should be anticipated. Follow-up measurements in subsequent (3 to 5) years provide more complete information (Omer, 1992; Omer and Pirela-Cruz, 1994).

RATING SCALES FOR FUNCTIONAL EVALUATION

Moberg (1978) made the valid point that all nerve sutures must be evaluated by a single meaningful method to permit

▼ **TABLE 36–9**

Comparison of the Moberg Scale and the British Research Council System

Moberg Scale	British Code	Sensory Grades
Good	S4	Complete recovery; Tactile gnosis—two-point discrimination distance of 12 mm or less
Fair		Sensibility of 12 to 15 mm
Poor	S3+	Sensibility for gross grip and slow protection—two-point discrimination distance of 15–20 mm
Bad	S3	Sensibility at 20 mm; reaction too slow for good protection
	S2	Hyperesthesia or paresthesia, producing impairment to gripping function
	S1	Feeling—the total field reacts to cotton wool and pinprick
	S0	Absent

From Moberg E: Sensibility in reconstructive limb surgery. *In* Fredericks S, Brody GS (eds): Symposium on the Neurologic Aspects of Plastic Surgery. St Louis, CV Mosby Company, 1978, pp 30–35.

proper comparison of techniques. Further, Moberg believed that the sensibility system adopted by the British Research Council in 1954 is inadequate. He believed that there should be additional ratings between S3+ and S4, and that all lower ratings are useless to the reconstructive surgeon (Table 36–9). Further, in order to use the British Research Council grading system, one must define proximal and distal muscles

▼ **TABLE 36–10**

Identification of Proximal and Distal Muscles for Each Nerve

Radial Nerve

Proximal Muscles	*Distal Muscles*
Brachioradialis	Abductor pollicis longus
Extensor carpi radialis longus	Extensor pollicis longus
Extensor digitorum communis	Extensor indicis
Extensor carpi ulnaris	

Median Nerve

Proximal Muscles	*Distal Muscles*
Pronator teres	Abductor pollicis brevis
Flexor carpi radialis	
Flexor digitorum superficialis	
Flexor pollicis longus	

Ulnar Nerve

Proximal Muscles	*Distal Muscles*
Flexor carpi ulnaris	Abductor digiti quinti
Flexor digitorum profundus (ring and little)	Interossei

Common Peroneal Nerve

Proximal Muscles	*Distal Muscles*
Tibialis anterior	Extensor digitorum brevis
Extensor digitorum longus	
Extensor hallucis longus	
Peronei	

Tibial Nerve

Proximal Muscles	*Distal Muscles*
Gastrocnemius and soleus	Intrinsic muscles of sole
Tibialis posterior	Abductor hallucis
Flexor digitorum longus	
Flexor hallucis longus	

▼ **TABLE 36–11**

Grading System for Each Nerve

Median Nerve (S scale according to Moberg; M scale according to Seddon)

Good	S4 or S3+	:M3
Fair	S3	:M2
Bad	S1 or S2	:M1 or M0

Ulnar Nerve (S scale according to Moberg; M scale according to Seddon)

Good	S3	:M4
Fair	S2	:M3
Bad	S1 or S0	:M2 or M1

Radial Nerve (M scale according to Seddon)

Good		:M4
Fair		:M3
Bad		:M2 or M1

Digital Nerve (S scale according to Moberg)

Good	S4 or S3+
Fair	S3
Bad	S2 or S1

Common Peroneal Nerve (M scale according to Seddon)

Good	:M4
Fair	:M3
Bad	:M2 or M1

Tibial Nerve (S and M scales according to Seddon)

Good	S4 or S3+	:M3
Fair	S3	:M2
Bad	S2 or S1	:M1 or M0

for each nerve (Table 36–10). The grading system must be able to combine motor and sensory findings to demonstrate a good clinical recovery (Table 36–11).

If possible, clinical results should be assessed by clinicians who did not participate in the surgical procedure. Clinical studies should be performed before the nerve is sutured, as well as postoperatively.

CORRELATION OF RATING SCALES WITH CLINICAL OUTCOME

Before routine magnification became widely used, the largest clinical series subjected to motor and sensory evaluation for functional recovery were the military injuries in World War II (Seddon, 1954; Woodhall and Beebe, 1956). This study was the stimulus for the M0 to M5 grading for motor recovery and S0 to S5 for sensory recovery. Reported results indicated that the potential for a good clinical result 5 years after secondary suture in a severe injury is as shown in Table 36–12 (Woodhall and Beebe, 1956).

No great accuracy can be claimed for these measurements because they relate to functions with fluctuating fortunes (Sunderland, 1995). For example, measuring reinnervated muscles acting solely as prime movers neglects the muscle's important role as an antagonist, synergist, and fixator in the execution of a wide range of movements. A residual paresis not only impairs a muscle's function as a prime mover but destabilizes the actions of other normally innervated muscles (Sunderland, 1995). The M0-M5:S0-S4 coding system has never been subjected to a critical examination to ascertain if

▼ **TABLE 36–12**
Results of Motor and Sensory Evaluation for Functional Recovery

Nerve	British Code (Good Result)	Total Nerves		Percent Good	
		U.S.	British	U.S.	British
Median	M3 to M5	233	290	51.1	32.7
	S3+ to S4	244	278	17.6	8.6
Ulnar	M4 to M5	433	384	12.9	4.9
	S3 to S4	441	390	31.4	30.8
Radial	M4 to M5	197	114	21.3	36.9
Tibial	M3 to M5	91	—	24.5	—
	S3 to S4	97	118	2.0	0.0
Common peroneal	M4 to M5	138	—	7.2	—

From Woodhall B, Beebe GW (eds): Peripheral Nerve Regeneration: A Follow-Up Study of 3,656 World War II Injuries. Veterans Administration Medical Monograph. Washington, D.C., U.S. Government Printing Office, 1956, pp 116, 257.

▼ **TABLE 36–14**
Brown's Results with Secondary Sutures

Nerve	Number Repaired	No Return (Percent)	Some Return (Percent)
Ulnar	68	44 (65)	24 (35)
Median	38	19 (50)	19 (50)
Radial	5	3 (60)	2 (40)
Digital	24	10 (40)	14 (60)
Totals	135	76 (56)	59 (44)

From Brown PW: The time factor in surgery of upper extremity peripheral nerve injury. Clin Orthop *68*:14–21, 1970. Copyright © 1970, John Wiley & Sons. Reprinted by John Wiley & Sons, Inc.

the code actually did equate with the restoration of useful function (Sunderland, 1995).

The British Research Council grading system was not retained for military injuries. Omer (1974) reported the results of 143 epineural sutures of upper extremity nerves during the Vietnam War that were followed for at least 12 months (Table 36–13). This study did not identify specific nerves with their proximal and distal muscles, and used a modification of the sensibility levels in reporting results (Omer, 1974). There were two criteria for clinical return: for the above-elbow lesion, progressive motor return with independent movement and point localization of 3.84 von Frey filament without overresponse (M3-S2); for the below-elbow lesion, progressive motor return with independent movement and two-point discrimination of 20 millimeters (M3-S3). In addition, Omer (1974) noted that none of his patients had recovery of the intrinsic muscles of the hand during the study period.

Brown (1970) recorded the results of 135 epineural sutures followed 6 to 24 months during the Vietnam War. This study did not report the level of nerve lesion, and there was no attempt to use the British Medical Research Council rating scale (Table 36–14).

Brown's (1970) rating scale was "no return" and "some return." This study was continued by Eversmann and con-

▼ **TABLE 36–13**
Neurorrhaphies Performed During the Vietnam War Related to Etiology and Level of Injury

Etiology	Adequate Follow-up	Clinical Return	Percentage
Lacerations			
9 above elbow	8	3	37
90 below elbow	67	30	45
High-Velocity Gunshot Wound			
24 above elbow	21	6	28
24 below elbow	14	6	43
Low-Velocity Gunshot Wound			
19 above elbow	18	9	50
16 below elbow	14	6	43
Fracture-Dislocations			
1 above elbow	1	0	0
1 below elbow	0	0	0

From Omer GE Jr: Injuries to nerves of the upper extremity. J Bone Joint Surg *56A*:1615–1624, 1974.

tained 681 patients, representing studies of 198 ulnar, 151 median, 39 radial, and 93 digital nerves (Omer and Eversmann, 1994). There was no documentation of results according to the British Research Council scales, but it was recorded that "several well-studied cases" had return of intrinsic muscle function of the hand more than 2 years after above-elbow suture of the ulnar nerve. The longest documented length of time to return of function was 8 years after suture.

Many others have modified a portion of the British Medical Research Council rating system. Sunderland (1978) graded sensory function in four grades of response to pinprick, six grades of response to light touch, five grades of response to temperature, and three grades of response to two-point discrimination. Millesi (1985) developed a scoring system based on three examination levels: anatomical, sensibility, and strength. The normal range of motion is scored. Sensibility testing is based on static two-point discrimination, plus a standardized picking-up test in the blindfolded patient. Strength measurements include power grip, pinch pinch, and key pinch. The achieved values may be converted to percent values and compared with 100% of normal hand function (Deutinger et al, 1993).

Kline and Hudson (1995) disagree with the Lovett method of muscle power grading because it was developed to measure patients with anterior poliomyelitis, in whom a trace of either retained function or recovery of function had great predictive importance. They used the Louisiana State University Medical Center (LSUMC) system, which is shown in Table 36–15. Sensory grades "were also changed to accommodate a more practical and readily carried out examination, concentrating on ability to localize various stimuli" (Kline and Hudson, 1995, p 89) (see Table 36–15). There is no precise rating of sensibility as presented by Moberg (1975). For grading whole nerve function, the LSUMC system devised a similar but altered scheme (Table 36–16). This grading system also must identify appropriate proximal and distal muscles for each nerve (Kline and Hudson, 1995).

The systems listed earlier for grading clinical results were published in 1970, 1974, 1978, 1985, and 1995, and illustrate the several modifications of the British 1954 rating scales or the several totally different systems that have been used for documenting outcomes. In general, the restoration of function for daily activities is the objective of nerve repair, yet most current grading systems provide an inadequate prognosis for the ultimate outcome (March, 1990; Sunderland, 1995).

Sensibility evaluation in these grading systems is less reliable than evaluation of motor strength and resistance.

▼ **TABLE 36–15**
The Louisiana State University Medical Center System of Grading

		Individual Muscle
Grade	*Evaluation*	*Description*
0	Absent	No contraction
1	Poor	Trace contraction
2	Fair	Movement against gravity only
3	Moderate	Movement against gravity and some mild resistance
4	Good	Movement against moderate resistance
5	Excellent	Movement against maximal resistance

		Sensory Grades
Grade	*Evaluation*	*Description*
0	Absent	No response to touch, pin, or pressure
1	Bad	Testing gives hyperesthesia or paresthesia; deep pain recovery in autonomous zones
2	Poor	Sensory response sufficient for grip and slow protection; sensory stimuli mislocalized with over-response
3	Moderate	Response to touch and pin in autonomous zones; sensation mislocalized and not normal with some over-response
4	Good	Response to touch and pin in autonomous zones; response localized but sensation not normal; no over-response

From Kline DG, Hudson AR: Nerve Injuries: Operative Results for Major Nerve Injuries, Entrapments, and Tumors. Philadelphia, W.B. Saunders Company, 1995, p 89.

Given the lack of stimulus control in many sensibility instruments and the known variables in measurement, these grading scales are not likely to be as repeatable as needed to properly evaluate improvement and worsening of peripheral nerve status following injury, but they are a start. They should be used within limits. In the end, all sensibility and motor tests need to be validated in measuring clinical morphology by correlation with loss and recovery of patient function.

With the exception of Moberg's sensibility study (1975), most grading systems published since the British Medical Research Council special report in 1954 have not provided additional or standardized evaluation methods for (1) mea-

▼ **TABLE 36–16**
The Louisiana State University Medical Center System for Grading Whole Nerve Injury

Grade	Evaluation	Description
0	Absent	No muscle contraction, absent sensation
1	Poor	Proximal muscles contract but not against gravity; sensory grade 1 or 0
2	Fair	Proximal muscles contract against gravity; distal muscles do not contract; sensory grade if applicable is usually 2 or lower
3	Moderate	Proximal muscles contract against gravity and some resistance; some distal muscles contract against at least gravity; sensory grade is usually 3
4	Good	All proximal and some distal muscles contract against gravity and some resistance; sensory grade is 3 or better
5	Excellent	All muscles contract against moderate resistance; sensory grade is 4 or better

From Kline DG, Hudson AR: Nerve Injuries: Operative Results for Major Nerve Injuries, Entrapments, and Tumors. Philadelphia, W.B. Saunders Company, 1995, p 90.

surement of individual muscle motor strength as a prime mover, antagonist, synergist, or stabilizer; (2) measurement of tactile gnosis sensibility level and associated pain interference; and (3) measurement of sensory mechanisms in motor performance and precise motor coordination in sensory discrimination/sensibility and stereognosis.

The recording of peripheral nerve recovery for now is based on primary elements of motor and sensory recovery. A variety of tests are now available for evaluating motor function and tactile discrimination. These tests need to be explored further regarding their value in recording functional recovery following peripheral nerve suture. Sunderland (1995) underscored the need for a grading scale with defined criteria that can convey a clear picture of the residual function of the extremity, as reflected in performance of a patient's daily activities. This could be used with confidence for comparing one set of results with another, one technique with another, and one management policy with another. A solution demands selection, standardization, and approval by some international body. The first step toward change was made by the Audit Committee of the British Society for Surgery of the Hand, who advanced measures of outcome in terms of movement, power, sensibility, pain, and activities of daily living (Macey and Burke, 1995).

AN IDEAL CLINICAL RESULTS STUDY

No one individual surgeon or specialist has a sufficient number of patients for statistically valid evaluation of all the factors involved in the repair of peripheral nerve injuries. Only the combined results from many surgical centers will provide answers, but to be useful, all must be measured on an identical scale with identical techniques.

An ideal clinical study would have the following features: (1) documentation of motor and sensory impairment, and of associated sudomotor loss, before the surgical procedure; (2) the nerve injury must be at the same level in a similar age group; (3) the nerve must be repaired with identical surgical techniques at approximately the same time after injury; (4) there should be a continuing study of the effect of spontaneous or planned re-education on the functional activities of the involved extremity; (5) there should precise and serial motor and sensibility tests to measure the regeneration of the involved nerve; (6) the "final" clinical evaluation should be delayed until 3 to 5 years after the nerve suture; and (7) all the nerve suture repairs should be performed by one surgeon, and all the clinical evaluations should be performed by another examiner.

References

Bell-Krotoski JA: Sensibility testing: Current concepts. *In* Hunter JM, Mackin EJ, Callahan AD (eds): Rehabilitation of the Hand, 4th ed. St. Louis, C. V. Mosby Company, 1995, pp 109–128.

Bowden REM, Napier JR: The assessment of hand function after peripheral nerve injuries. J Bone Joint Surg *43(B)*:481–492, 1961.

Brand PW, Hollister A: Clinical Mechanics of the Hand, 2nd ed. St. Louis, C. V. Mosby Company, 1993, pp 179–222, 223–253.

Brown PW: The time factor in surgery of upper extremity peripheral nerve injury. Clin Orthop *68*:14–21, 1970.

Daniels L, Williams M, Worthingham C: Muscle Testing: Techniques of Manual Examination. Philadelphia, W. B. Saunders Company, 1946.

Deutinger M, Girsch W, Burggasser G, Windisch A, Joshi D, Mayr N, Freilinger G: Peripheral nerve repair in the hand with and without motor sensory differentiation. J Hand Surg *18A*:426–432, 1993.

Dodge TC (ed): Guides to the Evaluation of Permanent Impairment, 4th ed. Chicago, The American Medical Association, 1993, pp 303–314.

Fess EE: Documentation: Essential elements of an upper extremity assessment battery. *In* Hunter JM, Schneider LH, Mackin EJ, Callahan AD (eds): Rehabilitation of the Hand, 3rd ed. St. Louis, C. V. Mosby Co., 1989, pp 53–81.

Fess EE: The need for reliability and validity in hand assessment instruments. J Hand Surg *11(A)*:621–623, 1986.

Greenseid DZ, McCormack RM: Functional hand testing: A profile evaluation. Plast Reconstr Surg *42*:567, 1968.

Kline DG, Hudson AR: Nerve Injuries: Operative Results for Major Nerve Injuries, Entrapments, and Tumors. Philadelphia, W. B. Saunders Company, 1995.

Macey AC, Burke FD: Outcomes of hand Surgery. J Hand Surg *20B*:841–855, 1995.

March D: The validation of measures of outcome following suture of divided peripheral nerves supplying the hand. J Hand Surg *15B*:25–34, 1990.

Millesi H: Microsurgical restoration of nerves and evaluation of results. *In* Delwaid PJ, Gorio A (eds): Clinical Neurophysiology in Peripheral Neuropathies. Amsterdam, Elsevier Science Publication, 1985, pp 67–90.

Moberg E: Objective methods for determining the functional value of sensibility in the hand. J Bone Joint Surg *40B*:454–476, 1958.

Moberg E: Criticism and study of methods for examining sensibility in the hand. Neurology *12*:8–19, 1962.

Moberg E: Surgical treatment for absent single-hand grip and elbow extension in quadriplegia, principles and preliminary experience. J Bone Joint Surg *57A*:196–206, 1975.

Moberg E: Sensibility in reconstructive limb surgery. *In* Fredricks S, Brody GS (eds): Symposium on the Neurologic Aspects of Plastic Surgery. St. Louis, C. V. Mosby Company, 1978, pp 30–35.

Omer GE, Jr: Evaluation and reconstruction of the forearm and hand after acute traumatic peripheral nerve injuries. J Bone Joint Surg *50A*:1454–1478, 1968.

Omer GE, Jr: Assessment of peripheral nerve injuries. *In* Cramer LM, Chase RA (eds): Symposium on the Hand. Educ Found Am Soc Plast Reconstr Surg, Vol. 3, 1971. St. Louis, C. V. Mosby Company, pp 1–11.

Omer GE, Jr: Injuries to nerves of the upper extremity. J Bone Joint Surg *56A*:1615–1624, 1974.

Omer GE, Jr: Sensory evaluation by the pickup test. *In* Jewett DL, McCarroll HR, Jr (eds): Nerve Repair and Regeneration: Its Clinical and Experimental Basis. St. Louis, C. V. Mosby Company, 1980, pp 250–251.

Omer GE, Jr: Physical diagnosis of peripheral nerve injuries. Orthop Clin North Am *12*:207–228, 1981a.

Omer GE, Jr: Methods of assessment of injury and recovery of peripheral nerves. Surg Clin North Am *61*:303–319, 1981b.

Omer GE, Jr: Report of the committee for evaluation of the clinical result in peripheral nerve injury. J Hand Surg *8*:754–759, 1983.

Omer GE, Jr: Evaluation of the extremity with peripheral nerve injury and timing for nerve suture, Part II. *In* Omer GE, Jr, Spinner M: Management of peripheral nerve problems. Instr Course Lect Am Acad Orthop Surg *33*:461–530, 1984.

Omer GE, Jr: Traumatic peripheral nerve injuries. *In* Benzel EC (ed): Practical Approaches to Peripheral Nerve Surgery. Park Ridge, IL, American Association Neurological Surgeons, 1992, pp 109–117.

Omer GE, Jr, Eversmann WW, Jr: Peripheral nerve problems. *In* Burkhalter WE (ed): Orthopedic Surgery in Vietnam. Washington, D.C., Center of Military History, United States Army, 1994, pp 155–188.

Omer GE, Jr, Pirela-Cruz M: Complications of peripheral nerve injuries. *In* Epps CH, Jr (ed): Complications in Orthopaedic Surgery, 3rd ed. Philadelphia, J. B. Lippincott Company, 1994, pp 811–856.

Omer GE, Jr, Spinner M: Peripheral nerve testing and suture techniques. Instr Course Lect Am Acad Orthop Surg *24*:122–143, 1975.

Omer GE, Jr, Spinner M: Management of peripheral nerve problems. Instr Course Lect Am Acad Orthop Surg *33*:461–530, 1984.

Porter RW: New test for fingertip sensation. Br Med J *2*:927, 1966.

Seddon HJ (ed): Peripheral Nerve Injuries. Medical Research Council Special Report Series, No. 282. London, Her Majesty's Stationery Office, 1954.

Seddon HJ: Surgical Disorders of the Peripheral Nerves, 2nd ed. Edinburgh, Churchill Livingstone, 1975.

Stromberg WB, Jr, McFarlane RM, Bell JL, Koch SL, Mason ML: Injury of the median and ulnar nerves. J Bone Joint Surg *43A*:717–730, 1961.

Sunderland S: Nerves and Nerve Injuries. 2nd ed. Edinburgh, Churchill Livingstone, 1978, pp 329–339.

Sunderland S: Nerve Injuries and Their Repair. Edinburgh, Churchill Livingstone, 1991, pp 413–430.

Sunderland S: Thirteen years down the track. *In* Kline DG, Hudson AR (eds): Nerve Injuries: Operative Results for Major Nerve Injuries, Entrapments, and Tumors. Philadelphia, W. B. Saunders Company, 1995, pp 593–596.

Swanson AB, Goran-Hagert C, Swanson G deG: Evaluation of impairment of hand function. *In* Hunter JM et al (eds): Rehabilitation of the Hand, 2nd ed. St. Louis, C. V. Mosby Company, 1984, pp 101–132.

Woodhall B, Beebe GW (eds): Peripheral nerve regeneration: A follow-up study of 3,656 World War II injuries. Veterans Administration Medical Monograph. Washington DC, U.S. Government Printing Office, 1956, pp 116, 257.

Wynn-Parry CB: Rehabilitation of the Hand, 3rd ed. London, Butterworths, 1973.

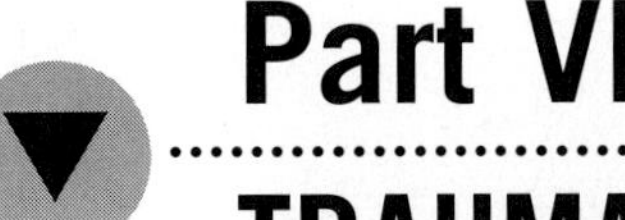

Part VI

TRAUMA: MISSILES, LACERATIONS, TRACTION, AND INJECTIONS

Chapter 37

• Göran Lundborg

• Lars Dahlin

Pathophysiology of Peripheral Nerve Trauma

The peripheral nerve trunk is a well-vascularized and anatomically complex stucture. The nerve fibers are well protected in connective tissue sheaths, and moderate trauma to the nerve may induce an inflammatory response in the connective tissue before the axons as such are damaged, leading to delayed nerve dysfunction. A more severe trauma, damaging the axons as well as the connective tissue sheaths, represents a very complex situation resulting in a local response with respect to Schwann cells, fibroblasts, macrophages, and endothelial cells (non-neuronal cells), as well as distant reactions in the nerve cell bodies situated in the spinal cord (motor neurones) or in the dorsal root ganglia (sensory neurons). Appropriate understanding of the pathophysiology of nerve trauma as well as the physiology of post-traumatic regeneration requires a good insight into the macroanatomy and microanatomy of nerve trunks, as well as the cellular, biochemical and molecular changes that occur in a nerve trunk following a trauma.

NORMAL ANATOMY AND PHYSIOLOGY

Microanatomy

Axons are closely packed in the endoneurial connective tissue of fascicles (Fig. 37–1). Fascicles are surrounded by the perineurial membrane—a multilaminated sheath of remarkable mechanical strength and it can act as a diffusion barrier. Several fascicles usually run together in fascicular groups, and they are embedded in the epineurial sheath—a protective and supporting connective tissue carrying a large number of epineurial vessels. The nerve trunk is surrounded by a conjunctiva-like, loose connective tissue, which allows a great deal of gliding. Normally, nerves are dynamic structures that slide over millimeters or centimeters with movements of the extremity (Millesi et al, 1990; Szabo et al, 1994; Wilgis and Murphy, 1986). For example, the median and ulnar nerves proximal to the wrist can move up to 15.5 mm, with the wrist ranged through full extension and flexion.

Intraneural Microcirculation

Nerves are well vascularized and exhibit a well-developed microvascular system in all layers (Lundborg, 1979, 1988). In the epineurium, large vessels form a characteristic longitudinal pattern in superficial as well as deeper layers between the fascicles (Fig. 37–2). Anastomosing vessels pass into the endoneurial space through the perineurium in a characteristic way. Such anastomosing vessels run between the lamella of the perineurium and pass in an oblique way through the inner layer, forming a weak spot where the vessels are easily

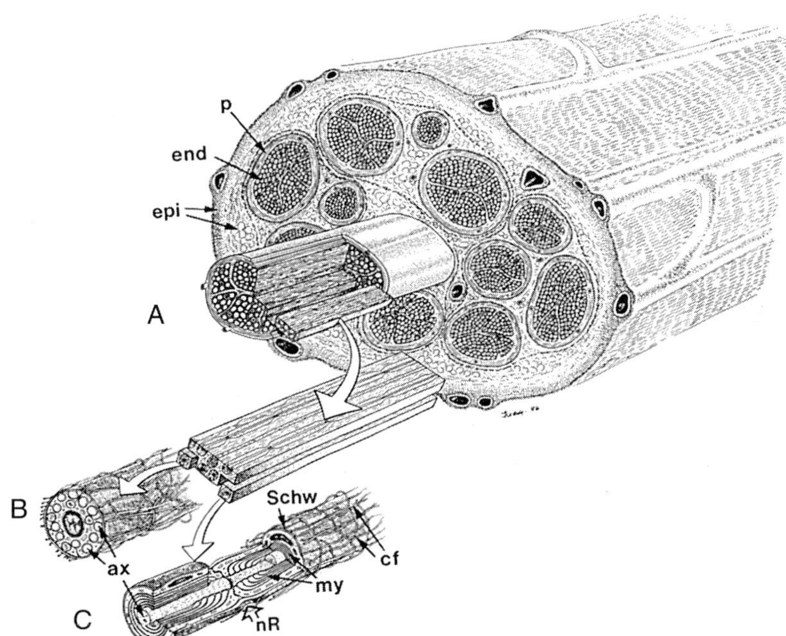

FIGURE 37–1. Microanatomy of the peripheral nerve trunk. *A,* The epineurium (epi) is the loose connective tissue and the fascicles are surrounded by the perineurium (p). The intrafascicular tissue is called endoneurium (end). *B* and *C* illustrate the appearance of nonmyelinated and myelinated fibers respectively. Schw, Schwann cell; my, myelin sheath; ax, axon; cf, collagen fibers; nR, node of Ranvier. (From Lundborg G: Nerve Injury and Repair. Edinburgh, Churchill Livingstone, 1988.)

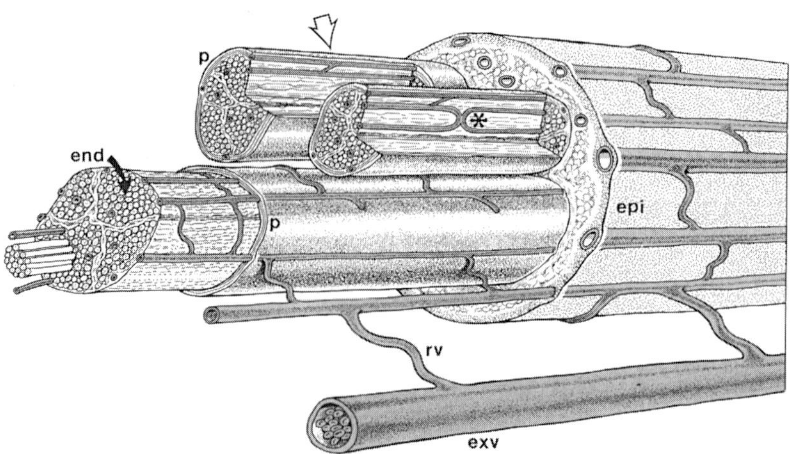

FIGURE 37–2. The vascularization of peripheral nerve. Abandoned vessels are seen in all layers of the nerve forming longitudinally oriented vessels. Extrinsic vessels (exv) are via regional feeding vessels (rv) supporting vascular plexa in the epineurium (epi), perineurium (p), and endoneurium (end). Note the oblique course of vessles penetrating the perineurium *(arrow)* and the intrafascicular double loop formation (*). (From Lundborg G: Nerve Injury and Repair. Edinburgh, Churchill Livingstone, 1988.)

closed as a result of compression or an increase in the intrafascicular pressure (Lundborg et al, 1983; Myers and Powell, 1981). Inside the fascicles, there is a longitudinal capillary network consisting mainly of capillaries.

Diffusion Barriers

The endothelium of the intrafascicular capillaries processes a blood-nerve barrier equivalent to the more well-known blood-brain barrier (Lundborg, 1988; Olsson, 1966a, 1966b). The structural basis for this barrier is so-called tight junctions between extremely closely opposed endothelial cells (Olsson, 1996a, 1996b). A diffusion barrier to proteins is also constituted in the perineurial membrane (Thomas and Olsson, 1984). Together with the blood-nerve barrier, this perineurial diffusion barrier is essential for the maintenance of a specialized endoneurial environment. Normally, there is a slightly positive tissue pressure inside fascicles, resulting in a certain degree of stiffness. This endoneurial fluid pressure (EFP) as measured in experimental animals is 2.1 ± 1.0 cm H_2O (Myers et al, 1978). Trauma may result in increased EFP, which may interfere with normal intrafascicular microvascular flow (Lundborg et al, 1983; Myers and Powell, 1981).

The Axon–Schwann Cell Complex and Axonal Transport

Axons represent extended processes from nerve cell bodies located in the anterior horn of the spinal cord (motor neurons), in the dorsal root ganglia (sensory neurons), or in the sympathetic trunk (sympathetic fibers) (Fig. 37–3). Axons are myelinated or nonmyelinated (Thomas and Olsson, 1984). However, the axons are surrounded by a chain of Schwann cells arranged in different ways in myelinated versus nonmyelinated axons. In nonmyelinated fibers, one Schwann cell can enclose a great number of axons, whereas in the myelinated fiber, one axon is associated with only one Schwann cell. This anatomical arrangement promotes a close contact between the axon and the Schwann cells (Bolin and Shooter, 1993; Rogister et al, 1993; Scherer et al, 1993) and makes the impulse propagation optimal along the axons (Galbraith and Myers, 1991). The Schwann cell basal lamina, together with adjacent parts of the endoneurial connective tissue, forms an endoneurial tube, also called the Schwann cell tube.

The metabolic machinery of neurons is concentrated in the cell bodies. Material synthesized in the cell bodies is transported distally via *anterograde* axonal transport; there is also a constant *retrograde* transport of material in the

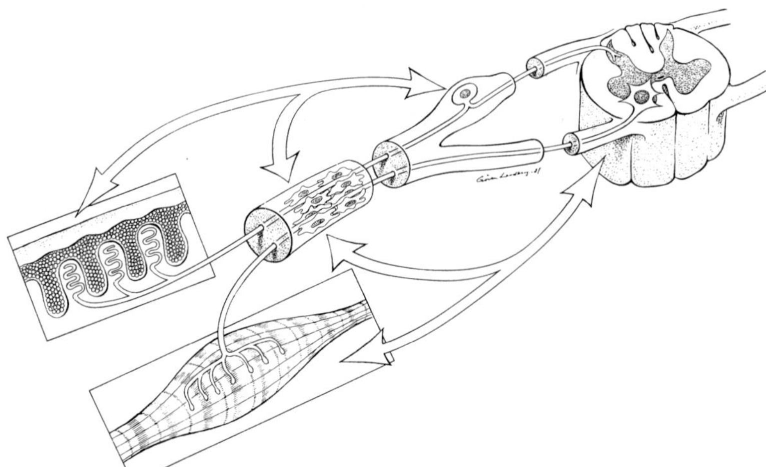

FIGURE 37–3. Schematic drawing of the neuron with the nerve cell body located in the anterior horn of the spinal cord or in the dorsal root ganglia. One process—the axon—is extended out to the periphery where the targets are located. The axon is supported by non-neuronal cells in the peripheral nerve trunk. There is an intimate contact between the axon and the Schwann cells, and a continuous flow of information from the periphery up to the nerve cell body and vice versa. (From Lundborg G: Nerve Injury and Repair. Edinburgh, Churchill Livingstone, 1988.)

opposite direction toward the cell body of materials for recycling. The anterograde transport can include fast (mainly membrane associated material) and slow (cytoskeletal proteins) components (Grafstein and Forman, 1980). Neurotrophic factors, synthesized in the peripheral targets (e.g., nerve growth factor [NGF]), are normally picked up by the nerve terminals and transported via the retrograde transport to the nerve cell body to maintain its viability and survival. Through changes in the retrograde axonal transport, peripheral damage may induce changes also in the nerve cell bodies. In such situations, the nerve cell body usually changes its morphology and it can modify its metabolism and build up a potential for regeneration (Archer et al, 1994).

COMPRESSION

Compression injuries may occur as acute or chronic lesions. The severity of the damage depends on the duration as well as the magnitude and type of the compression trauma. Functionally, the disorder may vary from slight paresthesia or motor weakness, or both, to complete sensory loss or muscle paralysis. The effect of compression depends on the microanatomy of the nerve: Small fascicles embedded a large amount of epineurium are less vulnerable to compression than large fascicles in a small amount of epineurium. Also, nerve fibers show varying levels of susceptibility to compression, with large fibers being more vulnerable than small fibers (Dahlin et al, 1989; Erlanger and Gasser, 1937; Gasser and Erlanger, 1929). Chronic compression may be a result of local irritation, resulting in an inflammatory response in the epineurial sheaths, impaired gliding resulting in microstretching injuries, further scarring, and finally an entrapment situation.

Intraneural Microcirculation

From experimental animal models, it is known that an extraneural pressure of 20 to 30 mm Hg may interfere with intraneural venular flow and that a pressure of at least 80 mm Hg may result in a complete circulatory arrest in the nerve (Ogata and Naito, 1986; Rydevik et al, 1981). However, the ischemic level may vary with the blood pressure of the object (Szabo et al, 1983). Thus, already at a low magnitude of compression intraneural microcirculation may be severely disturbed. With extended ischemia or increased pressure or both, endothelial cells may be damaged to such an extent that an endoneurial edema may occur when circulation is re-established. Such an increase in EFP may induce a no reflow phenomenon, which may jeopardize the oxygen supply to the axons, thereby inducing a closed compartment syndrome in miniature in the nerve (Myers et al, 1978; Lundborg et al, 1983; Rydevik et al, 1981).

Axonal Transport

Extraneural pressure may interfere with anterograde as well as retrograde axonal transport directly or secondarily via microvascular interference (Dahlin, 1986). In animal experiments, a pressure of 20 to 30 mm Hg, depending on the duration of pressure, has been found to block completely or partially anterograde fast axonal transport (Dahlin et al, 1984). Such a block is reversible within the first 24 hours, but after a pressure of 200 mm Hg is applied for 2 hours, the blockage could last for days. A pressure of 30 mm Hg is also sufficient to inhibit slow anterograde axonal transport as well as the retrograde transport (Dahlin and McLean, 1986; Dahlin et al, 1986). These pressures of low magnitude should be compared with the pressure known to be acting on the median nerve in the carpal tunnel in humans with carpal tunnel syndrome (Gelberman et al, 1981).

Disturbances in axonal transport following peripheral nerve compression may induce structural and biochemical changes in the corresponding nerve cell bodies (Dahlin et al, 1993). Functional changes as an increased regenerative capacity in the nerve following a test injury also have been reported following acute and chronic nerve compression (Dahlin and Kanje, 1992; Dahlin and Thambert, 1993). These alterations in the neuron may induce subsequent changes in anterograde axonal transport, thereby making other parts of the neuron more susceptible to additional compression due to the lack of cytoskeletal elements, for example (Dahlin and Lundborg, 1990; Dahlin et al, 1986). A similar mechanism has been proposed in subjects with diabetic neuropathy (Dahlin et al, 1986, 1987), in which an increased incidence of nerve entrapments has been reported (Mulder et al, 1961).

Nerve Fibers

Uniform compression of nerve fibers seems to cause little or no damage (Grundfest, 1936). The situation is different when a *segment* of a nerve trunk is compressed. In such situations, shear forces occur at the edges of the compressed segment due to distribution of the tissue from compressed to non-compressed areas (Rydevik et al, 1989). The myelin sheaths may be damaged locally in such situations. In experimental studies on primates using application of inflatable tourniquets, displacement of the nodes of Ranvier under the border zones of a tourniquet has been observed (Fowler et al, 1972; Ochoa et al, 1972). Activation and proliferation of non-neuronal cells as well as local Schwann cell necrosis have also been observed (Kanje et al, 1994; Powell and Myers, 1986).

CLASSIFICATION OF PERIPHERAL NERVE INJURIES

Nerve lesions may have various origins, such as mechanical (compression, vibration, stretching, severance), ischemic, thermal, or chemical trauma. Classification of nerve injuries may be based on functional consequences as well as structural changes in the nerve trunk.

Metabolic Conduction Block

If intraneural microcirculation is locally inhibited, such as by compression, a local metabolic or physiological conduction block may be induced. Examples of such metabolic blocks are the numbness of the foot when the peroneal nerve is compressed by one leg crossed over the knee at the opposite side or the conduction block induced by an inflated tourniquet around the nerve. This type of metabolic block, which is due to local circulatory arrest, is immediately reversible when the pressure is removed. Nerve fibers are fairly resistant to ischemia and can tolerate up to 6 hours of ischemia before they are irreversibly damaged (Dahlin et al, 1989; Lundborg, 1975). If the trauma induced edema in the fascicle, the resulting increase in EFP may compromise capillary flow for an extended time, thereby inducing a prolonged period of sensory disturbance. Because the perineurium is a diffusion barrier to proteins such edema can not easily be drained to extrafascicular layers (Shdanow, 1931).

Neurapraxia (Sunderland Lesion I)

Compression or stretching may induce a conduction block lasting for weeks or months before it is spontaneously reversed. Such a conduction block was named neurapraxia by Seddon (Seddon, 1943, 1972), suggesting preserved axonal continuity, but there is local damage to myelin sheaths. Neurapraxia often includes motor paralysis, although some sensory and sympathetic functions may be spared; these latter functions are confined to thin fibers, which are less vulnerable to compression (Dahlin et al, 1989; Gasser and Erlanger, 1929).

Saturday night palsy (a radial nerve lesion in the upper arm) is a good example of a neurapractic lesion. The radial nerve can be activated electrically *distal* to the lesion because no degeneration has taken place and axonal continuity is preserved.

The motor and sensory dysfunction sometimes observed following tourniquet application around the upper arm is another example of a neurapractic lesion. Such nerve dysfunction may occur after very short periods of tourniquet application and is usually due to too high pressure in the cuff, usually resulting from use of a faulty gauge. The pathoanatomical basis has been described by Ochoa and co-workers as a local invagination phenomena of the myelin sheath at the nodes of Ranvier (Ochoa et al, 1972).

Axonotmesis (Sunderland Lesion II)

A crush injury or traction injury may injure the axons so that their continuity is broken although the endoneurial tubes are still intact. The explanation is that the endoneurial tubes are mechanically more resistant to trauma compared with the axons. Regeneration of the axons is required to restore functional recovery, but because the preserved endoneurial tubes offer correctly oriented pathways, the growing axons arrive at the correct peripheral targets.

Neurotmesis (Sunderland Lesion III-V)

Neurotmesis means injury to the connective tissue elements of the nerve trunk in addition to loss of axonal continuity. According to Seddon's original classification (Seddon, 1972, p 32), neurotmesis is "a term used to describe the state of the nerve that has either been completely severed or is so disorganized by scar tissue that spontaneous regeneration is out of the question." Surgical repair is required to make possible axon regeneration.

Sunderland has described a more detailed classification of these lesions. Sunderland group III lesions entail loss of continuity of endoneurial tubes but preserved continuity of the perineurium. Sunderland lesion IV and V lesions include loss of perineurial and epineurial continuity, respectively.

The Carpal Tunnel Syndrome—a Model for Correlating Pathophysiological Levels with Clinical Signs

The carpal tunnel syndrome offers a good clinical model for understanding how clinical signs can reflect various pathological stages. Nocturnal paraesthesia represents an *early stage,* and it reflects microvascular dysfunction based on increased tissue pressure in the carpal tunnel. It is known that, on average, the tissue pressure in the carpal tunnel of these patients is 30 mm Hg (mean pressure in healthy individuals is 2.5 mm Hg [Gelberman et al, 1981]), a pressure that is known to disturb axonal transport as well as microvascular venular blood flow in the nerve (Dahlin 1986; Rydevik et al, 1981). Intracarpal tunnel pressure in patients suffering from carpal tunnel syndrome always exceeds the critical pressure of 30 mm Hg during nighttime, the highest being found in the early morning (Luchetti et al, 1994). During the day, these patients, who are suffering from the earliest stage of the syndrome, have no problems because the intracarpal pressure then goes down and the mean blood pressure rises. In the *intermediate stage,* when there are constant symptoms of permanent numbness and some motor weakness, there is an established pathoanatomical problem in the nerve, such as intrafascicular edema or damage to the myelin sheaths, or both. Thus, we are dealing not only with the metabolic problem but also with a neurapractic problem. In *later stages* of true sensory disturbances and muscle atrophy, axonotmesis with axonal degeneration are also present.

Also, the time course for relief of symptoms following compression reflects the pathological state of various fiber groups. More or less immediate relief of some problems reflect recovery of those fibers suffering from metabolic block only. Symptoms that disappear after days and weeks may reflect disappearance of intrafascicular edema, whereas symptoms that lasting for months arise from neurapractic lesions. Axonotmesis requires months or years before regeneration eventually takes place.

VIBRATION

Long-term work with handheld vibrating tools may induce a hand-arm vibration syndrome expressing itself in vibration-induced white fingers, sensorineural disturbances in the hand, and sometimes pain and muscle weakness (Agate, 1949; Brammer and Pyykkö, 1987; Lundborg et al, 1987; Narini, et al, 1993). The neurological problems may vary from slight paraesthesia to pain, sensory disturbances, impaired dexterity, and muscle weakness. Such symptoms may be interpreted as signs of a nerve entrapment because several studies have reported a higher prevalence of carpal tunnel syndromes in workers exposed to vibration than controls (Bovenzi and Zadini, 1991; Chatterjee et al, 1982; Silverstein and Fine, 1987; Wieslander et al, 1989). Decompression of a peripheral nerve may result in incomplete recovery with some remaining symptoms (Boström et al, 1994; Hagberg et al, 1991; Nilsson et al, 1993).

Vibration represents a type of rapidly iterated compression applied to the skin of the hand. The energy may be transmitted to the tissues of hand and more proximally in the extremity. Vibration may induce displacement of the tissues of various distances. The frequency, acceleration, and duration of the exposure is important for induction of the hand-arm vibration syndrome, although the expression in term of displacement may be more relevant (Necking et al, 1992; Strömberg et al, 1994). All tissues may be damaged, and in the peripheral nervous system, injuries may be induced in skin receptors as well as in the nerve trunk with its nerve fibers. It has been observed that plantar nerves in the feet of rats, which were experimentally subjected to vibration, exhibit obvious pathoanatomical changes as revealed by histological and ultrastructural techniques. Nonmyelinated fibers showed distinct changes, including deranged microtubuli in the axoplasm, which were reversible after a recovery period of 2 weeks (Lundborg et al, 1990) and even myelinated fibers showed morphological changes (Chang et al, 1994; Ho and Yu, 1989). Functional changes in vibration-exposed nerves have also been observed (Dahlin et al, 1992), and some studies indicate that non-neuronal cells as well as the neuron may be affected by the vibration trauma (Bergman et al, 1995; Dahlin et al, 1994; Strömberg et al, 1994). The functional changes are interesting in view of the reported increased prevalence of carpal tunnel syndrome (Bovenzi and Zadini, 1991; Chatterjee et al, 1982; Silverstein and Fine, 1987; Wieslander et al, 1989). Damage to nonmyelinated fibers is of special interest because sympathetic fibers belong to these fiber groups. Hypothetically, damage to such fibers explains the vascular dysfunction in vibration-exposed patients (Lundborg et al, 1990). Interestingly, changes in nonmyelinated as well as myelinated fibers have been observed in biopsies from fingers of vibration-exposed workers (Takeuchi et al, 1986, 1988).

Although occupational groups, such as concrete workers, grinders, and platers, are exposed to low or intermediate frequencies, other occupational groups, such as dental technicians, are exposed to vibration of extremely high frequencies. These patients may acquire local nerve lesions in the distal nerves and skin receptors as a result of the vibration exposure (Hjortsberg et al, 1989). These patients may suffer from impaired sensibility and dexterity, lost precision, clumsiness, and a tendency to drop small items.

POST-TRAUMATIC DEGENERATION AND REGENERATION

Changes in the Nerve Cell Body

An injury of the axons is followed by cellular and biochemical changes distally as well as proximally. The corresponding nerve cell body undergoes characteristic structural, biochemical and functional changes (Grafstein, 1975; Grafstein and McQuarrie, 1978; Lieberman, 1971; Rich et al, 1987; Torvik, 1976). Severance of an axon means amputation of a great deal of the neuron, and at this point, there is a metabolic preparation in the nerve cell body to replace the lost axoplasmic volume. There is an increase in cell body volume, displacement of the nucleus to the periphery, and a disappearance of basophilic material to the cytoplasm (chromatolysis). Such changes may be a nonspecific reaction, but it may also reflect changes in protein synthesis (Brattgård et al, 1957) based on alterations in the arrangement and concentration of RNA-containing material in the cell and subsequent changes in axonal transport aiming at restoring the axonal anatomy (Archer and McLean, 1985). For that reason, there is a change in the general mode of axonal transport expressed in a decrease of components associated with synaptic transmission (Boyle and Gillespie, 1970; Koo et al, 1988; Nandy, 1968; Ochs, 1976) and delivery of more components of the axon like the cytoskeletal component tubulin that are necessary for construction (Grafstein, 1975, 1986; Tetzlaff et al, 1988). Changes in the axonal transport occur as changes in the amount of material transported with no change in rate, but changes in rate may occur in some species and following a previous nerve injury (Archer et al, 1994; Frizell et al, 1976; Jacob and McQuarrie, 1993; Kreutzberg and Schubert 1971; McQuarrie and Jacob, 1991; Ochs, 1976). The cell body reaction can vary with the proximity of the lesion. A proximal lesion may lead to death of the cell body, but more distal lesions could also result in a considerable amount of proximal cellular death (Liss et al, 1994).

Different mechanisms have been proposed to explain the structural and biochemical changes in the cell body that occur following a severe nerve injury (Cragg, 1970). The signal could be mediated via changes in the axonal transport when some of the anterograde-transported material is reversed at the site of lesion and is incorporated in the retrograde transport, leading to a premature return of the material to the cell body (Bisby and Bulger, 1977). Another possible explanation may be arrest of supply of factors such as NGF, which is normally transported to the nerve cell body via retrograde axonal transport, and the lack of that support may lead to the observed central effects. Changes in the nerve cell bodies induced by axotomy can be reversed by local application of NGF (Hendry, 1975; Johnson et al, 1986; Otto, 1987; Purves and Njå, 1976; Rich et al, 1987).

Degeneration of the Distal Segment

After an axon is severed, its distal part undergoes degeneration. There is a granular disintegration of axoplasmic microtubules and neurofilaments due to proteolysis (Lubinska, 1982; Schlaepfer, 1974, 1977; Vial, 1958), and there is growing evidence that this protein disintegration is calcium dependent and mediated by calcium-activated enzymes in the axoplasm (Schlaepfer and Hasler, 1979). The myelin breaks up into droplets and is phagocytosed by Schwann cells and macrophages. In the peripheral nerve, macrophages are normally present and constitute approximately 2% to 4% of the endoneurial cells (Oldfors, 1980), but following an injury to the nerve, there is an immediate recruitment of macrophages to the nerve (Brown et al, 1991; Monaco et al,

1992; Stoll et al, 1989). These macrophages are of hematogenous origin (Olsson and Sjöstrand, 1969) and the breakdown of the myelin sheaths is prevented if the recruitment of the macrophages is inhibited (Beuche and Friede, 1984). The recruited macrophages are important not only for the degeneration process but may be of even more importance for the regeneration process (see The Role of Macrophages). Most of these changes that occur in the distal segment are completed within the first weeks, but disposal of old myelin sheaths may require a longer amount of time. The Schwann cells undergo mitosis (Kanje et al, 1995) and line up in characteristic Schwann cell columns (bands of Büngner). The multiplication of Schwann cells and degeneration starts 1 to 5 days after the nerve is severed, with the peak activity occurring at approximately the third day after surgery (Abercrombie and Johnson, 1946a, 1946b; Spencer et al, 1981; Weinberg, and Spencer, 1978). The proliferation may be stimulated by factors emanating from the recruited macrophages (Dahlin et al, 1996; Miyauchi et al, 1996). These cells produce many substances (Nathan, 1987), like the cytokin interleukin-1 and platelet-derived growth factor, which may regulate the synthesis of NGF in Schwann cells and induce the proliferation of these cells, respectively (Davis and Stroobant, 1990; Eccleston, 1992; Lindholm et al, 1988, 1987). Conversely, Schwann cells do produce interleukin-1 (Bergsteinsdottir et al, 1991), which increases the recruitment of macrophages. The Schwann cells also constitute a trophic source of regenerating fibers on their way to the periphery by providing trophic substances and create pathways by their basal lamina.

Axonal Regeneration

In experimental animal models, a crush injury, representing axonotmesis, is usually used as a test lesion. Such an injury leaves the endoneurial tube intact and, therefore, represents a favorable situation resulting in outgrowth of axons to their correct peripheral targets. A transection (neurotmesis) represents a much more complicated type of damage because there are no remaining guidelines across the zone of injury. Axonotmesis is followed by retrograde degeneration over one or several internodal segments and, later, by subsequent production of a great number of collateral and terminal sprouts from the distal stump of myelinated axons. Clusters of sprouts, confined to one single Schwann cell and originating from the same axon (the so-called regenerating unit) (Morris et al, 1972a, 1972b), are advanced distally after a short initial delay. There is a further reorganization of the nerve trunk into a large number of miniature compartments surrounded by new perineurium, each of them containing several regenerating units (Lundborg and Hansson, 1979). The reason for the constitution of such numerous small minifascicles (compartmentation) is probably to restore the normal endoneurial environment as soon as possible by restoring the perineurial barrier. A new nerve trunk with an intact perineurium can also be formed without nerve fibers present (Zhao et al, 1992).

In the distal segment, the advancing sprouts follow the Schwann cell tubes constituting appropriate pathways by their basal lamina (Fig. 37–4). Following transection and repair of the nerve trunk, there is a great deal of misdirection

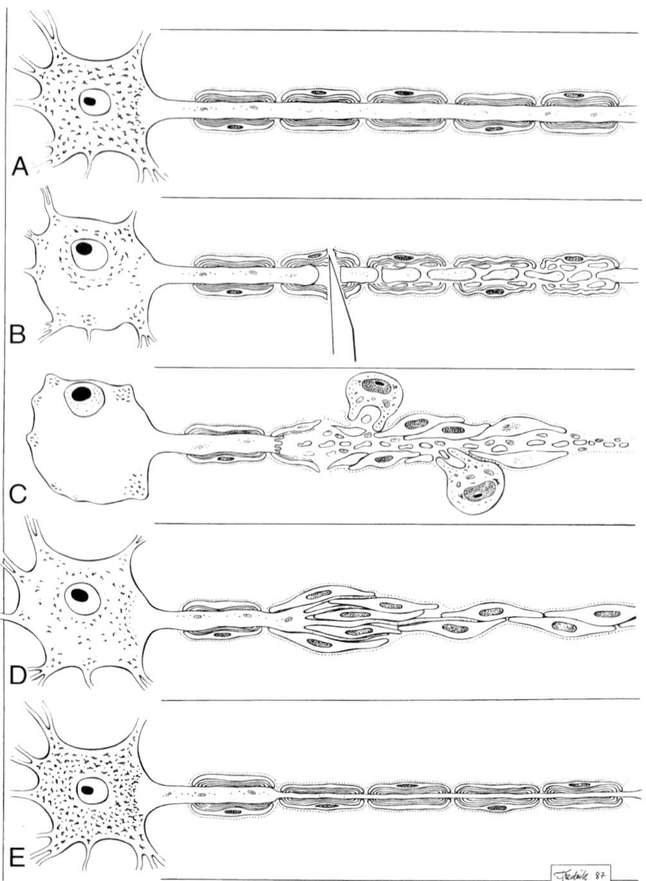

FIGURE 37–4. Degeneration and regeneration of myelinated nerve fiber. *A,* Normal appearance. *B,* Transection of the nerve fiber, which results in distal fragmentation of axon and myelin. Nerve cell body changes occur. *C,* Schwann cells proliferate in the distal nerve segment. Macrophages and Schwann cells phagocytose debris material. *D,* The Schwann cells line up in the bands of Büngner, and sprouts arise from the proximal axonal stump. *E,* Axonal connection with the periphery with maturation of nerve fiber. (From Lundborg G: Nerve Injury and Repair. Edinburgh, Churchill Livingstone, 1988.)

so that one endoneurial tube can contain sprouts from several different parent axons.

At the tip of each axon, there is a growth cone exhibiting a number of philopodia, which palpate and explore the environment. The growth cones are full of receptor sites and advance only on substrate presenting appropriate neurite-outgrowth promoting factors. The growth cones produce plasminogen activator as well as collagenase (Krystosek and Seeds, 1984; Patterson, 1985; Hawkins and Seeds, 1986), which facilitate their penetration through connective tissues and scars. The grow cones also pick up trophic factors, which are transported to the nerve cell body by retrograde axonal transport. Schwann cells at the front of the advancing growth cones are up regulated in terms of NGF production as well as the occurrence of NGF receptors on their surface, but when the growth cones have passed, this activity is down regulated (Taniuchi et al, 1988).

The rate of axonal outgrowth varies with species, type of injury, and level of occurrence. In experimental animals, regeneration falls within the range of 2 to 3 mm per day after transection and repair, and 3.0 to 4.5 mm per day after crush injury (Lundborg, 1988). Axonal regeneration in humans is nonlinear, with a gradually decreased regeneration rate in distal parts. On average, the outgrowth rate is about 1 to 2 mm per day (Buchthal and Kühl, 1979; Seddon, 1972).

Trophism and Tropism

The amount of growth-stimulating factors is substantially increased following an injury. Neurotrophic factors like NGF support survival of nerve cells (Meakin and Shooter, 1992) while neurotropic factors may influence the growth direction of axons by exerting an attraction at the distance (Lundborg et al, 1994a). In reality, it might be impossible to make a clear distinction between the two factors because substances that are secreted by the non-neuronal cells after an injury can act like a tropic factor, although they normally have a trophic influence (Kuffler, 1987). Advancing axons want an attractive environment with tropic and trophic influence as well as they should be provided by specific molecules for an optimal growth-cone formation and outgrowth, and examples of such neurite-promoting factors are laminin, fibronectin, and L1 (Schachner, 1992).

The Role of Macrophages

As pointed out earlier, macrophages may not only participate in the degeneration process by engulfing myelin debris but they may also influence the regeneration process because they release the factors that stimulate Schwann cell proliferation (Baichwal et al, 1988) and the production of NGF in non-neuronal cells (Brown et al, 1991; Heumann, 1987)—a process that may be controlled via interleukin-1 (Lindholm et al, 1987, 1988). External application of macrophages to a peripheral nerve increases the outgrowth of axons (Dahlin et al, 1996; Stolz et al, 1991), probably by factors that are secreted from the macrophages and that affect non-neuronal cells and the axon, leading to activation of the nerve cell bodies in the dorsal root ganglia (Kanje et al, 1995). Introduction of inflammation into the dorsal root ganglia can also promote the regeneration process (Lu and Richardson, 1991). Conversely, regeneration can be impeded if the recruitment of macrophages is hindered or if an antagonist to the interleukin-1 receptor is provided (Guénard et al, 1991; Tanaka et al, 1992).

Specificity

To express the accuracy of regeneration, it may be valuable to use the term specificity. Different types of specificity have been described in experimental models (Lundborg et al, 1994a). Tissue specificity refers to the preferential reinnervation of the distal nerve versus other types of tissue, whereas topographic specificity indicates preferential reinnervation of analogous distal pathways. An example of the topographic specificity is the preferential reinnervation of peroneal pathways by peroneal fibers versus tibial fibers. Motor axons may also preferentially reinnervate motor targets versus sensory targets (motor versus sensory specificity) (Brushart, 1988, 1990; Lundborg et al, 1994a).

Conditioning Lesions

The regeneration process in peripheral nerves can be manipulated by different procedures. It has been shown 20 years ago that the regenerative capacity in a peripheral nerve can be markedly improved if the nerve has been injured previously (i.e., a conditioning lesion) (McQuarrie and Grafstein, 1973; McQuarrie et al, 1977). If a test crush lesion was applied to the previously injured nerve 2 weeks after the initial injury, the axons started to grow early (initial delay; that is, time from injury to start of regeneration) and there was also an increased rate of regeneration. Such a phenomenon is called the conditioning lesion effect. This phenomenon has been observed when the nerve previously has been crushed or transected (Bisby and Pollock, 1983; McQuarrie and Grafstein, 1973; McQuarrie et al, 1977; Sjöberg and Kanje, 1990). Regenerative capacity after the test crush lesion can also vary with location of the conditioning lesion (Bisby and Pollock, 1983; Sjöberg and Kanje, 1990).

The conditioning lesion phenomenon can be used as a sign of injury to the peripheral nerve trunk, and the phenomenon also is observed after other types of conditioning lesions such as acute and chronic compression (Dahlin and Kanje, 1992; Dahlin and Thambert, 1993), vibration exposure (Bergman et al, 1995; Dahlin et al, 1992; Strömberg et al, 1994), and the application of electromagnetic fields (Kanje et al, 1993; Rusovan and Kanje, 1991).

THE ROLE OF THE CENTRAL NERVOUS SYSTEM IN PERIPHERAL NERVE INJURIES

Transection of a nerve trunk results in denervation of peripheral territories and also degeneration of corresponding cortical projectional areas. Normally, the hand is represented in areas 3B and 1 in the somatosensory cortex, where fingers are projected as well-defined bands (Jenkins et al, 1990a, 1990b). Following a nerve injury, these cortical areas undergo complete reorganization (Wall and Kaas, 1986; Wall, 1986). Following transection of the median nerve, there is a black hole in the brain corresponding to the area controlling the median nerve innervation territory. Soon this area becomes occupied by substitute tactile input from adjacent hand locations that remain innervated by other nerves. When the regenerating axons make a peripheral connection, unfortunately, to a great extent, with the wrong receptor sites, the result is total functional reorganization in the somatosensory cortex. This reorganization produces major topographical changes, with digit representation in small discontinuous patches in the cortex (Fig. 37–5). In the cortex, separate recording sites may be associated with multiple cutaneous receptive fields.

Clinically, this is the basis for the incomplete recovery of all qualities of functional sensibility following nerve repair. In specific sensibility training programs (Dellon, 1981; Imai et al, 1991), it is possible to reprogram the brain in a relearning process. By simultaneously touching and looking at structures, the mind can relearn by creating an image of the structures the hand is touching. Such a relearning process may involve phenomena such as long-term potentiation of

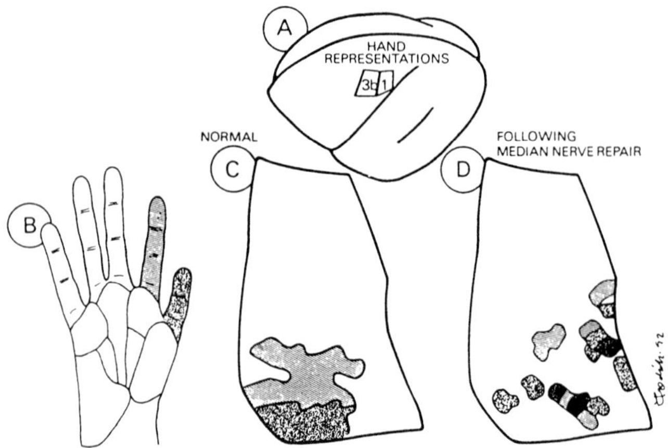

FIGURE 37–5. Functional reorganization of the somatosensory cortex *(A)* following a median nerve transection, repair and regeneration (in the owl monkey). *B* and *C*, Normal cortical representation of the thumb and index finger. *D*, Representation of these fingers following median nerve transection, microsurgical repair, and regeneration. Major topographic changes in the somatosensory cortex with the digit representation in small discontinuous patches. (Data from Lundborg G: Peripheral nerve injuries. Pathophysiology and strategies for treatment. (Editorial.) J Hand Therapy *6*:179–189, 1993.)

existing synapses and formation of new synaptic connections (Kandel and Hawkins, 1992).

CLINICAL PERSPECTIVES

Nerve trauma, especially transection of major nerve trunks usually results in considerable disability in adults. For a long time, interest has been focused on refinement and modification of suture techniques, but it seems that the results have reached a plateau at which functional recovery still is unsatisfactory in adults. The surgical technique cannot be further refined, and for that reason, there is a need for an alternative approach to peripheral nerve injuries to improve the results for the future.

Increased knowledge of molecular mechanisms regulating axonal outgrowth may prove to be the key factor in the future. At present, use of neurotrophic factors cannot be applied clinically, but this method may well be possible in the near future. There are reasons to believe that the current accelerating development of central nervous system research with special reference to brain plasticity may prove to be another key factor in the future. Improved techniques for relearning, including programs addressing specific brain functions, may be important. There are indications that factors like verbal learning capacity and visuospatial cognitive capacity are important for recovery of functional sensibility following nerve injury in adults (Lundborg et al, 1994b; Rosén et al, 1994).

References

Abercrombie M, Johnson ML: Collagen content of rabbit sciatic nerve during wallerian degeneration. J Neurol Neurosurg Psychiatry *9*:113–120, 1946a.

Abercrombie M, Johnson ML: A quantitative histology of wallerian degeneration: nuclear population in rabbit sciatic nerve. J Anat. *80*:37–50, 1946b.

Agate JN: An outbreak of cases of Raynaud's phenomenon of occupational origin. Br J Ind Med *6*:144–163, 1949.

Archer DR, Dahlin LB, Mclean WG: Changes in slow axonal transport of tubulin induced by local application of colchicine to rabbit vagus nerve. Acta Physiol Scand *150*:57–65, 1994.

Archer DR, McLean WG: Effects of temporary and permanent disruption on axonally transported proteins in rabbit vagus nerve. J Neurochem *44*(Suppl):123, 1985.

Baichwal RR, Bigbee JW, DeVries GH: Macrophage-mediated myelin-related mitogenic factor for cultured Schwann cells. Proc Natl Acad Sci *85*:1701–1705, 1988.

Bergman S, Widerberg A, Danielsen N, Dahlin LB: Nerve regeneration in nerve grafts conditioned vibration exposure. Restor Neurol Neuroscience *7*:165–169, 1995.

Bergsteinsdottir K, Kingston A, Mirsky R, Jessen KR: Rat Schwann cells produce interleukin-1. J Neuroimmunol *34*:15–23, 1991.

Beuche W, Friede RL: The role of non-resident cells in Wallerian degeneration. J Neurocytol *13*:767–796, 1984.

Bisby M, Pollock B: Increased regeneration rate in peripheral nerve axons following double lesions: Enhancement of the conditioning lesion phenomenon. J Neurobiol *14*:467–472, 1983.

Bisby MA, Bulger VT: Reversal of axonal transport at a nerve crush. J Neurochem *29*:313–320, 1977.

Bolin LM, Shooter EM: Neurons regulate Schwann cell genes by diffusible molecules. J Cell Biol *123*:237–243, 1993.

Boström L, Göthe CI, Hansson S, Lugnegård H, Nilsson BY: Surgical treatment of carpal tunnel syndrome in patients exposed to vibration from handheld tools. Scand J Plast Reconstr Surg *28*:147–149, 1994.

Bovenzi M, Zadini A: Occupational musculoskeletal disorders in the neck and upper limbs of forestry workers exposed to hand-arm vibration. Ergonomics *34*:547–562, 1991.

Boyle FC, Gillespie JS: Accumulation and loss of noradrenaline central to a constriction on adrenergic nerves. Euro J Pharmacol *12*:77–84, 1970.

Brammer AJ, Pyykkö I: Vibration-induced neuropathy: Detection by nerve conduction measurements. Scand J Work Environ Health *13*:317–322, 1987.

Brattgård SO, Edström JE, Hydén H: Chemical changes in regenerating neurons. J Neurochem *1*:316–325, 1957.

Brown MC, Perry VH, Lunn ER, Gordon S, Heumann R: Macrophage dependence of peripheral sensory nerve regeneration: Possible involvement of nerve growth factor. Neuron *6*:359–370, 1991.

Brushart TME: Preferential reinnervation of motor nerves by regenerating motor axons. J Neurosci *8*:1026–1031, 1988.

Brushart TME: Preferential motor reinnervation: A sequential double-labeling study. Restor Neurol Neurosci *1*:281–287, 1990.

Buchthal F, Kühl V: Nerve conduction, tactile sensibility, and the electromyogram after suture or compression of peripheral nerve: A longitudinal study in man. J Neurol Neurosurg Psychiatry *42*:436–451, 1979.

Chang KY, Ho ST, Yu HS: Vibration induced neurophysiological and electron microscopical changes in rat peripheral nerves. Occup Environ Med *51*:130–135, 1994.

Chatterjee DS, Barwick DD, Petrie A: Exploratory electromyography in the study of vibration-induced white finger in rock drillers. Br J Ind Med *39*:89–97, 1982.

Cragg BG: What is the signal for chromatolysis? Brain Res *23*:1–21, 1970.

Dahlin LB: Nerve compression and axonal transport. [Doctoral thesis]. Göteborg, Sweden, Göteborg University, 1986.

Dahlin LB, Archer DR, McLean WG: Treatment with an aldose reductase inhibitor can reduce the susceptibility of fast axonal transport following nerve compression in the streptozotocin-diabetic rat. Diabetologia *30*:414–418, 1987.

Dahlin LB, Archer DR, McLean WG: Axonal transport and morphological changes following nerve compression. An experimental study in the rabbit vagus nerve. J Hand Surg (Br) *18*:106–110, 1993.

Dahlin LB, Kanje M: Conditioning effect induced by chronic nerve compression. Scand J Plast Reconstr Hand Surg *26*:37–41, 1992.

Dahlin LB, Lundborg G: The neurone and its response to peripheral nerve compression. J Hand Surg *15B*:5–10, 1990.

Dahlin LB, McLean WG: Effects of graded experimental compression on slow and fast axonal transport in rabbit vagus nerve. J Neurol Sci *72*:19–30, 1986.

Dahlin LB, Meiri KF, McLean WG, Rydevik B, Sjöstrand J: Effects of nerve compression on fast axonal transport in streptozotocin-induced diabetes mellitus. Diabetologia *29*:181–185, 1986.

Dahlin LB, Miyauchi A, Danielsen N, Thomsen P, Kanje M: Stimulation of nerve regeneration by macrophages in granulation tissue. Rest Neurol Neurosci 9:141–149, 1996.

Dahlin LB, Necking LE, Lundström R, Lundborg G: Vibration exposure and conditioning lesion effect in nerves. An experimental study in rats. J Hand Surg (Am) 7:858–861, 1992.

Dahlin LB, Rydevik B, McLean WG, Sjöstrand J: Changes in fast axonal transport during experimental nerve compression at low pressures. Exp Neurol 84:29–36, 1984.

Dahlin LB, Shyu BC, Danielsen N, Andersson S: Effects of nerve compression or ischemia on conduction properties of myelinated and nonmyelinated nerve fibres. An experimental study in the rabbit common peroneal nerve. Acta Physiol Scand 136:97–105, 1989.

Dahlin LB, Sjöstrand J, McLean WG: Graded inhibition of retrograde axonal transport by compression of rabbit vagus nerve. J Neurol Sci 76:221–230, 1986.

Dahlin LB, Thambert C: Acute nerve compression at low pressure has a conditioning lesion effect on rat sciatic nerves. Acta Orthoped Scand 64:479–481, 1993.

Davis JB, Stroobant P: Platelet-derived growth factors and fibroblast growth factors are mitogens for rat Schwann cells. J Cell Biol 110:1353–1360, 1990.

Dellon AL: Evaluation of sensibility and reeducation of sensation in the hand. Baltimore, Williams and Wilkins, 1981.

Eccleston PA: Regulation of Schwann cell proliferation: Mechanisms involved in peripheral nerve development. Exp Cell Res 199:1–9, 1992.

Erlanger J, Gasser H: Electrical Signs of Nervous Activity. Philadelphia, University of Pennsylvania Press, 1937.

Fowler TJ, Danta G, Gilliatt RW: Recovery of nerve conduction after penumatic tourniquet observations on the hindlimb of the baboon. J Neurol Neurosurg Psychiatry 35:638–647, 1972.

Frizell M, McLean WG, Sjöstrand J: Retrograde axonal transport of rapidly migrating labelled proteins and glycoproteins in regenerating peripheral nerves. J Neurochem 27:191–196, 1976.

Galbraith JA, Myers RR: Impulse conduction. In Gelberman RH (ed): Operative Nerve Repair and Reconstruction, vol 1. Philadelphia, J.B. Lippincott Company, 1991, pp 19–46.

Gasser HS, Erlanger J: The role of fibre size in the establishment of a nerve block by pressure or cocaine. Am J Physiol 88:581–591, 1929.

Gelberman RH, Hergenroeder PT, Hargens AR, Lundborg G, Akeson WH: The carpal tunnel syndrome—a study of carpal canal pressure. J Bone Joint Surg (Am) 63:380–383, 1981.

Grafstein B: The nerve cell body response to axotomy. Exp Neurol 48:32–51, 1975.

Grafstein B: The retina as a regenerating organ. In Adler R, Farber DB (eds): The Retina: A Model for Cell Biology Studies, Part II. New York: Academic Press, 1986, pp 275–335.

Grafstein B, Forman DS: Intracellular transport in neurons. Physiol Rev 60:1167–1283, 1980.

Grafstein B, McQuarrie IG: Role of the nerve cell body in axonal regeneration. In Cotman CW (ed): Neuronal Plasticity. New York, Raven Press, 1978, pp. 155–195.

Grundfest H: Effects of hydrostatic pressures upon the excitability, the recovery and potential sequence of frog nerve. Cold Spring Harb Sympo Quant Biol 4:179–187, 1936.

Guénard V, Dinarello CA, Weston PJ, Aebischer P: Peripheral nerve regeneration is impeded by interleukin-1 receptor antagonist released from a polymeric guidance channel. J Neurosci Res 29:396–400, 1991.

Hagberg M, Nyström Å, Zetterlund B: Recovery from symptoms after carpal tunnel syndrome surgery in males in relation to vibration exposure. J Hand Surg (Am) 16A:66–71, 1991.

Hawkins RL, Seeds NW: Effect of proteases and their inhibitors on neurite outgrowth from neonatal mouse sensory ganglia in culture. Brain Res 398:63–70, 1986.

Hendry IA: The response of adrenergic neurons to axotomy and nerve growth factor. Brain Res 94:87–98, 1975.

Heumann R: Regulation of the synthesis of nerve growth factor. J Exp Biol 132:133–150, 1987.

Hjortsberg U, Rosén I, Örbaek P, Balogh I, Lundborg G: Finger receptor dysfunction in dental technicians exposed to high frequency of vibration. Scand J Work Environ Health 15:339–344, 1989.

Ho ST, Yu HS: Ultrastructural changes of the peripheral nerve induced by vibration: An experimental study. Br J Ind Med 46:157–164, 1989.

Imai H, Tajima T, Natsumi Y: Successful reeducation of functional sensibility after median nerve repair at the wrist. J Hand Surg 16A:60–65, 1991.

Jacob JM, McQuarrie IG: Acceleration of axonal outgrowth in rat sciatic nerve at one week after axotomy. J Neurobiol 24:356–367, 1993.

Jenkins WM, Merzenich NM, Ochs MT, Allard T, Guic-Robles E: Functional reorganization of primary somatosensory cortex in adult owl monkeys after behaviorally controlled tactile stimulation. J Neurophysiol 63:82–104, 1990a.

Jenkins WM, Merzenich NM, Recanzona G: Neocortical representational dynamics in adult primates: Implications for neurophysiology. Neuropsychologia 28:573–584, 1990b.

Johnson Jr EM, Rich KM, Yip HK: The role of NGF in sensory neurons in vivo. Trends Neurosci 1:33–37, 1986.

Kandel ER, Hawkins RD: The biological bases of learning and individuality. Sci Am 267:53–60, 1992.

Kanje M, Rusovan A, Sisken B, Lundborg G: Pretreatment of rats with pulsed electromagnetic fields enhance regeneration of the sciatic nerve. Bioelectromagnetics 14:353–359, 1993.

Kanje M, Stenberg L, Ahlin A, Dahlin L: Activation of non-neuronal cells in the rat sciatic nerve in response to inflammation caused by implanted silicone tubes. Rest Neurol Neurosci 8:181–187, 1995.

Koo EH, Hoffman PN, Price DL: Levels of neurotransmitter and cytoskeletal protein mRNAs during nerve regeneration in sympathetic ganglia. Brain Res 449:361–363, 1988.

Kreutzberg GW, Schubert P: Changes in axonal flow during regeneration of mammalian motor nerves. Acta Neuropathol (Berl) 5(Suppl):70–75, 1971.

Krystosek A, Seeds NV: Peripheral neurons and Schwann cells secrete plasminogen activator. J Cell Biol 98:773–776, 1984.

Kuffler DP: Long-distance regulation of regenerating frog axons. J Exp Biol 132:151–160, 1987.

Lieberman AR: The axon reaction: A review of the principal features of perikaryal responses to axonal injury. Int Rev Neurobiol 14:99–124, 1971.

Lindholm D, Heumann R, Hengerer B, Thoenen H: Interleukin 1 increases stability and transcription of mRNA encoding nerve growth factor in cultured rat fibroblasts. J Biol Chem 263:16348–16351, 1988.

Lindholm D, Heumann R, Meyer M, Thoenen H: Interleukin-1 regulates synthesis of nerve growth factor in non-neuronal cells of rat sciatic nerve. Nature 330:658–659, 1987.

Liss AG, af Ekenstam FW, Wiberg M: Cell loss in sensory ganglia following peripheral nerve injury. An anatomical study in the cat. Scand J Plast Reconstr Hand Surg 28:177–187, 1994.

Lu X, Richardson PM: Inflammation near the nerve cell body enhances axonal regeneration. J Neurosci 11:972–978, 1991.

Lubinska L: Pattern of wallerian degeneration myelinated fibres in short and long peripheral stumps and in isolated segments of rat phrenic nerve. Interpretation of the role of axoplasmic flow of the trophic factor. Brain Res 233:227–240, 1982.

Luchetti R, Schoenhuber R, Alfarano M, Deluca S, De Cicco G, Landi A: Serial overnight recordings of intracarpal canal pressure in carpal tunnel syndrome patients with and without wrist splinting. J Hand Surg 19B:35–37, 1994.

Lundborg G: Structure and function of the intraneural microvessels as related to trauma, edema formation and nerve function. J Bone Joint Surg 57-A:938–948, 1975.

Lundborg G: The intrinsic vascularization of human peripheral nerves: Structural and functional aspects. J Hand Surg 4:34–41, 1979.

Lundborg G: Nerve Injury and Repair. Edinburgh, Churchill Livingstone, 1988.

Lundborg G, Dahlin L, Danielsen N, Zhao Q: Trophism, tropism and specificity. J Reconstr Microsurg 5:345–354, 1994a.

Lundborg G, Dahlin LB, Danielsen N, Hansson HA, Necking LE, Pyykkö I: Intraneural edema following exposure to vibration. Scand J Work Environ Health 13:326–329, 1987.

Lundborg G, Dahlin LB, Hansson H-A, Kanje M, Necking LE: Vibration exposure and peripheral nerve fiber damage. J Hand Surg 15A:346–351, 1990.

Lundborg G, Hansson HA: Regeneration of peripheral nerve through a preformed tissue space. Preliminary observations on the reorganization of regenerating nerve fibres and perineurium. Brain Res 178:573, 1979.

Lundborg G, Myers R, Powell H: Nerve compression injury and increase in endoneurial fluid pressure: A miniature compartment syndrome. J Neurol Neurosurg Psychiatry 46:1119–1124, 1983.

Lundborg G, Rosen B, Abrahamsson SO, Dahlin LB, Danielsen N: Tubular repair of the median nerve in the human forearm. Preliminary findings. J Hand Surg 19B:273–276, 1994b.

McQuarrie IG, Grafstein B: Axonal outgrowth enhanced by a previous nerve injury. Arch Neurol 29:53–55, 1973.

McQuarrie IG, Grafstein B, Gershon MD: Axonal regeneration in rat sciatic nerve: Effect of a conditioning lesion and of dcb-AMP. Brain Res *132*:443–453, 1977.

McQuarrie IG, Jacob JM: Conditioning nerve crush accelerates cytoskeletal protein transport in sprouts that form after a subsequent crush. J Comp Neurol *305*:139–147, 1991.

Meakin SO, Shooter EM: The nerve growth factor family of receptors. Trends Neurosci *15*:323–332, 1992.

Millesi H, Zöch G, Rath T: The gliding apparatus of peripheral nerve and its clinical significance. Ann Hand Surg 9:87–97, 1990.

Miyauchi A, Kanje M, Danielsen N, Dahlin LB: Role of macrophages in the stimulation and regeneration of sensory nerves by transposed granulation tissue and temporal aspects of the response. Scand J Plast Reconstr Hand Surg *30*: 1996.

Monaco S, Gehrmann J, Raivich G, Kreutzberg GW: MHC-positive, ramified macrophages in the normal and injured rat peripheral nervous system. J Neurocytol *21*:623–634, 1992.

Morris JH, Hudson AF, Weddell G: A study of degeneration and regeneration in the rat sciatic nerve based on electron microscopy. II. The development of the "regenerating unit." Zeitschrift für Zellforschung *124*:103–130, 1972a.

Morris JH, Hudson AR, Weddel G: A study of degeneration and regeneration in the rat sciatic nerve using electron microscopy. I. Traumatic degeneration of myelin in the proximal stump of the divided nerve. Zeitschrift für Zellforschung. *124*:76–102, 1972b.

Mulder DW, Lambert LH, Bastrom JA, Sprague RG: The neuropathies associated with diabetes mellitus. A clinical and electromyographic study of 103 unselected diabetic patients. Neurology *11*:275–284, 1961.

Myers RR, Powell HC: Endoneurial fluid pressure in peripheral neuropathies. *In* Hargens A (ed): Tissue fluid pressure and composition. Baltimore, Williams & Wilkins, 1981, pp 193–207.

Myers RR, Powell HC, Costello ML, Lambert LW, Zweifach BW: Endoneurial fluid pressure: Direct measurement with micropipettes. Brain Res *148*:510–515, 1978.

Nandy K: Histochemical study on chromatolytic neurons. Arch Neurol *18*:425–434, 1968.

Narini P, Novak C, Mackinnon SE, Coulson-Roos C: Occupational exposure to hand vibration in Northern Ontario gold miners. J Hand Surg *18A*:1051–1058, 1993.

Nathan CF: Secretory products of macrophages. J Clin Invest *79*:319–326, 1987.

Necking LE, Fridén J, Dahlin L, Lundborg G, Lundström R, Thornell LE: Frequency-related muscle damage following vibration. VIth International Conference on Hand and Vibration, Bonn, Germany, 1992.

Nilsson T, Hagberg M, Burström L, Kihlberg S, Lundström R: Risk assessment of impaired nerve conduction at the carpal tunnel in relation to vibration among platers and assemblers. *In* Dupuis H, Christ E, Sandover J, Taylor W, Okada A (eds): Proceedings of the 6th international conference on hand-arm vibration. Bonn, Germany, Druckzentrum Sutter & Partner GmbH, 1993, pp 395–402.

Ochoa J, Fowler TJ, Gilliatt RW: Anatomical changes in peripheral nerves compressed by a pneumatic tourniquet. J Anat *113*:433–455, 1972.

Ochs S: Fast axoplasmic transport in the fibres of chromatolyzed neurons. J Physiol *255*:249–261, 1976.

Ogata K, Naito M: Blood flow of peripheral nerve. Effects of dissection, stretching and compression. J Hand Surg *11B*:10–14, 1986.

Oldfors A: Macrophages in peripheral nerves. Acta Neuropathol *49*:43–49, 1980.

Olsson Y: Studies on vascular permeability in peripheral nerves. 1. Distribution of circulating fluorescent serum albumin in normal, crushed and sectioned rat sciatic nerve. Acta Neuropathol (Berl) 7:1–15, 1966a.

Olsson Y: Studies on vascular permeability in peripheral nerves. 2. Distribution of circulating fluorescent serum albumin in rat sciatic nerve after local injection of 5-hydroxytryptamine, histamine and compound 48/80. Acta Physiol Scand *69*(Suppl. no. 284):1–22, 1966b.

Olsson Y, Sjöstrand J: Origin of macrophages in wallerian degeneration of peripheral nerves demonstrated autoradiographically. Exp Neurol *23*:102–112, 1969.

Otto EA: Pharmacological effects of nerve growth factor and fibroblast growth factor applied to the transectioned sciatic nerve on neuron death in adult rat dorsal root ganglia. Neurosci Lett *83*:156–160, 1987.

Patterson PH: On the role of proteases, their inhibitors and the extracellular matrix in stimulating neurite outgrowth. J Physiol (Paris) *80*:207–211, 1985.

Powell HC, Myers RR: Pathology of experimental nerve compression. Lab Invest *55*:91–100, 1986.

Purves D, Njå A: Effect of nerve growth factor on synaptic depression following axotomy. Nature *260*:535–536, 1976.

Rich KM, Luszcynski JR, Osborne PA, Johnson EMJ: Nerve growth factor protects adult sensory neurons from cell death and atrophy caused by nerve injury. J Neurocytol *16*:261–268, 1987.

Rogister B, Delrée P, Leprince P, Martin D, Sadzot C, Malgrange B, Munuat C, Rigo JM, Lefebvre PP, Octave JN, Schoenen J, Moonen G: Transforming growth factor β as a neuronoglial signal during peripheral nervous system response to injury. J Neurosci Res *34*:32–43, 1993.

Rosén B, Lundborg G, Dahlin LB, Holmberg J, Karlson B: Nerve repair: Correlation of restitution of functional sensibility with specific cognitive capacities. J Hand Surg (Br) *19B*:452–458, 1994.

Rusovan A, Kanje M: Stimulation of regeneration of the rat sciatic nerve by 50 Hz sinusoidal magnetic fields. Exp Neurol *112*:312–316, 1991.

Rydevik B, Lundborg G, Bagge U: Effects of graded compression on intraneural blood flow. An in vitro study on rabbit tibial nerve. J Hand Surg (Am) 6:3–12, 1981.

Rydevik B, Lundborg G, Skalak D: Biomechanics of nerves and nerve injuries—biomechanical aspects. *In* Frankel VF, Nordin M (eds): Basic Biomechanics of the Musculoskeletal System. Philadelphia, Lea & Febiger, 1989, pp 75–87.

Schachner M: Neural recognition molecules and their influence on cellular functions. *In* Letourneau PC, Kater SB, Macagno ER (eds): The Nerve Growth Cone. New York, Raven Press 1992, pp 237–244.

Scherer SS, Kamholz J, Jakowlew SB: Axons modulate the expression of transforming growth factor-Beta in Schwann cells. Glia 8:265–276, 1993.

Schlaepfer W: Calcium-induced degeneration of axoplasm in isolated segments of rat peripheral nerve. Brain Res 69:203–215, 1974.

Schlaepfer W: Structural alterations of peripheral nerve induced by a calcium ionophore A23187. Brain Res *136*:1–9, 1977.

Schlaepfer WW, Hasler MB: Characterization of the calcium-induced disruption of neurofilaments in rat peripheral nerve. Brain Res *136*:1–9, 1979.

Seddon H: Three types of nerve injury. Brain 66:237–288, 1943.

Seddon H (ed): Surgical Disorders of The Peripheral Nerves, 2nd ed. Edinburgh, Churchill Livingstone, 1972.

Shdanow DA: Die Lymphwege des peripherischen und Zentralnervensystems. Anat Anz 71:231–245, 1931.

Silverstein B, Fine L: Occupational factors and carpal tunnel syndrome. Am J Ind Med *11*:343–358, 1987.

Sjöberg J, Kanje M: The initial period of peripheral nerve regeneration and the importance of the local environment for the conditioning effect. Brain Res *529*:79–84, 1990.

Spencer PS, Politis MJ, Pellegrino RG, Weinborg HJ: Control of Schwann cell behavior during nerve degeneration and regeneration. *In* Gorio A, Millesi H, Minigrino S (eds): Post-traumatic nerve regeneration. New York, Raven Press, 1981, pp 411–426.

Stoll G, Griffin JW, Li CY, Trapp BD: Wallerian degeneration in the peripheral nervous system: Participation of both Schwann cells and macrophages in myelin degradation. J Neurocytol *18*:671–683, 1989.

Stolz B, Erulkar SD, Kuffler DP: Macrophages direct process elongation from adult frog motorneurons in culture. Proc R Soc Lond *244*:227–231, 1991.

Strömberg T, Lundborg G, Holmquist B, Dahlin LB: Impaired regeneration in rat sciatic nerves exposed to short term vibration. J Hand Surg *21B*:746–749, 1996.

Szabo R, Gelberman R, Williamson R, Hargens A: Effects of increased systemic blood pressure on the tissue fluid pressure. Threshold of peripheral nerve. J Orthop Res *1*:172–178, 1983.

Szabo RM, Bay BK, Sharkey NA, Gaut C: Median nerve displacement through the carpal canal. J Hand Surg *19A*:901–906, 1994.

Takeuchi T, Futatsuka M, Imanishi H, Yamada S: Pathological changes observed in the finger biopsy of patients with vibration-induced white finger. Scand J Work Environ Health *12*:280–283, 1986.

Takeuchi T, Takeya M, Imanishi H: Ultrastructural changes in peripheral nerves of the fingers of three vibration-exposed persons with Raynaud's phenomenon. Scand J Work Environ Health *14*:31–35, 1988.

Tanaka K, Zhang QL, Webster HF: Myelinated fiber regeneration after sciatic nerve crush: Morphometric observations in young adult and aging mice and the effects of macrophage suppression and conditioning lesions. Exp Neurol *118*:53–61, 1992.

Taniuchi M, Clark HB, Schweitzer JB, Johnson EMJ: Expression of nerve growth factor receptors by Schwann cells of axotomized peripheral nerves: Ultrastructural location, suppresion by axonal contact and binding properties. J Neurosci 8:664–681, 1988.

Tetzlaff W, Bisby MA, Kreutzberg GW: Changes in cytoskeletal proteins in the rat facial nucleus following axotomy. J Neurosci 8:3181–3189, 1988.

Thomas PK, Olsson Y: Microscopic anatomy and function of the connective tissue components of peripheral nerve. *In* Dyck PK, Thomas PK, Lambert EH, Bunge R (eds): Peripheral Neuropathy, Vol 1. Philadelphia, W. B. Saunders Company, 1984, pp 97–120.

Torvik A: Central chromatolysis and the axon reaction: A reappraisal. Neuropathol Appl Neurobiol 2:423–432, 1976.

Vial JD: The early changes in the axoplasm during wallerian degeneration. J Biophysical Biochemical Cytol 4:551–556, 1958.

Wall JT, Kaas JH: Long-term cortical consequences of reinnervation errors after nerve regeneration in monkeys. Brain Res 372:400–404, 1986.

Wall JT, Kaas JH, Sur M, Nelsen RJ, Felleman DJ, Merzenich MM: Functional reorganization in somatosensory cortical areas 3b and 1 of adult monkeys after median nerve repair: Possible relationships to sensory recovery in humans. J Neurosci 6:218–233, 1986.

Weinberg HJ, Spencer PS: The fate of Schwann cells isolated from axonal contact. J Neurocytol 7:555–569, 1978.

Wieslander G, Norbäck D, Göthe CJ, Juhlin L: Carpal tunnel syndrome (CTS) and exposure to vibration, repetitive wrist movements and heavy manual work: A case-referent study. Br J Ind Med 46:43–47, 1989.

Wilgis S, Murphy R: The significance of longitudinal excursions in peripheral nerves. Hand Clin 2:761–768, 1986.

Zhao Q, Dahlin LB, Kanje M, Lundborg G: The formation of a "pseudo-nerve" in silicone chambers in the absence of regenerating axons. Brain Res 592:106–114, 1992.

Chapter 38

• George E. Omer, Jr

The Prognosis for Untreated Traumatic Injuries

The more extensive and severe the injury to the involved extremity, the longer the time required for equilibrium (homeostasis) of the tissues. Nerves are only as functional as the pertinent sensory receptors and muscle-tendon motors. Multiple nerve involvement jeopardizes functional recovery of the entire extremity more than an isolated nerve injury. Severe vascular deficiency, chronic osteomyelitis, osseous nonunion, and articular incongruity all contribute to fibrotic infiltration, adhesions, and limited joint motion. Clinical studies of peripheral nerve recovery in humans show considerable variation because return of useful function depends as much on the total response of the extremity to the injury as on the regeneration of the injured nerve (Omer, 1974).

During World War II, Seddon (1943) introduced a simple classification of traumatic nerve injuries. In this classification, minimal injury is termed neurapraxia and may be secondary to localized ischemic demyelination. Moderate injury is termed axonotmesis. It is characterized by interruption of the axons and their myelin sheath; the endoneurial tubes remain intact and guide the regenerating axons to their appropriate peripheral connections. Severe injury, termed neurotmesis, involves a nerve that either has been completely severed or is so seriously disorganized that spontaneous regeneration is impossible. Most traumatic injuries, including fractures, dislocations, and gunshot wounds, can result in any one or combinations of these three types of injury patterns.

Sunderland (1951) has provided the following classification in relation to the internal structure of the nerve trunk. (1) First-degree trauma—loss of axon conduction; (2) second-degree trauma—transection of the axon with an intact endoneurial sheath; (3) third-degree trauma—transection of axon and endoneurial sheath inside an intact perineurium; (4) fourth-degree trauma—transection of many axons with their endoneurial sheath and the perineurium; nerve trunk continuity is maintained by epineurial tissue; and (5) fifth degree trauma—transection of the entire nerve trunk. Injuries may not be of uniform severity, either across or along the length of the nerve trunk. Partial and mixed lesions are produced by varying combinations of the first four degrees of injury.

It is clinically important to assess the percentage of nerves that will recover from various types of traumatic injuries and the time required for return of function.

LACERATIONS

Lacerations are low-velocity injuries that do not demonstrate significant spontaneous recovery. Lacerations usually result in neurotmesis (Seddon) or fifth-degree injury (Sunderland), and the total loss of nerve function resulting from this injury demands exploration and reconstruction of the affected nerve.

A problem is the injured major nerve with minimal involvement that is not diagnosed because most of the nerve's function can be demonstrated. The patient with a laceration in an extremity should have a complete examination, which includes assessment of all branches of a potentially involved peripheral nerve. Lacerations with associated loss of peripheral nerve function should be diagnosed as complete lesions (neurotmesis) until proved otherwise by intraoperative examination.

PROJECTILE INJURIES

Firearms are the second leading cause of injury-related death in the United States (Schwab et al, 1995). At present, there are 732 shootings per day, of which 75% result from handguns (Ordog et al, 1994a). Firearms lead to approximately 236,000 injuries per year, with 65,000 annual hospitalizations. Ordog and colleagues (1994b) recorded 28,150 patients with gunshot wounds over a 14-year period (1977–1991) seen in a big city emergency room. Following their evaluation, 16,892 (60%) were treated as outpatients. Rifles were involved in only 2% of the outpatient cases, and shotguns were involved in 4% of cases. Single missiles from handguns were involved in 91% of cases, whereas multiple missiles were evident in 3% of the outpatient cases. Peripheral nerve injuries were diagnosed in 114 (0.08%) patients, including injuries of the digital, radial, ulnar, and peroneal nerves. Only 19% of these patients returned for subsequent nerve repair.

Civilian handgun injuries are usually low velocity, with a smaller shock wave and temporary cavitation (neurapraxia or axonotmesis) and, therefore, may not require extensive debridement, surgical exploration and decompression, and delayed primary closure (Howland and Ritchey, 1971; Marcus et al, 1980; Ordog et al, 1994b). However, the reported incidence of peripheral nerve injuries as a result of civilian gunshot wounds ranges from 22% to 100% (Wiss and Gellman, 1992).

The incidence of peripheral nerve injuries associated with gunshot wounds has been relatively well documented in war wounds. After World War I, the incidence of peripheral nerve injuries in all nonfatal wounds was estimated to be 2% (Campbell, 1959). Total peripheral nerve injuries in

nerve lesions recovered spontaneously. If the diagnosis of an entrapped median nerve is made, surgical release is required.

The ulnar nerve has the highest incidence of injury related to dislocations of the elbow (Gurdjian and Smathers, 1945). Cubitus valgus resulting from trauma is the major cause of delayed ulnar palsy at the elbow, and surgical intervention has been the accepted treatment. The potential for full motor recovery after operation is reduced greatly in patients in whom neuropathy symptoms have been present for more than a year.

Radial nerve injuries at the elbow are often associated with Monteggia's fracture-dislocations, and the majority have spontaneous recovery of function. Boyd and Boals (1969) reported neurological deficits in 5 of 159 Monteggia's lesions, with total spontaneous recovery.

Hip

Epstein (1974) noted that the sciatic nerve was injured in approximately 13% of 282 patients with posterior fracture-dislocation of the hip. Two thirds involved only the peroneal division, and one third involved both components of the sciatic nerve. He also recorded a 6% incidence of neuropathy following simple posterior dislocations. Hunter (1969) reported 83% spontaneous recovery of sciatic nerve lesions, but Seddon (1975) recorded that only 73% had normal or slightly impaired function. Secondary sciatic neuropathy may develop within 24 to 72 hours when traction is applied to a dislocation without reduction (Derian and Bibighaus, 1974). Exploration of the clinically complete neuropathy resulting from fracture-dislocation is appropriate in 3 to 4 months.

Knee

The incidence of nerve injury is higher in dislocations and stretch injuries than in fractures. Nerve problems occur in approximately 18% of knee dislocations (usually traction injuries that vary from neurapraxia to neurotmesis) (Kennedy, 1963). Peroneal nerve palsy has an even greater incidence in an injury to the knee with disruption damage to the lateral ligamentous structures. Towne and co-workers (1971) recorded a 56% rate of injury to the peroneal nerve in 18 knees with lateral compartment syndromes. Meyers and associates (1975) recorded 14 peroneal palsies in 53 cases; 12 nerves did not regain function. Ottolenghi and Traversa (1974) described 22 cases in which the common peroneal nerve was injured; 12 did not regain function.

Peroneal nerve injury sometimes is associated with femoral traction. If the leg is maintained in external rotation to align fractures, the peroneal nerve may be compressed at the head of the fibula. Highet and Holmes (1943) reported eight cases of traction peroneal palsy; four had complete rupture, and four had macroscopic changes. Only one of six neurorrhaphies regained any function. However, White (1968) described six cases in which two nerves were sutured with functional recovery; the other four nerves had spontaneous recovery, with onset between 2 and 6 months and complete function between 4 and 12 months. Meyers and colleagues (1975) record 14 peroneal palsies in 53 patients, in whom 12 nerves did not regain function. Towne and co-workers (1971) used irradiated nerve homografts in four cases of peroneal nerve injury secondary to a lateral compartment syndrome of the knee; however, none of the nerve grafts were successful.

MANAGEMENT PROGRAM

Closed Traumatic Injuries

Closed nerve injuries associated with fractures of long bones should be observed for 4 to 5 months because approximately 85% of these lesions have spontaneous clinical recovery. The older the patient and the more severe the trauma, the less likely is spontaneous recovery. When manipulating fractures and dislocations, one should remember the potential additional injury to nerves, such as the spiral fracture with radial angulation involving the distal third of the humerus.

Nerve injuries associated with a dislocated joint or a fracture adjacent to a joint are suspect because fascial envelopes hold the nerves close to the bone near joints. These fracture-dislocation accidents often stretch the nerve, resulting in an axonotmesis lesion with spontaneous recovery that may require 4 to 9 months. The nerve lesion associated with a dislocation is less likely to have spontaneous recovery than is a nerve lesion associated with a fracture.

After a period of 3 to 4 months, it is not inappropriate to explore the clinically complete nerve lesion in stretch injuries from dislocated joints, severely comminuted fractures, and fractures adjacent to joints (Omer and Pirela-Cruz, 1994). An external neurolysis is recommended when an intact nerve is found. About 60% of these nerves will have a neuroma in continuity, however, and a decision regarding resection of the neuroma requires special equipment for recording nerve action potentials or other electrodiagnostic studies (Kline, 1980; Kline and Hudson, 1995).

Open Traumatic Injuries

Open wounds with associated nerve palsy require debridement. Incisions should be placed to directly observe the neurovascular structures. Although appropriate treatment for a severed nerve is neurorrhaphy, many factors prevent ideal treatment of gunshot wound injuries. The condition of the entire extremity, the level and extent of the nerve injury, and the time until definitive care can be provided influence the results of the initial operation. A problem during debridement is the potential nerve gap. Sharp lacerations without loss of nerve tissue that are allowed to persist for a number of weeks result in nerve gaps secondary to retraction and joint motion. In the complex injury with fractures and soft tissue loss, the nerve gap is associated with extensive scarring. If the disrupted nerve is not sutured, two fine wire sutures are aligned in the epineurium of the proximal and distal portions of the nerve. Each wire suture is then sutured to adjacent soft tissue to prevent retraction. Later, the disruption in the nerve can be identified radiologically, and the initial internal alignment of the nerve can be identified at the time of reconstruction (Omer, 1988, 1991). World War II studies indicate an average loss from optimal motor recovery following suture of gaps, of about 6% per cm up to a critical limit of 7.5 cm (Woodhall and Beebe, 1956).

In some cases, multiple nerve palsies resulting from high-velocity gunshot wounds but without disruption at the time of initial debridement may be observed up to 9 months, because 69% of these lesions undergo spontaneous recovery within 9 months. However, the proximal (high) injury presents a very difficult problem. It may be a considerable distance from the site of the nerve lesion to the first motor point to be reinnervated. From the time of injury, there is progressive distortion and degeneration of the distal motor and sensory end-organs, with associated slowing of the regenerative process for axon regrowth. Expectant management could be prolonged to the time when suture of a previously unrecognized severed nerve would be without hope of functional recovery (Omer, 1980).

At 3 to 4 months, it is appropriate to explore the clinically complete nerve lesion in gunshot wounds above the elbow or knee, stretch injuries from dislocated joints, and fractures adjacent to joints (Omer and Pirela-Cruz, 1994). Neurolysis is recommended when an intact nerve is found during exploration of a nonfunctioning nerve. Omer (1974) performed external neurolysis in 59 cases from the Vietnam War in which the injured nerve was found in continuity but bound in scar tissue. Nine of the cases were excluded secondary to short follow-up (less than 3 months), but the neurolysis procedure was successful in 60% of the remaining 50 nerves. When function of the extremity returns within the time frame for spontaneous recovery after injury, there is doubt concerning the efficacy of neurolysis, because the intact nerve in such a case might have recovered spontaneously without surgery (Omer, 1991). In the same study, of 45 gunshot wounds followed for 12 months or longer, 25 demonstrated clinical return of function. Ten of the nerves recovered during the time frame allotted for spontaneous recovery. Therefore, neurolysis was successful in restoring function in only 15 (33%) of 45 nerves injured by gunshot wounds. Kline (1980) subsequently developed an operating room technique for stimulating the involved nerve proximally and recording distal to the neuroma in continuity. The nerve action potential is related to axon population and myelin return. Significant spontaneous recovery is gained in approximately 90% of those nerves when a normal nerve action potential is recorded across a neuroma in continuity at 3 months after injury.

PROGNOSIS FOR FUNCTIONAL PERFORMANCE

Motor and sensory performance are greatly improved by practice and experience. In evaluating outcomes, it is important to consider that final function is improved by retraining that is directed at increasing the patient's ability to use new and altered patterns of motor and sensory innervation. It is difficult to put a time limit on this phase of recovery, because it depends on nerve regeneration plus other factors such as age, intelligence, patience, perseverance, and motivation (Al-Ghazal et al, 1994; Rosen et al, 1994). It is a slow process that certainly continues for at least 5 years following initial return of function.

References

Al-Ghazal SK, McKiernan M, Khan K, McCann J: Results of clinical assessment after primary digital nerve repair. J Hand Surg *19B:*255–257, 1994.

Barton NJ: Radial nerve lesions. Hand *3:*200–208, 1973.

Bjik KD, Bellamy RF: Editorial: A note on combat casualty statistics. Mil Med, *149:*229–230, 1984.

af Bjorkesten G: Suture of war injuries to peripheral nerves. Clinical studies of results. Acta Chir Scand *95*(suppl 119):1–188, 1947.

Blom S, Dahlback LO: Nerve injuries in dislocations of the shoulder joint and fractures of the neck of the humerus. Acta Chir Scand *136:*461–466, 1970.

Boyd HB, Boals JC: The Monteggia lesion. A review of 159 cases. Clin Orthop *66:*94–100, 1969.

Brown JT: Nerve injuries complicating dislocation of the shoulder. J Bone Joint Surg *34B:*526, 1952.

Campbell EH Jr: The Mediterranean (formerly North African) theater of operation. *In* Coates JB Jr, Spurling RG, Woodhall B (eds): Surgery in World War II. Washington, DC, Office of the Surgeon General, Department of the Army, 1959, pp 231–238.

D'Ambrosia RD: Supracondylar fractures of the humerus—prevention of cubitus varus. J Bone Joint Surg *54A:*60–66, 1972.

Derian PS, Bibighaus AJ: Sciatic nerve entrapment by ectopic bone after posterior fracture–dislocation of the hip. South Med J *67:*209–210, 1974.

Epstein HC: Posterior fracture-dislocations of the hip. J Bone Joint Surg *56A:*1103–1127, 1974.

Fowles JV, Kassab MT: Displaced supracondylar fractures of the elbow in children. J Bone Joint Surg *56B:*490–500, 1974.

Garcia A Jr, Maeck BH: Radial nerve injuries in fractures of the shaft of the humerus. Am J Surg *99:*625–627, 1960.

Goodall RJ: Nerve injuries in fresh fractures. Tex Med *52:*93–94, 1956.

Grant RE, Epps CH Jr, Cotler JM, Kim DD: Complications of treatment of fractures of the humeral shaft. *In* Epps CH Jr (ed): Complications in Orthopaedic Surgery, 3rd ed. Philadelphia, Lippincott-Raven, 1994, pp 257–284.

Gurdjian ES, Smathers HM: Peripheral nerve injury in fractures and dislocations of long bones. J Neurosurg *2:*202–211, 1945.

Hardin WD, O'Connell RC, Adinolfi MF, Kerstein MD: Traumatic arterial injuries of the upper extremity: Determinants of disability. Am J Surg *150:*226–270, 1985

Highet WB, Holmes W: Traction injuries to the lateral popliteal nerve and traction injuries to peripheral nerves after suture. Br J Surg *30:*212–233, 1943.

Holstein A, Lewis GB: Fractures of the humerus with radial nerve paralysis. J Bone Joint Surg *45A:*1382–1388, 1963.

Howland WS Jr, Ritchey SJ: Gunshot fractures in civilian practice. J Bone Joint Surg *53A:*47–55, 1971.

Hunter GA: Posterior dislocation and fracture-dislocation of the hip, a review of fifty-seven patients. J Bone Joint Surg *51B:*38–44, 1969.

Kelsey JL, Pastides H, Kreiger N, Harris C, Chernow RA: Upper Extremity Disorders. A Survey of their Frequency and Cost in the United States. St. Louis, C.V. Mosby, 1980, p 40.

Kennedy JC: Complete dislocation of the knee joint. J Bone Joint Surg *45A:*889–904, 1963.

Keon-Cohen BT: Fractures at the elbow. J Bone joint Surg *48A:*1623–1639, 1966.

Kettelkamp DB, Alexander H: Clinical review of radial nerve injury. J Trauma *7:*424–432, 1967.

Klenerman L: Fractures of the shaft of the humerus. J Bone Joint Surg *48B:*105–111, 1966.

Kline DG: Evaluation of neuroma-in-continuity. *In* Omer GE Jr, Spinner M (eds): Management of Peripheral Nerve Problems. Philadelphia, W. B. Saunders Company, 1980, pp 450–461.

Kline DG, Hudson AR: Nerve Injuries. Philadelphia, W. B. Saunders Company, 1995, pp 101–116.

Leffert RD: Brachial plexus injuries. N Engl J Med *291:*1059–1067, 1974.

Leffert RD, Seddon H: Infraclavicular brachial plexus injuries. J Bone Joint Surg *47B:*9–22, 1965.

Lewis D, Miller EM: Peripheral nerve injuries associated with fractures. Ann Surg *76:*528–538, 1922.

Luce EA, Griffin WO: Shotgun injuries of the upper extremity. J Trauma *18:*487–492, 1978.

Marcus NA, Blair WF, Shuck JM, Omer GE Jr: Low-velocity gunshot wounds to extremities. J Trauma *20:*1061–1064, 1980.

Mast JW, Spiegel RG, Harvey JP, Harrison C: Fractures of the humeral shaft. A retrospective study of 240 adult fractures. Clin Orthop *112:*254–262, 1975.

Matsen FA III, Thomas SC, Rockwood CA Jr: Anterior glenohumeral instability. *In* Rockwood CA Jr, Matsen FA III (eds): The Shoulder. Philadelphia, W. B. Saunders Company, 1990, pp 526–622.

McLaughlin HL, Cavallaro WV: Primary anterior dislocations of the shoulder. Am J Surg *80:*615–621, 1950.

Meyers MH, Moore TM, Harvey JP: Follow-up notes on articles previously published in the Journal: Traumatic dislocation of the knee joint. J Bone Joint Surg *57A:*430–433, 1975.

Omer GE Jr: Injuries to nerves of the upper extremity. J Bone Joint Surg *56A:*1615–1624, 1974.

Omer GE Jr: The results of untreated traumatic injuries. *In* Omer GE Jr, Spinner M (eds): Management of Peripheral Nerve Problems. Philadelphia, W. B. Saunders Company, 1980, pp 502–506.

Omer GE Jr: Nerve, neuroma, and pain problems related to upper limb amputations. Orthop Clin North Am *12:*751–762, 1981.

Omer GE Jr: Results of untreated peripheral nerve injuries. Clin Orthop *163:*15–19, 1982.

Omer GE Jr: Fractures and major nerve injuries in the fractured extremity. *In* Meyers MH (ed): The Multiply Injured Patient with Complex Fractures. Philadelphia, Lea & Febiger, 1984, pp 156–161.

Omer GE Jr: War injuries of the hand. *In* Tubiana R (ed): The Hand, Vol. 3. Philadelphia, W. B. Saunders Company, 1988, pp 903–924.

Omer GE Jr: Nerve injuries associated with gunshot wounds of the extremities. *In* Gelberman RH (ed): Operative Nerve Repair and Reconstruction. Philadelphia, J.B. Lippincott Company, 1991, pp 655–670.

Omer GE Jr, Eversmann WW Jr: Peripheral nerve problems. *In* Burkhalter WE (ed): Orthopedic Surgery in Vietnam. Washington, DC, Office of the U.S. Army Surgeon General and Center of Military History, 1994, pp 155–188.

Omer GE Jr, Pirela-Cruz M: Complications of peripheral nerve injuries. *In* Epps CH Jr (ed): Complications in Orthopaedic Surgery, 2nd edition. Philadelphia, J.B. Lippincott Company, 1994, pp 811–856.

Ordog GJ, Balasubramanium S, Wasserberger J, Kram H, Bishop M, Shoemaker W: Extremity gunshot wounds: Part one—identification and treatment of patients at high risk of vascular injury. J Trauma *36:*358–368, 1994a.

Ordog GJ, Wasserberger J, Balasubramanium S, Shoemaker W: Civilian gunshot wounds—outpatient management. J Trauma *36:*106–111, 1994b.

Ottolenghi CE, Traversa CH: Vascular and nerve complications in injuries of the knee. Reconstr Surg Traumatol *14:*114–135, 1974.

Rakolta GG, Omer GE Jr: Combat-sustained femoral nerve injuries. Surg Gynecol Obstet *128:*813–817, 1969.

Rich NM, Spencer FC: Vascular Trauma. Philadelphia, W. B. Saunders Company, 1978, pp 125–155.

Rosen B, Lundborg G, Dahlin LB, Holmberg J, Karlson B: Nerve repair: Correlation of restitution of functional sensibility with specific cognitive capacities. J Hand Surg *19B:*452–458, 1994.

Rothberg JM, Tahmoush AJ, Oldakowski R: The epidemiology of causalgia among soldiers wounded in Vietnam. Milit Med *148:*347–350, 1983.

Rowe CR: Instabilities of the glenohumeral joint. Bull Hosp Joint Dis *39:*180–186, 1978.

Schwab CW, Chairman, Violence Prevention Task Force of the Eastern Association for the Surgery of Trauma: Violence in America: A public health crisis—the role of firearms. J Trauma *38:*163–168, 1995.

Seddon HJ: Three types of nerve injury. Brain *66:*237–288, 1943.

Seddon HJ: Nerve lesions complicating certain closed bone injuries. JAMA *135:*691–694, 1947.

Seddon HJ: Surgical Disorders of the Peripheral Nerves, 2nd ed. Edinburgh, Churchill Livingstone, 1975, pp 691–694.

Shaw JL, Sakellarides H: Radial-nerve paralysis associated with fractures of the humerus. A review of forty-five cases. J Bone Joint Surg *49A:*899–902, 1967.

Simeone FA: Neurological complications of closed shoulder injuries. Orthop Clin North Am *6:*499–506, 1975.

Spar I: A neurologic complication following Monteggia fracture. Clin Orthop 122:207–209, 1977.

Spitzer AG, Paterson DC: Acute nerve involvement in supracondylar fractures of the humerus in children. Proceedings, Australian Orthopaedic Association. J Bone Joint Surg *55B:*227, 1973.

Sunderland S: A classification of peripheral nerve injuries producing loss of function. Brain *74:*491–516, 1951.

Sunderland S: Nerve and Nerve Injuries, 2nd ed. Edinburgh, Churchill-Livingstone, 1978, pp 505–507.

Towne LC, Blazina ME, Marmor L, Lawrence JF: Lateral compartment syndrome of the knee. Clin Orthop *76:*160–168, 1971.

Visser PA, Hemreck AS, Pierce GE, et al: Prognosis of nerve injuries incurred during acute trauma to peripheral arteries. Am J Surg *140:*596–599, 1980.

White J: The results of traction injuries of the common peroneal nerve. J Bone Joint Surg, *50B:*346–350, 1968.

Wiss DA, Gellman H: Gunshot wounds to the musculoskeletal system. *In* Browner BD, Jupiter JB, Levine AM, Trafton PG (eds): Skeletal Trauma. Philadelphia, W. B. Saunders Company, 1992, pp 367–400.

Woodhall B, Beebe GW (eds): Peripheral nerve regeneration. VA medical monograph. Washington, DC, U.S. Government Printing Office, 1956, pp 5, 191, 311–340, 498.

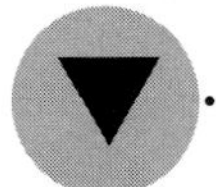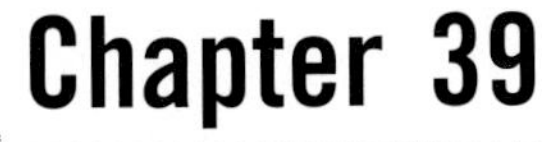

Chapter 39

• Madjid Samii

Diagnosis and Management of Intracranial Nerve Lesions

The introduction of the operating microscope into peripheral nerve surgery (Jacobson, 1963; Michon and Masse, 1964; Smith, 1964) brought a new dimension into the surgical treatment of cranial nerves. The satisfying results derived from the microsurgical techniques of neurolysis, nerve suture, and nerve graft after peripheral nerve lesions considerably enlarged the indication of operative treatment of cranial nerve lesions (Millesi, 1968; Samii 1970). During the past three decades, previously existing operative methods were refined, and new approaches have been put into practice.

With increasing experience, the preservation and functional reconstruction of cranial nerves became an important component of the operating concept of tumor surgery in the region of the cerebellopontine angle, the base of the skull, and the neck.

In this chapter, surgical possibilities with regard to specific cranial nerves are reviewed. A systematic record of the etiology of lesions, topographic anatomy, and clinical symptomatology would be too comprehensive. Special attention is given to the surgical methods of preserving and repairing cranial nerve function through nerve decompression, neurolysis, nerve suture, and nerve grafting.

OLFACTORY NERVE (FIRST CRANIAL NERVE)

The olfactory nerve may be damaged by frontobasal injuries with fractures in the region of the cribriform plate and by space-occupying processes in the region of the anterior cranial fossa. The neurosurgical approach to the anterior cranial fossa and the sella region may involve sectioning of the fila olfactoria, the bulb, or the tractus olfactorius. Therefore, in cases of frontobasal cerebrospinal fluid (CSF) fistulas without loss of the sense of smell, the question arises as to whether the rhinosurgical approach would be more advisable than the subfrontal to repair a dura leak and at the same time preserve the olfactory nerve. In pituitary gland surgery one has to think of similar aspects. Olfactory function can be saved by choosing either the subfrontal, the transseptosphenoidal, or the transethmoidosphenoidal approach. Until the present there has been no report on surgical restoration of a damaged olfactory nerve. For this reason, before each surgical procedure in the region of the anterior fossa, the surgeon should be certain that craniotomy is really the best available method.

OPTIC NERVE (SECOND CRANIAL NERVE)

The optic nerve as a rostrally situated part of the brain has no regeneration power after interruption of continuity;

therefore, surgical efforts are restricted to decompressive relief operations. The subfrontal approach may be given preference in cases of traumatic swelling within the bony canal, hematoma of the optic sheath, or retrobulbar hemorrhage. Early diagnosis and immediate surgical intervention may be of great significance for the prognosis (Fig. 39–1). The transethmoidal route to decompression of the optic canal has been favored by Japanese authors (Fukado, 1981).

It is possible to preserve existing visual function. Microsurgical technique is mandatory in the transsphenoidal procedure and is a great help in subfrontal procedures for the removal of inflammatory space-occupying processes or tumors in the sellar region and orbit.

Functional improvement of visual power and in the field of vision is frequently observed after decompression of the optic apparatus by any surgical approach (Fig. 39–2A and B). This occurs particularly when edema is the main cause of the optic nerve fiber dysfunction.

Among 155 treated cases of pituitary tumors, we found disturbances of the visual field in 5 patients, although the adenoma of the pituitary gland did not produce any compression of the optic nerve or the optic chiasm (Samii and Schürmann, 1978). In 1 patient, who appeared clinically to have a bitemporal hemianopsia, there was a vascular compression of the optic chiasm caused by anomalies of both anterior cerebral arteries (Fig. 39–3).

According to our cisternotomographic investigations, the position and course of the optic nerve in the craniocaudal direction showed considerable variations. These variations

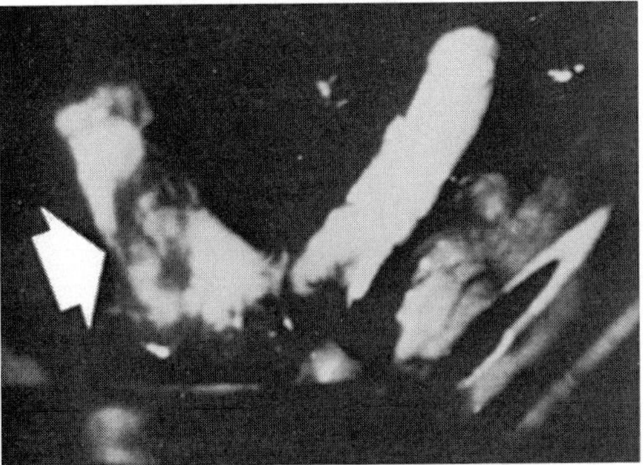

FIGURE 39–1. A 20-year-old patient. Amaurosis 3 hours after a head injury with fracture of the left optic canal. Decompression of the considerably swollen left optic nerve *(arrow)* in the optic nerve canal 3½ hours after the beginning of the amaurosis. Postoperatively, the patient had a satisfactory recovery.

371

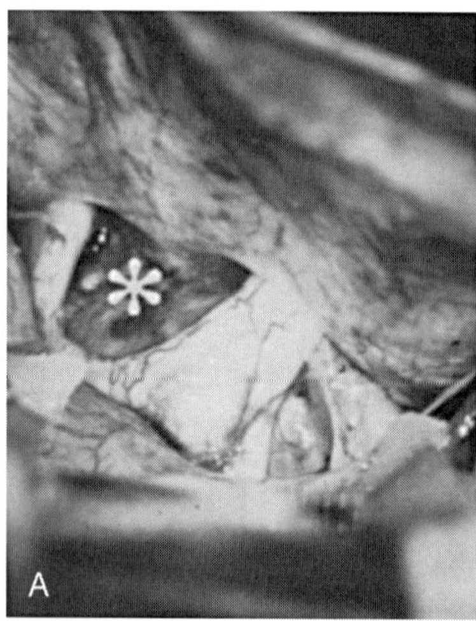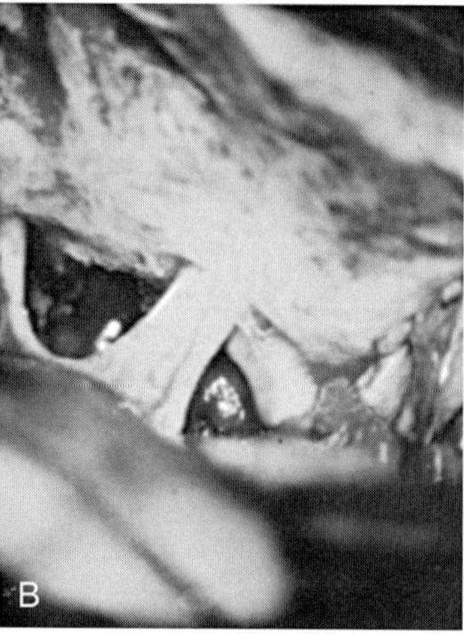

FIGURE 39–2. *A,* Compression of optic nerves and optic chiasm due to an intrasellar and suprasellar pituitary gland tumor *(asterisk). B,* Decompression of the optic nerves and the optic chiasm after removal of the pituitary gland tumor.

were revealed by a study of 50 normal pneumoencephalotomograms. The optic chiasm is located close to the diaphragma sellae or up to 10 mm from it. Knowing the possible variations in the course of the optic nerves to the craniocaudal line, we again studied the pneumoencephalographic films of 19 patients with visual disturbances in which an intracranial space-occupying process could be excluded with certainty. In 3 patients with visual field defect (temporal or bitemporal upper quadrantanopia), we found a low projection of the optic chiasm in the cistern picture. A noticeable compression of the optic chiasm was caused by the dorsum sellae (Samii, 1972). However, these examinations were retrospective studies, and the patients could not be recalled for operative treatment. In these cases, a partial resection of the dorsum sellae possibly would have also led to a functional improvement of the clinical syndrome (Fig. 39–4). Retrobulbar tumors in the region of the orbit, with increasing size, may cause a slow and progressive reduction of the visual power because of a compression of the optic nerve. This may especially occur if the optic sheath meningioma is compressing the nerve because the tumor grows all around it and continually constricts the nerve (Fig. 39–5A and B). Using microsurgical technique after transfrontal orbitotomy for the removal of the tumor, it is possible to free the optic nerve without injuring the bulb or other intraorbital

structures (Fig. 39–5C and D). At present, magnetic resonance imaging is the method of choice for the delineation of the optic nerve and chiasm, and of any compressing or infiltrating lesions.

OCULOMOTOR, TROCHLEAR, AND ABDUCENT NERVES (THIRD, FOURTH, AND SIXTH CRANIAL NERVES)

Lesions of the oculomotor, trochlear, and abducent nerves, as long as they are not nuclear in origin, often show complete regression after surgical intervention during the optimal time period. Supratentorial intracranial space-occupying processes of a different etiology lead to compression in the tentorial notch, the consequence of which is strain of the oculomotor nerves near the brain stem. An early elimination of the cause of the compression permits complete return of function. Direct compression of the oculomotor nerve in the tentorial notch may also occur from a tumor or aneurysm (Fig. 39–6A and B).

The very close relation of the oculomotor nerves to the sinus cavernosus explains their involvement in traumatic processes (e.g., carotid cavernosus fistula), inflammatory thrombosis of sinus cavernosus, and parasellar tumors. Retrobulbar tumors with increasing volume may lead to a neurogenic oculomotor lesion. Although previous experiences regarding relieving and decompressive interventions on the

FIGURE 39–3. Vascular compression of the optic chiasm *(asterisk)* with the clinical picture of a bitemporal hemianopsia caused by an anomaly of both anterior cerebral arteries *(arrow).*

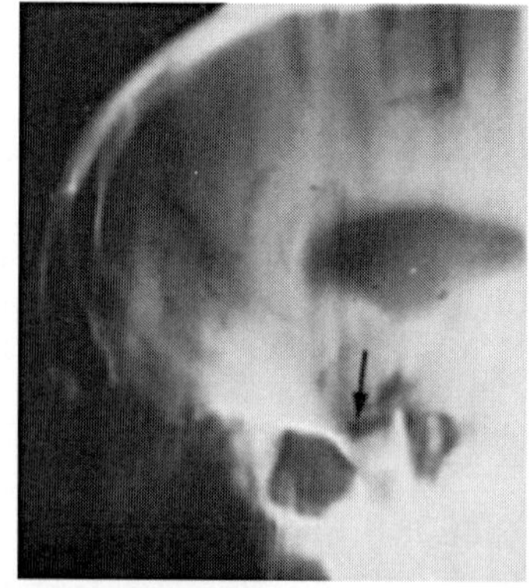

FIGURE 39–4. Midline pneumoencephalotomogram of a patient with bitemporal upper quadrantanopia. The soft tissue shadows of the optic chiasm *(arrow)* are distinctly visible. The chiasm is located very low and is compressed by the dorsum sellae.

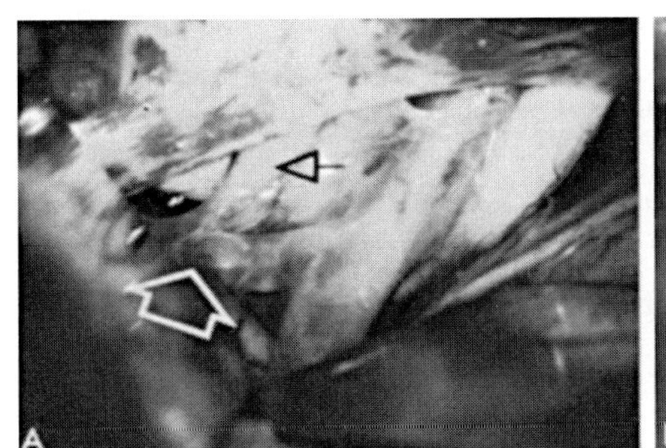

FIGURE 39–5. *A,* Computed tomogram of a retrobulbar optic nerve sheath meningioma. In contrast to a normal optic nerve on the left side, the nerve on the right side is encircled by the tumor *(arrow)*. *B,* Transfrontal orbitotomy and exposure of the retrobulbar optic nerve sheath meningioma. *C,* After transfrontal orbitotomy and partial removal of the tumor, the optic nerve is partially exposed. *D,* Total removal of a retrobulbar optic nerve sheath meningioma. The optic nerve is exposed from the optic canal up to the bulb.

oculomotor nerves were judged to be satisfactory, to our knowledge a few have succeeded in reconstruction (nerve grafting) after interruption of continuity. Yasargil (1977), Deruty and co-workers (1988), Grimson and colleagues (1984), and Lanzino and associates (1994) observed functional recovery of a severed oculomotor or trochlear nerve as a result of an end-to-end anastomosis or grafting. In the future, there should be more thought given to the reconstruction of injured cranial nerves III, IV, and VI.

TRIGEMINAL NERVE (FIFTH CRANIAL NERVE)

There are several indications for the surgical treatment of a traumatized trigeminal nerve (Samii, 1972b). Severe facial injuries may be accompanied by lesions of different branches of the trigeminal nerve, most of all at the forehead in the area of the frontal branches or in fractures of the mandible where the inferior alveolar nerves are located. Fractures of the base of the skull or intracranial space-occupying processes may lead to a lesion of the trigeminal nerve with partial or total loss of sensation on one part of the face and paralysis of the masticatory muscles.

Radical tumor extirpation of the lower jaw often requires the resection of the inferior alveolar nerve. The consequence is loss of sensation in the region of the mucosa, the lip, and the chin. Today we are able to perform an exact restoration of the trigeminal nerve.

Transection of the frontal nerve caused by an incised wound produces a relatively minor hypoesthesia in the region of the forehead. A trigeminal neuralgia resistant to any therapy may also appear, owing to the formation of a neuroma, and is of greater clinical importance. Neurolysis has been successful only in rare cases. Dissection of the trigeminal nerve in this region to re-establish the continuity of the nerve through an end-to-end suture or a nerve graft can be performed. As a result, pain is relieved and sensation is restored.

The loss of function of the ophthalmic nerve is a special problem and can have serious consequences. Keratitis neuroparalytica can lead to ulcer of the cornea and blindness of the patient, a possible result of sensory and trophic disorder of the cornea.

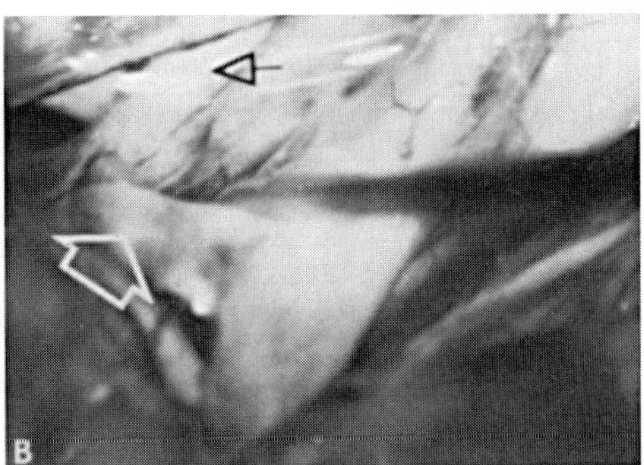

FIGURE 39–6. *A,* Supraclinoid aneurysm *(white arrow)* of the carotid artery on the left side with compression of the oculomotor nerve *(black arrow).* *B,* The aneurysm *(white arrow)* is kept away with an instrument from the oculomotor nerve *(black arrow).*

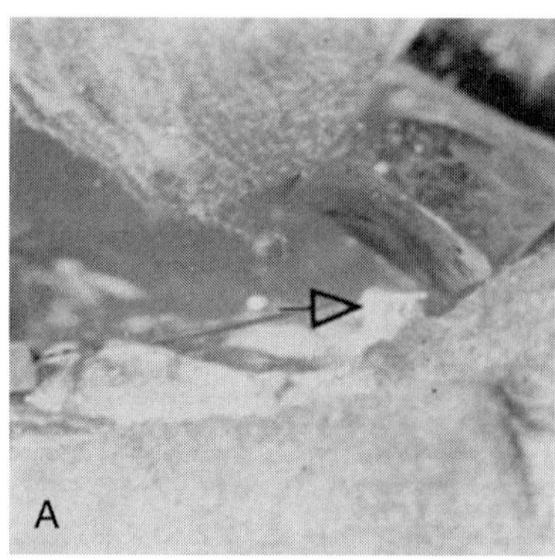
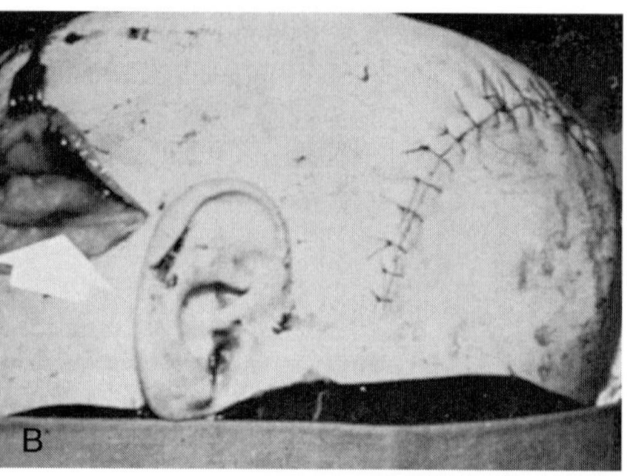

FIGURE 39–7. *A,* Transfrontal orbitotomy. Exposure of the ophthalmic nerve *(arrow)* in a patient with a retroganglionic trigeminal lesion. Amaurosis was caused by keratitis. *B,* After anastomosis of a 17-cm-long autologous nerve graft between the ophthalmic nerve and the major occipital nerve. The right-sided frontal craniotomy is closed again. The nerve graft is still visible behind the ear *(arrow).*

Disorders of the ophthalmic nerve occur in connection with retroganglionic injury or after surgical treatment of a trigeminal neuralgia, which may result in a complete loss of sensation. In this case, restoration of sensation in the cornea must be the surgical goal. Although a direct surgical approach to intracranial damage of the trigeminal nerve used to be technically impossible, an anastomosis between the ophthalmic nerve and a cutaneous nerve can be performed. The major occipital nerve seems to be most suitable; it is of the same diameter as the ophthalmic nerve and participates, as does the major ophthalmic nerve, in the sensory innervation of the galea.

Operative Technique

After exposure of the major occipital nerve, an osteoplastic frontal craniotomy is performed. The anterior cranial fossa is epidurally exposed, the roof of the orbit is opened, and, through an incision of the periorbital capsule, the ophthalmic nerve is exposed and proximally transected. The peripheral stump of the ophthalmic nerve is then anastomosed with a sural nerve graft. The transplant is led out of the skull and anastomosed with the major occipital nerve in the subgaleal layer (Fig. 39–7A and B). Recovery of sensa-

tion in the region of the cornea has been observed after about 6 months.

Resection of the inferior alveolar nerve is often unavoidable during surgery of benign or malignant tumors of the mandible (Fig. 39–8).

Anesthesia of the affected side of the lower lip is often a serious problem for the patient because of uncontrolled drooling and difficulty in drinking. Ulceration of the lower lip may appear when the anesthetic lip is traumatized between the teeth while chewing. Although for some patients this may not be irritating, others seem to suffer tremendously from this loss of sensation. For this reason, all attempts should be made to preserve this nerve, at least in cases of benign tumors of the lower jaw (Becker, 1967, 1970, 1972). However, this is only possible in patients in whom the nerve lies apart from the tumor.

The inferior alveolar nerve is endangered in a group of lower jaw fractures when the fracture lines cross the nerve canal. Because of its elasticity, the nerve may not be totally affected in many cases. The damage may be restricted to tension, contusion, or an edematous compression with temporary loss of sensibility. If there is a compound comminuted fracture or fracture defect, a loss of continuity of the nerve and a total sensory deficit follow (Greve, 1927; Hermann, 1958; Simpson, 1958).

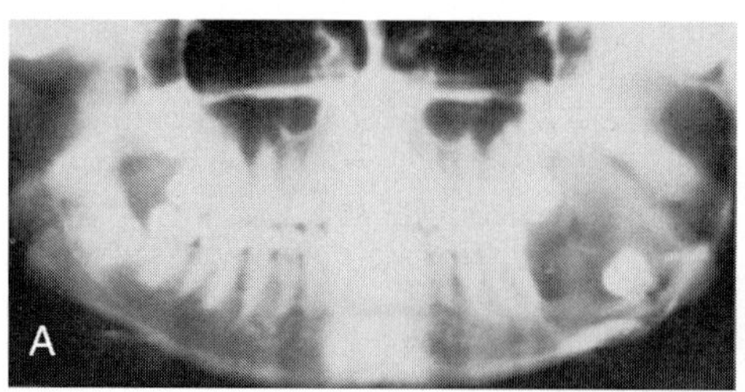
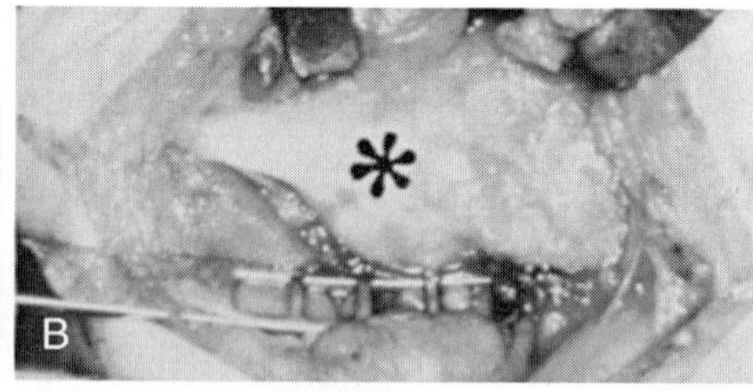
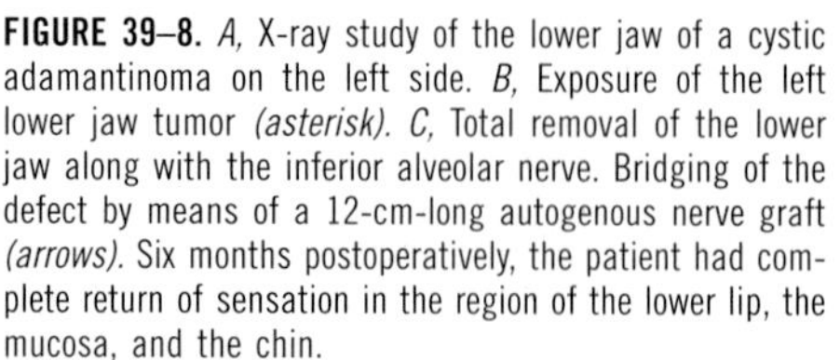
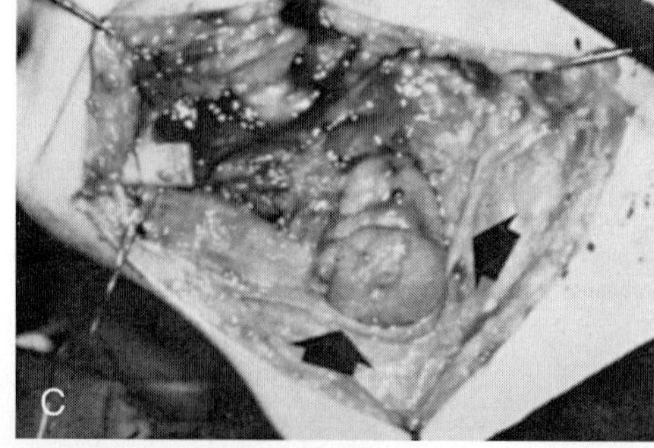

FIGURE 39–8. *A,* X-ray study of the lower jaw of a cystic adamantinoma on the left side. *B,* Exposure of the left lower jaw tumor *(asterisk). C,* Total removal of the lower jaw along with the inferior alveolar nerve. Bridging of the defect by means of a 12-cm-long autogenous nerve graft *(arrows).* Six months postoperatively, the patient had complete return of sensation in the region of the lower lip, the mucosa, and the chin.

For the reconstruction of the inferior alveolar nerve after resection of the lower jaw, it is advisable (Hausamen et al, 1973; Samii, 1972d) to mark and cut the proximal and distal nerve stumps at the mandibular and mental foramina. Thereafter, the tumor resection and the osteoplastic reconstruction may be performed. To restore the continuity of the inferior alveolar nerve, a neural graft is necessary. The sural nerve is the most suitable for bridging the defect (Cornelius et al, 1994). The transplant should be 12 to 15 cm long. The transplant needs to re-establish its connection with the blood circulation. Initially, it remains dependent on its surroundings via diffusion for nutrition. For this reason, we do not place the nerve graft in the avascular bony transplant but at a distance to it.

LINGUAL NERVE (A MAJOR BRANCH OF THE TRIGEMINAL NERVE)

The course of the peripheral part of the lingual nerve in the floor of the mouth is of special interest. After leaving the pterygomandibular space, the lingual nerve establishes very close contact with the mandible at the level of the third molar. Its branches are to be found under the mucosa before they enter the tongue. The nerve supplies the sensory innervation of the anterior two thirds of the tongue, the floor of the mouth, and the lingual side of the mandibular gingiva. In addition, it sends out the afferent and efferent parasympathetic fibers for the submandibular and sublingual glands.

The lingual nerve can be traumatized by careless extraction of the lower third molar, by improper intraoral incision of a sublingual abscess, and by injuries with drills during preparation of cavities of the lower molars. Furthermore, the lingual nerve has to be sacrificed in cases of tumors of the floor of the mouth that have invaded the nerve (Fig. 39–9). The sensory disorder of the tongue can lead to repeated bite injuries. In some patients, taste may be impaired.

Reconstruction of the lingual nerve may be successful if performed near its trunk and proximal to its divisions in the floor of the mouth. If an extraoral approach is used to resect the mandible, identification of the proximal and peripheral stumps and performance of nerve grafting do not present any special problems (Cornelius et al, 1994; Hausamen et al, 1974).

The intraoral approach to the nerve stumps of the pterygomandibular space and in the floor of the mouth is also not particularly difficult (Fig. 39–10A and B).

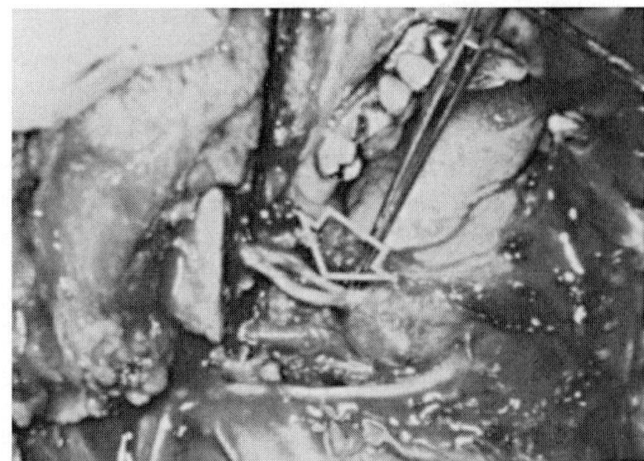

FIGURE 39–9. Reconstruction of the lingual nerve with two nerve grafts *(arrow)* after total removal of a large tumor in the floor of the mouth and the mandible.

In contrast, the nerve grafting is technically difficult, especially in patients with full dentition, because of the very narrow surgical field. Because of the superficial course of the lingual nerve, the transplant has to be bedded directly underneath the mucosa, and an exact wound closure is all-important.

FACIAL NERVE (SEVENTH CRANIAL NERVE)

In comparison with other cranial nerves, the facial nerve is the one most frequently afflicted by different types of lesions, such as tumors, trauma, and different processes in the area of the skull base and the face. The resulting paralysis of the muscles of the face results in a tragic situation for the patient.

Facial nerve paresis caused by tumors develops slowly. Paresis can be caused by tumors of the cells of the neurilemma or tumors in the environment that lead to compression of the nerve, as is the case with cerebellopontine angle tumors; tumors found in the region of the petrous bone (e.g., epidermoid, cholesteatoma, chordoma, carcinoma); and tumors of the parotid. Some malignant tumors can infiltrate the facial nerve.

Facial nerve paresis can also be caused by viral or bacterial infections. In particular, it can occur in meningitis and in acute or chronic middle ear infection.

Facial nerve paresis of traumatic origin is caused mostly by laterobasal fractures of the skull or severe facial injuries.

The etiology of Bell's palsy is not well understood. Ac-

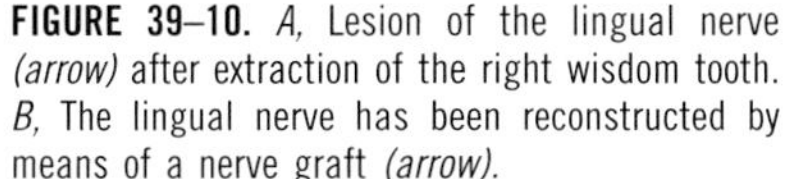

FIGURE 39–10. *A,* Lesion of the lingual nerve *(arrow)* after extraction of the right wisdom tooth. *B,* The lingual nerve has been reconstructed by means of a nerve graft *(arrow).*

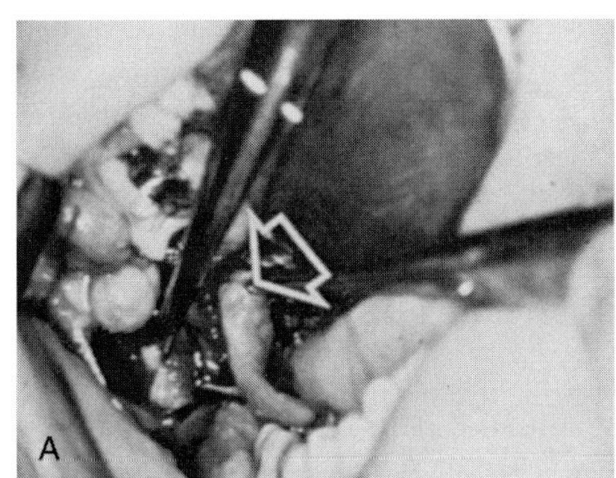

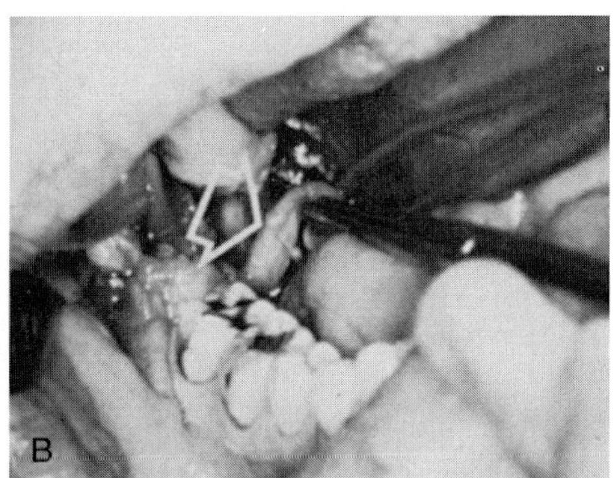

cording to Hilger (1949) and other authors, it may be the result of a spasm of the facial branch of the external carotid artery. The arterial spasm is followed by disturbances at the capillary level with ischemia and edema of the nerve. The edema itself causes a compression of the nerve, and this leads to an obstruction of the lymphatic and venous circulation, which again increases the edema. With that, a vicious circle is completed (Jongkees, 1958, 1961).

A vascular dysfunction does not appear to be the definitive cause. More favored is the hypothesis of an acute benign cranial neuritis caused by a neurotropic herpes simplex virus (Adour, 1977).

Since Jannetta (1977) was able to achieve good results in cases of Bell's palsy after exposure of the cerebellopontine angle and getting the nerve free from compression of a vascular loop, he holds the opinion that a sudden pathological change of the position of an artery loop within the cerebellopontine angle brings about a stretching of the nerve, with resulting paresis.

Hemifacial spasm represents another still unsolved problem. Opinions differ with regard to the etiology. Miehlke (1973) argues that the true cause of the idiopathic facial spasm cannot yet be explained satisfactorily. In his opinion, the therapy has to be symptomatic as long as the cause is unknown. According to Gardner and Sava (1962), Jannetta (1970, 1975), and Bertrand and co-workers (1977), the facial spasm is to be attributed to a vascular loop compressing the intracranial segment of the facial nerve at the brain stem. In other cases, however, a tumor may be the cause of the facial spasm. During regeneration of a damaged facial nerve a spasm is possible because of scar strangulation of the nerve fibers. This type of facial spasm may occur after nerve suture, nerve grafting, or blunt trauma or during regeneration with incomplete recovery. In the majority of cases, arterial (rarely venous) vascular compression will be identified at exposure at the cerebellopontine angle, and Jannetta's method of vascular decompression will lead to permanent cure in more than 80% of cases (Adams, 1989; Jannetta, 1981).

Surgical Treatment of the Facial Nerve

The present standard of surgical treatment of the facial nerve would not be conceivable without the pioneering work of Bunnel (1927), Martin (1931, 1936), Ballance and Duel (1932), Duel (1934), Cawthorne (1951, 1963, 1965), Maxwell (1951, 1954), Kettel (1957, 1959), Lathrop (1953, 1956, 1962), Conley (1955, 1961), Clerc and Batisse (1954), Dott (1958), Jongkees (1958, 1961), Wullstein (1958), Miehlke (1960, 1961), House (1961, 1963), and Fisch (1969, 1970b, 1977), among others. In consideration of the anatomical course of the facial nerve, one can distinguish among three different regions for surgical treatment:

1. The intracranial region.
   a. Surgical treatment of hemifacial spasm in the cerebellopontine angle.
   b. Preservation or reconstruction of the facial nerve in the cerebellopontine angle.
2. The intratemporal region.
3. The extratemporal region.

In addition, the surgical treatment of the loss of facial nerve origin (treated with reanimation procedures) of Bell's palsy will be discussed.

SURGICAL TREATMENT OF THE FACIAL NERVE IN THE INTRACRANIAL REGION

Surgical Treatment of Hemifacial Spasm in the Cerebellopontine Angle. Previous surgical methods for the correction of hemifacial spasm consisted of traumatizing the facial nerve at different levels. All these methods failed to produce satisfactory results. In eight patients treated by resection of the peripheral branches of the facial nerve, permanent healing was not achieved; although none of the patients showed immediate postoperative signs of a recurrent facial spasm, this occurred a few months later. The longest symptom-free interval was 18 months.

Vascular compression of the facial nerve in the cerebellopontine angle as a possible etiology of facial spasm was mentioned in 1947 by Campbell and Keedy and in 1962 by Gardner. In 1970, Jannetta reported on the microsurgical vascular decompression of facial spasm in the cerebellopontine angle. His long-term results in 45 patients operated on between 1966 and 1974 were published in 1977. The result was excellent in 38 cases, good in 2, fair in 3, and poor but improved in 2 (cases 3 and 16—persistent clinical spasm). Of great importance is that the motor disorders in the region of the facial muscles preoperatively ascertained by electromyography were postoperatively reversible in many cases.

The operative technique consists of suboccipital craniotomy and exposure of the cerebellopontine angle. After incision of the dura, the cerebellum is elevated, with the help of a retractor blade, and the facial nerve is exposed at the internal auditory meatus. Dissection of the facial nerve has to be carried out up to the brain stem. After craniomedial elevation of the cerebellar hemisphere, the chorioid plexus of the lateral recess of the fourth ventricle and the flocculus of the cerebellum must be held cautiously away with a retractor blade to expose the central part of the facial nerve. It is essential to expose the exit area of the nerve at the brain stem where the vascular decompression has to be carried out. All vessels in the region of the cerebellopontine angle—the vertebral, basilar, inferior posterior cerebellar, inferior anterior cerebellar, and cochlear arteries—may cause vascular compression. Vascular compression may also be the result of dilated veins or arteriovenous angiomas. Other etiological factors of facial spasm are small neurinomas or cholesteatomas. Decompression of the facial nerve is performed by changing the axis of the arterial loop and its relationship with the nerve root exit zone at the brain stem. The new position is maintained by placing a segment of muscle between the proximal and distal limbs of the vascular loop and the brain stem. The position of the muscle segment must not be changed by later rotations of the head. To ensure its firm position between the brain stem and the vascular loop, the head is turned intraoperatively in different directions. Jannetta's technique seems to be the operative treatment of choice for facial spasm, although the risk of inducing deafness has to be discussed with the patient. An essential prerequisite for the performance of such a surgical intervention is the mastery of the microsurgical technique.

Preservation and Reconstruction of the Facial Nerve in the Cerebellopontine Angle. The portion of the facial nerve in the cerebellopontine angle, with a length of 23 to 24 mm, is endangered by space-occupying processes. About 71%

of all tumors of the cerebellopontine angle are acoustic neurinomas. Meningiomas, epidermoids, and occasionally metastases occur. During the growth of a cerebellopontine angle tumor, the function of the facial nerve remains intact for a long time. Primary intrameatal tumors with extension into the cerebellopontine angle cause early paralysis, especially when arising from the facial nerve itself. In the cerebellopontine angle, the position and course of the facial nerve may be displaced in different directions by space-occupying processes. Identification of the facial nerve may prove extremely difficult during tumor surgery. Accurate exposure and preservation of the continuity of the facial nerve through microsurgical technique during the removal of cerebellopontine angle tumors should be part of the modern surgical concept.

The neurosurgical suboccipital approach of the cerebellopontine angle permits either dorsolateral or dorsocaudal exposure of the tumor. After retracting the cerebellum craniomedially, the caudal cranial nerves, often slightly compressed by the tumor, must be identified and freed from the tumor capsule. An immediate identification of the facial nerve in the cerebellopontine angle will be possible only in those cases in which the tumor is relatively small and, especially, when the tumor compresses the nerve in a more dorsal direction (Fig. 39–11).

The facial nerve is not visible at the brain stem or in the internal auditory meatus when the tumor is large (Fig. 39–12A). Starting from a 5- to 10-mm opening of the tumor capsule, the reduction of the tumor is performed under the operating microscope. Thus, the tumor capsule loses its primary tension (Fig. 39–12B). By gradual resection of the tumor capsule, the facial nerve can be identified at the brain stem (Fig. 39–12C).

Any direct manipulation of the facial nerve in the cerebel-lopontine angle will most probably lead to postoperative loss of function, although the continuity of the nerve may be preserved. The facial nerve, therefore, must be pursued from the brain stem to the internal auditory meatus under highest magnification and with extreme patience and caution (Fig. 39–12D).

The nerve may not be detached from the tumor capsule, but the tumor capsule itself must be dissected carefully, using microsurgical instruments, from the nerve. Stretching of the nerve, with its adhesion to the tumor capsule, must be strictly avoided. The tumor capsule may be slightly stretched with one hand while, with a microsurgical scissor in the other hand, the membrane between the tumor capsule and the nerve is precisely transected. Not infrequently, the nerve, owing to an expansion compression, is rolled out around the tumor capsule in a thin, broad surface of approximately 2 to 3 cm (Fig. 39–12E). The preservation of the facial nerve in such a case is quite difficult; however, it is technically possible (Fig. 39–12F).

Most frequently, the facial nerve is injured at the internal auditory meatus when the tumor grows in a cone shape into the internal auditory meatus. Removal of the tumor from this region, likewise, must be performed under direct vision. The internal auditory meatus is exposed by cutting away the posterior lip of the internal auditory meatus with the help of refined punches or a diamond drill (Fig. 39–13).

The facial nerve may remain preserved in its continuity in 80 to more than 90% of all cerebellopontine angle tumors by using the microsurgical technique and observing the above-mentioned principles (Bentivoglio et al, 1988; Drake, 1973; Glasscock et al, 1993; Haid and Wigand, 1992; Hitselberger and House, 1973; Koos et al, 1973; Samii 1979, 1981, 1989; Samii and Matthies, 1994, 1995a, 1995b; Samii et al, 1985; Symon et al, 1989; Torrens et al, 1994; Yasargil,

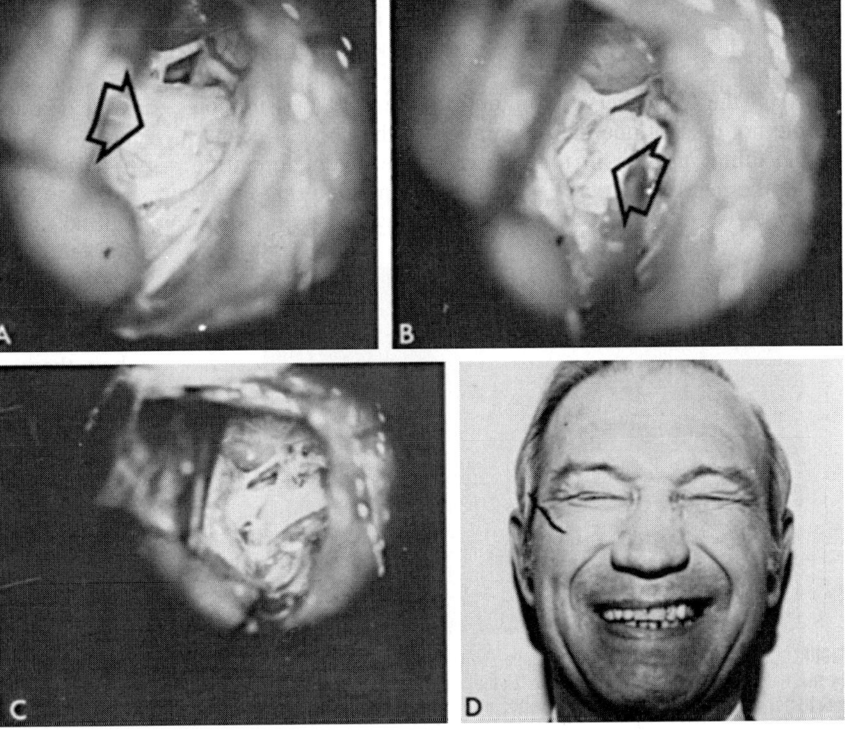

FIGURE 39–11. *A,* Small neuroma *(arrow)* of the cerebellopontine angle on the right side. The facial nerve is already visible when the tumor is exposed. *B,* The tumor *(arrow)* from the brain stem. *C,* Total removal of the neuroma of the cerebellopontine angle after opening the internal meatus. The facial nerve is preserved. *D,* Three months postoperatively.

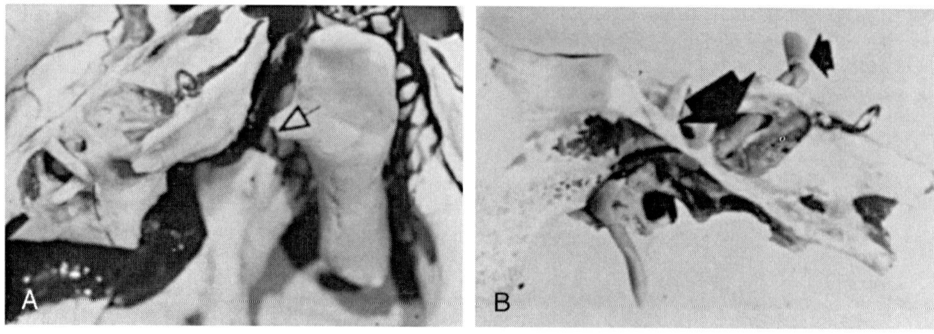

FIGURE 39–16. *A,* Model of a nerve defect of the facial nerve *(arrow)* in the cerebellopontine angle and internal auditory canal. *B,* Model of a reconstructed nerve in the cerebellopontine angle and internal auditory canal by means of nerve grafting *(large arrow)* between the central stump *(small arrow)* at the brain stem and the distal stump of the mastoidal course.

base or by a tumor, or the cause can be iatrogenic. In patients with craniocerebral injuries who exhibit paralysis of the facial nerve, one should investigate a possible fracture in the region of the petrous bone by use of special x-ray techniques, including tomography (Figs. 39–19 and 39–20).

Sometimes it is difficult to identify a fracture line radiologically. According to Fisch, laterobasal fractures of the skull damage the facial nerve in the meatal-labyrinthine area.

One third of patients with early paralysis of the facial nerve after pyramidal longitudinal fractures showed a complete loss of continuity in the proximal intratemporal course of the facial nerve. Paralysis of the facial nerve caused by pyramidal *longitudinal* fractures may be caused by compression of a bony fragment or by an interruption in continuity of the nerve. In 50% of the cases, a stretching of the geniculate ganglion with perineural or intraneural hemor-

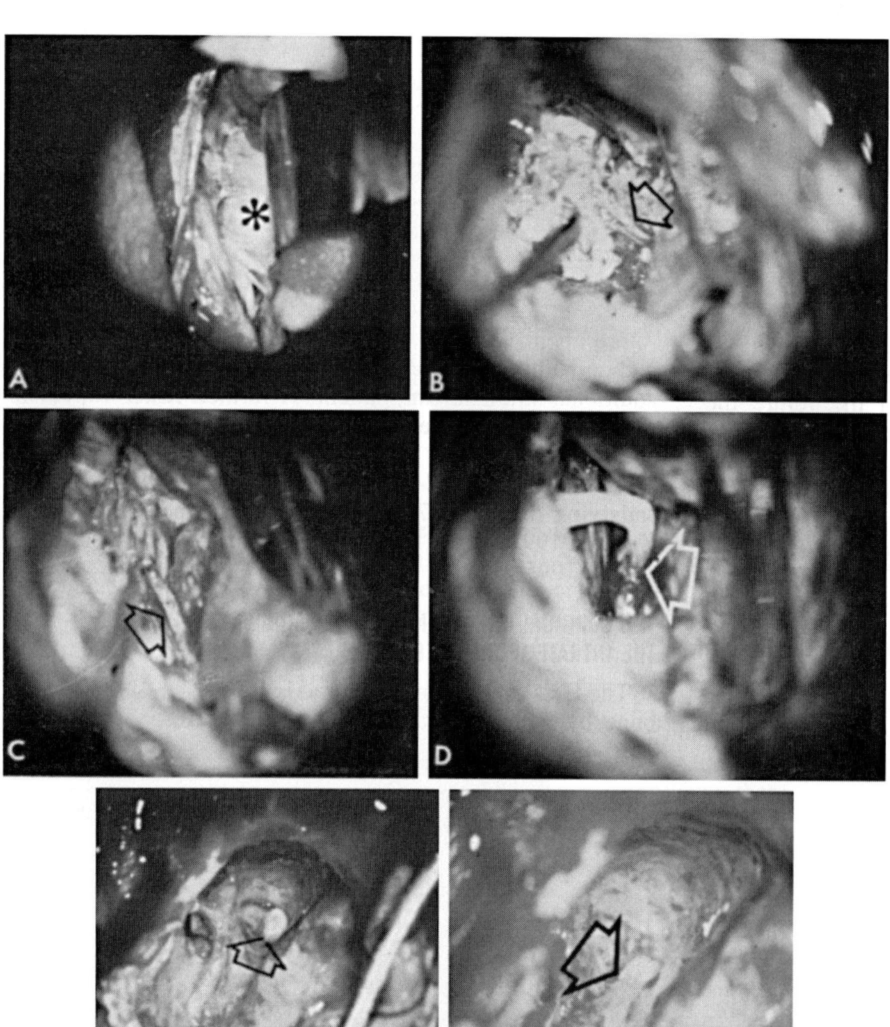

FIGURE 39–17. *A,* Suboccipital exposure of a left-sided acoustic neuroma *(asterisk).* The caudal cranial nerves are visible in the region of the lower tumor pole. *B,* After partial resection of the tumor. Exposure of the facial nerve at the brain stem *(arrow).* *C,* Total removal of the large tumor along with a part of the facial nerve. Exposure of the central stump of the facial nerve at the brain stem *(arrow).* *D,* Anastomosis between the central nerve stump of the facial nerve at the brain stem with a sural nerve graft *(arrow).* *E,* Mastoidectomy and translabyrinthine exposure of the internal auditory canal. Exposure of the facial nerve in the mastoidal and tympanal course. The rolled-up second end of the nerve graft in the internal auditory canal is visible *(arrow).* *F,* The facial nerve is transected below the geniculate ganglion. The distal stump is mobilized dorsally and anastomosed with the nerve graft *(arrow).*

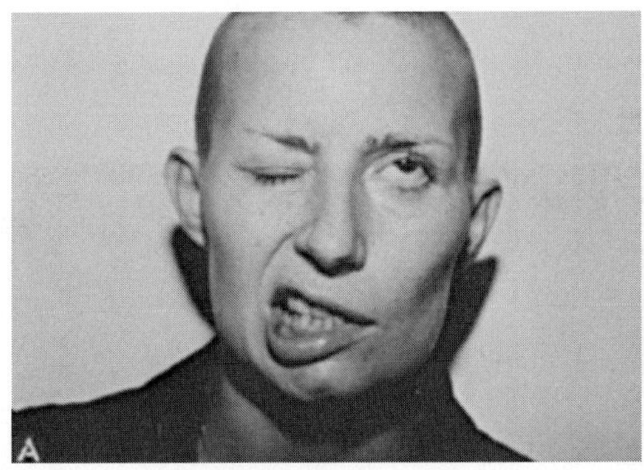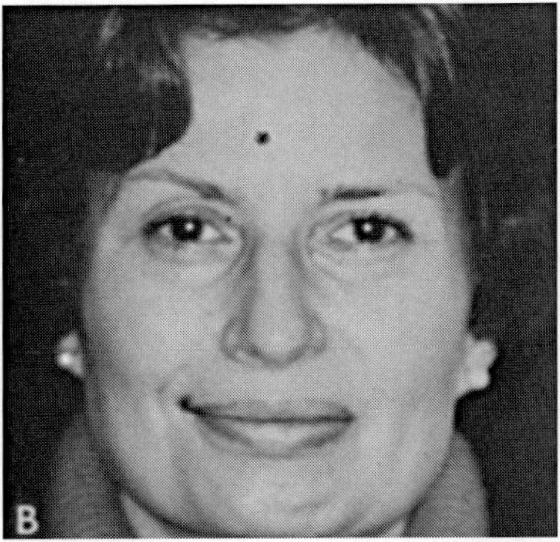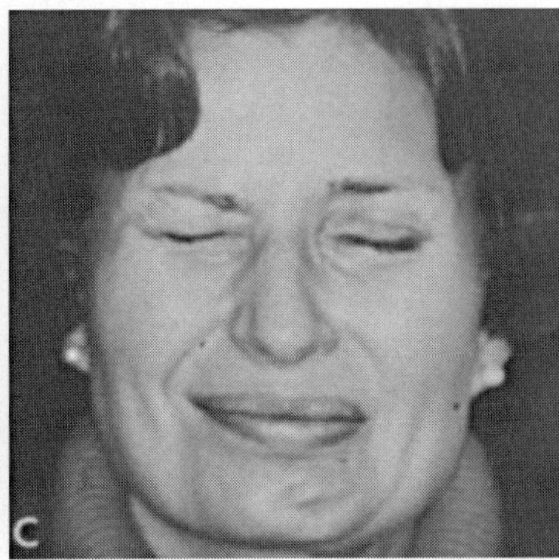

FIGURE 39–18. *A,* Ten days after removal of a large acoustic neuroma on the left side with reconstruction of the facial nerve by means of a 5-cm-long graft between the proximal stump at the brain stem and the mastoidal segment in the petrous bone. Total paralysis of facial nerve on the left side. *B* and *C,* Functional return 13 months after nerve grafting between the intracranial and intratemporal part of the facial nerve.

rhage may be the cause (Fisch, 1972). Pyramidal *transverse* fractures, occurring with much less frequency (in 30 to 50% of all cases), lead to early paralysis of the facial nerve. One differentiates between external transverse fractures, located distal to the internal auditory canal, and internal transverse fractures, situated proximal of the fundus meatus.

The surgical approach to the various segments of the intratemporal course of the facial nerve can differ. In the meatal and labyrinthine region, the facial nerve is reached on the transtemporal extradural approach to the middle fossa (Fisch, 1970a and b; House, 1961). The exposure extends from the porus acusticus internus up to the tendon of the tensor tympani muscle without opening the internal ear space (Fig. 39–21).

The transtemporal approach renders preservation of the ear function possible. In cases of deafness, the transmastoidal-translabyrinthine approach is chosen (Fig. 39–22).

If the mastoidal segment is injured, the facial nerve must be exposed by means of mastoidectomy up to the stylomastoid foramen. The nerve may be followed up to the lateral semicircular canal. In cases where the lesion is located in the tympanal segment, the preparation of the mastoidal segment can be continued in a central direction up to the geniculate ganglion without impairment of auditory function (Fig. 39–23*A* and *B*).

CROSSED FACIAL ANASTOMOSIS

A further development of anastomosis of the facial nerve to other cranial nerves is the faciofacial anastomosis, also known as *crossover cross-face anastomosis.* The advantage of this technique is that reinnervation of the paralyzed muscles can be partially achieved without sacrificing another cranial nerve and without loss of function. This technique was reported for the first time by Smith (1971) and Scaramella (1971). The method was improved by Anderl (1972) and Samii (1976a, 1979). The technical principle of the faciofacial anastomosis is based on the anatomical fact that the branches of the facial nerve within the face region build a kind of plexus—the pes anserinus—and that parts of these branches may be cut without risk of visible functional deficit. The central stumps of the transected branches in the healthy side of the face are anastomosed with nerve grafts crossing the face subcutaneously in the upper lip region to the damaged side. Here, they have to be sutured with the analogous branches (Fig. 39–24*A* and *B*).

Our experience has proved the sural nerve to be the most appropriate for transplantation. However, it must be taken into consideration that the course of the peripheral branches of the facial nerve is different in each individual. Fujita (1934) found irregularities in this pattern even when comparing the two sides of the face in one person. McCormack and co-workers (1945) established eight different types of facial nerve branch distribution in the face. According to their investigations, an anastomosis among the different groups of branches is lacking in only 13% of all people. In general, a more or less well-developed parotid plexus is found, whereas the mandibular branch is very seldom connected through anastomosis with the other branch groups, and the cervicalis colli branch never is.

According to Davis and co-workers (1956), this percentage varies. Intraoperative electrodiagnostic stimulation of

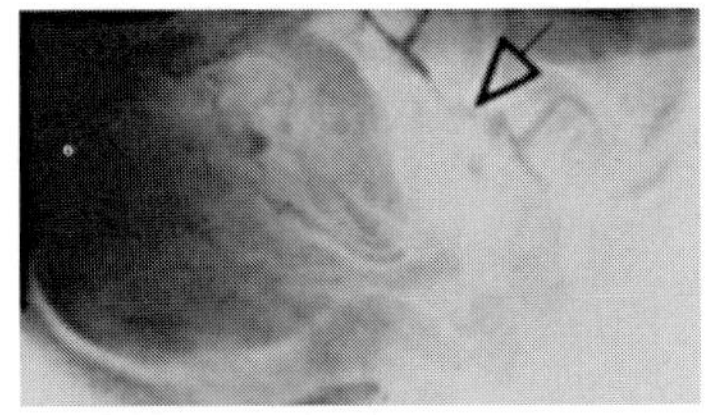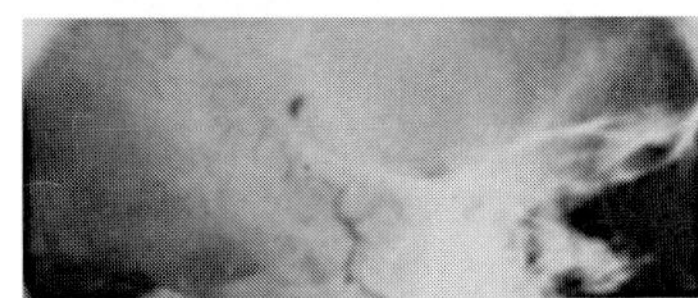

FIGURE 39–19. Combined longitudinal and transverse fracture *(arrow)* of the petrous bone.

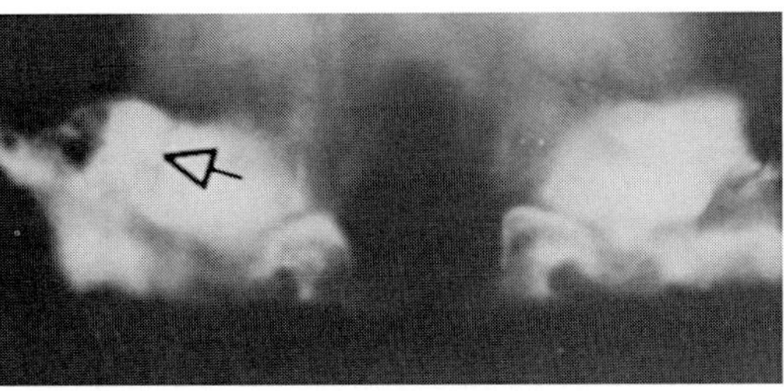

FIGURE 39–20. Medial pyramidal transverse fracture *(arrow)* on the right side reaching into the fundus of the internal auditory meatus and the vestibulum. Lateral to the fracture fissure one can recognize the upper and lateral semicircular canal.

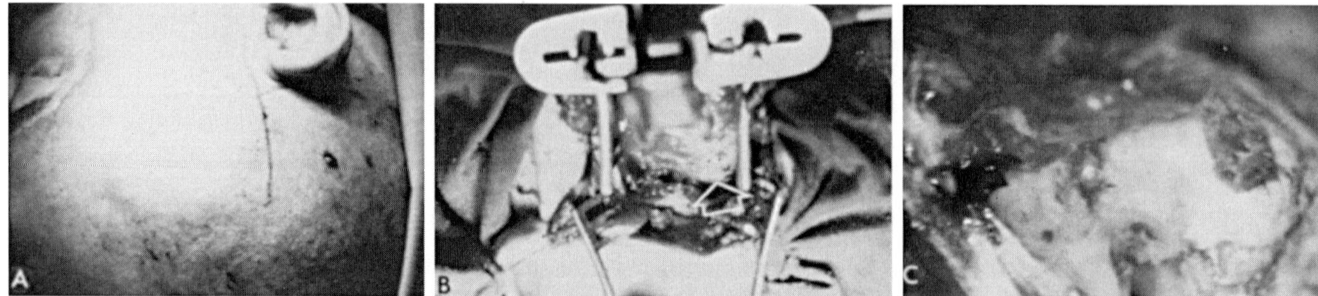

FIGURE 39–21. *A,* Skin incision line to the transtemporal and extradural approach to the middle fossa for the exposure of the facial nerve in the meatal and labyrinthine region. *B,* Temporal craniotomy and exposure of the dura *(arrow)* in the region of the middle fossa. *C,* Transtemporal decompression of the facial nerve proximal to the geniculate ganglion in a case of laterobasal skull fracture.

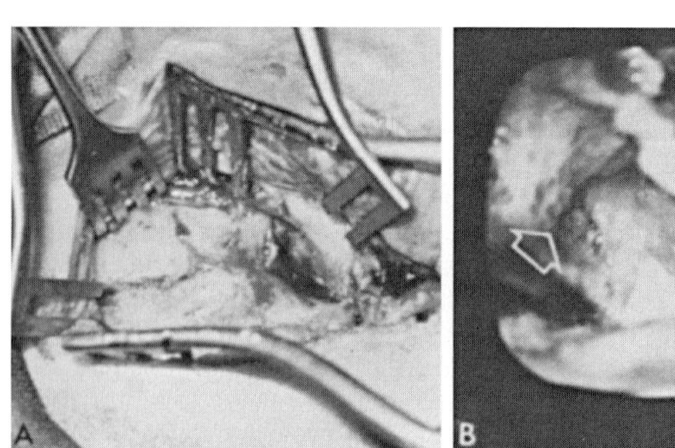

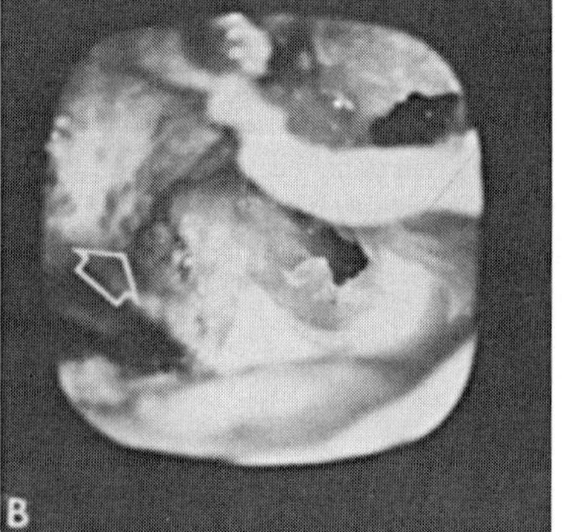

FIGURE 39–22. *A,* Operating feature: fracture of the mastoid and temporal bone. *B,* Operating feature: transmastoidal exposure of the facial nerve. The fracture line *(arrow)* is vertically crossing the facial canal at the level of the lateral semicircular canal.

FIGURE 39–23. *A,* Interposition of a 2.5-cm graft *(arrow)* in the region of the mastoidal and tympanal segments of the facial nerve. *B,* Functional return 1½ years after the operation.

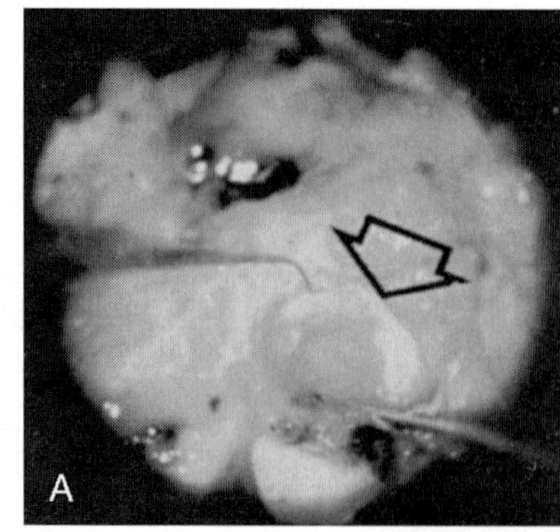

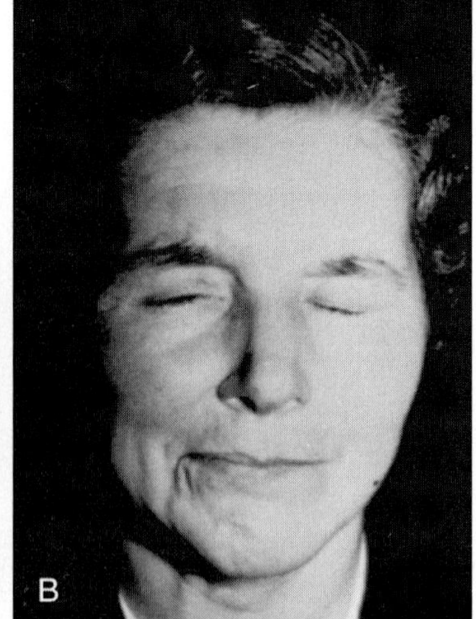

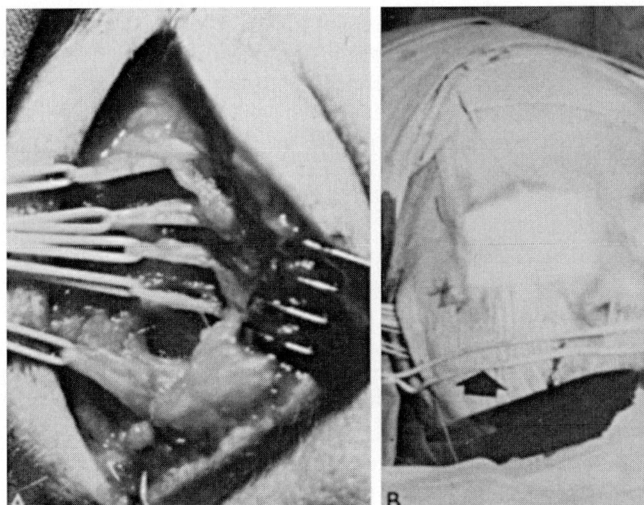

FIGURE 39–24. *A,* Exposure of the peripheral branches of the facial nerve (tapes) in the face as for a faciofacial anastomosis. *B,* Exposure of the peripheral branches of the facial nerve on both the intact and the damaged sides. Two grafts of sural nerve, which will be passed subcutaneously and anastomosed with both sides, are seen placed over the upper lip *(arrow).*

the individual branches of the facial nerve confirms these anatomical variations. With this technique, the innervation patterns of the facial nerve of each patient can be accurately evaluated. It is our impression that the zygomatic branch is the most important of all the facial nerve branches because electrical stimulation of it produces contraction of the orbicularis oculi and orbicularis oris muscles. Because of overlapping supply by the ocular and mandibular branches of the facial nerve, a complete transection of its zygomatic branch rarely produces a visible paralysis. To clarify these clinical observations, we counted the nerve fibers in the zygomatic branches in cadavers. We found that this branch makes up approximately 40% of the total fibers of the facial nerve. End result studies of faciofacial anastomosis, in which each branch was anastomosed with the analogous branch of the opposite side, revealed failure of reinnervation of the frontal branch. For this reason, we have now simplified the technique. We have abandoned the method of complete exposure of all peripheral branches of the facial nerve. Instead, we merely expose both zygomatic branches through two 2-cm-long incisions. These two branches are identified, transected, and anastomosed, using a sural nerve graft (Fig. 39–25*A* and *B*).

The results in 41 patients up to the present are satisfactory. In 90% of examined cases, we could observe electromyographic and clinical reinnervation of muscles. In 50% of patients, we could ascertain symmetry of the face in a state of repose. Although in the other 40% we could recognize a satisfying contraction of muscles, the paralysis of the facial nerve while in a state of repose was evident. In these cases, we regularly perform a skin correction in the sulcus nasolabialis to achieve a symmetrical position of the face in repose (Samii and Matthies, 1994).

In only a few cases could we achieve an ideal symmetrical function in connection with active contraction of face muscles. The cause arises from the fact that only 50% of the fibers of the facial nerve on the healthy side may be called on for reconstruction without the risk of loss of function. In my opinion, the technique of the faciofacial anastomosis therefore constitutes only an alternative to the accessory-facial anastomosis or hypoglossal-facial anastomosis. Faciofacial anastomosis is inadequate when direct exposure and treatment of the lesion are possible.

Faciofacial anastomosis is a good additional method when direct treatment of the facial nerve lesion results only in partial reinnervation.

Surgical Treatment of Bell's Palsy

Bell's palsy, the etiology of which is still uncertain, constitutes 58 to 88% of all facial nerve lesions (Adour, 1977; Cadena, 1977; Devriese, 1977; Gomez, 1977; Hosomi, 1977; Pietersen, 1977). The attitude toward an operative treatment has changed very much during the past years. According to Hilger's (1949) theory of a vascular dysregulation and ischemia with following edema and compression of the nerve, principally in the fallopian canal, the only reasonable therapy

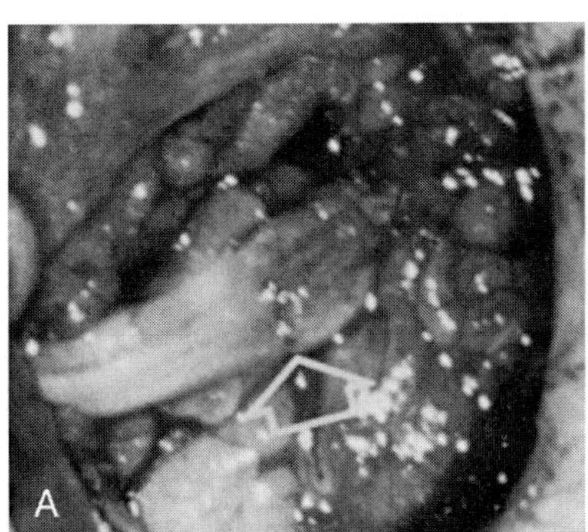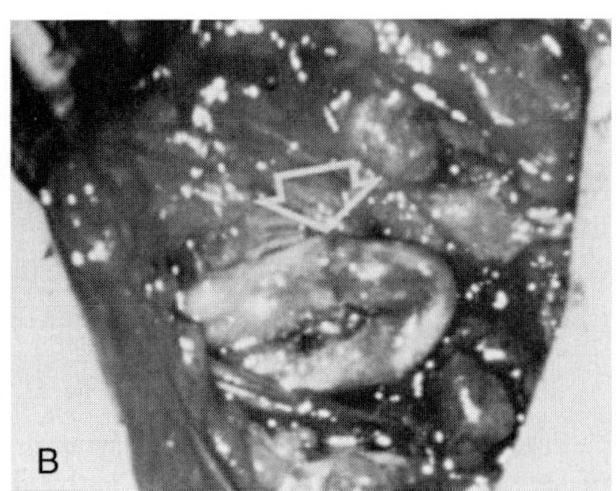

FIGURE 39–25. *A,* After a 2-cm skin incision below the zygomatic branch of the facial nerve on the intact side, the zygomatic branch is exposed and transected, and the central stump is already anastomosed with the sural nerve *(arrow). B,* The second end of the graft is anastomosed with the distal stump of the zygomatic branch of the facial nerve on the damaged side *(arrow).*

seemed to be early operative decompression with neurolysis in the facial canal. Other investigations emphasize the role of allergic factors or viral pathogenesis, with the result of a considerable decrease in the frequency of operative decompressions of the facial nerve. In about 70 to 90% of all cases a return of function was possible by means of conservative therapy (Gomez, 1977; Hosomi, 1977; Peitersen, 1977). The intensity of the disease may be substantially reduced by prednisone therapy. Jongkees reported that with prednisone therapy he was able to limit the number of operative decompressions to 10%.

An indication for intratemporal facial decompression, according to Esslen (1973), should be when electroneurographic examinations give the following results:

1. If more than 50% of the nerve fibers show signs of degeneration 4 days after occurrence of the facial paralysis.

2. If about 50% of the fibers are degenerated on the 4th day and a further 15 to 20% are degenerating during the following 2 days.

3. If 90% or more of the fibers have degenerated within 7 days.

Because electroneurography is being increasingly used, several authors suggest the 90% limit as the time for operative intervention. When surgical treatment is indicated, Fisch (1977) suggests exposure of the entire course of the facial nerve from the brain stem up to the stylomastoid foramen, not only the preparation of the mastoidal and tympanal segment. In 11 of 12 such interventions, he found either an exclusive or added involvement of the nerve proximal to the geniculate ganglion. About half of those cases with total decompression showed slight secondary ischemia in the mastoidal segment.

Based on experience with the decompression of the facial nerve in patients with Bell's palsy, Helms (1976) supported the view that an isolated transmeatal exposure of the geniculate ganglion may lead to satisfactory results. He performed decompression of the geniculate ganglion with local anesthesia. This technique, however, applies only in those cases where active muscle contraction is no longer ascertainable and electrical examinations establish a rapid decrease in muscle reaction. The period of time between onset of the paralysis and operation extends from 7 days to 12 weeks. In all patients on whom transmeatal decompression of the geniculate ganglion has been done, a return of motor function in the three branches of the facial nerve could be diagnosed.

Studies by Jannetta on the surgical treatment of Bell's palsy show that in some patients a sudden displacement of an arterial loop in the cerebellopontine angle can lead to extensive stretching of the facial nerve. Jannetta pointed out that in some cases this mechanism may be regarded as a cause of Bell's palsy. He has found in six patients that this vascular change in the cerebellopontine angle is the cause of Bell's palsy. In five cases, he could achieve satisfactory results by decompression of the facial nerve from an arterial loop. The surgical approach and the technique of vascular decompression correspond to the findings of Jannetta (1977) regarding facial spasm.

ACOUSTIC NERVE (EIGHTH CRANIAL NERVE)

The problem of functional preservation and reconstruction of the acoustic nerve is that after a short period of morpho-

logical interruption of this nerve, an irreversible loss of the corresponding sensory cells is unavoidable. In the past, the loss of the acoustic organ and the organ of equilibrium (vestibular apparatus) as a result of tumor surgery in the cerebellopontine angle was accepted as inevitable. Efforts have been made since 1979–1980 to preserve the acoustic nerve in the cerebellopontine angle as well as in the internal auditory meatus by early diagnosis and with the help of microsurgical technique (Rhoton, 1976; Wigand, 1976). For the patient, this is especially advantageous when the symmetry of hearing between the two ears is not good. Meanwhile, increasing rates of hearing preservation from 22% to 80% under special circumstances are being reported (Fig. 39–26) (Bentivoglio et al, 1988; Cohen, 1979, 1992; Cohen and Ransohoff, 1984; Cohen et al, 1986; Fischer et al, 1987, 1992; Gardner and Robertson, 1988; Glasscock et al, 1993; Haines and Levine, 1993; Harner et al, 1984, 1990; Helms, 1992; House and Shelton, 1992; Kanzaki et al, 1989; Maniglia et al, 1989; Nadol, 1993; Nedzelski and Tator, 1984; Ojemann et al, 1984; Post et al, 1995; Samii, 1988, 1989; Samii and Matthies, 1995a, 1995b; Shelton, 1992; Silverstein et al, 1986; Sterkers et al, 1986; Symon et al, 1989; Wigand, 1989).

Whether the attempt to preserve the vestibular nerve is justified seems to be open to question. Although a complete loss of this nerve may be compensated centrally, especially in younger patients, partial damage may cause constant, troublesome vertigo.

GLOSSOPHARYNGEAL, VAGUS, SPINAL ACCESSORY, AND HYPOGLOSSAL NERVES (NINTH THROUGH TWELFTH CRANIAL NERVES)

The lesions of cranial nerves IX–XII are classified in three descending topographical and anatomical sections according to the possibilities of surgical approach.

1. The intracranial cerebellopontine region.
2. The extradural area of the base of the skull (jugular foramen, canal of the hypoglossal nerve).
3. The neck region.

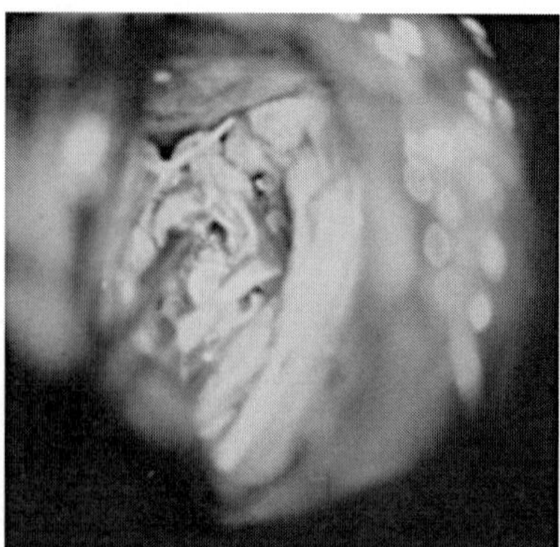

FIGURE 39–26. Cerebellopontine angle neuroma on the right side. After partial removal, one can clearly discern the tumor originating in the fascicle of the vestibular nerve. The facial nerve as well as the cochlear nerve in this case could be preserved. The preoperative extent of hearing remained unaltered after surgery.

The caudal cranial nerves in the first and second areas lie closely together. They are often affected by pathological processes, either one after the other or at the same time, whereas each nerve in the neck region requires individual attention. In our experience, preservation of the glossopharyngeal and vagus nerves for the patient (particularly if preoperative functions are intact) is almost as important as complete removal of the pathological process. Although a slowly proceeding loss of these nerves (e.g., because of the growth of a tumor) is less significant with regard to swallowing, the acute interruption of continuity of the nerve leads to severe dysphagia and aspiration. In such cases, only plastic reconstructive measures in the neck area, as mentioned by Denecke (1961), or partial closure of the glottis (personal communication, Draf, 1977) will allow physical rehabilitation for the patient.

In the region of the cerebellopontine angle, the protective sheath of connective tissue of the caudal cranial nerves is less thick than outside the base of the skull. Therefore, microsurgical manipulation, bipolar coagulation, and the avoidance of direct contact of the nerve are essential conditions for functional preservation. Because of the vital functions of the caudal cranial nerves, the first step after suboccipital exposure of the cerebellopontine angle during tumor operation should be the preparation and protection of the caudal cranial nerves (Figs. 39–27 and 39–28).

The jugular foramen, as the exit area of cranial nerves IX–XI, can be the place of origin of extradural space-occupying processes at the base of the skull (neurinomas, glomus tumors). Frequently, the jugular foramen is secondarily involved, as is the hypoglossal canal in processes that are located directly caudal to the base of the skull (tumors of the jugular glomus and of the tympanic glomus, as well as high lymphatic node metastases). From this point, penetration into the endocranium is also possible (Fig. 39–29).

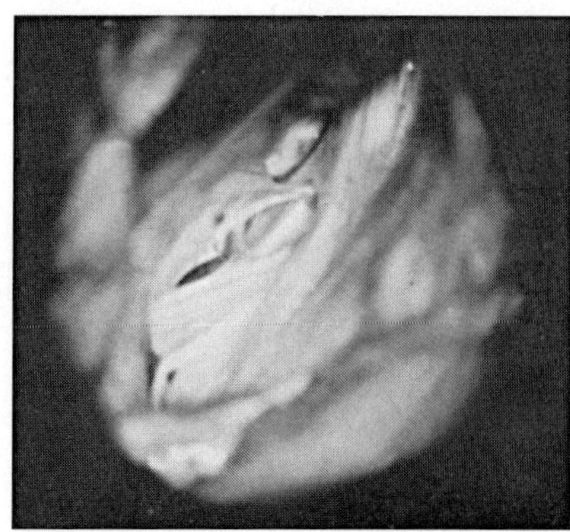

FIGURE 39–27. Demonstration of the normal condition of the caudal cranial nerves after suboccipital approach to the cerebellopontine angle. The dura has been opened and the cerebellum retracted.

Clinical and neuroradiological examination is absolutely necessary before embarking on any surgical intervention in this region to estimate the exact extension of the tumor. The exposure of this area of the base of the skull was developed by Grunert (1894), Rehn (1919), Zehm (1969), Arena (1974), Conley (1975), and Fisch (1976). Among others, Denecke (1969) published essential references regarding this surgical technique.

The approach to the middle and posterior base of the skull, including the jugular foramen, is performed dorsocaudally after turning the sternocleidomastoid muscle to the side. The field of operation can be enlarged: through a temporary splitting of the lower jaw and by pulling up the neighboring part of the joint; through tangential resection of the ascending branch of the lower jaw, including the processus articularis; through resection of the styloid process and, if necessary, of the lip of the mastoid; then the internal

FIGURE 39–28. *A,* Exposure of the cerebellopontine angle on the left side with a very extensive cholesteatoma *(asterisk).* The tumor capsule is adherent to the caudal cranial nerves. *B,* After dissection with preservation of the caudal cranial nerves, the tumor *(asterisk)* is seen partially removed. *C,* Extensive removal of the tumor. The caudal cranial nerves, the facial nerves, and the acoustic nerves as well as the vessels running to the brain stem are preserved. The hypoglossal nerve is visible. *D,* Total extirpation of the large cholesteatoma (measuring 6 × 5 cm). The cranial nerves and the brain stem as well as the vessels are preserved. The slight depression of the pons and the anterior cerebellar artery is distinctly demonstrated.

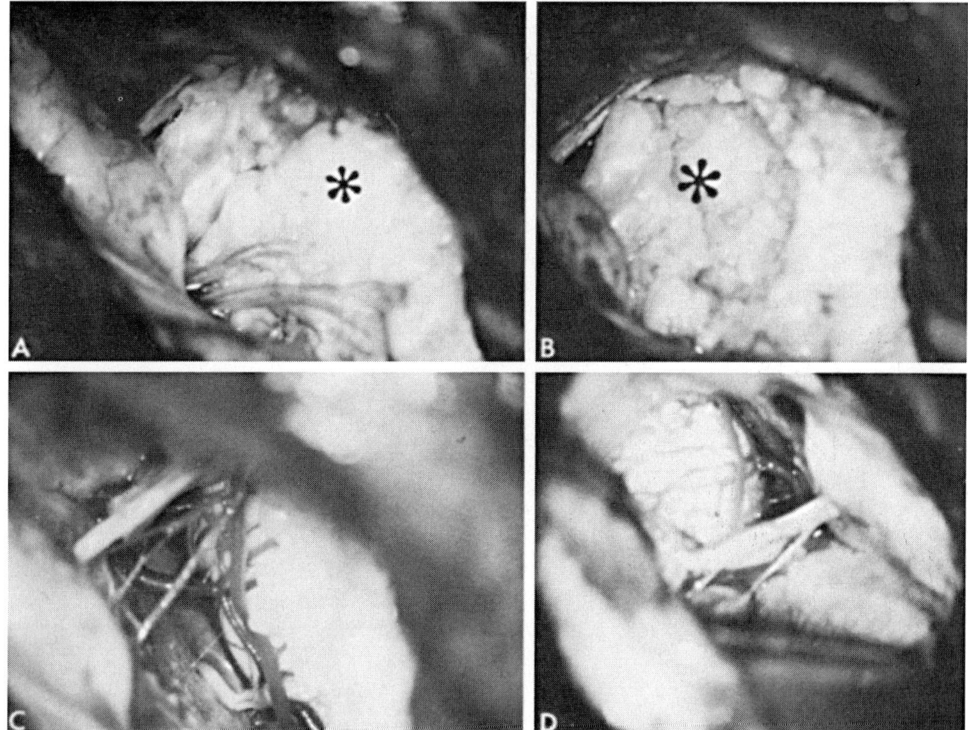

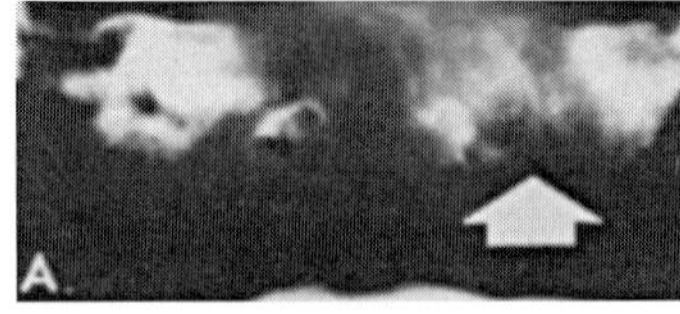

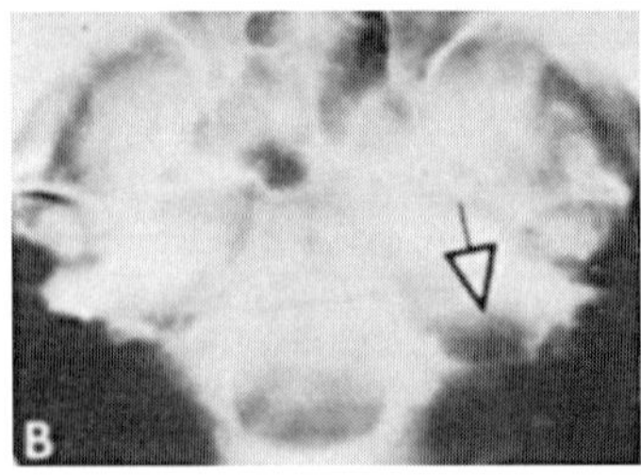

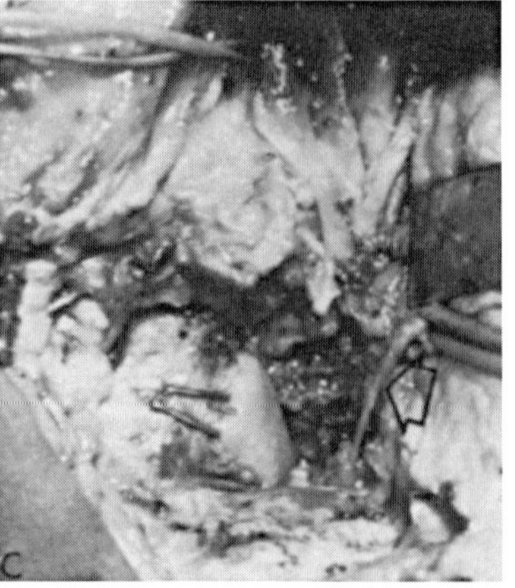

FIGURE 39–29. *A* and *B*, Roentgenograms of the base of the skull. Large glomus tumor with extensive destruction of the base of the skull *(arrows)* in the region of the jugular foramen and the petrous bone. *C*, After removal of the large glomus tumor of the base of the skull, exposure of the jugular foramen. The preserved caudal cranial nerves and the internal carotid artery are visible. A dura defect is bridged using lyophilized dura after resection because of tumor infiltration in the area of the middle and posterior fossa. The facial nerve *(arrow)* is exposed in the cerebellopontine angle up to its entrance into the parotid gland.

jugular vein in the bulb or sigmoid sinus as well as the internal carotid artery and the accompanying cranial nerves can be isolated and distinctly arranged (Draf and Samii, 1977; Samii and Draf, 1978).

Processes at the jugular foramen may require the exposure or resection of the jugular bulb after ligation of the sigmoid sinus. In such a manner, it is possible to prepare cranial nerves IX, X, and XI more distinctly in the anterior section of the jugular foramen and to preserve them in cases of expansive tumors, provided that the tumor does not originate in one of these cranial nerves (see Fig. 39–29). Injuries to the caudal cranial nerves in the neck region may be traumatic, tumorous, or iatrogenic.

Isolated glossopharyngeal nerve lesions in the neck region are comparatively rare and are of lesser significance because of the mixed innervation of the pharyngoglossal area. Additionally, this nerve is located in the neck region and reaches its supply area relatively cephalad. Besides, many anastomo-

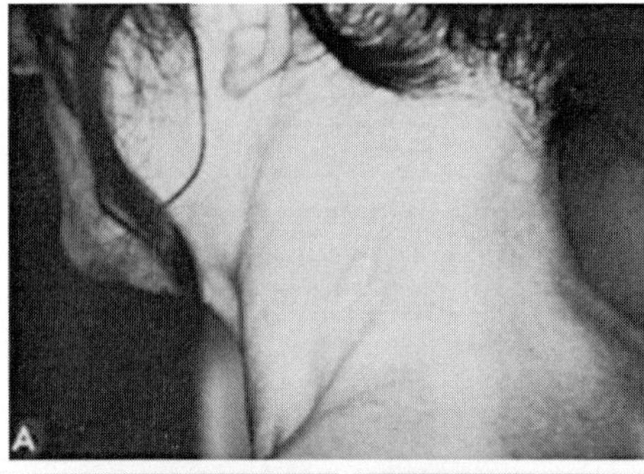

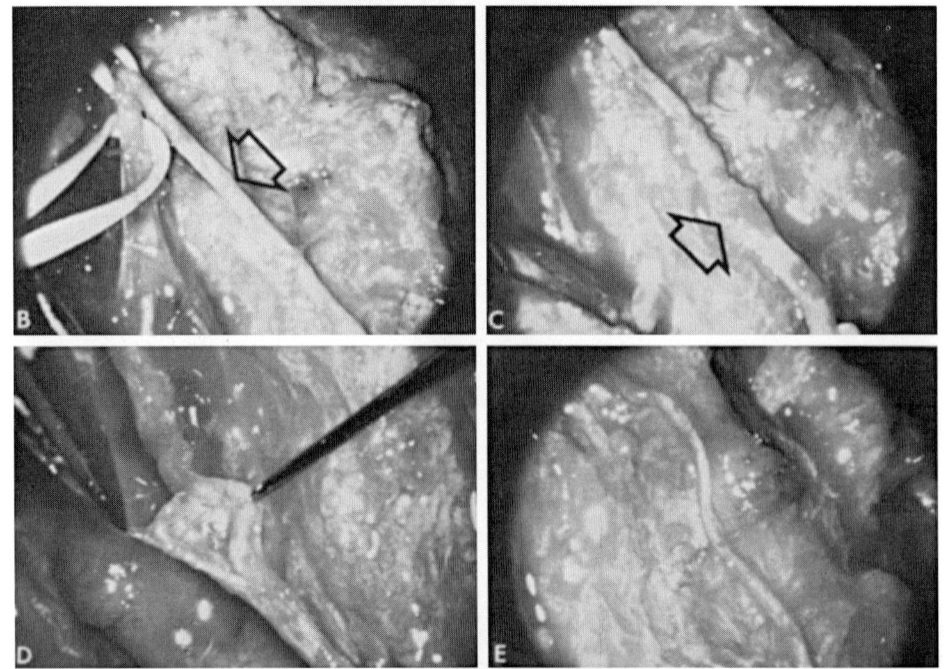

FIGURE 39–30. *A*, Typical scar to the lateral border of the sternocleidomastoid muscle after removal of a lymph node with injury of the accessory nerve. *B*, Exposure of the accessory nerve *(arrow)* at the lateral border of the sternocleidomastoid muscle. *C*, The lesion is exposed. The continuity of the nerve is preserved. One can observe a thickening of the nerve trunk *(arrow)*. *D*, Microsurgical epineurotomy. The fascicle of the nerve is exposed. *E*, A fascicular neurolysis has been performed. The fascicle is preserved in its continuity.

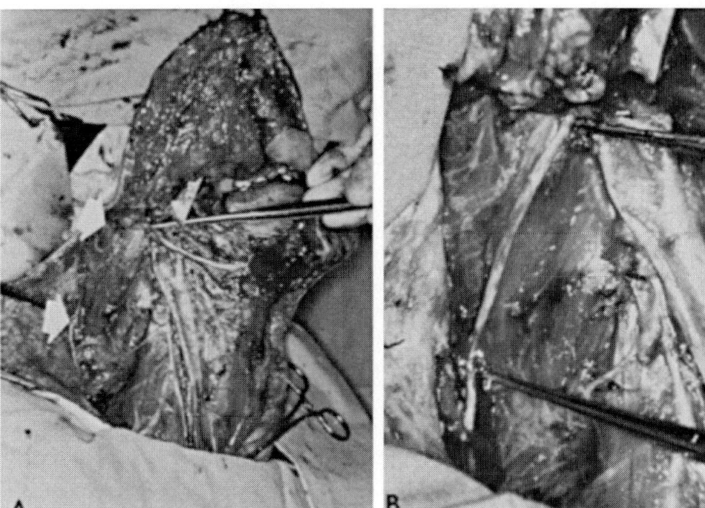

FIGURE 39–31. *A*, Operative field after neck dissection that included the resection of the accessory nerve. Exposure of the distal and central stumps *(arrows)*. *B*, Bridging of the nerve defect by means of a 12-cm nerve graft (between forceps).

ses exist between this nerve and the vagus nerve just caudal to the jugular foramen. Surgical interventions medial of its guide muscle (the stylopharyngeal) are performed rarely. Previously, some trials have been performed to use this nerve for reanimation procedures for the facial nerve (Ballance, 1924; Watson and Williams, 1927), a method that has been abandoned.

The clinical symptom of a vagus nerve disorder depends on the location of the lesion and is characterized by dysphagia, shifting of the velum palatinum toward the healthy side, loss of the coulisse phenomenon of the pharyngeal muscles, and paralysis of the vocal cord. Besides the disturbance of the swallowing reflex, the sensory disorder in the pharynx region, including the danger of aspiration, is especially high.

The clinical disturbances caused by the injury of the trunk of the vagus nerve distal to the posterior belly of the digastric muscle, with the exception of the recurrent nerve, are not significant. In respect to correction of vocal cord paralysis after injury of the recurrent nerve distal to its takeoff from the vagus nerve (most often after thyroidectomy), Miehlke (1976) elaborated in animal experiments the recurrence of decompression, an end-to-end anastomosis as well as an autograft. Hengerer and Tucker (1973) successfully performed, in animal experiments, an anastomosis of a muscle quadrant between the sternohyoid muscle still connected with a cervical branch of the hypoglossal nerve and the cricoarytenoid muscle.

The principle of this operation is that by blunt preparation, the cricoarytenoid muscle on one side, and, if necessary, at some further step on the second side, is exposed just on the

plate of the cricoid cartilage. A 1 × 1-cm large and about 5-mm thick cube-shaped piece of the sternohyoid muscle is prepared and kept attached to the innervating branch of the ansa hypoglossi. This piece of muscle is inserted like an inlay into the defect of the cricoarytenoid muscle.

SPINAL ACCESSORY NERVE (ELEVENTH CRANIAL NERVE)

A clinical diagnosis of a neurological deficit of the accessory nerve has serious impact. Preservation of function or reconstruction of the accessory nerve is very important. Patients with complete loss of function of this nerve with paralysis of the trapezius muscle are no longer able to perform strenuous physical activity. Damage to the accessory nerve caused by accidents is relatively rare, even though the nerve lies in the lateral neck triangle close under the skin. However, the accessory nerve may frequently get damaged during extirpation of a tumor or of a lymphatic gland lateral to the posterior border of the sternocleidomastoid muscle (Fig. 39–30A).

Excisions of lymphatic glands and small tumors in this region must be performed very carefully. During such an intervention, the accessory nerve in this area should always be exposed at the posterior border of the sternocleidomastoid muscle. Subsequently, the removal of a tumor or the lymphatic gland may be executed. If postoperative paralysis occurs, the accessory nerve must be operated on as soon as possible by means of neurolysis, nerve suture, or nerve grafting. When exposing the nerve, one must avoid the scar

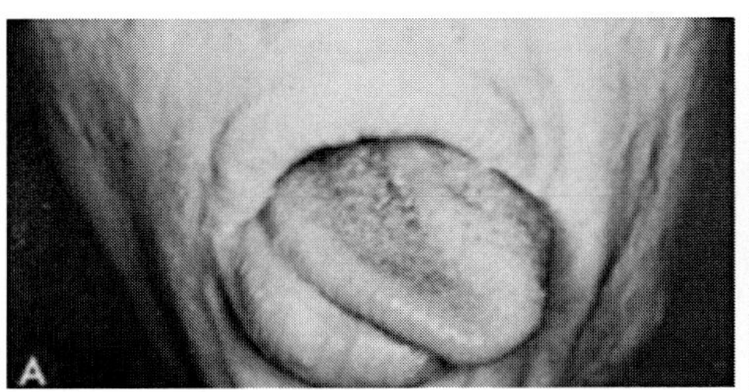
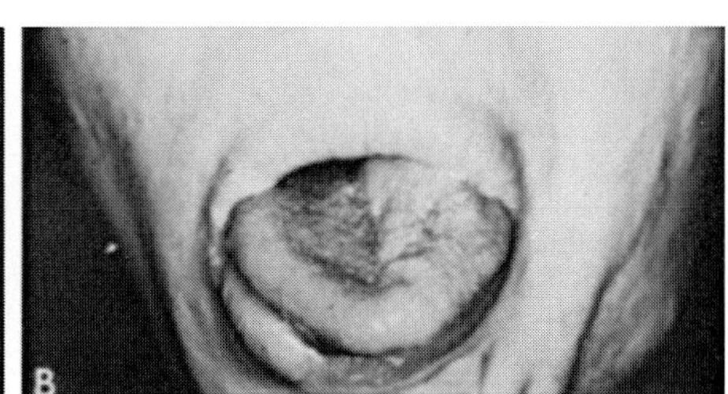

FIGURE 39–32. *A*, Paralysis of hypoglossal nerve on the left side after laceration of the neck in a 19-year-old patient. *B*, Functional improvement 4 days after a fascicular neurolysis.

region in the area of the lesion and start with its exposure in the healthy part at the posterior margin of the sternocleido-mastoid muscle. If the continuity is evident macroscopically, a fascicular neurolysis can be performed under the micro-scope. In some cases, there may be only a serious fibrosis with compression of the nerve, requiring the removal of the fibrotically changed epineurium (see Fig. 39–30).

In case of neuromatous change of the fascicles, even if the continuity is preserved, the neuroma should be resected and an end-to-end anastomosis or nerve grafting performed. If the accessory nerve is interrupted in its continuity and the neuroma of the proximal stump is located in a scar region with no relation to the distal stump, one must endeavor to trace the accessory nerve distal to the nerve lesion. Extensive damages, especially when the lesion is located at a great distance, may cause difficulties with regard to the exposure of the distal stump because the nerve at this point soon begins to branch off and ends in the anterior segment of the trapezius muscle.

Malignant tumors that involve the accessory nerve and cases that demand radical neck dissection require preopera-tive consideration of accessory nerve reconstruction. As soon as the skin flap is prepared for neck dissection, the central portion of the accessory nerve distal to the jugular foramen is marked and cut. The distal part also has to be traced and is cut before its entrance into the trapezius muscle (Fig. 39–31A and B). After neck dissection, the existing defect can be bridged by a graft approximately 12 cm long from the sural nerve.

HYPOGLOSSAL NERVE (TWELFTH CRANIAL NERVE)

Injuries to the hypoglossal nerve in the neck region rarely occur with penetrating injuries of the soft tissues of the neck. During tumor surgery in the neck region, especially when dissecting the carotid sheath, where the hypoglossal nerve often is surrounded by a venous plexus, it may be damaged during the management of bleeding vessels. Furthermore, damage may occur during a difficult extirpation of the sub-mandibular gland, especially when the nerve is adherent to the inflammatory mass or is infiltrated by the tumor. Tumors in the retrolingual region and on the floor of the mouth may grow around the hypoglossal nerve and cause paralysis. An important clinical symptom is a disturbance of articulation. Reconstruction of the hypoglossal nerve is demanded in traumatic cases and should be performed by microsurgical techniques. The spectrum of surgical treatment extends from neurolysis to nerve suture and nerve grafting, depending on the operative findings (Fig. 39–32A and B).

References

Adams CBT: Microvascular compression: An alternative view and hypothe-sis. J Neurosurg 57:1–12, 1989.

Adour K: Etiology and pathogenesis of Bell's palsy. Panel Discussion No. 10. In Fisch U (ed): Facial Nerve Surgery. Amstelveen, The Netherlands, Kugler Medical Publ, 1977, p 371.

Anderl H: A simple method for correcting the ectropion. Plast Reconstr Surg 49:156, 1972.

Arai H, Sato K, Yanai A: Hemihypoglossal-facial nerve anastomosis in treating unilateral facial palsy after acoustic neurinoma resection. J Neu-rosurg 82:51–54, 1995.

Arena S: Tumor surgery of the temporal bone. Laryngoscope 84:645, 1974.

Ballance CA, Duel AB: The operative treatment of facial palsy; by the introduction of nerve grafts into the fallopian canal and by other intra-temporal methods. Arch Otolaryngol 15:1, 1932.

Becker R: Die Kontinuitätsresektion des Unterkiefers unter Erhaltung des N. mandibularis. Dtsch Zahnärztl Z 22:929, 1967.

Becker R: Continuity resection of the mandible with preservation of man-dibular nerve. Br J Oral Surg 8:45, 1970.

Becker R: Behandlung und Behandlungsergebnisse bei 38 Ameloblastomen. Fortschr Kiefer Gesichtschir. 15:211, 1972.

Bentivoglio P, Cheeseman AD, Symon L: Surgical management of acoustic neuromas during the last five years. Part II: Results for facial and cochlear nerve function. Surg Neurol 29:205–209, 1988.

Bertrand RA, Molina P, Hardy J: Surgical treatment of hemi-facial spasm. In Fisch U (ed): Facial Nerve Surgery. Amstelveen, The Netherlands, Kugler Medical Publ, 1977, p 512.

Bunnell S: Surgery of the nerves of the hand. Surg Gynecol Obstet 44:145, 1927.

Cadena G: Incidence and management of Bell's palsy according to geo-graphic distribution. Panel Discussion No. 9. In Fisch U (ed): Facial Nerve Surgery. Amstelveen, The Netherlands, Kugler Medical Publ, 1977, p 328.

Campbell E, Keedy C: Hemifacial spasm: A note on the etiology in two cases. J Neurosurg 4:342, 1947.

Cawthorne T: The pathology and surgical treatment of Bell's palsy. J Laryngol 65:792, 1951.

Cawthorne T: Geniculate ganglion facial palsy. Arch Otolaryngol 81:502, 1965.

Cawthorne T, Wilson T: Indications for intratemporal facial nerve surgery. Arch Otolaryngol 78:429, 1963.

Clerc P, Batisse R: Abord des organes intra-pétreux par voie endocranienne. Ann Otolaryngol (Paris) 71:20, 1954.

Cohen NL: Acoustic neuroma surgery with emphasis on preservation of hearing. Laryngoscope 89:886–896, 1979.

Cohen NL: Retrosigmoid approach for acoustic tumor removal. Otolaryngol Clin North Am 25:295–310, 1992.

Cohen NL, Ransohoff J: Hearing preservation—posterior fossa approach. Otolaryngol Head Neck Surg 92:176–183, 1984.

Cohen NL, Hammerschlag P, Berg H, Ransohoff J: Acoustic neuroma surgery: An eclectic approach with emphasis on preservation of hearing. Ann Otol Rhinol Laryngol 95:21–27, 1986.

Conley JJ: Facial nerve grafting in treatment of parotid gland tumors. Arch Surg 70:359, 1955.

Conley JJ: Facial nerve grafting. Arch Otolaryngol 73:322, 1961.

Conley JJ: Salivary Glands and the Facial Nerve. Stuttgart, George Thieme Verlag, 1975.

Cornelius CP, Ehrenfeld M, Wiethölter H: Late results after reconstruction of the sensory branches of the mandibular nerve. In Samii M (ed): Skull Base Surgery. Basel, Karger, 1994, pp 639–646.

Cusimano MD, Sekhar L: Partial hypoglossal to facial nerve anastomosis for reinnervation of the paralyzed face in patients with lower cranial nerve palsies: Technical note. Neurosurgery 35:532–533, 533–534, 1994.

Davis RA, Anson BJ, Budinger JM, et al: Surgical anatomy of the facial nerve and parotid gland based upon a study of 350 cervicofacial halves. Surg Gynecol Obstet 102:385, 1956.

Denecke HJ: Operationstechnische Probleme bei der Entfernung großer Neurinoma im Bereich von Felsenbeinpyramide. N. facialis, Pharynx. Gefäßscheide, Osophagusmund und Zunge. H.N.O. (Berlin) 8:343, 1959/60.

Denecke HJ: Korrektur des Schluckaktes bei einseitiger Pharynx-Larynxläh-mung. 'HNO', Wegweiser für die fachärztl. Praxis 9:351, 1961.

Denecke HJ: Diskussionsbemerkung Nobel Symposion 10. Stockholm, Almquist and Wiksell, 1969.

Deruty R, Guyotat J, Mottolese C, et al: Partial recovery of the oculomotor nerve after section and repair during the excision of a tumor. Neurochirur-gie 34:287–292, 1988.

Devriese PP: Experimental compression of the facial nerve. In Fisch U (ed): Facial Nerve Surgery. Amstelveen, The Netherlands, Kugler Medi-cal Publ, 1977, p 344.

Dott NM: Facial paralysis. Restitution by extrapetrous nerve graft. Proc R Soc Med 51:900, 1958.

Draf W, Samii M: Otorhinolaryngologisch-neurochirurgische Probleme an der Schädelbasis. Laryngol Rhinol 56:1007, 1977.

Draf W, Samii M: Intracranial-intratemporal anastomosis of the facial nerve after cerebellopontine angle tumor surgery. In Graham MD, House WF (eds): Disorders of the Facial Nerve. New York, Raven, 1982, pp 441–449.

Drake CG: Acoustic neurinoma: Repair of facial nerve with autogenous graft. J Neurosurg 17:836, 1960.

Drake CG: Experiences and results with posterior approaches. In Schürmann K, Brock M, Reulen HJ, Voth D (eds): Brain Edema—Cerebellopontine Angle Tumors. Advances in Neurosurgery. New York, Springer Verlag, 1973, vol 1, p 240.

Duel AB: Clinical presentation of improvement in surgical repair of the facial nerve. Laryngoscope 44:599, 1934.

Esslen E: Electrodiagnosis of facial palsy. In Miehlke A (ed): Surgery of the Facial Nerve. Munich, Urban & Schwarzenberg, 1973, p 45.

Esslen E: Electromyography and electroneurography. In Fisch U (ed): Facial Nerve Surgery. Amstelveen, The Netherlands, Kugler Medical Publ, 1977, p 93.

Fisch U: Operations on the facial nerve. In Yasargil MG (ed): Microsurgery. Stuttgart, Thieme, 1969, p 208.

Fisch U: Transtemporal surgery of the internal auditory canal: Report of 92 cases, technique, indications and results. Adv Otorhinolaryngol 17:203, 1970a.

Fisch U: Die totale Freilegung des Nervus facialis bei laterobasalen Schädelfrakturen. Arch Klin Exp Ohren Nasen Kehlkopfheilkd 196:187, 1970b.

Fisch U: Die Verletzungen des Nervus facialis bei laterobasalen Schädelfrakturen. Med Mitteil Braun Melsungen 46:165, 1972.

Fisch U: Chirurgie im inneren Gehörgang und an benachbarten Strukturen. In Naumann HH (ed): Kopf- und Halschirurgie, Bd. III: Ohrregion. Stuttgart, Georg Thieme Verlag, 1976.

Fisch U: Facial Nerve Surgery. Amstelveen, The Netherlands, Kugler Medical Publ, 1977.

Fischer G, Morgon A, Fischer C, Bret P, Massini B, Kzaiz M, Charlot M: Total removal of acoustic neuromas: Facial nerve and hearing preservation. Neurochirurgie 33:169–183, 1987.

Fischer G, Fischer C, Remond J: Hearing preservation in acoustic neurinoma surgery. J Neurosurg 176(6):897–900, 910–917, 1992.

Fujita T: Über die periphere Ausbreitung des Nervus facialis beim Menschen. Gegenbaurs Morph Jb 73:578, 1934.

Fukado Y: Microsurgical transethmoidal optic nerve decompression: Experience in 700 cases. In Samii M, Jannetta P (eds): The Cranial Nerves. New York, Springer, 1981, pp 125–128.

Gardner G, Robertson JH: Hearing preservation in unilateral acoustic neuroma surgery. Ann Otol Rhinol Laryngol 97:55–66, 1988.

Gardner WJ: Concerning the mechanism of trigeminal neuralgia and hemifacial spasm. J Neurosurg 19:947, 1962.

Gardner WJ, Sava GA: Hemifacial spasm: A reversible pathophysiologic state. J Neurosurg 19:240, 1962.

Glasscock ME III, Hays JW, Minor LB, Haynes DS, Carrasco VN: Preservation of hearing in surgery for acoustic neuromas. J Neurosurg 78:864–870, 1993.

Gomez JG: Incidence and management of Bell's palsy according to geographic distribution. Panel Discussion No. 9. In Fisch U (ed): Facial Nerve Surgery. Amstelveen, The Netherlands, Kugler Medical Publ, 1977, p 319.

Greve K: Histologische Befunde bei komplizierten Kieferfrakturen mit besonderer Berücksichtigung des Mandibularkanals. Dtsch Mschr Zahnheilk 45:458, 1927.

Grimson BS, Ross MJ, Tyson G: Return of function after intracranial resuture of the trochlear nerve. Case Report. J Neurosurg 61:191–192, 1984.

Grunert KA: Die operative Ausräumung des Bulbus venae jugularis (Bulbusoperation). Arch Ohrenheilk 36:71, 1894.

Haid CT, Wigand ME: Advantages of the enlarged middle cranial fossa approach in acoustic neurinoma surgery: A review. Acta Otolaryngol Stockh 112:387–407, 1992.

Haines SJ, Levine SC: Intracanalicular acoustic neuroma: Early surgery for preservation of hearing. J Neurosurg 79:515–520, 1993.

Harner SG, Laws ER Jr, Onofrio BM: Hearing preservation after removal of acoustic neurinoma. Laryngoscope 94:1431–1434, 1984.

Harner SG, Beatty CW, Ebersold MJ: Pterosigmoid removal of acoustic neuroma: Experience 1978–1988. Otolaryngol Head Neck Surg 103:40–45, 1990.

Hausamen JE, Samii M, Schmidseder R: Repair of the mandibular nerve by means of autologous nerve grafting after resection of the lower jaw. J Maxillofac Surg 1:74, 1973.

Hausamen JE, Samii M, Schmidseder R: Indication and technique for the reconstruction of nerve defects in head and neck. J Maxillofac Surg 2:159, 1974.

Helms J: The transmeatal approach to the geniculate ganglion. Acta Otolaryngol Belg 30:84, 1976.

Helms J: Hearing preservation in acoustic neurinoma surgery. Otolaryngol Pol 46:533–537, 1992.

Hengerer S, Tucker HM: Restoration of abduction in the paralyzed canine vocal cord. Arch Otolaryngol 97:247, 1973.

Hermann M: Über die Verletzung der Gesichtsnerven. Zahnärztl Praxis 9:97, 1958.

Hilger JA: The nature of Bell's palsy. Laryngoscope 59:228, 1949.

Hitselberger WE, House WF: Experiences and results with the translabyrinthine approach and related techniques (Abstract). In Schuermann K, et al (eds): Advances in Neurosurgery, Volume 1: Brain Edema: Pathophysiology and Therapy; Cerebello Pontine Angle Tumors: Diagnosis and Surgery. New York, Springer-Verlag, 1973, p 239.

Hof E: Facial palsy of infectious origin in children. In Fisch U (ed): Facial Nerve Surgery. Amstelveen, The Netherlands, Kugler Medical Publ, 1977, p 414.

Hosomi H: Management of Bell's palsy. In Fisch U (ed): Facial Nerve Surgery. Amstelveen, The Netherlands, Kugler Medical Publ, 1977, p 382.

House WF: Surgical exposure of the internal auditory canal and its contents through the middle cranial fossa. Laryngoscope 71:1363, 1961.

House WF: Middle cranial fossa approach to the petrous pyramid. Arch Otolaryngol 78:460, 1963.

House WF, Shelton C: Middle fossa approach for acoustic tumor removal. Otolaryngol Clin North Am 25:347–359, 1992.

Jacobson JH: Microsurgical technique in the repair of the traumatized extremity. Clin Orthop 29:132, 1963.

Jannetta PJ: Microsurgical exploration and decompression of the facial nerve in hemifacial spasm. Curr Top Surg Res 2:217, 1970.

Jannetta PJ: Neurovascular compression of the facial nerve in hemifacial spasm: Relief by microsurgical technique. In Merei FT (ed): Reconstructive Surgery of Brain Arteries. Budapest, Publishing House of the Hungarian Academy of Sciences, 1974, p 193.

Jannetta PJ: The cause of hemifacial spasm: Definitive microsurgical treatment at the brainstem in 31 patients. Am Acad Ophthalmol Otolaryngol 30:319, 1975.

Jannetta PJ: Trigeminal neuralgia and hemifacial spasm: Etiology and definitive treatment. Trans Am Neurol Assoc 100:53, 1975.

Jannetta PJ: Etiology and definitive microsurgical treatment of hemifacial spasm. J Neurosurg 47:321, 1977.

Jannetta PJ: A theory as to aetiology. Observations in six patients. Laryngoscope 89:849, 1978.

Jannetta PJ: Hemifacial spasm. In Samii M, Jannetta PJ (eds): The Cranial Nerves. Berlin, Springer, 1981, pp 484–493.

Jongkees LBW: Die chirurgische Behandlung der intratemporalen Facialislähmung. Dtsch Med Wochenschr 83:865, 1958.

Jongkees LBW: Über die intratemporale Facialislähmung und ihre chirurgische Behandlung. Z Laryng Rhinol 40:319, 1961.

Jongkees LBW: Nerve excitability test. In Fisch U (ed): Facial Nerve Surgery. Amstelveen, The Netherlands, Kugler Medical Publ, 1977, p 83.

Kanzaki J, Ogawa K, Shiobara R, Toya S: Hearing preservation in acoustic neuroma surgery and postoperative audiological findings. Acta Otolaryngol Stockh 107:474–478, 1989.

Kanzaki J, Kunihiro T, O-Uchi T, Ogawa K, Shiobara R, Toya S: Intracranial reconstruction of the facial nerve: Clinical observation. Acta Otolaryngol Suppl Stockh 487:85–90, 1991.

Kettel K: Repair of the facial nerve in traumatic facial palsies: Results of decompression, nerve suture and nerve grafting in one hundred twenty-seven cases. Arch Otolaryngol 66:634, 1957.

Kettel K: Peripheral Facial Palsy, Pathology and Surgery. Copenhagen, Munksgaard, 1959.

Koos WT, Böck FW, Salah S: Experiences in microsurgery of acoustic neurinomas (Abstract). In Schuermann K, et al (ed): Advances in Neurosurgery, Volume 1: Brain Edema: Pathophysiology and Therapy; Cerebello Pontine Angle Tumors: Diagnosis and Surgery. New York, Springer-Verlag, 1973, p 251.

Lanzino G, Sekhar LN, Sen CN, Pomonis S: Reconstruction of cranial nerves III through VI during cavernous sinus surgery. In Samii M (ed): Skull Base Surgery. Basel, Karger, 1994, pp 477–481.

Lathrop FD: The facial nerve: Technique of exposure and repair. Surg Clin North Am 33:909, 1953.

Lathrop FD: Surgical repair of the facial nerve: Technique. Surg Clin North Am 36:583, 1956.

Lathrop FD: Management of the facial nerve during operations on the parotid gland. Ann Otol 72:780, 1962.

Chapter 40

• Giorgio A. Brunelli
• Giovanni R. Brunelli

Direct Muscle Neurotization

There are peculiar peripheral nerve lesions in which neither nerve suture nor grafts may be done because a traumatic agent or a surgical operation either has avulsed the motor nerve from the muscle or muscles or has destroyed the so-called neural part of the muscle (i.e., that part in which the distal motor nerve divisions form the neuromuscular junction: the motor plates). To overcome these conditions in the early 1970s, we carried out research to determine whether it was possible to achieve reinnervation of the denervated muscle by implanting a new nerve to it. Once the authors obtained promising experimental results, this procedure was used successfully in several patients.

HISTORY

The first experiments of direct muscular reinnervation were performed by Heineke (1914), Erlacher (1915), Steindler (1915), and Elsberg (1917). The clinical applications that followed had such inconsistent results that the technique was abandoned. In the 1950s and 1960s, research was carried out that focused on the effects of placing a nerve directly on the surface of denervated muscle (Aitken, 1950; Gutmann and Hanzlikova, 1967; Heineke, 1914; Katz and Miledi, 1964; Sakellarides et al, 1972). When the nerve was stimulated postoperatively, weak contractile responses from muscle were produced. Formation of new synapses at the contact of nerve with denervated muscle was thought to have been responsible (Bennet and Pettigrew, 1976; Bradley, 1977; Brenner and Sakmann, 1978; Brunelli et al, 1976; Engel, 1970; Frenk et al, 1975; Guth and Zalewski, 1963; Lomo and Slater, 1980; Sakellarides et al, 1972).

In 1970, the authors started experimental studies of directly implanting a foreign nerve into muscle: The tibial nerve was resected and removed from the triceps, and the peroneal nerve was implanted into the lateral head of this muscle, which is an aneural zone (i.e., devoid of nerve endings). Physiological muscle responses were obtained, and formation of new motor end-plates in aneural zones of muscle was noted (Brunelli et al, 1976; Brunelli, 1981). In 1972, Sakellarides and colleagues published similar results from experiments performed in dogs. In 1973, our experimental model was modified by dividing the nerve in several fascicles to obtain a larger area of reinnervation (Fig. 40–1).

In the following years, the wider distribution of these divisions both in width and in depth gave better and better results.

Histology demonstrated that these results were due to the formation of new motor end-plates between the nerve and the denervated muscular fibers (Brunelli et al, 1976; Brunelli, 1981, Brunelli and Monini, 1985, 1988; Brunelli, 1991).

Experimental studies demonstrated that denervated muscle is sensitive throughout its fibers to acetylcholine, whereas normally innervated muscle is not. The wide distribution of receptors for acetylcholine allows the formation of new motor end-plates, even in aneural, ectopic sites of the muscle.

MATERIAL AND METHODS

In the first series, which was composed of 21 rabbits, the distal part of the tibial nerve with its intramuscular branches was removed from the gastrocnemius muscle and the peroneal nerve was severed and implanted into the proximal portion of the lateral head. (This zone would not, under normal conditions, exhibit motor end-plates.) At 1- and 2-month intervals, the animals were sacrificed. The distal end of the transplanted nerve was identified and studied by light and transmission electron microscopy. The formation of new motor end-plates was noted; this is thought to be a functional adaptation of nerve branches, where they came into contact with the surface of the denervated muscular fibers.

A succeeding research study used a modified technique in rats. The epineurium of the peroneal nerve was removed, and the nerve was divided into several fascicles under the operating microscope. These small branches were implanted into muscle through small slits, spreading them as widely and deeply as possible in order to increase the number of neurotized muscle fibers. A large number of motor end-plates was found. The amount, in different microscopic fields, appeared to depend on the distance of the muscle field from the nerve implant.

Before sacrifice, electrical stimulation of the peroneal nerve demonstrated good functional reinnervation of the triceps as early as 1 month after surgery. Muscle fibers in which new motor end-plates had formed regained trophicity and showed normal morphology (Fig. 40–2); in contrast, the nonreinnervated fibers showed a typical dystrophic appearance. Transmission electron microscopy demonstrated normal motor end-plates with bare axon branches rich in presynaptic vesicles in direct contact with the membranes of muscle fibers that had normal-appearing folds. Presynaptic vesicles and mitochondria were noted in the axon branches, whereas only a single layer of Schwann cytoplasm was present over the axon on the opposite side of the muscle. There were no connective elements between the axon branches and the muscle (Fig. 40–3).

The nerve was stained for acetylcholine (Koelle and Tsuge

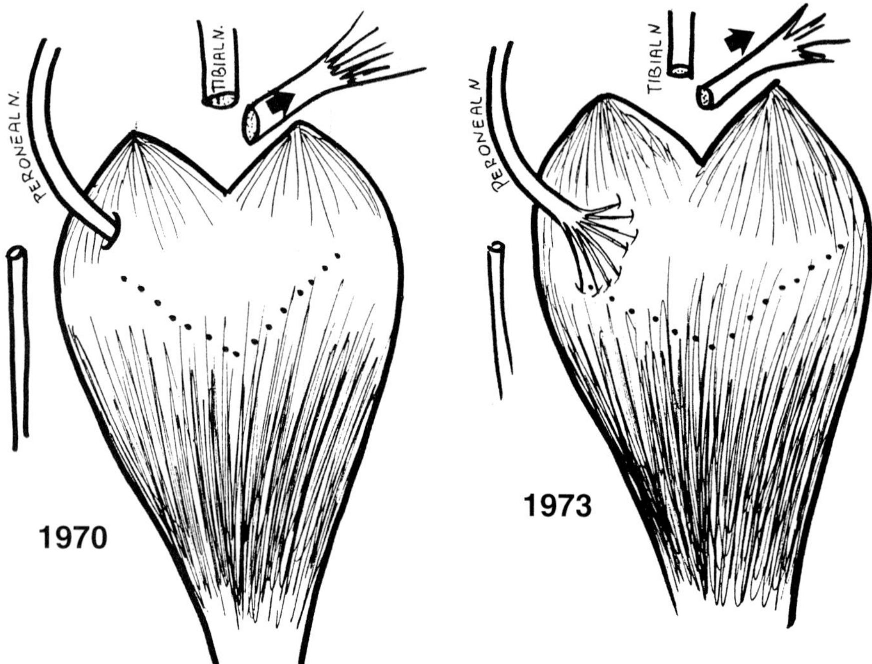

FIGURE 40–1. Scheme of the experimental surgery: The tibial nerve is cut, and its branches to the muscle removed from the so-called "neural zone" of the triceps (the zone where the nerve ends form motor end-plates). The peroneal nerve is then cut, divided in thin slips, and introduced in small slits in the proximal part of the muscle, the aneural zone where normally no motor end-plates exist.

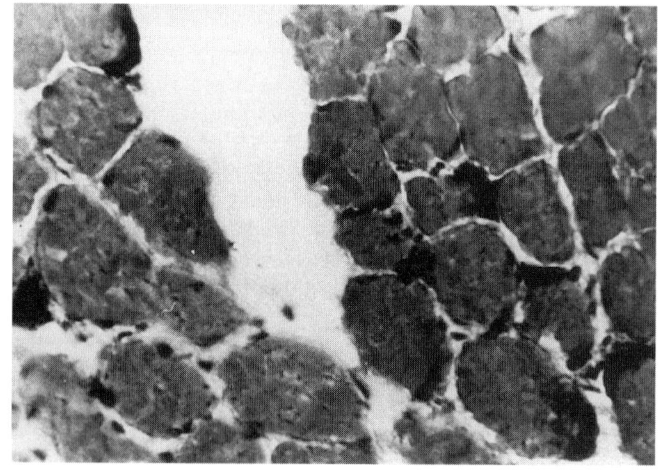

FIGURE 40–2. Motor end-plates are forming at 2 months after operation. The reinnervated muscle fibers show better appearance; the nonreinnervated ones are still dystrophic.

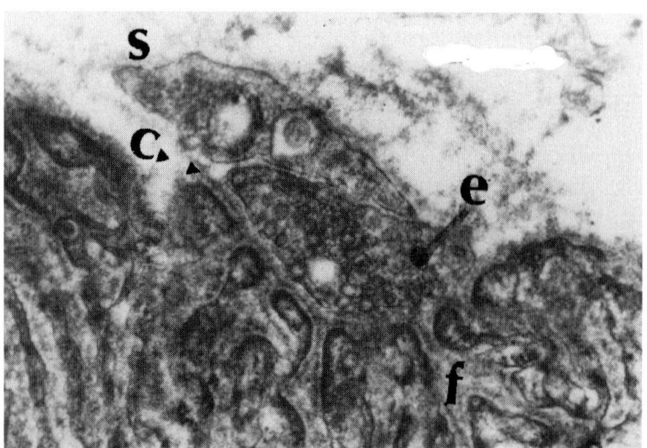

FIGURE 40–3. Newly formed motor end-plates after direct muscular neurotization in a previously aneural zone of the muscle. e, Nerve ending with synaptic vesicles; C, synaptic cleft; f, folding of the muscular membrane; S, cytoplasm of Schwann's cell.

technique). Some of the fibers did not take up the stain. This is probably indirect evidence that both afferent and efferent fibers are present.

Encouraging results may also have been due to the so-called adoption phenomenon, which depends on the chemotactic appeal exerted by the denervated muscle fibers on the surrounding regenerated axons. The axons send out sprouts (from a node of Ranvier, from the axon immediately above the motor end-plate, or even from the motor end-plate itself, reinnervating neighboring orphan muscle fibers.) In this way, giant motor units are formed. They are demonstrated by electromyography. These giant motor units constitute a large part of the newly functioning muscle.

CLINICAL INDICATIONS AND OPERATIVE TECHNIQUE

After obtaining encouraging experimental results, the authors began clinical direct muscular neurotization in 1975 (Brunelli and Monini, 1985, 1988; Brunelli, 1991). The candidates were patients who had sustained injuries in which the proximal nerve stump was available but the distal branches were missing owing to traumatic or surgical loss of that muscle portion in which the motor nerve branches and motor end-plates are located. A long interval of denervation such that the reparative ability of anterior horn cells is exhausted was considered a contraindication. The procedure is also inappropriate if too large a portion of muscle has been destroyed, if the remaining muscle is extremely fibrotic, or if other extramuscular limiting conditions, such as marked joint stiffness, exist.

We have performed 15 reinnervation operations of the extensor muscles of the forearm (Fig. 40–4) and 14 of the leg. In addition, the procedure has been performed in seven trapezium muscles (six of which were damaged by iatrogenic causes) (Fig. 40–5); six deltoid muscles (four were due to avulsion of C5–C6 roots of the brachial plexus, and one was due to avulsion of the muscle branches of the axillary nerve). Four thenar muscles (Fig. 40–6), two muscles of the tongue, and one extensor pollicis longus have also been reinnervated. In one case, the denervated biceps muscle was neurotized

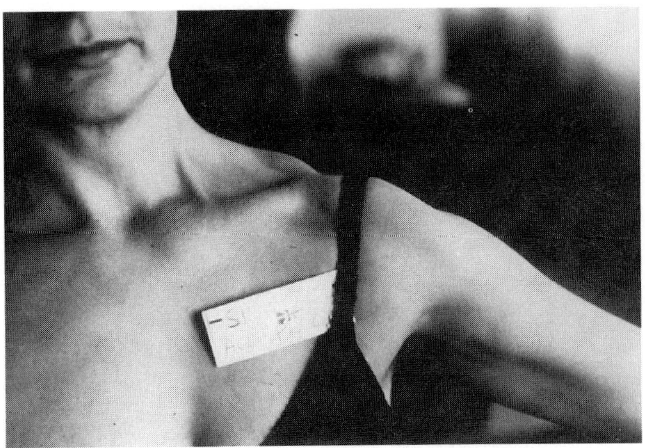

FIGURE 40–5. Result of direct muscle neurotization of the trapezium after iatrogenic avulsion during a lymph node biopsy.

by means of sural grafts connected with a branch for the triceps muscle of the radial nerve (Fig. 40–7).

The original nerve is always dissected from normal into scar tissue and up to the neuroma. This is resected, and the stump of the severed nerve is elongated by means of nerve grafts to muscle. As many grafts as necessary are used to match the fascicles of the proximal stump. The distal ends of the grafts are divided into as many thin slips as possible (Fig. 40–8), which are then introduced into the muscle through longitudinal slits made as atraumatically as possible in the distal portion of the muscle. If bleeding is noted following creation of a slit, a new atraumatic slit is created in another area. Bleeding is avoided to limit the formation of scar. The nerve branches are implanted in as wide an area as possible to increase the volume of reinnervated muscle. The epineurium is sutured to the muscle fascia with 6-0 nonabsorbable suture. In general, the slips stay in their slits and do not need sutures. Autogenous fibrin is sufficient to keep them at this place; if not, the grafts are sewn individually with 10-0 suture. The limb is immobilized, and the reinnervated muscle is kept at rest for 15 days after surgery. Local radiation therapy and steroids are administered to avoid scar formation.

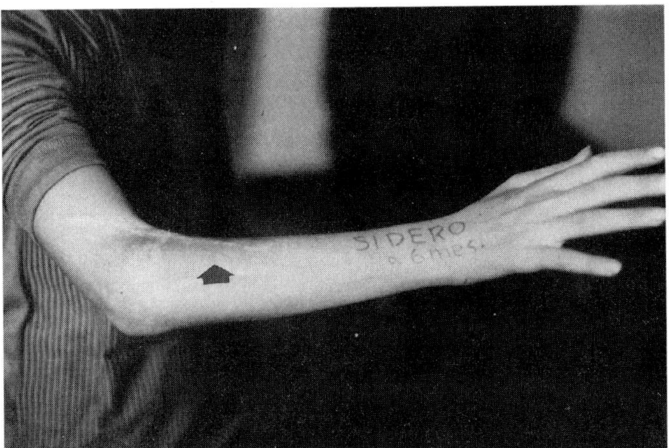

FIGURE 40–4. Very good result after direct muscular neurotization of the extensor muscles of the forearm, the proximal part of which had been removed by trauma. The arrow shows the loss of muscles.

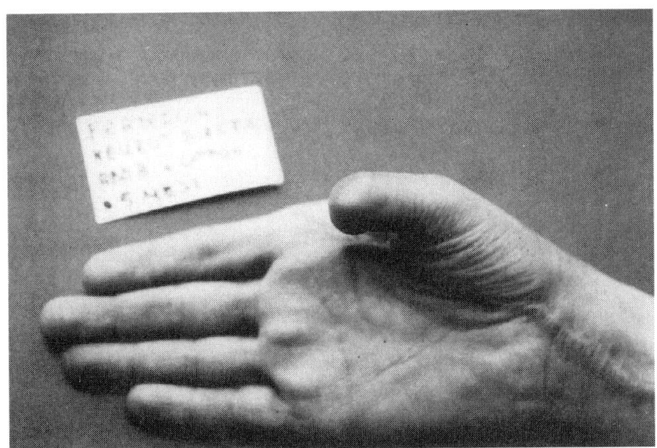

FIGURE 40–6. Good result of direct neurotization of thenar muscles after traumatic avulsion of the motor branch of the median nerve.

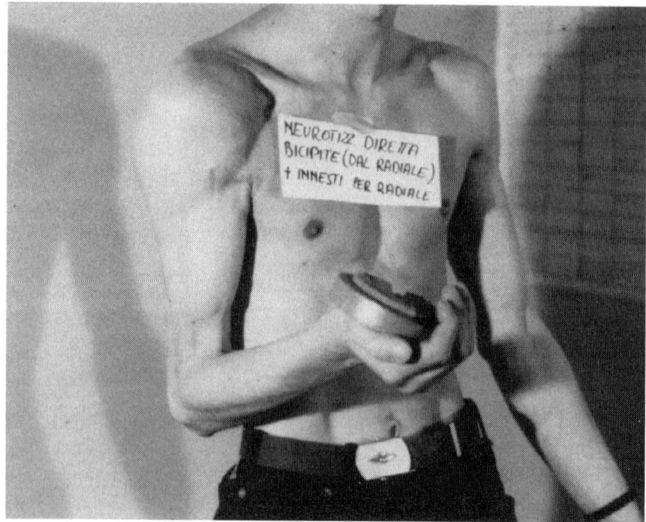

FIGURE 40–7. Good result of direct neurotization of the biceps muscle after traumatic removal of part of its proximal belly and avulsion of the musculocutaneous nerve. A branch to the triceps of the radial nerve was used for neurotization.

RESULTS

Results are shown in Table 40–1. They were good or very good in 50 clinical cases out of the 56 examined. The time for reinnervation to occur depends on the distance from the proximal nerve stump to the point of implantation (nerve regenerates on an average speed of 1 mm per day).

DISCUSSION

In the reported series, 53 of the 56 cases were operated on by connecting the originally innervating nerve with the muscle by means of sural nerve grafts inserted into the muscle. In three cases, connection was done with foreign motor donor nerves.

There are no current techniques by which reinnervation can be obtained when the distal segment of the nerve has been completely destroyed. In these cases, procedures such

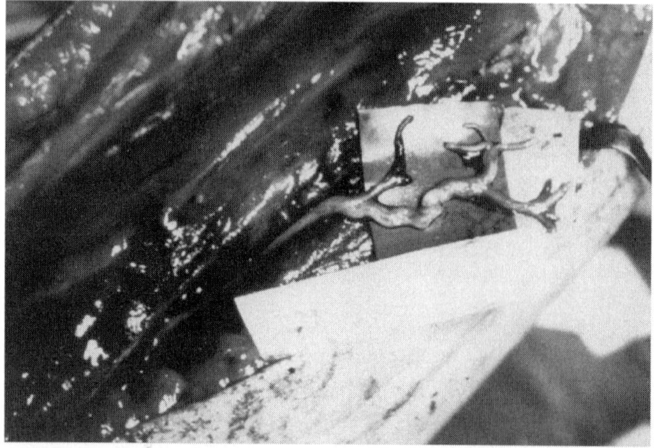

FIGURE 40–8. Surgical appearance of the graft of the sural nerve after its artificial division in several branches.

▼ **TABLE 40–1**
Results of Direct Muscle Neurotization

Muscle	Number of Cases	M-5*	M-4	M-3 +	M-3 or Less
Extensor muscles, forearm	15	10	4	1	0
Extensor muscles, leg	14	11	2	1	0
Trapezius	7	4	2	1	0
Biceps	7	4	2	1	0
Thenar	4	3	1	0	0
Extensor pollicis longus	1	0	1	0	0
Deltoid	6	1	3	1	1
Tongue (hypoglossal)	2	1	1	0	0
Total	56	34	16	5	1

*British Medical Research Council Grade. Very good (the majority of the muscles), M-5; good, M-4; fair, M-3 +; poor, M-3 or less.

as tendon transfers and arthrodeses are traditionally indicated.

We believe that meticulous microsurgical technique, as well as the so-called adoption phenomenon involving axonal branches and their reinnervation of neighboring orphan motor fibers (described above), have accounted for the good results that have been achieved with direct muscular neurotization.

In the recent survey of cases using direct muscular neurotization, which have been operated on by different surgeons using this technique, the percentage of good and very good results was not as high as that reported here. This is probably due to the fact that details of the operative technique were not rigorously and precisely carried out by the less-experienced clinicians. Others, with more extensive experience, have achieved similar results to ours.

CONCLUSION

Our experimental research and clinical application lasting over 25 years allow us to say that direct muscle neurotization is the only solution to the otherwise unsolvable problem of destruction of the neuromuscular junction.

References

Aitken JT: Growth of nerve implants in voluntary muscle. J Anat *84:*38, 1950.

Bennet MR, Pettigrew G: The formation of neuromuscular synapses. Cold Spring Harbor Symp Quant Biol *40:*409, 1976.

Bradley R: The morphology of the normal end plate in lambs as revealed by silver impregnation and light microscopy. Res Vet Sci *23:*250, 1977.

Brenner HR, Sakmann B: Gating properties of acetylcholine receptor in newly formed neuromuscular synapses. Nature *271:*366–368, 1978.

Brunelli G, Monini L, Antonucci A, Maraldi N: Neurotizzazione in zona aneurale di muscoli denervati. Il Policlinico *83:*611–616, 1976.

Brunelli G: Direct neurotization of severely damaged and denervated muscles. *In* Freilinger ER, Holle F (eds): Muscle Transplantation. Vienna, Springer Verlag, 1981, pp 283–286.

Brunelli G, Monini L: Direct muscular neurotization. J Hand Surg *10A:*993–997, 1985.

Brunelli G, Monini L: Direct muscular neurotization. Brunelli G (ed): *In* Textbook of Microsurgery. Milan, Masson, 1988, pp 683–685.

Brunelli G: Direct muscular neurotization. *In* Gelbermann R (ed): Operative Nerve Repair and Reconstruction. Philadelphia, J.B. Lippincott Company, 1991, pp 783–791.

Elsberg CA: Experiments on motor nerve regeneration and the direct neurotization of paralyzed muscles by their own and by foreign nerves. Science *45:*318, 1917.

Engel G: Locating motor end plates for electron microscopy. Mayo Clin Proc *45:*450, 1970.

Erlacher P: Direct and muscular neurotization of paralyzed muscles. Am J Orthop Surg *13:*22, 1915.

Frenk E, Jansen JKS, Lomo T, Westgaard RH: The interaction between foreign and original motor nerves innervating the soleus muscle of rats. J Physiol *247:*725–742, 1975.

Guth L, Zalewski AA: Disposition of cholinesterase following implantation of nerve into denervated muscle. Exp Neurol *7:*316, 1963.

Gutmann E, Hanzlikova V: Effects of accessory nerve supply to muscle achieved by implantation into muscle during degeneration of its nerve. Phisiol Bohemostaw *16:*244, 1967.

Heineke D: Die directs einflanzung des nerve in den muskel. Zentralb Chir *41:*465, 1914.

Katz B, Miledi R: The development of acetylcholine sensitivity in nerve free segments of skeletal muscle. J Physiol *170:*389, 1964.

Lomo T, Slater CR: Acetylcholine sensitivity of developing junctions in adult rat soleus muscle. J Physiol *303:*173–187, 1980.

Sakellarides HT, Sorbie C, James L: Reinnervation of denervated muscles by nerve transplantation. Clin Orthop *83:*194, 1972.

Steindler A: The method of direct neurotization of paralyzed muscles. Am J Orthop Surg *13:*33, 1915.

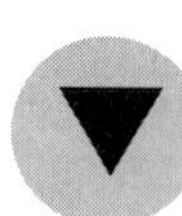

Chapter 41

• George E. Omer, Jr

Peripheral Nerve Injuries and Gunshot Wounds

The increase in violent crimes combined with the availability of handguns has resulted in a significant increase in the number of gunshot wounds in the United States. Firearms are the second leading cause of injury-related death in this country (Schwab et al, 1995). Over 1 million American civilians have been killed by firearms since 1933 (Wintemute, 1987), and at present, there are 732 shootings per day, of which 75% are with handguns (Ordog et al, 1994a). Firearms lead to approximately 236,000 injuries per year, with 65,000 annual hospitalizations. Firearm injuries are the leading cause of death in black males aged 15 to 34 years (Mock et al, 1994). The annual medical costs of firearm injuries in the United States exceed $4 billion (Martin et al, 1988). The estimated loss of income caused by gunshot wounds is 16 billion dollars annually (Ordog et al, 1994a).

Ordog and associates (1994b) recorded 28,150 patients with gunshot wounds over a 14-year period (1977–1991) seen in an urban emergency room. Following evaluation, 16,892 patients with wounds (60%) were treated as outpatients. Wounds were secondary to low-velocity missiles in 88%, medium velocity in 7%, and high velocity in 5%. Single missiles from handguns were involved in 91% of cases, whereas multiple missiles were evident in 3% of cases. Rifles were involved in only 2% of patients managed as outpatients, and shotguns were involved in 4% of cases. The most frequent areas hit were the thighs (22%), legs (16%), upper arms (13%), and hands (10%). The left side of the body was hit 12% more frequently than the right side. Medical histories showed that 12% of patients had a previous gunshot wound, and 5% had a previous stab wound. Peripheral nerve injuries were diagnosed in 114 patients (0.08%), including injuries of the digital, radial, ulnar, and peroneal nerves. Only 19% of these patients returned for subsequent nerve repair.

The reported incidence of peripheral nerve injuries as a result of either low-velocity or high-velocity gunshot wounds in civilian injuries ranges from 22% to 100% (Wiss and Gellman, 1992). Visser and colleagues (1980) found that 71% of patients with vascular injury to an upper extremity had a concomitant peripheral nerve injury. Hardin and associates (1985) reported that patients with nerve deficits associated with upper extremity arterial injuries had serious limitation of extremity function in 23% and moderate limitation in 23%; only 10% sustained nerve injuries that resolved.

The incidence of peripheral nerve injuries associated with gunshot wounds has been relatively well documented in reports of war wounds. After World War I, the incidence of peripheral nerve injuries in all nonfatal wounds was estimated to be 2% (Campbell, 1959). Total peripheral nerve injuries in World War II were about 40,000 (Woodhall and

Beebe, 1956), representing 6.6% of all wounds requiring hospitalization (Bjik and Bellamy, 1984). Final disposition data from Army hospitals in Vietnam indicate an incidence of peripheral nerve injuries of about 7.3% of the nonfatal wounds from 1964 to 1973 (Rothberg et al, 1983). The data indicated that 61% of 7138 peripheral nerve injuries involved the upper extremity. In patients with upper extremity injuries admitted to Brooke Army Medical Center from Vietnam between January 1966 and September 1970, 22% had lesions of major peripheral nerves (Omer, 1974). A study group of 681 patients admitted to Fitzsimons Army Medical Center from 1967 to 1983 included 17 with brachial plexus injuries, 198 with ulnar injuries, 151 with median injuries, 39 with radial injuries, 93 with isolated or multiple digital nerve injuries; 132 with injuries to the sciatic, posterior tibial, or the peroneal nerves; and 51 multiple nerve injuries in either the upper or lower extremity. Over 85% were combat-incurred injuries (Omer and Eversmann, 1994). The Vietnam Vascular Registry recorded concomitant nerve injury in 42.4% and fractures in 28.5% of 1000 acute major arterial injuries (Rich and Spencer, 1978).

WOUND BALLISTICS

The distinguishing feature of gunshot wounds is the pressure disturbance in the tissues, which often results in loss of function without gross disruption of peripheral nerves. Wound ballistics is the study of the effects on the body produced by penetrating projectiles (Fackler, 1988). Three factors, laceration and crushing, shock waves, and cavitation, determine the damage imparted by the bullet to the tissues (Rybeck and Janzon, 1976). In 1894, Horsley identified the explosive pattern of gunshot wounds and concluded that the cause of tissue disruption was the high velocity and spin of the bullet (Adams, 1982). In 1898, Woodruff reported that during the missile's passage, a cavity was created in the target into which air was sucked. Borrowing a marine engineering term, he called this effect cavitation (Adams, 1982). The theory was correct and was later confirmed by high-speed photography. Impacting projectiles, rather than weapons, are classified into velocity ranges that correlate with wound severity: low, less than 1200 ft/sec (370 m/sec); medium, 1200 to 2500 ft/sec (370–760 m/sec); and high, over 2500 ft/sec (760 m/sec) (Ragsdale, 1984).

Comparison of wound profiles illustrates the fallacy of attempting to judge wound severity on velocity alone (Lindsey, 1980). It is widely believed that high-velocity projectiles cause wounds that must be treated by extensive excision of tissue around the missile path (Whelan et al, 1968) and low-velocity missile wounds need little or no treatment (Marcus, et al, 1980). Studies performed at the wound ballistics laboratory of the Letterman Army Institute of Research have demonstrated that the tissue located along the missile path is injured by a crush from direct contact with the projectiles, or by stretching from temporary cavitation. Tissue disruption studies done at missile penetration depths of 12 and 24 cm emphasize that increased velocity is pertinent only with deeper tissue penetration (Fackler, 1986, 1988). The military M-16 has far more potential for damage than the civilian .22 long rifle, but this potential for damage generally is realized only with greater tissue penetration. In most soft tissue extremity wounds, with less than 12 cm of penetration, the high-velocity M-16 bullet would not be expected to cause more tissue disruption than the low-velocity .22 long rifle bullet. The potential for tissue disruption does depend on the mass and striking velocity of the projectile, but the actual amount, type, and location of disruption also depend on the projectile's shape and construction and target tissue type (Fackler, 1986). Therefore, marked tissue disruption is typical for abdominal perforations with the M-16 bullet, whereas soft tissue extremity wounds with the M-16 bullet may be minimal. Omer (1974, 1980) demonstrated the difficulty of rating wound severity on velocity alone when he recorded the same percentage (69%) of spontaneous recovery in peripheral nerves involved in low-velocity (227 of 331) and high-velocity (183 of 264) gunshot wounds of extremities during the Vietnam War.

However, shotgun injuries with multiple missiles are very different from single-missile gunshot wounds. The velocity of a charge of shotgun pellets may only range from 1100 to 1350 feet per second, but the weight of the shot in a 10-gauge shotgun shell is very high (1 5/8 to 2 oz), with very high kinetic energy at the muzzle. Most shotgun injuries to humans occur at close range while the shot is still tightly packed, leading to tremendous tissue destruction (Shepard, 1980) (Fig. 41–1). In addition, shotgun shells have plastic, felt, paper, or cork wadding between the powder and the shot charge. At close range, this wadding often remains in the wound, further complicating management (Paradies and Gregory, 1966). The rate of spontaneous recovery of nerves following shotgun wounds has been reported as only 45% (Luce and Griffin, 1978).

MANAGEMENT PRINCIPLES

If possible, information should be obtained concerning the type of weapon used and the distance from which the weapon was discharged. Contact wounds are produced when the barrel of a gun is held against the skin. Close-range wounds are defined as those in which the weapon is fired from 2.5 feet or less, and the bullet, along with the expelled gases, smoke, and gunpowder particles, are driven inside the skin. Shotgun injuries are often close-range wounds and usually result in extensive tissue damage and contamination. The range is a key variable in determining the severity of this wound, but in one study, it was difficult to obtain an accurate history of such important data as the distance of the patient from the weapon at the time of injury, the stance of the patient at the time of injury, or even the type of weapon involved (Letts and Miller, 1976). Wounds sustained in urban areas are even less predictable; in only one third of patients with gunshot wounds seen at the Louisiana State University Surgical Service in New Orleans was the weapon identified (Dugas and D'Ambrosia, 1985).

On admission, the patient should be carefully evaluated for multisystem injury or occult wounds (Omer, 1956). Deal with life-threatening injuries first, then treat the limb injuries that are lethal only with major bleeding. Do not start intravenous lines in the injured extremity. Do not use both saphenous veins for cutdowns, because one may be needed as a graft. Do not blindly clamp bleeding wounds. Avoid tourniquets, and use direct pressure to allow collateral blood flow. A careful and thorough evaluation of peripheral neurosensory status is mandatory. Documentation of deficits on admission is of medical-legal significance.

Patients with pulsatile hemorrhage, bruits or thrills, expanding or large hematomas, or absent or diminished distal pulses have clinically apparent vascular injuries that must be explored (Ordog et al, 1994a; Wiss and Gellman, 1992). Angiography is performed before surgery in the stable pa-

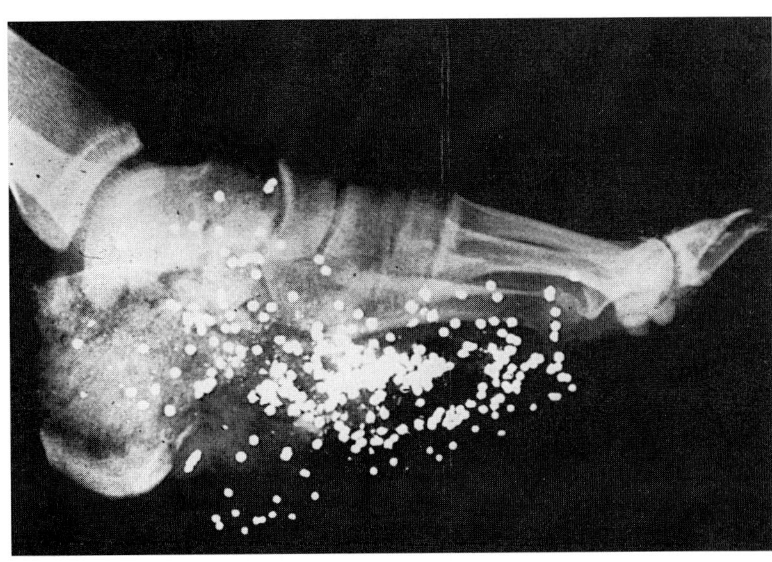

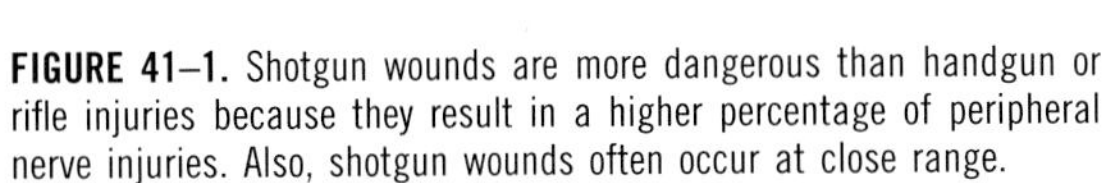

FIGURE 41–1. Shotgun wounds are more dangerous than handgun or rifle injuries because they result in a higher percentage of peripheral nerve injuries. Also, shotgun wounds often occur at close range.

tient, or intraoperative angiography is used in the unstable patient. Proximate injuries are those in which the missile track passes within a 1-inch radius of the known anatomical path of a major vessel. The wound may be investigated with Duplex Doppler Ultrasonography (Ordog et al, 1994a) and then referred for biplanar arteriography. Examples of positive results from arteriograms in patients with proximate injuries and palpable peripheral pulses are an intimal flap, arteriovenous fistula, and pseudoaneurysm (Shuck et al, 1972) (Fig. 41–2). If an extremity has been ischemic for over 4 hours, fasciotomy is indicated. Compartment pressures between 20 and 40 mm Hg in a swollen leg are observed with repeated pressures taken every 4 hours, and angiography is indicated by increased pressures. Fasciotomy and exploration is indicated by pressures over 40 mm Hg. The incision for fasciotomy is extensive and includes the overlying skin as well as the fascia. If evidence of a vascular injury is present, then intravenous antibiotics are given. Shotgun wounds have the highest incidence of vascular and nerve injury because there are multiple missiles with multiple trajectories, which result in multiple locations of injury.

Appropriate management of gunshot wounds of the penetrating or perforating type includes early operative intervention (Omer, 1991). The operative procedure termed debridement has two objectives: to excise necrotic tissue and to incise fascial sheets that inhibit the circulation of edematous muscle. The earlier French definition of the procedure (from the verb debrider, to unbridle) was the cutting of parts (fascia) that, like a bridle, constrict or strangulate the organs they cover and prevent the discharge of pus and hematoma (Ragsdale, 1984). In the American usage, which was initiated during World War II, debridement is the macroscopic cleaning of wounds by operative removal of nonviable tissue, foreign matter, and even tissue of questionable viability, with provision for ample drainage.

Exploration and debridement of gunshot wounds includes generous longitudinal skin incisions, economical skin excision, longitudinal incisions of deep fascia, decompression of compartments, excision of all devitalized tissue, and removal of foreign bodies and loose cortical bone fragments without soft tissue attachments. The shotgun charge wad, which may be composed of felt, plastic, or cardboard, should always be found and removed in close-range shotgun wounds. The high-velocity missile frequently damages tissue remote from the track of the bullet. Radical removal of all bone fragments often leads to delayed union or nonunion. Loose cancellous bone can be cleaned and used as bone grafts. Primary repair of major blood vessels is performed. The wound is not closed following initial debridement (Fig. 41–3). The surgeon aggressively incises the wound but does not empirically excise tissue more widely than clinical judgment normally dictates (Omer, 1988, 1991). In both low-velocity and high-velocity missile wounds, debridement should be rational rather than radical.

Debridement includes skin incisions planned for the direct observation of potentially involved neurovascular structures. The nature of the nerve deficit, such as total or partial transection versus contusion, is carefully documented. Magnification is indicated for the evaluation of the injury, and only those portions of peripheral nerves that are obviously damaged beyond salvage are excised. The remaining nerve is replaced in the best available bed of soft tissue. Primary repair of peripheral nerves usually is not performed in high-velocity or shotgun injuries. Because transected nerves retract with joint motion, the epineurium of the proximal and distal stumps is sutured to adjacent soft tissue with very fine monofilament wire suture to prevent retraction. The level and extent of disruption of the nerve may be identified later with roentgenograms (Omer, 1988).

Miniaturization of existing components of external fixation devices has been a significant step toward solving problems such as maintenance of length, alignment, and mobility (Calkins et al, 1987). If external fixation is chosen to stabilize the wound with associated fractures, fixation is best applied at the time of the initial debridement. Although microvascular composite flap reconstruction may be an appropriate alternative to conventional staged skin flaps and cancellous bone grafting (MacKennon et al, 1983; Salibian et al, 1984), it is performed only when the tissues are receptive to the transfer and the wound is clean. Unless it is done well, such surgery will further jeopardize a wound with marginal circulation.

Civilian handgun injuries are usually low velocity, with a smaller degree of shock wave and cavitation. Injuries from low-velocity missiles, such as .22 caliber, may be surprisingly minor, and extensive debridement, radical exploration, and decompression is usually unnecessary. However, thorough washing, nonclosure, a bulky dressing, and elevation is indicated (Howland and Ritchey, 1971; Marcus et al, 1980; Ordog et al, 1994b). Tetanus prophylaxis is pertinent, and a short course of antibiotics is advisable. Active motion is started early. Patients with these wounds can be treated as outpatients. Injuries from high-velocity missiles or shotgun blasts potentially are far more dangerous, and exploration, debridement, decompression, and evaluation of neurovascular structures are necessary procedures (Omer, 1981).

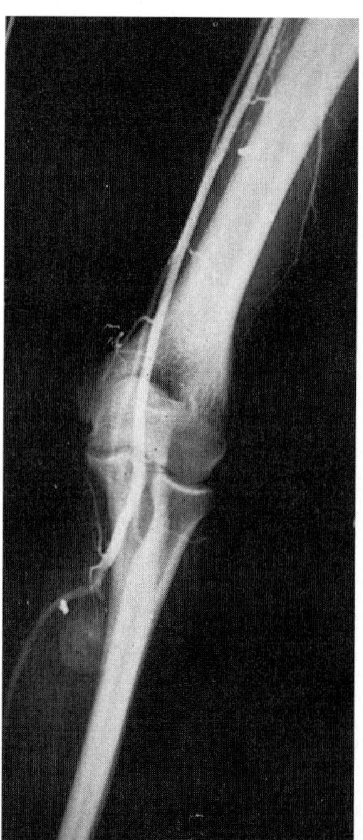

FIGURE 41–2. Pseudoaneurysm demonstrated with arteriogram following injury.

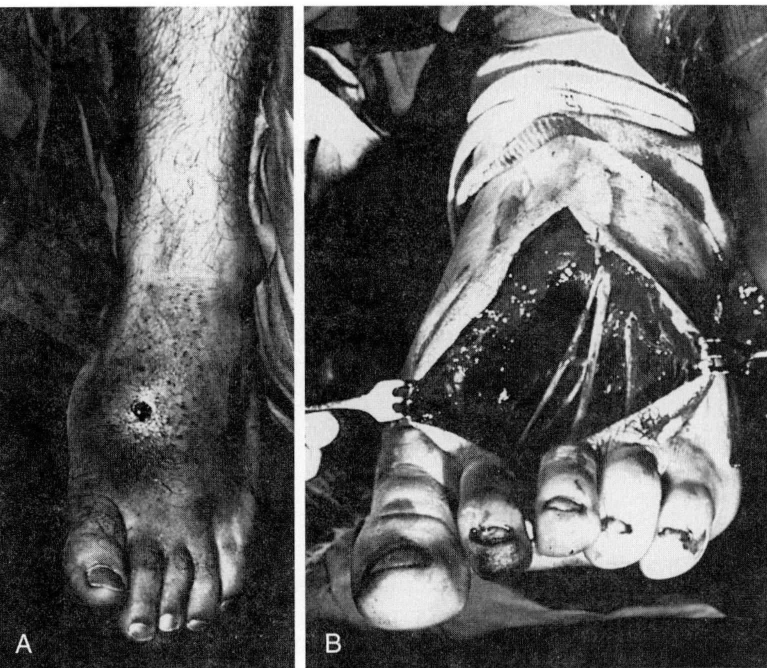

FIGURE 41–3. *A*, High-velocity gunshot wound of the foot. *B*, Debridement incision to incise deep fascia, decompress muscle compartments, and remove multiple loose bone fragments without soft tissue attachments.

Cleaning the wound, stabilizing any fractures, restoration of adequate circulation, and skin closure over neurovascular structures have priority over peripheral nerve repair. However, a disrupted nerve requires repair at the earliest opportunity. In the complex injury, with fractures and soft tissue loss, the nerve gap is associated with extensive scarring (Fig. 41–4). Techniques used to overcome a nerve gap associated with a gunshot wound include (1) mobilization of nerve trunks—a longitudinal release requires that the nerve survive on its internal longitudinal circulation; (2) skeletal shortening—this is potentially dangerous because all soft tissue structures, such as muscle-tendon units, are relatively lengthened and weakened; (3) transposition and rerouting—

if a choice is available, the distal portion of a nerve is rerouted because the proximal portion contains the regenerating axons and needs immediate blood supply (Fig. 41–5); (4) flexion of joints—the elbow or knee is not flexed beyond 90 degrees, and after the initial healing period of 3 to 6 weeks, the joints are extended only 10 degrees per week to prevent intrinsic ischemia; and (5) nerve grafts—the sural nerve and the medial or lateral antebrachial cutaneous nerves are the best sources (Fig. 41–6); the nerve pedicle graft was introduced after World War II in an attempt to maintain adequate circulation in a full-thickness graft (St. Clair Strange, 1947) (Fig. 41–7).

The proximal (high) injury presents a very difficult prob-

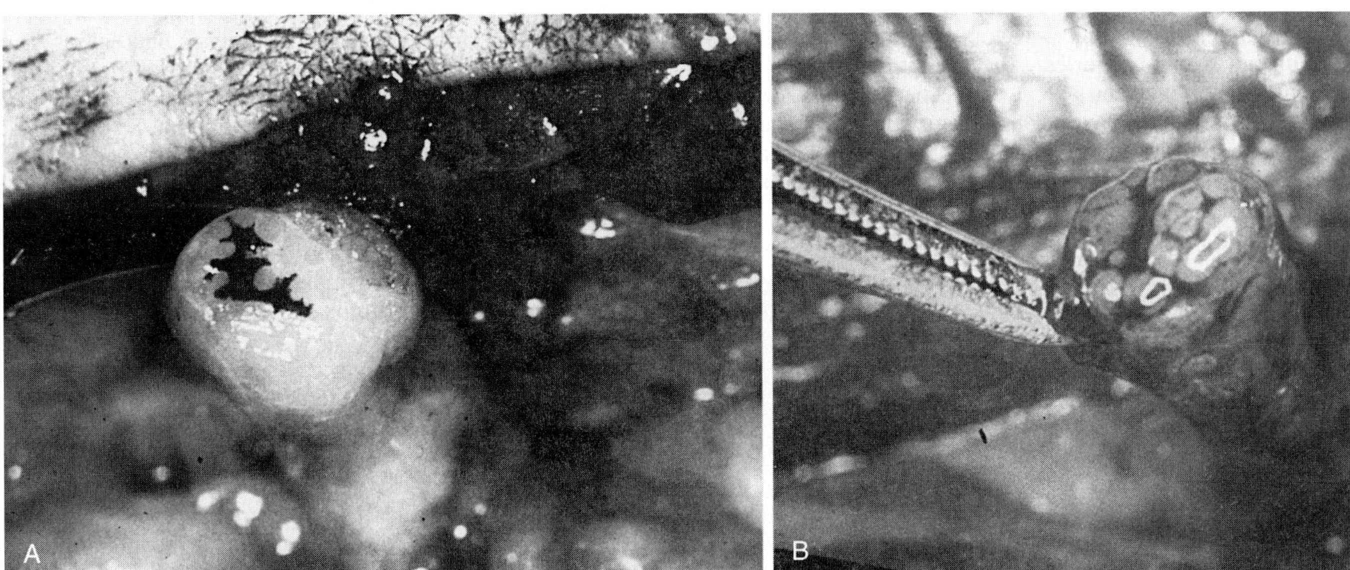

FIGURE 41–4. *A*, The scarred end of a peripheral nerve following severe injury. *B*, Same nerve following debridement. (From Grabb WC: Management of nerve injuries in the forearm and hand. Orthop Clin North Am *1*:419, 1970.)

injuries; there was 50% above-elbow and 43% below-elbow low-velocity gunshot nerve injuries. Both series of patients were followed for 6 to 24 months, and none of the above-elbow neurorrhaphies showed recovery of function of the intrinsic muscles of the hand during the period of study.

The results of these two series from Vietnam indicate that suture of nerves results in progressive functional return over the first 1 to 2 years after surgery in only 40% to 45% of gunshot wounds. However, the continued long-term study of Brown's series by Eversmann (Omer and Eversmann, 1994) demonstrated higher percentages of functional return. In several well-studied cases, a return of interosseous muscles with intrinsic function was clearly demonstrated more than 2 years after above-elbow suture of the ulnar nerve. The longest time elapsed before functional return was 8 years after nerve suture. These well-documented late returns of neurological function to the intrinsic muscles of the hand are contrary to all results previously reported in the medical literature.

It is difficult to place a time limit on functional retraining and recovery, because it depends on nerve regeneration plus other factors such as age, intelligence, patience, perseverance, and motivation (Al-Ghazal et al, 1994; Rosen et al, 1994). The patient's ability to use new and altered patterns of motor and sensory innervation is a slow process that continues for at least 5 years following initial return of function. Clinical studies of neural recovery following gunshot wounds in the human show considerable variation, because return of useful function depends as much on the total response of the extremity to the injury as the regeneration of the injured nerve (Omer, 1974, 1991; Wiss and Gellman, 1992).

References

Adams DB: Wound ballistics: A review. Milit Med *147:*831–835, 1982.

Al-Ghazal SK, McKiernan M, Khan K, McCann J: Results of clinical assessment ofter primary digital nerve repair. J Hand Surg *19B:*255–257, 1994.

Bjik KD, Bellamy RF: Editorial: A note on combat casualty statistics. Milit Med *149:*229–230, 1984.

Brown PW: The time factor in surgery of upper extremity peripheral nerve injury. Clin Orthop *68:*14–21, 1970.

Calkins MS, Burkhalter WE, Reyes F: Traumatic segmented bone defects in the upper extremity. J Bone Joint Surg *69A:*19–27, 1987.

Campbell EH Jr: The Mediterranean (formerly North African) theater of operation. *In* Coates JB Jr, Spurling RG, Woodhall B (eds): Surgery in World War II. Washington, DC, Office of the Surgeon General, Department of the Army, 1959, pp 231–238.

Dugas R, D'Ambrosia R: Civilian gunshot wounds. Orthopaedics *8:*1121–1125, 1985.

Fackler ML: Ballistic injury. Ann Emerg Med *15:*1451–1455, 1986.

Fackler ML: Wound ballistics, a review of common misconceptions. JAMA *259:*2730–2736, 1988.

Hardin WD, O'Connell RC, Adinolfi MF, Kerstein MD: Traumatic arterial injuries of the upper extremity: Determinants of disability. Am J Surg *150:*266–270, 1985.

Howland WS Jr, Ritchey SJ: Gunshot fractures in civilian practice. J Bone Joint Surg *53A:*47–55, 1971.

Kline DG: Evaluation of the neuroma-in-continuity. *In* Omer GE Jr, Spinner M (eds): Management of Peripheral Nerve Problems. Philadelphia, W.B. Saunders Company, 1980, 450–461.

Kline DG, Hackett ER: Reappraisal of timing for exploration of civilian peripheral nerve injuries. Surgery *78:*54–65, 1975.

Letts RM, Miller D: Gunshot wounds of the extremities in children. J Trauma *16:*807–811, 1976.

Lindsey D: The idolatry of velocity, or lies, damn lies, and ballistics. J Trauma *20:*1068–1069, 1980.

Luce EA, Griffin WO: Shotgun injuries of the upper extremity. J Trauma *18:*487–492, 1978.

MacKennon SE, Weiland AJ, Godina M: Immediate forearm reconstruction with a functional latissimus dorsi island pedicle myocutaneous flap. Plast Reconstr Surg *71:*706–710, 1983.

Marcus NA, Blair WF, Shuck JM, Omer GE Jr: Low-velocity gunshot wounds to extremities. J Trauma *20:*1061–1064, 1980.

Martin MJ, Hunt TK, Hulley SB: The cost of hospitalization for firearm injuries. JAMA *260:*3048, 1988.

Mock C, Pilcher S, Maier R: Comparison of the costs of acute treatment for gunshot and stab wounds: Further evidence of the need for firearms control. J Trauma *36:*516–522, 1994.

Omer GE Jr: The early management of gunshot wounds of the extremities. South Dakota J Med Pharm *9:*340–346, 1956.

Omer GE Jr: Evaluation and reconstruction of the forearm and hand after acute traumatic peripheral nerve injuries. J Bone Joint Surg *50A:*1454–1478, 1968.

Omer GE Jr: Assessment of peripheral nerve injuries. *In* Cramer LM, Chase RA (eds): Symposium on the Hand. Educational Foundation, American Society of Plastic and Reconstructive Surgeons, St. Louis, C. V. Mosby Company, 1971, pp 1–13.

Omer GE Jr: Injuries to nerves of the upper extremity. J Bone Joint Surg *56A:*1615–1624, 1974.

Omer GE Jr: The results of untreated traumatic injuries. *In* Omer GE Jr, Spinner M (eds): Management of Peripheral Nerve Problems. Philadelphia, W.B. Saunders Company, 1980, pp 502–506.

Omer GE Jr: The management of traumatic injuries of peripheral nerves in the extremities. Surgical Rounds *4:*22–32, 1981.

Omer GE Jr: Results of untreated peripheral nerve injuries. Clin Orthop *163:*15–19, 1982.

Omer GE Jr: War injuries of the hand. *In* Tubiana R (ed): The Hand, Vol. 3. Philadelphia, W.B. Saunders Company, 1988, pp 903–924.

Omer GE Jr: Nerve injuries associated with gunshot wounds of the extremities. *In* Gelberman RH (ed): Operative Nerve Repair and Reconstruction. Philadelphia, J.B. Lippincott Company, 1991, pp 655–670.

Omer GE Jr, Eversmann WW Jr: Peripheral nerve problems. *In* Burkhalter WE (ed): Orthopedic Surgery in Vietnam. Washington, DC, Office of the U.S. Army Surgeon General and Center of Military History, 1994, pp 155–188.

Ordog GJ, Balasubramanium S, Wasserberger J, Kram H, Bishop M, Shoemaker W: Extremity gunshot wounds: Part one—identification and treatment of patients at high risk of vascular injury. J Trauma *36:*358–368, 1994a.

Ordog GJ, Wasserberger J, Balasubramanium S, Shoemaker W: Civilian gunshot wounds—outpatient management. J Trauma *36:*106–111, 1994b.

Paradies LH, Gregory CF: The early treatment of close-range shotgun wounds to the extremities. J Bone Joint Surg *48A:*425–435, 1966.

Ragsdale BD: Gunshot wounds: A historical perspective. Milit Med *149:*301–315, 1984.

Rakolta GG, Omer GE Jr: Combat-sustained femoral nerve injuries. Surg Gynecol Obstet *128:*813–817, 1969.

Rich NM, Spencer FC: Vascular Trauma. Philadelphia, W.B. Saunders Company, 1978, pp 125–155.

Rosen B, Lundborg G, Dahlin LB, Holmberg J, Karlson B: Nerve repair: Correlation of restitution of functional sensibility with specific cognitive capacities. J Hand Surg *19B:*452–458, 1994.

Rothberg JM, Tahmoush AJ, Oldakowski R: The epidemiology of causalgia among soldiers wounded in Vietnam. Milit Med *148:*347–350, 1983.

Rybeck B, Janzon B: Absorption of missile energy in soft tissue. Acta Chir Scand *142:*201–207, 1976.

Salibian AH, Anzel SH, Mallerick M, Tesoro VE: Microvascular reconstruction for close-range gunshot injuries to the distal forearm. J Hand Surg *9A:*799–804, 1984.

Schwab CW: Violence in America: A public health crisis—the role of firearms. J Trauma *38:*163–168, 1995.

Seddon HJ: Three types of nerve injury. Brain *66:*237–288, 1943.

Shepard GH: High-energy, low-velocity close range shotgun wounds. J Trauma *20:*1065–1067, 1980.

Shuck JM, Omer GE Jr, Lewis C: Arterial obstruction due to intimal disruption in extremity fractures. J Trauma *12:*481–489, 1972.

St. Clair Strange FG: An operation for nerve pedicle grafting. Br J Surg *34:*423–425, 1947.

Visser PA, Hemreck AS, Pierce GE, et al: Prognosis of nerve injuries incurred during acute trauma to peripheral arteries. Am J Surg *140:*596–599, 1980

Vrettos RC, Rochkind S, Boome RS: Low velocity gunshot wounds of the brachial plexus. J Hand Surg *20B:*212–214, 1995.

Whelan RJ Jr, Burkhalter WE, Gomez A: Management of war wounds. Adv Surg *3:*227–350, 1968.

Wintemute GJ: Firearms as a cause of death in the United States, 1920–1982. J Trauma *27:*532–536, 1987.

Wiss DA, Gellman H: Gunshot wounds to the musculoskeletal system. *In* Browner BD, Jupiter JB, Levine AM, Trafton PG (eds): Skeletal Trauma. Philadelphia, W. B. Saunders Company, 1992, pp 367–400.

Woodhall B, Beebe GW (eds): Peripheral nerve regeneration. VA medical monograph. Washington, DC, U.S. Government Printing Office, 1956, pp 5, 191, 311–340, 498.

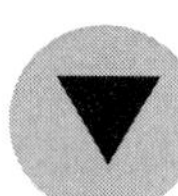

Chapter 42

• Rajiv Midha
• Abhijit Guha
• Fred Gentili
• David G. Kline
• Alan R. Hudson

Peripheral Nerve Injection Injury

Injury to peripheral nerves secondary to injection is a well-known complication of intramuscular drug administration. With the numerous agents delivered by deep intramuscular injection, this occurrence has come to be increasingly recognized as a cause of pain and disability in adults (Clark et al, 1970; Combes et al, 1960; Kline and Hudson, 1995). In children, as well as in adults, nerve injection injury may be responsible for permanent, severe paralytic deformities (Combes et al, 1960; Villarejo and Pascual, 1993). The iatrogenic basis of the majority of injection nerve injuries is of particular concern, because of both its clinical and medicolegal implications. Despite better clinical and pathological characterization of the problem, the management of injection nerve injury remains a controversial topic (Clark, 1972; Kline and Hudson, 1995).

LITERATURE REVIEW

Peripheral nerve injury resulting from the deep injection of therapeutic and prophylactic agents has been recognized for over three quarters of a century, starting with a report of two patients with sciatic nerve palsy due to the injection of quinine (Turner, 1920). The early cases most frequently occurred secondary to administration of sulfonamide and penicillin antibiotics (Broadbent et al, 1949; Elkington, 1942; Kolb and Gray, 1946). The localized neuritis resulting from multiple intramuscular injections of penicillin preparations adjacent to and distant from the involved peripheral nerve was initially ascribed to an allergic phenomenon (Kolb and Gray, 1946). In seven patients, the paralysis had a delayed onset (from 1 to 3 weeks after drug injection), involved motor more than sensory function, and was associated with significant recovery in five patients within 4 months. Subsequently, the clinical features of penicillin-induced peripheral nerve palsy were delineated as severe pain at the onset of injection radiating along the distribution of the injected nerve, followed rapidly by motor and sensory impairment of the nerve, and variable recovery of function over time (Broadbent et al, 1949).

Further reports of peripheral nerve injury after the injection of agents other than penicillin followed (Combes et al, 1960; Hudson et al, 1950; Matson, 1950). Numerous agents were implicated over the years, including antibiotics, analgesics, local anesthetics, steroid agents, vaccines, and vitamin preparations (Gentili et al, 1980; Mackinnon et al, 1982). In contrast to earlier authors, Combes and colleagues (1960) found recovery of neurological function to be disappointing in all but one of their 12 patients who had received a wide variety of intramuscular drugs. Therefore, they suggested that the site, volume, and type of injected material were important factors in determining the degree of injury. In addition to the direct neurotoxic effects of the injected agent on nerve tissue (Clark et al, 1970; Gilles and French, 1961), other pathogenetic mechanisms postulated include an allergic peripheral neuritis (Kolb and Gray, 1946), direct needle trauma (Berry and Wallis, 1977; Horowitz, 1994), ischemic injury (von Hochstetter, 1955), vascular embolization of drug (Hudson et al, 1950), and secondary constriction by scar (Combes and Clark, 1960).

Several authors stressed the increased frequency of sciatic nerve injuries in premature infants and pediatric patients following intragluteal injections (Combes et al, 1960; Curtiss and Tucker, 1960; Gilles and French, 1961; Villarejo and Pascual, 1993). The predisposition to injury in these patients was believed to be related to the relatively small area of the infant buttock and the relative paucity of muscle covering the sciatic nerve, factors accentuated in the premature infant (Curtiss and Tucker, 1960). On the basis of this information, it was recommended that the buttock be abandoned as a site of deep injection in pediatric patients, favoring the distal lateral thigh musculature as a preferred site for drug delivery (Gilles and French, 1961). In spite of increased awareness, the sciatic nerve remains the most commonly injured nerve by injection, owing to its size and to the frequency of intramuscular injections in the buttock (Kline and Hudson, 1995; Villarejo and Pascual, 1993). However, injection injury of virtually every major peripheral nerve, including radial (Broadbent et al, 1949; Elkington, 1942; Kline and Hudson, 1995; Ling and Loong, 1976), ulnar (Broadbent et al, 1949), median (Kline and Hudson, 1995), axillary (Clark et al, 1970), femoral, and lateral femoral cutaneous (Clark et al, 1970; Kline and Hudson, 1995), has been described.

The clinical characteristics of the nerve injection injury itself and the outcome over time in afflicted patients have been debated. In the majority of cases, an immediate onset of pain followed rapidly by paralysis and sensory dysfunction occurs on injection of the drug (Broadbent et al, 1949; Clark, 1972). In a subset of patients, the nerve damage manifests in a delayed fashion (Kolb and Gray, 1946). An exaggerated frequency of delayed onset may have been based on the large number of infant and pediatric cases, involving multiple injections and unreliable history, in the earlier reports (Combes et al, 1960; Gilles and French, 1961). This truly occurs in perhaps only 10% of cases (Kline and Hudson, 1995). Reports of both favorable (Curtiss and Tucker, 1960; Kolb and Gray, 1946) and disappointing (Combes et al, 1960; Gilles and French, 1961) neurological outcomes after nerve injection injury attest to the variable natural history. However, the majority of patients have residual motor deficit, with only 14% demonstrating complete recovery on follow-up examination (Clark et al, 1970; Clark, 1972). Early onset of return of function appears to be the only favorable prognostic factor (Clark et al, 1970).

There is considerable controversy regarding the treatment of nerve injection injury. If the complication is noted immediately, closed irrigation with 50 to 100 ml of normal saline or even open irrigation (Elkington, 1942) has been advocated in an attempt to dilute the drug and thereby prevent permanent neuropathy. Although this approach is logical, such treatment is rarely practical because the patients are infrequently seen in emergent situations, and experience with this method is lacking. Early exploration (within 3 to 4 weeks) has been advocated in order to perform a thorough external neurolysis (Matson, 1950). Others, citing the experimental work of Tarlov (1951), which implicated intraneural pathology, favor conservative management for 1 year in children before resorting to neurolysis (Gilles and French, 1961). If there is complete loss of function for a sufficient duration that spontaneous recovery is considered unlikely, the trend has been to explore the nerve and to resect and repair the nerve in the absence of an intraoperative nerve action potential (Clark, 1972; Kline and Nulsen, 1972). The authors recommend exploration of those nerve injection injuries that are complete and show no or little recovery at 8 to 16 weeks.

EXPERIMENTAL STUDIES AND PATHOLOGY

The results of experiments on various animal models have shed considerable light on the pathology and pathogenesis of nerve damage following injection. The two most important factors appear to be the exact location of the injection and the nature of the injected material. Early studies in rabbits demonstrated an intense inflammatory reaction, profound axonal and myelin damage, and associated connective tissue scarring after intraneural injection, versus mild inflammation and little or no neural damage after epineurial injection, and no pathological effect from injection adjacent to the nerve (Tarlov et al, 1951). An intrafascicular location of injection (Fig. 42–1) appears to be the major pathogenetic factor in a variety of animal models in several subsequent studies (Combes and Clark, 1960; Gentili et al, 1979; Woodhall et al, 1950).

The degree of neural damage following injection also appears to be related to the type and formulation of material administered (Clark et al, 1970; Gentili et al, 1979; Holbrook and Pilcher, 1950; Mackinnon et al, 1982; Woodhall et al, 1950). Certain agents are relatively well tolerated, whereas others are inherently more toxic than others, with penicillin and diazepam being the most hazardous (Gentili et al, 1979). Placement of the needle in the nerve and control injections of small volumes of normal saline and blood components appear innocuous (Clark et al, 1970; Combes and Clark,

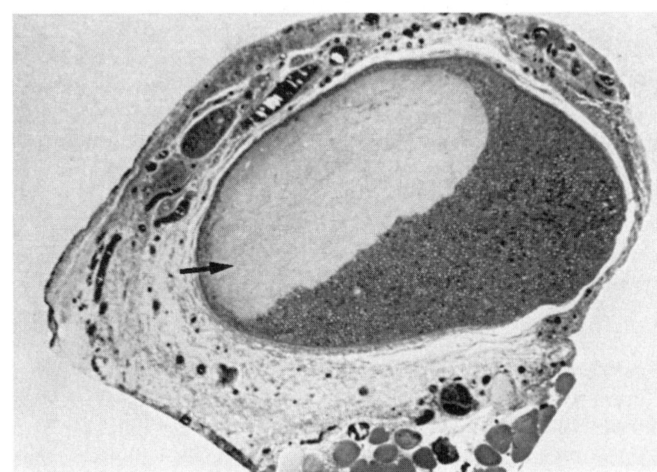

FIGURE 42–1. An intrafascicular locus of injection *(arrow)*, produced experimentally by direct injection of collagen in a primate nerve, is demonstrated. (Modified from Kline DG, Hudson AR: Nerve Injuries: Operative Results from Major Nerve Injuries, Entrapments, and Tumors. Philadelphia, W.B. Saunders Company, 1995.)

1960; Gentili et al, 1979; Tarlov et al, 1951). The interdependence of both site and agent as important variables is evident because extrafascicular injection of the more toxic drugs, especially in larger dosages, evokes mild injury in nerve fibers (Gentili et al, 1979, 1980). It is tempting to speculate that in the 10% or so of patients that manifest a delayed neuropathy after nerve injection, placement of the drug adjacent to the nerve or within the epineurium around the nerve fascicles from where it can diffuse to the nerve fibers is responsible for nerve damage. In summary, the locus of the nerve injection seems to be the most important factor, with the ultimate pathological effect considerably modified by the toxicity of the delivered drug.

The pathology of nerve injection injury is also dependent on the injection site and the agent administered. After intraneural injection, acute edema, inflammatory infiltrate, and necrosis of both axons and myelin occur (Gentili et al, 1979; Mackinnon et al, 1982; Tarlov et al, 1951). The blood-nerve barrier is profoundly altered at both the perineurial site and the endoneurial capillary level, contributing to endoneurial edema (Gentili et al, 1980). Grossly, the nerve demonstrates immediate internal swelling and petechial hemorrhages on its surface (Mackinnon et al, 1982). After the initial few days, the injected segment of the nerve may no longer appear swollen. With a longer period of time, the injected portion of the nerve may be of a normal diameter or even appear shrunken. Over time, at a cellular level, resolution of the inflammatory reaction and connective tissue proliferation within the nerve produce intrafascicular scar. This presents a formidable barrier to successful regeneration of axons, and the resulting intrafascicular neuroma contains a meshwork of connective tissue entwined with fine-caliber, poorly myelinated axons. The gross appearance may be deceiving because the external nerve is in excellent physical continuity and even intraneural dissection often demonstrates a good fascicular structure despite the presence of intrafascicular damage that is neurotmetic.

Depending on the toxicity of the agent, injection adjacent to the nerve or into the epineurium produces a variable degree of intrafascicular nerve fiber damage (Gentili et al,

1979). Dense adhesions between the nerve and surrounding tissue accompanied by discoloration of the nerve and inflammatory infiltrate within the nerve are found (Woodhall et al, 1950). The clinical correlate appears to be patients that often present in a delayed fashion with a variable amount of neurological dysfunction. Sometimes, patients manifest a severe pain syndrome that greatly exceeds the findings on neurological examination. Although earlier experimental studies did not discern damage at a light or electron microscopic level to nerve following simple needle penetration (Clark et al, 1970; Combes and Clark, 1960; Gentili et al, 1979; Tarlov et al, 1951), more recent reports provide subtle evidence of nerve fiber damage and dysfunction after penetration of the needle alone (Fried et al, 1989; Rice and McMahon, 1992). These injection injuries appear to represent one extreme of the clinical spectrum, in which patients present with painful symptoms in the absence of clinical or electrical evidence of neuropathy, following accidental puncture of the nerve with a sharp needle (Horowitz, 1994).

The gross findings at operation include inflammatory tissue, reactive changes, and scar about the nerve, as well as occasional extensive intraneural scarring (Clark et al, 1970; Clark, 1972; Kline and Hudson, 1995; Matson, 1950). Most frequently, one finds reactive changes around the nerve, with discoloration and increased local scar tissue (see Fig. 42–6). The nerve itself appears focally swollen as in a neuroma in continuity, which is usually firm but may be soft. The older injury may demonstrate severe atrophy and attenuation. In rare cases, no gross abnormality is evident. The lesion in continuity is often eccentric, reflecting the direction of the needle entry and injection. Damage to one part of the nerve may be greater, a finding particularly relevant with the sciatic nerve in the buttock, because the more lateral and superficial peroneal division is more prone to injury than the deeper tibial division.

PATIENT MANAGEMENT: GENERAL GUIDELINES

As in most clinical settings, the history and physical examination are key to the appropriate diagnosis and subsequent treatment of the patient with a nerve injection injury. The site of needle insertion predicts the nerve that may have been injured. Additional clinical factors besides the exact location of injection, which is the most important, underlie the possibility of nerve damage from injection and should be obtained in the history. These factors include the length of the needle used, the angle or trajectory of skin penetration, and the force with which the injection is delivered. Administration that is deeper than intended may result if long needles are used or if extra force is imposed where the hub of the needle inverts skin and underlying soft tissue. This may be compounded for a nerve such as the sciatic if the needle penetrates soft tissue at an angle headed toward the nerve rather than at a right angle to a horizontal plane through the body. Movement of the patient during the injection is another important consideration. The uncooperative, struggling infant or child receiving a buttock injection places the sciatic nerve at risk. A child or occasionally an adult may shrug or jerk the shoulder, perhaps in anticipation of pain, during a deltoid injection and damage the radial nerve. The incidence

of injection into the sciatic nerve may also be increased by a buttock administration if the patient is in a lateral and recumbent position or is standing and bent over. Finally, infusions or needles intended for veins can be inadvertently placed in nerves. The median and ulnar nerves at the elbow and wrist levels, the femoral nerve in the groin, the posterior tibial nerve at the ankle, and many cutaneous nerves in the forearm have been injured in this fashion (Horowitz, 1994; Kline and Hudson, 1995). The above-mentioned anatomical and clinical considerations need to be broadly advertised to all health care workers to facilitate primary prevention of nerve injection injuries.

The history associated with nerve injection injury is characteristic. In the typical scenario, needle placement results in an immediate electrical-like shock sensation down the extremity. Concomitantly, on injection of the agent, severe radicular pain and paresthesias result. The patient usually experiences severe pain, described with adjectives such as burning, searing, or electrical, or a numbing sensation along the course of the injected nerve (Ochs, 1989). In approximately 10% of cases, a delayed onset of the neuropathy occurs after injection injury (Kline and Hudson, 1995). In these cases, the symptoms are often less dramatic, described variously as a burning pain, a deep discomfort, or bothersome paresthesias down the limb and in the distribution of the affected nerve.

Following injection of the nerve, the neurological deficit frequently parallels the time course of the onset of symptoms. Therefore, in the majority of patients, an immediate nerve palsy occurs, whereas a delayed deficit evolves in the minority of patients. Neurological deficit may be complete or incomplete in the distribution of the injected nerve. Unfortunately, a frequent picture is a severe neuropathy with total or virtually complete motor and sensory deficit. When the injury is incomplete, motor loss is usually greater than sensory loss (Clark, 1972). Neuritic pain, which is of variable intensity, often accompanies the neurological deficit. Less severe injection nerve injuries produce one of two patterns. The first pattern is a neuropathy consisting of conductive abnormalities and reflex loss in the nerve distribution in the face of preserved motor and sensory function. The second pattern is a neurogenic pain syndrome, associated with no or little sensory and motor change. Increasingly recognized is the entity of chronic and severe painful nerve lesions that may occur after simple penetration of the nerve with the needle, as during attempted venipuncture, without the need for any injection (Berry and Wallis, 1977; Horowitz, 1994; Kline and Hudson, 1995).

The diagnosis of nerve injection injury is readily apparent from the above-mentioned clinical features. Further management of the patient with a peripheral nerve injection injury essentially follows the guidelines established for any patient with a nerve lesion in continuity (Kline and Nulsen, 1972). The exact date of nerve injury is usually available. Electrophysiological tests are useful, along with the initial neurological examination, as a baseline to assess the subsequent evolution of the neuropathy. It is reasonable to anticipate regeneration at approximately 1 inch per month. It is appropriate to examine the first distal target muscle clinically and with electrophysiological studies to determine whether or not there is any evidence of recovery after an appropriate duration of waiting. In the most common situation, profound clinical loss is associated with denervational changes on electromyography (EMG). Injuries of such a severe nature rarely reverse spontaneously despite maintenance of physical continuity of the nerve. If no recovery is appreciated within 2 to 4 months, surgical exploration is indicated. Most injuries that are partial to begin with and the occasional complete injury recover without operative intervention. Early return of function appears to be the most significant prognostic factor in these cases (Clark et al, 1970). The patient is best managed expectantly under these circumstances. While awaiting recovery, these patients are treated with vigorous physical therapy and pain medications. Some patients present primarily with a severe pain syndrome and minimal or no neurological deficit (Horowitz, 1994; Kline and Hudson, 1995). When the pain is medically intractable, surgical exploration of the injury site with external and internal neurolysis may be of great benefit in relieving pain in about half of these patients (Kline and Hudson, 1995).

The above-mentioned general management guidelines are based on the prior experience of the two senior authors. Over the past 25 years, the senior author at Louisiana State University Medical Center (LSUMC) has had the opportunity to manage 80 patients with nerve injection injuries (Table 42–1). Half of these patients have required surgical treatment, whereas the other half were managed expectantly. In the following sections, the management of nerve injection injuries of specific nerves, illustrated with case reports, is discussed.

RADIAL NERVE

Injury of the radial nerve at mid-humeral level is the second most frequent site, after sciatic nerve at buttock level, of nerve injection damage. In these cases, the injection is meant for the deltoid muscle, and a more lateral or inferior placement than intended can injure the nerve deep to the triceps and adjacent to the spiral groove. Triceps function is preserved, because the branches to that muscle are derived proximal to the point of injury. Wrist drop, weakness in supination, loss of thumb extension, and only limited finger extension by intrinsic hand muscles are usually present. Sensory deficit is variable and seldom a practical problem. If recovery occurs, it is heralded by return of brachioradialis function, as exemplified in the following case report.

▼ **TABLE 42–1**
LSUMC Nerve Injection Injury Experience

Nerve	Total Evaluated	Operated	Nonoperated
Radial	7	7	0
Median	18	10	8
Ulnar	2	2	0
Sciatic	50	20	30
Peroneal (knee)	2	0	2
Femoral	1	0	1
TOTAL	80	39	41

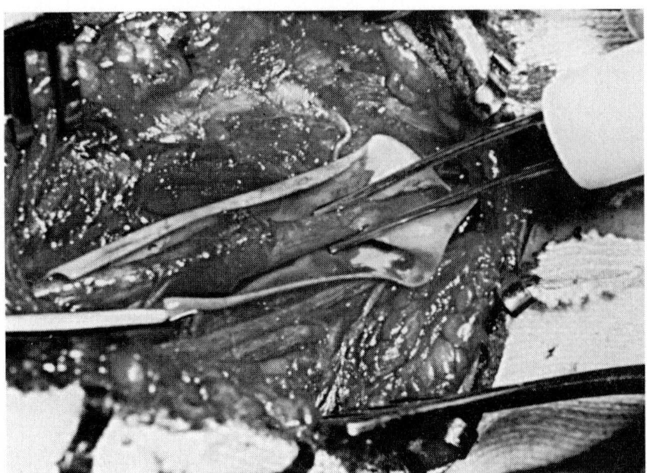

FIGURE 42–2. Neuroma in continuity resulting from injection injury of the radial nerve deep to triceps. The nerve is undergoing electrical evaluation 4 months after injury, with the stimulating electrode proximal to the damaged site. There was no brachioradialis contraction in response to stimulation either at or above the lesion, leading to resection and repair in this case. (Modified from Kline DG, Hudson AR: Nerve Injuries: Operative Results from Major Nerve Injuries, Entrapments, and Tumors. Philadelphia, W.B. Saunders Company, 1995.)

CASE 1

A 55-year-old right-handed male experienced extreme pain on receiving an injection of meperidine hydrochloride in the lateral aspect of his right arm, just distal to the spiral groove. Severe pain radiated down his forearm to the dorsal aspect of his thumb. Wrist drop followed immediately. Examination at the University of Toronto revealed a complete radial nerve palsy beyond the triceps. The patient was managed expectantly. Clinical and electrical evidence of brachioradialis reinnervation was detected at 20 weeks. Subsequent visits disclosed serial reinnervation of the forearm muscles supplied by the radial nerve, followed by eventual recovery of muscles supplied by the posterior interosseous nerve.

The pathology in the above-mentioned case was presumably axonotmesis with wallerian degeneration, followed by regeneration into Schwann cell tubes distal to the point of injury and subsequent muscle reinnervation. *Unfortunately, spontaneous recovery following radial nerve injection injury has been the exception in our experience. It is essential that surgical intervention not be unduly postponed in these patients.* In the LSUMC series, all seven patients referred with this diagnosis failed to exhibit spontaneous recovery, requiring surgical exploration from 3 to 7 (average 4) months following injury. The radial nerve is most easily found at operation in the trough between brachialis and brachioradialis (Sunderland, 1978). From here, the nerve is followed back to the injury site. After inspection of the neuroma in continuity, the nerve is stimulated proximal to the lesion, with recording electrodes placed distally. In many cases, this approach requires exposure of the proximal radial nerve on the inner or medial side of the arm. In five of the seven cases, the neuroma in continuity failed to conduct a nerve action potential (NAP), requiring resection of the lesion and repair (Fig. 42 2). The repair is performed by either suturing the two ends or placement of interfascicular nerve grafts, depending on the nerve gap that exists after trimming back the proximal and distal stumps to a normal fascicular pattern and mobilizing the nerve (Kline and Nulsen, 1972). All seven patients in the LSUMC experience went on to make a useful recovery (at least Grade 3), and four had excellent (Grade 5) restoration of radial nerve function, although finger and thumb extension remained weak (Kline and Hudson, 1995). The presence of an NAP in two cases mandated against resection of the lesion or indicated a partial repair, as illustrated in the next case report.

CASE 2 *(modified from Kline and Hudson, 1995)*

A 19-year-old male received a morphine injection below the deltoid muscle in the lateral arm. An electrical shock down the arm to the back of the hand preceded an immediate wrist drop. On EMG a week later, absence of motor units in the brachioradialis and more distal radial-innervated muscles was revealed. Radial sensory NAPs were present initially but diminished in amplitude on serial evaluation before finally disappearing. Clinical examination 1 month later disclosed a complete radial nerve palsy beyond the triceps, accompanied by a severe denervational pattern on EMG. At 2.5 months, no clinical or electrical evidence of reinnervation was detected, and therefore surgical exploration recommended. The radial nerve in the lateral arm between biceps and triceps was first exposed, demonstrating scar investing the somewhat atrophic nerve over several centimeters in and beyond the spiral groove. An NAP recording on the lateral arm portion produced a very small potential; therefore, proximal exposure of the radial nerve was carried out via a separate high medial arm incision. The radial nerve proximal to the spiral groove conducted a fast (80 meters per second) NAP of good amplitude. Across the spiral groove, recordings gave an NAP of much smaller amplitude, conducting at 30 meters per second. An internal neurolysis was performed on the injured portion, with removal of a scar and a small portion of the nerve that was severely affected, and the severely damaged section was repaired (Fig. 42–3). Histological assessment of the resected tissue demonstrated myxoid material forming a perineural halo surrounding degenerated nerve fibers. The patient has been followed for over 3.5 years and has made an excellent functional recovery, even in finger and thumb extension.

MEDIAN NERVE

As an etiological entity, damage by injection has formed a surprisingly large category of median nerve injuries at LSUMC. Out of 18 cases, the majority (13) have been at the elbow and forearm level, but the nerve has been injured by injection in the upper arm (1 case), wrist (1 case), and the anterior interosseous division in the proximal forearm in three instances (Kline and Hudson, 1995). Accidental entry into the nerve during attempted venipuncture, intravenous line insertion, or sampling or catheterization of the brachial artery has been the typical setting for median nerve injury. A severe pain syndrome was universally present in this group of patients and was the primary reason for referral in

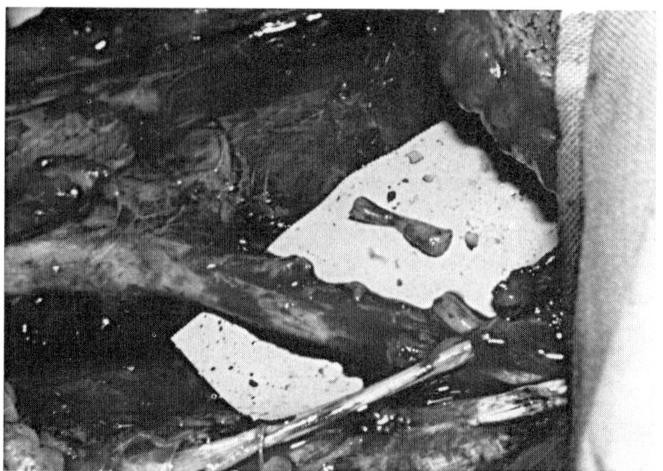

FIGURE 42–3. Radial nerve lesion resulting from injection injury, summarized in Case 2. The portion of nerve severely damaged by injection was eccentric in location, and is shown excised from the main nerve trunk. The resected portion was grafted, resulting in a split repair. (Modified from Kline DG, Hudson AR: Nerve Injuries: Operative Results from Major Nerve Injuries, Entrapments, and Tumors. Philadelphia, W.B. Saunders Company, 1995.)

the majority. Neurological deficits were partial in most of these patients. A few, including the individual shown in Figure 42–4, had profound neurological deficit, requiring surgical exploration. *However, the main indication for surgery in patients with injection injuries of the median nerve was severe pain and paresthesias that did not respond to conservative management.*

CASE 3 *(modified from Kline and Hudson, 1995)*

A 38-year-old male underwent open catheterization of the brachial artery for cardiac angiography. Following the procedure, the patient described neuritic pain in the median nerve distribution. This was in the form of painful dysesthesias that extended down the forearm to the hand. Only partial and temporary relief had been obtained from sympathetic blocks. On percussion and palpation over the healed angiography incision, pain and electrical shock–like stimuli radiating into the hand were evoked. Evaluation by EMG showed only mild denervational changes in median-innervated muscles, but conduction of sensory NAPs across the elbow was delayed. Surgical exploration at 3 months after injury demonstrated a slightly scarred median nerve beneath the lacertus fibrosus. Conduction velocity of the NAP across the lesion was 38.5 meters per second before and after external and partial internal neurolysis. The patient had substantial relief of pain, without any deterioration of function. He has been followed over 4 years.

The above-mentioned case demonstrates the benefit of neurolysis in patients with severe, noncausalgic, neuritic pain resulting from local nerve injection injury. Unfortunately, this is not always the case, especially if percussion over the injection site fails to produce distal radiation of paresthesias. In the 13 patients who had elbow and forearm nerve injection injuries, eight patients had severe pain and paresthesias that did not respond to nonoperative treatment. At surgery directed to the damaged nerve, seven patients

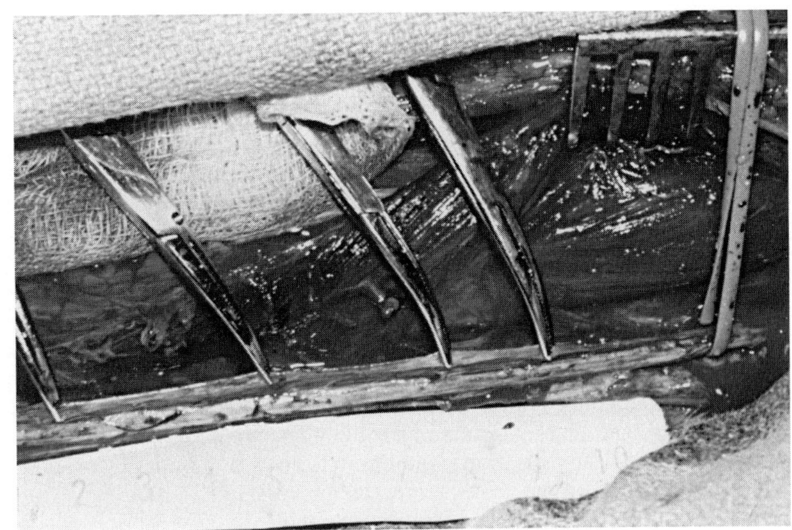

FIGURE 42–4. An injection injury involving the median nerve resulting from infusion of a local anesthetic drug, presumably into the nerve, during an axillary-level block. The great length of involved nerve illustrates that injection injuries are not always focal. This lesion required resection and long interfascicular grafts to repair. (Modified from Kline DG, Hudson AR: Nerve Injuries: Operative Results from Major Nerve Injuries, Entrapments, and Tumors. Philadelphia, W.B. Saunders Company, 1995.)

required neurolysis, whereas one needed resection and suture repair. Those who underwent neurolysis maintained preoperative function (Grade 4 or 5) and had some amelioration of pain. In the case involving resection and repair, pain was relieved, but only a Grade 3 functional result was achieved (Kline and Hudson, 1995). Similar outcomes were evident from median nerve injection injury of upper arm and anterior interosseous division. Even when the main indication for surgery is loss and nonrecovery of neurological function, a decrease in pain from preoperative levels sometimes follows neurolysis or resection of the neuroma in continuity.

ULNAR NERVE

Only two patients with ulnar nerve injury by injection were managed. Both patients had injuries that occurred at the elbow and forearm level, and both required surgical exploration after failing to demonstrate spontaneous recovery. Intraoperative NAP recordings assisted in deciding how to manage the lesion in continuity. One lesion failed to conduct an NAP and required resection and repair. This patient had partial recovery at follow-up, with Grade 3 function in the flexor profundus to little and ring fingers and adductor pollicis, and Grade 2 function in ulnar-innervated intrinsics. The other injury, which was explored 3.5 months after injury, demonstrated an NAP across the injury site, leading to neurolysis. The second patient had a very good recovery when evaluated at follow-up 1.5 years after surgery.

SCIATIC NERVE

The sciatic nerve at the buttock remains a distressingly frequent site of injury from nerve injection (Kline and Hudson, 1995; Villarejo and Pascual, 1993). Indeed, this is the most common etiology for sciatic nerve injury at the buttock level in our experience, outnumbering all other causes of sciatic injury at this site (Kline and Hudson, 1995). Patients with poor gluteal covering, including infants, children, and constitutionally thin or chronically ill and debilitated individuals, are predisposed to this type of injury. This is especially the case if the injection is given anywhere except the upper outer quadrant of the buttock (Fig. 42–5).

In the buttock, the sciatic nerve lies in a trough, between the bony boundaries of the ischial tuberosity and the greater trochanter. It is beneath the piriformis muscle and overlies the gemellus, quadratus, and obturator internus muscles. Drugs that are not injected directly into the nerve may pool in this trough and produce neuritis. Direct injection appears to be the typical cause of sciatic nerve injury, resulting in an almost immediate onset of pain, paresthesias, and deficit. The less frequent pattern, in about 10% of cases, is an onset delayed from minutes to many hours, of paresthesias and deficit, which appears to be related to injection adjacent to the nerve or into the epineurium.

In our most recent review of sciatic nerve injection injuries at LSUMC, 50 patients were identified (see Table 42–1). Of these patients, 30 (60%) were managed nonoperatively, with time, vigorous physical therapy, and pain medications. These patients usually had partial injuries that spared some function in both the tibial and peroneal divisions. In the 30 patients treated conservatively, two thirds (20) had neurological improvement to a level of useful (Grade 3 or better) function. Pain was a problem in most of these cases,

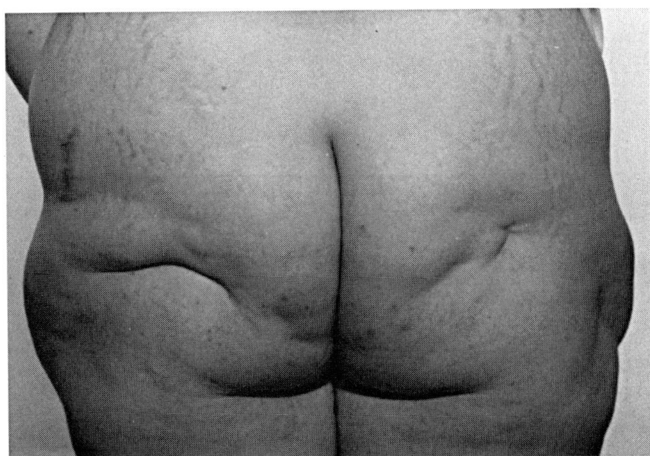

FIGURE 42–5. This patient received multiple buttock-level injections and unfortunately developed a sciatic palsy on the right. (Modified from Kline DG, Hudson AR: Nerve Injuries: Operative Results from Major Nerve Injuries, Entrapments, and Tumors. Philadelphia, W.B. Saunders Company, 1995.)

but fortunately, the majority responded to analgesic and tricyclic antidepressant drugs. A lesion with partial loss of function and severe pain not responding to analgesics may resolve to some degree with external or internal neurolysis. An occasional patient may have true causalgia. If recurrent sympathetic blocks have provided temporary relief, the patient may benefit from sympathectomy.

Both peroneal and tibial divisions of the sciatic nerve should be considered as a separate nerve during the preoperative assessment and during operative exploration. The peroneal division is injured with a much greater frequency than the tibial division by buttock-level injections to the sciatic nerve (Villarejo and Pascual, 1993). Injuries to the sciatic nerve that result in complete deficit of the whole nerve or either its peroneal or tibial divisions usually require surgical treatment. The best time for exploration is 3 to 5 months after the injection injury. The nerve can be exposed at the gluteal fold line and followed proximally, with division of the gluteus maximus laterally, leaving a generous pedicle for reattachment, and retraction of the muscle mass medially. The nerve is split into its two components so that each can be assessed independently with nerve stimulation and recording studies. The result of NAP recordings allow differential treatment of the two nerves, as illustrated in Figure 42–6 and in the following case study.

CASE 4 *(modified from Kline and Hudson, 1995)*

A 52-year-old woman received an injection of a narcotic drug in the right buttock. The patient felt pain radiate down her posterior thigh to the calf and foot, with the immediate onset of sciatic palsy. Partial dorsiflexion of the foot returned in a few days, but plantarflexion remained absent. At 4 weeks, EMG showed a severe denervational pattern in tibial muscles and partial changes in peroneal muscles. Clinically, 4 months after injury, hamstring function was normal and peroneal-innervated muscles below knee were evaluated as Grade 3. However, motor and sensory function related to the tibial nerve remained absent and EMG showed no nascent activity. Surgical exploration of the sciatic nerve at a buttock level revealed a swollen nerve along its medial aspect. An NAP was recorded across the lesion, and so the nerve was split into its peroneal and tibial divisions. Both divisions appeared to conduct an NAP. After dissection away from the tibial division of the main hamstring branch, which was very adherent to it, the tibial nerve no longer transmitted an NAP. As a result, this was resected and the gap repaired with three 5.8-cm–long sural nerve grafts. The peroneal division underwent only an external neurolysis. The resected segment demonstrated marked epineurial and interfascicular fibrosis, endoneurial thickening, and degenerated axons. Only fine axons were present, and they were mixed in with a moderately heavy proliferation of scar tissue. In follow-up after slightly over 2 years, the patient had maintained excellent peroneal-innervated function. Restoration of calf girth accompanied return of some function in the tibial distribution: plantar flexion and foot inversion were evaluated as being Grade 3, with no toe flexion but with protective sensation on the sole.

In the 20 patients requiring operation in our series, the presence of NAPs in 26 divisions led to neurolysis. Grade 3 or superior results were obtained in 21 of these 26 divisions. Lack of NAPs in the remainder of the cases led to resection of the lesion and either direct suture or graft repair of the involved division. Graft repairs were more common than suture because the lesions were rarely focal and usually required resection of several centimeters of injured, scarred nerve. As in the above-mentioned case, when tibial loss predominated and required repair (suture in two and grafting in five), the results were usually gratifying (six out of seven with at least Grade 3 recovery). On the other hand, the results of peroneal nerve suture or grafting at this level have been disappointing (Kline and Hudson, 1995).

In addition to the peroneal division injuries, which were frequent following buttock injections to the sciatic nerve, two patients with isolated peroneal nerve injury secondary to injections in the region of the knee were managed. In both cases, the neurological impairment was relatively mild and did not warrant surgical intervention.

FEMORAL NERVE

The most common etiology of femoral nerve injury is iatrogenic injury, related to various surgical procedures in

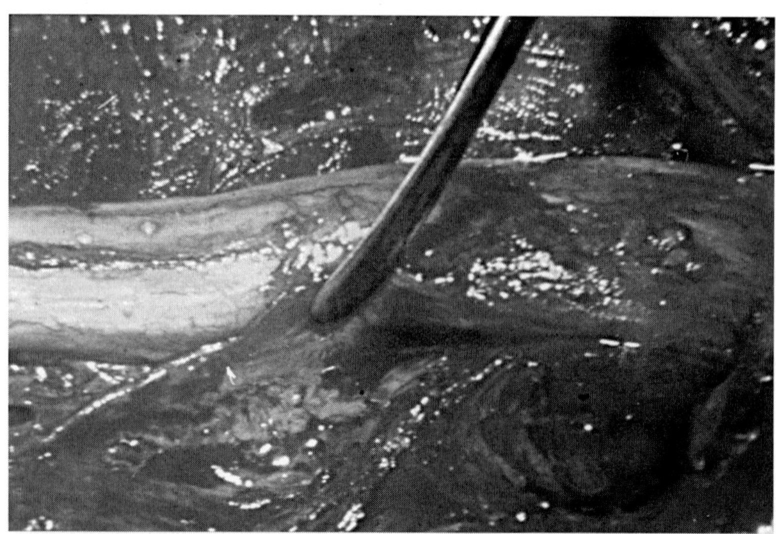

FIGURE 42–6. Intraoperative photo of sciatic nerve injured by injection of morphine, demonstrating abnormal reactive tissue adjacent to the injected segment of nerve. The tibial division failed to conduct a NAP, requiring resection and repair. (Modified from Kline DG, Hudson AR: Nerve Injuries: Operative Results from Major Nerve Injuries, Entrapments, and Tumors. Philadelphia, W.B. Saunders Company, 1995.)

the groin region. In some femoral neuropathies, which are seen following vascular procedures in the groin, femoral nerve damage may have occurred from accidental puncture of the nerve in the pelvis by a cannula or catheter. This possibility, as well as the need to explore the intrapelvic segment of the nerve, must be borne in mind when operating on these patients. A small subset of iatrogenic injuries to the femoral nerve result from catheters and needles inserted percutaneously to obtain vascular access for infusion and catheterization (Clark et al, 1970; Kline and Hudson, 1995). Iliopsoas muscle function, tested by hip flexion, is often intact because the location of nerve damage is distal to the branches to this muscle. Loss of quadriceps function (inability to extend the knee), absent knee reflex, and sensory loss in the saphenous distribution attest to a femoral nerve injury. In those patients not recovering spontaneously by 3 to 4 months, surgical exploration and intraoperative NAP assessment of the lesion is warranted. Another indication for operation is the patient with little neurological impairment but with a severe pain syndrome and disturbing paresthesias, because the pain and paresthesias may respond to surgical neurolysis.

References

Berry PR, Wallis WE: Venepuncture nerve injuries. Lancet *1*:1236, 1977.

Broadbent TR, Odom GL, Woodhall B: Peripheral nerve injuries from administration of penicillin. JAMA *140*:1008, 1949.

Clark K, Williams PEJ, Willis W, McGravan WA: Injection injury of the sciatic nerve. Clin Neurosurg *17*:111, 1970.

Clark WK: Surgery for injection injuries of peripheral nerves. Surg Clin North Am *52*:1325, 1972.

Combes MA, Clark WK: Sciatic nerve injury following intragluteal injection: Pathogenesis and prevention. Am J Dis Child *199*:579, 1960.

Combes MA, Clark WK, Gregory CF, James JA: Sciatic nerve injury in infants: Recognition and prevention of impairment resulting from intragluteal injections. JAMA *173*:1330, 1960.

Curtiss PHJ, Tucker HJ: Sciatic palsy in premature infants: A report and follow-up study of ten cases. JAMA 174:1586, 1960.

Elkington JSC: Peripheral nerve palsies following intramuscular injections of sulphonamides. Lancet 2:425, 1942.

Fried K, Frisen J, Mozart M: De- and regeneration of axons after minor lesions in the rat sciatic nerve. Effects of microneurography electrode penetrations. Pain *36*:93, 1989.

Gentili F, Hudson AR, Hunter D: Clinical and experimental aspects of injection injuries of peripheral nerves. Can J Neurol Sci *7*:143, 1980.

Gentili F, Hudson AR, Hunter D, Kline DG: Nerve injection injury with local anesthetic agents: A light and electron microscopic, fluorescent microscopic, and horseradish peroxidase study. Neurosurgery *6*:263, 1980.

Gentili F, Hudson AR, Kline DG, Hunter D: Peripheral nerve injection injury. An experimental study. Neurosurgery *4*:244, 1979.

Gilles FH, French JH: Post-injection sciatic nerve palsies in infants and children. J Pediatr *58*:192, 1961.

Holbrook TJ, Pilcher C: The effects of injection of penicillin, peanut oil and beeswax, separately and in combination, upon muscle and nerve. An experimental study. Surg Gynecol Obstet *90*:39, 1950.

Horowitz, SH: Peripheral nerve injury and causalgia secondary to routine venipuncture. Neurology 44:962, 1994.

Hudson FP, McCandless A, O'Malley AG: Sciatic paralysis in newborn infants. BMJ *1*:223, 1950.

Kline DG, Hudson AR: Nerve Injuries: Operative Results from Major Nerve Injuries, Entrapments, and Tumors. Philadelphia, W.B. Saunders Company, 1995.

Kline DG, Nulsen FE: The neuroma in continuity: its preoperative and operative management. Surg Clin North Am *52*:1189, 1972.

Kolb LC, Gray SJ: Peripheral neuritis as a complication of penicillin therapy. JAMA *132*:323, 1946.

Ling CM, Loong SC: Injection injury of the radial nerve. Injury *8*:60, 1976.

Mackinnon SE, Hudson AR, Gentili F, Kline DG, Hunter D: Peripheral nerve injection injury with steroid agents. Plast Reconstr Surg *69*:482, 1982.

Matson DD: Early neurolysis in the treatment of injury of the peripheral nerves due to faulty injection of antibiotics. N Engl J Med *242*:973, 1950.

Ochs G: Painful dysesthesias following peripheral nerve injury. A clinical and electrophysiological study. Brain Res *496*:228, 1989.

Rice ASC, McMahon SB: Peripheral nerve injury caused by injection needles used in regional anaesthesia: Influence of bevel configuration, studied in a rat model. Br J Anaesth *69*:433, 1992.

Sunderland S: Nerve and Nerve Injuries, 2nd ed. Edinburgh, Churchill Livingstone, 1978.

Tarlov IM, Perlmutter I, Berman AJ: Paralysis caused by penicillin injection; mechanism of complication—a warning. J Neuropathol Exp Neurol *10*:158, 1951.

Turner GG: The site for intramuscular injections. Lancet 2:819, 1920.

Villarejo FJ, Pascual AM: Injection injury of the sciatic nerve (370 cases). Childs Nerv Syst *9*:229, 1993.

von Hochstetter A: Problems and techniques of intragluteal injections. 1. Influence of medication and patient characteristics on the development of syringe injuries. Schweiz Med Wschr *85*:1138, 1955.

Woodhall B, Broadbent TR, Javer J: The neuropathology of antibiotic-induced peripheral nerve paralysis. Surg Forum *1*:394, 1950.

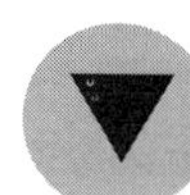

Chapter 43

• Moheb S. A. Moneim
• George E. Omer Jr

Clinical Outcome Following Acute Nerve Repair

Many factors affect the results of nerve repair. At the outset, it may be helpful to state that return of normal function following nerve injury and repair is not possible in adults. This is mainly secondary to the complexity of the nerve structure and regeneration. Sunderland (1945, 1991) initiated our understanding of such complexity by developing intraneural maps of major nerves at different levels in the extremity. Jabaley and associates (1980) determined the path and location of individual branches as they entered the nerve and what their position was relative to the rest of the nerve. These observations were confirmed by other authors (Chow et al, 1985; Williams and Jabaley, 1986).

Sunderland (1991) classified the anatomical factors that control recovery after nerve repair into three groups: central to the lesion, at the level of the repair, and at the periphery.

Central factors relate to the survival of the nerve cells and their ability to produce regenerating axons. The cells are more severely affected by lesions near the spinal cord, and the effect is more profound in sensory than in motor neurons. Therefore, sensory recovery is slower and less satisfactory than motor recovery.

Factors that affect recovery at the site of injury relate mainly to the scar tissue forming between the two nerve ends and the Schwann's cells with their endoneural tubes attracting the regenerating axons into the fasciculi of the distal nerve stumps. The only clinically applicable way to reduce connective tissue proliferation at the suture site is the resection of a strip of epineurium from the two stumps (Millesi, 1968). Millesi (1968) indicates that the resection increases the chances for a proper alignment of the fascicular cross sections by reducing the production of nonfascicular tissue. The gap between the two stumps should be reduced as much as possible for an optimal coaptation between the fascicular cross sections. By the fourth month following injury, the fascicular atrophy in the distal segment is at its peak, resulting in shrinkage and discrepancy between the two nerve stumps. The entry of regenerating axons into distal fasciculi depends on the fascicular patterns at the nerve ends, the cross-sectional area of the trunk occupied by the fasciculi, and the degree to which denervated fasciculi have atrophied; as a result, axons may be obstructed, lost, or misdirected into foreign endoneurial tubes. Only a cross-sectional analysis of biopsy material taken from the nerve ends during their preparation for nerve repair would reveal the extent of these potential problems (Sunderland, 1991).

The results of nerve repair are less satisfactory when a mixed nerve has been repaired at levels where the motor and sensory fibers are intermingled. Repairs of the median and ulnar nerves at the wrist do better than at the elbow. At the wrist, the median nerve is mainly sensory (90%),

whereas the motor fibers (45%) of the ulnar nerve have their own separate groups of fascicles. Above the elbow, where the fibers of other branches are included, the motor and sensory components are not as well segregated. In a fascicular cross section of the median nerve above the elbow, terminal sensory fibers (60%) are less segregated, and there are few thenar motor fibers (5%). In a fascicular cross section of the ulnar nerve above the elbow, terminal sensory fibers (35%) and the intrinsic motor fibers (28%) are not well segregated (Sunderland, 1991).

Anatomical factors that influence the quality of the nerve recovery at the periphery include recovery of muscles and the residual pattern of sensibility. Muscle fibers survive denervation for several years, providing the muscle receives passive exercise, is not exposed to cold, is not subjected to trauma, and its circulation is not impaired (Sunderland, 1991). Gaul (1982) and Omer and Eversmann (1994) have demonstrated recovery of intrinsic muscle action in adults up to 8 years after nerve repair. However, if denervation persists and muscle fibrosis results, recovery will not be possible and atrophy of the motor end-plates will occur. Sensory recovery can be a slow process that can extend into the fifth year, and in some patients, probably extends far beyond that time (Spinner, 1984). There is the possibility that the denervated area may be reduced by ingrowths from the sensory terminals of adjacent intact cutaneous nerves. Further improvement must be based on the capacity of the central nervous system to adjust and provide clinical function.

Other factors that influence the clinical outcome of nerve repair include the patient's age and motivation, the mechanism of injury, the time between injury and repair, and the surgical technique (Millesi, 1984; Spinner, 1984).

The younger the patient, the better the result because axonal growth and maturation is better. However, Almquist and Eeg-Olofsson (1970) believe that the better clinical results in the young are based on the greater adaptability of the central nervous system at that age. Rosen and co-workers (1994) have found correlation of restitution of functional sensibility with specific cognitive capacities. Children recover protective sensibility without education. Altissimi and colleagues (1991) found primary repair resulted in two-point discrimination less than 11 mm in 53% of patients aged 11 to 40 years but in only 27% in patients over 40 years of age. This pattern of sensibility would seem to indicate increased responsibility for the unmyelinated afferents and a changed priority of information for sensory cortex interpretation.

The nerve lesion is not an isolated event confined to an extremity, and it cannot be dissociated from the patient to whom it belongs. Recovery is a prolonged and tedious process, and it is during the long months of treatment that the personality of the patient determines whether he or she is going to make the most of the neurological recovery (Sunderland, 1991). For some patients, the reinnervated part will remain useless and the disability one to be exploited, whereas for other patients the disabled extremity will represent a challenge and through rehabilitation will be made to serve a useful purpose.

The nature of the injury, whether it be a clean laceration or an avulsion injury affecting a long segment of the nerve, has an obvious effect on the clinical outcome of nerve repair. Fibrosis will develop and result in poor prognosis after delayed repair. The quality of recovery declines if the repair is delayed, especially if it is delayed for longer than 6 months (Sunderland, 1991). Atraumatic technique, the vascularity of the bed, the intraneural anatomy of the nerve, excursion of the nerve, tension at the suture line, appropriate magnification and suture size (8–10/0 nylon) are important factors that relate to the technique of nerve repair (Omer and Pirela-Cruz, 1994; Spinner, 1984; Wilgis and Brushart, 1993).

Many of the harmful factors attributed to delayed repair are the result of severe wounding rather than the elective timing of the repair. The more severe and extensive the injury to the extremity, the longer the time required for homeostasis of the tissues (Omer, 1968). Severe vascular deficiency, chronic osteomyelitis, bony nonunion or articular incongruity all contribute to decreased function. Single or multiple nerve lesions with incomplete or multiple levels of laceration, contusion, stretch, crush, avulsion, or segmental loss present a recovery problem that is often complicated by extensive fibrotic reaction in all tissues of the involved extremity (Omer, 1983). Peripheral nerves are only as functional as the pertinent sensory receptors and musculotendinous motor units. Return of useful function depends as much on the total response of the extremity to the injury as on the regeneration of the injured nerve (Omer, 1974).

The results of nerve repair sometimes fall far short of expectations, prompting Sunderland's (1984) statement that "even in skilled hands the prognosis for repair remains unpredictable, while the results are far from good and in many cases, decidedly bad." However, there is ample evidence that the understanding of the complexity of the nerve structure and the introduction of microsurgical techniques have helped to improve the results of nerve repair (Sunderland, 1984).

TECHNIQUES FOR NERVE REPAIR

There are two basic techniques for nerve repair, end-to-end suture and nerve grafting. End-to-end suture is the preferred technique for repair, including acute or delayed repairs with minimal tension at the suture line (McEwan, 1962; Seddon, 1975) (Fig. 43–1). Tension at the suture line produces excessive scarring and traction injury to the repaired nerve as adjacent joints are mobilized (Highet and Sanders, 1943; Millesi, 1990; Omer, 1974; Omer et al, 1987; Rodkey et al, 1980; Walton and Finseth, 1977; Young et al, 1980). A nerve laceration is best dealt with by primary suture, because the growing axons cross only one suture line and fascicular matching is usually possible (Millesi, 1981, 1990). Results are largely influenced by the type of injury and the technique used by the surgeon, and can be different from one surgeon to another (Millesi, 1984). Many reports in the literature advocate primary end-to-end repair and assert better results with this approach than with nerve grafting (Birch and Raji, 1991; Jorgen and Van Twisk, 1988; Leclercq et al, 1985; Lijftogt et al, 1987; Mailander et al, 1987; Merle et al, 1986; Mitchell and Ostermann, 1991; Moneim and Omer, 1992).

The most commonly used technique for end-to-end suture is epineurial repair (Braun, 1980). Group fascicular repair has been recommended for some clinical situations (Chow et al, 1985, 1986; Hurst et al, 1991; Ito et al, 1976; Moneim and Omer, 1992; Urbaniak, 1982; Zong et al, 1988), especially the ulnar nerve at the wrist or the radial nerve at the elbow. The group fascicular repair technique is also indicated in partial nerve injuries (Tupper et al, 1980).

Repair of a major peripheral nerve laceration that is delayed for more than 3 weeks will result in excessive fibrosis at the level of the repair. The fibrosis must be cleared, which will dictate resection of more tissue from the nerve stumps and produce a defect that has to be bridged by grafts. Nerve grafting is indicated in a major peripheral nerve whenever there is a gap resulting from a failed primary repair, an unsutured nerve laceration more than 3 weeks old, or a primary loss of nerve substance (Barrios et al, 1990; Moneim, 1982; Terzis and Strauch, 1978; Young et al, 1980;

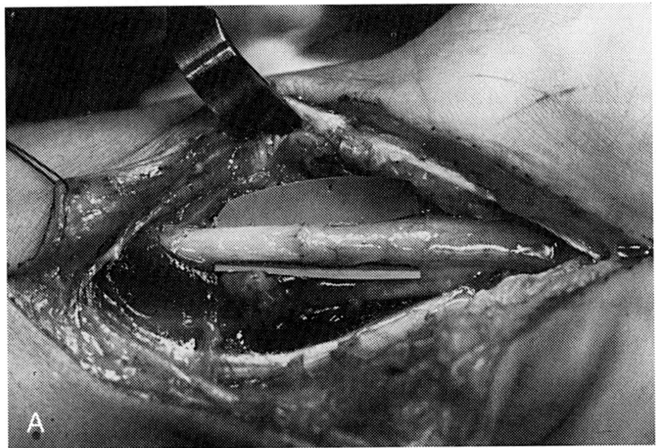

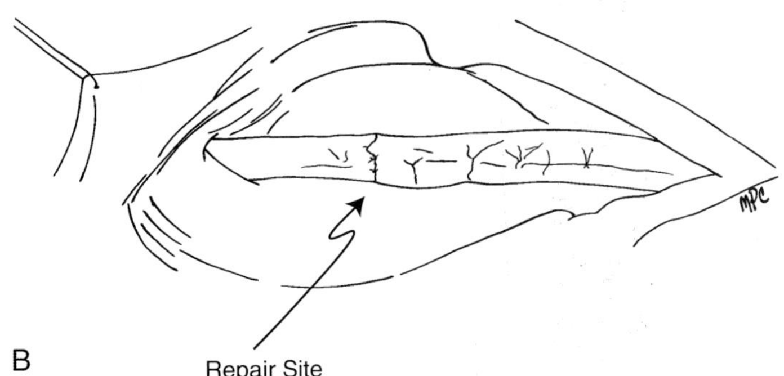

FIGURE 43–1. *A,* End-to-end suture of a median nerve laceration at the wrist. Technique was epineurial repair with anatomical fascicular alignment. *B,* Sketch highlighting key features.

Vastamaki et al, 1993). Millesi and associates (1972) introduced the concept of interfascicular nerve grafting (Fig. 43–2). Several studies have reported success with this technique (Haase et al, 1980; Kutz et al, 1981; Millesi, 1981; Millesi et al, 1976; Moneim, 1982; Stellini, 1982; Walton and Finseth, 1977).

EVALUATION OF CLINICAL RESULTS

A major problem in the evaluation of nerve repair is the definition of a good clinical result. There are no worldwide accepted criteria for evaluation of a functional recovery after nerve suture. A minimal evaluation of fuctional recovery should include (1) motor strength and range of motion, (2) sensibility level and associated pain interference, and (3) biomechanical balance and coordination of the extremity. Motor evaluation is based on examining muscle strength as it relates to gravity and resistance. Sensibility evaluation is based on return of superficial cutaneous pain, tactile sensibility, and two-point discrimination. The probable clinical outcome of nerve repair can be established after 2 years, but in order for results to be meaningful, a follow-up is needed of approximately 5 years in adults and 2 years in children (Omer, 1981a, 1981b, 1983; Omer and Spinner, 1975, 1984).

The British Medical Research Council introduced a grading system in 1954 that attempted to assess the recovery of an entire peripheral nerve in relation to total extremity function (Seddon, 1954; Table 43–1). It is rated in motor (M) and sensory (S) levels.

There have been several modifications of the British rating scales (see Chapter 36 on the Evaluation of Clinical Results), yet most grading systems published since the British Medical Research Council special report in 1954 have not provided additional or standardized evaluation methods for (1) measurement of individual muscle motor strength as a prime mover, antagonist, synergist, or stabilizer; (2) measurement of tactile gnosis sensibility level and associated pain interference, and (3) measurement of sensory mechanisms in motor performance, and precise motor coordination in sensory discrimination and sensibility, and stereognosis. We consider a Seddon M4 or better as a good level of motor recovery and a Seddon S3 or better as a good sensory recovery.

▼ **TABLE 43–1**
The British Medical Research Council Rating Scale

Level of Motor Recovery	Level of Sensory Recovery	Description
M5	S4	Complete recovery
M4	S3+	All synergetic and independent movements are possible
		Some recovery of two-point discrimination within autonomous area
M3	S3	All important muscles act against resistance
		Return of superficial cutaneous pain and tactile sensibility throughout the autonomous area with disappearance of any previous overreaction
M2	S2	Return of perceptible contraction in both proximal and distal muscles
		Return of some degree of superficial cutaneous pain and tactile sensibility within the autonomous area of the nerve
M1	S1	Return of perceptible contractions in proximal muscles
		Recovery of deep cutaneous pain sensibility within the autonomous area of the nerve
M0	S0	No contraction
		Absence of sensibility in the autonomous area

From Seddon HJ (ed): Peripheral Nerve Injuries, Medical Research Council Special Report Series, No. 282. London, Her Majesty's Stationery Office, 1954.

CLINICAL RESULTS

Earlier results following nerve repair came from England and the United States in reports on the experience from World War II. The British reported median nerve results of 33% M3 or better and 9% S3+ or better; ulnar nerve results were reported as 5% M4 or better and 31% S3 or better. The Americans reported median nerve results of 51% M3 or better and 18% S3+ or better; ulnar nerve results were reported as 13% M4 or better and 31% S3 or better. For the radial nerve, the British recorded 37% M4 or better, while the Americans recorded 21% M4 or better (Woodhall and Beebe, 1956). In both of these studies, median motor recovery was at or less than 50%, even when M3 recoveries were

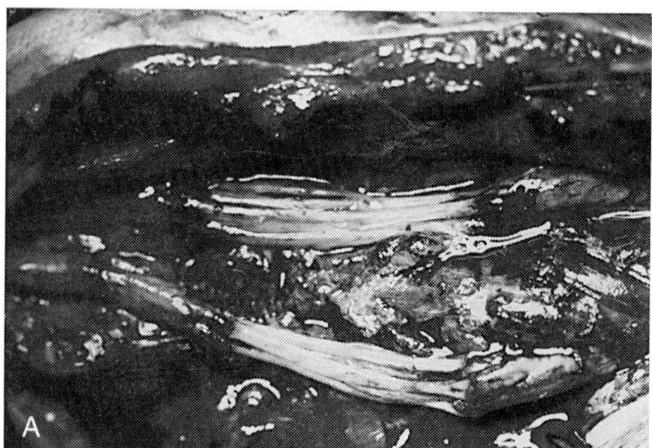

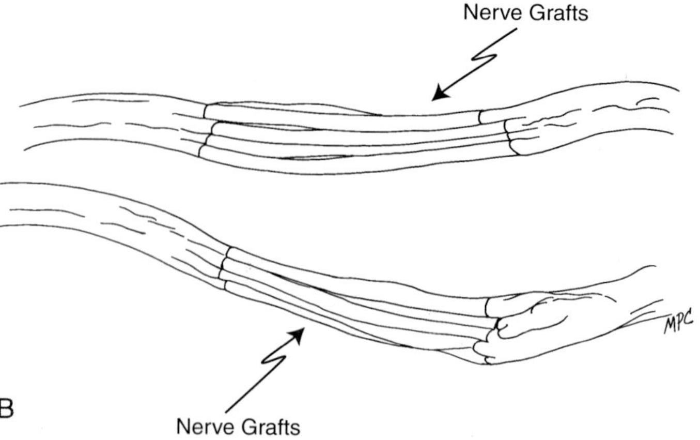

FIGURE 43–2. *A*, Median and ulnar nerve grafting. The lesion was a gunshot wound with extensive loss of nerve substance at a level above the elbow. The repair was performed 3 months after the injury. Note the interfascicular matching proximally and distally, using sural nerve grafts. *B*, Sketch highlighting key features.

RESULTS OF END TO END SUTURE
Motor Recovery

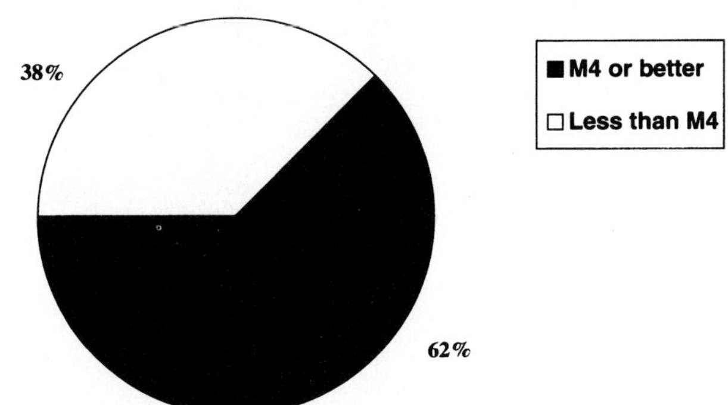

FIGURE 43–3. Combined results of median and ulnar nerve repairs are shown. Twenty of 32 nerves had M4 motor recovery or better.

included. The ulnar nerve motor and sensory recoveries were poor. These poor results occurred in military injuries, usually with delayed suture of the involved nerve, often in a severely damaged extremity. When the follow-up period was extended to 5 years after civilian injuries, somewhat better results were recorded: median motor recovery 65% M3 or better and sensory recovery 28% S3+ or better; ulnar nerve motor recovery 35% M4 or better and sensory recovery 69% S3 or better (Seddon, 1975).

There has been considerable improvement in reported outcome since microsurgical techniques have been introduced and surgeons have considered the complexity of the nerve structure. The use of electrical stimulation of the severed nerve ends to identify the motor from the sensory fascicles before repair was reported by Hakstian (1968), Terzis and Strauch (1978), and Gaul (1983). Gaul used electrical stimulation of the sensory fascicles in the proximal stump while the patient was awake. He reported on a group of 15 patients and rated the results as a percentage of the normal nonaffected side. In 10 median nerves, 50% had 75% motor recovery or better and 40% had S3+ or better; in five ulnar nerves, 20% had 75% motor recovery or better and 60% had S3+ or better. At present, techniques to achieve intraoperative motor or sensory differentiation of injured median and ulnar nerves have been reported to improve functional sensibility (Deutinger et al, 1993a, 1993b).

It is generally agreed that primary end-to-end repair yields better results than secondary reconstruction (LeClercq et al, 1985; McEwan, 1962; Merle et al, 1986; Mitchell and Ostermann, 1991; Sakellarides, 1962; Stromberg et al, 1961). Birch and Raji (1991) reviewed a series of 108 repairs in median and ulnar nerves between the elbow and wrist. All repairs were performed by the senior author and included 48 primary repairs, 25 delayed repairs, and 35 grafts. Excellent results were M5 motor recovery and normal sensibility. Good results were M4 or better motor recovery and two-point discrimination equal to or less than 8 mm. Assessment demonstrated that 39 of 48 primary repairs obtained good to excellent results; there were no excellent and only 7 good results in 25 patients who had delayed repairs; and only 11 of 35 patients who had grafts obtained good results. In this study, 19 of 26 median nerves (73%) and 20 of 22 ulnar nerves (91%) had good to excellent results; all but one of

the excellent results were in distal injuries in young people younger than 21 years of age. The authors emphasized that the experience of the surgeon was important and that the nerve repair should be delayed for timely referral and management if an experienced surgeon is not available initially. There were 35 nerves that had primary repair done at other institutions before being referred; revision revealed unacceptable technical errors in nerve repair, dense adhesions between tendons and nerves with nerve compression within the carpal canal, and in a few patients, the lacerated ulnar artery was not repaired and led to compression of the nerve. When the delayed repair was performed within 6 months of the injury, 3 of 32 failed; in those repaired after 6 months, 9 of 28 failed.

Primary nerve repair is not always possible. In a review of 1794 traumatic nerve injuries, De Medinaceli and co-workers (1993) found that primary end-to-end suture was possible in 87% of cases and graft repair in 2% of cases; repair was not possible in 11% of cases. A high proportion of the injuries involved digital nerves. The major reason for the inability to perform primary end-to-end repair was a nerve gap. There is general agreement that the outcome of digital nerve injuries is age related (Altissimi et al, 1991; Poppen et al, 1979; Sullivan, 1985).

Jacobson and Saurez are recognized for introducing the term microsurgery in 1960, and the operating microscope was first used in 1964 for peripheral nerve repair by several surgeons, including Kurtze, Michon, Masse, and Smith (Omer et al, 1987). Millesi applied microsurgical techniques as he introduced the concept of interfascicular nerve grafting, in which groups of fascicles are joined by grafts taken from a small cutaneous nerve (Millesi, 1981, 1990; Millesi et al, 1976). He stated that recovery from nerve grafts very closely approximated that of end-to-end suture.

The authors (Moneim and Omer, 1992) have had similar experience to that reported by Birch and Raji (1991), both with end-to-end epineurial suture and group fascicular suture nerve repair in adults. Following end-to-end suture of median and ulnar nerves, M4 or better motor recovery was recorded in 20 of 32 nerves (62%) (Fig. 43–3), and S3 or better sensibility was obtained in 27 of 32 nerves (84%) (Fig. 43–4). Following grafting of median and ulnar nerves, M4 or better motor recovery was recorded in only 7 of 25

RESULTS OF END TO END SUTURE
Sensory Recovery

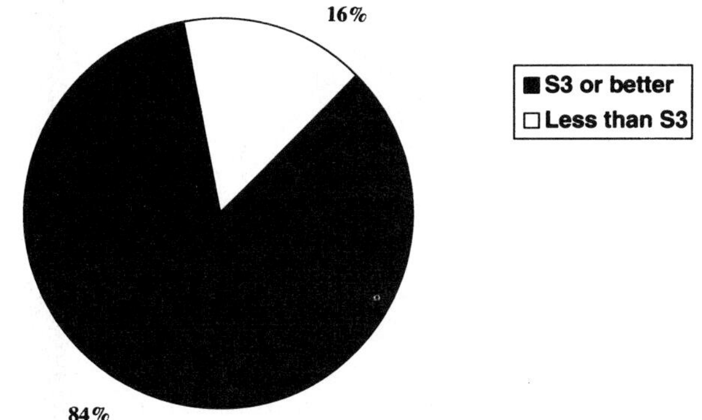

FIGURE 43–4. Combined results of median and ulnar nerve repairs are shown. Twenty-seven of 32 nerves had S3 sensibility recovery or better.

RESULTS OF GRAFTING
Motor Recovery

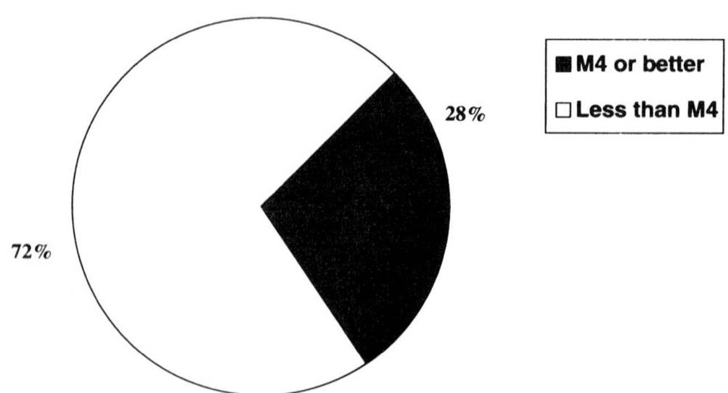

FIGURE 43–5. Combined results of median and ulnar nerve grafts are shown. Only 7 of 25 nerves obtained M4 motor recovery or better.

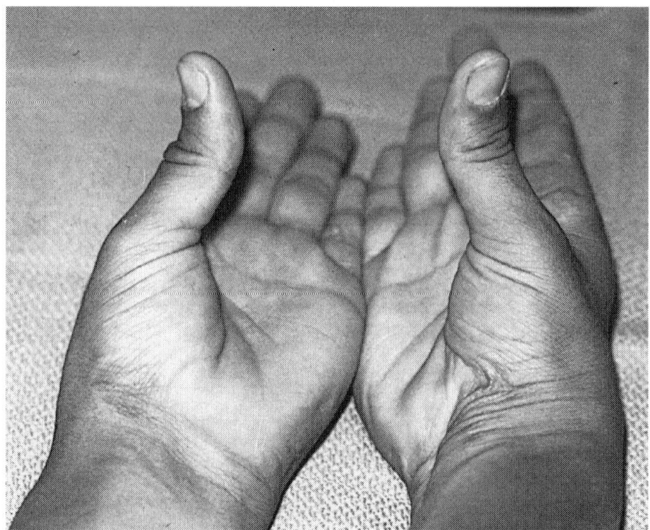

FIGURE 43–7. Recovery of thenar muscles to M5 motor level. Patient is shown 5 years following an end-to-end repair of the right median nerve at the wrist.

nerves (28%) (Fig. 43–5) and S3 or better sensibility was obtained in 15 of 25 nerves (60%) (Fig. 43–6). Analysis indicated that there was a statistical significance, with the suture group doing better in both motor and sensibility recovery.

In our study, when only distal forearm repairs were considered, the median nerve repairs demonstrated M4 or better recovery in 9 of 13 nerves (69%) (Fig. 43–7) and S3 or better sensibility in 12 of 13 nerves (92%). There were 15 distal repairs of the ulnar nerve, and 10 of 15 (67%) had M4 or better motor recovery and S3 or better sensibility in 13 of 15 (87%). Ulnar nerve repairs demonstrated M4 or better motor recovery in 83% of the group fascicular repairs, and only 45% of the epineurial repairs.

In the group that underwent the nerve graft procedure were 17 median and ulnar nerves with a defect of 5 cm or less; in this group, 6 nerves (35%) were evaluated at M4 or better motor recovery and 10 nerves (59%) demonstrated S3 or better sensibility. Only one nerve with a defect of more than 5 cm obtained M4 motor recovery. In the group that underwent the nerve graft procedure, there was only one

median nerve with recovery of S4 sensibility, and none of the ulnar nerves had any recovery of two-point discrimination.

M4 motor recovery or better was documented in 4 of 6 (67%) radial nerves. The two nerves with less than M4 recovery had repairs performed with loupe magnification, and one had the repair done 60 days after injury. Nine radial nerves were repaired by nerve grafting, and 7 of 9 (78%) obtained M4 or better motor recovery. Six nerves had defects more than 5 cm, and five (83%) demonstrated M4 or better recovery.

CONCLUSION

There is general agreement that acute nerve repair provides the best clinical result. Other factors that influence the outcome include the mechanism of injury, the time between injury and repair, the patient's age and motivation, and the surgical technique. Knowledge of fascicular group patterns and the use of microsurgical techniques have improved clinical outcomes. The most common technique for end-to-end suture is epineurial repair. Group fascicular repair is an advantage when motor and sensory components are well segregated, such as the ulnar nerve at the wrist. The surgeon who uses appropriate repairs, such as group fascicular or epineurial sutures, should obtain good to excellent results following nerve lacerations at the wrist.

RESULTS OF GRAFTING
Sensory Recovery

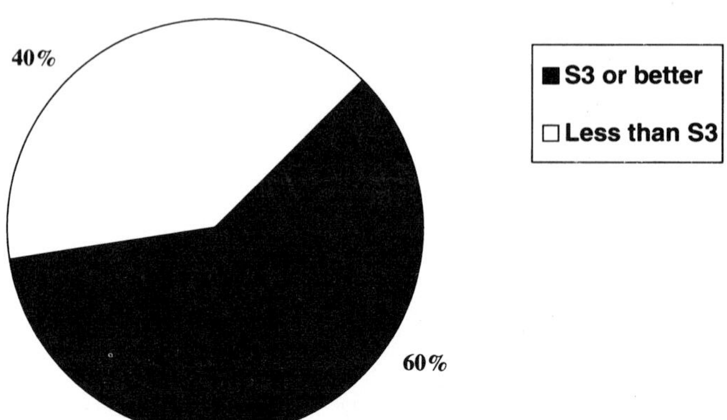

FIGURE 43–6. Combined results of median and ulnar nerve grafts are shown. Fifteen of 25 nerves obtained S3 or better sensibility recovery.

References

Almquist E, Eeg-Oloffsson O: Sensory-nerve-conduction velocity and two-point discrimination in sutured nerves. J Bone Joint Surg *52A*:791–796, 1970.

Altissimi M, Mancini GB, Azzara A: Results of primary repair of digital nerves. J Hand Surg *16B*:546–547, 1991.

Barrios C, Amillo S, de Pablos J, Canadell J: Secondary repair of ulnar nerve injury: 44 cases followed for 2 years. Acta Orthop Scand *61*:46–49, 1990.

Birch R, Raji ARM: Repair of median and ulnar nerves: Primary suture is best. J Bone Joint Surg *73B*:154–157, 1991.

Braun RM: Epineurial nerve repair. *In* Omer GE Jr, Spinner M (eds):

Management of Peripheral Nerve Problems. Philadelphia, W.B. Saunders Company, 1980, pp 366–379.

Chow JA, Van Beek AL, Meyer DL, Johnson MC: Surgical significance of the motor fascicular group of the ulnar nerve in the forearm. J Hand Surg *10A*:867–872, 1985.

Chow JA, Van Beek AL, Bilos ZJ, Meyer DL, Johnson MC: Anatomical basis for repair of ulnar and median nerves in the distal part of the forearm by group fascicular suture and nerve grafting. J Bone Joint Surg *68A*:273–280, 1986.

De Medinaceli L, Prayon M, Merle M: Percentage of nerve injuries in which primary repair can be achieved by end-to-end approximation: Review of 2,181 nerve lesions. Microsurgery *14*:244–246, 1993.

Deutinger M, Girsch W, Burggasser G, Windisch A, Joshi D, Mayr N, Frielinger G: Peripheral nerve repair in the hand with and without motor sensory differentiation. J Hand Surg *18A*:426–432, 1993a.

Deutinger M, Girsch W, Burggasser G, Windisch A, Joshi D, Mayr N, Frielinger G: Clinical application of motor sensory differentiated nerve repair. Microsurgery *14*:297–303, 1993b.

Gaul JS: Intrinsic motor recovery—A long-term study of ulnar nerve repair. J Hand Surg *7*:502–598, 1982.

Gaul JS: Electrical fascicle identification as an adjunct to nerve repair. J Hand Surg *8*:289–296, 1983.

Haase J, Bjerre P, Simesen K: Median and ulnar nerve transections treated with microsurgical interfascicular cable grafting with autogenous sural nerve. J Neurosurg *53*:73–84, 1980.

Hakstian RW: Funicular orientation by direct stimulation. J Bone Joint Surg *50A*:1178–1186, 1968.

Highet WB, Sanders FK: The effect of stretching nerves after suture. Br J Surg *30*:355–369, 1943.

Hurst LC, Dowd A, Sampson SP, Badalamente MA: Partial lacerations of median and ulnar nerves. J Hand Surg *16A*:207–210, 1991.

Ito T, Hirotani H, Yamamoto K: Peripheral nerve repairs by the funicular suture technique. Acta Orthop Scand *47*:283–289, 1976.

Jabaley ME, Wallace WH, Heckler FR: Internal topography of major nerves of the forearm and hand: A current view. J Hand Surg *5*:1–8, 1980.

Jongen SJ, Van Twisk R: Results of primary repair of ulnar and median nerve injuries at the wrist: An evaluation of sensibility and motor recovery. Neth J Surg *40*:86–89, 1988.

Kutz JE, Shealy G, Lubbers L: Interfascicular nerve repair. Orthop Clin North Am *12*:277–286, 1981.

Leclercq DC, Carlier AJ, Khue T, Depierreux L, Lejeune GN: Improvements in the results in 64 ulnar nerve sections associated with arterial repair. J Hand Surg *10A*(Supp):997–999, 1985.

Lijftogt HJ, Dijkstra R, Storm van Leeuwen JB: Results of microsurgical treatment of nerve injuries of the wrist. Neth J Surg *39*:170–174, 1987.

Mailander P, Berger A, Schaller E, Ruhe K: Results of primary nerve repair in the upper extremity. Microsurgery *10*:147–150, 1989.

McEwan LE: Median and ulnar nerve injuries. Aust N Z J Surg *32*:89–104, 1962.

Merle M, Amend P, Cour C, Foucher G, Michon J: Microsurgical repair of peripheral nerve lesions: A study of 150 injuries of the median and ulnar nerves. Peripheral Nerve Repair and Regeneration *2*:17–26, 1986.

Millesi H: Zum Problem der Ueberbruckung von Defekten peripherer Nerven. Wien Med Wschr *118*:182–187, 1968.

Millesi H: Nerve grafts: Indications, techniques, and prognosis. *In* Omer GE Jr, Spinner M (eds): The Management of Peripheral Nerve Problems. Philadelphia, W.B. Saunders Company, 1980, pp 410–430.

Millesi H: Reappraisal of nerve repair. Surg Clin North Am *61*:321–340, 1981.

Millesi H: Nerve grafting. Clin Plast Surg *11*:105–113, 1984.

Millesi H: Peripheral nerve surgery today: Turning point or continuous development? J Hand Surg *15B*:281–287, 1990.

Millesi H, Meissl G, Berger A: The interfascicular nerve grafting of the median and ulnar nerves. J Bone Joint Surg *54A*:727–750, 1972.

Millesi H, Meissl G, Berger A: Further experience with interfascicular nerve grafting of the median, ulnar, and radial nerves. J Bone Joint Surg *58A*:209–218, 1976.

Mitchell JR, Ostermann AL: Physiology of nerve repair: A research update. Hand Clin *7*:481–490, 1991.

Moneim MS: Interfascicular nerve grafting. Clin Orthop *163*:65–74, 1982.

Moneim MS, Omer GE Jr: Results of nerve repair under ideal conditions. Orthop Trans *16*:200–201, 1992.

Omer GE Jr: Evaluation and reconstruction of the forearm and hand after acute traumatic peripheral nerve injuries. J Bone Joint Surg *50A*:1454–1478, 1968.

Omer GE Jr: Injuries to nerves of the upper extremity. J Bone Joint Surg *56A*:1615–1624, 1974.

Omer GE Jr: Physical diagnosis of peripheral nerve injuries. Orthop Clin North Am *12*:207–228, 1981a.

Omer GE Jr: Methods of assessment of injury and recovery of peripheral nerves. Surg Clin North Am *61*:303–320, 1981b.

Omer GE Jr: Report of the committee for evaluation of the clinical result in peripheral nerve injury. J Hand Surg *8*:754–759, 1983.

Omer GE Jr, Eversmann WW Jr: Peripheral nerve problems. *In* Burkhalter SE (ed): Orthopedic Surgery in Vietnam. Washington, DC, Office of The Surgeon General and the Center of Military History, U.S. Army, 1994, pp 155–188.

Omer GE Jr, O'Brien WJ, Murray HM, Torkelson, EO, Orgel MG: Has microsurgical technique improved the results of epineurial repair of peripheral nerves? *In* Urbaniak, JR (ed): Microsurgery for Major Limb Reconstruction. St. Louis, C.V. Mosby Co., 1987, pp 372–385.

Omer GE Jr, Pirela-Cruz M: Complications of peripheral nerve injuries. *In* Epps CH Jr (ed): Complications in Orthopaedic Surgery, 3rd ed. Philadelphia, J.B. Lippincott Co., 1994, pp 811–856.

Omer GE Jr, Spinner M: Peripheral nerve testing and suture techniques. *In* Instructional Course Lectures, American Academy of Orthopaedic Surgeons, Vol. 24, 1975. St. Louis, C.V. Mosby Company, pp 122–143.

Omer GE Jr, Spinner M: Management of peripheral nerve problems. *In* Instructional Course Lectures, American Academy of Orthopaedic Surgeons, Vol. 33, 1984. St. Louis, C.V. Mosby Company, pp 461–530.

Poppen NK, McCarroll HR Jr, Doyle JR, Niebauer JJ: Recovery of sensibility after suture of digital nerves. J Hand Surg *4*:212–226, 1979.

Rodkey WG, Cabard EH, McCarroll RH Jr: Neurorrhaphy after loss of a nerve segment; comparison of ipineural suture under tension versus multiple nerve grafts. J Hand Surg *5*:366–371, 1980.

Rosen B, Lundborg G, Dahlin LB, Holmberg J, Karlson B: Nerve repair: Correlation of restitution of functional sensibility with specific cognitive capacities. J Hand Surg *19B*:452–458, 1994.

Sakellarides H: A follow-up study of 172 peripheral nerve injuries in the upper extremity in civilians. J Bone Joint Surg *44A*:140–148, 1962.

Seddon HJ (ed): Peripheral Nerve Injuries. London, Her Majesty's Stationery Office, Medical Research Council Special Report Series, No. 282, 1954.

Seddon H: Surgical Disorders of the Peripheral Nerves, 2nd ed. Edinburgh, Churchill Livingstone, 1975, pp 303–314.

Spinner M: Current concepts of nerve suture. *In* Instr. Course Lect., Amer. Acad. Orthop. Surg. St. Louis, C.V. Mosby Co., pp 487–498, 1984.

Stellini L: Interfascicular autologous grafts in the repair of peripheral nerves: Eight years' experience. Br J Plast Surg *35*:478–482, 1982.

Stromberg WB Jr, McFarlane RM, Bell JL, Koch SL, Mason ML: Injury of the median and ulnar nerves. J Bone Joint Surg *43A*:717–730, 1961.

Sullivan DJ: Results of digital neurorrhaphy in adults. J Hand Surg *10B*:41–44, 1985.

Sunderland S: The interneural topography of the radial, median, and ulnar nerves. Brain *68*:243–298, 1945.

Sunderland S: Editorial: Nerve repair. J Hand Surg *9A*:1–3, 1984.

Sunderland S: Nerve Injuries and Their Repair. Edinburgh, Churchill Livingstone, 1991, pp 31–40.

Terzis JK, Strauch B: Microsurgery of the peripheral nerve: A physiological approach. Clin Orthop *133*:39–48, 1978.

Tupper JW: Fascicular nerve repair. *In* Omer GE Jr, Spinner M (eds): Management of Peripheral Nerve Problems. Philadelphia, W.B. Saunders Company, 1980, pp 380–387.

Urbaniak JR: Fascicular nerve suture. Clin Orthop *163*:57–64, 1982.

Vastamaki M, Kallio PK, Solonen KA: The results of secondary microsurgical repair of ulnar nerve injury. J Hand Surg *18B*:323–326, 1993.

Walton R, Finseth F: Nerve grafts in the repair of complicated peripheral nerve trauma. J Trauma *17*:793–796, 1977.

Wilgis EFS, Brushart TM: Nerve repair and grafting. *In* Green DP (ed): Operative Hand Surgery, 3rd ed. New York, Churchill Livingstone, 1993, pp 1315–1340.

Williams HB, Jabaley ME: The importance of internal anatomy of the peripheral nerves to nerve repair in the forearm and hand. Hand Clin *2*:689–707, 1986.

Woodhall B, Beebe GW (eds): Peripheral nerve regeneration, a follow-up study of 3,656 World War II injuries. Veterans Administration Medical Monograph. Washington DC, U.S. Government Printing Office, 1956, pp 116–257.

Young LV, Wray CR, Weeks PM: The results of nerve grafting in the wrist and hand. Ann Plast Surg *5*:212–215, 1980.

Zong S, Wang G, He YS, Sun B: The relationship between structural features of peripheral nerves and suture methods for nerve repair. Microsurgery *9*:181–185, 1988.

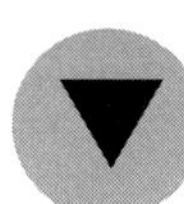

Chapter 44

- David G. Kline
- Robert Tiel
- Daniel Kim
- Carter Harsh

Lower Extremity Nerve Injuries

Since preparing this chapter for the first edition of this book, which was published in 1980, this series of patients with lower extremity nerve lesions has expanded considerably. This factor has permitted analysis of a relatively large group of patients and, from this, the development of some guidelines for management. The period of study extended from 1967 until 1991, or a total of 24 years, although some of the data to be presented are based on the proportion of cases cared for between only 1967 and 1987. Older civilian series of operated lower extremity nerve lesions (Clawson and Seddon, 1960a, 1960b; Fried et al, 1978; Johnson, 1969; Kline, 1980; Osgaard and Husby, 1977; Paradies and Gregory, 1966) have not been much more encouraging than series based on war injuries (Highet and Holmes, 1943; Rakolta and Omer, 1969; Rizzoli, 1965; Seddon, 1972; Sunderland, 1984). On the other hand, except for mild, partial injuries, nonoperative treatment can frequently fail as well (Kline, 1980; Kline and Hudson, 1995; Omer, 1982; Sunderland, 1984; Kim and Kline, 1995).

PERTINENT SURGICAL ANATOMY—SCIATIC COMPLEX

The sciatic nerve originates from both the anterior and posterior divisions of L4, L5, and S1, and the S2 spinal nerves or roots. The anterior division of S3 usually also contributes to this complex (Kopell, 1980). Anterior root divisions contribute mainly to the tibial division of the sciatic and its main hamstring branch. The posterior root divisions contribute to the peroneal division. Shortly after the lumbosacral plexus forms the whole sciatic nerve, the sciatic nerve exits the sciatic foramen to reach the level of the buttocks. There, the nerve penetrates or lies anterior to the piriformis muscle, and the nerve's divisions are sometimes split by this muscular structure. On rare occasions, the sciatic nerve can be spontaneously entrapped near the notch by hypertrophy of this muscle (Banerjee and Hall, 1976). Gluteal vessels and nerves exit the foramen with the sciatic nerve and take a posterior course to supply the gluteus major and minor muscles. In addition, the principal hamstring branch or nerve usually originates within the sciatic notch or soon after the nerve exits it. The sciatic nerve then passes over or posterior to the obturator internis and both the superior and inferior gemelli as it runs distally toward the thigh and beneath the glutei.

As the nerve enters the thigh, it is somewhat deep to and between the medial and lateral hamstring muscles. Meanwhile, the hamstring branch reaches the upper thigh by running parallel but medial to the sciatic nerve. In the proximal thigh, this hamstring branch supplies the long head of the biceps femoris, the semitendinosus, and the semimembranosus muscles. Another branch to the hamstrings, usually the lateral or short head, arises from lateral or peroneal division of the sciatic nerve. Lack of such hamstring function can sometimes place the peroneal lesion at a very proximal level (Rizzoli, 1965).

The level where the sciatic nerve bifurcates into the tibial and peroneal nerve varies but is usually at the junction of middle and lower thirds of the thigh (Kline, 1972; Kopell, 1980). As these nerves approach the popliteal space, they are increasingly surrounded by fat. The tibial nerve lies posterior to the popliteal artery and vein, and branches just proximal to its entrance into the gastrocnemius soleus muscle. For the most part, these branches supply this muscle, but a major portion of the nerve branch also runs deep to this muscle and eventually supplies sensation to the sole of the foot and motor input to the foot intrinsic muscles. At the popliteal or posterior knee level, the peroneal nerve runs obliquely from a medial to lateral direction and tends to lie beneath the lateral or short head of the biceps femoris tendon. In the popliteal fossa, the peroneal usually gives rise to the sural nerve, although in some cases, the sural nerve receives input from the tibial nerve as well. The sural nerve leaves the popliteal fossa under cover of the gastrocnemius soleus fascia to run down the posterior lower leg at a relatively superficial level. Usually at mid-calf level, the sural nerve leaves the cover of the gastrocnemius; there, the nerve lies in the subcutaneous tissues and usually is adherent or adjacent to vein or veins, especially as it approaches the underside of the lateral malleolus.

The peroneal nerve lies posterior and inferior to the head of the fibula and the neck, which it curves around somewhat to enter the anterior compartment of the leg. This portion of the nerve can usually be readily assessed by both clinical and electrophysiologic studies, especially those that evaluate conduction velocity (Berry and Richardson, 1976). In addition to fine branches to the joint, the peroneal nerve begins to split into a superficial and a deep cascade of branches as it overlies the head and posterior portion of the neck of the fibula. The deep branch enters proximal anterior compartment and quickly branches into inputs to anterior tibialis, extensor communis of the toes, and extensor hallucis longus. There is some variation in the length and number of deep branches associated with each of these muscles. By comparison, the superficial branches run more inferiorly and in a vertical fashion under cover of the laterally located peronei, which it innervates.

The posterior tibial nerve itself can be traced for a short distance into the gastrocnemius soleus by elevating the superior edge of this muscle. Branches running beneath this edge of the calf supply the plantaris, popliteus, and tibialis posterior, as well as the gastrocnemius soleus (Sedel and Nizard, 1993). Inputs to the flexor digitorum and hallucis longus leave the nerve further distally in more lower leg.

Retraction of the superior edge of the gastrocnemius can expose an inch or so of the calf level of the nerve, but a different approach is necessary for more distal leg level lesions. Such injuries can be approached by an incision on the medial leg posterior to tibia and yet anterior to the bulk of the gastrocnemius soleus. Dissection at this level is a deep one and usually requires isolation and control of posterior tibial artery and vein, as well as healthier proximal and distal tibial nerve. This, then, permits a safer dissection of the scarred or neuromatous portion of the nerve. Once located at this level, the tibial nerve can then be traced proximally toward popliteal fossa or distally toward the ankle.

Exposure of the tibial nerve at the ankle is more straightforward than at leg level but not as readily performed as exposure of median nerve at wrist and hand for carpal tunnel syndrome. As the posterior tibial nerve approaches the ankle, it lies beneath the medial collateral ligaments and inferior to the medial malleolus. In addition to a calcaneal branch heading inferiorly toward the heal, the tibial nerve provides medial and lateral plantar branches. Intertwined in these branches are the tibial artery and vein, and this makes dissection much more difficult than that for exposure or neurolysis of median nerve in the hand. Nerve branches then travel deep to the plantar musculature in the instep or the region of the true tarsal tunnel. Structures overlying the nerve in the region of the instep must thus be sectioned to unroof what is termed the true tarsal tunnel.

Anatomy of the peroneal nerve at the level of the lower leg and distal to the fibular head and neck is more straightforward for superficial than deep branches (Wood, 1991a). The superficial branches descend the lower leg beneath the fascia and some of the musculature of the peronei. At the mid-level of the lower leg, either one or two anterior tibial branches arise. These nerves are almost always destined for sensory sites. The anterior tibial branches are superficial, lying beneath subcutaneous tissues. Branches become more anterolateral as they approach ankle, where they divide to supply sensory fibers to the dorsum of the foot.

By comparison, the deep branch of the peroneal nerve passes over the head and neck of the fibula and then into the anterior compartment, where it quickly divides to supply the anterior tibialis, extensor digitorum longus, and extensor hallucis longus. Dissection at the level of the knee is difficult but is aided by magnification, use of the bipolar cautery and gentle retraction of nerve branches. The posterior edge of the peroneus fascia and muscle is cleared by sharp dissection, retracted, and partially split to expose the superficial peroneal branch. A Penrose drain is placed around the peroneal nerve proximal to the level of the head of the fibula so that it and its proximal branches can be gently elevated. Dissection is then performed on the underside or anterior side of the deep branch, which is then traced as best as possible into the anterior compartment.

RESULTS OF BUTTOCK-LEVEL SCIATIC NERVE SURGERY

Lesions selected for operation were those with either tibial loss alone or, more commonly, tibial loss as well as peroneal division loss that was complete clinically and electrically. Included were also less complete lesions, in which neuritic pain could not be managed pharmacologically. The surgical approach is through a curvilinear, lateral buttocks incision. Glutei were transected laterally but medial enough to leave a cuff of muscle with which to repair the muscle (Kline, 1972) (Fig. 44–1). The more superior gluteus was split in the direction of its fibers. Then, both the gluteus maximus and minimus were retracted medially by rakes and the sciatic complex was approached from a lateral to medial direction. The submuscular plane thus developed is somewhat avascular. Once the sciatic nerve was encountered at mid-buttock level, it was dissected in a circumferential fashion down to the thigh distally and up and into the sciatic notch region proximally. Even at this level, the nerve can be divided into its two divisions and evaluated individually by nerve action potential (NAP) recordings (Fig. 44–2). Dissection within the notch required isolation of the sciatic and splitting away gluteal and hamstring nerve branches with preservation of as many gluteal vessels as possible.

Table 44–1 includes results for both divisions of the nerve

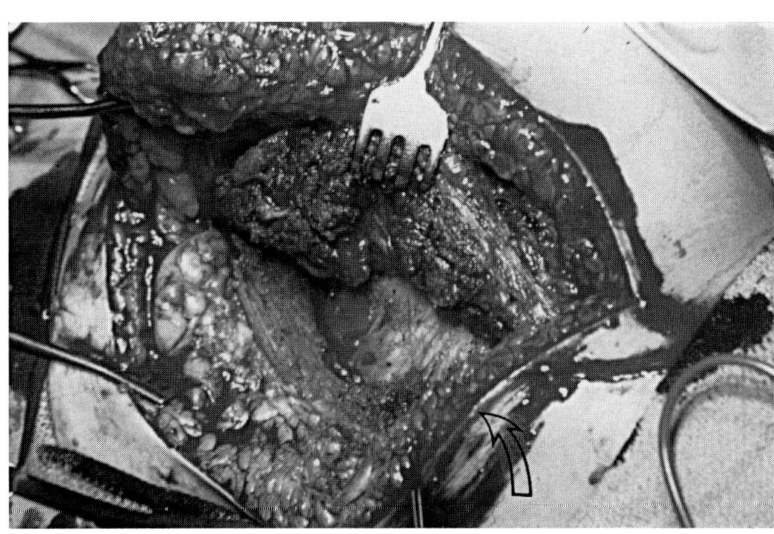

FIGURE 44–1. Initial steps in exposure of the sciatic nerve at the buttock level. Arrow points to skin areas of the buttock crease. Rake is reflecting the glutei, which have been detached laterally and medially. A cuff of muscle has been left laterally to sew the muscle back. More superior gluteal fibers will be split in the direction they run. Dissection, then, proceeds medially and beneath muscle until the sciatic nerve is encountered superficial to the gemelli and quadratus. (From Kline D, Hudson A: Nerve Injuries: Operative Results for Major Nerve Injuries, Entrapments, and Tumors. Philadelphia, W. B. Saunders Company, 1995.)

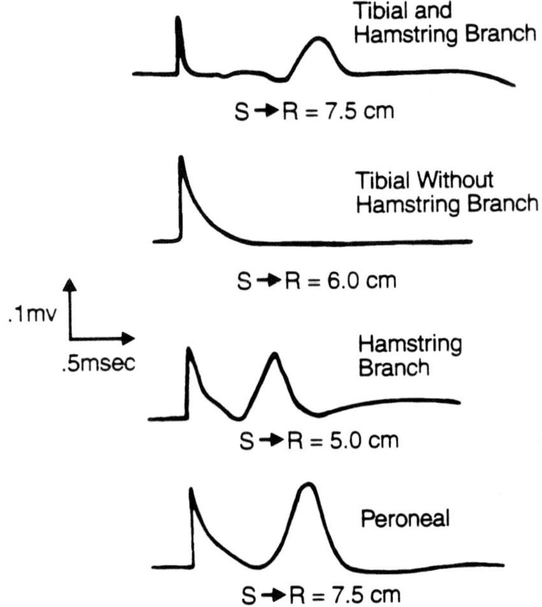

FIGURE 44–2. Intraoperative NAP recording from the sciatic nerve at the proximal buttock level. Before the hamstring branch was split away from the tibial division, there was an NAP. Once the hamstring branch was split away, there was no NAP. A length of this division required resection and repair. Fortunately, it was clear by the recording from the hamstring branch that this section did have an NAP, as did the peroneal division, so they were spared resection. (From Kline D, Hudson A: Nerve Injuries: Operative Results for Major Nerve Injuries, Entrapments, and Tumors. Philadelphia, W. B. Saunders Company, 1995.)

and for the various lesions operated on by category of injury or involvement. A minimal period of 3 years of follow-up was necessary for inclusion in this table; tracking patients for follow-up was difficult, so not all patients seen or operated on during the period studied are included. In any case, the present data are based on those cases so evaluated with follow-up and managed at one institution, Louisiana State University Medical Center (LSUMC), and by one surgeon (DGK).

One of the largest buttock level categories was that due to injection injury (Clark et al, 1970; Hudson et al, 1980; Villarejo and Pascual, 1993). Only about 40% of the patients with injection injury were selected for operation. Some of these patients had severe deficits persisting for 3 or more months and for that reason were operated on. In a few other cases, deficit was incomplete but had neuritic pain that did not respond to pharmacologic management. Once surgical exploration was decided on, neurolysis was used rather than repair because there was either a positive NAP across a lesion, indicating regeneration despite severe loss, or an NAP in a lesion in which loss in the distribution of that element was known to be mild beforehand. Either suture or graft repair, particularly for the peroneal division in which only 3 of 12 (25%) gained significant recovery in that distribution, was less reliable in providing recovery of function, whereas, 8 of 11 (73%) with tibial division repair did regain function. When repair was necessary and pain was present preoperatively in the distribution of the element repaired, there was almost always significant pain relief. Neurolysis was less reliable in relieving pain.

The vulnerability of the sciatic complex with bony hip injury has been described by a number of authors (Adams, 1964; Gentili and Hudson, 1985; Johnson, 1969; McLean, 1986; Solheim and Hagen, 1980; Weber et al, 1976). Sixteen patients in this series with hip fracture or dislocation were selected for operation, whereas 15 were followed without operation. Lesions associated with hip fracture were usually in continuity, although prior instrumentation of the fracture site had inadvertently divided sciatic nerve in several patients. When NAPs were not conducted across the lesions in continuity, grafts were usually necessary (13 elements), although end-to-end sutures were possible on four lesions. Again, repairs fared well when they were performed on the tibial division but less so on the peroneal division.

As can be seen in Table 44–1, more than half of the patients with gunshot wounds (GSWs) involving the buttock level of the sciatic nerve did not have evidence of significant clinical or electrical recovery in the early months after wounding and required an operation. Either end-to-end suture or graft repair was necessary for eight elements, whereas neurolysis sufficed for 13. Recovery was not ensured, especially when repair was necessary. Recovery was also incomplete in many patients followed without surgery primarily because the peroneal division was less likely to gain a grade of 3 over time, although tibial division often did.

Most of the patients with lacerations or stab wounds involving the sciatic nerve required operation because loss was either complete or near-complete to one or both divisions. Repair, as opposed to neurolysis was more likely to be needed than in other categories of injury. Even so, as can be seen in Table 44–1, one case was still in continuity despite severe distal loss. NAPs transmitted through both divisions of this lesion, which underwent neurolysis and achieved an excellent recovery. Despite the relatively focal nature of lacerations to nerves, only about one quarter of the peroneal divisions requiring repair had enough recovery of dorsiflexion to no longer need a kick-up foot brace. Thus, use of a posterior tibialis transfer or other procedure is indicated fairly frequently in this group of proximal injuries. This, of course is only feasible in patients in whom tibial division is spared to begin with or recovers over time (Bourrel, 1967; Millesi, 1987).

RESULTS OF THIGH-LEVEL SCIATIC NERVE SURGERY

A combination of sharp dissection by scalpel and blunt dissection by Metzenbaum scissors was used to split the hamstring muscles and to dissect out the sciatic complex at this level. Divisions were usually split apart by working in a proximal direction from the tibial and peroneal nerves and splitting them under magnification using microinstruments (Kline, 1972) (Fig. 44–3). The leading mechanism providing sciatic injury at this level was GSW (Kopell, 1980). Stretch associated with fracture was the next largest category (Aldea and Shaw, 1986). Transection in association with soft tissue laceration or stab wounds also occurred fairly frequently.

Table 44–2 includes the results of surgery at the thigh level and further differentiates tibial from peroneal division outcomes. It remained important to evaluate each division of the nerve operatively because sometimes there was a spectrum of severity of injury involving each even in a given patient. Neurolysis was based on NAP recordings, which suggested that repair was not necessary because potentials

▼ **TABLE 44–1**
Sciatic Complex—Buttock Level (1967–1987)

	Neurolysis		Suture		Graft		No Operation Sciatic
	T	*P*	*T*	*P*	*T*	*P*	
Injection (n = 66)	12/10*	11/8	3/2	3/1	8/6	9/2	38/23
Hip f(x)–disloc (n = 36)	5/5	3/1	1/1	3/1	7/4	6/1	15/6
GSW (n = 26)	8/7†	5/3	1/1	2/0	2/1†	3/1†	9/6
Lac/Sta (n = 12)	1/1	1/1	3/2	4/1	4/4	3/1	2/0
Compression/Contusion (n = 9)	3/2	3/1	0/0	2/1	0/0	1/0	2/1
Totals	29/25	23/14	8/6	14/4	21/15	22/05	66/36

*Number of cases operated on and number of cases gaining a grade 3 or better result. Not included in this table are outcomes in nine patients with tumors of or involving sciatic nerve at the buttock level.
†Sympathectomies (lumbar) were done in several patients.
F(x)–disloc, fracture dislocation; GSW, gunshot wound; Lac/stab, laceration and stab wounds; n, cases evaluated in each category; T, tibial; P, peroneal.
Adapted from Kline D, Hudson A: Nerve Injuries: Operative Results of Major Nerve Injuries, Entrapments, and Tumors. Philadelphia, W.B. Saunders Company, 1995.

were recorded across the lesion. Repairs by suture or by grafts were performed on those lesions that did not conduct an NAP or that were transected. Figure 44–4 compares relative outcome for neurolysis, suture, and grafts for both tibial and peroneal divisions. Figure 44–5 provides a similar analysis for just GSWs at the thigh level. As at the buttock level, the tibial division at the thigh also had better outcomes than the peroneal division. Nonetheless, the peroneal repairs fared somewhat better at thigh than at buttock level. Distraction of the repair site was a possibility, especially if sutures were used rather than grafts.

GSWs and fracture-associated sciatic palsies at the thigh

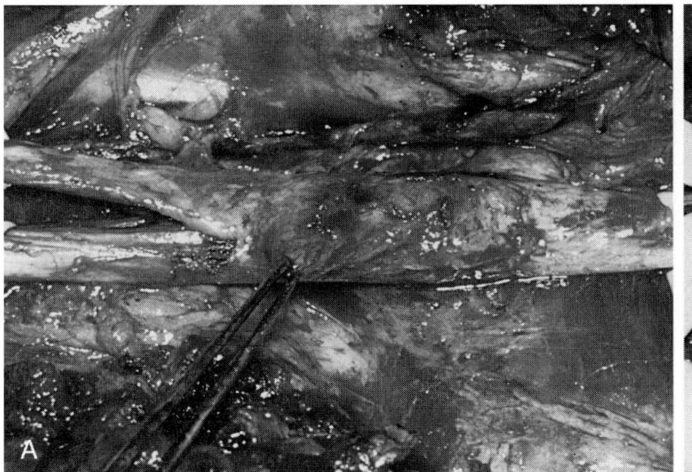

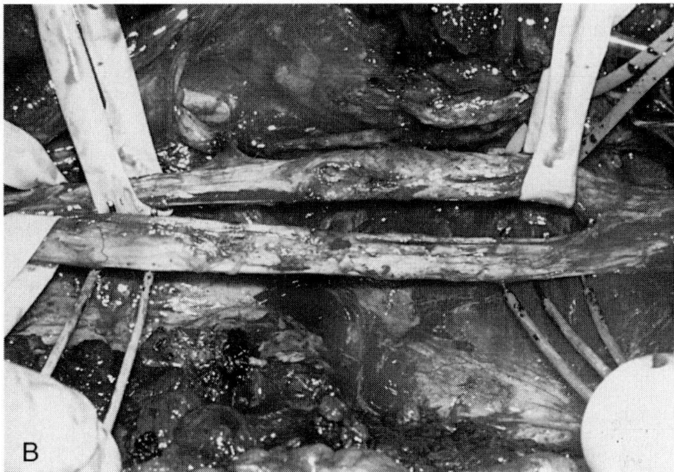

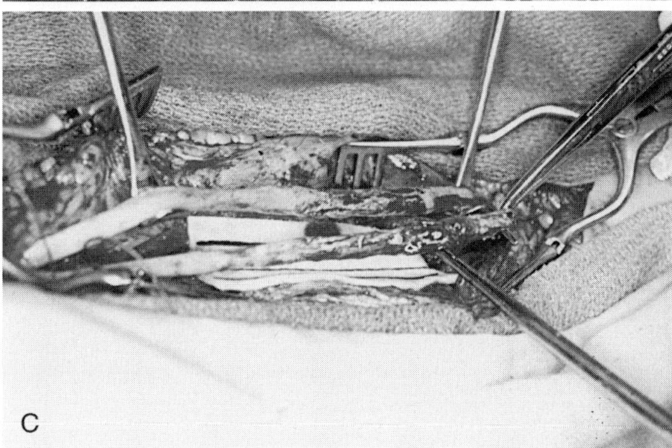

FIGURE 44–3. Sciatic nerve at the level of the thigh injured by GSW fragments *(A)*. Divisions distal to the left of the photograph have been partially split because the sciatic lesion conducted an NAP. After completion of the split, each division was tested for an NAP *(B)*. Both conducted an NAP, so only an external neurolysis was performed. Thigh-level shotgun injury to the sciatic nerve in a child. Divisions have been split apart *(C)*. Both divisions appeared to be equally injured, but one conducted an NAP and one did not, even though the extent of injury to both seemed to be the same. Resection and repair were necessary on one division and neurolysis on the other.

▼ TABLE 44–2
Operative Results—Sciatic Nerve at the Thigh Level* (1967–1987)

	Neurolysis		Suture		Graft		No Operation	
	T	*P*	*T*	*P*	*T*	*P*	*T*	*P*
GSW (n = 48)	17/17†	16/15	8/8	9/5	8/5	8/2	4/4	5/4
Fracture (n = 34)	11/10	9/9	1/1	1/0	4/4	8/2	9/7	10/2
Contusion (n = 16)	3/3	2/2	0/0	1/1	0/0	1/1	8/7	8/6
Laceration/Stab (n = 26)	1/1	2/1	5/5	6/4	11/10	9/4	2/1	2/0
Compression (n = 6)	4/4	4/3	0/0	0/0	0/0	0/0	1/0	1/0
Iatrogenic (n = 6)	2/1	1/1	0/0	0/0	2/2	3/1	3/2	3/2
TOTALS	38/36	34/31	14/14	17/10	25/21	29/10	27/21	29/14

*Table does not include three sympathectomies, 14 resected tumors, and one sciatic nerve repair for a recluse spider bite.
†Divisions operated and those reaching a grade 3 or better result.
GSW, Gunshot wound; T, tibial division; P, peroneal division; n, number of cases evaluated.
Adapted from Kline D, Hudson A: Nerve Injuries: Operative Results of Major Nerve Injuries, Entrapments, and Tumors, Philadelphia, W.B. Saunders Company, 1995.

level were usually operated on 3 to 5 months after wounding because of failure to improve function of one or both divisions (Marcus et al, 1980; Omer, 1982, 1991; White, 1960). Transected nerves were operated on earlier, if possible. For example, the latter category included four patients with five transected sciatic nerves as well as transected hamstring muscles resulting from falling, being thrown, or pushed through glass windows or doors. Each of these injuries were repaired during the early hours or days after they occurred. These were relatively sharp injuries, and the transected nerve stumps could usually be re-opposed after relatively minimal

trimming. Retraction was also minimal since surgery was early. In only one of these nerves was graft repair necessary. This is in contrast to other injuries to the sciatic nerve in which distraction with suture is more common (Whitcomb, 1946) and the need for grafts is more likely (Kline, 1972; Millesi, 1980).

RESULTS OF TIBIAL NERVE SURGERY

Table 44–3 indicates the numbers of patients with tibial nerve injuries evaluated in the various categories, whereas

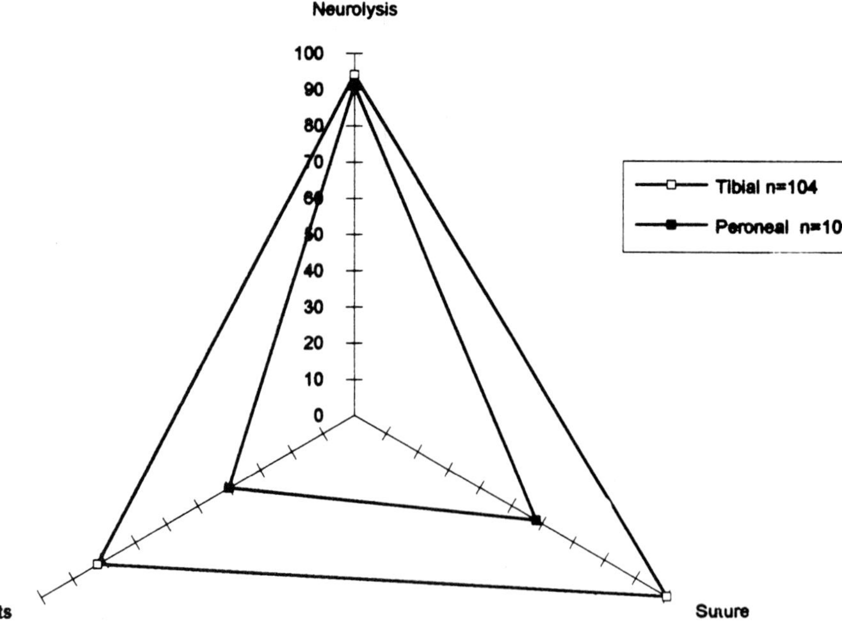

FIGURE 44–4. Operative results of sciatic repair at the thigh level, 1967–1987.

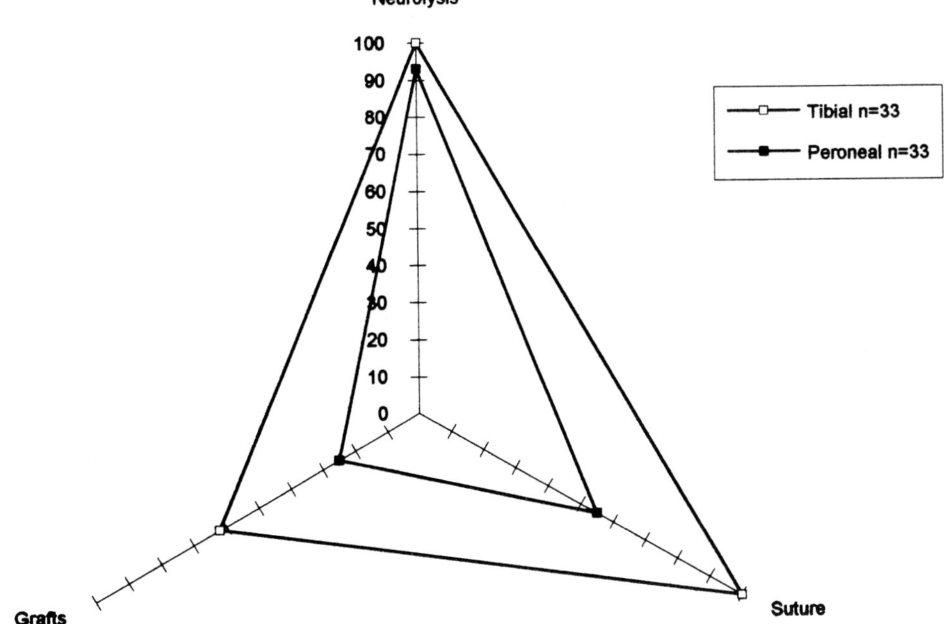

FIGURE 44–5. Results of treatment of GSW of the sciatic nerve at the thigh level, 1967–1987.

Table 44–4 provides the overall results of treatment with neurolysis, suture, grafts, or no operation. Table 44–5 provides a separate analysis of ankle-level tibial nerve injuries.

Provided the decision for or against surgery was correct, tibial was one of the most favorable nerves in the whole body to manage. As expected, when injury was partial or the nerve shown to be regenerating according to NAP recordings, outcomes in terms of plantar flexion and usually inversion as well as plantar sensation were excellent. Outcome was also favorable when repair was necessary, and indeed even when grafts were used, results were excellent. Pain associated with lesions involving this nerve was usually helped by surgery. There were exceptions, however. In one such case, lengthy tibial involvement led to resection without repair because of severe pain persisting for many years. In several other cases, internal as well as external neurolysis was believed to be necessary in an attempt to help alleviate neuritic pain.

Categories of injury at the level of the knee included contusion and stretch with or without associated fracture, GSW, laceration or stab wound, and iatrogenic injury related to popliteal vascular procedures, open knee operations, or in several cases, arthroscopy. Although it is seen less frequently in recent years, in the past, injury could be a secondary complication of placement of implanted stimulating electrodes for pain (Nielson et al, 1976).

Lacerations, contusion, and occasional GSW and fracture-associated injuries involved 29 tibial nerves at the level of the ankle. When selected for operation because of severe sensory deficit on the sole of the foot or severe pain, or both, dissection was not easy because of scarred plantar branches intertwined with injured or scarred vessels. When repair was indicated because of poor physical continuity or lack of a transmitted NAP, grafts rather than sutures were necessary because lesions and thus gaps after resection were relatively long.

There were also 20 other patients believed to have tarsal tunnel syndrome who had appropriate enough clinical and conductive findings for operation. Symptoms included paresthesias and sometimes burning discomfort on the sole as well as toes of the foot (Borges et al, 1981; Edwards et al,

▼ **TABLE 44–3**
Injuries to Tibial (Posterior Tibial) Nerve (1967–1991)

Type of Injury	Number Evaluated	Number Operated
Stretch/Fracture	12	8
Stretch/No Fracture	10	5
Laceration	15	13
GSWs	6	4
Iatrogenic	5	4
Other	3	8
	51	36

GSW, Gunshot wounds.

▼ **TABLE 44–4**
Results of Tibial Nerve Surgery (1967–1991)

Type of Surgery	Cases Operated/ Cases Improved*	Percent
Neurolysis	15/14	92
Suture	5/5	100
Grafts	16/13	81
No Operation	15/12	80

*Grade 3 or better result. Does not include those at an ankle level.

▼ TABLE 44–5
Surgery on Ankle-Level Tibial Injuries (1967–1991)

	(Positive) NAP, External Neurolysis	(Positive) NAP, Internal Neurolysis	Grafts	Resection
Contusion with fracture (14)	7/5*	2/1†	5/3‡	1/1
Contusion without fracture (7)	4/2*	2/1†	1/1	1/0
Blunt transection (3)	—	—	3/2	—
GSW (2)	1/1	—	1/1	—
Iatrogenic (1)	—	—	1/0	—
TOTALS (27)	12/8	4/2	11/7	2/1

*Improvement in these cases where neurolysis was done included at least partial relief of pain.
†One patient with internal neurolysis which failed had excision with partial relief of pain.
‡Cases done and cases with significant sensory recovery as well as relief of pain if significant preoperatively.

1969). Sensory conduction studies were abnormal (DeSeze, 1970; Johnson and Ortiz, 1966). A history of an associated systemic neuropathy due to diabetes or alcohol misuse was sought (Lam, 1967). Such a history was not a contraindication to neurolysis of the nerve if Tinel's sign was present along medial ankle and especially in the instep region and entrapment was felt to be superimposed. Nerves entrapped in the tarsal canal had complete external neurolysis with a 360-degree exposure of plantar and calcaneal branches rather than the simpler but less effective unroofing or exposure without neurolysis. Instep musculature over plantar branches was also divided without placing an incision on the plantar surface of the foot.

RESULTS OF PERONEAL NERVE SURGERY

This has been a difficult category in which to produce good results, although this as well as other series provide some hope (Demuynck and Zuker, 1987; Millesi, 1980; McMahon and Craig, 1994; Sedel and Nizard, 1993; Trumble and Vanderhooft, 1994; Wood, 1991a, 1991b). Table 44–6 provides results both by category of injury and operation performed or not performed for a relatively large group of 153 peroneal nerve injuries. One hundred and four injuries were selected for operation. The largest category was stretch and contusion injuries, which are usually associated with knee injury, either with or without concomitant fracture of

femur, tibia, or fibula (Krackow et al, 1993; Nobel, 1966) (Fig. 44–6). Nineteen lacerations, eight GSWs, and nine entrapments were also operated on. When NAPs across the lesion were present, only a neurolysis was performed and 31 of 34 patients recovered significant function. End-to-end sutures could be performed only in a few nerves with focal lesions, but seven of these 10 nerves reached a Grade 3 or better result. Graft repairs did not fare as well because many were performed for stretch and contusive injuries, and in most of those cases, the grafts had to be relatively lengthy. One third of these patients had distractions of their nerves, whereas two thirds had lesions in continuity. Data from a larger group of operated peroneal stretch injuries not included in Table 44–7 have been analyzed (Kim and Kline, 1996; Kline and Hudson, 1995). Patients with grafts 2 inches or less in length fared much better (close to 50% recovery to Grade 3) than those more than 3 inches in length (only 18% recovery to grade 3 level). By contrast, when either significant sparing or regeneration was shown by NAP studies, recovery to Grade 3 was good in over 90% of patients. Decompression without repair has been advocated by others when injury is associated with knee surgery (Krackow et al, 1993). The authors' own experience indicates the need for operative electrophysiologic testing before relying on neurolysis to provide recovery under these circumstances. As with peroneal division injury, reconstructive procedures reported by others were used regularly by our orthopedic collaborators (Cozen, 1969; Ninkovic et al, 1994; Wood, 1991a,

▼ TABLE 44–6
Injuries and Surgical Results—Peroneal Nerve at the Knee Level* (1967–1987)

	Neurolysis	Suture	Graft	No Surgery	Other	Total
Stretch/Contusion	11/10†	0/0	35/6	25/6	0	71
Stretch/Fracture	3/3	2/2	5/2	5/5	0	15
Laceration/Stab	5/5	5/3	9/4	4/4	0	23
GSW	2/2	3/2	3/1	6/6	1‡	15
Entrapment	7/6	0/0	2/1	1/0	0	10
Iatrogenic	1/1	0/0	1/0	0/0	0	2
Injection	0/0	0/0	0/0	2/2	0	2
Compression	5/4	0/0	4/2	6/5	0	15
TOTALS	34/31	10/7	59/16	49/28	1	153

*Eleven of 12 tumors were operated on and are not included in this table; 6 were ganglion cysts; 2 required repair by grafts.
†Nerves operated on and nerves recovering grade 3 or better function.
‡Sympathectomy.
From Kline D, Hudson A: Nerve Injuries: Operative Results of Major Nerve Injuries, Entrapments, and Tumors. Philadelphia, W.B. Saunders Company, 1995.

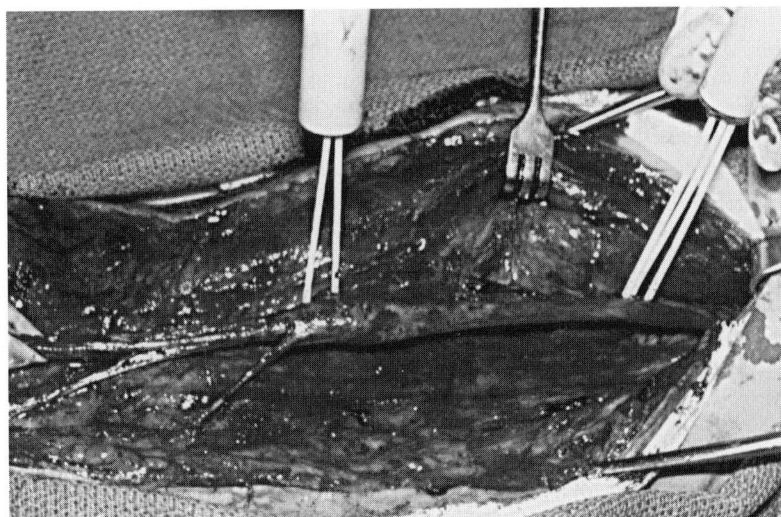

FIGURE 44–6. Severely stretched peroneal nerve injured behind the knee and over the head of the fibula. Even the more normal-appearing portion of the nerve between stimulating electrodes *(right)* and recording electrodes *(left)* did not conduct an NAP. A lengthy resection and lengthy grafts were necessary.

1991b). The authors have not had an operative experience with Hansen's disease, but others have found external neurolysis alone to be a useful approach (Chaise and Roger, 1985; Sedel, 1985).

In other peroneal categories, not all soft tissue lacerations associated with severe peroneal deficits divided a nerve. Such lesions had to be evaluated operatively with NAP recordings just like other in-continuity injuries. In addition, not all entrapments recovered with only neurolysis and partial fibulectomy. A large number of our entrapments (53%) were seen in runners or joggers, as reported by Leach and colleagues (1989). Most of these patients had external neurolysis and improved as reported by others (Vastamaki, 1986). Owing to the need for repetitive surgery, as well as severe associated neuropathy, a few entrapped nerves did, however, need repair.

FEMORAL NERVE—RESULTS OF INTRAPELVIC AND EXTRAPELVIC SURGERY

The femoral nerve innervates iliopsoas, the major hip flexor, as well as quadriceps, and extends the leg or the hip.

▼ **TABLE 44–7**
Iatrogenic Femoral Lesions (1967–1987)

	Number Evaluated	Number Undergoing Surgery
Hernia repair	9	7
Hip replacement	10	8
Vascular repair	9	5
Angiography	6	3
Gynecologic surgery	4	3
Abdominal laparoscopy	2	0
Abdominal surgery	2	0
Lumbar sympathectomy	3	1
Appendectomy	1	1
Injection	1	0
	47	28

In addition to lack of knee extension, the knee jerk reflex is lost and there is sensory loss over anterior thigh with severe femoral injury (Fig. 44–7). The femoral nerve was usually approached initially by a vertical incision in the femoral triangle parallel but lateral to femoral artery. Iliacus fascia was opened to expose the nerve, which branches profusely 1 to 1½ inches below the inguinal ligament. If the injury or lesion extended proximally or originated or was confined to the pelvic level, the nerve was traced into the pelvis by

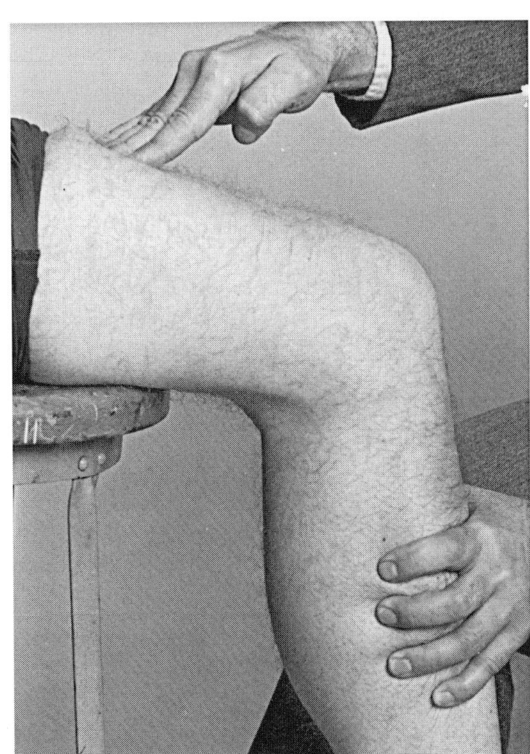

FIGURE 44–7. Testing a subject for quadriceps function. The patient is asked to straighten out or extend the leg or thigh as the examiner palpates the muscle. At times, the tensor fascia lata can straighten out the leg even when the quadriceps is totally paralyzed. (From Kline D, Hudson A: Nerve Injuries: Operative Results for Major Nerve Injuries, Entrapments, and Tumors. Philadelphia, W. B. Saunders Company, 1995.)

dividing abdominal musculature close to but superior to the ilium, finding the retroperitoneal fat and then sweeping posterior peritoneum and more anterior abdominal contents medially with a large abdominal retractor. This method provided exposure of intrapelvic femoral nerve, as well as the lateral femoral cutaneous and the more medial genitofemoral nerve. Originating near the region of the superior course of femoral were the ilioinguinal and iliohypogastric nerves. The relationships of pelvic level femoral nerve and its branches to iliacus and psoas muscles could then be readily worked out.

The largest category of femoral injury was iatrogenic and included those associated with hernia or vascular repairs, various pelvic and abdominal operations, and even lumbar sympathectomy. This observation was the same in other smaller civilian series (Gentili and Hudson, 1985; Hudson et al, 1979; Osgaard and Husby, 1977). In times of war, GSWs or shell fragment injuries are, of course, much more frequent (Rakolta and Omer, 1969; Rizzoli, 1965; Seddon, 1972). Smaller numbers of cases were due to GSWs and laceration or stab wounds and contusive injury unassociated with an operation (Fig. 44–8). Occasional compression due to an intrapelvic or iliopsoas hematoma was also seen, as has been reported elsewhere (Calvery and Mulder, 1960; Young and Norris, 1976).

When the femoral nerve was involved by direct injury, scar, or suture associated with hernia repair, the lesion was usually at the level of the inguinal ligament. Assessment as well as repair required exposure at a pelvic as well as femoral triangle level. Neurolysis helped pain in several patients in whom loss was incomplete. In other patients in whom preoperative loss was more complete and an NAP was not transmitted across the lesion, resection and usually graft repair were necessary.

Femoral palsy associated with hip replacement also occurred and has been reported before (Solheim and Hagen, 1980). This was sometimes due to investment with methyl methacrylate but was more often due to stretch and contusion associated with retraction. Exploration was necessary in a number of cases. Neurolysis based on a positive NAP led to excellent results, and also, more than 50% of the suture repairs had significant recovery. Experience was similar with

▼ **TABLE 44–8**
Operative Results: Femoral Lesions

Neurolysis*	25/23	(92%)
Grafts*	36/27†	(75%)

*Cases operated on/cases reaching a grade 3 or better result.
†Includes grafts 2.5 to 14 cm in length.

angiographic and vascular bypass complications involving femoral nerve as well as in most of the other iatrogenic categories.

Lacerations or stab wounds involving the femoral nerve occurred at both the femoral triangle and intrapelvic levels. Recovery was excellent after either suture or graft repair. Operation was often necessary with GSWs involving femoral nerve. Repair was necessary in two thirds of those who underwent surgery. Results were good. In the category of contusion or stretch associated with hip fracture, three out of three who underwent neurolysis and one of two of the repairs recovered.

Overall, surgical results with operation on the femoral nerve were favorable and this included pelvic as well as thigh level lesions (Table 44–8).

Sixteen patients with injury to the sural nerve required operation. Mechanisms of injury included laceration by glass, knife wounds, metal wire made ballistic by a lawn mower, and GSWs. Iatrogenic causes included sural nerve biopsy, venous stripping and ligation operations, and orthopedic procedures to repair fracture of the tibia.

Patients presented because of painful neuromas. Although not always palpable, neuromas were suspected because percussion or tapping elicited Tinel's sign in a sural distribution and usually reproduced the patient's symptoms. Repair of such injuries by suture or graft led with time to another painful neuroma. As a result, after this initial experience, we elected wide resection of nerve both well proximal and distal to the injury site. Some attempt was made to discourage new neuroma symptoms by leaving the sharply divided proximal stump of the nerve deep to muscle and by sealing shut fasciculi with the use of fine-tipped bipolar forceps and a bipolar current. A similar approach was used with five saphe-

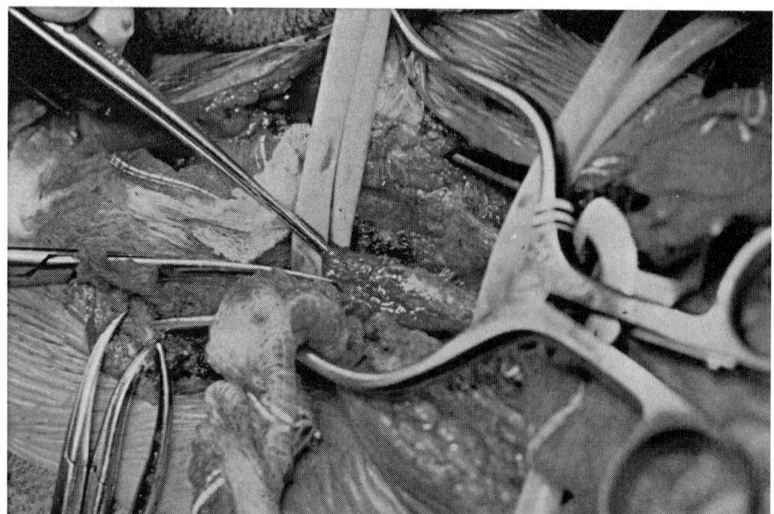

FIGURE 44–8. Femoral nerve injury in continuity due to severe contusion in the region of the pelvic brim. This lesion required resection and repair by sural grafts, which extended from the distal pelvis to the upper thigh level.

nous neuromas. These were of iatrogenic origin having been associated with stripping and ligation operation for venous varicosities (two cases), as reported previously by Cox (1974), or operations on the knee (three cases). Success with either sural or saphenous neuromas was not uniform but, in most cases, was close to curative, so management has remained the same.

LATERAL FEMORAL CUTANEOUS NEUROPATHY

The lateral femoral cutaneous nerve originates from high lumbar roots and takes a retroperitoneal route to reach the brim of the pelvis. It exits the pelvis beneath the lateral portion of the inguinal ligament and just medial to the anterior inferior spine of the ileum. Deep to fascia in its proximal course through thigh, this sensory nerve rapidly branches to supply skin over lateral thigh (Stevens, 1957).

Entrapment or injury to the lateral femoral cutaneous nerve causes meralgia paresthetica. This condition produces a zone of hyperesthesia that is sometimes combined with hypesthesia and is located over lateral thigh. Pain can be spontaneous and often is described as burning paresthesias. The most frequent surgical procedures for this disorder have included release of the presumed entrapment at the level of the iliac crest or resection of the nerve (Sunderland, 1984; Williams and Trail, 1991). The authors prefer to resect the nerve and furthermore try to resect enough of the intrapelvic and extrapelvic portion so that a large gap exists between the ends. The nerve is most readily found medial to the anterior inferior spine of the ilium and then can be traced both intrapelvically and extrapelvically following resection. The fasciculi of the proximal stump is then bipolared, similar to that in the treatment of sural and saphenous neuromas.

Results with resection have been good. Table 44–9 categorizes outcomes in terms of the patient's evaluation of relief of the most severe component of pain as good, fair, or poor. Nonetheless, it is difficult in some patients to alleviate all sensory symptoms, even when lateral thigh is made hypesthetic.

PELVIC PLEXUS INJURIES

The anatomy of both the lumbar and sacral portion of the pelvic plexus is well recorded elsewhere (Kline and Hudson, 1995; Kopell, 1980; Sunderland, 1984) and thus is not repeated here. Excellent papers concerning pelvic plexus injury with pelvic fracture (Byrnes et al, 1977; Harris, 1974; Huttinen, 1972; Patterson, 1972) and other agents (Gilden, 1977)

have been published. In a 20-year period (1967 to 1987), the authors evaluated 49 injuries and 18 tumors involving the pelvic plexus and operated on 32 of these patients; all 18 tumors and 14 of the pelvic plexus injuries. Included in the operative injury category were three involving the plexus secondary to fractures of the pelvis or sacrum, or both. At the same time, 15 other fracture-associated lesions were managed without operation. Four of 10 GSWs, three of four stab wounds, only one of six stretch injuries, and three of eight iatrogenic injuries were operated on. Tumors treated surgically included 11 neurofibromas, five schwannomas, one ganglioneuroma, and one neurogenic sarcoma.

Pan pelvic plexus involvement combines femoral or obturator nerve involvement with that of the sciatic nerve. There may also be gluteal, ilioinguinal, iliohypogastric, genitofemoral or lateral femoral cutaneous nerve losses. Surgery may be indicated for persisting and severe femoral outflow deficit or tibial distribution sciatic loss, or both. Repair at the level of the plexus level seldom changes peroneal distribution loss. Fortunately, most pelvic plexus injuries associated with stretch and fracture are either incomplete or improved with time. If surgery is to be performed because of failure to improve, then, myelography is necessary.

The lumbar plexus was approached in this series by a muscle-splitting flank incision and then a retroperitoneal dissection similar to that used for a lumbar sympathectomy. A transabdominal approach was used to approach the sacral plexus. This latter type of approach was used in conjunction with general or gynecologic surgery.

References

Adams JC: Vulnerability of the sciatic nerve in closed ischiofemoral arthrodesis by nail and graft. J Bone Joint Surg (Br) 46:748–753, 1964.

Aldea PA, Shaw WA: Lower extremity nerve injuries. Clin Plast Surg 14:691–699, 1986.

Banerjee T, Hall CD: Sciatic entrapment neuropathy. J Neurosurg 45:216–217, 1976.

Berry H Richardson PN: Common peroneal nerve palsy: A clinical and electrophysiological review. J Neurol Neurosurg Psychiatry 39:1162–1171, 1976.

Borges LF, Hallett N, Selkoe DJ, Welch K: The anterior tarsal tunnel syndrome. J Neurosurg 54:89–92, 1981.

Bourrel P: Transfer of the tibialis posterior to tibialis anterior, and of flexor hallucis longus to the extensor digitorum longus in peroneal palsy. Ann Chir 21:1451–1456, 1967.

Byrnes O, Russo GL, Ducker TB, Cowley RA: Sacrum fractures and neurological damage. J Neurosurg 47:459–462, 1977.

Calvery JR, Mulder DW: Femoral neuropathy. Neurology 10:963–967, 1960.

Chaise F, Roger B: Neurolysis of the common peroneal nerve in leprosy. A report on 22 patients. J Bone Joint Surg (Br) 67:426–429, 1985.

Clark K, Williams P, Willis W, McGavran WL: Injection injuries of sciatic nerve. Clin Neurosurg 17:111–125, 1970.

Clawson DK, Seddon HJ: The results of repair of the sciatic nerve. J Bone Joint Surg (Br) 42B:205–213, 1960a.

Clawson DK, Seddon HJ: The late consequences of sciatic nerve injury. J Bone Joint Surg 42B:213–225, 1960b.

Cox SJ: Saphenous nerve injury caused by stripping of long saphenous vein. BMJ 1:415–417, 1974.

Cozen L: Management of foot drop in adults after peroneal nerve loss. Clin Orthop 67:151–158, 1969.

Demuynck N, Zuker RN: The peroneal nerve: Is repair worthwhile? J Reconstr Microsurg 3:193–197, 1987.

DeSeze S: Electromyography of the tarsal tunnel syndrome. Rev Rheum Mal Osteoartic 37:189–195, 1970.

Edwards WG, Lincoln CR, Bassett FH, Goldner JL: The tarsal tunnel syndrome. JAMA 207:716–720, 1969.

▼ **TABLE 44–9**
Results of Lateral Femoral Cutaneous Resection (1967–1991)

	Good	Fair	Poor
Entrapment	10	4	1
Injury during bone graft removal	2	1	0
Laceration	3	0	0
Injection	1	0	0
	16	5	1

Fried G, Salerno T, Brown HC, et al: Management of the extremity with combined neurovascular and musculoskeletal trauma. J Trauma *18*:481–486, 1978.

Gentili F, Hudson AR: Peripheral nerve injuries: Types, causes, grading. *In* Wilkins RH, Rengachary SS (eds): Neurosurgery, Vol 2. New York, McGraw-Hill Book Company, 1985, pp 1802–1812.

Gilden DH, Eisner J: Lumbar plexopathy caused by disseminated intravascular coagulation. JAMA *237*:2846–2847, 1977.

Harris WR: Avulsion of lumbar roots complicating fracture of the pelvis. J Bone Joint Surg *55A*:1436, 1974.

Highet WB, Holmes W: Traction injuries to the lateral popliteal and traction injuries to peripheral nerves after suture. Br J Surg *30*:212, 1943.

Hudson AR, Hunter GA, Waddell JP: Iatrogenic femoral nerve injuries. Can J Surg *22*:62–66, 1979.

Hudson AR, Kline DG, Gentili F: Peripheral nerve injection injury. *In* Omer GE Jr, Spinner M (eds): Management of Peripheral Nerve Problems. Philadelphia, W. B. Saunders Company, 1980, pp 639–653.

Huttinen V: Lumbosacral nerve injury in fracture of the pelvis. A postmortem radiographic and pathoanatomical study. Acta Chir Scand *429*(Suppl):7–41, 1972.

Johnson EW: Nerve injuries in fractures to the lower extremity. Minn Med *52*:627–633, 1969.

Johnson EW, Ortiz PR: Electrodiagnosis of tarsal tunnel syndrome. Arch Phys Med *47*:776–780, 1966.

Kim D, Kline D: Management and results of peroneal nerve lesions. Neurosurgery *39*:313–320, 1996.

Kline DG: Operative management of major nerve lesions of the lower extremity. Surg Clin North Am *52*:1247–1265, 1972.

Kline DG: Operative experience with a major lower extremity nerve lesion. *In* Omer GE Jr, Spinner N (eds): Management of Peripheral Nerve Problems. Philadelphia, W. B. Saunders Company, 1980, pp 607–625.

Kline D, Hudson A: Nerve Injuries: Operative Results of Major Injuries, Entrapments, and Tumors. Philadelphia, W. B. Saunders Company, 1995.

Kopell HP: Lower extremity lesions. *In* Omer GE Jr, Spinner N (eds): Management of Peripheral Nerve Problems. Philadelphia, W. B. Saunders Company, 1980, pp 626–638.

Krackow KA, Maar DC, Mont NA, Carroll C: Surgical decompression for peroneal nerve palsy after total knee arthroplasty. Clin Orthop *292*:223–228, 1993.

Lam SJ: Tarsal tunnel syndrome. J Bone Joint Surg *49B*:87–92, 1967.

Leach RE, Purnell NB, Saito A: Peroneal nerve entrapment in runners. Am J Sports Med *17*:287–291, 1989.

Marcus NA, Blair WF, Shuck JN, et al: Low-velocity gunshot wounds to extremities. J Trauma *20*:1061–1064, 1980.

McLean N: Total hip replacement and sciatic nerve trauma. Orthopedics *9*:1121–1127, 1986.

McMahon NS, Craig SN: Interfascicular reconstruction of the peroneal nerve after knee ligament injury. Ann Plas Surg *32*:642–644, 1994.

Millesi H: Nerve grafts: Indications, techniques and prognosis. *In* Omer GE Jr, Spinner N (eds): Management of Peripheral Nerve Problems. Philadelphia, W. B. Saunders Company, 1980, pp 410–430.

Millesi H: Lower extremity nerve lesions. *In* Terzis J (ed): Microreconstruction of Nerve Injuries. Philadelphia, W. B. Saunders Company, 1987, pp 239–251.

Nielson KD, Watts C, Clark WK: Peripheral nerve injury from implantation of chronic stimulating electrodes for pain control. Surg Neurol *5*:51–53, 1976.

Ninkovic N, Sucur D, Starovic B, Markovic S: A new approach to persistent traumatic peroneal nerve palsy. Br J Plast Surg *47*:185–189, 1994.

Nobel W: Peroneal palsy due to hematoma in the common peroneal nerve sheath after distal torsional fractures and inversion ankle sprains. J Bone Joint Surg *48A*:1484–1495, 1966.

Omer GE Jr: Results of untreated peripheral nerve injuries. Clin Orthop *163*:15–19, 1982.

Omer GE: Nerve injuries associated with gunshot wounds of the extremities. *In* Gelberman R (ed): Operative Repair and Reconstruction. Philadelphia, J. B. Lippincott Company, 1991, pp 655–670.

Osgaard O, Husby J: Femoral nerve repair with nerve autografts. Report of two cases. J Neurosurg *47*:751–754, 1977.

Paradies LH, Gregory CF: The early treatment of close-range shotgun wounds to the extremities. J Bone Joint Surg *48A*:425–428, 1966.

Patterson FP: Neurological complications of fractures and dislocations of the pelvis. J Trauma *12*:1013–1023, 1972.

Rakolta GG, Omer GE: Combat-sustained femoral nerve injuries. Surg Gynecol Obstet *128*:813–817, 1969.

Rizzoli HV: Treatment of peripheral nerve injuries. *In* Coates JB, Meirowsky AN (eds): Neurological Surgery of Trauma. Washington DC, Office of the Surgeon General, Department of the Army, 1965, pp 565–579.

Seddon HJ (ed): Surgical Disorders of the Peripheral Nerves. Baltimore, Williams & Wilkins, 1972.

Sedel L: The surgical management of nerve lesions in the lower limbs: Clinical evaluation, surgical technique and results. Int Orthop *9*:159–170, 1985.

Sedel L, Nizard RS: Nerve grafting for traction injuries of the common peroneal nerve. A report of 17 cases. J Bone Joint Surg (Br) *75*:772–774, 1993.

Solheim LF, Hagen R: Femoral and sciatic neuropathies after total hip arthroplasty. Acta Orthop Scand *51*:531–534, 1980.

Stevens H: Meralgia paresthetica. Arch Neurol Psychiatry *77*:557–574, 1957.

Sunderland S: Nerves and Nerve Lesions, 2nd ed. Edinburgh, Churchill Livingstone, 1984.

Trumble T, Vanderhooft E: Nerve grafting for lower-extremity injuries. J Pediatr Orthop *14*:161–165, 1994.

Vastamaki N: Decompression for peroneal nerve entrapment. Acta Orthop Scand *57*:551–554, 1986.

Villarejo FJ, Pascual AN: Injection injury of the sciatic nerve (370 cases). Childs Nerv Syst *9*:229–232, 1993.

Weber ER, Daube JR, Coventry NB: Peripheral neuropathies associated with total hip arthroplasty. J Bone Joint Surg *58A*:66–69, 1976.

Whitcomb BB: Separation at the suture site as a cause of failure in regeneration of peripheral nerves. J Neurosurg *3*:399–406, 1946.

White JC: Timing of nerve suture after gunshot wound. Surgery *48*:946–951, 1960.

Williams P, Trail KP: Management of meralgia paresthetica. J Neurosurg *74*:76–80, 1991.

Wood NB: Peripheral nerve injuries to the lower extremity. *In* Gelberman R (ed): Operative Nerve Repair and Reconstruction. Philadelphia, J. B. Lippincott Company, 1991a.

Wood N B: Peroneal nerve repair. Surgical results. Clin Orthop *267*:206–210, 1991b.

Young NR, Norris JW: Femoral neuropathy during anticoagulant therapy. Neurology *26*:1173–1175, 1976.

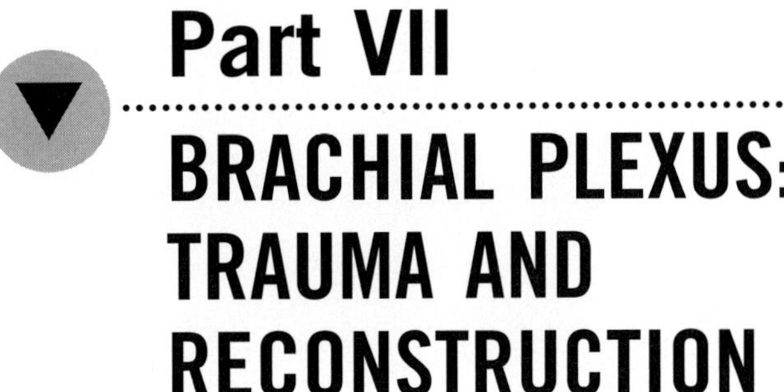

BRACHIAL PLEXUS: TRAUMA AND RECONSTRUCTION

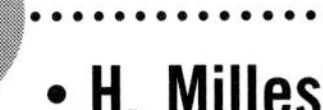

Chapter 45

• H. Millesi

Trauma Involving the Brachial Plexus

BASIC CONSIDERATIONS

A severe loss of function suffered in brachial plexus injuries leads to serious consequences for the family and professional life of the patient and his future. A short time ago, the chances of improvement by surgery of the root lesions were regarded as minimal (Seddon, 1972). Today significant improvement can be achieved, but expectations must not be too high. Return of function is far from being satisfactory from an objective point of view; however, for the patient it means a significant improvement and helps him to resume a somewhat normal social life. The great expenditure that is necessary for such an improvement is therefore highly justified.

Brachial plexus injuries can be caused by direct trauma leading to an open injury, or by foreign bodies being thrust into the neck area during an accident. Gunshot wounds are, at least in our country, infrequent causes during peace time. Most often the lesion is caused by traction in a longitudinal direction, or by compression, or by a combination of both. The distance between the intervertebral foramina and the upper arm is increased and the brachial plexus is elongated if the head is moved and turned to the contralateral side while the shoulder joint and the thorax are depressed. The distance is further increased if the arm is moved away from the body by luxation of the shoulder joint or by a fractured humerus.

The scalenus muscles and the connective tissue of the infraclavicular area act to prevent the elongation. Under sufficient force, the scalenus muscles themselves are partially elongated and the protection is lost. As a result of this damage, these muscles may undergo fibrotic changes. Sometimes there are fractures of the transverse processus of the corresponding cervical vertebra. The elongation leads to ruptures within the part of the brachial plexus until continuity is lost, either partially or completely.

Compression of the brachial plexus occurs between the first rib and the clavicle. This compression is caused by an external force that presses the clavicle onto the first rib. The compression occurs on the distal part of the trunks and the proximal parts of the cords. It can cause various degrees of damage.

If the brachial plexus is compressed *and* the arm is moved in a caudal or a lateral direction, the greatest damage will occur within the cords (damage of level IV).

If the compression is between the clavicle and the first rib, and the head is moved to the contralateral side, the trunks and the roots will be under stress and will suffer a traction lesion (lesion of level III and II).

If trauma causes movement of the head mainly to the lateral side and there is compression of the brachial plexus, a root avulsion is likely to occur (lesion of level I).

Roots are exposed to traction in various degrees according to the position of the arm at the moment of the accident. If the arm is in a pendulous position, the greatest traction will occur in roots C5 and C6. If the arm is in lateral abduction, all roots are under great stress, with the greatest stress being on C7. If the arm is in an elevated position, the greatest traction is exerted on C8 and T1. If the traction force is limited, then only these specific roots are avulsed, while the others remain intact or remain minimally damaged. If, of course, the traction force is severe and excessive, all roots can be damaged, regardless of the position of the arm.

THE BRACHIAL PLEXUS PATIENT

A patient with a brachial plexus injury usually receives the first treatment at an emergency facility, where the saving of his life is the first concern. The patient has suffered a major accident with cerebral concussion, shock, and other injuries. The brachial plexus lesion is noted, but not very much is to be done at this moment. After the patient's other problems have been attended to and he is no longer in immediate danger, he is presented for consultation in relation to the brachial plexus lesion. This relates to *closed* brachial plexus lesions.

It is a completely different situation if there is an *open wound*, which has to be treated immediately. If the brachial plexus lesion was caused by stabbing and the individual elements have been transected in a clean way, then an end-to-end repair as a primary repair is indicated.

A concomitant lesion of the subclavian artery or vein is an emergency indication for surgery, and the vascular damage has to be repaired. The question arises, whether in the same stage the brachial plexus repair should be performed to deal with the whole injury immediately. If not only a vascular surgeon, but also a surgeon experienced in brachial plexus surgery is available, and if the patient's state is well enough that he can sustain an 8-hour operation, then an attempt to repair the brachial plexus may be undertaken. The author's personal view is, however, that it is much better to concentrate at this stage on the vascular repair and leave the brachial plexus for an early secondary repair. In order to avoid too much scarring, it is also much better not to undertake an attempt to define the lesion of the brachial plexus at this stage, because this might increase the damage and the following scarring. Therefore, Bonney and Birch (1982) recommended an early operation of all cases with the argument that this stage creates too much scarring and surgery may be

Sunderland's scheme is based on loss or preservation of continuity of individual structures. It does not take into account the reaction of the nerve tissue in the form of fibrosis, which influences, as already mentioned, the prognosis. It seems, therefore, adequate to add an evaluation of the amount of fibrosis.

Millesi (1984, 1986) distinguishes several degrees of fibrosis, according to the location and the overall situation.

Type A fibrosis means that the superficial layers of the epineurium, the epifascicular epineurium, has become fibrotic and constricts the nerve like a stocking that is too tight. This fibrosis of type A may be combined with a lesion of degree I (IA), II (IIA), and III (IIIA) of Sunderland. This constriction may prevent the spontaneous recovery that otherwise can be expected. Epifascicular epineuriotomy or, in extended cases, an epifascicular epineuriectomy is the treatment of choice for this lesion.

Type B fibrosis is defined by involvement of not only the epifascicular epineurium but also the interfascicular epineurium. Again, compression of the fascicular tissue may interfere with spontaneous recovery, which otherwise could be expected. Type B fibrosis can be combined with a lesion of degree I (IB), II (IIB), or III (IIIB) according to the scheme of Sunderland. In these cases, not only epifascicular epineuriectomy but also partial interfascicular epineuriectomy has to be performed.

Type C fibrosis is defined by intrafascicular fibrosis and loss of the endoneurial structure. In these cases, the fascicles themselves are fibrotic and regeneration is unlikely to occur. By definition, a fibrosis of type C can occur only in a lesion of third degree of Sunderland (3C). Resection of such fascicles or fascicle groups is recommended with restoration of continuity by nerve grafting.

In a fourth-degree lesion, we may differentiate between a lesion of grade IV-S (S for scar), which means that the continuity is preserved only by scar tissue, or grade IV-N (N for neuroma), which means that in the weeks following the injury, the connective tissue that still preserves the continuity has been invaded by axon sprouts (N, neuroma).

The combination of these two evaluation systems allows a relatively precise definition of the severity of the lesion for each segment.

Extension of the Lesion

LONGITUDINAL EXTENSION

Level I

Level I is a lesion of the rootlets or a preganglionic lesion. In these lesions there is a complete loss of motor and sensory function. Motor conduction has been lost. The motor fibers undergo wallerian degeneration, but there is no wallerian degeneration in the sensory fibers because they are still in continuity with their neurons in the spinal ganglion. Therefore, sensory conduction is preserved. The paralysis extends also to the very proximal muscles including the deep muscles of the neck, supplied by the dorsal branch of the root.

The serratus anterior muscle, supplied by the long thoracic nerve and the muscles supplied by the dorsal scapular nerve are also involved. The degeneration of these muscles can be proved by electromyography. There is no Tinel-Hoffmann sign with irradiation of parasthesias to the arm and the hand, because the sensory fibers are not separated from their ganglion cells or from their neurons and they do not form a neuroma. One must avoid misinterpretation of a Tinel-Hoffmann sign owing to a lesion of one of the branches of the cervical plexus. The presence of Horner's syndrome, spinal cord symptoms, and fractures of transverse processes supports the assumption that a supraganglionic lesion is present. By CT myelography, a meningocelia can be demonstrated. These facts speak strongly for an avulsion of this root; however, there are well-documented cases with a positive myelogram and *no* avulsion.

If the myelogram is negative and does not show a meningocelia, the presence of a root avulsion cannot be completely excluded. It is not uncommon that some roots are avulsed and others are ruptured or have preserved continuity.

In the MRI scan, the loss of continuity of the rootlets may be visible.

Level I/II

Level I/II is a combined lesion of the roots and spinal nerves. In case of a supraganglionic lesion, sympathetic functions such as sweat production and vascular response should be normal. But this is true only in very well defined lesions. The symptoms can be difficult to interpret if there is a combined rupture and avulsion of different roots or if a lesion extends in a longitudinal direction to involve both the supraganglionic and infraganglionic areas.

Level II

A postganglionic (infraganglionic) lesion inolving the spinal nerve is considered level II lesion. In these lesions, there is a complete loss of continuity peripherally to the spinal ganglion, with complete loss of motor and sensory function and loss of conductivity of motor and sensory fibers, which are completely separated from the neurons and undergo wallerian degeneration. The dorsal branches of the spinal nerve are not involved and the deep muscles of the neck are fully innervated. The Tinel-Hoffmann sign is positive, with radiation to the hand and fingers.

Level III

Level III lesions are lesions of the trunk. The symptoms are similar to an infraganglionic lesion, but the very proximal muscles, such as the serratus anterior, are spared.

Level IV

The level IV lesion is localized at the cord. There is a complete loss of motor and sensory function with loss of conductivity, Tinel's sign is present, and the infraganglionic area, and the supraspinatus and infraspinatus muscles supplied by the suprascapular nerve are not involved.

Level III/IV

A level III/IV lesion is a combined lesion of cords and trunks. A fracture of the clavicle can cause a brachial plexus lesion at this level by direct pressure of a bony fragment.

LATERAL EXTENSION OF THE LESION

A complete brachial plexus lesion means that all parts of the brachial plexus are involved: In a root lesion, all five roots; in a lesion of the supraclavicular fossa, all three trunks; and in a lesion of the infraclavicular fossa, all three cords. Frequently, the roots do not all suffer the same amount of damage. As already mentioned, we may differentiate a complete brachial plexus lesion C5, C6, C7, C8, and T1; an upper brachial plexus lesion involving C5 and C6; an extended upper brachial plexus lesion involving C5, C6, and C7; a middle brachial plexus lesion focused on C7; and a lower brachial plexus lesion involving C8 and T1.

PLAN OF TREATMENT

Phase One

During the first weeks or months following the injury in patients with closed lesions, conservative treatment is performed and a diagnosis is established. If loss of continuity is proved, the surgical exploration of the brachial plexus should be performed as soon as the patient's situation permits. Cases with the possibility of spontaneous recovery should be excluded.

The first-degree lesions are easy to recognize because motor and sensory conduction is continuously present and there are early signs of recovery.

In second-degree lesion, the return of regeneration potentials in proximal muscles and the advancement of the Tinel's sign can be observed. In these cases, conservative treatment is continued until full recovery occurs, or the spontaneous regeneration stops. In this event, the indication for surgery is reconsidered. This might be true in cases of a degree of damage identified as IA, IB, IIA, or IIB. In these cases, exploration and neurolysis are indicated. If regeneration does not occur, one might consider a lesion of level III, IV, or V. In this case, exploration is indicated and surgery should be performed according to the local situation.

Phase Two

If the indication for surgery is established, the brachial plexus should be explored and the local treatment performed according to the situation.

Phase Three

After the postoperative treatment is finished and the wounds are healed, all forms of conservative treatment should be applied to encourage maximum regeneration. Passive exercises are necessary to maintain the joints in good condition until recovery occurs. This period may be extended over 1 year or more.

Phase Four

If recovery occurs and has reached a peak, an analysis of present function is performed and reconstructive techniques are applied to achieve the best use of the regenerated muscles. This phase may also extend over years.

It cannot be emphasized enough that useful recoveries can be achieved only by a combination of direct repair and reconstructive surgery. In contrast, very often the direct repair is already planned with consideration of special reconstructive procedures, as will be shown later. In recent years, the possibility of free muscle grafting has enlarged the possibilities to achieve useful return of function. In inveterate cases, when no regeneration within the local muscles can be expected owing to irreversible atrophy, special functions like elbow flexion can be provided by free muscle grafting.

SURGICAL TREATMENT

Attempts to repair the brachial plexus by surgery have been made already in the last century. In the 1940s and 1950s, Seddon, Merle d'Aubigne, Bateman, and Yeoman and others tried to improve the outcome of brachial plexus lesions by surgery. The problem was that they had no reliable technique to deal with the long defects created by brachial plexus injuries. Attempts to shorten the distance between the proximal and distal stumps by resecting large segments from the humerus bone failed. However, it is important to note that two cornerstones of our present armamentarium in brachial plexus surgery have been developed during this period of time.

Seddon (1972, 1975) reported in his book that he had tried to repair the continuity of transected segments in upper brachial plexus lesions by nerve grafting in five cases and there was regeneration in three of them. The intention was to achieve elbow flexion. Unfortunately he did not follow this promising way because Clark (1946) published the possibility of pectoralis muscle transfer in order to regain elbow flexion and, therefore, he gave up this approach.

Following the suggestion of Yeoman, Yeoman and Seddon (1961) published a new approach consisting of elongating a nerve outside of the brachial plexus (in this particular case, the intercostal nerve) by nerve grafts in order to transfer axons into a denervated nerve of the brachial plexus to neurotize this nerve. A successful case was described with a patient having had a complete brachial plexus lesion and amputation of the forearm. The intercostal nerves were elongated by nerve grafts and connected with the musculocutaneous nerve. Active elbow flexion was achieved.

This is the classic case of transfer of axons from a nerve outside the plexus to a denervated nerve within the plexus, in order to neurotize this nerve. Unfortunately, the term neurotization has become a term for all nerve transfer procedures, which is not correct. The term neurotization is used for other procedures, and the application to brachial plexus surgery in this form may lead to misinterpretations.

Neurotization is what we want to achieve if measures are undertaken to bring axons into a denervated tissue. This is actually the aim of different procedures. If a continuity of a transected peripheral nerve is restored, we want to achieve neurotization of the denervated distal stump by fibers coming from the proximal stump after the neurorrhaphy. This can be called nerve-to-nerve neurotization.

If a proximal nerve stump containing motor fibers is brought into contact with a denervated muscle, axon sprouts are growing into this muscle and neurotize it. This is the well-known procedure of nerve-to-muscle neurotization.

If a denervated muscle is brought into contact with an innervated muscle, axon sprouts from the innervated muscle are growing to the denervated muscle. This is called muscle-to-muscle neurotization.

There is even the situation when a nerve graft with one end is put into an innervated muscle and the other end is brought into a denervated muscle. Axons will grow from the innervated muscle via the nerve graft to the denervated muscle. This is called muscle-nerve-muscle neurotization.

If we connect one proximal stump of an innervated nerve with a distal stump of another nerve, we transfer the nerve fibers from the innervated nerve into the denervated nerve. The aim of this procedure is to achieve neurotization of the denervated nerve. The procedure is, however, a nerve transfer.

In spite of all these attempts, in the 10th SICOT Congress in Paris (1966) a symposium was held attended by Seddon, Merle d'Aubigne, Yeoman, Bateman, and others. The result of this symposium was that so far surgery has nothing to offer in cases of root lesion, featuring a loss of continuity, except clarifying the diagnosis. At that time, neurolysis was performed with considerable success in the form of external neurolysis. I attended this symposium and I certainly would have been discouraged if I would not have had results already with a new grafting technique.

Different Suggestions To Solve the Problem

The first approach involves exposure of the brachial plexus with application of all available means and sources to neurotize important segments of the denervated brachial plexus. This method was resumed by Millesi and followed by Narakas, applying microsurgical techniques and the new interfascicular nerve grafting technique, which provided a safe technique to manage even long defects (Millesi, 1977; Millesi et al, 1966, 1972, 1973, 1976).

Again two different ways to attack the lesion have developed.

The patient is placed in the sitting position, with the surgeon approaching from in front of the patient. This technique was mainly used by Narakas (1972) and others. It is evident that in this case, the clavicle is an obstacle, and consequently, an osteotomy of the clavicle was performed, followed by osteosynthesis using a plate and screws at the end of surgery.

Another method involves the patient lying on his back and the surgeon approaching the brachial plexus from the cranial direction. The surgeon is sitting between the upper arm and the head, and isolates and lifts the clavicle by a proper pull on this bone. He is able to enter the supraclavicular and infraclavicular fossa from the cranial direction. No osteotomy of the clavicle is necessary.

The major part of this surgery is to clarify the anatomical situation—in other words, to expose the cords, the trunks, and the roots; to identify avulsed roots; and to make a clear diagnosis of the amount of damage for each individual segment. Having done this, accordingly, in lesions of levels I to III, neurolysis is performed; in cases of level IV or V lesions, the involved segment is resected and the defect

managed by nerve grafts. In case of root avulsion, a nerve transfer is performed.

In the vast majority of cases, a root avulsion can be clarified by external dissection. There are few cases in which there is an avulsion of the rootlets; however, the spinal nerve is not extracted from the intervertebral canal. These cases may be misinterpreted as intact continuity.

For such cases, it was suggested to perform a laminectomy from behind in a primary step, in order to visualize the rootlets. I do not think this is necessary because during the operation, we can prove the continuity of fibers in the dorsal root by evoked potentials and for the ventral roots by central stimulation with great reliability (Turkof et al, 1989, 1995).

Based on this approach, in recent years, it was suggested to provide nerve grafts with open ends for later free muscle grafting to increase the functional result (Terzis, unser Symposium, dann gibt es eine Arbeit von Berger und dann gibt es noch eine Arbeit von einem Inder oder Perser, beide müßten im grünen Buch stehen).

A completely different approach was elected by Tsujama (1968), followed by a sequence of other surgeons (Kotani et al, 1971, 1972). If a root avulsion was diagnosed by myelography, an immediate nerve transfer of intercostal nerves to neurotize the musculocutaneous nerve and to achieve biceps muscle function was performed. An exploration of the brachial plexus was not done. Results of this technique have reached a high level of reliability (Hara et al, 1995). Nothing is done for other functions. Avulsion of all five roots is rather rare, and in the case of avulsion of only four or three roots, respectively in a case of prefixation with an important contribution of C4, available axons are wasted.

Following this line, Doi (1996) has introduced another strategy: If a root avulsion is indirectly proved, he suggests to proceed in two stages. In the first stage, a free microvascular gracilis muscle transfer is performed in a way to achieve elbow flexion and finger extension. The muscle is neurotized by transfer of the accessory nerve. At the same time, sensible nerve fibers are transferred from the cervical plexus to the median nerve. In the second stage, the other gracilis muscle is transferred to achieve elbow flexion and finger flexion. This muscle is innervated by the motor fibers of the intercostal nerves 2, 3, and 4. The sensory fibers of the intercostal nerves 2, 3, and 4 are connected to the ulnar nerve. The motor part of the intercostal nerves 5 and 6 are transferred to the triceps muscle.

Incisions

Longitudinal incisions give regularly bad scars and must be avoided. Over the years, a zig-zag incision was widely used. This incision starts on the neck behind the sternocleidomastoideus muscle, turns at the level of the clavicle, and follows the clavicle to the lateral extremity, turns again, and traverses the area over the greater pectoralis muscle. At the level of the anterior axillary fold, it turns again, follows the fold, turns again to reach the medial surface of the upper arm, and follows this line as long as necessary. With these long incisions, all parts of the brachial plexus can be exposed, including the nerves emerging from the brachial plexus. It is obvious that in particular cases, only a segment of this incision is opened. However, there is always the potential to elongate this incision according to this suggestion.

Frequently, this incision ends with a keloidal or an atrophic scar. Sometimes the edge between the incision in the neck and the clavicle becomes too acute, and skin necrosis may develop. Therefore, several suggestions have been made to modify this incision.

For the author, the main disadvantage of this incision is the fact that a triangular flap is created between the incision on the neck and the incision following the clavicle bone. This flap is lifted and reversed in a cranial direction. It is the base of this flap that does not allow an optimal access to the dorsal aspect of the spinal nerves and to the trunks with the patient in supine position and the surgeon approaching from a cranial direction. This consideration and the sometimes unpleasant aspect of the scar was the reason to perform a study about the tension pattern of the skin of the neck and the supraclavicular and infraclavicular fossa in different functional situations (Eberhard et al, 1993; Eberhard and Millesi, 1996). The result of this study outlined incisions optimally adapted to the tension pattern.

A transverse incision following the tension lines on the neck gives access to spinal nerves C5 and C6. A sagittal incision across the supraclavicular fossa following the minimal tension pattern gives access to the trunks, and the spinal nerves C7, C8, and T1 from the front and from behind.

A third incision starts at the coracoid process, proceeds in a curved line, again following the tension pattern to the anterior axillary fold, and then follows the same line as the above-mentioned incision to the median aspect of the medial upper arm, if necessary.

The skin between these incisions is lifted as a bipedicled flap and tracted accordingly to provide optimal access. In case of emergency, these skin flaps between incisions can be transected immediately to have a wider access. This was necessary only in one case of our series. We used this incision since 1989 in 65 cases. As far as the scars are concerned, the results are optimal. We had no problem except in the above-mentioned case with the access in contrast. Using the sagittal incisions, we have a better access to spinal nerves and trunks from behind.

Surgical Technique

In the following section, the technique is described as we use it. As already mentioned, the patient is in the supine position and the area of the scapula is lifted to get better access to the lateral thoracic wall in case of intercostal nerve transfer. The arm is completely cleansed and included in the operative field in order to be able to move the arm in different directions during surgery. We must have good access to the whole ipsilateral side of the neck, the supraclavicular and infraclavicular fossa, anterior and lateral part of the thoracic wall, the shoulder, the axillary grove, and the whole arm. The surgeon is sitting between the arm and the head, approaching the brachial plexus from a cranial direction. The assistant is sitting between the thorax and the arm. Only when the exposure is extended to the axillary groove and medial aspect of the upper arm, the surgeon changes the position and is sitting between the arm and the thorax. We

start with the incision from the coracoid process to the ventral axillary fold. The sulcus deltoideus pectoralis is defined, and we enter the sulcus and isolate the cephalic vein. Entering between the muscles, the minor pectoralis muscle is met including the fascia medially and laterally from this muscle. The fascia is incised, and the minor pectoralis muscle is isolated so that it can be drawn in a medial and lateral direction. We then enter the space lateral to the minor pectoral muscle. Here, we meet the lateral cord as the first structure. Dorsally the dorsal cord, below and medially the artery, and further down the medial cord and the axillary vein are located. This area is usually normal. In this way, we can define all the structures within normal tissue. One can then proceed in a cranial direction to the infraclavicular space.

If, however, this area is also fibrotic and scarred, we do not lose time with a difficult dissection here. In this case, the incision is extended to the upper arm, the peripheral nerves are defined in normal tissue of the upper arm, and the dissection proceeds again in a cranial direction from normal to pathological tissue.

The next step is to perform the sagittal incision to isolate the clavicle and to lift the clavicle accordingly to provide access. The clavicular origin of the major pectoralis muscle is detached. Also, the subclavius muscle is isolated.

The dissection now enters the supraclavicular fossa. The external jugular vein is lifted. Between the scalenus anterior and the scalenus medius muscle, we meet the superior trunk and beneath it the intermedius trunk.

In similar way, following the intermedius trunk, we define C7, and following the superior trunk, we define C5 and C6. At the site of the distal division of the superior trunk, the suprascapular nerve is isolated. Originating from the lateral and from the medial cord, we locate the lateral and the medial pectoralis nerve.

In order to achieve this, it is necessary to isolate the omohyoideus muscle, the transversa colli artery and vein, the clavicle, the subclavius muscle, and the fascia behind the clavicle. All of these tissues are isolated, and windows are created between them. Accordingly, they can be shifted in a cranial or caudal direction to provide the desired approach.

If there is a lot of scar tissue at the level of the superior trunk, the spinal nerve C5 and C6 including the scalenus muscle, the phrenic nerve is defined. Following the phrenic nerve, one finds the main source of its fibers from C4, the branches of C4 can be isolated. From C4, one steps down to where C5 should be expected.

If the resection is continued along the surface of the middle scalene muscle, the dorsal nerve of the scapula and more caudally the long thoracic nerve can be defined after having penetrated this muscle. By electric stimulation, the conductivity of these nerves is tested.

The inferior trunk is more difficult to explore. It is best explored from the infraclavicular fossa, following the medial cord. Further dissection here leads to the exposure of T1 and C8.

After all structures have been defined, the amount of damage is estimated.

PRESERVED CONTINUITY (LEVEL I TO III)

If continuity is preserved, an external neurolysis is performed to remove all constricting scar tissue. If a fibrosis of the epifascicular epineurium is present, a longitudinal epifascicular epineuriotomy is performed. Sometimes after this step, the compressed fascicles expand and complete decompression is achieved. In this case, the diagnosis of a fibrosis of type A is obvious and no further step is necessary. If the fibrosis extends between the fascicles into the nerve, an epifascicular epineuriectomy is performed. Very often this is sufficient. In this case, a fibrosis of type B is diagnosed. Sometimes the interfascicular fibrosis is so advanced that a partial interfascicular epineuriectomy is necessary. If decompression is achieved, no further step is necessary. If the fascicles are fibrotic without turgor, most probably a fibrosis of type C is present. In this case, the involved segment is resected. The same is done if the fascicular pattern has been lost due to a level IV lesion. Sometimes there is a partial level III, a partial level IV lesion. In this case, it is the judgment of the surgeon which part he or she thinks is overwhelming. Accordingly, the surgeon will do an interfascicular epineuriectomy or a resection with grafting. In this situation, electrical stimulation helps establish the diagnosis. All of these different changes can be present at different sites along the brachial plexus.

LEVEL IV OR V

If there is level IV damage or a complete loss of continuity (level V), the involved segment including the stumps are resected. If we have to deal with a rather short segment, the continuity is restored by nerve grafts. One has to use as many nerve grafts as necessary to cover the cross section completely.

If there is a long defect, it might be better to connect the proximal stump directly with peripheral nerves, for example, with the musculocutaneous nerve from the anterior division of the superior trunk or the radial and axillary nerve from the posterior division of the superior trunk.

In the vast majority, the avulsed roots can be identified and the diagnosis is established.

Sometimes, however, the rootlets are avulsed but the roots are still in the intervertebral canal. In this case, by dissection from outside, the spinal nerve can be followed to the intervertebral canal and one still does not know whether the root is avulsed or not. Careful dissection into the canal may expose the dorsal branch leading to the muscles of the neck, which should be conducting if the rootlets are not avulsed. In C5, C6, and C7, the origin of the long thoracic nerve may be encountered. Also, conductivity would exclude an avulsion of this root. By testing evoked potentials, the conductivity of the dorsal root can be clarified, and by central stimulation, the conductivity of the ventral rootlets can be tested. Sometimes even using these techniques, the situation cannot be completely clarified. If one sees the condition of the spinal nerve becoming better as one enters the intervertebral canal and if not only the motor fibers but also the sensory fibers are seemingly intact but demyelinated, the author tends to finish the operation as a neurolysis. Then the author waits for 2 or 3 months to determine whether Tinel's sign appears and regeneration starts. Otherwise the author would explore the plexus again and perform a nerve transfer.

In cases with *avulsion of four or five roots,* the author attempted to neurotize as many nerves as possible with the same axon donor, for example, the intercostal nerves. In time, with follow-up studies, it turned out that this does not provide results because if antagonistic nerves are neurotized by the same kind of axon donors, even under optimal conditions the functional result will be poor because of contraction of muscle groups. The limited number of fibers in the intercostal nerve makes it necessary to use several intercostal nerves to neurotize one musculocutaneous nerve.

For the author, there is only one exception for neurotizing antagonistic muscles and it is the triceps brachii. In this situation, one has to face co-contractures, which, even after good nerve regeneration, prevent a good functional result. However, the neurotization of both biceps and triceps, by intercostal nerves was performed with the intention of transfer of the triceps to the biceps tendon and create an elbow flexor from both. In this case the co-contraction of these muscles is wanted. Several advantages are offered. If the biceps does not regenerate well but the triceps does, it can be transfered to the biceps tendon and can act as an elbow flexor. If biceps function returns well, the triceps can be transferred to the finger flexors and act as finger flexor. If biceps and triceps are weak, there is still the possibility of performing a triceps transfer and having both muscles act as flexors of the elbow. The combination of the two weak muscles might achieve enough force for a useful elbow flexion.

ELECTION OF RECIPIENT NERVES IN CASE OF FOUR OR FIVE ROOT AVULSIONS

The *musculocutaneous* nerve has absolute priority, and the best axon donor should be used for this nerve. It is still debated whether one should use three intercostal nerves or the accessory nerve for the musculocutaneous nerve. If after four root avulsions, one spinal nerve has a good proximal stump (most frequently C5), this proximal nerve is used for the musculocutaneous nerve.

The next priority is *shoulder function.* First, we tend to neurotize the suprascapular nerve, sometimes both the suprascapular and the axillary nerves, and in a few cases only the axillary nerve. If the shoulder function is too weak, a transfer of the horizontal fibers of the trapezius helps stabilize the shoulder joint. The pectoralis major muscle is always neurotized. If this function returns, its insertion at the humerus is detachted and the muscle reinserted in a way that it continues to adduct but performs external rotation. This pectoralis transfer in phase 4 always follows a rotational osteotomy to achieve about 45% of external rotation.

We always have to neurotize the long thoracic nerve, and we do this by using motor branches of the cervical plexus or by end-to-end neurorrhaphy of the second intercostal nerve with the long thoracic nerve. Occasionally, also the thoracodorsal nerve is neurotized via the second or third intercostal nerve.

Whenever possible, *forearm muscles* are also neurotized, if we succeed and have one, two or three muscles innervated a primitive gripping function can be restored using arthrodesis of the wrist joint and other joints in the finger and the thumb.

If only three roots are avulsed, the situation is much better and one can use one of the root stumps to neurotize the median nerve–innervated muscles of the forearm.

In case of avulsion of *one or two roots,* we tend to restore continuity of the interrupted nerves to the greatest degree possible and do not perform a nerve transfer.

Donor Nerves for Axons

INTERCOSTAL NERVES

Transfer of the intercostal nerves can be performed in three different ways:

1. The intercostal nerve is isolated and followed as far as possible into the periphery. It is then transected. By electric stimulation, the motor part is defined. The isolated nerve is then reversed and brought directly in contact with the distal stump at the nerve to be neurotized (Hara et al, 1995).

2. The intercostal nerve along with its artery and vein can be isolated and transferred as a vascularized nerve graft.

The big advantage of this technique is that there is only one line of coaptation. The disadvantage is that the nerve has to be rather long in order to reach the distal stump, which means that the number of motor fibers is not as great as with the more proximal segments.

3. In order to avoid a long pedicled nerve segment and to maximize the number of motor axons, one can also transect the intercostal nerve in the midaxillary line, extend the proximal stump by a nerve graft, and reach the distal nerve via a nerve graft. The big disadvantage is the fact that there are two lines of coaptation to cross. The advantage is that the nerve is more proximally transected where the number of motor fibers is greater.

The author has always preferred an elongation of the intercostal nerve by a nerve graft, and we have had satisfactory results. The functional result was not better if we used the longer segment of the intercostal nerve and had only one line of coaptation.

If we use the more caudal intercostal nerves VI, VII, and VIII, we have to elongate them with a nerve graft because the distances are too long. We have neurotized musculocutaneous nerve with good results. We could improve our results by neurotizing the triceps muscle as well and transferring the triceps muscle to augment the force. As mentioned earlier, we were not much successful with transferring intercostal nerves on the median or the ulnar nerve.

ACCESSORY NERVE

The accessory nerve is transected after the first branch has left to innervate the trapezius muscle. In this way, the trapezius muscle remains innervated. Narakas (1984) has developed a technique to achieve an end-to-end coaptation between the accessory nerve and the suprascapular nerve. Frequently we have to use a nerve graft. We used the accessory nerve in the majority of cases for the shoulder function innervating the suprascapular or the axillary nerve, or both. We have also excellent results in a certain number of cases in which the accessory nerve was an axon donor for the musculocutaneous nerve and the biceps muscle.

PLEXUS CERVICALIS

It was Brunelli (1980), and Brunelli and Monini (1984) who elaborated a technique of using motor branches or sensory branches of the cervical plexus as axon donors. The proximal stump of the supraclavicular nerve was connected to the median nerve to bring sensory fibers into the median nerve. Motor branches of the cervical plexus have to be defined carefully by electrical stimulation. They have been used to neurotize the long thoracic nerve and, the dorsalis scapular nerve if it does not function, and even the medial or lateral pectoralis nerve. It is extremely important to neurotize these nerves and the greater pectoralis muscle because they are used for a transfer to achieve external rotation.

PHRENIC NERVE

It was also suggested to use the phrenic nerve. The author has done this occasionally but with great reluctance. The author does not feel comfortable in sacrificing this nerve and accepting the paralysis of the ipsilateral diaphragm. The nerve was employed as a donor if an accessory phrenic nerve was available.

HYPOGLOSSAL NERVE

Also the hypoglossal nerve has been transferred with good success.

C7 TRANSFER

Gu and colleagues (1992) and Chuang and co-workers (1993) exploited the fact that a transection of C7 does not cause too much functional loss. They elongated the C7 root from the contralateral side with a vascularized nerve graft to innervate certain structures on the paralyzed side. By electric stimulation, the motor and sensory part is differentiated. By electric stimulation, it is recognized to which extent C7 innervates the musculature in order to estimate the eventual loss of function. Usually the functional loss is limited to reduction of sensibility. At the index finger reduction of force in the triceps muscle and the finger extension. In a few weeks this functional loss is compensated. In case of an innervation anomaly, however, an unexpected loss may occur and this, of course, would be a catastrophe for the patient. By electric stimulation, the amount of innervation from C7 can be estimated. The author has ligated the C7 root in a first step in order to be able to evaluate the functional loss. If this loss would have been more than expected, one could have immediately transected the ligature with a good chance of recovery. If the patient accepted the functional loss, as it was in all five cases we have done so far, we proceeded with the transfer mainly using an ulnar nerve as a vascularized nerve graft and the median nerve as the recipient nerve. The patients retained finger and wrist flexion in a useful way but they have to perform a trick movement with the contralateral hand in order to move the fingers of the paralyzed hand.

Donor Nerves for Nerve Grafts

Sural Nerve. The sural nerve was most frequently used. If both are harvested a total length of 60 to 80 cm can be obtained.

Medial Cutaneous Nerve of the Forearm. The medial cutaneous nerve of the forearm nerve is part of the brachial plexus and is denervated. A segment of about 20 cm can be obtained. In case of necessity, the same nerve of the contralateral arm may be harvested. This nerve has a greater cross section area than the sural nerve.

Superficial Radial Nerve. The superficial radial was also used in certain cases. Because the nerve is also denervated, we are not afraid of the development of a painful neuroma in brachial plexus cases.

Lateral Cutaneous Nerves of the Thigh. The lateral cutaneous nerves of the thigh are used rarely in brachial plexus cases. They would provide a segment of 20 cm each.

Saphenous Nerve. We do not use the saphenous nerve in brachial plexus cases because we do not like to harvest both the sural and the saphenous nerve of the same extremity.

Ulnar Nerve. If C8 and T1 are avulsed, function in the ulnar nerve territory can be obtained only by a nerve transfer to this nerve. Because the chances of useful recovery are not very good, the ulnar nerve is available in this situation as a donor graft. It can be used in two ways. Bonney and associates (1984) suggested using the ulnar nerve, along with the brachial artery and vein, as a free vascularized nerve graft. Breidenbach and Terzis (1983, 1984) transferred the ulnar nerve pedicled on the superior collateral ulnar artery, which is able to nourish the whole length of the ulnar nerve. The ulnar nerve can be transferred as a free vascularized nerve graft or as an island flap on this pedicle. After local splitting of the perineurium and after isolation of the nerve within the perineurial entourage, the nerve trunk can be transected without endangering the circulation. Thus, the ulnar nerve can be arranged in U-shaped or S-shaped fashion, providing two or three parallel running segments, all based on the same pedicle. Excellent results can be achieved by this technique, and actually, the vascularized nerve grafts were very much favored for a long of time because everyone expected a better result (Alnot et al, 1984; Bonney et al, 1984; Merle, 1986, 1988).

Our approach to neurotize the biceps and the triceps simultaneously provided the opportunity to study this question clinically. In a series of cases, the biceps was neurotized by a vascularized ulnar nerve graft and the triceps by free sural nerve grafts. The evaluation of the results did not show a significant difference. Sometimes the biceps was better than the triceps, indicating a better regeneration across the vascularized nerve graft, but sometimes the reverse was true. In some cases, there was no difference. It was one vascularized nerve graft that did not show any recovery. This was apparently because of a vascular problem. If the pedicle is not well developed and the ulnar nerve cannot be used as a vascularized nerve graft, the nerve can be split into minor units approximately the size of the sural nerve; the units are then transplanted as free grafts (Eberhard and Millesi, 1996). The same is done with remaining segments of the ulnar nerve after the major segment has been used as a vascularized nerve graft.

POSTOPERATIVE TREATMENT

After nerve grafting, the patient is immobilized by a head-arm-trunk plaster device in the position he or she was in during the operation. This position is maintained for 8 days. After 8 days, limited passive motion is possible, and after 3 weeks, the full physiotherapy program can begin.

The postoperative treatment consists of passive kinesitherapy in order to preserve joint mobility. Contractures are avoided by active splinting.

In order to prevent elongation of paralyzed muscles, a support against gravity is provided by different orthoses.

Electric stimulation of the denervated muscles by a triangular stimuli and an exponential slope has proved useful. Electric stimulation using biofeedback is especially useful in cases of nerve transfers.

RECONSTRUCTIVE SURGERY

In phase 4, after regeneration is basically terminated, the careful analysis of the available function is performed and plans are designed for further improvement of function. Some of these procedures have been already mentioned and we provide a summary here.

Arthrodesis of the Shoulder Joint. This is an intervention that the author does only if the serratus anterior function is good.

Trapezius Transfer. The transfer of the horizontal portion of the trapezius including a bony segment of the acromion to the surgical neck of the humerus provides stability of the shoulder joint and avoids subluxation. In some cases, abduction of up to 20 degrees may be achieved.

Transfer of the Greater Pectoral Muscle. The transfer of the major pectoralis muscle insertion to the dorsal side of the humerus across a rotational osteotomy has proved very useful. Good external rotation can be achieved, and the major pectoralis muscle should preserve its adduction force.

Transfer of the Lateral Portion of the Greater Pectoral Muscle to Obtain Elbow Flexion. In the author's experience, this operation was not very successful. For more information, see the article by Clark (1946).

Transfer of the Latissimus Dorsi Muscle to Achieve Elbow Flexion. This operation was performed with great success in selected cases of partial lesion. (Zancolli and Mitre, 1973). However, after complete paralysis, the latissimus dorsi muscle is usually not strong enough for this purpose.

Transfer of the Triceps Muscle to Achieve Elbow Flexion. This operation was discussed earlier in detail. In our hands, it is a very good procedure and it may help obtain good elbow flexion even in cases in which the regeneration of the biceps and the triceps is weak. The big disadvantage, of course, is loss of active extension. Elbow extension is provided by gravity alone. For a patient with a complete brachial plexus lesion and limited function of the shoulder joint this is not really a problem and, therefore, this operation is strictly reserved for a case with a complete brachial plexus lesion. This operation was, however, also performed in cases in which a co-contraction of the biceps and the triceps developed with a weak biceps. In this case, the biceps and the triceps neutralize their function. If there is a strong biceps in a similar situation, we perform a lengthening of the triceps tendon in order to weaken this muscle and to allow the patient to learn to use the biceps alone as an elbow flexor.

Transposition of the Common Head of the Forearm Flexors to the Humerus Shaft to Achieve Elbow Flexion. This is a good operation to manage upper brachial plexus lesions in patients with strong forearm muscles (Steindler, 1918).

Transposition of Flexor Muscles and of the Pronator Teres to Restore Wrist Extension, Finger Extension, and Thumb Adduction, as in Radial Paralysis. This operation is indicated in cases of extended upper brachial lesions (C5, C6, C7) if radialis function does not recur.

Arthrodesis of the Wrist. Arthrodesis is achieved after removal of the cartridge within the wrist joint by a plate introduced between the radius and the third metacarpal bone. Pronation and supination is preserved. If there is no forearm muscle available, the wrist arthrodesis gives stability, and the patient with external rotation and good elbow flexion can use the hand and the forearm as a supporting limb.

Palliative Surgery at Finger Levels. When continuity has been lost, intrinsic muscle function does not return. Therefore, normal hand function is never achieved. This is one of the main reasons why the results still remain unsatisfactory from the objective point of view. However, in many cases it is possible to obtain primitive grip function by fixing the thumb in opposition to the fingers; using a bone graft between the first and second metacarpal bone; performing an arthrodesis of the interphalangeal joint of the thumb and the proximal interphalangeal and distal interphalangeal joints of the fingers; and concentrating the available muscle power on the metacarpal joint of the thumb and the metacarpal joints of the fingers to achieve pinch-and-hook function.

RESULTS

It is not possible in this limited space to report on the results of all cases. The progress that has been achieved in brachial plexus surgery becomes visible if one compares the results in the treatment of complete brachial plexus lesions at root level, as far as the elbow flexion is concerned. In the period of 1963 to 1972, among 31 cases of complete brachial plexus lesions, the author operated on 18 patients with root lesions. Elbow flexion of M3 or better was achieved in 11 out of the 18 cases (60%). From 1973 to 1980, the author operated on 73 complete brachial plexus lesions with 58 root lesions. Elbow flexion of M3 or better was achieved in 40 out of the 58 cases (69%). From 1980 to 1986, the author operated on 64 complete brachial plexus lesions. We could achieve elbow flexion of M3 or better in 52 out of the 64 cases (81%). This improvement is partially due to the new

approach that also used the triceps as an elbow flexor. From the last series with sufficiently long follow-up, the author report, on 13 cases with avulsion of four or five roots. Eleven of the 13 cases achieved a biceps muscle function of M3 and better with an average of 3.6. In eight of the cases, the biceps was the main contributor, and in three more cases, the triceps was the main contributor. Useful shoulder function was achieved in eight of 12 patients (one patient did not have sufficiently long follow-up), with an average of M2.8. Pectoralis major function was achieved in 9 of 10 patients (average 2.95), and forearm muscle function was achieved in 7 out of 10 patients (average M2).

References

Alnot JY, Oberlin CH, Bellaicke H: Vascularized ulnar nerve transfer in total palsy of the brachial plexus. Presented at the Joint Meeting of the Groupe pour I'Avancement de la Microchirurgie (GAM) and the DAM für Mikrochirurgie der peripheren Nerven und Gefäße. Strasbourg, May 2–4, 1984.

Bonney G, Birch R: Surgical aspects. Presented at the Symposium on Brachial Plexus Injuries by the British Society for Surgery of the Hand, Barbicane Center, London, November 1982.

Bonney G, Birch R, Jamieson AM, Eames RA: Experience with vascularized nerve grafts. Clin Plast Surg *11*:137, 1984.

Breidenbach WC, Terzis JK: Vascularized nerve grafts. A.S.P.R.S. Scholarship Contest, 1983.

Breidenbach WC, Terzis JK: The anatomy of free vascularized nerve grafts. Clin Plast Surg *11*:65–71, 1984.

Brunelli G: Neurotization of the avulsed roots of the brachial plexus by means of anterior nerves of the cervical plexus. Int J Microsurg *2*:55–58, 1980.

Brunelli G, Monini L: Neurotization of avulsed roots of brachial plexus by means of anterior nerves of cervical plexus. Clin Plast Surg *11*:149–152, 1984.

Chuang CCD: Remark at Panel Brachial Plexus Surgery, 11th Symposium of International Society of Reconstructive Microsurgery, Vienna, June 5–8, 1993.

Chuang CCD, Wei FC, Noordhoff MS: Cross-chest C7 nerve grafting followed by free muscle transplantation for the treatment of avulsed brachial plexus injuries: A preliminary report. Plast Reconstr Surg *92*:717–727, 1993.

Clark JPM: Reconstruction of the biceps brachii by pectoral muscle transplantation. Br J Surg *34*:180, 1946.

Doi K: Double-free muscle transfer for reconstruction of prehension following complete avulsion of brachial plexus: Long term results in reconstructive microsurgery current trends. Proceedings of the 12th Symposium of the International Society of Reconstructive Microsurgery, Singapore, September 6–8, 1996.

Eberhard D, Millesi H: Split nerve graft. J Reconstr Microsurg *12*:71–76, 1996.

Eberhard D, Millesi H, Knabl J, Reihsner R: Functional anatomy of skin and subcutaneous tissue in relation to tension distribution. Presented at 11th Symposium of the International Society of Reconstructive Microsurgery, Vienna, June 5–8, 1993.

Eberhard D, Reihsner R, Millesi H: A new approach to the brachial plexus. In Vastamäki M (ed): Current Trends in Hand Surgery. Amsterdam, Elsevier Science BV, 1995, pp 283–288.

Gu YD, Zang GM, Yan JG, Cheng XM, Chen L: Seventh cervical root transfer from the lateral healthy side for treatment of the brachial plexus. J Hand Surg *17B*:518–521, 1992.

Hara T, Nagano A, Akasaka Y, Takahashi M, Nakagawa T: The present and future of the intercostal nerve crossing as a treatment of brachial plexus injuries. *In* Vastamäki M (ed): Current Trend in Hand Surgery Proc. 6th Congr. of IFSSH, Helsinki, July 1995. Amsterdam, Elsevier 1995, pp 289–295.

Kotani PT, Matsuda H, Suzuki T: Trial of surgical procedures of nerve transfer to avulsion injuries of plexus brachialis. Abstracts SICOT XII, Israel, Oct. 9–13, 1972, p 520.

Kotani PT, Toyoshima Y, Matsuda H, Suzuki T, Ishizaki H, Ivani H, Yamano H, Inoue T, Moriguchi S, Ri K, Asada J: The postoperative results of nerve transfer for the brachial plexus injury in root avulsion. 14th Meeting of the Japanese Society for Surgery of the Hand, Osaka, 1971, Abstract, p 34.

Merle M: Neurotization of brachial plexus lesions with the spinal accessory nerve–function results. Presented at Annual Meeting of the American Society for Surgery of the Hand, Las Vegas, February 15, 1986.

Merle M: Vascularized nerve grafts. Presented at 9th Meeting International Microsurgical Society. Brescia, July 27–Aug. 1, 1986. Peripheral Nerve Regeneration 4,77, 1988.

Millesi H: The healing of nerves. Clin Plast Surg *4*:459, 1977.

Millesi H: Microsurgery of peripheral nerves, neurolysis, nerve grafts, brachial plexus injuries. *In* Buncke HJ, Furnas DW (eds): Proceedings Symposium on Clinical Fontiers in Reconstructive Microsurgery. St. Louis, C.V. Mosby 1984, pp 353–373.

Millesi H: Eingriffe an den peripheren Nerven. *In* Gschnitzer F, Kern E, Schweiberer L (eds): Chirurgische Operationslehre. Baltimore, Urban & Schwarzenberg, 1986, pp 1–88. (S.11)

Millesi H, Berger A, Meissl G: The interfascicular nerve grafting of the median and ulnar nerves. J Bone Joint Surg *54A*:727–750, 1972.

Millesi H, Berger A, Meissl G: Further experiences with interfascicular grafting of the median, ulnar, and radial nerves. J Bone Joint Surg *58A*:227–230, 1976.

Millesi H, Ganglberger J, Berger A: Erfahrungen mit der Mikrochirurgie peripherer Nerven. Chir Plastica *3*:47, 1966.

Millesi H, Meissl G, Katzer H: Zur Behandlung der Verletzungen des Plexus brachialis. Vorschlag zur integrierten Therapie. Bruns Beitr Klin Chir *220*:429–446, 1973.

Narakas A: Plexo braquial. Terapeutica quirurgica directa. Técnica, indicacion operatoria. Resultados in Cirurgia de los nervios perifericos. Madrid 1972, pp 339–404.

Narakas A: Thoughts on neurotization or nerve transfer in irreparable nerve lesions. Clin Plast Surg *11*:153–159, 1984.

Samii M: Personal communication at the Symposium on Brachial Plexus Lesions. Lindau, June 9–11, 1983.

Seddon HJ: Peripheral Nerve Injuries. Medical Research Council, Special Report, Her Majesty's Stationary Office, London 1954. (S 18)

Seddon HJ: Surgical Disorders of the Peripheral Nerves. London, Churchill Livingstone, 1972.

Seddon HJ: Surgical Disorders of the Peripheral Nerves, 2nd ed. London, Churchill Livingstone, 1975.

Sunderland S: A classification of peripheral nerve injuries producing loss of function. Brain *74*:491, 1951.

Steindler A: Reconstruction work on hand and forearm. N Y Med J *108*:117, 1918.

Tsujama NR, Sagakuchi T, Har T, Kondo S, Kaminuma M, Tjichi M, Ryn D: Reconstructive surgery in brachial plexus injuries. Proc. 11th Annual Meeting, Japanese Society for Surg of the Hand, Hiroshima, 1968, p 39.

Turkof E, Mayer N, Deecke L, Millesi H: Central stimulation to prove motor roots in brachial plexus surgery. Presented at 4th Congress of the International Federation of Societies for Surgery of the Hand, Jerusalem, April 9–14, 1989.

Turkof E, Monivais J, Dechtyar I, Belloia H, Millesi H: Motor evoked potential as a reliable method to verify the conductivity of anterior spinal roots in brachial plexus surgery: An experimental study on goats. J Reconstr Microsurgery *11*:5:357–362, 1995.

Yeoman PM, Seddon HJ: Brachial plexus injuries: Treatment of the flail arm. J Bone Jt Surg *43B*:493–500, 1961.

Zancolli E, Mitre H: Latissimus dorsi transfer to restore elbow flexion. An appraisal of eight cases. J Bone Jt Surg *55A*:1265, 1973.

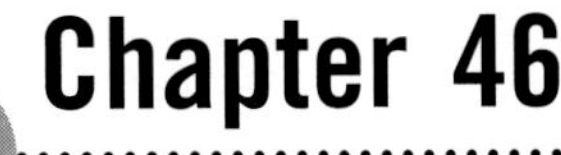

Brachial Plexus Injuries

Associated with the development of microneurosurgical techniques have been advances in the clinician's ability to diagnose the extent of complex and devastating peripheral nerve lesions, especially those that would benefit from early surgical intervention. The application of these techniques in dealing with several complex peripheral nerve lesions has resulted in significant changes in the philosophy of management of challenging problems such as injuries to the brachial plexus in both infants and adults.

The typical patient with a brachial plexus injury is a young man who is injured when thrown from a motorcycle. Although his helmet saves his life, it cannot prevent his shoulder from being driven downward and posteriorly, and his neck driven in the opposite direction as he strikes the ground, guardrail, or fencepost.

Before modern microneurosurgical techniques, there was little enthusiasm for operating on the nerves of such patients. If the palsy was complete, amputation of the arm was recommended. Today, with modern surgical techniques, useful function frequently can be restored, even to completely paralyzed limbs.

PATHOLOGY OF THE LESION

The extent of injury is primarily due to the level of energy and somewhat to the direction of the force relative to the limb and shoulder. Low-energy injuries, such as a fall onto the shoulder, typically cause mostly reversible injuries, such as neuropraxia (Seddon, 1947) (Sunderland [Sunderland, 1978] level I) or various degrees of axonotmesis (Sunderland levels II to IV.) High-energy injuries, for example, in a person thrown from a speeding motorcycle, are associated with more significant injuries, including rupture of plexal segments at any level (Sunderland level V) or avulsions of nerve roots from the spinal cord.

The force of the blow is imparted first to those structures having the most direct or straightest course from spine to arm, in this case the C-8 and T-1 roots and their continuation as the inferior trunk. The energy is imparted last to those structures having the longest anatomical course from fixed points in the neck to fixed points in the shoulder and arm; in this case the sigmoid course of the C5 and C6 roots and their superior trunk affords these structures some protection. The C7 root and associated middle trunk are intermediate in its course. The lower structures of the brachial plexus suffer more significant injuries, such as root avulsion, than more proximally located roots, trunks, and cords (Table 46–1). In the same patient, essentially every Sunderland level of injury as well as root avulsion can occur (Fig. 46–1). The same energy may also fracture the transverse processes of the cervical vertebrae (although this is more likely to be an avulsion of the origins of scalenus muscles), the clavicle, and the scapula. All are associated with a high-energy injury and, concomitantly, significant injury to the brachial plexus.

EVALUATION OF THE PATIENT

The goal of the examination is to determine as accurately as possible the extent of the nerve injury and, from this, determine whether or not the patient is a candidate for either early surgical reconstruction of the brachial plexus or a period of further observation.

Special Physical Signs

One important indicator of severity of injury is the presence of a Horner's sign on the affected side. This sign may be present immediately but occasionally is not readily apparent for 3 to 4 days following injury. The presence of Horner's sign indicates severe injury to the C8 and T1 roots and has been strongly correlated with avulsion of one or both of these roots. Severe pain in an anesthetic extremity is also a sign of poor prognosis, indicating some degree of deafferentation of the limb, again strongly correlated with root avulsion injuries.

Motor and Sensory Examination

A standard motor and sensory examination based on the known metameric levels of innervation is performed. Usually it is not necessary to test all individual muscles; rather, it is more helpful to assess functional groups of muscles, such as the external or internal rotators of the shoulder and flexors of the elbow. Two important indicators of the level of injury for the patient with near-total palsy are the presence or absence of activity of the rhomboids and serratus anterior muscles. Rapidly accomplished tests such as sharp-dull discrimination provide sufficient sensory testing. A study of several systems that are useful in recording the result of the

▼ TABLE 46–1
Operative Findings for Each Root from a Series of 114 Patients Presenting with Total or Near-Total Brachial Plexus Palsy

Root	Ruptured	Avulsed	Other
C5	59	14	40
C6	44	35	35
C7	39	53	20
C8	11	67	31
T1	11	61	37

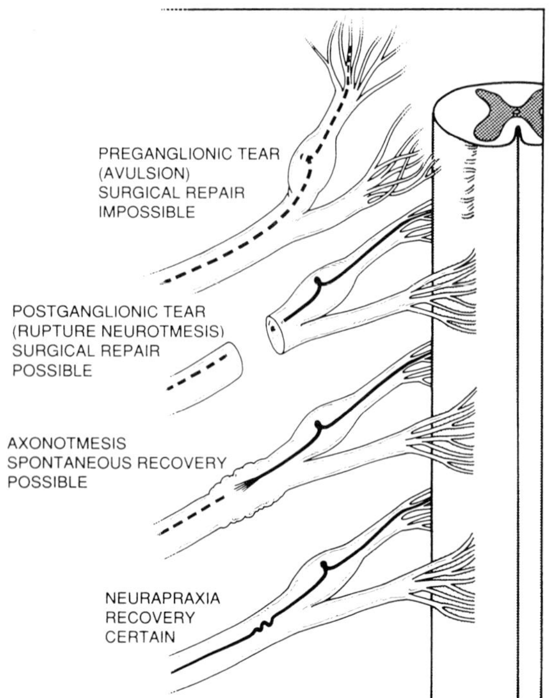

FIGURE 46–1. A severe traction injury to the brachial plexus may cause nerve injuries of varying severity including avulsion of the nerve root from the spinal cord (nonreparable), extraforaminal rupture of the root or trunk (surgically reparable), and an intraneural rupture of fascicles (some spontaneous recovery possible) in a single patient.

examination of the injured brachial plexus has been published (Narakas, 1977). It must be kept in mind that these charts represent the idealized or average situation and that individual variations in the anatomy of the plexus exist. For example, significant innervation may come from the C4 root, termed a prefixed plexus, or from the T2 root, termed a postfixed plexus.

Radiography

X-ray studies of the cervical spine, chest, clavicle, and scapula are necessary The chest x-ray study should include an inspiration and expiration anteroposterior view to determine the activity of the diaphragm. A paralyzed diaphragm is an indicator of severe injury to the upper roots of the plexus. The presence of fractures of the transverse processes is also strong evidence of a high-energy injury.

Special Diagnostic Examinations Including Computerized Tomography, Magnetic Resonance Imaging, and Myelography

Modern imaging techniques have improved the clinician's ability to predict what the microneurosurgeon will find at exploration. Traditional myelography using metrizamide contrast has been largely supplanted by computed tomography (CT) and magnetic resonance imaging (MRI) examinations, performed with and without contrast agents (Fig. 46–2). Both CT and MRI may be useful. MRI reformatting

provides a better picture of the soft tissues, particularly the T2-weighted images that highlight the fat content of the cervical spinal cord and nerve roots, and also the T1-weighted images that highlight the water content associated with a pseudomeningocele. The presence of a pseudomeningocele has been strongly associated with avulsion of the corresponding root. When these tests are performed within a few days of injury, especially with contrast, there may be a higher incidence of false-positive results because the contrast agent may leak through small tears in the dura, not necessarily associated with avulsion of the root.

Other evidence of significant injury include empty-appearing root sleeves or a shift of the cord in one direction or another away from the mid-line.

Sensory and Motor Evoked Potentials

These tests should be carried out after several weeks following injury to allow wallerian degeneration to proceed. Standard electromyography is not as helpful in the diagnosis and management of severe injuries as are sensory evoked potentials, corticosensory evoked potentials, and spinograms. Stimulating the area over Erb's point in the supraclavicular fossa and recording from the cortex using scalp electrodes is evidence that some roots may still be in continuity with the spinal cord. The spinogram can provide information about the level of innervation of the paraspinous muscles. Because these muscles are innervated by the posterior primary rami of the plexus, paralysis of these muscles indicates a very proximal injury but does not tell the examiner whether the injury is asociated with avulsion, rupture, or axonotmesis.

No one test can serve as the conclusive basis for surgical decision-making. All of the information must be assimilated and, most importantly, be viewed within the context of the presumed energy of the trauma.

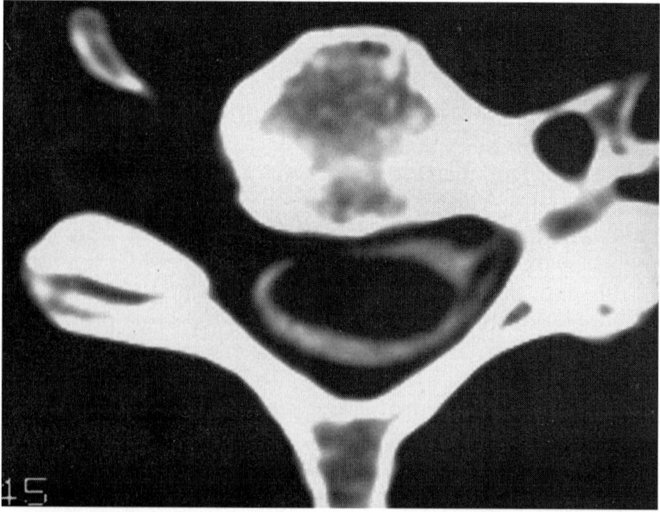

FIGURE 46–2. Computed tomography of the cervical spine with contrast demonstrates avulsion of a part of the transverse process and absence of the root shadow at the C6 level. This appearance suggests that the C6 root has been avulsed.

INDICATIONS FOR SURGERY

Most of the modern series describing the surgical experience in brachial plexus reconstruction attest to the inverse relationship between time from injury to operation to outcome. In cautious and skilled hands, exploration seldom results in extension of the injury. Even when total palsy exists, fewer than 20% of patients demonstrate avulsions of all five roots of the plexus, meaning that for the great majority, the surgeon will find something to repair or graft and, if this is not possible, reinnervate with a non-plexus nerve source (nerve transfer). If nerve transfer is included, then theoretically virtually all patients might benefit from microneural reconstruction. These factors imply that when there is a strong suspicion of significant damage to the plexus in the form of root avulsions and nerve ruptures, surgical exploration is warranted.

TIMING OF SURGERY

Immediate Surgery

Immediate surgery is indicated for essentially any patient with a plexus injury of almost any degree of severity secondary to a penetrating injury, such as a stab wound, or following an iatrogenic injury, such as known or suspected injury to the plexus at the time of first rib resection for the treatment of thoracic outlet syndrome. Occasionally, the reconstructive surgeon is afforded the opportunity to make an early assessment of the degree of damage, for example, when vascular reconstruction of a ruptured subclavian or axillary artery is to be performed by the vascular surgeon at the time of injury. In this instance, the vascular surgeon's incisions may be extended (as described later), the supraclavicular fossa explored, the degree of damage mapped, various structures tagged by metal markers such as vascular clips, and preliminary plans for secondary reconstruction begun. It is critical that the reconstructive surgeon be involved in this emergency procedure, both to take advantage of the opportunity afforded to assess nerve damage and also to guide the vascular surgeon in the dissection of the distal vessel in its intimate association with the components of the plexus and in the placement of any vein grafts that might be necessary in vascular reconstruction. Few surgical procedures are more tedious than reopening a wound after several weeks or months and dissecting a relatively thin-walled vein graft that has been placed in the most direct and convenient (for the vascular surgeon) spot, that is, always superficial to the plexus. With the reconstructive surgeon's help and guidance, the vascular surgeon can pass the vein graft deep to the injured elements of the plexus, keeping this structure out of the reconstructive surgeon's eventual path to the plexus and thus out of harm's way.

There are many good arguments against immediate reconstruction of the plexus in traction injuries. Most surgeons believe that some period of time must pass to permit delineation of injured from noninjured nerve.

Early Surgery (3 Weeks to 3 Months)

Early surgery is indicated for patients who present with total or near-total palsy, or an injury associated with high-

energy levels. It is also indicated for high-velocity, large-caliber gunshot wounds to the plexus. For those injuries associated with lower levels of energy, viz., low velocity and small caliber or those associated with partial upper level palsy, it is preferable to follow the course of recovery for 3 to 6 months. Surgery should be considered if recovery seems to plateau as determined by several successive evaluations carried out at monthly intervals. The presence or absence of advancing Tinel's sign can be a useful guide. The absence of Tinel's sign in the supraclavicular fossa in the face of a nearly complete C5–C6 level palsy is a poor indicator for spontaneous recovery and warrants early exploration with the likelihood that C5 and C6 nerve roots may be avulsed. In this case, nerve transfer is necessary. If events convince the author that exploration is indicated after the typical motorcycle accident, the author prefers to wait about 6 to 8 weeks following injury, both to allow time for diagnostic tests and to permit the patient some period of time in which he or she must adjust to living with his injury. Because the functional results of reconstruction of severe plexus injuries are on average so disappointing when compared with the function of the normal limb, when the patient has lived with a flail limb for some time, he or she may accept the ultimate functional limitations of microneural reconstruction.

Controversial Indications

An occasional patient presents with a partial C8 and complete T1 lesion, with some finger flexors working but with essentially an intrinsic palsy and anesthesia in the C8 or T1 distribution, or both. This represents somewhat of a dilemma in decision-making because it seems almost impossible to recover intrinsic muscle function in the adult and, when they are injured, the C8 and T1 nerve roots are so often avulsed from the spinal cord that it is unlikely that anything even worth repairing will be found at surgery.

The patient and family must be made aware of the relatively low level of performance expected following surgery. They also must be made aware of the long period of waiting for reinnervation of muscles when essentially nothing happens that the patient can appreciate. Before surgery, the patient should have been taught the exercises necessary to maintain a normal range of motion of the paralyzed joints rather than depending on another person such as the therapist to perform these exercises for him or her. The therapist can teach, advise, and record progress, but the patient must accept responsibility for performing the exercises.

SURGICAL FINDINGS

A relatively standard incision is employed by most surgeons and is shown in Figure 46–3. The author routinely infiltrates the proposed line of the incision with a 1:200,000 solution of epinephrine before the skin is prepared and scratches a few cross hatch marks at key points to assist in closing the incision properly. The skin is so lax in the neck and axilla that accurate closure can be difficult without these marks for guidance. Cross hatching the line of incision with a marking pen is usually fruitless. The marks have long since disappeared when it is time to close the wound.

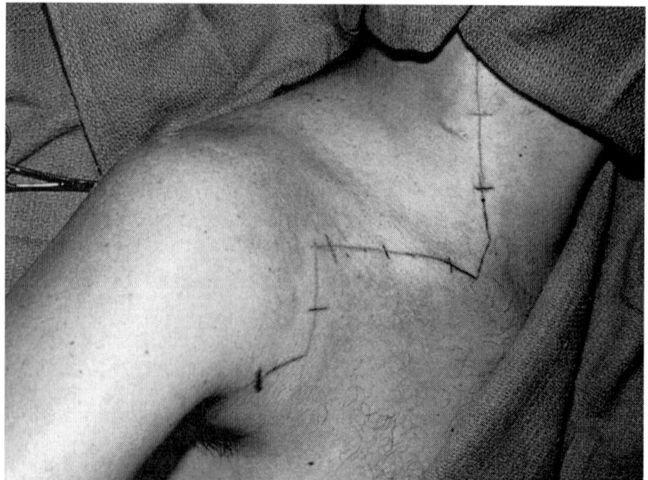

FIGURE 46–3. The standard incision is outlined. This allows exploration of both the supraclavicular and infraclavicular portions of the brachial plexus. The incision can be extended into the axilla and then parallels the medial intermuscular septum to allow exposure to the distal elements. The cross hatchings should be scored lightly with a knife blade because ink markings fade rapidly during the course of the procedure and the lax skin of the neck defies easy accurate reapproximation without these guides.

The superior limb of the incision parallels the posterior border of the sternocleidomastoid muscle but angles away from the inferior border. The incision then parallels the clavicle, crossing it at the level of the coracoid process. A slightly zigzagged limb more or less parallels the deltopectoral groove to the anterior axillary fold, where it parallels the axillary fossa to the midpoint of the medial upper arm. At this point, it turns distally, paralleling the brachial artery.

Unless the injury is clearly limited to one area of the plexus, for example, as following a stab wound, the entire plexus from neck to axilla may need to be exposed by this relatively standard technique. A variety of presentations may be seen. If the upper roots are avulsed, the rootlets and swollen dorsal root ganglion may be found twisted and lying either behind the clavicle or slightly above it in the region of the C8 root (Fig. 46–4). If the upper roots, superior trunk, or the middle trunk has ruptured, the distal ends typically lie behind the clavicle. The avulsed (often) or ruptured (infrequently) C8 and T1 structures are usually found much closer to their respective foramina than is the case with C5 or C6.

Essentially any combination of injuries may occur, including avulsion, rupture, and a neuroma in continuity. The supraclavicular dissection usually allows this assessment (Fig. 46–5). However, it is critical to complete the remainder of the dissection if the above-mentioned findings favor some type of reconstruction by nerve grafting because there exist a sufficient number of lesions occurring at two levels—for example, rupture of the superior trunk in combination with avulsion of the axillary nerve from the deltoid, or rupture of the musculocutaneous nerve at the level of the shoulder.

The helpful landmark in identifying the location of the C5 root stump in cases of rupture is the phrenic nerve. This nerve is found on the surface of the anterior scalene muscle running parallel to its fibers. A nerve stimulator is helpful in identifying this small nerve. It receives contributions from the C5 root, and by following the nerve superiorly, one may encounter the C5 root or superior trunk. Another approach is to follow the large cervical rami medially, which leads to the C4 or occasionally the C5 root level. The author has found it useful to bring a sterilized drawing of the normal plexus and on this make a sketch of the operative findings. The author uses the same map in planning the priorities in reconstruction; this map also is useful in describing what reconstruction was performed. It is a mistake to depend on memory in dictating the operative note.

Intraoperative Evoked Potentials

Intraoperative evoked potentials (Fig. 46–6 A and B) are helpful (though not foolproof) in determining when, for example, an intraforaminal avulsion (uncommon) versus a rupture has occurred, or in determining whether there exists only an empty root sleeve, that is, only connective tissue with no axons therein (more common.) By 2 to 3 months after injury, evoked potentials across a neuroma in continuity are reliable in assisting in decision-making. When stimulat-

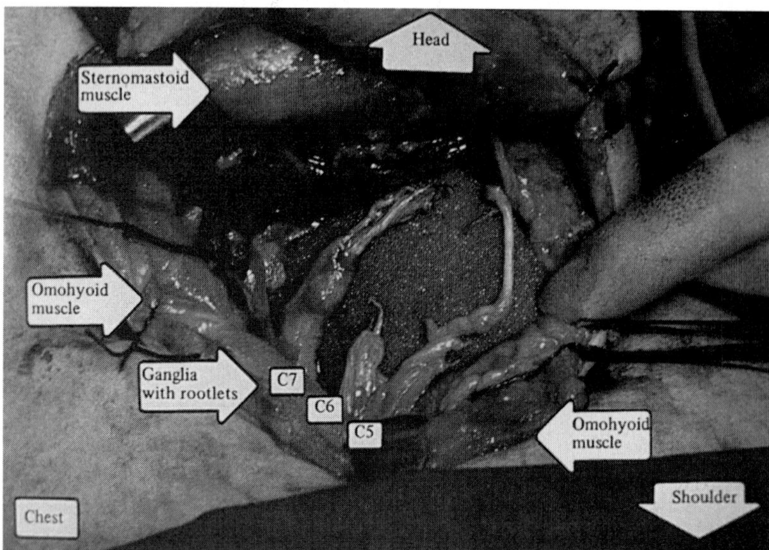

FIGURE 46–4. Operative findings in a case of total palsy. Avulsion of all roots is indicated by the presence of large dorsal root ganglia and avulsed rootlets. (With the kind permission of Mr. Rolfe Birch, Royal National Orthopedic Hospital.)

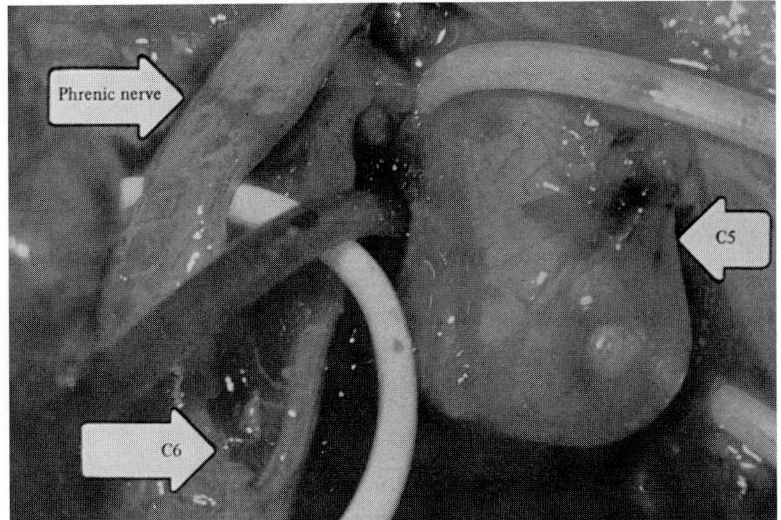

FIGURE 46–5. Intraoperative appearance of a ruptured C5 root. The contribution of C5 to the phrenic nerve remains intact. The phrenic nerve, if not avulsed, is an important guide to the location of the C5 root. (With the kind permission of Mr. Rolfe Birch, Royal National Orthopedic Hospital.)

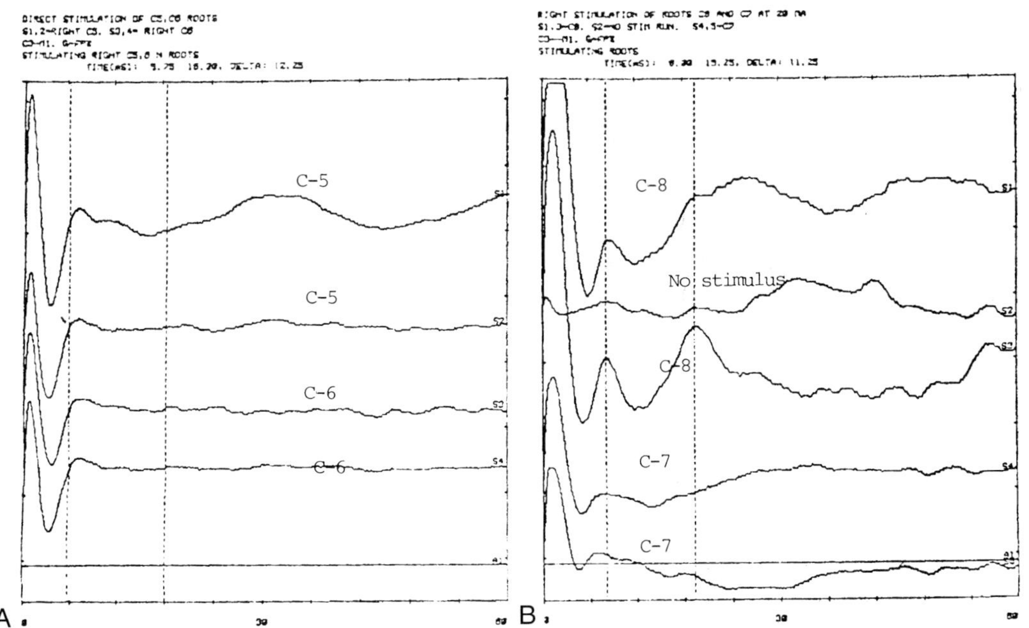

FIGURE 46–6. *A* and *B*, The results of intraoperative corticosensory evoked potential tests are demonstrated in a patient with a C5, C6, and C7 palsy. At exploration, all roots could be found exiting their foramina but the C5, C6, and C7 roots appeared somewhat firm compared with the C8 and T1 roots. The upper three tracings in *B* are the result of stimulating (or recording but not stimulating) the C8 root. With C8 root stimulation, a large response could be measured with the scalp recording electrodes. Stimulation of the C5, C6, and C7 roots (as indicated on the tracings in *A*) resulted in no measurable brain response, indicating probable avulsion of these roots proximal to the point of stimulation.

ing and recording across a neuroma in continuity, it is unnecessary to average a large number of stimulations. If there exists no easily discernible response above the noise level without averaging, the neuroma and adjacent damaged nerve are resected using the microscope to assist in determining when debridement is adequate, and nerve grafts are placed in the resultant defect. If a clear signal is identified above the noise, then only neurolysis under magnification is performed.

INTRAOPERATIVE DECISIONS AND PRIORITIES OF REPAIR

When the patient presents with essentially total brachial plexus palsy, the priorities of repair include

Provisions for elbow flexion—by biceps or brachialis muscle reinnervation, provisions for shoulder stabilization, abduction and external rotation—by suprascapular nerve reinnervation,

Provisions for brachiothoracic pinch (adduction of the arm against the chest)—by reinnervation of the pectoralis major muscle,

Sensation below the elbow in the C6–C7 area, by reinnervation of the lateral cord, and

Provisions for wrist extension and finger flexion—by reinnervation of the lateral and posterior cord.

These priorities have been chosen for three reasons. The first is their functional significance, and the second relates to the likelihood of obtaining the chosen function by nerve reconstruction (more proximal muscles are reinnervated more successfully than very distal muscles), and the third relates to the degree of difficulty in achieving the individual functions listed earlier by secondary surgery.

SURGICAL TECHNIQUES FOR PLEXO-PLEXAL NERVE RECONSTRUCTION

The neurologic surgeon should take advantage of the knowledge gained by others in internally mapping the plexus. At the root level, the areas bound by the posterior and anterior divisions are delineated in an attempt to guide these axons to appropriate target nerves. Next the distal targets are dissected. These targets usually include the suprascapular nerve, which is frequently difficult to find; the lateral cord; and posterior cord. Typically, there are far more targets for nerve grafts than proximal resources.

Technical Choices for Nerve Grafts—Conventional and Vascularized

The author uses both standard fascicular grafts and, for certain cases, vascularized nerve grafts. The typical first choice's are the two sural nerves. Other donor sites for standard grafts include both medial brachial and medial antebrachial cutaneous nerves. Standard microsuture techniques are typically used, although some surgeons now use autologous derived fibrinogen as a tissue adhesive to glue

together nerve ends more rapidly, apparently with equal success. If sutures are to be used, the author prefers to measure and precut the sural nerve segments. The author dyes both ends of the grafts destined for the posterior cord with methylene blue to assist in orientation of the infraclavicular part of the junctures and then begins the supraclavicular neurorraphies with the most distally situated root and trunk, working superiorly. The posterior grafts are placed before the anterior ones. The author finds it helpful to thread the distal ends of the grafts that are bound for similar subclavicular sites into a large-bore catheter. When all the proximal junctures are completed, the first catheter is passed deep to the clavicle, toward the destination for the grafts contained within. This has helped keep the multiple strands of graft separated into functional destinations. After the grafts have been passed under the clavicle, the superior junctures are checked a final time to be certain that no inadvertent disruption has occurred in passing the grafts under the clavicle. The microscope is moved over the subclavicular repair site, and these nerve junctures are performed (Fig. 46–7).

Once plexoplexal nerve grafting or extraplexal neurotization (see later) has been completed, the surgical wounds are closed as follows: the subclavius and omohyoid muscles are repaired because these muscles act as a buffer between nerve grafts and the clavicle; the supraclavicular fat pad is replaced, further protecting the nerve grafts; and a suction

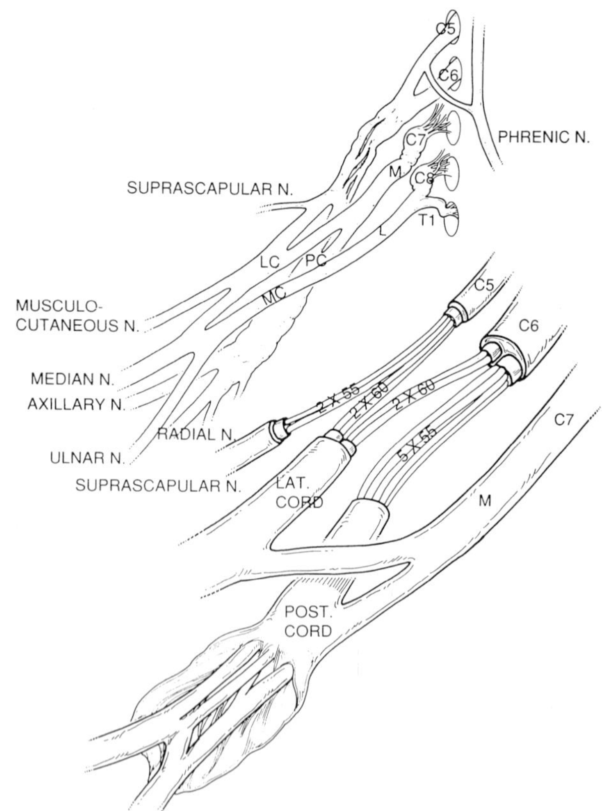

FIGURE 46–7. Operative findings in a case of total plexus palsy following a motorcycle accident. There was a neuroma in continuity of the superior trunk. The C7, C8, and T1 roots were avulsed. Reconstruction involved multiple sural nerve grafts from the healthy C5 and C6 roots to the suprascapular nerve, lateral cord, and the C5–C6 contributions to the posterior cord. The value of exploring the entire plexus in the adult injury is illustrated by the findings of a second, more distal lesion involving the posterior cord, which required neurolysis.

drain is placed somewhat away from the course of the grafts so that they are not dislodged when the drain is removed. The platysma is reapproximated and the skin closed. Subclavicularly, the pectoralis minor is repaired, as is the clavipectoral fascia, and the skin incisions are closed.

VASCULARIZED NERVE GRAFTS

The principal reason to consider a vascularized nerve graft in plexus reconstruction is to maximize the amount of nerve graft material for reconstruction. The best indication for a vascularized graft in plexus reconstruction is a case involving proven avulsion of C8 and T1 in association with large root stumps of the remaining plexus. In this case, there is no possibility of spontaneous recovery of the structures innervated by the ulnar nerve, and it makes little sense to waste precious proximal axons to recover some sensibility in the ulnar side of the hand (intrinsic muscle recovery is essentially never seen in the adult when C8 and T1 have been badly injured). In this instance, the best source of a vascularized nerve graft is the ulnar nerve itself, based in the upper arm on one of several branches of the brachial artery, usually the superior ulnar collateral artery. The dorsal sensory branch of the radial nerve has been described as a source of a vascularized nerve graft, as has the sural, the anterior tibial, the superficial peroneal, and the saphenous nerves.

Surgical Techniques for Nerve Transfer

In the most severe injuries, those with all or most of the nerve roots avulsed, there are insufficient numbers of proximal axon resources from the remaining parts of the plexus still in continuity with the spinal cord. In these cases, it has been necessary to turn to extraplexal sources of especially motor and also sensory axons. Many different nerves have been advocated by knowledgeable surgeons; however, the most common sources of extraplexal motor axons have been the spinal accessory nerve and the intercostal nerves from C3–C6. Additionally, motor branches of the cervical rami or even cross chest grafts from branches of the contralateral plexus, such as a branch from the lateral pectoral nerve, are used. The Chinese have described using the contralateral C7 root as a source of healthy axons. They describe using a vascularized nerve graft passed subcutaneously across the neck to the involved plexus. Other unique sources of healthy motor axons include the medial pectoral nerve in palsies involving C5 and C6. This has typically been transferred onto the musculocutaneous nerve to restore elbow flexion. Also described is the transfer of motor fascicles of an intact ulnar nerve onto fascicles innervating the biceps at the level of the upper arm (Fig. 46–8).

The most appropriate targets for neurotization are the suprascapular nerve (shoulder abduction and external rotation), the musculocutaneous nerve (elbow flexion), or the lateral pectoral nerve (thoracicohumeral pinch).

Neurotization in the Neglected Plexus Injury

In very select circumstances, it is possible to combine microneural reconstruction with free vascularized functional

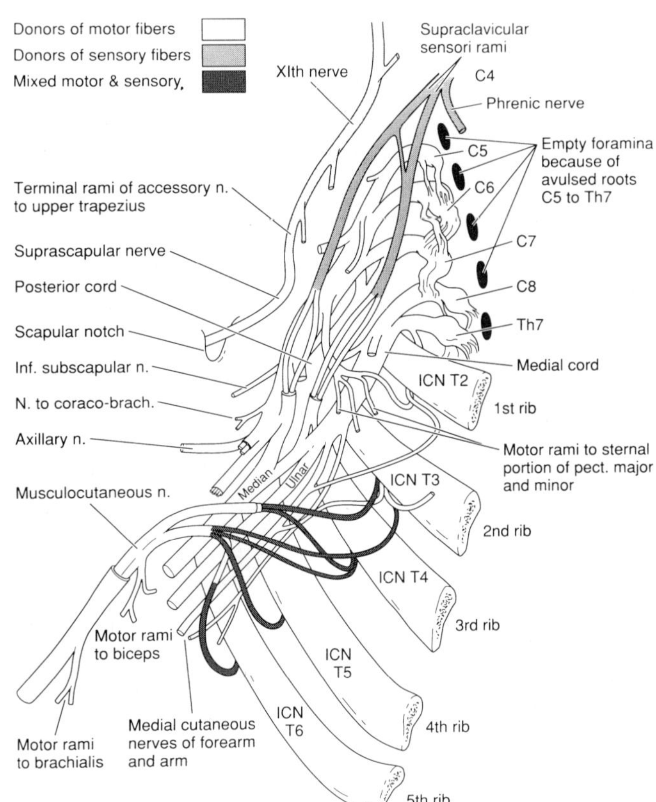

FIGURE 46–8. The findings and method of reconstruction in a case involving avulsion of all elements of the plexus are illustrated. The terminal rami of cranial nerve II was led to the suprascapular nerve to restore some shoulder abduction and perhaps some external rotation. Four intercostal motor rami were anastomosed to the musculocutaneous nerve to regain some elbow flexion. Sensory cervical rami were led to the lateral cord to provide some distal sensibility. These functions have the highest reconstructive priority in these most serious cases.

muscle transfers for unrepaired cases of total brachial plexus palsy. In these cases, the time since injury is too long (in the adult, certainly beyond 2 years) for successful neurotization or reinnervation of long-term denervated muscles. Either the opposite latissimus dorsi, the gracilis, or another muscle is transferred to the shoulder and arm by microvascular free transfer. The motor nerve of the transferred muscle is joined to the donor motor nerve, usually an extraplexal motor nerve such as the spinal accessory or intercostal nerve. Many unique anatomic arrangements have been described, including passing the transfer across the elbow and fixing it into the tendons of the radial wrist extensors in an attempt to provide both elbow flexion and some wrist extension.

▼ TABLE 46–2
Results of Reconstruction with Total Supraclavicular Palsy

Author	Number of Patients	Developed Useful Function
Millesi (1977)	20	10/20*
Sedel (1982)	26	22/26†

*Shoulder 5/8, elbow flexion 9/18, wrist/finger 2/18. An additional six patients were explored surgically, but nothing was repaired.
†Grade 3, 11; Grade 4, 12; Grade 5, 3.

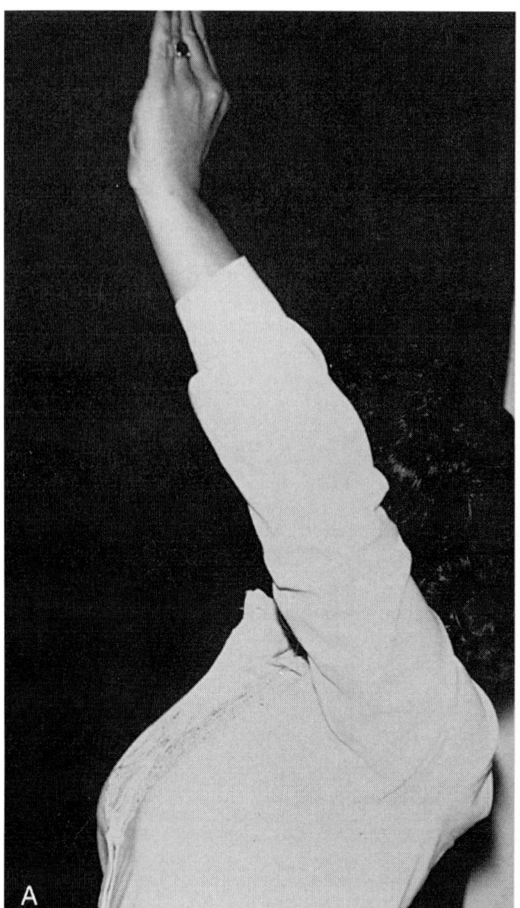
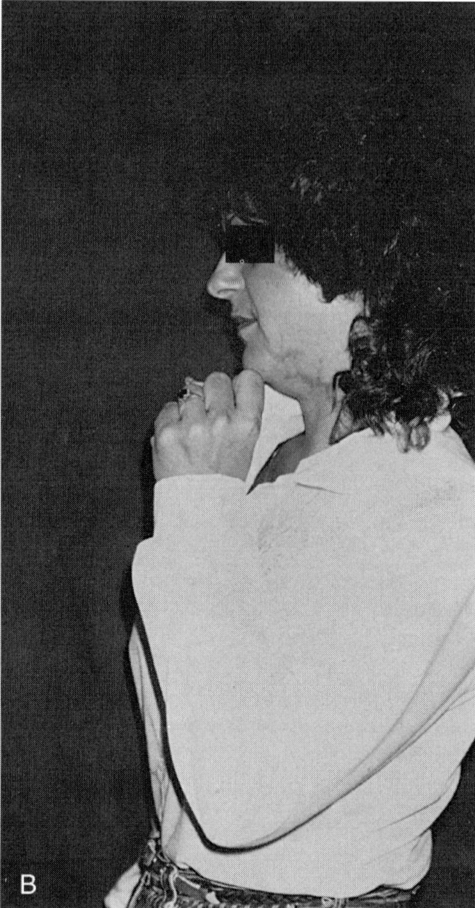

FIGURE 46–9. *A* and *B*, This young woman suffered a shotgun injury to the upper plexus area leaving her with a C5, C6, and C7 palsy. At surgery, the C6 root had been avulsed. The C5 and C7 lesions were nerve grafted. Two years following surgery she had regained near-normal shoulder control and motor grade 4⁺ elbow flexion and extension.

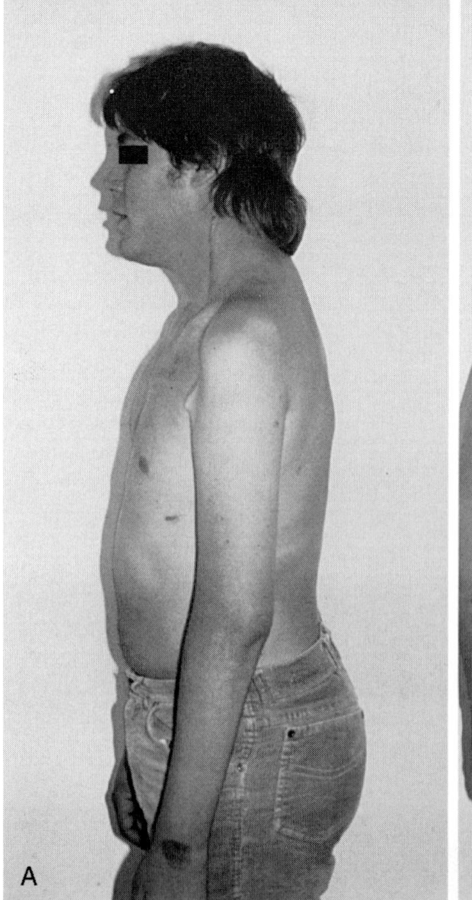
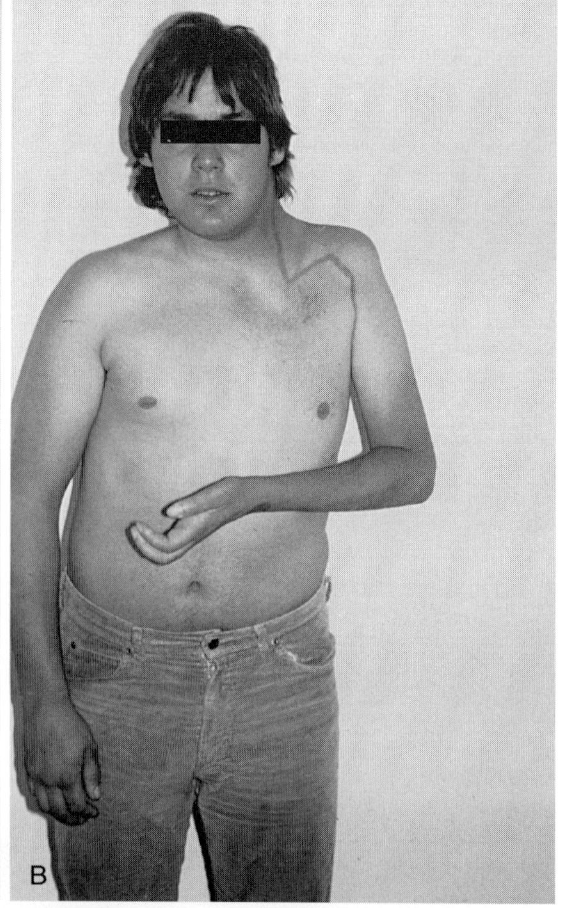

FIGURE 46–10. *A* and *B*, The results of extraplexal neurotization in a case of total avulsion. The spinal accessory nerve was led to the musculocutaneous nerve to provide some elbow flexion, and the cervical motor rami was led to the lateral pectoral nerve to provide some brachiothoracic pinch between the arm and the chest wall. Minimal but important (more than academic) function has been restored.

▼ TABLE 46–3
Results of Reconstruction with Partial Palsy

Author	Number of Patients	Developed Useful Function
Millesi (1977)	11 supraclavicular lesions	9/11
	12 infraclavicular lesions	10/12
Sedel/Narakas (1982)	23	20/23

▼ TABLE 46–4
Results of Nerve Transfer for Elbow Flexion

Nerve	Author	Number of Patients	Good Results	Bad Results
Spinal Accessory Nerve	Allieu (1984)	15	3	12
	Narakas (1988)	3	2	1
	Merle (1986)	7	3	4
Intercostal Nerve	Millesi (1987)	22	11	11
	Narakas (1988)	24	9	15
	Nagano (1987)	117	80	37

Postoperative Care

At the completion of the operation, a cervical collar is fitted about the neck to restrict neck motion. The shoulder and elbow are immobilized, the shoulder in adduction and the elbow in 90 degrees of flexion, for 2 weeks; range of motion exercises are then renewed without restrictions. After initial healing, the progress of nerve regeneration is assessed about every 3 months. At least 2 and perhaps 3 years are necessary before the results of nerve reconstruction can be assessed.

Results of Nerve Reconstruction by Graft and Neurotization

In his 1963 address to the Royal College of Surgeons, Seddon (1947) stated that repair of traction injuries of the brachial plexus was sufficiently disappointing as to essentially preclude it. More modern thought regarding the potential of reconstruction began with more favorable reports by Samii and Kahl (1972), Millesi (1977), and Narakas (1977, 1981). These authors and others (Hentz and Narakas, 1988; Sedel, 1982) reported their results following neural reconstruction of traction injuries to the brachial plexus. However, no systematic scheme of outcome analysis was employed, and it is difficult to compare one series with another. Tables 46–2 and 46–3 summarize the results of several published series for repair by both plexoplexal grafts, including, where necessary, by neurotization. Table 46–4 summarizes the results as compiled by Narakas and Hentz (1988) for neurotization using either spinal accessory nerve or intercostal neurotization.

Analysis of these series leads to several conclusions. Repair does improve the prognosis. Infraclavicular injuries have a better prognosis than supraclavicular injuries. Supraclavicular injuries associated with at least two repairable roots have good prognosis, and partial injuries have a better prognosis than do complete injuries. The results of neurotization have been more mixed. Figure 46–9 demonstrates the functional outcome in a patient with an upper root injury secondary to a shotgun wound, while Figure 46–10 demonstrates the functional result in a case of total root avulsion.

Further innovations in the management of plexus injuries can be anticipated as greater numbers of surgeons become convinced that surgical reconstruction leads to improved functional outcomes.

References

Hentz VR, Narakas A: The results of microneurosurgical reconstruction in complete brachial plexus palsy. Assessing outcome and predicting results. Orthop Clin North Am 19:107–114, 1988.

Millesi H: Surgical management of brachial plexus injuries. J Hand Surg 2:367–379, 1977.

Narakas A: Les lesions dans les elongations du plexus brachial. Differentes possibilities et associations lesionnelles. Rev Chir Orthop 63:44–54, 1977.

Narakas A: Brachial plexus surgery. Orthop Clin North Am 12:303–323, 1981.

Narakas AO, Hentz VR: Neurotization in brachial plexus injuries. Indication and results. Clin Orthop 237:43–56, 1988.

Samii M, Kahl R: Clinische resultate der autologen nerven transplantation. Meslssunger Med Mittel 46:197, 1972.

Seddon H: Surgical Disorders of the Peripheral Nerves, 2nd Ed. Edinburgh, Churchill Livingstone, 1975.

Seddon HJ: The use of autogenous grafts for the repair of large gaps in peripheral nerves. Br J Surg 35:151–167, 1947.

Sedel L: Results of surgical repair in brachial plexus injuries. J Bone Joint Surg 64B:54–66, 1982.

Sunderland S: Nerves and Nerve Injuries, 2nd Ed. Edinburgh, Churchill Livingstone, 1978.

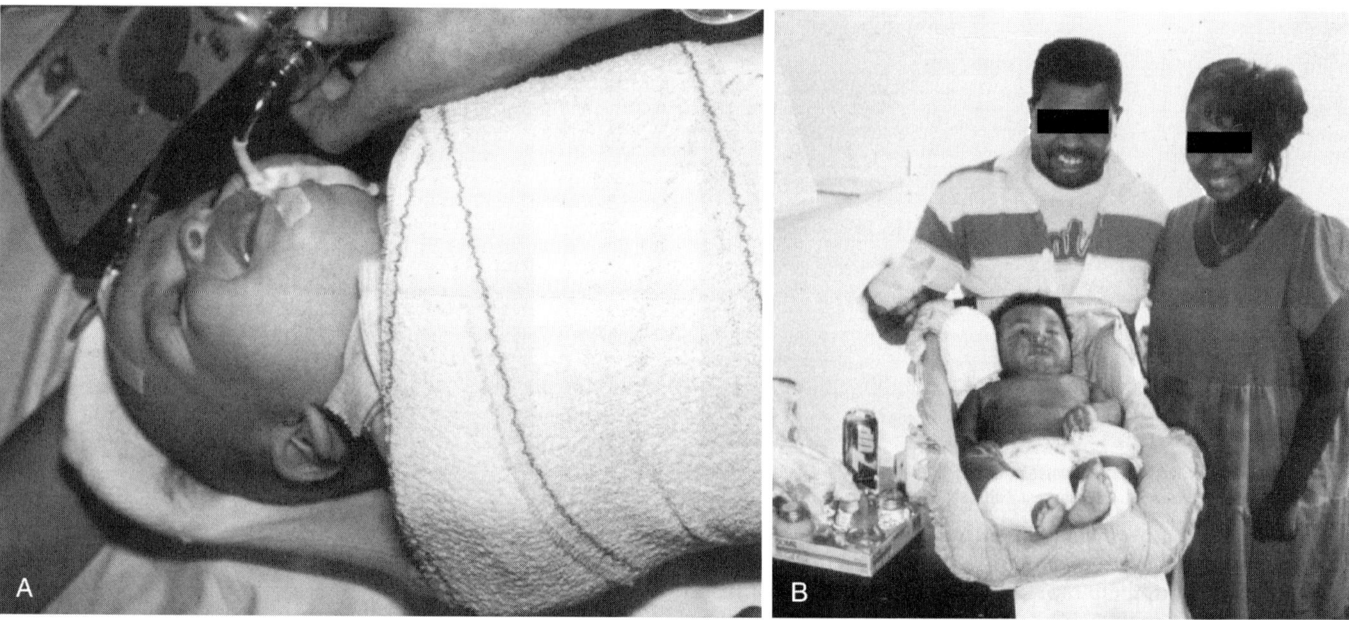

FIGURE 47–5. Postoperative appearance. *A*, A plaster shell may be used to immobilize the infant. *B*, Alternatively, a car seat may be used.

and posteriorly to a point on the trapezius in the midclavicular line. This incision gives excellent exposure to the supraclavicular plexus and is cosmetically superior to the classic incision. If infraclavicular exposure is needed, an additional incision is made from the axilla proximally, joining in a T fashion (Fig. 47–7). Subcutaneous epinephrine (1/100,000 dilution) injected before the incision will control bleeding considerably.

Dissection is taken through the supraclavicular fat, dividing the omohyoid muscle and both superficial and deep transverse cervical vessels. It is very important to look for, identify, and protect the phrenic and spinal accessory nerves in the superior aspect of the incision. If the lower roots are involved, the subclavian artery is mobilized and retracted medially and inferiorly. The intervening roots and proximal plexus can then be safely dissected (Fig. 47–8).

The distal aspect of the neuroma is then mobilized. It is not necessary to divide the clavicle in the infant. Frequently by elevating the clavicle with a towel clip, the uninvolved cords can be mobilized and identified. If there is any doubt, the infraclavicular portion is exposed. Now the pathology can be determined exactly and the course of repair chosen.

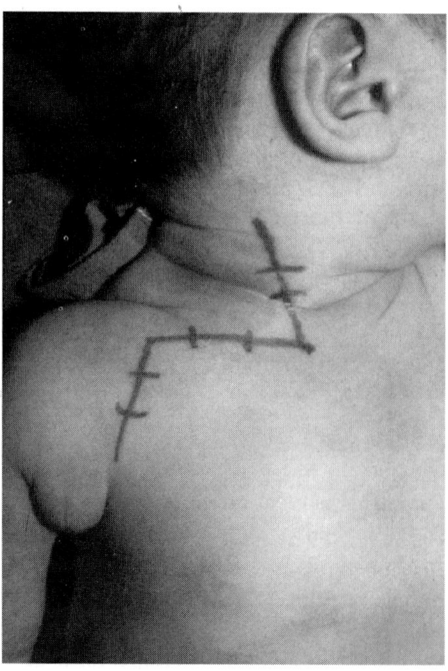

FIGURE 47–6. The classic incision follows the sternomastoid to the clavicle, then turns laterally to the coracoid and, if necessary, to the axillary fold.

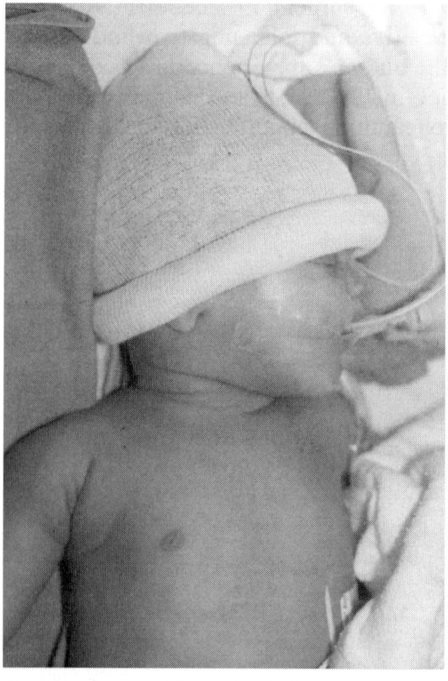

FIGURE 47–7. Transverse neck incision—gives better cosmetic results, especially if only a suprascapular approach is needed.

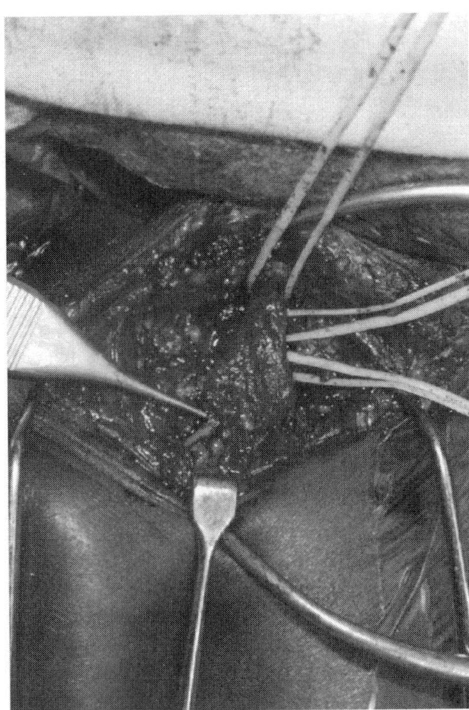

FIGURE 47–8. Neuroma mobilized with nerve roots dissected proximally, and suprascapular nerve and divisions and cords dissected distally.

If all roots are present, neurolysis or excision, or both, of the neuroma and grafting can be performed. The roots should be stimulated, and if a good evoked response is obtained and there is a high percentage of myelinated fibers present, it is a good root. Myelination is determined by sending a thin piece of proximal nerve root for frozen section from the site at which the grafts will be placed (Meyer et al, 1995).

When it is apparent that grafting is necessary, a second surgeon should begin harvesting a sural nerve while mobilization of the neuroma is proceeding. The other sural nerve can be harvested (if necessary) while closing the first leg. We prefer a longitudinal incision starting at the ankle and continuing to the popliteal fossa to ensure the maximal length (Fig. 47–9). Closure is performed with a running subcutaneous absorbable suture. The legs are then dressed, and attention is turned to the neck. While finishing the

harvesting of graft, the staining of sections of the proximal nerve root should be completed (Meyer et al, 1995).

Myelineated fibers stain red, so a nerve with a high percentage of so-called red fibers is generally a good root and a source of axons. If there is a very poor evoked response with few myelinated fibers, it is a poor root and should be given a low priority when grafting.

If there is no signal and no or very few myelinated fibers, it should be abandoned. If there is no signal and a moderate number of myelinated fibers, it may represent an avulsed root ganglion. Either it should not be used or also given a low priority.

Unlike the adult with a complete palsy, the highest priority in the infant is to reinnervate the hand.* If the hand is not reinnervated, the infant does not recognize or use the arm. Thus, when there are multiple avulsions, neural input from the remaining roots should go to the lower trunk first. The biceps and shoulder are innervated next, and last, if there are enough good proximal roots, the posterior cord is innervated.

If just C5 and C6 are involved, simple excision and grafting will suffice; likewise, if C7 is involved as a rupture, it will be grafted as well. In cases of multiple avulsion, primary neurotization should be performed. Intercostal nerves 3, 4, and 5 can be used to innervate the biceps. The distal spinal accessory nerve can be coapted to the suprascapular nerve. Using just the distal part leaves the superior trapezius functioning to stabilize the scapula. Forces generated by the biceps and supraspinatus and infraspinatus muscles will stabilize the shoulder, leaving the one or two roots to innervate (or supply) the lower trunk and distal lateral cord, innervating the hand.

Postoperatively, the infant is immobilized either in the plaster shell (see Fig. 47–5A and B) or, alternatively, a car seat. Padding is added to keep the head from deviating away from the operated side. The babies are discharged generally on the morning of the second postoperative day. Immobilization is maintained for 3 weeks. The baby may be removed for bathing but should be watched closely when out of the restraint to prevent significant movement of the head away from the involved shoulder.

After the 3-week postoperative interval, passive stretching exercises (similar to the preoperative regimen) are reinsti-

---

*Gilbert A: Personal communication.

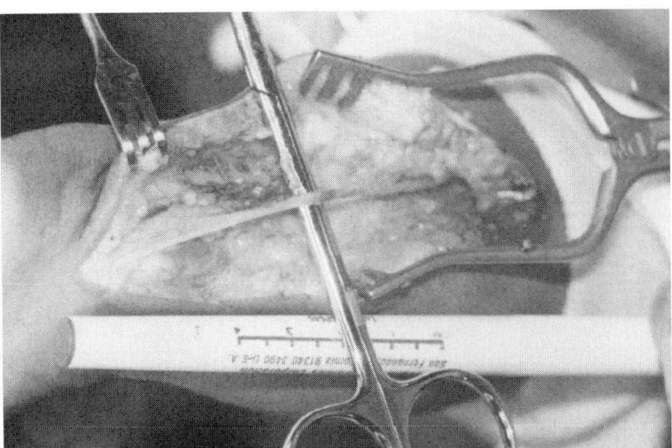

FIGURE 47–9. A longitudinal incision is used from the ankle to the popliteal fossa. Approximately 8 to 9 cm can usually be obtained.

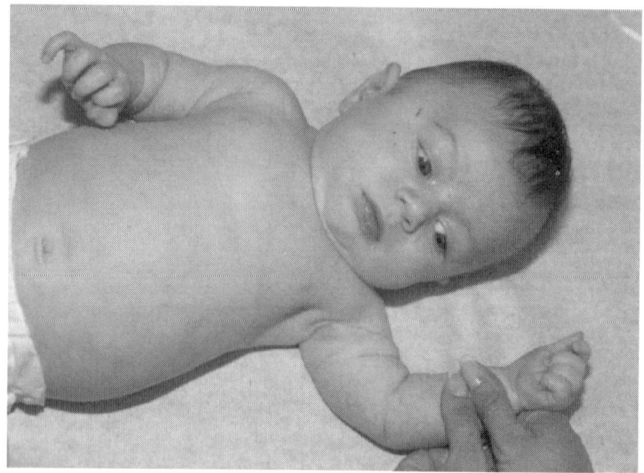

FIGURE 47–10. With every diaper change, the arm should be abducted, and externally rotated, and the hand placed flat on the bed. If the joints are tight, the normal side will elevate.

tuted (Fig. 47–10). At this time, there are no data to support that splints or electrical stimulation have any significant effect, and these methods are not used. Other generalized exercises to increase the awareness of the limb or the strength of the remaining muscles, or both, may be used, but again there are no data to support any benefits from this approach.

RESULTS

Return of weak function may be seen as early as 3 to 4 months in the suprascapular nerve. the biceps generally takes 6 months to function. The return of distal function may require up to 2 years. Certainly tendon transfers should not be considered for at least 2 to 3 years. However, even if function does not return as well as expected, Terzis has shown that limb length discrepancies are much less in babies who have undergone surgical intervention. Gilbert has also shown that his best results (in which arms are almost normal) are in babies who have subsequently had tendon transfers after plexus repair.

In the author's original series, babies treated nonoperatively average almost one grade less in function (according to the Mallet scale) than those treated operatively. To date, these babies have not lost any motor function that was already present. With neurotization, sensation and function can be obtained in the hand even in multiple level avulsions. Babies with C5–C7 lesions can expect to have good shoulder function. These babies, according to Gilbert, will have almost normal shoulders after tendon transfers are performed.

References

Clark LP, Taylor AS, Prout TP: A study on brachial birth palsy. Am J Med Sci *130*:670–707, 1905.

Duchenne GB: De l'électrisation localisée et de son application à la pathologie et à la thérapeutique, 3rd ed. Bailliere, Paris, 1872, p 357.

Erb W: On a characteristic site of injury in the brachial plexus. (Translated by Brody & Wilkins). Arch Neurol *21*:443, 1969.

Fairbank HAT: Birth palsy: Subluxation of shoulder joint in infants and young children. Lancet *1*:217, 1913.

Gjorup L: Obstetrical lesion of the brachial plexus. Acta Neurol Scand *18*(42):9–280, 1966.

Johnson EW Jr: Brachial palsy at birth. International Abstracts of Surgery *111*:409–416, 1960.

L'Episcopo JB: Tendon transplantation in obstetrical paralysis. Am J Surg *25*(1):122, 1934.

Lauwers ME: Le traitement chirurgical de la paralysie obstetrical. J Chir *36*:161, 1930.

Meyer RD, Claussen GC, Oh SJ: Modified trichrome staining technique of the nerve to determine proximal nerve viability. Microsurgery *16*(3):129–132, 1995.

Narakas A: Brachial plexus surgery. Orthop Clin North Am *12*(2):303–323, 1981.

Sever JW: A research on obstetrical paralysis, its causation and anatomy. Boston Med Surg J *174*:327, 1916.

Sharpe W: The operative treatment of brachial plexus paralysis. JAMA *66*:876–881, 1916.

Smillie W: Collection of preternatural cases and observations in midwifery completing the design of illustrating his first volume on that subject, Vol III. London, 1764, p 504.

Tassin JL: Paralysies obstetricales du plexus brachial: Evolution spontanée, résultats des interventions réparatrices précoces. Paris, France, Thesis, Université de Paris, 1983.

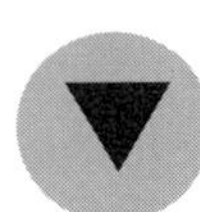

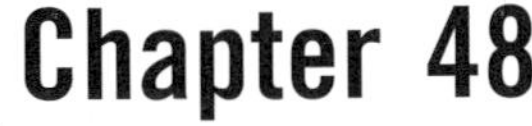

Chapter 48

• Panupan Songcharoen

Neurotization in the Treatment of Brachial Plexus Injuries

The pattern of injury of the brachial plexus has changed gradually over the past 2 decades. The incidence of severe brachial plexus injuries presenting with root avulsions has increased in many centers throughout the world (Allieu et al, 1984; Azze, 1994; Brandt and Mackinnon, 1993; Brunelli, 1982). The higher incidence of this kind of injury is mainly due to the rapidly growing number of motorcycle accidents. The young motorcyclist falls off the vehicle with his or her head forcefully separated from the shoulder, causing cervical nerve root avulsions. This injury has become a great challenge to peripheral nerve surgeons because it cannot be repaired by neurorrhaphy or nerve grafting, it has no possibility of spontaneous recovery, and occurs most often in individuals who are in their productive age. Carlstedt and associates (1995) have tried repairing roots into the ventral spinal cord, which they believed produced an improved result. At present, the only method of surgical treatment of a brachial plexus root avulsion is neurotization.

In general, neurotization means reinnervation of a denervated motor or sensory end-organ. Theoretically, there are five types of neurotization: musculomuscular, cutaneocutaneous, neurocutaneous, neuromuscular, and neuroneural (Narakas, 1985). Only neuroneural and neuromuscular neurotization have been used in the treatment of traumatic lesions of the brachial plexus. The attempt of neuroneural neurotization dates back to 1873, when Letiévant proposed an end-to-side coaptation of the distal stump of an irreparable nerve to a nearby healthy nerve. In 1903, Harris and Low reported the first attempt of intraplexal neurotization by implanting the distal stump of the ruptured C5 spinal nerve into the healthy C6 spinal nerve. In 1913, Tuttle introduced the method of extraplexal neurotization. He neurotized a ruptured upper trunk with branches of the uninjured deep cervical plexus. Since then, different types of neuroneural neurotizations have been used. Yeoman and Seddon first reported intercostal neurotization for the restoration of elbow flexion in 1963. Their technique was later modified and popularized by Tsuyama, Hara, and Nagano (Nagano et al, 1989, 1992). Brunelli (1982, 1984) popularized the use of the motor branch of the deep cervical plexus as a donor for neurotization and the method of neuromuscular neurotization. Allieu et al (1984), Narakas (1984, 1985, 1991), and Songcharoen (1995, 1996) successfully used spinal accessory neurotization on various recipients. In 1989, Gu and colleagues (1989) first reported the use of the phrenic nerve as a donor for motor neurotization of the brachial plexus lesion. He later reported the contralateral C7 nerve root transfer for the brachial plexus root avulsion in 1992.

PRINCIPLES OF NEUROTIZATION AND BASIC CONSIDERATIONS

Although the methods of neurotization have been widely used for decades, in general, the results have been less reliable than nerve grafting. At present, neurotizations are considered to be the last choice to restore the functions of the injured brachial plexus that cannot be operated on with other methods of neural repair. In order to maximize the total function of the patient, the following factors should be considered.

Neurotization involves sacrificing the donor nerve to restore the recipient nerve or muscle function. The expected gain in function must be more important to the affected limb than the function that is lost.

Restoration of motor or sensory function can be accomplished by neurotization. Theoretically, transferring a pure motor donor nerve to a motor recipient nerve gives the best result of motor neurotization, for example, spinal accessory–suprascapular neurotization or deep cervical plexus–suprascapular neurotization. However, not all of the available donor nerves are pure motor nerves. Some donors, such as the intercostal nerve, which is one of the most widely used donor nerves, contains a significant amount of sensory fibers. In this instance, its motor rami should be identified before it is connected to the motor recipient. The method of identification includes intraoperative electrical stimulation (Sugioka et al, 1982), topographical dissection from the motor endplate toward the proximal trunk, and histochemical staining (Carson and Terzis, 1985).

The numbers and types of donor nerve fascicles should be in good proportion to or, if possible, match the requirement of the recipient nerve. The inadequacy of donor fascicles will jeopardize the functional result of the reinnervated organ. A commonly used donor nerve such as the intercostal nerve contains approximately 1300 myelinated nerve fibers, and the spinal accessory nerve 1700 fibers (Narakas, 1984, 1985, 1991). Concerning the recipient side, the musculocutaneous nerve contains approximately 6000 fibers; the suprascapular nerve, 3500 fibers; the axillary nerve, 6500 fibers; the median nerve, 18,000 fibers; the ulnar nerve, 16,000 fibers; and the radial nerve, 19,000 fibers (Narakas, 1984). Assuming that there is no loss of axonal sprouts at the suture site or in the nerve pathway, an ideal motor neurotization of the musculocutaneous nerve that has 60% motor fiber would require two spinal accessory nerves or five intercostal nerves. However, in clinical situations, only one spinal accessory nerve or two intercostal nerves can reinnervate biceps to a functional level (British Medical Research Council gr. III or more) in 70% of patients (Songcharoen et al, 1996; Nagano et al, 1992; Chuang, 1992). This phenomenon is partly due to an increasing number of nerve fibers from the proximal stump at the suture site. This compensatory mechanism of collateral sprouting (Lundborg, 1988) can produce an excess of approximately 30% of the nerve fiber traveling to the distal stump of the nerve. In spite of this mechanism, a significant discrepancy between proximal and distal nerve segments still remains in extraplexal neurotization. Therefore, a meticulous exploration of the whole plexus must be made in order to identify the lesion in the proximal part. If the lesion is found to be extraforaminal, the uninjured nerve fibers in the remaining roots can be used as an intraplexal donor for neurotization. In general, the number of surviving axons in these roots is far greater than the number in all other extraplexal donors.

Neurotization to a recipient at the peripheral part of the plexus such as the musculocutaneous nerve, the suprascapular nerve, or the axillary nerve is more effective than a recipient in the central part such as the posterior cord or the lower trunk. In the instance of a recipient in the central part, the donor fibers are dispersed through branches to several nerves. Scattering of donor fibers over a large area not only makes neurotization insufficient but also causes simultaneous contraction of antagonistic muscles.

The use of nerve fibers from the same donor (C5, C6) or from several donors with the same function (e.g., the third, fourth, fifth, and sixth intercostal nerves) to neurotize several recipients must be well planned in order to avoid antagonistic co-contraction. If two intercostal nerves are neurotized to the musculocutaneous nerve to restore elbow flexion, the other intercostal nerves should not be connected to the radial nerve, which controls elbow extension.

The motor neurotization should not be aimed toward the restoration of complicated functions. Because most of the available donor nerves control relatively simple functions of shoulder elevation or thorax expansion, it is impractical to use them to control sophisticated hand function. Apart from several peripheral factors, the success of motor neurotization depends largely on the convertibility of the donor neurons to the new functions.

AVAILABLE DONOR NERVES FOR NEURONEURAL NEUROTIZATION

Spinal Accessory Nerve

The spinal accessory, or the eleventh cranial nerve, arises from two separate origins. One origin is in medulla oblongata (cranial part); the other origin is in cervical spinal cord (spinal part). Only the spinal portion of the nerve is used in neurotization of the brachial plexus. This portion of the nerve is purely motor. It supplies the sternocleidomastoid and trapezius muscles. It leaves the cranial cavity through the jugular foramen and extends into the neck. It lies obliquely downward under the posterior belly of the digastric. It pierces or lies close to the deep surface of the sternocleidomastoid muscle and supplies it. It runs obliquely downward underneath the cervical fascia in the posterior

triangle of the neck and gives off 2 to 3 muscular branches for the upper trapezius. It then passes under and supplies the middle and lower portions of the muscle in conjunction with branches of the cervical plexus. Even though the trapezius muscle is dually innervated, the spinal accessory nerve should be transected for neurotization after it gives off the first one or two branches, in order to minimize denervation of the trapezius muscle. At this level, the spinal accessory nerve usually contains 1300 to 1600 myelinated nerve fibers.

The spinal accessory nerve can be transferred to a number of different recipients. In the author's experience with 270 spinal accessory neurotizations, the musculocutaneous, axillary, and suprascapular nerves have been successfully neurotized. The percentages of useful motor recovery (MRC grade III or more) after spinal accessory nerve transfers to suprascapular, musculocutaneous, and axillary nerves are 80%, 74%, and 60%, respectively. In contrast to Allieu's experience (1984), the suprascapular nerve seems to be the best recipient for spinal accessory neurotization, in the author's opinion. The spinal accessory nerve can be directly transferred to the suprascapular nerve without using an intermediate nerve graft. The direct nerve coaptation not only reduces axonal sprout loss at suture sites or in the nerve graft but also shortens regeneration distance and recovery time. In patients with good results from spinal accessory suprascapular neurotization, the shoulder abduction of 70 degrees, flexion of 60 degrees, and external rotation of 30 degrees are usually obtained. The musculocutaneous nerve is almost equally as good as a recipient (Fig. 48–1). Its main drawbacks are, first, the necessity for interposition nerve graft. Although Kotani and associates (1972) were able to make a direct coaptation of the spinal accessory nerve and the lateral cord by elevating the shoulder to the neck, the method was found to be impractical. The other drawback of using the musculocutaneous nerve is the mixture of both motor and sensory fibers within the same recipient. The donor motor sprouts from the spinal accessory nerve are partly diverted

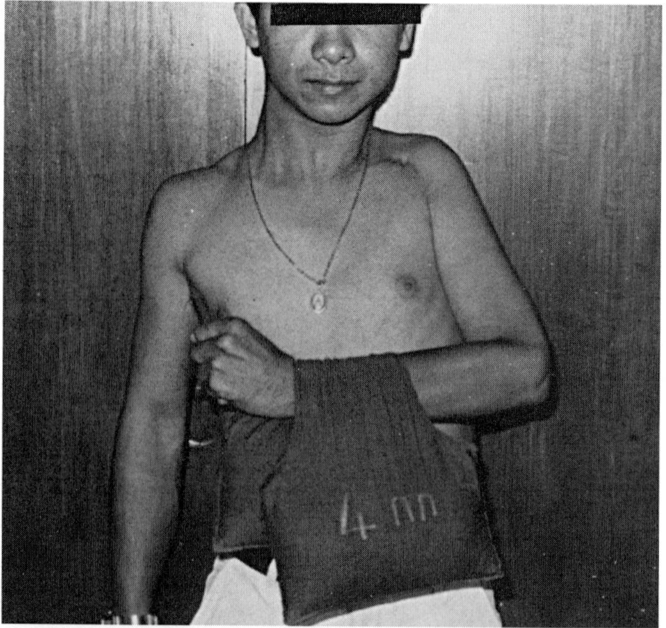

FIGURE 48–1. Three years after the spinal accessory musculocutaneous neurotization. The patient could lift a 4-kg weight from 0 to 90 degrees elbow flexion.

to sensory receptors through the lateral cutaneous nerve of the forearm. To prevent the motor fiber loss, a much longer intermediate graft is needed in between the spinal accessory nerve and the motor branch of the musculocutaneous nerve. The other alternative in dealing with motor fiber loss is rerouting all these fibers back by performing a direct neuromuscular neurotization of the lateral cutaneous nerve of the forearm to the biceps muscle (Brandt and Mackinnon, 1993). The best result in the author's series of a spinal accessory musculocutaneous neurotization allowed patients to lift a weight of 5 kg to 90 degrees of flexion of elbow and 2 kg to 90 degrees of flexion for 100 times. The spinal accessory axillary neurotization is a moderately good alternative for the spinal accessory suprascapular neurotization for restoration of shoulder abduction. The patient can have 60 degrees of shoulder abduction and 45 degrees of flexion without external rotation. An intermediate nerve graft is also needed. Neurotizations of the spinal accessory nerve to the radial and the median nerve give an unsatisfactory result.

Intercostal Nerves

Intercostal nerves are the anterior branches of the thoracic spinal nerves. An intercostal nerve contains both motor and sensory fibers. The percentage of motor fibers ranges from 15% to 45% along the course of the nerve (Freilinger et al, 1978). The anterior ramus contains approximately 3000 to 4000 myelinated fibers, and each intercostal nerve carries a different amount of motor and sensory fibers. The first and sometimes part of the second intercostal nerves are parts of the plexus. The second intercostal nerve contains mostly sensory fibers and should not be used for motor neurotization. The third and fourth intercostal nerves contain a significant amount of motor fiber. The fibers in the fifth and sixth intercostal nerves are mostly motor fibers. They can be effectively used as donors for motor neurotization. Their sensory branches, which innervate the breast, must be preserved. The lower intercostal nerves (seventh to the eleventh) innervate intercostal and abdominal muscles. They should be alternately harvested to minimize massive denervation of the abdominal muscles.

The intercostal neurotization can be performed by several methods. The point of intercostal nerve resection, which determines the necessity of intermediate nerve graft, varies in each method. In the author's experience, the method proposed by Tsuyama and Hara (1972) is the most practical one and gives the best result. In their technique, the third and fourth intercostal nerves are exposed and mobilized from the axilla to the tip of the rib. The nerves are cut at the costochondral junction and passed subcutaneously to the proximal part of the arm, where they are anastomosed directly to the musculocutaneous nerve nearest to its motor point without using nerve graft. The intercostal nerve can be transferred to the axillary, radial, median, and ulnar nerves. In the author's experience of 22 intercostal-musculocutaneous neurotizations, 65% of the patients gained a good (MRC III or more) biceps recovery. This figure is comparable to the other series. The average time to an MRC gr. III motor recovery is 12 months. At that time, the patients with the best recovery could lift a weight of 5 kg to 90 degrees of flexion. During the first 2 years after the operation, biceps

function synchronizes with the respiratory cycle. Although more action potentials are detected on inspiration, the voluntary biceps contraction occurs at the same time as an expiratory motion (Lundborg, 1988; Takahashi, 1983). In the third postoperative year, voluntary biceps control is usually attained but involuntary contraction while coughing and sneezing still persists. Sensory recovery in the musculocutaneous nerve area is also obtained. During the first 4 years, sensation is perceived only in the chest. Later, some sensation is also noted in the neurotized area. The results of intercostal nerve transfers to the other recipients are generally much poorer. Nagano and co-workers (1989) reported only one patient with an MRC III and four with an MRC II motor recovery of extensor carpi radialis out of 30 intercostal radial neurotizations (Lundborg, 1988; Nagano et al, 1989). Kawai and colleagues (1988) reported on five patients who had regained a fair motor recovery (MRC II–III) of wrist flexion out of 15 intercostal median neurotizations (by using three intercostal nerves). Dolenc (1987) reported on two patients with a MRC III recovery of intrinsic muscles of the hand after intercostal nerves were transferred for avulsion of the root C8 and T1.

Phrenic Nerve

The phrenic nerve originates mainly from C4 nerve root, with additional branches arising from the C3 and C5 nerve roots. The main trunk of the phrenic nerve was formed at a point midway between the mandible and the clavicle. It runs downward on the scalene anterior muscle posterolateral to the internal jugular vein. At the root of the neck, it passes in front of the subclavian artery and behind the vein. It then enters the thorax and the mediastinum to reach the diaphragm. The phrenic nerve contains both efferent and afferent fibers. It innervates the diaphragm, the diaphragmatic pleura, the pericardium, and the diaphragmatic peritoneum. An accessory phrenic nerve is occasionally present in 25% to 38% of cases (Narakas, 1991). It may arise from C3–C4, C5, C5–C6 nerve roots, or from the nerve to the subclavius muscle. The accessory phrenic nerve usually joins the main nerve in the distal part of the neck or in the thorax.

Before a phrenic nerve transfer is considered, diaphragmatic and pulmonary function must be assessed. The impairment of the hemidiaphragmatic movement is an absolute contraindication for a phrenic neurotization. In patients who sustain a severe chest injury with multiple rib fractures, the pulmonary function must be carefully evaluated. Even though the diaphragmatic movement is still intact, the use of the phrenic nerve in these patients will greatly jeopardize pulmonary function because respiratory movement depends mainly on the diaphragm. In these patients, the phrenic neurotization should be delayed until the fractures are well healed. Early postoperative restriction of pulmonary function can be seen in patients who undergo both phrenic and intercostal neurotization in the same setting (Gu et al, 1989). Although the respiratory function recovers, this procedure should be avoided. Phrenic neurotization is contraindicated in young infants, owing to the fact that the infant who was born with diaphragmatic paralysis usually had severe respiratory complications. In the author's experience with 30 phrenic neurotizations in 29 adults and one 6-year-old boy, during the 2-year follow-up period, none of the patients had any clinical signs or symptoms of respiratory insufficiency or postoperative respiratory complications. Postoperatively, 27% of the patients had normal diaphragmatic movement with normal pulmonary function tests, and 73% of the patients had diminished pulmonary function that gradually recovered after 8 months. In the author's experience, the phrenic nerve has been successfully neurotized to the musculocutaneous, axillary, and suprascapular nerve. The percentages of the useful motor recovery (MRC gr. III or more) after the phrenic nerve was transferred to the suprascapular, musculocutaneous, and axillary nerves were 75%, 66%, and 66%, respectively.

In the author's opinion, the suprascapular nerve is the best recipient for phrenic neurotization. This procedure can generally be performed without an interposition nerve graft. Patients with good results obtain 70 degrees of shoulder abduction with 30 degrees of external rotation. The average time of MRC III motor recovery was 8 months. The phrenic nerve transfers to the axillary nerve, and the musculocutaneous nerve needs an intermediate nerve graft. Patients with good results from phrenic axillary neurotization obtain 70 degrees of shoulder abduction and forward flexion, whereas patients with good results of phrenic musculocutaneous neurotization can lift a 2-kg weight to 90 degrees of flexion. The activity in the recovered muscle synchronizes with the inspiratory motion. The involuntary movement of the neurotized biceps muscle gradually changes to a voluntary movement after 2 years.

Although the phrenic nerve has been successfully used as a donor for neurotization, a long-term follow-up of changes in the patients' pulmonary function is still needed.

The Fifth to Sixth Cervical Spinal Nerve Stump

In complete brachial plexus paralysis with avulsion of C6–T1 or C7–T1 roots, the extraforaminally ruptured C5 or C5 and C6 roots can be used as donors for neurotization. The atrophied C7 root is directly sutured to the C6 stump in addition to the grafts connecting C6 to its distal stump. Because a normal C5 or C6 root contains a much larger amount of nerve fibers than other available extraplexal donors, this type of nerve transfer usually yields a higher percentage of motor recovery. The most frequently encountered problem with this method of intraplexal neurotization is a co-contraction of the antagonistic muscles. To reduce co-contraction, the author uses a longer intermediate graft to connect the available donor stumps (C5 or C6) to the recipient nerve or motor branches of the nerve at the peripheral part of the plexus. By this method, the fibers from the donor go directly to the designated muscle or the group of muscles with synergistic functions. In the author's experience of performing 16 plexoplexal neurotizations, 12 patients had gained more than MCR III motor recovery after 2 years. The successfully neurotized recipients were the posterior cord, suprascapular nerve, musculocutaneous nerve, axillary nerve, and median nerve. Another commonly encountered problem of plexoplexal neurotization is the method used to determine whether the ruptured root stump is appropriate to be a donor. Because the amount of donor axon in the proximal stump is a vital factor to a successful neurotization, the

quantitative evaluation of a viable axon in the donor stump should be carried out intraoperatively. Although histochemical staining has been proved to be useful, the method has not been widely used owing to its difficulties. At present, the use of the microscopic appearance of the proximal stump seems to be the most practical approach to this problem. The plexoplexal neurotization can be performed in combination with other extraplexal neurotizations in treating complete brachial plexus injury with a highly successful result.

Cervical Plexus

The cervical plexus is formed by branches arising from the anterior rami of C1–C4 nerves. According to Brunelli, the cervical plexus has eight branches: four motor and four sensory. The motor branches contain an average of 4090 fibers, which innervate the sternocleidomastoid, the rhomboid, the trapezius, the levator scapulae, and the deep cervical muscles. The sensory branches contain an average of 3250 fibers, which innervate an area of skin along the ear down to the acromion. Brunelli first neurotized the C5 and C6 root with all the available fibers from the cervical plexus without success. Later he found that a better result can be achieved by selective neurotizations of terminal branches of the brachial plexus, such as the suprascapular and the musculocutaneous nerve (Brunelli and Monini, 1984). The sensory neurotization can also be performed by transferring the supra-acromial and the supraclavicular branches to the median nerve. The author's experience with three cervical plexus musculocutaneous neurotizations was disappointing. None of the patients gained a MRC III motor recovery. Brunelli reported that all of the 18 patients who had motor neurotization of the cervical plexus to the suprascapular and the musculocutaneous had active shoulder abduction and elbow flexion. Ten out of 15 sensory neurotizations of the median nerve had some degree of protective sensation. He concluded that, in his experience, the cervical plexus neurotization yielded a better result than the intercostal neurotization (Brunelli and Monini, 1984). The combined use of motor branches of the cervical plexus and the spinal accessory nerve as donors for neurotization must be carefully planned in order to avoid the risk of denervation of the scapulothoracic muscles.

Long Thoracic Nerve

The long thoracic nerve arises from C5, C6, C7, and occasionally, C4 nerve roots as they leave the intervertebral foramina. It is also called Bell's nerve. The contributing rami pierce the scalene medius, and pass in front of the scalene, behind the cords of the brachial plexus, and downward over the first rib. It enters the axilla between the serratus anterior and the axillary artery. The nerve continues downward and pierces the axillary surface of the serratus anterior muscle to supply it. The use of the long thoracic nerve in brachial plexus injury is rather limited. The long thoracic nerve cannot be used in upper root avulsions because it originates from these roots. Only one or two of its terminal rami can be used to avoid a complete paralysis of the serratus anterior, which leads to a gross dissociation of scapulothoracic motion.

Seventh Cervical Nerve Root from the Contralateral Side

In 1991, Brunelli observed that an isolated avulsion of the C7 nerve root produced only a minimal degree of morbidity in the affected limb. In 1986, Gu first transferred a C7 nerve root from the contralateral side to treat a completely avulsed brachial plexus. Theoretically, this surgical procedure greatly helps plexal surgeons solve the problem of donor axon inadequacy because the C7 root contains 18,095 to 40,576 fibers. This amount is far greater than the number of fibers from all other extraplexal donors together. According to Gu, this procedure is indicated in patients with root avulsion injury when other donor nerve cannot be used, or offer poor material. The contralateral normal C7 nerve root can be severed at the trunk or at the origin of the posterior or the anterior division. The donor stump is connected via a vascularized ulnar nerve graft taken from the affected side to the median, the radial, or the musculocutaneous nerve of the injured plexus. Although Gu's early result of motor and sensory recovery in 49 patients seems to be encouraging, a number of patients have some degree of donor-side motor or sensory deficiency. This deficiency includes muscular weakness (latissimus dorsi, triceps brachii, flexor digitorum communis, and flexor carpi ulnaris), reduction of grip and pinch strength, and numbness and pain in the fingers. Gu reported that all of the deficiencies were only temporary. They completely disappeared within a few weeks after surgery. In the author's early experience of two cases, triceps weakness and reduction of endurance of the donor limbs persisted after the fourth month after surgery. In the author's opinion, the contralateral C7 neurotization can be selectively used in patients who sustain a complete root avulsion brachial plexus injury with concomitant spinal accessory nerve, intercostal nerve, phrenic nerve, and cervical plexus injury (Fig. 48–2). This combined nerve lesion can occasionally be seen in a person involved in a severe motorcycle accident, resulting in neck and chest injury. The author would perform the contralateral C7 neurotization only after the preoperative evaluation of the loss of C7 function. The evaluation was performed by recording the neurological changes after an open selective normal C7 block with bupivacaine (Marcaine). If the patient has significant neurological loss, the operation is not carried out.

NEUROMUSCULAR NEUROTIZATION (DIRECT MUSCULAR NEUROTIZATION)

In addition to neuroneural neurotization, neuromuscular neurotization, or direct muscular neurotization, has found its role in the treatment of brachial plexus injury.

Neuromuscular neurotization is a procedure in which healthy nerve fibers are directly implanted into a denervated muscle. Experimental studies in animals were successfully performed by Heineke, Steindler, and Elsberg. In 1982, Brunelli reported successful clinical cases using this procedure. Originally, neuromuscular neurotization was indicated only in patients who had sustained avulsion injury of terminal muscular branches from muscle. Later it was used to enhance recovery of biceps function in brachial plexus reconstruction. Brandt and Mackinnon (1993) found that nearly one half of the fibers entering the musculocutaneous nerve terminate in the lateral antebrachial cutaneous nerve. They reported successful results with biceps renervation in brachial plexus injury by combining neuroneural (medial pectoral to musculocutaneous) and neuromuscular (lateral antebrachial cutaneous nerve directly into biceps) neurotization in the same operation. In the author's experience with four cases of neuromuscular neurotization, the lateral antebrachial cutaneous nerve was implanted into the biceps muscle 3 years after the initial operation in which nerve grafting or neuroneural neurotization to the musculocutaneous was performed with no or poor results. Two out of four patients had MRC III biceps recovery within 6 months. Although it is far too early to make a conclusion on the effectiveness of direct muscular neurotization in brachial plexus injury, early results of these procedures were encouraging.

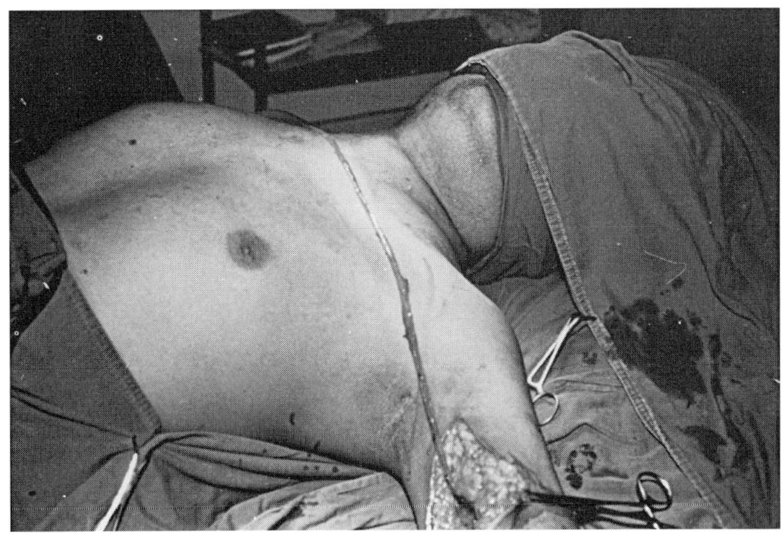

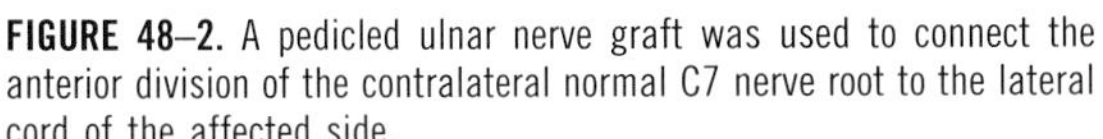

FIGURE 48–2. A pedicled ulnar nerve graft was used to connect the anterior division of the contralateral normal C7 nerve root to the lateral cord of the affected side.

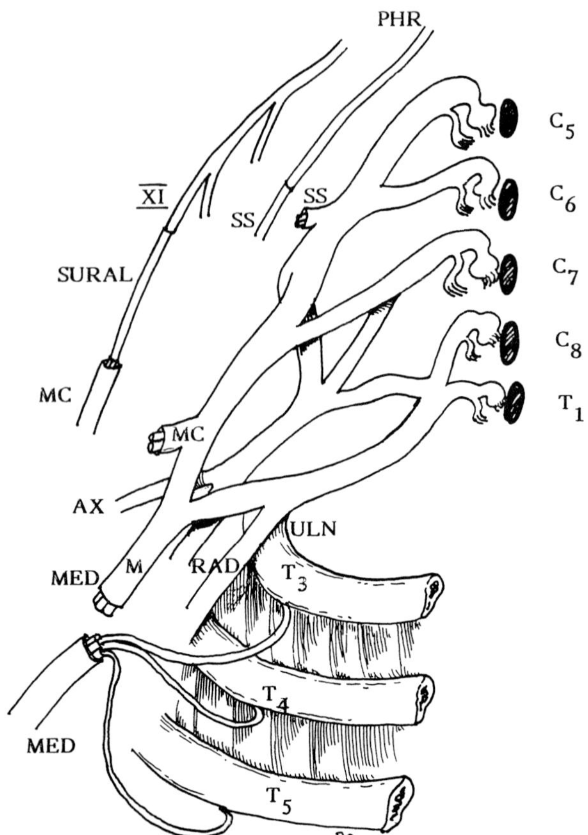

FIGURE 48–3. Avulsion of C5 to T1. The affected extremity function can be partially restored by spinal accessory–musculocutaneous neurotization for elbow flexion, phrenic-suprascapular neurotization for shoulder abduction, and intercostal-median neurotization for wrist flexion and palmar sensation.

CONCLUSION

Neurotizations have given some hope to a previously hopeless patient with a nerve root avulsion injury (Fig. 48–3). Certain types of neurotizations provide predictable results in the restoration of nonsophisticated functions. The selective combination of neurotizations gives a moderate degree of shoulder and elbow control. Even though some wrist and finger movements can occasionally be achieved by the current method of neurotization, the result of restoration of useful hand function is still far from satisfactory. The use of intraplexal and contralateral plexal neurotization, along with the better understanding of central-peripheral functional integration, may provide purposeful hand function in the future.

References

Allieu Y, Privat JM, Bonnel F: Paralysis in root avulsion of the brachial plexus. Neurotization by spinal accessory nerve. Clin Plast Surg *11*:133–136, 1984.

Azze RJ, Mattar R, Ferreira MC, Starck R, Canedo AC: Extraplexual neurotization of brachial plexus. Microsurgery *15*:28–32, 1994.

Brandt KE, Mackinnon SE: A technique for maximizing biceps recovery in brachial plexus reconstruction. J Hand Surg *18*:726–733, 1993.

Brunelli G: Direct neurotization of severely damaged muscles. J Hand Surg *7*:572–579, 1982.

Brunelli GA, Brunelli GR: The fourth type of brachial plexus lesion. J Hand Surg (Br) *16*(5):492–494, 1991.

Brunelli G, Monini L: Neurotization of avulsed roots of brachial plexus by means of anterior nerves of cervical plexus. Clin Plast Surg *11*:149–152, 1984.

Carlstedt T, Grane P, Hallin RG, Norén G: Return of function after spinal cord implantation of avulsed spinal nerve roots. Lancet *346*:1323–1325, 1995.

Carson KA, Terzis JK: Carbonic anhydrase histochemistry: A potential diagnostic method for peripheral nerve repair. Clin Plast Surg *12*:227–229, 1985.

Chuang DCC, Yeh MC, Wei FC: Intercostal nerve transfer of the musculocutaneous nerve in avulsed brachial plexus injuries: Evaluation of 66 patients. J Hand Surg *17*:822–828, 1992.

Dolenc VV: Intercostal neurotization of the peripheral nerves in avulsion plexus injuries. *In* Terzis JK (ed): Microreconstruction of nerve injury. Philadelphia, W. B. Saunders, 1987, pp 425–434.

Elsberg CA: Experiments on motor nerve regeneration and the direct neurotisation of paralyzed muscles by their own and foreign nerves. Science *45*:318–320, 1917.

Freilinger G, Holle J, Sulzbruger SC: Distribution of motor and sensory fibers in the intercostal nerves. Plast Reconstr Surg *62*:240–244, 1978.

Gu YD, Wu MM, Zhen YL, Zhao JA, Zhang GM, Chen DS, Yan JG, Cheng XM: Phrenic nerve transfer for brachial plexus motor neurotization. Microsurgery *10*:287–289, 1989.

Gu YD, Zhang GM, Chen DS, Yan JG, Cheng XM, Chen L: Seventh cervical nerve root transfer from the contralateral healthy side for treatment of brachial plexus root avulsion. J Hand Surg *17*B:518–521, 1992.

Harris W, Low VW: On the importance of accurate muscular analysis in lesions of the brachial plexus and the treatment of Erb's palsy and infantile paralysis of the upper extremity by cross-union of nerve roots. BMJ *2*:1035–1038, 1903.

Heineke D: Die direkte einpflanzung des nerven in den muskel. Zentralbl Chir *41*:465–467, 1914.

Kawai H, Kawabata H, Masada K, Ono K, Yamamoto K, Tsuyuguchi Y, Tada K: Nerve repairs for traumatic brachial plexus palsy with root avulsion. Clin Orthop *237*:75–86, 1988.

Kotani PT, Matsuda H, Suzuki T: Trial surgical procedures of nerve transfers to avulsion injuries of plexus brachialis. Excerpta Med (Int 12th Congress Series *291*):348–350, 1972.

Letiévant JJE: Traité des sections nerveuses. Paris, Ballière, 1875.

Lundborg G: Nerve Injury and Repair. Edinburgh, Churchill Livingstone, 1988.

Nagano A, Ochiai N, Okinaga S: Restoration of elbow flexion in root lesions of brachial plexus injuries. J Hand Surg *17*:815–821, 1992.

Nagano A, Tsuyama N, Ochiai N, Hara T, Takahashi M: Direct nerve crossing with the intercostal nerve to treat avulsion injuries of the brachial plexus. J Hand Surg *14*:980–985, 1989.

Narakas AO: Neurotization in the treatment of brachial plexus injuries. *In* Gelberman RH (ed): Operative Nerve Repair and Reconstruction. Philadelphia, J. B. Lippincott Company, 1991, pp 1329–1358.

Narakas AO: Neurotization or nerve transfer in traumatic brachial plexus lesions. *In* Tubiana R (ed): The Hand, Vol 1. Philadelphia, W. B. Saunders Company, 1985, pp 656–683.

Narakas AO: Thoughts on neurotization or nerve transfers in irreparable nerve lesions. Clin Plast Surg *11*:153–159, 1984.

Seddon H: Nerve grafting. J Bone Joint Surg *45*:447–461, 1963.

Songcharoen P: Brachial plexus injury in Thailand: a report of 520 cases. Microsurgery *16*:35–39, 1995.

Songcharoen P, Mahaisavariya B, Chotigavanich C: Spinal accessory neurotization for restoration of elbow flexion and avulsion injuries of the brachial plexus. J Hand Surg *21*:387–390, 1996.

Songcharoen P, Chotigavanich C: Brachial plexus injury: A report of 289 neurotizations. J Jpn Orthop Assoc *68*:S513, 1994.

Steindler A: Direct neurotization of paralyzed muscle. Further studies of the question of direct implantation. Am J Orthop Surg *14*:707–719, 1916.

Sugioka H, Tsuyama N, Hara T, Nagano A, Tachibana S, Ochiai N: Investigation of brachial plexus injuries by intraoperative corticol somatosensory evoked potentials. Arch Orthop Trauma Surg *99*:143–151, 1982.

Takahashi M: Studies on conversion of motor function in intercostal nerves crossing for complete brachial plexus injuries of root avulsion type. J Jpn Orthop Assoc *57*:139, 1983.

Tsuyama N, Hara T: Intercostal nerve transfer in the treatment of brachial plexus injury of root avulsion type. Excerpta Med (Int 12th Congress Series 291):351–353, 1972.

Tuttle H: Exposure of the brachial plexus with nerve transplantation. JAMA *61*:51, 1913.

Yeoman PM, Seddon HJ: Brachial plexus injuries: Treatment of the flail arm. J Bone Joint Surg [Br] *43*:493–500, 1961.

Reconstruction of the Shoulder and Elbow Following Brachial Plexus Injury

The shoulder and elbow provide the "reach" without which "grasp" is impossible. When loss of power or control of these joints due to a nerve lesion occurs, the individual's ability to manipulate the environment is severely compromised. The surgical literature devoted to reconstruction of the limb under such circumstances is large and varied. Until the second half of this century, the most common cause of such incapacity was poliomyelitis. The tremendous experience gained from patients with this disease allows for transfer of many of the technical considerations to the management of patients with brachial plexus injuries.

However, there are important differences in the two groups that require further consideration in the treatment alternatives for the brachial plexus injury. The functional loss in the upper extremities of the brachial plexus–injured patients is usually greater than those that occur with polio because of the lack of sensation and proprioceptive feedback in those with brachial plexus injuries. Although both conditions may produce profound paralysis, the brachial plexus injury tends to conform to one or two patterns in an "all-or-nothing" distribution. In general, the shoulder and elbow are paralyzed by postganglionic lesions of C5 and C6. If the C7 root is included, then a functional radial palsy results in addition. The trapezius, being cranially innervated, is almost always spared, even in severe traction injuries to the brachial plexus. The serratus anterior, because it comes from root collaterals of C5, C6, and C7, is usually preserved unless the patient has sustained an unusual series of preganglionic avulsions of the upper roots or the long thoracic nerve has sustained direct injury.

TIMING OF PERIPHERAL RECONSTRUCTION

Patients with brachial plexus injuries acquired in adulthood have usually lost the function of the limb that is crucial to their established way of life. The timing of their peripheral reconstruction takes on an urgency usually not present in those with obstetrical palsies.

Following the initial assessment in adult plexus injuries, as accurate a prognosis for functional recovery as can be formulated must be conveyed to the patient. In closed traction injuries, it is unusual for preganglionic root avulsion of C5 and C6 to occur, and although it may happen, it is more common in the lower roots. The combination of clinical examination, electrodiagnostic techniques and CT myelography can clarify this issue, whereupon peripheral reconstruction can begin immediately if the roots are avulsed and there is enough preserved function to allow for tendon transfer. Neurotization may also be considered as an alteration in such cases. Because the neurological reconstruction of these lesions has been discussed elsewhere in this volume, we will assume either that neural continuity cannot be restored surgically, or that sufficient time has elapsed so that spontaneous recovery is unlikely to occur. This judgment is based on carefully documented recovery statistics (Barnes, 1949; Bonney, 1959; Leffert and Seddon, 1965) compared with regular clinical and electromyographic examination of the particular patient under consideration. In general, if functional shoulder control is not present at 1 year after the injury, it is unlikely to improve with time. For the elbow, and especially after nerve suture or graft in the supraclavicular fossa, useful recovery may not be appreciated for as long as 1 1/2 years. With these time periods in mind, one may proceed with reconstruction, according to the needs of the individual patient. In the case of the growing child, not only must the possibility of evolving bone and joint deformity be anticipated but also whatever normal growth is possible must not be thwarted by ill-conceived or ill-executed surgery.

THE SHOULDER

Tendon Transfers

Although a number of ingenious tendon transfer procedures have been described for the treatment of the paralytic shoulder due to polio, they are usually not applicable to the adult traumatic brachial plexus patient (Saha, 1967). Most of the patients that are seen with upper trunk traction lesions have completely lost the function of both the deltoid and the rotator cuff because they share the same root innervation. Although it may be possible to reinnervate the suprascapular nerve or the axillary nerve by means of nerve grafting, there are usually insufficient axons available to attain a level of function of the muscles they innervate to allow for adequate control of abduction and external rotation of the weighted limb in activities of daily living. If neurological reconstruction succeeds in restoring some power of contraction of the deltoid in the absence of rotator cuff function, the shoulder will be weak in abduction or forward flexion. If the limb is positioned in forward flexion to assist the sound side, as is often required, it will tend to rotate medially even under its own weight, thus compromising its mission. For these reasons, the results of nerve grafting to restore function of the shoulder must be critically examined in terms of the criteria for a successful result. A patient who reportedly can voluntarily reduce the interior subluxation of the glenohumeral joint, or who "has some abduction" should not be considered as having attained a satisfactory functional result.

Despite reports of successful transfer of the trapezius to the shaft of the humerus, the complex nature of shoulder function mitigates against use of this technique. In 1990, Aziz and associates, reported on 27 such patients and advocated trapezius transfer as an alternative to fusion. However, despite the fact that the preoperative subluxation was corrected, these patients averaged 45 degrees of abduction postoperatively. Because multiple force couples control the glenohumeral joint, one muscle cannot realistically be expected to replace or partially substitute for them. This point was emphasized by Itoh when he reported on the use of latissimus transfer to replace the paralyzed anterior deltoid (Itoh et al, 1987).

In those patients in whom partial function of the scapulohumeral musculature remains, tendon transfer of adjacent muscles may provide gratifying results. As described by Harmon (1950), the procedure may be adapted to use in the brachial plexus–injured patient. The clavicular origin of the pectoralis major is moved laterally to the acromion, and any intact part of the posterior or middle deltoid is rotated anteriorly. The long head of the triceps may be brought to the acromion posteriorly and the short or long head of biceps

to the acromion. These transfers augment shoulder flexion, extension, and abduction. The teres major and latissimus dorsi are rerouted posterolaterally for lateral rotation. Eight such patients were reported by Leffert and Pess (1988) (Fig. 49–1). Most of the patients had an individual and distinct muscle picture preoperatively, so that the combinations of transfers varied according to what was available. At follow-up, the results were classified as good in three, whereas five were improved. Of the five patients who were improved following their surgery, two required reoperations to adjust muscle tension and to achieve their final result. Nevertheless, these patients had mobile shoulders that added appreciably to their function.

However, it must be emphasized that the patient with a birth palsy who is seen as an adolescent or an adult has had the factor of growth to modify the deformity. Thus, important considerations of static and dynamic nature must be entertained.

Patients with obstetrical palsy involving the upper trunk or C5-6 have deficient shoulder abduction and external rotation, which may result in internal rotation-adduction contractures and skeletal deformity with growth. The anterior structures that are contracted are released or lengthened as needed (usually pectoralis major and subscapularis), and the latissimus dorsi and teres major are then transferred posterolaterally to convert their function from medial rotators and adductors to lateral rotators (Chen, 1990; D'Aubigne et al, 1956; Freund et al, 1986; L'Episcopo, 1939; Zachary, 1957) (Fig. 49–2). It is most important to obtain preoperative radiographs to verify that there is no evidence of shoulder subluxation, because this problem would necessitate preliminary humeral osteotomy. The use of osteotomy as a means of

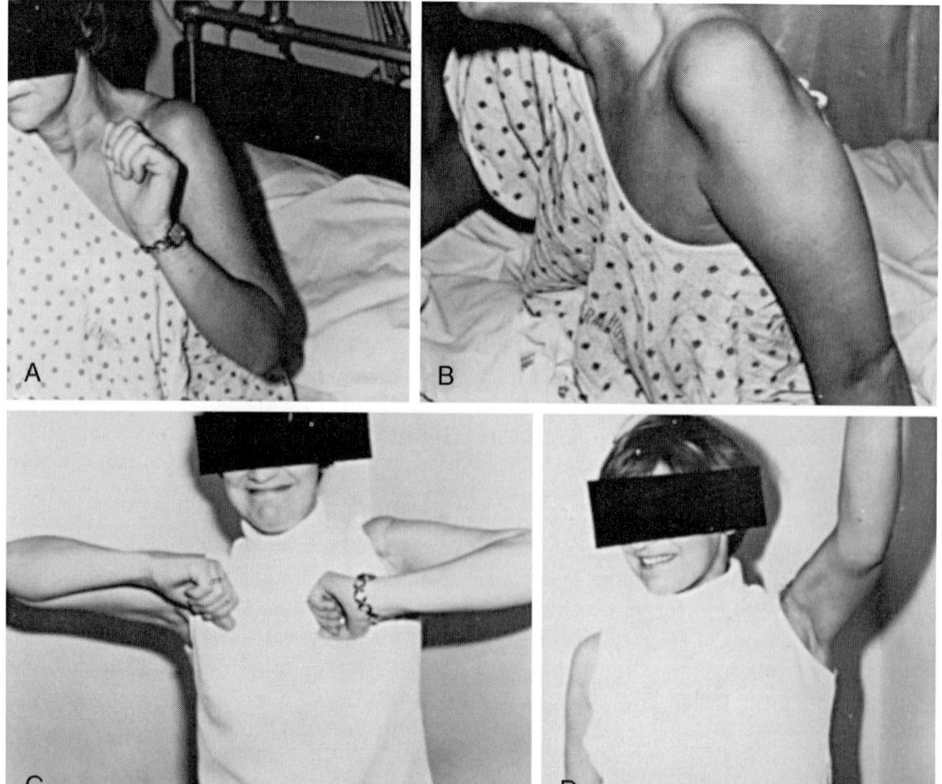

FIGURE 49–1. Shoulder paralysis due to a partial laceration of the upper trunk of the left brachial plexus. *A,* Elbow flexion is possible but no abduction. *B,* Only the posterior deltoid is intact. The middle and anterior portions are atrophic. *C* and *D,* Function following extensive tendon transfer, which included (1) posterior deltoid rotated anteriorly to the position of the middle deltoid; (2) posterolateral transfer of the latissimus dorsi and teres major; (3) transfer of the long head of the biceps to the anterior acromion; and (4) transfer of the origin of the clavicular head of the pectoralis major laterally to the acromion.

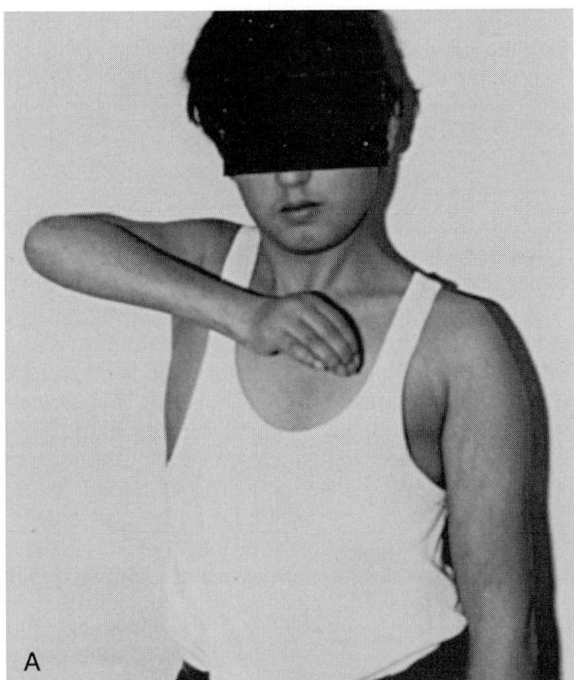

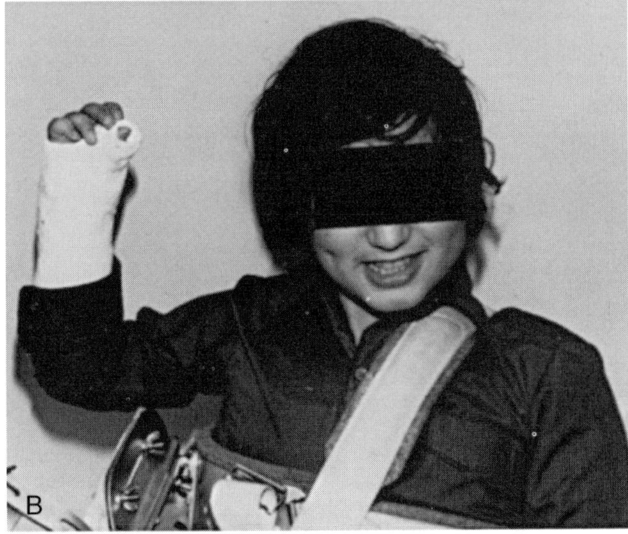

FIGURE 49–2. *A,* Preoperative appearance of abduction and attempt at lateral rotation. *B,* Following Zachary's tendon transfer of latissimus dorsi and teres major.

restoring function in children with external rotation weakness has been reported on favorably by Goddard and Fixsen (1984).

In my opinion, children younger than the age of 4 years are usually too young to cooperate in the postoperative program of rehabilitative exercises so that their surgery should be delayed. Fortunately, the improvement in availability of physical therapeutic services and appreciation of the need to maintain passive range of motion in the shoulders of children with obstetrical palsy have reduced the incidence of established contractures requiring surgical correction. Nevertheless, for children with very severe weakness of lateral rotators, the need for augmentation of this function may dictate tendon transfer even if contractures have not developed with growth and development.

Of 10 such patients reported by Leffert and Pess (1988),

there were seven rated as good and three as improved at final evaluation.

Arthrodesis of the Shoulder

As stated, the adult patient with a flail or paretic shoulder due to a lesion at C5–6 usually has weakness of lateral rotators of the humerus and deltoid as well as the clavicular pectoralis major and elbow flexors. Because of the predictable results of shoulder fusion in this group with few alternate motors and shoulder instability, arthrodesis remains the most often used technique at this time in our clinic.

Fusion is, ordinarily, a dependable salvage procedure for these cases of paralysis. It provides a relatively strong shoulder girdle, albeit limited in range, and it is durable. The pain that patients experience because of unrelieved paralytic subluxation of the glenohumeral joint will usually be relieved by arthrodesis, but many patients have pain that is neurogenic, and as such, some will continue to have pain even after a bony fusion has been obtained (Richards et al, 1985). Although the procedure is lasting, it is also practically irreversible, and the motion that is obtained can be awkward. Errors in positioning at the time of surgery may result in permanently poor position if internal fixation is used, as it usually is. Some patients may not be able to sleep on the fused side, and there is a predisposition to fracture if the humerus is subjected to excessive forces, particularly in torsion.

Obviously, unless there is good scapular control, with an intact trapezius and serratus anterior, the ultimate function of the scapulohumeral complex will be deficient. Fortunately, this is unusual in the uncomplicated case.

The preoperative discussions with the patient should review all of the alternatives, as well as the pros and cons of the procedure. The needs of the individual regarding activities of daily living will influence the final position chosen for fusion, and the postoperative program should be reviewed and be clear to all concerned. It is helpful to arrange a meeting of the prospective fusion patient with someone who has already had the operation so that all issues can be discussed in the absence of the surgeon.

Assuming normal scapular control and sound fusion, all postoperative functions should depend on proper choice of position for the fusion. However, it is not a simple matter to determine. Not only is the optimal position in three planes still undecided but also even the reference points are not always agreed on. In addition, determining the exact position of the fusion at the operating table is still an inexact procedure (Jonsson et al, 1989). One can use the "arm-at-the-side" (a somewhat arbitrary guideline) or the relationship of the axis of the humeral shaft with each of three bony landmarks: the spine of the scapula, its lateral (axillary) border, or the vertebral border. If internal fixation is used at the time of the procedure, then the position at operation is permanent, so the landmarks used for angular measurements should definitely be accessible to the surgeon. The author finds that the vertebral border of the scapula is easily palpable using the posterior approach and has proved to be most convenient.

The position recommended by the Research Committee of the American Orthopaedic Association in 1942 (Barr et al, 1942) requires careful analysis to avoid misinterpretation.

With the patient supine, the arm was placed in the desired degree of abduction, which was 45 degrees to 50 degrees from the vertebral border and forward flexion of 15 degrees to 25 degrees from the plane of the scapula. With the elbow flexed at 90 degrees, the forearm was then vertical. The humerus was then externally rotated 25 to 30 degrees, which leaves the shoulder in 25 degrees of internal rotation when the forward flexed arm is returned to the side. It should be noted that the majority of these patients were children who ultimately lost some of their abduction with growth, because internal fixation was not used at that time. Furthermore, the recommendation never was to fuse the shoulders in external rotation. Nevertheless, the interpretation of this work led to many fusions in a position of excessive abduction. Many patients experienced pain in their periscapular musculature due to the strain when attempting to position the arm at the side. This was noted by Rowe, who, in 1974, redefined the recommended position for shoulder fusion. He suggested using the resting position, with the arm at the side of the body in only 20 degrees of abduction; enough forward flexion, usually 30 degrees, to allow the hand to reach the face with the elbow flexed; and enough internal rotation to allow the patient to reach the midline of the body (usually 40 to 45 degrees). Richards and associates (1985) have recommended a 30-30-30 degree position, whereas Cofield (1985) believed that a range of positions was compatible with satisfactory function.

Although it should be clear that fusion inherently must impose functional compromises on the ultimate range of motion that is obtained postoperatively, the patient should be able to reach the midline in front as well as the back pocket and perineum. In the sagittal plane, the arm should come to the horizontal and thereby allow the hand to reach the head and mouth. At rest, the arm should lie in a naturally appearing position at the side, without causing undue strain on the scapulothoracic musculature or winging of the scapula (Rowe, 1983) (Fig. 49–3). The author's own experience has been that as long as excessive abduction is avoided, then the pain of muscular strain is not a problem. The degree of flexion and internal rotation should be determined by the

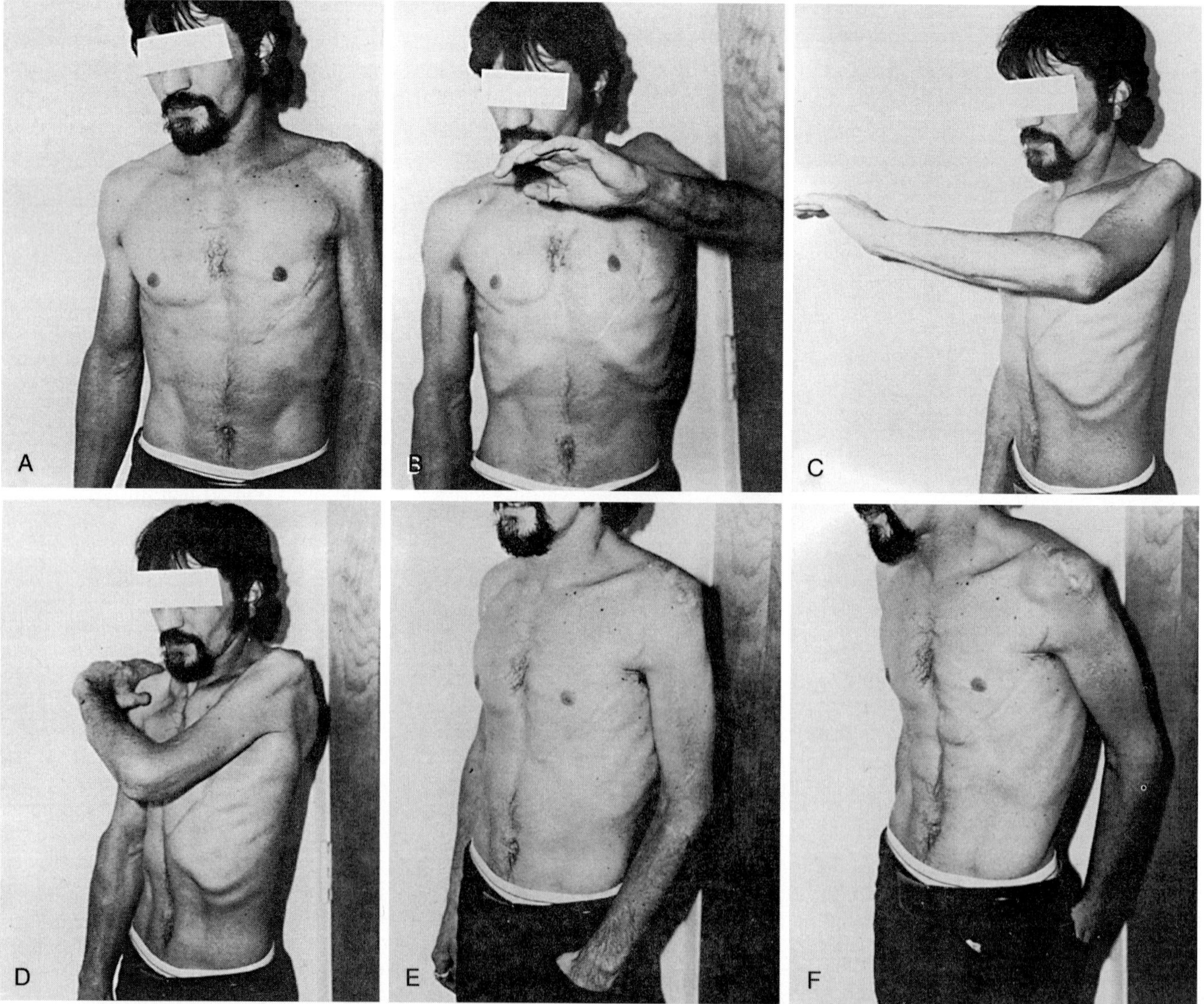

FIGURE 49–3. *A* to F, C5, C6, C7 traction injury of the left brachial plexus with flail shoulder and elbow, as well as wrist and finger extensor paralysis. Shoulder fusion and pectoral transfer have been done, as well as tendon transfers in the hand. (From Leffert RD: Brachial Plexus Injuries. New York, Churchill Livingstone, 1985.)

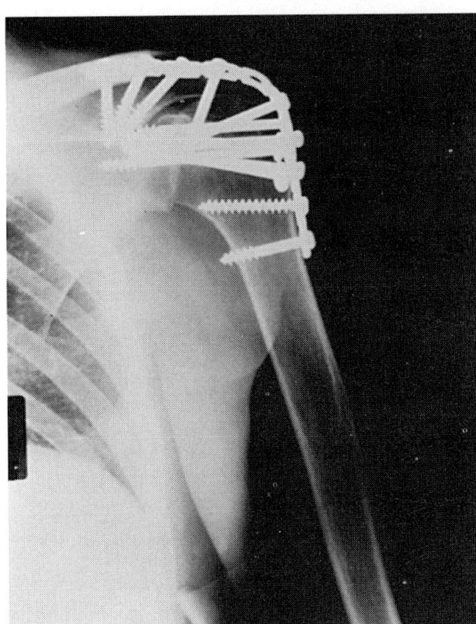

FIGURE 49–4. Radiograph of a shoulder fusion using compression screws and pelvic reconstruction plate.

functional needs of the patient. However, patients who cannot reach the midline of the body for dressing and personal hygiene are considerably less pleased with their results than those who can accomplish these tasks.

The surgical technique for shoulder fusion has evolved according to the pathology that necessitated it. Whereas infection, particularly tuberculosis, required sometimes elaborate maneuvers to remain extra-articular, the paralytic shoulder has no such requirement, but extra-articular sites are welcomed as additional "insurance." In the author's experience, the posterior approach is convenient, no more bloody than the anterior, and has the advantage of easy access to the spine of the scapula for application of a long plate that then runs caudad to the shaft of the humerus (Leffert, 1988). The arm is supported on a padded stand that permits maintenance of the position that is finally determined for the fusion. The glenoid is decorticated before the humeral head because to do the reverse would obscure vision due to bleeding. If the head can be translocated cephalad, or the overlying acromion partially osteotomized so that it can be bent down to the head, then a secondary site of fusion can be obtained. The bone from the resected head can be used as local graft, and usually, no additional bone graft is needed.

The author prefers to use a broad osteotome to prepare the fusion site rather than power tools to avoid overheating the bone. Seventy-five to eighty millimeter 1/3 threaded cancellous screws are used to secure the head to the glenoid, with care to ensure that the threads are all within the glenoid for maximal compression. Although the author formerly used a dynamic compression plate over the scapular spine and lateral aspect of the proximal humerus (Riggins, 1976), the pelvic reconstruction plate serves the same purpose and is considerably easier to conform to the bone (Richards et al, 1988) (Fig. 49–4).

Postoperative immobilization may, in some very reliable patients, be limited to a sling. However, I continue to employ a shoulder spica cast for most patients 4 or 6 weeks following surgery. Most patients achieve solid fusion by 3 months,

although the degree of compression that the system of fixation affords, plus the amount of metal that it requires, make radiographic assessment difficult. Tomography may be used to clarify the issue.

THE ELBOW

The adult patient with a lesion of the upper trunk of the brachial plexus will have lost the major power of active elbow flexion, although if the arm can be raised to or above the horizontal, elbow flexion can be achieved by trick motion using gravity. It is obvious, then, that the status of the shoulder is crucial in the function of the weak or paralyzed elbow. If the flexor-pronator forearm muscles are intact, and especially with the arm at the horizontal, the patient may pronate the forearm, strongly clench the fist, and achieve elbow flexion by supplementary motion (called the Steindler effect). This led Steindler, in 1917 to design the flexorplasty that bears his name (Steindler, 1944). It has been performed in countless polio patients with gratifying functional results. In this procedure, the origin of the flexor-pronator muscles is detached from the medial epicondyle of the humerus and advanced proximally to the intermuscular septum to increase the moment for flexion at the elbow. Obviously, passive elbow motion must be free preoperatively. There are two disadvantages of the procedure, however.

The first disadvantage is that the combined work capacity of the transfer is about 20% of the combined capacity of the brachialis, biceps, and brachioradialis, and the second disadvantage is that there is a tendency for the forearm to pronate when the elbow is flexed (Fig. 49–5).

Kettlekamp and Larsen's analysis of 15 Steindler flexorplasties (Kettlekamp and Larsen, 1963) revealed that nine patients could lift 1 lb through 110 degrees, and the maximal weight that could be lifted by the strongest transfer in the series was 6 lb. The tendency to forearm pronation can be reduced by a modification introduced by Mayer and Green (1954). The muscle pedicle is detached, along with 0.75 cm

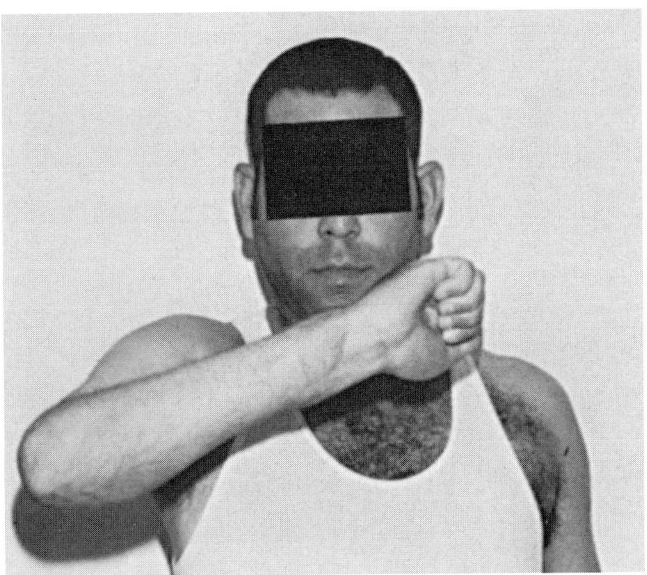

FIGURE 49–5. Elbow flexion using the Steindler effect.

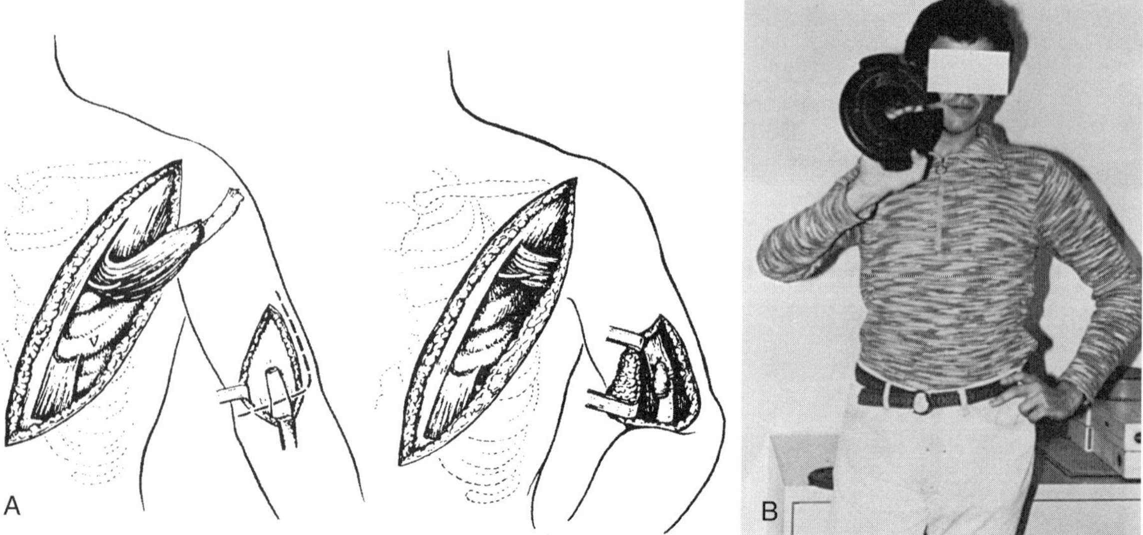

FIGURE 49–6. Clark's pectoral transfer. *A,* Schema of the procedure. Note the preservation of the lateral pectoral branch to the pedicle. *B,* Appearance following shoulder fusion and pectoral transfer. The patient is holding a 10-lb weight. (From Leffert RD: Brachial Plexus Injuries. New York, Churchill Livingstone, 1985.)

of bone from the medial epicondyle, and the muscles are then mobilized so that the pedicle and bone can be attached to the anterior cortex of the humerus by nonabsorbable sutures through drill holes. In most patients, the advancement proximally is 5 to 7 cm. The elbow is immobilized at 100 degrees of flexion for a month, following which gentle exercises are begun, and a sling is used for 3 months at night to create a flexion contracture. It is important that the elbow retain a slight flexion contracture, because initiation of flexion is facilitated from this position. Alnot and Abols reported on 22 Steindler flexorplasties in 1984 and reported that five had poor results.

It is because of this problem of strength that the Clark's

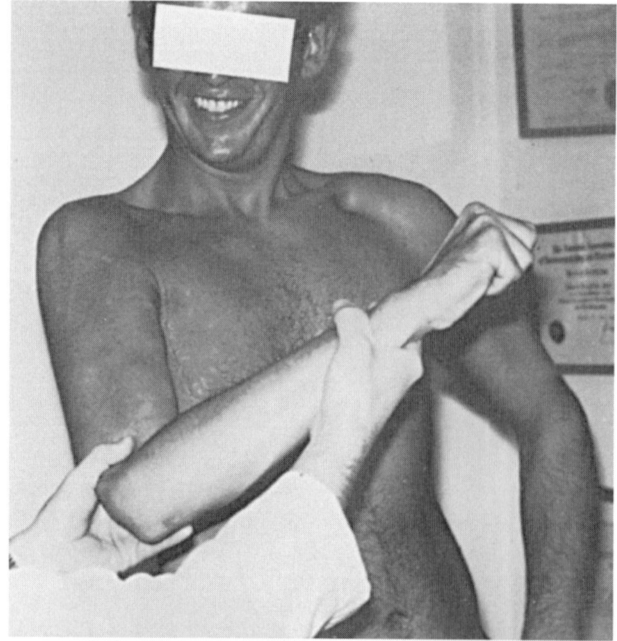

FIGURE 49–7. Good elbow flexion, which allows moderately heavy use of the arm. (From Leffert RD: Brachial Plexus Injuries. New York, Churchill Livingstone, 1985.)

pectoral transfer has become my procedure of choice for the restoration of active elbow flexion (Clark, 1946). The prerequisites are, in addition to free passive elbow motion, a fused shoulder or one under excellent control and an essentially normal sternal head of the pectoralis major. Even though the clavicular head will be paralyzed by a lesion of C5 and C6, the sternal head will still be functioning, and a pedicle of about 2 inches in width can be raised from the chest and turned with its blood and nerve supply to be re-routed down the arm. The tunnel is made subcutaneously, and attachment is to the biceps tendon in the antecubital fossa. There must be no scarring in the proposed site of transfer (hence no anterior shoulder fusions) and the length of the pedicle can be adequate only if additional tissue from the rectus sheath is included in continuity when the dissection is performed. It is absolutely essential to identify the lateral anterior thoracic nerve and protect it throughout the procedure. This can be greatly facilitated by the use of a nerve stimulator at operation. Postoperatively, the elbow is maintained in flexion for 4 weeks before gentle, guarded exercises are begun. It is kept in a sling between exercise periods for 3 months to encourage a permanent flexion contracture of about 30 degrees. The active power of the transfer is good, because the tendency to medial rotation or to adduction of the humerus is prevented by shoulder fusion.

It is these mechanical points that have resulted in extremely satisfactory results in the patients we have so treated, as opposed to early published evaluations of this procedure in the literature (Segal et al, 1959) (Fig. 49–6). I believe that the poorer results in that series resulted from failure to ensure control of the shoulder. If the shoulder is flail or weak, the pull of the pectoral transfer will be dissipated in adducting the humerus or medially rotating it rather than flexing the elbow. In our series of 15 patients (Leffert and Pess, 1988), there were eight good results and four patients who were improved. One patient with a poor result following this operation had not had a fusion. Of the other two poor results, the tendon was torn in a fall in one, and the other simply stretched out.

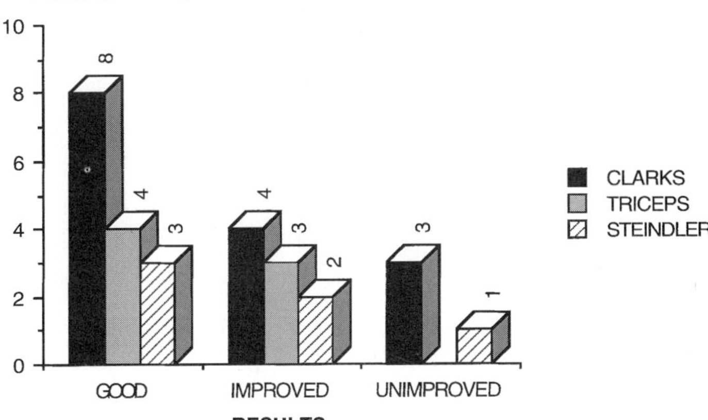

FIGURE 49–8. Results of tendon transfers for restoration of elbow flexion. (From Leffert RD, Press GM: Tendon transfers for brachial plexus injury. Hand Clin North Am 4:273–288, 1988.)

Clark's operation has been modified, mostly to improve the line of pull of the muscle by attaching it to the acromion (D'Aubigne et al, 1956; Schottstaedt et al, 1955). In 1979, Carroll and Kleinman presented a further modification, with good results reported.

The use of the latissimus to restore active elbow extension was described by Lange in 1930, and for either extension or flexion by Schottstaedt and associates in 1955. Hovnanian (1956) and Zancolli and Mitre (1973) have reported favorably on this transfer. Although the muscle is equivalent in power and excursion to the pectoralis major, its root innervation (C5–7) is the same as that of the muscles for elbow flexion. It has been either paralyzed or severely weakened in most of our patients who have needed restoration of elbow flexion. The author's personal experience with this transfer for flexion has been only two cases, both producing poor results.

In 1986, Moneim and Omer reported on five patients after latissimus dorsi muscle transfer to restore elbow flexion. The active range of flexion did not exceed 115 degrees in any patient. Two patients could lift 4 lb, whereas two others could lift 1 and 1.5 lb, respectively. Evaluation of activities of daily living by a standardized test revealed disappointing results. They concluded that this procedure should not be performed unless the latissimus dorsi muscle is normal preoperatively.

The triceps brachii may be used to replace a paralyzed biceps and brachialis. The technique of Carroll and associates (1952, 1953, 1970), which is a modification of the procedure described by Bunnell (1951), can provide excellent elbow flexion. The entire triceps is detached from its insertion, which is prolonged by elevating several inches of the deep fascia of the proximal forearm with the pedicle. This allows the muscle to be routed subcutaneously and to be inserted directly into the biceps tendon without having to interpose a fascial graft. The procedure has been particularly gratifying when there has been confused reinnervation with simultaneous co-contraction of the triceps when the patient attempts to flex the elbow. Although the operation works well (and thereafter gravity extends the elbow), there are several problems that must be anticipated preoperatively. Obviously, this procedure should not be performed bilaterally because it would cause significant disability in activities

such as getting out of a deep chair or turning over in bed. Crutch walking is hindered by lack of a triceps, and pushing a revolving door or working overhead is impossible. Nonetheless, it is a very useful procedure, and phase conversion has not been a problem (Leffert and Meister, 1976) (Fig. 49–7).

Of the seven triceps transfers in my series, four were good, and three were improved at last evaluation (Leffert and Pess, 1988).

The results of tendon transfers performed for restoration of elbow flexion in 28 patients using three different techniques in our clinic is shown in Figure 49–8

References

Alnot JY, Abols Y: Restoration of elbow flexion by tendon transfer in traumatic paralysis of the brachial plexus in adults. Apropos of 44 injured patients. Rev Chir Orthop 70:313–323, 1984.

Aziz W, Singer RM, Wolff TW: Transfer of the trapezius for flail shoulder after brachial plexus injury. J Bone Joint Surg 72B:701–704, 1990.

Barnes R: Traction injuries of the brachial plexus in adults. J Bone Joint Surg 31B:10, 1949.

Barr JS, Freiberg JA, Colonna PC, Pemberton PA: A survey of end results of stabilization of the paralytic shoulder. (Report of the Research Committee of the American Orthopaedic Association.) J Bone Joint Surg 24:699, 1942.

Bonney G: Prognosis in traction lesions of the brachial plexus. J Bone Joint Surg 41B:4–35, 1959.

Bunnell S: Restoring flexion to the paralytic elbow. J Bone Joint Surg 33A:566–571, 1951.

Carroll RE: Restoration of flexor power to the flail elbow by transplantation of the triceps tendon. Surg Gynecol Obstet 95:685, 1952.

Carroll RE, Hill NA: Triceps transfer to restore elbow flexion: A study in 15 patients with arthrogryposis and paralytic lesions. J Bone Joint Surg 52A:239–244, 1970.

Carroll RE, Gartland JJ: Flexorplasty of the elbow. An evaluation of a method. J Bone Joint Surg 35A:706–710, 1953.

Carroll RE, Kleinman WB: Pectoralis major transplantation to restore elbow flexion to the paralytic limb. J Hand Surg 4:501–507, 1979.

Chen WS: Sever-L'Episcopo transfers in obstetrical palsy: A retrospective review of twenty cases. J Pediatr Orthop 10:442–444, 1990.

Clark JMP: Reconstruction of biceps brachii by pectoral muscle transplantation. Br J Surg 34:180, 1946.

Cofield RH: Shoulder arthrodesis and resection arthroplasty. Instr Course Lect 34:268–277, 1985.

D'Aubigne M, Benassy J, Ramadieu JO: Chirurgie Orthopaedique des Paralysies. Paris, Masson, 1956, pp 122–139.

Freund RK, Terzis JK, Jordan L, Taylor G: Modified latissimus dorsi and teres major transfer for external rotation deficit of the shoulder. Orthopedics 9:505–506, 1986.

Goddard NJ, Fixsen JA: Rotation osteotomy of the humerus for birth injuries of the brachial plexus. J Bone Joint Surg 66B:257–9, 1984.

Harmon PH: Surgical reconstruction of the paralytic shoulder by multiple muscle transplantation. J Bone Joint Surg 32A:583–595, 1950.

Hovnanian AP: Latissimus dorsi transplantation for loss of flexion or extension at the elbow. A preliminary report of technique. Ann Surg 143:493, 1956.

Itoh Y, Sasaki T, Ishiguro T, et al: Transfer of latissimus dorsi to replace a paralyzed anterior deltoid. A new technique using an inverted pedicled graft. J Bone Joint Surg 69B:647–651, 1987.

Jonsson E, Lidgren L, Rydholm U: Position of shoulder arthrodesis measured by Moire photography. Clin Orthop 238:117–121, 1989.

Kettlekamp DB, Larsen CB: Evaluation of the Steindler flexorplasty. J Bone Joint Surg 45A:513–518, 1963.

L'Episcopo JB: Restoration of muscle balance in the treatment of obstetrical paralysis. NY J Med 39:357–363, 1939.

Lange F: Die epidemische Kinderlahmung. Munich, Lehmann, 1930.

Leffert RD: Compression-plate fusion of a flail shoulder. Strategies in Orthopaedic Surgery-Upjohn, Vol. 7. New Scotland, NY, LTI Medica, 1988.

Leffert RD, Meister M: Patterns of neuromuscular activity following tendon transfers in the upper limb—a preliminary study. J Hand Surg 1:181–189, 1976.

Leffert RD, Pess GM: Tendon transfers for brachial plexus injury. Hand Clin 4:273–288, 1988.

Leffert RD, Seddon HJ: Infraclavicular brachial plexus injuries. J Bone Joint Surg 47B:9–22, 1965.

Mayer L, Green W: Experiences with the Steindler flexorplasty at the elbow. J Bone Joint Surg 36A:775–789, 1954.

Moneim MS, Omer GE: Latissimus dorsi muscle transfer for restoration of elbow flexion after brachial plexus disruption. J Hand Surg 11A:135–139, 1986.

Richards RR, Sherman RM, Hudson AR, Waddell JP: Shoulder arthrodesis using a pelvic-reconstruction plate. A report of eleven cases. J Bone Joint Surg 70A:416–421, 1988.

Richards RR, Waddell JP, Hudson AR: Shoulder arthrodesis for the treatment of brachial plexus palsy. Clin Orthop 198:250–258, 1985.

Riggins R: Shoulder fusion without external fixation. A preliminary report. J Bone Joint Surg 58A:1007–1008, 1976.

Rowe CR: Arthrodesis of the shoulder used in treating painful conditions. Clin Orthop 173:92–96, 1983.

Rowe CR: Re-evaluation of the position of the arm in arthrodesis of the shoulder in the adult. J Bone Joint Surg 56A:913, 1974.

Saha AK: Surgery of the paralyzed and flail shoulder. Acta Orthop Scand (Suppl) 97:5–90, 1967.

Schottstaedt ER, Larsen LJ, Bost FC: Complete muscle transposition. J Bone Joint Surg 37A:897–919, 1955.

Segal A, Brook DM, Seddon HJ: Treatment of paralysis of the flexors of the elbow. J Bone Joint Surg 41B:44–50, 1959.

Steindler A (ed): Muscle and tendon transplantation at the elbow. Thompson, JEM (ed): Instructional Course Lectures on Reconstructive Surgery, Vol 2. Chicago, AAOS, 1944, pp 276–283.

Zachary RB: Transplantation of the teres major and latissimus dorsi for loss of external rotation at the shoulder. Lancet 2:757, 1957.

Zancolli E, Mitre H: Latissimus dorsi transfer to restore elbow flexion. An appraisal of eight cases. J Bone Joint Surg 55A:1265–1275, 1973.

Part VIII

COMPRESSION LESIONS

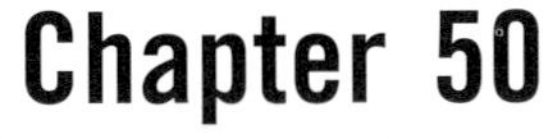

Chapter 50

• José L. Ochoa

Nerve Fiber Pathology in Acute and Chronic Compression

Many adults, both ill and healthy, harbor subclinical local lesions of one kind or another within their peripheral nerves or spinal nerve roots. At present, many of us have or will develop clinical manifestations, such as muscle weakness and atrophy, sensory loss, or paresthesias and pains in various combinations, from such lesions. Such symptoms motivate frequent neurological and orthopedic consultations.

When one is not familiar with the pathology of local nerve lesions, one somehow tends to assume that the nerve looks thickened, or narrowed, and contains the carcasses of nerve fibers asphyxiated in collagen. The real picture is not as tragic and is certainly not uniform. There are nerve lesions and nerve lesions, with different mechanisms of production, histopathological features, electrophysiology, clinical manifestations, and prognoses. When electron microscopy was applied to the study of abnormal nerves, the histopathology behind local nerve injuries stopped being the dull chapter in the story of nerve disease. What follows is an attempt to describe the more lively aspects of the subject, emphasizing those areas that allow correlation with abnormal physiology and with clinical manifestations.

FOCAL NERVE LESIONS WITH ACUTE INTERRUPTION OF AXONS

When a nerve is cut, crushed, or infarcted, the distal stump dies. However, until about the third or fourth day after injury, the structure of the disconnected distal nerve fibers remains grossly preserved. The fibers in the distal stump then become fragmented into ovoids, and become unexcitable when stimulated directly. In other words, before 3 or 4 days, one cannot tell whether paralysis or sensory loss following nerve injury is due to physiological block (neurapraxia) or anatomical interruption of nerve fibers (axonotmesis and neurotmesis). Nerve fibers in the distal stump undergo a series of changes involving active disintegration of axons and myelin, together with proliferation of Schwann cells. Such changes, best described by Cajal (1928) and by Williams and Hall (1971a, 1971b), culminate with the organization of solid columns made of Schwann cells, which eventually welcome regenerated axons and direct them to the peripheral tissues. Meanwhile, the neuronal cell body is engaged in synthesis of macromolecules (chromatolysis), which are transported at various rates down the axon and added at the tip of the stump to build new nerve fibers. Elongation of regenerating axons in tissue culture requires certain dynamics at the tip of the growth cones, which involves ameboid movements dependent on a contractile apparatus of actin microfilaments (Yamada et al, 1970, 1971). Despite adequate synthesis and transport, nerve regeneration may become arrested if growth cone dynamics are interfered with (Yamada et al, 1971; Wessells et al, 1971). So-called gigantic clubs attest to the arrested progress of regeneration (Cajal, 1928; Ochoa and Morgan-Hughes, 1974). An example is given in Figure 50–1.

Each parent axon regenerates several thin branches, like a pruned trunk. Anatomical and functional restitution following a nerve lesion characterized by axonal division is much more complete when the nerve trunk retains continuity (axonotmesis) than when it is interrupted (neurotmesis). Decisive factors are the helpful guidance of regenerated fibers toward appropriate terminals along the scaffold provided by surviving endoneurial tubes of basal lamina and the reduced opportunity for fibers to escape their perineurial continent (Gutmann and Sanders, 1943; Thomas, 1964; Young, 1949). After functional contact with the periphery is re-established, only select fibers will mature in diameter and, therefore, approach normal conduction velocity. Failure to establish peripheral contact results in an overproduction of regenerated fibers, which remain of immature caliber (Aitken et al, 1947; Evans and Murray, 1956; Sanders and Young, 1945; Weiss and Taylor, 1944; Weiss et al, 1945). Regenerated fibers may go astray and end in the wrong target, especially when they are required to grow across a gap in a divided nerve, or across a scar. The consequences of aberrant reinnervation are particularly dramatic in facial muscles (Nielsen, 1984; Sanders, 1989). It is common knowledge that regenerating fibers advance about 1 mm per day in human nerves. The progress of sensory fiber regeneration can be roughly monitored clinically by following the advance of Tinel's sign with the passage of time.

Such are some of the events that follow anatomical interruption of nerve fibers, which is, of course, their major pathological catastrophe. It leads to prolonged paralysis with atrophy and anesthesia. Recovery is slow and incomplete.

TRANSIENT ISCHEMIC NERVE BLOCK

On the mild end of the spectrum of consequences of local mechanical injury is the transient paralysis and anesthesia that may follow acute compression of a nerve, as, for example, when an arm or a leg "go to sleep" or 20 to 30 minutes after application of a suprasystolic cuff to a limb. In the case of the application of a suprasystolic cuff, the deficit is almost

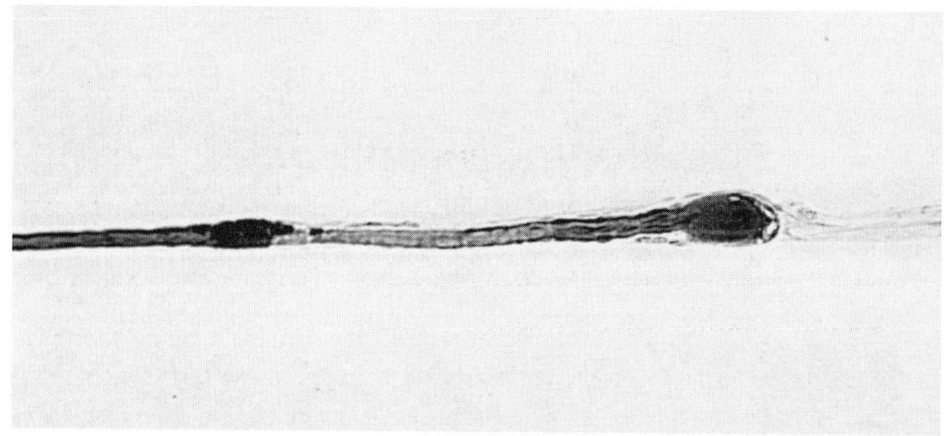

FIGURE 50–1. Single microdissected myelinated fiber from rat sciatic nerve, many weeks after onset of acrylamide intoxication. Acrylamide causes a so-called dying back type of neuropathy. The fiber shows neither signs of active degeneration nor regenerating axon sprouts. Its features are similar to those of the "gigantic clubs" described by Cajal (1928) in arrested regeneration.

immediately reversible on release of the cuff, and when the nerve is fixed instantaneously, there is no recognizable microscopic or ultramicroscopic pathology (Ochoa, unpublished observations). From the classic experiments by Lewis, Pickering, and Rothschild (1931), most practitioners in the field accept that such an immediately reversible defect is the result of nerve ischemia. One key experiment involved reversible paralysis and anesthesia in the upper limb of human volunteers induced by means of a pneumatic cuff inflated above systolic pressure, but just before releasing the cuff, a second suprasystolic cuff was placed further proximally. Thus, the original local pressure on the nerves was removed but the circulation remained arrested. In contrast to the single-cuff experiment, paralysis and anesthesia did not recover until the second cuff, maintained for various periods of time, was released. This indicates that ischemia of the limb and not direct local mechanical pressure is responsible for such type of transient nerve dysfunction.

NEURAPRAXIA

The author has referred to the two extremes in the scale of severity of acute local nerve disorders. A fascinating intermediate level was defined electrophysiologically over a century ago by Erb (1876).

Following some forms of acute nerve injury, particularly in so-called Saturday night paralysis and tourniquet paralysis, there is motor deficit with only mild sensory loss and little or no muscle atrophy. The nerve distal to the site of the injury remains excitable throughout. In the terminology of Sir Herbert Seddon (1943) this is neurapraxia. This type of intermediate lesion caught the interest of Denny-Brown and Brenner in the 1940s. They demonstrated that in experimental tourniquet paralysis, the local nerve lesion selectively affected the myelin sheaths, sparing axons. That was probably the first revival of the idea of demyelinating disease in the twentieth century. In 1880, Gombault had described demyelination in experimental lead poisoning, but the phenomenon was then forgotten. Transcendental as it was, the work of Denny-Brown and Brenner (1944a, 1944b) reached an equivocal conclusion for reasons that in retrospect can be qualified as misleading coincidences. Their conclusion was that the local demyelinating lesion that follows local nerve compression is a result of ischemia and would merely represent a complication of the immediately reversible ischemic nerve block reported by Lewis and colleagues (1931). In support of their hypothesis, and against the alternative of a direct mechanical effect, Denny-Brown and Brenner cited a classic by Grundfest (1936), who had, for different purposes, compressed portions of nerve within pressure chambers. Grundfest had found that, even under enormous pressures, nerves continued to conduct, provided there was oxygen within the chamber. From the data to be described later, it becomes clear why the apparently legitimate extrapolation by Denny-Brown and Brenner was inaccurate.

In a series of papers from Queen Square, Gilliatt, Fowler, Rudge, and Ochoa re-examined demyelinating lesions caused by acute nerve compression in the baboon. Using the tourniquet paralysis model and also a model akin to Saturday night paralysis, the authors confirmed demyelination but failed to confirm three important features of the lesion described originally by Denny-Brown (Fowler, 1975; Ochoa et al, 1971, 1972a, 1972b; Rudge et al, 1974).

First, it was found that small-diameter fibers are spared (the original description implicated fibers of all diameters). The sparing of small fibers is a very consistent feature and affords a coherent explanation for sparing of pain and temperature sensation and of autonomic function in tourniquet paralysis (Moldaver, 1954). Second, it was found that the nerve fiber defects do not extend throughout the compressed area. Instead, they are concentrated under the edges of the cuff, with sparing under the center. In the narrower lesion seen in the model of Saturday night paralysis, the center was again spared. But the most dramatic incongruence with the original report concerned the nodes of Ranvier, which were said to be normal soon after compression; nevertheless, a spectacular distortion of the nodes can be demonstrated consistently in large-diameter nerve fibers with modern histologic techniques. In myelinated nerve fibers fixed for electron microscopy, osmicated and microdissected in fluent epoxy resin, one can see by light microscopy that the nodal gaps are occluded and a dark area is present toward one side at a gradual distance from the original site of the node. Single-fiber electron microscopy (Ochoa, 1972) explains the lesion: One myelin segment invaginates the next (Fig. 50–2). The polarity of invagination is reversed on either edge of the compressed region (Fig. 50–3).

How does this come about? Pressure differences between compressed and uncompressed nerve at the edges generate

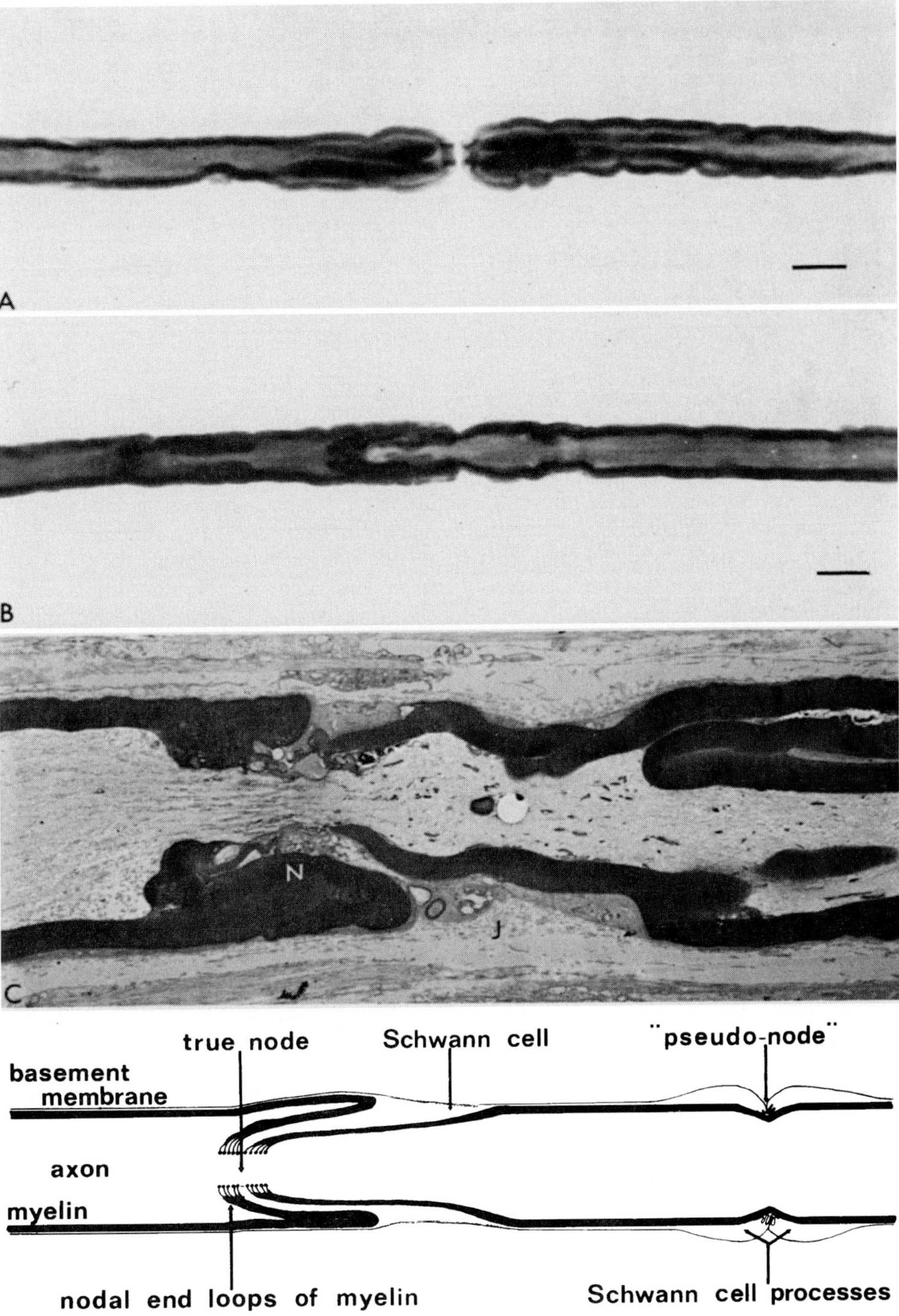

FIGURE 50–2. *A,* Normal microdissected myelinated fiber showing node of Ranvier. Baboon tibial nerve. (Bar = 10 μm.) *B,* Abnormal fiber, early after acute compression. The nodal gap is occluded due to intussusception from right to left. An indentation (pseudonode) marks the original site of the node. (Bar = 10 μm.) *C,* Low-power electron micrograph of abnormal myelinated fiber, cut longitudinally after microdissection. Note indentation at Schwann cell junction, J, and new position of the node, N, under infolded myelin (From Rudge P, Ochoa J, Gilliatt RW: J Neurol Sci *23*:403, 1974, with kind permission from Elsevier Science—NL, Sara Bergerhartstraat 25, 1055, KV Amsterdam, The Netherlands.) *D,* Diagram of affected fiber showing invagination of one paranode by the adjacent one, movement occurring from right to left. (From Ochoa J, Fowler TJ, and Gilliatt RW: *In* Desmedt JE (ed): New Developments in Electromyography and Clinical Neurophysiology, vol 2. Basel, Karger, 1973, pp 166–173.)

longitudinal driving forces that tend to extrude axoplasm like toothpaste from a tube. The nodes of Ranvier, where the axon is normally narrowed, offer resistance to axoplasmic prolapse, and so progressively, the axon becomes stretched at the paranodal region and the node of Ranvier becomes dislocated from a few to several hundred microns, depending on the duration and amount of pressure applied. Myelin is relatively firmly tethered to the axon and hence stretches passively. Axon and myelin in the adjacent paranode infold as they receive the dislocated neighboring structures. The whole picture is strongly reminiscent of an intussusception of the bowel. Unlike myelin, the Schwann cells do not follow the dislocated axon; they seem to be more firmly tethered to the basal lamina and surrounding collagen than to the myelin and axon. Thus, both the infolded and the stretched paranodal myelin become extracellular with respect to their stationary Schwann cells. An apparently rigid collar at the Schwann cell junction retains its original position and indents the intruding nerve fiber elements (becoming a pseudo-node), thus providing a point of reference to measure the extent of nodal dislocation. No such longitudinal forces are generated under the middle of the compressed region

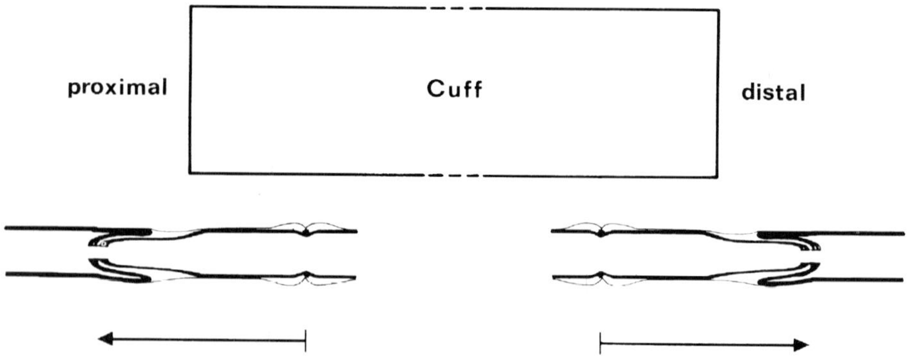

FIGURE 50–3. Diagram describing the direction of dislocation of the nodes of Ranvier in relation to the compressed zone. (From Ochoa J, Fowler TJ, Gilliatt RW: J Anat *113*:433, 1972.)

because there are no pressure gradients there. Grundfest's experiment compressing segments of nerves within a pressure chamber does not apply, because pressure gradients could not develop under those physical conditions.

Small fibers are spared because greater amounts of force are required to displace the viscous contents of the increasingly narrower diameter tubes: Nerve fibers are probably crushed before the required force is met. Indeed, if pressure is excessive or is sustained for too long, then axons get crushed or overstretched and degenerate: The wallerian component becomes prominent (Fowler and Ochoa, 1975; Ochoa et al, 1972a).

Paranodal demyelination and, occasionally, demyelination of complete segments follow within a few days after the injury, with the peak occurring during the second week. Repair is achieved by Schwann cells, which proliferate and migrate toward the injured paranodes, and intercalated remyelinated segments are formed (Fig. 50–4).

Remyelination parallels clinical and electrical recovery, which is usually fastest between the third and the sixth week (Fowler et al, 1972). Onset of recovery may be delayed and its time course protracted following severe compression. Under these circumstances, the development of intramyelin and periaxonal edema, perhaps due to anoxia, complicates recovery (Ochoa et al, 1972a). How does the early lesion (invagination of myelin segments) cause nerve conduction block? Presumably through occlusion of the nodes of Ranvier and blockade of ionic currents; however, this remains to be explored. Subsequent demyelination, of course, can also produce a conduction block; its mechanism has been elucidated by McDonald (1963a, 1963b) and by Rasminsky and Sears (1972).

CHRONIC NERVE ENTRAPMENT

Is chronic entrapment the result of cumulative subclinical acute compressions? In other words, is the pathogenesis of acute compression similar to that of chronic entrapment? A negative answer emerges from plain histopathology. Indeed, in chronic entrapment, there exists a distinct and peculiar anatomical lesion, with a fine structure that practically reveals its pathogenesis.

In 1913, Marie and Foix discovered that a cause for some forms of thenar wasting in patients was an anatomical lesion of the median nerve at the wrist. Using vintage stains, they noticed that myelin disappeared under the carpal tunnel, but they did not examine the nerves distal to the wrist. Fifty

years later, in London, Thomas and Fullerton (1963) obtained another postmortem specimen from a proven case of carpal tunnel syndrome. Again, myelin disappeared in the region under the tunnel but reappeared distally. Thus, there was an element of focal demyelination in the lesion, which accounts for focal slowing of nerve conduction.

In the 1960s, Fullerton and Gilliatt and their associates discovered that guinea pigs aged 2 years and older consistently express a carpal tunnel syndrome (Anderson et al, 1970; Fullerton and Gilliatt, 1967). They confirmed local demyelination under the wrist in guinea pigs and also described a peculiar distortion of the myelin segments proximal to the wrist, but, like Marie and Foix, they did not focus on the changes distal to the wrist.

While working with Gilliatt at Queen Square, Ochoa and Marotte (1973) adopted the guinea pig model of chronic nerve entrapment, expecting to find evidence of invagination of nodes of Ranvier, as seen following acute compression. Acute changes were never found. However, the authors confirmed that, along stretches of up to 20 mm or more, proximal to the wrist, myelin segments were deformed, resembling tadpoles, being bulbous at one end and tapered at the other. The abnormal segments were consistently polarized, the bulb pointing away from the wrist. Interestingly, distal to the carpal tunnel the same distorted internodes were present as found proximally but with a reversed polarity. In young animals, there is merely asymmetry without demyelination, and the turning point can be shown under the tunnel. With age, the lesions become grotesque, and demyelination and remyelination follow. Eventually, axons get interrupted and their distal portions degenerate (Fig. 50–5).

Examination of the abnormal myelin segments by electron microscopy revealed that internal myelin lamellae had slipped away at the tapered ends and that these displaced lamellae had buckled at the bulbous ends (Fig. 50–6). Ochoa and Marotte (1973) suggested that there is nothing peculiar about demyelination in this model: Initially, it is simple slippage of myelin lamellae, followed by disintegration of the contorted myelin at the bulbs. In support of this concept is the observation that loss of myelin is initially confined to the tapered ends. Sunderland (1976) proposed that nerve fiber damage in the carpal tunnel syndrome is due to ischemia caused by local obstruction of venous return resulting from increased pressure in the tunnel. The authors believe that repeated minor trauma, or perhaps repeated stretching or friction against flexor tendons, elicits pressure waves that propagate in opposite directions, causing detachment of myelin lamellae, which slip away. The unrolled myelin

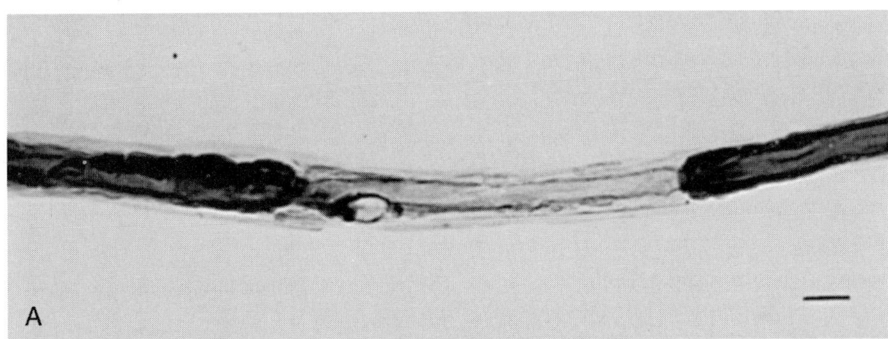

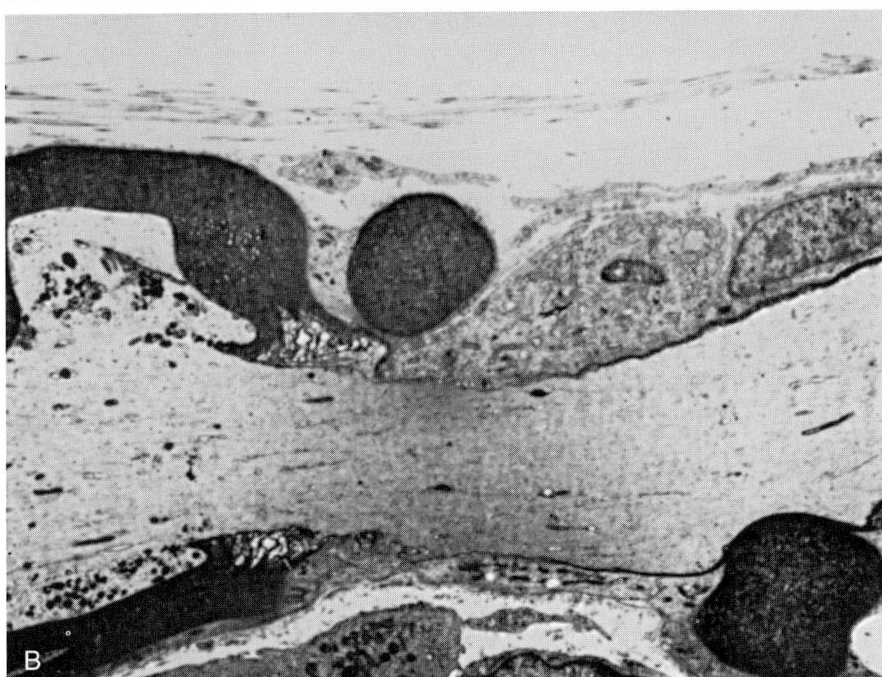

FIGURE 50–4. *A*, Thinly remyelinated segment intercalated in fiber microdissected from baboon sciatic nerve during repair of paranodal invagination and demyelination (Bar = 10 μm.) *B*, Low-power electron micrograph after ultra-thin sectioning of the fiber shown in *A*. It shows detail of the node on the left. (× 5500) (From Ochoa J: J Neurol Sci *17*:103, 1972, with kind permission from Elsevier Science—NL, Sara Bergerhartstraat 25, 1055, KV Amsterdam, The Netherlands.)

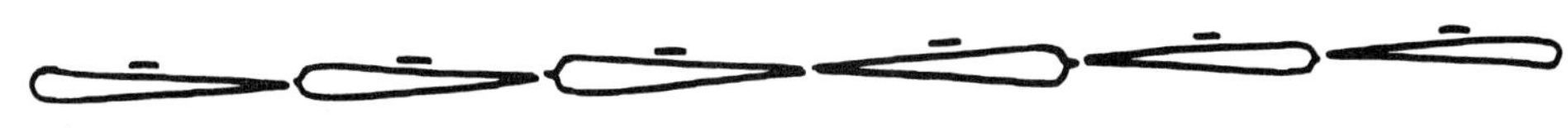

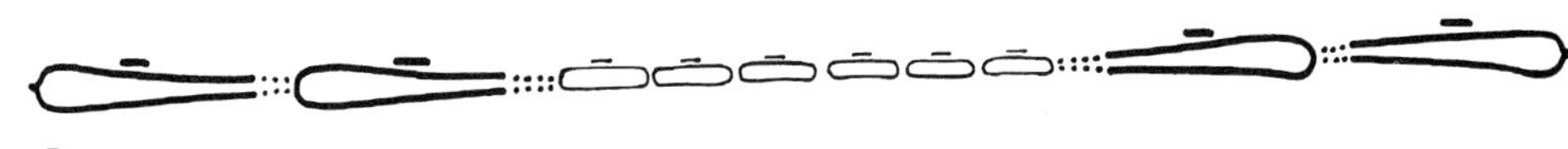

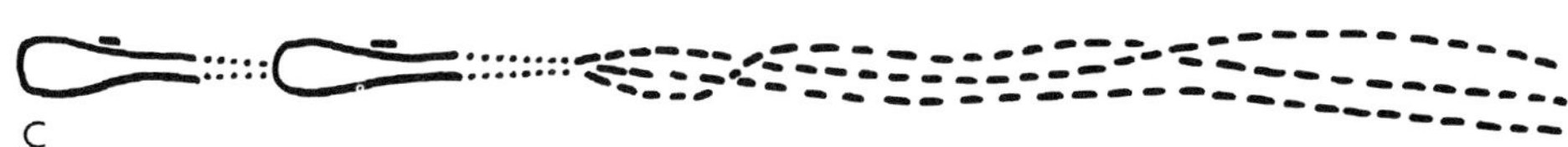

FIGURE 50–5. *A*, Diagram showing distorted myelin segments from median nerve of young guinea pig. Note reversal of polarity at the wrist. *B*, Further distortion and exposure of the axon proximal and distal to the site of entrapment. The median nerve under the carpal tunnel has lost its original myelin segments. Multiple short remyelinated internodes repair the lesion. *C*, Advanced lesion with massive bulbs and axonal wallerian degeneration and regeneration.

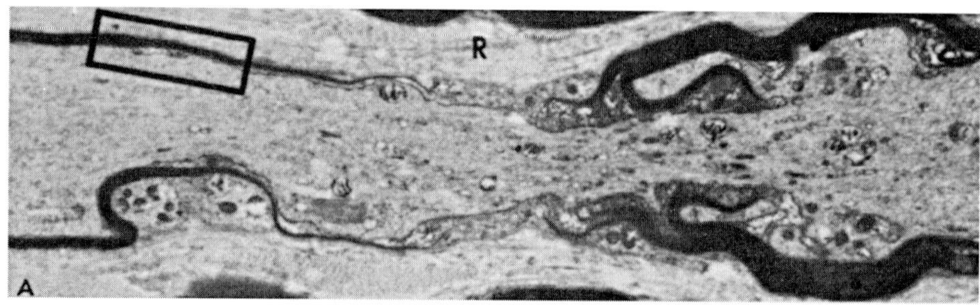

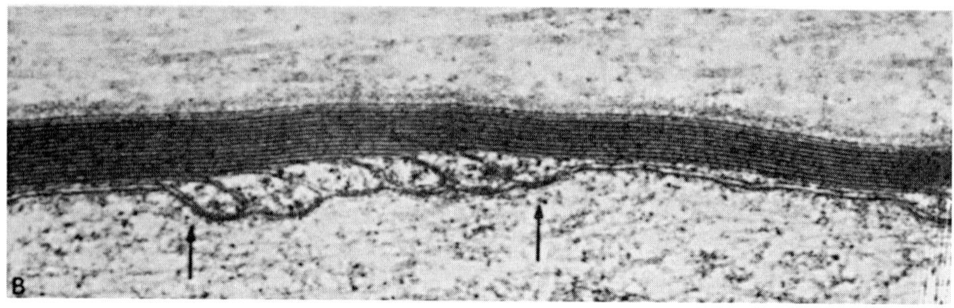

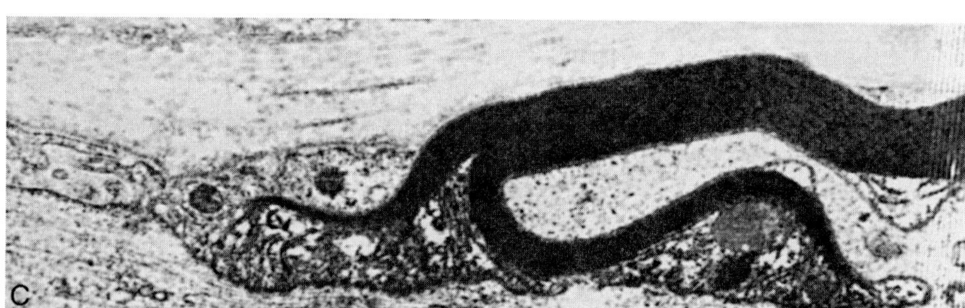

FIGURE 50–6. *A,* Low-power electron micrograph of a moderately abnormal fiber taken from a guinea pig median nerve above the wrist. The paranode on the left is tapered. The bulbous paranode on the right shows inturning of a group of inner lamellae. (R = node of Ranvier.) (× 7000.) *B,* Enlargement of the area enclosed in the rectangle in *A.* Six myelin lamellae end in cytoplasmic loops between the arrows. (× 48,000.) *C,* Detail of the bulbous paranode. (× 20,000.) (From Ochoa J, Marotte L: J Neurol Sci *19*:491, 1973, with kind permission from Elsevier Science—NL, Sara Bergerhartstraat 25, 1055, KV Amsterdam, The Netherlands.)

sheath, which is normally symmetrical, becomes skewed (Fig. 50–7).

Neary, Ochoa, and Gilliatt (1975) confirmed, in human median nerves at the wrist and ulnar nerves at the elbow, all the findings described earlier in the guinea pig; identical changes have been found in the lateral cutaneous nerve of the thigh under the inguinal ligament in a case of meralgia paresthetica (Ochoa, 1977, unreported data), which seems to consolidate the lesions described by Ochoa and Marotte (1973) as the primary pathology of myelinated fibers underlying chronic entrapment in general. Unmyelinated fibers resist until late in the course of entrapment, when evidence of their degeneration and regeneration becomes increasingly apparent (Marotte, 1974). It is conceivable that similar lesions occur at other common sites of local entrapment, the posterior interosseus nerve being strongly suspect at the elbow in the vicinity of the supinator muscle (Spinner, 1968), where it may be macroscopically enlarged and microscopi-

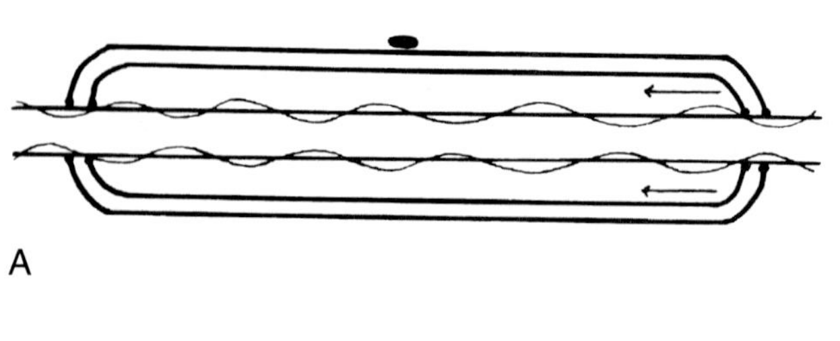

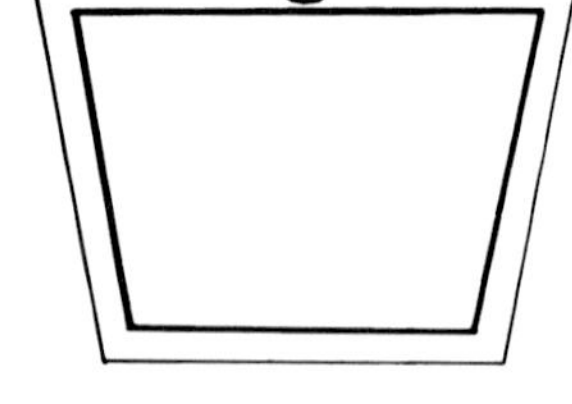

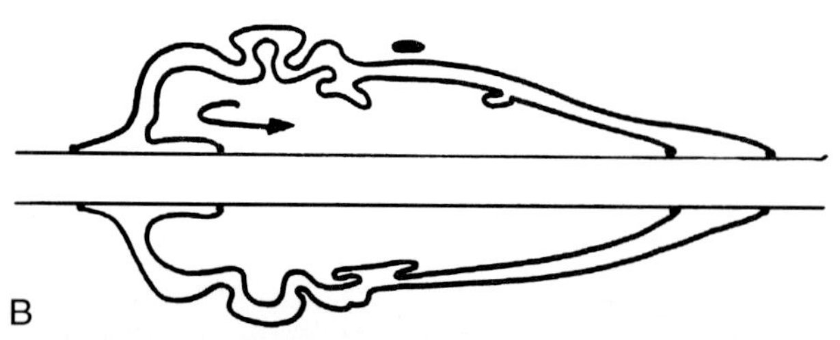

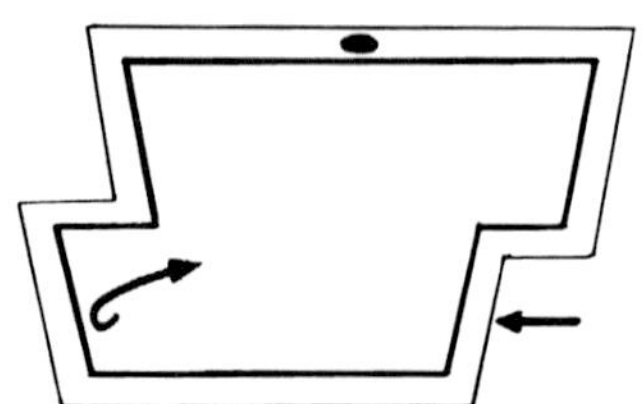

FIGURE 50–7. *A,* Normal myelin segment and unrolled myelin sheath *(right),* which is trapezoid shaped. Hypothetical pressure waves in the direction of the arrows along the axon. *B,* Distorted segment with tapered end caused by myelin slippage, and bulbous end containing inturned redundant myelin lamellae. If the myelin were unrolled, it would be altered as indicated *(right).*

cally so modified that distinction from a neoplasm may be difficult (Ochoa and Neary, 1975).

There should be no doubt that severe acute and chronic ischemia can cause primary damage to nerves (Asbury, 1970; Eames and Lange, 1967; Gairns et al, 1960; Korthals and Wisniewski, 1975). Further, ischemia can contribute to modified function in diseased nerves, in both diabetic polyneuropathy (Seneviratne and Peiris, 1968) and mononeuropathies, particularly in the carpal tunnel syndrome, in which ischemia is known to precipitate or exaggerate symptoms (Gilliatt and Wilson, 1953; Fullerton, 1963). It is also conceivable that chronic ischemia may play some role in the pathogenesis of chronic entrapment, because vasa nervorum eventually suffer prominent local damage in plantar neuromas (Lassman et al, 1976). Vascular damage in chronic entrapment may be more frequent than it would appear from the study of epineurial arterioles and venules alone. Endoneurial vessels appear to be reduced in numbers locally, and it seems possible to the author that Renaut bodies (Asbury, 1973) may represent the residue of injured small-caliber endoneurial vessels. Although there are good grounds to suspect a secondary role for ischemia in the pathogenesis of the nerve lesion underlying chronic entrapment, it seems overwhelmingly clear that the polarized changes described in myelinated fibers, involving graded displacement of structures away from the site of entrapment, must be mechanical in origin.

PAINFUL NERVE LESIONS: PHYSIOLOGICAL CLUES FROM MORPHOLOGY

Too many patients suffer chronic pain from local nerve lesions, and yet we know little about the mechanisms involved and even less about the underlying histopathology in humans. This is not a trivial subject, because current conflicting theories to explain neuralgia presuppose different pathological substrates.

For example, Noordenbos (1959) believed that selective loss of large-diameter afferents releases the inputs from small fibers that conduct impulses related to pain. Noordenbos' concept was based on clinical and histological observations in postherpetic neuralgia and was inspired by Henry Head's ideas of two conflicting peripheral sensory systems. Such is the fiber dissociation theory, which was subsequently embraced by the gate control theory of pain (Melzack and Wall, 1965). Another theory, not individually championed but formerly popular, implicates a so-called artificial synapse created at the level of the injury, where pain fibers would be ephaptically cross-excited by normal, ongoing ascending or descending (somatic or autonomic) impulses. Ephaptic excitation at the artificial synapse has been shown electrophysiologically in acute experimental local nerve injuries in animals (Granit and Skoglund, 1945) and in dysmyelinated spinal roots of dystrophic mice (Rasminsky, 1978), but Wall and colleagues (1974) failed to confirm long-lasting cross-excitation following acute experimental local nerve injury. No comparable studies are available in painful nerve lesions in humans. On the morphological side, there has been no serious attempt to identify the structural correlates of artificial synapses. A third relevant theory to explain neuralgia incriminates the spontaneous generation of impulses in abnormal nerve fibers. For Wall and Gutnick (1974a, 1974b), the abnormal generators would be immature axon sprouts from small diameter afferent fibers. Their electrophysiological studies on experimental amputation neuromas in the rat are convincing and invite extrapolation to human disease. Similarly, Rasminsky (1978) has claimed spontaneous impulse generation in nerve fibers with defective myelin, and it is conceivable and theoretically sound that other structural deviations in nerve fibers may also behave as abnormal pacemakers (Calvin et al, 1977).

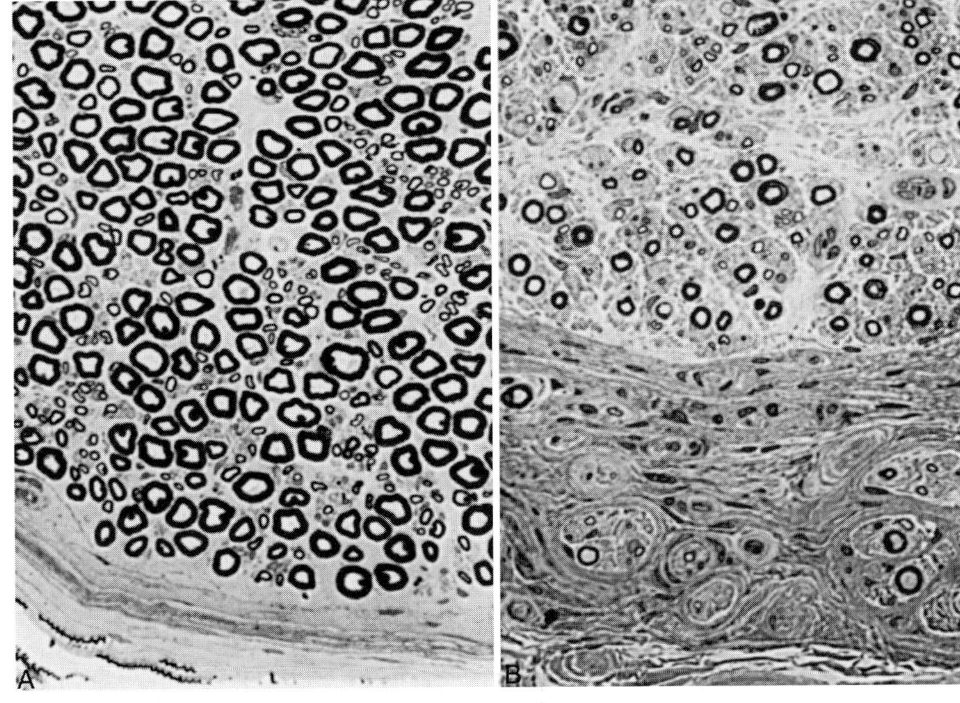

FIGURE 50–8. *A*, Normal portion of human superficial radial nerve, above the site of the injury. *B*, At the site of the lesion, note the drop out of the large diameter fibers. Miniature fascicles are seen external to the perineurium *(bottom half)*. Magnification is similar for *A* and *B*.

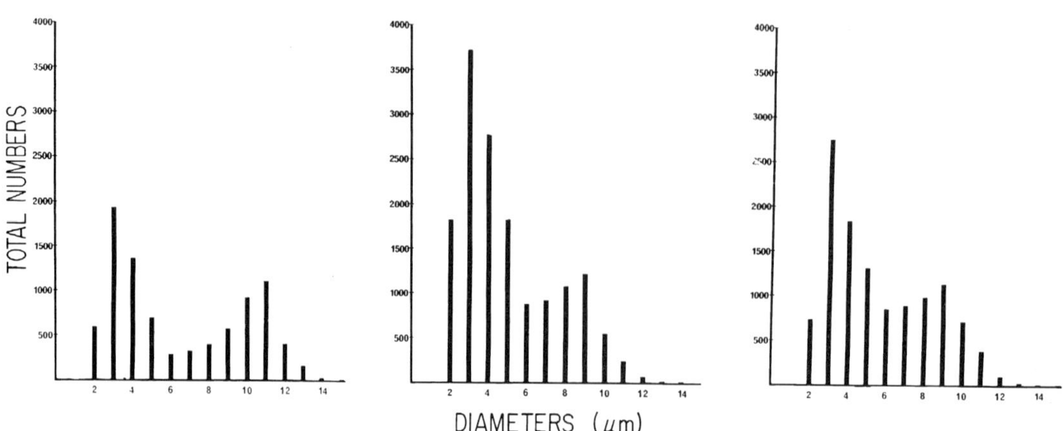

FIGURE 50–9. Myelinated fiber spectra of a painful neuroma in continuity after total counts proximal to the lesion *(left)*, at the level of the lesion *(center)*, and distal to the lesion *(right)*. Note the increase in the number of small fibers at the level of the lesion: Many were immature sprouts. Note further, that in this case, there is no selective loss of large diameter fibers.

Because only a small proportion of local nerve lesions cause chronic pain, any attempt to define the elusive histopathology underlying painful nerve lesions must use human material because we still depend on communication of the sensory experience as the single measure of pain. Obviously, a morphological study is unlikely to provide answers on mechanisms but should contribute toward the authentication of current theories to explain neuralgia.

Painful amputation neuromas in humans, studied by classic histology, are characterized by a focal increase in volume, largely due to deposition of fibrous tissue, and the presence of many tangled nerve fibers. Fiber counts and size frequency histograms obtained from various levels are not available, and it remains unknown whether nonpainful neuromas show any distinctive features when compared with painful neuromas. Amputation neuromas in experimental animals were thoroughly studied by Spencer (1971), who emphasized the formation of small fascicles within or outside the original perineurial limits, as well as nerve fiber branching, the predominance of small sized axons, and the swollen growth cones and retrograde-regenerated fibers previously described by Cajal (1928).

Quantitative studies from human painful nerve lesions in continuity are available (Ochoa, 1977; Ochoa and Noordenbos, 1978). In selected cases in which samples of the whole nerve trunk could be examined proximal to, at, and distal to the local lesion, the common denominator was the presence of an increased total number of fibers, many of them immature, confined to the level of the lesion itself (Fig. 50–8). The myelinated fiber spectrum distal to the lesion was often distorted but not universally so (Fig. 50–9). A similar pattern was found to apply to unmyelinated fibers. If sprouts from small diameter afferents concerned with nociceptive (painful) impulses are represented in the local fiber excess (and this is likely), then such excess of fibers demonstrated at the level of the painful lesions seems to support the theory of abnormal pacemakers in preference to so-called fiber dissociation. As to the artificial synapse, current morphological techniques are not suited for its assessment.

Substantial new knowledge has accumulated over the past decade about the complexities of neuropathic pain (see Ochoa, 1993, 1994).

References

Aitken JT, Sharman M, Young JZ: Maturation of regenerating nerve fibers with various peripheral connections. J Anat *81*:1, 1947.

Anderson MH, Fullerton PM, Gilliatt RW, Hern JEC: Changes in the forearm associated with median nerve compression at the wrist in the guinea-pig. J Neurol *33*:70, 1970.

Asbury AK: Ischemic disorders of peripheral nerve. *In* Vinken PJ, Bruyn GW (eds): Handbook of Clinical Neurology, Vol. 8. Amsterdam, Holland, North-Holland Publishing Company, 1988, p 154.

Asbury AK: Renaut bodies: A forgotten endoneurial structure. J Neuropathol Exp Neurol *32*:334, 1973.

Cajal SR: Degeneration and Regeneration of the Nervous System. London, Oxford University Press, 1928.

Calvin WH, Loeser JD, Howe JF: A neurophysiological theory for the pain mechanism of tic douloureux. Pain *3*:147, 1977.

Denny-Brown D, Brenner C: Paralysis of nerve induced by direct pressure and by tourniquet. Arch Neurol Psychol *51*:1, 1944a.

Denny-Brown D, Brenner C: Lesion in peripheral nerve resulting from compression by spring clip. Arch Neurol Psychol *52*:1, 1944b.

Eames RA, Lange LS: Clinical and pathological study of ischaemic neuropathy. J Neurol Neurosurg Psychiatry *30*:215, 1967.

Erb W: Diseases of the peripheral cerebrospinal nerves. *In* Ziemssen H von (ed): Cyclopedia of the Practice of Medicine, Vol. XI. London, Samson Low, Marston, Searle and Rivington, 1876.

Evans DHL, Murray JG: A study of regeneration in a motor nerve with unimodal fiber diameter distribution. Anat Rec *126*:311, 1956.

Fowler TJ: Tourniquet Paralysis in the Baboon. D.M. Thesis. London, University of Oxford, 1975.

Fowler TJ, Danta G, Gilliatt RW: Recovery of nerve conduction after a pneumatic tourniquet: Observations on the hind-limb of the baboon. J Neurol Neurosurg Psychiatry *35*:638, 1972.

Fowler TJ, Ochoa J: Unmyelinated fibers in normal and compressed peripheral nerves of the baboon; a quantitative electron-microscopic study. Neuropathol Appl Neurobiol *1*:247, 1975.

Fullerton PM: The effect of ischaemia on nerve conduction in the carpal tunnel syndrome. J Neurol Neurosurg Psychiatry *26*:385, 1963.

Fullerton PM, Gilliatt RW: Median and ulnar neuropathy in the guinea-pig. J Neurol Neurosurg Psychiatry *30*:393, 1967.

Gairns FW, Garven HSD, Smith G: The digital nerves and the nerve endings in progressive obliterative vascular disease of the leg. Scot Med J *5*:382, 1960.

Gilliatt RW, Wilson TG: A pneumatic-tourniquet test in the carpal tunnel syndrome. Lancet 2:595, 1953.

Gombault A: Contribution a l'étude anatomique de la nevrite parenchymateuse subaigüe et chronique—nevrite segmentaire periaxile. Arch Neurol 1:11, 1880,

Granit R, Skoglund CR: Facilitation, inhibition and depression at the artificial synapse formed by the cut end of a mammalian nerve. J Physiol 103:435, 1945.

Grundfest H: Effects of hydrostatic pressures upon the excitability, the recovery, and the potential sequence of frog nerve. Cold Spring Harb Symp Quant Biol 4:179, 1936.

Gutmann E, Sanders FK: Recovery of fiber numbers and diameters in the regeneration of peripheral nerves. J Physiol 101:489, 1943.

Korthals JK, Wisniewski HM: Peripheral nerve ischemia: Part 1. Experimental model. J Neurol Sci 24:65, 1975.

Lassmann G, Lassmann H, Stockinger L: Morton's metatarsalgia: Light and electron microscopic observations and their relation to entrapment neuropathies. Virchows Arch A Pathol Anat Histopathol 370:307, 1976.

Lewis T, Pickering GW, Rothschild P: Centripetal paralysis arising out of arrested bloodflow to the limb, including notes on a form of tingling. Heart 16:2, 1931.

McDonald WI: The effects of experimental demyelination on conduction in peripheral nerve: A histological and electrophysiological study. I. Clinical and histological observations. Brain 86:481, 1963a.

McDonald WI: The effects of experimental demyelination on conduction in peripheral nerve: A histological and electrophysiological study. II. Electrophysiological observations. Brain 86:501, 1963b.

Marie P, Foix C: Atrophie isolée de l'eminence thenar d'origin nevritique, role du ligament annulaire anterieur du carpel dans la pathogénie de la lesion. Rev Neurol 26:647, 1913.

Marotte LR: An electron microscope study of chronic median nerve compression in the guinea-pig. Acta Neuropathol 27:69, 1974.

Melzack R, Wall PD: Pain mechanisms: A new theory. Science 150:971, 1965.

Moldaver I: Tourniquet paralysis syndrome. Arch Surg 68:136, 1954.

Neary D, Ochoa J, Gilliatt RW: Sub-clinical entrapment neuropathy in man. J Neurol Sci 24:283, 1975.

Nielsen VK: Pathophysiology of hemifacial spasm. I. Ephaptic transmission and ectopic excitation. Neurology 34:418–426, 1984.

Noordenbos W: Pain. Amsterdam, Elsevier, 1959.

Ochoa J: Ultrathin longitudinal sections of single myelinated fibres for electron microscopy. J Neurol Sci 17:103, 1972.

Ochoa J: Neuralgia and hyperalgesia from local nerve lesions: Pathophysiology. Electroencephalogr Clin Neurophysiol 43:97, 1977.

Ochoa J: Guest Editorial: Essence, investigation, and management of "neuropathic" pains: Hopes from acknowledgement of chaos. Muscle Nerve 16:997–1008, 1993.

Ochoa J: Pain mechanisms in neuropathy. Current Science 7:407–414, 1994.

Ochoa J, Danta G, Fowler TJ, and Gilliatt RW: Nature of the nerve lesion caused by a pneumatic tourniquet. Nature 233:265, 1971.

Ochoa J, Fowler TJ, Gilliatt RW: Anatomical changes in peripheral nerves compressed by a pneumauc tourniquet. Anatomy 113:433, 1972a.

Ochoa J, Gilliatt RW, Fowler TJ: Tourniquet paralysis in the baboon. Trans Am Neurol Assoc 97:52, 1972b.

Ochoa J, Marotte L: Nature of the nerve lesion underlying chronic entrapment. J Neurol Sci 19:491, 1973.

Ochoa J, Morgan-Hughes JA: Arrested peripheral nerve regeneration in acrylamide neuropathy—an ultrastructural study. Excerpta Medica. International Congress Series, 1974. Vllth international Congress of Neuropathology—Budapest.

Ochoa J, Neary D: Localised hypertrophic neuropathy, intraneural tumour, or chronic nerve entrapment? Lancet, March 15, 632–633, 1975.

Ochoa J, Noordenbos W: Pathology and disordered sensation in local nerve lesions: An attempt at correlation. In Bonica J, Liebeskind CJ, Albe-Fessard DG (ed): Advances in Pain Research and Therapy, Vol 3. New York, Raven Press, 1978, p 67–90.

Rasminsky M: Ectopic generation of impulses and cross-talk in spinal nerve roots of "dystrophic" mice. Ann Neurol 3:351–357, 1978.

Rasminsky M, Sears TA: Internodal conduction in undissected demyelinated nerve fibers. J Physiol 227:323, 1972.

Rudge P, Ochoa J, Gilliatt RW: Acute peripheral nerve compression in the baboon. Anatomical and physiological findings. J Neurol Sci 23:403, 1974.

Sanders DB: Ephaptic transmission in hemifacial spasm: A single-fiber EMG study. Muscle Nerve 12:690–694, 1989.

Sanders FK, Young JZ: Effect of peripheral connection on diameter of nerve fibers. Nature 155:237, 1945.

Seddon HJ: Three types of nerve injury. Brain 66:237, 1943.

Seneviratne KN, Peiris 0A: The effect of ischaemia on the excitability of sensory nerves in diabetes mellitus. J Neurol Neurosurg Psychiatry 31:348, 1968.

Spencer PS: Light and electron microscopic observations on localised peripheral nerve injuries. Thesis. London, University of London, 1971.

Spinner M: The arcade of Frohse and its relation to posterior interosseous nerve paralysis. J Bone joint Surg 50B:809, 1968.

Sunderland S: Nerve lesion in the carpal tunnel syndrome. J Neurol Neurosurg Psychiatry 39:615, 1976.

Thomas PK: Changes in the endoneurial sheaths of peripheral myelinated nerve fibers during Wallerian degeneration. J Anat 98:175, 1964.

Thomas, PK, Fullerton PM: Nerve fiber size in the carpal tunnel syndrome. J Neurol Neurosurg Psychiatry 26:520, 1963.

Wall PD, Gutnick M: Ongoing activity in peripheral nerves: The physiology and pharmacology of impulses originating from a neuroma. Exp Neurol 43:580, 1974a.

Wall PD, Gutnick M: Properties of afferent nerve impulses originating from a neuroma. Nature 248:740, 1974b.

Wall PD, Waxman S, Basbaum AI: Ongoing activity in peripheral nerve: Injury discharge. Exp Neurol 45:576, 1974.

Weiss P, Edds MV, Cavanaugh M: The effect of terminal connections on the caliber of nerve fibers. Anat Rec 92:215, 1945.

Weiss P, Taylor AC: Further experimental evidence against "neurotropism" in nerve regeneration. J Exp Zool 95:233, 1944.

Wessells NK, Spooner BS, Ash JF, Bradley MO, Luduena MA, Taylor EL, Wrenn JT, Yamada KM: Microfilaments in cellular and developmental processes. Science 71:135, 1971.

Williams PL, Hall SM: Prolonged in vivo observations of normal peripheral nerve fibers and their acute reactions to crush and deliberate trauma. J Anat 108:397, 197la.

Williams PL, Hall SM: Chronic wallerian degeneration—an in vivo and ultrastructural study. J Anat 109:487, 1971b.

Yamada KM, Spooner BS, Wessells NK: Axon growth: Roles of microfilaments and microtubules. Proc Natl Acad Sci U S A 66:1206, 1970.

Yamada KM, Spooner BS, Wessells NK: Ultrastructure and function of growth cones and axons of cultured cells. J Cell Biol 49:614, 1971.

Young JZ: Factors influencing the regeneration of nerves. Adv Surg 2:165, 1949.

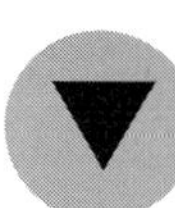

Chapter 51

• Ghazi M. Rayan
• Nabih R. Asal
• Paula C. Bohr

Epidemiology and Economic Impact of Compression Neuropathy

Over the last two decades, there has been a noticeable increase in the incidence of compression neuropathy (CN). All indications lead to the conclusion that this increase will continue and approach epidemic proportions. The causes of this increase are multifactorial. Few studies have attempted to investigate the cause of this complex problem. Some studies have attributed CN to repetitive motion, excessive force, and poor work habits or posture in a stressed and automated industrial setting. Others have attributed the increase in incidence to antiquated workers' compensation laws and changing work ethics. The condition is now recognized as a major public health problem. It has profound impact on many aspects of the individual's life. No one is immune because CN may affect people of all ages and walks of life, including the blue-collar workers on assembly lines, white-collar workers using computer keyboards, athletes, musicians, and housewives. CN is one of the most frequently encountered conditions in the hand surgeon's daily practice, which contributed to the evolution of industrial hand surgery. The media has intensified public awareness of one aspect of the problem, carpal tunnel syndrome (CTS). Carpal tunnel surgery is among the most commonly performed surgical procedures in the United States.

The purpose of this chapter is to review the recent literature on the public health aspects of CN, including studies on the epidemiology, economic costs, and prevention strategies. Carpal tunnel syndrome is the most prevalent of all compression syndromes and has received most of the attention from reported epidemiologic studies. This chapter focuses on CTS as a prototype of CN. The chapter includes definitions of epidemiologic terms, a discussion of the incidence and prevalence in the general population, demographics, etiology, and risk factors. Special emphasis is placed on the problem among athletes, musicians, and occupational groups. The last two sections deal with the economic costs and prevention. It is hoped that the reader will have a good appreciation of CN as a public health problem and will understand the many faceted etiology and factors that may affect its occurrence, diagnosis, treatment, and control.

DEFINITIONS

Epidemiology

Epidemiology studies the distribution and determinants of health-related states and events in certain populations. This is accomplished by using disease frequency measures (inci-

dence and prevalence) and measures of association (odds ratio and relative risk) to establish links between exposures and outcomes, and to assess the value of prevention and control programs. The epidemiologic approach has been used sparingly in the study of CN.

Disease incidence is defined as the number of new events that occur in a population. The incidence rate applies to a specified at-risk population and measures the probability of developing a disease in such a population during a given time. The incidence measure, usually derived from prospective cohort studies of individuals exposed to risk factors, has not been used extensively to study the incidence of CN.

Disease prevalence is defined as the number of existing cases in a specified population at a given time. It is often used in conjunction with the incidence rate and is more applicable to chronic conditions. The prevalence rate is estimated from cross-sectional surveys of special population groups. The prevalence measure has been frequently reported in CN.

The measures of association are derived from analytic studies, which compare the prevalence of specific risk factors between cases and controls or the incidence of disease outcome between exposed and nonexposed groups. The odds ratio is used in case-control studies, whereas the relative risk is used in prospective cohort studies, and often, both are used interchangeably.

Clinical Types

Cumulative trauma disorders (CTDs), also known as overuse syndromes or repetitive strain injury, are a group of soft tissue symptoms caused by repeated exertions and movements of the body (Armstrong, 1986). In the upper extremity, they include CN and tendonopathy that is often referred to as "tendinitis." CTD has emerged as a controversial term. The American Society for Surgery of the Hand (1996) has expressed concern about using this term as a diagnosis and the tendency to assign causal relationship to work, on the basis of subjective complaints only and without epidemiologic evidence. CN may occur at any level, from the hand to the thoracocervical region. It may affect more than one nerve in the same upper extremity, that is, double and multiple entrapment, or a single nerve at more than one level, that is, double crush and multiple crush injuries. The most frequently encountered CN is the median nerve at the wrist (Omer, 1992), followed by ulnar nerve at the elbow (Rayan, 1992). Other neuropathies affect the brachial plexus at the thoracic outlet, radial and median nerves in the forearm, ulnar nerve at the wrist, and digital nerves in the hand. Examples of rarely encountered neuropathies are those of the musculocutaneous and suprascapular nerves.

THE GENERAL POPULATION

The overall incidence and prevalence rates of CN in the general population are not known or documented. However, it is generally observed that CN has become one of the most common disorders encountered in a hand surgeon's daily practice. The clinical impression is that an increase in the incidence of CN has taken place over the last two decades. This increase may have resulted from the refinement of diagnostic tools, availability of better treatment modalities, increased mechanization and stressful work settings, and the heightened awareness of CN as a workers' compensation disorder. Compression neuropathy may affect people of any age, race, sex, or socioeconomic status. Perhaps there is a potential for overdiagnosing CTS. It is believed, however, that CN in general is underreported (Zimmerman et al, 1992). Attempts at evaluating the extent of morbidity of CN from workers' compensation claims underestimate the problem because not all cases of CN are attributed to "injuries" in the workplace and not all individuals with CN seek workers' compensation (Bleeker et al, 1985). Another reason to suggest that the incidence and prevalence of CN may be greater than reported is the difficulty in diagnosing certain atypical neuropathies and those associated with musculoskeletal pathology.

The Kelsey report in 1980 was not specific for CN but was the first attempt to use national data to describe the problem (Kelsey et al, 1980). It is estimated that each year in the United States, there are about 16 million upper extremity injuries of sufficient severity that bring about either a restriction of activity or a visit to a physician. These injuries affect the musculoskeletal or nervous system, and two thirds of these injuries occur in working people. These injuries are responsible for about 90 million days of restricted activity and 16 million days lost from work annually. They result in half a million inpatient hospitalizations, six million visits to emergency rooms, and 12 million visits to physicians annually.

The second Kelsey report* gathered recent data on the estimated number and percent of nerve related upper extremity outpatient visits and procedures in the United States for 1992. There were 2,699,602 outpatient visits, which accounted for 12.5% of the total outpatient visits. Using International Classification of Diseases codes, about 90% of these visits are attributed to CTS and 8% to other upper extremity nerve lesions. The number of visits ranked 4th and was exceeded only by disorders of joints, cartilage, tendons, and bursae; open wounds; and fractures.

The number of outpatient nerve-related procedures involving the upper extremities was 2,341,790, which accounted for 32.8% of the total operations. These include 2,186,811 for carpal tunnel release and 154,979 operations for other peripheral nervous system problems, such as decompression, transposition and neurolysis. The number of operations

*Kelsey J: Personal communication, 1994.

ranked second to the musculoskeletal system, and about 93.4% of the operations were associated with carpal tunnel syndrome (Table 51–1). In her recent report, Kelsey* also estimated the annual average number and percent of nerve-related hand and upper extremity inpatient operative procedures in the United States between 1989 and 1991. There were 44,000 procedures, 18,000 (40.9%) for men and 26,000 (59.1%) for women. About 25,000 procedures were performed for carpal tunnel release. The percent distribution by age did not differ much between men and women except for the low number of procedures performed in men in the group aged 65 and over. Inpatient operations involving the carpal tunnel accounted for 4.3% of the total upper extremity procedures and 56.8% of the nervous system procedures (Table 51–2).

Although these data provide information about the magnitude of the problem, they are not precise for calculating incidence and prevalence rates because during outpatient visits, each patient may have had more than one visit or procedure.

*Kelsey J: Personal communication, 1994.

▼ TABLE 51–1

Estimated Number of Outpatient Visits and Procedures for Nervous System–Related Upper Extremity Conditions in the United States, 1992

Variable	Number of Nerve-Related Visits	Percent of Total Disease Categories	Rank
Visits	2,699,602	12.5	4th*
ICD-9 Code 354.0			
Carpal tunnel syndrome	2,430,496	11.2	
Operations	2,341,790	32.8	2nd†
ICD-9 Code 4.43			
Carpal tunnel syndrome	2,186,811	30.6	

*Exceeded by the categories (1) disorders of joints, cartilage, tendon, and bursa; (2) open wounds; and (3) fractures.
†Exceeded by operations on the musculoskeletal system.
Adapted from data provided by Kelsey J: Personal communication, 1994.

▼ TABLE 51–2

Hand and Upper Extremity Nervous System–Related Inpatient Procedures by Age and Gender in the United States, Annual Average, 1989–1991

Gender		<18	18–44	45–64	65 and Over	Total
Total	#	*	19,000	15,000	9,000	44,000
	(%)		(43.2)	(34.1)	(20.5)	(100.0)
Male	#	*	8,000	7,000	2,000	18,000
	(%)		(44.4)	(38.9)	(11.1)	(100.0)
Female	#	*	11,000	8,000	7,000	26,000
	(%)		(42.3)	(30.8)	(26.9)	(100.0)
Release of Carpal Tunnel						25,000
Total Procedures (including the nervous system)						587,000

*Estimate does not meet standard of reliability or precision source: National Center for Health Statistics, National Hospital Discharge Survey, Data Tapes, 1989–91. Data from Kelsey J: Personal communication, 1994.

Demographics, Etiology, and Risk Factors

Some compression neuropathies are more common among women than men such as CTS and thoracic outlet syndrome. Carpal tunnel syndrome is more frequent in women than in men. The reported female:male ratio varies from 2:1 to 6.6:1 (Garland et al, 1957; Heathfield, 1957; Phalen, 1970, 1972; Tanzer, 1959; Yamaguski et al, 1965). The condition appears to present a bimodal age distribution at diagnosis, with peaks at ages 25 to 30 and 40 to 60 years (Garland et al, 1957; Kendall, 1960; Litchman et al, 1984; Phalen, 1970, 1972; Yamaguski et al, 1965). The first peak appears to affect the occupational group. The second peak in age of onset for CTS in women has been explained by the influence of exogenous and endogenous hormonal factors associated with the perimenopausal period. These factors include artificial menopause, estrogen replacement therapy, gynecological surgery, and use of oral contraceptives (Bjorkquist et al, 1977; Cannon et al, 1981; Layton, 1958; Reid, 1956; Sabour and Fadel, 1970; Schiller and Kolb, 1954). A population-based study on CTS found the average age of diagnosis to be 50 years for men and 51 for women, and 58% had bilateral involvement (Stevens et al, 1988). The incidence of CTS showed a sharp increase in the last 5 years. Multiplying the age-adjusted rates by the average life expectancy of 70 years, the cumulative lifetime probability of being diagnosed with CTS in this population is 3.5% for men and 11% for women. One study showed that patients older than 70 years of age are at high risk for developing severe CTS (Seror, 1991). Approximately 60% of such patients had severe CTS, and more than 95% of these patients had severe sensory and motor denervation.

CN may be idiopathic, or it may be due to extrinsic or intrinsic causes, such as blunt trauma and fractures. It may be caused by neoplastic conditions such as myeloma and neurofibromatosis or by space occupying lesions, such as ganglion, lipoma, and fibroma. Congenital causes of CN include vascular anomalies such as persistent median artery, aberrant muscles in the carpal tunnel, bony malformation of the elbow, or cervical rib in the thoracic outlet region.

CTS has been reported in association with a number of medical conditions. It is not clear what role these conditions play in the etiology of this neuropathy. In a review of 915 cases of CTS seen at the Mayo Clinic (Blodgett et al, 1962), the most frequently associated conditions were cervical spine and wrist degenerative arthritis (18.4%), rheumatoid arthritis (10.5%), thyroid disease (9.0%), previous trauma (6.4%), diabetes (6.4%), localized tenosynovitis (5.4%), shoulder arthritis (4.1%) other neurological disorders (3.4%), miscellaneous disorders (2.2%), hematological disorders (2.2%), pregnancy (1.2%), and gout (0.7%). In 30.6% of the cases, there were no systemic diseases reported.

Other conditions that may be associated with CTS include scleroderma, systemic lupus erythematosus, renal disease, alcoholism, acromegaly, myeloma, hemophilia, and amyloidosis (Grokoest and Demactini, 1954; Grossman et al, 1961). Individuals on hemodialysis are at high risk for developing CTS (Holtmann and Anderson, 1977; Jain et al, 1979). These patients may have amyloidosis from nondialyzable serum protein and may develop polyneuropathy (Bickness et al, 1991). The incidence of median neuropathy in dialysis patients is reported to vary between 4% and 31% (Naito et

al, 1987), and usually occurs on the side of the fistula (Minami and Ogino, 1987; Naito et al, 1987). One study found smoking and obesity to be statistically significant risk factors in developing CTS (Vessey et al, 1990).

CN may also be predisposed by physiologic conditions or hormonal changes, such as malnutrition, pregnancy, obesity, menustral disorders and menopause. A number of studies suggested that reproductive factors explain the higher prevalence of CTS in women. These studies have found such a trend during and after pregnancy (Benson and Inman, 1956; Crisp and Defrancesco, 1964; Downie, 1964; Gould and Wissinger, 1978; Guly, 1959; Layton, 1958; Massey, 1978; Melvin et al, 1969; O'Duffy et al, 1973; Soferman et al, 1964; Tobin, 1967; Wilkinson, 1960). The association between CTS and pregnancy is intriguing, and a number of hypotheses have been proposed to explain this association. These include fluid retention, weight gain, and poor posture during pregnancy, which may cause cervical nerve root compression (Benson and Inman, 1956; Downie, 1964; Guly, 1959; Phalen, 1972; Wilkinson, 1960). Other investigators have been unable to support these hypotheses (Bjorkquist et al, 1977; Crisp and Defrancesco, 1964; Gould and Wissenger, 1978). Wand (1990) suggested that CTS during pregnancy and lactation appears to be two separate entities. In both, the syndrome affects older primiparous women, but unlike CTS in pregnancy, CTS of lactation is not associated with pre-eclampsia or peripheral edema. Clinical observations suggest that CTS and tendonopathy in lactating mothers occur frequently on the side the mother carries her infant and is more common among primiparous mothers. A valid reference on the epidemiology of CTS is a publication by Kelsey in 1982.

CTS may be an expression of cumulative trauma due to occupational, recreational, or household activities. There is strong evidence to suggest that CTS is caused by repetitive hand motions, especially of the digits and wrist (Garland et al, 1957; Phalen, 1972; Tanzer, 1959; Yamaguski et al, 1965). Gelberman showed that the carpal canal mean pressure with the wrist in neutral position is 32 mm Hg. With 90 degrees of each wrist flexion and extension, the pressure increased to 94 mm Hg and 110 mm Hg, respectively (Gelberman et al, 1981).

One study showed that CTS in the workplace occurred twice as often bilaterally than on the dominant hand alone, which confirms the importance of nonoccupational risk factors (Loslever and Ranaivosoa, 1993). The higher frequency of CTS in women than in men may be explained partly by the repetitive motion activities that are executed by women in some occupations, such as typing, sewing, knitting, scrubbing, and polishing. These activities are found to increase the risk of CTS (Garland et al, 1957; Kendall, 1960; Phalen, 1972; Tanzer, 1959; Yamaguski et al, 1965). A number of case-control studies have shown that patients with CTS are more likely than controls to engage in tasks involving repetitive motion and exposure to vibration (Cannon et al, 1981).

The carpal tunnel cross-sectional area as a risk factor for CTS particularly in women is a controversial issue. Bleecker and colleagues (1985, 1987) reported on their findings from two studies that investigated the size of the carpal canal in the workplace using computerized tomography. They found that workers with CTS had a smaller carpal tunnel cross-sectional area than controls. Workers with subclinical syndrome had an area that was similar to the symptomatic group. Wrist circumference was not a predictor of smaller carpal canal area.

Wrist ratio, calculated by dividing the anteroposterior by the mediolateral diameters of the wrist and taken during pre-employment testing, was a predictor of symptoms associated with CTS. Gordon and co-workers (1988) took such measurements at a large midwestern manufacturing plant and noted that over a 3-year period, one half of the symptomatic employees had wrist ratios greater than or equal to 0.7. This same ratio was found among three fourths of the asymptomatic employees who displayed abnormal nerve conduction studies. There was also a significant positive correlation between distal motor median latency and wrist ratio. One study found that small carpal tunnel size was not a risk factor in the development of CTS and, therefore, it was considered of questionable value as a screening tool for industries (Winn and Habes, 1992).

SPECIAL GROUPS

The Musician

Musicians are sensitive even to mild degrees of nerve compression because their performance suffers. They may become disabled more easily than nonmusicians. Secondary gain, litigation, and malingering are rarely an issue among musicians. The excessive wrist flexion often acquired during performance in violinists and guitarists, excessive gripping of bows or strings, and carrying heavy instruments may be predisposing factors for CTDs and CN. Using keyboard, string, wind or percussion instruments can also predispose an individual to CN.

Musculoskeletal problems were more common among female (70%) than male (52%) musicians and among string players than woodwind or brass players. The prevalence of nonmusculoskeletal problems is not strongly related to gender or instrument (Middlestadt and Fishbein, 1989). Reports from clinics reflect a predominance of symptoms among keyboard players, followed by string players (Brandfonbrener, 1990; Hochberg et al, 1983).

The International Conference of Symphony Orchestra Musicians (ICSOM) conducted a membership survey regarding the prevalence of medical problems and risks related to playing instruments (Fishbein et al, 1988). There was an overall occurrence of performance-related problems of 76%. Recent studies showed significant gender-associated risk, with women reporting more medical complaints related to playing than men (Brandfonbrener, 1990). In the ICSOM study, female musicians had greater risk of injury associated with playing a large string instrument such as the viola and cello. Adolescent female musicians are particularly vulnerable to playing-related injuries (Fry et al, 1988). Female students reported a significantly higher rate of injuries than male students, as did players of large instruments when compared with players of small instruments (Lockwood, 1988). Among university-level students, the incidence is twice as high in women as in men. The incidence among keyboard and string players was three times that of woodwind and brass players (Manchester and Fielder, 1991).

Studies reported peripheral nerve disorders in 18%

(Hochberg, 1983) and 29% (Lederman, 1989) of musicians. The Mayo Clinic reported that 22% of musicians complaints were related to CN, including CTS, cubital tunnel syndrome, thoracic outlet syndrome, and pronator syndrome (Amadio and Russotti, 1990). Entrapment neuropathy was the most common disorder (48%) among 200 consecutively examined musicians with upper extremity symptoms (Charness, 1992). The distribution of upper extremity disorders in order of frequency was free lance, professionals, orchestra, students, and lastly, amateur musicians. The causative musical instruments in order of frequency were piano, violin, flute, guitar, cello, clarinet, viola, bass, saxophone, and drums. In their order of frequency, the following nerve entrapments were observed: ulnar nerve at the elbow, brachial plexus at the thoracic outlet, and median nerve at the wrist. Less common types of entrapment neuropathy involved radial nerve in forearm, digital nerves, radiculopathy, ulnar nerve at the wrist, medial cutaneous nerve of the forearm, and axillary and median nerves in the forearm.

Examples of measures to prevent playing-related injuries include the following (Charness, 1992): practice time should be increased gradually before recitals and auditions; increased playing intensity should be compensated by reducing total playing time; return to play after layoff should be gradual; overworking one group of muscles and excessive muscle contraction should be avoided; the weight of instrument on the upper extremity can be minimized by using supports for the instruments. Other preventive measures include musculoskeletal conditioning and body relaxation, acquiring sound playing postures, taking frequent breaks, and lastly, performing stretching and warming up exercises (Brandfonbrener, 1990).

The Athlete

CN can develop in professional or recreational athletes. The incidence of these injuries, especially among recreational athletes, has been on the rise. Enthusiastic, and ill-prepared young athletes are prone to injuries. Long hours of repetitive motion during practice fueled by parental pressure may also contribute to that increase. Approximately 25% to 50% of sports injuries are attributed to overuse (Pinter, 1990). Most peripheral nerve injuries in athletes occur in the upper extremity. Hirasawa and Sakakeda found that sports-related neuropathies account for approximately 6% of all nerve injuries (Hirasawa and Sakakeda, 1983). The involved nerves, in order of frequency, were brachial plexus, radial, ulnar, axillary median, and digital nerve. Most sports-related nerve injuries are caused by repetitive trauma to the palmar aspect of the hand and wrist, with median and ulnar nerves most frequently affected at the wrist (Rettig, 1990). In a comprehensive review article Sicuranza and McCue (1992) found that throwing sports are most frequently associated with ulnar neuropathy at the elbow, median nerve in the forearm and wrist, and radial nerve in the forearm. Cyclists' palsy or ulnar neuropathy in bicycle riders is one of the most common athletic CNs. Bowler's thumb, or ulnar digital nerve compression, is one of the most frequently reported hand injuries among bowlers. Digital neuropathy is also caused by mountain climbing, gymnastics, and baseball. Other sports associated with CN are archery (Rayan, 1992), racquet sports, swimming, contact collision, and intensive gripping and catching sports, such as gymnastics and weight-lifting (Sicuranza and McCue, 1992).

THE WORKPLACE

The overall incidence and prevalence rates of CN in the workforce are unknown. The recently reported increase in frequency of CN is most likely due to the more repetitive nature and the rapidly increased work cycle. Technological advancements and the shift from an industrial to a service-oriented society have resulted in jobs becoming fast paced and more repetitive. The link between neuropathy and tendonopathy to cumulative trauma in the workplace has been facilitated by increased clinician awareness of the problem. Repeated sustained exertion of the upper extremity is a major ergonomic risk factor for developing "CTDs." This is enhanced by force, localized mechanical stress, postural stress, low temperature, and vibration (Armstrong, 1986). Other factors that might contribute to CN include sociopolitical and economic forces, liberalized workers' compensation laws, litigious society, and psychological factors (Millender, 1992). CN of the upper extremity has become a major cause of workers' compensation claims. Most reported epidemiologic and demographic data are related to CTS, and little, if any, are available on the remaining compressive syndromes. Therefore, the following discussion is restricted for the most part to CTS. Individuals in occupations that require repetitive or forceful hand motion, or both, are considered to be at high risk for developing CN, particularly carpal tunnel and cubital tunnel syndrome.

CTS is the most frequently encountered and most studied of all upper extremity CNs and is now considered the most prevalent occupational disease. Katz and colleagues (1991) estimated the prevalence of CTS to be about 1% in the general population and up to 15% in workers in high-risk industries. There are an estimated 20 million workers on assembly lines or at other jobs requiring repetitive and continuous upper extremity motions or awkward wrist positions that increase their risk for developing CN (Blair and Bear-Lehman, 1987).

Workers at risk of developing CTS include butchers, poultry workers, assembly line workers, garment workers or seamstresses, carpenters, packers, pneumatic tool operators, checkout and cash register operators, computer operators, journalists, and telegraphers (Armstrong et al, 1982; Louis, 1992; Margolis and Krause, 1987). Armstrong and colleagues (1982) reported an incidence rate of CN in poultry processing plant workers that ranged from 6.2 to 129.6 per 200,000 work hours. The rates varied depending on the specific tasks performed. In an electronic assembly plant, a rate of 6.6 cases per 200,000 hours worked was reported among less physically demanding occupations (Hymovich and Lindholm, 1966). Poultry processors were found using extremes of wrist flexion and ulnar deviation to manipulate the straight-handled knife (Armstrong et al, 1982). Two studies found that women with CTS tended to hold the wrist in positions that deviated from the neutral position and exerted greater force than did the control groups performing the same job (Armstrong and Chaffin, 1979; Masear et al, 1986).

A report from the Bureau of Labor Statistics noted a 50% increase in new occupational illness associated with repeated trauma during a 5-year period (1980 to 1984) (Blair and Bear-Lehman, 1987). The National Institute of Occupational Safety and Health (NIOSH) estimated the annual incidence and prevalence of CTS among U.S. laborers to be about 23,000 and 230,000 cases, respectively (Sager, 1982). The California Occupational Health Program surveyed health care practitioners for the occurrence of CTS in Santa Clara County. The respondent providers cared for a total of 7214 patients with CTS during 1987 alone, which equals a prevalence rate of 529/100,000 population. About 47% of these cases were considered to be work related, producing a prevalence rate of 244/100,000 population. The low overall response rate (30%) suggests that the overall prevalence rate may be underestimated by 70% (Centers for Disease Control, 1989).

Franklin and associates (1991) conducted a Washington State population-based study to assess the incidence rate of occupational CTS from the State Workers' Compensation data base. During a 5-year period, (1984 to 1988) they identified 7926 incident claims or about 1585 new claims per year. The 5-year incidence rate was about 1.74 claims/ 1000 FTEs. The female-to-male ratio was 1.2:1 in the occupational group, with mean age of 37.4 years. The nonoccupational CTS mean age was 51 years, and the female-to-male ratio was 3:1. Furthermore, the highest industry-specific rates were found in the food processing, carpentry, egg production, wood products, and logging industries.

Overseas countries have also recognized CTDs as a cause for workers' disabilities. Repetitive wrist flexion was documented as a risk factor in a study from the Netherlands (De Krom, 1990). The increased incidence of CTS was associated with an increase in flexion and extension of the wrist, and the duration of exposure. Hagberg and colleagues (1992) in Sweden reviewed the findings from 15 cross-sectional studies on CTS involving 32 occupational or exposure groups and six case-control studies. The prevalence of CTS in the occupational groups varied from 0.6% to 61%. The highest prevalence rates were reported for grinders, butchers, grocery store workers, frozen food factory workers, platers, and workers with high-force, highly repetitive manual movements. Liss and co-workers (1992) used billing data for the Province of Ontario, Canada to estimate CTS morbidity and surgery rates at a plant manufacturing ice cream novelties. Among the 150 employees on the plant's seniority lists (1979 to 1990), CTDs had been diagnosed in 17 workers, 9 of whom required carpal tunnel surgery. There were about six workers' compensation billings for "tendinitis" and CTS among plant employees during a 3-year period (1987 to 1989). This frequency was about 68 times that of the entire Ontario labor force. In a study from China, repetitive use of the hand and local exposure to cold were identified as risk factors for CTS among frozen food factory employees (Chiang et al, 1990). Ireland (1992) found that in Australia, repetitive strain injury bears the hallmark of a sociopolitical phenomenon rather than a medical problem, and therefore, its incidence has declined in that country.

The prevalence of self-reported CTS from a mailed survey among 1345 female supermarket checkers ages 18 to 49 was estimated to be 62.5% (Margolis and Kraus, 1987). Prevalence rates were related to use of laser scanners, age, years on the job, and average weekly work hours. The prevalence of CTS for those using scanners was significantly different when compared with that of nonusers.

Accumulated evidence supports the relationship between work-related repetitive and forceful tasks and the development of CTS. In a doctoral dissertation that included an extensive literature review, Silverstein studied 574 workers in 6 plants (Silverstein, 1985). Jobs were categorized according to the forcefulness and repetitiveness of tasks performed. Each job was classified into high or low force and high or low repetition, producing four job categories; low force/low repetition, low force/high repetition, high force/high repetition, and high force/low repetition. Thirty-three percent of the workers interviewed had CTDs compared with 19.5% on physical examination plus interview. The high-force/high-repetition group had the highest risk of all hand-wrist CTDs, including "tendinitis" and CTS. Repetitiveness was more important as a risk factor in CTS, whereas force was more important in hand-wrist CTDs. Gender was a factor, with a 2:1 female-to-male ratio in CTDs but not in CTS.

Silverstein and co-workers (1987) investigated the prevalence of CTS among 652 workers in 39 jobs in seven different industries. When the workers were divided into four groups according to the job's amount of hand force and repetition requirements, the group with the lowest force and repetition categories had the lowest CTS prevalence rate (0.6%), whereas the group with the highest force and repetition had the highest prevalence rate (5.6%). When the highest group was compared with the lowest group using the odds ratio as a measure of association, it resulted in a value of 15, which was statistically significant. Furthermore, the authors found that repetitiveness was a greater risk factor than force for the development of CTS.

Arndt (1987) used electromyography to study the relationship of the work pace and CTDs. A link was established between fast work pace and CTDs, and this factor was suggested to be partly due to job pressures associated with faster pace. In another study of 700 electronics assembly workers, Feldman (1987) reported that more workers in the highly repetitious tasks (17.9%) had complaints of hand paresthesias than did workers in the less repetitious group (8.7%). The high-risk group reported more nocturnal and daytime paresthesias (22.6%) than the low-risk group (14.8%).

Dental hygienists are reported to be at risk of developing CTS (Gerwatowski et al, 1992). In a survey of 493 hygienists, 7% were diagnosed to have CTS and 63% had experienced symptoms of CTS (Osborn et al, 1990). Conrad and co-workers (1990), using vibrometry for early detection of nerve compression among hygienists, found 25.9% to have CTS. The high-frequency vibrating tools used by hygienists was suggested to be the cause of demyelinating nerve lesions (Hjortsberg et al, 1989). The respondents to a survey among cardiac sonographers reported symptoms of CTS in 86%, but only 3% were diagnosed as such (Vanderpool et al, 1993). In an experimental study Lundborg and associates (1990) confirmed that vibration produces nerve fiber damage.

Cannon and co-workers (1981) used a case-control study to evaluate the relationship between low-frequency hand-held vibrating tools and the development of CTS. He compared 30 cases of CTS among employees of an aircraft corporation with 90 controls matched by sex but randomly selected from employees of the same plant. The odds ratio was 13.8, which was statistically significant, indicating a 13.8-fold risk increase for workers in tasks involving hand-held or vibrating tools. Another case-control study from Sweden investigated the relationship between hand-held tools and CTS, and compared 34 CTS cases with a matched number of controls (Weislander et al, 1989). The odds ratio for vibration exposure from hand-held tools was 3.3 and for more repetitive wrist motions was 2.7. Both values were statistically significant. The data indicate about a three-fold increase in risk for the development of CTS for tasks involving either vibration exposure or repetitive wrist motion. A study from Italy showed significantly higher prevalence rates of persistent upper limb symptoms and CTS among forestry workers than among controls (Bovenzi et al, 1991). The prevalence increased with increasing vibration exposure. NIOSH estimated that 1.2 million workers in the United States have vibration exposure (National Institute for Occupational Safety and Health, 1989). Miller and associates (1994) considered hand-arm vibration syndrome to be a separate entity that can be associated with CTS or misdiagnosed as CTS. He quoted several studies on the prevalence of hand-arm vibration syndrome among vibration-exposed workers worldwide and the prevalence varied from 10% to 70%. Another study found the incidence of vibration-induced CTS to be 5%, approximately 50% were bilateral, the mean age was 33 years, and 81% were males (Conner and Kolisek, 1986). Boyle and colleagues (1988) found that 63% of patients with vibration white fingers had CTS. Gupta and McCabe (1993) listed several studies that found the prevalence of vibration white finger to vary from 7% to 84%. From these studies, it became clear that the prevalence of this problem is decreasing. This is probably due to improved design of vibrating tools such as the chain saw (Gupta and McCabe, 1993).

ECONOMIC COSTS

The economic impact has been highlighted as current political agendas focus on medical services cost containment and changing health care delivery models. Traditionally, medical management has focused on tangible costs, with the understanding that the intangible benefits often influence decisions on care. The economic costs of CN is not easily identified. Generally, CN is included in a broader category of upper extremity injuries. Upper extremity injuries account for approximately 30% of the total number of work-related injuries (Clifton, 1993). Reports from therapists indicate that at least 40% of their cases involve "cumulative trauma," primarily CTS (Schachner, 1990). Some data are available for the costs of CTS, but little or no data are currently defined for other types of CNs.

In 1991, the estimated costs of occupational injuries and illnesses ranged from $1.96 billion to $2.82 billion annually for medical care and lost wages (Neumark et al, 1991). In the workers' compensation system alone, the estimated costs of injury were nearly $70 billion by 1993 (Clifton, 1993). Medical and rehabilitation service costs consume between 40 and 50% of workers' compensation expenditures (Clifton, 1993). In 1990, it was estimated that more than 100,000 carpal tunnel surgeries were performed (Schachner, 1990).

The average CTS case potentially reaches $40,000 in medical costs and about $3000 in benefits to the injured worker (Slattery, 1992). Current estimates by the Chubb Corporation indicate that the amount paid for cases involving repetitive motion injuries averages between $35,000 and $75,000 on the East and West coasts of the United States and between $12,000 and $20,000 in the Midwest (Marley, 1994). Marley indicated that only about 5% of repetitive motion injuries are full-blown cases of CTS, but they account for the largest portion of the paid claims. When surgery does not resolve the symptoms, these cases are often reopened and the payouts for treatment can reach as high as $200,000 per case (Marley, 1994). Carpal tunnel release was the 10th most frequently performed procedure in the older age group with regard to monies spent under Medicare B with total cost of $15.5 million (AAOS, 1996).

Lost earnings have the most profound effect on the injured worker (Neumark et al, 1991). Estimates from 1980 indicate that upper extremity injuries correspond to 16 million work days lost, with an additional 90 million days of restricted activity (Kelsey et al, 1980). With five-fold increasing incidence of CNs reported by the Bureau of Labor Statistics in recent years, the days of lost work and restricted activity have increased dramatically. The average length of time away from work because of cumulative trauma disability is 8 to 10 weeks (Clifton, 1993). Statistics from the Pacific Northwest of the United States indicate the average lost time was 12 weeks, with 3 weeks of postoperative hand therapy exceeding $8500 per case (Schachner, 1990). In some cases in which the lost time nears 1 year, the medical costs alone could range from $5000 to $11,000 without consideration for time lost wages (Schachner, 1990). These losses may be born directly by the worker or, to a lesser extent, by workers' compensation or medical insurance. Workers' compensation indemnity benefits averaged $15,000 annually in East coast states (Schachner, 1990). Early intervention can decrease medical costs and minimize time away from work. Rehabilitation can be sometimes overutilized; however, independent studies indicate that every dollar invested in rehabilitation services will return between $8 and $14 in claims savings (Madeja, 1991). Ergonomics programs can reduce the overall expenditure for work injuries. Marley (1994) reports that the number of reported cases and the company costs per case increase in the first year, level off in the second year, and pay off in the third year as new cases are being recognized in earlier stages, when treatment is less costly. Finally, Pasque and Rayan (1995) studied the results of surgical management for cubital tunnel syndrome and noted that legal representation, especially active litigation, has an adverse relationship to the outcome and prolonged the time of recovery, which can have an impact on the total cost.

PREVENTION STRATEGIES

Prevention of occupationally related CN must address both medical and nonmedical aspects, along full continuum of primary, secondary, and tertiary prevention. At the primary level, reducing injury is achieved by controlling the conditions likely to cause symptoms or by decreasing the individual's vulnerability to develop CN. Secondary prevention focuses on early identification of symptoms and providing medical management to alter the pathological process. In secondary prevention, it is believed that impairment leads to disability over time and that the processes can be halted or reversed with prompt medical care. If medical management is effective at the secondary prevention level, the need for tertiary prevention is reduced. Tertiary prevention becomes necessary when CN results in permanent or irreversible disability. At this level, the individual is often faced with work restrictions or must be accommodated at some level on the job and while performing self-care and during leisure activities. Prevention should be a team approach including the patient, physician, rehabilitation therapist, nurse, and the employer.

Primary Prevention

Primary prevention must address concerns for the individual's general health, the work force, increasing age, and identification of CN predisposing factors. General fitness programs that address an individual's predisposing factors are part of primary prevention. Although these programs may be effective in reducing workers' physical and emotional stresses, their effectiveness in preventing work-related injuries has not been documented.

Educational programs on injury prevention allow workers and supervisors to identify job-specific risk factors that can be modified before injury results. Modifications could involve alterations in worker performance traits, the success of which is dependent on the individual's willingness to learn and implement new methods of task performance. Supervisors can observe workers to ensure that proper task performance procedures are used, but ultimately the worker is responsible for avoiding risky behaviors and for ongoing compliance with the recommendation. Worker motivation to comply is influenced by incentive pay systems, job satisfaction, and advancement opportunities.

Although many individuals have short-term favorable responses, administrative measures such as job rotation or sharing may not be effective primary prevention strategies. If the physical demands of the job tasks are contributing to development of CN, job rotation may only delay identification of the problem or expose more workers to the problem.

Plant visits by physicians and ancillary health professionals with on-site job analysis and modification of the job environment allow control of job-related risk factors. Work performance videotapes are a valuable tool in the overall management of the "injured" worker and a useful alternative to plant visits. Modifications are based on evaluation of job performance associated with tool use, the impact of technology on work skills, and individual adaptations to the work area. Temporary alterations in the work environment such as the use of sorbothane-padded gloves to minimize pressure and vibration are short-term measures to address environment problems. Long-term solutions require engineering controls. The type and design of tools and equipment used can be altered to decrease the forces required, vibration, contact trauma, or awkward postures often associated with CNs development. Rearrangement of the work area is effective in minimizing postural stresses. Redesign of a work area allows easy task performance without maintaining stressful postures or acquiring awkward movement patterns. Altering the relationship of the worker to the work surface results in maintaining neutral positions of the worker's joints or the use of gravity as an assist rather than a resistance to task motions.

A variety of products are being marketed with claims of reducing the incidence of work-related problems. In general, most products are designed to adapt current environments. Biomechanical principles should be applied to the use of products, otherwise the product may not alleviate the problem. Many companies, for example, now market wrist rests to be placed between the computer keyboard and the worker. The intent is for the pad to serve as a supportive surface for resting the wrists periodically during data entry. If, however, the wrist rest is used permanently to support the wrist during typing the worker often develops the habit of working with the wrist in hyperextension rather than in the neutral position. The pressure over the carpal tunnel area from the pad may produce or exacerbate the symptoms of CTS. Use of ergonomically designed products should be carefully evaluated for each individual to determine whether the product is likely to produce the desired preventive results. It is unlikely that a single product will meet the needs of every worker.

Matching the worker to the job provides the greatest opportunity for primary prevention. This aspect of prevention involves thorough evaluation of each job to determine the essential tasks and the physical and emotional demands each places on the worker. Also, the individual worker's capacities should be assessed specifically as they relate to the proposed job assignment. Establishing a preplacement screening program will match the workers abilities to the job demands. The risk of injury is minimized if the worker's capabilities are not being exceeded by the job demands. Periodic reviews must be part of ongoing follow-up activities if the balance between worker capacity and the job demands are to be maintained. Fitness programs such as warming exercises, muscle stretching before work, and periodic breaks were also suggested as measures of primary prevention.

Secondary Prevention

Symptoms identification is a prerequisite to secondary prevention; hence, a surveillance system must be in place. The surveillance system, whether it is active or passive, can record and track developing symptoms so that early management is possible. Referral for evaluation and possible medical care should be provided as soon as symptoms are identified. Unfortunately, some workers expect a great deal of aches and pains as a normal part of working life or the result of aging. Reporting of symptoms is often delayed until the impairments begin to have an impact on functional performance. Medical management should be directed toward alleviating symptoms and preventing permanent nerve damage. This is accomplished by nonoperative or operative means. Education on predisposing risk factors and risky behaviors should be part of medical intervention.

Job tasks should be re-evaluated regarding the cognitive, social, sensorial and perceptual, and physical demands to isolate the aspects that have contributed to the development of symptoms. It may be necessary to introduce administra-

tive or engineering measures, or both, that alleviate the problematic areas. Administrative measures are directed toward altering worker behaviors. Diminishing incentive pay systems, rotating workers, and establishing training programs to instruct workers on proper technique are examples of common administrative measures. As with any type of intervention, the long-term impact of the administrative measure must be anticipated. For example, rotating workers to limit exposure to risk factors may at some level be a logical solution, but if worker rotation results in more workers developing symptoms over a longer period of time, the solution is ineffective. The effectiveness of administrative controls vary depending on the systems in place to ensure compliance with established administrative procedures.

Engineering controls generally use information and physical ergonomics. Information ergonomics addresses issues related to the processing of data from the work environment (location of displays or controls, illumination, automation). Physical ergonomics relates to use of space, equipment design and physical stresses such as vibration, weights and sizes of objects. Engineering modifications should reflect anticipated facility development and new technology implementations, and should incorporate established ergonomic principles. Modifications should be evaluated before they are implemented to anticipate potential problems.

Tertiary Prevention

When the condition results in an individual's impairment to perform functional activities, tertiary prevention is necessary. Tertiary prevention focuses on the individual's interaction with the social, cognitive, and physical environment. Management becomes an issue of whether or not the individual is able to perform instrumental tasks associated with self-care, work, and leisure activities. In addition to limited task performance, there may be structural and attitudinal barriers that interfere with the individual's ability to fulfill occupational roles.

Return to work may take one of the several forms. The worker may return to previous work, adapted work, alternative work, or referred to vocational training. Whether a worker is able to return to work is a decision that must be addressed early in the intervention process. Return to work depends on the functional and healing ability of the individual because these factors relate to the critical demands of the job. Only when the individual's functional performance matches the critical demands of the job is return to full duty possible. In cases in which functional output does not match critical job demands, consideration should be given to work-conditioning and work-hardening programs. A short-term work-hardening program allows a worker to achieve a higher physical capacity level by simulating the actual work environment. The return-to-work process should be initiated immediately following early intervention. Early initiation minimizes the opportunity for the worker to learn adverse illness behaviors that may delay the actual return to work. Even with aggressive management, it may be necessary to release the individual to work with a restricted status. When it is necessary to place restrictions on the worker's performance, issues of work environment accommodations must be addressed. Careful assessment is an integral part of physical accommodation in the work environment. Use of adapted equipment or alternative techniques to perform tasks may be necessary.

References

Amadio P, Russotti G: Evaluation and treatment of hand and wrist disorders in musicians. Hand Clin 6:405–416, 1990.

American Society for Surgery of the Hand: Editorial: Repetitive strain injuries and cumulative trauma disorders. J Hand Surgery 21A:337, 1996.

Armstrong TJ: Ergonomics and cumulative trauma disorders. Hand Clin 2:553–565, 1986.

Armstrong TJ, Chaffin DB: Carpal tunnel syndrome and selected personal attributes. J Occup Med 21:481, 1979.

Armstrong TJ, Foulke JA, Joseph BS, et al: Investigation of cumulative trauma disorders in a poultry processing plant. Am Ind Hyg Assoc J 43:103–115, 1982.

Arndt R: Work pace, stress, and cumulative trauma disorders. J Hand Surg 12A:866–869, 1987.

Benson RC, Inman VT: Brachialgia statica dysesthetica in pregnancy. West J Surg 64:115–130, 1956.

Bickness JM, Lim A, Raroque H, et al: Carpal tunnel syndrome subclinical median mononeuropathy and peripheral polyneuropathy: Common early complications of chronic peritoneal dialysis and hemodialysis. Arch Phys Med Rehabil 72:378–381, 1991.

Bjorkquist SE, Lang AH, Punnoner R, Rauramo L: Carpal tunnel syndrome in ovariectomized women. Acta Obstet Gynecol Scand 56:127–130, 1977.

Blair S, Bear-Lehman J: Editorial comment: Prevention of upper extremity occupational disorders. J Hand Surg 12A:821, 1987.

Bleecker M: Medical surveillance of carpal tunnel syndrome in workers. J Hand Surg 12A:845–848, 1987.

Bleecker ML, Bohlman M, Moreland R, et al: Carpal tunnel syndrome: Role of carpal canal size. Neurology 35:1599–1604, 1985.

Blodgett RC, Lipschomb PR, Hill RW: Incidence of hematologic disease in patients with carpal tunnel syndrome. JAMA 182:814–815, 1962.

Bovenzi M, Zadini A, Franzinelli A, et al: Occupational musculoskeletal disorders in the neck and upper limbs of forestry workers exposed to hand-arm vibration. Ergonomics 34:547, 1991.

Boyle JC, Smith NJ, Burke FD: Vibration white finger. J Hand Surg [Br]13:171–176, 1988.

Brandfonbrener A: The epidemiology and prevention of hand and wrist injuries in performing artists. Hand Clinics, Hand Injuries in Sports and Performing Arts 6:365–377, 1990.

Cannon LJ, Bernacki EJ, Walter SD: Personal and occupational factors associated with carpal tunnel syndrome. J Occup Med 23:255, 1981.

Centers for Disease Control: Occupational disease surveillance: Carpal tunnel syndrome. JAMA 262:886–889, 1989.

Charness M: Unique upper extremity disorders of musicians. In Millender L, Louis D, Simmons B (eds): Occupational Disorders of the Upper Extremity. New York, Churchill Livingstone, 1992, pp 227–252.

Chiang HC, Chen SS, Yu HS, et al: The occurrence of carpal tunnel syndrome in frozen food factory employees. Kao Hsiung I Hsueh Ko Hsueh Tsa Chih 6:73–80, 1990.

Clifton, D: Reimbursement for and Case Management of Carpal Tunnel Syndrome. Low Back Injury and Carpal Tunnel Syndrome: Proceedings of Project Focus '93 Conference on Work-Related Injury, August 28, 1993, Alexandria, Virginia (published by the American Physical Therapy Association for the Foundation for Physical Therapy, Inc.)

Conrad JC, Osborn JB, Conrad KJ, et al: Peripheral nerve dysfunction in practicing dental hygienists. J Dent Hygiene 64:382–387, 1990.

Conner D, Kolisek F. Vibration-induced carpal tunnel syndrome. Orthopaed Rev 15:49–54, 1986.

Crisp WE, Defrancesco S: The hand syndrome of pregnancy. Obstet Gynecol 23:433–437, 1964.

De Krom M, Kester A, Knipschild P, et al: Risk factors for carpal tunnel syndrome. Am Med J Epidemiol 132:1102–1110, 1990.

Downie AW: Carpal tunnel syndrome during pregnancy. JAMA 190:689, 1964.

Feldman RG, Travers PH, Chirico-Post J, et al: Risk assessment in electronic assembly workers: Carpal tunnel syndrome. J Hand Surg 12A:849–855, 1987.

Fishbein M, Middlestadt S, Ottati V, et al: Medical problems among ICSOM musicians: Overview of a national survey. Med Prob Perform Art 3:1, 1988.

Franklin GM, Haug J, Heyer N, et al: Occupational carpal tunnel syndrome in Washington State, 1984–1988. Am J Public Health 81:741–746, 1991.

Fry H, Ross P, Rutherford M: Music-related overuse in secondary schools. Med problem Perform Art 3:133, 1988.

Garland H, Bradshaw T, Clark J: Compression of median nerve in carpal tunnel and its relation to acroparesthesia. BMJ 1:730–734, 1957.

Gelberman RH, Hergenroeder PT, Hargens AR, et al: The carpal tunnel syndrome: A study of carpal canal pressure. J Bone Joint Surg 63A:380–383, 1981.

Gerwatowski LJ, Mcfall DB, Stach DJ: Carpal tunnel syndrome. Risk factors and preventive strategies for the dental hygienist. J Dent Hygiene 66:89–94, 1992.

Gordon C, Johnson EW, Gatens PF, et al: Wrist ratio correlation with carpal tunnel syndrome in industry. Am J Phys Med Rehabil 67:270–272, 1988.

Gould JS, Wissinger, HA: Carpal tunnel syndrome in pregnancy. South Med J 71:144–145, 1978.

Grokoest AW, Demactini FE: Systemic disease and the carpal tunnel syndrome. JAMA 155:635–637, 1954.

Grossman LA, Kaplan HJ, Ownby FD, et al: Carpal tunnel syndrome—initial manifestation of systemic disease. JAMA 176:259–261, 1961.

Gully PJ: Carpal tunnel syndrome (letter). BMJ 1:1184, 1959.

Gupta A, McCabe S: Vibration white fingers. Hand Clin 2:325–337, 1993.

Hagberg M, Morgenstern H, Kelsh M: Impact of occupations and job tasks on the prevalence of carpal tunnel syndrome. (Review.) Scand J Work Environ Health 18:337–345, 1992.

Heathfield K: Acroparthesia and carpal tunnel syndrome. Lancet 2:663–666, 1957.

Hirasawa Y, Sakakeda K: Sports and peripheral nerve injury. Am J Sports Med 11:420–426, 1983.

Hjortsberg U, Rosen I, Orbaek P, et al: Finger receptor dysfunction in dental technicians exposed to high-frequency vibration. Scand J Work Environ Health 15:339, 1989.

Hochberg F, Leffert R, Heller M, et al: Hand difficulties among musicians. J Am Med Assoc 294:14, 1983.

Holtmann B, Anderson CB: Carpal tunnel syndrome following vascular shunts for hemodialysis. Arch Surg 112:65–66, 1977.

Hymovich L, Lindholm M: Hand, wrist and forearm injuries. J Occup Med 8:573–577, 1966.

Ireland D: The Australian experience with cumulative trauma disorders. In Millender L, Louis D, Simmons B (eds): Occupational disorders of the upper extremity. New York, Churchill Livingstone, 1992, pp 79–88.

Jain VJK, Cestero RVM, Baum J: Carpal tunnel syndrome in patients undergoing maintenance dialysis. JAMA 242:2868–2869, 1979.

Katz J, Larson M, Sabra A, et al: The carpal tunnel syndrome, diagnostic utility of the history and physical examination findings. Ann Inter Med 112:321–327, 1991.

Kelsey JL: Epidemiology of musculoskeletal disorders. New York, Oxford University Press, 1982.

Kelsey J, Pastides H, Kreiger N, et al: Upper Extremity Disorders: A Survey of Their Frequency and Cost in the United States. St Louis, CV Mosby, 1980.

Kendall D: Etiology, diagnosis and treatment of paresthesias in the hands. Br Med J 2:1633–1640, 1960.

Layton, RB: Acroparesthesia in pregnancy and the carpal tunnel syndrome. J Obstet Gynecol Br Emp 65:823–825, 1958.

Lederman R: Peripheral nerve disorders in instrumentalists. Ann Nerol 26:640, 1989.

Liss GM, Armstrong C. Kusiak RA, et al: Use of provincial health insurance plan billing data to estimate carpal tunnel syndrome morbidity and surgery rates. Am J Ind Med 22:395–409, 1992.

Litchman H, Silver C, Simon S, et al: Carpal tunnel release efficiency as an ambulatory outpatient procedure done under local anesthesia. Orthopaed Rev 13:93–97, 1984.

Lockwood A: Medical problems in secondary school–aged musicians. Medical Problem Perform Art 4:129, 1988.

Loslever P, Ranaivosoa A: Biomechanical and epidemiological investigation of carpal tunnel syndrome at workplaces with high risk factors. Ergonomics 36:537, 1993.

Louis D: The carpal tunnel syndrome in the work place. In Millender L, Louis D, Simmons B (eds): Occupational Disorders of the Upper Extremity. New York, Churchill Livingstone, 1992, pp 145–154.

Lundborg G, Dahlin LB, Hansson HA, et al: Vibration exposure and peripheral nerve fiber damage. J Hand Surg 15A:346–351, 1990.

Madeja P: Cumulative trauma disorders: As claims increase, firms eye prevention and early diagnosis. Business Insurance, 25:19, 1991.

Manchester R, Fielder D: Further observation on the epidemiology of hand injuries in music students. Med Problem Perform Art 6:11, 1991.

Margolis W, Kraus JF: The prevalence of carpal tunnel symptoms in female supermarket checkers. J Occup Med 29:953, 1987.

Marley S: Repetitive motion claims increase: Employees report more injuries as information widens. Business Insurance 28:3, 1994.

Masear VR, Hayes JM, Hyde AG: An industrial cause of carpal tunnel syndrome. J Hand Surg 11A:222–226, 1986.

Massey EW: Carpal tunnel syndrome in pregnancy. Obstet Gynecol Surv 33:145–148, 1978.

Melvin JL, Burnett CN, Johnson E. Median nerve conduction in pregnancy. Arch Phys Med Rehab 50:75–80, 1969.

Middlestadt S, Fishbein M: The prevalence of severe musculoskeletal problems among male and female symphony orchestra string players. Med Prob Perform Art 4:41, 1989.

Miller R, Lohman W, Maldonado G, et al: An epidemiologic study of carpal tunnel syndrome and hand-arm vibration syndrome in relation to vibration exposure. J Hand Surg 19A:99–105, 1994.

Millender L: Orthopedic, psychosocial and legal implications. In Millender L, Louis D, Simmons B (eds): Occupational Disorders of the Upper Extremity. New York, Churchill Livingstone, 1992, pp 1–14.

Minami A, Ogino T: Carpal tunnel syndrome in patients undergoing hemodialysis. J Hand Surg 12:93–97, 1987.

Naito M, Ogata K, Goya T: Carpal tunnel syndrome in chronic renal dialysis patients. Clinical evaluation of 62 hands and resulting operative treatment. J Hand Surg (Br) 12:366–374, 1987.

National Institute for Occupational Safety and Health: Criteria for a recommended standard: Occupational exposure to hand-arm-vibration. Cincinnati, Ohio, US Dept of Health and Human Services, DHHS No 89–106, 1989.

Neumark D, Johnson R, Breznitx E, et al: Costs of Occupational Injury and Illness in Pennsylvania. J Occu Med 33:971–976, 1991.

O'Duffy JD, Randall RV, MacCarty C: Median neuropathy (carpal tunnel syndrome) in acromegaly. A sign of endocrine overactivity. Ann Intern Med 78:379–383, 1973.

Omer G Jr: Median nerve compression at the wrist. Hand Clin 8:317–324, 1992.

Osborn JB, Newell KJ, Rudney JD, et al: Carpal tunnel syndrome among Minnesota dental hygienists. J Dent Hygiene 64:79–85, 1990.

Pasque C, Rayan G: Anterior submuscular transposition of the ulnar nerve for Cubital Tunnel Syndrome. J Hand Surg (Br) 20:447–453, 1995.

Phalen GS: Reflection on 21 years' experience with carpal tunnel syndrome. JAMA 212:1365, 1970.

Phalen GS: The carpal-tunnel syndrome. Clin Orthop 83:29–40, 1972.

Pinter MA: Pathophysiology of overuse injuries in the hand and wrist. Hand Clin 6:355–364, 1990.

Rayan GM: Proximal ulnar nerve compression; cubital tunnel syndrome, nerve compression syndromes. Hand Clin 8:325–334, 1992.

Rayan GM: Archery related injuries of the hand, forearm and elbow. Southern Medical Journal 3:961–964, 1992.

Reid S: Tenovaginitis stenosis at the carpal tunnel. Aust N Z J Surg 25:204–213, 1956.

Rettig AC: Neurovascular injuries in the wrists and hands of athletes. Clin Sports Med 9:389, 1990.

Sabour M, Fadel H: The carpal tunnel syndrome—a new complication ascribed to the bill. Am J Obstet Gynecol. 107:1265–1267, 1970.

Sager M: Hazards in the workplace. The Washington Post Feb 22:D1, 1982.

Schachner M: Treat symptom before it worsens: Experts. Business Insurance 24:30–31, 1990.

Schiller F, Kolb FO: Carpal tunnel syndrome in acromegaly. Neurology 4:271–282, 1954.

Seror P: Carpal tunnel syndrome in the elderly. Annales de Chirurgie de la Main et du Membre Superieur 10:217–225, 1991.

Sicuranza MJ, McCue FC: Compressive neuropathies in the upper extremity of athletes. Hand Clin 8:263–273, 1992.

Silverstien B: The prevalence of upper extremity cumulative trauma disorders in industry. Ph.D. Dissertation. Ann Arbor, Michigan, University of Michigan, 1985.

Silverstein BA, Fine LJ, Armstrong TJ: Occupational factors and carpal tunnel syndrome. Am J Ind Med 11:343–358, 1987.

Slattery TJ: Back, Carpal Tunnel Claims Mounting. Risk & Insurance Management Society Annual Meeting, Anaheim, California. National Underwriter 96:1042–6841, 1992.

Soferman N, Weissman S, Haimov M: Acroparesthesias in pregnancy. Am J Obstet Gynecol 89:528–531, 1964.

Stevens JC, Sun S, Beard C, et al: Carpal tunnel syndrome in Rochester Minnesota 1961 to 1980. Neurology 38:134–138, 1988.

Tanzer R: The carpal tunnel syndrome. J Bone Joint Surg 41:626–634, 1959.

Tobin SM: Carpal tunnel syndrome in pregnancy. Am J Obstet Gynecol 97:493–498, 1967.

Vanderpool HE, Friis EA, Smith BS, et al: Prevalence of carpal tunnel syndrome and other work-related musculoskeletal problems in cardiac sonographers. J Occup Med 35:604–610, 1993.

Vessey MP, Villard-Mackintosh L, Yeates D: Epidemiology of carpal tunnel syndrome in women of childbearing age. Findings in a large cohort study. Int J Epidemiol 19:655–659, 1990.

Wand S: Carpal tunnel syndrome in pregnancy and lactation. J Hand Surg 15B:93–95, 1990.

Weislander G, Norback D, Gothe C-J, et al: Carpal tunnel syndrome (CTS) and exposure to vibration, repetitive wrist movements, and heavy manual work: A case-referent study. Br J Ind Med 46:43–47, 1989.

Wilkinson M: The carpal tunnel syndrome in pregnancy. Lancet 1:453–454, 1960.

Winn F, Habes D: Carpal tunnel area as a risk factor for carpal tunnel syndrome. Muscle Nerve 13:254–258, 1992.

Yamaguski DM, Lipscomb PR, Sonle EH: Carpal tunnel syndrome. Minn Med 48:22–33, 1965.

Zimmerman NB, Zimmerman SI, Clark GL: Neuropathy in the workplace. Hand Clin 8:255–262, 1992.

Thoracic Outlet Syndrome

The signs and symptoms of thoracic outlet syndrome (TOS) result from proximal compression of the nerves and vessels supplying the upper limb. It is important to understand the varied clinical manifestations of this entity which commonly presents with a clinical picture that may be difficult to differentiate from other causes of peripheral nerve compression. Failure to consider it in the differential diagnosis may deprive the patient of an opportunity for relief, or worse, subject him or her to unnecessary surgical procedures in the limb, to be followed by the label ''neurotic'' when the complaints continue.

The compression occurs in the anatomic area where these structures join in their path from the spinal cord and mediastinum, respectively, and can take place in the interscalene area, between the clavicle and the first rib, or less commonly, further distally beneath the coracoid process.

ANATOMY

The anatomy of the thoracic outlet extends from the intervertebral foramina and superior mediastinum to the axilla (Nichols, 1967; Pollack, 1980; Troeng, 1987). The apex of the axilla is bounded by the clavicle and subclavius muscle anterolaterally, and the upper border of the scapula and subscapularis muscle dorsally. The anterolateral border of the first rib is medial. The brachial plexus and subclavian vessels leave this area and pass beneath the coracoid process.

The first rib is divided into three parts. The first, or articular portion, extends from the head to the neck, and the second is oriented almost perpendicular to it and serves as the attachment for the middle scalene, the first digitation of the serratus anterior, and the muscles of the first intercostal space. The third, or vascular segment, contains the scalene tubercle, the attachment of the anterior scalene muscle, the costoclavicular ligaments, and the subclavius muscle. The subclavian vein is usually found between the costoclavicular ligaments and the anterior scalene, which is attached to the tubercle. The subclavian artery is located posterior to the anterior scalene and, immediately adjacent to it, the lower trunk of the brachial plexus crosses the first rib after the eighth cervical and first thoracic nerves unite (Fig. 52–1). Unfortunately, the anatomy as described is not always what is encountered at surgery, so that the surgeon must be prepared to appreciate variations in arrangement (Nichols, 1967).

PATHOGENESIS

The anatomy must be considered not only in one plane but in three dimensions to appreciate the potential mechanisms of compression.

In 1912, Todd described the dynamic relationship of the first thoracic nerve and the first rib, and explained why the lower trunk of the plexus is vulnerable to compression at this point. In normal growth and development, because the vertebral column grows faster than the upper limb, the scapula descends, dragging the nerves and vessels with it. Ordinarily, this does not present a problem, but if the scapular supporting musculature, particularly the trapezius, is weakened due to injury or disuse, this will further increase the descent of the scapula and cause compression. Additional aggravating factors are obesity and excessively large breasts in women (Kaye, 1972). Todd described the relationship between the angles of the clavicle and first rib and their differences in the two sexes at different ages, which explains the striking demographics of TOS. The costoclavicular interval, which is narrowed by abduction of the arm and bracing the shoulders, is another mechanism for neurovascular compression. Clavicular abnormalities, both congenital and posttraumatic, may further narrow this interval. Not only will malformations of the clavicle cause the costoclavicular interval to be narrowed, but because the normal clavicle is S shaped and rotates during abduction of the arm, both the military brace position and hyperabduction will produce symptoms in susceptible individuals.

Although the anterior scalene muscle has been indicted as the primary villain in pathogenesis and has been the target of many surgical procedures in the past (Adson, 1947, 1951), it alone is rarely the cause. Variations in the manner of insertion of the scalenes on the first rib, as well as the occurrence of congenital fibrous bands and adventitious ribs, are of importance in some but not all patients. Roos has described nine types of congenital bands as producing compression of the nerves and vessels within the thoracic outlet (Roos, 1976). The most common of these is one that stretches across the concavity of the first rib from the neck to the scalene tubercle, where it can irritate the lower trunk of the brachial plexus. The anterior scalene muscle, which normally inserts on the scalene tubercle, may extend to cover the surface of the first rib and thereby narrow the interscalene interval and compress the nerves and vessels. The anterior and middle scalenes may insert in the form of a conjoined and fibrous edge that can cause compression with scapular ptosis. Such variations as overlapping, hypertrophy of the muscles, or fusion of their insertions by a fibrous falciform band are only diagnosed at the time of surgery.

The scalene muscles, which are flexors and rotators of the neck, were formerly considered major causes of compression, leading not only to the term scalenus anticus syndrome, but to therapy directed solely at their release (scalenotomy) (Adson, 1951), a relatively simple procedure with a high failure rate (Claggett, 1962). Because the anterior and middle scalenes both insert on the first rib, and the subclavian artery and brachial plexus must pass between them, anything that

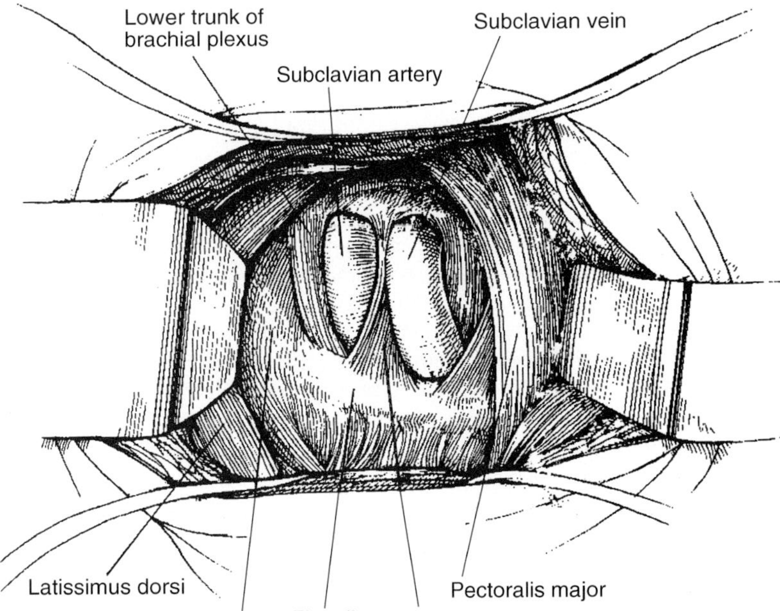

FIGURE 52–1. The anatomy of the thoracic outlet as seen from the axillary surgical approach. (From Leffert RD: Thoracic outlet syndrome. J Am Acad Ortho Surg 2:317–325, 1994. © 1994 American Academy of Orthopaedic Surgeons. Reprinted from the *Journal of the American Academy of Orthopaedic Surgeons: A Comprehensive Review*, Volume 2 (6), pp. 317–325 with permission.)

alters the funnel-shaped interscalene tunnel can produce compression. However, when there are long cervical transverse processes or rudimentary cervical ribs present, one may sometimes anticipate the presence of a fibrous band extending from the adventitious bone to the region of the scalene tubercle, where it may cause compression. Although the incidence of cervical ribs in the general population is about 1% (Pollack, 1980), the mere presence of such a bony variation should not lead a priori to a diagnosis of thoracic outlet syndrome, because this may be merely an incidental finding. If a cervical rib is long enough, it may indeed directly impinge on nerves or vessels.

Several authors have commented on the relationship between vascular abnormalities such as subclavian aneurysm and cervical ribs (Blank and Conner, 1974; Short, 1975). Needless to say, any space-occupying lesion, whether it is hypertrophy of a muscle or an expanding Pancoast's tumor, has the potential for mechanical mischief and must be considered in the differential diagnosis in all patients.

SYMPTOMS AND SIGNS

It is obvious that with a multiplicity of potential causes for compression, the three structures at risk, the subclavian artery, the vein, and the lower trunk of the brachial plexus, may be affected to significantly different degrees. The designation of various types of TOS as being either vascular or purely neural really serves no purpose, because in most cases, there is some compression of all structures, although one may predominate.

As has been suggested, the typical patient is likely to be a woman, usually aged 20 to 40 years, and in our experience, the ratio of women to men is approximately 4 to 1. Complaints are often vague and difficult to define. The patient may experience nocturnal paresthesias, leading to confusion with carpal tunnel syndrome. However, careful history taking

in the thoracic outlet group will usually correctly identify their locus of complaint as the medial forearm, little, and ring fingers. Commonly, they experience similar symptoms with overhead use of the arm such as reaching to a high shelf or holding a hair dryer. Sometimes, driving or lifting weight provokes symptoms. Many patients will also describe discomfort felt in the posterior hemithorax, anterior chest or breast, and upper arm. If this is on the left side, it may be confused with angina (Campbell and Simel, 1988; Urschel et al, 1972), and several of the author's patients have had multiple cardiac evaluations before the true nature of the problem was realized.

Some patients report that they feel as though the blood is being shut off to the arm, which may reflect arterial compression. A most elusive complaint, that of intermittent swelling of the limb with exercise, may not be accepted as real until the venous hypertension becomes sufficiently great to produce measurable asymmetry or a pronounced superficial venous pattern due to the formation of collaterals. Some patients present with acute thrombosis of the subclavian vein, or so-called effort-thrombosis, which should be treated aggressively with intravenous catheterization using thrombolytic agents and then anticoagulation (Shuttleworth et al, 1987).

Although it is not common for patients to complain of gross motor weakness, changes in manual dexterity or handwriting may be appreciated. In these cases, careful manual muscle testing often detects hypothenar, interosseous, or adductor pollicis weakness of a subtle degree. The profundi to the little and ring fingers may be weak, and less commonly, the median motor nerve distribution of the lower trunk may be affected. However, it is usually not observed in the absence of weak ulnar innervated musculature. Some patients present with significant weakness and atrophy of hand muscles. However, about half the patients have no motor deficit at all.

The sensory deficit, if present, usually affects the medial forearm, hypothenar eminence, and little and ring fingers. It is essentially that of the ulnar nerve sensory distribution plus that of the medial cutaneous nerve of the forearm. Knowledge of the anatomical boundaries aids in differential diagnosis of ulnar neuropathy. As with the motor findings, those of the sensory deficit may be subtle or even absent in symptomatic patients.

The vascular symptoms have already been eluded to, and these may be spontaneous and noted by the patient or provoked by the examiner in a series of diagnostic positions of the arm and neck. The provocative maneuvers must be carefully interpreted to avoid overdiagnosis. It is not significant to be able to merely obliterate the pulse by some position of the arm, because many women who are asymptomatic exhibit this phenomenon. A test cannot be considered to be positive unless the patient, without prompting, reports reproduction of the symptoms when the arm is placed in the provocative position.

The classic Adson maneuver is performed with the patient seated and the examiner palpates the radial pulse with the patient's arm dependent. The neck is turned toward the side of the lesion and extended while a deep breath is taken. In the author's experience, this test has a low yield.

In order to perform Wright's maneuver, the arm is placed in the abducted and externally rotated position (Wright, 1945). This test has a higher rate of positivity, which may, in some cases, be increased by having the patient inspire deeply, or turn the head to the other side. As with all the other provocative maneuvers, not only is the pulse palpated at the wrist, but the patient must spontaneously reproduce her symptoms in order for the test to be considered positive. A potential pitfall is the possibility of ulnar neuropathy at the elbow. Therefore, the maneuver should be repeated with the elbow in full extension so that a positive elbow flexion test does not confuse the issue. Assuming the shoulder braced position produces symptoms in patients with narrowing of the costoclavicular interval. Those with ptosis of the scapula as a cause of the compression will exacerbate their symptoms with downward pressure on the shoulder girdle. The overhead exercise test requires the patient to flex and extend the fingers with the arms elevated, and in those with significant compression, symptoms of fatigue and cramping will occur within 30 seconds (Fig. 52–2). With all of these tests, the examiner should auscultate the subclavian artery for the presence of a bruit.

In some cases, color changes indicating pallor or cyanosis may be observed with the various maneuvers, depending on whether the compression is predominantly arterial or venous. It is unusual for TOS to present with acute arterial insufficiency because of sudden occlusion of the subclavian artery. This may be associated with an aneurysm and requires immediate vascular surgery. In all patients being screened for TOS, it is wise to palpate and auscultate the supraclavicular fossa for the presence of a mass or bruit.

ANCILLARY DIAGNOSTIC MANEUVERS

Plane films of the cervical spine and chest are required of all patients. Because a significant percentage of unselected patients have some evidence of degenerative change in the cervical spine and cervical radiculopathy is considerably more common than TOS, this entity must be ruled out. However, it should be remembered that although cervical radiculopathy is a major cause of brachialgia, it is unusual for it to affect the C8–TI outflow and produce the corresponding sensory loss and intrinsic atrophy in the hand. The cervical spine radiographs should be scrutinized for the presence of cervical ribs or other osseous abnormalities such as long transverse processes at C7. Although the incidence of cervical ribs in the general population is about 1% (Pollack, 1980), less than 20% of our operative cases have significant osseous abnormalities. A chest radiograph that clearly shows the apices is also important.

Although it was reported that the measurement of conduction velocity of the ulnar nerve through the thoracic outlet was a reliable indicator (Urschel et al, 1972) of compression, this work has been seriously questioned (Wilbourn and Lederman, 1984). In my opinion, the test is not useful in TOS unless one is concerned about the possibility of a coexisting lesion such as a double crush syndrome (Wood and Biondi, 1990). Whereas somatosensory evoked potentials may be abnormal, they are not invariably so for this purpose (Veilleux et al, 1988). Digital plethysmography does not reflect the state of the nerves.

Both arteriography and venography have been recommended for the study of these patients. However, we find that in most cases, they are unnecessary. Angiography is

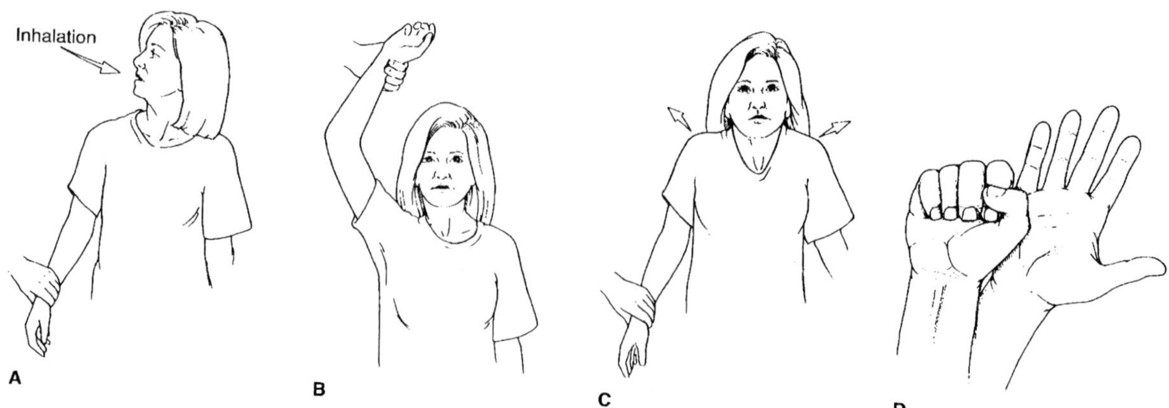

FIGURE 52–2. The provocative maneuvers. *A,* Adson's maneuver. *B,* Wright's maneuver. *C,* Costoclavicular or military brace maneuver. *D,* Overhead exercise test maneuver. (From Leffert RD: Thoracic outlet syndrome. J Am Acad Ortho Surg 2:317–325, 1994. © 1994 American Academy of Orthopaedic Surgeons. Reprinted from the *Journal of the American Academy of Orthopaedic Surgeons: A Comprehensive Review,* Volume 2 (6), pp. 317–325 with permission.)

ordinarily reserved for those patients who have significant cervical ribs and in whom the possibility of subclavian aneurysm exists (Judy and Heymann, 1973). In 20 such cases over the past 21 years, I have not found an aneurysm. Patients who have had multiple unsuccessful previous operations in the area and who are potential operative candidates might be studied with arteriography if it appears to be indicated.

Venography is mandatory in the diagnostic workup for those patients who are suspected of having acute thrombosis of the subclavian vein (Sanders and Haug, 1990). These patients have the acute onset of severe pain in the arm, accompanied by swelling and cyanosis. Immediate treatment is essential because initial treatment with intravenous catheterization, thrombolytic agents, and anticoagulation can reverse the process. Subsequent elective first rib resection prevents rethrombosis (Gloviczki et al, 1986; Shuttleworth et al, 1987). In the author's opinion, digital plethysmography should be used in the evaluation of patients with the provisional diagnosis of TOS if there is serious concern over the possibility of intrinsic vascular disease.

TREATMENT

Conservative Therapy

It is not rare, once the patient learns that the symptoms have an anatomical basis and that they can be alleviated, for her to want something dramatic done as soon as possible. However, unless there is significant vascular compromise or motor loss, most patients are best treated initially by conservative methods. A thorough explanation of the problem is useful in enlisting the patient's cooperation in a therapeutic program. Sometimes, there are factors in the activities of daily living that are aggravating the condition. The conditions and ergonomics of the work station must be examined and modified if they are irritating. Some occupations that involve repetitive or overhead use of the arms must be avoided if the patient is to get well.

As stated previously, many of the patients who are seen with symptoms and signs of TOS have no evidence of adventitious ribs or long transverse processes, or any other static skeletal abnormalities. These patients usually have poor posture and, in particular, ptosis of the scapula on the involved side. The trapezius muscle is often atrophic and weak, and this allows the scapula to droop. Hence, any injury or condition that causes disuse of the limb, even if it does not directly affect this muscle, tends to induce atrophy and weakness. Habitually poor posture or overuse with some occupations can produce similar changes in the scapular musculature. Pain and spasm of the periscapular muscles will then develop, and the patient will have both local and peripheral complaints.

Each patient must be evaluated individually to determine the proper course of conservative treatment. A knowledgeable physical therapist is of tremendous benefit, because many of the protocols that are available in the literature are general and may not be applicable to a particular patient. In addition, those exercises that include overhead use of the arms or shoulder bracing will, in most cases, prove to be aggravating to the patient (Peet et al, 1956). The use of forceful stretching or deep massage in the supraclavicular fossa to mobilize the first rib is often poorly tolerated. What is needed is a program of gently progressive strengthening exercises for the scapular suspensory muscles that the patient can learn to perform at home. These exercises are varied depending on the degree of irritability of the structures in the thoracic outlet when the patient is initially evaluated by the therapist. Some patients can only tolerate gentle upward shrugging of the shoulders, whereas others are able to do their exercise while holding a 1- or 2-pound weight in their hands. All exercises are performed with the arms below shoulder height, and bracing the shoulders back is avoided. There must be close communication between the patient and the therapist so that mid-course corrections can be made when necessary. Ultimately, when the patient becomes stronger and more confident, water exercises and swimming are a good way to keep up conditioning and avoid recurrences.

For those patients who are obese, weight reduction helps improve posture and lessen drag on shoulder girdles. If these measures are unsuccessful and patient comes to surgery, the procedure will be rendered easier and safer. Improved breast support or in rare cases, reduction may be indicated for those women in whom the weight of the breast is problematical.

The conservative course of treatment should be pursued, faithfully for 3 to 4 months unless symptoms are worsened, which sometimes happens, or until it is readily apparent that there has been no improvement. In the author's experience, if there is significant compression, as indicated by severe muscle atrophy, conservative therapy will not suffice and surgery is indicated.

Operative Therapy

The indications for surgery in TOS are as follows:

1. Failure of a carefully supervised exercise and postural program
2. Intractable pain
3. Significant neurological deficit
4. Impending vascular catastrophe
5. Following successful initial treatment of subclavian vein thrombosis

Which procedure to perform for decompression of the thoracic outlet is controversial. Scalenotomy, although of historic interest, has a high incidence of recurrence and is not recommended.

Some surgeons consider scalenectomy an alternative to first rib resection, and some employ a combined approach (Qvarfordt et al, 1984; Roos, 1982; Sanders et al, 1979; Sanders and Pearce, 1989; Sanders and Raymer, 1985). Roos has described an upper type of TOS that involves compression in the interscalene area and that may be benefited by anterior scalenectomy. Claviculectomy is rarely indicated unless the clavicle cannot be saved or a wide exposure is needed to manage a patient who has had prior surgery and in whom the subclavian vein is adherent to a retained anterior rib fragment. Pectoralis minor release has the allure of simplicity. However, the surgeon must be certain that this is the only point of compression, which would be unusual.

Owing to the interest of surgeons of different specialty orientations in the treatment of TOS, there have been and remain divergent preferences for the anatomical approach. The transaxillary route, as originally described by Roos (Roos, 1966, 1971), has become increasingly popular because it transects no important muscles. The degree of muscular relaxation of the patient under general anesthesia is critical to safe access within the operative field, and the short-acting muscle relaxants are ideal for this purpose.

The patient is placed in the lateral decubitus position, with the affected arm held up by a scrubbed assistant, who can raise and lower it as the surgeon requires (Fig. 52–3). A horizontal skin incision is made in the axilla, just caudad to the lower border of the axillary hairline, from the pectoralis major to the latissimus dorsi muscle. The intercostobrachial nerve is preserved and retracted if possible. Full muscular relaxation and a proper line of pull on the arm opens the thoracic outlet. Dissection is carried out bluntly along the rib cage until the first rib can be palpated. The supreme thoracic branch of the axillary artery is ligated and divided to allow for full mobilization of the vessels. These vessels must be constantly kept under direct vision to avoid injury. Because the field is a pyramid, with the apex 10 to 12 cm beneath the skin, it is necessary to use either lighted retractors or an operating headlight for illumination. The areolar tissue surrounding the upper surface of the first rib and neurovascular structures is gently cleared by blunt dissection, and the anterior scalene is identified as it attaches to the scalene tubercle between the artery and vein. Although the phrenic nerve is not at risk at this level, the pleura is, and pneumothorax will result if the anterior scalene muscle is not separated from it before section. The outermost edge of the first rib may be cleared with an elevator to free the attachments of the scalenus medius. Blunt dissection is used

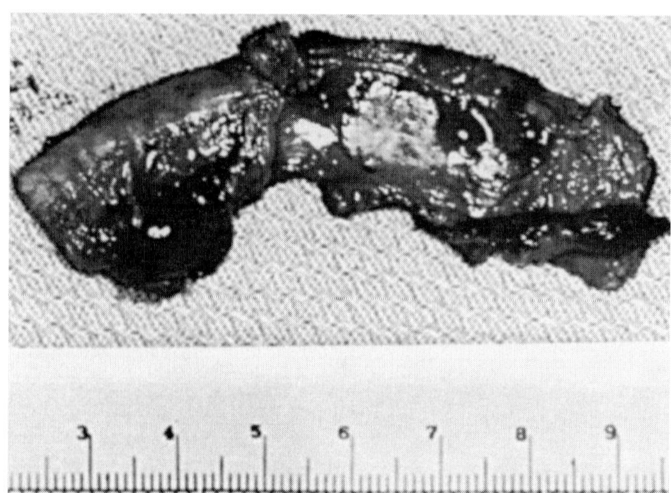

FIGURE 52–4. The resected rib and attached soft tissues. (Scale in centimeters.)

to avoid injury to the long thoracic nerve. When working on the under surface of the rib to separate it from the suprapleural membrane and pleura, it is helpful to have the anesthetist hypoventilate the patient. If a pneumothorax results, it may not be obvious until the wound is flooded with irrigating solution, which will then bubble owing to the air leak. This occurs in about 30% of our cases and is easily managed by inserting a chest tube through the rent in the pleura and leading it out through a small stab wound to underwater suction.

When the rib has been sufficiently cleared, the proposed line of section should lie at least 2 cm behind the lower trunk of the brachial plexus. Then, with all structures under direct vision, the Roos rib cutter is placed around the rib, almost closed, and pushed posteriorly to cut the rib. Any bands coming from it should be sectioned. The rib is then detached anteriorly from the sternum. As much of the periosteum as possible must be removed or disrupted to prevent re-growth of bone (Fig. 52–4). The thoracic outlet is then gently explored digitally with the arm and shoulder in the provocative positions to determine if adequate decompression has been achieved. If not, then a portion of the second rib may have to be removed to provide more space, although this is not commonly required. The wound is then irrigated to test for air leaks, and the muscles are allowed to fall back into place. The subcutaneous tissues are approximated, and the skin is closed without a drain, usually by means of a subcuticular suture (Fig. 52–5).

The constraints of space do not permit a detailed description of all of the operative techniques available for decompression of the thoracic outlet. For more information on these techniques, the reader is referred to the bibliography (Adson, 1947; Claggett, 1962; Pollack, 1980; Qvarfordt et al, 1984; Roos, 1982; Sanders et al, 1979; Sanders and Raymer, 1985).

Complications

Some of the potential complications of first rib resection and their management have already been described. There is

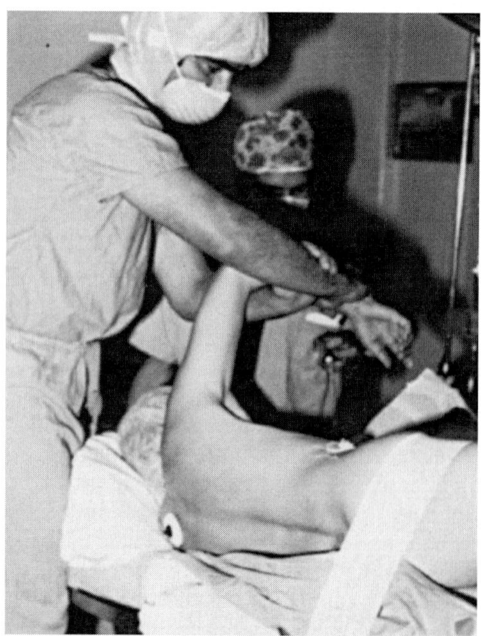

FIGURE 52–3. The correct position of the assistant supporting the arm during the procedure.

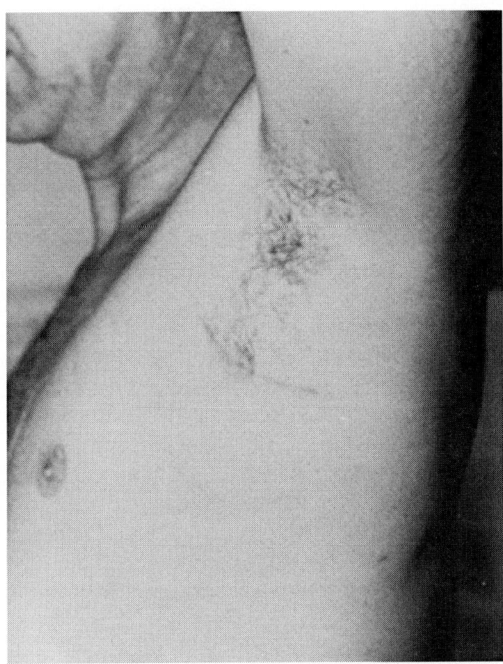

FIGURE 52–5. A healed axillary incision. This patient developed signs and symptoms of TOS after he sustained a traction injury of his spinal accessory nerve in a fall. Owing to the paralysis of the trapezius, the droop of his scapula caused neurovascular compression. Although the muscle recovered substantially, his symptoms ultimately required first rib resection. Thereafter, he was asymptomatic.

a significant risk to the vessels and nerves in the field, and one must be prepared with backup for all eventualities. Laceration of the brachial plexus at this level would be irrevocable, and it should be remembered that the plexus has little excursion here. Hence, anything more than the most gentle retraction on the nerves creates a risk of injury.

Some patients experience transient aching about the shoulder and winging of the scapula due to traction on the long thoracic nerve supplying the serratus anterior. Unless the nerve has actually been cut, it usually recovers within a few weeks or months. The possibility of permanent damage is, however, very real. Because the first digitation of the muscle must be detached from the first rib as part of the procedure, this also contributes to transient weakness.

The numbness of the axilla and posterior aspect of the arm caused by traction on the intercostobrachial nerve gradually fades over a few months if continuity has been preserved.

Postoperative Management

Although the potential for serious and even life-threatening complications from this surgery must not be forgotten, the usual morbidity from transaxillary first rib resection is not great in the hands of an experienced operator because no major muscles are cut and blood loss is often negligible. A sling usually is not needed and the dressing may be removed after 4 or 5 days. Patients must be cautioned against resumption of normal activities involving heavy lifting for 3 or 4 weeks. Moderate intrinsic hand muscle weakness may be reversed, although significant atrophy may be permanent.

In the author's experience, about 35% of patients are totally asymptomatic at follow-up, and an equal number have substantial relief and require no analgesics. About 15% derive no benefit from surgery. However, the evaluation of outcome in this group of patients is extremely difficult because one must rely on the subjective assessment and reporting of a complex group of patients. Nevertheless, the overall results of the operation in properly selected patients can be very gratifying, and in a number of cases, the so-called functional overlay has completely disappeared.

References

Adson AW: Surgical treatment for symptoms produced by cervical ribs and the scalenus anticus muscle. Surg Gynecol Obstet 85:687, 1947.

Adson AW: Symptoms, differential diagnosis for section of the insertion of the scalenus anticus muscle. J Int Coll Surg 16:546, 1951.

Blank RH, Conner RG: Arterial complications associated with thoracic outlet syndrome. Ann Thorac Surg 17:315–324, 1974.

Campbell PT, Simel DL: Left arm pain isn't always angina. N C Med J 49:564–567, 1988.

Claggett OT: Presidential address: Research and prosearch. J Thorac Cardiovasc Surg 44:153, 1962.

Gloviczki P, Kazmier FJ, Hollier LH: Axillary-subclavian venous occlusion: The morbidity of a nonlethal disease. J Vasc Surg 4:333–337, 1986.

Judy KL, Heymann RL: Vascular complications of thoracic outlet syndrome. Am J Surg 123:521–531, 1973.

Kaye BL: Neurologic changes with excessively large breasts. South Med J 65:177–180, 1972.

Nichols HM: Anatomic structures of the thoracic outlet. Clin Orthop 51:17–25, 1967.

Peet RM, Henricksen JD, et al: Thoracic outlet syndrome: Evaluation of a therapeutic exercise program. Staff Meet Mayo Clin 31:281, 1956.

Pollack EW: Surgical anatomy of the thoracic outlet syndrome. Surg Gynecol Obstet 150:97–103, 1980.

Qvarfordt PG, Ehrenfeld WK, Stoney RJ: Supraclavicular radical scalenectomy and transaxillary first rib resection for the thoracic outlet syndrome. A combined approach. Am J Surg 148:111–116, 1984.

Roos DB: Transaxillary approach for first rib resection to relieve thoracic outlet syndrome. Ann Surg 163:354, 1966.

Roos DB: Experience with first rib resection for thoracic outlet syndrome. Ann Surg 173:429–442, 1971.

Roos DB: Congenital anomalies associated with thoracic outlet syndrome. Anatomy, symptoms, diagnosis, and treatment. Am J Surg 132:771–778, 1976.

Roos DB: The place for scalenectomy and first-rib resection in thoracic outlet syndrome. Surgery 92:1077–1085, 1982.

Sanders RJ, Haug C: Subclavian vein obstruction and thoracic outlet syndrome: A review of etiology and management. Ann Vasc Surg 4:397–410, 1990.

Sanders RJ, Monsour JW, Gerber WF, et al: Scalenectomy versus first rib resection for treatment of the thoracic outlet syndrome. Surgery 85:109–121, 1979.

Sanders RJ, Pearce WH: The treatment of thoracic outlet syndrome: A comparison of different operations. J Vasc Surg 10:626–634, 1989.

Sanders RJ, Raymer S: The supraclavicular approach to scalenectomy and first rib resection: Description of technique. J Vasc Surg 2:751–756, 1985.

Short DW: The subclavian artery in 165 patients with complete cervical ribs. J Cardiovasc Surg 16:135, 1975.

Shuttleworth RD, van der Merwe DM, Mitchell WL: Subclavian vein stenosis and axillary vein 'effort thrombosis'. Age and the first rib bypass collateral, thrombolytic therapy and first rib resection. S Afr Med J 71:564–566, 1987.

Todd WW: The descent of the shoulder after birth. Anatomischer anzeiger centralblatt fur die gesamte Wissenschaftliche Anatomie 41:385–397, 1912.

Troeng T: The anatomy of the thoracic outlet and the causes of thoracic outlet syndrome. Vasa 16:149–152, 1987.

Urschel HC Jr, Razzuk MA, Hyland JW, Matson JL, Solis RM, Wood RE, Paulson DL, Galbraith NF: Thoracic outlet syndrome masquerading as coronary artery disease (pseudoangina). Ann Thorac Surg 16:239–248, 1973.

Urschel HC Jr, Razzuk MA, Wood RE, et al: Objective diagnosis (ulnar nerve conduction velocity) and current therapy of the thoracic outlet syndrome. Ann Thorac Surg *12*:608–620, 1972.

Veilleux M, Stevens JC, Campbell JK: Somatosensory evoked potentials: Lack of value for diagnosis of thoracic outlet syndrome. Muscle Nerve *11*:571–575, 1988.

Wilbourn A, Lederman R: Evidence for conduction delay in thoracic outlet syndrome is challenged. N Engl J Med *310*:1052–1053, 1984.

Wood VE, Biondi J: Double-crush nerve compression in thoracic-outlet syndrome. J Bone Joint Surg *72A*:85–87, 1990.

Wright IS: The neurovascular syndrome produced by hyperabduction of the arms. Am Heart *29*:1, 1945.

Chapter 53

• Morton Spinner
• Robert J. Spinner

Management of Nerve Compression Lesions of the Upper Extremity

Nerve compression lesions are a major and significant cause of spontaneous neural dysfunction. In view of the many contributions over the past century, there has been an improved understanding of clinical entities as well as anatomic explanations for previously considered idiopathic or cryptogenic conditions.

In the management of a neural compression lesion, early recognition of the etiology and timely treatment are essential in order to obtain optimal recovery. It is critical that the precise level of the lesion be identified in order to accurately plan effective treatment. This can be accomplished by careful serial clinical examinations and confirmed by electroneuromyographic and imaging techniques. The physician who directs his or her attention to the wrong pathological process, the incorrect neural localization, or to both, leaves the patient essentially untreated.

A detailed understanding of the normal and variant anatomy—both gross and microscopic—is thus vital for success in diagnosing, localizing, and managing the common and rare nerve compression lesions. A physician, armed with this knowledge, is well equipped to tackle the difficult challenges of patients with nerve compression syndromes.

This chapter is intended to be a brief introduction to the management of peripheral nerve compression syndromes in the upper extremity (Gelberman et al, 1994). For further detailed descriptions on these subjects, I recommend the works of Gelberman (1991) and Kline and Hudson (1995).

CLASSIFICATION OF NEURAL COMPRESSION LESIONS

There are two recognized methods of classifying neural injuries (Seddon 1972; Sunderland, 1978), each of which represents an attempt to correlate the degree of injury with the characteristic symptoms and localized neural pathology. Sir Herbert Seddon's classification employs three terms to describe the degree of the severity of the injury—neurapraxia, axonotmesis, and neurotmesis. Sir Sydney Sunderland has a five-fold system of classifying nerve injuries. They can be compared in the manner shown in Figure 53–1.

Seddon's neurapraxia is analogous to Sunderland's first degree of injury. Neurapraxia is characterized by complete motor paralysis with little sensory or autonomic involvement and is a transient syndrome. Segmental demyelination occurs in some cases and is followed by segmental remyelination; wallerian degeneration does not occur. Recovery is excellent.

The next level of severity is called axonotmesis by Seddon

and includes all second-degree and some mild third-degree injuries in the Sunderland classification. In this type of nerve injury, the axon fiber is damaged at the point of compression, resulting in complete motor, sensory, and autonomic dysfunction. Muscle atrophy is progressive. The nerve fibers are separated into proximal and distal sections, but the continuity of the basement membrane is maintained (Thomas, 1964, 1966). The distal fibers are phagocytized. Restoration of muscle-nerve continuity by wallerian regeneration occurs and leads to motor and sensory recovery. Regeneration is influenced by contact guidance, neurotropism, and neurotrophism and occurs at the rate of about 1 mm/day. The interval of recovery depends on the distance between the muscle to be reinnervated and the site of axonotmesis. Prognosis is good.

Sunderland's third-degree lesion corresponds to Seddon's axonotmesis or to neurotmesis, depending on the extent of the neural injury. In a third-degree injury, the nerve fibers, along with their Schwann tubes, are damaged within intact nerve fascicles. Some of these lesions are reversible, and these fall into the axonotmetic group. However, in the more severely involved group of third-degree neural lesions, the process may be irreversible because of the number of axons damaged and the extent of the irreversible fibrotic process within the fasciculi.

The fourth-degree lesion is a neuroma in continuity. There is no gross separation of the nerve and no retraction of nerve ends, but microscopically, the axons are in complete disarray and are not structurally in continuity.

Loss of continuity of the nerve trunk is designated as a fifth-degree injury. This neural lesion occurs when the nerve is actually severed and the ends retract. This degree of injury is not seen with compression lesions.

Recently, some (Mackinnon and Dellon, 1988) have suggested the possibility of a sixth-degree lesion, referring to a neuroma in continuity. This lesion is a mixed one, which may include many or all of Sunderland's five degrees of injury reflected in various fascicles of the peripheral nerve.

It is important to note that although classification of nerve injury is useful to the clinician, each of the methods yields only an approximation of the true degree of nerve injury. A lesion, even in experimentally controlled situations, seldom produces a single pattern of nerve fiber damage. In one fascicle, different fibers may suffer neurapraxia, axonotmesis, or neurotmesis. In general, the extent of the nerve fiber damage increases in severity with time as the mechanical forces continue to influence the lesion (Spinner and Spencer, 1974). Peripheral nerve fibers are involved initially,

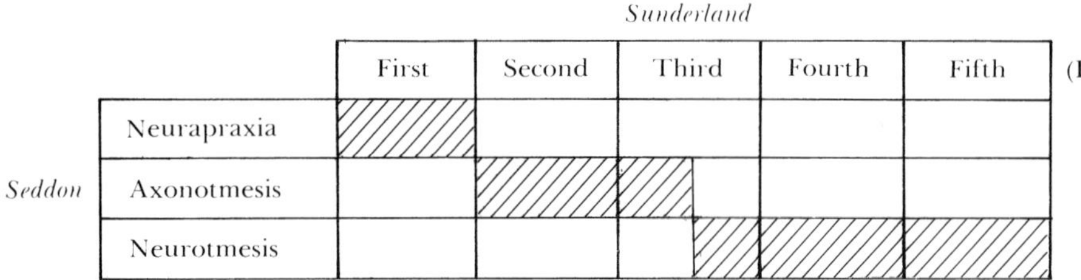

FIGURE 53–1. Correlation of Seddon's and Sunderland's classification of nerve injuries.

and central fibers are involved subsequently. Nature has created a large functional reserve in the number of motor and sensory axons present so that with recovery of 50% of the total, function can clinically be nearly normal.

CLINICAL CORRELATION OF THE DEGREE OF NERVE INJURY

The Lesions of Neurapraxia

There appear to be three types of neurapractic lesions: ionic, vascular, and mechanical. Ionic changes occurring at the node of Ranvier may cause electrolyte imbalance (Kuczynski, 1974). Vascular causes, once thought to be due to ischemia (Denny-Brown and Brenner, 1944), are now thought to be due to fascicular anoxia at the capillary level from venous obstruction in the epineurium (Lundborg, 1970; Sunderland, 1978). The third type of neurapractic lesion is mechanical, with structural changes of the myelin sheath in a short segment of the nerve fibers due to compression-shear forces (Gilliatt et al, 1974; Ochoa, 1974). Two types of ultrastructural mechanical lesions have been demonstrated away from the site of the compression: paranodal myelin intussusception at the node of Ranvier in acute focal compression and bulbous myelin lesions with segmental tapering of internodal segments in chronic nerve compression.

A classic example of a neurapraxia may be seen in a limb following the passage of a low-velocity bullet close to a major nerve (Mitchell, 1872). In general, the lesion may be complete or partial, and recovery after an episode of neurapraxia is often rapid and complete.

Most neurapractic lesions respond to nonoperative treatment within 3 months. If the patient has neural compression persisting for more than 3 months without signs of recovery, then the lesion may well be a mixed one or a local block may be present and surgical exploration of the nerve at the level of the lesion is indicated. If a neurapractic lesion is left untreated, it can increase in severity.

Clinically, the speed of return of function suggests the type of neurapractic lesion. A rapid recovery, within hours of neurolysis, suggests the ionic or vascular type, whereas if recovery occurs 1 to 2 months afterward, a structural neurapractic lesion seems most likely. This segmental structural type is independent of the distance of the compression to its motor or sensory end-organ. Recovery time is identical whether the lesion is high or low. No distal wallerian degeneration occurs. The length of the recovery time after surgery for a neurapractic lesion depends on whether the nerve must undergo a process of segmental demyelination and

remyelination. If such a process is necessary, recovery usually takes 1 to 2 months rather than hours or days, as observed with a nonstructural neurapractic lesion.

Axonotmetic Lesions

In a pure axonotmetic lesion, owing to wallerian degeneration distal to the level of the compression, the time of recovery is based on the distance of the motor end-plates and sensory end-organs from the lesion. With neural healing, new axonal sprouting and growth occurs from the point of injury, along with the formation of a new myelin sheath. The closer to the end-plates, the faster the recovery. Thus, recovery following neurolysis of an axonotmetic neural lesion may occur more than 6 months later, depending on the level of the lesion and the location of the closest motor end-plate to be reinnervated.

Neurotmetic Lesions

When severe or complete fibrosis of a segment occurs, a nonfunctioning, nonconductive neuroma in continuity exists. Excision of the neuroma and epineural repair is indicated. If direct approximation cannot be performed owing to the size of the gap, then interfascicular grafting is necessary. The prognosis depends on the specific nerve involved, the duration of the paralysis, the age of the patient, and the level of the complete neurotmetic lesion. If paralysis has been present for more than 10 months, recovery after nerve repair is usually poor, because the motor fibers atrophy and may become fibrotic. Sensory recovery may be successful long after 10 months and may occur more than 2 to 3 years after repair. This occurs owing to the viability of the sensory organelles and the thinly myelinated axons, which are capable of late regeneration (provided the distal endoneural tubes are patent).

When a nerve is lacerated and the ends retract, this lesion, too, is neurotmetic and falls into a lesion of the fifth degree, according to Sunderland's classification.

Example: Application of Degree Lesions to Carpal Tunnel Syndrome

The neurapractic nerve lesion that responds immediately following surgical release may reveal only locally increased or decreased vascular markings. In the carpal tunnel region, the neural injection is due to increased venous markings characteristic of the neurapractic lesion of the carpal tunnel syndrome (Sunderland, 1978). Lysis of the flexor retinaculum alone is sufficient to relieve symptoms and to restore function in this first-degree group of cases.

Frequently, when dissecting the proximal and distal portions of the normal component of the nerve to the area of the compression, the nerve may be suddenly liberated. A fibrotic band or thrombosed blood vessel is released; the nerve is freed and is found to have a narrow area of indentation. There is no visible neuroma. The recovery pattern typically follows an axonotmetic course; the time for the first sign of motor recovery is related to the closeness to its first motor end-plate.

With elderly patients, the symptoms of the carpal compression often have been permitted to exist for a prolonged period. In this group, second- and third-degree lesions are common. Depending on the patient's predominant symptoms, such as dysesthesias in the long finger or thumb, specific internal neurolysis, liberating only those fasciculi involved clinically, can be performed. Indiscriminate internal neurolysis can result in excessive local interfascicular fibrosis (Rydevik et al, 1976) and should not routinely be performed. In severe recurrent carpal tunnel problems, in which the median nerve becomes thickened and adherent to the radial side of the carpal canal and the residual flexor retinaculum, limited internal neurolysis along with the use of a Silastic sheath can be of help in relieving the patient's symptoms. Because traction has added to compressive forces, we have placed the wrist in dorsiflexion for 10 to 14 days. It is important to note that the Silastic should not buckle with wrist motion. On occasion, the Silastic has to be removed at a later procedure, when necessary. Others have recommended local muscle flaps (Mackinnon and Dellon, 1988), vascularized fat (Urbaniak, 1991), or nerve wrapping (Gould, 1991) if recurrent symptoms occur. Even in the severest of carpal tunnel syndromes with marked median nerve pathology (with advanced third-degree lesions), the senior author has not needed to resect and perform a neurorrhaphy or nerve graft the lesion to relieve the patient's major complaints.

PRINCIPLES IN EVALUATION OF NEURAL LESIONS

Early, accurate diagnosis and treatment is essential for the most favorable results in compression lesions. Understanding the underlying disease process and the etiology is equally as critical.

A mechanical lesion of a peripheral nerve or one of its major branches is reflected by a disturbance of a specific motor, sensory, or autonomic function within the extremity. Although any peripheral nerve may become compressed, certain anatomic considerations make particular nerves at specific sites more vulnerable, leading to clinical patterns or syndromes. In addition, certain groups of people, including those with diabetes or renal disease (Redfern and Zimmerman, 1995) (Fig. 53–2) are more vulnerable to developing these compressive lesions. A group of patients with a hereditary predisposition to pressure palsies has been identified, and specific DNA tests can confirm the diagnosis.

The precise level of the lesion must be identified in order to accurately plan effective treatment. This can be

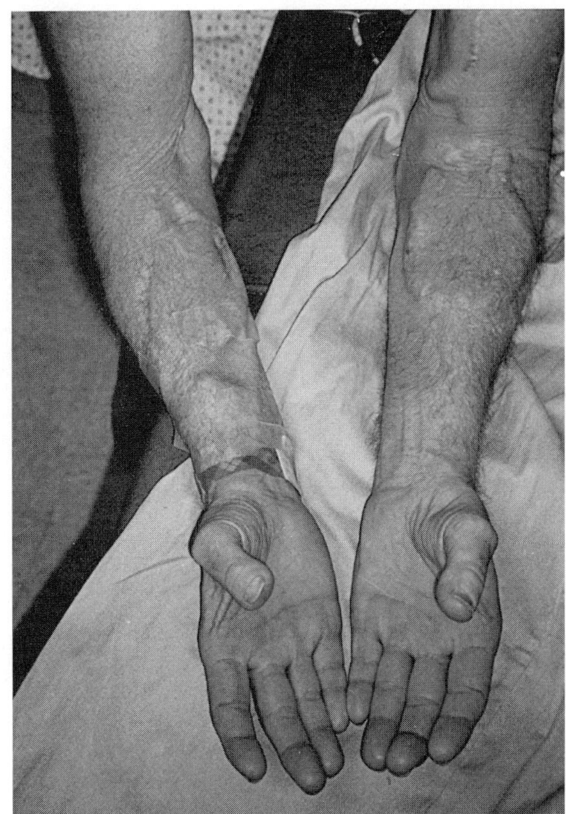

FIGURE 53–2. A 50-year-old man with a history of chronic renal insufficiency and bilateral carpal tunnel syndrome. Photograph demonstrates left greater than right thenar atrophy and bilateral forearm shunts.

accomplished by a careful history and clinical examination in combination with adjuvant electrical and radiographic studies. Although localizing neural lesions associated with masses (such as lipomas, fibromas, hemangiomas, and ganglia) may be relatively easy, often few such tell-tale signs are present and thus a systematic approach is necessary to tackle all cases. Atypical presentations can occur from partial lesions and anatomic variations as well as compression at unusual sites (for example, ulnar nerve compression in the forearm [Holtzman, 1984]). If the diagnosis is unclear, repeat clinical examination and electrical studies are indicated until the diagnosis becomes clear. Assessment of a neural lesion may require several quantitative tests, which are repeated at regular intervals for comparison and prognosis (Omer and Spinner, 1975).

Focus should be directed at determining the precise details of the neurologic deficit. Knowledge of anatomic variants in the upper limb (such as Martin-Gruber or Riche-Cannieu anastomoses and neural loops) should always be considered (Tountas and Bergman, 1993). The intraneural topography should be correlated with the clinical findings (Chow et al, 1985; Gunther et al, 1992; Jabaley et al, 1980; Slinghuff et al, 1987; Sunderland, 1978; Terzis et al, 1984; Watchmaker et al, 1991; Williams and Jabaley, 1986).

In all cases, the percussion test, when present, serves to pinpoint the site of compression (Moldaver, 1978). Pain is usually an early symptom but is often transient and diffuse. The resting functional attitudes of the afflicted hand as in cases of posterior or anterior interosseous nerve syndrome

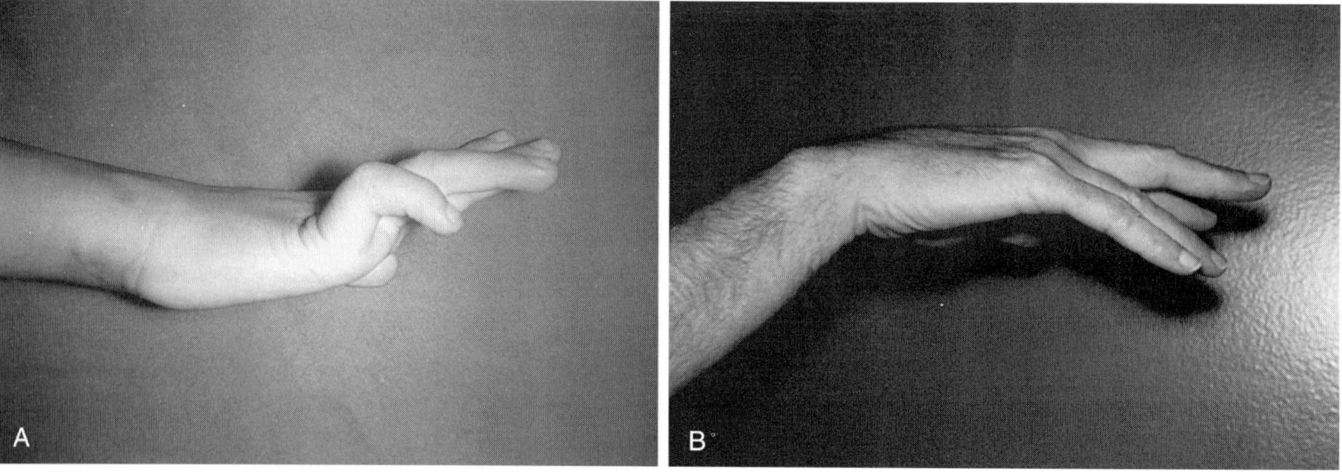

FIGURE 53–3. Functional attitude of the hand. *A,* Clawing with hyperextension at the metacarpophalangeal joint characteristic of an ulnar nerve lesion. *B,* Pseudoulnar clawing of ring and little fingers, with extension lag at metacarpophalangeal joints characteristic of a partial posterior interosseous nerve compression.

or ulnar nerve compression can be the first clue to the localization (Figs. 53–3*A* and *B*). A multitude of provocative tests (such as the tourniquet, Phalen's or reverse Phalen's, elbow flexion, and Adson's tests) are often helpful, but the sensitivity and specificity of each test varies. Additional provocative testing may be necessary to document dynamic neural compression (Braun et al, 1989). The diagnosis of a nerve compression syndrome is relatively easy to make when all symptoms, signs, and confirmatory tests are present. It takes an especially astute clinician to recognize and localize the problem when symptoms persist despite few if any confirmatory findings. Sometimes, an isolated symptom of night pain in the hand is the only complaint given in a patient with carpal tunnel syndrome without any findings. Electrical studies, when positive, are helpful in confirming the diagnosis in this case scenario.

Serial electrical studies are important both in the diagnosis of an entity and the differentiation from others. Many surgeons use them in every case of nerve compression. Communication between the referring physician and the electromyographer is vital. The treating surgeon should pose specific questions for the problem involved that need to be addressed. For example, in the case of a posterior interosseous paralysis—Is there a conduction block across the elbow in this nerve? Are there fibrillations in the extensor digitorum communis? Is the extensor carpi radialis longus normal? Is the paralysis complete? Is there any evidence of spontaneous recovery with the appearance of nascent potentials? Although false-negative findings do exist (Louis et al, 1987), these rates have decreased with improving electromyographic technologies and techniques.

Imaging studies can also be beneficial and may include plain films, arthrography (Roth, et al, 1986), CT (Ogino, et al, 1991), and magnetic resonance imaging (MRI) (Hems et al, 1997; Rosenberg et al, 1993; Subin et al, 1989). Using short-tau inversion recovery (STIR) sequences, MRI can demonstrate deinnervated muscles that can be correlated anatomically in the same manner as when an electromyogram (EMG) was used in the past (West et al, 1994). Three-dimensional reconstruction and dynamic imaging are being used by some in helping establish diagnoses. As resolution

continues to improve, the use of MRI may play an increasing role in spontaneous compression syndromes.

The differential diagnosis of any lesion is extensive and may include more generalized neuropathies, musculoskeletal causes for pain (lateral epicondylitis versus posterior interosseous nerve syndrome [Roles and Maudsley, 1972] or shoulder pain and suprascapular nerve entrapment), Parsonage-Turner syndrome (1948), amyotrophic lateral sclerosis, radiculopathy, or a central nervous system lesion. One must always rule out the presence or coexistence of a more proximal lesion. For example, pseudo–anterior interosseous nerve syndromes have been described (England and Sumner, 1987; Katirji, 1985; Rennels and Ochoa, 1980; Wertsch et al, 1985) that may involve the median nerve proximal to the take-off of the anterior interosseous branch and may affect the anterior interosseous nerve fibers as well as neighboring nerve fibers (such as the flexor carpi radialis). An isolated flexor pollicis longus weakness (Fig. 53–4) may be due to an incomplete anterior interosseous nerve lesion, a median

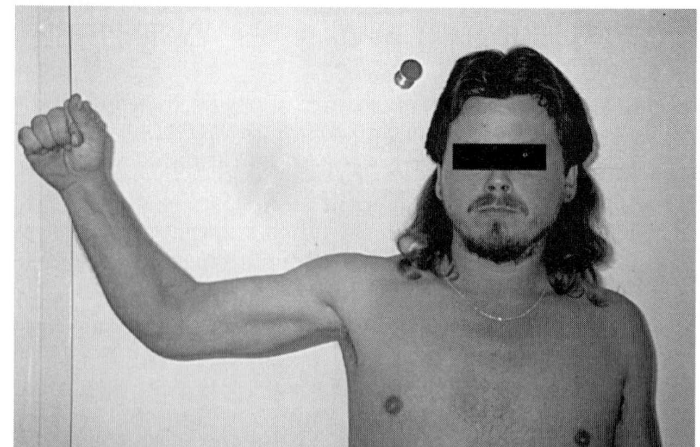

FIGURE 53–4. This 30-year-old man presented with spontaneous, flexor pollicis longus paralysis without other symptoms or clinical findings. At this time, the differential diagnosis included congenital absence of the flexor pollicis longus, tendon and muscle rupture, partial anterior interosseous nerve paralysis, high median nerve lesion, cryptogenic brachial neuritis (Spinner, 1976), and Parsonage-Turner syndrome. He developed rhomboid and other shoulder girdle weakness 1 month later and was diagnosed with Parsonage-Turner syndrome. Contrast with Figure 53–20*A-F.*

nerve lesion in the axilla (Spinner, 1976), a tendon rupture (Mody, 1992), or a manifestation of Parsonage-Turner syndrome. Preoperatively the use of succinylcholine (Doyle et al, 1981) may be useful in making the correct diagnosis. Succinylcholine paralyzes normal skeletal muscle by blocking transmission at the myoneural junction. In deinnervated muscle, one may see sustained muscle contractions that last several minutes (deinnervation hypersensitivity) after injection of succinylcholine. In injured muscle or tendon, one may see fasciculations that last only a few seconds. In addition, the entity of a double-crush lesion (such as a cervical radiculopathy combined with carpal tunnel syndrome) is well established and needs to be considered in appropriate cases (Osterman, 1988; Upton and McComas, 1973; Wood and Biondi, 1990).

Each nerve lesion can be clinically described as a high or low neural lesion—that is a high or low median, radial, or ulnar lesion. In addition, there are further refinements and localizations within this gross classification. For example, a complete low ulnar nerve lesion at the pisiform should bring to mind a mixed lesion with a clawed ring and little finger, with sensory loss of these digits. However, when the ulnar lesion is at the hook of the hamate, sensation is normal throughout the fingers. The motor intrinsic muscle paralysis is usually complete, or the hypothenar muscle may be spared. There can be many subtleties to intrinsic paralysis (Hirooka et al, 1997). For example, the intrinsic muscles of the first web space alone may be atrophic, as in a case reported due to a bifurcated deep branch of the ulnar nerve at the hook of the hamate (Fenning, 1965; Lanz, 1974; Lassa and Shrewsbury, 1975). Similar localized atrophy of the first web space intrinsic musculature has been described as being caused by a ganglion in juxtaposition to the deep branch of the ulnar nerve at the level of the third metacarpal (McDowell and Henceroth, 1977). An unusual presentation of an ulnar nerve lesion with the absence of Froment's test, presence of Wartenberg's sign, normal sensation, and isolated paralysis with clawing of the little and ring fingers was due to penetration of the deep branch of the ulnar nerve by the passage of an aberrant tendon (Fig. 53–5*A* to *D*) (Spinner et al, 1996). Therefore, atrophy of the muscles of the first web space can occur without ulnar nerve sensory disturbance, or other intrinsic muscle involvement can be observed when entrapment of the deep branch of the ulnar nerve occurs at variable locations. The pathology does not have to be at the spinal cord (anterior horn cell) level when purely intrinsic muscle involvement is found. Recognition of this isolated peripheral nerve problem is critical to patients with isolated intrinsic paralysis. The difference in the prognosis between amyotrophic lateral sclerosis and entrapment of the deep branch of the ulnar nerve is marked. A relatively simple neurolysis of the deep branch of the ulnar nerve in the palm can be curative.

The choice of therapy and the timing of necessary surgical intervention must be individualized. A thorough evaluation of the injured nerve and its peripheral end-organs, muscle fibers, and sensory organelles dictates the localization and optimal therapeutic approach. At times, a trial of nonoperative therapy may reverse the process. If the symptoms do not subside or if they recur, then prompt surgical intervention is indicated. Complete spontaneous paralysis due to an entrapment lesion should not be left untreated surgically for more than 3 months because the degree of injury to the nerve may worsen with the passage of time. If the total paralysis is permitted to exist without relief for 18 months, the pathological process most often becomes irreversible, because internal fibrosis occurs within the nerve and the deinnervated muscles. The final pathological event is a fourth-degree neural lesion, a neuroma in continuity. This does not apply to partial lesions, in which complete recovery may ensue following neurolysis 2 to 3 years after the onset of the compressive process. High complete lesions require earlier treatment because the prognosis is less favorable than low complete ones. Tendon transfers may be necessary either to act as an internal splint or to augment function.

The advanced age of a patient is not a factor affecting recovery following neural compression because older patients do recover well following appropriate neurolysis. In general, age is not a factor in the prognosis and to deny surgical relief to the older age group is unjustified. However, in this age group, when the neural lesion is of the fourth-degree type, the results of nerve repair are unpredictable and often poor.

On occasion, patients do not allow surgery to be performed. At these times, the treating surgeon is frustrated by the fact that he or she knows what to do but the patient does not wish to have any invasive procedure performed. These patients so often accept weakness in the hand or numbness as long as they do not have pain. Their wishes must be respected.

MANAGEMENT OF NERVE COMPRESSION LESIONS

Nonoperative Management

Frequently, patients with nerve compression syndromes may respond favorably to nonoperative measures. These may include simple measures such as avoidance of exacerbating activities or therapeutic positions and weight reduction. Completing a pregnancy or treating an underlying endocrine disorder or systemic disease may help. A trial of full-time or part-time splinting is often worthwhile. Some recommend the use of pyridoxine (vitamin B_6, 100 mg twice daily by mouth for a few months) (Amadio, 1985), although others do not (Spooner et al, 1993). Megadoses of pyridoxine are contraindicated and can cause a peripheral neuropathy in a dose level as low as 500 mg per day (Schaumburg et al, 1983). Diuretics and local steroid injections may also be effective.

Surgical Management

Surgery is often indicated after a trial of several months without clinical or electrical improvement. Surgery should be directed at a thorough neural decompression at obvious defined sites of potential compression (e.g., ligaments, tendinous bands, and fibrotic arch). In cases of anatomic variation, such as accessory muscles and bands, these should be resected or rerouted to restore or recreate a more normal anatomy.

On occasion, surgery must be performed within the first week because of the severe, unrelenting pain and numbness

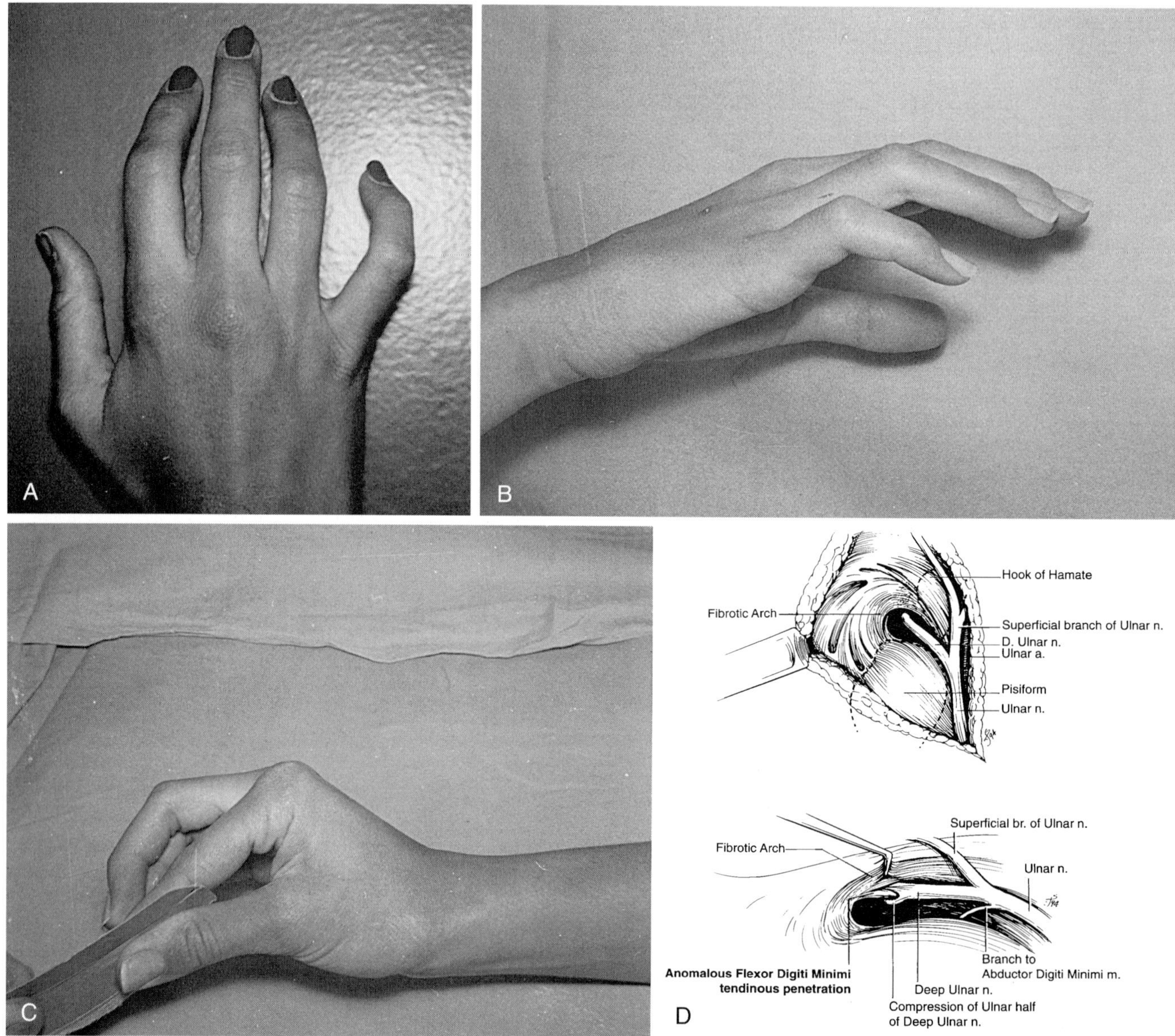

FIGURE 53–5. Isolated intrinsic atrophy *A,* A 20-year-old woman presented with isolated motor deficit and deformity involving the right ring and little fingers without sensory abnormality. Physical examination demonstrated mild clawing of these two digits and the presence of Wartenberg's sign. The differential diagnosis at this time included a partial lesion of the deep motor branch of the ulnar nerve as well as amyotrophic lateral sclerosis (From Spinner RJ, Lins RE, Spinner M: Compression of the medial half of the deep branch of the ulnar nerve by an anomalous origin of the flexor digiti minimi. J Bone Joint Surg *78A:*427, 1996.) *B,* Lateral view shows the clawing as well as atrophy of the third and fourth web spaces. *C,* Note the normal bulk in the first web space; Froment's sign is absent. *D,* Surgical exploration demonstrated an anomalous tendinous penetration of the deep branch of the ulnar nerve. A neural loop created compression of its medial half. Clawing resolved in the recovery room, and muscle tone and strength normalized within 3 months. (*B* to *D* From Khoo D, Carmichael SW, Spinner RJ: Ulnar nerve anatomy and compression. Orthop Clin North Am *27:*317, 1996.)

that is not responsive to nonoperative measures. Furthermore, following traumatic injury (especially with an impending Volkmann's ischemia) to the wrist or elbow—sites where fibro-osseous tunnels exist—surgery may need to be performed within hours for best recovery if sensory and motor deficits are present.

The surgical exposure must be adequate. The actual extent of the surgery is always much greater than the lesion itself. Approaches should use internervous planes (Spinner, 1978) (Fig. 53–6 to 53–10) and be extensile when appropriate (Henry, 1970). Skin incisions, however, should be planned to avoid cutaneous neuromata.

The nerve must be handed gently. It is necessary to identify the normal proximal and distal regions of the nerve adjacent to the pathology in normal anatomic planes. By dissecting toward the lesion from both directions, the neural lesion is exposed. During this phase of the external neurolysis, one must be certain to avoid conversion of a first or second-degree neural lesion to one of a more advanced degree by further intraoperative injury.

Before separating the involved nerve segment from its scarred bed, electrical stimulation proximal and distal to the lesion can be performed. The response to this bipolar stimulation is evaluated by observing the muscle reaction distally, or by recording the distal evoked nerve action potential (Fig. 53–11*A*). Axons of sufficient maturity to conduct nerve action potentials must extend well into the distal segment of the nerve weeks before intraoperative electroneu-

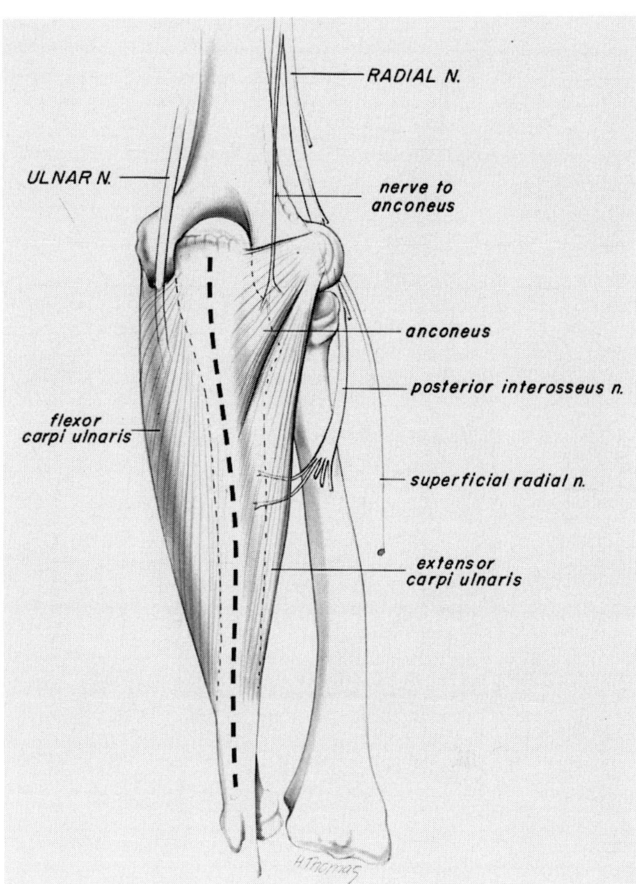

FIGURE 53–6. The first internervous plane, which lies on the subcutaneous border of the ulna, separates the ulnar innervated flexor carpi ulnaris from the radial innervated muscles (From Spinner M: Injuries to the Major Branches of Peripheral Nerves of the Forearm, 2nd ed. Philadelphia, W. B. Saunders, 1978.)

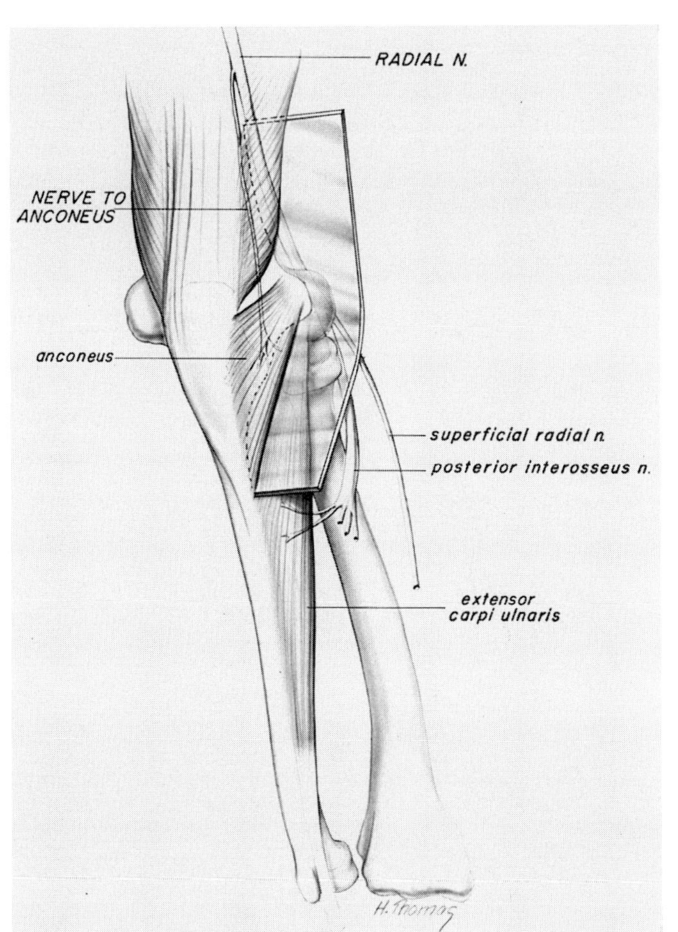

FIGURE 53–7. The second internervous plane is between the anconeus (radial nerve) and the extensor carpi ulnaris (posterior interosseous nerve). (From Spinner M: Injuries to the Major Branches of Peripheral Nerves of the Forearm, 2nd ed. Philadelphia, W. B. Saunders, 1978.)

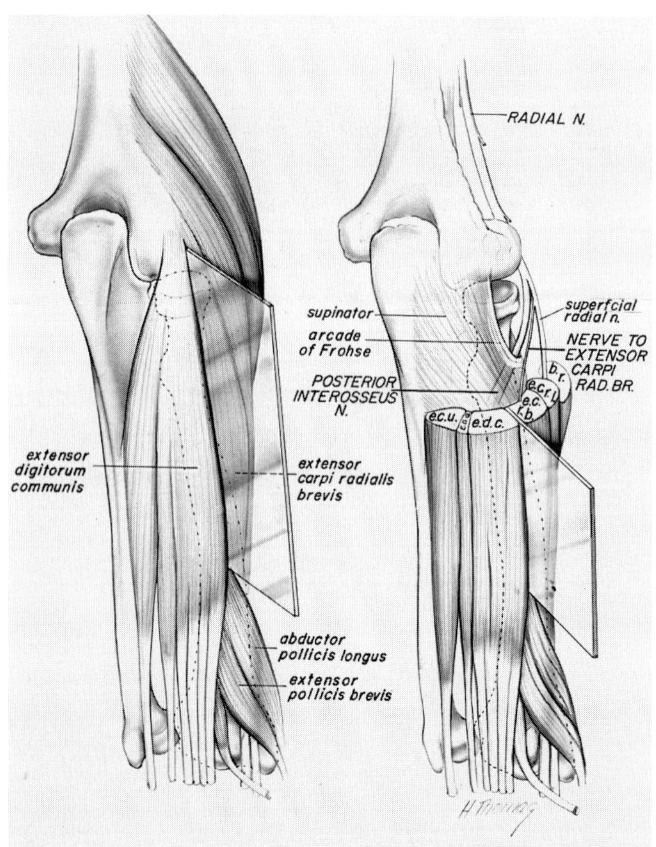

FIGURE 53–8. The third internervous plane (Thompson approach to the forearm) is between the extensor digitorum communis (posterior interosseous nerve) and the extensor carpi radialis brevis (separate branch from the superficial radial nerve or at the bifurcation of the superficial radial and posterior interosseous nerves). Ecu, extensor carpi ulnaris; edq, extensor digitorum quinti; edc, extensor digitorum communis; ecrb, extensor carpi radialis brevis; ecrl, extensor carpi radialis longus; br, brachioradialis. (From Spinner M: Injuries to the Major Branches of Peripheral Nerves of the Forearm, 2nd ed. Philadelphia, W. B. Saunders Company, 1978.)

FIGURE 53–9. The fourth internervous plane (Henry approach) lies between the brachioradialis (radial nerve) and the lateral border of the flexor-pronator muscles (median nerve). Br, brachioradialis; pt, pronator teres; fcr, flexor carpi radialis. (From Spinner M: Injuries to the Major Branches of Peripheral Nerves of the Forearm, 2nd ed. Philadelphia, W. B. Saunders Company, 1978.)

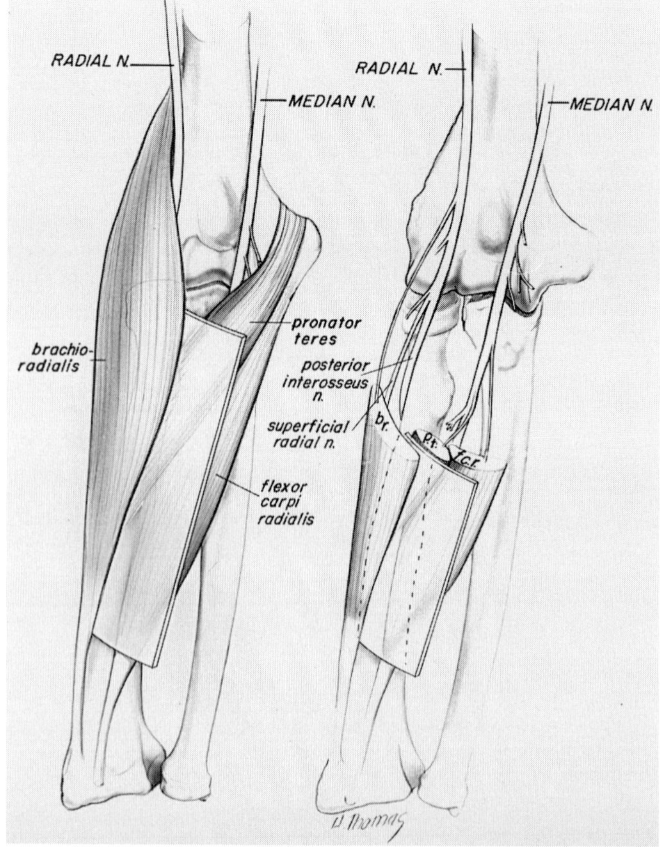

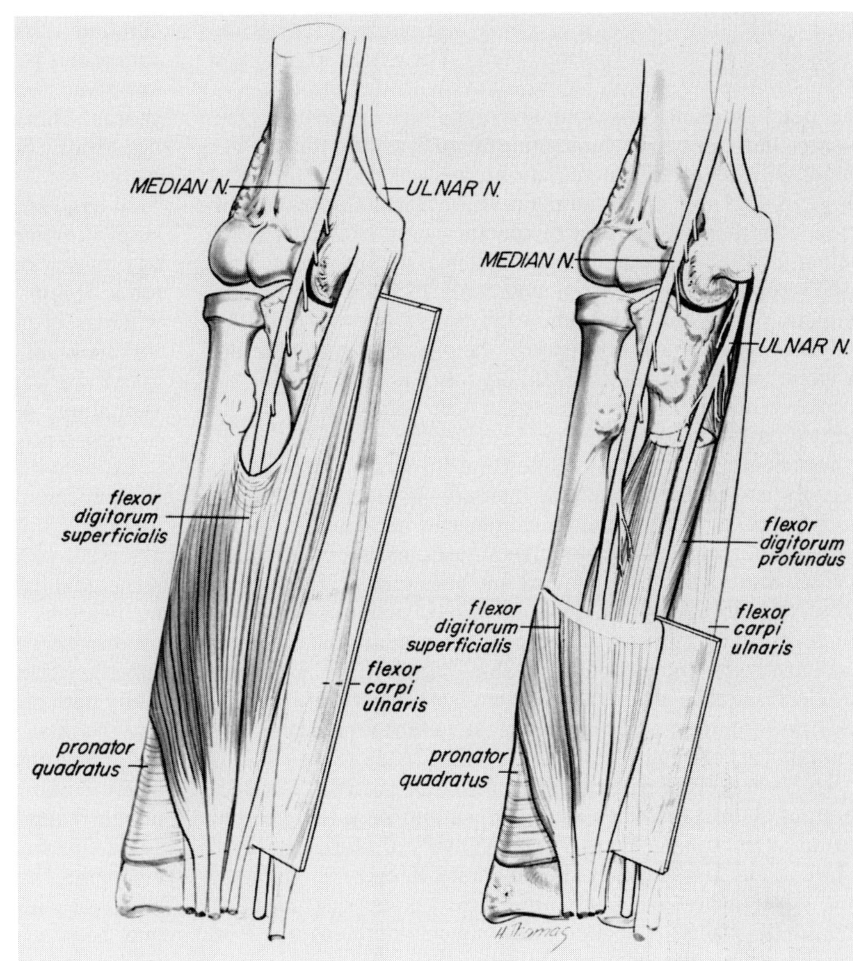

FIGURE 53–10. The fifth internervous plane lies between the medial border of the flexor digitorum superficialis (median nerve) and the flexor carpi ulnaris (ulnar nerve). (From Spinner M: Injuries to the Major Branches of Peripheral Nerves of the Forearm, 2nd ed. Philadelphia, W. B. Saunders Company, 1978.)

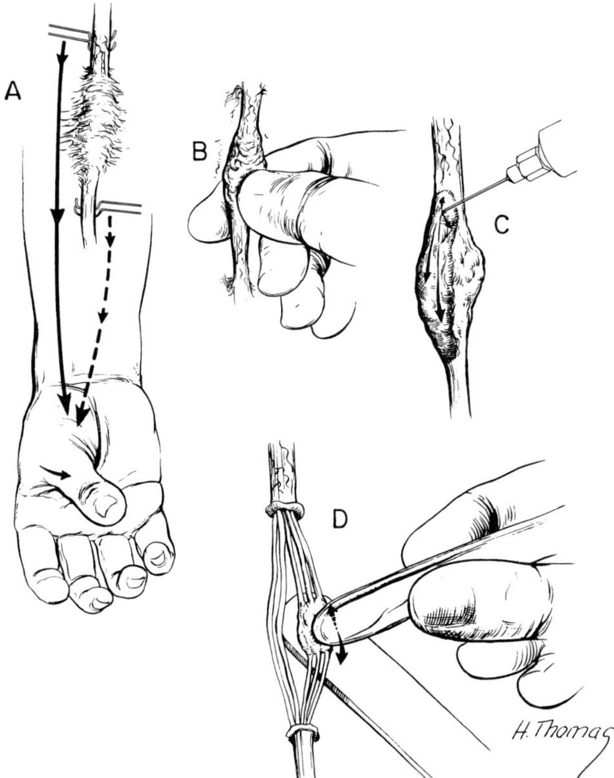

FIGURE 53–11. Intraoperative evaluation of a neuroma in continuity. *A*, Electrical stimulation of the nerve proximal and distal to the site of injury before the neuroma is separated from its bed. *B*, Palpation of the entire neural lesion. *C*, Saline injection followed by internal neurolysis if indicated. *D*, Palpation of several fasciculi using a scalpel handle.

romyographic evidence of recovery can be recorded (Kline et al, 1969; Kline and Hudson, 1972). The extent of the axon population recovery can be correlated with the amplitude of the potential both proximal and distal to the lesion. The greater the number of conducting mature axons, the greater the amplitude of the nerve action potential that is recorded (Fig. 53–12*A* and *C*). Intraoperative electrical studies can be of help in the management of specific nerve lesions (Campbell et al, 1988), especially in the brachial plexus. Some have used somatosensory evoked potentials (SSEPs) in fracture reduction or fixation, or both.

Palpation of the lesion may be helpful in the evaluation. A stone-hard neuroma in continuity has a poor prognosis for recovery by neurolysis, whereas a soft enlargement of the nerve is a favorable sign (Fig. 53–11*B*).

Intraneural injection of saline (Fig. 53–11*C*), followed by neurolysis—both external and internal—using the operating microscope or ocular magnification, can be a helpful technique in dealing with some of these lesions (Brown, 1972).

The nerve can be evaluated on a fascicular level. The gross appearance of the fasciculi under magnification and intraoperative firmness of the fascicular neuromata can be evaluated with the aid of the scalpel handle (Fig. 53–11*D*). Single fascicular electrical recordings (Williams and Terzis, 1976) offer a most critical intraoperative technique for evaluation of partial neural lesions (Fig. 53–12*B*).

Thickened epineurium can be opened or partially excised. Internal neurolysis, when indicated, should be limited to the neural segment and internal region involved clinically (Fig. 53–13). The perineurium should rarely if ever be violated, and never when it is unscarred. Nerves in scarred beds should be placed in better positions without tension. Bed reconstruction may also be necessary.

During postoperative care, early mobilization has been encouraged in an effort to promote neural gliding. The period of immobilization is shorter, for example, with the Learmonth procedure (submuscular transposition of the ulnar nerve at the elbow). For many years, immobilization was

continued for 3 to 4 weeks; now, gradual controlled mobilization can be instituted within the first week. The results are improved in that the period of elbow stiffness is much shorter. Similar principles have been applied to carpal tunnel syndrome, but we would recommend avoidance of wrist flexion for 2 to 3 weeks.

In evaluating a patient with persistence of symptoms after surgical treatment, one must consider the intraneural pathology that was present and its natural history. High axonotmetic lesions may take 1 to 2 years for maximal recovery, whereas even lesions at the wrist may take 6 to 9 months for maximal recovery. During this recovery time, it is frequent for patients to experience some of the preoperative symptoms. An advancing Tinel's sign can be monitored and is a good prognostic sign.

Re-exploration must not be taken lightly. With each operative procedure, the chance for further fibrosis with irreversible nerve injury increases. Each patient must be individually assessed. Nonoperative measures should be attempted, and some advocate a trial of transcutaneous stimulation and pain medications (such as Elavil, Sinequan, or Paxil). Factors that need to be considered include the experience of the primary surgeon, whether the initial procedure was open or endoscopically performed, and the underlying etiology. Re-exploration may be necessary in certain situations: (1) cases in which serial examinations and electrical studies reflect progression of the compression in spite of conservative care, (2) spontaneous recurrence years after a good result, (3) following some cases of failed endoscopic release, (4) cases in which cutaneous neuromata are clinically suspected. For example, a patient with persistent pain following carpal tunnel release may have a neuroma of the palmar cutaneous branch of the median nerve. This patient has numbness in the skin of the thenar eminence and tenderness to percussion in the course of the median palmar cutaneous branch. If conservative therapy including local steroid injections at the site of the neuroma fails, he or she may benefit from excision of the neuroma.

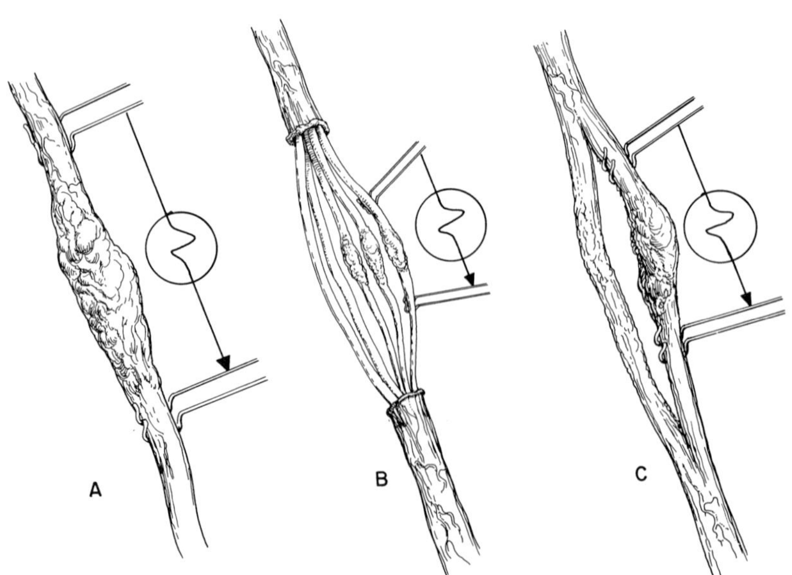

FIGURE 53–12. Intraoperative nerve action potentials can aid in the determination of the viability of the neuroma in continuity. This can be performed on *A*, the whole nerve; *B*, at the fascicular level; *C*, on the entire partial lesion.

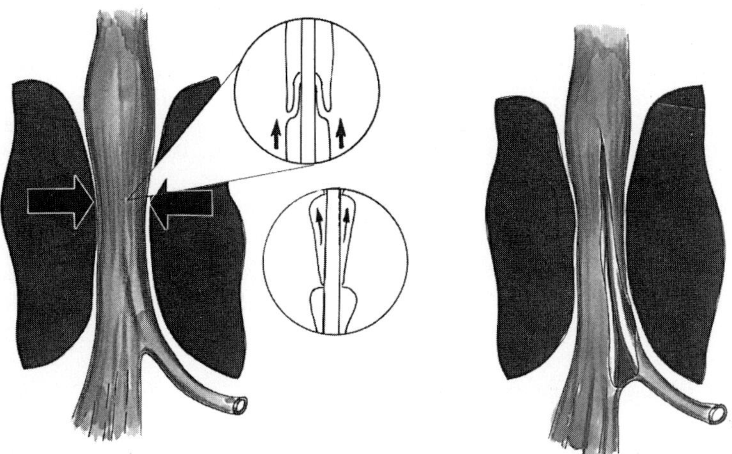

FIGURE 53–13. Internal neurolysis, when indicated, during the operative procedure should be limited to those fasciculi that are clinically involved. This is correlated with the preoperative observations and the intraoperative findings, as well as with knowledge of the internal topography of the nerve. Even the neurapractic structural lesions *(inserts)*, consisting of myelin intussusception or bulbous myelin formation, can heal following release of the neural compression.

NEURAL ENTRAPMENT LESIONS IN THE UPPER EXTREMITY

Median Nerve Syndromes

WRIST

Carpal tunnel syndrome (Amadio, 1992; Marie and Foix, 1913; Paget, 1854; Phalen, 1951, 1966, 1970, 1981) is the most common nerve compression lesion. This syndrome is the result of median nerve compression at the volar aspect of the wrist. As in other tunnel syndromes, predisposing causes may be intrinsic or extrinsic in that the nerve or the other contents within the tunnel may be enlarged or the passage through the carpal tunnel may be narrowed. It is most frequently seen in females between the ages of 40 and 60 as a chronic disorder. However, it may be seen in patients of all ages, including children, and may also occur in an acute fashion.

There are many presentations of carpal tunnel syndrome. Pain and paresthesias in the median nerve distribution of the hand are the usual symptoms. Nocturnal burning pain, relieved by shaking the hand, is frequently reported. Pain may radiate proximally. The symptoms, signs, and findings may include sensory or autonomic disturbances of the radial 3 1/2 digits, weakness or atrophy of the thenar muscles, a positive percussion sign at the wrist, the presence of Phalen's sign, and motor and sensory electroneuromyographic abnormalities. All need not be present in any one case. The presentation of carpal tunnel syndrome may include a combination of classic symptoms, but rarely are all symptoms and signs involved (Spinner et al, 1989; Stevens et al, 1988). For example, patients may have isolated numbness of the middle finger, or children may present with atrophy of the index finger; there may be no thenar muscle atrophy and percussion, and Phalen's signs may not be present. In addition, up to 5% of patients with this syndrome may have a normal electrical studies.

Sensitivity to cold may be a major presenting symptom. Sympathetic overflow related to reflex sympathetic dystrophy may be associated with carpal tunnel syndrome (Grundberg and Regan, 1991; Linscheid et al, 1967). Median and ulnar nerve compression following fractures or dislocations of the wrist can be a cause of reflex sympathetic dystrophy of the hand. It may be necessary to release one or both of these nerves in order to prevent or relieve the stiffness of the digits characteristic of reflex sympathetic dystrophy. In this instance, early diagnosis of the neural entrapment can be confirmed by electrical studies, and with appropriate surgical intervention, the reflex sympathetic dystrophy can be aborted.

The causes of median nerve compression at the wrist are extensive and relate specifically to the anatomy of the carpal canal, physiologic conditions, and systemic disease or overuse. Likewise, its differential diagnosis is also extensive (Spinner et al, 1989).

According to personal observations, 50% of patients with carpal tunnel syndrome respond to conservative treatment measures. Splinting the wrist in a neutral position and avoidance of exacerbating activities is often effective in these patients. On occasion, treatment of an arthritic neck alone can improve concomitant symptoms of carpal tunnel syndrome. However, with these double-crush problems, it is most appropriate to treat both areas simultaneously. Treatment of any underlying systemic disease, if present, should be performed. If conservative methods do not provide relief or if patients present late with thenar atrophy, it may be necessary to release the transverse carpal ligament. Acute carpal tunnel syndrome should be addressed early. Overuse syndromes should be treated with avoidance of excessive activity or exacerbating positions.

In general, the transverse carpal ligament can be released through an open or endoscopic technique. In either case, care must be taken to avoid injury to proximate neurovascular structures, including the recurrent branch (Bennett and Crouch, 1982), the median palmar cutaneous branch (Carroll and Green, 1972; Taleisnik, 1973), ulnar nerve (Chow, 1994), ulnar nerve–median nerve palmar communicating branch (May and Rosen, 1981), and the superficial palmar arch. The advantages and disadvantages of these techniques are discussed in Chapters 54 and 55.

THE RECURRENT MOTOR BRANCH OF THE MEDIAN NERVE

The recurrent motor branch of the median nerve may be involved by itself or in combination with the median nerve under the transverse carpal ligament. It frequently passes through a discrete tunnel at the distal end of the transverse carpal ligament (Johnson and Shrewsbury, 1970). The recurrent motor branch of the median nerve may be entrapped in the flexor retinaculum (Papathanassiou, 1968) or compressed by a ganglion (Katon et al, 1991) or an anomalous muscle (Yamanaka et al, 1994). With specific involvement of the thenar branch, there is isolated weakness of abduction of the thumb and thenar atrophy; no sensory disturbance is present in the hand. Recognition of the localization and neurolysis of this motor branch is essential. Knowledge of its variations is also important (Lanz, 1977).

THE MEDIAN PALMAR CUTANEOUS NERVE

The median palmar cutaneous nerve, which usually arises 5 cm proximal to the radial styloid and innervates the thenar eminence, may be entrapped or injured, leading to pain and sensory disturbance (Al-Qattan, 1997). Anatomic variants may be present, including two separate branches, and may have clinical significance. A discrete tunnel within the superficial layers of the transverse carpal ligament has been described at the tubercle of the scaphoid (Naff et al, 1993). Compression has been described due to anatomic variants such as the palmaris longus (Stellbrink, 1972), ganglia (Al-Qattan and Robertson, 1993; Buckmiller and Rickard, 1987; Haskin, 1994), and fascial edge of the brachioradialis (Shimizu et al, 1988). Laceration of this branch due to its subcutaneous course and its vulnerability in explorations of the wrist may lead to painful neuromata.

PROXIMAL FOREARM/ELBOW

Anterior Interosseous Nerve Syndrome

The anterior interosseous nerve syndrome (Fearn and Goodfellow, 1965; Kiloh and Nevin, 1952; Nakano, et al, 1977; Schantz and Riegels-Nielsen, 1992; Sood and Burke, 1997; Spinner, 1970) is caused by compression of the anterior interosseous branch of the median nerve, typically at a site close to its origin (the nerve branch usually arises 6 cm below the lateral epicondyle). The syndrome is characterized by an inability to flex the terminal phalanges of the thumb,

index, and the long fingers. Paralysis of the pronator quadratus muscle is also observed. There is a typical pinch attitude seen with this paralysis. The remaining muscles innervated by the median nerve in the hand and forearm are intact. Sensation is undisturbed in the hand. With this localized paralysis, the patient can still oppose his thumb and can flex the proximal interphalangeal joints of the index and long fingers because the opponens pollicis and flexor digitorum superficialis are unaffected. Furthermore, there can be partial lesions of this major nerve branch (Hill et al, 1985), in which case isolated paralysis of the flexor pollicis longus or flexor digitorum profundus of the index or long finger may occur. Pain in the proximal forearm frequently may be a harbinger of these localized paralyses.

Important relevant anatomic variants may apply to the presentation of patients with the anterior interosseous nerve syndrome. If a Martin-Gruber connection is present (Leibovic and Hastings, 1992; Spinner, 1970; Uchida and Sugioka, 1992), there are variations in the clinical pattern. This neural variant, occurring in approximately 15% of limbs, transports ulnar fibers via the median nerve to the ulnar nerve in the proximal forearm. It connects frequently via the anterior interosseous branch of the median nerve. With this anatomic variation, entrapment of the anterior interosseous nerve may produce some intrinsic muscle paralysis in the hand. Furthermore, through a connection within the substance of the flexor digitorum profundus muscle between the anterior interosseous branch of the median nerve and a motor branch of the ulnar nerve, the flexor digitorum profundus muscle is innervated to a variable degree by the median and ulnar nerves (Sunderland, 1978). Thus, flexion of the terminal phalanges can be variably disturbed in an anterior interosseous nerve syndrome (Spinner, 1970, 1978).

When surgery is performed, the median nerve should be identified proximal to the bicipital aponeurosis (lacertus fibrosus) and traced distally through the region of the pronator teres. Decompression of the median nerve should include all potential compressive sites. The most common restraining structure is the tendinous origin of the deep head of the pronator teres, which crosses the anterior interosseous nerve at its hilum from the median nerve. Other causes of compression include variant tendinous structures (Fig. 53–14*A* and

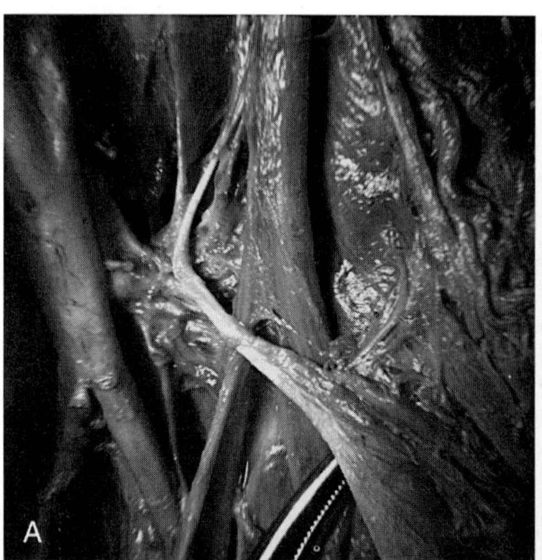
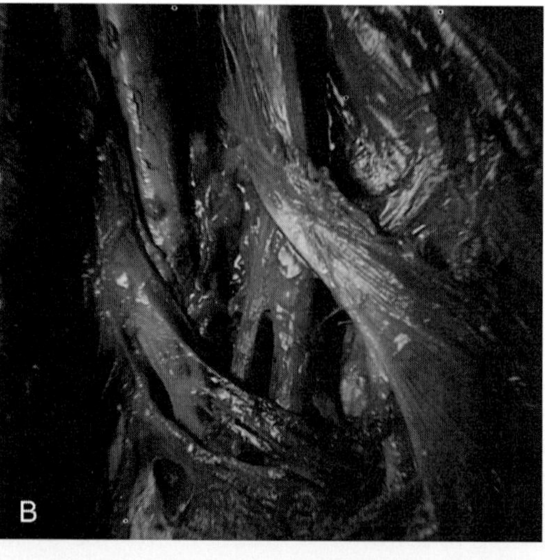

FIGURE 53–14. Right anatomical specimens demonstrating some variations of the deep head of the pronator teres and the anterior interosseous nerve. *A,* A thin tendinous origin of the deep head of the pronator teres is demonstrated crossing the median nerve and its anterior interosseous branch. *B,* The tendinous origin of the deep head of the pronator teres crosses the median nerve, and the ulnar collateral vessels traverse the branches more distally. (From Spinner M: Injuries to the Major Branches of Peripheral Nerves of the Forearm, 2nd ed. Philadelphia, W. B. Saunders Company, 1978.)

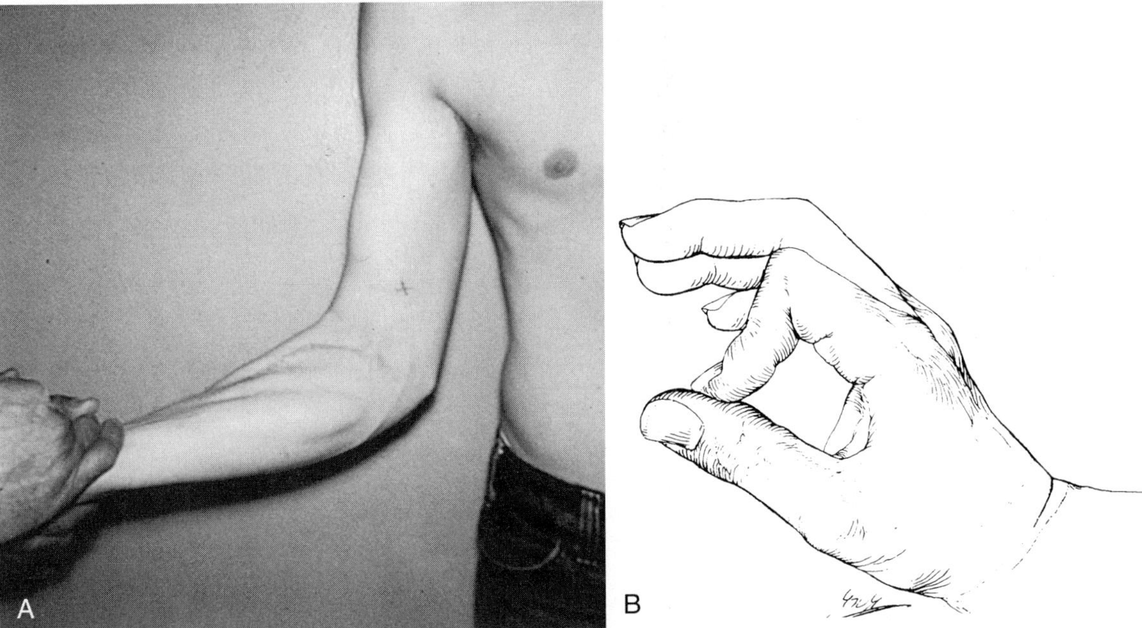

FIGURE 53–15. Pseudoanterior interosseous nerve syndrome. *A,* A 28-year-old man presented following injury to his dominant antecubital fossa with paralysis of his anterior interosseous nerve innervated muscles as well as more proximal median nerve innervated muscles (namely, flexor carpi radialis and pronator teres). Sensibility was normal in the hand. He underwent surgical decompression of the anterior interosseous branch in his proximal forearm with mild improvement only in the flexor digitorum profundus to the index finger. He was referred at that time. Pain was elicited on percussion of the median nerve in the distal arm (X) and an anomalous fascial expansion (an accessory bicipital aponeurosis) was noted on resistance to elbow flexion. A diagnosis of a pseudoanterior interosseous nerve syndrome was made. (From Spinner RJ, Carmichael SW, Spinner M: Partial median nerve entrapment in the distal arm because of an accessory bicipital aponeurosis. J Hand Surg *16A*:236, 1991. ©1991, Churchill Livingstone, New York.) *B,* A square pinch is present when a patient is unable to flex the terminal phalanges of the thumb and index finger. Although characteristic of an anterior interosseous nerve paralysis, a square pinch (Spinner, 1969) may also be present in cases of more proximal median nerve compression. (From Spinner M: Injuries to the Major Branches of Peripheral Nerves of the Forearm, 2nd ed. Philadelphia, W. B. Saunders Company, 1978.)

B), thrombosed ulnar collateral vessels, old penetrating forearm scars, anomalous radial artery passage, and casts.

Other entities need to be considered in the differential diagnosis of anterior interosseous nerve syndrome, including more proximal lesions of the median nerve, which may also present with paresis or paralysis of the anterior interosseous nerve-innervated muscles, as well as the flexor carpi radialis, pronator teres, palmaris longus, or flexor digitorum superficialis (Fig. 53–15). This is an important differential diagnosis, especially when pain is not initially present in the forearm. When an accessory bicipital aponeurosis causes median nerve compression in the distal arm, it must be released and neurolysis of the median nerve should be performed in the distal arm and proximal forearm (Spinner et al, 1991a). The Parsonage-Turner Syndrome also should be considered.

PRONATOR SYNDROME

The pronator syndrome (Hartz et al, 1981; Johnson et al, 1979; Kopell and Thompson, 1958; Olehnik et al, 1994) occurs when the median nerve is compressed in the proximal forearm most commonly at the pronator teres, then the flexor superficialis arch, and the bicipital aponeurosis (lacertus fibrosus). Usually the patient has chronic symptoms with a 9- to 24-month history of nonlocalized forearm pain. Frequently, the pronator teres is believed to be abnormally thickened, tubular-shaped, and firm, running obliquely from the medial epicondyle to the radius in the proximal forearm. Patients may have vague numbness in some digits innervated by the median nerve. Although a positive percussion test

can localize the level of the pathology, it may not appear for 4 to 5 months after the initial examination. The percussion test is positive more proximally in the forearm when the bicipital aponeurosis is the site of median nerve compression when compared with the other two localizations.

A frequent clinical finding is reproduction of the proximal forearm pain when forearm pronation is resisted. The pain is intensified when the flexed, pronated forearm is extended. This test is reliable for localizing the lesion to the pronator teres (Fig. 53–16*A*). Pain in the proximal forearm, reproduced by resistance to flexion of the flexor digitorum superficialis of the long finger, helps localize the pathology to the flexor superficialis arch (Fig. 53–16*B*). One must consider the site of entrapment at the bicipital aponeurosis (lacertus fibrosus) when resistance to flexion of the elbow and supination of the forearm reproduces the pain (Fig. 53–16*C*).

EMG evaluation can aid in the diagnosis, particularly when several serial studies are compared. It would be extremely helpful if a conduction delay were found. However, frequently all that can be found electrically is the appearance of some positive sharp waves or fibrillations in some of the forearm median nerve–innervated muscles (Buchtal et al, 1974). It is important that these muscles be the ones innervated distal to the pronator teres to be of confirmatory value. If more proximal median innervated muscles, such as the pronator teres, flexor carpi radialis, and palmaris longus, have these findings, then a more proximal median nerve problem must be considered.

A more acute, so-called lacertus syndrome may occur following a traumatic event, such as venipuncture or excr-

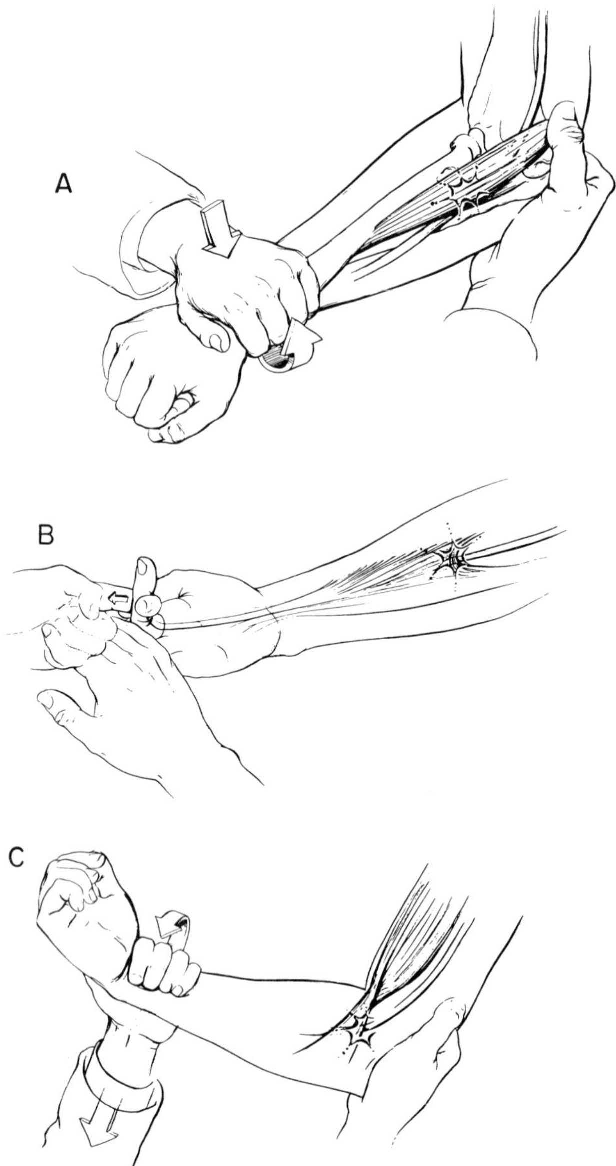

FIGURE 53–16. Tests for the site of compression in a pronator syndrome. *A,* When the forearm pain is reproduced by resistance to pronation of the forearm, and is aggravated by extending the elbow, the localization is at the pronator teres. *B,* When the pain occurs on resistance to flexion of the flexor digitorum superficialis of the long finger, the examiner's fingers keep the patients' remaining fingers in extension, and resistance to flexion of the proximal interphalangeal joint of the long finger. This test localizes the compression to the flexor superficialis arch. *C,* When the forearm pain is reproduced by resistance to flexion of the elbow and supination of the forearm, the bicipital aponeurosis (lacertus fibrosus) is the offending fibrous structure. (From Spinner M: Injuries to the Major Branches of Peripheral Nerves of the Forearm, 2nd ed. Philadelphia, W. B. Saunders Company, 1978).

cise, resulting in a complete or partial but rapidly progressing median nerve lesion at the antecubital fossa (Swiggett and Ruby, 1986).

Conservative management of patients with pronator syndrome should be performed initially. This approach consists of physical therapeutic measures, local steroid injections, immobilization, transcutaneous nerve stimulation, and anti-inflammatory medication. When surgery is necessary, the median nerve is identified, first, proximal to the bicipital

aponeurosis (which is released). Then the deep tendinous origin of the pronator teres should be released, and the median nerve can be traced as it passes deep to the flexor superficialis bridge. To accomplish this tracing, it is necessary to develop the plane between the lower border of the pronator teres and the proximal margin of the flexor carpi radialis. Then the median nerve is traced between these two sites proximally and distally in the forearm, releasing all restraints on it, including the bicipital aponeurosis, bands within the pronator teres, the deep tendinous origin of the pronator teres, hypertrophied pronator teres, thickened flexor superficialis arch, and accessory tendinous origin of the flexor carpi radialis from the ulna (Fig. 53–17*A* and *B*).

On occasion, with recurrent cases or with specific anomalies, such as a hyptertrophied superficial head of the pronator teres, the median nerve may be transposed subcutaneously. This is accomplished by lengthening the pronator teres at its musculotendinous junction and by bridging the lengthened pronator teres tendon posterior to the median nerve. The flexor superficialis bridge is released (Fig. 53–18*A* to *C*). Branches of the median nerve are preserved and usually require mobilization in order to permit easy passage through its new subcutaneous course.

COMPRESSION AT THE LIGAMENT OF STRUTHERS

The median nerve may be compressed by the ligament of Struthers complex (Al-Qattan and Husband, 1991; Crotti et al, 1981; Laha et al, 1977; Smith and Fisher, 1973; Struthers, 1881; Suranyi, 1983). This ligament is typically but not uniformly found with a supracondylar process (Fig. 53–19*A* and *B*). This anomalous spur is located 3 to 5 cm proximal to the medial epicondyle and connects these two bony prominences. It is found in approximately 1% of normal limbs and may be bilateral or familial (Terry, 1929). Other anatomic variations include a high division of the brachial artery, a high origin of the flexor-pronator group, and anomalous insertion of the coracobrachialis. The median nerve passes through this tunnel, usually with the ulnar artery. Typically, the spur is found incidentally on routine elbow radiographs and no neurovascular symptoms are present. However, after local trauma especially, high median nerve symptoms may appear. The brachial artery or ulnar artery also runs through the foramen and may be compressed (Talha et al, 1986); several authors have described ulnar nerve compression (Fragiadakis and Lamb, 1970; Mittal and Gupta, 1978).

INFRACLAVICULAR MEDIAN NERVE ENTRAPMENT

The median nerve can be compressed at the level of the axilla. Several causative factors have been identified, including anomalous axillary arch muscles, anomalous vascular perforations of the median nerve or its roots, the pectoralis minor, and thickening of the deltopectoral fascia.

All of these factors have a common mechanism for the production of paralysis, namely, abduction of the shoulder. Compression of the median nerve is aggravated by this repetitive motion because the offending anatomical structures cross anteriorly or penetrate the nerve. Some of the cases previously considered to be idiopathic or viral causes of brachial plexitis, may be related to the above-mentioned factors.

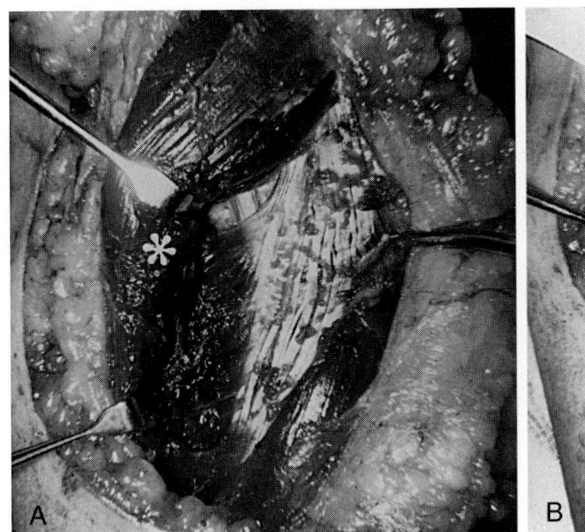
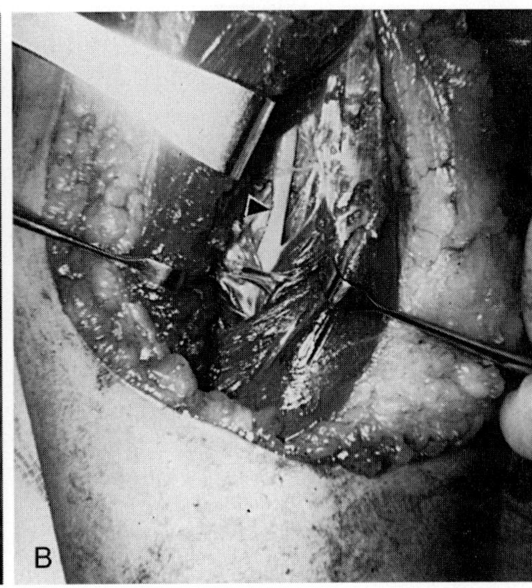

FIGURE 53–17. Pronator syndrome. *A,* The flexor superficialis arch was found to be the compressing structure in this patient with a pronator syndrome of the right forearm. The inferior margin of the pronator teres (*) is retracted radially. The median nerve is seen passing posterior to the flexor superficialis arch. *B,* On release and excision of a portion of the flexor superficialis arch, the median nerve was found to be narrowed and devoid of vascular markings in the region. (From Spinner, M.: Injuries to the Major Branches of Peripheral Nerves of the Forearm, 2nd ed. Philadelphia, W. B. Saunders Company, 1978.)

Langer's muscle which arises from the tendon of insertion of the latissimus dorsi and crosses anterior to the axillary neurovascular bundle to insert into the tendon of the pectoralis major (Narakas, 1991), is an example of an axillary arch muscle. According to Langer, this muscle has a 3% occurrence rate. It may occur in association with other anomalous pectoral muscles. Langer's muscle is capable of producing median nerve symptoms.

Six patients with either partial or complete median nerve paralysis caused by anomalous vascular perforations or vascular arches compressing or tethering the median nerve in the axilla have been treated by the senior author (Fig. 53–20). The associated vascular anomalies were either arterial or venous in origin. When the lesion was partial, sensation was unaffected and some of the forearm median-innervated muscles were paralyzed. On occasion, an isolated muscle such as the flexor pollicis longus may alone be paralyzed. More commonly, the flexor pollicis longus, pronator teres, pronator quadratus, flexor carpi radialis and palmaris longus were nonfunctioning, whereas the remaining median innervated intrinsic and extrinsic musculature was uninvolved clinically or electrically.

Subclavian arteriography, with the arm at the side and repeated with the arm abducted, is helpful in confirming the diagnosis of a vascular penetration of the median nerve. With the arm at the side, the arterial tree is visualized, whereas, in abduction, the vessel that may have an aberrant course does not fill. Brachial venography, with similar posi-

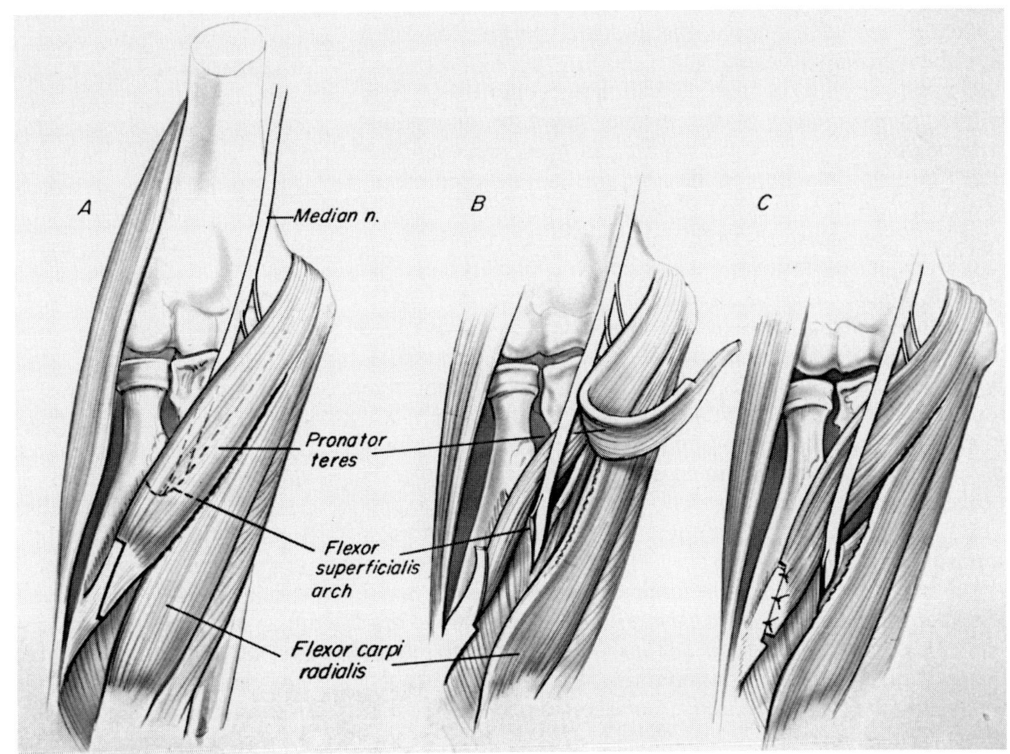

FIGURE 53–18. Translocation of the median nerve. *A,* When the median nerve is to be translocated into a subcutaneous bed in the proximal forearm, the median nerve is identified proximally and is traced through the two heads of the pronator teres. After opening the plane between the pronator teres and the flexor carpi radialis, the median nerve is identified at its entrance to the flexor superficialis bridge. The tendon of the pronator teres is then detached in a step-cut manner. On elevating the pronator teres, the median nerve is traced through the region and its numerous branches are preserved. *B,* The flexor superficialis arch is incised. *C,* The median nerve is elevated. When necessary, its motor branches are liberated by opening the epineurium. The superficial head of the pronator teres is then passed posterior to the median nerve and is resutured.

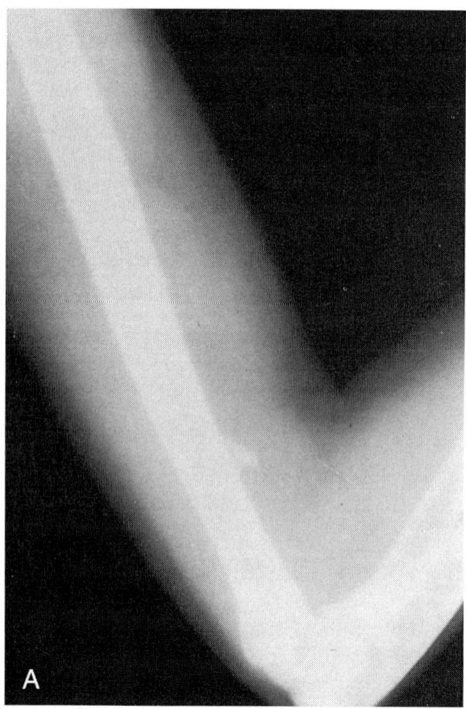

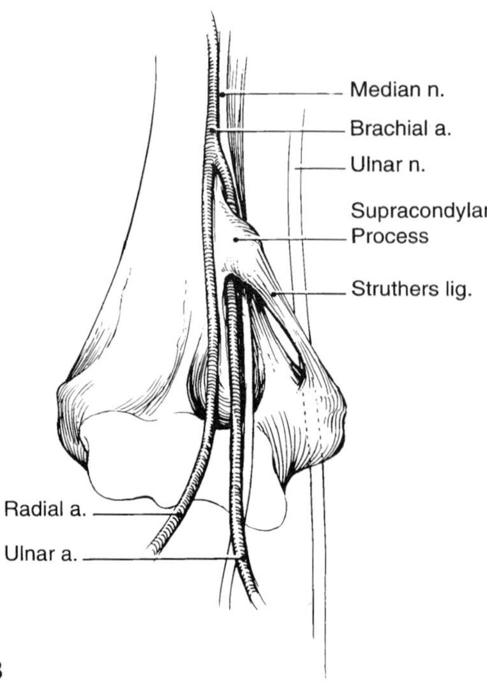

FIGURE 53–19. Supracondylar process of the humerus. *A,* A supracondylar process was an incidental finding on this patient's radiograph and is seen in 1% to 2% of the normal population. It is associated with other anatomical variations, including a ligament of Struthers, high division of the brachial artery, anomalous origin of the pronator teres, and insertion of the coracobrachialis. However, a supracondylar process along with the ligament of Struthers may produce neurovascular symptoms from median nerve, ulnar nerve, or brachial or ulnar artery compression. *B,* Drawing of the anatomic relationships of the supracondylar spur, the ligament of Struthers and the neighboring neurovascular structures. (From Spinner RJ, Lins RE, Jacobson SR, Nunley JA: Fractures of the supracondylar process of the humerus. J Hand Surg *19A*:1038, 1994. © 1994, Churchill Livingstone, New York.)

tioning of the arm, may reveal venous penetration of a nerve. Venography should be performed using the basilic vein rather than the cephalic system in order to visualize details of the venous system of the region. The most common variant perforation of the median nerve that is correlated with symptoms is found with abnormalities of the posterior humeral circumflex artery or vein. The subscapular and anterior thoracic vessel have been reported to follow anomalous paths. In a study of 480 human extremities, an 8% aberrant relationship between the axillary artery, its major branches, and elements of the brachial plexus has been described (Miller, 1939).

Thus, some cases of high median nerve compression may be due to perforation of the median nerve by anomalous branches of the axillary vessels. It has been proposed that with repeated abduction of the arm, median nerve compression or traction is produced (Spinner, 1976). Isolated flexor pollicis longus paralysis from this cause must be differentiated from partial anterior interosseous nerve palsy and an isolated rupture of the flexor pollicis longus tendon.

The pectoralis minor, with the coracoid process, can cause compression of the neurovascular bundle when the arm is hyperabducted (Mayfield, 1970). Sleeping in an abnormal position or working continuously with the arm fully abducted in a cramped position can produce neural symptoms in the limb. With abduction of the arm, the radial pulse is frequently obliterated. Conservative management is preferred, but on occasion, surgical release of the pectoralis minor is necessary.

The deltopectoral fascia becomes thickened, and its distal edge becomes fibrotic after trauma to the shoulder or brachial plexus. We have seen lesions of the brachial plexus and arm in which the distal fibrotic edge of the thickened deltopectoral fascia produced a compression of the median nerve.

A tumor can also cause high median nerve compression (Weinzweig and Browne, 1988).

Ulnar Nerve Syndromes

WRIST

The ulnar nerve is vulnerable to compression at the level of the wrist, resulting in a wide spectrum of motor or sensory symptoms, or both (Hayes et al, 1969; Mannerfelt, 1966; Shea and McClain, 1969; Uriburu et al, 1976). The clinical presentation relates to the specific zone of compression within the distal ulnar tunnel (Gross and Gelberman, 1985; Kuschner et al, 1988). Clinically relevant anatomical studies of the distal ulnar tunnel have defined three zones: Zone 1 consists of the ulnar nerve proximal to its bifurcation, and lesions herein predominantly result in a combination of motor and sensory symptoms, although pure motor or sensory symptoms may occur depending on the internal topography affected. Zone 2 includes the deep branch of the ulnar nerve, and such lesions nearly exclusively result in motor deficits. Lesions in Zone 3, which encompasses the superficial branch, result in sensory abnormalities. The most common sites for compression occur in Zones 1 and 2. The most common causes are masses such as ganglia or anatomical variations. Patients with complete ulnar nerve lesions at the wrist typically have sensory abnormalities in the palmar aspect of the ring and little fingers, and weakness and atrophy of the ulnar-innervated intrinsic muscles of the hand. Sensory abnormalities in the dorsoulnar hand or paralysis of ulnar innervated extrinsic muscles indicate a more proximal site of compression. Specific signs, such as Froment's, Wartenberg's or Mannerfelt's signs, are classically present. If surgical decompression is deemed necessary, the fibrotic arch (Dellon and Mackinnon, 1988; Lotem et al, 1973)

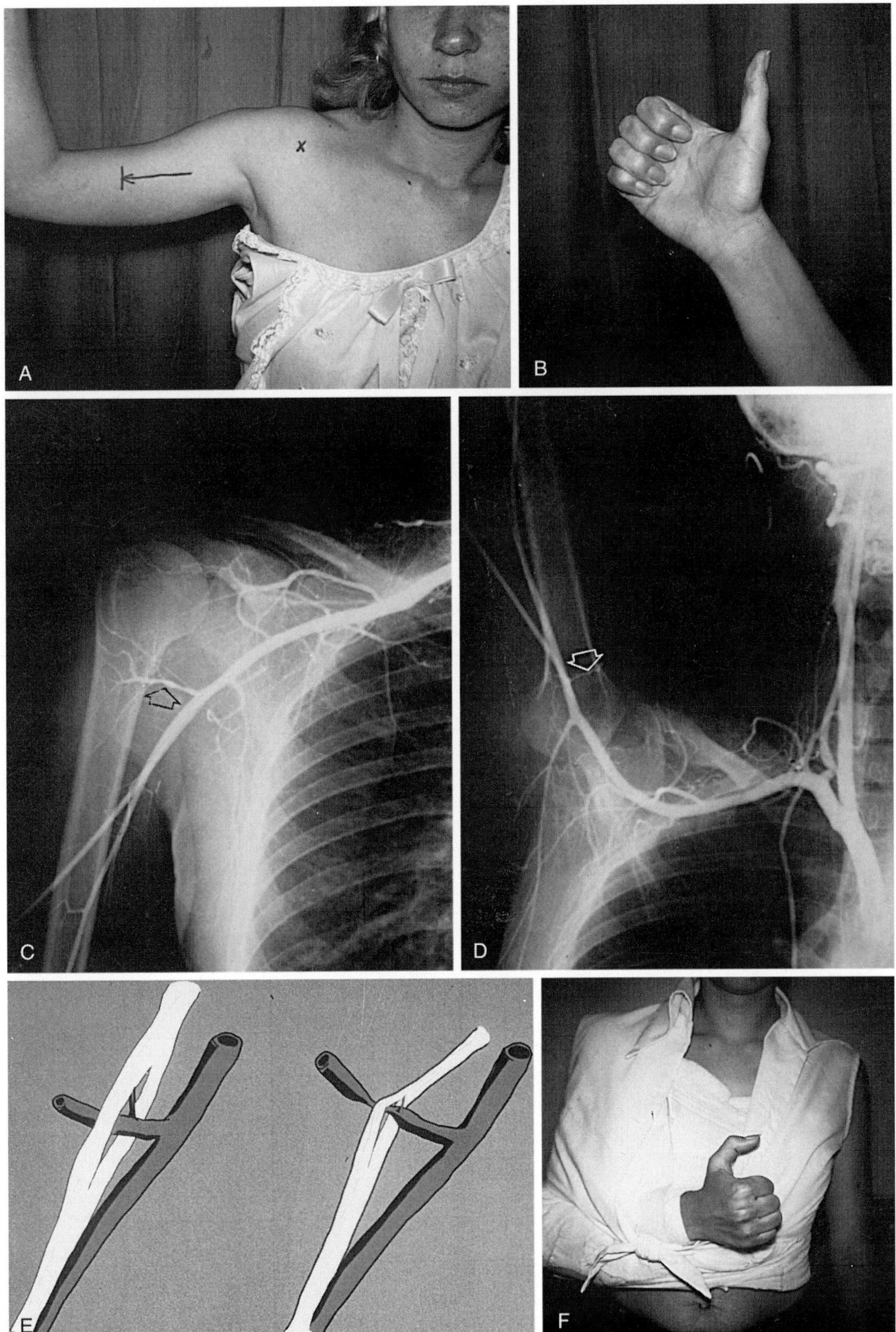

FIGURE 53–20. Cryptogenic infraclavicular brachial plexus neuritis. *A,* This 25-year-old woman presented with right shoulder pain and an inability to flex the terminal phalanx of the thumb. Maximal tenderness to percussion of the neurovascular bundle (X) was noted over the coracoid process. *B,* Isolated paralysis of the flexor pollicis longus was detected without sensory abnormality. *C,* The posterior humeral circumflex artery *(arrow)* is seen to be wavy. *D,* The second subclavian arteriogram, with the arm abducted, reveals only the anterior humeral circumflex artery *(arrow).* The posterior humeral circumflex artery is not visualized with the arm in this position. At surgery, the posterior humeral circumflex artery was found to penetrate the median nerve. *E,* Artistic rendition demonstrates vascular penetration of a nerve with dynamic compression of the vessel, the nerve, or both. (Courtesy of Goran Lundborg.) *F,* Flexion of the terminal phalanx of the thumb improved immediately postoperatively (patient seen in Velpeau dressing) and normalized 4 months after surgery.

should be released when present. If a mass is present, it should be removed at the time of neurolysis of the ulnar nerve.

DORSAL CUTANEOUS BRANCH OF THE ULNAR NERVE

Patients may present with isolated sensory abnormalities in the dorsoulnar aspect of the hand and proximal portion of the ring and little fingers due to compression of or injury to the dorsal sensory branch of the ulnar nerve. The dorsal cutaneous branch of the ulnar nerve usually arises 6 to 8 cm proximal to the wrist joint. However, many variations have been described. It can arise as proximal as near the elbow. This ulnar sensory branch is less vulnerable to trauma than the superficial radial nerve. Blunt trauma or extrinsic compression from casts may result in isolated lesions; spontaneous entrapment may also occur (McCarthy and Nalebuff, 1980). We have seen several left-handed patients who were symptomatic due to direct pressure of a firm writing surface on the ulnar border of the wrist. In these people, pain was exacerbated with active flexion or extension of the digit because the neuroma had become adherent to the extensor tendon of the little finger.

FOREARM

Unusual sites of compression of the ulnar nerve in the forearm have been described resulting from masses, anatomical variations (such as a hypertrophied flexor carpi ulnaris), fibrovascular bands, and penetrating vessels. Sensory abnormalities in the dorsoulnar aspect of the hand signify a lesion proximal to the take-off of the dorsal cutaneous branch of the ulnar nerve in the forearm. In these several reports, the site of maximal pain on percussion proved to be critical to the localization of the lesion.

ELBOW

The ulnar nerve is most commonly compressed at the elbow. Compression typically occurs at one of the following sites: Arcade of Struthers (Al-Qattan and Murray, 1991; Kane et al, 1973; Ochiai et al, 1992), medial intermuscular septum (Spinner and Kaplan, 1976), cubital tunnel (O'Driscoll et al, 1991; Osborne 1957, 1970), arcade of the flexor carpi ulnaris, and the flexor-pronator aponeurosis (Amadio and Beckenbaugh, 1986; Inserra and Spinner, 1986). Primary compression is usually localized to one site within the cubital tunnel or flexor carpi ulnaris aponeurosis; in contrast, secondary compression frequently is multilevel and typically include the medial intermuscular septum, arcade of Struthers, and the deep flexor-pronator aponeuroses. The dynamic role of the ulnar nerve and the triceps muscle in causing compression, especially with flexion of the elbow, has been clarified (Apfelberg and Larson, 1973; Dreyfuss and Kessler, 1978; Hayashi et al, 1984; Macnicnol, 1979; Reis, 1980; Rolfsen 1970; Spinner and Goldner, 1995; Vanderpool et al, 1968). The ulnar nerve may also be compressed by the ligament of Struthers associated with a supracondylar spur (Fragiadakis and Lamb, 1970).

Patients typically present with motor weakness, predominantly in the intrinsics of the hand or sensory abnormalities in the ulnar nerve distribution, both in the dorsal and palmar aspects of the hand. Patients have difficulty crossing and snapping their fingers. The early sparing of the flexor carpi ulnaris and flexor digitorum profundus in ulnar nerve compression at the elbow can be understood in terms of the internal topography (Sunderland, 1978). The ulnar intrinsics and the sensory fibers are more peripherally located than the central fibers of the flexor carpi ulnaris and flexor digitorum profundus.

Most frequent causes of ulnar nerve compression at the elbow include external pressure; compression by synovitis,

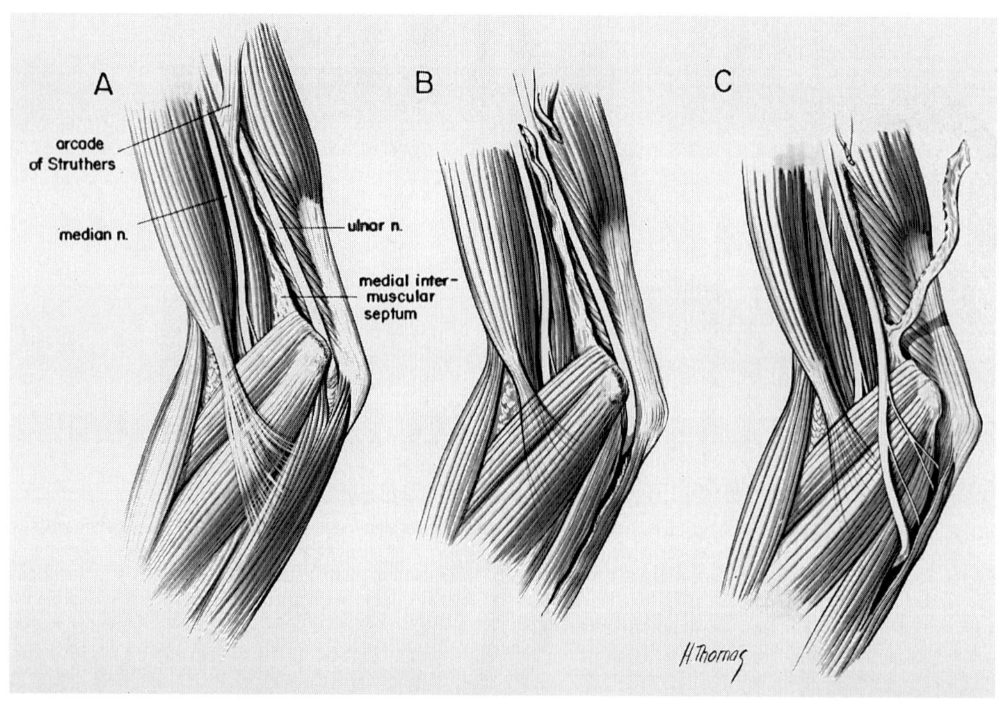

FIGURE 53–21. Subcutaneous transposition of the ulnar nerve. *A,* The relationship of the ulnar nerve to the intermuscular septum and arcade of Struthers is noted. *B,* Release of the ulnar nerve proximally to the arcade of Struthers is performed. *C,* The medial intermuscular septum is released. Decompression of the ulnar nerve is performed distally so that with anterior transposition it is not kinked. (From Spinner M: Injuries to the Major Branches of Peripheral Nerves of the Forearm, 2nd ed. Philadelphia, W. B. Saunders Company, 1978.)

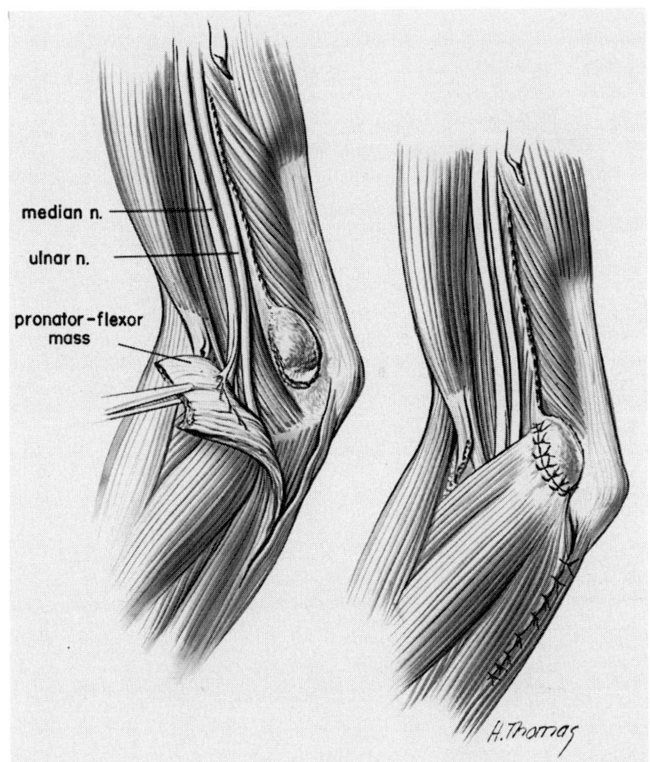

FIGURE 53–22. In any transposition of the ulnar nerve, a thorough decompression of the ulnar nerve must be performed. In a submuscular transposition, the ulnar nerve is translocated anterior and deep to flexor-pronator muscles. The ulnar nerve is placed adjacent and parallel to the median nerve. The flexor-pronator muscles are loosely resutured to their origin. (From Spinner M: Injuries to the Major Branches of Peripheral Nerves of the Forearm, 2nd ed. Philadelphia, W. B. Saunders Company, 1978).

osteophytes, masses, anomalous muscles, fracture callus, perineural adhesions, and hematomas; or nerve instability.

Patients with ulnar nerve compression at the elbow should be treated with a trial of nonoperative therapy, and surgery should not be taken lightly. The elbow can be immobilized in a long arm orthoplast splint. The elbow is kept at 70 degrees, the wrist at neutral, and the forearm in mid-position for 6 weeks full time and an additional 6 weeks part time. In refractory cases, surgery is indicated. The choice of surgical procedure depends largely on the surgeon's preference, and results have been nicely reviewed by Dellon (1989). In general, procedures may be divided into local ones (which attempt to release the offending structure from the nerve's anatomical course) and anterior transposition (movement of the nerve to an uninvolved bed in a more favorable environment). Surgical options include in situ decompression; medial epicondylectomy; and subcutaneous (with or without a fasciodermal flap; Eaton et al, 1980) (Fig. 53–21), intramuscular (Kleinman and Bishop, 1989) or submuscular transpositions (Fig. 53–22) (Learmonth, 1942; Leffert, 1982; Spinner, 1994). Internal neurolysis may be used as an adjuvant procedure. The authors do not employ medial epicondylectomy or intramuscular transposition. In situ decompression can be used in mild cases of ulnar nerve compression that are localized to the flexor carpi ulnaris arcade when the patient has persistent symptoms without electrical findings. The ulnar nerve should not subluxate or dislocate after in situ decompression. Other local procedures relate

to the simple excision of masses; when an anomalous muscle (anconeus epitrochlearis) or supracondylar ligament of Struthers is present, it frequently is the offending structure. During cases of transposition, the ulnar nerve should be released thoroughly, and the arcade of Struthers should be released. The medial intermuscular septum should be excised in order to prevent a secondary potential entrapment compression (Gabel and Amadio, 1990). Care must be taken to avoid injury to the branch of the ulnar nerve to the flexor digitorum profundus and to the sensory branches (Dellon and Mackinnon, 1985).

The authors favor submuscular transposition in cases of resistant or recurrent ulnar neuropathy and, in many instances, primary neuropathy (Spinner, 1994). When the ulnar nerve is transposed anteriorly, it is unwise to place it in a groove within the flexor-pronator group of muscles, because postoperative nerve traction produces ulnar neuritis and frequently complicates this technique (Seddon, 1972). In this instance with recurrence, it is best to mobilize the nerve completely and to transpose it deep to the entire flexor-pronator muscle mass; the traumatized ulnar nerve is placed in a favorable bed parallel to the median nerve. The nerve should be in a straight line without kinks or angles as viewed anteriorly or laterally. The Learmonth procedure (submuscular transposition of the ulnar nerve) is contraindicated in patients with advanced osteoarthritis or traumatic arthritis involving the ulnohumeral aspect of the elbow, or an unstable elbow from rheumatoid disease; in these cases, anterior subcutaneous transposition is indicated. Failed ulnar nerve surgery may be due to inadequate release, iatrogenic compression (due to inadequate proximal [Fig. 53–23] or distal dissection [Fig. 53–24A to C] or a constrictive environment, such as an overly tight fasciodermal sling), or improper localization (Bednar et al, 1994; Rogers et al, 1991). Persistent postoperative snapping (Fig. 53–25A and B) may also complicate ulnar nerve surgery, and the elbow should be examined intraoperatively in flexion and extension to ensure that mechanical causes for compression (including the dynamic role of the medial head of the triceps) are addressed adequately.

ARM AND AXILLA

Several descriptions of ulnar nerve compression in the arm and axilla exist in the literature, and extrinsic compression by masses or from blunt or direct trauma have been responsible for the compression. We have seen one case of infraclavicular compression due to a chondroepitrochlearis muscle, an anomalous pectoral muscle (Spinner et al, 1991b). Similarly, the authors have used conservative treatment in a patient with high median and ulnar nerve paralysis who, while inebriated, fell asleep in a chair sitting backward. The inner aspect of his arm was compressed between his head and the edge of the unpadded wooden chair. It took 6 months for full spontaneous recovery. This is a variant of the Saturday night paralysis (high radial nerve compression).

Radial Nerve Syndromes

POSTERIOR INTEROSSEOUS NERVE

The posterior interosseous nerve (Fuss and Wurzl, 1991) may be compressed in the elbow region by a fibrous band

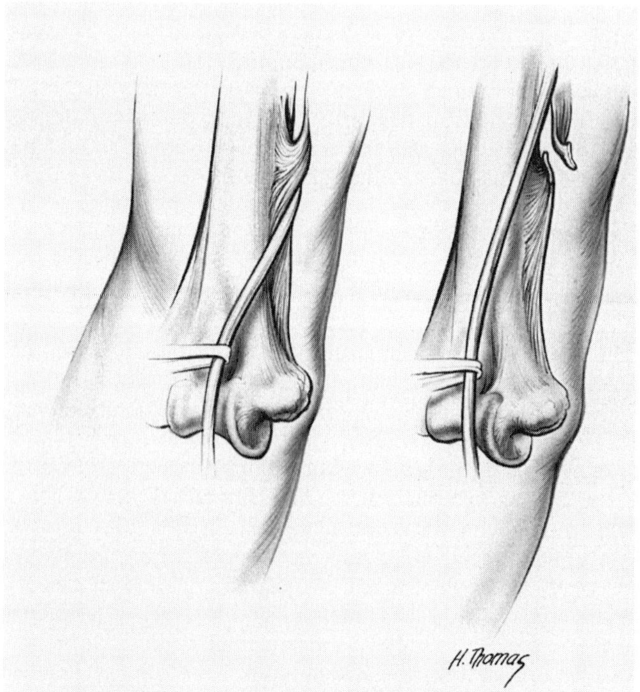

FIGURE 53–23. Entrapment of the ulnar nerve at the arcade of Struthers 8 cm proximal to the medial epicondyle can be a cause for a secondary ulnar neuritis following incomplete translocation of this nerve. (From Spinner M: Injuries to the Major Branches of Peripheral Nerves of the Forearm, 2nd ed. Philadelphia, W. B. Saunders Company, 1978.)

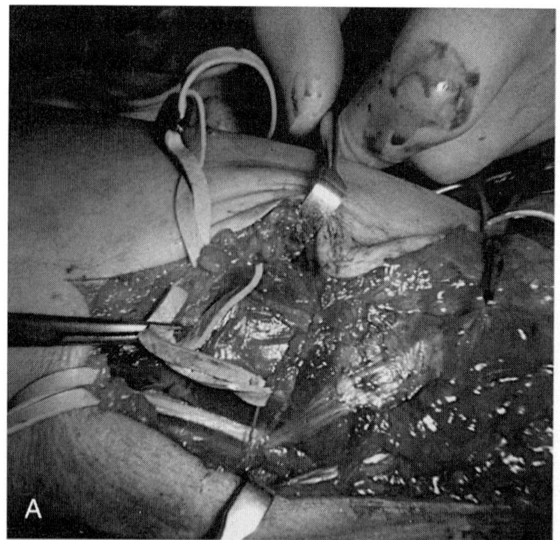

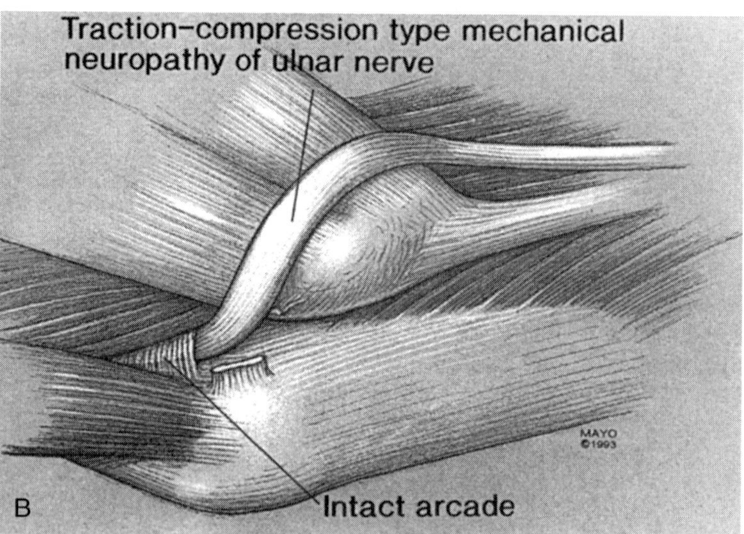

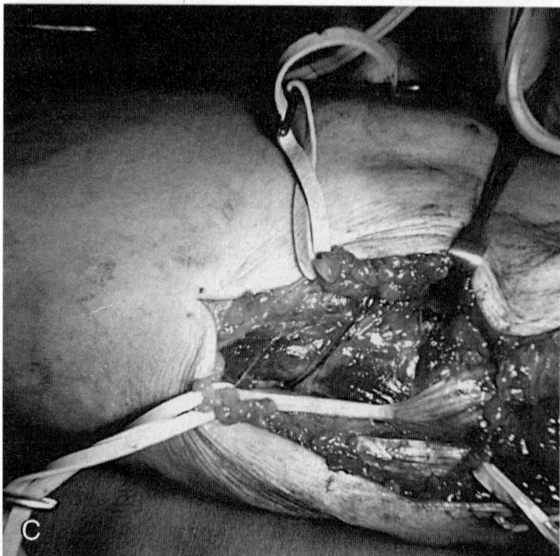

FIGURE 53–24. Resistant ulnar neuropathy due to incomplete distal decompression. *A,* Tethering of the ulnar nerve distal to the elbow is demonstrated in this patient with persistent symptoms following a subcutaneous transposition. *B,* Artistic rendition. (By permission of Mayo Foundation.) *C,* Decompression of the ulnar nerve with release of this mechanical block led to clinical recovery. (From Spinner M: Nerve decompression. *In* Morrey BF (ed): Master Techniques in Orthopaedic Surgery. The Elbow. New York, Raven Press, 1994, p 196.)

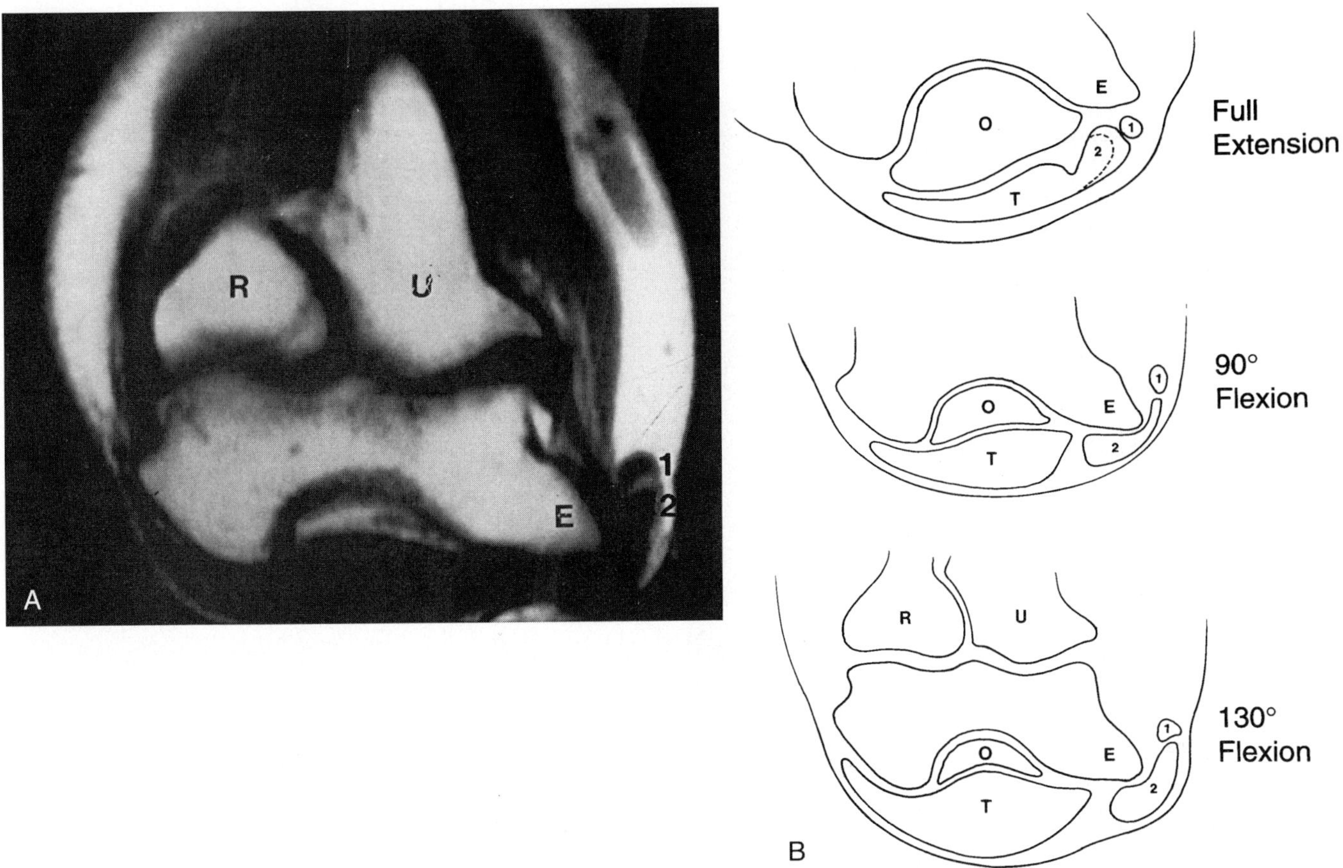

FIGURE 53–25. Snapping triceps and ulnar neuropathy. *A,* Magnetic resonance imaging study performed with the elbow fully flexed demonstrates a dislocating ulnar nerve (1) and medial triceps (2) over the medial epicondyle (E) in a patient with a snapping elbow and ulnar nerve symptoms. R, radius; U, ulna. (Spinner RJ, Goldner RG: Snapping triceps and ulnar neuropathy: Anatomic and dynamic factors. American Orthopaedic Association annual meeting, White Sulphur Springs, WV, June, 1995.) *B,* Drawing based on magnetic resonance imaging studies performed with the elbow extended and flexed in different positions in this patient with snapping triceps and ulnar neuropathy. O, olecranon; T, triceps. (From Khoo D, Carmichael SW, Spinner RJ: Ulnar nerve anatomy and compression. Orthop Clin North Am *27*:317, 1996.)

at the radiocapitellar joint (Roles and Maudlsey, 1972), a portion of the vascular leash of Henry (from the radial recurrent artery), the leading proximal tendinous edge of the extensor carpi radialis brevis, and a band in the proximal, middle, or distal supinator (Comtet and Chambaud, 1975; Derkash and Niebauer, 1981). Most frequently, the level of compression is at the arcade of Frohse, the proximal edge of the supinator (which is fibrotendinous in 30% of limbs; (Papadopoulos et al, 1989; Prasartrirtha et al, 1993; Spinner 1968, 1978). The tendinous origin of the extensor carpi radialis brevis places additional force on the proximal edge of the supinator in pronation.

Entrapment can occur spontaneously, or compression may be due to an extrinsic mass such as a soft tissue tumor (Fig. 53–26) (Weinberger, 1939) or related to trauma (Cravens and Kline, 1990; Young et al, 1990). Iatrogenic injuries may result from so-called blind procedures, such as elbow arthroscopy or injections, or from open procedures such as radial head resection (Capener, 1966), tennis elbow release, fracture stabilization (Figs. 53–27 and 53–28) and total elbow arthroplasty; neural symptoms in these cases may result from direct injury to the nerve or from surrounding compression from edema or hematoma.

Patients may present with complete or partial paralysis. In complete paralysis, all of the muscles supplied by the posterior interosseous nerve are not functioning. The patient can-

not extend the thumb, index, long, ring, and little fingers at the metacarpophalangeal joints. The wrist can dorsiflex but does so in a dorsoradial direction. This occurs as a result of a muscular imbalance of the wrist extensors due to paralysis of the extensor carpi ulnaris and the extensor digitorum communis; the extensor carpi radialis longus and brevis are spared because they are usually innervated at a site proximal to the compression. Pain in the proximal forearm, which may be present in the early phases, usually is not a major complaint in late presentations. Sensation in the hand is intact.

The second pattern is characterized by a lack of extension of the thumb or one or more of the digits at the metacarpophalangeal level. Paresis or paralysis of the remaining digits often develops.

The symptom complex known as radial tunnel syndrome is recognized frequently to be due to posterior interosseous nerve compression in the region of the arcade of Frohse (Lister et al, 1979; Lister, 1991; Roles and Maudsley, 1972). This syndrome is characterized by pain about the lateral aspect of the elbow without motor loss and can be recognized by pain on resistance to extension of the long finger at the metacarpophalangeal joint and is associated with localized tenderness on direct pressure over the arcade of Frohse noted anteriorly over the radial head and neck region. In the authors' experience, up to 10% of patients with lateral epicondylitis have a coexistent radial tunnel syndrome. We

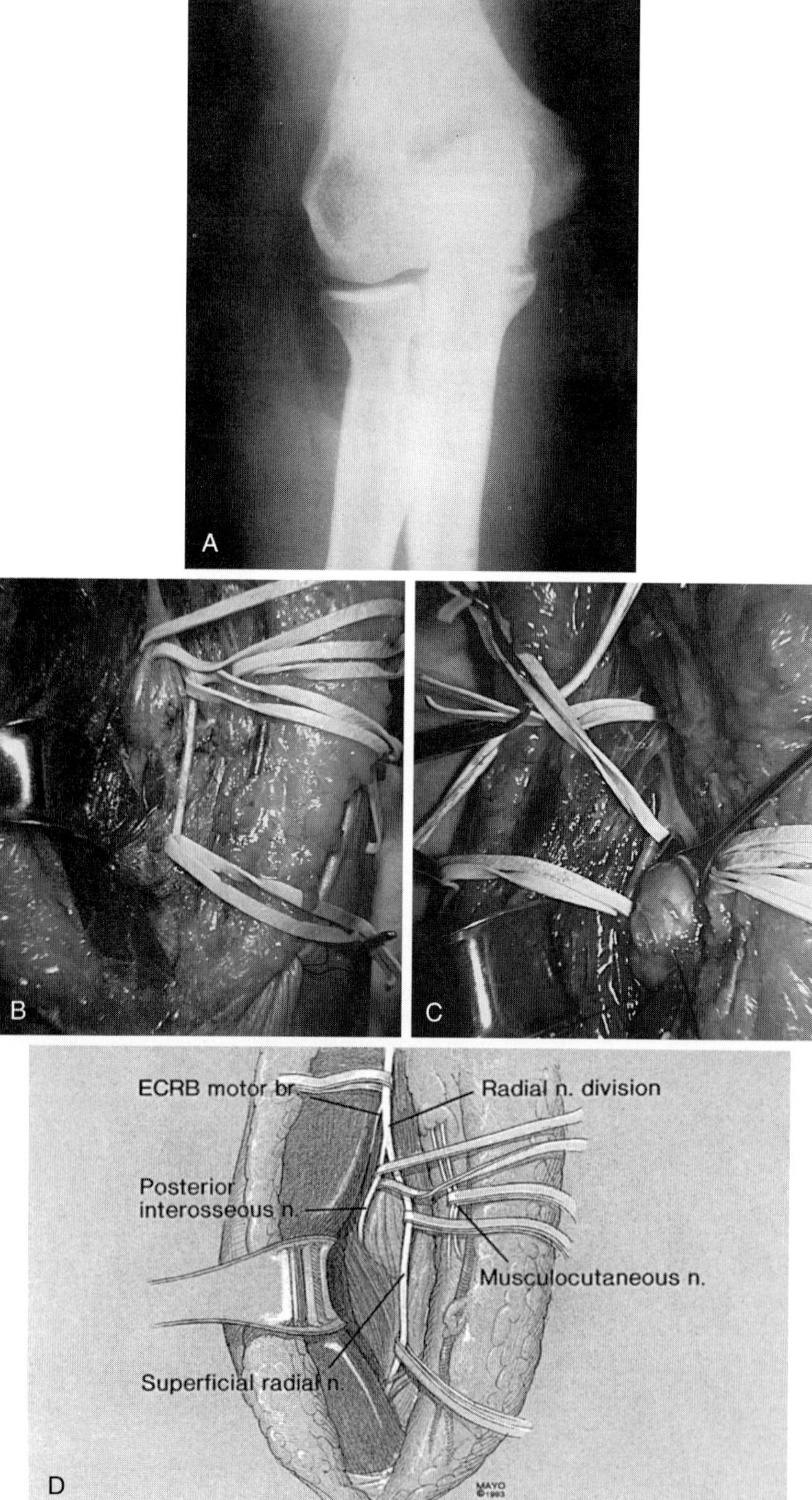

FIGURE 53–26. Partial posterior interosseous nerve compression due to a lipoma. See clinical presentation in Figure 53–2B. *A,* Radiograph demonstrates a soft tissue lucency adjacent to the radial head consistent with a lipoma. *B,* An anterior (Henry) approach was used to expose the lipoma. The relationship of the lipoma to the posterior interosseous nerve can be appreciated. *C,* Traction sutures were placed to deliver the mass. *D,* Corresponding artistic drawing. (By permission of the Mayo Foundation.)

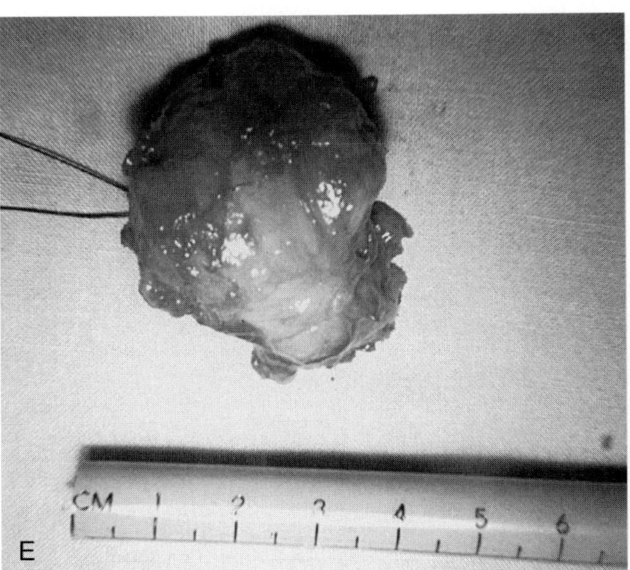

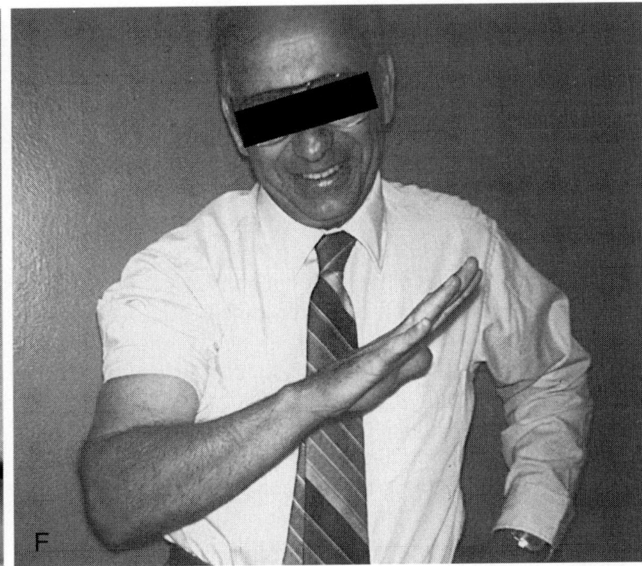

FIGURE 53–26 *Continued E,* The excised lipoma is demonstrated. *F,* Full recovery occurred by 6 weeks. (From Spinner M: Nerve decompression. *In* Morrey BF [ed]: Master Techniques in Orthopaedic Surgery. The Elbow. New York, Raven Press, 1994, p 196.)

believe that the combination of radial tunnel syndrome along with lateral epicondylitis is due to radiocapitellar bursitis; with recurrent inflammation, the arcade of Frohse contracts. It becomes narrowed and encroaches on the posterior interosseous nerve. In these cases, at surgery, the arcade of Frohse was found to be narrowed and was displaced radially. To manage this group of patients, both conditions must be treated simultaneously with tennis elbow release and neurol-

ysis of the posterior interosseous nerve to obtain optimal results. In patients who have not responded to conservative care and who have not had prior surgery, the authors use the modified Thompson approach. One can strip the epicondyle and drill it, and then the posterior interosseous nerve can be released. A significant number of patients who have not responded to conservative treatment, release of the lateral epicondylar soft tissues, or excision of a portion of the orbicular ligament have been relieved by neurolysis of the posterior interosseous nerve. If pain persists following the customary surgery for tennis elbow, posterior interosseous

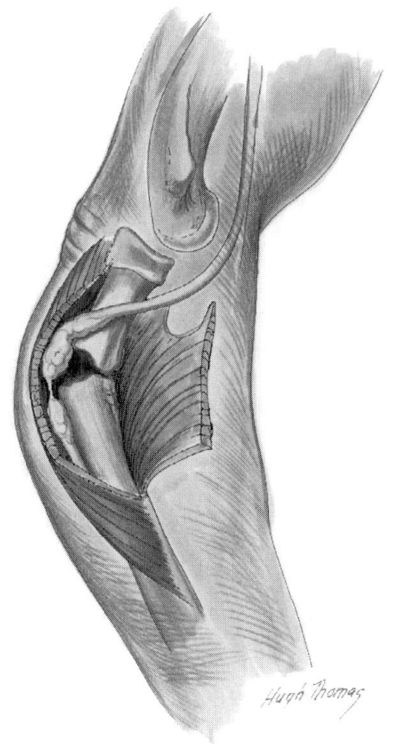

FIGURE 53–27. Fracture of the proximal radius can be associated with posterior interosseous nerve paralysis, especially if there is posterior angulation of the fracture site.

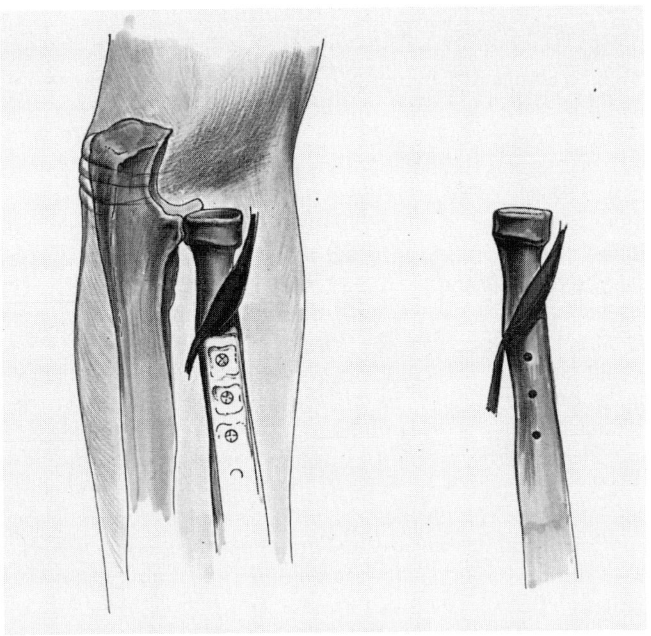

FIGURE 53–28. Open reduction with plate and screw fixation of a fracture of the proximal half of the radius can be complicated by a posterior interosseous nerve paralysis. Early removal of the plate and replacement with a shorter plate or, if the fracture is healed, neurolysis alone can restore neuromuscular function.

nerve compression should be suspected as a possible cause. In these patients, if surgery is elected, a separate anterior Henry incision is used.

Common surgical approaches to the posterior interosseous nerve include anterior (Henry, 1970), posterior (Thompson, 1918), brachioradialis splitting (Lister et al, 1979), and brachioradialis–extensor carpi radialis longus interval (Hall et al, 1984). Depending on the localization of the entrapment and whether there had been prior surgery or injury in the area, the following method is recommended. In primary cases, the best operative approach can be selected based on the clinical findings and localization aid of electromyographic and imaging studies. If there is a posterior interosseous nerve lesion confirmed on electromyography and if the supinator muscle has fibrillations throughout, then the entrapment is at the proximal edge of the supinator and the anterior Henry approach is recommended.

If there is a posterior interosseous nerve lesion confirmed on EMG, and the studies of the supinator muscle are normal, then the lesion is at the distal end and the best operative approach is the modified Thompson approach. This includes release of the origin of the extensor carpi radialis brevis and a portion of the extensor carpi radialis longus from the distal humerus. This gives full exposure of the posterior interosseous nerve. The anterior Henry approach does not give adequate exposure of the distal half of the supinator and posterior interosseous nerve, and is not recommended in this instance.

On occasion when there is a large tumor or prior scarring from shotgun pellets or proximal radial plating, both the anterior Henry and the posterior Thompson approaches are necessary to gain control of the distal radial nerve as well as the proximal and distal portion of the posterior interosseous nerve.

SUPERFICIAL RADIAL NERVE

The superficial radial nerve (Wartenberg's syndrome [1932]) is usually compressed at one of two sites: 8 cm proximal to the radial styloid at the fascial edge of the brachioradialis and extensor carpi radialis longus (Dellon and Mackinnon, 1986; Lanzetta and Foucher, 1993; Turkof et al, 1995), or at its subcutaneous position at the radial styloid, where it is vulnerable to external compression. In addition, the superficial radial nerve may be compressed in the proximal forearm by soft tissue masses, sometimes in association with the posterior interosseous nerve or anterior interosseous nerve of the median nerve (Agnew, 1867). Compression in the distal forearm typically occurs spontaneously. Compression at the wrist is usually related to constrictive bands (Fig. 53–29), tight surgical gloves, cuffs (Massey and Pleet, 1978), casts, jewelry, and so on. Symptoms may also be aggravated by fluid retention or with weight gain. Patients present with pain (cheiralgia paresthetica) and sensory abnormalities in the dorsoradial part of the hand. Variations in the sensory pattern are due to overlapping patterns with the lateral antebrachial cutaneous nerve (Mackinnon and Dellon, 1985). Lesions of the superficial radial nerve compression must be differentiated from De Quervain's tenosynovitis, although the two may coexist; in fact, a Finkelstein sign may be present with either condition. Nonoper-

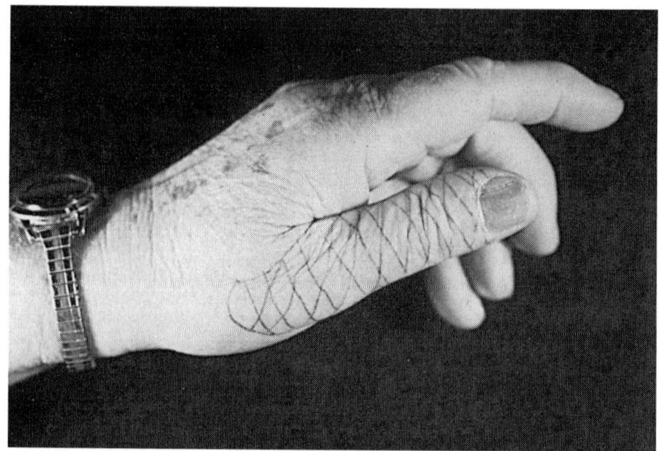

FIGURE 53–29. Superficial radial nerve compression by a watchband (From Spinner M: Injuries to the Major Branches of Peripheral Nerves of the Forearm, 2nd ed. Philadelphia, W. B. Saunders Company, 1978.)

ative therapy is successful in many cases, but surgical neurolysis is recommended in refractory cases.

POSTERIOR CUTANEOUS BRANCH OF THE FOREARM

Several cases of isolated sensory abnormalities in the dorsolateral forearm, at times associated with pruritus, have been described due to lesions of the posterior antebrachial cutaneous nerve (Chang and Oh, 1990; Massey and Massey, 1986). They occurred either spontaneously or following surgical procedures (fracture manipulation or flap harvesting). Residual pain following lateral epicondylar surgery may be due to a neuroma of this neural branch. Removal of the neuroma and allowing the proximal end to retract into normal fat can relieve the symptoms.

HIGH RADIAL NERVE COMPRESSION IN THE ARM OR AXILLA

Spontaneous radial nerve compression may occur in the mid-arm, usually at the level of the lateral head of the triceps (Lotem et al, 1971; Lubahn and Lister, 1983; Manske, 1977; Nakamichi and Tachibana, 1991). Patients have often presented with a history remarkable for strenuous muscular exercise. High radial nerve palsy may also occur from other well-defined etiologies such as humeral diaphyseal fractures, external compression (Saturday night palsy), and masses. In addition, a more proximal spontaneous compression lesion may occur in the axilla due to vascular penetrations of the terminal portions of the plexus. The senior author has treated 12 patients with this entity.

Unlike a posterior interosseous nerve paralysis at the level of the elbow, which leads to wrist dorsiflexion in a radial direction (and extension lag of the digits), a lesion at the mid-arm level produces complete wrist drop, along with finger and thumb extension lag. Elbow extension is normal, and there is anesthesia of the dorsal basilar aspect of the thumb and first web space (Fig. 53–30A and B). With radial nerve lesions of the mid-arm, there is additional sensory loss on the lateral aspect of the distal arm (involvement of the lower radial sensory branch) as well as the radial nerve autonomous zone of the dorsoradial aspect of the hand. If, however, in addition to a drop of the wrist, fingers, and thumb, there is partial or complete paralysis of the triceps, then a higher lesion is probably present. If the lesion is of the posterior cord, not only are there the above-mentioned problems present but there is further proximal loss of sensation in the arm and paralysis of the deltoid muscle, as well as loss of extension of the elbow.

To demonstrate the location and the etiology of a lesion of the radial nerve at the axilla, subclavian arteriography and basilic venography, with the arm at the side and abducted, can be helpful. An aberrant subscapular artery can penetrate the radial nerve and, with repeated abduction, can produce radial nerve dysfunction. On the posterior axillary wall, an aberrant muscle, the accessory subscapularis-teres-latissimus, may cross all or a portion of the radial nerve (Kameda, 1976). This anomalous muscle can involve the axillary nerve as well.

If a patient has a spontaneous radial nerve paralysis in the arm that does not reveal clinical or electrical evidence of recovery by 3 to 4 months following onset, then exploration is indicated. If the paralytic lesion is complete for 18 months, the procedure of choice is primary tendon transfers. If, in addition to the paralysis, pain is a persistent complaint, neurolysis of the radial nerve to relieve the chronic pain is indicated.

Musculocutaneous Nerve

The musculocutaneous nerve may be compressed at various levels resulting in a mixed motor and sensory or a pure sensory presentation. The terminal branch of the lateral cord is specifically vulnerable to entrapment where it penetrates the coracobrachialis (Pecina and Bojanic, 1993). There are many variations in both the anatomy of the coracobrachialis and the levels where the musculocutaneous nerve penetrates the muscle. A complete lesion of this nerve results in paralysis of the biceps and brachialis muscles with atrophy, and

there is a sensory loss on the lateral aspect of the forearm. Tenderness on percussion over the course of the nerve is often present. Typically, this lesion occurs following heavy exercise (Braddom and Wolfe, 1978). The musculocutaneous nerve may also be compressed or stretched following positioning, trauma (including shoulder dislocation and clavicle fracture) (Jerosch et al, 1989), or after shoulder procedures (Richards et al, 1987). The relationship of the musculocutaneous nerve to the coracoid has received the attention of several reports (Flatow et al, 1989), which are important to study to avoid its injury during open (Caspi et al, 1987; Dundore and DeLisa, 1979; Katznelson et al, 1976) or arthroscopic surgery (Wolf, 1989). Electrical studies generally are diagnostic and help differentiate more proximal lesions. Symptoms that develop spontaneously usually improve over several months with nonoperative therapy. However, if symptoms of a musculocutaneous nerve lesion develop after a surgical procedure and do not improve within 3 to 4 months, exploration should be performed because a reversible mechanical cause of neurologic injury may be responsible and has been identified in a high percentage of cases.

Lateral Cutaneous Nerve of the Forearm

The lateral cutaneous nerve of the forearm, the terminal sensory branch of the musculocutaneous nerve, may be compressed at the level just proximal to the elbow. Here, the nerve is particularly vulnerable as it emerges lateral to the bicipital tendon at its musculotendinous junction (Bassett and Nunley, 1982; Patel et al, 1991; Davidson et al, 1995). The sharp edge of the biceps tendon has been demonstrated to tighten with elbow extension and pronation or with resisted elbow flexion and pronation. A positive percussion test is usually present in the anterolateral aspect of the distal arm just proximal to the elbow. Patients present with isolated sensory disturbance in the distal volar radial forearm. The

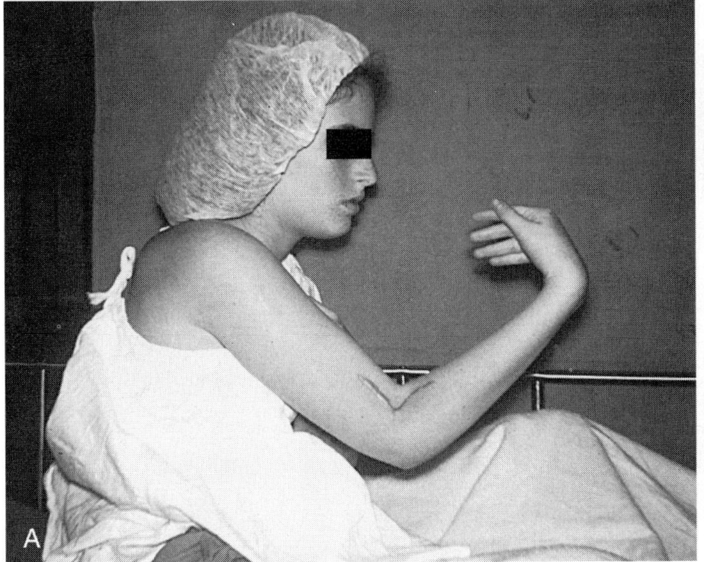
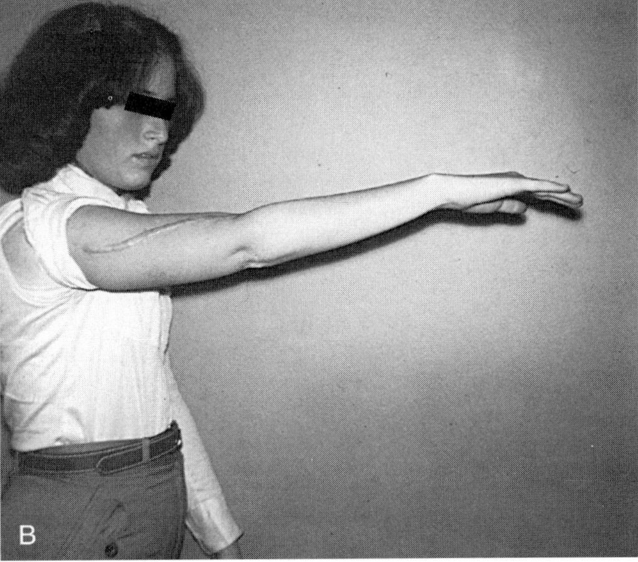

FIGURE 53–30. High radial nerve palsy. *A,* Preoperative photograph shows wrist drop. This patient previously underwent an unsuccessful posterior interosseous nerve decompression at the elbow. *B,* The patient, after decompression of the radial nerve in the proximal arm, regained full wrist extension. A fibrous band from the lateral head of the triceps was compressing the nerve.

distribution can be limited to a 4-inch region at the volar radial aspect of the forearm just distal to the junction of its middle and distal third. The sensory pattern may vary due to anatomical variations, especially given the overlap pattern of the cutaneous nerves of the forearm. Symptoms may be exaggerated with pronation. Pain may be acute and follow a discrete event, usually with forceful elbow extension. The pain may also be more vague and follow repetitive elbow overuse. Tenderness can usually be pinpointed to the compression site in the antecubital fossa. In addition, in the authors' experience, compression of other peripheral nerves may co-exist along with this entrapment, leading to an atypical presentation. Compression may involve the anterior interosseous and the musculocutaneous or the median nerve at the elbow due to thickened brachial and antebrachial fascia as seen following trauma. In these cases, especially, electrical studies can confirm the clinical diagnoses.

Nonoperative measures including rest, splintage, a sling, analgesics, corticosteroid injections, or transcutaneous electrical nerve stimulation (TENS) units have been recommended and frequently suffice. Surgical decompression of the terminal nerve branch of the musculocutaneous nerve with partial excision of the offending bicipital tendon and thickened fascia is indicated in refractory cases and has had excellent results. When there are multiple entrapments in this area, all of the localizing sites must be released at the time of surgery.

Axillary Nerve

Isolated axillary nerve palsy may follow shoulder fractures or dislocations or from blunt trauma without associated shoulder fracture or dislocation. It may also occur following shoulder reconstructive surgery (Richards et al, 1987). Patients with this condition typically present with inability to abduct the shoulder or weakness related to deltoid paresis or paralysis (Fig. 53–31A) and sensory disturbance in the outer aspect of the shoulder. Patients must be followed clinically and electrically. Often, spontaneous resolution occurs. The earliest sign of recovery occurs in the posterior deltoid, then the middle deltoid, and lastly the anterior deltoid. The deltoid

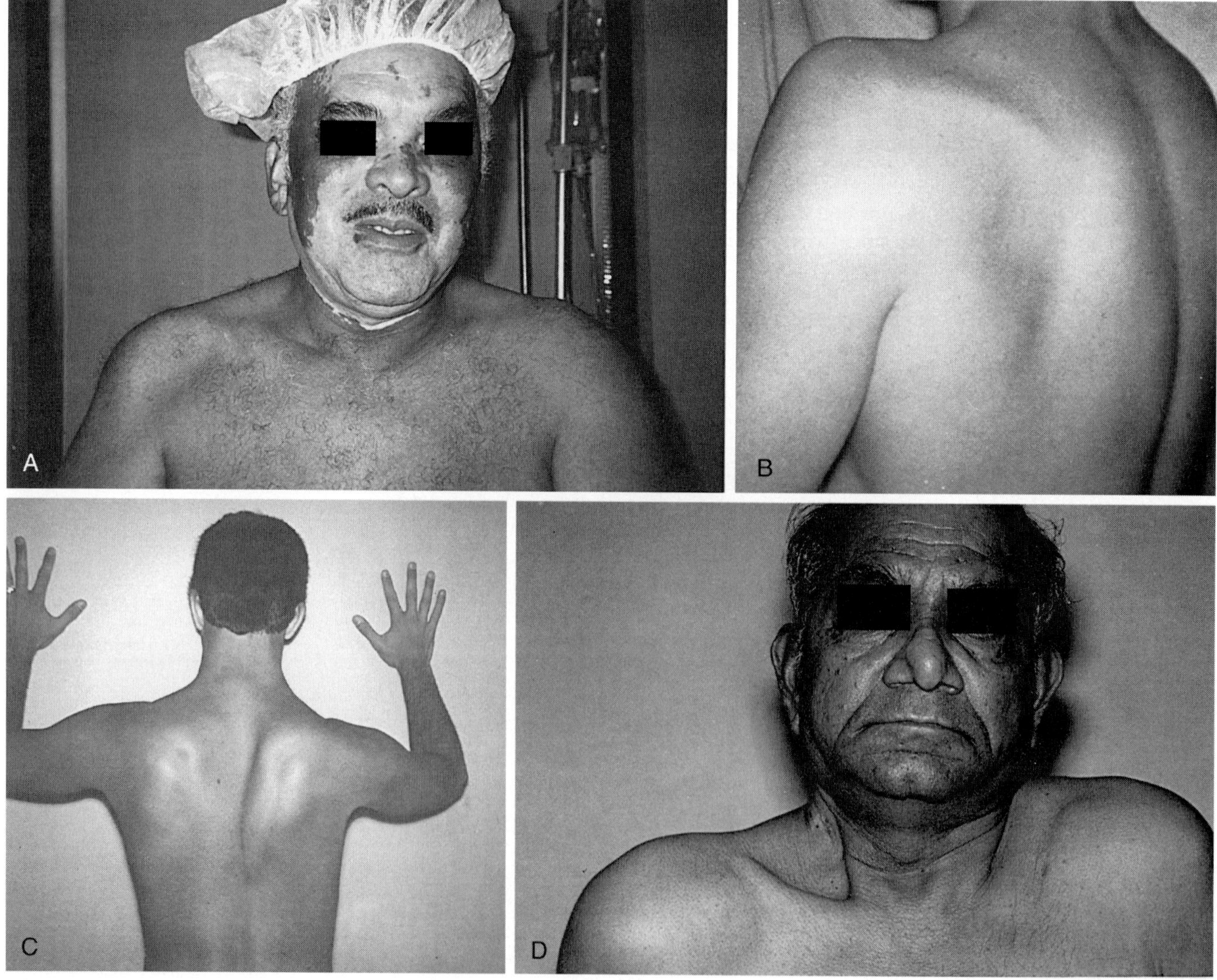

FIGURE 53–31. Nerve injuries about the shoulder. *A,* Right axillary nerve compression in a patient with vitiligo resulting in deltoid atrophy. *B,* Left suprascapular nerve compression in an athlete with marked spinati atrophy. *C,* Right long thoracic nerve compression with serratus anterior paralysis resulting in scapular winging. *D,* Inability to shrug right shoulder in a patient with trapezius atrophy following cervical lymph node biopsy and iatrogenic injury to the spinal accessory nerve.

is best tested with the patient flexed at the waist 90 degrees and holding the examination table in his or her good arm with the elbow extended. Improving extension of the shoulder against resistance is a good harbinger of recovery. The appearance of nascent potentials on EMG studies supports the recovery. Physical therapy is important in maintaining range of motion and strengthening the shoulder. If no clinical or electrical improvement is noted by 3 months, then operative intervention is indicated. A combined anteroposterior approach is often necessary because the injury is frequently diffuse. Nerve repair is often impossible owing to difficulty mobilizing the ends of the axillary nerve, and often, nerve grafting without tension is the procedure of choice (Nunley and Gabel, 1991).

In contrast, in the quadrilateral space syndrome, the axillary nerve or the posterior humeral circumflex artery, or both, may be compressed (Cahill, 1980; Cahill and Palmer, 1983; Francel et al, 1991; Linker et al, 1993; McKowen and Voorhies, 1987). Patients typically are between 20 and 40 years of age. Symptoms include diffuse type shoulder pain (which is aggravated with abduction, external rotation, or overhead activities) as well as shoulder paresthesias. Athletes who engage in sports involving throwing may have a proclivity toward developing this syndrome (Cahill and Palmer, 1983; Cormier et al, 1988; Redler et al, 1986). Patients typically have tenderness posteriorly in the quadrilateral space. Deltoid weakness is only present in 1% of cases, and neurological examination is typically normal. Electrodiagnostic studies are rarely helpful. If this diagnosis is being considered, subclavian arteriography is recommended. Quadrilateral space syndrome must be differentiated from other mechanical shoulder diagnoses and other neurologic conditions affecting the neck and shoulder. Its diagnosis remains somewhat controversial. Conservative therapy is successful in improving symptoms in over 75% of cases. Surgery may be indicated in refractory cases. A posterior approach is recommended by Cahill (1980, 1983). Surgery may reveal compression due to hypertrophy of the teres minor or fibrous bands, although often little pathology is visualized at the time of surgery. Good to excellent results have been reported in 80% of patients.

Suprascapular Nerve

The suprascapular nerve may be compressed at one of two sites at the scapula. More commonly, the suprascapular nerve is compressed at the suprascapular notch, producing combined supraspinatus and infraspinatus weakness (Vastamaki and Goransson, 1993), than at the spinoglenoid notch, which produces isolated infraspinatus weakness (Aiello et al, 1982; Kaspi et al, 1988). Altered relationships in the bony and ligamentous anatomy of the scapula from congenital causes or related to trauma frequently are responsible for symptoms. A relationship to athletic activities with exertion, such as that seen with volleyball players, wrestlers, and windsurfers, has been noted, leading to compression or traction injuries. Masses, including ganglia, may lead to extrinsic compression. Entrapment may be bilateral. Several detailed anatomic descriptions of the suprascapular nerve exist that should be especially useful to surgeons for avoidance of

iatrogenic injury during open or arthroscopic shoulder procedures (Bigliani et al, 1990; Rengachary et al, 1979).

Patients typically present with shoulder pain and weakness. Physical examination is notable for weak external rotation, especially against resistance and tenderness over the site of compression. In full-blown cases of suprascapular compression, with the elbow at the side, the patient is unable to resist an internal rotational force when the arm is positioned in external rotation. If atrophy of one or both of the spinati is present (Fig. 53–31*B*), the diagnosis of suprascapular nerve entrapment is easier to make. However, other shoulder diagnoses must always be considered and in fact, may at times overlap. Often, however, patients present late, having failed other shoulder procedures. Electrical studies are often helpful in establishing, confirming, or localizing a lesion, and MRI may establish an etiology (Fritz et al, 1992). In a lesion at the suprascapular notch, there would be a conduction delay of the suprascapular nerve across the suprascapular ligament, along with fibrillations of both of spinati; in a lesion at the spinoglenoid notch, there is a conduction delay to the infraspinatus (but not to the supraspinatus), along with fibrillations only in the infraspinatus. Plain films and studies such as CT scans or arthrograms may be part of the evaluation to rule out other differential diagnoses. A suprascapular notch view is a preoperative study to evaluate the potential need of enlargement of the suprascapular notch.

If atrophy is not present, treatment can initially be conservative for 3 to 4 months concentrating on pain management and physical therapy. We prefer a posterior trapezial elevating approach for the proximal lesion (Post and Grinblat, 1993) rather than a muscle-splitting approach. The transverse scapular ligament is carefully released without bony enlargement of the notch (Rask, 1977). The distal lesion is approached by elevating a portion of the posterior deltoid and adjacent trapezius from the spine of the scapula to expose the infraspinatus fossa. Surgical results have been good, especially for pain relief. In the authors' experience, when the diagnosis is made within the first 3 to 4 months of onset, the recovery of function in both the spinati has been excellent. The literature, however, has reported better return of muscle function for the supraspinatus than the infraspinatus. Patients who present more than 1 year with a complete lesion with significant atrophy may have poorer results.

Long Thoracic Nerve

Injury to the long thoracic nerve may occur, producing shoulder pain with serratus anterior muscle weakness or paralysis (Narakas, 1991; Overbeck and Gromley, 1940). Physical examination demonstrates true winging of the scapula (Fig. 53–31*C* and *D*), which can be exaggerated by flexion of the arm or being pushed against a wall. Mechanisms for injury are thought to be from compression, stretch, traction, or friction, or a combination of these factors. Common etiologies include exertion (from repetitive activities or strenuous work), acute trauma, direct pressure, and positioning (Gregg et al, 1979; Vastamaki and Kauppila, 1993). The long thoracic nerve is commonly affected in Parsonage-Turner syndrome. Still many cases remain in the idiopathic category. The relationship of the long thoracic nerve to the first rib also explains its potential for iatrogenic injury following procedures such as transaxillary first rib resections (Wood and Frykman, 1980) or mastectomy.

Patients should be treated conservatively with nonsteroidal anti-inflammatory agents and avoidance of any provocative activities. After the pain has ceased, gradual physical therapy for range of motion and strengthening exercises to maintain other shoulder muscles is appropriate. The majority of patients recover, but recovery can take 1 to 2 years and may not be complete. Prognostic evaluation with serial electrical studies relative to the appearance of nascent (recovery) potentials in the proximal two thirds of the serratus anterior can be helpful to the treating physician and can be a good prognostic sign. For those with no clinical or electrical recovery, tendon transfers may be indicated (Goldner, 1983).

Dorsal Scapular Nerve Compression

Isolated dorsal scapular lesions are extremely rare (Kopell and Thompson, 1976). Spontaneous (compressive) lesions are even rarer but usually relate to extrinsic pressure from masses (Narakas, 1991). The dorsal scapular nerve is vulnerable to iatrogenic injury during procedures such as thoracic outlet surgery or from trauma such as in stab wounds. It may also be injured following radiation therapy.

The dorsal scapular nerve innervates the levator scapulae and rhomboids. Patients with this lesion may present with shoulder pain localized to the medial scapula. They have rhomboid weakness and winging of the scapula. The winging is less prominent than that from serratus anterior palsy and may be best seen with slowly lowering the arms from the forward flexed elevated position. Symptoms of shoulder weakness may be masked by function of other synergistic shoulder muscles. Neurolysis of the dorsal scapular nerve is indicated in the presence of these symptoms and signs if there is no clinical recovery or electrical evidence of nascent (recovery) potentials in the levator and rhomboids. Erect plain films may reveal lateral displacement of the scapula. Isolated dorsal scapular lesions may be the presenting findings in cases of Parsonage-Turner syndrome, brachial plexus lesions (Malessy et al, 1993) and C5 lesions.

Thoracic Outlet Syndrome

Thoracic outlet syndrome is discussed in detail by Dr. Leffert in Chapter 52.

Bowler's Thumb

Bowler's thumb results from digital nerve compression (Fig. 53–32*A* to *C*). It is characterized by pain in the thumb; numbness, especially on the ulnar aspect; a palpable mass at the base of the thumb; and a positive percussion test over the mass. It may be seen in bowlers (Dobyns et al, 1972), baseball batters or catchers, or cherry pitters (Viegas and Torres, 1989). In addition, digital nerve compression may be due to a thrombosed aneurysm of the ulnar digital artery (Pons, 1983), hyperplastic pacinian corpuscles (Zweig and Burns, 1968), or fibrous bands (Berlemann and Dunkerton,

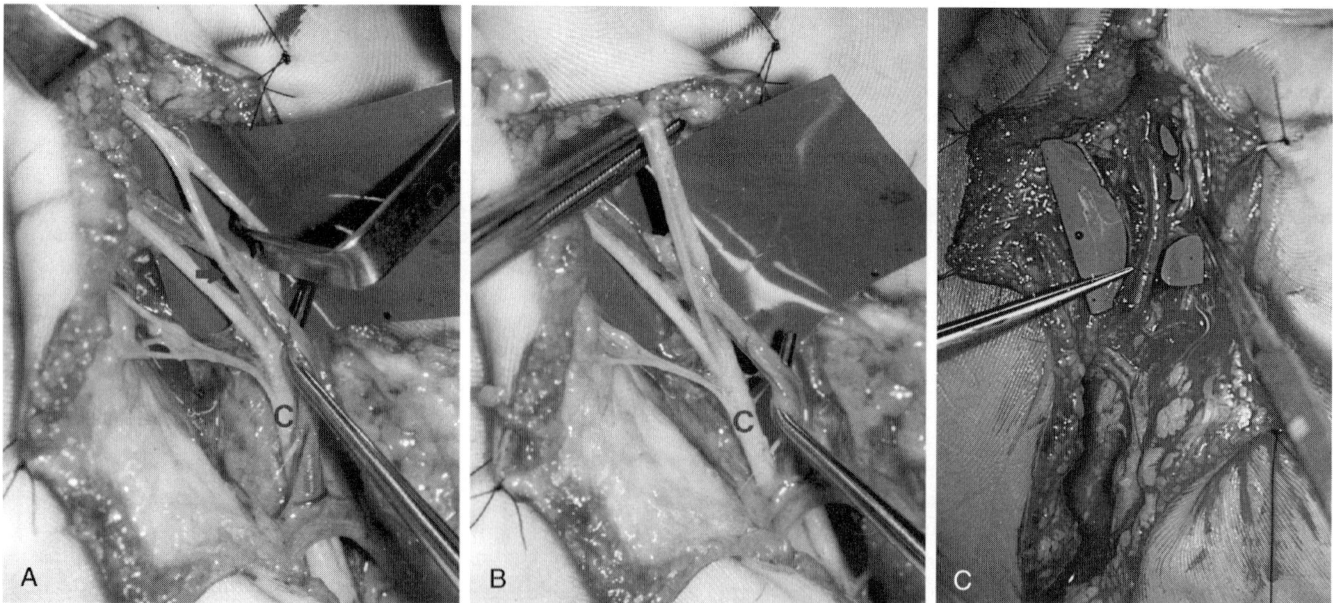

FIGURE 53–32. Neural penetration by an artery at the digital level. See other reports of similar neural penetration at other levels in the upper extremity in patients with evidence of nerve compression (Spinner, 1976; Gainor and Jeffries, 1987; Jones and Ming, 1988; Proudman and Menz, 1992). *A,* A 26-year-old man presented following a crush injury with palmar pain, intermittent numbness in the webspace between the index and long fingers, and cold intolerance in the hand. He had diminished two-point discrimination in the ulnar aspect of the index finger and radial aspect of the long fingers. The sweat test showed decreased coloration in the common digital nerve distribution to the index and long fingers. The Digital Allen test filled normally. At surgery, the common digital artery was noted to penetrate the proper digital nerve to the radial aspect of the long finger. A portion of the proper digital nerve was compressed and was slightly discolored *(arrow)*. The common digital nerve (C) and the superficial palmar arch can be seen. *B,* The tight "resting" relationship of the common digital artery (probe) and the two halves of the proper digital nerve to the long finger can be appreciated. Dynamic compression of the common digital artery probably also occurred. *C,* The common digital artery was transposed and reanastomosed microscopically. The suture line is demonstrated by the forceps. Neurolysis of the median nerve and the digital nerves was performed. (From Spinner RJ, Varela CD, Urbaniak JR: Digital nerve penetration by a digital artery in a patient with neurovascular symptoms. J Hand Surg *21A*:1101, 1996. © 1996, Churchill Livingstone, New York.)

1994), or related to poorly fitting thumb splints (Rayan and O'Donoghue, 1983). Often, it is the direct pressure on a firm edge of an object that produces this digital compression. The authors have seen a variant of the bowler's thumb in two morticians who had numbness in all the pulps of the fingers (with normal thumbs); when they stopped lifting and carrying the caskets, their digital numbness resolved spontaneously.

Multiple Entrapment Lesions

Simultaneous, co-existent, or sequential compression may affect one or more peripheral nerves at different levels. That one nerve can be trapped simultaneously at two levels (i.e., double-crush injury) has been shown both experimentally and clinically (Osterman, 1988; Upton and McComas, 1973). This is most frequently seen with cervical radiculopathy or thoracic outlet syndrome (Hurst et al, 1985; Wood and Biondi, 1990) as the proximal site of compression and carpal tunnel syndrome. At times, it may be necessary to explore a peripheral nerve at more than one level. However, in addition, one must remember that a thorough decompression is critical at each level in order to avoid resistant or recurrent compression (Gabel and Amadio, 1990; Sponseller and Engber, 1983).

Multiple compressive neuropathies may also occur and may be present in certain types of individuals susceptible to compression neuropathies, such as those with systemic diseases like diabetes or metabolic diseases like porphyria. Familial and hereditary neuropathies (Behse et al, 1972; Earl et al, 1964; Karpati et al, 1973; Lubahn and Lister, 1983) exist that are predisposed to pressure; other syndromic diseases may have an underlying biochemical problem with resultant neuropathies (Dellon et al, 1984).

One must remember also that patients can have two completely separate neurological conditions, such as syringomyelia of the cervical cord and a compressed peripheral nerve (Spinner and Spencer, 1974). EMG studies may be helpful but are not always sensitive enough to localize accurately all sites of compression.

CONCLUSION

1. Any nerve can be compressed. However, owing to anatomical constraints, individual nerves may be vulnerable at certain sites. A standard pattern of common neural entrapments has led to certain well-defined syndromes. The clinical presentation can be classic when there is normal anatomy and the lesion is complete. Likewise, there can be variations in presentation based on variant anatomy or a partial lesion. Knowledge of normal and variant anatomy, along with correlation of the intraneural topography, is critical in understanding these lesions fully.

2. If the diagnosis or localization of a lesion is unclear, repeated clinical examinations and electromyography at 4- to 6-week intervals are indicated until the diagnosis is clear.

3. Early accurate diagnosis and treatment are essential for the most favorable results in compression lesions.

4. Age is not a prognostic factor for recovery with entrapment lesions, and it is unjustified to deny surgical relief to the older age group. Factors affecting nerve recovery in compression lesions include nerve fiber pathology, the level of the injury, duration of the injury, and the status of the end-organs.

5. The neural pathology of compression lesions is most often a mixed lesion. Pure first-, second-, third-, or fourth-degree neural lesions are unusual; one lesion type frequently predominates. Clinical studies usually define the variable nature of the neural pathology.

6. Surgery is indicated if there is no progressive improvement in function within 3 to 4 months. Prompt surgical intervention is indicated for acute presentation following trauma or infection, impending Volkmann's ischemia, or in cases of unrelenting pain and neurological symptoms despite nonoperative care.

7. Complete nerve compression lesions that have been present for 18 months or longer have an extremely poor prognosis. Appropriate tendon transfers should be performed either by themselves or in conjunction with local neural exploration. Partial neural compression lesions may obtain functional recovery well beyond the 18-month period, and tendon transfers often can be avoided.

References

Agnew DH: Bursal tumour producing loss of power of forearm. Proceedings of the Pathological Society of Philadelphia, 1860–1867, 2:139, 1867.

Aiello I, Serra G, Traina GC, Tugnoli V: Entrapment of the suprascapular nerve at the spinoglenoid notch. Ann Neurol 12:314, 1982.

Al-Qattan MM: Anatomical classification of sites of compression of the palmar cutaneous branch of the median nerve. J Hand Surg 22B:48, 1997.

Al-Qattan MM, Husband JB: Median nerve compression by the supracondylar process: A case report. J Hand Surg 16B:101, 1991.

Al-Qattan MM, Murray KA: The arcade of Struthers: An anatomical study. J Hand Surg 16B:311, 1991.

Al-Qattan MM, Robertson GA: Entrapment neuropathy of the palmar cutaneous nerve within its tunnel. J Hand Surg 18B:465, 1993.

Apfelberg DB, Larson SJ: Dynamic anatomy of the ulnar nerve at the elbow. Plast Reconstr Surg 51:76, 1973.

Amadio PC: Pyridoxine as an adjunct in the treatment of carpal tunnel syndrome. J Hand Surg 10A:237, 1985.

Amadio PC: The Mayo Clinic and carpal tunnel syndrome. Mayo Clin Proc 67:42, 1992.

Amadio PC, Beckenbaugh RD: Entrapment of the ulnar nerve by the deep flexor-pronator aponeurosis. J Hand Surg 11A:83, 1986.

Bassett FH, Nunley JA: Compression of musculocutaneous nerve at elbow. J Bone Joint Surg 64:1050, 1982.

Bednar MS, Blair SJ, Light TR: Complications of the treatment of cubital tunnel syndrome. Hand Clin 10:83, 1994.

Behse F, Buchthal F, Carlsen F, Knappeis GG: Hereditary neuropathy with liability to pressure palsies: Electrophysiological and histopathological aspects. Brain 95:777, 1972.

Bennett JB, Crouch CC: Compression syndrome of the recurrent branch of the median nerve. J Hand Surg 7A:407, 1982.

Berlemann U, Dunkerton MC: Compression of the radial digital nerve of the thumb. J Hand Surg 19B:288, 1994.

Bigliani LU, Dalsey RM, McCann PD, April EW: An anatomical study of the suprascapular nerve. Arthroscopy 6:301, 1990.

Braddom RL, Wolfe C: Musculocutaneous nerve injury after heavy exercise. Arch Phys Med Rehabil 59:290, 1978.

Braun RM, Davidson K, Doehr S: Provocative testing in the diagnosis of dynamic carpal tunnel syndrome. J Hand Surg 14A:195, 1989.

Brown BA: Internal neurolysis in traumatic peripheral nerve lesions in continuity. Surg Clin North Am 52:1167, 1972.

Buchtal F, Rosenfalck A, Trojaborg W: Electrophysiological findings in entrapment of the median nerve at wrist and elbow. J Neurol Neurosurg Psychiatry 37:340, 1974.

Buckmiller JF, Richard TA: Isolated compression neuropathy of the palmar cutaneous branch of the median nerve. J Hand Surg 12A:97, 1987.

Cahill BR: Quadrilateral syndrome. *In* Omer GE Jr, Spinner M: Management of Peripheral Nerve Problems. Philadelphia, W. B. Saunders Company, 1980, p 602.

Cahill BR, Palmer RE: Quadrilateral space syndrome. J Hand Surg 8:65, 1983.

Campbell WW, Sahni SK, Pridgeon RM, Riaz G, Leshner RT: Intraoperative electroneurography: Management of ulnar neuropathy at the elbow. Muscle Nerve *11*:75, 1988.

Capener N: The vulnerability of the posterior interosseous nerve of the forearm. J Bone Joint Surg *48B*:770, 1966.

Carroll RE, Green DP: The significance of the palmar cutaneous nerve at the wrist. Clin Orthop *83*:24, 1972.

Casey PJ, Moed BR: Fractures of the forearm complicated by palsy of the anterior interosseous nerve caused by a constrictive dressing. J Bone Joint Surg *79A*:122, 1997.

Caspi I, Ezra E, Nerubay J, Horoszovski H: Musculocutaneous nerve injury after coracoid process transfer for clavicle instability. Acta Orthop Scan *58*:294, 1987.

Chow JCY: Ulnar nerve transection as a complication of two-portal endoscopic carpal tunnel release. J Hand Surg *19A*:522, 1994.

Chow JA, Sunderland S, Van Beek AL: Surgical significance of the motor fascicular group of the ulnar nerve in the forearm. J Hand Surg *9A*:605, 1985.

Comtet JJ, Chambaud D: Paralysie "spontanee" du nerf inter-osseux posterieur par lesion inhabituelle. Rev Chir Orthop *61*:533, 1975.

Cormier PJ, Matalon TAS, Wolin PM: Quadrilateral space syndrome: a rare cause of shoulder pain. Radiology *167*:797, 1988.

Cravens G, Kline DG: Posterior interosseous nerve palsies. Neurosurgery *27*:397, 1990.

Crotti FM, Mangiagalli EP, Rampini P: Supracondyloid process and anomalous insertion of pronator teres as sources of median nerve neuralgia. J Neurosurg Sci *25*:41, 1981.

Davidson JJ, Bassett FH III, Nunley JA: Musculocutaneous nerve entrapment revisited. American Orthopaedic Association Annual Meeting, White Sulphur Springs, West Virginia, June, 1995.

Dellon AL: Review of treatment results for ulnar nerve entrapment at the elbow. J Hand Surg *14A*:688, 1989.

Dellon AL, Mackinnon SE: Injury to the medial antebrachial cutaneous nerve during cubital tunnel surgery. J Hand Surg *10B*:33, 1985.

Dellon AL, Mackinnon SE: Radial-sensory nerve entrapment in the forearm. J Hand Surg *11A*:199, 1986.

Dellon AL, Mackinnon SE: Anatomic investigations of nerves at the wrist: II. Instance of fibrous arch overlying the motor branch of the ulnar nerve. Ann Plast Surg *21*:36, 1988.

Dellon AL, Trojak JE, Rochman GM: Median nerve compression in Weill-Marchesani syndrome. Plast Reconstr Surg *74*:127, 1984.

Denny-Brown D, Brenner C: Paralysis of nerve induced by direct pressure and by tourniquet. Arch Neurol Psychol *51*:1, 1944.

Derkash RS, Niebauer JJ: Entrapment of the posterior interosseous nerve by a fibrous band in the dorsal edge of the supinator muscle and erosion of a groove in the proximal radius. J Hand Surg *6*:524, 1981.

Dobyns JH, O'Brien ET, Linscheid RL, Farrow GM: Bowler's thumb. Diagnosis and treatment. A review of seventeen cases. J Bone Joint Surg *54A*:751, 1972.

Doyle JR, Semenza J, Gilling B: The effect of succinylcholine on denervated skeletal muscle. J Hand Surg *6*:40, 1981.

Dreyfuss U, Kessler I: Snapping elbow due to dislocation of the medial head of the triceps. A report of two cases. J Bone Joint Surg *60B*:56, 1978.

Dundore DE, DeLisa JA: Musculocutaneous nerve palsy: An isolated complication of surgery. Arch Phys Med Rehabil *60*:130, 1979.

Earl CJ, Fullerton PM, Wakefield GS, Schutta HS: Hereditary neuropathy with liability to pressure palsies. A clinical and electrophysiological study of four families. Quart J Med *33*:481, 1964.

Eaton RG, Crowe JF, Parkes JC III: Anterior transposition of the ulnar nerve with a non-compressing fasciodermal sling. J Bone Joint Surg *62A*:820, 1980.

England JD, Sumner AJ: Neuralgic amyotrophy: An increasingly diverse entity. Muscle Nerve *10*:60, 1987.

Fearn CB, Goodfellow JW: Anterior interosseous nerve palsy. J Bone Joint Surg *47B*:91, 1965.

Fenning JB: Deep ulnar-nerve paralysis from an anatomical abnormality. J Bone Joint Surg *47A*:1381, 1965.

Flatow EL, Bigliani LU, April EW: An anatomic study of the musculocutaneous nerve and its relationship to the coracoid process. Clin Orthop *244*:166, 1989.

Fragiadakis EG, Lamb DW: An unusual cause of ulnar nerve compression. Hand *2*:14, 1970.

Francel TJ, Dellon AL, Campbell JN: Quadrilateral space syndrome: Diagnosis and operative decompression technique. Plast Reconstr Surg *87*:911, 1991.

Fritz RC, Helms CA, Steinbach LS, Genant HK: Suprascapular nerve entrapment: Evaluation with MR imaging. Radiology *182*:437, 1992.

Fuss FK, Wurzl GH: Radial nerve entrapment at the elbow: surgical anatomy. J Hand Surg *16A*:742, 1991.

Gabel GT, Amadio PC: Operation for failed decompression of ulnar nerve in the region of the elbow. J Bone Joint Surg *72A*:213, 1990.

Gainor BJ, Jeffries JT: Pronator syndrome associated with a persistent median artery. A case report. J Bone Joint Surg *69A*:303, 1987.

Gelberman RH (ed): Operative Nerve Repair and Reconstruction. Philadelphia, J. B. Lippincott, 1991.

Gelberman RH, Eaton RG, Urbaniak JR: Peripheral nerve compression. *In* Schafer M (ed): Instructional Course Lectures, Vol 33. Rosemont, IL, American Academy of Orthopaedic Surgeons, 1994, p 31.

Gilliatt BW, Ochoa J, Rudge P, Neary D: The cause of nerve damage in acute compression. Trans Am Neurol Assoc *99*:71, 1974.

Goldner JL: Muscle-tendon transfers for partial paralysis of the shoulder girdle. *In* Evarts CM (ed): Surgery of the Musculoskeletal System, Vol 3. Philadelphia, Churchill Livingstone, 1983, p 145.

Gould JS: Treatment of the painful injured nerve incontinuity. *In* Gelberman RH: Operative Nerve Repair and Reconstruction. Philadelphia, J. B. Lippincott, 1991, p 1541.

Gregg JR, Labosky D, Harty M, et al: Serratus anterior paralysis in the young athlete. J Bone Joint Surg *61A*:825, 1979.

Gross MS, Gelberman RH: The anatomy of the distal ulnar tunnel. Clin Orthop *196*:238, 1985.

Grundberg AB, Regan DS: Compression syndromes in reflex sympathetic dystrophy. J Hand Surg *16A*:731, 1991.

Gunther SF, DiPasquale D, Martin R: The internal anatomy of the median nerve in the region of the elbow. J Hand Surg *17A*:648, 1992.

Hall HC, Mackinnon SE, Gilbert RW: An approach to the posterior interosseous nerve. Plast Reconstr Surg *74*:435, 1984.

Hartz CR, Linscheid RL, Gramser RR, Daube JR: The pronator teres syndrome. Compressive neuropathy of the median nerve. J Bone Joint Surg *63A*:885, 1981.

Haskin JS: Ganglion-related compression neuropathy of the palmar cutaneous branch of the median nerve: a report of two cases. J Hand Surg *19A*:827, 1994.

Hayashi Y, Kojima T, Kohno T: Case of cubital tunnel syndrome caused by the snapping of the medial head of the triceps brachii muscle. J Hand Surg *9A*:96, 1984.

Hayes JR, Mulholland RC, O'Connor BT: Compression of the deep palmar branch of the ulnar nerve. J Bone Joint Surg *51B*:469, 1969.

Hems TEJ, Burge PD, Wilson DJ: The role of magnetic resonance imaging in the management of peripheral nerve tumours. J Hand Surg *22B*:57, 1997.

Henry AK: Extensile Exposure, 2nd ed. Baltimore, Williams & Wilkins, 1970.

Hill NA, Howard FM, Huffer BR: The incomplete anterior interosseous nerve syndrome. J Hand Surg *10A*:4, 1985.

Hirooka T, Hashizume H, Nagoshi M, Shigeyama Y, Inoue H: Guyon's canal syndrome. A different clinical presentation caused by an atypical fibrous band. J Hand Surg *22B*:52, 1997.

Holtzman R, Mark M, Patel M, Weiner L: Ulnar nerve entrapment in the forearm. J Hand Surg *9A*:576, 1984.

Hurst LC, Weissberg D, Carroll RE: The relationship of the double crush to carpal tunnel syndrome (an analysis of 1,000 cases of carpal tunnel syndrome). J Hand Surg *10B*:202, 1985.

Inserra A, Spinner M: An anatomic factor significant in transposition of the ulnar nerve. J Hand Surg *11A*:80, 1986.

Jabaley ME, Wallace WH, Heckler FR: Internal topography of major nerves of the forearm and hand: A current view. J Hand Surg *5*:1, 1980.

Jerosch J, Castro WH, Colemont J: A lesion of the musculocutaneous nerve. A rare complication of anterior shoulder dislocation. Acta Orthop Belg *55*:230, 1989.

Johnson RK, Shrewsbury MM: Anatomical course of the thenar branch of the median nerve—usually in a separate tunnel through the transverse carpal ligament. J Bone Joint Surg *52A*:269, 1970.

Johnson RK, Spinner M, Shrewsbury MM: Median nerve entrapment syndrome in the proximal forearm. J Hand Surg *4*:48, 1979.

Jones NF, Ming NL: Persistent median artery as a cause of pronator syndrome. J Hand Surg *13A*:728, 1988.

Kameda Y: An anomalous muscle (accessory scapularis-teres-latissimus muscle) in the axilla penetrating the brachial plexus in man. Acta Anat 96:513, 1976.

Kane E, Kaplan EB, Spinner M: Observations on the course of the ulnar nerve in the arm. Ann Chir 27:470, 1973.

Karpati G, Carpenters S, Eisen AA, Feindel W: Familial multiple peripheral nerve entrapments—an unusual manifestation of a peripheral neuropathy. Trans Am Neurol Assoc 98:267, 1973.

Kaspi A, Yanai J, Pick CG, Maun G: Entrapment of the distal suprascapular nerve—an anatomic study. Int Orthop 12:273, 1988.

Katirji MB: Pseudo-anterior interosseous nerve syndrome (letter). Muscle Nerve 9:266, 1985.

Katon H, Ogino T, Nanbu T, Nakamura K: Compression neuropathy of the motor branch of the median nerve caused by palmar ganglion. J Hand Surg 16A:751, 1991.

Katznelson A, Nerubay J, Oliver S: Dynamic fixation of avulsed clavicle. J Trauma 16:841, 1976.

Kiloh LG, Nevin S: Isolated neuritis of the anterior interosseous nerve. BMJ 1:850, 1952.

Kleinman WB, Bishop AT: Anterior intramuscular transposition of the ulnar nerve. J Hand Surg 14A:972, 1989.

Kline DG, Hackett ER, May PR: Evaluation of nerve by evoked potentials and electromyography. J Neurosurg 31:128, 1969.

Kline DG, Nulsen FE: The neuroma in continuity. Its preoperative and operative management. Surg Clin North Am 52:1189, 1972.

Kline DG, Hudson AR: Nerve Injuries. Operative Results for Major Nerve Injuries, Entrapments and Tumors. Philadelphia, W. B. Saunders Company, 1995.

Kopell HP, Thompson WAI: Pronator syndrome: A confirmed case and its diagnosis. N Engl J Med 259:712, 1958.

Kopell HP, Thompson WAI: Peripheral entrapment neuropathies, 2nd ed. New York, Robert E. Kreiger Publishing Company, 1976.

Kuczynski K: Functional microanatomy of the peripheral nerve trunks. Hand 6:1, 1974.

Kuschner SH, Gelberman RH, Jennings C: Ulnar nerve compression at the wrist. J Hand Surg 13A:577, 1988.

Laha RK, Dujovny M, DeCastro C: Entrapment of median nerve by supracondylar process of the humerus. A case report. J Neurosurg 46:252, 1977.

Lanz U: Lähmung des tiefen Hohlhandastes des nervus ulnaris, bedingt durch eine anatomische Variante. Handchirurgie 6:83, 1974.

Lanz U: Anatomical variations of the median nerve in the carpal tunnel. J Hand Surg 2:44, 1977.

Lanzetta M, Foucher G: Entrapment of the superficial branch of the radial nerve (Wartenberg's syndrome). A report of 52 cases. Internat Orthop 17:342, 1993.

Lassa R, Shrewsbury MM: Variation in the path of the deep motor branch of the ulnar nerve at the wrist. J Bone Joint Surg 57A:990, 1975.

Learmonth JR: Technique for transplanting the ulnar nerve. Surg Gynecol Obstet 75:792, 1942.

Leffert RD: Anterior submuscular transposition of the ulnar nerve by the Learmonth technique. J Hand Surg 7:147, 1982.

Leibovic SJ, Hastings H, II: Martin-Gruber revisited. J Hand Surg 17A:47, 1992.

Linker CS, Helms CA, Fritz RC: Quadrilateral space syndrome. Radiology 188:675, 1993.

Linscheid RL, Peterson LFA, Juergens JL: Carpal tunnel syndrome associated with vasospasm. J Bone Joint Surg 49A:1141, 1967.

Lister GD, Belsoe RB, Kleinert HE: The radial tunnel syndrome. J Hand Surg 4:52, 1979.

Lister GD: Radial tunnel syndrome. In Gelberman RH: Operative Nerve Repair and Reconstruction. Philadelphia, J. B. Lippincott, 1991, p 1023.

Lotem N, Fried A, Levy M, Solzi P, Najenson T, Nathan H: Radial palsy following muscular effort. A new compression syndrome possibly related to a fibrous arch of the lateral head of the triceps. J Bone Joint Surg 53B:500, 1971.

Lotem M, Gloobe H, Nathan H: Fibrotic arch around the deep branch of the ulnar nerve in the hand. Anatomical observations. Plast Reconstr Surg 52:553, 1973.

Louis DS, Hankin FM: Symptomatic relief following carpal tunnel decompression with normal electroneuromyographic studies. Orthopedics 10:434, 1987.

Lubahn JD, Lister GD: Familial radial nerve entrapment syndrome: A case report and literature review. J Hand Surg 8:297, 1983.

Lundborg G: Ischemic nerve injury. Experimental studies on intraneural microvascular pathophysiology and nerve function in a limb subjected to temporary circulatory arrest. Scand J Plast Reconstr Surg (Suppl) 6:1, 1970.

Mackinnon SE, Dellon AL: The overlap pattern of the lateral antebrachial cutaneous nerve and the superficial branch of the radial nerve. J Hand Surg 10A:522, 1985.

Mackinnon SE, Dellon AL: Surgery of the Peripheral Nerve. New York, Thieme, 1988.

Macnicol MF: The results of operation for ulnar neuritis. J Bone Joint Surg 61B:159, 1979.

Malessy MJ, Thomeer RT, Marani E: The dorsoscapular nerve in traumatic brachial plexus lesions. Clin Neurol Neurosurg 95:S17, 1993.

Mannerfelt L: Studies in ulnar paralysis. Acta Orthop Scand 87(Suppl):19, 1966.

Manske PR: Compression of the radial nerve by the triceps muscle. A case report. J Bone Joint Surg 59A:835, 1977.

Marie P, Foix C: Atrophie isolee de l'eminence thenar d'origin neuritique, role du ligament annulaire anterieur du carpal dans la pathogenie de la lesion. Rev Neurol 26:647, 1913.

Massey EW, Massey JM: Forearm neuropathy and pruritus. South Med J 79:1259, 1986.

Massey EW, Pleet AB: Handcuffs and cheiralgia paresthetica. Neurology 28:1312, 1978.

May JW, Rosen H: Division of sensory ramus communicans between the ulnar and median nerves: A complication following carpal tunnel release: case report. J Bone Joint Surg 63A:836, 1981.

Mayfield FH: Compression syndromes of the shoulder girdles and arms. In Vinken PJ, Bruyn GW (eds): Handbook of Clinical Neurology. Diseases of Nerves, Vol 7. New York, Elsevier, 1970, p 441.

McCarthy RE, Nalebuff EA: Anomalous branch of the dorsal cutaneous nerve: A case report. J Hand Surg 5:19, 1980.

McDowell CL, Henceroth WD: Compression of the ulnar nerve in the hand by a ganglion. J Bone Joint Surg 59A:980, 1977.

McKowen HC, Voorhies RM: Axillary nerve entrapment in the quadrilateral space. J Neurosurg 66:932, 1987.

Miller R: Observations upon the arrangement of the axillary artery and brachial plexus. Am J Anat 64:143, 1939.

Mitchell SW: Injuries of Nerves and Their Consequences. London, Smith Elder, 1872.

Mittal RL, Gupta BR: Median and ulnar nerve palsy: An unusual presentation of the supracondylar process. J Bone Joint Surg 60A:557, 1978.

Mody BS: A simple clinical test to differentiate rupture of flexor pollicis longus and incomplete anterior interosseous paralysis. J Hand Surg 17B:513, 1992.

Moldaver J: Brief Note. Tinel's sign. Its characteristics and significance. J Bone Joint Surg 60A:412, 1978.

Naff N, Dellon AL, Mackinnon SE: The anatomical course of the palmar cutaneous branch of the median nerve, including a description of its own unique tunnel. J Hand Surg 18B:316, 1993.

Nakamichi K, Tachibana S: Radial nerve entrapment by the lateral head of the triceps. J Hand Surg 16A:748, 1991.

Nakano KK, Lundergan C, Okihiro MM: Anterior interosseous nerve syndrome. Arch Neurol 34:477, 1977.

Narakas AD: Compression and Traction Neuropathies about the shoulder and arm. In Gelberman RH: Operative Nerve Repair and Reconstruction. Philadelphia, J. B. Lippincott, 1991, p 1147.

Nunley JA, Gabel G: Axillary nerve. In Gelberman RH: Operative Nerve Repair and Reconstruction. Philadelphia, J. B. Lippincott, 1991, p 437.

Ochiai N, Hayashi T, Ninomiya S: High ulnar nerve palsy caused by the arcade of Struthers. J Hand Surg 17B:629, 1992.

Ochoa J: Schwann cell and myelin changes caused by some toxic agents and trauma. Proc Roy Soc Med 67:3, 1974.

O'Driscoll SW, Horii E, Carmichael SW, Morrey BF: The cubital tunnel and ulnar neuropathy. J Bone Joint Surg 73B:613, 1991.

Ogino T, Minami A, Katon H: Diagnosis of radial nerve palsy caused by ganglion with use of different imaging techniques. J Hand Surg 16A:230, 1991.

Olehnik WK, Manske PR, Szerzinski J: Median nerve compression in the proximal forearm. J Hand Surg 19A:121, 1994.

Omer G, Spinner M: Peripheral nerve testing and suture techniques. In Instructional Course Lectures of the American Academy of Orthopaedic Surgeons, Vol 24. St. Louis, C. V. Mosby Company 1975, p 122.

Osborne G: The surgical treatment of tardy ulnar neuritis. J Bone Joint Surg 39B:782, 1957.

Osborne G: Compression neuritis of the ulnar nerve at the elbow. Hand 2:10, 1970.

Osterman AL: The double crush syndrome. Orthop Clin North Am 19:147, 1988.

Overbeck D, Gromley R: Paralysis of the serratus magnus muscle. JAMA 114:1904, 1940.

Paget J: Lectures on Surgical Pathology. Philadelphia, Lindsay and Blakiston, 1854.

Papadopoulos N, Paraschos A, Pelekis P: Anatomical observations on the arcade of Frohse and other structures related to the deep radial nerve. Anatomical interpretation of deep radial nerve entrapment neuropathy. Folia Morphol 37:319, 1989.

Papathanassiou BT: A variant of the motor branch of the median nerve in the hand. J Bone Joint Surg 50B:156, 1968.

Parsonage MJ, Turner JWA: Neuralgic amyotrophy. The shoulder-girdle syndrome. Lancet 1:973, 1948.

Patel MR, Bassini L, Magill R: Compression neuropathy of the lateral antebrachial cutaneous nerve. Orthopedics 14:173, 1991.

Pecina M, Bojanic I: Musculocutaneous nerve entrapment in the upper arm. Int Orthop 17:232, 1993.

Phalen GS: Spontaneous compression of the median nerve at the wrist. JAMA 145:1128, 1951.

Phalen GS: The carpal tunnel syndrome. Seventeen years experience in diagnosis and treatment of six-hundred forty-four hands. J Bone Joint Surg 48A:211, 1966.

Phalen GS: Reflections on 21 years' experience with the carpal tunnel syndrome. JAMA 212:1365, 1970.

Phalen GS: The birth of a syndrome, or carpal tunnel revisited (editorial). J Hand Surg 6:109, 1981.

Pons RK: Bowler's thumb. J Hand Surg 8:630, 1983.

Post M, Grinblat E: Suprascapular nerve entrapment: Diagnosis and results of treatment. J Shoulder Elbow Surg 2:190, 1993.

Prasartrirtha T, Liuopolvanish P, Rojanakit A: A study of the posterior interosseous nerve (PIN) and the radial tunnel in 30 Thai cadavers. J Hand Surg 18A:107, 1993.

Proudman TW, Menz PJ: An anomaly of the median artery associated with the anterior interosseous nerve syndrome. J Hand Surg 17B:507, 1992.

Rask MB: Suprascapular nerve entrapment—a report of two cases treated with suprascapular notch resection. Clin Orthop 123:73, 1977.

Rayan GM, O'Donoghue DH: Ulnar digital compression neuropathy of the thumb caused by splinting. Clin Orthop 175:170, 1983.

Redfern AB, Zimmerman NB: Neurologic and ischemic complications of upper extremity vascular access for dialysis. J Hand Surg 20A:199, 1995.

Redler MR, Ruland JL III, McCue FC III: Quadrilateral space syndrome in a throwing athlete. Am J Sports Med 14:511, 1986.

Reis ND: Anomalous triceps tendon as a cause for snapping elbow and ulnar neuritis: a case report. J Hand Surg 5:361, 1980.

Rengachary SS, Neff JP, Singer PA, Brackett CF: Suprascapular entrapment neuropathy. A clinical, anatomical and comparative study, part I. Neurosurgery 4:441, 1979.

Rennels GD, Ochoa J: Neuralgic amyotrophy manifesting as anterior interosseous palsy. Muscle Nerve 3:160, 1980.

Richards RR, Hudson AR, Bertoia JT, Urbaniak JR, Waddell JP: Injury to the brachial plexus during Putti-Platt and Bristow procedures. A report of eight cases. Am J Sports Med 15:374, 1987.

Rogers MR, Bergfield TG, Aulicino PL: The failed ulnar nerve transposition. Etiology and treatment. Clin Orthop 269:193, 1991.

Rolfsen L: Snapping triceps tendon with ulnar neuritis. Acta Orthop Scand 41:74, 1970.

Roles NC, Maudsley RH: Radial tunnel syndrome. Resistant tennis elbow as a nerve entrapment. J Bone Joint Surg 54B:499, 1972.

Rosenberg ZS, Beltran J, Cheung YY, Ro SY, Green SM, Lenzo SR: The elbow: MR features of nerve disorders. Radiology 188:235, 1993.

Roth AI, Stulberg BN, Fleegler EJ, Belhobek GH: Elbow arthrography in the evaluation of posterior interosseous nerve compression in rheumatoid arthritis. J Hand Surg 11B:120, 1986.

Rydevik B, Lundborg G, Nordberg G: Intraneural tissue reactions induced by internal neurolysis. Scand J Plast Reconstr Surg 10:3, 1976.

Schantz K, Riegels-Nielsen P: The anterior interosseous nerve syndrome. J Hand Surg 17B:510, 1992.

Schaumburg H, Kaplan J, Windebank A, Vick N, Rasmus S, Pleasure D, Brown MJ: Sensory neuropathy from pyridoxine abuse: A new megavitamin syndrome. N Engl J Med 309:445, 1983.

Seddon H: Surgical Disorders of the Peripheral Nerves. Edinburgh, Churchill Livingstone, 1972.

Shea JD, McClain EJ: Ulnar nerve compression syndromes at and below the wrist. J Bone Joint Surg 51A:1095, 1969.

Shimizu K, Iwasaki R, Hoshikawa H, Yamamuro T: Entrapment neuropathy of the palmar cutaneous branch of the median nerve by the fascia of flexor digitorum superficialis. J Hand Surg 13A:581, 1988.

Slingluff CL, Terzis JK, Edgerton MT: The quantitative microanatomy of the brachial plexus in man—reconstructive relevance. In Terzis JK (ed): Microreconstruction of Nerve Injuries. Philadelphia, W. B. Saunders Company, 1987.

Smith RV, Fisher RG: Struthers ligament, a source of median nerve compression above the elbow. J Neurosurg 38:778, 1973.

Sood MK, Burke FD: Anterior interosseous nerve palsy. A review of 16 cases. J Hand Surg 22B:64, 1997.

Spinner M: The arcade of Frohse and its relationship to posterior interosseous nerve paralysis. J Bone Joint Surg 50B:809, 1968.

Spinner M: The functional attitude of the hand afflicted with an anterior interosseous nerve paralysis. Bull Hosp Joint Dis 30:21, 1969.

Spinner M: The anterior interosseous nerve syndrome, with special attention to its variations. J Bone Joint Surg 52A:84, 1970.

Spinner M: Cryptogenic infraclavicular brachial plexus neuritis (preliminary report). Bull Hosp Joint Dis 37:98, 1976.

Spinner M: Injuries to the Major Branches of Peripheral Nerves of the Forearm, 2nd ed. Philadelphia, W. B. Saunders Company, 1978.

Spinner M: Nerve decompression. In Morrey BF (ed): Master Techniques in Orthopaedic Surgery. The Elbow. New York, Raven Press, 1994, p 196.

Spinner RJ, Bachman JW, Amadio PC: The many faces of carpal tunnel syndrome. Mayo Clin Proc 64:829, 1989.

Spinner RJ, Carmichael SW, Spinner M: Partial median nerve entrapment in the distal arm because of an accessory bicipital aponeurosis. J Hand Surg 16A:236, 1991a.

Spinner RJ, Carmichael SW, Spinner M: Infraclavicular ulnar nerve entrapment due to a chondroepitrochlearis muscle. J Hand Surg 16B:315, 1991b.

Spinner RJ, Goldner RG: Snapping triceps and ulnar neuropathy: Anatomic and dynamic factors. American Orthopaedic Association Annual Meeting, White Sulphur Springs, West Virginia, June, 1995.

Spinner RJ, Lins RE, Spinner M: Compression of the medial half of the deep branch of the ulnar nerve by an anomalous origin of the flexor digiti minimi. J Bone Joint Surg 78A:427, 1996.

Spinner M, Kaplan EM: The relationship of the ulnar nerve to the medial intermuscular septum in the arm and its clinical significance. Hand 8:239, 1976.

Spinner M, Spencer PS: Nerve compression of lesions of the upper extremity. A clinical and experimental review. Clin Orthop 104:46, 1974.

Sponseller PD, Engber WD: Double-entrapment radial tunnel syndrome. J Hand Surg 8:420, 1983.

Spooner GR, Desai HB, Angel JF, Reeder BA, Donat JR: Using pyridoxine to treat carpal tunnel syndrome. Randomized control trial. Can Fam Physician Med Fam Con 39:2122, 1993.

Stellbrink G: Compression of the palmar branch of the median nerve by atypical palmaris longus muscle. Handchirurgie 4:155, 1972.

Stevens JC, Sun S, Beard CM, O'Fallon WM, Kurland LT: Carpal tunnel syndrome in Rochester, Minnesota, 1961–1980. Neurology 38:134, 1988.

Struthers J: On the processus supra-condyloideus humeri of man. Trans Int Med Congr London 1:148, 1881.

Subin GD, Mallon WJ, Urbaniak JR: Diagnosis of ganglion in Guyon's canal by magnetic resonance imaging. J Hand Surg 14A:640, 1989.

Sunderland S: Nerves and Nerve Injuries. Edinburgh, Churchill Livingstone, 1978.

Suranyi L: Median nerve compression by Struthers ligament. J Neurol Neurosurg Psychiatry 46:1047, 1983.

Swiggett R, Ruby LK: Median nerve compression neuropathy by the lacertus fibrosus: Report of three cases. J Hand Surg 11A:700, 1986.

Taleisnik J: The palmar cutaneous branch of the median nerve and the approach to the carpal tunnel: An anatomic study. J Bone Joint Surg 55:1212, 1973.

Talha H, Enon B, Chevalier JM, L'Hoste P, Pillet J: Brachial artery entrapment: Compression by the supracondylar process. Ann Vasc Surg 1:479, 1986.

Terry RJ: A study of the supracondyloid process in the living. Am J Phys Anthropol 4:129, 1929.

Terzis JK, Feeker BL, Sismour EN: A computerized study of the intraneural organization of the median nerve. J Hand Surg 9:605, 1984.

Thomas PK: Changes in the endoneural sheaths of peripheral myelinated nerve fibers during wallerian degeneration. J Anat 98:175, 1964.

Thomas PK: The cellular response to nerve injury. 1: The cellular outgrowth from the distal stump of transected nerve. J Anat *100*:287, 1966.

Thompson JE: Anatomical methods of approach in operations on the long bones of the extremities. Ann Surg *68*:309, 1918.

Tountas CP, Begman RA: Anatomic Variations of the Upper Extremity. New York, Churchill Livingstone, 1993.

Turkof E, Puig S, Choi S-S, Zoch G, Dellon AL: The radial sensory nerve entrapped between the two slips of a split brachioradialis tendon: A rare aspect of Wartenberg's syndrome. J Hand Surg *20A*:676, 1995.

Uchida Y, Sugioka YL: Electrodiagnosis of Martin-Gruber connection and its clinical importance in peripheral nerve surgery. J Hand Surg *17A*:54, 1992.

Upton ARM, McComas AJ: The double crush in nerve entrapment syndromes. Lancet *2*:359, 1973.

Urbaniak JR: Complications of median nerve decompression. *In* Gelberman RH: Operative Nerve Repair and Reconstruction. Philadelphia, J. B. Lippincott, 1991, p 794.

Uriburu IJF, Morchio FJ, Marin JL: Compression syndrome of the deep motor branch of the ulnar nerve (pisohamate hiatus syndrome). J Bone Joint Surg *58A*:145, 1976.

Vanderpool DW, Chalmers J, Lamb DW, Whiston TR: Peripheral compression lesions of the ulnar nerve. J Bone Joint Surg *50B*:792, 1968.

Vastamaki M, Goransson H: Suprascapular nerve entrapment. Clin Orthop *297*:135, 1993.

Vastamaki M, Kauppila LI: Etiologic factors in isolated paralysis of the serratus anterior muscle: A report of 197 cases. J Shoulder Elbow Surg *2*:240, 1993.

Viegas SF, Torres FG: Cherry pitter's thumb: Case report and review of the literature. Orthop Rev *18*:336, 1989.

Wartenberg R: Cheiralgia paresthetica. Z Neurol Psychiatry *141*:145, 1932.

Watchmaker GP, Gumucio CA, Crandall RE, Vannier MA, Weeks PM: Fascicular topography of the median nerve: A computer based study to identify branching patterns. J Hand Surg *16A*:53, 1991.

Weinzweig N, Browne EZ Jr: Infraclavicular median nerve compression caused by a lipoma. Orthopedics *11*:1077, 1988.

Weinberger LM: Nontraumatic paralysis of the dorsal interosseous nerve. Surg Gynecol Obstet *69*:358, 1939.

Wertsch JJ, Sanger JR, Matloub HS: Pseudo-anterior interosseous nerve syndrome. Muscle Nerve *8*:68, 1985.

West GA, Haynor DR, Goodkin R, Tsuruda JS, Bronstein AD, Kraft G, Winter T, Kliot M: Magnetic resonance imaging signal changes in denervated muscles after peripheral nerve injury. Neurosurgery *35*:1077, 1994.

Williams NB, Terzis JK: Single fascicular recordings. An intraoperative diagnostic tool for the management of peripheral nerve lesions. Plast Reconstr Surg *57*:562, 1976.

Williams HB, Jabaley ME: The importance of internal anatomy of the peripheral nerves to nerve repair in the forearm and hand. Hand Clin *2*:689, 1986.

Wolf EM: Anterior portals in shoulder arthroscopy. Arthroscopy *5*:201, 1989.

Wood VE, Biondi J: Double crush nerve compression in thoracic-outlet syndrome. J Bone Joint Surg *72A*:85, 1990.

Wood VE, Frykman GK: Winging of the scapula as a complication of first rib resection: A report of six cases. Clin Orthop *149*:160, 1980.

Yamanaka K, Horiuchi Y, Yabe Y: Compression neuropathy of the motor branch of the median nerve due to an anomalous thenar muscle. J Hand Surg *19B*:711, 1994.

Young C, Hudson A, Richards R: Operative treatment of palsy of the posterior interosseous nerve of the forearm. J Bone Joint Surg *72*:1215, 1990.

Zweig J, Burns H: Compression of digital nerves by pacinian corpuscles. J Bone Joint Surg *50A*:999, 1968.

Chapter 54

- George E. Omer, Jr
- Moheb S. A. Moneim

Conventional (Open) Carpal Tunnel Release

The best-known compression syndrome is carpal tunnel syndrome. Conventional (open) carpal tunnel release is the most commonly performed operation on the hand; 90% of operated upper extremity nerve lesions result from carpal tunnel syndrome.

Kaplan et al (1990) indicated five factors in predicting response to nonsurgical treatment: (1) patient older than 50 years; (2) symptom duration longer than 10 months; (3) constant paresthesias; (4) stenosing flexor tenosynovitis; and (5) positive Phalen's test. Nonsurgical treatment resulted in failure in 60% of patients with one factor, in 83% with two factors, and in 93% with three factors.

A diagnostic open operative approach is indicated in those patients with (1) rheumatoid arthritis or other significant tenosynovitis; (2) a distorted carpal tunnel secondary to trauma or degenerative arthritis; (3) a suspected tumor of soft tissue or bone, such as lipoma, aberrant muscle, or giant cell tumor; (4) concurrent ulnar tunnel syndrome at the wrist; (5) recurrent carpal tunnel syndrome; (6) thenar muscle atrophy; and (7) inability to hyperextend the wrist. An open operative approach may be elected in all other patients in whom there is symptomatic compression without a specific diagnosis. We prefer to use magnification with tourniquet control and either general or regional anesthesia.

DIAGNOSTIC INCISION

A diagnostic incision is indicated in the patient who has a potential diagnostic problem or a distorted carpal tunnel. This longitudinal incision begins on the ulnar side of the thenar crease at a point that would be intersected by a line drawn along the ulnar side of the extended thumb. This incision is placed between the palmar branches of the median and ulnar nerves and follows the thenar crease to a point approximately 1.5 to 2 cm distal to the wrist flexion crease. There it moves ulnar to reach the wrist flexion crease at a point in line with the long axis of the ring finger and then radially to reach the ulnar side of the palmaris longus at a point approximately 1.5 to 2 cm proximal to the wrist flexion crease (Omer, 1992). The incision extends to the subcutaneous tissue along its entire length, and then dissection is done from proximal to distal for the deeper structures. The superficial fascia of the forearm may be divided longitudinally.

The ulnar border of the median nerve is identified, and a blunt freer elevator is introduced for a short distance (0.5 cm) between the ulnar border of the median nerve and the transverse carpal ligament. The transverse carpal ligament is then divided. The dissection is done in layers, first dividing the fascia and then slowly extending the incision in the transverse carpal ligament, with the blunt instrument to protect the median nerve, until the median nerve is exposed from the forearm to the superficial vascular arch in the palm. If indicated, a step-cut incision can be made in the transverse carpal ligament that will permit closure after exploration. The approach is close to Guyon's canal at the base of the palm, and Guyon's canal can also be decompressed if its release is indicated.

If the carpal canal is oppressed with proliferative synovia, a tenosynovectomy should be performed. The dorsal floor of the canal can be explored if there are bony abnormalities or neoplasms. If indicated, the motor branch of the median nerve may be explored (Lilly and Magnell, 1985) (Fig. 54–1). If a transligamentous course of the motor branch is identified, the branch should be freed by further dissection of the ligament. On occasion, a ligamentous arch compresses the motor branch as it enters the thenar space, which requires release of the ligamentous arch. If the palmar cutaneous branch of the median nerve has been cut in a previous injury, it is better to dissect it proximally and section it at its origin from the median nerve than it is to repair it. A repair usually results in a painful neuroma.

An internal neurolysis is rarely indicated in the primary release of carpal tunnel syndrome. On occasion, there is a bluish red discoloration of the median nerve under the proximal edge of the transverse carpal ligament that suggests internal compression and inadequate circulation. When this pathology is present, the tourniquet should be released and

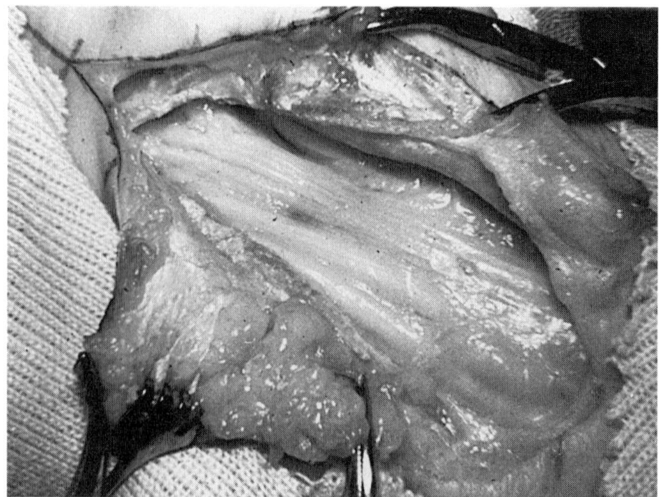

FIGURE 54–1. Exposure of the median nerve. The motor branch of the median nerve is at the top of the picture, beneath and distal to the transverse carpal ligament.

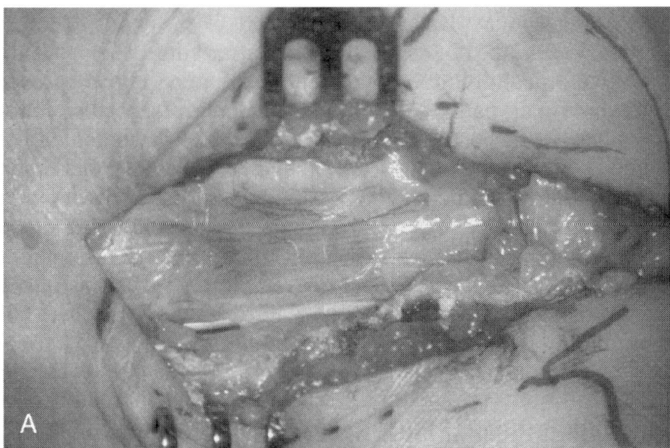
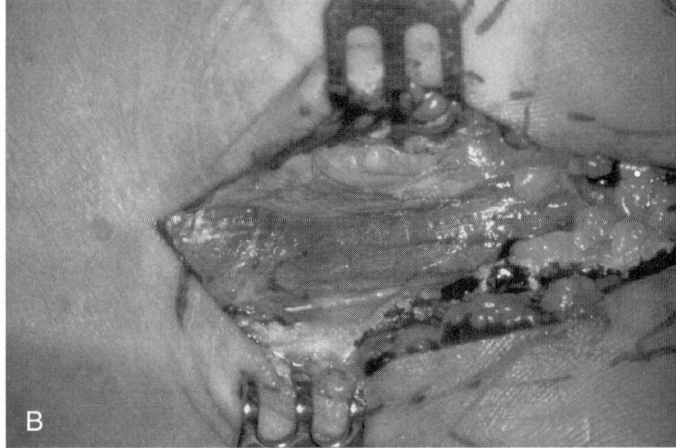

FIGURE 54–2. *A,* Compression of the median nerve under the proximal edge of the transverse carpal ligament, with discoloration and hourglass-shaped compression. *B,* Improved circulation usually occurs when the tourniquet is released for a short period (one minute) of time.

the nerve observed for at least 1 minute (Omer, 1992); usually there is improved circulation and the tourniquet can be reinflated (Fig. 54–2; see Color Plate as well). Continued controversy concerning internal neurolysis of the median nerve during the secondary release of carpal tunnel syndrome exists because there are paresthesias related to chronic tenosynovitis, so-called pillar pain with weakness (Jakab et al, 1991), and double-crush syndrome (Eason et al, 1985) as well as local ischemia and fibrosis in the nerve. It is difficult to predict which patients would benefit from internal neurolysis.

LIMITED INCISION

This is the appropriate incision for adequate decompression of the median nerve under direct vision. The straight longitudinal incision is 2 to 3 cm long, in line with the radial border of the ring finger and distal to the palmar crease. The palmaris longus can also be used as a landmark. The incision should always remain ulnar to the thumb thenar crease. It begins 1 cm distal to the wrist flexion crease and extends distally short of a line drawn transversely across the palm from the ulnar side of the thumb metacarpophalangeal joint (Fig. 54–3).

Sharp dissection is taken through the skin to incise the palmar fascia. The adipose tissue from the hypothenar eminence should be retracted ulnad. A self-retaining retractor is introduced into the wound to identify the transverse fibers of the flexor retinaculum (Fig. 54–4). The flexor retinaculum is incised and the carpal tunnel is entered midway through the incision. A blunt instrument or freer elevator is introduced deep to the flexor retinaculum through the opening, and further sharp retinacular release is done proximally and distally. The median nerve is then identified (Fig. 54–5). Blunt dissection is carried out proximally and distally to identify and protect any cross-communicating branches between the median and ulnar nerves. The rest of the flexor retinaculum is released as is the forearm fascia. Distal dissection is carried out until the superficial palmar arch is identified. The tourniquet is then released, bleeding is arrested, and only skin closure is done.

POSTOPERATIVE CARE

The forearm and wrist are immobilized in a bulky compressive dressing. The wrist is held in 10 to 20 degrees of extension with a plaster splint external to the dressing. The splint is on the volar surface and extends from the distal palmar crease to the mid-third of the forearm. Bowstringing of the flexor tendons must be avoided, as should be adherence of the tendons or the median nerve to the healing subcutaneous tissues (Kiritsis and Kline, 1995). A stockinette tube tied around the thorax and enclosed around the dressing may be used to hold the forearm and hand in elevation at night. Digital motion is encouraged. After 72 hours, the compression dressing is removed, and the patient is fitted with a palmar-to-forearm molded wrist plaster splint and lighter dressing. During this period, nighttime elevation of the forearm and hand should be achieved with a stockinette tube dressing. Digital motion is emphasized and supervised as necessary during this entire time, because stiffness of the nonoperated parts of the hand from edema and pain can be more disabling than the original condition.

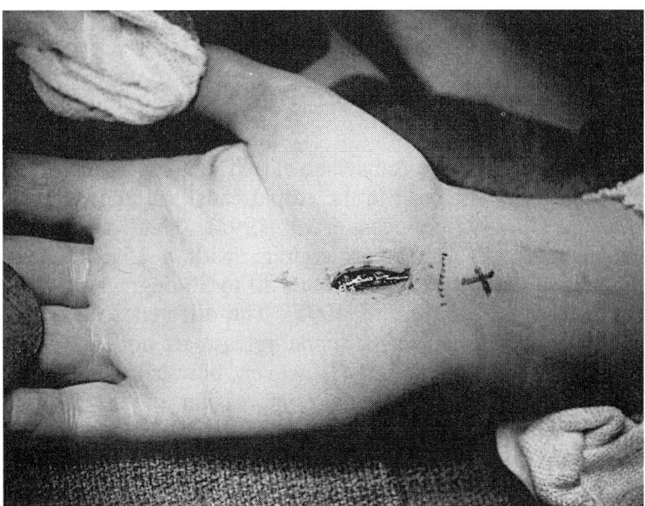

FIGURE 54–3. Limited carpal tunnel incision. It starts 1 cm distal to the wrist crease and extends distally in line with the palmaris longus tendon and the radial border of the ring finger.

Chapter 55

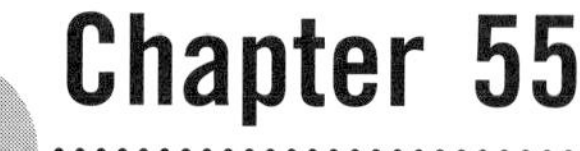
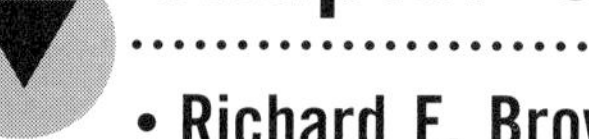

• Richard E. Brown

Endoscopic Carpal Tunnel Release

The management of carpal tunnel syndrome, including open carpal tunnel release (OCTR), is discussed in chapter 54. Although the open release has been the standard of surgical care since it was popularized by Phalen in the 1950s, the postoperative morbidity from OCTR (i.e., prolonged palmar pain and recovery time) has led many surgeons to look for less invasive means of decompressing the median nerve. Paine (1983) described division of the transverse carpal ligament (TCL) using a retinaculotome placed through a small incision in one of the volar wrist creases. However, incomplete division occurred in 2% to 3% of patients and about 1% had palmar hematomas possibly secondary to superficial palmar arch injury. Subsequently, several surgeons independently developed and described endoscopic techniques for division of the TCL. Their techniques have been enthusiastically endorsed and used by some and just as enthusiastically denounced by others. The role of endoscopic carpal tunnel release (ECTR) is still evolving, and its ultimate place in the management of carpal tunnel syndrome is yet to be determined. This chapter focuses on the indications and rationale for ECTR, the most common techniques, and the results and complications thus far reported.

RATIONALE AND INDICATIONS

Division of the TCL by open or endoscopic methods has been shown to increase the volume (Richman et al, 1989; Viegas et al, 1992) and to decrease the pressure within the carpal tunnel (Gelberman et al, 1981; Okutsu et al, 1989a). In addition, simple epineurotomy (Goetz et al, 1994; Leinberry et al, 1994) or internal neurolysis (Mackinnon et al, 1991) has been shown to provide no additional benefit over simple decompression. Also, carpal tunnel release alone has been shown to alleviate 89% of paresthesias in the ulnar nerve distribution (Silver et al, 1985). Therefore, with a few exceptions, the indications for ECTR are essentially the same as for OCTR. Endoscopic carpal tunnel release should not be performed in patients with rheumatoid arthritis or other significant tenosynovitis, recurrent carpal tunnel syndrome, or concurrent ulnar tunnel syndrome at the wrist or in those suspected to have a mass within the carpal tunnel.

TECHNIQUES

Several techniques for ECTR have been described. All have in common release of the TCL under direct vision via an endoscopic camera. They differ, however, in the actual instruments used and the number of portals. The four most commonly used techniques are the Agee (3M) inside job, the Chow two-portal (Dyonics) technique, the Okutsu universal subcutaneous endoscope method, and the Menon (Linvatec Concept) method. In a recent survey of American Society for Surgery of the Hand members, 157 surgeons (in 185 surgical series) reported using the Chow technique in 58%, the Agee technique in 34%, and other techniques in 8% (Schenck, 1995).

Chow (Dyonics) Two-Portal Method

The Chow method uses a proximal portal 1 cm proximal and 1 cm radial to the pisiform and a second portal just distal to the distal edge of the TCL (Chow, 1989) (Fig. 55–1A). The extrabursal (or subligamentous) approach of Resnick and Miller (1991) has replaced the original transbursal approach, which had a higher incidence of ulnar nerve and flexor tendon injuries. The antebrachial fascia is incised, and the undersurface of the TCL is cleared of synovium. A slotted canula and trocar are placed under the ligament via the proximal portal and then out the distal portal at the point, where the tip of the trocar is palpable (Fig. 55–1B). The trocar is removed and the camera is placed in the proximal sheath, giving visualization of the entire ligament (Fig. 55–1C). The distal half of the TCL is incised using a series of three knives available in the ECTRA Disposable Kit (i.e., a probe or push knife, a triangular knife, and a retrograde or pull knife) (Fig. 55–1D). The scope is then placed distally and the proximal half is incised. The slotted canula is then rotated, allowing visualization of both cut edges. After closure, a light dressing is applied (Fig. 55–1E), and the patient is allowed to use the hand for light activities.

Lewicky (1994) described another modification of the Chow technique to "improve patient safety and provide good ligament visualization" (p 39). In this modification, the undersurface of the TCL is cleared with a so-called recessed-neck dissector that is then passed out the distal portal. A plastic guide tube is then attached to the end of the dissector distally and pulled through the carpal tunnel and out the proximal portal. The obturator is then attached to the plastic guide tube, and both the obturator and slotted canula are guided distally through the proximal and distal portals. The remainder of the procedure is as Chow described.

Agee (3M) Method

The Agee method uses a single-portal technique and a pistol-grip device that includes the attached endoscopic cam-

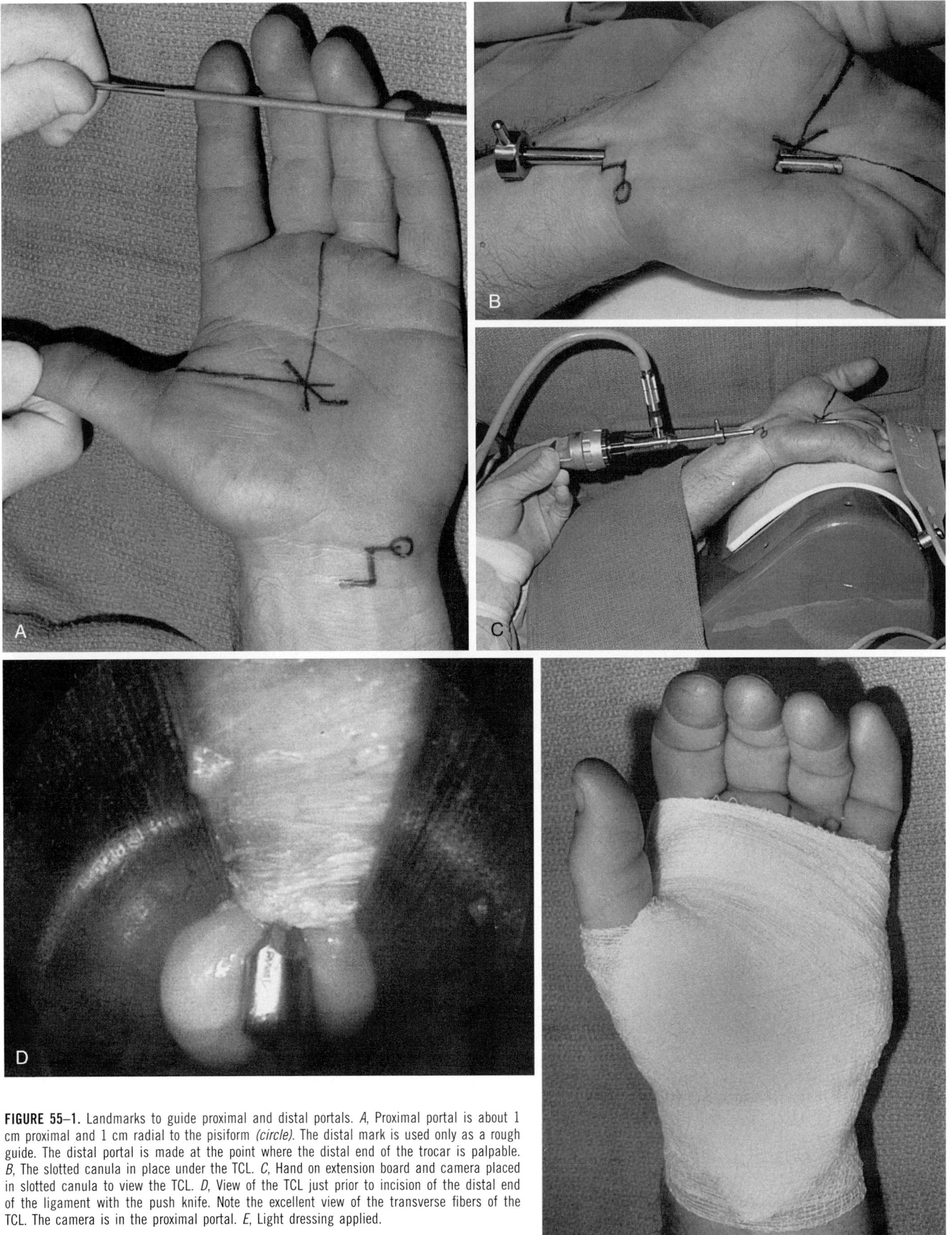

FIGURE 55–1. Landmarks to guide proximal and distal portals. *A,* Proximal portal is about 1 cm proximal and 1 cm radial to the pisiform *(circle).* The distal mark is used only as a rough guide. The distal portal is made at the point where the distal end of the trocar is palpable. *B,* The slotted canula in place under the TCL. *C,* Hand on extension board and camera placed in slotted canula to view the TCL. *D,* View of the TCL just prior to incision of the distal end of the ligament with the push knife. Note the excellent view of the transverse fibers of the TCL. The camera is in the proximal portal. *E,* Light dressing applied.

era and a disposable blade assembly (Agee et al, 1992). A 2- to 3-cm transverse incision is made in a volar flexion crease between the flexor carpi radialis tendons and the flexor carpi ulnaris tendons. A distally based flap of antebrachial fascia is raised, and the undersurface of the TCL is cleared as in the modified Chow method. The retractable blade device is passed distally under the ligament in line with the ring finger. The endoscopic camera allows a view of the retractable blade and the under surface of the ligament. With identification of the fat pad at the end of the ligament, the trigger is fired, elevating the blade. The distal end of the ligament is cut and inspected, and the device is withdrawn proximally, cutting the remainder of the TCL. Full-thickness division is verified by noting clifflike edges of the divided ligament.

Okutsu Universal Subcutaneous Endoscope Method

The Okutsu method was the first endoscopic method used (Okutsu et al, 1987). This technique uses a clear plastic canula placed through a proximal portal through which is passed a standard 30-degree oblique forward-viewing arthroscope. The undersurface of the TCL is cleared by passing a probe along the plastic canula. Similarly, a retrograde hook knife is then placed along the canula and used to incise the ligament in a distal-to-proximal direction.

Menon (Linvatec Concept) Method

The Menon technique also uses a single-portal technique through which is passed a boat-shaped hollowed-out canula (Menon, 1993). A 25-gauge needle is then percutaneously placed at the distal end of the TCL into the canula. The undersurface is cleared and a 30-degree scope inserted. A concave knife is placed through the canula just distal to the end of the scope. The ligament is cut in a proximal-to-distal direction by simultaneously advancing the scope and knife distally until the end of the ligament is reached (marked by the 25-gauge needle).

CADAVER AND ANATOMIC STUDIES

Several cadaver studies have investigated the proximity of endoscopic devices to structures in and about the carpal tunnel as well as the efficacy of endoscopic release of the transverse carpal tunnel. Rotman and Manske (1993) studied the relationship of the Agee device to surrounding structures by doing serial sections of cadaver wrists with the disposable blade apparatus in place. The average distance between the elevated blade and the median nerve was 3.1 mm, and the distance between the end of the TCL and the superficial arch was 4.8 mm. Two more recent studies, one using fresh-frozen cadavers (Cobb et al, 1994) and one using in vivo magnetic resonance scans (Polsen et al, 1994), have also noted that the ulnar neurovascular bundle running through Guyon's canal extends radially to the hook of the hamate. These three studies point out the vulnerability of surrounding

structures during ECTR and the need for accurate placement of the endoscopic device.

Four cadaver studies have also looked at the efficacy of ECTR. Lee and colleagues (1992) noted a 50% incidence of incomplete division of the TCL in 24 fresh cadaver hands. However, the releases were done by five different surgeons all newly trained on the two-portal technique. Seiler and co-workers (1992) similarly noted an incomplete release in two of 10 fresh cadaver wrists using Chow's original technique. However, using a modified subligamentous technique and identification of the arch and the distal end of the TCL through the distal portal before passing the trocar, no incomplete releases occurred in the next 10 cadaver wrists. In a similar study, Rowland and Kleinert (1994) reported a 38% incomplete release as well as multiple neurovascular complications in 24 fresh or fresh-frozen wrists. Again, numerous recently trained surgeons participated. Schwartz and associates (1993) reported results of TCL releases in 13 fresh-frozen cadaver wrists using the Agee technique by a surgeon "specifically trained in the technique and with a large clinical experience." No nerve, vessel, or tendon lacerations were noted, but four questionable and four definite incomplete releases were noted.

Having participated in cadaver laboratories as a student and as an instructor, the author has noted similar difficulties. Yet, it is believed that cadavers, whether fresh or fresh-frozen, are more difficult to work with than the actual patient. Therefore, the results from these cadaver studies must be taken at face value only and do not correlate with reported clinical studies. They do indicate the learning curve for ECTR and again the need for accurate placement of whatever endoscopic device is used.

CLINICAL RESULTS

Chow (1989) and Okutsu and colleagues (1989b) reported excellent results in their early experience using their respective techniques, including complete resolution of symptoms and no complications. Chow (1990) updated his series a year later, including 149 carpal tunnel releases with complete resolution of symptoms, earlier return to work, but one partial ulnar nerve palsy that resolved spontaneously. Early results with the Agee device from a multicenter randomized prospective study were presented at the 1990 ASSH meeting and published in 1992 (Agee et al, 1992). Eighty-two ECTRs were compared with 65 OCTRs. Overall, the median return-to-work time for those having unilateral surgery was 25 days for those in the ECTR group and 46.5 days for those in the OCTR group. However, in the worker's compensation group, the difference was only 7 days (71 versus 78). Grip and pinch returned to normal faster in those in the ECTR group and complaints of pain were less. Two had persistent symptoms after ECTR that required open exploration; one was found to have an incomplete release. Two transient ulnar neuropraxias occurred in the ECTR group, and one ulnar deep motor branch injury occurred in the open group. Subsequent to this study, the original Agee device was taken off the market because of difficulties with the blade assembly. It was redesigned and remarketed.

Numerous other reports have since been published. Menon (1994), using the Linvatec method, reported resolution of symptoms in 92% of 100 cases, with three transient neuropraxias of the common digital nerve to the ring and middle fingers. Brown and associates (1993) reported the results of a prospective randomized study comparing OCTR to a two-portal ECTR. Scar tenderness and return-to-work time were less in the ECTR group, but overall outcome and patient satisfaction were similar. However, four complications occurred in the ECTR group of 78 hands, including one partial transection of the superficial palmar arch, one digital nerve contusion, one ulnar nerve neuropraxia, and one wound hematoma. Also, despite the earlier return-to-work time, there were few worker's compensation claim patients.

Other comparative studies have noted similar results. McDonough and Gruenloh (1993) compared 50 consecutive OCTRs with 50 consecutive ECTRs (five Agee, 45 Chow method). Resolution of symptoms occurred in all patients, however, in each group one patient had recurrence of symptoms. There was one patient in the ECTR group who had persistence of paresthesias in the common digital nerve distribution to the ring and middle fingers. Return-to-work time was markedly shorter in the ECTR group, even for those on worker's compensation (32.4 versus 56 days). In England, Erdmann (1994) likewise reported an earlier return-to-work time (14 vs 39 days), but no details about the patients' type of employment were given. Overall, complications were higher in the ECTR group. However, when the transbursal cases were excluded, the complication rate in the ECTR group was actually less than that in the open group. Palmer et al (1993) noted a faster recovery of pinch and grip and a earlier return-to-work time in a prospective clinical study comparing open technique with either the Agee or Chow endoscopic techniques. The earliest return-to-work time occurred in the Agee group. In contrast, Brown and associates (1992) noted no major differences in a prospective study comparing the single-portal and two-portal techniques.

Several other retrospective studies of the Chow or modified Chow technique have noted excellent results, but the incidence of complications has varied. Pennington and Davies (1993) reported 550 ECTRs with no neurovascular or tendon injury. Similarly, Slattery (1994) in Australia noted no nerve or tendon injuries in 215 cases, but did have two cases of reflex sympathetic dystrophy and two cases without resolution of symptoms. In contrast to these, Kelly and colleagues (1994) noted less satisfactory results in 83 cases, with five incomplete releases and six nerve problems, including two median nerve lacerations. Likewise, Feinstein (1993), in a community-based series using the Agee method, noted good functional results but voiced reservation with the technique because of one median nerve laceration toward the end of his series. In contrast, Chow updated his series of ECTRs in 1993, again noting a fast return-to-work time and no permanent nerve, tendon, or vessel injury and only two transient neuropraxias (Chow, 1993).

COMPLICATIONS

As noted earlier, the complications from ECTR have varied and some have been significant. The most common have been incomplete release, nerve lacerations, digital nerve neuropraxias, superficial arch injury, and tendon lacerations. However, in a recent survey of ASSH members, the complication rate for 6,833 ECTRs was similar to that published for a collective review of OCTRs (Schenck, 1995). The overall complication rate for ECTR was 2.6%, and for OCTR, 9.2%. When scar tenderness was excluded from the OCTR group, the rate was 3.2%. More importantly, when transient nerve complications were excluded, the overall incidence of nerve, artery, and tendon complications was 1.2% for ECTR and 0.8% for OCTR.

AUTHOR'S EXPERIENCE AND IMPRESSIONS

In more than 150 ECTRs using the two-portal subligamentous modified Chow method, the author has noted good relief of symptoms and few minor complications. Two patients were converted to the open method because of an inability to adequately visualize the TCL. One patient was re-explored about 4 months after the operation for persistence of preoperative symptoms. Complete resolution occurred after the open release. No major neurovascular or tendon injuries have occurred, although there have been two transient neuropraxias of the common digital nerve to the ring and middle fingers.

The role of ECTR will undoubtedly continue to evolve. Having had the opportunity to teach ECTR to several residents, it is clear that the learning curve for endoscopic methods differs from that of the open release. Some technically superb residents struggle with endoscopic techniques. This is also true of experienced hand surgeons taking endoscopic courses. This steep learning curve will no doubt continue to fuel the debate about the role of endoscopic methods versus the standard open technique.

In safe hands, ECTR has potential benefits: less postoperative pain, faster return of grip and pinch strength, and less time out of work. Whether these potential benefits will continue to justify its use remains to be seen. In addition, if prospective studies continue to show faster return-to-work times, especially in the industrial sector, insurance carriers may eventually dictate the use of endoscopic methods. Clearly, this is not the final chapter on ECTR.

References

Agee JM, McCarroll HR, Tortosa RD, Berry DA, Szabo RM, Peimer CA: Endoscopic release of the carpal tunnel: A randomized prospective multicenter study. J Hand Surg *17A*:987–995, 1992.

Brown MG, Keyser B, Rothenberg ES: Endoscopic carpal tunnel release. J Hand Surg *17A*:1009–1011, 1992.

Brown RA, Gelberman RH, Seiler JG, Abrahamsson S, Weiland AJ, Urbaniak JR, Schoefeld DA, Furcolo D: Carpal tunnel release. J Bone Joint Surg *75A*:1265–1275, 1993.

Chow JCY: Endoscopic release of the carpal ligament: A new technique for carpal tunnel syndrome. Arthroscopy *5*:19–24, 1989.

Chow JCY: Endoscopic release of the carpal ligament for carpal tunnel syndrome: 22-Month clinical result. Arthroscopy *6*:288–296, 1990.

Chow JCY: The Chow technique of endoscopic release of the carpal ligament for carpal tunnel syndrome: Four years of clinical results. Arthroscopy *9*:301–314, 1993.

Cobb TK, Carmichael SW, Cooney WP: The ulnar neurovascular bundle at the wrist. J Hand Surg *19B*:24–26, 1994.

Erdmann MWH: Endoscopic carpal tunnel decompression. J Hand Surg *19B*:5–13, 1994.

Feinstein PA: Endoscopic carpal tunnel release in a community-based series. J Hand Surg *18A*:451–454, 1993.

Gelberman RH, Hergenroeder PT, Hargens AR, Lundborg GN, Akeson

WH: The carpal tunnel syndrome: A study of carpal canal pressures. J Bone Joint Surg Am *63A*:380–383, 1981.

Goetz DD, Ross MA, Blair WF, Steyers CM: Carpal tunnel release with and without epineurotomy. Presentation at the American Association for Surgery of the Hand, Cincinnati, October, 1994.

Kelly CP, Pulisetti D, Jamieson AM: Early experience with endoscopic carpal tunnel release. J Hand Surg *19B*:18–21, 1994.

Lee DH, Masear VR, Meyer RD, Stevens DM, Colgin S: Endoscopic carpal tunnel release: A cadaveric study. J Hand Surg *17A*:1003–1008, 1992.

Leinberry CF, Hammond NL, Siegfried JW: Epincurotomy: Its role in chronic carpal tunnel syndrome. Presentation at the American Association for Surgery of the Hand, Cincinnati, October 1994.

Lewicky RT: Endoscopic carpal tunnel release: The guide tube technique. Arthroscopy *10*:39–49, 1994.

Mackinnon SE, McCabe S, Murray JF, Szalai JP, Kelly L, Novak C, Kin B, Burke GM: Internal neurolysis fails to improve the results of primary carpal tunnel decompression. J Hand Surg *16A*:211–218, 1991.

McDonough JW, Gruenloh TJ: A comparison of endoscopic and open carpal tunnel release. Wis Med J *92*:675–677, 1993.

Menon J: Endoscopic carpal tunnel release: A single portal technique. Contemp Orthopaed *26*:109–116, 1993.

Menon J: Endoscopic carpal tunnel release: Preliminary report. Arthroscopy *10*:31–38, 1994.

Menon J, Etter C: Endoscopic carpal tunnel release: Current status. J Hand Therapy, April/June 139–144, 1993.

Okutsu I, Ninomiya S, Takatori Y, et al: Subcutaneous operation under the universal subcutaneous endoscope. Arthroscopy *12*:77–81, 1987.

Okutsu I, Ninomiya S, Hamanaka I, Kuroshima N, Inanami H: Measurement of pressure in the carpal canal before and after endoscopic management of carpal tunnel syndrome. J Bone Joint Surg *71A*:679–683, 1989a.

Okutsu I, Ninomiya S, Takatori Y, Ugawa Y: Endoscopic management of carpal tunnel syndrome. Arthroscopy *5*:11–18, 1989b.

Paine KWE, Polyzoidis KS: Carpal tunnel syndrome: Decompression using the paine retinaculotome. J Neurosurg *59*:1031–1036, 1983.

Palmer DH, Paulson JC, Lane-Larsen CL, Peulen VK, Olson JD: Endoscopic carpal tunnel release: A comparison of two techniques with open release. Arthroscopy *9*:498–508, 1993.

Pennington GA, Davies BW: Two portal, direct view endoscopic carpal tunnel release. Plast Surg Forum, New Orleans, *16*:274–277, 1993.

Polsen C, Netscher DT, Thornby J: Anatomical delineation of the ulnar nerve and artery in relation to the carpal tunnel. Presentation at the American Society for Surgery of the Hand, Cincinnati, October, 1994.

Resnick CT, Miller BW: Endoscopic carpal tunnel release using the subligamentous two-portal technique. Contemp Surg *22*:269–277, 1991.

Richman JA, Gelberman RH, Rydevik BL, Hajek PC, Braun RM, Gylys-Morin VM, Berthoty D: Carpal tunnel syndrome: Morphologic changes after release of the transverse carpal ligament. J Hand Surg *14A*:852–857, 1989.

Rotman MB, Manske PR: Anatomic relationship of an endoscopic carpal tunnel device to surrounding structures. J Hand Surg *18A*:442–450, 1993.

Rowland EB, Kleinert JM: Endoscopic carpal-tunnel release in cadavera. J Bone Joint Surg *76A*:266–268, 1994.

Schenck RR: The role of endoscopic surgery in the treatment of carpal tunnel syndrome. *Adv Plas Reconstr Surg 11*:17–43, 1995.

Schwartz JT, Waters PM, Simmons BP: Endoscopic carpal tunnel release: A cadaveric study. Arthroscopy *9*:209–213, 1993.

Seiler JG, Barnes K, Gelberman RH, Chalidapong P: Endoscopic carpal tunnel release: An anatomic study of the two-incision method in human cadavers. J Hand Surg *17A*:996–1002, 1992.

Silver MA, Gelberman RH, Gellman H, Rhoades CE: Carpal tunnel syndrome: Associated abnormalities in ulnar nerve function and the effect of carpal tunnel release on these abnormalities. J Hand Surg *10A*:710–713, 1985.

Slattery PG: Endoscopic carpal tunnel release use of the modified Chow technique in 215 cases. Med J Aust *160*:104–107, 1994.

Viegas SF, Pollard A, Kaminksi K: Carpal arch alteration and related clinical status after endoscopic carpal tunnel release. J Hand Surg *17A*:1012–1016, 1992.

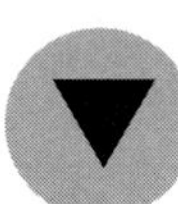

Chapter 56

- Richard M. Braun
- Sandra Doehr
- Nancy Leonard

Quantitative Measurement of Hand Function:
Application to Medical Decision-Making and Return to the Workplace After Cumulative Nerve Trauma

The alarming increase in the number of patients afflicted with cumulative trauma disorders has focused our attention on functional evaluation of the working hand. The term "dynamic carpal tunnel syndrome" was created to describe those patients with negligible complaints at rest who developed significant symptoms and hand dysfunction associated with measured swelling when the hand was used for pinching, grasping, twisting, and holding activities that simulated requirements in the workplace (Braun et al, 1989). Similar measurements may assist physicians responsible for medical decision-making when the hand is evaluated during or after treatment. Dynamic measurements do not replace standard single experience testing such as grip strength measurement, subjective sensory testing, or manual muscle grading. Functional studies such as quantitative measurements of work, power output, or endurance capacity add comparatively to the information gained from static tests. The hand is measured repeatedly, over a period of time, in patients who are receiving conservative or operative treatment. Serial determinations as recovery proceeds identify the pattern or pathway of clinical recovery. The patient, physician, and therapist may then decide when the functional tests scores indicate that the patient is ready to return to a modified job or to full duty. Reasonable accommodation in the workplace may allow a partially recovered hand to perform activities that are compatible with the patient's abilities. This will avoid functional decompensation and failure because of premature, unrealistic work demands. Appropriate functional data collection and intelligent medical decision-making will promote a congenial relationship between the functional abilities of the worker and the requirements of the job.

BIOLOGICAL BASIS OF RECOVERY AS RELATED TO FUNCTIONAL TESTING

Progressive tissue healing after injury is an inherent property of living systems. Biological healing models have been studied by investigators who measured tensile strength of experimental wounds. These early studies serve as the scientific basis for our current patient management decisions

(Dunphy and Van Winkle, 1969; Forrester et al, 1969). Functional recovery of the hand after cumulative trauma injury and subsequent treatment occurs in a similar pattern to that seen in wound healing experiments. This is no coincidence. Healing mechanisms of biological systems are expected to perform along lines that are genetically regulated and predictable. Inappropriate tension on a fresh suture line causes dehiscence, whereas balanced mechanical stress will cause strengthening and early tissue remodeling with enhanced functional recovery. Functional recovery curves plotted after carpal tunnel release have demonstrated an orderly pattern of improvement that may assist therapists and physicians in designing controlled exercise programs that enhance recovery and prevent decompensation caused by premature overload demands. The basis for these curves is the underlying legacy of scientific knowledge regarding the wound healing mechanism that is dependent on species specificity, character and degree of injury, and the ability of the particular host to respond to the injury with unimpaired healing.

TECHNOLOGY OF FUNCTIONAL MEASUREMENT

Functional measurements can be obtained with an entire spectrum of technological assistance. Our experience involves the Baltimore Technology and Engineering Company (BTE) work simulator (Fig. 56–1). The device involves an electronic brake to adjust resistance and a series of tools that are inserted into the hub of the circular brake mechanism (Curtis and Engalitacheff, 1981). Angular displacement of the tools is registered on a record that may be saved for serial comparison of performance over time. Our patients are studied before treatment or operation and are tested after treatment or postoperatively at monthly intervals. Measurements are recorded for static grip and pinch as well as BTE measurements for work (force × distance), power (work per unit of time), and endurance (work to the point of fatigue). Tools are selected for repetitive pinch, grasp, twisting, holding, and similar activities that simulate the work experience (Fig. 56–2). In some cases, work simulation may include actual job activities such as manipulating small parts, key-

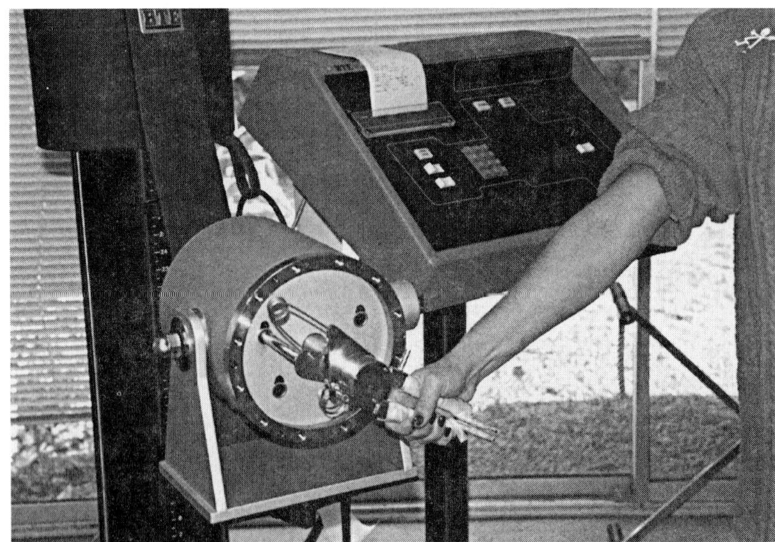

FIGURE 56–1. We have used the Baltimore Technology and Engineering Company (BTE) work simulator to measure hand function for activities that require strength and repetitive motion. Values for work (force times distance), power (work performed in a measured time), and endurance (work until fatigue) are recorded over the anticipated recovery time.

board work, or even such strenuous activities as shoveling sand.

Sensory testing is advisable in assessing any nerve disorder. Monofilament sensory mapping of the hand is a standard technique that is used in our facility. This test is less sophisticated than electronic vibrometry, but the results of monofilament sensory determination are reproducible and useful (Bell-Krotoski and Tomanick, 1987). Monofilament testing values enable us to document the sensory status of the hand. The test can be administered readily with simple, portable, and inexpensive equipment (Szabo et al, 1984). Serial examinations are recorded. Standard interpretation of the sensory monofilament test is presented in Figure 56–3 and Table 56–1.

Assembly tests are also used occasionally and correlate directly with sensory recovery (Fig. 56–4A) if the remainder of the musculoskeletal system is relatively normal. This is frequently the case in cumulative trauma disorders that do not involve direct mutilating injuries, vascular insufficiency, or traumatized joints. Assembly tasks are measured for productivity associated with time and the number of errors that are produced during the test time.

Volumetric measurements are used to evaluate and monitor the mechanical stress-strain relationship in the hand (Fig. 56–4B). Volumetric measurement produces a direct record of swelling and allows assessment of the functional capability and biological response in the hand. Major swelling in the hand, often associated with increasing symptoms and reduced sensation, is cause for concern. Treatment may be altered because of this direct evidence of hydrostatic imbalance in the working hand.

The most important consideration for functional testing is that the same test is followed serially over time and data are recorded to document performance. The performance data may be compared to values obtained before treatment, during treatment, or to average values for a similar condition in a diagnostic-specific group.

BTE work simulation data provide a simple record of performance for each patient. It is understood that BTE data may vary from one machine to another. We rely on the fact that a single patient uses a single machine. Data are compared on a time scale that relates one current test to a previous test performed at an earlier date. The values are expressed in percentages, which allows each patient to serve as his or her own control. This produces a functional recovery curve that permits tracking of the ability of that particular person to perform a specific repetitive task.

THE FUNCTIONAL RECOVERY CURVE

A composite curve was created for 300 patients who had undergone carpal tunnel nerve release surgery over a 6-year period. These serial BTE measurement values were used

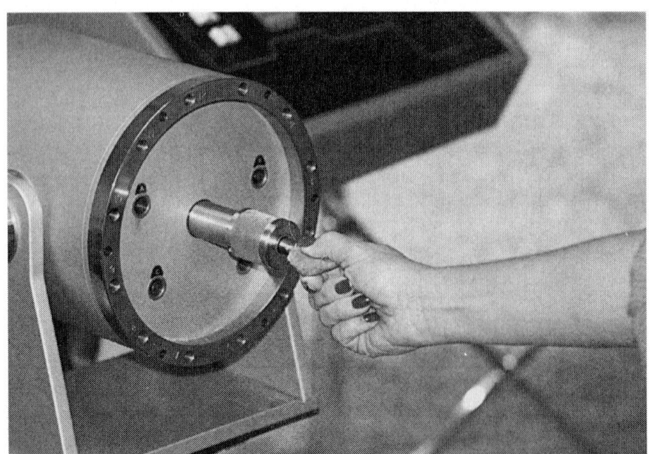

FIGURE 56–2. Specific tool inserts, placed in the chuck of the BTE device, allow for specific functional evaluation of pinching, gripping, or twisting activities.

▼ **TABLE 56–1**
Scale of Interpretation for Monofilament Sensory Testing

Monofilaments	Filament Markings
Normal	1.65–2.86
Diminished light touch	3.22–3.61
Diminished protective sensation	3.84–4.31
Loss of protective sensation	4.56–6.65
Untestable	>6.65

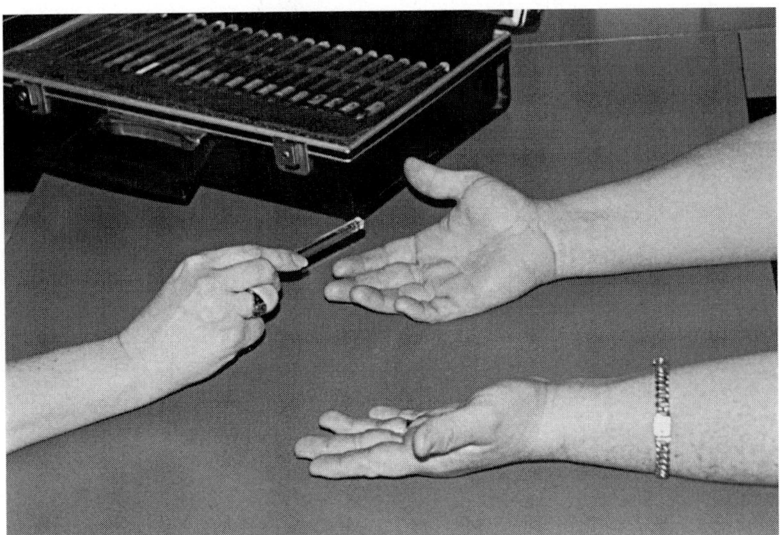

FIGURE 56–3. The therapist applies the monofilament test to the skin of the finger in determining threshold sensation. A sensory map is obtained in this simple reproducible study, which may be repeated to document a changing clinical condition. Sensory monofilament values may be generally considered to have these narrative descriptors (See Table 56–1).

to create graphs that plot functional recovery after nerve decompression. Each activity produced a curve that could be used for comparing the recovery of an individual patient with the anticipated normal recovery process. This curve now serves as our standard anticipated recovery pathway (Fig. 56–5).

Without complications or additional medical problems, we expect general compliance with this pattern of recovery. If functional recovery is delayed, we look for a reason in the medical or social environment to explain the delay, and we attempt to initiate an activity that will enhance progress. Some patterns that were initially considered troublesome are now accepted because of the inherent weakness in the system that assumes that all patients will behave alike. It is recognized that the initial baseline established by a particular individual will affect later measurement and the development of that individual's functional recovery curve. An unusually high initial effort may result in all future measurements falling short of the initial value; nevertheless, the individual

patient's recovery curve may show a parallel path that matches the slope of the average curve for this group of patients. In these situations, the individual patient curve is considered to be a reasonable response because it produces a similar shape as the standard curve. This lower output curve with a normal shape is used in similar fashion to a standard curve to evaluate and predict recovery. Similar patterns are seen in patients who give an initially weak performance. They may show a higher comparative recovery percentage after treatment or operation, but they will usually create a similar shape to their individual graph when compared to the standard graph (Fig. 56–6A).

A totally irregular series of measurements may define a noncompliant patient. Delay in recovery, as identified on the functional recovery curve, may indicate a significant medical problem or a complication that requires the attention of the treating physician or therapist. Without medical complication, a flat or low level of measured function after treatment may define a noncooperative patient (Fig. 56–6B).

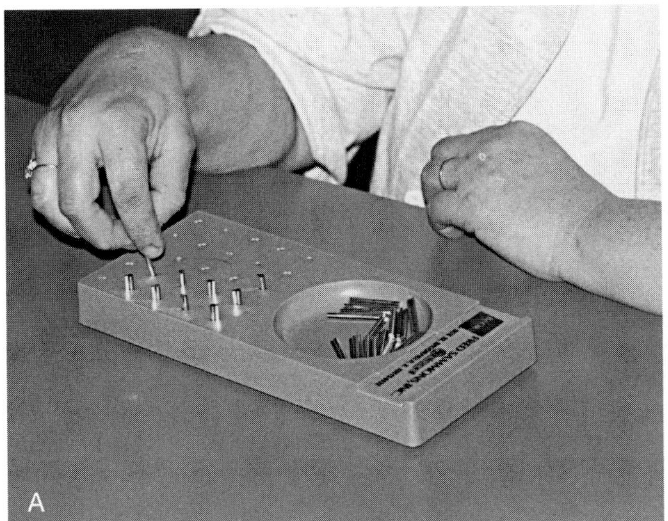

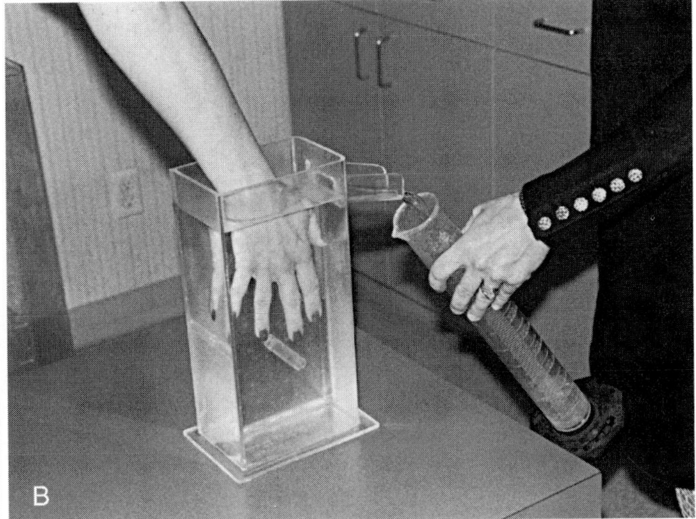

FIGURE 56–4. A, Assembly tests simulate fine manipulative activities that are frequently required in the workplace. Measured efficiency in assembly tasks correlates with sensory and mechanical status of the hand. B, Volumetric measurements are used to evaluate swelling that appears in the hand after a standardized provocative work simulation test. Resting volume measurements may also indicate residual swelling in a hand that is not under immediate load but is not ready to resume unrestricted work.

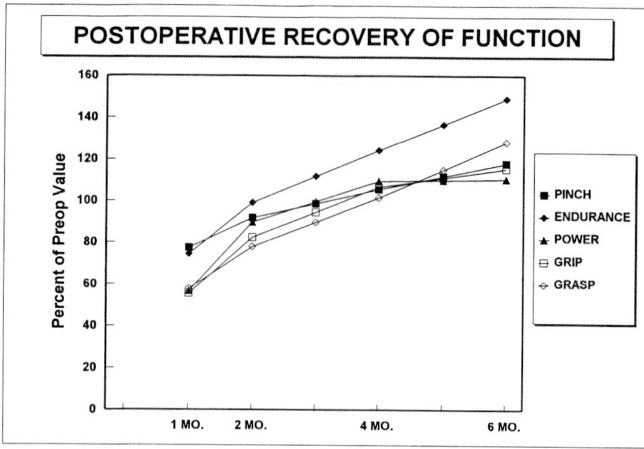

FIGURE 56–5. A functional recovery curve was established for 300 patients who have undergone carpal tunnel release. This composite graph serves as an anticipated clinical pathway of recovery. Physicians, therapists, case managers, and patients may use this graph to monitor functional recovery of a patient who has undergone carpal tunnel release.

FUNCTIONAL RECOVERY AND RETURN TO WORK

Many factors involve an individual worker's ability to return to the job. Some of these factors are out of the physician's control, and some can be controlled partially by the medical treatment team (Table 56–2). Functional recovery is the only area where the patient, physician, and hand therapist remain virtually the sole determinants of success. It is important for the physician to remain an active participant in the decision-making process regarding the patient's return to work. Functional recovery measurement enhances physician participation in this decision by providing data that can be understood by all parties who participate in allowing the patient to return to work. Three workers with the same diagnosis, treatment, and functional recovery pattern may be expected to return to their jobs at different times depending on the accommodation available in the workplace. Functional recovery data provide the rational link to this matching problem. An illustration of this concept is presented with a narrative review of three similar patients.

Degree of Physician Involvement in Return-to-Workplace Variables*

Major	Minor
Functional recovery	Employer motivation
Moderate	Economic motivation
Worker motivation	Job availability
Job requirements	Litigation
Job modification	Secondary gain
Rehabilitation	

*Functional recovery represents a significant factor in return to the workplace. Nevertheless, workers may not return to work unless all areas are conducive to recovery and re-employment. Each significant area requires individual evaluation in the decision-making process.

CASE STUDIES

 CASE 1:

A secretary for a neurologist returned to work 2 to 3 weeks after her carpal tunnel release operation. Her functional scores indicated that she had recovered about one third of her preoperative functional capacity. Her employer modified her job to allow one-handed work and limited requirements for the postoperative hand. Functional improvement was documented over the next month on serial BTE testing. Resumption of hand work activities was gradually increased to about two thirds of normal anticipated productivity. Full functional recovery to about 120% of preoperative measurement levels was obtained at 6 months after carpal tunnel release. During the 3- to 6 month postoperative period, the patient gradually resumed all required activities of employment, including the use of her computer. She has remained at work without modifications and has used the computer keyboard throughout the entire workday for a period of over 1 year (Fig. 56–7A).

CASE 2:

A self-employed anesthesiologist was concerned about when he could return to work after carpal tunnel release. The safety of his patients was of paramount importance. He demonstrated functional recovery to 100% of preoperative measurement levels

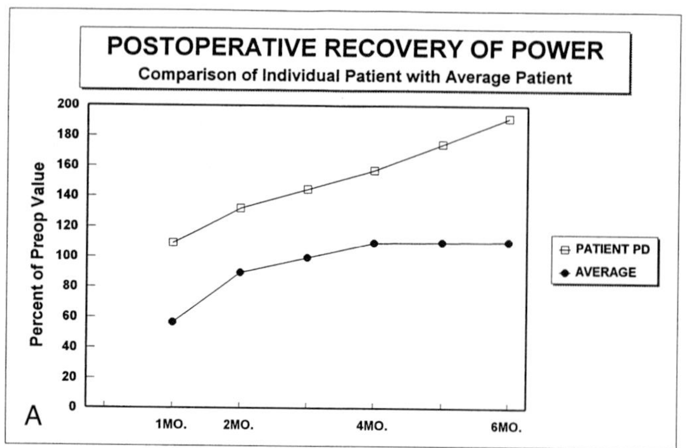

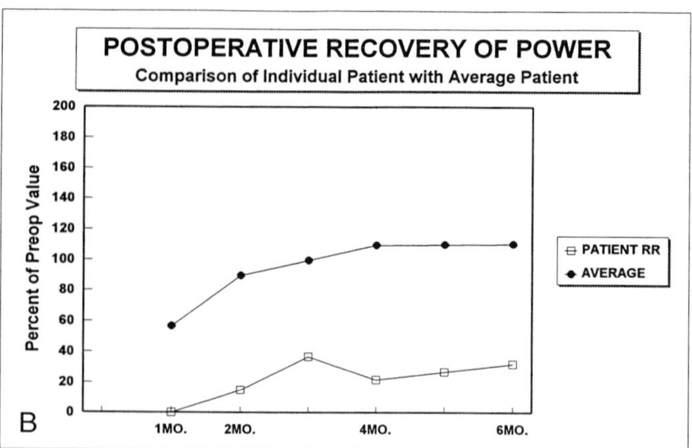

FIGURE 56–6. *A*, A "high curve" occurred in a worker with a low initial baseline measurement due to a hand that was painful prior to operation. Normal progression was measured following postoperative pain relief and functional recovery. *B*, This patient is not performing in a compliant or predictable fashion. Therapy should not be continued indefinitely in a case of this type.

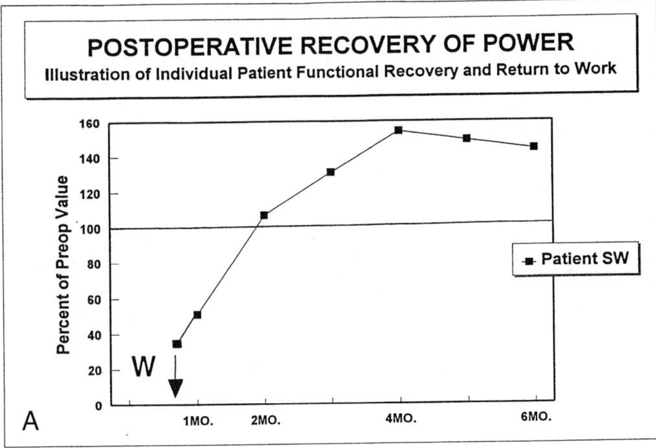

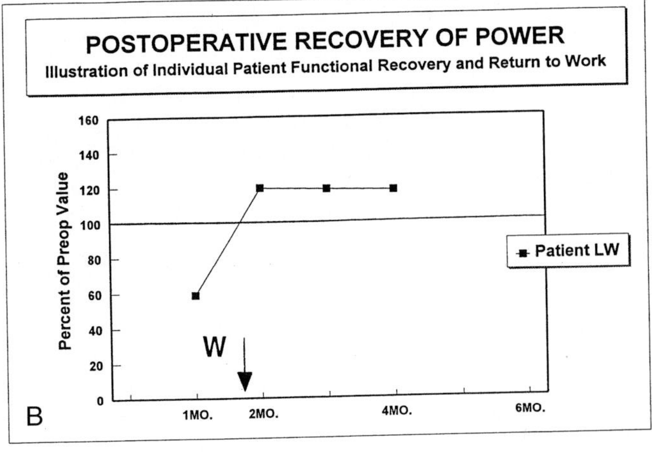

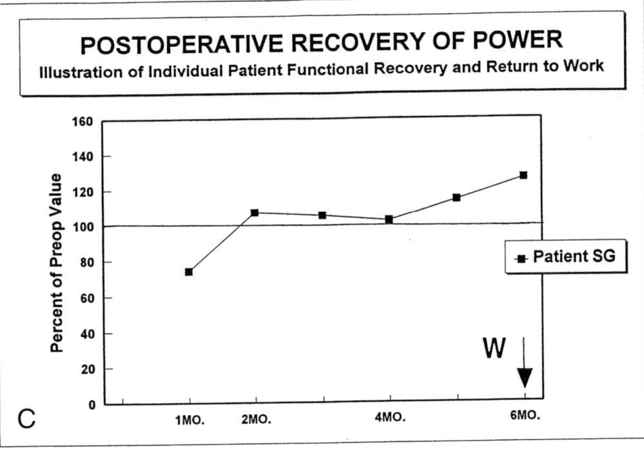

FIGURE 56–7. *A*, The patient returned to work (W) early because of major modifications in the workplace that required only minimal use of her operated hand. Because of this accommodation to the patient, early successful return to work was possible. Job requirements increased as functional recovery was documented. *B*, An anesthesiologist could not return to work without some assurance of safety on the job. He returned to work (W) when his data showed functional recovery to preoperative levels measured while he was working before his operation. *C*, A grocery checker required maximum power and endurance on the job that provided no accommodation for any functional impairment. Her reconditioning program required 6 months before she successfully returned to work (W).

at 6 to 7 weeks after operation. He returned to his regular job shortly thereafter, but selected his cases carefully during the next 6 weeks. He gradually recovered 120% of his initial preoperative test values. He now works without symptoms and without any job modifications 1 year after his operation (Fig. 56–7*B*). He expressed his gratitude that we had obtained hard data that validated his decision to return to work safely, 6 weeks after nerve decompression.

CASE 3:

An athletic, middle-aged, grocery checker tolerated significant symptoms of carpal tunnel syndrome for over 1 year. She requested surgical treatment when her pain became intolerable and she could no longer work. After operation, her functional abilities recovered slowly. Despite nerve decompression, this patient required a prolonged physical reconditioning program to allow her to return to a strenuous job. Her employer offered no reasonable accommodation in the workplace. Her therapy program was designed to gradually improve her power and endurance as well as upper body strength. Stretching and postural exercises were added to her program. Reasonable productivity goals were set based on measured functional recovery, symptom thresholds, and volumetric hand measurements. She finally produced BTE work simulator scores indicating reasonable recovery of function and returned to work 6 months after her operation (Fig. 56–7*C*). She remains employed 1 year later in a job that was not modified and is considered

strenuous. Mild symptoms occur occasionally with very heavy work periods.

These individual cases illustrate the value of objective data in considering appropriate balance between the ability of the worker and the demands of the job.

FUNCTIONAL RECOVERY DATA AND THE DEVELOPMENT OF CLINICAL PATHWAYS

Return to work is a reasonable milestone on a functional recovery pathway. Employers, insurance carriers, workers, and physicians may set goals based on reasonable anticipated recovery for a large group of workers with a similar diagnosis (or clinical presentation) treated in a standardized fashion. We applied this theory to a group of injured workers seen in a private office practice.

A composite graph was developed for 300 workers who underwent surgical treatment for carpal tunnel syndrome during a 7-year period. All patients were managed through the worker's compensation system of our state, and all were considered to have a causal relationship between the repetitive use of their hands at work and the presence of significant symptoms. All patients had conservative care for 3 months before operation. We excluded some patients who had severe symptoms because of use of vibratory or pneumatic tools, performed extremely heavy work, showed major atrophy in the hand musculature, or demonstrated profound numbness. The reason to exclude this small group with severe involvement is that we wished to plot a clinical pathway for the majority of our patients who had a more common pattern of involvement. Our patients were basically healthy adults with common symptoms of pain and numbness, modest sensory loss, and with a positive Tinel's or Phalen's test, or both. The symptoms were considered moderate in that they significantly reduced productivity and therefore prevented the worker from returning to the job or competing on the open labor market. A composite functional recovery curve and a bar graph for return-to-work dates were prepared on the same format (Fig. 56–8). The composite graph demonstrates that the functional recovery curve and the return-to-work date have a positive correlation. This represents the usual anticipated association of recovery and return to work in a large (more than 100 patients) group of workers. It demonstrates real experience in returning injured workers to the workplace in our community, and it is used to counsel and monitor all patients of this type that receive treatment in our facility. The time for functional recovery and return to work was longer than the employers' often expected; however, the data represented by the functional recovery curve allowed us to show employers and case managers that reasonable accommodation in the workplace would allow an earlier match for the ability of the hand and the demands of the job. This composite functional recovery curve and return-to-work bar graph has promoted a more intelligent and sensitive approach to the interface of a previously disabled patient with the demands that are associated with return to the workplace.

FUNCTIONAL RECOVERY DATA AND EVALUATION OF MEDICAL MANAGEMENT

Analysis of cost-effective medical care requires some type of outcome measurement. Functional recovery data allow comparison of recovery rates as well as absolute measurements. Functional recovery data can be used to compare a

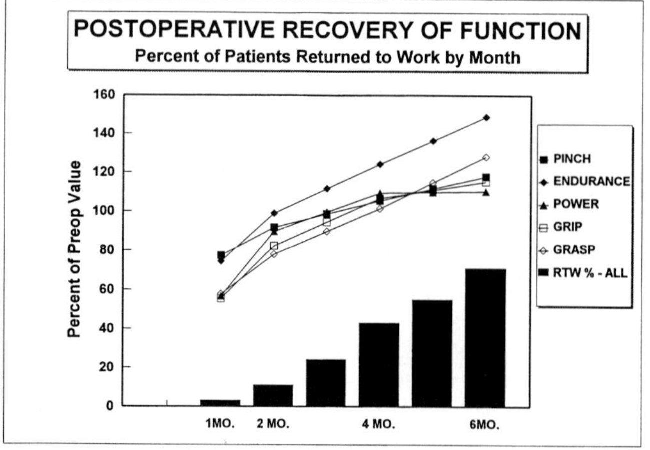

FIGURE 56–8. Functional recovery (line graphs) and return to work (bar graphs) show good correlation. Reasonable accommodation in the workplace will allow patients with hands with less recovery of function to return to work at an earlier date.

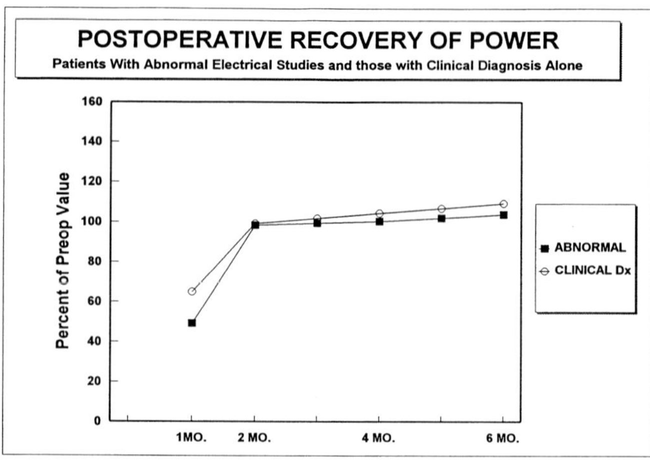

FIGURE 56–9. This graph documents functional recovery for two groups of patients who underwent carpal tunnel release. A group of patients with a clinical diagnosis of carpal tunnel syndrome was compared with a similar group that showed abnormal electrodiagnostic studies. There is no statistically valid functional difference in the recovery pathways demonstrated by each of these groups. Electrodiagnostic studies of a threshold type do not afford prognostic information regarding functional recovery rates in patients undergoing carpal tunnel release.

pathway achieved by one group of patients measured against another similar group used as a standard. A measured variable in diagnostic procedures or treatment options can be subjected to analysis of the pathway that was achieved when each variable entered the system. A brief illustration of this type of analysis will be presented for a diagnostic procedure and for a method of surgical treatment.

The prognostic significance of threshold electrodiagnostic studies was subjected to functional recovery study (Braun and Jackson, 1994). A group of patients with a clinical diagnosis of carpal tunnel syndrome was compared with a similar group that showed abnormal electrodiagnostic studies. The functional recovery rate for each group was similar. The functional recovery graphs and serial measurements showed no statistical difference. Although we still advise electrodiagnostic testing, we are now more inclined to operate on a patient with a firm clinical diagnosis (Fig. 56–9).

Changes in treatment variables can also be followed with similar graphic pathway mapping. Endoscopic carpal tunnel release was subjected to this method of analysis using functional recovery curve measurements. A series of patients who underwent endoscopic release were plotted on a functional recovery curve. Comparison with the previously established case management data showed no advantage in recovery rates of grip, power, or endurance functions in endoscopic cases. For this reason, we have not adopted the endoscopic procedure for our standard patient population. The endoscopic procedure may be used occasionally on an individual or selective basis.

FUNCTIONAL RECOVERY DATA AND PROSPECTIVE PROGRAM PLANNING

Clinical mapping, as demonstrated by the creation of functional recovery curves, allows for prospective planning for similar patients who experience similar treatment. It is reasonable to use a case manager to assist with patient placement in reasonable job positions before full recovery is measured. Employers may anticipate return of the worker to a modified position at a future point in time. A good match will balance the functional ability of the worker and reasonable job demands. The established recovery pattern may be anticipated as a generalization while understanding that an individual patient may vary in his or her recovery rate. Nevertheless, advanced planning is more likely to produce a reasonable match than are arbitrary decisions made in an environment that is already charged with the personal interest of each participant. This prospective use of data is very helpful when an injured patient whose environment is controlled by the doctor becomes a re-employed worker whose environment is controlled by the employer. Accommodation in the workplace is an essential element of the Americans With Disabilities Act, a law that will continue to influence our country's workplace in the 21st century.

SUMMARY

Functional testing and measurement may now be added to previously accepted standard procedures for examination of the hand. Functional evaluation relates directly to the practical demands of our working society. Statistically correct pathways have been defined for large series of patients who received surgical treatment for median neuritis or carpal tunnel syndrome. This study serves as an initial model for recovery pathway mapping. Each individual treatment facility may develop a similar model that is appropriate for the geographic and socioeconomic factors present in the patients treated in that area. Retrospective study data and prospective planning for appropriate use of this data have been presented as a learning tool, not as a rigid protocol. Functional recovery data allow all parties involved to use rational decision-making in an effort to match the ability that is available to the task at hand.

References

Bell-Krotoski J, Tomanick E: The repeatability of testing with Semmes-Weinstein monofilaments. J Hand Surg *12A:*155–161, 1987.

Braun RM, Davidson K, Doehr S: Provocative testing in the diagnosis of dynamic carpal tunnel syndrome. J Hand Surg *14A:*195–197, 1989.

Braun RM, Jackson W: Electrical studies as a prognostic factor in the surgical treatment of carpal tunnel syndrome. J Hand Surg *19A:*893–900, 1994.

Curtis R, Engalitacheff J Jr: A work simulator for rehabilitating the upper extremity: Preliminary report. J Hand Surg *6:*449–500, 1981.

Dunphy JE, Van Winkle W: Repair and Regeneration: The Scientific Basis for Surgical Practice. New York, McGraw Hill, 1969, pp 349–359.

Forrester J, Zederfeldt B, Hayes T, Hunt T: Mechanical, biochemical, and architectural features of repair. *In* Dunphy JE, VanWinkle HR: Repair and Regeneration: The Scientific Basis for Surgical Practice. New York, McGraw Hill, 1969, pp 71–85.

Szabo R, Gelberman R, Dimick M: Sensibility testing in patients with carpal tunnel syndrome. J Bone Joint Surg *66A:*61–64, 1984.

origins or over the course of the specific tendons directly. The symptoms may be exacerbated by resistive motions. In the early phases of these problems, simple measures for early management are of paramount importance to prevent progression to later, more difficult, stages (Furth et al, 1994; Louis, 1992; Szabo and Madison, 1991).

Early treatment may involve rest, splints, casts, and work cessation or modification where indicated. All avocational pursuits that may have an additive effect on the symptoms should be avoided, such as bowling, weight lifting, racket sports, etc. A careful look at the patient's job and body mechanics is important to control potential ergonomic stressors, i.e., work station height if standing; chair height if sitting; forearm, arm, and wrist positions (Armstrong, 1986).

In the early symptomatic stage, these measures, along with other reasonable alterations, should usually result in the cessation of symptoms. Job rotation (Schultz and Schkade, 1992), frequent work breaks, analgesics, and nonsteroidal anti-inflammatory medications may also be helpful accommodations. There may be a gradual progression of symptomatic states depending on the duration or chronicity of the symptoms. In general, those individuals with long-standing complaints usually will have more significant physical findings, and management (Herbin, 1987; Schultz-Johnson, 1987) is usually correspondingly difficult.

Late Symptomatic Stage

Individuals in this stage usually have ignored their early symptoms and have sought treatment late in the evolution of their complaint. It is not surprising, then, that a person in this situation with carpal tunnel syndrome will have abnormal electrophysiologic studies when initially seen (Anthony, 1993; Bell-Krotoski et al, 1993; Szabo et al, 1984). Likewise, it is not unusual that a person with tendon irritation, such as de Quervain's syndrome, will have a markedly positive Finkelstein's test. The manifestations of other forms of muscle and tendon irritation are likewise more obvious, flagrant, and increasingly painful.

Individuals who are seen at this advanced stage require more vigorous and restricting measures to effect maximal rehabilitation. Work cessation and interdiction of all potentially aggravating recreational pursuits are necessary (Lowe, 1992). In addition to a job analysis, permanent job restrictions (Baxter-Petralia, 1990; Johnson, 1993; King, 1990; King, 1994), rotation, or modifications may be necessary (Hart et al, 1993; Herbin, 1987; Rivet, 1992). This, of course, is not easy and in some circumstances may be impossible. Although surgery may be a temporary symptomatic solution (e.g., carpal tunnel syndrome), not all patients will remain asymptomatic if they return to their previous jobs. This is one of the most frustrating aspects of patient management for physicians, employers, and workers (Matheson, 1988). At times, there is no ideal solution, and vocational rehabilitation is the most effective way of returning the worker to gainful, although modified, activity.

A CURRENT DILEMMA

One of the most difficult diagnostic and therapeutic problems that physicians face today is the lack of diagnostic specificity and rampant therapeutic expediency. Patients are told that their symptoms are the result of *tendonitis* or *tenosynovitis*—inappropriate, nonspecific terms that have no correlation to actual pathology (Ireland, 1992). After they are treated for these problems, they begin to believe that they have a disease. The same is true when the terms *reflex sympathetic dystrophy, cumulative trauma disorders,* or *repetitive strain injury* are used (Hadler, 1990; Williams and Westmorland, 1994). An unsophisticated patient may become fearful of the term used and believe that it has far more importance than is in fact the case (Wolfe et al, 1991).

It is unfortunate that patients are often given specific diagnoses when there is no objective evidence (Hadler, 1990, Ireland, 1992) and when all that is present is a symptomatic state without an explanation. A simple diagnosis of limb pain (HICDA code 729.5) would be sufficient and not misleading. Unfortunately, failure to use this very specific designation has probably led to countless inappropriate insurance payments, work days missed, unnecessary operations, and other treatments.

Rehabilitation for conditions that appear to be workplace-related is a complex management exercise. It requires a specific diagnosis based on objective findings and a persistent evaluation of the patient and his or her job, personal circumstance, and motivation to effect a beneficial outcome.

References

Anthony MS: Sensory evaluation. *In* Clark GL, Shaw Wilgis EF, Aiello B, Eckhaus D, Eddington LV (eds): Hand Rehabilitation: A Practical Guide. New York, Churchill Livingstone, 1993, pp 55–67.

Armstrong TJ: Ergonomics and cumulative trauma disorders. Hand Clin 2:553–565, 1986.

Baxter-Petralia PL: Therapist's management of carpal tunnel syndrome. *In* Hunter JM, Schneider LH, Mackin EJ (eds): Rehabilitation of the Hand, 3rd ed. St. Louis, Mosby, 1990, pp 640–646.

Baxter-Petralia PL, Bruening L, Blackmore S: Work therapy program of the Hand Rehabilitation Center in Philadelphia. *In* Hunter JM, Schneider LH, Mackin EJ (eds): Rehabilitation of the Hand, 3rd ed. St. Louis, Mosby, 1990, pp 1155–1164.

Bell-Krotoski J, Weinstein S, Weinstein C: Sensibility, including touch-pressure, two point discrimination, point localization, and vibration. J Hand Ther 6:114–122, 1993.

Berryhill BH: Returning the worker with an upper extremity injury to industry: A model for the physician and therapist. J Hand Ther *3*:56–63, 1990.

Furth H, Holm M, James A: Reinjury prevention follow-through for clients with cumulative trauma disorders. Am J Occup Ther *48*:890–898, 1994.

Hadler NM: Cumulative trauma disorders: An iatrogenic concept. J Occup Med 32:38–41, 1990.

Hart DL, Isernhagen SJ, Matheson LN: Guidelines for functional capacity evaluation of people with medical conditions. J Orthop Sports Phys Ther *18*:682–686, 1993.

Herbin ML: Work capacity evaluation for occupational hand injuries. J Hand Surg *12A*:960, 1987.

Ireland DCR: The Australian experience with cumulative trauma disorders. *In* Millender LH, Louis DS, Simmons BP (eds): Occupational Disorders of the Upper Extremity. New York, Churchill Livingstone, 1992, pp 79–88.

Johnson SL: Therapy of the occupationally injured hand and upper extremity. Hand Clin 9:289–298, 1993.

King JW: An integration of medicine and industry. J Hand Therapy *3*:45–50, 1990.

King JW: Upper extremity cumulative trauma disorders: Returning the CTD-injured worker to work. Presented at the meeting of the American Society for Surgery of the Hand Therapists on Upper Extremity Cumulative Trauma Disorders, San Diego, February 1994.

Lane C: Therapy for the occupationally injured hand. Hand Clin 2:593–602, 1986.

Louis DS: Evolving concerns relating to occupational disorders of the upper extremity. Clin Orthop *254*:140–143, 1990.

Louis DS: The carpal tunnel syndrome in the work place. *In* Millender LH, Louis DS, Simmons BP (eds): Occupational Disorders of the Upper Extremity. New York, Churchill Livingstone, 1992, pp 145–153.

Lowe C: Treatment of tendinitis, tenosynovitis, and other cumulative trauma disorders of musicians' forearms, wrists, and hands: Testing function with hand therapy. J Hand Ther *5*:84–90, 1992.

Matheson LN: How do you know that he tried his best? The reliability crisis in industrial rehabilitation. Industrial Rehabilitation Quarterly *1*:1–12, 1988.

Mosely LH, Kalafut RM, Levinson PD, Mokris SA: Cumulative trauma disorders and compression neuropathies of the upper extremities. *In* Kasdan ML (ed): Occupational Hand and Upper Extremity Injuries and Diseases. Philadelphia, Hanley and Belfus, 1991, pp 353–402.

Petralia PB, Penney V: Cumulative trauma. *In* Stanley BG, Tribuzi SM (eds): Concepts in Hand Rehabilitation. Philadelphia, F. A. Davis, 1992, pp 420–425.

Rivet L: Functional capacity evaluation. *In* Casanova JS (ed): Clinical Assessment Recommendations. Chicago, American Society of Hand Therapists, 1992, pp 123–130.

Schultz S, Schkade J: Occupational adaptation: Toward a holistic approach for contemporary practice. Part 2. Am J Occup Ther *46*:917–925, 1992.

Schultz-Johnson K: Assessment of upper extremity-injured persons' return to work potential. J Hand Surg *12A*:950–957, 1987.

Semple CS: Tenosynovitis, repetitive strain injury, cumulative trauma disorders and overuse syndromes, et cetera. J Bone Joint Surg *73B*:536–538, 1991.

Szabo RM, Gelberman RH, Williamson RV, et al: Vibratory testing in acute peripheral nerve compression. J Hand Surg *9*:104–109, 1984.

Szabo RM, Madison M: Management of carpal tunnel syndrome. *In* Kasdan ML (ed): Occupational Hand and Upper Extremity Injuries and Diseases. Philadelphia, Hanley and Belfus, 1991, pp 341–352.

Williams R, Westmorland M: Occupational cumulative trauma disorders of the upper extremity. Am J Occup Ther *48*:411–420, 1994.

Wolfe TL, DiPlacido MS, Lubahn JD: Unable to return to work—now what? *In* Kasdan ML (ed): Occupational Hand and Upper Extremity Injuries and Diseases. Philadelphia, Hanley & Belfus, 1991, pp 483–488.

• J. Leonard Goldner
• Reginald L. Hall

Chapter 58

Nerve Entrapment Syndromes of the Low Back and Lower Extremities

GENERAL PRINCIPLES OF NERVE ENTRAPMENT SYNDROMES

Nerve Roots and Peripheral Nerves

Peripheral nerve entrapment, compression, or irritation of nerve roots forming the lumbosacroplexus may cause lower extremity pain, burning, or uncomfortable feelings that affect the dermatomes, myotomes, or sclerotomes (Goldner, 1956). The dermatome involvement is characterized by hypesthesia or hyperesthesia that provides a clue to the site of origin of pain. If there is no dermatome change but only myotome or sclerotome pain, the site of the primary lesion may be in the organ complex such as in muscle or bone rather than in a compressive proximal nerve lesion.

Referred pain originating from a more central neural lesion such as the conus or the proximal spinal cord may be difficult to localize because of a vague pain pattern. Thus, the importance of a detailed history, physical examination, and determination of the characteristics of pain are necessary for an accurate diagnosis. Special imaging studies may be required in certain situations.

Differential Diagnosis of Back and Lower Extremity Pain

Several lesions occur that simulate nerve root irritation. The complaints are somewhat different than those that arise from a primary peripheral nerve entrapment (Goldner, 1956). Also, peripheral nerve entrapment lesions due to external compression or trauma should be differentiated from spontaneous or internal compressive lesions. The external or visible causes are recognized by the force of an object that compresses or damages the nerve; the internal or nonvisible compressive lesion may require special diagnostic studies to recognize a pathological process; or the patient may require surgical exploration to document a suspected entrapment lesion that is recognized by an intermittent or persistent pattern of pain and paresthesias, a specific relationship to the circadian cycle, and aggravation by physical activities. A positive percussion test and an abnormal electrical study provide additional evidence that the nerve is trapped and irritated.

Neurophysiological Terminology Associated with Nerve Entrapment Syndromes (Goldner, 1983; Wall and Melzack, 1984)

Anesthesia—no recognition of external stimuli other than movement of the part or extreme pressure on the part.

Hypesthesia—diminished recognition of a sharp or dull object on the skin. The affected area varies in size and may not follow a nerve root dermatome.

Dysesthesia—an uncomfortable, unpleasant sensation that results from stimulation of a cutaneous area affected by peripheral nerve trauma or a regenerating nerve. Stimulation of one side of the digit may be interpreted as occurring in an adjacent digit—the so-called split axon phenomenon. This noxious sensation is not well tolerated.

Paresthesias—uncomfortable tingling, aching, or burning sensations frequently described as "pins and needles" along the course of a peripheral nerve while the nerve is being percussed. Also, stimulation of the skin in the autonomous zone of the injured nerve may cause similar sensations. This may be felt continuously or intermittently and is described as feeling like an electric shock.

Hyperesthesia—an unpleasant excessive sensibility resulting from stimulation of skin or hair in the distribution of a cutaneous nerve. A hyperesthetic digit shows areas of skin or a fingernail with excessive sensitivity.

Hyperpathia—an unpleasant painful sensation aggravated by tapping, rubbing, scraping, or irritating the involved skin. These maneuvers result in an unpleasant painful sensation that causes a withdrawal action.

Causalgia—a sustained burning pain that is also described as searing, cutting, firelike, and hot (Mitchell, 1872). This sensation may be associated with a complete or incomplete peripheral nerve injury and involves, particularly, the tibial nerve. In the upper extremity, the median nerve is most frequently involved and accounts for the description of St. Anthony's fire that referred to the burning extremity associated with a toxic neuritis from ergot poisoning due to moldy rye bread.

Deafferentation—a state of dysesthetic pain resulting from a neural injury. Certain syndromes cause intractable dysesthesia with incomplete alteration of sensitivity.

Allodynia—pain that results from non-noxious stimulation of normal skin, such as stroking of the skin.

Neuropathology of Nerve Compression

The nerve may be compressed acutely by a thigh tourniquet at a specified higher pressure than is usually used for a specific length of time. Or the nerve may be subject to chronic compression by persistent abnormal pressure from an external force, such as an excessively tight knee immobilizer that is not released for 24 hours. The nerve entrapment implies that there is a disproportion between the volume of the peripheral nerve and the space through which it passes. For example, as it enters the plantar surface of the foot, the tibial nerve is crossed by the fibrous edge of the origin of the abductor hallucis muscle, making a relatively small space that may result in pain and paresthesias.

A mixed nerve is a highly differentiated, well-defined system of axons arranged in groups of different thickness with different functions. Abnormal compression may depend on the relative amount of epineurium compared with axoplasm (Lyons and Woodhall, 1949). Small nerve fascicles with a large epineurial covering are less likely to be abnormally compressed than are nerves with large fascicles and small amounts of epineurium surrounding the fascicles. The resulting pattern of clinical involvement varies according to the topographical location of the myelinated motor or sensory fibers. The effect of compression on the outer fibers is determined by either eccentric or symmetrical location of the compressing force. The peripheral heavily myelinated fibers include motor, sensory, proprioceptive, light touch, and vibratory axons, whereas the thinly myelinated pain and sympathetic fibers, and regenerating sensory and motor fibers are deeper within the nerve (Ochoa, et al, 1972) (Fig. 58–1).

Other important factors are related to the intraneural vascular injury, the pressure gradient within the nerve between its compressed and uncompressed parts, and the deprivation that is occurring at the periphery of the compression zone (Lundborg and Rydevik, 1973).

Systemic conditions affecting peripheral nerves cause nerve sensitivity that may result in earlier compressive or entrapment syndromes that otherwise might not occur. For example, diabetics or chronic alcoholics have hypersensitive peripheral nerves that are more readily susceptible to compressive forces than are normal nerves (Baba, et al, 1987; Brown and Ashburg, 1984). A mechanical factor such as a recent neurapraxia from a fracture may sensitize the nerve to a pneumatic tourniquet of average pressure and time, and result in a compressive neuropathy that would not occur with a healthy nerve. External pressure to a peripheral nerve in the range of 20 to 30 mm Hg causes retardation of venular blood flow in the epineurium, whereas pressures of 60 to 80 mm Hg cause a complete standstill of intraneural blood flow in compressed nerve segments (Rydevik et al, 1981).

Axonal transport is affected adversely by excessive high and prolonged pressure. These conditions affect antegrade and retrograde axonal transport. Pressures of 130 to 150 mm Hg applied for a specified time result in an acute block of conduction in peripheral nerves. Large-diameter fibers are more susceptible to compression than small-diameter fibers.

Both low and high pressures cause capillary permeability changes in intraneurial blood vessels. Endoneurial fluid pressure increases and causes a miniature closed compartment syndrome (Lundborg et al, 1983)

Ionic electrolytic imbalance related to potassium, sodium, adenosine, and diphosphatase disturbances occurs at the node of Ranvier.

The current terminology used to describe the severity of compressive and shear forces based on the structural changes that have been described were initiated by Seddon, who used neurapraxia, axonotmesis, and neurotmesis; Sunderland categorized nerve injuries in terms of first through fifth

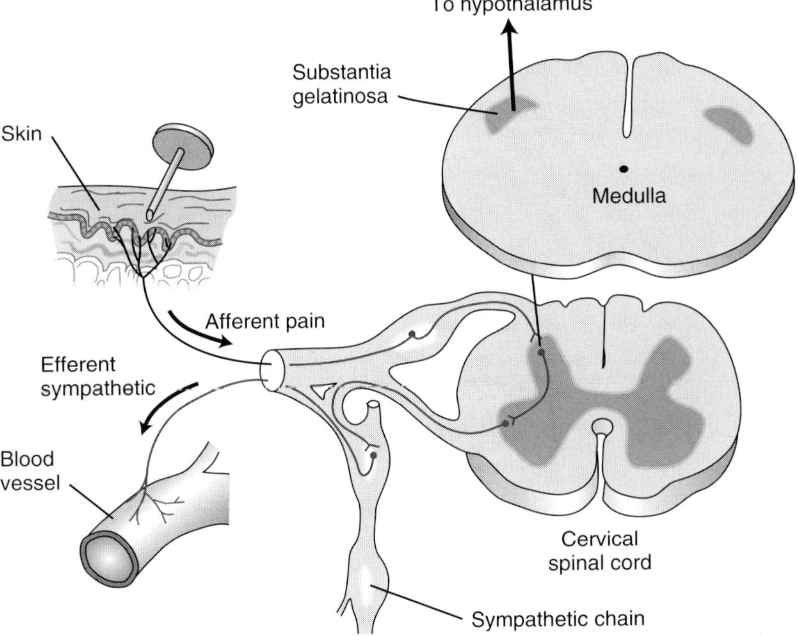

FIGURE 58–1. Diagram of the spinal cord, the anterior and posterior horns, the dorsal and ventral roots, and the main nerve trunk. Also, the afferent sensory fibers from the skin with the cell body in the posterior ganglions; the efferent sympathetic fibers from the anterior horn through the white ramus; a synapse in the sympathetic ganglion; and a postganglionic fiber through the peripheral nerve to the blood vessels. The preganglionic fibers reach the sympathetic ganglion through the white ramus, and the postganglionic fibers rejoin the major nerve through the gray matter.

degree. The varying gradations of compressive force and the amount of time that the nerve is compressed affect the severity of sensory and motor changes. If severe entrapment or compression persists for several weeks, recovery may be delayed and incomplete (Seddon, 1972; Sunderland, 1978) (Fig. 58–2).

Minimal and mild mechanical nerve compression of relatively short duration results in momentary changes in the nerve that are due to both a mechanical and ionic alteration of conduction. Recovery is usually complete. A more severe form of mechanical compression is associated with structural changes due to both compressive and shear forces, resulting in paranodal myelin intussusception at the nodes of Ranvier. This is an acute focal compression as seen in a systemic condition with bulbous myelin lesions with segmental tapering of the internodal segments that occurs in chronic long-standing nerve entrapment. This change occurs away from the actual site of compression and may be either proximal or distal. After segmental demyelinization, there is healing and segmental remyelinization. The basement membrane is intact, and in a first-degree compressive lesion, total degeneration of the proximal area does not occur. After a compressive injury, speed of recovery of anatomical realignment and function correlates with severity and duration of the initial and subsequent injury (Baba et al, 1982; Lundborg, 1970; Mackinnon and Dellon, 1986; Ochoa, et al., 1972) (Fig. 58–3).

When or if to decompress an entrapped nerve depends

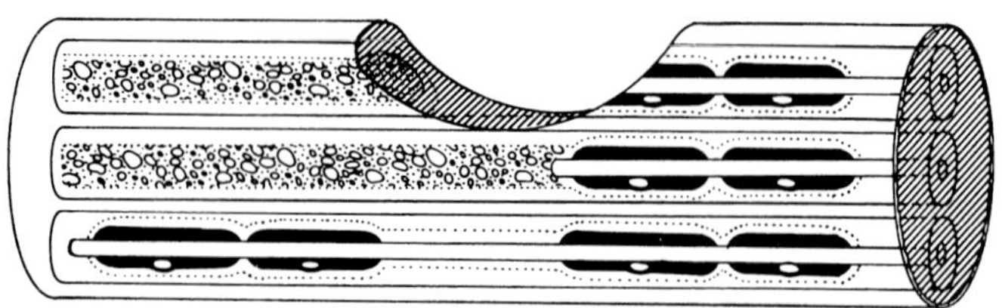

FIGURE 58–3. Diagram of a complex nerve injury. Three fascicles are represented, each with a single myelinated nerve fiber within a connective tissue sheath. Varying degrees of damage have occurred to each fascicle. Axon 1 shows a missing segment that may require a nerve graft or an orientation tube, axon 2 shows wallerian degeneration, and axon 3 shows neuropraxia without wallerian degeneration. (From Jabalay M, Williams HB [eds]: Stewart JD: Electrodiagnostic techniques in the evaluation of nerve compressions and injuries in the upper limb. Hand Clin North Am 2:685, 1986.)

primarily on frequent clinical assessment, and in certain instances, electrical studies are necessary and helpful. The severity of the problem must be assessed from time to time, the author's and "severity classification" includes that of Seddon, Sunderland, and the prognosis factor that we have included that considers the length of time necessary for recovery once the compressive force is eliminated (Seddon, 1975; Sunderland, 1968).

Group 1—a momentary compressive force occurs that lasts for seconds or minutes (Seddon system—neurapraxia; Sunderland system—first-degree lesion). Sensory fibers

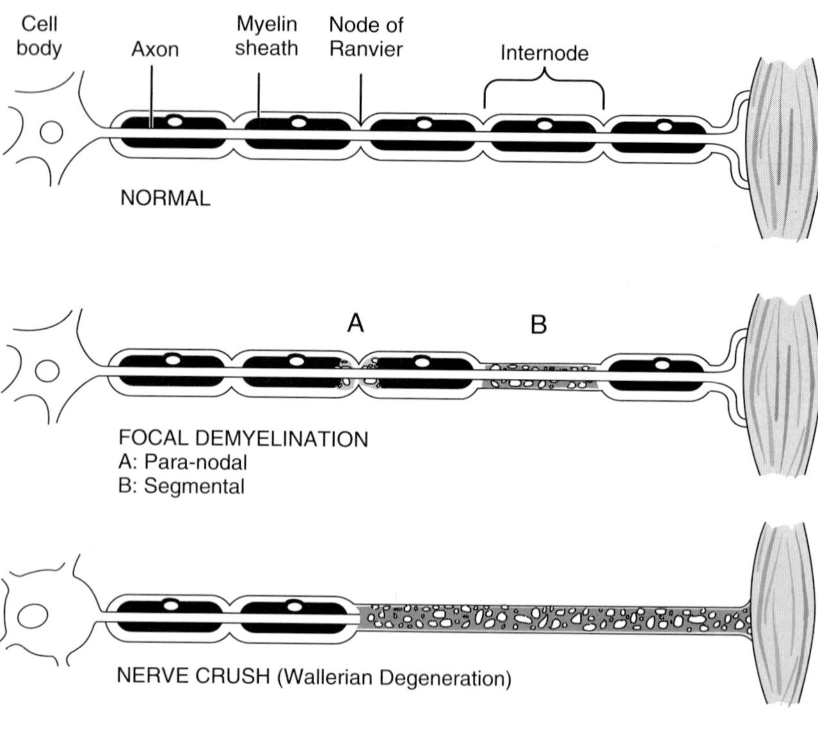

FIGURE 58–2. Diagram of a single myelinated nerve fiber showing the kinds of damage that may occur with focal demyelinization, either from nerve crush or laceration. In the nerve crush or laceration, there is complete wallerian degeneration from the point of trauma distally. A certain degree of regeneration occurs in the nerve crush lesion, but the quantity depends on the severity and duration of the crush and the extent of damage to the blood supply.

Regeneration after a nerve laceration depends on end-to-end repair of axonal tissue, blood supply, and the amount of fibrosis. (Modified from Stewart JD: Focal Peripheral Neuropathies. New York, Elsevier, 1987, p 9.)

are usually affected initially because the patient complains of varying degrees of tingling. Hypesthesia may be mild, moderate, or severe but quickly disappears as compressive forces are eliminated.

Group 2—nerves in this group undergo brief temporary compression due to mechanical and vascular causes that lasts for hours and days. Recovery is eventually complete (Seddon system—neurapraxia; Sunderland system—first-degree lesion). Electromyographic studies are normal, but sensory conduction is frequently delayed and motor conduction may or may not be affected.

Group 3—nerves in this group show a temporary delay of conduction with diminished motor and sensory function that may last for weeks or months even though the nerve is intact (Seddon system—axonotmesis; Sunderland system—second- or third-degree lesion). The conduction alterations are mechanical, ionic, and ischemic. Electrical conduction is delayed, and latency is prolonged.

Group 4—these nerves show a prolonged, partial permanent interruption of nerve conduction even though the nerve is intact. These lesions may persist for months or years, and complete recovery usually does not occur (Seddon system—neurotmesis; Sunderland system—third- or fourth-degree lesion). The electrical studies show abnormal action potentials, delayed conduction velocity, and prolonged latency. The prognosis for full recovery is poor, although partial recovery does occur.

Group 5—a total permanent lesion because the nerve is not in continuity. (Seddon system—neurotmesis; Sunderland system—fifth-degree lesion). All electrical studies are abnormal. There are denervation action potentials, and conduction times and latency are not recordable.

Nerve lesions in groups 1 and 2 show complete recovery; group 3 may have a moderate residual alteration that is not severe; groups 4 and 5 are complete lesions without significant recovery unless the nerves are repaired (Goldner, 1984).

Differentiation of Entrapment Lesions

The more severe the compression and the longer the duration of compression, the greater is the change in axons and their surrounding myelin sheaths and perineural tissues. Ischemic and mechanical alterations occur simultaneously (see Fig. 58–3).

A True Neuroma. A true neuroma is a mass of entangled axons and fibroblasts from epineurium, perineurium, and endoneurium. The lesion is caused by a contusion, constriction, or partial or complete laceration accompanied by varying degrees of ischemia. The lesion is called a neuroma in continuity, a spindle neuroma, or a partial neuroma in continuity. These lesions allow incomplete or no conduction associated with varying degrees of axoplasm flow (Matthews and Osterholm, 1972).

A Bulb Neuroma. A bulb neuroma is a complete neuroma arising from the proximal segment of a completely lacerated nerve. Axons and fibrous tissue proliferate in the proximal segment, and in the distal segment a fibroma occurs. The proximal neuroma and distal fibroma (bulbs) may be joined by a heavy strand of fibrous tissue that gives the nerve the appearance of continuity. Palpation of the bulbs between the examiner's thumb and index fingernails, however, readily demonstrates the bulbs and the fibrous interval between them. There is no axon flow and no electrical conduction in this segment.

A Pseudoneuroma. A pseudoneuroma lesion is secondary to external compression and ischemia that results in thickening of the epineurium and secondary changes in the perineurium. The axons are uniform, and they show no proliferation or irregularities. The lesion has the gross appearance of a spindle neuroma in that the epineurium and perineurium are thick but the axons are uniform as seen in perineural fibrosis of a plantar digital nerve (Morton's neuroma).

Diagnosis of Nerve Entrapment Syndromes

Subjective and objective data referable to the involved region of the musculoskeletal system is obtained from the patient in a logical sequence.

Presenting Symptom. The patient describes the anatomical location, and the examiner attempts to determine whether this is a conventional anatomical distribution, if the pain is referred, or if both possibilities exist. Causative factors are obtained by encouraging the patient to recall any incidents that were unusual. The examiner then gives suggestions that might remind the patient about possible causes of the symptom.

Historical Information. The patient's occupation, daily activities, the pain pattern, localization of the symptom, and the intensity of pain based on a scale of 1 (minimal) to 10 (severe) are determined. Was there a specific injury or surgical operative procedure that preceded the onset? The details of onset of pain as it relates to a particular event are clarified. A daily diary that reflects work; sleep pattern; standing, sitting, and sleeping postures; driving, walking, running, and other physical or sedentary activities is prepared, and the examiner attempts to determine whether these activities affect the complaint. The severity of the current complaints is compared with prior complaints at specified times to determine whether the condition is progressive.

Medications. Pharmacological agents may cause paresthesias, vasospasm, excessive sweating, or other complaints that are similar to or may augment a peripheral neuropathy. The physician should document patient's chronic use of analgesic or anti-inflammatory medications.

Physical Examination. A meticulous clinical assessment is performed by examining the skin texture, sensibility of the area involved and by determining hypesthesia, hyperesthesia, and hyperpathia, or areas that show allodynia and paresthesias with stroking or light percussion. Regardless of the symptom, the patient is unrobed, and an overview of the general musculoskeletal system is conducted. Range of neck motion is determined, movement of the upper extremities is observed, intrinsic muscles of the hand are tested, and the joints are palpated and put through a range of motion to determine whether there is evidence of systemic disease.

When lower extremity pain is the presenting symptom, the range of back motion is tested, the spine is percussed, chest expansion is measured, and range of motion of the hip joints is tested and recorded.

Muscle tone, strength, and size of the glutei, hamstrings, quadriceps, and triceps surae and anterior compartment muscles are determined. Sciatic and femoral stretch tests are done, and muscle strength during active motion and resistance is determined in the thigh, the calf, and the hips. Tiptoe and heel walking quickly demonstrate areas of local muscle weakness.

The peripheral vascular pulses in the groin, popliteal area, medial ankle region, and the dorsum of the foot are palpated. The knee and ankle reflexes are tested with and without reinforcement and dermatome topography is outlined.

Foot and knee stability are observed, pertinent tendon sheaths are palpated, and the vascular status of the extremity is tested. The patient's gait is observed to determine if there is a leg length discrepancy, muscle weakness, or an antalgic gait.

Regional and Local Tests Used to Determine Nerve Sensitivity

A *stretch test* affects nerve gliding and implies entrapment if the usual range of motion of the segment is limited because of pain or paresthesias. The nerve being assessed for possible tethering or compression is tested with the extremity in different positions. For example, the L5 nerve root nerve is evaluated using the following tests.

Straight leg raising is performed with the patient in a sitting position. Physiological lordosis is determined, and the extremity is adducted to place maximum tension on the sciatic nerve and its nerve roots. With the knee joint straight, the extremity is flexed without allowing the patient to round the back to a point at which extremity or back pain are recognized by the patient. If pain occurs at 40 degrees of flexion with the knee straight, *foot dorsiflexion* is then performed passively, and if pain is aggravated, there is probable tethering or excessive tension on the nerve or a block of nerve root gliding, or a segment of the lumbosacroplexus or the sciatic nerve is affected by a lesion. Once pain is recognized with foot elevation, *head flexion* is performed to determine if pain is worsened or improved. If the pain is worsened, the enlargement or fibrosis that is tethering the nerve root is directly under the nerve or superior to it. Conversely, if head flexion diminishes the pain, the disc fragment or osteophyte is below the nerve root in the axilla and the nerve gliding is cephalad away from the mass. The same test is repeated in the supine position; the knee is straight, the extremity is adducted and flexed at the hip, and the position of the extremity when pain is reproduced is noted. *Forced elevation of the foot,* depending on the location of the mass that is tethering the nerves, will either alleviate or aggravate the pain. *Head flexion* is then performed to determine whether cephalad motion of the spinal cord and nerve roots relieves the pain. These positions of pain production should be consistent whether the patient is *sitting, supine,* or *standing.*

The *femoral stretch test* is performed when the patient is prone. In this test, the *thigh is adducted* and extended, after which the leg is slowly flexed on the thigh. This test applies traction to the L2 and L3 roots, which are not tested during *straight leg raising.*

Tendon reflexes at the knee and ankle are graded according to their activity by direct tapping below the patella and above the calcaneus. *Reinforcement* by minimal contraction of the quadriceps or calf muscle is used if ordinary tapping does not elicit a response. If neither activity results in involuntary movement of the foot or leg, the *muscle belly* is tapped directly.

Sensibility of the skin of the thigh, calf, and foot is determined by having the patient slowly and gently pass his or her fingertips circumferentially around the extremity at several different levels from the thigh to the dorsum of the foot. The patient will detect asymmetrical sensibility such as hypesthesia, hyperesthesia, or hyperpathia much quicker, and at times, more accurately than the examiner. However, if this test is performed with a sharp pin point, the patient receives several pin punctures and the test is not always accurate. If a straight pin is placed through a tongue blade, and this is used as a method of circumferentially testing the extremity without puncturing the skin, variations in sensibility are readily determined and the areas are marked off so that the *dermatomes* are visible.

The patient's *gait* is observed for several steps while he or she does toe walking and heel walking to place the calf muscles and the dorsiflexor muscles under tension and fatigue. A single test of strength in dorsiflexion may be spurious, whereas after the patient walks several steps on the heels, the dorsiflexor muscles may weaken if they are not normal.

The *nerve percussion test* is done. If it is lightly tapped, an exposed, normal, or a sensitive abnormal peripheral nerve may result in paresthesias in the autonomous zone of the nerve. The *percussion test* has different significance than determining whether *Tinel's sign* is present or absent. The terms are incorrectly used interchangeably. A *positive percussion test* may be obtained by tapping a healthy normal nerve in the ulnar groove when the elbow is flexed. Paresthesias (the sensation of an electrical shock) occur distally in the ring and little fingers, but retrograde percussion of that nerve is usually negative. The uncomfortable sensations occur only at the point of subcutaneous exposure. The positive percussion test is frequently present in a normal person over the median nerve at the wrist, the tibial nerve at the ankle, the peroneal nerve at the knee, and the ulnar nerve at the elbow.

When the examiner attempts to determine whether there is a *positive percussion* test associated with a pathological lesion, the test should be performed distal to proximal and then directly over the area of a sensitive cutaneous or a major mixed nerve. The percussion test localizes the position of the nerve, whether it is pathological or not, and gives information about the degree of sensitivity and whether or not the nerve is sensitive to retrograde percussion, antegrade tapping, or only directly over the nerve.

Nerve Excursion (Gliding)

One way of localizing an entrapped nerve is to stretch it by moving the joints distal to the area of entrapment and thereby producing increased pressure or irritation of the nerve reflected by paresthesias as stretch occurs. If entrapment is present, maximum stretch should be applied for a long enough time to produce paresthesias. This time varies from a few seconds to a minute.

Nerves undergo excursion because of the outer epineurium and the inner layers of perineurium and endoneurium. If fibrosis occurs external to the nerve and limits gliding, sensory receptors are stimulated and pain occurs. If fibrosis is extensive, the nerve may be compressed if the foot is stretched. If a ruptured disc is located under a nerve root, the somatic and autonomic fibers are compressed and ischemia also occurs locally. This factor aggravates pain. This same mechanism of fibrosis, entrapment by a small opening in the bone or fascia, or diminished elasticity of collagen occurs at many different locations in the body. Compression or entrapment of the nerve may occur with or without ischemia. If collagen elasticity diminishes rapidly, nerve excursion may be diminished and compression and entrapment worsen. Surgical decompression may be necessary, and the purpose is to lessen external compression on the nerve and improve excursion and, indirectly, to eliminate the mechanical irritation and to improve the nerve vascularity.

The Significance of Tinel's Sign

Tinel described a "formication sign" related to axon regeneration (Tinel, 1918). "When percussion is lightly applied to the injured nerve trunk, we find in the cutaneous region of the nerve a creeping sensation usually compared by the patient to that caused by electricity" (Tinel, 1918). The patient best understands this sensation if the examiner asks "do you feel pins or needles or do you feel anything like your funny bone was hit?." These sensations are not readily determined in the child, but if the examiner watches the child's expression and interprets the withdrawal of the extremity properly, a positive percussion test may be elicited in the child as well as in the adult. Percussion should begin distally and progress proximally to avoid the unpleasant sensation that occurs when the point of nerve fibrosis, entrapment, injury, or repair is tapped directly. The term Tinel's sign should be reserved for regenerating nerves after a nerve laceration has been repaired or after a severely compressed nerve has been decompressed. Conversely, the term percussion test should be used for nerves that are subject to irritation from compression or from normal exposure, but the test does not determine if axons are regenerating at a specific rate. The average speed of regeneration of a peripheral nerve is 1 mm a day or 25 mm a month in the adult and two or three times that speed in the child.

External Pressure Applied to a Nerve to Determine Abnormal Nerve Sensitivity or Compression

If the examiner applies about 10 lb of direct pressure at a point of 1 to 2 cm proximal to an area of suspected entrapment or compression, distal paresthesias occur. In this location, axoplasm is congregated and enlarged, and compression or percussion demonstrates hypersensitivity. At least two changes occur with the compression test:

1. Compression of the peroneal nerve at the knee, for example, bowstrings the nerve. This causes nerve gliding proximally at the point of fibrosis or compression and results in stimulation of pain receptors at the site of entrapment.

2. Digital pressure on an area of enlarged axoplasm causes irritation and temporary ischemia of a sensitive nerve that produces distal paresthesias. A patient with a known tibial nerve compression or entrapment lesion at the fibrous origin of the abductor hallucis muscle demonstrates a positive compression test about 2 cm proximal to the point of entrapment. Continuous firm pressure applied at that proximal location causes a rapid onset of paresthesias, whereas the same test performed on the opposite uninvolved side does not cause the same sensation.

NERVE COMPRESSIVE OR ENTRAPMENT LESIONS OF THE LOW BACK

Nerve root compression or entrapment may occur distal to the posterior sensory ganglion in the common nerve root after the motor and sensory fibers have joined and the autonomic nerve fibers have formed the sympathetic nerve chain. The subjective complaints may be back pain; referred buttock pain; anterior, lateral, or posterior thigh numbness; or hyperesthesia and paresthesias into the lower extremity in a dermatome distribution. If L2–3 roots are involved, the pain pattern or the dermatome may be in the groin and the anterior thigh; pain from the fourth lumbar nerve root radiates to the inner distal thigh and knee region; and pain from the fifth lumbar root is in the buttock, lateral thigh, and the great toe. The S1 nerve root pain distribution is posterior thigh, calf, and plantar surface of the foot. Motor weakness varies with the severity of the entrapment.

Mechanisms of Nerve Root Entrapment

See Figure 58–4.

Intervertebral Disc

A bulge of the annulus due to moderate displacement of the nucleus pulposus may be central, lateral, or far lateral location. The location of pain, whether it be dermatome, myotome, or sclerotome, depends on the particular nerve roots involved and the affected interspace.

Hypermobile Posterior Bone Elements or a Neural Arch Defect

In spondylosis or spondylolisthesis, hypermobile posterior bone elements and a neural arch defect show a minimal dermatome pain pattern but a greater myotome and sclerotome pain distribution. If the spinal instability involves L4 on L5, the L4 nerve root may be affected. If operation is necessary, that root is decompressed by opening the L3–4

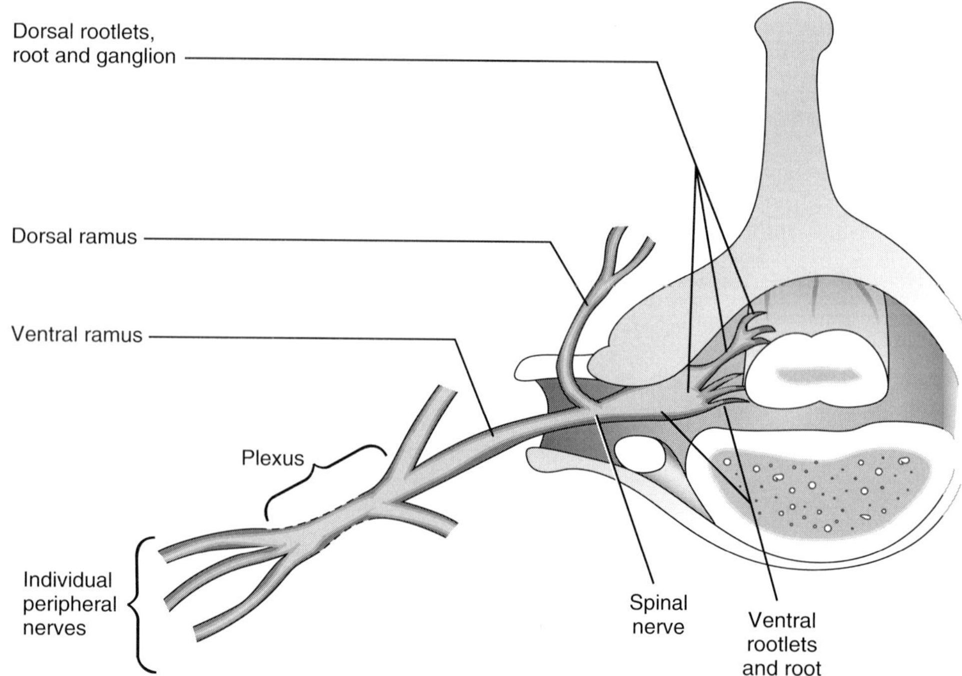

FIGURE 58–4. Diagram of a cross section of a vertebral body, posterior elements, cauda equina, and nerve roots. The rootlets are the motor fibers that are released in certain patients with muscle spasticity. Diminution of spasticity may occur after this operation. The nerve roots join to form a plexus, which, in turn, gives rise to a peripheral nerve. (Modified from Stewart JD: Focal Peripheral Neuropathies. New York, Elsevier, 1987, p 219.)

posterior interspace to approach the L4 root adjacent to the abnormal neural arch.

Facet Hypertrophy with Osteophytes

Facet hypertrophy with osteophytes constrict the nerve root foramina and irritate the root in flexion, lateral bending, or extension.

Radicular Canal

The radicular canal is smaller because of degeneration of the intervertebral disc, narrowing of the intervertebral interspace, and osteophyte formation that cause nerve root compression in certain patients. If this compression occurs slowly and if the nerve has adequate elasticity, the patient's symptoms may be minimal.

Large Sensory Ganglion or a Conjoined Nerve Root

A large sensory ganglion or conjoined nerve root within or proximal to the foramen results in compression of the enlarged neural structures and pain that follows an aberrant distribution.

Far Lateral Extruded Intervertebral Disc

The far lateral extruded intervertebral disc may not be seen on the magnetic resonance imaging (MRI) scan, myelogram, or computed tomography (CT) scan; but the CT-myelogram or the discogram demonstrates the defect in the annulus, and the ruptured nucleus will be localized in an aberrant position.

Herniation of the Dural Sac

Hermation of the dural sac due to trauma or prior operation distorts the nerve root so that it is angled or entrapped, and this problem may cause pain. Intradural rupture of the intervertebral disc occurs occasionally, and this rupture compresses the cauda equina.

Dural Cyst or a Neurilemmoma

A dural cyst, neurilemmoma or neurofibroma may compress or involve the nerve root. There are many clinical diagnoses that describe these problems. The most frequent are (Fig. 58–5)

1. A bulging intervertebral disc.
2. A ruptured intervertebral disc.
3. Radicular canal stenosis.
4. Central-radicular canal spinal stenosis.
5. Soft tissue lesions or anomalies affecting the nerve roots.

THE LOW BACK—NERVE ROOT CLINICAL SYNDROME

The problem is analyzed and the diagnosis determined in a logical sequence (Goldner and Bright, 1980a). The history of onset, duration, distribution, and localization of pain during a 24-hour cycle is determined, and questions concerning the pain pattern are posed. These are concerned with how

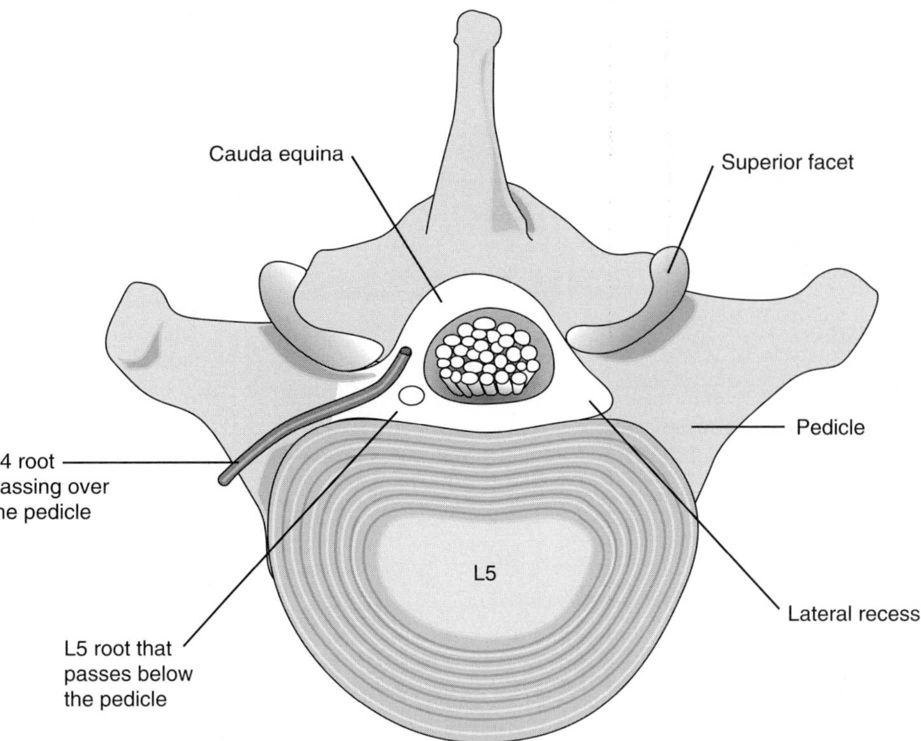

FIGURE 58–5. Cross section of the 5th lumbar interspace, with the intervertebral disc between L4 and L5 designated. The L5 root is medial to the L4 root and opposite the intervertebral disc at the L4–L5 interspace. At this space, the L4 root is lateral to the L5. L4 is more central opposite the L3–L4 interspace. Surgically, the L5 root is exposed after the ligamentum flavum is removed at the L4–L5 interspace posteriorly. The L5 root passes below the pedicle of L5 and the L4 root passes over or above the pedicle. Thus, the L4 root is below the pedicle of L4 and the L5 root is below the pedicle of L5. (Modified from Stewart JD: Focal Peripheral Neuropathies. New York, Elsevier, 1987, p 219.)

the pain is relieved, the effect of rest on the pain, how activity may aggravate the pain, and how posture whether in flexion or extension affects the pain pattern.

Age Group. Patients from 20 to 40 years of age are usually affected by problem with the intervertebral disc or spondylolisthesis; patients aged 40 to 60 years may have radicular canal stenosis, spinal stenosis, intervertebral disc disease, or vascular insufficiency.

Cauda equina stenosis results in ischemia that causes pain. Claudication from iliac artery disease is differentiated by exercise pattern, position of relief, and vascular studies.

Physical Examination. This examination includes range of back motion, attempted pain production by *percussion,* right and left *lateral bending,* and trunk *flexion* and *extension* to produce pain. In spondylolisthesis, extension rather than flexion usually causes pain. If the intervertebral disc in the axilla of the nerve root is compressing the left root, right lateral bending aggravates and left lateral bending decreases pain. If the intervertebral disc is outside the left axilla, right lateral bending may relieve pain and left lateral bending may aggravate pain.

Straight leg raising is performed (see earlier discussion).

Popliteal compression is performed if the straight leg raising test is positive. The examiner compresses the peroneal nerve in the popliteal area just medial to the biceps tendon with the extremity straight and under tension. If nerve compression causes back pain or paresthesias, this bowstringing results in a selective positive test and differentiates nerve root pain from hamstring tightness. The tibial nerve may be compressed in the same way, but the distribution of pain is the posterior calf and the plantar surface of the foot.

Femoral nerve stretch is performed (see earlier discussion).

Potential atrophy of the buttock is determined if an S1 nerve root compressive lesion is present, the gluteus maximus will show loss of tone and atrophy on the involved side.

Material and Methods

The primary source of this material is the authors' clinical experience during the past 45 years. An accurate diagnosis was the guide to successful treatment. Iatrogenic lesions are discussed, and methods of prevention are suggested. Other lesions are described in order to guide the clinician through a logical assessment for an accurate diagnosis.

Clinical Material—Examples of Entrapment Syndrome

Demographics. The true incidence of specific entrapment lesions is difficult to determine because almost all patients with this condition were referred to our tertiary care center. Prevalence, however, was determined by a trend. There were more patients with common peroneal nerve compression than with primary sciatic nerve compression. However, the largest number of patients had lumbar and lumbosacral nerve root compression syndromes.

Lumbosacral Nerve Root Compression

SYMPTOMS

Pain is the primary symptom. Pain may occur in the back, the buttock, or the lower extremity. The dermatome distribution varies according to the root involved and the location of the compressive material. There are usually two categories of pain or discomfort:

1. The dermatome hypesthesia, hyperesthesia, or paresthesias.

2. The deep dull aching pain that represents the myotome or the sclerotome. The pain usually varies according to the patient's activities.

Diagnosis

The diagnosis is determined based on the history; a daily diary listing conditions that aggravate or alleviate the pain; and a clinical examination that includes muscle strength, nerve stretch tests, sensibility alterations, gait changes, and range of spine, hip, and knee and ankle motion.

IMAGING STUDIES

These studies include routine radiographs with oblique exposures to show neural arch status; lateral flexion extension radiographs if stability is questioned; and an anteroposterior image of the pelvis to observe the hip joints, sacroiliac joints, or other critical areas of the pelvis. Additional studies include CT, myelogram with CT, discogram followed by a CT, and MRI with or without gallium. A technetium-99m bone scan is helpful.

ELECTRICAL STUDIES

Electrical studies include sensory, motor nerve conduction, needle, and cutaneous electromyography in order to localize the site of nerve entrapment. Inching determinations give better localization of entrapment than routine nerve conduction alone. Somatosensory evoked potential may detect a proximal lesion when the distal findings are not positive other than pain radiation.

PATHOLOGICAL LESIONS—VARIATIONS (Fig. 58–6)

The most common intervertebral disc pathology is at L4–5 involving the L5 nerve root unilaterally, bilaterally, or centrally. The annulus may be partially or completely torn, and the nucleus migrates peripherally. The annulus may bulge in the center, medial to the root, or directly under the root, or lateral to the root (Fig. 58–7). Part of the nucleus may be extruded, and part may remain in the center of the interspace. A free fragment of nucleus is separated from the annulus and may migrate directly opposite the interspace or above or below the interspace. A fragment of nucleus may rupture through the dura.

Other lesions may compress the nerve root such as osteophytes, a trifoil thickened posterior canal, and a diffuse spinal stenosis. If the entire cauda equina is compressed, claudication occurs. Radicular canal stenosis may affect only one nerve root.

Incongruity of the interspace reduces the size of the foramina and the radicular canal, and indirectly compresses the nerve root. Hypermobility of the vertebral bodies may be due to intervertebral disc disease that weakens the disc bond. The posterior elements may be hypermobile and cause direct compression of the nerve roots or cauda equina. Sclerosis or hypertrophy of the facet joints may indirectly compress a nerve root.

TREATMENT

Treatment begins once the severity of the clinical syndrome is determined and the stability of the spine is assessed. Moderate pain unaccompanied by neurological deficit is managed by limited activity, diminished axial loading, lessening of sitting, and a mild exercise program. The patient either stands or lies down, but avoids sitting and axial loading. Several weeks of limited activity may concur with shrinkage of the bulging or displaced nucleus. Dermatome changes and reflex alterations with minimal muscle weakness are reversible. The decision either to operate or to observe depends on the patient's occupation, age, and

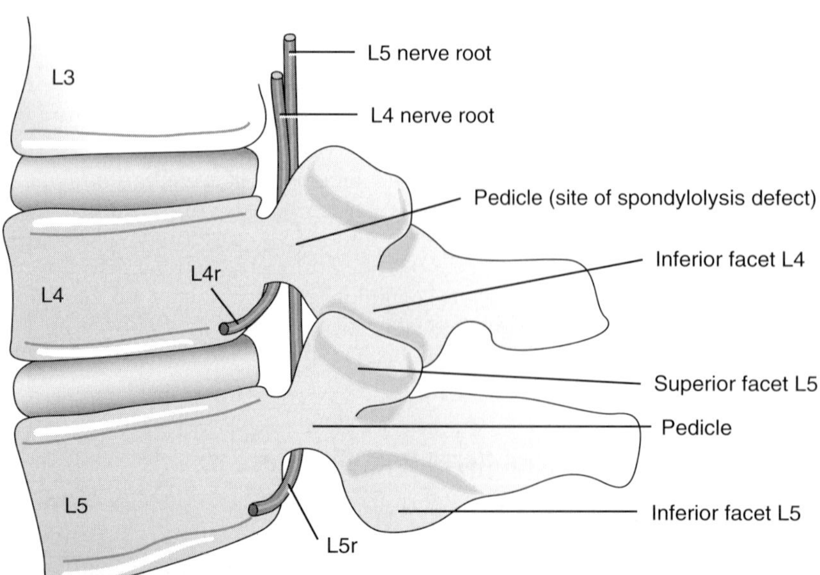

FIGURE 58–6. A lateral diagram showing the anatomical relationships between the nerve roots, the vertebral bodies, the intervertebral discs, and the pedicles. A posterior disc rupture at the L4–L5 interspace compresses the L5 root. A far lateral disc rupture at the L4–L5 interspace may compress the L4 root rather than the L5 root. Similarly, a posterior disc rupture at L3–L4 interspace compresses the L4 root and affects the quadriceps muscle. The examiner must then depend on a femoral stretch test rather than a sciatic stretch to provoke thigh pain.

Spondylolisthesis at L4 on L5 requires decompression of the L4 nerve root by entering the L3–L4 posterior interspace and following the L4 root under the fibrocartilage pedicle of L4. (Modified from Stewart JD: Focal Peripheral Neuropathies. New York, Elsevier, 1987, p 219.)

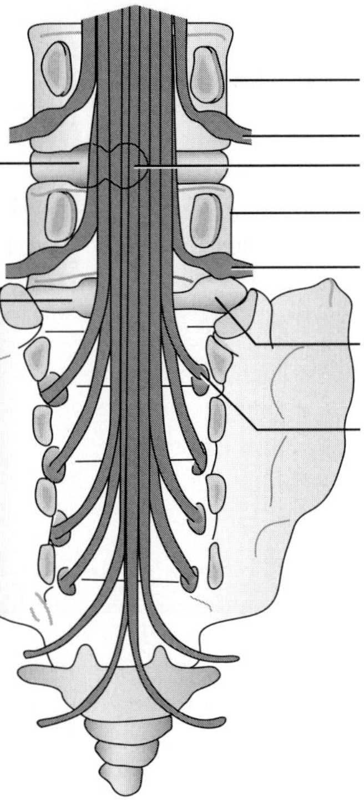

FIGURE 58–7. Diagram of the dorsal view of the lumbar and sacral intervertebral discs, vertebral bodies, and the relationship of the spinal nerves to these structures. There is a central disc protrusion at the L4–L5 interspace, which affects primarily the L5 and the S1 nerve roots. The lesion is transverse, and affects the lower and central roots. This diagram shows the reasons for different roots being compressed even though the disc protrusion is at a specific interspace. The far lateral protrusion of the L5–S1 disc, in particular, affects the L5 nerve root rather than the S1 root because of the far lateral position. (Modified from Stewart JD: Focal Peripheral Neuropathies. New York, Elsevier, 1987, p 220.)

whether or not the motor and sensory changes are stationary, regressing, or progressive.

If the patient has spondylolysis or spondylolisthesis, the method of management is similar to that described. A displaced vertebra or a loose posterior element are not an indication for surgery. However, if nerve root compression persists, if motor weakness increases, and if pain is not relieved by limited activity, then surgical treatment is indicated (Leonard, 1967).

Nerve root irritation alone is usually managed by decompression of the nerve root without fusion. An unstable spine, however, is best managed by arthrodesis in conjunction with nerve root decompression.

Selection of Approach for Decompression. Uncomplicated intervertebral disc disease with nerve root irritation is usually managed by localized intervertebral discectomy and minimal laminectomy. Microdiscectomy is acceptable if one is trained in performing that procedure. Macrodiscectomy is acceptable.

Alternative Methods of Managing Nerve Root Compression. Suction discectomy has not yet reached a consensus of all surgeons who treat intervertebral disc disease. More data are necessary to determine if this procedure is equivalent to open discectomy.

Chymopapain continues to be used by some surgeons. The dosage of the chymopapain has been reduced, the technique for inserting the material has been altered, and there are many series that are successful. However, there have been complications associated with the procedure, even though the exact cause of the complication has not always been determined.

Anterior discectomy and fusion are reserved for recurrent persistent nerve root compression after failed prior discectomy. Occasionally an abnormal intervertebral disc is removed primarily from the anterior approach after the lesion has been documented by discography. The anterior approach is also useful if there has been prior posterior infection or causalgia affecting the nerve roots.

Posterior lumbar interbody fusion is used by some surgeons. The major disadvantage is the extensive laminectomy needed to expose the cauda equina, the dura, and the nerve roots. An option to the interbody fusion is an anterior retroperitoneal removal of the disc and bone grafting complemented by a direct posterior decompression and posterolateral fusion. Minimal additional decompression of the cauda equina and the nerve roots may be necessary. The extent of the decompression depends on the pathology.

Incisions. The lumbar spine and lumbosacral region may be exposed from a posterior vertical incision or a horizontal incision. There are several different ways to perform the operation using the anterior approach: (1) a paramedian retroperitoneal approach; (2) a flank incision for anterior only or for combined anteroposterior exposure; (3) a transabdominal incision for anterior exposure (Hollingshead, 1969).

LOW BACK—CUTANEOUS NERVE COMPRESSIVE LESION OF THE GLUTEAL REGION AND THIGH

Anterior Division of the Twelfth Thoracic Nerve

This nerve communicates with the first lumbar nerve and also with the iliohypogastric nerve of the lumbar plexus. The lateral cutaneous branch of the last thoracic nerve is large and does not divide into an anterior and posterior branch. It descends over the iliac crest in front of the lateral cutaneous branch of the iliohypogastric and is distributed to the skin of the front part of the gluteal region. Some of its elements extend as low as the greater trochanter.

CLINICAL SYNDROME

The twelfth thoracic nerve may be affected by surgical procedures around the posterior and lateral aspects of the pelvis or the trunk. If the nerve is lacerated or forcibly retracted, postoperative hypesthesia or hypersensitivity, or both, may result. Other conditions that affect the nerve are constricting bands around the waist such as a belt or elastic in either a thin individual or in a diabetic person with a sensitive nerve.

TREATMENT

If a surgical procedure preceded the onset of the complaint, a period of observation, percussion tests, and a local nerve block of sensitive areas will usually determine if progressive improvement is occurring or if hypersensitivity persists because of a neuroma. If nonoperative treatment for several months is unsuccessful, then either a neurolysis or a neurectomy and bipolar cauterization of the distal segment usually relieves the pain. The area of hypesthesia will gradually diminish, and the patient learns to cope.

Anatomy—Posterior Cutaneous Branches

POSTERIOR DIVISIONS OF THE SPINAL NERVES
(Gray, 1936; Hollingshead, 1969)

The *superior cluneal nerves* give off cutaneous nerves that descend across the posterior part of the iliac crest to the skin of the buttock. Some of these nerves run as far as the level of the greater trochanter. This combination of cutaneous nerves from T12 and L1–3 form the cluneal nerves (Goldner, 1956; Goldner and Bright, 1980).

The *inferior cluneal nerves* arise from the lesser sciatic nerve, which is distributed to the skin of the perineum and the posterior surface of the thigh and leg. It arises from the dorsal divisions of the first and second sacral nerves, and from the ventral divisions of the second and third sacral nerves. It passes through the greater sciatic foramen below the piriformis muscle (Arnoldussen and Korten, 1980).

CLUNEAL NERVE SYNDROME

The cluneal nerves are involved most frequently during a surgical incision for a bone graft from the posterior superior iliac spine and the iliac crest through a separate skin incision. Postoperatively, these areas may be hypersensitive due to nerve laceration or forcible retraction. Sensation may be diminished or an area of hyperesthesia may occur. Occasionally, the hypersensitivity, paresthesias, and posterior buttock and thigh pain may be severe enough to warrant aggressive treatment. This is managed by local injections, protection from external compression, a transcutaneous nerve stimulator (Goldner and Hendrix, 1977), and the administration of doxepin (Sinequan), carbamazepine (Tegretol), tricyclics,

and phenytoin (Dilantin). If the local management and the central depressant pain medications do not produce positive results, then surgical excision of the damaged nerves and cauterization of the proximal and distal segments is usually successful.

POSTERIOR PRESACRAL NERVE COMPRESSION SYNDROME

Posterior presacral nerve compression syndrome is a distinct condition that is amenable to treatment. The history indicates that the patients spend several hours a day in the automobile, that their activities may require intermittent forward flexion, and they may have areas of painful fat (Dercum's disease). The area of painful fat compression over the sacrum is usually temporarily relieved by injections of lidocaine and a steroid. The injections alone may diminish the pain, and the problem may gradually improve. If nonoperative treatment is unsuccessful, the painful area remains localized, and other clinical findings are not present, then the lesion is exposed through a horizontal incision under local anesthesia and the lipoma or irregular fatty mass is removed. Usually, there is a blood vessel and a deep nerve in the region where the mass has been removed (Goldner, 1956).

PERINEAL BRANCHES OF THE CLUNEAL (PUDENDAL) NERVE (Fig. 58–8)

The perineal branches of the cluneal (pudendal) nerve are distributed to the skin at the upper and medial side of the thigh. One long perineal branch, the inferior pudendal nerve, curves forward and below and in front of the ischial tuberosity, pierces the fascia lata, and runs forward beneath the superficial fascia to the perineum to the skin of the scrotum and to the labium majus in the female. This nerve may be affected by pressure while riding a bicycle.

ANTERIOR CUTANEOUS NERVES—THIGH

Iliohypogastric Nerve

The iliohypogastric nerve arises from the first lumbar nerve and divides into a lateral and anterior cutaneous branch (Fig. 58–9). The lateral cutaneous branch exits immediately above the iliac crest and is distributed to the skin of the gluteal region behind the lateral cutaneous branch of the last thoracic nerve. The *anterior cutaneous branch* perforates the aponeurosis of the obliquus externus about 2.5 cm. above the subcutaneous inguinal ring and is distributed to the skin of the hypogastric region. This nerve communicates with the last thoracic and the ilioinguinal nerves.

CLINICAL SYNDROME

Trauma, groin incisions in the flank or the retroperitoneal area, or a gridiron incision for an appendectomy may affect the iliohypogastric nerve adversely. Occasionally, herpes zoster follows the course of one or several of these cutaneous nerves.

If an area of hypesthesia or hyperesthesia is recognized,

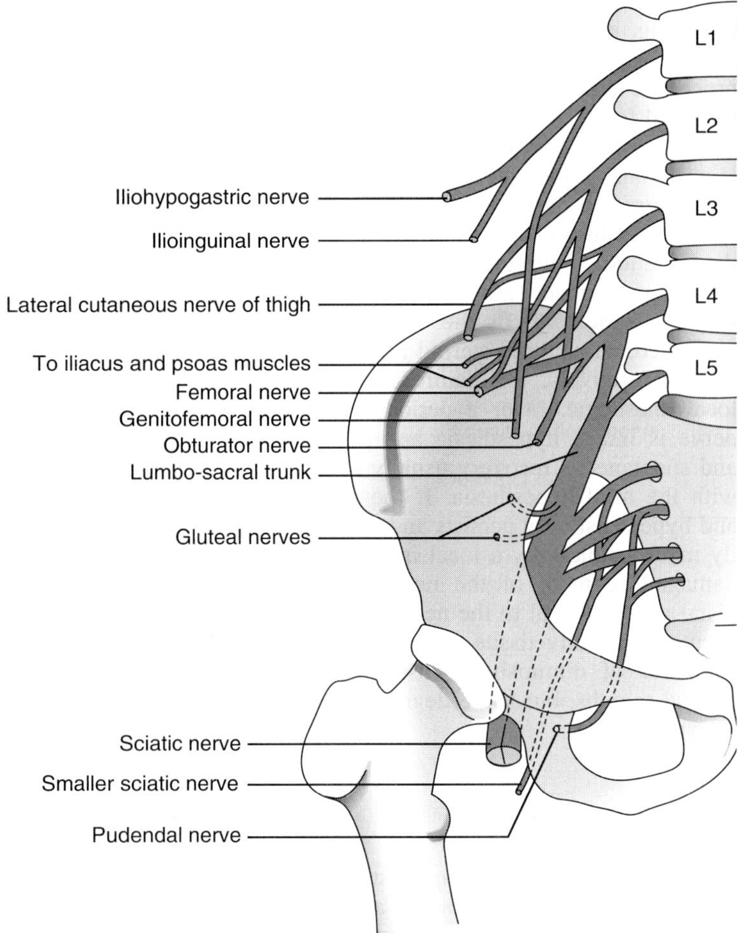

FIGURE 58–8. This diagram shows the nerves involved in peripheral entrapment rather than those adjacent to the vertebral body. The three major nerves arising from L1 are the iliohypogastric, the ilioinguinal, and the genitofemoral nerves. They originate in the retroperitoneal space and exit at the rim of the pelvis. Note the pudendal nerve and the posterior cutaneous nerve of the thigh. (Modified from Stewart JD: Focal Peripheral Neuropathies. New York, Elsevier, 1987, p 253.)

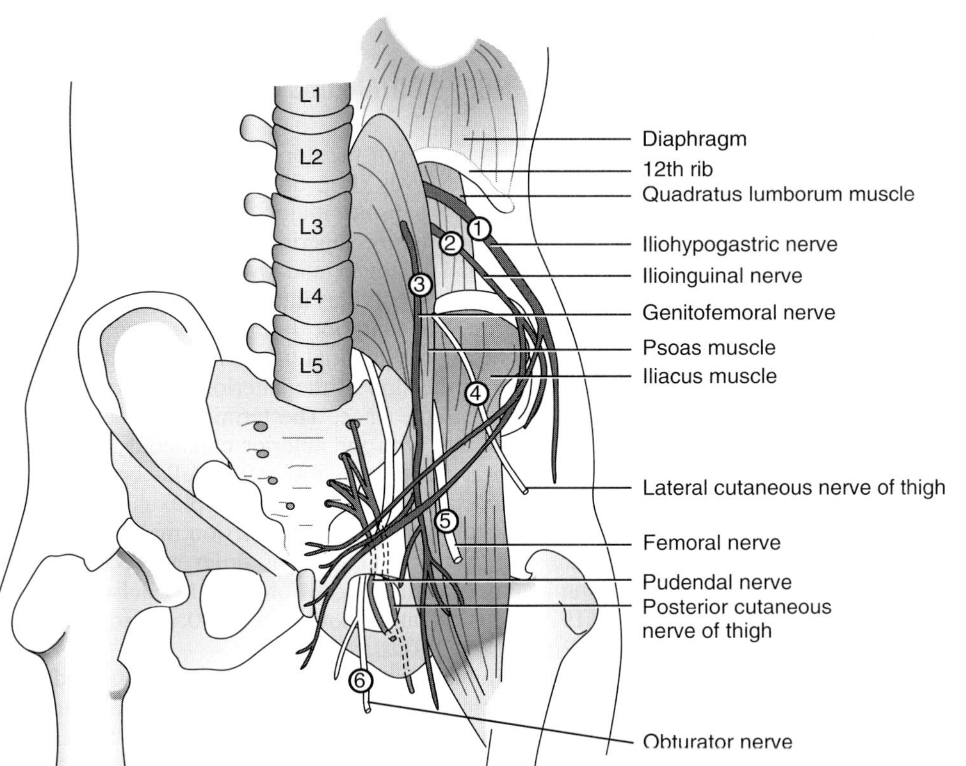

FIGURE 58–9. This diagram emphasizes the major nerves to the groin: iliohypogastric, ilioinguinal, genitofemoral, lateral femoral cutaneous, femoral nerve, obturator nerve. (Modified from Stewart JD: Focal Peripheral Neuropathies. New York, Elsevier, 1987, p 323.)

External Compression

Compression may occur in *obese* individuals, or from a *tight belt* or tight clothing. A prolonged abnormal sitting posture or a *constricting elastic* around the anterior spine region may cause damage to the nerve. Once the compression is recognized and relieved, regeneration usually occurs in several weeks. The hypesthesia and burning are gradually replaced by physiologic sensations (Manicol and Thompson, 1990; Williams and Trzil, 1991).

Removal of a bone graft from the ilium is the most common cause of damage to the lateral femoral cutaneous nerve in the patient undergoing a surgical procedure (see Fig. 58–11). The nerve may be stretched by a self-retaining or hand-held retractor, or it may be compressed or entrapped by fascia as the nerve exits from behind the ilium to its exit foramen. Damage to the nerve during an operative procedure may result in a causalgic syndrome (Goldner and Fleming, 1992).

If pain and paresthesias persist longer than 6 months after the injury and if hypesthesia is present and the percussion test is strongly positive, then nerve decompression or resection, depending on the local pathology, usually lessens the patients reports of pain (Nelson and Ivins, 1965).

FEMORAL CUTANEOUS NERVE—COMPRESSION

The femoral nerve gives off *anterior cutaneous* branches that form the intermediate and medial cutaneous nerves. The intermediate cutaneous nerve pierces the fascial lata about 7.5 cm below the inguinal ligament and divides into two branches, which descend along the forepart of thigh to supply the skin as low as the front of the knee. These branches communicate with the medial cutaneous nerve and the infra-patella branch of the saphenous nerve to form the *patellar plexus* (Hemler et al, 1991). In the upper part of the thigh, the lateral branch of the intermediate cutaneous end communicates with the lumboinguinal branch of the genitofemoral nerve.

The *medial cutaneous* nerve divides into an anterior branch that perforates the fascia lata at the lower third of the thigh and supplies the skin as low as the medial side of the knee and crosses to the lateral side of the patella.

The *posterior branch descends* along the medial border of the sartorius, where it pierces the fascia lata, communicates with the saphenous nerve, gives off subcutaneous branches, and supplies the skin on the medial side of the leg.

The *posterior division of the femoral nerves* gives off the saphenous nerve (Katz, 1989).

SAPHENOUS NERVE ENTRAPMENT—GONALGIA PARESTHETICA (Wartenberg, 1943)

This is the largest cutaneous branch of the femoral nerve. It emerges from behind the lower edge of the aponeurotic covering of the adductor canal (Hunter's canal), where it may be compressed or entrapped. The nerve may be damaged by direct external trauma or internally from a fracture to the femur. Where the nerve pierces the fascia lata between the tendons of the sartorius and gracilis muscles, it becomes subcutaneous and may be damaged at this point. One branch of the nerve courses along the margin of the tibia and ends

at the ankle and the other passes in front of the ankle, and is distributed on the medial side of the foot and communicates with the superficial peroneal nerve. The large infrapatella branch is distributed to the skin in front of the patella. The nerve may be damaged by an incision made to enter the knee joint or one used to isolate the sartorius, gracilis, or semitendinosus muscle. The infrapatellar branch may be damaged during direct arthroscopy, varicose vein stripping, or a displaced fracture of the proximal tibia (Hemler et al, 1991; Kopell and Thompson, 1960; Murayama et al, 1991).

A pes anserine bursa may be large enough to irritate the infrapatellar branch and cause paresthesias. The nerve courses anterior to the medial malleolus and may be damaged in this location when a vein is being isolated for intravenous use. After a Syme amputation, a painful neuroma may develop; or after open reduction of an ankle with incision on the medial side, the saphenous nerve may be injured.

OBTURATOR NEUROPATHY

The obturator nerve is primarily a motor nerve arising from the ventral divisions of the second, third, and fourth lumbar nerves. Entrapment may occur associated with a fracture of the ilium or an injury involving the bone surrounding the obturator foramen. An obturator node dissection and methyl methacrylate that enters the pelvis because of a defect in the acetabulum may affect this nerve. Neoplasms involving the obturator canal may affect both the motor and the sensory branches of the nerve (Siliski and Scott, 1985).

FEMORAL NEUROPATHY

As the femoral nerve leaves the pelvis under the inguinal ligament it may be damaged by a fracture of the underlying bone, compression of the nerve from a hematoma, direct trauma, or retraction (Fig. 58–12). If the nerve has been affected by a false aneurysm or insertion of a catheter for angiography, or by lymph node dissection for lymphoma or retroperitoneal biopsy, an entrapment syndrome may result. A hematoma in the iliacus muscle either from trauma or from anticoagulation or from spontaneous bleeding is suspected when the clinical history and physical findings indicate quadriceps muscle paralysis from femoral nerve compression. CT provides helpful information in making the diagnosis (Eustace et al, 1994; Giuliani et al, 1990; Kumar et al, 1992; Miller and Benedict, 1985; Simon and Goodrich, 1984; Susins et al, 1968; Warfel et al, 1993).

Clinical Syndrome

Anterior thigh pain, paresthesias, and hypesthesias are noted. Weakness of the quadriceps muscle mass prevents straight leg raising and thigh support during standing. Thigh muscle weakness may be overlooked if straight leg raising is not tested each day.

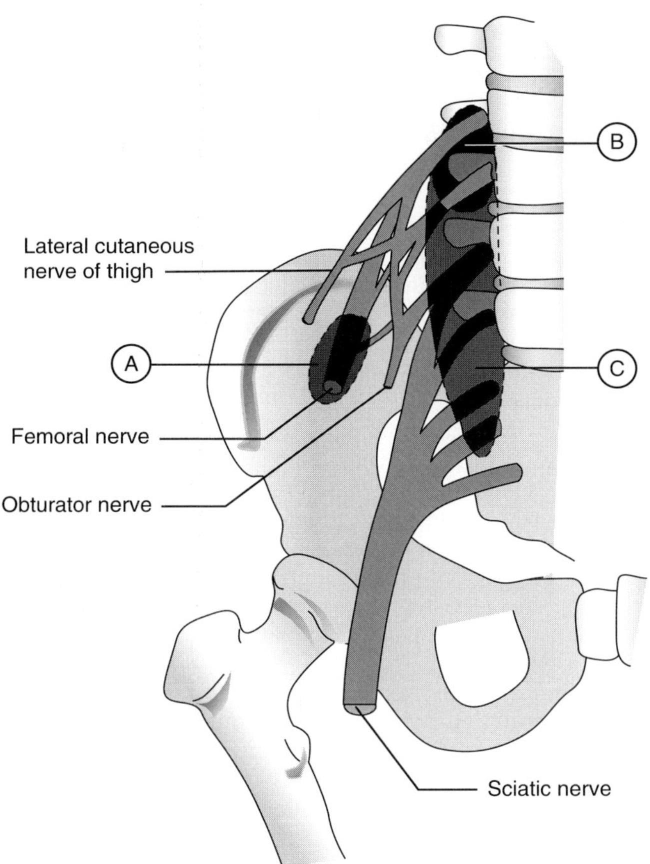

FIGURE 58–12. Areas of hematoma associated with spontaneous bleeding from fracture, vascular injury, or anticoagulation are shown. *A,* An iliacus hematoma producing femoral neuropathy. *B,* Retroperitoneal hematoma of iliopsoas associated with fractured vertebrae. *C,* Fractured pelvis with retroperitoneal hemorrhage causing a secondary lumbosacral plexus neuropathy. (Modified from Stewart JD: Focal Peripheral Neuropathies. New York, Elsevier, 1987, p 259.)

Treatment

If hematoma from anticoagulation is suspected, recovery is usually spontaneous but slow once the clotting profile has been determined and abnormal bleeding stops. If a surgical procedure has occurred and there is a possibility of direct damage, then exploration of the nerve is necessary. If a displaced pelvic fracture has resulted in femoral nerve compression, then neurolysis is appropriate.

LUMBOSACROPLEXUS NERVE COMPRESSIVE LESIONS ARE RARE

A patient with a sudden onset of severe pain, distal paresthesias in the thigh and leg, and some degree of motor weakness probably has the Spillane-Parsonage-Turner syndrome (Fig. 58–13). However, this is frequently a diagnosis of exclusion (Sander and Sharp, 1981). The sudden onset and the characteristics of the symptoms, however, do not necessarily warrant extensive diagnostic studies until the patient has been observed for a few weeks. Usually, this inflammatory neuropathy defines itself. Recovery is slow, and the relief of pain may require carbamazepine (Tegretol)

or similar medications and, occasionally, an epidural block for temporary relief or diminution of the central pain syndrome (Evans et al, 1981; Hardaker et al, 1989; Huittinen, 1972; Sander, 1981; Thomas et al, 1985; Wagner, 1989; Whittaker and Sharp, 1958).

Other Causes of Lumbosacroplexus Compression

Other conditions that may involve the lumbosacroplexus before the nerves exit the pelvis are fractures, radiation plexopathy, tumor compression of the plexus, obstetrical injuries to the plexus, and direct trauma due to gunshot wounds or crush injuries.

Treatment of each of these problems is determined by the clinical assessment, imaging findings, and evidence of progression of the neurological deficit.

PUDENDAL NERVE COMPRESSION OR ENTRAPMENT

The pudendal nerve arises from the second, third, and fourth sacral nerves, first exiting the pelvis and then re-entering under the sacrotuberous ligament. The nerve gives off three branches—the inferior rectal nerve, the perineal nerve, and the dorsal nerve of the penis. The functional deficits associated with pudendal nerve compression are

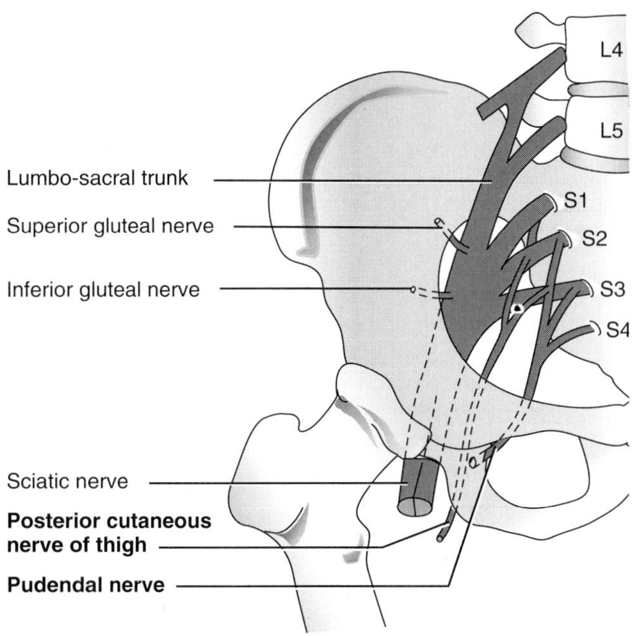

FIGURE 58–13. This diagram shows the formation of the sciatic nerve from L4, L5, S1, S2, and S3 nerves. Fractures of the pelvis or hemorrhage may damage these nerves. External compression of the pudendal nerve, the posterior cutaneous nerve of the thigh, and the perineal branches to the upper thigh deserve special attention in attempting to isolate clinical complaints of paresthesias and hypesthesia associated with compression or entrapment mechanisms. (Modified from Stewart JD: Focal Peripheral Neuropathies. New York, Elsevier, 1987, p 271.)

great. They affect urethral control, genital sensation, and erection (Goodson, 1979; Silbert et al, 1991) (Fig. 58–14).

Clinical Syndromes. Possible damage to the pudendal nerve may occur associated with hip joint injuries or other pelvic fractures. Surgical procedures to correct pelvic fractures, acetabular injuries, or hip fractures that require the center post for counter traction may damage the pudendal nerve. Operative procedures or trauma to the ischial tuberosity or osteotomy of the pelvis in children for acetabular deformity may affect the pudendal nerve.

Traction and Perineal Pressure. The pressure exerted in the perineal region during actual and simulated closed femoral reaming has been simulated on patients undergoing treatment and volunteers on a fracture table in the lateral position. The larger the diameter of the post and the better the padding, the less the perineal pressure. A 9-cm post without padding had a 100% less pressure on the perineum than a 3-cm post with 1.5-cm padding.

Preoperative management of the fractured femur is accomplished by maintaining length, thereby not requiring excessive traction during the procedure, or femoral distractors may be used during treatment of pelvic fractures rather than longitudinal traction. If the fracture table is used to carry part of the load from the torso, there will be less compression of the perineum by the post. Anesthetic agents that provide total muscle paralysis will also lessen the amount of external traction necessary to realign fractured fragments (Bray and Leighton, 1989; Oberpenning et al, 1994).

Bicycle Rider's Syndrome. direct compression of the pudendal nerve affecting one or more of its branches may occur during bicycle riding or similar activities that require a rigid stationary positioning (see Fig. 58–14).

SCIATIC NERVE COMPRESSION OR ENTRAPMENT
(Fig. 58–15A and B)

This nerve is vulnerable as it exits through the sciatic notch. Fractures of the sacrum or ilium may traumatize or entrap the nerve. Firm fixation of the nerve before leaving the pelvis causes stretch of both the peroneal and the tibial components if the extremity is manipulated beyond the individual's tolerance (Adams, 1964; Claussen and Geddon, 1960; Leonard, 1972; McClane, 1986; Wagner, 1989).

Posterior dislocation of the femur or a fractured dislocation of the femur and acetabulum may contuse, compress, or entrap the nerve either mildly or severely. Recognition of the distal motor and sensory deficit should be made early and before any manipulation or treatment is attempted so that the baseline condition of the nerve is established as occurring from the force that caused the femoral displacement rather than from the treatment that attempts to realign the joint components.

Fractures of the proximal one third of the femur with posterior displacement of the distal fragment may contuse or spear the nerve and cause varying degrees of damage. The immediate onset of motor and sensory deficits suggests that the nerve has been damaged, and the method of management of both the fracture and the nerve lesion requires careful assessment. If the fracture fragments are widely separated and nerve damage has occurred, *operative exploration of the nerve is indicated.* Surgical exploration of the sciatic nerve in all three of the conditions mentioned may

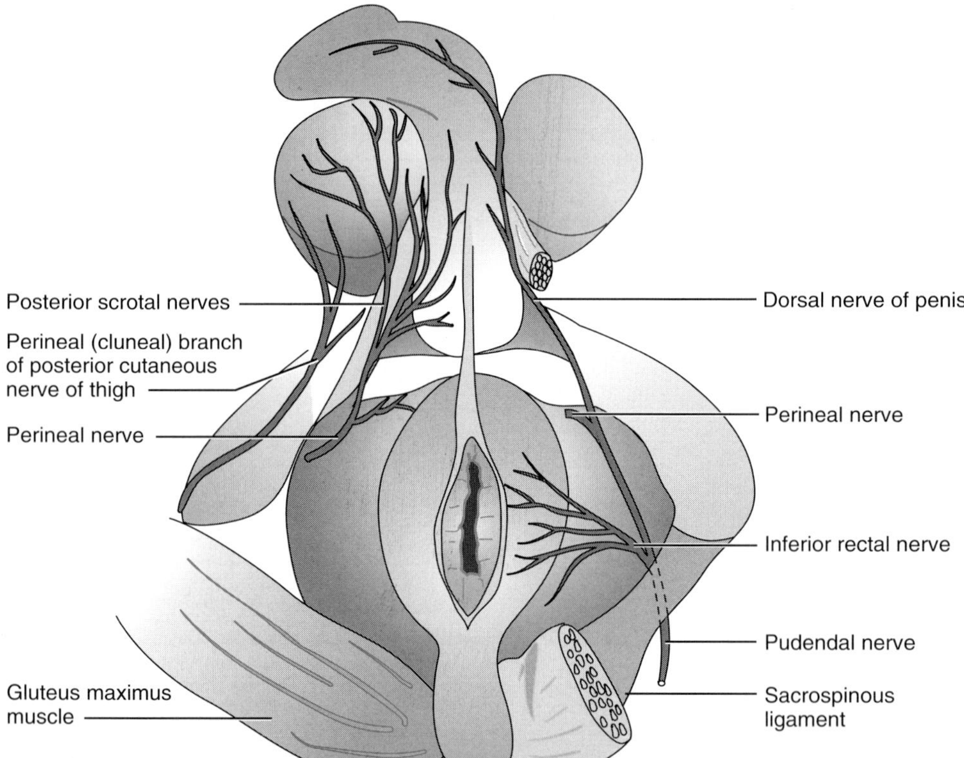

FIGURE 58–14. Diagram of the rectum and genitalia. Note the pudendal nerve, the perineal nerve, and the dorsal nerve to the penis or analogous nerves in the female. Each of these nerves is subject to compression or entrapment from indirect or direct trauma or hemorrhage. (Modified from Stewart JD: Focal Peripheral Neuropathies. New York, Elsevier, 1987, p 275.)

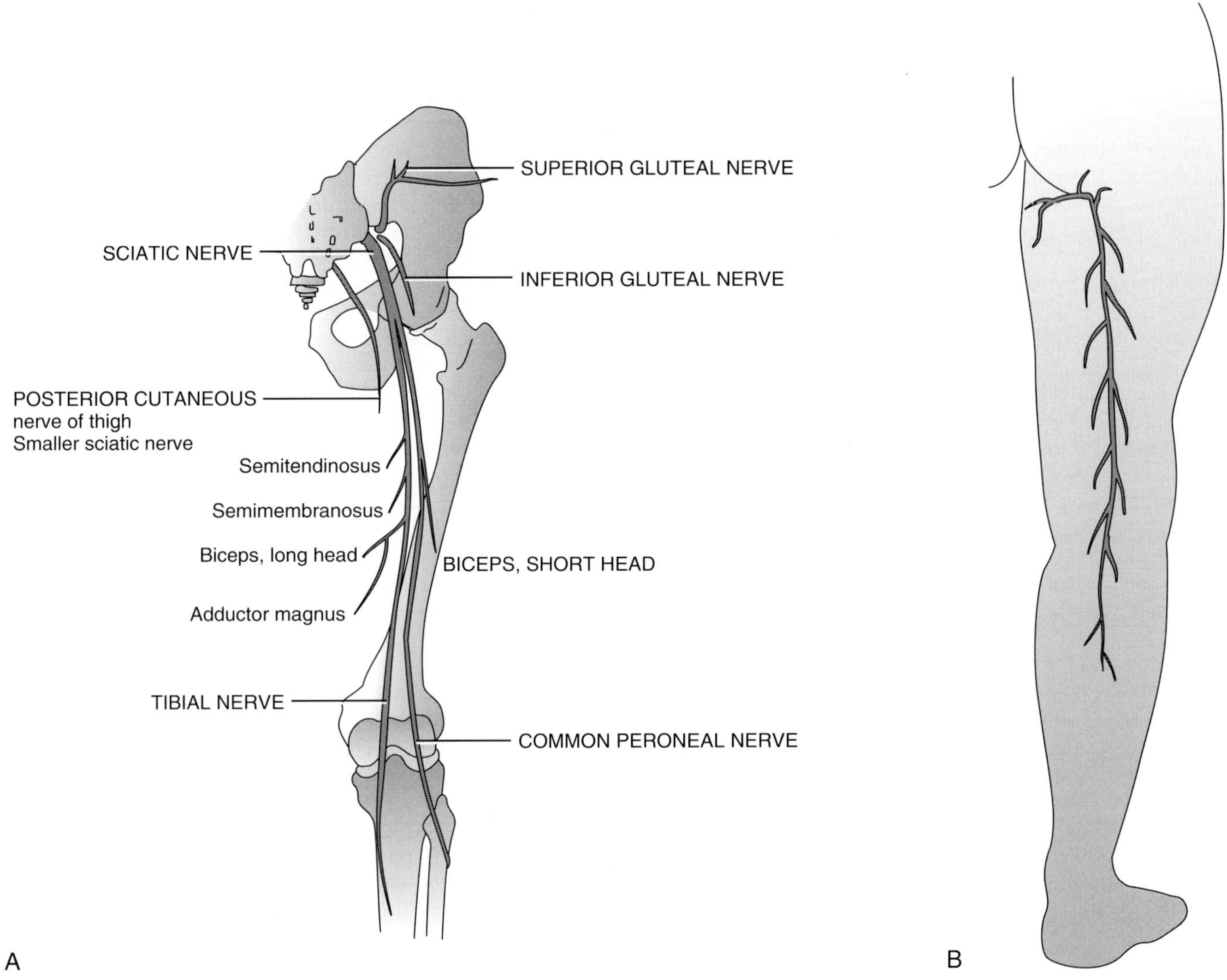

FIGURE 58–15. *A,* This diagram shows two critical areas related to the greater and smaller sciatic nerves. Any or all of the nerves seen may be damaged by trauma or by retraction. The sciatic nerve near the notch may be damaged by a fractured pelvis; a posterior dislocation of the hip may result in damage to the nerve by the displaced femur. Also, the nerve is exposed to infections and external trauma.

The single motor branch that arises laterally on the sciatic nerve is the motor supply to the biceps brevis. This fact aids in determining whether a peroneal palsy affecting the foot arises at the knee or the hip level.

B, The posterior cutaneous nerve of the thigh (smaller sciatic nerve) is shown. This nerve supplies primarily the skin, as illustrated. Damage to this nerve may be confused with a direct injury to the sciatic nerve. Differential sensibility testing will usually aid in the diagnosis. The posterior cutaneous nerve of the thigh does not radiate into the foot, whereas the common sciatic nerve does. (Modified from Stewart JD: Focal Peripheral Neuropathies. New York, Elsevier, 1987, pp 273–274.)

prevent further damage to the nerve by persistent trauma from displaced bone segments. Once the status of the nerve is recognized, the continuity is determined, and the subsequent management is based on known pathology of the nerve rather than hoping for the nerve to recover when the condition of the nerve is not known (Adams, 1964).

Sciatic nerve compression may occur when coagulopathy results with anticoagulation. There may be bleeding around the nerve, into the nerve, or both (Leonard, 1972). Once the clotting mechanism is controlled and a physiological condition returns, the nerve regains its physiological condition. This may require weeks or months but occurs in a regular predictable way.

The sciatic nerve may be compressed by a direct blow such as a fall from a height or when the individual misses the chair and sits on the floor. This condition may result in what is frequently referred to as the piriformis syndrome.

CT imaging shows swelling of the muscle and indirect compression of the nerve from both the edema and the initial direct contusion. The clinical findings vary in severity from momentary paresthesias to sensory and motor deficiencies that may take several months to resolve. A differential diagnosis of intervertebral disc disease and nerve root irritation from direct sciatic nerve contusion may require electrical studies and additional imaging studies if the clinical findings are not sufficient to arrive at an accurate diagnosis. Sciatic nerve compression in a thin person may occur from prolonged sitting that causes pressure of the ischium on the nerve, or an object in the back pocket such as a wallet may compress the nerve against the pelvic bone. This is referred to as "hip pocket" or "credit card" sciatica.

Other specific pathological conditions such as an osteochondroma of the pelvic ring, an angiolipoma of the gluteus maximus, or an endometrial implant directly on the sciatic nerve near the notch may cause excessive compression on the nerve.

The sciatic nerve may also be compressed by a neurilemmoma in the region of the pelvis, the mid-thigh, or just proximal to the popliteal area where the nerve branches. The lesion itself compresses the nerve, and the surrounding fascia, tendons, and muscle tissue add to the compression and the clinical symptoms.

The Piriformis Syndrome

The piriformis syndrome has been mentioned by several authors (Barton, 1991; Jankiewicz et al, 1991) (Fig. 58–16). The senior author's experience has not documented a specific patient with a true compressive lesion of the sciatic nerve by the piriformis muscle. Four patients have been assessed for possible piriformis syndrome after prior surgery elsewhere for buttock pain and posterior radiation. The sciatic nerve had been explored for persistent buttock pain after a prior spine operation had been done. All four patients proved to have an L4 nerve root lesion. The relationship of the sciatic nerve to the piriformis was determined in all these patients. Relief was not obtained by releasing the piriformis or by sectioning the fascia and muscle fibers over the nerve. All four patients proved to have an L4 nerve root lesion caused by either a neural arch defect, far lateral intervertebral disc compression, or an osteophyte. The referred pain and sensory distribution were in the buttock and the posterior thigh, but the actual cause of the pain was from a proximal nerve root irritation. A proximal nerve root block is helpful in the preoperative assessment. If it eliminates the buttock pain, this suggests that the pain may be arising proximally. However, even if it eliminates the pain, the site of the pain could be from the sciatic nerve distally, but the nerve root block eliminates sensory conduction along those fibers that arise at the site of compression within the piriformis. Various clinical maneuvers such as adduction and internal rotation are used to test sciatic nerve tethering. A differential epidural or spinal anesthetic with low-dose novocaine may give information about the primary site of a compressive lesion. Although mechanical compression of the sciatic nerve as it passes through the piriformis muscle would intuitively relate to compression, the number of patients with a well-documented lesion is very small.

Patients who are most likely to have direct contusion of the sciatic nerve because of edema of the piriformis are those who have had a direct fall on the buttock from a height. A slip and fall on the stairway, missing a chair when sitting down, or similar kinds of accidents may cause immediate paresthesias in the thigh and calf, and result in persistent sciatic nerve irritation for several weeks.

The *differential diagnosis* is between nerve root irritation or sciatic nerve contusion in the region of the piriformis. Both sites of pathology may exist. The history and the physical findings usually determine the exact site of the pathology, but CT scan of the sciatic nerve and the piriformis provides additional information about localized edema of the muscle.

Treatment. If the muscle is edematous and causes compression of the sciatic nerve, a direct injection of corticosteroid into the muscle (but not the nerve) may diminish edema sufficiently to reinforce the diagnosis and serve as supportive treatment.

Sciatic nerve tethering and compression may occur after hamstring lengthening in a spastic extremity (Fig. 58–17). After the hamstring muscles are lengthened in the child, adolescent, or adult, and while the tourniquet is still elevated and in place, the sciatic nerve may be stretched when the

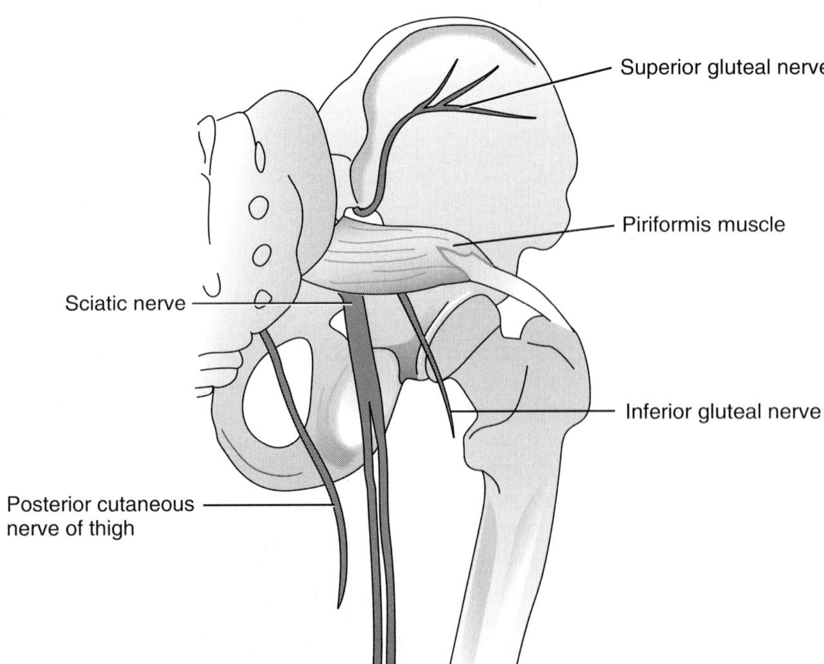

FIGURE 58–16. The piriformis muscle exits from the pelvis and attaches to the greater trochanter of the femur. It covers the sciatic nerve and is adjacent to the superior and inferior gluteal nerves. The reported occurrence of the piriformis syndrome is very low. MRI or CT scanning may document localized edema associated with hemorrhage or contusion. (Modified from Stewart JD: Focal Peripheral Neuropathies. New York, Elsevier, 1987, p 272.)

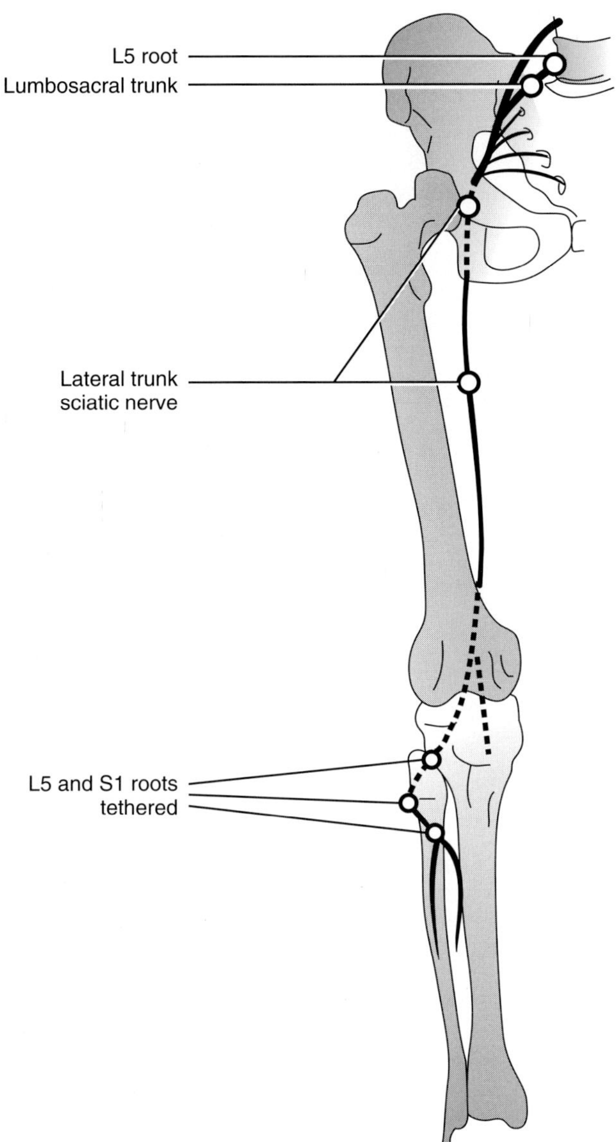

FIGURE 58–17. This anteroposterior diagram of the pelvis and lower extremity shows the areas of tethering of the lumbosacral nerve roots and sacral nerves that form the two segments of the sciatic nerve. The lateral trunk of the sciatic nerve gives off the peroneal nerve, which is damaged most frequently during dislocation of the hip, retraction during hip operations, or severe adduction-flexion of the extremity. For this reason, the knee joint should be flexed during hip operations and the hip joint extended and the knee flexed postoperatively. The extended hip and the flexed knee relax the tethered sciatic nerve. (Modified from Stewart JD: Focal Peripheral Neuropathies, New York, Elsevier, 1987, p 298.)

leg is straightened to determine if adequate lengthening has occurred. The nerve is temporarily tethered by the tourniquet, and having been shortened previously due to the hamstring contracture, the nerve undergoes sudden elongation and stretch. Postoperatively, the patient has paresthesias, dysesthesia, and a causalgic syndrome that usually improves over a period of several months. However, occasionally neurolysis is necessary as the nerve becomes compressed and entrapped by adjacent fascia bands.

Sciatic nerve contusion or stretch caused by temporary compression of a retractor or manipulation of the femur may occur in association with a posterior approach to the hip joint. If the nerve is seen and identified with a Penrose drain

without a clamp on the suture and if retractors are placed carefully, compression damage may be prevented. Actually seeing the nerve is safer than theoretically knowing where it is.

CLINICAL SYNDROME

The physical examination shows involvement of both the posterior tibial and peroneal nerve branches of the sciatic nerve. The site of pathology depends on the dermatome pattern and proximal muscle weakness. If clinical examination is insufficient to determine obvious weakness in the hamstrings, electrical studies are helpful. The short head of the biceps femoris is innervated by a proximal lateral motor branch from the sciatic nerve. The medial hamstrings are innervated by the tibial nerve.

Management of Sciatic Nerve Compressive or Entrapment Lesions

The major aspect of management depends on a detailed history and an accurate diagnosis. If external forces have caused the damage, spontaneous regeneration usually occurs. Percussion tests, Tinel's sign, manual muscle testing, dermatome assessment, and electrical studies provide information about progressive recovery or lack of recovery.

Internal lesions should be defined and the decision made concerning immediate or early exploration of the nerve versus frequent and careful observation.

The surgeon should be prepared to handle the lesion depending on the grade of severity (Sunderland grades 1 to 5), which requires appropriate electrical stimulation during surgery, determination of action potentials in the adjacent muscles, neurolysis, direct resection and nerve repair, or nerve grafting.

SURAL NERVE NEUROPATHY

The sural nerve is formed by the junction of the medial sural cutaneous with the peroneal anastomotic branch and extends distally between the lateral malleolus and the calcaneus (Docks and Salter, 1979; Gould and Trevino, 1981; Pringle et al, 1974). It ends in the lateral dorsal cutaneous nerve along the lateral border of the foot and the little toe. It communicates with the dorsum of the foot with the intermediate dorsal cutaneous nerve, a branch of the superficial peroneal nerve. Proximal involvement of the sural nerve may be associated with exercise-induced compartment syndrome affecting the calf muscles. Entrapment would be proximal between the two heads of the gastrocnemius. The nerve pierces the fascia about the mid-leg. The nerve may be compressed in this location by a thigh band of a brace or by direct trauma. Specific pathological lesions around the foot and ankle are proliferative tenosynovitis of the peroneal tendons that secondarily compress the nerve. More distal compression by a ganglion from the fibular talar joint or a ganglion or villonodular synovitis arising from the calcaneocuboid joint.

Fractures of the fifth metatarsal or postsurgical treatment

of this fracture may affect the lateral dorsal cutaneous branch of the sural nerve.

Distal involvement of the sural nerve may occur from external causes such as shoes, boots, or direct trauma. Most lesions, however, are due to internal entrapment related to post-traumatic or postsurgical incidents. We have treated several patients who have had prior surgical procedures and subsequent entrapment of the sural nerve. The procedures were heel cord lengthening displaced fractures of the calcaneus requiring open reduction lateral incision for clubfoot release subtalar joint osteotomy peroneal tendon repair or laceration lateral ankle reconstruction using peroneal tendon triple arthrodesis and sural nerve autologous graft. These lesions varied in severity from local hypesthesia and sensitivity, to percussion to constant pain from shoe pressure to a major causalgic syndrome. The youngest patient with causalgia was a 4-year-old child who had undergone a subtalar arthrodesis, during which a partial laceration of the sural nerve had occurred. Nerve block relieved the pain temporarily, and repair of the nerve alleviated the complaints. A 7-year-old child developed a causalgic syndrome after lateral incision for clubfoot surgery in which the lateral cutaneous branch was partially lacerated (Goldner and Bright, 1980). This patient was managed by resection of the involved segment and bipolar cauterization.

When treatment was resection, the proximal end was treated with bipolar cauterization and placed in either muscle or adjacent fat. If adequate nerve was present and the damage was not severe, a suture of the nerve segments was done.

Our observations of several hundred patients who have had sural nerve taken for nerve grafts indicate that resuture of an old injury is not necessary because the sensory deficit gradually diminishes as time passes and the patients tolerate the hypesthesia very well. We have performed neurolysis on several patients who have had an area of fibrosis without neuroma incontinuity, and these procedures have been reasonably successful.

The patient's complaints relative to this lesion should not be ignored, nor should they be considered as minor until some form of assessment relative to the severity of pain has been conducted and appropriate treatment completed.

COMMON PERONEAL NEUROPATHY

This nerve is one of the two major segments of the sciatic nerve, which is the largest nerve in the body, measuring about 2 cm in breadth usually passes out of the pelvis through the greater sciatic foramen below the piriformis muscle (Grant, 1947; Gray, 1940; Hollingshead, 1969) (Fig. 58–18). Occasionally, if the division between the tibial nerve and the peroneal nerve occurs at the sacroplexus level, the common peroneal nerve usually pierces the piriformis (Gray, 1936). The peroneal nerve is about half the size of the tibial nerve. During hip surgery, if the knee joint is maintained in flexion and particularly when the nerve is being retracted, there is less likelihood that the peroneal segment of the sciatic nerve that is relatively static at the sciatic notch and around the fibular neck will be damaged (Kopell and Thompson, 1960a).

Compression or entrapment of the peroneal nerve may be

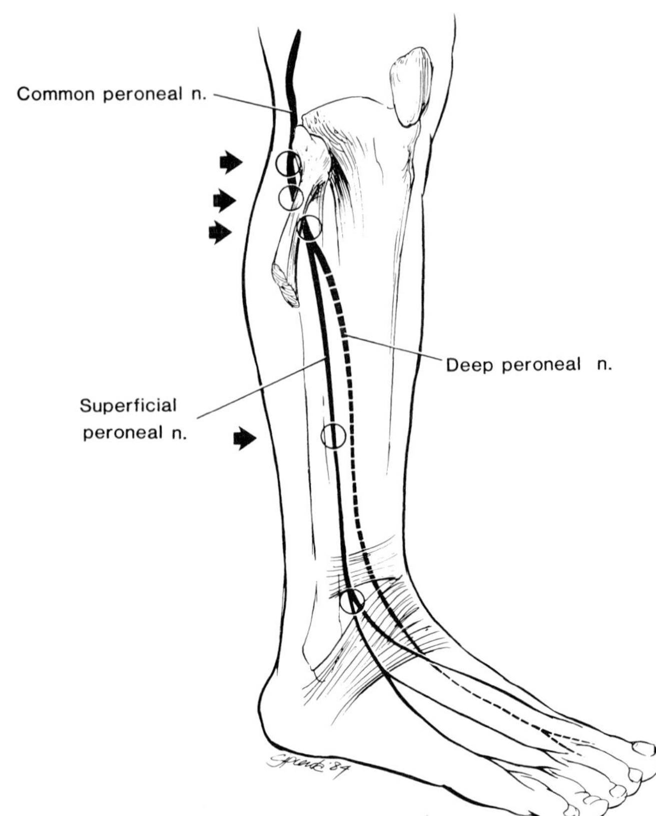

FIGURE 58–18. The common peroneal nerve as it passes posterior to the fibula, through the peroneal muscles, and divides into superficial and deep branches. The arrows and the circles represent the locations of most frequent compression. (From Goldner JL: Nerve Entrapment Syndromes of the Foot, Ankle, and Leg. The Jefferson Orthopaedic Journal 13:1, 1984.)

due to external or internal causes (Berry and Richardson, 1976; Brooks, 1952) (see Fig. 58–18).

External Compression

External compression may be caused by a firm or flexible wrapping or an object that compresses the nerve against underlying fascia or bone. Examples are (1) an elastic wrapping that rolls on itself and tightens around the knee region or over the head of the fibula causes compression, and (2) a plaster cast, fiberglass splint, or knee immobilizer applied with the knee joint hyperextended or slightly flexed may result in direct pressure on the nerve against the bone. The ribs in the knee immobilizer or a tight Velcro strap may be the specific cause of the compression. If this compression persists for several minutes or an hour, nerve conduction may be impaired. (3) Nerve compression by a calf or thigh band of a limb orthosis may interrupt conduction. (4) Knee crossing repeatedly and for a prolonged period by a person who has lost a large amount of weight recently may result in nerve compression and sensory and motor alterations (Waltman, 1929). (5) Suspension slings used for traction or elevation of the extremity may compress the nerve (White, 1968). (6) If it is applied just above the knee, the edge of a pneumatic tourniquet may compress the nerve excessively while the tourniquet is elevated. Also, if the extremity is spastic, the hamstrings are tight, and the tourniquet is applied with the knee in flexion, the nerve may be stretched or compressed as it is extended with the tourniquet still elevated. (7) Ice packs applied to the lateral knee for cryotherapy may cause complete motor paralysis that requires several months to resolve (Bassett et al, 1992).

Internal Compression

Internal causes of peroneal nerve compression proximally or distally may be either spontaneous or traumatic. Traumatic incidents occur during a high tibial osteotomy (Kettelkamp and Leach, 1975), a leg lengthening procedure in which the nerve is compressed by the fascia origin of the peroneus longus, or by fracture of the proximal fibula or of the distal femur. Other traumatic lesions, such as complete dislocation of the knee joint, forced hyperextension of the knee from trauma, or prolonged sitting with the heel higher than the hyperextended knee, may compress or damage the nerve.

A special problem associated with inversion of the foot and ankle may result in stretch of the tethered peroneal nerve at the origin of the peroneus longus, and a partial or complete motor and sensory deficit may result (Meals, 1977). This problem is easily overlooked during the early examination but should be recognized during the course of treatment.

Other internal lesions related to surgical procedures are (1) partial or complete laceration of the nerve in the region of the fibular head or peroneus longus origin; (2) excessive intraoperative retraction, which causes temporary damage to the nerve (Rose et al, 1982); (3) compression of the nerve by manual manipulation or displaced bone fragments.

Other pathological lesions that may result in nerve compression or entrapment are a ganglion of the tibiofibular joint (Evans et al, 1994; Fransen et al, 1991), a false aneurysm of the peroneal vessels, a true aneurysm associated with a developmental or traumatic incident, an osteochondroma of the proximal tibia or fibula affecting the nerve, or a synovial cyst (Baker's Cyst) (Cobb and Maiel, 1974; Garland and Moorhouse, 1952; Marivah, 1964; Nakano, 1978).

We have observed a hypermobile chronic dislocation of the proximal tibiofibular joint with secondary compression of the peroneal nerve. Also, a neurilemmoma of the peroneal nerve interferes with conduction in the region of the fibular head (Kars et al, 1992; Parkes, 1961; Stack et al, 1965; Watson and Torch, 1993).

Clinical Experience

In our clinical practice, more than 100 patients have been diagnosed with either external or internal compression of the common peroneal nerve. Diagnosis was made by obtaining reports of symptoms, clinical examination, and electrical studies, as necessary. Treatment depended on the cause, the duration of compression, and the probability of spontaneous regeneration. In most patients, relief of the external pressure and a period of observation resulted in spontaneous recovery. We used a percussion test, Tinel's sign, and appropriate electrical studies to observe motor and sensory recovery.

Treatment of Internal Compression

The senior author has had a great deal of experience with this problem, and the choice of treatment depended on the circumstances. If a leg-lengthening procedure was being performed and motor weakness in the dorsiflexors of the foot occurred, the lengthening procedure was temporarily halted, the traction partially relieved, and the patient observed for 24 to 48 hours. Frequently, that was sufficient to allow motor recovery. However, if additional lengthening was necessary and motor weakness persisted or recurred, decompression of the V-shaped fascial bands of the peroneus longus origin that compressed the nerve was performed.

If a peroneal palsy occurs immediately after a high tibial osteotomy, the decision to operate or observe depends on the surgeon's knowledge of how the procedure was performed. If forcible retraction is necessary and if the nerve is visualized or if the nerve is not seen but only palpated, the surgeon will determine whether re-exploration is necessary or whether a period of observation is relatively safe. Our experience has been that reoperation is a safe approach because the edematous nerve and the fascia over the nerve are decompressed and the condition of the nerve is known immediately. Following that, spontaneous regeneration is observed with the knowledge that the nerve has not been lacerated or that it is not being severely compressed by bone, fascia, or sutures. If there has been an open operative procedure for joint replacement or removal of a soft tissue mass for correction of a deformity, and if a peroneal nerve lesion occurs postoperatively, there is justification for reoperating on the nerve to relieve persistent compression or to determine if partial or complete laceration of the nerve has occurred (Mann and Plattner, 1989).

SUPERFICIAL PERONEAL NEUROPATHY

External Lesions

Compressive lesions of the superficial peroneal nerve may be caused by external blunt trauma from a direct fracture of the fibula or tibia, or compression from shoe tops, straps, or external bands around the lower leg, the ankle, or the foot (Lindenbaum, 1979) (Fig. 58–19). The thinner the individual, the more likely is the compression. The subjective symptoms usually include direct pain at the site of compression, burning and tingling distal to the compression site, or combinations of these (Lusskin, 1982).

Internal Lesions

This nerve becomes superficial as it penetrates the lateral fascia of the leg. Along with the nerve, a segment of fat may herniate and cause both nerve compression and local fat necrosis (Garfin et al, 1977). Also, as a result of direct trauma or muscle tear, a bundle of muscle fibers may be entrapped in the fascial opening and compress the nerve. The superficial peroneal nerve divides into a medial and intermedial dorsal cutaneous nerve (see Fig. 58–19). The medial branch divides into two dorsal digital branches, one of which supplies the medial side of the great toe and the

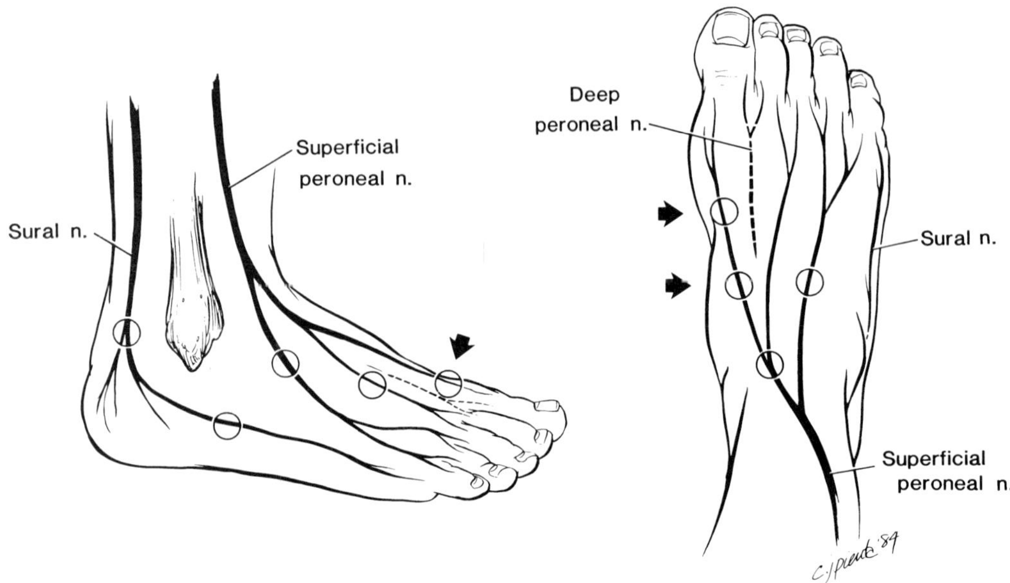

FIGURE 58–19. Lateral and dorsal view of the foot. The circles represent the most frequent sites of nerve compression. (From Goldner JL: Nerve entrapment syndromes of the foot, ankle, and leg. The Jefferson Orthopaedic Journal *13*:1, 1984.)

other the adjacent side of the second and third toes. It also supplies the skin on the medial side of the foot and ankle, and communicates with the saphenous nerve and with the deep peroneal nerve. This nerve may be entrapped or compressed by a bony exostosis of the first tarsometatarsal joint or a tenosynovitis of the extensor digitorum longus to the medial toes. The intermedial dorsal cutaneous (external or lateral branch of the superficial peroneal (supplies the skin on the lateral side of the foot and ankle and communicates with the sural nerve). Branches of the superficial peroneal nerve supply the skin of the dorsal surfaces of all the toes except the lateral side of the little toe and the adjoining sides of the great and second toes, with the little toe being supplied by the lateral dorsal cutaneous branch of the sural nerve. These nerves vary considerably in their terminal branches (Banerjee and Koons, 1981; Kernohan et al, 1985; Sridhara and Izzo, 1985).

There is an anomalous accessory branch of the superficial peroneal nerve that may supply a motor branch to the extensor digitorum brevis or an aberrant sensory branch over the lateral malleolus. Unexplained pain in this region may arise from trauma or irritation of the aberrant branch (Massey, 1978; Meharg, 1984).

The most frequent internal entrapment or compressive lesions are postsurgical and associated with branches of the superficial peroneal nerve. These branches would be affected in open reduction of ankle fractures from the lateral side, triple arthrodesis, soft tissue ankle reconstruction, or arthrodesis of the ankle. All of these cutaneous nerve branches should be taken into consideration when the examiner evaluates the patient's symptoms of pain after surgical procedures (Styf, 1989; Mann, 1989).

We have treated over 50 patients with painful lesions of the lower leg and ankle and dorsum of the foot associated with superficial peroneal nerve compression or entrapment. About half of these lesions were related to both external and internal compression, and the remainder were associated with prior surgical procedures.

Great Toe Branch of the Superficial Peroneal Nerve

This entrapment lesion is usually a combined external and internal lesion caused by an exostosis of the first metatarsal from within and compression of the shoe on the nerve from without. Neurogenic pain usually stops when the shoe is off (see Fig. 58–19). Other internal compression lesions occur during a hallux valgus procedure. About 50 patients have been examined and treated for a painful, great toe superficial peroneal nerve trauma. In several patients, the lesion was bilateral. The cutaneous nerve lesions varied from fibrosis of the nerve branches to a complete laceration and bulb neuroma. The complaints varied from mild to severe and depended on the location of the injury, the extent of fibrosis, and the amount of tethering (see Figs. 58–2 and 58–4). The more distal the lesion, the less severe were the complaints. These variations were probably related to overlap of sensation from the plantar digital nerves and from the arborization of the distal segments of the nerve. Some sensory segments were spared, whereas a more proximal lesion included all segments of the nerve (Kosinski, 1926; Szabo, 1989).

TREATMENT

The specific method of management depends on the complaints. Hypersensitivity, exquisite tenderness associated with a neuroma, or chronic fibrosis of the nerve is usually managed by resection, bipolar cautery of the proximal segment, and placement of the proximal segment in muscle or fat. Occasionally, neurolysis is possible, and a thin layer of fat is used to cover the nerve before closure. The tethered nerve is released from adjacent collagen or bone and re-routed to avoid compression of the shoe.

Areas of hypersensitivity and hypesthesia may respond spontaneously as time passes; betamethasone (Celestone) injections may be helpful and protection of the sensitive area by padding may be beneficial.

Time does not heal all hypersensitive areas or eliminate all painful neuromas. Many areas of hyperpathia recede with time, but the problem in certain patients may last for years unless it is treated aggressively (Goldner et al, 1975).

Lateral Branch of the Superficial Peroneal Nerve (Intermediate Cutaneous Branch of the Foot)

External lesions are usually associated with compression from the edge of a shoe, a shoe strap, boot, or an equinus inversion cutaneous stretch (see Fig. 58–19). This anatomical area of the dorsal lateral aspect of the foot is called the anterior tarsal region and accounts for the designation of the anterior tarsal tunnel syndrome as compared with the tarsal tunnel syndrome affecting the tibial nerve (see Figure 58–19). Compression or entrapment of the deep branch of the peroneal nerve in the anterior ankle region is also referred to as anterior tarsal syndrome (Borges et al, 1981; Dellon, 1990; Gessini et al, 1984; Krause et al, 1977; Zonghao et al, 1991).

Internal entrapment of the lateral branch of the peroneal nerve usually occurs after a triple arthrodesis, a lateral ankle reconstruction, or an operation in the region of the sinus tarsi. Hypersensitivity of the dorsum of the foot and ankle region have been observed after open operation of a fractured ankle. In our series, 25 patients have been diagnosed and treated by resection, neurolysis, and covering the nerve with fat, or resection and resuture. The method of treatment depends on the severity of the lesion, age of the patient, duration of the complaint, and whether or not a local nerve block at the proximal peroneal branch eliminate's most of the pain. If there is an *autonomic nervous system problem,* sympathetic nerve blocks may be necessary in addition to other forms of treatment for complete relief. Pharmacological agents affecting the adrenergic receptors and calcium channel blockers are also helpful.

DEEP PERONEAL NEUROPATHY

An area of hypesthesia or hyperesthesia between the great and the second toes is usually associated with *compression of the common peroneal nerve proximally* (Jutmann, 1970) (see Fig. 58–19). The deep branch of the peroneal nerve courses under the extensor retinaculum and ends in the skin at the base of the first three digits. Thus, although the common peroneal nerve if compressed may cause this altered sensibility, a compressive lesion of the deep peroneal nerve may occur in the region of the distal tibia, the ankle, or the dorsum of the foot. This nerve may be affected by external compression over the first and second cuneiforms by a direct blow; constant firm compression by a cast; or an internal lesion resulting from surgical incisions anterior to the ankle joint, exposure of the tarsometatarsal joints, or incision just lateral to the extensor hallucis longus. Open reduction of a Lisfranc's fracture or an incision about the base of the metatarsals may affect the deep branch of the peroneal nerve. Also, a transmetatarsal amputation necessarily exposes this nerve, and it should be resected and allowed to retract so that it does not become entrapped and cause distal phantom pain. We have diagnosed and treated at least 25 patients

with symptomatic lesions of entrapment of the deep branch of the peroneal nerve from the anterior aspect of the ankle joint to the base of the great toe.

An accessory lateral branch from the deep branch of the peroneal nerve occurs occasionally, may innervate the extensor digitorum brevis, and supplies sensation to a skin zone on the lateral side of the foot. Thus, the extensor digitorum brevis, if active, does not necessarily mean that the entire peroneal nerve is conducting motor fibers (Lambert, 1969).

TIBIAL NEUROPATHY

The tibial nerve as the medial segment of the sciatic nerve is a separate entity within the epineurial sheath of the sciatic nerve (Fig. 58–20). The actual separation of peroneal and tibial segments may occur in the mid- or distal thigh. Compressive or entrapment lesions may affect the tibial nerve anywhere along its course, but particularly in the mid- or distal thigh, the popliteal region, the proximal calf, or the distal leg and foot. These lesions are divided into proximal and distal.

Proximal Lesions

We have treated patients with an osteochondroma of the femur, a myositis ossificans that compresses the nerve, and

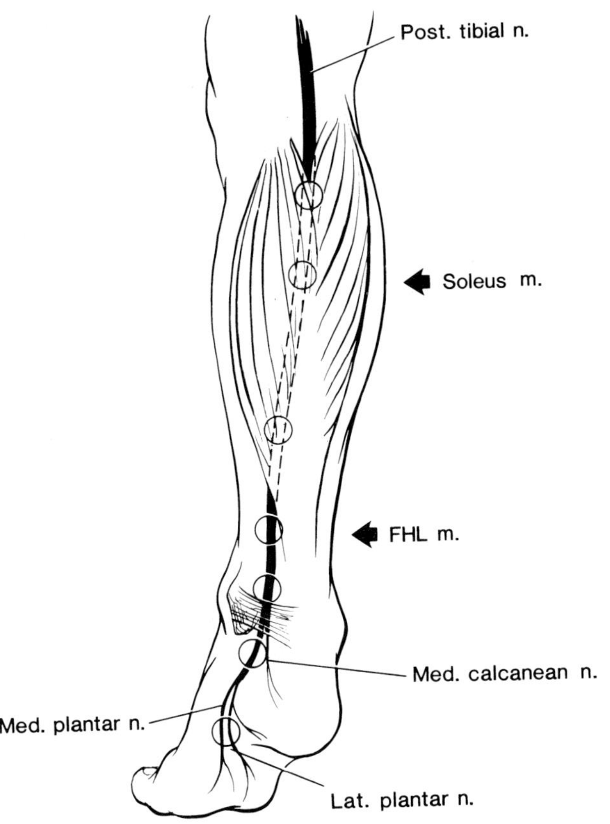

FIGURE 58–20. The tibial nerve as it passes under the gastrocnemius soleus. The circles represent sites of nerve compression that the authors have treated. (From Goldner JL: Nerve entrapment syndromes of the foot, ankle, and leg. The Jefferson Orthopaedic Journal *13*:1, 1984.)

a neurofibroma or neurilemmoma that affects the tibial segment of the nerve in the knee and upper calf region. A large popliteal cyst originating within the knee joint may compress the tibial nerve and cause distal paresthesias and weakness of the large or small foot muscles (Kashani et al, 1985; Millesi, 1987). An aneurysm of the popliteal or tibial artery may directly compress the nerve. A compartment syndrome affecting the proximal calf muscles may cause a rapid painful compression of the tibial nerve with resulting hypesthesias, paresthesias, and hyperpathia, as well as distal motor weakness in the toe flexors and the posterior tibial muscle.

An *exercise compartment syndrome* involving the calf muscles has resulted in compression of the deep motor and sensory branches of the gastrocnemius and soleus. Decompression of the compartment and neurolysis of segmental nerves, and ligation of capillary and venous vessels compressing the nerve have been successful in eliminating pain.

A *chronic compartment syndrome* with contracted residual fibrotic muscle and collagen causes nerve compression and limited excursion that causes distal pain, paresthesias, hypesthesias, and hyperpathia.

Treatment of the Proximal Lesions of the Tibial Nerve

The treatment depends on the clinical symptoms, the physical findings, and an accurate diagnosis. Clinical examination, supplemented by electrical studies in certain situations, should provide an accurate diagnosis. If the proximal lesion is related to hematoma or anticoagulation, spontaneous regeneration of the nerve usually occurs once the bleeding tendency is reversed. A compressive or entrapment lesion requires removal of the pathological mass that is causing compression or relief of the fascia or vascular or muscular tissue that is interfering with conduction. Fibrosis of the proximal calf muscles or compression of the nerve by acute compartment pressure requires decompression of the compartment and neurolysis.

Tibial Neuropathy—Mid-Leg to the Malleolus
(see Fig. 58–20)

The history and physical findings will aid in localizing the tibial nerve compressive or entrapment lesion in the deep compartment of the leg down to the flexor retinaculum at the level of the medial malleolus (see Fig. 58–20). The conditions that affect the tibial nerve in this second segment are (1) fracture of the mid- or distal tibia, (2) chronic tenosynovitis of the posterior tibial or flexor digitorum longus tendons, (3) anomalous muscles on the medial aspect of the lower leg and ankle, (4) postsurgical tibial nerve entrapment, and (5) specific pathological lesions.

Fracture of the mid- or distal tibia may result in hemorrhage, edema, and increased compartmental pressure in the deep compartment of the leg. This syndrome affects nerve conduction because of direct compression of and ischemic alteration of the nerve. This is recognized by pain on attempted dorsiflexion of the foot and toes, hypesthesia and hyperesthesia on the plantar surface of the foot, and measurable increase of compartment pressure by mechanical means.

In the acute phase of this syndrome, compartmental decompression is essential to preserve the muscle and decompress the nerve. In the chronic phase, neurolysis relieves the compressive lesion and allows nerve regeneration.

Chronic tenosynovitis of the posterior tibial or flexor digitorum longus tendons just proximal to the malleolus may affect the tibial nerve by local compression. Swelling of these tendon sheaths fills the area under the retinaculum, and retinacular compression of the nerve may occur. In this region also, flexor hallucis longus tenosynovitis or partial rupture from trauma may irritate the tibial nerve.

Anomalous muscles on the medial aspect of the lower leg and ankle arising from the soleus or gastrocnemius may also compress the tibial nerve during exercise. The anomalous mass, although not compressing the nerve during childhood and adolescence, may cause compression as the muscle enlarges or as collagen becomes less elastic (Sammarco and Conti, 1994). The diagnosis of an anomalous muscle is made by physical examination of a palpable mass, aggravation of the tibial nerve compression symptoms by running in place for 3 to 5 minutes, and in certain patients, by dorsiflexion forced abduction of the foot. The latter maneuver compresses the stretched nerve. In at least 10 patients, we have confirmed this diagnosis by inserting an electromyographic needle into the mass and detecting action potentials as the calf muscle is contracted.

Other pathological lesions such as gouty tophi located in the skin or in the synovium of adjacent tendon sheaths may compress the tibial nerve.

There are several postsurgical causes of tibial nerve entrapment. Tibial nerve entrapment may occur from prior attempts to treat proximal tarsal tunnel, open reduction of ankle joint injury, attempted repair of partially or completely ruptured posterior tibial tendon, prior surgical treatment of congenital clubfoot, prior surgical treatment of a relaxed flat foot, surgical attempts at removing a talocalcaneal coalition, triple arthrodesis from the lateral side causing unrecognized damage to the tibial nerve on the medial aspect of the subtalar joint, and perineurial fibrosis of the tibial nerve after tibiotalar arthrodesis. We have diagnosed and treated patients with all of these conditions. The diagnosis is made primarily by clinical assessment. Electrical studies may be helpful, but if they are negative, one should not rule out the nerve compression syndrome. MRI has been somewhat helpful but not essential in most patients.

Specific pathological lesions may compress the tibial nerve. Neurilemmoma just proximal to the medial malleolus was an enlarged lesion visible on physical examination, was exquisitely tender to percussion, and caused paresthesias on the plantar surface of the foot. This lesion was excised successfully without damage to the fascicles. Occasionally, there are fascicles running over or around the lesion and these should be observed with magnification and severing them should be avoided. Otherwise, a causalgic syndrome may occur.

Tibial Neuropathy from the Malleolus to the Distal Foot (see Figs. 58–20 and 58–21)

Internal Lesions Affecting the Tibial Nerve. Severe acute trauma with massive swelling and increased compartmental

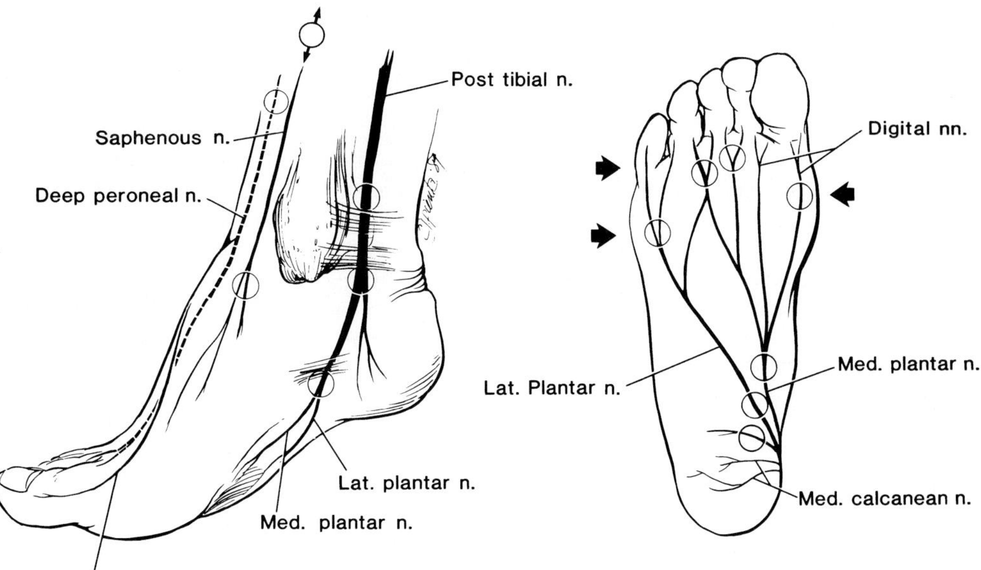

FIGURE 58–21. The medial and plantar view of the tibial and plantar nerves. The circles on the medial diagram show sites of compression of the tibial, the saphenous, and the deep peroneal nerves. The plantar view shows several areas of compression that resulted in entrapment lesions that we have recognized and treated. (From Goldner JL: Nerve entrapment syndromes of the foot, ankle, and leg. The Jefferson Orthopaedic Journal *13*:1, 1984.)

pressure on the medial and plantar aspect of the foot. This condition occurs more frequently than is recognized. We have seen at least 100 patients during the past 30 years who have plantar muscle fibrosis, claw toes, and sensory neuropathy after an episode of severe trauma. The compartment syndrome was not recognized, and residual tibial nerve compression persisted.

Treatment of the acute problem depends on early diagnosis by palpation and observation of massive firm swelling on the plantar and medial aspect of the foot. This may be documented by compartmental pressure readings, and the appropriate decompression should be performed early. This should begin at the point where the tibial nerve divides into medial and lateral plantar nerves and should extend along the medial plantar aspect of the foot, at least to the level of the first metatarsal head. The medial and lateral plantar nerves and vessels are identified, the fascia is split, and the individual muscle layers are opened.

Tarsal Tunnel Syndrome. This condition may be spontaneous and slowly progressive associated with obesity, decreased elasticity of collagen, or a progressive flat foot in an adult (Edwards et al, 1969; Keck, 1962) (see Fig. 58–21). The first patient we treated in 1953 had a fractured calcaneus and a residual osteophyte that compressed the nerve. Other internal causes of the syndrome are a deep medial ganglion from the subtalar joint, or an adjacent *chronic tenosynovitis* or partial *rupture of the posterior tibial tendon* with secondary compression of the nerve (Henricson and Westlin, 1984).

DIAGNOSIS

An accurate diagnosis depends on a detailed history, a meticulous clinical examination, electrical studies, and occasionally, detailed imaging (Goodgold et al, 1965). A positive percussion test from proximal to distal and distal to proximal usually reproduces paresthesias in the digits distal to the point of percussion. A positive percussion test proximal to the point of severe compression usually means that the nerve

is compressed about 2 cm distal to the enlarged tibial nerve. A perineurial injection of 1% lidocaine (Xylocaine) diminishes paresthesias and pain with weightbearing and, although anesthesia occurs, the relief of pain and discomfort adds diagnostic information (Kaplan and Kernahan, 1981). The clinical findings of diminished sweating, hypesthesia, decreased vibratory sense, and unilateral sensibility changes compared with the uninvolved opposite side are all helpful diagnostic findings. Electrical studies, if positive, as a prolonged nerve conduction velocity, or a positive electromyogram of the abductor hallucis muscle belly reinforces the clinical diagnosis. However, it is not *unusual to have negative electrical studies unless the patient undergoes 15 or 20 minutes of walking, standing, or tiptoeing before the tests are performed.* If exercise causes paresthesias, compression is usually present (Edwards et al 1969; Oh et al, 1979).

TARSAL TUNNEL

The tarsal tunnel should be divided into a *proximal zone,* which extends from the retinaculum to the origin of the abductor muscle and a *distal zone,* which begins at the fibrous origin of the abductor muscle and extends through this muscle (see Fig. 58–21). The tibial nerve usually divides into medial and lateral plantar nerves about 1 cm proximal to the fibrous leash of the abductor hallucis muscle. The lesions noted in the distal part of the tarsal tunnel are a congenital hypertrophy of the abductor muscle that may affect both medial and lateral plantar nerves, a deep medial ganglion from the subtalar joint compressing the nerve, a proliferative plantar fibromatosis affecting the medial plantar nerve, and a plantar calcaneal exostosis compressing the lateral plantar nerve (Baxter and Thigpen, 1984; Edwards et al, 1969; Schon et al, 1993).

A pigmented villonodular synovitis of the flexor hallucis longus in the tarsal canal caused primary compression of the nerve, and chronic tenosynovitis of the adjacent flexor tendons also affects this nerve (Johnson et al, 1992).

Accessory and anomalous muscles (Sammarco and Conti,

1994), gouty tophi, and villonodular synovitis from the subtalar joint also compress the tibial nerve.

Compressive Medial Plantar Neuropathy

This branch of the nerve may be compressed by extensive fibromatosis, a progressive hemangioma, a neurilemmoma, or a synovial cyst (see Fig. 58–21). We have treated all of these lesions. Direct trauma by a foreign body and subsequent retained segments of foreign bodies such as glass, a toothpick, a sliver of lumber, or an oyster shell either compressed or lacerated the medial plantar nerve.

Digital paresthesias may also be caused by marching, unusual shoe design, and excessive repetitive trauma or misuse of the foot (Massey, 1978; Meharg, 1984; Stein et al, 1989).

TREATMENT

Treatment of these lesions requires a spectrum of methods of management after exploration is performed under a tourniquet. Neurolysis and removal of the foreign body; resection of a localized neuroma and resuture; resection and nerve grafting if the defect is larger and the patient is young; or in a chronic area of extensive fibrosis where grafting is unlikely to succeed, resection and bipolar cauterization of the proximal nerve segment will give satisfactory results. The area of hypesthesia will diminish during a 2- to 3-year period.

Other more distal lesions are compression of the first plantar digital nerve by an exostosis of the first metatarsal head constriction of the first plantar nerve by a plantar fascial compartment (Joplin's neuroma) and compression of this same nerve by a displaced sesamoid bone. The entrapped nerve is treated by realigning the metatarsals, removing the exostosis, and releasing the fascial compartment.

Postsurgical entrapment of the medial plantar digital nerve of the great toe may occur with blind surgical treatment when the nerve has been either wound up in an electric drill, lacerated and avulsed by an air drill, or damaged during blind mini-incisional surgery to remove an exostosis of the first metatarsal head.

Treatment. The damaged nerve is managed either by neurolysis or resection and cauterization of the proximal and distal segments. The treatment decision depends on the patient's age, the severity and duration of the lesion, the intensity of the pain, and the patient's requests.

Lateral Plantar Neuropathy (see Fig. 58–21)

External Compression. Proximally, the lateral plantar nerve is compressed or entrapped under the calcaneus by an exostosis or the origin of a short flexor (Schon et al, 1993).

Treatment. This compression may be managed by diminishing repetitive trauma, appropriate pads or orthotics, unloading the heel with a plastic heel cup, or increasing the shock absorber effect of the shoes.

Occasionally, neurolysis of the branch of the lateral plantar nerve to the short flexors may be necessary to diminish the local pain. This is achieved by either removing soft tissue around the nerve or removing a local exostosis. Also, excision of the proximal attachment of the plantar fascia and excision of the origin of the short flexors may also accomplish the same purpose. However, plantar fasciotomy is performed more logically in the cavus foot rather than in a flat foot.

Lateral Plantar Nerve—Distal Compression
(see Fig. 58–21)

Internal Compression
Nonoperative Treatment. Compression of the common plantar digital nerves occurs at the junction between the third and fourth digital nerves. Because of the cross connection, the common digital nerve is tethered and compressed by the transverse metatarsal ligament. We have treated, nonoperatively, over 100 patients with perineural fibrosis due to entrapment caused by conjoined nerves of the third and fourth digital nerves that are tethered by the plantar aponeurosis as the nerves course from the plantar surface to their digital location. The pseudotumor is distal to the edge of the transverse metatarsal ligament. Treatment varied according to the severity. Wider shoes, lower heels, metatarsal pads, metatarsal bar on the shoe, and injection of steroid and lidocaine directly into the pseudotumor were usually successful in alleviating the symptoms.

Operative Treatment. If clinical symptoms persisted in spite of this treatment, the pseudotumor was resected through a web space incision. Magnification was used by the surgeon, the blood vessels were separated from the nerve, and the enlargement of the nerve was identified. With this technique, the intermetatarsal ligament was not incised. The operation was performed under tibial nerve block and minimal local infiltration. An ankle tourniquet was applied. The digital nerves were identified and followed proximally to the pseudotumor, which was resected without cutting the ligament or resecting the digital vessels. Once the enlargement was recognized, lidocaine was injected directly into the nerve proximal to the tumor and the nerve was resected. The proximal segment was allowed to retract to prevent the nerve from adhering to the transverse metatarsal ligament, the metatarsal head, or the short flexor tendons.

The site of occurrence of perineural fibrosis in our large series of patients has been third to fourth interspace, 84%; second to third interspace with a long skin web, 12%; great toe, tibial side, 3%; and first and last interspaces, 1%.

Recurrent Digital Nerve Pain After Prior Nerve Excision

We have treated over 30 patients who have had prior resection of the perineural pseudotumor but had persistent plantar pain and paresthesias (see Fig. 58–21). These patients had a preoperative nerve block as a diagnostic study. If their pain was relieved, we used a plantar incision to identify the nerve and localize the site of adhesions. Once the fibrotic segment of nerve was identified and dissected distally, it was then followed proximally to the junction of the digital nerves, where they form the common nerves to the third and fourth digits.

If preoperative testing indicated that there was more proximal tethering of the tibial nerve, a condition that had been noted in 12 of our 30 patients, the dissection was continued proximal to the origin of the abductor hallucis muscle (Sunderland, 1978; Upton and McComas, 1973).

Causalgia Syndrome Associated with Tibial Neuropathy

Nerves referred to as being causalgic, are the median, sciatic, obturator, and optic. They all have a central artery for their major blood supply. Other nerves may also be involved in this syndrome, but these particular nerves have an extensive dermatome distribution and a large autonomic nerve component. Trauma or entrapment affects afferent receptors, limits axon flow, interferes with ion membrane transfer, and causes relative segmental ischemia (Lundborg et al, 1983; Mackinnon and Dellon, 1986). These insults cause neuromas in continuity, perineural fibrosis, and abnormal afferent stimuli through the sensory ganglia and autonomic nerves. If the pathological state persists, the peripheral segment of the extremity shows objective evidence of both autonomic and somatic nerve involvement (Levine et al, 1985). Objective findings such as vasospasm, mottling, coolness, hyperhidrosis, slow growth of nails, hypesthesias, hyperpathia, and allodynia have been observed. All of these characteristics are not necessarily present in each patient with causalgia (Goldner and Bright, 1980). Some patients have only hypesthesia and a constant burning, searing, or tearing sensation. Others have symptoms only with lower or higher temperature alterations (Goldner and Bright, 1980). Thermography is helpful in the diagnosis and management of indications used to treat this pain syndrome (Herrick, 1987).

A differential diagnosis is made by the historical pattern, the objective findings, local anesthetic infiltrations, proximal mixed nerve block, and autonomic paravertebral block of the lumbar sympathetics. Each procedure is observed, and the alteration in objective and subjective findings is correlated with the defined syndrome (Levine et al, 1985).

TREATMENT

If the affected nerve has been contused but no fascicles are lacerated, autonomic nerve blocks may be sufficient to alter the afferent stimuli and decrease the intensity and severity of pain and reverse the condition. Supplementary management with a transcutaneous stimulator (Goldner and Hendrix, 1980), active exercise program, warm gloves or stockings, and protection of the sensitive lesion site may be sufficient to manage the syndrome. These methods are supplemented by pharmacological agents that affect the alpha- and beta-adrenergic and parasympathetic receptors. Occasionally, in resistive situations, a microelectrical stimulator placed directly on or directly adjacent to the involved nerve proximal to the lesion may relieve symptoms (Goldner and Bright, 1980).

If nonoperative methods are unsuccessful, surgical treatment is helpful. Neurolysis improves nerve gliding and may diminish ischemia by improving intraneural and extraneural vascularity. Also, a fat or muscle covering is provided for the nerve. Resection of a neuroma or re-establishment of continuity of the nerve with or without nerve grafting may be helpful.

There is a spectrum of lesions from minimal entrapment that responds spontaneously to moderate entrapment that requires local decompression and neurolysis, and severe compressive lesions that require local treatment, pharmacological agents, and microelectrical stimulator to diminish the intensity of central afferent stimuli (Goldner et al, 1975).

NERVE COMPRESSION AND ENTRAPMENT—WHEN TO OPERATE?

Surgical treatment of a compressive lesion requires accurate data from clinical assessment, evidence of improvement or regression reflected by nerve regeneration or degeneration, and occasionally, electrical evidence of interference with sensory and motor conduction.

Clinical Examples

Immediate surgical relief of a compression lesion is required in a compartment syndrome.

Postoperative Progressive Loss of Dorsiflexion of the Foot. Another example of an acute compressive problem is a patient with a *common peroneal nerve-muscle palsy after completion of a high tibial osteotomy.* The decision to re-explore the wound to examine the common peroneal nerve depends on the surgeon's knowledge of the factors that affected the nerve during the operation. If the preoperative deformity was in severe valgus and if the alignment was changed to neutral position postoperatively, the nerve may be stretched and compressed by the fascia of the peroneal muscles. Re-exploration decompression of the nerve is appropriate. Although most stretched or compressed nerves recover spontaneously, the small percentage that do not justify the re-exploration to determine if the nerve has been lacerated, compressed by fascial bands, or impaled on a bone fragment. If forcible retraction was done and was unrecognized, compression or manipulation will cause temporary interference with conduction. At re-exploration, the surgeon determines whether the nerve is intact. Regeneration is then followed in an orderly predictable fashion. Furthermore, if a laceration had unknowingly occurred during the operation, the nerve is repaired within a few days of the incident rather than several weeks or months later, at which time nerve grafting would probably be necessary and the end result would be less satisfactory than a direct early repair.

Another situation that requires a decision exists when immediately after surgery, active dorsiflexion of the foot and physiological sensation were present, but 24 hours later, peroneal nerve function was diminished and the aggressive muscle weakness was caused by either external compression of the nerve or internal edema and hemorrhage with resulting compression. In that situation, a brief period of observation is justified if all external compression is removed, the blood clotting profile is determined, and detailed observation is continued. This delay is not harmful in observing peripheral nerve lesions so long as there is evidence of progressive improvement or, at least, no severe progression.

LOW BACK PAIN WITH SCIATICA—ONSET AND MANAGEMENT

The patient who has a *sudden onset of severe back pain,* sciatica, positive clinical findings, a diminished ankle reflex, and a weak calf demonstrates objective evidence of impairment of the S1 nerve root. If imaging studies show that a large extruded intervertebral disc is compressing the nerve root, an early operation is indicated. This is particularly true if progressive weakness occurs during a short period of observation of the patient's progress.

If a person has a chronic back pain, intermittent sciatica and gradual onset of muscle weakness and sensory alteration in the S1 nerve root distribution, and if the clinical findings are stable but the imaging studies show that only moderate compression of the nerve root exists, it is safe to observe this patient for several weeks before a decision is made whether to operate or not.

MISCELLANEOUS LESIONS

A patient with a severe open lateral subtalar dislocation accompanied by a tear of the posterior tibial tendon and trauma to the tibial nerve should have that nerve decompressed and freed of any constricting bands and assessment of the continuity of the nerve at the time that the open wound is irrigated and surgically excised. A similar concept holds if the lateral subtalar dislocation is closed and severe sensory impairment and a causalgic syndrome occur during the 3- to 5-day period after the injury. The tibial nerve should be decompressed because our experience has shown that the nerve is entrapped by the transverse retinacular ligament, the swollen traumatized abductor hallucis muscle, fibrous bands, and the edema of the nerve from direct contusion. Decompression of the nerve proximally, in the central area, and distally diminishes ischemia and chronic fibrosis of the nerve.

The patient who has had a *fracture of the distal one third of the tibia* treated by closed reduction and application of a long leg cast and who has severe pain, hypesthesia on the plantar surface of the foot, and weakness of toe flexion should be treated as if there is a deep fourth compartment syndrome of the leg. Wick catheter measurements should be obtained to confirm this problem, and decompression of the compartment and of the tibial nerve and the flexor hallucis longus muscle belly should be performed.

A patient who has had a *posterior fracture dislocation of the hip* and a temporary compressive lesion of the sciatic nerve, and immediate evidence of motor and sensory deficit in the foot, leg, and thigh requires immediate realignment of the joint, removal of material that is compressing the nerve, and release of any fibrous constricting bands affecting the nerve. Spontaneous regeneration is then observed for several months by monitoring by percussion tests, the presence or

absence of Tinel's sign, the varying amount of pain, and electrical studies.

The *chronic entrapment lesion such as the lateral femoral cutaneous nerve after a bone graft,* the *obturator nerve* irritation after a fracture of the pelvis into the obturator foramen, irritation of the infrapatellar branch of the saphenous nerve after arthroscopy, posterior tibial nerve entrapment associated with progressive rupture of the posterior tibial tendon are lesions that may be observed for weeks or months so long as there is evidence of axon regeneration. Surgical treatment directed toward decompression of the nerve is done when there is evidence that the lesion is persistent and that improvement is not occurring. The intensity and severity of pain, persistent hypesthesia, and progressive motor weakness are the major reasons for surgically decompressing and entrapped or compressed nerve.

Double Compressive Nerve Lesions (Double Crush Syndrome). Double compressive nerve lesions (double crush syndrome), according to our experience, and that of others (Matsumato et al, 1987; Sunderland, 1978; Upton and McComas, 1973) indicate that proximal compression of a specific nerve lessens that nerve's ability to withstand distal compression. The nerve becomes "sensitive" distally when two or more isolated compressive lesions, each insufficient to greatly impair nerve function, together demonstrate an additive effect on axon flow and nerve conduction (Neary et al, 1976). An example of double crush injury is, compression of the first sacral nerve root and concomitant compression of the tibial nerve at the ankle by a lesion that would ordinarily not cause a tarsal tunnel syndrome. Nonoperative treatment of a tibial nerve that is mildly compressed and causes moderate complaints is frequently successfully. However, this same distal compressive lesion in the presence of a proximal S1 root lesion may require surgical decompression of both sites of nerve compression.

References

Adams JC: Vulnerability of the sciatic nerve inclosed ischiofemoral arthrodesis by nail and graft. J Bone Joint Surg (Br) *46:*748–753, 1964.

Arnoldussen WJ, Korten JJ: Pressure neuropathy of the posterior femoral cutaneous nerve. Clin Neurol Neurosurg *82:*57–60, 1980.

Baba M, Fowler CJ, Jacobs JM, Gilliatt RW: Changes in peripheral nerve fibers distal to a constriction. J Neurol Sci *54:*197–208, 1982.

Baba M, Ozaki I, Watahiki Y, et al: Focal conduction delay at the carpal tunnel level and the cubital fossa in diabetic polyneuropathy. Electromygr Clin Neurophysiol *27:*119–123, 1987.

Banerjee T, Koons DD: Superficial peroneal nerve entrapment: Report of two cases. J Neurol Surg *55:*991–994, 1981.

Barton PM: Piriformis syndrome: A rational approach to management. Pain *47:*345–352, 1991.

Bassett FH, Kirkpatrick JS, Engelhardt D, Malone TR: Cryotherapy—induced nerve injury. Am J Sports Med *20:*516–518, 1992.

Baxter DE, Thigpen CM: Heel pain: Operative results. Foot Ankle *5:*16, 1984.

Beresford HR: Meralgia paresthetica after seatbelt trauma. J Trauma *11:*629–636, 1971.

Berry H, Richardson P: Common peroneal nerve palsy: A clinical and electrophysiological review. J Neurol Neurosurg Psychiatry *30:*1162–1171, 1976.

Borges LF, Hale HM, Selkoed J, Welch K: The anterior tarsal tunnel syndrome: Report of two cases. J Neurosurg *54:*89–90, 1981.

Bray TJ, Leighton RK: Pudendal and peroneal nerve compression. *In* Szabo RM (ed): Nerve Compression Syndromes: Diagnosis and Treatment. Thorofare, NJ, Slack, Inc., 1989, pp 309–317.

Brooks DM: Nerve compression by simple ganglia. J Bone Joint Surg (Br) *34:*391–400, 1952.

Brown MJ, Ashbury AK: Diabetic neuropathy. Ann Neurol *15:*2–12, 1984.

Claussen DK, Geddon HJ: The late consequences of sciatic nerve injury. J Bone Joint Surg (Br) *42:*213–225, 1960.

Cobb CA, Maiel RH: Ganglion of the peroneal nerve. J Neurosurg *41:*255–259, 1974.

Dellon AL: Deep peroneal nerve entrapment on the dorsum of the foot. Foot Ankle *11:*73–80, 1990.

Docks GW, Salter, MS: Sural nerve entrapment: An unusual report. J Foot Surg *18:*42–43, 1979.

Edelson JG, Nathan H: Meralgia paresthetica. Clin Orthop *122:*255–262, 1977.

Edwards WG, Lincoln CR, Bassett FH III, Goldner JL: The tarsal tunnel syndrome. JAMA *207:*716, 1969.

Eustace S, McCarthy C, O'Byrne J, Breatmach E, Fitzgerald E: Computed tomography of the retroperitoneum in patients with femoral neuropathy. Can Assoc Radiol J *45:*277–282, 1994.

Evans BA, Stevens JC, Dyck PJ: Lumbosacral plexus neuropathy. Neurology *31:*1327–1330, 1981.

Evans JD, Neumann L, Frostick SP: Compression neuropathy of the common peroneal nerve caused by a ganglion. Microsurgery *15:*193–195, 1994.

Fransen P, Thauvoy C, Sindic CJ, Stroobandt G: Intraneural ganglionic cyst of the common peroneal nerve: Case report and review of the literature. Acta Neurol Belg *91:*231–235, 1991.

Garfin S, Mubarak SJ, Owen CA: Exertional anterolateral compartment syndrome: Case report with fascial defect, muscle herniation, and superficial peroneal nerve entrapment. J Bone Joint Surg (Am) *59:*404–405, 1977.

Garland H, Moorhouse D: Compressive lesions of the external popliteal (common peroneal) nerve. BMJ *2:*1373–1378, 1952.

Gessini L, Jandolo B, Peitrangel A: The anterior tarsal tunnel syndrome: Report of four cases. J Bone Joint Surg (Am) *66:*786–788, 1984.

Giuliani G, Poppi N, Acciarri N, Forti A: CT scan and surgical treatment of traumatic iliacus hematoma with femoral neuropathy: Case report. J Trauma *30:*229–231, 1990.

Goldner JL: Lesions of the low back and lower extremities simulating ruptured discs. N C Med J *17:*260–267, 1956.

Goldner JL: Pain: General review and selected problems affecting the upper extremity. J Hand Surg *8:*740–745, 1983.

Goldner JL: Nerve entrapment syndromes of the foot, ankle, and leg. The Jefferson Orthopaedic Journal 8:6–16, 1984.

Goldner JL, Bright DS: Pain: Extremities and spine—Evaluation and differential diagnosis. *In* Omer G, Spinner M (eds): Management of Peripheral Nerve Problems, 1st ed., Philadelphia, W.B. Saunders Company, 1980a, pp 119–175.

Goldner JL, Bright DS: The effect of extremity blood flow on pain and cold tolerance. *In* Omer G, Spinner M (eds): Management of Peripheral Problems, 1st ed., Philadelphia, W.B. Saunders Company, 1980b, pp 176–194.

Goldner JL, Bright DS, Nashold BS Jr: Electrical stimulation of peripheral nerves for relief of intractable chronic pain. J Bone Joint Surg *57A:*729, 1975.

Goldner JL, Fleming L: Lateral femoral cutaneous nerve affected by iliac bone graft for spine fusion. Unpublished data, 1993.

Goldner JL, Hendrix PC: Use of transcutaneous electrical stimulation in the management of chronic pain syndromes. *In* LeRoy PL (ed): Current Concepts in the Management of Pain, Miami, FL, Symposia Specialists Medical Books, 1977, pp 111–725.

Goodson JD: Pudendal neuritis from biking. Letter to the Editor. N Engl J Med *304:*365, 1979.

Goodgold J, Kopell HP, Spielholt NJ: The tarsal tunnel syndrome: Objective diagnostic criteria. N Engl J Med *273:*742, 1965.

Gould N, Trevino S: Sural nerve entrapment by avulsion fracture of the base of the fifth metatarsal bone. Foot Ankle *2:*153–155, 1981.

Grant JC: An Atlas of Anatomy, 2nd ed. Baltimore, Williams & Wilkins Company, 1947.

Gray H: Anatomy of the Human Body, 23rd ed. Philadelphia, Lea and Febiger, 1936.

Hardaker WT, Aymond JK, Goldner JL: Neuralgic amyotrophy. Orthop Rev *18:*1275–1279, 1989.

Harms BA, DeHaas DR, Starling JR: Diagnosis and management of genito-femoral neuralgia. Arch Surg *119:*339–341, 1984.

Hemler DE, Ward WK, Karstetter KW, Bryant PM: Saphenous nerve entrapment caused by pes anserine bursitis mimicking stress fracture of the tibia. Arch Phys Med Rehabil *72:*336–337, 1991.

Henricson AS, Westlin NE: Chronic calcaneal pain in athletes: Entrapment of the calcaneal nerve? Am J Sports Med *12:*152, 1984.

Herrick RT, Herrick SK: Thermography in the detection of carpal tunnel syndrome and other compressive neuropathies. J Hand Surg (Am) *12A:*943–949, 1987.

Hollingshead WH: Anatomy for Surgeons: The Back and Limbs, 2nd ed. New York, Harper and Row, 1969.

Huittinen VM: Lumbosacral nerve injury in fracture of the pelvis. A postmortem radiographic and pathoanatomical study. Acta Clin Scand 429(Suppl):1–43, 1972.

Jankiewicz JJ, Hennrikus WL, Houkom JA: The appearance of the piriformis muscle syndrome in computed tomography and magnetic resonance imaging: A case report and review of the literature. Clin Orthop *262:*205–209, 1991.

Johnson ER, Kirby K, Lieberman JS: Lateral plantar nerve entrapment: Foot pain in a power lifter. Am J Sports Med *20:*619–620, 1992.

Jutmann L: A typical deep peroneal neuropathy. J Neurol Neurosurg Psychiatry *33:*453, 1970.

Kaplan PE, Kernahan WT: Tarsal tunnel syndrome. J Bone Joint Surg (Am) *63:*96–99, 1981.

Kars HZ, Topaktas S, Dogan K: Aneurysmal peroneal nerve compression. Neurosurgery *30:*930–931, 1992.

Kashani SR, Moon AH, Gaunt WD: Tibial nerve entrapment by a Baker cyst: Case report. Arch Phys Med Rehabil *66:*49–51, 1985.

Katz RT: Nerve entrapments: An update. Orthopedics *12:*1097–1107, 1989.

Keck C: The tarsal tunnel syndrome. J Bone Joint Surg *44A:*180, 1962.

Kernohan J, Levack B, Wilson JN: Entrapment of the superficial peroneal nerve (three case reports). J Bone Joint Surg *57B:*60–61, 1985.

Kettelkamp DB, Leach RE, Wasca R: Pitfalls of proximal tibial osteotomy. Clin Orthop *106:*232–238, 1975.

Kopell HP, Thompson WA: Peripheral entrapment neuropathies of the lower extremity. N Engl J Med *252:*56–58, 1960a.

Kopell H, Thompson WA: Knee pain due to saphenous nerve entrapment. N Engl J Med *263:*351–353, 1960b.

Kopell HP, Thompson WA: Peripheral Entrapment Neuropathies. Baltimore; Williams & Wilkins Company, 1963.

Kosinski C: The course, mutual relations, and distribution of the cutaneous nerves of the metazonal region of leg and foot. J Anat *60:*274–297, 1926.

Krause KH, Witt T, Ross A: The anterior tarsal tunnel syndrome. J Neurol *217:*67–74, 1977.

Kumar S, Anantham J, Wan Z: Post traumatic hematoma of the iliacus muscle with paralysis of the femoral nerve. J Orthop Trauma *6:*110–112, 1992.

Lambert EH: The accessory deep peroneal nerve: A common variation in innervation of extensor digitorum brevis. Neurology, *19:*1169, 1969.

Leonard M: Immediate improvements of sensation on relief of extraneural compression. J Bone Joint Surg *51A:*1282, 1967.

Leonard MA: Sciatic nerve paralysis following anticoagulant therapy. J Bone Joint Surg (Br) *54:*152–153, 1972.

Levine JD, Dardick SJ, Basbaum AI, Scipio E: Reflex neurogenic inflammation, I. contribution of the peripheral nervous system to spacially remote inflammatory responses that follow injury. J Neurol Sci *5:*1380–1386, 1985.

Lindenbaum BL: Ski boot compression syndrome. Clin Orthop *140:*19, 1979.

Lundborg G: Ischemic nerve injury: Experimental studies on intraneural, microvascular, pathophysiology, and nerve function in a limb subjected to temporary circulatory arrest. Scand J Plast Reconstr Surg 6(Suppl):1–113, 1970.

Lundborg G, Myers R, Powell H: Nerve compression injury and increased endoneurial fluid pressure: A "miniature compartment syndrome." J Neurol Neurosurg Psychiatry *46:*1119–1124, 1983.

Lundborg G, Rydevik B: Effects of stretching the tibial nerve of the rabbit: A preliminary study of the intraneural circulation and the barrier function of the perineurium. J Bone Joint Surg (Br) *55:*390–401, 1973.

Lusskin R: Peripheral neuropathies affecting the foot. *In* Jahss MH (ed): Disorders of the Foot. Philadelphia, W.B. Saunders Company, 1982, pp 1169–1204.

Lyons WR, Woodhall B: Atlas of Peripheral Nerve Injuries. Philadelphia; W.B. Saunders Company, 1949.

Mackinnon SE, Dellon AL: Experimental study of chronic nerve compression. Hand Clin *2:*639–650, 1986.

Maigne JY, Maigne R, Guerin-Surville H: Anatomic study of the lateral

• Lewis H. Millender*
• Andrew L. Terrono
• Martin J. O'Malley

Chapter 59

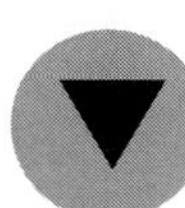

Neurological Involvement of the Extremities Associated with Rheumatoid Arthritis

Pain, weakness, and sensory loss are prominent symptoms in patients with rheumatoid arthritis and can be caused by neuropathy, but the diagnosis can be difficult. The most frequent cause of pain, of course, is the arthritis itself, which can affect virtually all of the synovial joints in the body. Additionally, the inflammatory process can affect tendon sheaths and can lead to a painful tenosynovitis, such as flexor tenosynovitis associated with carpal tunnel syndrome. Destruction of the joints can lead to deformity, restriction of range of motion, and disuse, all of which produce weakness. Tendon rupture is another cause of weakness without neurological involvement. The clinical assessment of true muscle weakness can be impossible in the face of significant joint pain and deformity. Because sensory symptoms can be experienced as a kind of pain, it is not surprising that, in this setting, they may be ascribed initially to the arthritis. When weakness is out of proportion to the joint disease, and when numbness and paresthesias are recognized, neurological involvement is clear. However, even then one is faced with the differential diagnosis of myopathy, radiculopathy, and myelopathy as well as neuropathy. The authors discuss the details of the several varieties of neuropathy encountered in patients with rheumatoid arthritis and then touch on the major features of the principal differential diagnostic entities.

NEUROPATHIES

There are three main classes of neuropathies in rheumatoid arthritis: (1) entrapment neuropathies; (2) a typically severe mononeuropathy multiplex; and (3) a mild, distal, mainly sensory polyneuropathy. The relative incidence of each type is not well established. Neuropathy does not seem to be an inevitable concomitant of the disease, as it is, for example, in diabetes mellitus or uremia. On the other hand, nerve biopsies or electromyographic studies of asymptomatic patients may be abnormal (Beckett and Dinn, 1972).

Entrapment Neuropathies

Compression neuropathies are a frequent manifestation of rheumatoid arthritis, which is seen frequently in the upper extremity. Their incidence has been reported to be as high as 45% (Nakano, 1975b). The most frequent cause of the compression is a proliferative rheumatoid tenosynovitis or

synovitis that causes local compression over a segment of the nerve as it passes through a fibrous or fibro-osseous canal. In addition to this, bony protrusion, joint subluxations, and joint deformities can cause the syndrome. Chapters 53, 54, 55, and 58 are focused on compression neuropathies; therefore, in this section the authors discuss only the specific characteristics that the rheumatoid patient presents.

UPPER EXTREMITY COMPRESSION NEUROPATHIES

Median Nerve

Carpal tunnel syndrome is the most common rheumatoid compression neuropathy, which is seen in approximately 23% of rheumatoid patients (Chamberlain and Corbett, 1970) (Fig. 59–1). It may be the initial manifestation of the disease, and it is not uncommon to have the diagnosis of rheumatoid arthritis made by the pathologist after carpal tunnel release for what was thought to be an idiopathic carpal tunnel syndrome.

The early signs and symptoms of rheumatoid carpal tunnel syndrome are identical to those of carpal tunnel syndrome of other causes. These include nocturnal symptoms, paresthesias in the median nerve distribution, and pain that extends both proximally and distally. As with idiopathic carpal tunnel syndrome, a high percentage of cases may present bilaterally. As the condition progresses, involvement of the flexor tendons plus thenar atrophy can significantly affect hand function.

Wrist flexor tenosynovitis initially causes only symptoms of median nerve compression. However, as the proliferation continues, flexor tendon function becomes affected (Millender and Nalebuff, 1975a). The early effects of this proliferation are minimal loss of active digital flexion, with passive flexion preserved. However, as the disease progresses, severe limitation of digital flexion may be seen. In addition to the wrist flexor tenosynovitis, the tenosynovium may extend into the palm and digits, and one should evaluate these areas (Nalebuff and Potter, 1968). Digital fullness, palpable tendon nodules, and triggering are the common signs of palmar and digital flexor tenosynovitis.

Another complication of wrist flexor tenosynovitis is tendon rupture (Nalebuff, 1969). Although not common, tenosynovium can infiltrate into the flexor tendons, resulting in their rupture. When a tendon rupture is diagnosed, one must

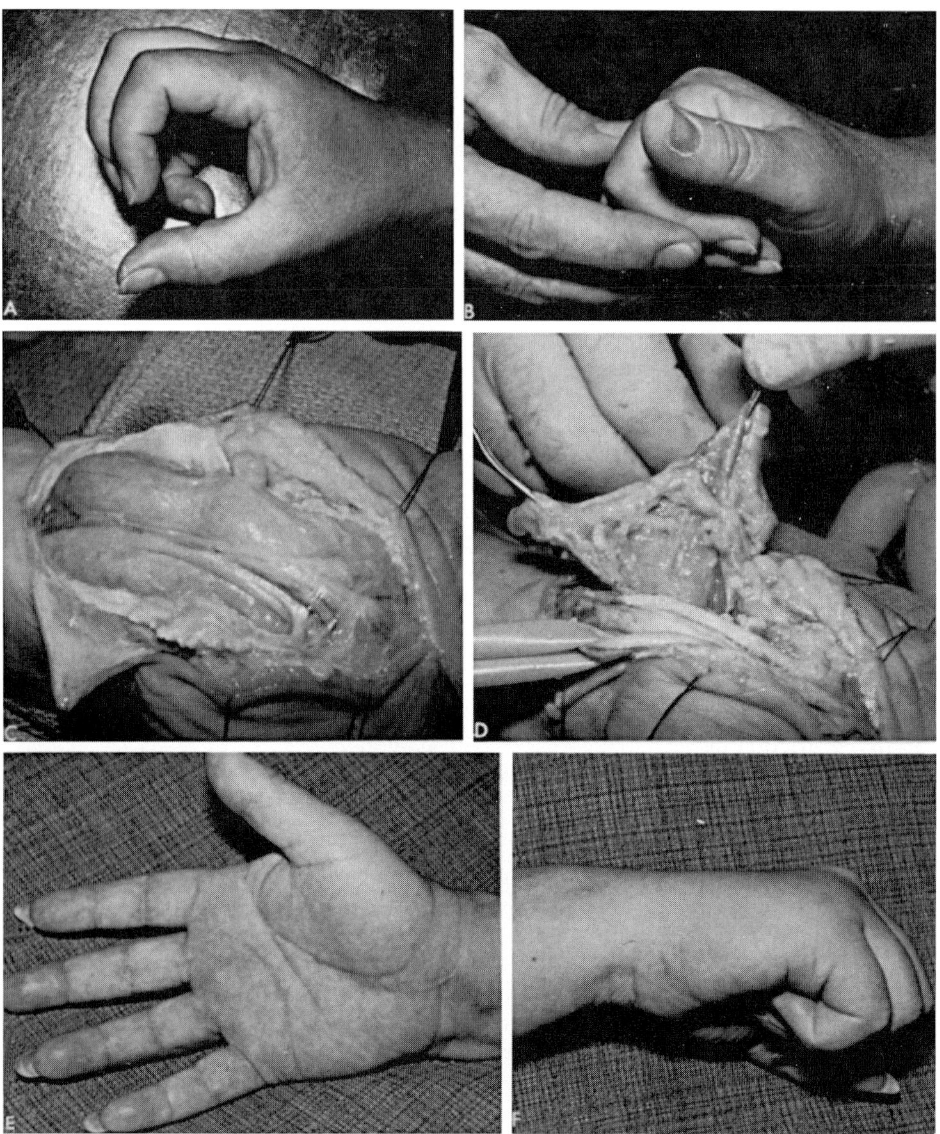

FIGURE 59–1. *A*, Patient complains of numbness in the median nerve distribution and limited active digital flexion. *B*, Passive digital flexion preserved. *C*, Carpal tunnel exposed, and the median nerve seen surrounded by large amount of flexor tenosynovitis. *D*, Median nerve retracted with a Penrose drain. Flexor tenosynovium plus large bursa exposed prior to tenosynovectomy. *E* and *F*, Full digital motion restored.

differentiate whether the rupture occurred at the wrist, palm, or digital level.

An interesting manifestation of tendon rupture that must be differentiated from anterior interosseous nerve paralysis is the Mannerfelt's syndrome (Fig. 59–2). In this condition, there may be rupture of the flexor pollicis longus alone or of the flexor pollicis longus plus the flexor digitorum profundus to the index and long digits from a sharp spur that develops on the anterior aspect of the scaphoid (Nalebuff, 1969). When a patient presents with inability to flex the interphalangeal joint of the thumb and the distal interphalangeal joint of the index finger, anterior interosseous nerve paralysis must be suspected (Spinner, 1978). Although anterior interosseous nerve paralysis is no more common in the rheumatoid patient than in the general population, the condition must be considered in differential diagnosis and ruled out. Oblique films of the wrist sometimes show an erosion of the scaphoid. Additionally, electromyography can help confirm the diagnosis of anterior interosseous nerve paralysis.

The other serious complication of wrist flexor tenosynovi-tis and subsequent median nerve compression is involvement of the thenar muscles. Generalized intrinsic muscle atrophy is commonly seen in the rheumatoid patient. It is associated with cervical spine disease, median and ulnar nerve involvement, and disuse atrophy from pain and joint involvement. Thenar atrophy can significantly affect the rheumatoid thumb, especially if there is associated joint involvement (Millender and Nalebuff, 1975b). As thenar atrophy progresses, there is loss of active opposition that leads to a fixed supination contracture with loss of effective pulp or key pinch. The end result of this ineffective side pinch is destruction of the interphalangeal joint or the metacarpophalangeal joint, or both.

The diagnosis of rheumatoid carpal tunnel syndrome usually can be established clinically, especially if there is wrist fullness and limited active digital flexion. One must be careful not to attribute all thenar atrophy to carpal tunnel syndrome, because of the multiple factors that can cause its appearance. When the clinical diagnosis is in doubt, electromyography and nerve conduction velocity studies should be obtained to confirm the diagnosis.

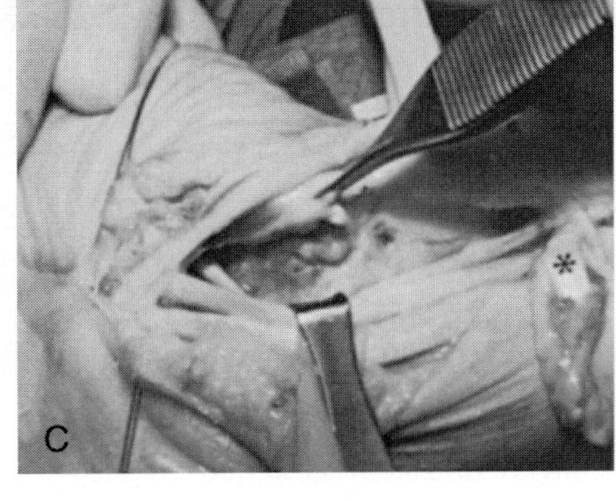

FIGURE 59–2. *A,* Patient with inability to actively flex interphalangeal joint of the thumb or distal interphalangeal joint of index finger. Anterior interosseous nerve palsy suspected. Note arrow pointing to localized area of tenderness. *B,* Roentgenogram of the wrist demonstrates punched out lesion in the scaphoid often seen with ruptured flexor pollicis longus. *C,* Carpal tunnel exposed. Ruptured flexor pollicis longus held with forceps. The synovium from the wrist joint can be seen bulging through the capsule. The proximal end of the flexor pollicis longus has also been identified (asterisk).

In addition to tenosynovitis, carpal tunnel syndrome can be associated with both wrist joint subluxation and lateral or fixed flexion contractures. One manifestation of rheumatoid arthritis is volar wrist dislocation associated with wrist destruction. This can cause symptoms of both median and ulnar nerve compression. Correction of the deformity by wrist arthrodesis or arthroplasty usually alleviates the symptoms, although carpal tunnel release may be necessary (Millender and Nalebuff, 1975b). However, median nerve compression has been seen after wrist arthrodesis. This is seen more commonly if severe volar subluxation of the carpus has been corrected. The volar surface of the radius may project into the carpal tunnel. This should be treated with decompression of the median nerve with resection of the bone prominence from the volar aspect of the distal radius (Ekerot et al, 1983).

For early carpal tunnel syndrome associated with flexor tenosynovitis, steroid injection plus wrist splinting may give temporary or long-term remission, depending on the general condition of the disease. However, for persistent symptoms, especially if the condition is associated with tendon function or thenar atrophy, carpal tunnel release with flexor tenosynovectomy is indicated. In addition to the wrist flexor tenosynovectomy, palmar or digital flexor tenosynovectomy, or both, should be carried out, if indicated (Millender and Nalebuff, 1975b). If flexor tendon ruptures are present, tendon transfers or intercalary tendon grafts may be necessary.

Ulnar Nerve

Ulnar nerve compression at the elbow is not especially common in rheumatoid arthritis (Nakano, 1975a). Upton and co-workers (1978) have diagnosed cubital tunnel syndrome by electrophysiological testing in 12% of their patients.

However, the diagnosis is mainly a clinical one. Electrophysiological testing may be helpful, but often there is a poor correlation between clinical evaluation and electrodiagnostic testing (Balagtas-Balmaseda et al, 1983). Ulnar nerve compression can be seen secondary to elbow synovitis or cyst (Mainard et al, 1991), which bulges medially and compresses the nerve as it passes through the tunnel behind the medial epicondyle (Fig. 59–3). It can also be associated with scarring and narrowing of the ulnar tunnel secondary to the inflammatory process and destruction of the elbow joint. A less frequent cause is bony deformity. Moore and Weiland (1980) have reported one case of bilateral attritional ruptures of the ulnar nerve at the elbow, possibly on eroded bone ends. Rarely, ulnar nerve compression has been seen in association with a large olecranon bursa that has extended medially. Although many rheumatoid patients have elbow flexion contractures and cubitus valgus, few of them manifest symptoms of ulnar nerve compression. Even in cases of elbow instability due to joint destruction with ligamentous laxity, ulnar nerve involvement is not especially common.

Additional cases of ulnar nerve compression are seen after lower extremity surgery and after total elbow replacement. Good and associates (1965) have demonstrated that a diffuse peripheral neuropathy with pre-existing marginal nerve function may predispose patients to having an increased incidence of ulnar nerve symptoms postoperatively (Boyd and Thornhill, 1989). Following major lower extremity surgery, such as total hip or total knee replacement, patients with weak hands sometimes tend to push themselves up on their elbows. If done excessively, this can result in symptoms of ulnar nerve irritation. Also, patients using platform crutches can develop ulnar nerve symptoms if the crutches are inadequately padded or do not fit properly.

A postoperative complication of total elbow replacement

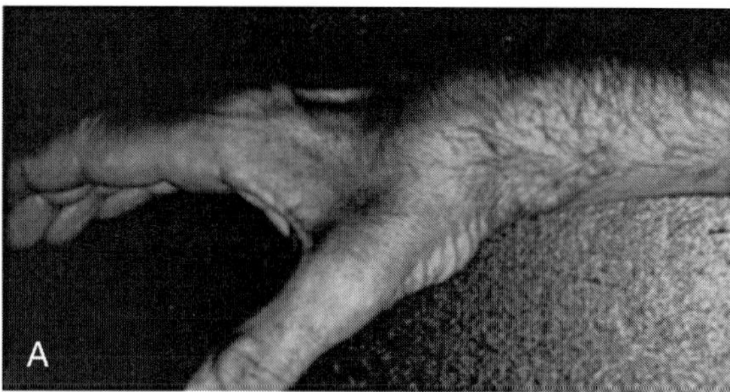

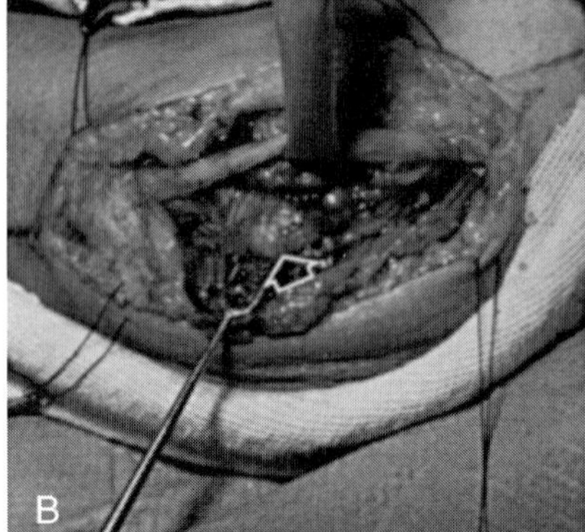

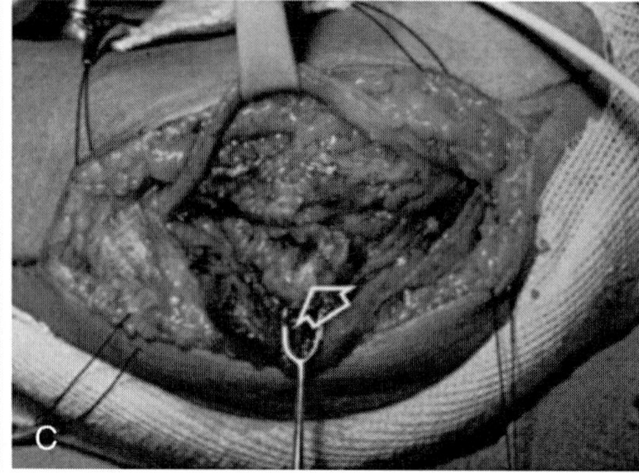

FIGURE 59–3. Ulnar nerve palsy associated with elbow joint synovitis. *A*, Interosseous muscle atrophy. *B*, The ulnar nerve is retracted and the synovium *(arrow)* is demonstrated bulging from the medial elbow joint. *C*, The capsule of the elbow joint is opened, demonstrating the proliferative synovitis *(arrow)*.

is the presence of ulnar nerve irritation symptoms. These symptoms are seen especially when the nerve is not completely mobilized and retracted before the joint resection or introduction of the methyl methacrylate. The symptoms are usually transient, and are probably related to traction on the nerve during surgery. They also may be associated with the heat of the methyl methacrylate. Permanent symptoms of ulnar nerve compression may be related to postoperative compression of the nerve, especially if it was not completely mobilized at the time of the total joint replacement. The use of the lateral subperiosteal approach instead of the posterior approach has decreased the incidence of ulnar nerve compression after total elbow replacement (Ewald et al, 1993).

When ulnar nerve symptoms are associated with elbow joint synovitis, steroid injections into the joint and immobilization often alleviate the condition. If elbow synovectomy is indicated, a separate medial incision should be made to release the ulnar nerve. In cases of ulnar nerve involvement associated with severe elbow destruction, decompression of the ulnar nerve with total joint replacement is indicated.

Ulnar nerve entrapment at the wrist in Guyon's canal is seen much less frequently than median nerve compression associated with carpal tunnel syndrome (Shea and McClain, 1969; Spinner, 1978). This is understandable, because there are no tendons, and therefore no tenosynovium, within Guyon's canal. Rarely, ulnar nerve compression at the wrist level can be associated with large amounts of wrist flexor tenosynovitis. Swanson (1973) has stated that he has seen several cases of ulnar nerve motor impingement within Guyon's canal associated with flexor tenosynovitis. Taylor (1974) has reported a case of tenosynovium from the flexor digitorum sublimis to the ring and little fingers. It displaced the ulnar nerve against the flexor carpi ulnaris tendon and extended into the canal of Guyon. Ulnar nerve involvement at the wrist can also be associated with wrist dislocation and wrist joint deformities similar to median nerve involvement (Millender and Nalebuff, 1973).

When patients present with symptoms of ulnar nerve compression, the diagnosis may not be easily established. Many of these patients have multiple joint involvements and can have, in addition to wrist and elbow involvement, cervical spine disease (Nakano, 1975a). As with the median nerve, the ulnar nerve may become entrapped concomitantly with lower cervical spine disease or with thoracic outlet syndrome. When compression of the ulnar nerve in the wrist is diagnosed, standard decompression of the ulnar nerve in the hand with tenosynovectomy as needed is indicated.

Posterior Interosseous Nerve Paralysis

Posterior interosseous nerve paralysis is a rare but well-documented complication of rheumatoid arthritis (Millender et al, 1973; Marshall and Murray, 1974) (Fig. 59–4). It results from elbow synovitis bulging anteriorly and compressing the posterior interosseous nerve as it enters into the supinator muscle. Depending on the degree of nerve compression, either a partial or complete paralysis of the muscles innervated by the posterior interosseous nerve is seen. The clinical appearance of compression neuropathy, especially when it is partial, is similar to extensor tendon ruptures. In two cases reported in the literature, patients were initially explored for extensor tendon ruptures (Marmor et al, 1967; Millender et al, 1973). Fernandez and associates (1979) have reported one case of radial nerve compression at the elbow with only sensory symptoms and abnormal electrodiagnostic testing of the sensory radial nerve but a normal electromyogram. The patient responded to a cortisone injection into the elbow joint.

The presenting manifestation is inability to extend either all or some of the digits and thumb. In two of the three cases, we have seen that there was inability to extend the ulnar three digits at the metacarpophalangeal joint. Extension was preserved in the index finger, and extension and abduction were preserved in the thumb (Millender et al, 1973).

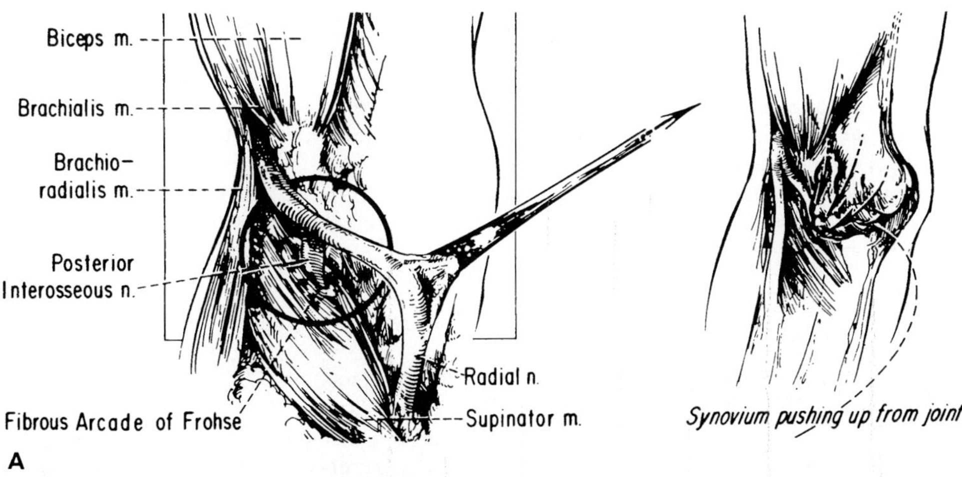

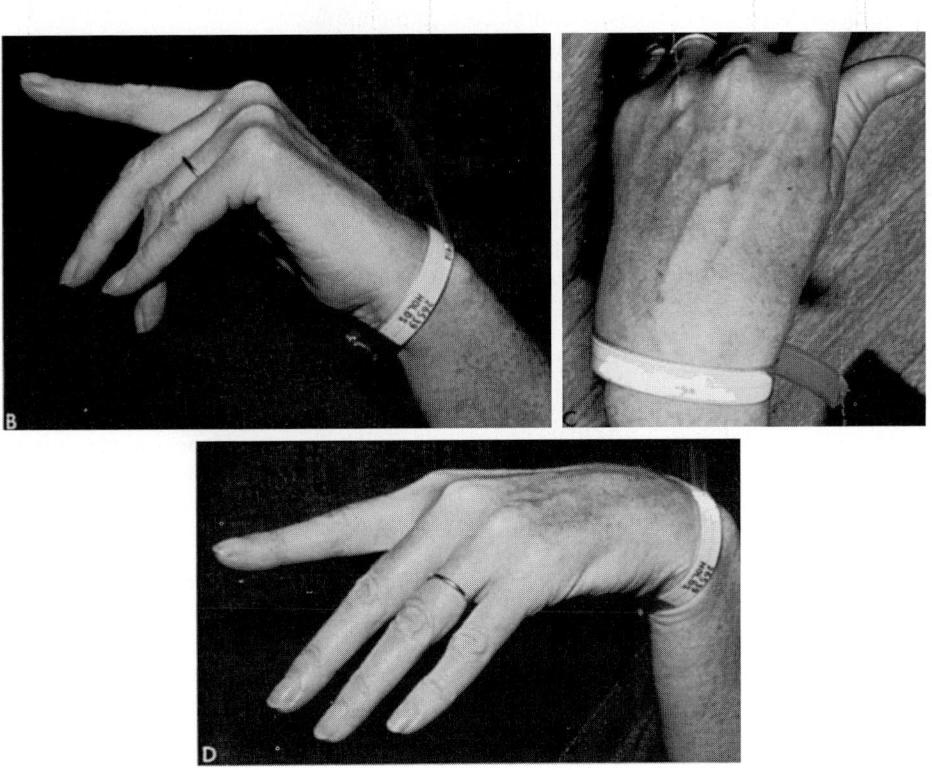

FIGURE 59–4. Posterior interosseous nerve paralysis associated with rheumatoid arthritis. *A,* Diagram demonstrates the elbow synovitis bulging anteriorly and compressing the posterior interosseous nerve as it penetrates the two heads of the supinator muscle. *B,* Partial posterior interosseous nerve paralysis with inability to extend ulnar three digits. *C,* Wrist extension is associated with radial deviation due to paralysis of the extensor carpi ulnaris. *D,* Positive tenodesis effect demonstrating that the extensor tendons are intact.

The proper diagnosis is readily established by careful clinical examination. The patient shows evidence of elbow synovitis with pain, limitation of digital extension, and tenderness over the anterior aspect of the elbow joint. There is usually absence of dorsal tenosynovitis, which would tend to rule out extensor tendon rupture. When the wrist is passively flexed, the metacarpophalangeal joints extend, demonstrating that the extensor tendons are intact (see Fig. 59–4*B* and *D*). In tendon rupture, the distal ends usually retract distal to the wrist joint, thereby giving a loss of tenodesis effect when the wrist is flexed. The most important physical findings are radial deviation of the wrist on active extension due to paralysis of the extensor carpi ulnaris with preservation of the extensor carpi radialis longus and brevis (Popelka and Vaino, 1974). In addition, any digital extensor tendons that are functioning show definite weakness. Electromyography can be used to confirm the diagnosis.

The treatment depends on the degree of involvement and the length of time the compression has existed. In one of the cases that we treated with a steroid injection into the elbow joint, the patient showed partial recovery of extensor tendon function in 2 weeks, with full recovery in 6 weeks. In another case, anterior exploration of the posterior interosseous nerve with elbow synovectomy was carried out. The patient showed return of extensor tendon function within 24 hours and full return of function within 4 days. In a case that was explored for ruptured extensor tendons, tendon transfer was carried out because the patient had shown inability to extend the digits for approximately 2 years (Millender et al, 1973).

LOWER EXTREMITY COMPRESSION NEUROPATHIES

Lower extremity compression neuropathies associated with rheumatoid arthritis are usually confined to the tibial and peroneal nerves. This is secondary to compression from popliteal cysts plus tarsal tunnel syndrome and lateral and medial plantar nerve syndrome (Nakano, 1975a). Bedridden patients or patients with cast immobilization can develop common peroneal nerve palsies secondary to external pressure over the vulnerable area at the proximal fibula. Although these neuropathies are seen with rheumatoid arthritis and must be differentiated from popliteal cysts, they are not a direct complication of rheumatoid arthritis.

Sciatic Nerve Entrapment

Sciatic nerve entrapments are uncommon. Most patients with rheumatoid arthritis with symptoms in the sciatic nerve distribution are caused by the intervertebral discs or other structures of the lumbar spine (e.g., spinal stenosis, degenerative disease). Sciatic nerve palsies can be seen as a complication of hip surgery or following improperly administered intramuscular injections but are not directly associated with rheumatoid arthritis. Rarely, true compression of the nerve may occur from the piriformis muscle, causing piriformis syndrome. Treatment of piriformis syndrome consists of releasing the insertion of the muscle into the greater trochanter and any other constricting bands. (Nakano, 1993). In addition, excessive lengthening of the extremity following total hip arthroplasty can cause sciatica nerve palsy.

Popliteal Space (Baker's Cyst)

Rheumatoid synovitis of the knee joint may cause a popliteal cyst (Baker's cyst; Fig. 59–5) that can result in compression of either the posterior tibial or peroneal nerve (Gardner, 1972). Numerous bursae are located in the popliteal space. These include bursae between the hamstring tendons and the collateral ligaments or condyles of the tibia, and a bursa is also located deep to each head of the gastrocnemius muscle. In nonrheumatoid adult patients, most popliteal cysts are associated with internal derangement of the knee, and the cyst may recur if the intra-articular pathology is not corrected (Justis, 1987). Although these cysts are common in rheumatoid arthritis, they rarely cause compressive neuropathy. Giant synovial cysts in patients with rheumatoid arthritis have been reported, and cause a syndrome that presents similarly to acute thrombophlebitis. Arthrography has documented that these cysts arise from and communicate with the knee (Hollingsworth, 1968). The diagnosis of these cysts is easily confirmed with an MRI scan. Treatment consists of posterior exploration with removal of the cyst and either open or arthroscopic knee joint synovectomy.

Peroneal Nerve Palsy

Peroneal nerve palsy has been reported in a patient with rheumatoid arthritis who had bilateral posterior dislocation of the proximal tibia-fibula joint (Ishikawa, 1984). Decompression by excision of the head of the fibula resulted in resolution of the symptoms. More commonly, the peroneal nerve can be stretched following total knee arthroplasty. This is seen most often when a significant valgus or flexion deformity is corrected; the physician and patient must be aware of this risk preoperatively (Rose et al, 1982).

Posterior Tibial Nerve/Tarsal Tunnel Syndrome

Tarsal tunnel syndrome is the resultant neuropathy from extrinsic or intrinsic compression of the posterior tibial nerve as it courses beneath the medial malleolus (Cimino, 1990). This is analogous to carpal tunnel syndrome, although it is much less common. The roof of the tarsal tunnel is formed by the flexor retinaculum or lacinate ligament. This fan-shaped ligament spreads out posteriorly from the medial malleolus to attach to the medial wall of the calcaneus and abductor hallucis fascia. The contents of the tunnel are the posterior tibial nerve, artery, vein, and tendon as well as the flexor hallucis and digitorum longus.

The posterior tibial nerve, a branch of the sciatic nerve, passes between the two heads of the gastrocnemius muscle, deep to the soleus muscle, and forms three terminal branches in the tarsal tunnel: the median plantar nerve, lateral plantar nerve, and calcaneal branch. A report of cadaver dissection showed 93% of the branching occurring in the tarsal tunnel and the remaining 7% proximal to it (Havel et al, 1988).

The etiology of tarsal tunnel syndrome is variable. Space-occupying lesions such as ganglions, varicosities, lipomas, and neurilemmomas account for one half of the cases (Cimino, 1990). Approximately 50% of the patients have a history of previous sprain, fracture, crush injury, or flatfoot (Schon and Baxter, 1994). Proliferative rheumatoid synovitis may cause posterior tibial nerve compression. In addition, patients with rheumatoid arthritis often have a valgus hindfoot deformity that can alter the cross-sectional area of the tunnel and compress the nerve (Lian, 1994). It has been reported that 25% of rheumatoid arthritis patients had electrodiagnostic evidence of posterior tibial nerve compression, although only two patients were symptomatic (Lian, 1994). For many patients with tarsal tunnel syndrome, no specific cause is found even after exploration.

The symptoms of tarsal tunnel syndrome are burning pain in the sole of the foot, which is often worse at night, with decreased sensitivity to light touch. Sensory symptoms predominate over motor symptoms (intrinsic weakness) because the sensory nerves are more sensitive to ischemia. Tinel's sign (percussion along the course of the nerve) has been reported in 50% to 100% of the patients (Schon and Baxter, 1994)

The diagnosis of tarsal tunnel syndrome is made by combining a positive history and physical examination with electrodiagnostic studies. The distal motor latencies of the medial (>6.2 milliseconds) and lateral (>7.0 milliseconds) plantar nerves have been the traditional tests employed, although distal sensory latency may be more sensitive (Lian, 1994). Both feet must be evaluated because none of the electrodiagnostic tests by themselves are absolute. MRI may be helpful in localizing a lesion in surgical candidates, but its role has not been clearly defined.

The treatment of tarsal tunnel syndrome in rheumatoid arthritis depends on the etiology. Proliferative synovitis may respond to immobilization, nonsteroidal anti-inflammatory drugs (NSAIDs), or a steroid injection. An orthotic device has been shown to be effective in patients with a hyper-mobile flatfoot and should be tried in all rheumatoid patients. If surgical intervention is indicated, decompression from above the medial malleolus to the two terminal branches is performed. Decompression has produced mixed results

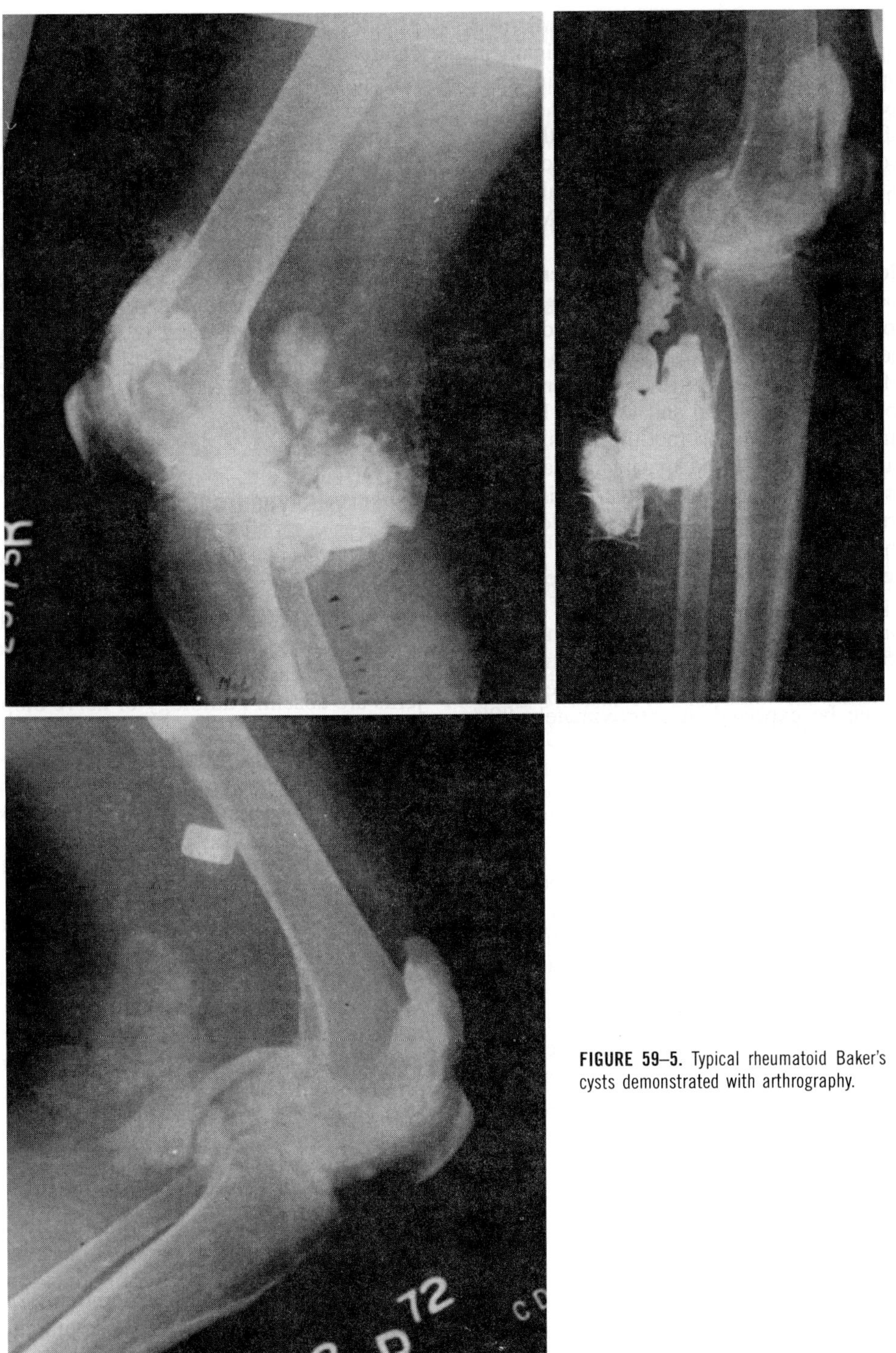

FIGURE 59–5. Typical rheumatoid Baker's cysts demonstrated with arthrography.

(<75% have satisfactory pain relief). If no specific cause of compression can be found, the results are worse (Lian, 1994). An even less favorable outcome can be anticipated if the symptoms existed for a long period of time before decompression. Symptoms may improve gradually over the course of several months after decompression.

Interdigital Neuroma (Morton's Neuroma)

Interdigital neuroma is the most common nerve problem of the foot and ankle (Mann and Reynolds, 1993). Most authors believe that Morton's neuroma is caused by an entrapment of the interdigital nerve as it passes under the intermetatarsal ligament (Schon and Baxter, 1994). In the last stage of gait, weight is transferred to the ball of the foot and the toes dorsiflex. The nerve is subsequently compressed between the plantar aspect of the foot and the edge of the intermetatarsal ligament. Tight shoes or high heels can aggravate this condition by holding the metatarsophalangeal joint in chronic dorsiflexion.

Studies in patients with rheumatoid arthritis suggest that,

Millender LH, Nalebuff EA: Preventive surgery—tenosynovectomy and synovectomy. Orthop Clin North Am 6:765, 1975a.

Millender LH, and Nalebuff EA: Reconstructive surgery in the rheumatoid hand. Orthop Clin North Am 6:709, 1975b.

Millender LH, Nalebuff EA, Holdsworth DE: Posterior interosseous nerve syndrome secondary to rheumatoid synovitis. J Bone Joint Surg 55A:753, 1973.

Miller HG, Abodesco L, Hey JP: Morton's neuroma symptoms from a rheumatoid nodule. J Am Podiatry Assoc 73:311–312, 1983.

Moore JR, Weiland AJ: Bilateral attritional rupture of the ulnar nerve at the elbow. J Hand Surg 5:358–360, 1980.

Nakano KK: Neurologic complications of rheumatoid arthritis. Orthop Clin North Am 6:861, 1975a.

Nakano KK: The entrapment neuropathies of rheumatoid arthritis. Orthop Clin North Am 6:837, 1975b.

Nakano KK: Entrapment neuropathies and related disorders. *In* Kelley W, Harris E, Ruddy S, Sledge CB (eds): Textbook of Rheumatology. Philadelphia, W. B. Saunders Company, 1993, p 1712.

Nakano KK, Schoene WC, Baker RA, Dawson DM: The cervical myelopathy associated with rheumatoid arthritis. Ann Neurol 3:144, 1978.

Nalebuff EA, Potter TA: Rheumatoid involvement of tendons and tendon sheaths in the hand. Clin Orthop 39:147, 1968.

Nalebuff EA: Surgical treatment of tendon rupture in the rheumatoid hand. Surg Clin North Am 49:811, 1969.

Pallis CA, Scott JT: Peripheral neuropathy in rheumatoid arthritis. BMJ 1:1141, 1965.

Popelka S, Vaino K: Entrapment of the posterior interosseous branch of the radial nerve in rheumatoid arthritis. Acta Orthop Scand 45:370–372, 1974.

Rasmussen M, Kitaotia M, Patzer G: Nonoperative treatment of plantar interdigital neuroma with a single cortisone injection. Presented at American Orthopaedic Foot and Ankle Society 25th Meeting, Orlando, 1995.

Rose HA, Hood RW, Otis JC, et al: Peroneal nerve palsy following total knee arthroplasty. A review of the Hospital for Special Surgery. J Bone Joint Surg 64A:347, 1982.

Schon LE, Baxter D: Heel pain syndrome and entrapment neuropathies about the foot and ankle. *In* Gould J (ed): Operative Foot Surgery. Philadelphia, W. B. Saunders Company, 1994, pp 192–207.

Shea JD, McClain EJ: Ulnar-nerve compression syndromes at and below the wrist. J Bone Joint Surg 51A:1095, 1969.

Spinner M: Injuries to the Major Branches of Peripheral Nerves of the Forearm, 2nd ed. Philadelphia, W. B. Saunders Company, 1978.

Stevens JC, Cartlidge NEF, Saunders M, Appleby A, Hall M, Shaw DA: Atlanto-axial subluxation and cervical myelopathy in rheumatoid arthritis. J Med 40:391, 1971.

Swanson AB: Flexible Implant Resection Arthroplasty in the Hand and Extremities. St. Louis, C. V. Mosby Company, 1973.

Taylor AR: Ulnar nerve compression at the wrist in rheumatoid arthritis. J Bone Joint Surg 56B:142–143, 1974.

Thompson F, Deland, J: Occurrence of two interdigital neuromas in one foot. Foot Ankle 3:238–243, 1993.

Upton ARM, Darracott J, Bianchi FA: Ulnar neuropathies in rheumatoid arthritis. Hand 10:77–81, 1978.

Upton ARM, McComas AJ: The double crush in nerve entrapment syndromes. Lancet 2:359–361, 1973.

Williams RC: Rheumatoid Arthritis as a Systemic Disease. Philadelphia, W. B. Saunders Company, 1974.

Management of Peripheral Nerve Tumors

Peripheral nerve tumors of the extremities are uncommon. Although the true incidence of these tumors is unknown, the reported incidence of hand and arm peripheral nerve tumors varies from 1% to 4.9% of all upper-extremity tumors (Boyes, 1970; Butler et al, 1960; Harkin and Reed, 1969; Stack, 1960; Strickland and Steichen, 1977). Non-neoplastic or reactive processes, including neuromas, are more frequently encountered, but their incidence is even less well documented.

An adequate preoperative assessment of peripheral nerve tumors is needed. The history should include the rate of growth of the lesion, the presence or absence of pain or neurological deficits, a history of neurofibromatosis, and the presence of other masses. The physical examination should determine, if possible, the size and location of the lesion, the presence of localized tenderness, Tinel's sign, and any neurologic deficits. In general, rapidly growing, deeply located masses should be suspected of malignancy. Patients with neurofibromatosis with a rapidly growing painful mass should also be suspected of having a malignant tumor.

Staging of the tumor is performed by determining the histologic grade of the tumor (low or high), anatomical location (intracompartmental or extracompartmental), tumor size (lesser or greater than 5 cm) and the presence of metastases (Enneking et al, 1980; Mankin, 1991). A diagnostic work-up of the tumor should include plain radiographs of the involved area and plain radiographs and a computed tomography (CT) scan of the chest. Computed tomography and magnetic resonance imaging (MRI) are used to help determine the anatomical location, the tumor margins, and the relationship of structures adjacent to the tumor (Chui et al, 1988; Levine et al, 1987; Mankin, 1991; Powers et al, 1983; Stull et al, 1991; Suh et al, 1992). Technetium bone scanning is used if bone metastases are suspected, and angiography, although not commonly performed, can be used to determine tumor vascularity and the relationship of vessels surrounding the tumor (Mankin, 1991).

A biopsy of the lesion should be carefully planned. Communication among the treating surgeon, radiologist, and pathologist aids in determining the appropriate area to biopsy, determining whether an adequate biopsy has been taken, and obtaining a definitive diagnosis. Communication with the pathologist also aids in determining whether adequate margins around the tumor have been obtained at the time of definitive treatment of the tumor. Occasionally, a needle biopsy can be used, but frequently an open biopsy is needed to obtain sufficient tissue for light microscopy, electron microscopy, immunohistochemistry, and cytogenetic studies. Longitudinally placed incisions, especially in the extremities, should be used. Transverse incisions should be avoided (Simon, 1982). The incision should be placed in a location where the tumor can be excised later, if needed. Hemostasis with the biopsy is essential to minimize the potential for spreading the tumor with the biopsy. The use of a tourniquet is debatable. If a tourniquet is used, gravity drainage of the limb, as opposed to Esmarch exsanguination, is preferred. If drains are used, they are to be placed in line with the biopsy incision (Mankin et al, 1982; Mankin, 1991).

Controversy exists between the use of an incisional or excisional biopsy. Superficial masses or tumors that appear to be clearly benign on imaging studies may be treated by excisional biopsy. Any mass appearing questionable should undergo an incisional biopsy to obtain a histological diagnosis before definitive treatment. Frozen sections of biopsy specimens can be used to determine adequacy of the biopsied specimens, but definitive treatment should not be based on results of the frozen section. Cultures of the wound should be taken at the time of biopsy (Mankin, 1991).

Resection of soft tissue tumors can be described as intralesional, marginal, wide, or radical (Enneking et al, 1980; Mankin, 1991). Intralesional resections include excision of a tumor, leaving visible tumor behind. Marginal resections include excision of a tumor with its surrounding capsule or reactive zone. Wide resections include removal of a tumor and reactive zone with a cuff of normal surrounding tissue, usually 1 cm or more in width. Radical resections include removal of the tumor and the entire anatomical compartment in which the tumor occurs. Intralesional and marginal resections are usually used for the treatment of benign tumors. Wide and radical resections are reserved for malignant lesions.

Although peripheral nerve tumors can frequently be diagnosed by light microscopy, additional studies are often needed, including electron microscopy, immunohistochemistry, and cytogenetics (Enneking et al, 1980; Rosenberg et al, 1991; Woodruff, 1993). Electron microscopy of the ultrastructural characteristics of soft tissue tumors is used to confirm the findings of light microscopy. Sampling error and the presence of relatively few ultrastructural markers in soft tissue tumors may, however, limit the usefulness of electron microscopy (Enzinger, 1988a, 1988b). Immunohistochemical methods use markers coupled with antibodies directed at specific antigens found in various areas of tumor cells. Detection of these antigens, usually proteins such as vimentin, cytokeratin, Leu-7, and S-100 protein, aids in the diagnosis of peripheral nerve tumors. Cytogenetic studies include the analysis of chromosomal abnormalities found in some peripheral nerve tumors (Enzinger, 1988a, 1988b; Rosenberg et al, 1991).

Peripheral nerve tumors have been commonly classified

according to their histogenesis or to the cell of origin of the tumor (Harkin and Reed, 1969; MacKinnon and Dellon, 1988; Rosenberg, 1991). However, there is no uniformly accepted classification system for these tumors. Different classification schemes have been previously proposed (Table 60–1) (Harkin and Reed, 1969; MacKinnon, 1988; Rosenberg, 1991). Harkin and Reed (1969) proposed a system dividing peripheral nerve lesions as non-neoplastic lesions, benign or malignant tumors of nerve sheath origin, neurocutaneous phakomatoses, neuroectodermal tumors, unclassified neural tumors, and tumors secondarily involving the peripheral nervous system.

Of clinical importance is the differentiation between non-neoplastic and neoplastic lesions and between benign and malignant peripheral nerve tumors.

BENIGN PERIPHERAL NERVE TUMORS

Neurofibroma

Clinical Presentation. Neurofibromas are one of the most common benign peripheral nerve tumors, accounting for approximately 1% to 3% of all hand tumors (Louis and Hankin, 1985). They occur in the third and fourth decades of life and equally affect the sexes (Enzinger, 1988a, 1988b; Rosenberg et al, 1991). The tumor arises from the nerve sheath and is composed primarily of Schwann cells. Neurofibromas can occur in the solitary form or in association with neurofibromatosis (von Recklinghausen's disease).

Only 10% of patients with solitary neurofibromas are thought to have neurofibromatosis (Geschickter, 1935). Therefore, the finding of a solitary neurofibroma is not considered to be diagnostic of neurofibromatosis. Superficial neurofibromas, occasionally called localized cutaneous neurofibromas, usually grow slowly as painless, soft masses that produce few symptoms. They can occur anywhere on the body and usually arise from small cutaneous nerve fibers (Rosenberg et al, 1991). They are located in the dermal and subcutaneous tissues and are usually evenly distributed over the body. These tumors are usually not encapsulated. Deeply occurring neurofibromas or localized deep neurofibromas

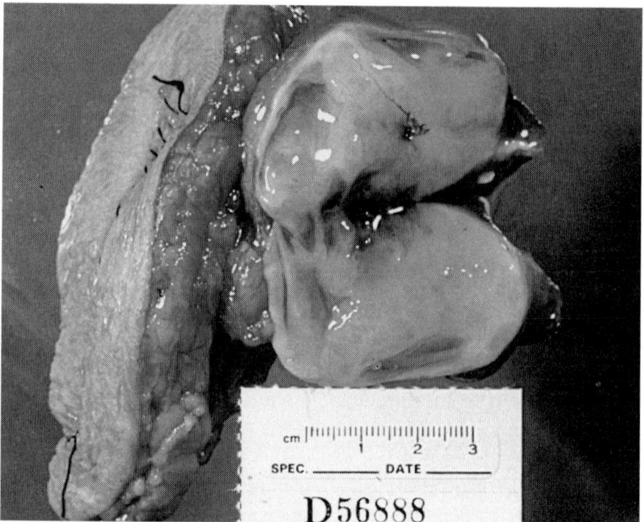

FIGURE 60–1. Myxoid neurofibroma of the thigh. (Courtesy of Dr. May Parisien.)

that remain confined and become encapsulated by the epineurium may produce symptoms (Harkin and Reed, 1969; Louis and Hankin, 1985).

Pathology. Grossly, the solitary tumor appears ovoid or fusiform in shape (Fig. 60–1). The tumor may appear pale gray, white-gray, or translucent (Harkin and Reed, 1969, Enzinger, 1988a, 1988b; Woodruff, 1993). In contrast to the neurilemmoma, the nonencapsulated neurofibroma is intimately associated to peripheral nerve fibers. Occasionally, a nerve can be found entering into the neurofibroma. The nerve fibers disappear, however, into the substance of the tumor, making separation of nerve fibers from the tumor difficult. The tumor is composed of a varying mixture of nerve sheath cells, collagen fibrils, mucoid material, mast cells, lymphocytes, and xanthoma cells. The tumor consists of intertwined bundles of elongated cells with wavy appearing, dark staining nuclei between wirelike strands of collagen (Enzinger, 1988a, 1988b) (Fig. 60–2). Variable amounts of mucoid matrix and relatively few Schwann cells can make the tumor appear similar to nerve sheath myxomas (Fig. 60–3). Areas of increased cellularity in some neurofibromas can also resemble the Antoni type A tissue of a neurilemoma (Harkin and Reed, 1969).

Neurofibromas have been noted to be immunohistochemically positive for S-100 protein and vimentin. Occasionally, the tumor is also positive for Leu-7 and glial fibrillary acid protein (Enzinger, 1988a, 1988b; Gray et al, 1989; Perentes and Rubenstein, 1985; Rosenberg et al, 1991; Weiss et al, 1983). Occasionally, some variants of neurofibromas may contain specialized receptors, including Wagner-Meissner bodies (tactile) or pacinian corpuscles (pressure) (Prichard and Custer, 1952; Schuler and Adamson, 1978). Several unusual types of neurofibromas, primarily of pathologic interest, have been described. These include storiform perineural, pacinian, epithelioid, and pigmented forms of neurofibromas (Enzinger, 1988a, 1988b).

Treatment. Most superficial subcutaneous neurofibromas do not require treatment. Staging studies for superficial neurofibromas are generally not needed. Magnetic resonance im-

▼ **TABLE 60–1**
Classification Schemes for Peripheral Nerve Tumors

Harkin and Reed	Rosenberg	MacKinnon and Dellon
Non-neoplastic lesions	Reactive processes	Benign neoplasms of nerve sheath origin
Benign nerve sheath tumors	Hamartoma	
	Choristoma	Malignant neoplasms of nerve sheath origin
Tumors of neurofibromatosis and other neurocutaneous phakomatoses	Benign tumors	
	Malignant tumors	Neoplasms of nerve cell origin
Malignant nerve sheath tumors		Tumors metastatic to peripheral nerves
Neuroectodermal tumors		Neoplasms of non-neural origin
Tumors of uncertain classification		Non-neoplasms
Tumors secondarily involving the peripheral nervous system		

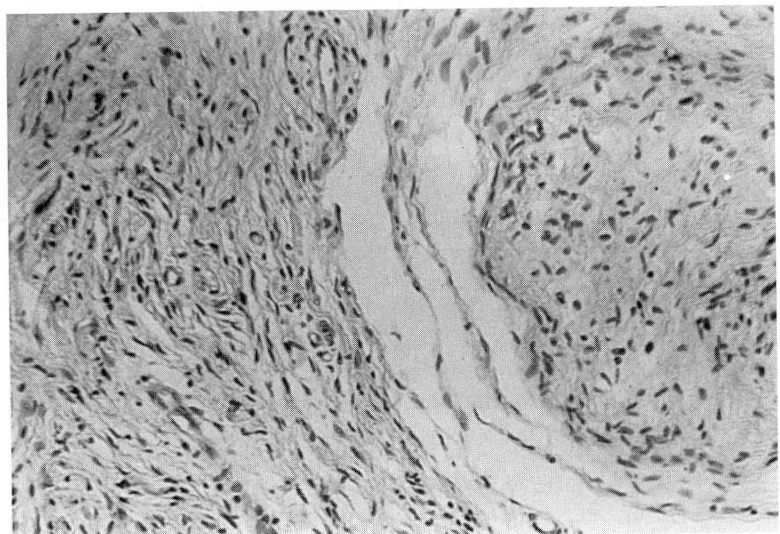

FIGURE 60–2. Histologic appearance of a neurofibroma. (Courtesy of Dr. May Parisien.)

aging has been used to determine the size and margins of the lesion (Levine et al, 1987). The indications for surgical excision of a neurofibroma include rapid tumor growth, pain, nerve dysfunction, or skin ulceration or infection associated with a superficial tumor (Rosenberg et al, 1991). Treatment usually includes an excisional biopsy of the mass (Ariel, 1980; Gaisford, 1960; Louis, 1987; Smith and Lipke, 1980).

Deeply located neurofibromas generally involve major peripheral nerves. Sometimes with the use of loupe or microscope magnification, an attempt is made to separate nerve fibers from the tumor mass. Although possible with the neurilemoma, this is generally not possible with the neurofibroma. Treatment can vary depending on the type of nerve involved, the location of the tumor, and the potential residual neurological deficit left after removal of the tumor. An incisional biopsy to obtain histological diagnosis before definitive treatment may be preferred for lesions involving major peripheral nerves. In general, tumor resection and nerve repair is usually performed (Louis, 1987; Rinaldi, 1983; Rosenberg et al, 1991). A direct end-to-end anastomosis after mobilization of the nerve or nerve grafting are

options for nerve reconstruction. Incomplete removal of the tumor, preserving some nerve fascicles and some nerve function, may be preferable to complete tumor and nerve excision (Healy and McCormack, 1993).

Malignancy can be suspected in tumors larger than 2 to 6 cm in diameter, irregularly shaped tumors, tumors adherent to surrounding soft tissue, and tumors where nerve fascicles are found to traverse the lesion (Rosenberg et al, 1991). An incisional biopsy should be considered. Treatment should then be based on the histological diagnosis of the tumor.

Results. Recurrence of a solitary neurofibroma after resection is rare. Surgical excision of the lesion is usually curative (Ariel, 1980; Smith and Lipke, 1980). Local recurrence of neurofibromas is more likely to occur in patients with neurofibromatosis (Mackinnon and Dellon, 1988).

Neurofibromatosis (von Recklinghausen's Disease)

Clinical Presentation. Neurofibromatosis is classified in the category of neurocutaneous syndromes or phakomatoses

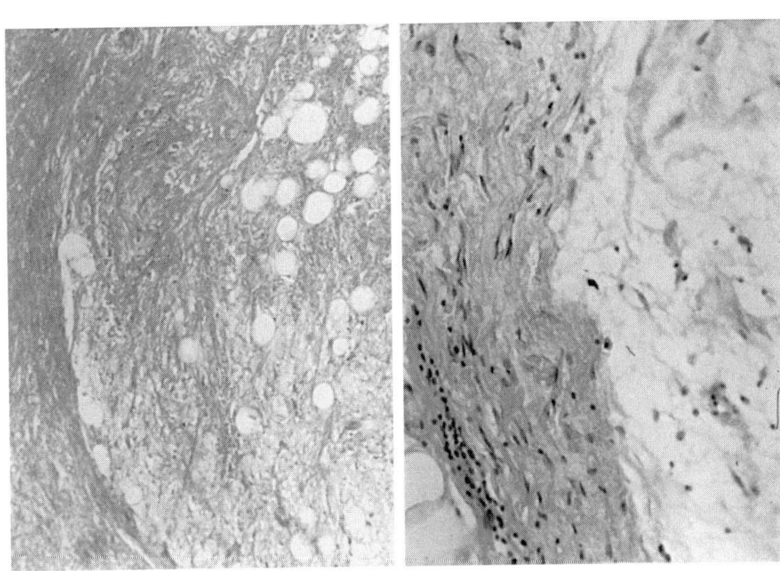

FIGURE 60–3. Histologic appearance of a myxoid neurofibroma. (Courtesy of Dr. May Parisien.)

(Enzinger, 1988a, 1988b). It is a disorder of neural crest–derived cells and is inherited as an autosomal dominant trait with variable expression (Bolande, 1981; Crowe et al, 1956; Lott and Richardson, 1981). The disease has been estimated as occurring in 1 of every 2500 to 3300 live births (Crowe et al, 1956). Half of patients with the disease are thought to be secondary to new mutations (Enzinger, 1988a, 1988b). Cytogenetic studies have shown that alterations of chromosomes 17 (type 1 neurofibromatosis) and 22 (type 2 neurofibromatosis) have been identified as responsible for the disorder (Barker et al, 1987; Cawthon et al, 1990; Viskochil et al, 1990; Rouleau et al, 1987; Wallace et al, 1990; Westelek et al, 1988). Neurofibromatosis appears in all races and has been reported to affect the sexes equally (Brasfield and Das Gupta, 1972) or to predominate in males (Canale and Bebin, 1972).

Two forms of neurofibromatosis have been described: peripheral and central. Peripheral neurofibromatosis (type 1 or NF-1) consists of the variable presence of neurofibromas, café-au-lait spots, pedunculated cutaneous tumors, pigmented hamartomas of the iris, skeletal abnormalities, and gynecomastia (Dell, 1985; Enzinger, 1988a, 1988b; Healy and McCormack, 1993; Woodruff, 1993).

Neurofibromas can appear variably during life, but they usually develop during childhood or adolescence and after the appearance of the café-au-lait spots (Enzinger, 1988a, 1988b). They can occur anywhere on the body but can be restricted to one area of the body. Internal organs, e.g., gastrointestinal tract, larynx, blood vessels, and heart, have also been reported to be involved (Cornell and Kirkendall, 1967; Greene et al, 1974; Hochberg et al, 1974; Merck and Kindblom, 1975; Pleasure, 1967; Pung and Hirsch, 1955; Salyer and Salyer, 1974; Schorn et al, 1974). An increase in the growth of neurofibromas has been noted during pregnancy and at puberty (Enzinger, 1988a, 1988b). However, a sudden change in size, pain, and the production of neurological symptoms should alert the clinician of the possibility of malignant transformation of the tumor. The reported incidence of malignant transformation has varied between 2% and 13% (Ghosh et al, 1973).

Café-au-lait spots, caused by increased melanin in the basal layer of the epidermis, usually appear in the first few years of life. The presence of six or more spots, greater than 1.5 cm in diameter, is seen in patients with von Recklinghausen's disease (Crowe et al, 1956). The number of café-au-lait spots tends to increase with age. The axilla and unexposed area of the body are common locations for these lesions. Palmar melanotic macules have been frequently noted in patients with neurofibromatosis (Yseudian and Premalatha, 1984).

Molluscum fibrosum or pedunculated cutaneous tumors are frequently found (Fig. 60–4). Lisch nodules or pigmented hamartomas of the iris are common in patients with neurofibromatosis (Riccardi, 1981).

Skeletal abnormalities, occurring in approximately 40% of patients, include external bone erosions by the soft tissue tumors (vertebral erosions) and primary skeletal abnormalities, including scoliosis, intrathoracic meningocele, congenital pseudoarthrosis and bowing of long bones, orbital malformations, and cystic bone lesions (Canale and Bebin, 1972; Crowe et al, 1956; Sagel and Forrest, 1975; Westelek et al, 1988; Zorab and Edwards, 1972).

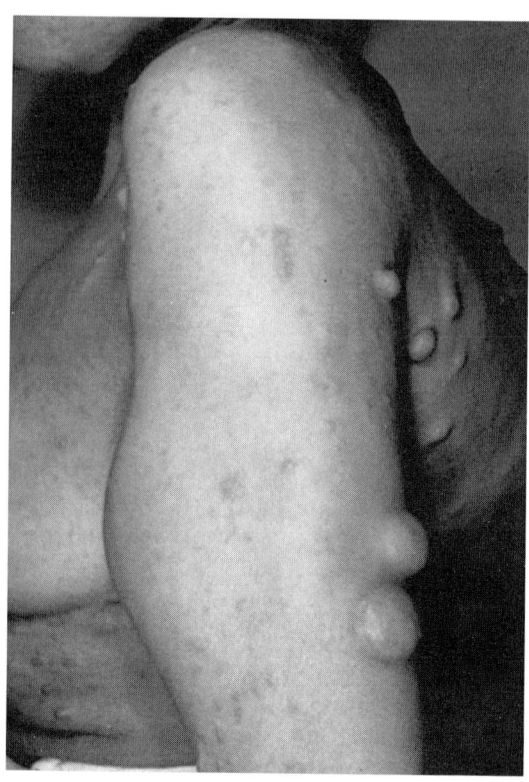

FIGURE 60–4. Molluscum fibrosum of pedunculated cutaneous tumors found in the peripheral form of neurofibromatosis. (Courtesy of Dr. May Parisien.)

Macrodactyly (digital enlargement) and extremity enlargement are known to be associated with neurofibromatosis (Chung et al, 1973; Dell, 1985; Healy and McCormack, 1993; Shereff et al, 1980). Pseudogynecomastia in young male patients with neurofibromatosis has also been noted (Enzinger, 1988a, 1988b).

Central neurofibromatosis (type 2 or NF-2) usually lacks the clinical findings seen in the peripheral form of the disease. Tumor involvement of the central nervous system is common. Neurilemomas, astrocytomas, meningiomas, and ependymomas may be intracranial or intraspinal in location. Acoustic neuromas (eighth cranial nerve) are commonly seen with von Recklinghausen's disease (Canale and Bebin, 1972; Lictenstein, 1949; Rodriguez and Berthong, 1966).

Pathology. Pathologically, several types of neurofibromas have been noted to occur. These include localized, plexiform, and diffuse neurofibromas. The localized form is the most common type and is identical to the solitary neurofibroma. They are usually located in the dermis and subcutaneous tissues but can occur in deeper tissues. They are usually larger than those tumors seen with solitary neurofibromas.

The diffuse form of neurofibromas is uncommon, occurring in children and young adults. A conservative estimation of 10% of patients with the diffuse form of neurofibroma are thought to have neurofibromatosis (Enzinger, 1988a, 1988b; Healy and McCormack, 1993). The tumor is more common in the head and neck regions. The tumor is ill-defined and diffusely infiltrates cutaneous and subcutaneous tissues. It is seen as a plaquelike mass with thickening of the subcutaneous region of the skin. Short fusiform tumor cells lie within a uniform matrix of fine fibrillary collagen,

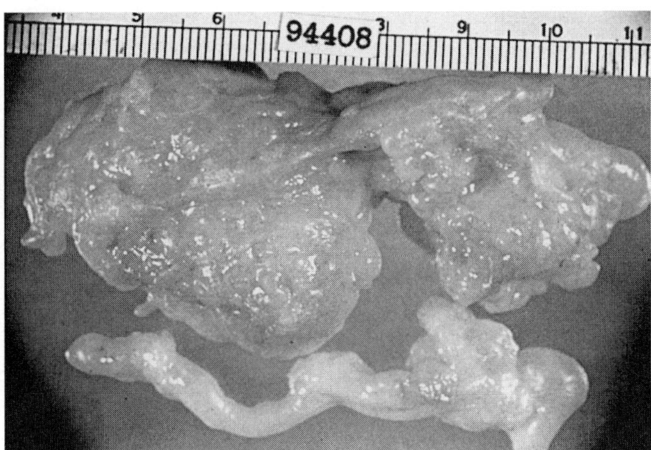

FIGURE 60–5. Plexiform neurofibroma of the wrist. (Courtesy of Dr. May Parisien.)

and clusters of Meissner's bodies may be seen within the tumor (Enzinger, 1988a, 1988b).

The plexiform neurofibroma is typically seen in and is pathognomonic of the neurofibromatosis (Harkin and Reed, 1969). Both small cutaneous and major nerves may become involved. When the tumor involves small cutaneous nerves, ill-defined nodules are noted. Major nerve involvement can cause enlargement of the entire extremity (elephantiasis neuromatosa) secondary to extremely large plexiform neurofibromas (Enzinger, 1988a, 1988b). Grossly, the tumor is a thick convoluted mass likened to a bag of worms (Enzinger, 1988a, 1988b) (Fig. 60–5). Histologically, a tortuous mass of nerve branches separated by increased endoneurial matrix with a proliferation of Schwann cells and wavy collagen bundles is noted (Enzinger, 1988a, 1988b) (Fig. 60–6).

Treatment. Most tumors associated with neurofibromatosis do not require surgical treatment. As with solitary neurofibromas, rapidly growing tumors causing pain or producing nerve dysfunction, especially in patients with neurofibromatosis, should be suspected of undergoing malignant transformation (Ariel, 1980; Harkin, 1980; Rosenberg et al, 1991; Smith and Lipke, 1980; Williams et al, 1984). Malignant transformation of neurofibromas is estimated to occur in 2%

to 29% of cases (Brasfield and Das Gupta, 1972; Charache, 1939; Crowe et al, 1956; Enzinger, 1988a, 1988b; Ghosh et al, 1973; Hosoi, 1931; Preston et al, 1952).

Because of the diffuse nature of the disease process, complete excision of neurofibromas is difficult. Potentially malignant tumors should undergo open biopsy. Frozen sections are obtained at the time of biopsy, but definitive treatment should be delayed until permanent histological studies have been obtained. If a malignant tumor is found, wide resection or amputation is needed (see discussion on treatment of malignant tumors).

Debulking, epiphysiodesis, osteotomies, shortening procedures, arthrodesis, and amputations have been advocated in treating enlarged digits and extremities (Dell, 1985; Match and Leffert, 1987).

Results. Because of the diffuse nature of nerve involvement, recurrence after the local excision of neurofibromas associated with neurofibromatosis is common (Enzinger, 1988a, 1988b; Healy and McCormack, 1993; MacKinnon and Dellon, 1988). However, removal of a benign neurofibroma does not appear to result in increased tumor growth (Ariel, 1980).

Neurilemoma (Schwannoma)

Clinical Presentation. Neurilemomas or schwannomas are benign, slowly growing, encapsulated peripheral nerve tumors. They occur between the ages of 20 and 50 (Geschickter, 1935) and have been variably reported to either equally affect the sexes (Enzinger, 1988a, 1988b) or predominate in females (Woodruff, 1993). There is some predilection for the flexor surfaces of the upper and lower extremities, head, and neck (Stout, 1935). Forearm and hand involvement is more common than digital involvement (Phalen, 1976). In 20% of cases, the tumor arises from the median, radial, or ulnar nerves (Enzinger, 1988a, 1988b; Rinaldi, 1983). The ulnar nerve appears to be particularly susceptible (Lassmann et al. 1977). Neurilemomas have been reported to comprise 0.8% to 2.1% of all hand tumors (Bogumill et al, 1975; Posch, 1991). Most neurilemomas occur as a solitary lesion, but they can occur as multiple lesions and can affect one or several nerves (Barre et al, 1987). A plexiform or multinodu-

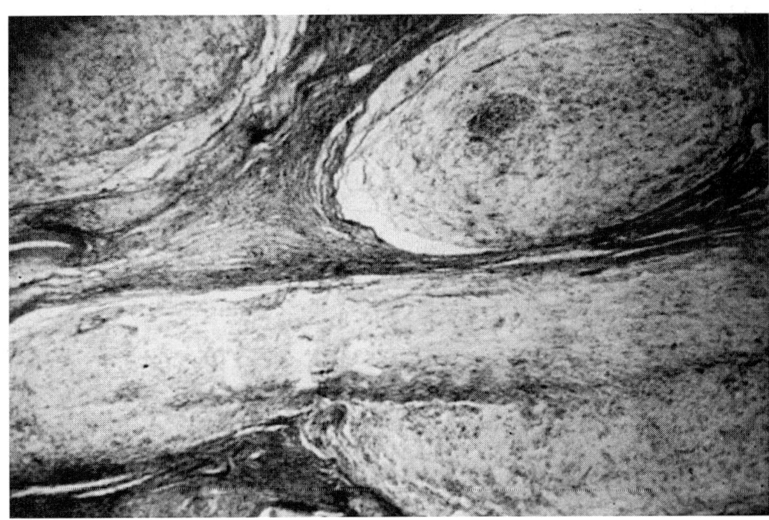

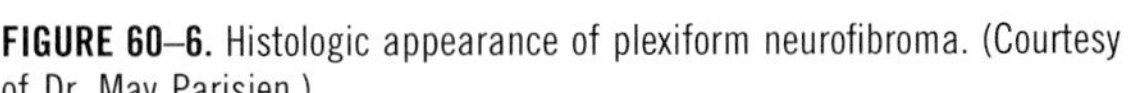

FIGURE 60–6. Histologic appearance of plexiform neurofibroma. (Courtesy of Dr. May Parisien.)

lar form of the tumor occurs in approximately 5% of cases (Enzinger, 1988a, 1988b; Fletcher et al, 1987; Iwashita and Enjoji, 1987; Woodruff et al, 1983). The tumor can also occur in association with neurofibromatosis (Izumi et al, 1971; MacKinnon and Dellon, 1988; Stout, 1935). A less common melanotic form of the tumor, most commonly involving spinal nerve roots, has also been described (Carney, 1990; Killeen et al, 1988).

The tumor usually is first seen as a painless, asymptomatic mass and is present several years before it is noticed. The mass may be mobile or relatively fixed, depending on the size and location of the tumor and the nerve involved. The tumor is usually less than 5 cm in size and varies from a round to oval to fusiform shape (Enzinger, 1988a, 1988b; Healy and McCormack, 1993; Holdsworth, 1985). Pain and paresthesias may occur when the tumor reaches sufficient size to compress the involved nerve. External pressure may produce localized tenderness, especially when the tumor is located in the hand (Healy and McCormack, 1993).

Pathology. Neurilemomas also arise from the nerve sheath. The tumor is usually located eccentrically within the nerve. They are usually surrounded by a fibrous capsule consisting of epineurium and residual nerve fibers (Enzinger, 1988a, 1988b). On sectioning, the tumor color may vary from a pink, white, tan, yellow to grayish appearance (Fig. 60–7). There also may be areas of hemorrhage or cyst formation (Das Gupta, 1983; Enzinger, 1988a, 1988b; Healy and McCormack, 1993; Rosenberg et al, 1991). Histologically, the tumor consists almost entirely of Schwann cells and is described as having two components. Antoni A areas consist of regions of dense, highly ordered spindle cells arranged in short bundles, interlacing fascicles, palisades, or Verocay bodies (an oval-shaped arrangement of two rows of well-aligned nuclei and cell processes). Antoni B areas consist of loose, myxoid matrix and collagen fibers with only occasional spindle or oval cells and inflammatory cells (Enzinger, 1988a, 1988b; Woodruff, 1993) (Figs. 60–8A to C). Cellular schwannoma, a benign form of schwannoma, is particularly difficult to pathologically differentiate from the malignant form of the tumor (Fletcher et al, 1987; Lodding et al, 1990; White et al, 1990, Woodruff et al, 1981).

Ultrastructurally, the Schwann cells have long thin processes that emanate from the cell body and are arranged in

layers. Basal lamina surround the cells; primitive intercellular junctions are present; and long-spacing collagen is found in the stroma (Dickersin, 1987; Erlandson and Woodruff, 1982; Fisher and Vuzevski, 1968; Lassman et al, 1977; Waggener, 1966). Immunohistochemically, the tumor is positive for vimentin, S-100 protein, and Leu-7. Less commonly, the tumor is positive for glial fibrillary acidic protein and keratin (Gray et al, 1989; Perentes and Rubenstein, 1985; Rosenberg et al, 1991; Weiss et al, 1983).

Malignant transformation has been reported only on rare occasions (Carstens and Schrodt, 1969; Louis et al, 1987; Rasbridge et al, 1989; Yousem et al, 1985).

Treatment. The treatment of a neurilemoma is surgical excision. A longitudinal incision should be made overlying the mass. The tumor should be well encapsulated. An incision is made into the epineurium. In contrast to the neurofibroma, the neurilemoma can be separated from the involved nerve. Initially, the tumor may appear intimately attached to nerve fibers, and on occasion, a few nerve fibers may need to be resected with the tumor (Barrett and Cramer, 1963; Phalen, 1976). The nerve should be inspected for the possibility of additional tumors (Barre et al, 1987; Lewis et al, 1981; Phalen, 1976). If the tumor is suggestive of a tumor other than a neurilemoma, an incisional biopsy should be performed.

Results. An excision of a neurilemoma is usually curative. Recurrence is rare, and relief of symptoms is common (Ariel, 1980; Barrett and Cramer, 1963; Lewis et al, 1981; Rinaldi, 1983; Smith and Lipke, 1980; Stout, 1935; Strickland, 1977). Occasionally, a neurological deficit is noted after excision of the tumor (Barrett and Cramer, 1963; Phalen, 1976).

Granular Cell Tumor

Clinical Presentation. Granular cell tumors are relatively uncommon (Aspisarnthanarax, 1981). They can occur at any age, but they are common during the fourth through sixth decades of life and are found rarely in children (Papageorgiou et al, 1967). Women are twice more often affected than men, and black persons more often than white persons (Garancis et al, 1970; Vance and Hudson, 1969).

The tumor is first seen as a small (< 3 cm), superficial, solitary, painless nodule located in the dermis or subcutaneous tissues. It has been found in submucosa, smooth or striated muscle, larynx, bronchus, stomach, bile duct, intestines, and anogenital region (Campagno, 1975; Enzinger, 1988a, 1988b; Fust and Custer, 1948; Horn and Stout, 1943; Tsuneyoshi and Enjoji, 1978; Vance and Hudson, 1969). Multiple lesions occur in approximately 10% to 15% of patients. Common sites of involvement include the tongue, chest wall, head and neck, and upper limbs (Enzinger, 1988a, 1988b; Strong et al, 1970; Woodruff, 1993).

Pathology. Granular cell tumors are small, poorly circumscribed masses. There is a close association between the tumor and peripheral nerves. The tumor may encompass small peripheral nerves, replacing the nerve. The tumor can also invade muscle, fibrous tissue (tendon, fascia, ligaments) and lymphoid tissue (Enzinger, 1988a, 1988b). On cut sec-

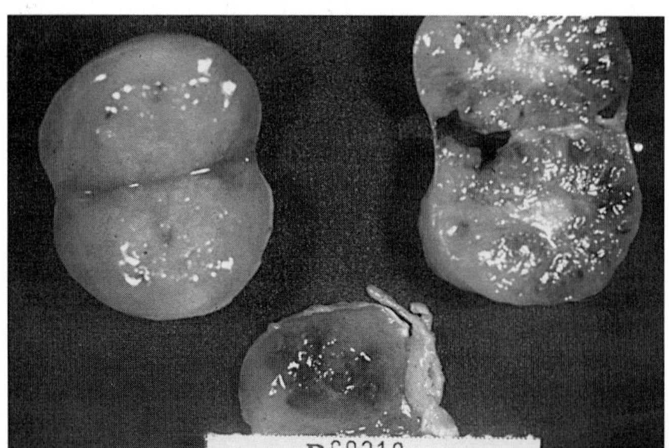

FIGURE 60–7. Neurilemomas. (Courtesy of Dr. May Parisien.)

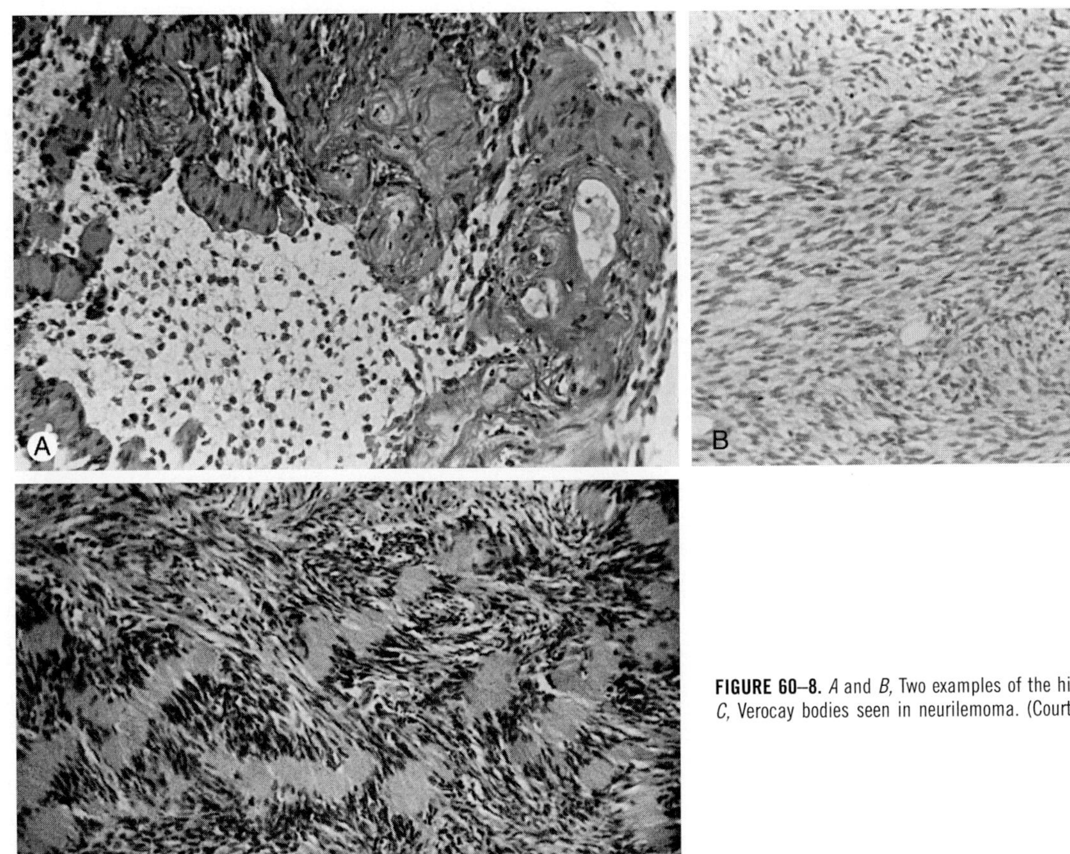

FIGURE 60–8. *A* and *B,* Two examples of the histologic appearance of neurilemoma. *C,* Verocay bodies seen in neurilemoma. (Courtesy of Dr. May Parisien.)

tion, they appear yellow-tan or yellow-gray. Histologically, the tumor consists of rounded or polygonal-shaped cells with coarsely granular eosinophic cytoplasm. The tumor cells are periodic acid–Schiff stain–positive. The nuclei are uniform in size, centrally placed and vesicular. Nuclear pleomorphism may be present but is usually not associated with increased mitotic activity (Enzinger, 1988a, 1988b). The cells are arranged in compact interlacing fascicles and are surrounded by a variable amount of collagenous stroma (Harkin and Reed, 1969; Rosenberg et al, 1991). Ultrastructurally, intracellular granules consisting of large membrane-bound autophagocytic vacuoles containing cellular debris surrounded by a basal lamina are seen (Fisher and Wechsler, 1962; Garancis et al, 1970; Sobel et al, 1973). The tumor is immunohistochemically positive for S-100 protein, neuron specific enolase (NSE), laminin, and vimentin (Enzinger, 1988a, 1988b; Miettinin et al, 1984; Nathrath and Remberger, 1986).

Included in the differential diagnosis of granular cell tumors are rhabdomyoma, fibroxanthoma, hibernoma, epithelioid smooth muscle tumors, vascular tumors, rhabdomyosarcoma, paraganglioma, alveolar soft part sarcoma, renal cell carcinoma, collections of granular histiocytes, granular cell leiomyosarcoma, and reactive changes associated with surgical trauma or injury (Enzinger, 1988a, 1988b; Robertson et al, 1981; Rosenberg et al, 1991).

The malignant form of granular cell tumors may be difficult to distinguish from the benign form. Histologically, the malignant form tends to be slightly more cellular and have increased mitotic figures. The cells tend to be smaller and more elongated (Enzinger, 1988a, 1988b). Clinically, there is a greater tendency for local recurrence, rapid growth, and larger size (> 3 to 5 cm) (Enzinger, 1988a, 1988b; Mackenzie, 1967).

Treatment. Treatment usually includes excisional biopsy. Often, no nerve is found entering into the mass, or if a small sensory nerve is found, it is excised with the mass (Blair, 1980; Fisher and Wechsler, 1962; Strong et al, 1970; Vance and Hudson, 1969). Larger masses should undergo incisional biopsy with definitive treatment being delayed until histological diagnosis is made.

Results. Local surgical excision is usually curative, with rare recurrences (Enzinger, 1988a, 1988b; Strong, 1970).

Neurothekeoma (Nerve Sheath Myxoma)

Clinical Presentation. Neurothekeomas are rare tumors that arise from the nerve sheath, particularly the endoneurium of peripheral nerves (Gallager and Helwig, 1980; Harkin and Reed, 1969). The tumors have also been called nerve sheath myxomas, pacinian neurofibromas, and bizarre cutaneous neurofibromas (Enzinger, 1988a, 1988b; Harkin and Reed, 1969; MacDonald and Wilson-Jones, 1977; Pulitzer and Reed, 1985).

The tumors normally occur in childhood and early adult

life. They have a predilection for the upper portion of the body, i.e., head, neck, shoulder, and upper extremity. They are probably most closely related to the neurofibroma (Enzinger, 1988a, 1988b). They are slow-growing tumors and have usually been present for several years; they occur more often in women than in men (Fletcher and Davies, 1986; Gallager and Helwig, 1980; Pulitzer and Reed, 1985). The mass usually presents as a small (1 cm), soft, nontender mass, located in the dermis and subcutis (Rosenberg et al, 1991).

Pathology. Grossly, the tumor appears lobular and gray-white or translucent (Rosenberg et al, 1991). The tumor is divided into distinct nodules by fibrous connective tissue resembling perineurium. The tumor cells may appear epithelioid, stellate, or spindle-shaped. The stromata may appear abundant in some areas, giving the tumor its myxoid appearance, and contain acid mucopolysaccharides, including chondroitin sulfate and hyaluronic acid (Angervall et al, 1984; Blumberg et al, 1989; Fletcher et al, 1986; Gallager and Helwig, 1980; Pulitzer and Reed, 1985). Some areas may have little stromata, consisting of compactly arranged tumor cells. Multinucleated giant cells may also be seen (Harkin and Reed, 1969). Ultrastructurally, the tumor cells contain basal lamina and form tight junctions with adjacent cells, supporting either a perineural or Schwann cell line of differentiation. Immunohistochemically, the tumor is S-100 positive (Angervall et al, 1981; Blumberg et al, 1989; Fletcher et al, 1986; Pulitzer and Reed, 1985).

Possible differential diagnoses are myxoid cysts of the skin, cutaneous focal mucinosis, mucinous ganglion cysts of peripheral nerve, myxoid neurofibroma, and myxoid malignant fibrous histiocytoma (Enzinger, 1988a, 1988b; Harkin and Reed, 1969; Woodruff, 1993).

Treatment. As with other peripheral nerve tumors, masses causing pain, increasing in size, or causing nerve dysfunction are candidates for surgical excision. Usually an excisional biopsy is performed. Because the tumor is relatively superficial, the overlying skin may be excised with the tumor (Rosenberg et al, 1991).

Results. Excision of this tumor is usually curative. Recurrence of the tumor is rare after resection, occurring in only 3 of a reported 123 cases. Metastases or local aggressive growth have not been reported (Enzinger, 1988a, 1988b; Gallager and Helwig, 1980; Pulitzer and Reed, 1985; Rosenberg et al, 1991).

MALIGNANT PERIPHERAL NERVE TUMORS

Malignant Schwannoma

Clinical Presentation. Malignant schwannomas are malignant peripheral nerve tumors arising from the nerve sheath. They are one of the most common malignant peripheral nerve tumors, accounting for approximately 10% of all soft tissue sarcomas. This tumor has also been called malignant neurilemoma, malignant peripheral nerve sheath tumor (MPNST), perineural fibrosarcoma, neurogenic sarcoma, neurofibrosarcoma, fibromyxosarcoma of nerve, sarcoma of nerve, malignant peripheral glioma, myxosarcoma of nerve sheath (Das Gupta, 1983; Enzinger, 1988a, 1988b; Rosenberg et al, 1991).

About one half of cases occur in patients with NF-1 (Ducatman et al, 1986; Enzinger, 1988a, 1988b; Hruban et al, 1990; Sordillo et al, 1981). Between 2% and 5% of patients with neurofibromatosis develop malignant schwannoma (Ducatman et al, 1983; Ducatman et al, 1986; Guccion and Enzinger, 1979; Riccardi, 1981; Sorensen et al, 1986). A long latent period of about 10 to 20 years before the development of the tumor has been noted, and multiple lesions may be found (Guccion and Enzinger, 1979; Sordillo et al, 1981). The tumor may arise from a pre-existing neurofibroma; arise de novo; or, rarely, develop from ganglioneuromas, ganglioblastomas, or schwannomas (Carstens and Schrodt, 1969; Ricci et al, 1984; Stout, 1935; Woodruff, 1993; Yousem et al, 1985). A genetic predisposition to develop malignant schwannoma has been postulated (Ducatman et al, 1986; Enzinger, 1988a, 1988b; Nambisan et al, 1984). About 11% of malignant schwannomas are thought to occur after radiation exposure, with a latency period averaging 15 years (range, 4 to 41 years) (Ducatman and Scheithauer, 1983; Ducatman et al, 1986; Foley et al, 1980).

Most malignant schwannomas occur between the ages of 20 and 50 years (Enzinger, 1988a, 1988b). Patients with neurofibromatosis appear to be affected at a younger age than those without the disease: 20 to 30 versus 40 to 50 years (Ducatman et al, 1986; Hruban et al, 1990; Wanebo et al, 1993). The reports vary concerning either a male or female propensity for the tumor (D'Agostino et al, 1963a, 1963b; Ducatman et al, 1986). Because of the propensity of males for neurofibromatosis, studies that include a high percentage of patients with neurofibromatosis have a higher male population with malignant schwannoma (D'Agostino et al, 1963a, 1963b; Guccion and Enzinger, 1979; Enzinger, 1988a, 1988b). In studies reporting only sporadic cases of malignant schwannoma, males and females are roughly equally affected (D'Agostino et al, 1963a, 1963b; Enzinger, 1988a, 1988b; Ghosh et al, 1973).

The tumor is usually noted as an enlarging mass, often present for several months. Pain, occurring more commonly in patients with neurofibromatosis, is variable. The tumor usually arises deeply within soft tissues, but can involve superficial neurofibromas (Enzinger, 1988a, 1988b). Those tumors involving major peripheral nerves usually produce neurological deficits, including paresthesias and motor weakness (Ducatman, 1986; Enzinger, 1988; Hruban, 1990; Nambisan, 1984; Thomas, 1983) (Fig. 60–9). Most tumors arise in association with major peripheral nerves, including brachial, sacral plexus, and sciatic nerves (Enzinger, 1988a, 1988b; Guccion and Enzinger, 1979; Woodruff, 1993).

Pathology. The tumor appears as a large (> 5 cm) fusiform, ovoid, or eccentric mass within a major peripheral nerve (Enzinger, 1988a, 1988b; Rosenberg et al, 1991) (Fig. 60–10A and B). The nerve from which the tumor arises can be identified in 45% to 90% of cases (Ducatman et al, 1986; Guccion and Enzinger, 1979; Hruban et al, 1990). The tumor may spread proximally and distally along the epineurium and perineurium. The tumor appears white-tan or yellow, with areas of hemorrhage and necrosis (Enzinger, 1988a,

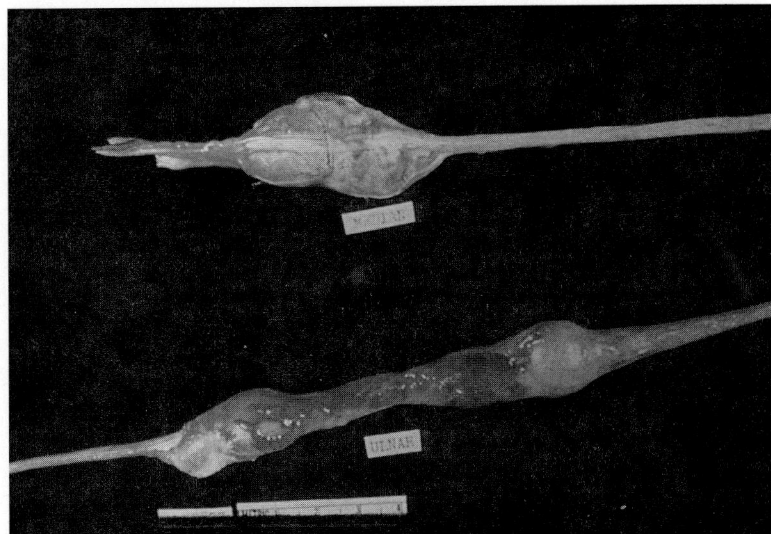

FIGURE 60–9. Malignant schwannomas of the median and ulnar nerves. (Courtesy of Dr. May Parisien.)

1988b; Hruban et al, 1990). A pseudocapsule may develop around the tumor.

Histologically, the tumor cell has the features of the normal Schwann cell. It is distinguished from its benign counterpart by the appearance of increased cellularity, nuclear hyperchromasia, pleomorphism, mitotic activity, tumor necrosis, and infiltrative growth pattern (Enzinger, 1988a, 1988b; Rosenberg et al, 1991). The pattern of the tumor varies from densely cellular fascicles to hypocellular myxoid areas. The spindled cells can be arranged in whorling patterns to palisades (Fig. 60–11). The nuclei appear wavy, buckled, or comma-shaped, with pointed ends (Enzinger, 1988a, 1988b).

Malignant schwannomas are so varied in appearance that they can resemble fibrosarcomas, monophasic synovial sarcomas, leiomyosarcomas, and malignant fibrous histiocytomas (Enzinger, 1988a, 1988b; Rosenberg et al, 1991; Woodruff, 1993). Other variations of the malignant schwannoma include the malignant epithelioid schwannoma and malignant schwannoma with rhabdomyoblastic differentiation or malignant Triton tumor.

Ultrastructurally, the tumor cells have many of the features of benign tumors, including cytoplasmic processes con-taining microtubules and neurofilaments, junctional complexes, basal lamina, and long-spacing collagen (Dickersin, 1987; Enzinger, 1988a, 1988b; Erlandson and Woodruff, 1982).

Immunohistochemistry shows variable degrees of positive staining for S-100 protein, Leu-7, myelin basic protein, neuron specific enolase, glial fibrillary acidic protein, and epithelial membrane antigen (Daimaru et al, 1985; Enzinger, 1988a, 1988b; Giangaspero et al, 1989; Gray et al, 1989; Hirose et al, 1992; Matsunou et al, 1985; Rosenberg et al, 1991; Swanson et al, 1987; Wick et al, 1987).

The differential diagnoses of malignant schwannomas include fibrosarcomas, monophasic synovial sarcoma, malignant fibrous histiocytoma, and leiomyosarcoma (Enzinger, 1988a, 1988b; Rosenberg et al, 1991; Woodruff, 1993).

Treatment. Preoperative assessment of the tumor should include plain radiographs of the area involved, chest radiographs, chest CT, and technetium bone scan (Rosenberg et al, 1991). Computed tomography and MRI are used to determine tumor margins and the relationship of surrounding soft tissues (Powers et al, 1983; Stull et al, 1991; Suh et al, 1992). Angiography may be used to determine the relation-

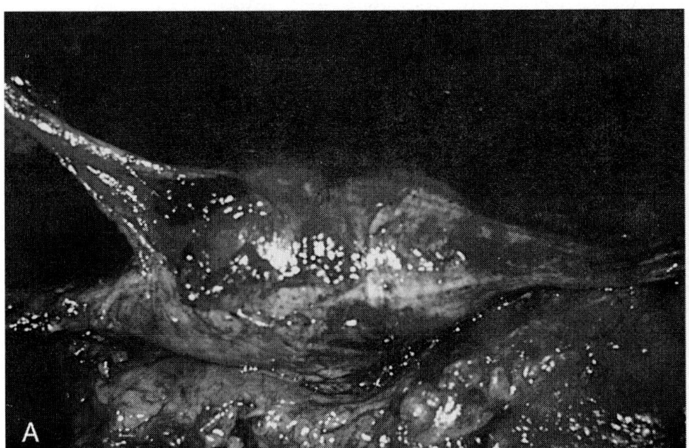
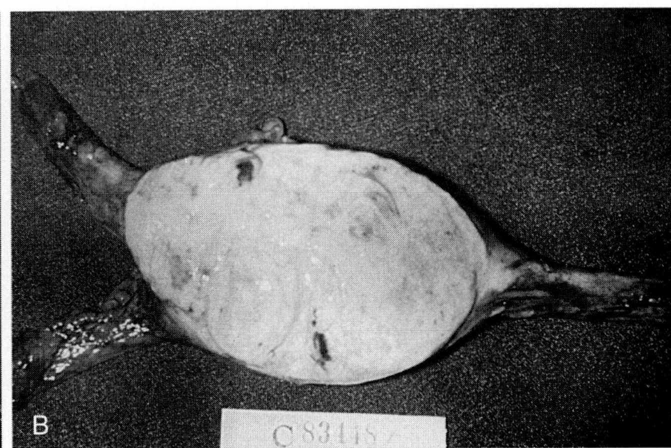

FIGURE 60–10. *A,* Malignant schwannoma of popliteal nerve. *B,* Cut section of malignant schwannoma. (Courtesy of Dr. May Parisien.)

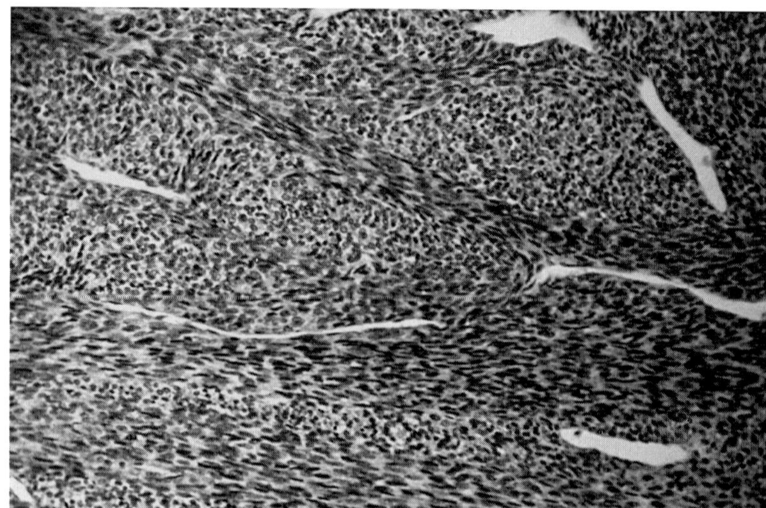

FIGURE 60–11. Histologic appearance of malignant schwannoma. (Courtesy of Dr. May Parisien.)

ship of surrounding vessels to the tumor. Magnetic resonance imaging (Suh et al, 1992) and gallium-67 citrate scintigraphy (Levine et al, 1987) can potentially differentiate between benign and malignant nerve tumors. These imaging techniques, however, should not be the sole diagnostic study used to determine treatment of the tumor.

A tumor suggestive of malignant schwannoma should initially undergo an open biopsy. Frozen sections can be obtained at the time of biopsy to ensure adequate tumor sampling, but definitive treatment should be delayed until histological diagnosis has been obtained with permanent pathological studies.

The treatment of malignant schwannomas includes either wide resection or amputation combined with radiation therapy and/or chemotherapy (Ariel, 1980, 1988; Basso-Ricci, 1989; D'Agostino et al, 1963a, 1963b; Ghosh et al, 1973; Giannestras and Bronson, 1975; Hruban et al, 1990; Karakousis et al, 1988; Lindberg et al, 1981; Nambisan et al, 1984; Raney et al, 1987; Smith and Lipke, 1980; Sordillo et al, 1981; Storm et al, 1980; Vieta and Pack, 1951; Wanebo et al, 1993). The type of tumor resection depends on the location and size of the tumor and the presence of metastases. A wide resection of the tumor may be performed if adequate margins can be obtained. An amputation may be the best option if resection of the tumor requires resection of the main arterial and nerve supply to the limb (Ariel, 1980; D'Agostino et al, 1963a, 1963b; Ghosh et al, 1973; Giannestras and Bronson, 1975; Smith and Lipke, 1980; Vieta and Pack, 1951). Because of the presence of multifocal lesions along the nerve, frozen sections of the margins of the resected nerve may help determine adequacy of the tumor resection. Some tumors located in close proximity to the trunk, e.g., brachial or sacral plexus lesions, cannot be resected with adequate margins. Forequarter amputation or palliative treatment may be the only option with these tumors (Healy and McCormack, 1993).

Radiation therapy has been used either as an adjunctive procedure after tumor resection or as a palliative procedure to decrease tumor size or reduce pain from an inoperable tumor (Ariel, 1980; Brennan et al, 1987; Shiu et al, 1984; Woodruff, 1993). Chemotherapy, including combinations of Adriamycin, methotrexate, Aleran, and actinomycin D, has been used for high-grade tumors. The efficacy of radiation

and chemotherapy together is not clearly defined (Ariel, 1980; Mankin, 1991; Rosenberg et al, 1991; Sordillo et al, 1981).

Results. The 5-year survival rate appears to be worse in patients with neurofibromatosis (16% to 23%) than in patients with sporadic malignant schwannoma (47% to 53%) (Dabski et al, 1990; D'Agostino et al, 1963a, 1963b; Ducatman et al, 1986; Ghosh et al, 1973; Giangaspero et al, 1989; Sordillo et al, 1981). Ten-year survival decreases to 23%. The median survival from the time of diagnosis is 3 years (Ducatman et al, 1986). Survival for solitary malignant schwannomas appears somewhat better, around 50% (Guccion and Enzinger, 1979; Sorensen et al, 1981). The poorer prognosis is thought to be a result of the tendency of these tumors to arise in difficult areas, including the trunk and proximal extremity, making early detection more difficult. The tumors also tend to be larger and more poorly differentiated, and they can be multifocal, involving long segments of the involved nerve or several nerves (Bojsen-Moller and Myrhe-Jensen, 1984; Dabski et al, 1990; Ducatman et al, 1986; Rosenberg et al, 1991; Sordillo et al, 1981).

Local recurrence occurs in 40% to 76% of cases (Ariel, 1980; Ducatman et al, 1986; Guccion and Enzinger, 1979; Hruban et al, 1990; Wanebo et al, 1993). Tumor metastases, occurring in 20% to 63% of cases, usually occur within 2 years of initial diagnosis and involve the lung, liver, subcutaneous tissue, and bone (Ariel, 1980; Enzinger, 1988a, 1988b; Guccion and Enzinger, 1979; Sorensen et al, 1981). Proximal migration of the tumor along the nerve trunk to involve the brain and spinal cord can also occur (Stewart and Copeland, 1931; Rosenberg et al, 1991). Metastases to regional lymph nodes appear to be uncommon (Ghosh et al, 1973; Sorensen et al, 1981; Stewart and Copeland, 1931). Amputation after local recurrence may be performed for resectable tumors with some success (Ariel, 1980).

Primitive Neuroectodermal Tumor

Clinical Presentation. Primitive neuroectodermal tumors are rare, aggressive malignant tumors of neural crest origin. The tumor is categorized in a group of other neuroectodermal tumors, including extraosseous Ewing's sarcoma, neuroepithelioma, Askin's tumors, and peripheral neuroblastoma (Bolen and Thorning, 1980; Das Gupta, 1983; MacKay et al, 1976; Marina et al, 1989; Nesbitt and Vidone, 1976; Rosenberg et al, 1991; Voss et al, 1984). The tumor appears in children and young adults, with a slight propensity for males (Rosenberg et al, 1991).

Patients normally have symptoms from a rapidly growing mass or metastasis. Locations of the tumor include the chest wall, pelvis, and proximal extremities. Peripheral nerves are involved in approximately 20% to 30% of cases (Enzinger, 1988a, 1988b, Fletcher, 1990; Jurgens et al, 1988; Llombart-Bosch et al, 1989; Marina et al, 1989; Miser et al, 1989). Metastases to the lung and regional lymph nodes are noted in approximately 25% to 50% of patients at the time of diagnosis (Enzinger, 1988a, 1988b, Jurgens et al, 1988; Marina et al, 1989).

Pathology. The tumors are generally large (> 9 cm) and appear tan-white. They are composed of sheets of densely packed small round to oval cells with similarly shaped nuclei (Enzinger, 1988a, 1988b; Rosenberg et al, 1991). A small amount of cytoplasm, occasionally containing glycogen, is noted within the cells; fibrovascular septa may subdivide the tumor (Rosenberg et al, 1991) (Fig. 60–12). Occasionally, the tumor cells can coalesce to form rosettes (Homer-Wright rosettes).

Pathologically, the tumor can resemble metastatic neuroblastoma, small cell carcinoma, and medulloblastoma (Das Gupta, 1983; Enzinger, 1988a, 1988b).

Ultrastructurally, primitive junctional complexes, cell processes with microtubules, and basal laminae are seen (Enzinger, 1988a, 1988b; Fletcher, 1990; Linnoila et al, 1986; Llombart-Bosch et al, 1989; Marina et al, 1989). Immunohistochemistry shows positive vimentin, neurofilament, neuron-specific enolase, chromogranin, synaptophysin, and Leu-7 staining (Enzinger, 1988a, 1988b; Fletcher, 1990; Giacobbe et al, 1988; Linnoila et al, 1986; Llombart-Bosch et al, 1989; Marina et al, 1989; Trojanowski, 1988). Cytogenetic studies showing a consistent translocation between chromosomes 11 and 21 suggest a close relationship between primitive neuroectodermal tumors and Ewing's sarcoma, but not with neuroblastomas (Rosenberg et al, 1991; Thiele et al, 1987; Whang-Peng et al, 1984, 1986).

Treatment. Treatment includes an open biopsy to obtain a diagnosis of the tumor. Definitive treatment should include either a wide resection or amputation. Radiotherapy and chemotherapy, including anthracyclines and alkylating agents, have been used after resection of the tumor or for treating unresectable tumors (Jurgens et al, 1988; Marina et al, 1989; Miser et al, 1987; Rosenberg et al, 1991).

Results. Although the tumor is thought to be sensitive to chemotherapy and radiotherapy, overall long-term survival appears to be poor (Enzinger, 1988a, 1988b, Rosenberg et al, 1991). Fewer than 40% of patients appear to survive long-term (Giacobbe et al, 1988; Jurgens et al, 1988; Marina et al, 1989). Recurrence rates vary from 15% to 45% (Dehner, 1986; Marina et al, 1989).

OTHER NEOPLASMS INVOLVING NERVE

Nerve Sheath Ganglion

Clinical Presentation. Nerve sheath ganglions are ganglia that occur in an intraneural location. They may form as a result of chronic mechanical irritation and are found frequently in the peroneal nerve. Other involved nerves include the ulnar and median nerves (Barrett and Cramer, 1963; Cobb and Moiel, 1974; Enzinger, 1988a, 1988b; Gurdjian et al, 1965; Hartwell, 1965). Compression of the nerve can cause sensory and motor loss. Peroneal nerve ganglia appear to affect mostly males in all age groups (Gurdjian et al, 1965).

Pathology. Grossly, localized swelling of the nerve is noted. Single or multiple lesions can be noted. The ganglia can extend along the nerve for several centimeters (Rosenberg et al, 1991). Marked displacement of the nerve fascicles by the cyst can be noted. The unlined cyst contains clear viscous fluid seen in ganglia from other areas of the body and represents a degenerative process as opposed to a neoplasm

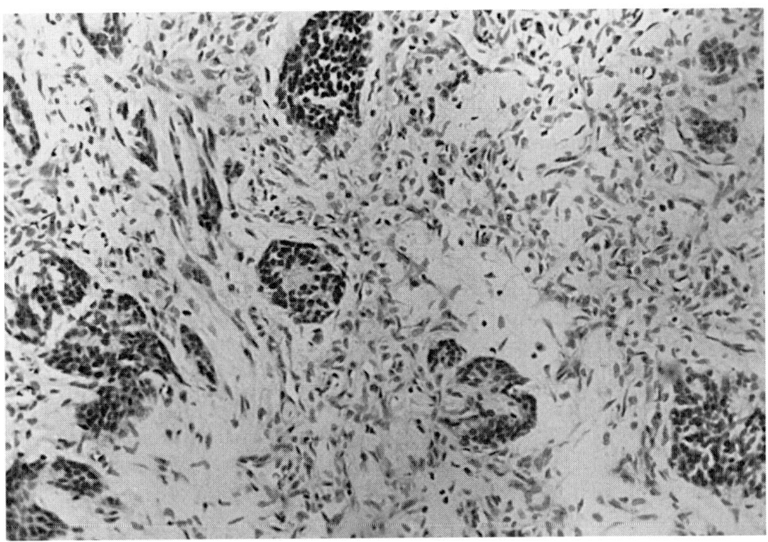

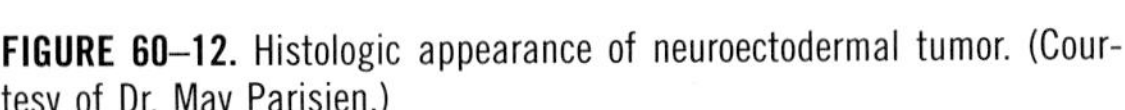

FIGURE 60–12. Histologic appearance of neuroectodermal tumor. (Courtesy of Dr. May Parisien.)

(Enzinger, 1988a, 1988b; Rosenberg et al, 1991). Areas of myxoid stroma can be mistaken for a nerve sheath myxoma.

Treatment. Needle aspiration or injection of nerve sheath ganglions has not proved effective (Rosenberg et al, 1991). Indications for surgery include loss of nerve function (e.g., foot drop with peroneal nerve involvement) of 6 weeks' to 3 months' duration, pain, localized nerve swelling, and presence of Tinel's sign (Cobb and Moiel, 1974; Rosenberg et al, 1991). Treatment usually includes local excision of the ganglion through a longitudinal incision of the epineurium. The ganglion can be dissected from nerve fascicles and excised under magnification. If nerve injury is a potential problem, especially with multiple lesions, decompression may be an option (Cobb and Moiel, 1974; Enzinger, 1988a, 1988b; Rosenberg et al, 1991). Care should be taken not to perform extensive unnecessary dissection of the nerve to remove the ganglion.

Results. Excision of the ganglion is usually curative for the lesion. Recurrences after resection of large lesions with severe neurological symptoms have been noted (Rosenberg et al, 1991, Strickland and Steichen, 1977). Recovery of nerve function is variable, and a worse prognosis is seen with severe preoperative neurological deficits from extensive involvement of the nerve by the ganglion (Cobb and Moiel, 1974; Parkes, 1961).

Lipofibromatous Hamartoma

Clinical Presentation. Lipofibromatous hamartomas are tumorlike lesions consisting of proliferative fibrofatty tissue invading peripheral nerves. Other terms used to describe the tumor include neural fibrolipomas, neurolipomatosis, infiltrating lipoma of nerve, perineural lipoma, and intraneural lipoma. The tumor usually involves the volar aspects of the hand, wrist, and forearm, particularly the median nerve and occasionally the ulnar and radial nerves (Goldman and Kaye, 1977; Louis, 1987; Paletta and Senay, 1981). A predilection for both males and females has been reported (Enzinger, 1988a, 1988b; Rosenberg, et al, 1991). The tumor occurs most commonly in children, usually within the first to third decade of life (Enzinger, 1988a, 1988b; Louis, 1987; Woodruff, 1993). About one third of the cases are associated with overgrowth of the limb (Silverman and Enzinger, 1985). Digital enlargement is more common than forearm or arm enlargement, and multiple-digit involvement is greater than single-digit enlargement (Amadio et al, 1988; Dabski et al, 1990; Dell 1985). Several terms have been used to describe limb enlargement, including macrodystrophia lipomatosa, macrodactyly, megalodactyly, local gigantism, and neural fibrolipoma with macrodactyly.

This slow-growing tumor may be seen as a simple mass or cause a combination of pain, tenderness, paresthesias, and signs of a compressive neuropathy with muscle denervation, e.g., carpal tunnel syndrome (Amadio et al, 1988; Goldman and Kaye, 1977; Silverman and Enzinger, 1985).

Pathology. Grossly, this soft tumor appears fusiform and grayish yellow. The tumor consists of fat and fibrous tissue that diffusely infiltrates into and around outside the nerve and its branches. Because of prolonged compression of the nerve, atrophy of neural elements are seen. With digital enlargement, the skeleton is enlarged and the subcutis infiltrated with fat. The tendons and vessels are usually normal (Dell, 1985; Rosenberg et al, 1991).

Treatment. An open biopsy of the tumor will help establish the diagnosis. Treatment options include nerve decompression, nerve decompression and neurolysis, nerve excision, and microscopic intraneural dissection of the tumor (Amadio et al, 1988; Bergman et al, 1970; Frykman and Wood, 1978; Jamra and Rebeiz, 1979; Louis, 1987; Louis and Hankin, 1985; Paletta and Rybka, 1972; Paletta and Senay, 1981; Patel, 1979; Rosenberg et al, 1991; Rowland, 1977; Smith and Lipke, 1980; Strickland and Steichen, 1977; Terzis et al, 1978). Because of the diffuse infiltrative nature of the tumor, complete excision of the tumor is generally not indicated. With median or ulnar nerve involvement, a decompression of the carpal or Guyon's canal, nerve decompression with an epineurotomy, and nerve biopsy to confirm the diagnosis are recommended (Barsky, 1967; Enzinger, 1988a, 1988b; Louis, 1987; Rosenberg et al, 1991). Microsurgical intraneural dissection and tumor resection generally results in some loss in nerve function. It is usually reserved for large painful tumors interfering with hand function or with recurrence of symptoms. Repeat nerve decompression may also be performed with recurrence of symptoms (Rosenberg et al, 1991; Smith and Lipke, 1980). Digital nerve involvement can be treated with partial or complete excision of the nerve and overlying skin. Debulking of macrodactylous digits can be performed with digital nerve excision. With excision of the nerve, nerve grafting can be performed in critical areas of digits requiring sensation, i.e., thumb, index, the radial aspect of the long finger, and the ulnar aspect of the little finger (Rosenberg et al, 1991).

Results. Relief of neurological symptoms, such as those of carpal tunnel syndrome, has been achieved with nerve decompression. Occasional recurrence of symptoms can occur. Nerve excision usually limits recurrence of the tumor (Amadio et al, 1988; Patel, 1979; Strickland and Steichen, 1977).

Neuromuscular Hamartoma

Clinical Presentation. Neuromuscular hamartomas are rare tumors composed of a combination of skeletal muscle and neural elements. They are also referred to as neuromuscular choristomas and benign triton tumors. They can be associated with a major peripheral nerve causing compression and neurological symptoms. The tumors are seen during infancy, occurring equally in males and females, and may occur during limb development (Bonneau and Brochu, 1983; Enzinger, 1988a, 1988b; Louhimo and Rapola, 1972; Markel and Enzinger, 1982; O'Connell and Rosenberg, 1990; Rosenberg et al, 1991).

Pathology. The tumor is firm and appears red-tan in color. The tumor is divided by fibrous septa into small lobules or nodules. The nodules are composed of randomly arranged, well-differentiated skeletal muscle fibers and myelinated and nonmyelinated nerve fibers (Enzinger, 1988a; 1988b; Rosenberg et al, 1991).

Treatment. Complete excision of the tumor is difficult without causing nerve injury. Initial treatment should include an incisional biopsy. Complete excision will result in a neurological deficit. Because of the benign nature of the tumor, partial removal is indicated for large tumors causing pain, causing neurological deficit, or interfering with surrounding structures (Rosenberg et al, 1991).

Results. Incomplete excision has resulted in resolution of some symptoms and has resulted in a decrease in the size of the tumor (Bonneau and Brochu, 1983; Enzinger, 1988a, 1988b). Recurrence of the tumor after excision has not been reported.

Hemangioma of Peripheral Nerve

Clinical Presentation. Hemangiomas of peripheral nerves are very rare tumors, with secondary involvement of the nerve by the hemangioma being more common (Enzinger, 1988a, 1988b; Healy and McCormack, 1993). Most tumors occur before the age of 40 without any specific anatomical predilection. Clinically, the presence of a mass, pain, and neurological symptoms is noted (Enzinger, 1988a, 1988b; Kojima et al, 1976; Kon and Vuursteen, 1981; Losli, 1952; Louis, 1987; Peled et al, 1980; Prosser and Burke, 1987; Wood, 1980).

Pathology. Histologically, benign cavernous–type hemangiomas are noted within or around the peripheral nerve (Enzinger, 1988a, 1988b).

Treatment. Local resection of the tumor or intralesional resection combined with nerve decompression appears to be successful in relieving symptoms (Kojima et al, 1976; Louis, 1987; Peled et al, 1980; Prosser and Burke, 1987). Intrafascicular excision of the tumor with magnification may minimize the morbidity of tumor resection (Prosser and Burke, 1987; Wood, 1980). Nerve resection and nerve grafting may be indicated with involvement of digital nerves (Healy and McCormack, 1993; Kon and Vuursteen, 1981).

Result. Tumor resection and nerve decompression appear to relieve symptoms (Louis, 1987). Local recurrence can occur (Healy and McCormack, 1993).

REACTIVE PROCESSES

Neuromas

Clinical Presentation. Neuromas can occur as the result of injury, such as an amputation, avulsion, or transection of a nerve (traumatic neuroma), or secondary to a chronic pressure, crush, or compression of a nerve (neuroma-in-continuity) (Herndon and Hess, 1991; Sunderland, 1978).

A neuroma is a proliferative, non-neoplastic mass formed at the site of a trauma (Harkin and Reed, 1969). They develop as the result of nerve regeneration. With an injury,

the continuity of the nerve is re-established by the growth of axons from the area proximal to the site of injury, across the site of injury, and into tubes of proliferating Schwann cells distal to the site of injury. Axons grow in a haphazard fashion in the absence of or with injury to distal endoneurial or Schwann cell tubules or in the presence of large gap between proximal and distal ends of nerve stumps.

With complete transection of the nerve, an enlarged stump (amputation stump neuroma or neuroma of a completely severed nerve) is generated by this axonal regeneration. With an incomplete transection of the nerve or with compression injuries to the nerve, a neuroma-in-continuity may form. Two types of neuromas-in-continuity can occur. A lateral neuroma occurs with regeneration of a partially transected nerve. A spindle neuroma, although not a true neuroma, occurs with a compressive nerve injury in which the perineurial sheath remains intact, e.g., Morton's neuroma. The injury results in edema formation and intraneural fibrosis of the nerve (Enzinger, 1988a, 1988b; Herndon, 1993; Herndon and Hess, 1991).

The true incidence of traumatic neuromas is unknown, but they are estimated to occur in 4% of patients after digital amputations and in up to 30% of patients after nerve injury (Fisher and Boswick, 1983; Nelson, 1977).

Clinically, the neuroma presents as a firm, tender, painful mass. Symptoms consist of dysesthesias, hyperalgesia, or burning sensations. Tapping over the nerve may cause pain or paresthesias (Healy and McCormack, 1993; Herndon and Hess, 1991). Lidocaine injection around the mass should relieve symptoms.

Pathology. Grossly, amputation neuromas appear as oblong, rounded masses at the end of a nerve stump (Fig. 60–13). They appear gray-white and are relatively firm. Histologically, they consist of a disorganized mass of nerve fascicles, Schwann cells, axonal processes, and fibroblasts in a dense collagenous matrix (Enzinger, 1988a, 1988b; Harkin and Reed, 1969; Rosenberg et al, 1991). Neuromas-in-continuity usually appear as a firm, fusiform enlargement of the nerve (Fig. 60–14). Intraneural edema and fibrosis involving the epineurium and perineurium are noted (Enzinger, 1988a, 1988b) (Fig. 60–15).

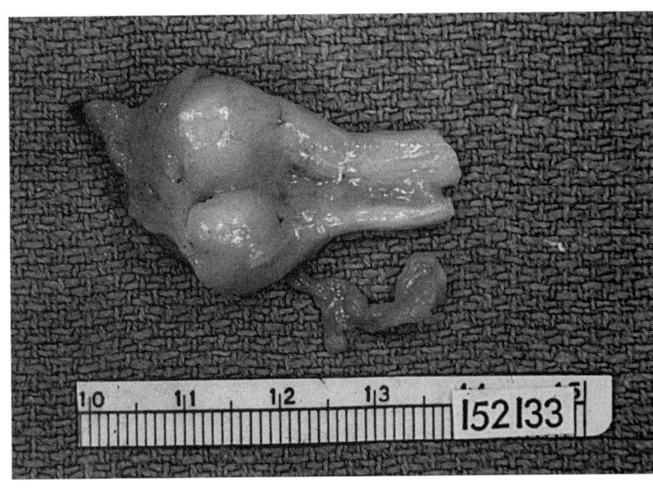

FIGURE 60–13. Amputation stump neuroma. (Courtesy of Dr. May Parisien.)

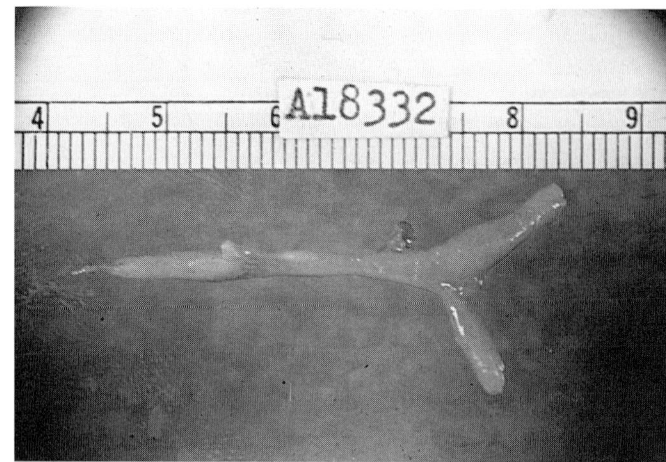

FIGURE 60–14. Interdigital neuroma. (Courtesy of Dr. May Parisien.)

Treatment. Nonoperative treatment of neuromas includes desensitization techniques such as percussion, local massage, and ultrasound; transcutaneous electrical nerve stimulation; and corticosteroid injections (Grant, 1951; Herndon and Hess, 1991; Omer, 1981; Russell, 1950; Smith and Gomez, 1970; Whipple and Unsell, 1988).

The operative treatment of amputation stump neuromas includes methods to prevent neuroma formation, resection of the neuroma, or transfer the neuroma to a new location (Eaton, 1980; Herndon, 1993; Herndon and Hess, 1991; Tupper and Booth, 1974).

Prevention techniques include crushing, ligation, coagulation, or sclerosis of the nerve. Physical methods used to occlude the ends of transected nerves include, among others, cauterization, freezing, and laser coagulation. A variety of chemical solutions, including formalin, alcohol, cortisone, phenol, acid, and chemotherapeutic agents, have been used to try to prevent neuroma formation. Many synthetic materials, including silicone, methylmethacrylate, gold foil, vitallium, and a variety of other materials, have been used to cap nerve endings.

Implantation of the nerve end into the same nerve (neuro-campsis) and suturing of the terminal ends of two nerves (cross-union) or two nerves of central origin (centrocentral anastomosis) have been used to prevent neuroma formation. Relocation methods include the implantation of nerve ends into bone or muscle or translocation of the nerve end into an area of healthy soft tissues (Eaton, 1980; Herndon, 1993; Herndon and Hess, 1991; Tupper and Booth, 1974).

The nonoperative treatment of neuromas-in-continuity includes the use of systemic medications (e.g., dipyridamole, pentoxifylline) to increase peripheral circulation, or calcium-channel blockers (e.g., nifedipine, diltiazem) and nonsteroidal medications. Corticosteroids and local anesthetics have been used locally. Densensitization techniques similar to those used for amputation stumps are also used. Surgical options include neurolysis, nerve transposition into healthy areas, and nerve coverage with nonvascularized barriers (vein wrapping) and vascularized flaps (muscle, fascia, omentum). The use of implantable electrical stimulators, nerve resection with or without nerve grafting, relocation of the resected nerve, and wandering nerve grafts has been described (Gould, 1991).

Nonoperative methods should initially be used for the

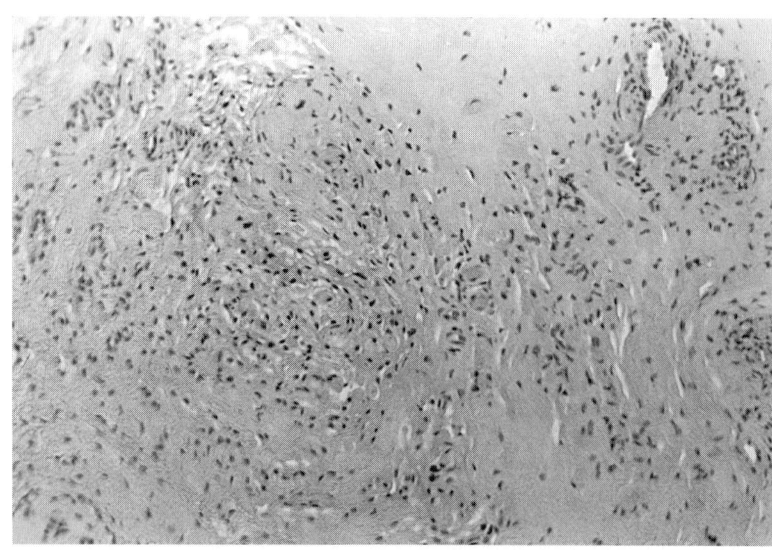

FIGURE 60–15. Microscopic appearance of an interdigital neuroma. (Courtesy of Dr. May Parisien.)

treatment of neuromas. The choice of surgical technique depends on the location of the neuroma, type of neuroma, and the quality of the surrounding tissue.

Results. No single method of treatment has proved universally successful (Healy and McCormack, 1993; Sunderland, 1978). Better results appear to occur with earlier operative management. Poorer results are expected in patients with worker's compensation, patients with radial sensory neuromas, and patients who have had three or more operative procedures (Herndon and Hess, 1991; MacKinnon and Dellon, 1988; Rosenberg et al, 1991).

References

Amadio PC, Reman HM, Dobyns JH: Lipofibromatous hamartoma of nerve. J Hand Surg *13A*:67–75, 1988.

Angervall L, Kindblom L, Haglid K: Dermal nerve sheath myxoma. Cancer *53*:1752–1759, 1984.

Ariel IM: Current concepts in the management of peripheral nerve tumors. *In* Omer GE, Spinner M (eds): Management of Peripheral Nerve Problems. Philadelphia, WB Saunders, 1980, pp 669–693.

Ariel IM: Tumors of the peripheral nervous system. Semin Surg Oncol *4*:7–12, 1988.

Aspisarnthanarax P: Granular cell tumor. J Am Acad Dermatol *5*:171–182, 1981.

Barker D, Wright E, Nguyen L, et al: Gene for von Recklinghausen neurofibromatosis is in the pericentromeric region of chromosome 17. Science *236*:1100–1102, 1987.

Barre PS, Schaffer JW, Carter JR, Lacey SH: Multiplicity of neurilemmomas in the upper extremity. J Hand Surg *12*:307–311, 1987.

Barrett R, Cramer F: Tumors of the peripheral nerves and so-called "ganglia" of the peroneal nerve. Clin Orthop *27*:135–146, 1963.

Barsky AJ: Macrodactyly. J Bone Joint Surg *49A*:1255–1266, 1967.

Basso-Ricci S: Therapy of malignant schwannomas: Usefulness of an integrated radiologic surgical therapy. J Neurosurg Sci *33*:253–257, 1989.

Bergman FO, Blom SEG, Stenstrom SJ: Radical excision of a fibro-fatty proliferation of the median nerve, with no neurological loss symptoms. Plast Reconstr Surg *46*:375–380, 1970.

Blair WF: Granular cell schwannoma of the hand. J Hand Surg *5*:51–52, 1980.

Blumberg AK, Kay S, Adelaar RS: Nerve sheath myxoma of digital nerve. Cancer *63*:1215–1218, 1989.

Bogumill GP, Sullivan DJ, Baker GI. Tumors of the hand. Clin Orthop *108*:214–222, 1975.

Bojsen-Moller M, Myrhe-Jensen O: A consecutive series of 30 malignant schwannomas: Survival in relation to clinicopathological parameters and treatment. Acta Pathol Microbiol Scand (Sect A) *92*:147–155, 1984.

Bolande RP: Neurofibromatosis: The quintessential neurocristopathy. Adv Neurol *29*:67–75, 1981.

Bolen JW, Thorning D: Peripheral neuroepithelioma: A light and electron microscopic study. Cancer *46*:2456–2462, 1980.

Bonneau R, Brochu P: Neuromuscular choristoma. Am J Surg Pathol *7*:521–528, 1983.

Boyes JH: Bunnell's Surgery of the Hand, eds. Philadelphia, JB Lippincott, 1970, pp 666–704.

Brasfield RD, Das Gupta TK: Von Recklinghausen's disease: A clinicopathological study. Ann Surg *175*:86–104, 1972.

Brennan MF, Hilaris B, Shiu MH, et al: Local recurrence in adult soft tissue sarcoma: A randomized trial of brachytherapy. Arch Surg *122*:1289–1293, 1987.

Butler D, Hamill JP, Seipel RS, et al: Tumors of the hand. Am J Surg *100*:293–303, 1960.

Canale DJ, Bebin J: Von Recklinghausen disease of the nervous system. *In* Vinken PJ, Bruyn GW (eds): Handbook of Clinical Neurology. New York, American Elsevier Publishers, 1972, pp 132–162.

Carney JA: Psammomatous melanotic schwannoma: A distinctive, heritable tumor with special associations, including cardiac myxoma and the Cushing syndrome. Am J Surg Pathol *14*:206–222, 1990.

Carstens PH, Schrodt GR: Malignant transformation of a benign encapsulated neurilemoma. Am J Clin Pathol *51*:144–149, 1969.

Cawthon RM, Weiss R, Xu G, et al: A major segment of the neurofibromatosis type 1 gene: cDNA sequence, genomic structure and point mutations. Cell *62*:193–201, 1990.

Charache H: Multiple neurofibroma with sarcomatous transformation and skeletal involvement. Arch Dermatol Syph *40*:185, 1939.

Chui MC, Bird BL, Rogers J: Extracranial and extraspinal nerve sheath tumors: Computed tomographic evaluation. Neuroradiology *30*:47–53, 1988.

Chung IH, Kim NH, Choi IY: Macrodactylism associated with neurofibroma of the median nerve: A case report. Yonsei Med J *14*:49, 1973.

Cobb AC, Moiel RH: Ganglion of the peroneal nerve. J Neurosurg *41*:255–259, 1974.

Compagno J, Hyams VJ, Ste-Marie P: Benign granular cell tumors of the larynx: A review of the 36 cases with clinical pathologic data. Ann Otol Rhinol Laryngol *84*:308, 1975.

Cornell SH, Kirkendall W: Neurofibromatosis of the renal artery, an unusual cause of hypertension. Radiology *88*:24–28, 1967.

Crowe FW, Schull WJ, Neel JV: A Clinical, Pathological and Genetic Study of Multiple Neurofibromatosis. Springfield, IL, Charles C Thomas, 1956.

Dabski C, Reiman HM, Muller SA: Neurofibrosarcoma of skin and subcutaneous tissues. Mayo Clin Proc *65*:164–172, 1990.

D'Agostino AN, Soule EH, Miller RH: Primary malignant neoplasm of nerves (malignant neurilemmomas) in patients without manifestations of multiple neurofibromatosis (von Recklinghausen's disease). Cancer *16*:1003–1027, 1963a.

D'Agostino AN, Soule EH, Miller RH: Sarcomas of the peripheral nerve and somatic soft tissues associated with multiple neurofibromatosis (von Recklinghausen's disease). Cancer *16*:1015–1027, 1963b.

Daimaru Y, Hashimoto H, Enjoji M: Malignant peripheral nerve-sheath tumors (malignant schwannomas): An immunohistochemical study of 29 cases. Am J Surg Pathol *9*:434–444, 1985.

Das Gupta TK: Pathology of soft tissue sarcoma. *In* Das Gupta TK (ed): Tumors of the Soft Tissue. Norwalk, Appleton-Century-Crofts, 1983, pp 22–183.

Dehner LP: Peripheral and central primitive neuroectodermal tumors. Arch Pathol Lab Med *110*:997–1005, 1986.

Dell PC: Macrodactyly. Hand Clin *1*:511–524, 1985.

Dickersin GR: The electron microscopic spectrum of nerve sheath tumors. Ultrastruct Pathol *10*:478–490, 1987.

Ducatman BS, Scheithauer BW: Post-irradiation neurofibrosarcoma. Cancer *51*:1028–1033, 1983.

Ducatman BS, Scheithauer BW, Piepgras DG: Malignant peripheral nerve sheath tumors: A clinicopathological study of 120 cases. Cancer *57*:2006–2021, 1986.

Eaton RG: Painful neuromas. *In* Omer GE Jr, Spinner M (eds): Management of Peripheral Nerve Problems. Philadelphia, WB Saunders, 1980, p 180.

Enneking WF, Spanier SS, Goodman MA: Current concepts review: The staging of musculoskeletal sarcoma. J Bone Joint Surg *62A*:1027–1030, 1980.

Enzinger FM, Weiss SW: Benign tumors of peripheral nerves. *In* Enzinger FM, Weiss SW (eds): Soft Tissue Tumors, ed 2. St. Louis, Mosby, 1988a, pp 719–780.

Enzinger FM, Weiss SW: Malignant tumors of peripheral nerves. *In* Enzinger FM, Weiss SW (eds): Soft Tissue Tumors, ed 2. St. Louis, Mosby, 1988b, pp 781–815.

Erlandson RA, Woodruff JM: Peripheral nerve sheath tumors: An electron microscopic study of 43 cases. Cancer *49*:273–287, 1982.

Fisher ER, Vuzevski VD: Cytogenesis of schwannoma (neurilemmoma), neurofibroma, dermatofibroma, and dermatofibrosarcoma as revealed by electron microscopy. Am J Clin Pathol *49*:941–954, 1968.

Fisher ER, Wechsler H: Granular cell myoblastoma—a misnomer. EM and histochemical evidence concerning its Schwann cell derivation and nature (granular cell schwannoma). Cancer *15*:936–943, 1962.

Fisher GT, Boswick JA: Neuroma formation following digital amputations. J Trauma *23*:136–142, 1983.

Fletcher CDM: Peripheral nerve sheath tumors: A clinicopathologic update. Pathol Annu *25*:53–74, 1990.

Fletcher CDM, Chan J-C, McKee PH: Dermal nerve sheath myxoma: A study of three cases. Histopathology *10*:135–145, 1986.

Fletcher CD, Davies SE: Benign plexiform (multinodular) schwannoma: A rare tumor unassociated with neurofibromatosis. Histopathology *10*:971–980, 1986.

Fletcher CD, Davies SE, McKee PH: Cellular schwannoma: A distinct pseudosarcomatous entity. Histopathology *11*:21–35, 1987.

Foley KM, Woodruff JM, Ellis FT, Posner JB: Radiation induced malignant and atypical peripheral nerve sheath tumors. Ann Neurol 7:311–318, 1980.

Frykman GK, Wood VE: Peripheral nerve hamartoma with macrodactyly in the hand: Report of three cases and review of the literature. J Hand Surg 3:307–312, 1978.

Fust JA, Custer RP: Granular cell "myoblastoma" and granular cell neurofibromas: Separation of the neurogenous tumors from the myoblastoma group. Am J Pathol 24:674, 1948.

Gaisford JC: Tumors of the hand. Surg Clin North Am 40:549–566, 1960.

Gallager RL, Helwig EM: Neurothekeoma: A benign cutaneous tumor of neural origin. Am J Clin Pathol 74:759–764, 1980.

Garancis JC, Komorowski RA, Kuzma JF: Granular cell myoblastoma. Cancer 25:542–550, 1970.

Geschickter CF: Tumors of peripheral nerve. Am J Cancer 25:377–410, 1935.

Ghosh BC, Ghosh L, Huvos AG: Malignant schwannoma: A clinicopathologic study. Cancer 31:184–190, 1973.

Giacobbe A, Facciorusso D, Conoscitore P, Spirito F, Squillante MM, Bisceglia M: Granular cell tumor of the esophagus. Am J Gastroenterol 83:139–140, 1988.

Giangaspero F, Fratamico FCM, Ceccaselli C, Brisiotti M: Malignant peripheral nerve sheath tumors and spindle cell sarcomas: An immunohistochemical analysis of multiple markers. Appl Pathol 7:134–144, 1989.

Giannestras NJ, Bronson JL: Malignant schwannoma of the medial plantar branch of the posterior tibial nerve (unassociated with von Recklinghausen's disease). J Bone Joint Surg 57A:701–703, 1975.

Goldman AB, Kaye JJ: Macrodystrophia lipomatosa: Radiographic diagnosis. AJR 128:101–105, 1977.

Gould JS: Treatment of the painful injured neuroma in-continuity. In Gelberman, RH (ed): Operative Nerve Repair and Reconstruction. Philadelphia, JB Lippincott, 1991, pp 1541–1550.

Grant GH: Methods of treatment of neuromata of the hand. J Bone Joint Surg 33A:841–848, 1951.

Gray MH, Rosenberg AE, Dickerson GR, Bhan A: Glial fibrillary acidic protein and keratin expression by benign and malignant nerve sheath tumors. Hum Pathol 20:1089–1096, 1989.

Greene J, Fitzwater J, Burgess J: Arterial lesions associated with neurofibromatosis. Am J Clin Pathol 62:481–487, 1974.

Guccion JG, Enzinger FM: Malignant schwannoma associated with von Recklinghausen's neurofibromatosis. Virchows Arch 383:43–57, 1979.

Gurdjian ES, Larsen RD, Linder DW: Intraneural cyst of the peroneal and ulnar nerves. J Neurosurg 23:76–78, 1965.

Harkin JC. Differential diagnosis of peripheral nerve tumors. In Omer GE, Spinner M (eds): Management of Peripheral Nerve Problems. Philadelphia, WB Saunders, 1980, pp 657–668.

Harkin JC, Reed RJ: Tumours of the Peripheral Nervous System. Washington, DC, Armed Forces Institute of Pathology, 1969.

Hartwell AS: Cystic tumor of median nerve. Boston Med Surg J 144:582–583, 1901.

Healy JH, McCormack RR: Nerve tumors. In Bogumill GP, Fleegler EJ (eds): Tumors of the Hand and Upper Limb. Edinburgh, Churchill Livingstone, 1993, pp 205–223.

Herndon JH: Neuromas. In Green, DP (ed): Operative Hand Surgery. New York, Churchill Livingstone, 1993, pp 1387–1400.

Herndon JH, Eaton RG, Littler JW: Management of painful neuromas in the hand. J Bone Joint Surg 58A:369–373, 1976.

Herndon JH, Hess AV: Neuromas. In Gelberman RH (ed): Operative Nerve Repair and Reconstruction. Philadelphia, JB Lippincott, 1991, pp 1525–1540.

Hirose T, Hasegawa T, Kudo E, Seki K, Sano T, Hizawa K: Malignant peripheral nerve sheath tumors: An immunohistochemical study in relation to ultrastructural features. Hum Pathol 23:865–870, 1992.

Hochberg FH, DaSilva AB, Galdabini J, et al: Gastrointestinal involvement in von Recklinghausen's neurofibromatosis. Neurology 24:1144–1151, 1974.

Holdsworth BJ: Nerve tumors in the upper limb: A clinical review. Br J Hand Surg 10:236–238, 1985.

Horn RC Jr, Stout AP: Granular cell myoblastoma. Surg Gynecol Obstet 76:315–318, 1943.

Hosoi K: Multiple neurofibromatosis (von Recklinghausen's disease) with special reference to malignant transformation. Arch Surg 22:258, 1931.

Hruban RH, Shiu MH, Senie RT, Woodruff JM: Malignant peripheral nerve sheath tumors of the buttock and lower extremity: A study of 43 cases. Cancer 66:1253–1265, 1990.

Iwashita T, Enjoji M: Plexiform neurilemmoma: A clinicopathological and immunohistochemical analysis of 23 tumors from 20 patients. Virchows Arch 411:305–309, 1987.

Izumi AK, et al: Von Recklinghausen's disease associated with multiple neurilemmomas. Arch Dermatol 104:172–176, 1971.

Jamra FNA, Rebeiz JJ: Lipofibroma of the median nerve. J Hand Surg 4:160–163, 1979.

Jurgens H, Bier V, Harms D, et al: Malignant peripheral neuroectodermal tumors: A retrospective analysis of 42 cases. Cancer 61:349–357, 1988.

Karakousis CP, Velez AF, Emrich LJ: Management of retroperitoneal sarcomas and patient survival. Am J Surg 150:376–380, 1985.

Killeen RM, Davy CL, Bauserman SC: Melanocystic schwannoma. Cancer 62:174–183, 1988.

Kojima T, Yoshita I, Marumo E, et al: Hemangioma of median nerve causing carpal tunnel. Hand 8:62–65, 1976.

Kon M, Vuursteen PJ: An intraneural hemangioma of a digital nerve. J Hand Surg 6:357–358, 1981.

Lassmann H, Jurecka W, Lassmann W: Different type of benign nerve sheath tumors: Light microscopy, electron microscopy, and autoradiography. Virchows Arch 375:197–210, 1977.

Levine E, Huntrakoon M, Wetzel, LH: Malignant nerve sheath neoplasms in neurofibromatosis: Distinction from benign tumors by using imaging techniques. AJR 149:1059–1064, 1987.

Lewis RC, Nannini LH, Cocke WM: Multifocal neurilemmomas of median and ulnar nerves of the same extremity. J Hand Surg 6:406–408, 1981.

Lictenstein BW: Neurofibromatosis (von Recklinghausen's disease of nervous system): Analysis of a total pathologic picture. Arch Neurol Psychiatry 62:822–839, 1949.

Lindberg RD, Martin RG, Romsdahl MM, Barkley T: Conservative surgery and postoperative radiotherapy in 300 adults with soft tissue sarcomas. Cancer 47:2391–2397, 1981.

Linnoila RI, Tsokos M, Triche TJ, Marongos PJ, Chondra RS: Evidence for neural origin and PAS-positive variants of the malignant small cell tumor of thoracopulmonary region ("Askin tumor"). Am J Surg Pathol 10:124–133, 1986.

Llombart-Bosch A, Terrier-Lacombe J, Peydro-Olaya A, Contesso G: Peripheral neuroectodermal sarcoma of soft tissue (peripheral neuroepithelioma). Hum Pathol 20:273–280, 1989.

Lodding P, Kindblom L, Angervall L, et al: Cellular schwannoma: A clinicopathologic study of 29 cases. Virchows Archiv 416:237–248, 1990.

Losli EJ: Intrinsic hemangiomas of the peripheral nerves. Arch Pathol 53:226–232, 1952.

Lott IT, Richardson EP: Neuropathological findings in the biology of neurofibromatosis. Adv Neurol 29:23–32, 1981.

Louhimo I, Rapola J: Intraneural muscular hamartoma: Report of two cases in small children. J Pediatr Surg 7:696–699, 1972.

Louis DS: Peripheral nerve tumors in the upper extremity. Hand Clin 3:311–318, 1987.

Louis DS, Hankin FM: Benign tumors of the upper extremity. Bull NY Acad Med 61:611–620, 1985.

Louis DS, Hankin FM, Green TL, Dick HM: Lipofibromas of the median nerve: Long-term follow-up of four cases. J Hand Surg 10A:403–408, 1985.

MacDonald DM, Wilson-Jones E: Pacinian neurofibroma. Histopathology 1:247–255, 1977.

MacKay B, Luna MA, Butler JJ: Adult neuroblastoma: Electron microscopic observations in nine cases. Cancer 37:1334–1351, 1976.

MacKenzie DH: Malignant granular cell myoblastoma. J Clin Pathol 20:739–742, 1967.

MacKinnon SE, Dellon AL: Surgery of the Peripheral Nerve. New York, Thieme Med, Publishers, 1988, pp 535–549.

Mankin HJ: Principles of soft-tissue tumor management. In Gelberman RH (ed): Operative Nerve Repair and Reconstruction. Philadelphia, JB Lippincott, 1991, pp 1587–1625.

Mankin HJ, Lange TA, Spanier SS: The hazards of biopsy in patients with malignant primary bone and soft tissue tumors. J Bone Joint Surg 64A:1121–1127, 1982.

Marina NM, Etcubanas E, Parha DM, Bowman LC, Green A: Peripheral primitive neuroectodermal tumor (peripheral neuroepithelioma) in children. Cancer 64:1952–1960, 1989.

Markel SF, Enzinger FM: Neuromuscular hamartoma: A benign "Triton tumor" composed of mature neural and striated muscle elements. Cancer 49:140–144, 1982.

Match RM, Leffert RD: Massive neurofibromatosis of the upper extremity with paralysis. J Hand Surg 12A:718–722, 1987.

Matsunou H, Shimoda T, Kakimoto S, Yamashida H, Ishikawa E, Mukai

M: Histopathology and immunohistochemical study of malignant tumors of peripheral nerve sheath (malignant schwannoma). Cancer *56:*2269–2279, 1985.

Merck C, Kindblom LG: Neurofibromatosis of the appendix in von Recklinghausen's disease. Acta Pathol Microbiol Scand *83A:*623–627, 1975.

Miettinen M, Lehtonen E, Lehtola H, et al: Histogenesis of granular cell tumour: An immunological and ultrastructural study. J Pathol *142:*221–229, 1984.

Miser JS, Kinsella TJ, Triche TJ, et al: Treatment of peripheral neuroepithelioma in children and young adults. J Clin Oncol *5:*1752–1758, 1987.

Nambisan RN, Rao V, Moore R, Karakousis CP: Malignant soft tissue tumors of nerve sheath origin. J Surg Oncol *25:*628–272, 1984.

Nathrath WBJ, Remberger K: Immunohistochemical study of granular cell tumors. Virchows Arch *408:*421–434, 1986.

Nelson AW: The painful neuroma: The regenerating axon vs the epineurial sheath. J Surg Res *23:*215–221, 1977.

Nesbitt KA, Vidone RA: Primitive neuroectodermal tumor (neuroblastoma) arising in sciatic nerve of a child. Cancer *37:*1562–1570, 1976.

O'Connell JX, Rosenberg AE: Multiple cutaneous neuromuscular choristomas. Am J Surg Pathol *14:*93–96, 1990.

Omer GE: Nerve neuroma and pain problems related to upper limb amputations. Orthop Clin North Am *12:*751–763, 1981.

Paletta FX, Rybka FJ: Treatment of hamartomas of the median nerve. Ann Surg *176:*217–222, 1972.

Paletta FX, Senay LC Jr: Lipofibromatous hamartomas of median nerve and ulnar nerve: Surgical treatment. Plast Reconstr Surg *68:*915–921, 1981.

Papageorgiou S, Litt JZ, Pomeranz JR: Multiple granular cell myoblastomas in children. Arch Dermatol *96:*168–171, 1967.

Parkes A: Intraneural ganglion of the lateral popliteal nerve. J Bone Joint Surg *43B:*784–790, 1961.

Patel ME, Silver JW, Lipton DE, Pearlman HS: Lipofibroma of the median nerve in the palm and digits of the hand. J Bone Joint Surg *43B:*784–790, 1961.

Peled D, Josipovich Z, Rousso M, Wexler MR: Hemangioma of the median nerve. J Hand Surg *5:*363–365, 1980.

Perentes E, Rubenstein LJ: Immunohistochemical recognition of human nerve sheath tumors by anti-leu-7 (HNK-1) monoclonal antibody. Acta Neuropathol *68:*319–324, 1985.

Phalen GS: Neurilemmomas of the forearm and hand. Clin Orthop *114:*219–223, 1976.

Pleasure J, Geller SA: Neurofibromatosis in infancy presenting with congenital stridor. Am J Dis Child *113:*390–393, 1967.

Posch JL: Tumors of the hand. *In* Jupiter JB (ed): Flynn's Hand Surgery, ed 4. Baltimore, Williams & Wilkins, 1991, pp 935–978.

Powers SK, Norman D, Edwards MSB: Computerized tomography of peripheral nerve lesions. J Neurosurg *59:*131–136, 1983.

Preston FW, Walsh WS, Clarke TS: Cutaneous neurofibromatosis (von Recklinghausen's disease). Arch Surg *64:*813–827, 1952.

Prichard RW, Custer RP: Pacinian neurofibroma. Cancer *5:*297–301, 1952.

Prosser AJ, Burke FD: Hemangiomas of the median nerve associated with Raynaud's phenomenon. J Hand Surg *12B:*227–228, 1987.

Pulitzer DR, Reed RJ: Nerve-sheath myxoma (perineural myxoma). Am J Dermatopathol *7:*409–421, 1985.

Pung S, Hirsch EF: Plexiform neurofibromatosis of the head and neck. Arch Pathol *59:*341–346, 1955.

Raney B, Schnaufer L, Ziegler M, Chatten J: Treatment of children with neurogenic sarcoma: Experience at Children's Hospital of Philadelphia. Cancer *59:*1–5, 1987.

Rasbridge SA, Browse NL, Tighe JR, Fletcher CD: Malignant nerve sheath tumor arising in benign ancient schwannoma. Histopathology *14:*525–528, 1989.

Riccardi VM. Von Recklinghausen neurofibromatosis. N Engl J Med *305:*1617–1627, 1981.

Ricci A Jr, Parham DM, Woodruff JM, et al: Malignant peripheral nerve sheath tumors arising from ganglioneuromas. Am J Surg Pathol *8:*19–29, 1984.

Rinaldi E: Neurilemmomas and neurofibromas of the upper limb. J Hand Surg *8:*1617–1627, 1983.

Robertson AJ, McIntosh W, Lamont P, Guthrie W: Malignant granular cell tumor (myoblastoma) of the vulva: A report of a case and review of the literature. Histopathology *5:*69–79, 1981.

Rodriguez HA, Berthong M: Multiple primary intracranial tumors in von Recklinghausen's neurofibromatosis. Arch Neurol *14:*467–475, 1966.

Rosenberg AE, Dick HM, Botte MJ: Benign and malignant tumors of peripheral nerve. *In* Gelberman RH (ed): Operative Nerve Repair and Reconstruction. Philadelphia, JB Lippincott, 1991, pp 1587–1625.

Rouleau GA, Wertelecki W, Haines JL, et al: Genetic linkage of bilateral acoustic neurofibromatosis to a DNA marker on chromosome 22. Nature *329:*246–248, 1987.

Rowland SA: Case report: Ten-year follow-up of lipofibroma of the median nerve in the palm. J Hand Surg *2:*316–317, 1977.

Russell WR: Painful amputation stumps: Treatment by percussion. Br Med J *2:*68–73, 1950.

Sagel SS, Forrest JV: Interstitial lung disease in neurofibromatosis. South Med J *68:*647–649, 1975.

Salyer WR, Salyer DC: The vascular lesions of neurofibromatosis. Angiology *25:*510–519, 1974.

Schorn D, Griessel PJ, Ziaday F: Neurofibromatosis with renovascular hypertension. S Afr Med J *48:*1537–1539, 1974.

Schuler FA III, Adamson JE: Pacinian neuroma, an unusual case of finger pain. Plast Reconstr Surg *62:*576–579, 1978.

Shereff MJ, Posner MA, Gordon MH: Upper extremity hypertrophy secondary to neurofibromatosis: A case report. J Hand Surg *5:*355–357, 1980.

Shiu MH, Turnbull AD, Nori D, et al: Control of locally advanced extremity soft tissue sarcomas by function: Saving resection and brachytherapy. Cancer *47:*1385–1392, 1984.

Silverman TA, Enzinger FM: Fibrolipomatous hamartoma of nerve: A clinicopathologic analysis of 26 cases. Am J Surg Pathol *9:*7–14, 1985.

Simon MA: Biopsy of musculoskeletal tumors. J Bone Joint Surg *64A:*1253–1257, 1982.

Smith JR, Gomez NH: Local injection therapy of neuromata of the hand with triamcinolone acetonide: A preliminary study of twenty-two patients. J Bone Joint Surg *52A:*71–83, 1970.

Smith RJ, Lipke RW: Surgical treatment of peripheral nerve tumors of the upper limb. *In* Omer GE, Spinner M (eds): Management of Peripheral Nerve Problems. Philadelphia, WB Saunders, 1980, pp 694–711.

Sobel HJ, Schwarz R, Marquet E: Light and electron microscopic study of the origin of granular cell myoblastoma. J Pathol *109:*101–111, 1973.

Sordillo PP, Hadju SI, et al: Malignant schwannoma: Clinical characteristics, surgery, and response to therapy. Cancer *47:*2503–2509, 1981.

Sorensen SA, Mulvihill JJ, Nielsen A: Long-term follow up of von Recklinghausen neurofibromatosis. N Engl J Med *314:*1010–1015, 1986.

Stack HG: Tumors of the hand. Br Med J *1:*919–922, 1960.

Stewart FW, Copeland MM: Neurogenic sarcoma. Am J Cancer *15:*1235–1320, 1931.

Storm FK, Eilber FR, Mirra J, Morton DL: Neurofibrosarcoma. Cancer *45:*129–129, 1980.

Stout AP: The peripheral manifestation of specific nerve sheath tumor (neurilemmoma). Am J Cancer *24:*751–796, 1935.

Strickland JW, Steichen JB: Nerve tumors of the hand and forearm. J Hand Surg *2:*285–291, 1977.

Strong EW, McDivitt RW, Brasfield RD: Granular cell myoblastoma. Cancer *25:*415–421, 1970.

Stull MA, Moser RP, Kransdorf MJ, Bogumill GP, Nelson MC: Magnetic resonance appearance of peripheral nerve sheath tumors. Skeletal Radiol *20:*9–14, 1991.

Suh JS, Abenoza P, Galloway HR, Everson LI, Griffiths HJ: Peripheral (extracranial) nerve tumors: Correlation of MR imaging and histologic findings. Radiology *183:*341–346, 1992.

Sunderland S: Nerves and Nerve Injuries, ed 2. Edinburgh, Churchill-Livingstone, 1978.

Swanson AB, Boeve NR, Lumsden RM: The prevention and treatment of amputation neuromata by silicone capping. J Hand Surg *2:*70–78, 1977.

Swanson PE, Manivel JC, Wick MR: Immunoreactivity for Leu-7 in neurofibrosarcoma and other spindle cell sarcomas of soft tissue. Am J Pathol *126:*546–560, 1987.

Terzis JK, Daniel RK, Williams HB, Spencer PS: Benign fatty tumors of peripheral nerve. Ann Plast Surg *1:*193–216, 1978.

Thiele CJ, McKeon C, Triche TJ, et al: Differential protooncogene expression characterizes histopathologically indistinguishable tumors of the peripheral nervous system. J Clin Invest *80:*804–811, 1987.

Thomas JE, Piepgras DG, Scheithauer BW, Manivel JC: Malignant peripheral nerve sheath tumor: A clinicopathologic study of 35 cases. Mayo Clin Proc *5:*640–647, 1983.

Trojanowski JQ: Cytoskeletal proteins and neuronal tumors. *In* Colvin RB, Bhan AK, McCluskey RT (eds): Diagnostic Immunopathology. New York, Raven, 1988, pp 225–243.

Tsuneyoshi M, Enjoji M: Granular cell tumor: A clinicopathological study of 48 cases. Fukuoka Acta Medica *69:*495, 1978.

Tupper JW, Booth NM: Treatment of painful neuromas of sensory nerves in the hand: A comparison of traditional and newer methods. J Hand Surg *1:*144–151, 1976.

Vance S, Hudson R: Granular cell myoblastoma. Am J Clin Pathol *52:*208–211, 1969.

Vieta JO, Pack JT: Malignant neurilemmomas of peripheral nerves. Am J Surg *82:*416–431, 1951.

Viskochil D, Buchberg AM, Xu G, et al: Deletions and a translocation interrupt a cloned gene at the neurofibromatosis type 1 locus. Cell *62:*187–192, 1990.

Voss BL, Pysher TJ, Humphrey GB: Peripheral neuroepithelioma in childhood. Cancer *54:*3059–3064, 1984.

Waggener JD: Ultrastructure of benign peripheral nerve sheath tumors. Cancer *19:*699–709, 1966.

Wallace MR, Marchuck DA, Andersen LB, et al: Type 1 neurofibromatosis gene: Identification of a large transcript disrupt in three NF-1 patients. Science *249:*181–249, 1990.

Wanebo JE, Malik JM, VandenBerg SR, et al: Malignant peripheral nerve sheath tumors. Cancer *71:*1247–1253, 1993.

Weiss SW, Langloss JM, Enzinger FM: Value of S-100 protein in the diagnosis of soft tissue tumors, with particular reference to benign and malignant Schwann cell tumors. Lab Invest *49:*299–308, 1983.

Westelek W, Roulou GA, Superneau DW, Forehand LW: Neurofibromatosis 2: Clinical and DNA linkage studies of a large kindred. N Engl J Med *319:*278–283, 1988.

Whang-Peng J, Triche TJ, Knutsen T, et al: Chromosome translocation in peripheral neuroepithelioma. N Engl J Med *311:*584–585, 1984.

Whang-Peng J, Triche TJ, Knutsen T, et al: Cytogenetic characterization of selected small round cell tumors of childhood. Cancer Genet Cytogenet *21:*185–208, 1986.

Whipple RR, Unsell RS: Treatment of painful neuromas. Orthop Clin North Am *19:*175–185, 1988.

White W, Shiu MH, Rosenblum MK, et al: Cellular schwannoma: A clinicopathological study of 57 patients and 58 tumors. Cancer *66:*1266–1275, 1990.

Wick MR, Swanson PE, Scheithauer W, Manivel JC: Malignant peripheral nerve sheath tumor: An immunohistochemical study of 62 cases. Am J Clin Pathol *87:*425–433, 1987.

Williams GD, Hoffman S, Schwarts IS: Malignant transformation in a plexiform neurofibroma of the median nerve. J Hand Surg *9A:*583–587, 1984.

Wood MB: Intraneural hemangioma: Report of a case. Plast Reconstr Surg *65:*74–76, 1980.

Woodruff JM: The pathology and treatment of peripheral nerve tumors and tumor-like conditions. CA Cancer J Clin *43:*290–308, 1993.

Woodruff JM, Godwin TA, Erlandson RA, et al: Cellular schwannoma: A variety of schwannoma sometimes mistaken for a malignant tumor. Am J Surg *5:*733–744, 1981.

Woodruff JM, Marshall ML, Godwin TA, et al: Plexiform (multinodular) schwannoma: A tumor simulating the plexiform neurofibroma. Am J Surg Pathol *7:*691–697, 1983.

Yousem SA, Colby TV, Urich H: Malignant epithelioid schwannoma arising in a benign schwannoma: A case report. *55:*2799–2803, 1985.

Yseudian P, Premalatha S, Thambiah AS: Palmar melanotic macules: A sign of neurofibromatosis. Int J Dermatol *23:*468, 1984.

Zorab P, Edwards H: Spinal deformity in neurofibromatosis. Lancet *2:*823, 1972.

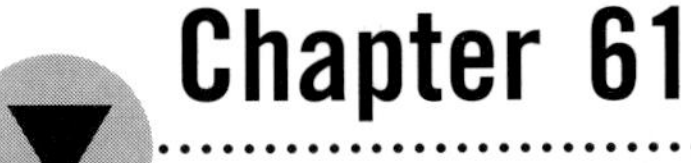

Chapter 61

• Carl Damian Enna

The Management of Leprous Neuritis

The management of leprous neuritis requires knowledge of the pathogenesis of the infection, the pathology of neural involvement, and the timing for instituting methods of prevention and treatment.

Three factors are related to the pathology: (1) the host response to the invasion of *Mycobacterium leprae,* the causative organism; (2) the sensitization and damage to the nerves by autoantigens; and (3) anatomical and physiological factors that predispose peripheral nerves to trauma or provide a temperature-related environment that is optimal for the growth of *M. leprae.*

The primary objectives of treatment are to halt the disease activity to prevent the loss of sensation and the development of deformity and to provide an environment in which the organisms do not grow. The sine qua non of treatment is specific antileprosy drug therapy to control, inactivate, and cure the disease. Certain anatomical and physiological features can contribute to failure in the management of leprous neuritis.

PATHOGENESIS AND HISTOPATHOLOGY

Leprosy (Hansen's disease) is caused by *M. leprae,* an acid-fast staining bacillus. A subclinical disease may be present for several years before it is diagnosed. The development of paralysis early in the course of the disease may be reversible after administering specific antileprosy drug therapy (Fig. 61–1). Numerous organisms are usually disseminated throughout the nerve as a result of an inadequate cell-mediated immune response. A localized fusiform enlargement may exist at potential sites of entrapment (Fig. 61–2). Generalized edema that exists during the early process of the disease is of short duration because it either subsides or progresses with the development of intraneural fibrosis.

In paucibacillary (tuberculoid) leprosy, the pathology involving peripheral nerves consists of a granulomatous caseation necrosis that destroys both the fasciculi and organisms. The involvement may be focal, affecting multiple sites, or more extensive, involving the entire cross section of the nerve, whereby it is transected to produce a total paralysis (Fig. 61–3).

The disease begins as an ascending centripetal infection affecting the peripheral nerves. The *M. leprae* initially infect fine sensory nerves and progress to involve larger nerve trunks possessing mixed sensory and motor fibers. The bacilli infect the Schwann cells, confined initially within the endoneurium. They spread along the length of the nerve before the perineurium is penetrated at any point where it

produces localization of the disease. Patients with multibacillary (lepromatous) leprosy react differently than patients with paucibacillary (tuberculoid) leprosy. The organisms survive apparently in symbiosis and grow freely throughout the entire length of the nerve. Although the nerve becomes thickened, paralysis is deferred until late when the axons are destroyed by extensive intraneural fibrosis (Fig. 61–4).

LOCALIZED SITES OF PREDILECTION

The common peripheral nerves affected and their sites of predilection to develop localized enlargements are as follows, in order of their frequent occurrence.

1. The ulnar nerve is the most frequent mixed nerve affected at the medial aspect of the elbow proximal to the cubital tunnel (Fig. 61–5). It is subsequently encountered at or proximal to the pisohamate tunnel (Enna, 1974).

2. The median nerve is commonly involved proximal to the carpal tunnel (Fig. 61–6). It is less often affected in the region of the elbow. Involvement in leprosy is never isolated. It is usually associated with involvement of the ulnar nerve and rarely with the radial nerve.

3. The common peroneal nerve is affected at the lateral aspect of the knee as it winds around the neck of the fibula.

4. The tibial nerve is usually affected at the medial aspect of the ankle proximal to the tarsal tunnel. The terminal plantar branches, however, are liable to be entrapped at the

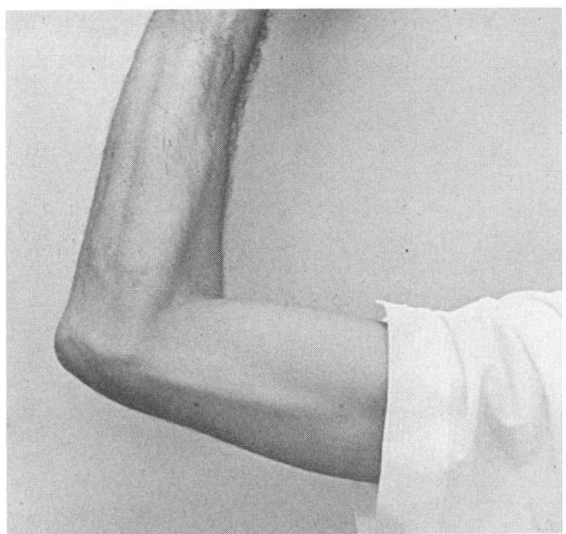

FIGURE 61–1. Asymptomatic enlarged ulnar nerve in patient with multibacillary disease, discovered on examination of patient contact.

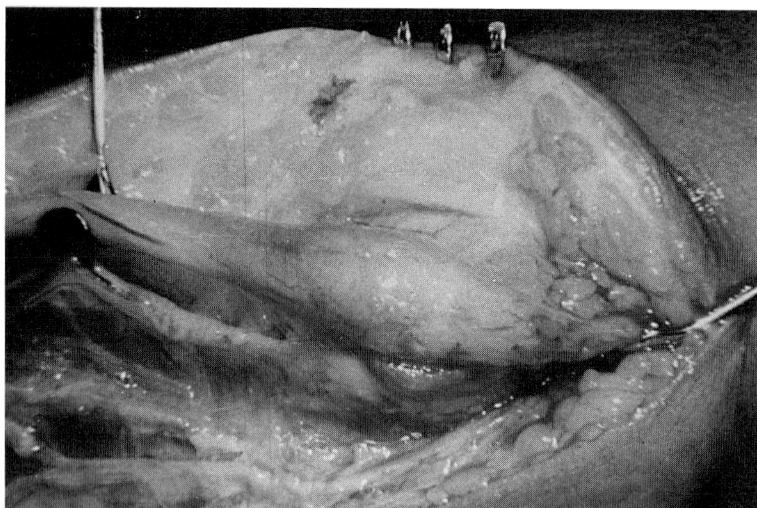

FIGURE 61–2. Localized fusiform enlargement of ulnar nerve in a patient with lepromatous leprosy.

portis pedis, through which they pass into the plantar aspect of the foot.

5. The zygomatic branch of the facial nerve lies superficial as it passes over the zygomatic arch, where it is subject to compression (Antia, 1974). It innervates the orbicularis oculi muscle, the paralysis of which when associated with loss of corneal sensation is the common cause of blindness in leprosy (Karat, 1974).

6. The radial nerve is the least affected peripheral nerve in leprosy. Infrequent involvement is attributed to the nerve assuming a position deep within muscles, where the environment is warm and lends protection from external forces. It is usually involved at the elbow, where it bifurcates proximally to the arcade of Frohse.

Certain features of the sites of predilection contribute to aggravation of the diseased nerve locally. Their superficial subcutaneous position makes them liable to injury from extrinsic sources. It also provides a favorable temperature for the growth of *M. leprae* (Shepard, 1975). The proximity

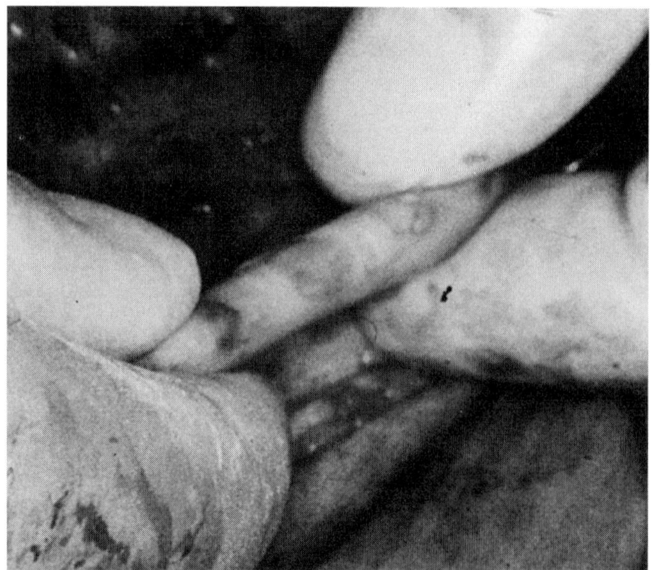

FIGURE 61–3. Focal deposits of caseation necrosis in a patient with tuberculoid leprosy.

of the nerve to bone and joints makes them vulnerable to injury from compression against unyielding bone or to the stretch incidental to movement of joints (Pandey, 1974). Grooves, tunnels, fibrous bands, and anomalous structures are associated with entrapment of peripheral nerves. Associated with increased intraneural tension, producing ischemia of the nerve, they become increasingly vulnerable to the cumulative effects of repetitive actions that occur with movements.

PREVENTION OF LEPROUS DEFORMITIES

Deformity is the main obstacle in the total rehabilitation of patients with leprosy. The various complications are preventable if adequate treatment directed to the disease is undertaken early. Once deformity has developed, it may be corrected by methods used for similar deformities resulting from other causes (Riordan, 1960). Although restitution is adequate, it is never absolutely complete. Residual minor degrees of deformity continue to contribute disability. This is well illustrated by surgical correction of deformities of the feet. Supplemental care is required, such as providing appropriate footwear fabricated to fit the foot. This consists of adjusting the external contour of the shoe as well as molding the insole to distribute weightbearing forces evenly to the plantar surface. Although one is prompted to institute prophylactic measures that prevent leprous neuritis and its deformities, this is unnecessary because effective drug therapy to control the disease is now available.

MEDICAL TREATMENT OF LEPROUS NEURITIS

Whatever medication or surgery is planned for leprous neuritis, specific drug therapy (diaminodiphenylsulfone [DDS]) must be given concomitantly to control the disease. The immediate treatment for acute leprous neuritis initially consisted of steroids. The value of prednisolone as an anti-inflammatory agent that diminishes nerve edema and controls the hyperactive cell mediated immune response of hypersensitivity is well recognized. Prednisone is usually effective, with minimal side effects. Unsuccessful or incom-

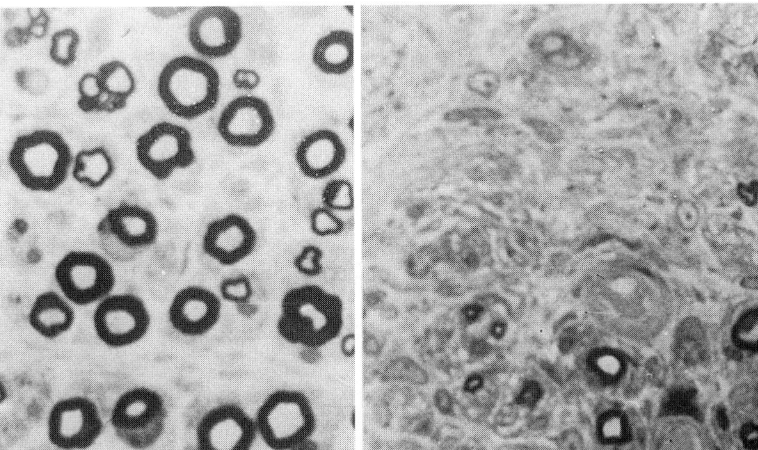

FIGURE 61–4. Microscopic cross section of the nerve. Normal nerve with intact axons, compared with nerve destroyed by extensive fibrosis in patient with lepromatous leprosy.

plete recovery may occur with delayed or inadequate treatment. Therapy is started with 60 mg/day of prednisone, which is gradually decreased over a period of 2 weeks. The patient's response is immediate, with fever and neuritis pain and tenderness subsiding within 24 to 48 hours. The dosage of 60 mg is continued for an additional 2 or 3 days, after which it is decreased every other day if symptoms do not recur.

The treatment is not as simple in patients with chronic disease of several years' duration. Although they improve with such treatment, the reaction tends to recur when attempting to discontinue the steroids. A maintenance dosage is necessary until the steroids can be withdrawn without recurrence of symptoms, which may take more than a year (Joplin and Cochrane, 1957). The prolonged administration of steroids causes serious side effects, including osteoporosis of the spine, producing multiple compression fractures. To avoid the side effects, steroids have been replaced by thalidomide or clofazimine. The dosage of either drug is 100 to 200 mg daily. The drug is given with the steroids until its effectiveness is evident and the steroids may be discontinued. Clofazimine is slower acting than thalidomide; therefore, before prednisone is discontinued, clofazimine is administered for a slightly longer period than thalidomide

(Karat and Karat, 1973; Pfaltzgraff, 1972). Thalidomide is teratogenic and should not be given to women of childbearing age unless they are protected against pregnancy (Sabin, 1974). Clofazimine stains the skin and conjunctiva a reddish brown discoloration.

Intraneural Injections

Steroids, hyaluronidase, and tolazoline have been injected into the nerve to relieve acute leprous neuritis (Antia, 1974; Joplin and Cochrane, 1957; Ramanujan, 1964; Sepaha and Sharma, 1964; Tio, 1966). Pain is relieved after the injection of 12.5 to 25 mg of hydrocortisone acetate. Repeated injections given at weekly intervals may be required to obtain complete relief. Other drugs are given to supplement steroids to enhance their effect.

The intraneural injection of steroids is not without harmful effects. Injection directly into the nerve may increase the intraneural pressure that produces ischemia and further damages the nerve. Rarely, the procedure may result in an iatrogenic abscess. Because relief from leprous neuritis is

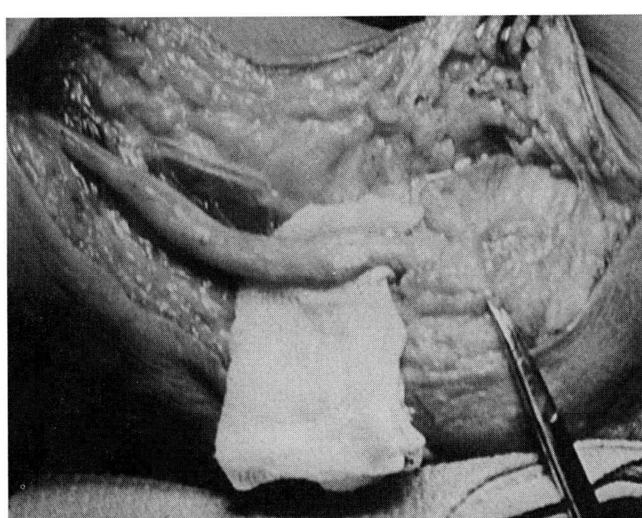

FIGURE 61–5. Chronic ulnar neuritis showing abrupt narrowing before the nerve enters the cubital tunnel.

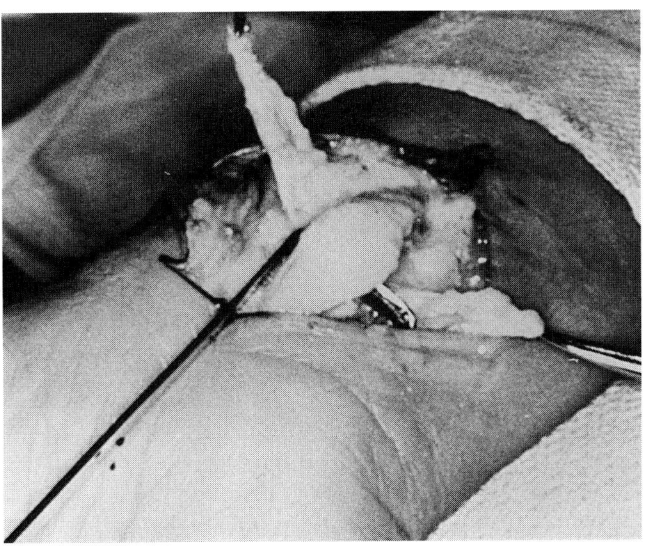

FIGURE 61–6. Localized swelling of median nerve proximal to entering the carpal tunnel. Process due to chronic leprous neuritis.

obtainable from appropriate medical therapy, the intraneural injection of steroids is reserved for chronic leprous neuritis in patients with advanced deformities in whom additional damage to the nerve is unlikely or inconsequential.

Role of Physical Therapy

Dry anesthetic skin is a common problem of sensory impairment that requires care. Educating the patient about the seriousness of the problem, the potential dangers of failing to care for himself or herself, and how the problem may be avoided are essential for motivating the patient to participate in his or her own preservation.

The painful extremity is splinted in optimal functional position for 4 to 6 weeks, or longer if necessary. Although several methods of therapy were used at the U.S.P.H.S. Hospital (National Leprosarium), Carville, Louisiana, for acute leprous neuritis, including diathermy, microthermy, ultrasound, and hot paraffin baths, none were of benefit.*

To combat anesthetic dry skin syndrome, the extremity is soaked in warm water, and an emollient is applied to the wet surface. The method retains water to maximize hydration. Daily inspections of the hands, feet, and stockings for wet spots can reveal otherwise unrecognized wounds. To maintain noninjured feet, inspection of footwear every 6 months can determine whether repair or substitution of a different kind of footwear is needed.

Passive and active exercises are performed regularly to maintain mobility of the joints. The patient's employment is reviewed to ascertain the nature of work and whether repetitive actions are involved, the accumulative actions of which may be harmful. The objective is to enable the patient to undertake a gainful occupation within the limitations of his or her disabilities without risk of injury.*

SURGICAL PROCEDURES

There are two methods of surgery for leprous neuritis and related problems: external and internal neurolysis. The objectives are primarily to release the nerve by freeing it from inflammatory adhesions and to relieve the nerve of caseation deposits and liquified abscesses. The course of the nerve is altered to prevent replacing it in its original bed and to provide a warm environment that is adverse to the growth of *M. leprae.* In accomplishing these objectives, anatomical features that predispose the nerve to injury are corrected.

The indications for the methods of neurolysis and the extent that each procedure is carried out remain controversial, because of the varying degrees of pathology encountered and the different experiences and opinions among the several physicians performing the surgery (Carayon and Giraudeau, 1976; Enna and Jacobson, 1974; McLeod et al, 1975; Pandey and Singh, 1974; Riordan, 1960; Vaidyanathan and Vaidyanathan, 1968). Our indications established at Carville for performing neurolysis are (1) failure to relieve acute pain after 48 to 72 hours of specific anti-inflammatory treatment; (2) the development of progressive signs of denervation in spite of apparent control of the disease with specific

medical therapy; (3) the persistence of a tender localized swelling; and (4) recurrent episodes of neuritis that interferes with a normal life (Enna, 1974; Enna et al, 1974; Enna and Brand, 1970; Enna et al, 1970).

External Neurolysis

This method mobilizes and frees the nerve from its bed. It is rarely recommended as the sole procedure returning it to its original bed (Vaidyanathan and Vaidyanathan, 1968). It is usually done as the first of multiple steps coping with the problems encountered during the operation. The most frequent nerve and involved site is the ulnar nerve at the elbow. In this situation, transposition of the nerve or medial epicondylectomy is done (Enna, 1974; King and Morgan, 1950). Other extrinsic causes may be responsible for compression of an adjacent nerve (Fig. 61–7) (Basombrio and Malbran, 1941; Enna and Calloway, 1964; Harrison and Nurick, 1970).

Perineurolyses is seldom adequate because of the usual involvement of the endoneurium. A single or multiple incision splitting the sheath longitudinally may be performed to decompress the nerve. Best results are obtained with release of adhesions, decompression of an edematous involvement, evacuation of abscess, and removal of caseous deposits (Fig. 61–8). Care is taken during release of the sheath from underlying funiculi to avoid injury to the small intraneural arteries.

Epineurectomy (decapsulation) consists of stripping segments of thickened epineurium (Gramberg, 1955). Difficulty is encountered due to parafascicular scarring and fibrosis. The procedure is reserved for relieving cicatricial constrictions caused by previous surgery and for those in whom there is less likelihood that unexpected damage will be inflicted. The procedure is considered technically dangerous and therefore is rarely done.

Transposition of the Ulnar Nerve

This procedure was advocated by Riordan (1960) at Carville and is applied to neurolysis of the ulnar nerve involved

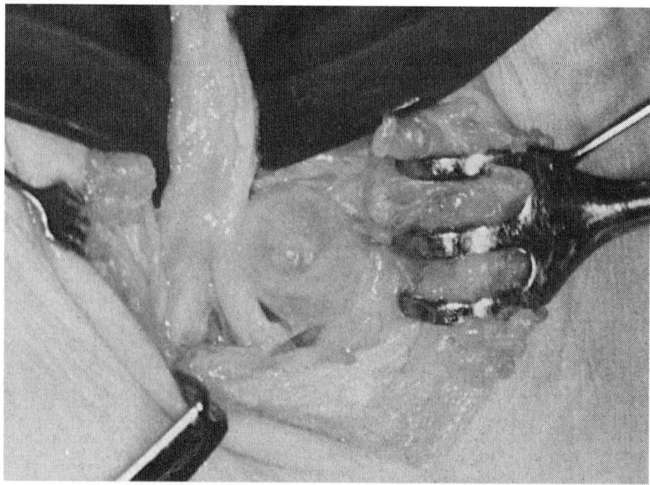

FIGURE 61–7. Tendon sheath ganglion compressing the nerve at the level prior to entering the tarsal tunnel.

---

*Shipley D: Personal communication, 1964.

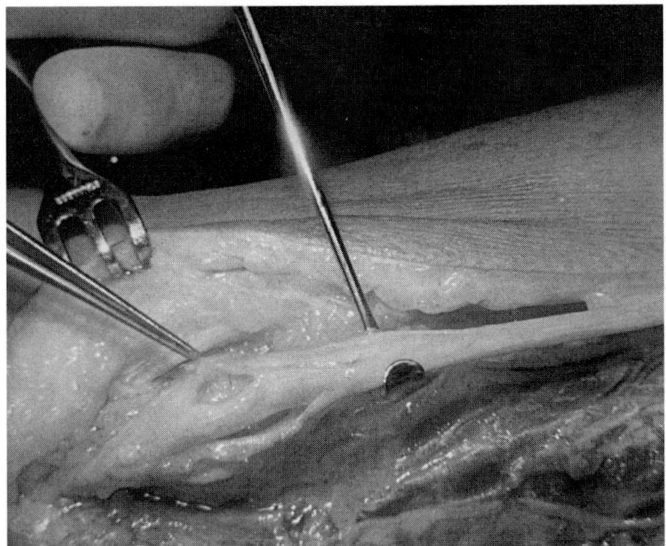

FIGURE 61–8. Evacuated liquified abscess cavity in patient with lepromatous leprosy.

Internal Neurolysis

This method requires incisions into the perineurium that in some instances extend to isolate fasciculi. A simple incision into the epineurium is inadequate for patients with chronic leprous neuritis. Carayon has recommended endoneurial dissection that isolates fasciculi (Carayon and Huet, 1974). The procedure is considered dangerous, with a high risk of injury to the nerve, because of the difficulty in isolating fasciculi that interweave and crisscross in a field of excessive fibrosis (Sunderland, 1973). The procedure is recommended only when the nerve has an irremediable lesion. The interfascicular splitting is carried out concentrically, sparing the margins of the mesoneurium. Limits are imposed on endoneurolysis by the complex branching of the nerve. Extensive neurolysis is recommended by Carayon only to eradicate antigenic foci when the nerve is already irreparably damaged. It has not been determined that there are benefits that will alter the course of the disease.

Partial Neurectomy

Localized caseous abscesses are removed by scooping them out with a blunt instrument, whereas liquified abscesses are evacuated by a simple incision. A fasciculus of nerve may be incised as a biopsy without significant augmentation of clinical manifestations. Excision of a fasciculus may be preceded by determining that the segment is electrically inactive. Biopsy specimens are preferably obtained from sensory nerves or of fasciculi affected with leprous disease, depending on the purpose of the procedure. The sural nerve is used for biopsy to determine disease activity when it is found to be inactive by skin biopsy (Enna et al, 1970). Biopsy incisions are always closed primarily, or a sinus will develop postoperatively that requires secondary excision. Segmental excision of a localized enlargement of a totally destroyed nerve is rarely indicated for relief of pain in patients with chronic leprous neuritis who possess multiple advanced deformities.

at the elbow. It avoids replacing the nerve in its original bed, which is the site of inflammatory reaction, and places it in a warm environment that is unfavorable to *M. leprae*. It obviates the problem of apparent redundancy by placing the nerve along the median nerve between the biceps and brachialis muscles, avoiding the stretching and compression that occurs with flexion of the elbow.

The proper performance of certain steps of the procedure is essential for a successful operation, as listed below.

1. Technical errors are encountered when surgical exposure is limited. (Exposure must be adequate. The incision extends from the upper arm distally into the proximal forearm. This is facilitated because the ulnar nerve does not innervate any muscle in the arm.

2. Increased mobilization is obtained distally by sacrificing the articular branch to the elbow joint and dissecting the nerve as it enters the flexor carpi ulnaris muscle. Extensive mobilization is necessary to permit a gradual alteration in the course of the nerve; otherwise, an abrupt angulation of the nerve may result (Fig. 61–9). The problems of inadequate exposure and mobilization often indicate a secondary procedure (Lluch, 1975). In our experience, extensive mobilization of the nerve is deemed necessary and has not resulted in additional injury to the nerve (Enna and Jacobson, 1974).

3. The medial intermuscular septum is excised to eliminate the ridge of taut fibers that the nerve would cross with transposition.

4. Dissection is carried out between the biceps brachii and brachialis muscles, exposing the median nerve along the side of which the ulnar nerve is placed (Fig. 61–10).

5. A transverse incision is made through the common origin of the forearm flexors just below the epicondyle. Several fibrous septa are divided to create a soft bed into which the nerve is placed.

6. The extremity is immobilized postoperatively with the elbow extended 165 to 180 degrees. Movement is activated early. This measure is undertaken to prevent harmful adaptive shortening of the ulnar nerve.

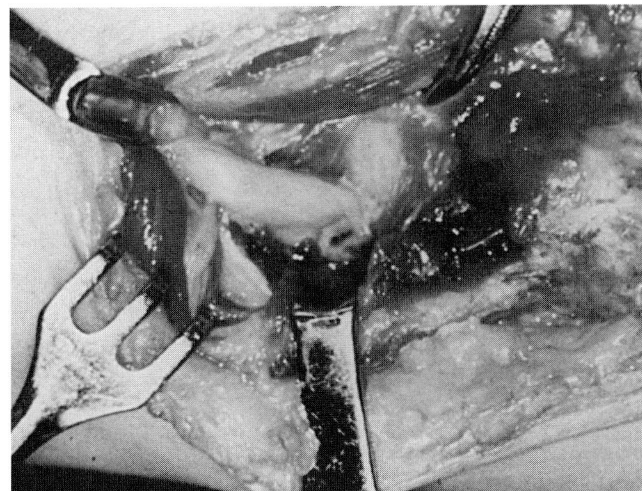

FIGURE 61–9. Acute angulation of ulnar nerve due to inadequate transposition following previous surgery performed with limited exposure.

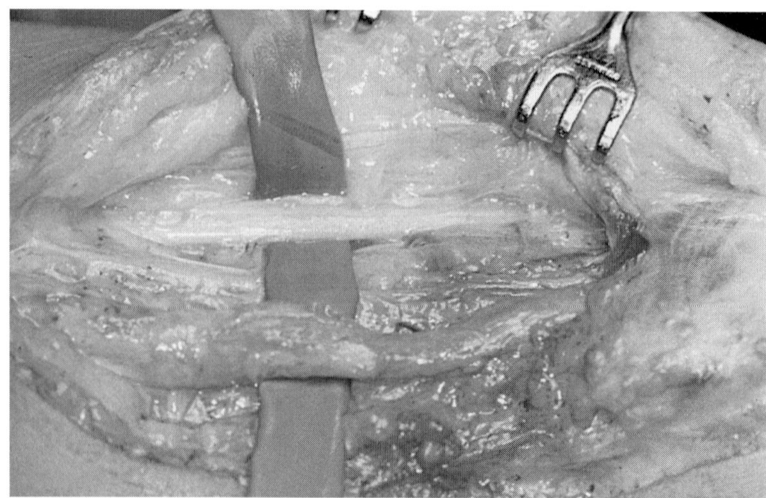

FIGURE 61–10. The ulnar nerve being transposed alongside the median nerve. The normal median nerve exposed between the biceps brachii and brachialis muscles. The ulnar nerve with lepromatous disease being translocated from its original bed.

Nerve Grafting in Leprosy

McLeod and colleagues studied excision and grafting segments of nerves (1975). Although there were no harmful effects from the procedures, benefits were described as limited to recovery of "useful protective sensation" in only a few patients. However, the procedure has not been continued nor recommended in leprosy because it is impossible to determine the length of nerve to replace. Studies by Sunderland demonstrated that *M. leprae* infiltrates the entire length of the nerves, even those that appear unaffected grossly (1973). It is uncertain that the remaining axons will unite to bridge the graft. Nerve grafting for leprosy is in the experimental stage and is considered only for volunteers who wish to participate in research studies.

Complementary Surgical Procedures

Medial Epicondylectomy. This procedure is recommended as an independent method for the treatment of ulnar neuritis in certain patients (Carayon and Giraudeau, 1976; King and Morgan, 1950). It is indicated for the relief of increased pressure on the nerve within the cubital tunnel when the elbow is flexed. The pressure interferes with the neural circulation, contributing to the development of intraneural hypertension besides inflicting injury to the nerve.

The question has been raised as to the indication for epicondylectomy versus neurolysis with transposition of the ulnar nerve. Its application is based on the production of pain associated with the mobility of the nerve as it relates to the cubital tunnel (Gore and Larson, 1966). If the nerve remains within the cubital tunnel when the elbow is flexed and pain is produced, the unyielding epicondyle is considered causative and its removal is recommended. However, when the mobility of a recurrent luxating nerve is subject to friction during movement, it is suggested that greater relief of pain and aggravation of pathology would be obtained by neurolysis and transposition of the nerve. Epicondylectomy has been used as the sole procedure in the treatment of leprous ulnar neuritis; however, it has not been used as a prophylactic procedure.

Reconstructive Procedures. The enigma of leprous neuritis is the production of deformities of the face, hands, and feet. Although the deformities are correctible by reconstructive procedures, best results are obtained when reconstruction is performed during the early phases of the disease when the skin is supple, the soft tissues flexible, and the joints mobile. Reconstructive procedures are more difficult when the deformities are complicated with rigid contractures.*

Basic muscle transfer procedures are used to correct the deformities. The temporalis transfer is performed to activate closure of the eyelids. The muscle segment transferred to the denervated orbicularis oculi muscle is activated by applying the bite mechanism. Gradually, the patient learns to close the eyelids without performing the bite exercise (Karat, 1974; Ranney and Furness, 1974). The tendons transferred from the forearm to correct the claw hand deformity are easily re-educated because they are phasic in their actions with the paralyzed muscles in the hand. Greater difficulty is encountered with transfer of the posterior tibialis muscle used to correct the drop foot deformity because it is aphasic to the paralyzed muscles. Patient concentration and repeated exercises using the muscle transfer generally result in a slightly longer time before the re-education conversion is accomplished.

SUMMARY

The management of leprous neuritis poses a greater challenge in leprosy than does peripheral neuritis from other causes because there is the added problem of first controlling the underlying disease. The treatment depends not only on the severity of its manifestations but also on the timing of administration of the treatment, which generally is not undertaken until the underlying disease is controlled.

Surgical indications for leprous neuritis are established; however, the chosen procedure depends on the nature of the pathology and the extrinsic factors that are contributing to the pathology.

The use of surgery to treat leprous neuritis is decreasing. The incidence of reactions and occurrence of neuritis is

---

*Shipley D: Personal communication, 1964.

becoming less frequent and less intense because most patients respond to appropriate medical and antireactional therapy. Although surgical methods for prophylaxis and definitive treatment are still used, their use remains controversial in view of the absence of long-term controlled studies.

References

Antia NH: Surgery of the nerves. *In* McDowell F, Enna CD (eds): Surgical Rehabilitation in Leprosy. Baltimore, Williams & Wilkins, 1974, p 31.

Basombrio G, Malbran C: Pseudomembranous neuritis of the cubital nerve with osteoarthritis of the elbow. Rev Argent Dermatosif 25:87, 1941.

Carayon A, Giraudeau P: Valeur de la resection de l'epitroclee dans la decompression et le derontement de 87 neurites cubitales Hanseniennes. Med Trop 36:163, 1976.

Carayon AE, Huet R: The value of peripheral neurosurgical procedures in neuritis. *In* McDowell F, Enna CD (eds): Surgical Rehabilitation in Leprosy. Baltimore, Williams & Wilkins, 1974, p 37.

Enna CD: Neurolysis and transposition of the ulnar nerve in leprosy. J Neurosurg 40:734, 1974.

Enna CD, Brand PW: Peripheral nerve abscess in leprosy. Lepr Rev 41:175, 1970.

Enna CD, Berghtholdt HT, Stockwell F: A study of surface and deep temperature along the course of the ulnar nerve in the pisohamate tunnel. Int J Lepr 42:43, 1974.

Enna CD, Calloway JC: Tarsal tunnel syndrome. Case report: Tibial leprous neuritis associated with tendon sheath ganglion. Int J Lepr 32:279, 1964.

Enna CD, Jacobson RR: A clinical assessment of neurolysis for leprous involvement of the ulnar nerve. Int J Lepr 42:162, 1974.

Enna CD, Jacobson RR, Mansfield RE: An evaluation of sural nerve biopsy in leprosy. Int J Lepr 38:278, 1970.

Garrett AS: Hyalaze injection for lepromatous nerve reaction. Lepr Rev 27:61, 1956.

Gore D, Larson S: Medical epicondylectomy for subluxating ulnar nerve. Am J Surg 111:851, 1966.

Gramberg KPCA: Nerve decapsulation in the leprosy patient. Int J Lepr 23:115, 1955.

Harrison MJG, Nurick S: Results of anterior transposition of the ulnar nerve for ulnar neuritis. Br Med J 1:27, 1970.

Joplin WH, Cochrane RG: The place of cortisone and corticotropin in the treatment of certain acute phases in leprosy. Lepr Rev 28:5, 1957.

Karat ABA, Karat S: A controlled clinical trial of clofazamine in the management of acute neurological problems in leprosy. Tenth International Leprosy Congress, Mexico City, Mexico, 1973.

Karat S: Correction of lagopthalmos by temporalis transfer. *In* McDowell F, Enna CD (eds): Surgical Rehabilitation in Leprosy. Baltimore, Williams & Wilkins, 1974, pp 85–94.

King J, Morgan FT: Treatment of traumatic ulnar neuritis by mobilization of nerve at elbow and removal of medial epicondyle. Aust N Z J Surg 20:95, 1950.

Lluch ASL: Ulnar nerve entrapment after anterior transposition at elbow. N Y State J Med 75:75, 1975.

McLeod JG, Hargrave JC, Gye RS, et al: Nerve grafting in leprosy. *Brain* 98:203, 1975.

Pandey S, Singh AK: Treatment of neural involvement in leprosy. Lepr India 46:83, 1974.

Pfaltzgraff RE: The control of neuritis in leprosy with clofazamine. Int J Lepr 40:4, 1972.

Ramanujan K: The use of intraneural corticosteroids in acute leprosy neuritis. Lepr India 36:261, 1964.

Ranney DA, Furness MA: Results of temporalis transfer for lagopthalmos. *In* McDowell F, Enna CD (eds): Surgical Rehabilitation in Leprosy. Baltimore, Williams & Wilkins, 1974.

Riordan DC: The hand in leprosy: A seven year clinical study. J Bone J Surg 42A:661, 1960.

Sepaha GC, Sharma DR: Intraneural cortisone and priscol in the treatment of leprosy. Lepr India 36:264, 1964.

Shepard CC: Temperature optimum for Mycobacterium leprae in mice. J Bact 90:1271, 1975.

Sunderland S: The internal anatomy of nerve trunk in relation to the neural lesions of leprosy: Observations on pathology, symptomatology and treatment. Brain 96:865, 1973.

Tio TH: Neural involvement in leprosy: Treatment with intraneural injection with prednisolone. Lepr Rev 37:93, 1966.

Vaidyanathan EP, Vaidyanathan ST: Treatment of ulnar neuritis and early ulnar paralysis. Lepr Review 39:217, 1968.

Chapter 62

• Roger E. Salisbury
• A. Griswold Bevin
• Aldo A. Lombardo

Burn-Induced Peripheral Nerve Injury

One does not often relate nerve damage to burn injury, because the latter is virtually considered a purely cutaneous injury. However, the extremely variable etiology of a burn—thermal, chemical, electrical, or radiation—may result in transient neuropraxia or large masses of necrotic tissue, requiring extirpation of muscle groups and peripheral nerves, perhaps even amputation. The purpose of this chapter is to define the peripheral nerve problems that result from burn injury and how to manage them.

THERMAL INJURY

Fire, hot liquids, or steam heat may result in peripheral nerve loss on the basis of (1) ischemic necrosis secondary to undiagnosed vascular insufficiency after a circumferential burn or (2) the heat itself causing coagulation necrosis. For instance, the patient in Figure 62–1 had a circumferential deep second- and third-degree burn to his arm and was transferred to our burn unit 4 days after the injury. Diminished radial sensation, wrist drop (Fig. 62–1C), and a questionable pulse at the wrist made it obvious that a compression injury had occurred. Exploration and debridement revealed deep second- and third-degree burns of the skin; in addition, ischemic necrosis of the whole extensor muscle compartment, including the radial nerve, was noted.

The mechanism of this injury is the tourniquet effect of the nondistensible, unyielding burn eschar. As edema increases after loss of capillary integrity, first venous and then arterial flow is compromised, resulting in a vascular emergency. The ensuing gangrene, Volkmann's contracture of the upper extremities, or compartment syndrome of the lower extremity can be prevented by the physician who considers this compression phenomenon when seeing a patient with a circumferential burn.

Progressive tissue ischemia is mediated through both systemic and local factors. Volume depletion, myocardial depression, and a constrictive burn eschar lead to reduced perfusion of injured tissues (Moncrief, 1970). Local factors such as leukocyte margination, platelet microthrombi, erythrocyte agglutination, direct and chemically mediated vasoconstriction, and interstitial edema add to the vascular insult (Robson, 1984).

To counteract local factors, Raine has shown that cooling the burned extremity within 30 minutes of injury will help maintain homeostasis between prostaglandin E_2 and prostaglandin $F_{2\alpha}$, thereby preventing the formation of thromboxane-mediated vasoconstriction and minimizing leukocyte margination (Raine et al, 1980).

Immediate elevation of the extremity with frequent exercise of the hand or foot may help reduce edema (Moylan, 1971) and maintain circulation. If the palpating finger cannot detect a pulse, however, the examiner should use a Doppler flowmeter, which is extremely sensitive in detecting blood flow. If no arterial flow is heard, the physician must first be sure intravenous resuscitation is adequate. If urine output is 30 to 50 ml per hour in an adult or proportionately less in a child, the state of hydration is satisfactory, and an absent pulse means vascular compression secondary to burn edema. The treatment is immediate escharotomy. This procedure can be done at the bedside or in the emergency room with a scalpel or electrocautery. The incision should be made laterally (Fig. 62–2) or medially through the constrictive eschar into unburned soft tissue along the entire length of the wound (Pruitt, 1968). After waiting several minutes to allow resumption of blood flow, Doppler evaluation is repeated. If arterial flow is still unsatisfactory, escharotomy along the other side should be performed. The extremity should be elevated to aid venous flow. No anatomical structures are at risk during escharotomy as long as the incisions are lateral

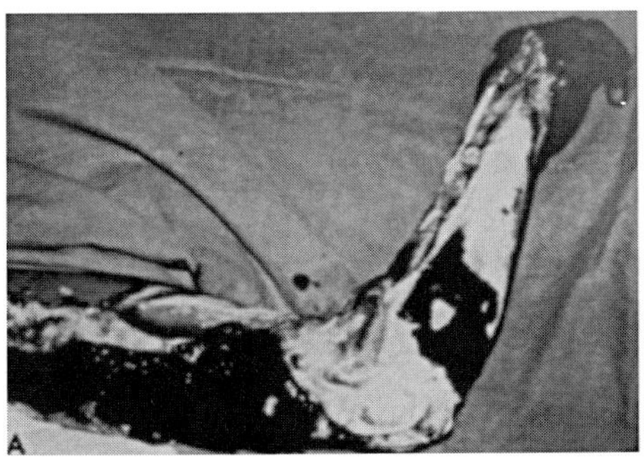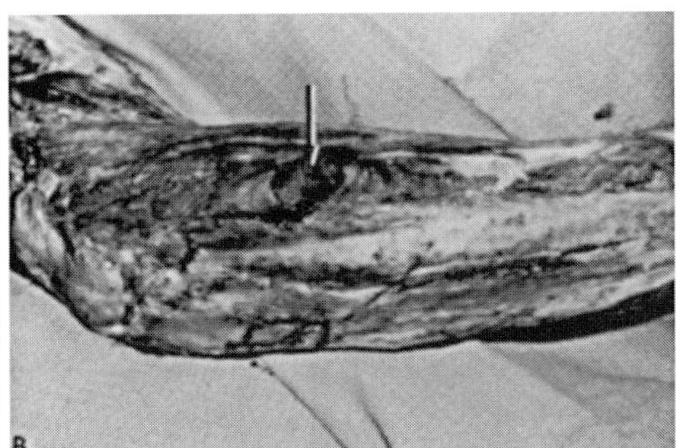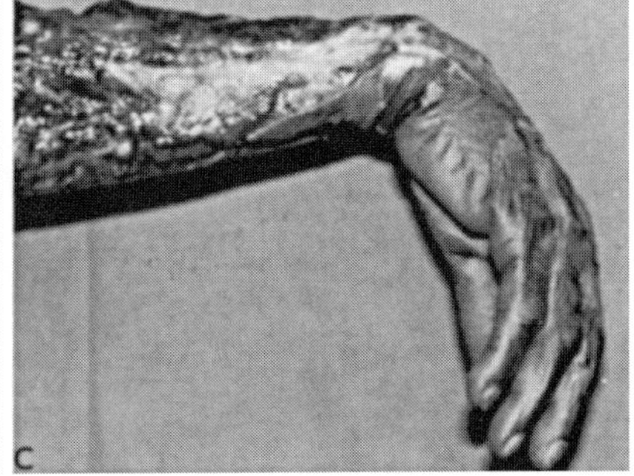

FIGURE 62–1. Delayed escharotomy (A) following a circumferential burn of the upper extremity revealed ischemic muscle; excision of necrotic extensor muscle (B) and radial nerve secondary to ischemia resulted in wrist drop (C).

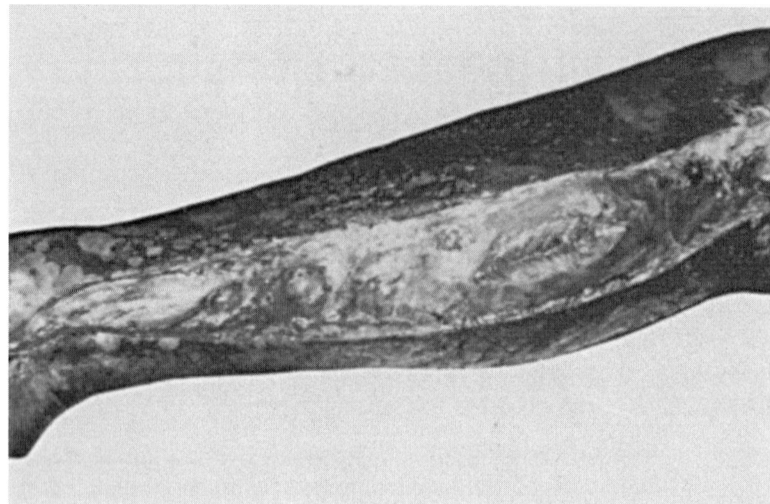

FIGURE 62–2. A single lateral incision may be enough to fully decompress the edematous extremity. In electrical burns, fasciotomy may be one way to decompress injured muscle.

and extend only into the interface between eschar and viable tissue. Care should be taken at the elbow, however, to make the incision anterior to the medial epicondyle, because the ulnar nerve lies in the soft tissue posteriorly.

An alternative to surgical escharotomy is the application of an enzymatic debriding agent. Travase (Flint Laboratories, Deerfield, Ill.) is an inactivated enzyme of *Bacillus subtilis* in sutilains ointment. This agent causes proteolytic degradation of the constrictive eschar while preserving viable dermis below (Krizek et al, 1975). The ointment is applied in a wet dressing for 1 hour and circulation is reassessed. If circulation has not been restored, the procedure is repeated. Disadvantages of this technique include localized pain and potential early burn wound sepsis.

Direct thermal injury of peripheral nerves is not rare and is seen in patients who have prolonged contact with hot objects, such as occurs with an unconscious driver after an automobile or motorcycle wreck or with an inebriate who is found in a burning house. The ulnar nerve at the elbow, the radial nerve at the distal humerus, and the peroneal nerve at the fibular head are especially at risk. The ulnar nerve, shielded by the flexor carpi ulnaris in the arm, and the median nerve (except at the wrist, where it is superficial) are well protected. Although diagnosis of sensory loss may be masked because of generalized pain of the deep burn, motor loss is obvious.

Treatment of the nerve lesion must frequently be delayed until the burn wound has healed (Falcone, 1990). Necrotic tissue, high bacterial counts, and the necessity for early and aggressive splinting and exercise make immediate nerve reconstruction impractical. The physician may elect to treat the wounds with topical antibiotics, daily debridement of eschar, and, finally, skin grafting of the granulating wound. In selected cases, the physician may opt for the more rapid course of primary excision and grafting of the burn wound. A good wound bed for further nerve reconstruction is not characteristic of either treatment.

Recent studies by Lister, Godina (1986), Xue-mei and Krizek have shown advantages to early aggressive wound debridement and coverage with free tissue transfer. This technique minimizes the need for prolonged local wound care, thereby limiting additional tissue destruction by desiccation and infection. Furthermore, it provides excellent soft tissue coverage for future nerve repair and grafting. Unquestionably, early tendon transfer in appropriate cases is the best solution for the patient with a motor deformity, because it is the fastest and least expensive path to rehabilitation (Bevin, 1976).

CHEMICAL INJURY

Chemical burns infrequently cause nerve injury because the wounds rarely cause more than full-thickness skin loss (Belliapoa et al, 1990; Bentivegna et al, 1990). Although different acids and alkalis have specific neutralizing agents (Table 62–1) (Salisbury et al, 1976a, b), valuable tissue is often lost until this can be obtained. Copious lavage with water remains the single best immediate treatment for most chemical burns. Phosphorus burns are an exception in that the particles continue to destroy tissue and may erode below the skin and into soft tissue (Curreri et al, 1970). White phosphorus ignites on exposure to air and is oxidized to phosphorus pentoxide. The reaction is more destructive than the inorganic acids of phosphorus formed, and the particles should be removed immediately in the operating room to prevent further damage. The particles may be located easily if they are smoking or by washing the wounds with 1% copper sulfate, which colors the particles black and permits easy identification. It is emphasized that the copper wash is not definitive treatment but removal of the particles is. The phosphorus creates ulcers of variable thickness that, if debrided and treated with topical antibiotics so no infection results, usually heal by contraction.

ELECTRICAL INJURY

Electrical burns cause the highest incidence of nerve injury. In a review of electrical burns of the upper extremity in 84 patients (Salisbury, 1976), there were 17 different peripheral nerve lesions. Electricity follows the path of least resistance and thus often destroys neurovascular bundles.

▼ **TABLE 62–1**
Treatment of Chemical Injury

Agent	Reaction	Treatment
Acids		
Chromic acid	Coagulates protein, ulcerates	Dilute, wash with dilute Na hyposulfite
Hydrochloric acid	Coagulation necrosis, shallow ulcers	Avoid lavage; neutralize with soda lime with soap magnesium
Formic acid	Firm, hard eschar, may be absorbed hepato/nephrotoxicity	Water lavage, may be absorbed, cover with oil Demulcent
Oxalic acid	Chalk white ulcer; acts by binding calcium	Lavage, administer calcium salt solution, intravenous calcium
Hydrofluoric acid	Deep ulceration, tough coagulum	Boric acid wash, hyamine 0.2% soaks. $NaHCO_3$ wash. Local Ca gluconate infilt. Local mag. sulfate paste
Sulfuric acid	Dessicant, hard eschar, ulcer	Avoid water lavage. Neutralize mag. oxide, lime water soap. Demulcents
Alkali		
Potassium hydroxide	Liquefaction necrosis; soft, gelatinous, friable tissue destruction	Dilute with lavage Neutralize with weak acid (0.5-5% acetic acid) Demulcents
Sodium hydroxide		
Ammonium hydroxide		
Lithium hydroxide		
Barium hydroxide		
Calcium hydroxide		
Sodium	In presence of water, forms NaOH and heat, may explode	Cover with oil, avoid water, excise
Other Chemical Injuries		
Na-hypochlorite	Coagulates protein	Sodium thiosulfate 1%; internally give milk, egg whites, starch, pasta, lavage
Potassium permanganate	Coagulates; thick brown-purple eschar	Lavage egg whites
Phenol	Rapid absorption, white coagulum, denatures protein	Dilute with water or cover with oil. Avoid alcohol. Demulcents
Phosphorus		Lavage with $KMnO_4$ or $Cu(SO_4)$ or cover with oil
DMSO	Hemolysis, edema, ischemia; histamine and serotonin release	Water lavage
Mustard gas	Severe blistering, partial-thickness necrosis	Wash with oil, kerosene, or gasoline, then soap and water
Cantharides	Severe partial-thickness skin loss	Water lavage, avoid oils
Tear gas		Lavage with water; neutralize with sodium bicarbonate

The resulting defect is frequently permanent and is secondary to irreversible destruction of the nerve.

The main physiological mechanism for tissue destruction in electrical injury remains unclear (Zachary, 1990). We know that there are at least two mechanisms responsible for cellular damage in electrical injury. The most widely accepted theory, joule heating, pertains to the thermal energy released when current passes through tissues that offer resistance. A second theory involves cell membrane lysis by electroporation (Lee and Kolodney, 1987a). In this process, pores or defects are created in the cell membrane by strong electrical fields. Lee and Kolodney have postulated that these electrical forces contribute to rhabdomyolysis. Large cells such as muscle and nerve cells experience greater transmembrane potentials and are thus more vulnerable to electroporation. Clinically, electroporation occurs before joule heating becomes significant; however, these processes have been shown to act synergistically (Zimmerman, 1986).

After the initial evaluation and adequate resuscitation, patients with high-voltage electrical injuries should be taken to the operating room. Escharotomy as well as fasciotomy should be performed. Nerves should be released from any areas of potential compression, including Guyon's canal, the carpal tunnel, and the cubital tunnel. A cornerstone of early management is the excision of nonviable musculature so that gas gangrene does not occur. The debridement of necrotic muscle should be complete. There has been a reluctance to radically debride and resurface severe thermal and electrical burns early because of the concept of progressive tissue necrosis. This idea has led surgeons to perform repetitive conservative debridement in an attempt to conserve all viable tissue. Recent evidence disputes the concept of progressive necrosis; what we are in fact experiencing is failure of early recognition of nonviable tissue (Zelt, 1988). Chick and colleagues (1992) recommend radical debridement of nonviable or questionably viable tissue. Muscle should be excised if it fails to contract when pinched with forceps. Nerves, tendons, and bones are left in place with minimal debridement if they are structurally intact, regardless of their appearance of questionable viability (Chick et al, 1992). Gottlieb and Krizek have supported the concept that marginally viable tissue can often be salvaged if covered immediately with vascularized tissue (Gottlieb and Krizek, 1990). Chick and colleagues have demonstrated this fact with early free flap coverage of electrical and thermal burns. This has been further supported by separate studies from Silverberg (1986) and Shen. In those cases not amenable to early debridement and coverage, the physician must protect viable structures from dessication. Biological dressings such as cadaver autograft or porcine xenograft would preserve viability by simulating a normal internal environment (Levine and Salisbury, 1976). The wound should then be covered and irrigated with a suspension of silver sulfadiazine and changed daily until the patient is stable to undergo surgery or the wound is free of all necrotic debris and ready for split-thickness grafting.

Although the techniques of nerve repair are beyond the scope of this chapter, preparation of the patient for reconstruction is of paramount importance. As in other extremity problems, all viable tissue should be conserved initially. The importance of this principle cannot be overemphasized. In an isolated finger injury, it is often stated that it is better to amputate if any three tissues are permanently damaged (skin, nerve, tendon, or bone); however, it is more common to have involvement of multiple fingers after electrical trauma. Thus, only obviously nonviable fingers should be amputated before the plan for the patient's reconstruction is formulated. For example, the patient in Figure 62–3 lost the index finger of both hands and sustained damage to other fingers as well. The radial neurovascular bundle of the long finger was coagulated, and thus effective pinch was impaired. The proximal interphalangeal (PIP) joint of the long finger was exposed, and the radial collateral ligament was destroyed. The flexor tendons, however, were perfect, as was the ulnar digital bundle. The obvious necrotic tissue was debrided, the PIP joint pinned in moderate flexion, and the bone rongeured to stimulate granulation tissue. The finger was then grafted to achieve wound closure. Moderate radial instability of the PIP joint caused overriding of the ring finger, which could be corrected by arthrodesis, and neurovascular island transfer from the ulnar to the radial portion of the long finger should render satisfactory pinch sensation. If the outcome of these combined procedures is unsuccessful, amputation is still a viable alternative. The point is that the reconstructive surgeon and the patient have a choice that would not exist if early, thoughtless debridement had been performed.

Nerve reconstruction may have to be delayed if the patient's general condition presents other priorities (Robson, 1992). For example, the current entered through the feet and exited through the arm and posterior skull of the patient shown in Figure 62–4. Debridement revealed a nonviable ulnar nerve at the condyle for a distance of 6.0 cm. Early nerve grafting would have been desirable except that bilateral above-knee amputations were followed by deep vein phlebitis. The patient presently requires crutches to walk, and upper extremity surgery would confine him to a bed or wheelchair, making him a prime risk for recurrent phlebitis or pulmonary embolus. Thus, nerve reconstruction will be delayed until the patient is independent from crutches.

RADIATION INJURY

The increased use of various radiation sources in the twentieth century led initially to a large number of injuries, frequently with hand and peripheral nerve involvement. X-rays and radium were common agents. As newer and more powerful radiation sources were developed, they were treated with extreme care, and only a few peripheral injuries in the arms, hands, and feet have been recorded. The damage from these various sources is similar, varying only in degree, and may be acute, subacute, chronic, or degenerative, leading to malignant change.

Biologically, electromagnetic radiations follow the laws of quantum mechanics, and injury is the result of application of excessive energy into the normal biochemical systems of cells. Longer wavelength sources, such as electricity, various radio waves, and light, promote an excitation phenomenon in which the high energy causes electrons to become displaced from inner to outer orbits in the affected atoms. Shorter wavelength radiation sources, such as certain x-rays and atomic particles, deliver their energy by causing atoms to yield an electron, forming negative-positive ion pairs, or by striking an atom and producing various secondary radiations. The result of these mechanisms may be disorganization of nucleic acid synthesis, prevention of enzyme synthesis, interference with normal cellular division, or alterations in membrane permeability. These injuries may be reversible or irreversible, causing temporary or permanent changes in cellular function.

Low-energy radiations, such as alpha and beta particles, ultraviolet light, and others, injure the superficial tissue most, the injurious effect being reduced as depth increases. Sources with high energy, such as supervoltage x-ray and products of linear type accelerators, cause secondary radiant energy primarily; thus, the deeper tissues are most affected. This principle, which allows relative sparing of the normal, nonsuperficial tissues, forms the basis for modern solid tumor therapy.

Tissues that have a high metabolic rate or that have high reproductive capability are vulnerable to radiation injury because of the effects on mitosis. The extremities, particularly the hand, are relatively radiosensitive because of their small size and variety of functional tissue, including sweat and sebaceous glands, fingernails, marrow-containing bones, blood vessels, nerves, and soft tissues. Generally, hemopoietic tissues are most sensitive to higher energy radiation, followed by the skin and the appendages, the vascular endothelium, connective tissue, fat, bone, and nerve and muscle.

Nerve tissue is rather resistant to radiant injury because of its depth, its low cellular reproduction, and its metabolic characteristics. Nerve injury may ensue, however, because

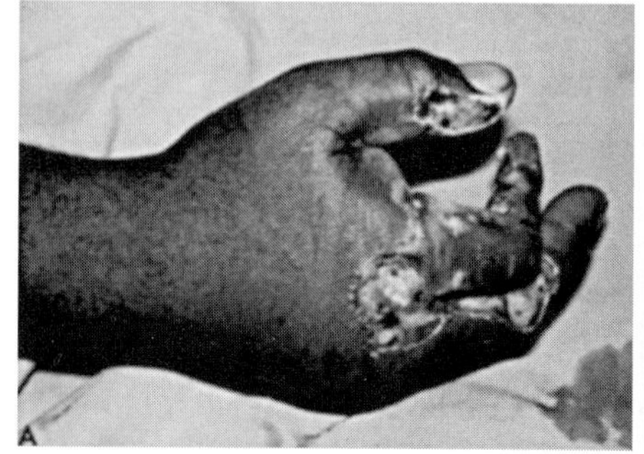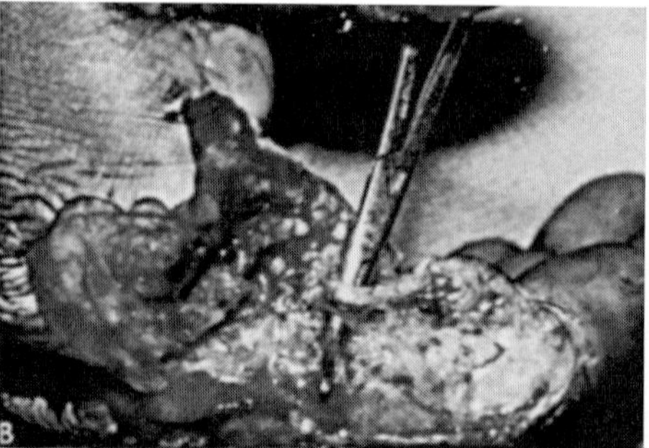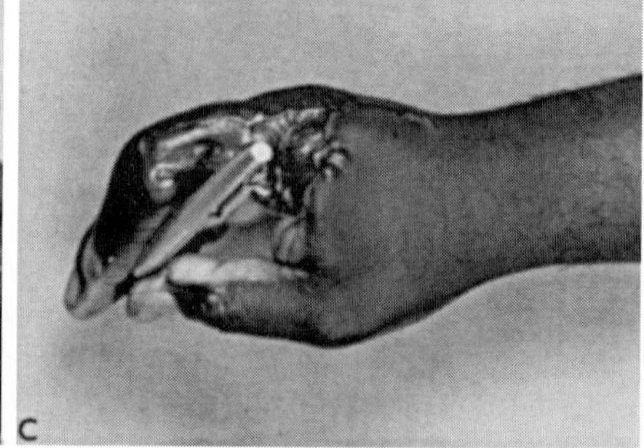

FIGURE 62–3. An obviously devitalized index finger *(A)* and the radial aspect of the long finger were debrided, including the neurovascular bundle *(B)*. Satisfactory range of motion and strength could be complemented with a neurovascular island transfer to provide sensation.

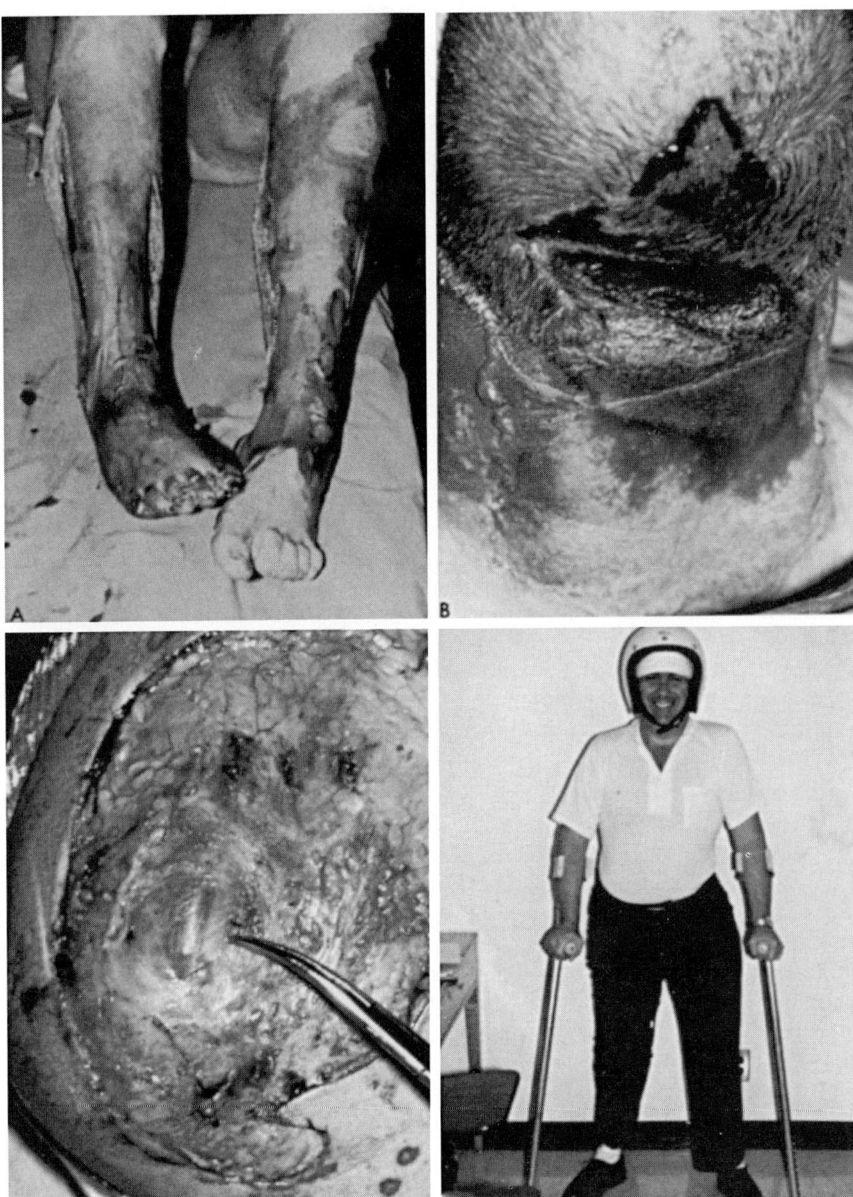

FIGURE 62–4. In the severe electrical burn, nerve repair may not be the top priority. Entrance *(A)* and exit *(B)* wounds resulted in bilateral AK amputations and the loss of posterior skull in addition to the ulnar nerve *(C)*. Mobilizing the patient on crutches to help prevent recurrent deep vein thrombosis took precedence over early ulnar neurorrhaphy *(D)*.

of proximity to affected structures that yield or transmit heat. As a corollary, in denervated tissues the vulnerability to radiant energy increases because of cellular turnover, changes in vascularity, and diminution of sensory feedback to the patient. Although infrared, visible, and ultraviolet light sources cause no unique injuries to nerve tissue itself, they often cause pronounced injury to denervated tissues. In the hands and feet, for example, peripheral nerve injury frequently results in soft tissue changes. Because of exposure and impaired sensory feedback, protective measures and patient education are necessary to prevent further injury by these energy sources. Very high energy sources such as x-ray and gamma radiation may injure some or all of the tissues in the extremities, and because of the smaller bulk of these structures, considerable damage may ensue.

The partially damaged cells constitute the major clinical radiation problem, because lethally injured tissues become necrotic and separate. In damaged tissue, the initial hyper-emia or early response to injury gradually diminishes after 3 to 4 weeks, caused by arteritis characterized by thrombosis and obstructive endothelial proliferation with unyielding diminution of fibroplasia and capillary proliferation. Even if such wounds eventually epithelialize, they are atrophic, ischemic, and vulnerable to further mechanical injuries. These cellular injuries are similar to those caused by certain biochemical materials, often called radiomimetic drugs.

In acute radiation injury, there may only be erythema of the skin and little or no pain, with resolution in a few days, although skin pigment changes may remain for months to years. In more severe acute exposure, necrosis and painful ulceration may ensue. Usually the ulcerations do not heal, and the likelihood of malignant degeneration in the skin and soft tissues is high over a long period of time. There have been two reported instances (Andrews, 1968) of fatal massive exposure to the hands alone, with destruction of all soft tissues, but usually massive exposure is to the whole body.

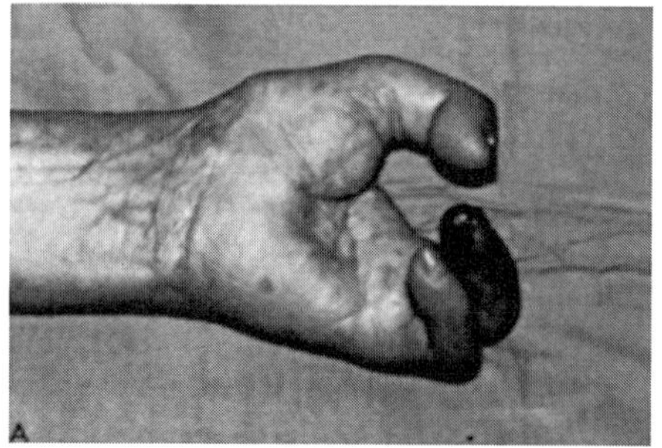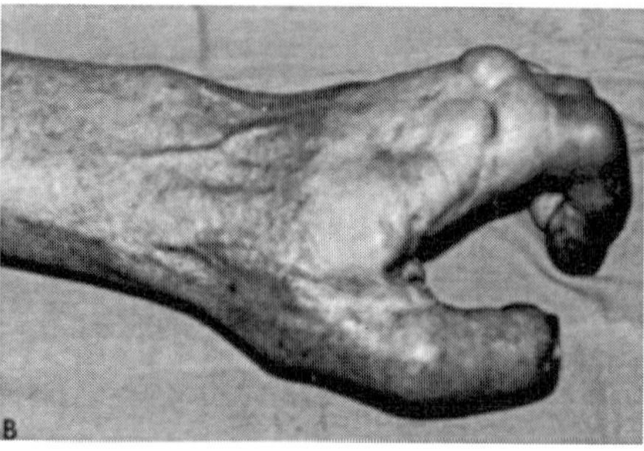

FIGURE 62–5. Chronic repetitive debridement, grafting, and serial amputations *(A and B)* reveal why nerve reconstruction is rarely a viable option following radiation injury.

Malignant degeneration commonly occurs in the skin, but no instances of selective malignant peripheral nerve degeneration have been noted.

In the treatment of radiation-injured tissues, the general principles of wound management (including excision), dressing, resurfacing, antisepsis, and revascularization must be practiced. Radiation wounds of significance rarely heal primarily and are subject to chronic degenerative changes. Wound excision, usually with wide margins to include all injured tissue, is indicated. Debridement is often required, because inadequate excision with graft coverage alone commonly fails. The injury is more diffuse than may be appreciated initially, and a recipient area must be appropriately vascularized or have the capability for vascularity before definitive wound coverage can be successful. Adherent dressings for debridement and, later, nonadherent dressings are applicable. Split- or full-thickness graft coverage may be useful at this point if evidence of vascularization of the recipient site is present. Often, however, local cutaneous skin flaps may be required for coverage. Direct or free muscle flaps with skin graft coverage or myocutaneous flaps may be required in the extensive injury, especially where neovascularization or reinnervation of a particular area is critical. When muscle flap coverage has failed, the omentum with immediate or delayed meshed skin grafting may be lifesaving. The omentum can protect exposed vital structures and bring excellent blood supply to the area. Pain caused by wound ischemia and neuritis or exposure of nerve tissue is associated with the more serious injuries. Because denervation from any cause renders the tissue more vulnerable to injury at all times, consideration must be given to reinnervation techniques such as neurorrhaphy, nerve grafts, or neurovascular pedicle methods. If these are not possible, protection of the reconstructed but denervated area by means of patient education and mechanical assistance, as in paraplegic patients, is required.

The handling of hazardous radioactive materials is becoming increasingly common; therefore, caution and prevention must be stressed. Patients with implanted materials, such as sutures or prosthetic devices, must be educated to avoid energy sources such as diathermy. If basic wound management principles are practiced by responsible clinicians, chronic changes, such as malignant degeneration, and susceptibility to further injury in the patient with previously denervated extremities may be reduced. Clinicians must be increasingly aware of the causes, time factors involved, and certain special characteristics of radiation injuries so that prevention and efficient rehabilitation can be achieved.

CONCLUSION

Under the general topic of burn injury reside several different etiologic agents. Although total nerve destruction may be immediate, as in some electrical injuries, and thus defy intervention, many patients may be helped. An awareness of the specific biological result rendered by radiation, electricity, fire, or chemical agent, a concern for early diagnosis, and a knowledge of specific treatments may lessen the incidence of crippling deformities (Fig. 62–5).

References

Andrews JR: Radiobiology of Human Cancer Radiotherapy. Philadelphia, WB Saunders, 1968.

Belliapoa PP, McCabe SJ: The burned hand. Hand Clin 6:313–324, 1990.

Bentivegna PE, Deane LM: Chemical burns of the upper extremities. Hand Clin 6:233–259, 1990.

Bevin AG: Early tendon transfer for radial nerve transection. Hand 8:134, 1976.

Chick LR, Lister GD, Sowder L: Early free-flap coverage of electrical and thermal burns. Plast Reconstr Surg 89:1013–1021, 1992.

Curreri WP, Morris M Jr, Pruitt BA Jr: The treatment of chemical burns: Specialized diagnostic, therapeutic, and prognostic considerations. J Trauma 10:634, 1970.

Falcone PA, Edstrom LE: Decision making in the acute thermal hand burn: An algorithm for treatment. Hand Clin 6:233–238, 1990.

Godina M: Early microsurgical reconstruction of complex trauma of the extremities. Plast Reconstr Surg 78:285–292, 1986.

Gottlieb CJ, Saunders J, Krizek TJ: Surgical technique for salvage of electrically damaged tissue. In Lu RC, Cravallios EG, Burke JF: Electrical Trauma: Pathophysiology and Clinical Management. Cambridge, Cambridge University Press, 1990.

Harrison DH, Parkhouse DM: Experience with upper extremity burns: The Mount Vernon experience. Hand Clin 6:191–209, 1990.

Krizek TJ, Robson MC, Koss N, et al: Emergency nonsurgical escharotomy in the burned extremity. Orthop Rev 4:53, 1975.

Lee PC, Kolodney MS: Electrical injury mechanisms: Dynamics of the thermal reconstruction. Plast Reconstr Surg 80:633–671, 1987a.

Lee PC, Kolodney MS: Electrical injury mechanisms: Electrical breakdown of cell membranes. Plast Reconstr Surg 80:672–681, 1987b.

Levine NS, Salisbury PE: Early removal of eschar in upper extremity burns. *In* Salisbury RE, Pruitt BA Jr: Burns of the Upper Extremities. Philadelphia, W. B. Saunders, 1976.

Moncrief JA, Pruitt BA Jr: Electrical injuries. Postgrad Med 48:189, 1970.

Moylan JA, Inge WW, Pruitt BA Jr: Circulatory changes following circumferential extremity burns evaluated by ultrasound flow meter. J Trauma 11:763, 1971.

Pruitt BA Jr, Moncrief JA: Escharotomy in early burn care. Arch Surg 96:502, 1968.

Raine TJ, Heggers JP, Robson MC, London MD, Johns L: Cooling the burn wound to maintain microcirculation. J Trauma 21:394–397, 1980.

Report of the U.N. Scientific Committee on the Effects of Atomic Radiation. Supplement No. 16 (A/5216). Washington, DC, GPO.

Robson MC, Murphy RC, Heggers JP: A new explanation for the progressive tissue loss in electrical injuries. Plast Reconstr Surg *73*:431–437, 1984.

Robson MC, Smith DJ Jr, Vanderzee AJ, Robert L: Making the burned hand functional. Clin Plast Surg *19*:663–671, 1992.

Salisbury RE, Hunt JL, Warden GD, Pruitt BA Jr: Management of chemical burns of the upper extremities. Plast Reconstr Surg *51*:648, 1976a.

Salisbury RE, Pruitt BA Jr: Burns of the Upper Extremity. Philadelphia, W. B. Saunders, 1976b.

Silverberg B, Banis JC Jr, Verdi GD, Acland RD: Microvascular reconstruction after electrical and deep thermal injury. J Trauma *26*:128–134, 1986.

Xue-mei W, Jia-ning W, Yung-hua S, et al: Early vascular grafting to prevent upper extremity necrosis after chemical burns. Burns *8*:303–312, 1981.

Zachary LM, Lee RC, Gottlieb LJ: Evolving chemical and scientific concepts of upper extremity electrical trauma. Hand Clin *6*:243–252, 1990.

Zelt R, Daniel RK, Ballard PA, Brisete T, Heroux P: High voltage electrical injuries: Chronic wound evolution. Plast Reconstr Surg *82*:1027–1030, 1988.

Zimmerman V: Electrical breakdown: Electropermeabilization and electrofusion. Rev Physiol Biochem Pharmacol *105*:176, 1986.

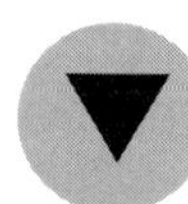

Chapter 63

• Robert E. Lins
• Michael J. Botte
• Richard H. Gelberman

Management of the Cerebral Palsy Patient

Cerebral palsy comprises a group of nonprogressive, nonhereditary central nervous system disorders characterized by varying degrees of paralysis, spasticity, coordination deficits, sensibility loss, and cognitive impairment (Bleck, 1987; Gelberman, 1991; Hoffer and Koffman, 1992). Mental retardation, learning defects, emotional or behavioral problems, and seizure disorders are common when patients have associated organic brain damage. The encephalopathy accompanying cerebral palsy is static. The neurological deficits seen are congenital, arising from a brain insult that occurred in the prenatal, perinatal, or postnatal periods. It is the most common neuromuscular disorder in the pediatric population in the United States, with reported prevalence rates of approximately 2.0 per 1000. This includes about 25,000 new domestic patients per year and 450,000 currently existing with cerebral palsy (Bleck, 1987; Gelberman, 1991; Goldner, 1979; Hoffer and Koffman, 1992; Pharoah, 1981; Tachdijian, 1972).

Classifications have been used to characterize clinical presentations, including those based on topographical involvement (monoplegia, hemiplegia, diplegia, quadriplegia); muscle tone (isotonic, hypertonic, hypotonic); severity (mild, moderate, severe); etiology (prenatal, natal, postnatal); and physiological motor status (spastic, dyskinetic, ataxic). A frequently used classification system based on the nature of observed motor deficit includes the four commonly described types: (1) spasticity (tetraplegia, paraplegia, hemiplegia, monoplegia); (2) extrapyramidal (athetosis, dystonia, tremor, choreiform, rigidity); (3) atonic (atonic diplegia, ataxia); and (4) mixed (Barnett and Einhorn, 1972; Barolat-Ramona and Davis, 1980; Bleck, 1987; Gelberman, 1991; Gschwind and Tonkin, 1992; Nelson et al, 1969; Omer and Capen, 1976).

The spastic type of cerebral palsy is the most common (65%), followed by the dyskinetic (25%), mixed (10%), and atonic (3%). Spastic hemiplegia accounts for about one third of children with cerebral palsy, and homonymous hemianopsia and a hemisensory deficit on the ipsilateral hemiplegic side are often present (O'Reilly and Walentynowicz, 1981). Twenty-five percent of patients have seizures, 20% have significant visual problems, and many, especially those with athetosis, have auditory deficits. Although the patients' intellectual abilities depend largely on the location and confinement of cerebral involvement to one hemisphere, significant learning problems are common. At least half are considered mentally retarded (Nelson et al, 1969; Paine, 1965).

The diagnosis is often delayed during the first year. Key diagnostic criteria include delay of developmental milestones, fluctuations of muscle tone, asymmetry of motor development, persistence of primitive reflexes, delays in balance or coordination, and pattern type of motion (simultaneous firing of muscle groups) as opposed to selective muscle control. The perinatal tonic neck reflexes are usually gone by 6 months, and sitting balance will usually have been achieved. By 1 year, a refined pinch with opposition of the thumb to the index finger normally develops. Handedness is present by 18 to 24 months; however, earlier hand preference may be a sign of poor function in the opposite hand. Selective muscle control, which can be graded in strength, should be developed by about age 5 years.

Recent studies that investigate the pathophysiological mechanisms underlying spasticity have provided information relevant to the planning of upper extremity operative treatment (Barolat-Ramona and Davis, 1980; Burman, 1938; Jensen and Alderman, 1963; Milner-Brown and Penn, 1979; Steindler, 1900). Electromyography (EMG) evaluation from agonist and antagonist muscles during passive involuntary alternating flexion and extension movements have demonstrated a diversity of patterns, varying from complete asynchrony with a reciprocal relationship between flexion and extension, to complete synchronous activity. In patients with mild cerebral palsy, normal alternating activity between flexors and extensors may be preserved during voluntary movements, whereas in those with moderate deficits, there are normal patterns with low-frequency movements and abnormal reciprocal patterns as movements become more rapid. In severely affected patients, continual muscle firing is noted, with both fast and slow attempts at alternating flexion and extension.

Based on this greater incidence of continuous muscle firing as the degree of involvement increases, a paradox in the treatment and outcomes of patients with spastic cerebral palsy has been observed. Operative management is more predictable and useful in patients with mild to moderate spasticity than in those with severe spasticity or those with motion disorders (ataxia, athetosis, dyskinesia, and tremors) (Hoffer, 1982; Hoffer et al, 1979). A conservative attitude toward operative reconstruction of the upper limb has resulted (especially in those with the most severe involvement), which is reflected by the observation that only 3% to 5% of patients are considered candidates for upper-extremity surgery (Boyes, 1962; Carroll and Craig, 1951; Keats, 1965, 1970; Koman et al, 1990; Matev, 1970; McCarroll, 1949; Phelps, 1951; Sherk, 1977; Stelling and Meyer, 1959).

PATIENT EVALUATION AND DIAGNOSTIC PROCEDURES

Patients classified as having spastic, athetoid, ataxic, or the mixed form of cerebral palsy can be subdivided by degree of involvement and assigned as mild, moderate, or severe. Classification requires sequential motor examination, reflex testing, elicitation of stretch reflexes, and evaluation for clonus. Predicted effectiveness of operative management is based on the patient's extent of involvement, age, limb sensibility, muscle strength and control, intelligence, and motivation (Bleck, 1987; Gelberman, 1991; Goldner, 1955, 1961, 1966, 1971a, 1971b, 1974, 1975, 1979, 1983; Goldner and Ferlic, 1966; Green, 1988). Parents, nurses, teachers, physical and occupational therapists, and hand therapists provide information concerning the patient's functional level, ability to perform daily activities, level of motivation, and capacity for learning.

Motivation is usually considered a higher priority than intelligence in selecting patients for operative management. An IQ of 70 to 80 has been suggested as necessary to obtain a patient's cooperation and assistance postoperatively. However, an IQ as low as 50 can still be compatible with a successful outcome (Goldner, 1961, 1971a, 1971b; Green, 1988). A patient's IQ should therefore be obtained and considered along with other factors in preoperative planning (Bleck, 1987; Green and Banks, 1962). In addition, in the evaluation of intelligence or motivation, the effect of the patient's motor impairment on intelligence testing should be appreciated (Gelberman, 1991; Samilson, 1966; Samilson and Morris, 1964).

MOTOR EVALUATION

Motor strength evaluation is difficult to assess in the patient with spastic paralysis and cognitive deficits. Sequential examination is often required. Additional evaluation and observation is obtained by the team occupational therapist, physical therapist, or hand therapist. Gross functional assessment is obtained by having the patient grasp and release objects, transfer them from hand to hand, and attempt to place or stack objects. Release may be difficult because of spasticity of digital flexors or weakness of digital extensors, and grasp may be difficult because of weak wrist extensors, thumb-in-palm deformity, weak extrinsic digital flexors, or a combination of these. Evidence for lateralization of hand function and assessment of the patient's ability to bring the hand across the mid-line should also be assessed.

Individual muscle strength testing is obtained by serial examination, performed days or weeks apart. Because the patient's perceived strength may change slightly throughout the day as a result of fatigue or muscle irritability, evaluation at different times of the day, especially after periods of splinting or stretching, may provide a more accurate overall assessment. The American Orthopaedic Association criteria for muscle strength is used, grading muscles from 0 to 5. Findings are recorded in a similar manner as that used for evaluation of peripheral nerve injury (Goldner, 1971).

Determination of the severity of spasticity and relative amounts of fixed soft tissue contracture is a prerequisite for planning upper-extremity operative management (Gelberman, 1991; Jensen and Alderman, 1963; Keenan et al, 1987). These determinations are accomplished by examination of the hand with palpation and passive stretch of individual muscles. Assessment of the digits in different positions, use of the tenodesis effect for extrinsic muscle contracture

evaluation, and examination using the intrinsic tightness tests are helpful. Peripheral lidocaine nerve blocks, an important diagnostic adjuvant, will effectively eliminate contributions of spastic muscles to deformity, but will not affect components of fixed soft tissue contracture.

Flexion deformities of the wrist, metacarpophalangeal (MP) joints, and interphalangeal (IP) joints result from spasticity of the extrinsic flexors and intrinsic muscles of the hand. To determine deformities caused by the extrinsic muscles, the wrist is passively extended and flexed. Deformities caused by the extrinsic muscles (flexor digitorum superficialis and flexor digitorum profundus) will increase with passive wrist extension (caused by the tenodesis effect of the tight extrinsic flexors) and decrease with passive wrist flexion. If the extrinsic muscles are involved, relative contributions of the flexor digitorum superficialis versus the flexor digitorum profundus can be evaluated by individual digital testing. With the wrist and MP joints placed in neutral position, resistance to extension of the proximal IP joints will indicate spasticity or contracture of the flexor digitorum superficialis (Bleck, 1987; Hoffer, 1982; Page, 1923). With the wrist and MP joints held in the same position, the proximal IP joint is brought into extension. Subsequent resistance to extension of the distal IP joint demonstrates spasticity or contracture of the flexor digitorum profundus muscle (Gelberman, 1991). Once it has been determined that the extrinsic muscles are causing the deformity, spasticity versus myostatic contracture is determined by median nerve and ulnar nerve block proximal to the elbow. Fixed myostatic contractures will remain after the nerve block, whereas deformity caused by spasticity will be eliminated. The median nerve block is accomplished by locating the nerve at the elbow 2 cm proximal and 2 cm lateral to the medial epicondyle. The brachial artery is palpated, and 10 cc of 1% lidocaine without epinephrine is injected 5 mm medial to the brachial artery. To block the ulnar nerve, the nerve is identified in the fossa between the olecranon and medial epicondyle. Three cc of 1% lidocaine without epinephrine is injected in the vicinity of the nerve.

If digital deformities do not change with passive wrist motion, the deformities are caused by either intrinsic muscle spasticity or fixed myostatic or joint contracture. Lidocaine nerve blocks to the ulnar and median nerve will help delineate deformities caused by intrinsic spasticity versus fixed soft tissue contracture and will further help separate contributions from the extrinsic muscles. If spasticity of the intrinsic muscles is present (with flexion deformities at the MP joints), a lidocaine ulnar nerve block at the wrist will decrease the deformity by eliminating tension from the interosseous muscles and from the two ulnar lumbrical muscles. A subsequent median nerve block at the wrist will further decrease any remaining deformity of the index and long-finger MP joints, because of spasticity of the two radial lumbrical muscles. Fixed soft tissue contracture will not change after lidocaine nerve blocks.

If digital and wrist flexor deformities are present, evaluation of the strength and control of digital and wrist extensors is aided by proximal median nerve block (to eliminate tension of the flexors). The wrist, finger, and thumb extensors are re-examined after nerve block. Passive and active motion of the hand and wrist are compared before and after nerve block. This information helps determine the necessity for digital or wrist flexor lengthening or soft tissue contracture release before, or in lieu of, tendon transfer (Goldner, 1971a; Goldner and Ferlic, 1966; Keenan, 1987).

Evaluation of the thumb is complex and requires careful assessment of intrinsic and extrinsic muscles. Spasticity of the thumb intrinsics and extrinsic flexor leads to thumb adduction and flexion, resulting in the thumb-in-palm deformity (Botte et al, 1989; Gelberman, 1991; Hoffer et al, 1983; Matev, 1963, 1970). Muscles contributing to this deformity include the flexor pollicis longus, flexor pollicis brevis, abductor pollicis brevis, opponens pollicis, adductor pollicis, and the first dorsal interosseous (Botte et al, 1989). Acute flexion at the IP joint of the thumb during rest usually indicates involvement of the flexor pollicis longus. This is verified if progressive passive wrist extension causes further flexion of the IP joint while the MP joint is held in neutral. Acute resting flexion of the MP joint usually indicates contributions from the flexor pollicis brevis, abductor pollicis brevis, and adductor pollicis. Spasticity of the abductor pollicis brevis, flexor pollicis brevis, adductor pollicis, and first dorsal interosseous can be further assessed from muscle palpation and web space measurement during passive abduction or palmar flexion of the thumb from the palm. Adduction of the metacarpal against the palm can be caused in part by the opponens pollicis and first dorsal interosseous. A lidocaine median nerve block given at the wrist eliminates spastic contributions from the flexor pollicis brevis, abductor pollicis brevis, and opponens pollicis. An ulnar nerve block at the wrist eliminates contributions from the adductor pollicis and first dorsal interosseous. A subsequent median nerve block given in the arm or proximal forearm will eliminate contribution from the flexor pollicis longus. Remaining deformity will be secondary to fixed ligamentous, myotendinous, or skin contracture.

Fine-motor coordination is evaluated by manual dexterity tests. These include the patient's ability to touch each fingertip to the thumb in rapid succession, to open and close the hand, and to place small objects in proper position or arrangement. Rapid pronation and supination of the forearm is assessed to reveal dysdiadochokinesia, and mirror movements are elicited by having the patient mimic the examiner's hand movements in a variety of simple maneuvers. Abnormal movements are also noted in the opposite resting hand. Although motion errors may be seen in normal children up to age 6 years, they are seen more frequently in children who have hemiplegia (Bleck, 1987).

The elbow and shoulder are examined as to resting position, passive and active range of motion, and manual muscle strength testing. Assessment of individual muscles or muscle groups is made using careful palpation while the elbow or shoulder is passively moved or positioned. Proximal to the elbow, sequential lidocaine nerve blocks to the musculocutaneous nerve and radial nerve help isolate contributions to elbow flexion from the biceps and brachialis, and from the brachioradialis, respectively. Accurate infiltration of lidocaine adjacent to the desired motor nerve is aided by use of a nerve stimulator connected to the hub of the needle used to administer the lidocaine.

Dynamic EMGs are useful for further assessing muscle control, and will help elucidate muscles with continuous activity (spastic), those with little or no activity (paretic or paralytic, respectively), or those with normal or volitional activity (phasic). An EMG is especially useful when physical examination alone cannot adequately determine activity of a deeply situated, hard-to-palpate muscle or when the activity of a muscle is difficult to assess during a specific activity. Standard electromyographic techniques and video analysis are performed while a patient undertakes various activities (Hoffer et al, 1979; Mowery, 1985). In preoperative planning and selection of the optimal muscle for tendon transfer, the EMGs help determine which muscles exhibit similar phasic activity to the ones requiring augmentation. Postoperatively, EMGs can assess activity of a transferred muscle. Studies using EMG evaluation have suggested that muscles that fire continuously before transfer can possibly become phasic postoperatively (Samilson, 1966). Synchronous activity of the flexor carpi ulnaris has been shown to be of special benefit if the muscle is transferred to either the extensor carpi radialis brevis or extensor digitorum communis (Samilson, 1966). Mowery and associates (1985) used electromyography to evaluate muscles of patients before and after tendon transfer, and demonstrated that muscles that were predominantly phasic could be transferred predictably and usually continued to function in phase. However, it was not conclusively determined whether muscles with continuous activity preoperatively could become phasic after transfer. Although the EMGs are a useful adjuvant in the planning of operative procedures in cerebral palsy, they are not consistently essential to decision making. Goldner (1974, 1975) has suggested that individual muscle testing and repeated observation of patient activities, including grasp and release, are more important factors in decision making.

In general, the most effective tendon transfers in cerebral palsy are those using muscles with retained volitional control, have grade 5 strength, and are phasic with the activity for which they are being transferred. Muscles that are out of phase or fire continuously may also be useful; however, they are not as predictable (Gelberman, 1991).

SENSIBILITY EVALUATION

Significant sensibility deficits are present in almost half of patients with cerebral palsy (Tachdijian and Minear, 1958; Van Heest et al, 1993). Approximately 30% of these have defects in stereognosis, 25% with abnormal two-point discrimination, and 10% to 15% have loss of proprioception. As in other neuromuscular disorders, a correlation between functional status and presence of sensory deficits exists in cerebral palsy. A high incidence of sensory loss is present in patients with severely dysfunctional upper extremities (Tachdijian and Minear, 1958).

Assessment of sensibility includes evaluation of stereognosis, two-point discrimination, and proprioception (Goldner, 1971b). Stereognosis is evaluated by having the patient raise one hand over the head with eyes closed. Different objects with varying shapes, sizes, and textures (i.e., metal coins, wooden pegs or pencils, rubber balls) are placed in the patient's hand and the patient's fingers are moved actively or passively over the object's surface. The patient's ability to describe the surface of the object is assessed (Fig. 63–1).

Two-point discrimination is assessed using the tips of a paper clip applied along the longitudinal axis of the digit depressed just to the point of blanching the skin (Moberg,

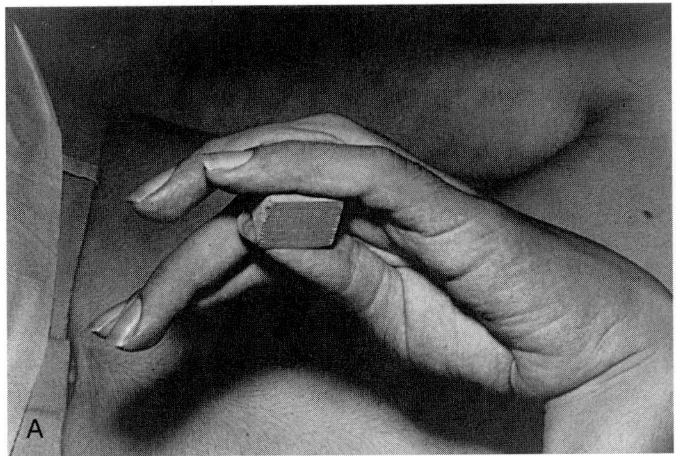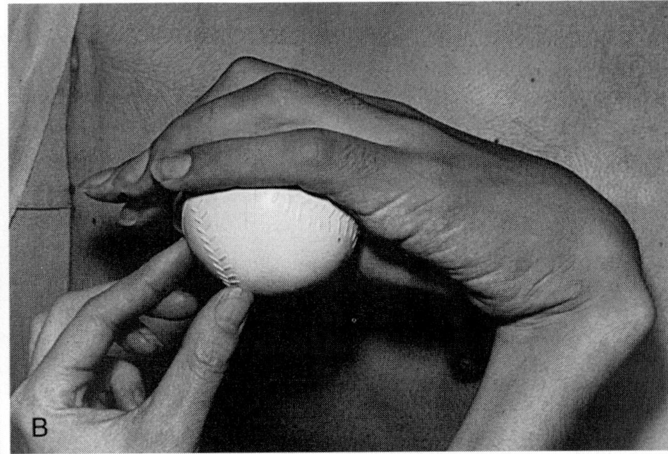

FIGURE 63–1. Stereognosis is assessed by having the patient identify the size, shape, and texture of objects placed in the hand (*A*). If the patient has limited active motion, the object is moved passively in the palm or over the fingers (*B*). (Illustration by Elizabeth Roselius, © 1991. Reprinted with permission from Gelberman RH: Cerebral palsy. *In* Gelberman RH [ed]: Operative Nerve Repair and Reconstruction. Philadelphia, J.B. Lippincott Company, 1991, pp 1455–1475.)

1976). Normal and good values for the median and ulnar nerves are 6 and 10 mm, respectively. Inability to discriminate greater than 15 mm is considered absent two-point discrimination. In the cooperative patient with normal or good two-point discrimination, further assessment can be obtained with monofilament testing.

Proprioception is evaluated by assessment of the patient's ability to correctly identify the position of the passively flexed or extended digit with eyes closed. In addition, the patient is observed for ability to touch the examiner's finger in space followed by touching his or her own nose, or ability to move the hand from the top of the head to the opposite knee and back to the top of the head.

In the very young or cognitively impaired patient, sensibility assessment is difficult. Attempts may be made to have the child differentiate shapes and sizes of objects or toys during play. Of special concern is the detection of the presence of body neglect, denial, or dissociation. Children with denial will lack stereognosis and will not benefit significantly from reconstructive surgery. Denial and athetosis are among the few abnormalities thought to be absolute contraindications to operative treatment (Goldner, 1971b, 1974, 1975).

Limb sensibility provides a reasonable predictor of expected results from operative management, and the results of surgical reconstruction have been shown to correlate closely with stereognosis (Green and Banks, 1962). Green noted that only 2 of 14 patients with improvement after tendon transfer lacked stereognosis. Of 16 patients with marginal improvement, 14 showed significant disturbances in sensibility (Green and Banks, 1962).

AGE CONSIDERATIONS

There are no specific age limitations for reconstructive surgery of the upper limb in cerebral palsy. Adults with long-standing upper limb deformities and young children under the age of 6 years with poorly controlled deformities can often benefit from operative management. In general, however, operative strategies usually follow a temporal sequence, and most surgery is delayed until the age of 4 to 6 years.

In the first few years of life, thumb-in-palm deformities, wrist and digital flexion, and elbow flexion are managed nonoperatively with home therapy programs, which include passive stretching and continuous or intermittent splinting. Patients are evaluated specifically at age 4 for refractory deformities that might benefit from operative treatment.

Although thumb-in-palm deformities may be corrected early and tendon transfers may be performed to provide grasp and release, the optimal age for tendon transfers is usually between 6 and 12 years of age.

In the child with severe pronation deformity of the forearm, posterior subluxation of the head of the radius can occur if correction is delayed; therefore, surgery in these patients is often considered early, before the age of 4 years (Bleck, 1987).

FUNCTIONAL CLASSIFICATION

A functional classification scheme allows comparison of preoperative and postoperative status and provides an objective method of assessing results of operative procedures. A classification scheme has been provided by Mowery and colleagues (1985) based on previous systems devised by Green and Banks (Table 63–1) (Gelberman, 1991; Green, 1942; Green and Banks, 1962; Swanson, 1960; Zancolli, 1979). This classification divides function into four groups: excellent, good, fair, and poor.

An *excellent* rating identifies a patient with functional use of the hand in dressing and eating, effective grasp or release,

▼ **TABLE 63–1**
Functional Classification

Excellent	Good use of hand, effective grasp and release, voluntary control
Good	Helper hand, effective grasp and release, some voluntary control
Fair	Helper hand, no effective use, moderate grasp and release, fair control
Poor	Paperweight, absent grasp and release

Courtesy of Mowery CA, Gelberman RH, Rhoades CE: Upper extremity tendon transfers in cerebral palsy: Electromyographic and functional analysis. J Pediatr Orthop 5:69, 1985. Used by permission.

and excellent control. Dorsiflexion of the wrist is possible to 45 degrees, and full digital extension is possible with the wrist extended 30 degrees or more. The patient can supinate to at least 50 degrees, and there is no ulnar deviation deformity of the wrist.

A *good* rating describes a patient whose hand is used as an aid for dressing and eating. There is effective grasp and release with good control, and active wrist dorsiflexion is possible from 15 degrees to 45 degrees. Digital extension is possible with the wrist dorsiflexed from zero degrees to 30 degrees. Supination of 10 to 50 degrees is possible, and there is minimal ulnar deviation deformity of the wrist.

A *fair* classification indicates a patient whose hand is used as a helper but is not effective in dressing. Grasp and release is possible with fair control when the wrist is at neutral. Active digital extension with the wrist in neutral is possible. Active supination to neutral is possible, and there may be an ulnar deviation deformity of the wrist.

A *poor* rating describes a patient whose hand is used only as a paperweight. Grasp and release are absent and the wrist is fixed in flexion. Digital extension is impossible unless the wrist is held in maximal palmar flexion. Pronation deformity of the forearm and ulnar deviation deformity of the wrist are present.

After surgical reconstruction, patients can be expected to improve at least one functional level. Occasionally, a patient may improve two levels. Operative management is not expected to achieve an excellent functional rating from a patient with a preoperative poor functional level.

GENERAL PRINCIPLES OF MANAGEMENT

Management of the patient with cerebral palsy is optimized with the team approach using the many rehabilitation disciplines for comprehensive assessment and treatment. Coordinated efforts are needed from those in pediatrics, neurology, physical therapy, occupational therapy, hand therapy, psychology, psychiatry, speech therapy, audiology, ophthalmology, sociology, vocational counseling, orthotic/prosthetics, and orthopedic surgery. Management requires evaluation and treatment of the patient as a whole, taking into consideration the medical, functional, and social aspects. Specialized teaching programs, therapy sessions, and operative procedures are coordinated with other disciplines and in accordance with the patient's schooling and family considerations.

Although spasticity in cerebral palsy is static, the deformities and associated problems may change over time. The deformities increase with the growth of the limb, with the development and maturation of the central nervous system, or as a result of chronic muscle imbalance on the immature skeleton. Nonsurgical and surgical treatment may span years, and operative procedures may have to be repeated, especially those involving muscle lengthening or the release of contracted soft tissues. In a patient with functional capabilities, the goals of surgery are to augment or maximize function, usually accomplished using soft tissue lengthening or release, tendon transfer, or joint arthrodesis. In the more severely impaired or minimally functional patient, surgical goals are more limited, directed toward correcting contractures to facilitate hygiene, dressing, and nursing care.

The characteristic upper-limb deformities in spastic hemiplegia consist of shoulder adduction, flexion, and internal

rotation; elbow flexion; forearm pronation; wrist flexion; digital flexion or hyperextension (including swan-neck deformities); and thumb-in-palm deformity (Fig. 63–2). Initial management consists of a comprehensive therapy program that incorporates passive joint mobilization and muscle stretching, static or progressive splinting, and strengthening of antagonist muscles.

Medical therapy for spasticity includes diazepam or dantrolene sodium. These medications can effectively decrease spastic muscle tone, diminish the startle response, relieve anxiety, and help control tremors. However, there are potential side effects of fatigue and somnolence. Possible hepatotoxicity requires periodic liver function testing.

Operative management is usually initiated with release or lengthening of fixed contractures, using muscle origin releases (recession), myotendinous lengthening, or Z-lengthening.* These procedures can effectively improve shoulder adduction internal rotation, elbow flexion, forearm pronation, wrist and digital flexion, and thumb-in-palm deformity. Once fixed contractures have been corrected, tendon transfers to augment function are considered if satisfactory passive motion exits and adequate, expendable donor muscles are available.† Common transfers include those to augment wrist extension (for inadequate grasp), transfers to reinforce digital and thumb extension (for inadequate release), and transfers or extensor realignment to provide thumb extension. Additional procedures include thumb or digital capsulodesis, tenodesis, or arthrodesis for joint instability or deformity (Bleck, 1987; Botte et al, 1989; Braun, 1988; Filler et al, 1976; Gelberman, 1991; Hoffer, 1982; Keats, 1965; Moberg, 1976; Tachdijian, 1972).

General anesthesia is usually preferable to regional anesthesia in upper-extremity surgery, because of the young age, emotional instability, and immaturity of many of these patients.

Several surgical procedures can be performed at the same time, and staging different procedures is not usually necessary. Thumb and wrist deformities can be corrected simultaneously. If severe deformity of the shoulder exists, this should be corrected first so that subsequent procedures can be performed with the limb flat on the operative table. Surgical drains are usually used when multiple muscles are released or lengthened because of the dead space created.

SHOULDER DEFORMITY

Adduction, flexion, and internal rotation deformity of the shoulder is caused by spasticity or contracture of the pecto-

---

*Bleck, 1987; Botte et al, 1987, 1989; Braun, 1988; Braun and Vise, 1973; Carrol and Craig, 1951; Gelberman, 1991; Goldner, 1955, 1961, 1966, 1971a, 1971b, 1974, 1975, 1979, 1983; Goldner and Ferlic, 1966; Gschwind and Tonkin, 1992; Hoffer, 1982; Hoffer et al, 1983; Inglis and Cooper, 1966; Keats, 1965; Keenan et al, 1987a, 1987b; Koman et al, 1990; McCarroll, 1949; Mital, 1979; Page, 1923; Pharoah, 1981; Sakellarides and Mital, 1976; Sherk, 1977; Strecker et al, 1988; Swanson, 1968; Tachdijian, 1972; Tonkin and Gschwind, 1992; White, 1972.

†Beach et al, 1991; Bleck, 1987; Botte et al, 1987; Boyes, 1962; Braun and Vise, 1973; Gelberman, 1991; Goldner, 1955, 1961, 1966, 1971a, 1971b, 1974, 1975, 1979, 1983; Goldner and Ferlic, 1966; Green, 1988, 1942a, 1942b; Green and Banks, 1962; Gschwind and Tonkin, 1992; Hoffer, 1978, 1982; Hoffer et al, 1986; Koman et al, 1990; McCarroll, 1949; McCue et al, 1970; Moberg, 1976; Mowery et al, 1985; Nelson, 1969; Omer and Capen, 1976; Phelps, 1957; Samilson and Morris, 1964; Samilson, 1966; Tachdijian, 1972; Wenner and Johnson, 1988; Zancolli, 1979.

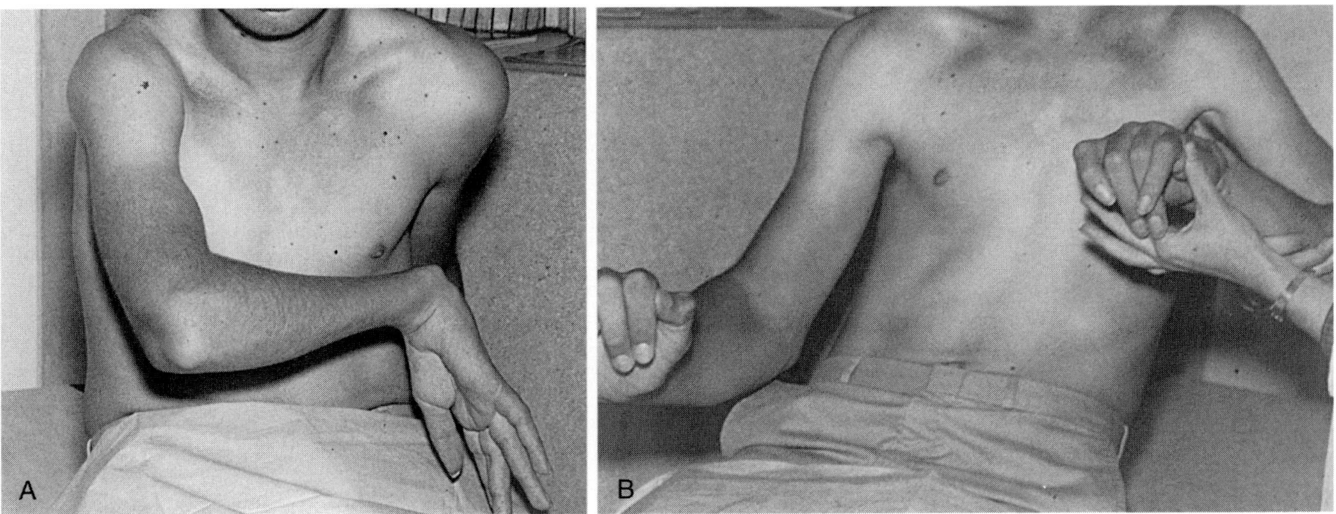

FIGURE 63–2. The characteristic upper limb deformity in spastic hemiplegia is shoulder adduction and internal rotation, elbow flexion, forearm pronation, wrist flexion, thumb-in-palm deformity, and digital flexion or extension (*A*). Spastic quadriplegia involving both upper extremities (*B*). (Illustration by Elizabeth Roselius, © 1991. Reprinted with permission from Gelberman RH: Cerebral palsy. *In* Gelberman RH [ed]: Operative Nerve Repair and Reconstruction. Philadelphia, J.B. Lippincott Company, 1991, pp 1455–1475.)

ralis major, subscapularis, teres major, and/or latissimus dorsi. If treatment using passive stretching and mobilization does not control deformity, resulting problems include functional impairment, difficulty dressing, or hygienic problems in the axilla. Surgery is directed toward release or lengthening of the offending muscles, usually including the pectoralis major and subscapularis, and, occasionally, the teres major and latissimus dorsi. The modified Sever procedure, as described by Green, has proved effective in reducing shoulder deformity (1942a).

Technique: Shoulder Contracture Release (Fig. 63–3). A deltopectoral incision is made from the anterior aspect of the acromioclavicular joint along the anterior margin of the deltoid muscle to a point just lateral to the anterior axillary fold. The fascia overlying the interval is incised and the cephalic vein and deltoid branches of the thoracoacromial are artery identified. The cephalic vein may be ligated or retracted laterally, along with a few fibers of the deltoid muscle. The U-shaped tendon of the pectoralis major is isolated along the crest of the greater tuberosity of the humerus, and either divided 3 to 4 cm from its insertion or lengthened using the Z-lengthening incision. The subscapularis tendon is isolated on the lesser tuberosity of the humerus just proximal to the circumflex humeral vessels. The interval between the subscapularis and anterior shoulder capsule is bluntly developed. The tendon is divided, taking care to avoid the leash of veins that course along the inferior border of the subscapularis. The capsule of the shoulder joint is usually not divided, in order to maintain shoulder

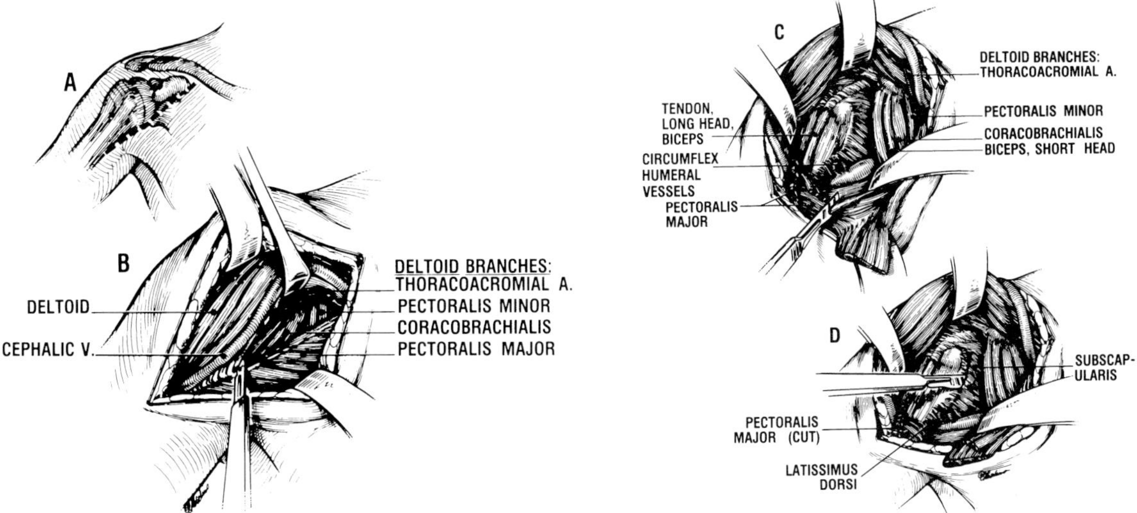

FIGURE 63–3. Shoulder contracture release: *A*, A deltopectoral incision is made from the anterior aspect of the acromioclavicular joint along the anterior margin of the deltoid muscle. The fascia overlying the deltopectoral interval is incised, and the cephalic vein is retracted laterally. *B*, The U-shaped tendon of the pectoralis major is incised sharply 3 to 4 cm from its insertion, along the intertubercular groove of the humerus. *C* and *D*, The subscapularis muscle is divided. Care is taken to avoid opening the capsule of the shoulder joint. (Illustration by Elizabeth Roselius, © 1991. Reprinted with permission from Gelberman RH: Cerebral palsy. *In* Gelberman RH [ed]: Operative Nerve Repair and Reconstruction. Philadelphia, J.B. Lippincott Company, 1991, pp 1455–1475.)

stability. If the shoulder deformity is not adequately corrected after release of the pectoralis major and subscapularis, and the latissimus dorsi and teres major are palpably tight during passive shoulder abduction or external rotation, release of these muscles is carried out. The interval lateral to the short head of the biceps and medial to the anterior deltoid is developed. This exposes the insertions of the latissimus dorsi and teres major onto the humerus. Each muscle is released near its insertion. The wound is irrigated, drains are placed, and subcutaneous tissues and skin are closed (Gelberman, 1991).

An external rotation abduction splint is worn postoperatively for 3 weeks, followed by a therapy program that includes active-assistive abduction, extension, and external rotation as well as shoulder strengthening and passive mobilization to maintain motion.

ELBOW FLEXION DEFORMITY

Flexion is the most common deformity of the elbow. The deformity interferes with function, limits extension for two-handed activities, and causes walking difficulties when crutches are required. Severe contractures cause skin maceration, hygienic problems, and difficulty with dressing. In some patients, a mild elbow flexion deformity becomes exaggerated during physical or mental stress and causes dynamic functional and balancing problems. Most deformities are less than 45 degrees and can be treated nonoperatively in a rehabilitation program using passive mobilization, strengthening, intermittent splinting, and muscle relaxant medication.

For refractory or severe deformities, operative management is usually indicated and includes either musculocutaneous neurectomy, flexor origin release (flexor-pronator slide), or elbow release (which consists of a combination of selective muscle lengthening and release). Operative release is usually indicated for contractures greater than 60 degrees. Operative release can improve general function, hygiene, and dressing. The procedures promote two-handed activities and have proved effective in facilitating independent crutch walking in patients with spastic quadriplegia (Mital, 1979).

Musculocutaneous Neurectomy

Musculocutaneous neurectomy is usually successful for minor contractures when increased muscle tone is the primary problem (Hoffer, 1982). Prerequisites for neurectomy are absence of fixed soft tissue contractures and a functioning brachioradialis that can provide adequate elbow flexion. The procedure is contraindicated when elbow flexion depends on the biceps and brachialis. To distinguish myostatic contractures from spasticity, a musculocutaneous nerve block is given, using lidocaine hydrochloride 1% without epinephrine injected along the proximal medial border of the biceps muscle. Accurate infiltration is aided with a nerve stimulator connected to the needle hub. The nerve block, which simulates a neurectomy, eliminates flexion contributions from the biceps and brachialis and demonstrates the ability of the brachioradialis to flex the elbow.

Technique: Musculocutaneous Neurectomy. The musculocutaneous nerve can be surgically exposed through an axillary approach or through a medial brachial incision. General anesthesia is recommended. A tourniquet is not used because it does not afford adequate exposure to the axilla and proximal arm. For the axillary approach, the biceps and lateral cord of the brachial plexus are located through direct axillary dissection. The axillary sheath is incised, the lateral cord identified, and the musculocutaneous nerve isolated before its entry into the biceps. A portion of nerve is transected in this location. Alternatively, an incision can be placed more distally on the medial arm, along the palpable interval between the biceps and brachialis. Dissection between the interval will expose the musculocutaneous nerve as it courses in a medial to lateral direction. A portion of nerve is excised in the proximal part of the incision, before the exit of motor branches to the biceps and brachialis. Wounds are irrigated and closed.

A therapy program for elbow mobilization is initiated postoperatively as soon as patient comfort and wound conditions permit. Splinting is continued to assist with gains in motion, and continued intermittently as needed to maintain long-term correction.

Although musculocutaneous neurectomy results in anesthesia along a portion of the lateral forearm (in the distribution of the lateral antebrachial cutaneous nerve), this is usually not a functional problem.

Flexor-Pronator Slide

The flexor-pronator slide is well proved and effective for patients with spasticity resulting in fixed elbow contractures that cause hygiene problems (Inglis and Cooper, 1966; Page, 1923; White, 1972). The procedure can, however, cause weakness of digital flexors and is not as effective functionally as selective elbow release and tendon lengthening. The flexor-pronator slide is indicated in selected patients who also have digital flexion and forearm pronation deformities.

In a hand with a clenched fist deformity, the flexor-pronator slide provides an adequate amount of tendon length for satisfactory correction. Braun has observed that if the digits are held tightly within the palm with the wrist extended and if the digits can be fully extended with the wrist flexed, then about 4 to 5 cm of additional tendon length is needed to allow extension of the digits with the wrist in 10 degrees of extension (Braun, 1988; Braun and Vise, 1973). The flexor-pronator slide provides this amount of tendon length for correction.

Technique: Flexor-Pronator Slide (Fig. 63–4). Under general anesthesia, the limb is exsanguinated and the tourniquet is inflated. A sterile tourniquet is applied. A medial elbow incision is placed 4 cm proximal to the medial epicondyle and extended into the proximal medial forearm. The ulnar nerve is isolated and protected proximally, and tagged with a rubber drain in preparation for anterior transposition later in the procedure (see Fig. 63–4). The lacertus fibrosus is incised, and the median nerve and brachial artery are identified and tagged medial to the biceps tendon. The flexor-pronator muscles are isolated along the anterior aspect of the medial epicondyle and elbow joint. A plane is carefully

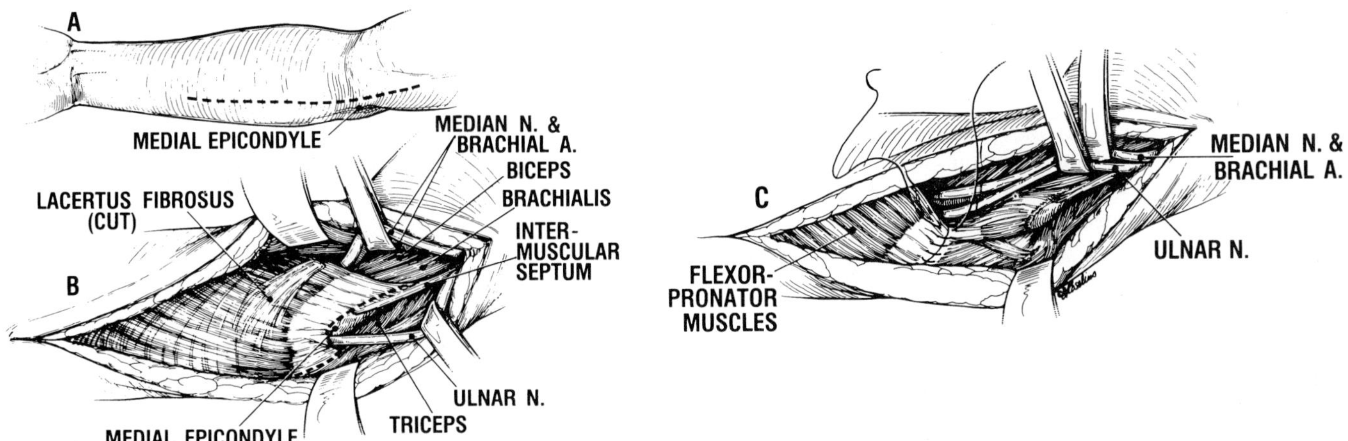

FIGURE 63–4. Flexor-pronator slide: *A,* A long medial arm incision is placed 4 cm proximal to the medial epicondyle and carried into the proximal forearm. *B,* The ulnar nerve is isolated and tagged; the median nerve and brachial artery are also isolated. The flexor-pronator muscles are delineated, and the plane beneath them is developed. *C,* Dissection is carried distally along the proximal motor branches of the median and ulnar nerves. The muscles are divided at their origin, elevated from the proximal ulna, and allowed to displace 3 to 5 cm distally. The origin of the flexor-pronator muscles may then be sutured to the periosteum of the ulna to maintain some pronation power. (Illustration by Elizabeth Roselius, © 1991. Reprinted with permission from Gelberman RH: Cerebral palsy. *In* Gelberman RH [ed]: Operative Nerve Repair and Reconstruction. Philadelphia, J.B. Lippincott Company, 1991, pp 1455–1475.)

developed deep to the flexor-pronator muscles on the anterior aspect of the elbow joint, carefully detaching the muscles from their origins. Dissection is continued distally along the medial intermuscular septum. Care is taken to preserve the proximal motor branches of the median and ulnar nerves. Once the muscle origins are released, the digits and wrist are passively corrected, thus pulling the muscles to a new, more distal position. Five centimeters of distal slide is generally obtained. The pronator teres can be sutured to the ulna in the lengthened position to retain some forearm pronation ability and to help prevent an overcorrection supination deformity. The tourniquet is deflated, hemostasis obtained, drains placed, and a bulky long-arm dressing applied with plaster splints.

The elbow, forearm, and digits are immobilized in the corrected position for 3 weeks to allow muscle reattachment. This is followed by a therapy program incorporating progressive active and passive mobilization and gentle strengthening. The extremity is splinted for an additional 6 weeks or as necessary to maintain correction.

Possible complications of the flexor-pronator slide include overcorrection, sometimes because of the unmasking of occult extensor spasticity, with resulting wrist and digital extension deformities and forearm supination.

Elbow flexor release and selective lengthening comprise lengthening the biceps brachii, myotomy or fractional lengthening of the brachialis, and release of the origin of the wrist flexors and pronator teres. Because of its long tendon, the biceps lends itself to Z-lengthening. Because of the relatively short tendon, the brachialis is difficult to Z-lengthen, and is therefore myotomized or lengthened using fractional lengthening. Elbow flexor release and selective muscle lengthening are indicated in patients with 60-degree flexion deformities of the elbow, especially those with deformities exaggerated with walking or running. Co-existing wrist flexion deformities may also be improved, because the wrist flexor origins are released.

Technique: Elbow Flexor Release With Selective Muscle Lengthening (Authors' Preferred Method). A curved incision is placed anterior to the medial epicondyle of the humerus. The ulnar nerve is isolated and tagged with a

rubber drain. The origin of the flexor carpi ulnaris, pronator teres, palmaris longus, and flexor carpi radialis are released from the medial epicondyle. The median nerve, brachial artery, and biceps tendon are isolated. The median nerve is protected and the biceps tendon is lengthened by Z-lengthening. Myotomy of the brachialis muscle is performed near its tendinous insertion using electrocautery. Alternatively, if a long myotendinous junction is encountered (especially in a relatively mild elbow deformity), fractional lengthening of the muscle can be performed by placement of three to four incisions in the tendinous portion, leaving the muscle fibers in continuity. The ulnar nerve is transferred anteriorly. The arcade of Struthers is incised, a portion of the medial intermuscular septum excised, and the cubital tunnel released. The flexor carpi ulnaris origin is released. It is important to release the vertical septum that extends between the flexor digitorum superficialis and overlying pronator teres to avoid compression in this area (Inserra and Spinner, 1986). The tourniquet is released, hemostasis obtained, and subcutaneous tissues and skin closed.

The elbow is immobilized for 3 weeks in a long arm plaster cast placed in 15 to 20 degrees of flexion. An elbow extension splint is used for an additional 3 to 6 months while a therapy program incorporating active-assisted mobilization and gentle strengthening is carried out.

FOREARM PRONATION

Pronation is the most common forearm deformity in spastic hemiplegia. Besides the functional and hygienic problems, posterior dislocation of the radial head may occur with persistent, severe deformity. Dislocation occurs most frequently between the ages of 5 and 8 years, and is caused by spasticity of the pronator teres and contracture of the interosseous membrane (Pletcher et al, 1976). Tenotomy of the pronator teres has been shown to improve active supination and reduce risk of radial head subluxation and has been recommended for a child as young as 3 to 5 years with fixed deformity (Bleck, 1987; Sakellarides and Mital, 1976; Strecker et al, 1988).

Technique: Pronator Teres Release. A straight 6-cm incision is placed on the palmar forearm along the distal portion of the pronator teres. The subcutaneous tissues and deep forearm fascia are incised. The tendon of the pronator teres is isolated and excised to the level of the myotendinous junction. The limb is passively mobilized to a corrected, supinated position. The tourniquet is released, hemostasis obtained, and subcutaneous tissues and skin closed.

The limb is immobilized in a plaster cast for 3 weeks. A therapy program is then initiated, incorporating active-assisted mobilization and gradual strengthening exercises. Intermittent splinting may be required to maintain correction.

Forearm pronation deformities will improve spontaneously in many patients after treatment of wrist and digital deformities, particularly when transfers for wrist and digital extension are passed subcutaneously around the ulnar border of the distal forearm and wrist. If pronation deformity persists after tendon transfer, isolated release of the pronator teres may be indicated.

WRIST AND DIGITAL FLEXION DEFORMITIES

The most common deformities of the wrist and digits are wrist flexion and MP and PIP flexion. Thumb-in-palm deformity often co-exists. Wrist flexion usually results in weak digital grasp. Co-existing weakness of the digital extensors leads to concomitant weakness of digital release.

With severe digital flexor spasticity, a clenched fist deformity is produced. Besides functional impairment, hygienic problems with skin maceration occur within the palm and wrist crease. Constant pressure of the digits and fingernails against the palm can cause skin ulceration. Limb positioning problems impair patient dressing.

The relative contributions of extrinsic and intrinsic muscles to digital deformities are determined by limb examination with the wrist in different degrees of flexion and extension. If extrinsic myostatic contractures are present, the digital flexion deformities are increased by passive extension of the wrist and decreased with passive wrist flexion. Intrinsic digital muscle contracture or fixed digital joint contracture will not change with passive wrist positioning. Determination of intrinsic muscle contracture is made with the intrinsic tightness test, where passive extension of the MP joint causes increased resistance to passive flexion at the PIP joint (caused by placement of the interosseous and lumbrical muscles on stretch). Fixed PIP joint contracture will not change with changes in position of the MP joint. Fixed contractures of the MP and PIP joints are not as common as extrinsic myostatic contracture.

Initial management of digital and wrist flexion deformities consists of a therapy program that incorporates passive stretching, strengthening of antagonist muscles, corrective serial casting, and static splinting to preserve gains in motion or position. Muscle relaxant medication (diazepam or dantrolene sodium) and lidocaine nerve blocks to the median and ulnar nerves proximal to the elbow facilitate limb mobilization and serial casting. Serial casting is accomplished with specific stretching of the digital or wrist flexor, followed by casting in progressively corrected positions. Stretching and recasting is repeated at weekly intervals. After 4 to 6 weeks of gradual extension, a bivalved cast or custom-molded splint is used intermittently with continued passive stretching exercises. Active exercises and strengthening are performed daily to stimulate voluntary finger control.

Operative management is indicated for refractory deformities that have not responded to a comprehensive therapy program. Operative correction of flexion deformities can be carried out using several methods, including fractional lengthening of digital and wrist flexors at the myotendinous junction in the forearm, superficialis-to-profundus transfer in the forearm, flexor-pronator slide procedure at the elbow, or Z-lengthenings of individual flexor tendons in the distal forearm (Botte et al, 1987; Braun, 1988; Braun and Vise, 1973; Keenan et al, 1987a, 1987b; Tonkin and Gschwind, 1992). Fractional lengthening is indicated in the patient with mild or dynamic deformities, who has retained functional control, and when the amount of needed correction is not as great as can be accomplished with the other methods (Keenan et al, 1987a). The superficialis-to-profundus transfer is effective when there are significant hygienic problems in the minimally functional hand; however, volitional control or functional improvement is not consistently obtained (Botte et al, 1987; Braun and Vise, 1973; Keenan et al, 1987b). The flexor-pronator origin release, though effective in achieving correction, requires more soft tissue dissection, creates dead space in the antecubital fossa and proximal forearm, and may lead to a supination, extended-wrist overcorrection deformity (Tachdijian, 1972). Individual Z-lengthening of the tendons is indicated if the amount of individual tendon lengthening needed varies between the digits (i.e., when spastic involvement differs greatly between the digits).

Technique: Fractional Lengthening of Wrist and Digital Flexor Tendons (Fig. 63–5). A 12-cm palmar mid-line incision is placed on the mid-forearm. Subcutaneous and antebrachial fascia are subdivided. The ulnar neurovascular bundle, the median nerve, radial artery, and superficial branch of the radial nerve are isolated and protected. Fractional lengthening of the flexor carpi radialis and flexor carpi ulnaris is carried out by incision of the tendinous portions of these muscles at their myofacial junction. Two incisions are placed into each muscle, spaced 1.5 to 2 cm apart, leaving the muscle portions intact. The incisions are oriented at differing angles, with the proximal incision transverse and the distal incision oblique. Alternatively, if either muscle, especially the flexor carpi radialis, has a short myotendinous portion and a long tendinous portion, Z-lengthening can be carried out. The palmaris longus is incised or fractionally lengthened with transverse incisions. The flexor digitorum profundus and superficialis are fractionally lengthened with transverse incisions. The wrist and digits are passively extended. The tendinous portions of the muscles will separate, and the muscular portions remain in continuity. If persistent pronation contracture remains after fractional lengthening of forearm muscles, the pronator teres is released or similarly lengthened with two oblique incisions 1.5 to 2 cm apart. The tourniquet is released, hemostasis obtained, and subcutaneous tissues and skin closed. A bulky dressing incorporating long-arm splints is fabricated, maintaining the elbow in 90 degrees of flexion, the wrist in 30 degrees of extension, the forearm in supination, and the digits and thumb in extension (Keenan et al, 1987a; Tachdijian, 1972).

Cast immobilization is carried out for 4 weeks, followed

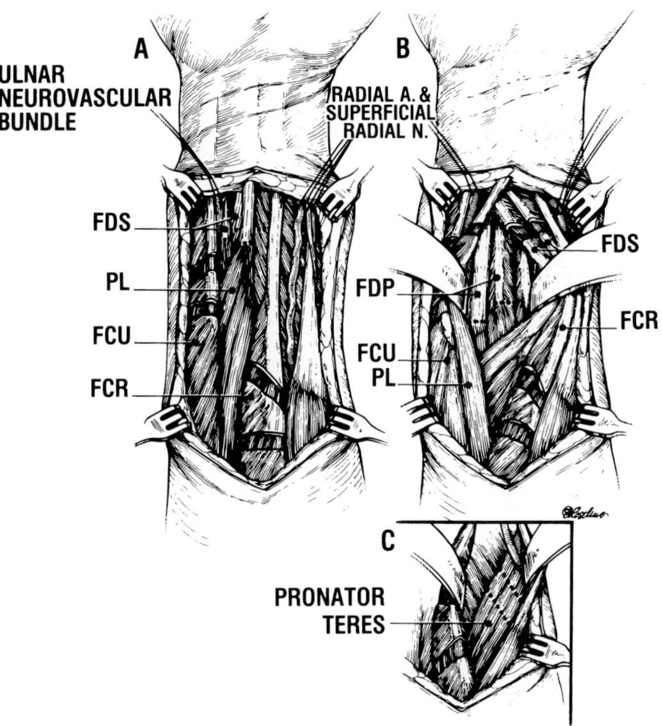

FIGURE 63–5. Fractional lengthening of wrist and digital flexor tendons: *A,* Lengthening of the flexor carpi radialis (FCR) and flexor carpi ulnaris (FCU) at their musculotendinous junctions is carried out with proximal transverse and distal oblique incisions. *B,* The deep flexors are lengthened by two transverse incisions. PL, Pollicis longus; FDS, flexor digitorum superficialis. (Illustration by Elizabeth Roselius, © 1991. Reprinted with permission from Gelberman RH: Cerebral palsy. *In* Gelberman RH [ed]: Operative Nerve Repair and Reconstruction. Philadelphia, J.B. Lippincott Company, 1991, pp 1455–1475.)

by protection with a molded splint. Gentle active-assisted and functional exercises are initiated at 4 weeks and are performed four or five times daily. Long-term night splinting is usually required, because recurrences of flexion deformity are common in the growing child.

Tendon Transfer to the Wrist Extensors (Inadequate Grasp)

The relationships between wrist position and the strength of digital grasp and release are well established (Hoffer, 1978; Hoffer and Koffman, 1992; Hoffer et al, 1979). With the wrist in a flexed position, the digital flexor tendons are slack, and grasp is weak. Therefore, transfers to augment wrist extension will usually improve grip strength (Beach et al, 1991; Bleck, 1987; Gelberman, 1991; Green, 1942; Hoffer et al, 1986; Koman et al, 1990; Tachdijian, 1972). However, wrist extension may also cause tightness of the extrinsic digital flexors, and reconstruction procedures that result in overextension of the wrist may cause digital release to be impaired (Gelberman, 1991; Goldner, 1983). These interrelationships must be carefully assessed before considering tendon transfers to improve wrist extension. The wrist should be passively held in extension to determine whether the patient can actively release the grip by active extension of the digits. If the digits cannot be actively extended with the wrist held in extension, digital release may be a greater problem than weak grasp if tendon transfer to augment wrist extension is carried out (Goldner, 1983).

In the patient with weak grasp and weak wrist extension who can still release the digits with the wrist passively extended, a tendon transfer to augment wrist extension is usually indicated. The flexor carpi ulnaris, pronator teres, extensor carpi ulnaris, flexor digitorum superficialis, and brachioradialis muscles have been used for this purpose (Beach et al, 1991; Gelberman, 1991; Goldner, 1971a; Goldner and Ferlic, 1966; Green, 1988; McCue et al, 1970; Wenner and Johnson, 1988). The selected muscle is transferred into the extensor carpi radialis brevis. The most appropriate transfer is selected by muscle testing.

Technique: Flexor Carpi Ulnaris Transfer for Wrist Extension (Figs. 63–6 and 63–7). A palmar-ulnar incision is placed on the forearm, beginning at the wrist flexion crease and extending proximally to the junction of the middle and proximal thirds of the forearm. Subcutaneous tissue is incised and the tendon of the flexor carpi ulnaris exposed. The ulnar neurovascular bundle, lying deep to the tendon in the distal forearm, is isolated and tagged. The tendon is incised at its attachment to the pisiform and mobilized to the proximal third of the forearm (Fig. 63–6). In mobilizing the muscle proximally, the most distal fibers are stripped extraperiostially from the underlying ulna. Mobilization is carried out proximal enough to allow straight-line transfer to the dorsum of the wrist. The tendon may be passed between the radius and ulna by excising a large rectangular portion of

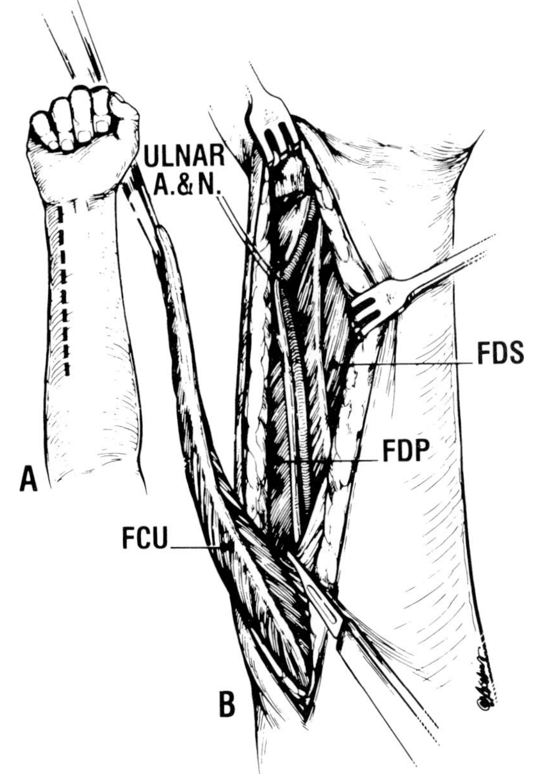

FIGURE 63–6. Flexor carpi ulnaris (FCU) transfer for wrist extension: *A,* A volar-ulnar incision is made from the wrist flexion crease to the proximal mid-third of the forearm. *B,* The FCU is isolated and divided proximal to the pisiform. The muscle is mobilized proximally with the most distal fibers elevated from the underlying ulna. FDP, Flexor digitorum profundus; FDS, flexor digitorum superficialis. (Illustration by Elizabeth Roselius, © 1991. Reprinted with permission from Gelberman RH: Cerebral palsy. *In* Gelberman RH [ed]: Operative Nerve Repair and Reconstruction. Philadelphia, J.B. Lippincott Company, 1991, pp 1475–1477.)

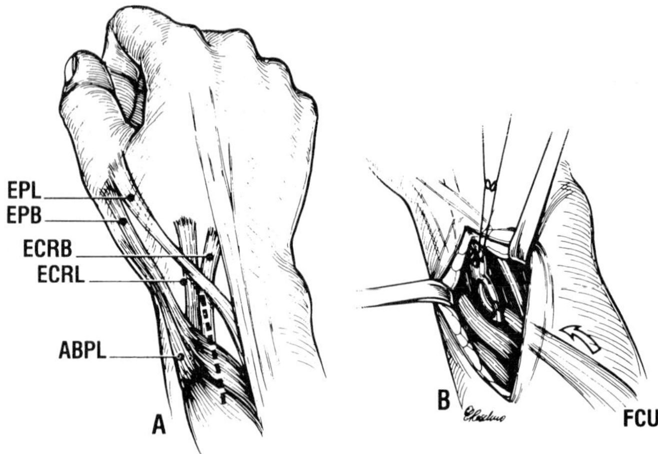

FIGURE 63–7. Flexor carpi ulnaris (FCU) transfer for wrist extension, *continued: A,* A longitudinal 4-cm incision is made over the dorsum of the wrist, centered over the second dorsal compartment. The extensor carpi radialis brevis (ECRB) tendon is isolated at the long-finger metacarpal base. *B,* A subcutaneous tunnel is created extending from the volar-ulnar incision to the dorsal wrist. The FCU tendon is passed through the tunnel to the second dorsal compartment and sutured into the ECRB with the Pulvertaft side-weave technique. ABPL, Abductor pollicis longus; ECRL, extensor carpi radialis longus; EPB, extensor pollicis brevis; EPL, extensor pollicis longus. (Illustration by Elizabeth Roselius, © 1991. Reprinted with permission from Gelberman RH: Cerebral palsy. *In* Gelberman RL [ed]: Operative Nerve Repair and Reconstruction. Philadelphia, J.B. Lippincott Company, 1991, pp 1475–1477.)

the interosseous membrane. Alternatively, the tendon may be passed subcutaneously around the ulnar border of the forearm.

A longitudinal incision is placed on the dorsum of the wrist over the second dorsal compartment, lateral to the dorsal radial tubercle (Fig. 63–7). The incision is extended proximally for 4 cm and continued through subcutaneous tissue to the extensor carpi radialis longus and brevis tendons. The flexor carpi ulnaris is passed through the interosseous space or around the ulnar border of the forearm to the dorsum of the wrist. If passed subcutaneously, care is taken to avoid injury or compression to the ulnar neurovascular bundle. With the forearm in supination and the wrist in 45 degrees of dorsiflexion, the flexor carpi ulnaris tendon is sutured to the extensor carpi radialis brevis using the Pulvertaft side-weave technique (Fig. 63–8). Nonabsorbable, 4-0

braided sutures are used. A resting posture of 15 to 20 degrees of extension is appropriate tension.

After placement of surgical drains and wound closure, a long-arm bulky dressing with plaster splints is applied, immobilizing the extremity with the forearm in supination and the wrist in extension. Sutures are removed at 10 days, and a long-arm is cast applied. Immobilization is continued for a total of 6 weeks. Active exercises are then initiated in a therapy program to stimulate wrist dorsiflexion, ulnar deviation, and forearm supination. Therapy is continued three or four times a day, with the limb maintained in a splint between therapy sessions for an additional 4 weeks. At 10 weeks, splinting is used at night only. Splinting is discontinued when the flexor carpi ulnaris strength is sufficient to maintain the wrist in the dorsiflexed position. Continued observation for early detection of recurrence of wrist flexion deformity is necessary, because additional long-term splinting may be required.

Technique: Pronator Teres Transfer for Wrist Extension (Fig. 63–9). A 6-cm longitudinal incision is placed over the middle third of the radius at the insertion of the pronator teres, just distal to the supinator. The superficial nerve branches are isolated and protected. The pronator teres is detached from its insertion along with a strip of periosteum extending along the radius toward the wrist (Bleck, 1987; Colton et al, 1976). The muscle is mobilized proximally and transferred superficially to the extensor carpi radialis brevis. It is sutured using a Pulvertaft side-weave technique, while holding the wrist in 30 degrees of extension. Nonabsorbable, 4-0 braided sutures are used. Sufficient tension of the transfer should maintain the wrist in 20 degrees of extension. The wrist is positioned in 20 to 30 degrees of extension, and a bulky, long-arm dressing with plaster splints is applied. Postoperative care is as described for the flexor carpi ulnaris transfer.

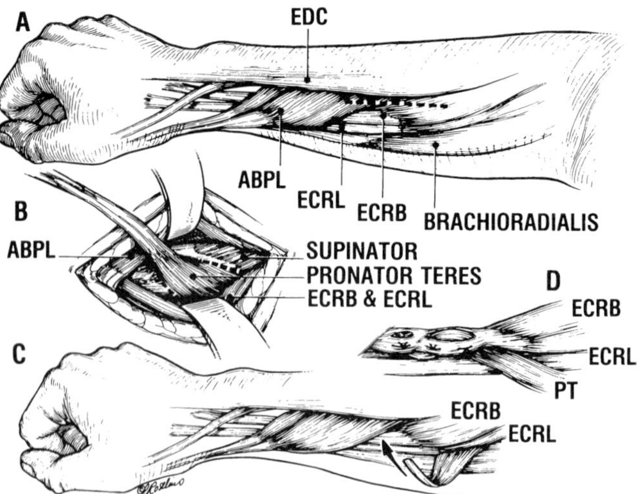

FIGURE 63–9. Pronator (PT) transfer for wrist extension: A 6-cm longitudinal incision is made over the middle third of the radius and the PT insertion is isolated. The PT is elevated with strips of periosteum to ensure adequate length for transfer. The muscle is mobilized proximally, transferred superficially to the extensor carpi radialis longus (ECRL), and sutured into the extensor carpi radialis brevis (ECRB), with the side-weave technique. APBL, Abductor pollicis longus; EDC, extensor digitorum communis. (Illustration by Elizabeth Roselius, © 1991. Reprinted with permission from Gelberman RH: Cerebral palsy. *In* Gelberman RH [ed]: Operative Nerve Repair and Reconstruction. Philadelphia, J.B. Lippincott Company, 1991, pp 1455–1475.)

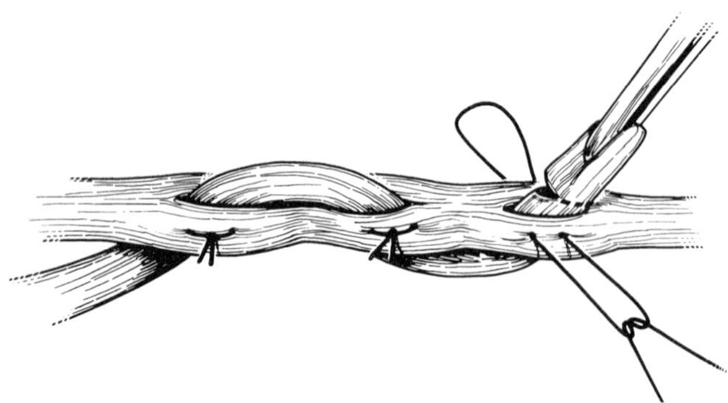

FIGURE 63–8. The Pulvertaft side-weave technique. Two 4-0 braided Dacron horizontal mattress sutures are passed through the tendons at each weave. (Illustration by Elizabeth Roselius, © 1991. Reprinted with permission from Gelberman RH: Cerebral palsy. *In* Gelberman RH [ed]: Operative Nerve Repair and Reconstruction. Philadelphia, J.B. Lippincott Company, 1991, pp 1455–1475.)

Technique: Extensor Carpi Ulnaris Transfer for Wrist or Digital Extension (Authors' Preferred Method) (Gelberman, 1991). The extensor carpi ulnaris is an effective muscle for transfer to the central wrist, thumb, or finger extensor if the wrist can be partially and actively extended (Goldner, 1983). A straight 12-cm dorso-ulnar incision is placed over the distal aspect of the forearm. The tendon of the extensor carpi ulnaris is incised at the base of the little finger metacarpal. The tendon is withdrawn from the extensor retinaculum proximally and mobilized to the proximal mid-forearm. A second incision is made over the second dorsal compartment, and the extensor carpi radialis brevis is identified. A subcutaneous tunnel is made from the extensor carpi ulnaris to the second dorsal compartment. The extensor carpi ulnaris is transferred to the second dorsal compartment and sutured to the extensor carpi radialis brevis, with the wrist held in 30 degrees of extension. The Pulvertaft side-weave technique using 4-0 nonabsorbable braided sutures is used. Sufficient tension should maintain the wrist in 20 degrees extension.

Postoperatively, the wrist is immobilized in extension for 6 weeks. Active-assisted motion is initiated, alternated with extension splinting. Three months postoperatively, a molded plaster splint holds the wrist in 20 degrees of extension at night.

Wrist Arthrodesis

Arthrodesis of the wrist is only rarely indicated in the growing child. It should not be considered if tendon transfers can be performed instead to improve wrist function. Arthrodesis is contraindicated if digital extension or flexion is dependent on wrist motion using the tenodesis effect. Wrist arthrodesis may be a reasonable alternative if there is severe wrist deformity with generalized poor muscle control and strength that precludes active flexion and extension of the digits, or a fixed deformity that is so severe that correction cannot be obtained with tendon lengthening or transfer alone (Hoffer and Zeitzew, 1988). Arthrodesis may also be considered as a salvage procedure when tendon transfers have failed (Bleck, 1987). Though generally contraindicated in a growing child, arthrodesis may be an option when the wrist and digits are severely flexed and have no volitional control (Bleck, 1987). In general, it is preferable to postpone surgery until the child is no longer growing and then perform arthrodesis using standard techniques as used in adults.

Digital and Thumb Extensor Transfers (Inadequate Release)

In the patient with inadequate digital or thumb release, reinforcement of the digital and thumb extensors can often be accomplished with tendon transfers. For inadequate digital release, the flexor digitorum superficialis to the long or ring finger or the flexor carpi ulnaris is transferred to the extensor digitorum communis. For inadequate thumb release, the flexor digitorum superficialis or brachioradialis is transferred to the extensor pollicis longus. Muscle selection for transfer is based on muscle testing. Patients must have adequate passive extension of the digits before extensor transfer, because a transfer will not overcome severely spastic or contracted flexors. Appropriate therapy or lengthening of the flexors to achieve adequate passive extension must precede extensor transfer.

Technique: Flexor Digitorum Superficialis Transfer to the Extensor Digitorum Communis (Authors' Preferred Method) (Gelberman, 1991). The flexor digitorum superficialis tendon to the long or ring finger is isolated through a transverse palmar incision placed proximal to the proximal digital crease. Common digital neurovascular bundles are protected and the selected tendon is divided proximal to the chiasm tendinum of Camper. A 4-cm longitudinal distal palmar forearm incision is made in line with the longitudinal axis of the ring finger. The superficialis tendon is delivered into this proximal incision. A third incision, 3 cm long, is placed along the distal ulnar mid-axial line of the distal forearm. A subcutaneous tunnel from the second incision to the third incision is made with a blunt hemostat. The flexor digitorum superficialis tendon is passed from the second incision to the third incision. Care is taken to avoid injury or compression to the ulnar neurovascular bundle. A fourth incision, 4 cm long, is placed longitudinally over the fourth dorsal compartment. The extensor digitorum communis tendons are isolated, and a subcutaneous tunnel is bluntly made connecting the ulnar and mid-dorsal incisions. The flexor digitorum superficialis is passed around the ulnar border of the forearm to the fourth dorsal compartment. The transferred tendon is sutured into the tendons of the extensor digitorum communis in a side-weave fashion. Appropriate tension is set to maintain the MP joints at zero degrees with the wrist held in neutral position. Immobilization is continued for 4 to 6 weeks, followed by gentle mobilization and strengthening in a progressive therapy program. Protective splinting is continued for an additional 4 to 6 weeks.

Alternatively, the flexor carpi ulnaris may be used to transfer to the digital extensors. The flexor carpi ulnaris is harvested as described previously for transfer for wrist extension (Green, 1942b; Green and Banks, 1962). The tendon is passed subcutaneously around the ulnar border of the forearm and sutured to the extensor digitorum communis in the same manner and with the same tension as that described for the flexor digitorum superficialis (Fig. 63–10).

Postoperatively, the limb is immobilized for 6 weeks with the wrist in 30 degrees extension and the digits extended. Wrist extension is then continued for an additional 2 weeks while the digits are mobilized. Subsequently, splinting is alternated with active-assisted range-of-motion exercises of the wrist and digits.

Technique: Flexor Digitorum Superficialis Transfer for Thumb Extension. The flexor digitorum superficialis to the long or ring finger is identified through a 4-cm straight palmar distal forearm incision along the longitudinal axis of the ring finger. Traction applied to the selected flexor digitorum superficialis tendon with the wrist and fingers flexed will allow maximal length to be harvested. The tendon is incised in the distal part of the incision. A large rectangular segment of the pronator quadratus is excised. A second longitudinal incision, 6 cm long and located dorsally over the dorsoradial tubercle, is placed and the extensor pollicis longus is identified and tagged. A communication between the two incisions is made through the interosseous membrane

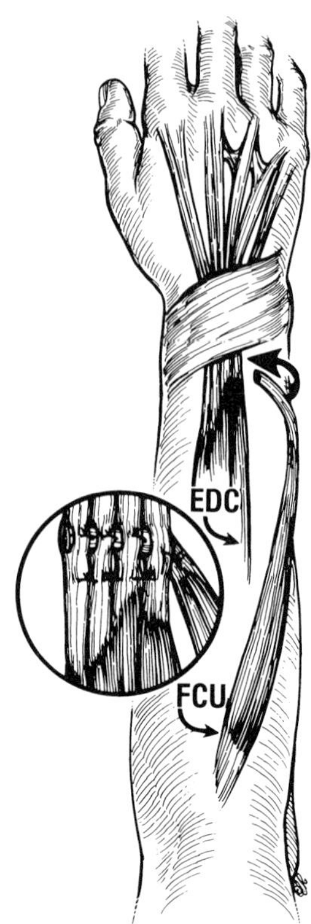

FIGURE 63–10. Flexor carpi ulnaris (FCU) transfer for digital extension: The FCU is passed subcutaneously around the ulnar border of the forearm and sutured to the tendons of the extensor digitorum communis (EDC) just proximal to the extensor retinaculum. (Illustration by Elizabeth Roselius, © 1991. Reprinted with permission from Gelberman RH: Cerebral palsy. *In* Gelberman RH [ed]: Operative Nerve Repair and Reconstruction. Philadelphia, J.B. Lippincott Company, 1991, pp 1455–1477.)

by bluntly passing a large hemostat from the dorsal incision through the defect in the pronator quadratus to the palmar aspect of the wrist. The flexor digitorum superficialis is delivered into the dorsal wrist incision. Care is taken to avoid injury or compression to the median nerve. The extensor pollicis longus is released from its tunnel and the flexor digitorum superficialis sutured to it in a side-weave fashion with 4-0 braided nonabsorbable horizontal mattress sutures. The wrist is splinted in 20 degrees of extension and the thumb in full extension for 6 weeks. A therapy program for progressive mobilization and strengthening is then initiated. Protective splinting is continued for an additional 4 to 6 weeks.

THUMB-IN-PALM DEFORMITY

Thumb-in-palm deformity is caused by spasticity or contracture of the adductor pollicis, flexor pollicis brevis, abductor pollicis brevis, opponens pollicis, first dorsal interosseous, and/or flexor pollicis longus (Bleck, 1987; Botte et al, 1989; Hoffer et al, 1983; Matev, 1963, 1970). Operative management is directed toward release, recession, or lengthening of the specifically offending muscles. Deepening of the thumb web space may also be indicated if skin contracture has developed. Determination of specific muscles involved is based on observation of the presenting deformity, examination with passive stretch of individual muscles, and,

as needed, selected diagnostic lidocaine nerve blocks or dynamic electromyogram analysis.

Goals of operative management are to allow the thumb to come out of the palm to promote grasp and pinch. Although true opposition may not be obtained, lateral pinch may be adequate and will greatly improve function. In the nonfunctional hand, operative management may still be indicated to allow hygiene care in the palm.

Realignment and Reinforcement of the Extensor Pollicis Longus

For mild deformities in a patient with retained volitional control of the thumb, realignment and reinforcement of the extensor pollicis longus can be considered, using transfer of either the flexor digitorum superficialis or brachioradialis. Thumb realignment can also be performed by imbrication of the abductor pollicis longus and flexor pollicis brevis (Goldner, 1983).

Technique: Realignment and Reinforcement of the Extensor Pollicis Longus (Fig. 63–11). In a thumb with volitional control and mild adduction deformity, function can be improved by rerouting the extensor pollicis longus and reinforcement by tendon transfer. A curved incision is placed over the extensor pollicis longus, centered over the dorsal radial tubercle. The extensor retinaculum adjacent to the tubercle is divided. The extensor pollicis longus is elevated from its tunnel and displaced radially. If the flexor digitorum superficialis of the long or ring finger is suitable for thumb reinforcement, it is detached distally as described above, mobilized, and transferred around the radial border of the forearm. The tendon is sutured to the extensor pollicis longus using the Pulvertaft technique. Tension of the transfer is adjusted so that with the wrist in neutral, the tip of the thumb lies 2 to 3 cm lateral to the edge of the index finger.

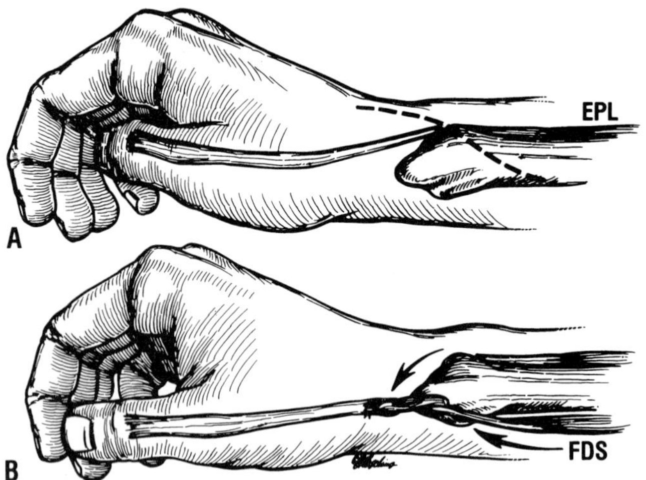

FIGURE 63–11. Rerouting of the extensor pollicis longus (EPL): The flexor digitorum superficialis (FDS) is mobilized and transferred around the radial aspect of the forearm to the rerouted EPL. The EPL tendon may be tenotomized at the fibro-osseous canal, with the distal segment placed in line with the radial styloid. The FDS tendon is interwoven with the distal tendon of the EPL. (Illustration by Elizabeth Roselius, © 1991. Reprinted with permission from Gelberman RH: Cerebral palsy. *In* Gelberman RH [ed]: Operative Nerve Repair and Reconstruction. Philadelphia, J.B. Lippincott Company, 1991, pp 1455–1477.)

With wrist flexion, the thumb should extend maximally, and with wrist extension, the thumb should lie just inside the radial border of the index metacarpal.

Alternatively, the brachioradialis may be used for transfer to the extensor pollicis longus, especially if the flexor digitorum superficialis is too weak for transfer or is unavailable. The brachioradialis tendon is isolated through a mid-axial distal forearm incision and mobilized along its distal portion. Because adequate brachioradialis excursion is necessary for satisfactory transfer, a second incision is placed in the mid-forearm to allow proximal muscle mobilization. The brachioradialis tendon is sutured to the extensor pollicis longus using the side-weave technique with 4-0 nonabsorbable interrupted horizontal sutures.

For either flexor digitorum superficialis or brachioradialis transfer, the hand and wrist are immobilized for 6 weeks with the thumb in the corrected extended position, followed by gentle mobilization and strengthening in a progressive therapy program. Protective splinting is continued for an additional 6 to 12 weeks.

Technique: Imbrication of the Abductor Pollicis Longus and Extensor Pollicis Brevis. Additional correction of mild thumb-in-palm deformity can be achieved with the plication of the abductor pollicis longus and extensor pollicis brevis (Goldner, 1983). A radial incision is placed over the first dorsal compartment along the distal aspect of the radius, taking care to protect the superficial branches of the radial nerve. The extensor retinaculum over the first dorsal compartment is incised, and the tendons are elevated from the fibro-osseous tunnel. The abductor pollicis longus and extensor pollicis brevis tendons are then plicated over each other by winding a portion of the intact tendons onto each other with a hemostat and suturing them together in the shortened position. Nonabsorbable 4-0 sutures are used. The thumb is splinted in extension for 6 weeks, followed by active mobilization in a therapy program.

Thenar Origin and Adductor Pollicis Recession for Thumb-in-Palm Deformity

In the more severe deformities, especially those with fixed myostatic contracture, thenar origin and adductor pollicis recession is effective. These procedures retain muscle continuity, although the entire muscle is allowed to displace to correct the position of the thumb. The muscle origin reattaches in a more radial location and can retain some function.

Specific involvement of the adductor pollicis may be treated by release (recession) of the muscle from the long finger metacarpal. If the thenar muscles are also involved, the origins of the flexor pollicis brevis, abductor pollicis brevis, and opponens can also be released as needed to obtain correction (thenar origin recession). Alternatively, if the MP joint is stable or has been previously fused, the adductor tendon may be released or Z-lengthened near its insertion or be transferred proximally (Bleck, 1987; Botte et al, 1988; Hoffer et al, 1983; Matev, 1963, 1970).

Technique: Thenar Origin and Adductor Pollicis Recession for Thumb-in-Palm Deformity (Fig. 63–12) (Bleck, 1987; Botte et al, 1988; Hoffer et al, 1983; Matev, 1963,

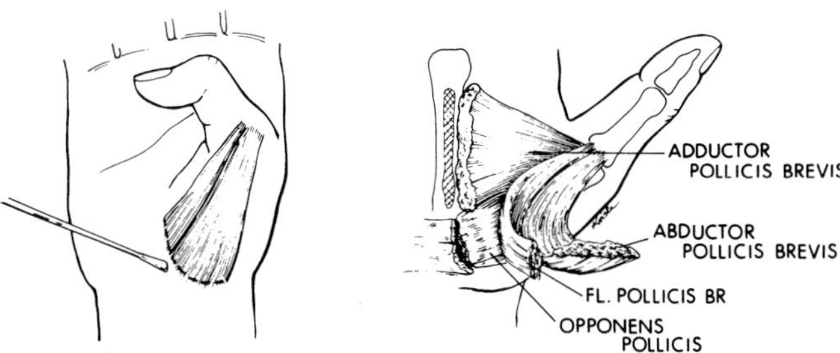

FIGURE 63–12. Thenar origin and adductor pollicis recession for thumb-in-palm deformity: The origins of the abductor pollicis brevis, flexor pollicis brevis, and opponens pollicis are gently freed from their attachments on the transverse carpal ligament. If needed, the adductor pollicis is released. The distal portion of the transverse carpal ligament often requires release to afford adequate access to the most proximal origin of the adductor pollicis. Following thumb position correction, the muscles are allowed to reattach in a more radial and distal position. (From Botte MJ, Keenan MA, Gellman H, Garland DE, Waters RL: Surgical management of spastic thumb-in-palm deformity in adults with brain injury. J Hand Surg [Am] *14*:174–182, 1989. © 1989, Churchill Livingstone, New York.)

1970). A curved incision is placed in the palm along the thenar crease. Dissection is extended to the base of the thenar muscles. The flexor pollicis brevis and abductor pollicis brevis are identified at their origin from the transverse carpal ligament. The muscles are elevated from their ligamentous attachments, taking care to protect the recurrent motor branch and palmar cutaneous branch of the median nerve. The proximal phalanx of the thumb is extended, allowing the released thenar muscles to slide radially and distally. Exposure of the opponens pollicis is provided, and its origin is released in a similar fashion. The thumb is immobilized in a corrected position for 4 weeks, followed by a hand therapy program for mobilization and progressive strengthening.

If the adductor pollicis also contributes to the deformity, it is released at the time of thenar origin release. The muscle is identified in the distal aspect of the incision, deep and distal to the flexor pollicis brevis. The adductor pollicis is released either from its origin on the third metacarpal or near its insertion. To release the muscle from its origin, the digital neurovascular bundles and flexor tendons to the index and long fingers are identified and retracted. The adductor pollicis is traced to its origin on the third metacarpal. The deep palmar vascular arch and the deep branch of the ulnar nerve penetrate the muscle between its transverse and oblique heads. The neurovascular structures are protected and the muscle is freed from the origin on the third metacarpal. If the adductor pollicis is to be released from its tendinous insertion, the muscle is traced radially and incised.

Recession of the origin of the adductor pollicis has the advantage of preserving some function. Release at the insertion, although technically simpler, obliterates the muscle's function.

Release of the First Dorsal Interosseous

If the first dorsal interosseous is palpably tight or the thumb metacarpal remains adducted against the index metacarpal, release of the first dorsal interosseous is considered. The muscle can be released from its origin along the thumb metacarpal and/or index metacarpal.

Technique: Release of the First Dorsal Interosseous and Insertion of the Adductor Pollicis (Fig. 63–13) (Bleck, 1987; Botte et al, 1989; Hoffer et al, 1983; Matev, 1963, 1970). A longitudinal incision is placed on the palpable dorso-ulnar margin of the thumb metacarpal. Branches of the superficial radial nerve are protected. The tendon of the extensor pollicis longus is identified along the radial margin of the incision. The dissection is continued ulnar to the extensor pollicis longus tendon to expose the broad origin of the first dorsal interosseous from the ulnar margin of the thumb metacarpal. The muscle is freed from its origin and the thumb metacarpal abducted in the plane of the palm to a corrected position. The insertion of the adductor pollicis can be released at this time if the incision is extended distal to the MP joint. The tendinous insertion is visible at the ulnar margin of the base of the proximal phalanx, distal to the first dorsal interosseous muscle. The tendon is released through this tendinous portion, including release of the attachments to the ulnar sesamoid. The thumb is immobilized for 4 weeks, followed by a therapy program for mobilization and strengthening.

Flexor Pollicis Longus Lengthening

If hyperflexion is present at the IP joint of the thumb, and the deformity is increased or decreased by the tenodesis effect of extending and flexing the wrist, respectively, lengthening the flexor pollicis longus should be considered. The flexor pollicis can be lengthened either by Z-lengthening in its tendinous portion or by fractional lengthening in its myotendinous junction (Botte et al, 1989).

Technique: Flexor Pollicis Longus Lengthening (Fig. 63–14). A curved longitudinal incision is placed on the distal third of the radiopalmar forearm. The flexor carpi radialis tendon, the median nerve with its palmar cutaneous branch, and the radial artery are identified and protected. The flexor pollicis longus tendon is isolated deep to the flexor carpi radialis tendon. The tendon is lengthened either by fractional lengthening at the myotendinous junction or by Z-lengthening through the tendinous portion, depending on the length of coexisting tendon and muscle in the myotendinous junction. Fractional lengthening is performed by placement of two or three incisions into the tendinous portion at the myotendinous junction, leaving the connecting muscle fibers

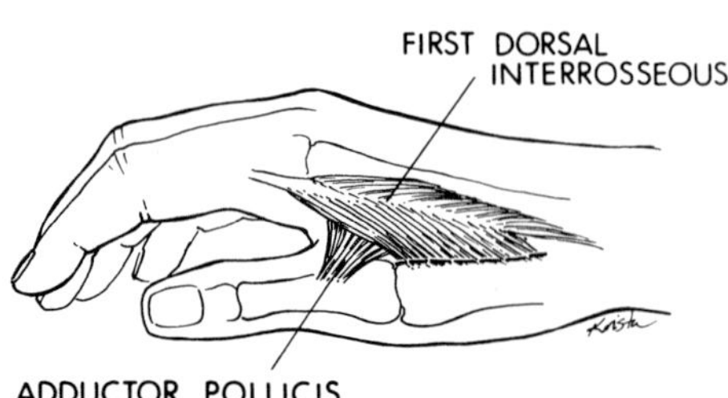

FIGURE 63–13. First dorsal interosseous and adductor pollicis release for thumb-in-palm deformity: Release of the first dorsal interosseous is performed through a dorsal incision along the ulnar margin of the thumb metacarpal. The muscle is released from its origin from the metacarpal. The insertion of the adductor pollicis can be released at the distal margin of the incision. (From Botte MJ, Keenan MA, Gellman H, Garland DE, Waters RL: Surgical management of spastic thumb-in-palm deformity in adults with brain injury. J Hand Surg [Am] *14*:174–182, 1989. © 1989, Churchill Livingstone, New York.)

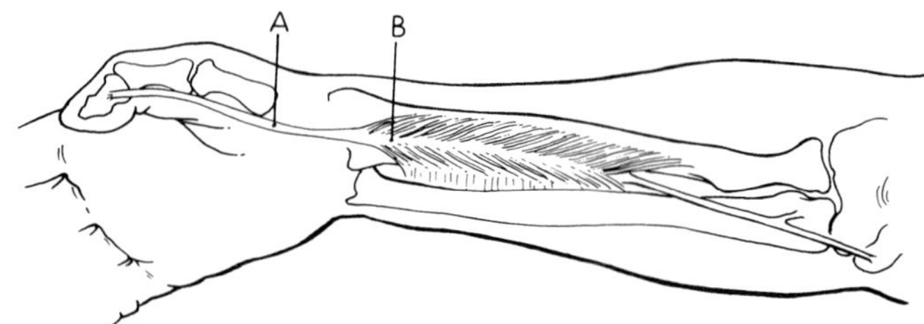

FIGURE 63–14. Flexor pollicis lengthening: Lengthening of the flexor pollicis longus is performed through its tendinous portion by Z-lengthening *(A)* or by fractional lengthening *(B)* if there is an adequate myotendinous junction. (From Botte MJ, Keenan MA, Gellman H, Garland DE, Waters RL: Surgical management of spastic thumb-in-palm deformity in adults with brain injury. J Hand Surg [Am] *14*:174–182, 1989. © 1989, Churchill Livingstone, New York.)

intact to preserve continuity of the muscle. The thumb is extended to the desired corrected position, creating gaps at the incision of the tendinous portion and thereby lengthening the muscle-tendon unit. Alternatively, if the muscle has a long tendinous portion, Z-lengthening can be performed to obtain desired length. With either fractional lengthening or Z-lengthening, care is taken to avoid overcorrection. Residual flexion of 10 to 20 degrees is desirable. A bulky hand dressing with plaster splints is applied, and the thumb is immobilized in the corrected position for 4 weeks. A therapy program for mobilization and progressive strengthening is then initiated.

Thumb Web Space Deepening

In severe deformities, where the metacarpal is adducted against the index finger metacarpal and the web is contracted, the web is deepened by four-quadrant Z-plasty (Fig. 63–15) (Gelberman, 1991). The procedure is usually combined with additional procedures such as thenar origin and adductor pollicis recession and first dorsal interosseous release (Bleck, 1987; Botte et al, 1989; Hoffer et al, 1983; Matev, 1963, 1970).

Thumb Volar Plate Advancement

If the MP joint is hypermobile in extension, particularly in the patient with an adducted metacarpal, a volar plate advancement or MP joint fusion is indicated (Bleck, 1987; Filler et al, 1976; Gelberman, 1991). If the MP joint hyperextends only mildly (less than 15 to 20 degrees), volar plate advancement is carried out as described by Filler. If hyperextension is severe, arthrodesis is indicated. The procedure can be performed in a child as young as 4 years old; however, the physis must be protected (Bleck, 1987; Gelberman, 1991; Goldner, 1983).

Technique: Thumb Volar Plate Advancement (Gelberman, 1991). Through a palmar thumb incision over the thumb MP joint, the neurovascular bundles are identified and protected. The flexor tendon sheath of the flexor pollicis longus is identified and opened over the A1 pulley. Care is taken to protect the radial digital nerve of the thumb, which may cross from ulnar to radial over the tendon in this area. The

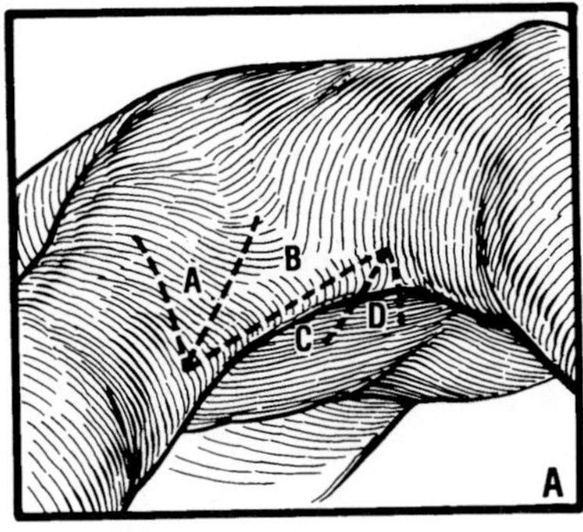

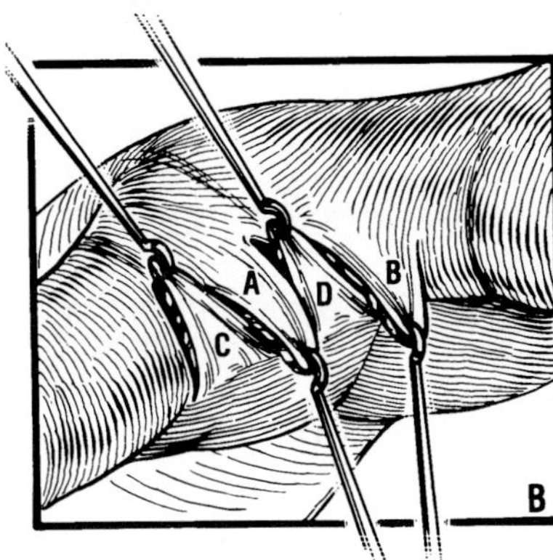

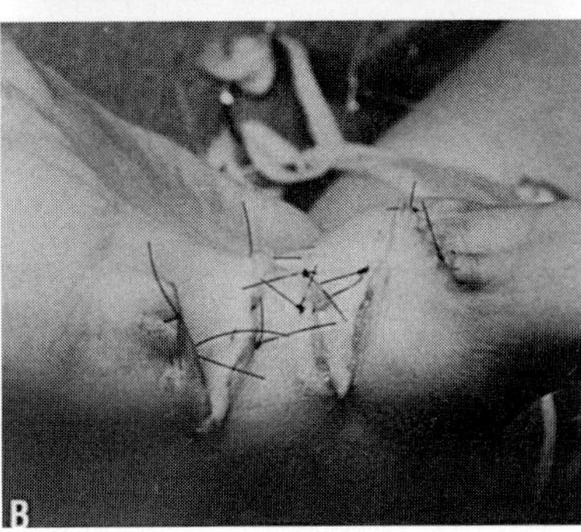

FIGURE 63–15. The four-flap Z-plasty. Four flaps are created with equal sides and with tip angles of 45 degrees. They are labeled A, B, C, and D, and after transposition, they should read C, A, D, and B. (Illustration by Elizabeth Roselius, © 1991. Reprinted with permission from Gelberman RH: Cerebral palsy. *In* Gelberman RH [ed]: Operative Nerve Repair and Reconstruction. Philadelphia, J.B. Lippincott Company, 1991, pp 1455–1475.)

flexor pollicis is retracted and volar capsule identified. The volar plate is detached from the metacarpal and advanced proximally into a grove place into the bone. Fixation is accomplished using a pull-out suture, and the suture is threaded through the capsule and then through two drill holes directed dorsally in the neck of the metacarpal. The sutures are tied over a button on the dorsum of the thumb. Thirty degrees of flexion is recommended. The joint is immobilized in a plaster cast for 6 weeks. A therapy program is initiated to mobilize neighboring joints and progressively increase thumb strength.

Thumb Arthrodesis

For fixed, isolated contracture or related instability of the IP or MP joint of the thumb, arthrodesis may be an alternative, especially in the older child or adult (Botte et al, 1989; Goldner, 1983). Growth plates must be protected in the growing child.

Technique: Arthrodesis of the MP Joint of the Thumb. An ulnar mid-axial incision is made along the MP joint of the thumb. The ulnar collateral ligaments are identified and incised. The accessory collateral ligament is released, and the joint is opened and visualized. Articular cartilage is removed from the metacarpal head and proximal phalanx. Although subchondral bone is exposed on both sides of the joint, little bone is removed. A 0.045-inch smooth pin, pointed on both ends, is drilled in retrograde fashion through the proximal phalanx. The MP joint is positioned in 10

degrees of flexion and 10 degrees of pronation and the pin passed across the fusion site. A second pin is then inserted. Care is taken to avoid the physis with the oblique pins. Pins are removed at 4 to 6 weeks.

Technique: Arthrodesis of the IP Joint of the Thumb. Arthrodesis of the IP joint of the thumb is usually reserved for the older adolescent or adult after growth plates have closed.

A curved dorsal incision is placed over the flexed IP joint. The dorsal capsule is incised, the articular surfaces of the IP joint are denuded of cartilage, and the joint is positioned in 10 to 15 degrees of flexion and 10 degrees of pronation. Internal fixation is accomplished using crossed 0.035- or 0.045-inch smooth pins. The joint is immobilized for 6 weeks or until fusion is evident. Pins are removed at 4 to 6 weeks.

SWAN-NECK DEFORMITY

Swan-neck deformities of the digits are common in cerebral palsy. The deformity is usually caused, in part, by the tenodesis effect of the extensor digitorum communis when the wrist is positioned in chronic flexion. Spasticity of the intrinsic muscles (interossei and lumbricals) also contributes to hyperextension of the PIP joint. With either mechanism, tension on the central slip produces hyperextension of the PIP joint, whereas the DIP joint is allowed to flex. The volar plate of the PIP joint becomes elongated and the lateral bands displace dorsally (Kaplan, 1962). Occasionally, swan-neck deformity is precipitated by harvest of the flexor digitorum superficialis, in which the flexion tension on the PIP joint is decreased and the hyperextension deformity allowed to develop (Swanson, 1960).

Surgery is indicated when functional grasp is inhibited, especially if the fingers lock in hyperextension at the PIP joints and voluntary flexion cannot unlock them.

PIP Tenodesis or Capsulorrhaphy for Swan-Neck Deformity

A successful method for correction of the swan-neck deformity uses the flexor digitorum superficialis for tenodesis of the PIP joint (Bleck, 1987; Gelberman, 1991; Hoffer, 1982; Swanson, 1960), producing a permanent mild flexion PIP contracture. The procedure is especially useful when the proximal portion of the flexor digitorum superficialis is harvested for transfer and is released from a digit that has a tendency to hyperextend at the PIP joint. Correction of a coexisting wrist flexion deformity should also be performed (Beach et al, 1991; Bleck, 1981; Swanson, 1960). Alternatively, a volar capsulorrhaphy of the PIP joint can be performed to correct hyperextension of the PIP joint (Bleck, 1987).

Technique: PIP Tenodesis (Fig. 63–16). A radial mid-lateral incision is placed along the PIP joint. The transverse retinacular ligament is divided and the flexor sheath isolated. The sheath is incised between the A2 and A4 pulleys. The flexor digitorum profundus tendon is retracted palmarly and the flexor digitorum superficialis isolated. The radial half of the flexor digitorum superficialis is located, and a 3-cm-long segment is mobilized and divided proximally. The free end of the superficialis tendon is either sutured to the fibro-osseous canal or passed through an incision in the distal aspect of the A2 pulley. Alternatively, the free tendon end can be anchored to the distal end of the proximal phalanx

using sutures passed through drill holes in the phalanx and tied over a dorsal button. Sufficient tension is applied to maintain the PIP joint in 20 to 30 degrees of flexion. The joint is immobilized with smooth-pin fixation for 4 weeks to protect the tenodesis. At 4 weeks, the pin is removed, and active mobilization in a therapy program is initiated. Protective splinting is continued at night for 3 to 6 months.

Technique: PIP Joint Volar Capsulorrhaphy. Radial and ulnar mid-lateral incisions are placed along the PIP joint, the flexor sheath between the A2 and A4 pulleys is incised, and tendons are retracted to expose the volar joint capsule. The volar plate is detached from the distal end of the proximal phalanx and advanced proximally to flex the joint. The volar plate is anchored to the new position with sutures passed through the proximal phalanx and tied to a dorsal button. The retinaculae are repaired, and the digit is immobilized with smooth-pin fixation for 4 weeks. Postoperative care is as that described for PIP tenodesis.

References

Barnett HL, Einhorn AH: Pediatrics. New York, Appleton-Century-Crofts, 1972.

Barolat-Ramona G, Davis R: Neurophysiological mechanisms in abnormal reflex activities in cerebral palsy and spinal spasticity. J Neurol Neurosurg Psychiatry 43:333–342, 1980.

Beach WR, Strecker WB, Coe J, Manske PR, Schoenecker PL, Dailey L: Use of the Green transfer in treatment of patients with spastic cerebral palsy: 17-Year experience. J Pediatr Orthop 11:731–736, 1991.

Bleck EE: Orthopaedic Management in Cerebral Palsy. Philadelphia, JB Lippincott, 1987.

Botte MJ, Keenan MA, Gellman H, Garland DE, Waters RL: Surgical management of spastic thumb-in-palm deformity in adults with brain injury. J Hand Surg 14A:174–181, 1989.

Botte MJ, Keenan MA, Korchek JI, Waters RL: Modified technique for the superficialis-to-profundus transfer in the treatment of adults with spastic clenched fist deformity. J Hand Surg 12A:639–640, 1987.

Boyes JH: Selection of a donor muscle for tendon transfers. Bull Hosp Joint Dis Orthop Inst 23:1, 1962.

Braun RM: Stroke rehabilitation. In Green DP (ed): Operative Hand Surgery, vol 1, ed 2. New York, Churchill-Livingstone, 1988.

Braun RM, Vise GT: Sublimis to profundus transfers in the hemiplegic upper extremity. J Bone Joint Surg [Am] 55:873, 1973.

Burman MS: The spastic hand. J Bone Joint Surg 20:133–145, 1938.

Carroll RE, Craig FS: Surgical treatment of cerebral palsy: The upper extremity. Surg Clin North Am 30:385–396, 1951.

Colton CL, Ransford AO, Lloyd-Roberts GC: Transposition of the tendon of pronator teres in cerebral palsy. J Bone Joint Surg [Br] 58:220–223, 1976.

Filler BC, Stark HH, Boyes JH: Capsulodesis of the metacarpophalangeal joint of the thumb in children with cerebral palsy. J Bone Joint Surg [Am] 58:667–670, 1976.

Gelberman RH: Cerebral palsy. In Gelberman RH (ed): Operative Nerve Repair and Reconstruction. Philadelphia, JB Lippincott, 1991, pp 1455–1475.

Goldner JL: Reconstructive surgery of the hand in cerebral palsy and spastic paralysis resulting from injury to the spinal cord. J Bone Joint Surg [Am] 37:1141–1154, 1955.

Goldner JL: Upper extremity reconstructive surgery in cerebral palsy or similar conditions. In AAOS Instructional Course Lectures, vol 18. St. Louis, Mosby, 1961, pp 169–177.

Goldner JL: Reconstructive surgery of the upper extremity affected by cerebral palsy or brain or spinal cord trauma. Curr Pract Orthop Surg 3:125–138, 1966.

Goldner JL: Cerebral palsy: Part I. General principles. In AAOS Instructional Course Lectures, vol 20. St. Louis, Mosby, 1971a, pp 20–34.

Goldner JL: Outline of operative procedures for reconstruction of the upper extremity in cerebral palsy. In Keats S (ed): Operative Orthopaedics in Cerebral Palsy. Springfield, IL, Charles C Thomas, 1971b, 50–99.

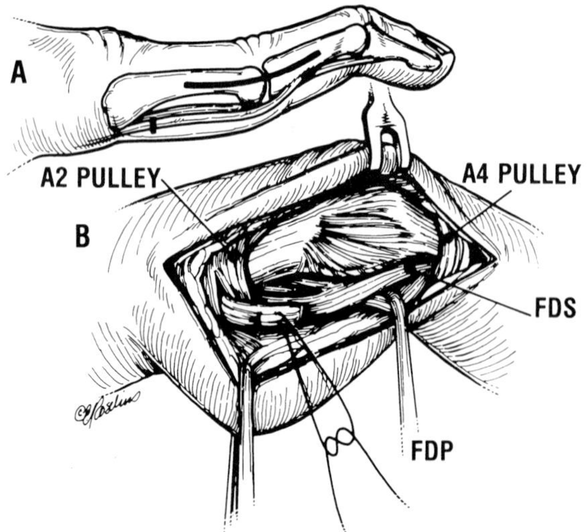

FIGURE 63–16. Proximal interphalangeal (PIP) tenodesis for swan-neck deformity: The radial flexor digitorum superficialis slip is mobilized proximally and sutured to the fibro-osseous canal or the A2 pulley with the PIP joint in 30 degrees of flexion. (Illustration by Elizabeth Roselius, © 1991. Reprinted with permission from Gelberman RH: Cerebral palsy. In Gelberman RH [ed]: Operative Nerve Repair and Reconstruction. Philadelphia, J.B. Lippincott Company, 1991, pp 1455–1475.)

Goldner JL: Upper extremity tendon transfers in cerebral palsy. Orthop Clin North Am 5:389–414, 1974.

Goldner JL: The upper extremity in cerebral palsy: Orthopedic aspects of cerebral palsy. In Samilson R (ed): Philadelphia, JB Lippincott, 1975, pp 221–257.

Goldner JL: Upper extremity surgical procedures for patients with cerebral palsy. In AAOS Instructional Course Lectures, vol 28. St. Louis, Mosby, 1979, pp 37–66.

Goldner JL: Surgical treatment for cerebral palsy. In Everts CM (ed): Surgery of the Musculoskeletal System, vol 1. New York, Churchill-Livingstone, 1983.

Goldner JL, Ferlic DC: Sensory status of the hand as related to reconstructive surgery of the upper extremity in cerebral palsy. Clin Orthop Rel Res 46:87–92, 1966.

Green DP: Operative hand surgery, vol 1, ed 2. New York, Churchill-Livingstone, 1988.

Green WT: Operative treatment of cerebral palsy of spastic type. JAMA 118:434, 1942a.

Green WT: Tendon transplantation of the flexor carpi ulnaris for pronation-flexion deformity of the wrist. Surg Gynecol Obstet 75:337–342, 1942.

Green WT, Banks HH: Flexor carpi ulnaris transplant and its use in cerebral palsy. J Bone Joint Surg [Am] 44:1343–1352, 1962.

Gschwind C, Tonkin M: Surgery for cerebral palsy: Part 1. Classification and operative procedures for pronation deformity. J Hand Surg 17(B):391–395, 1992.

Hoffer MM: The upper extremity in cerebral palsy. In Fredericks S, Brady GS (eds): Neurological Aspects of Plastic Surgery, vol 17. St. Louis, Mosby, 1978, pp 133–137.

Hoffer MM: Cerebral palsy. In Green DP (ed): Operative Hand Surgery. New York, Churchill-Livingstone, 1982, pp 185–194.

Hoffer MM, Koffman M: Cerebral palsy. In Nickel VL, Botte MJ (eds): Orthopaedic Rehabilitation. New York, Churchill-Livingstone, 1992, pp 329–335.

Hoffer MM, Zeitzew S: Wrist fusion in cerebral palsy. J Hand Surg 13:667–670, 1988.

Hoffer MM, Lehman M, Matani M: Long-term follow-up on tendon transfers to the extensors of the wrist and fingers in patients with cerebral palsy. J Hand Surg 11:836, 1986.

Hoffer MM, Perry J, Garcia M, Bullock D: Adduction contracture of the thumb in cerebral palsy. J Bone Joint Surg 65A:755–759, 1983.

Hoffer MM, Perry J, Melkonian GJ: Dynamic electromyography and decision-making for surgery in the upper extremity of patients with cerebral palsy. J Hand Surg 4:424–431, 1979.

Inglis AE, Cooper W: Release of the flexor-pronator origin for flexion deformities of the hand and wrist in spastic paralysis. J Bone Joint Surg [Br] 48:847–857, 1966.

Inserra S, Spinner M: An anatomic factor significant in transposition of the ulnar nerve. J Hand Surg [Am] 11:80, 1986.

Jensen GD, Alderman ME: The prehensile grasp of spastic diplegia. Pediatrics 31:470–477, 1963.

Kaplan EB: Surgical treatment of spastic hyperextension of the proximal interphalangeal joints accompanied by flexion of the digital phalanges. Bull Hosp Joint Dis Orthop Inst 23:35, 1962.

Keats S: Surgical treatment of the hand in cerebral palsy: Correction of the thumb-in-palm and other deformities—Report of 14 cases. J Bone Joint Surg [Am] 47:274–284, 1965.

Keats S: Operative Orthopaedics in Cerebral Palsy. Springfield, IL, Charles C Thomas, 1970.

Keenan MAE, Abrams RA, Garland DE, Waters RL: Results of fractional lengthening of the finger flexors in adults with upper extremity spasticity. J Hand Surg 12A:575–581, 1987.

Keenan MAE, Korchek JI, Botte MJ, Garland DE: Results of transfer of the flexor digitorum superficialis tendons to flexor digitorum profundus tendons in adults with acquired spasticity of the hand. J Bone Joint Surg 69A:1127–1132, 1987.

Keenan MAE, Todderud EP, Henderson R, Botte MJ: Management of intrinsic spasticity in the hand with phenol injection or neurectomy of the motor branch of the ulnar nerve. J Hand Surg 12A:734–739, 1987.

Koman LA, Gelberman RH, Toby EB, Peohling GG: Cerebral palsy: Management of the upper extremity. Clin Orthop Rel Res 253:62–74, 1990.

Matev L: Surgical treatment of spastic "thumb-in-palm" deformity. J Bone Joint Surg [Br] 45:703–708, 1963.

Matev L: Surgical treatment of flexion-adduction contracture of the thumb in cerebral palsy. Acta Orthop Scand 41:439–445, 1970.

Matsuo R, Lai T, Tayama N: Combined flexor and extensor release for activation of voluntary movement of the fingers in patients with cerebral palsy. Clin Orthop Rel Res 250:193–195, 1990.

McCarroll HR: Surgical treatment of spastic paralysis. In AAOS Instructional Course Lectures, vol 6. St. Louis, Mosby, 1949, pp 134–151.

McCue FC, Honner R, Chapman WC: Transfer of the brachioradialis for hands deformed by cerebral palsy. J Bone Joint Surg [Am] 52:1171–1180, 1970.

Milner-Brown HS, Penn RD: Pathophysiological mechanisms in cerebral palsy. J Neurol Neurosurg Psychiatry 412:606–618, 1979.

Mital MA: Lengthening of the elbow flexors in cerebral palsy. J Bone Joint Surg [Am] 61:515–522, 1979.

Moberg IE: Reconstructive hand surgery in tetraplegia, stroke and cerebral palsy: Some basic concepts in physiology and neurology. J Hand Surg 1:29–34, 1976.

Mowery CA, Gelberman RH, Rhoades CE: Upper extremity tendon transfers in cerebral palsy: Electromyographic and functional analysis. J Pediatr Orthop 5:69, 1985.

Nelson WE, et al: Textbook of Pediatrics, ed 9. Philadelphia, WB Saunders, 1969.

Omer GE, Capen DA: Proximal row carpectomy with muscle transfers for spastic paralysis. J Hand Surg 1:197–204, 1976.

O'Reilly DE, Walentynowicz JE: Etiology factors in cerebral palsy. Dev Med Child Neurol 23:633–642, 1981.

Page CM: An operation for the release of flexor contracture in the forearm. J Bone Joint Surg 5:233, 1923.

Pharoah P: Epidemiology of cerebral palsy: A review. J R Soc Med 74:516–521, 1981.

Paine RS: Early recognition of cerebral palsy and prognostic signs: Instructional course lecture. Cleveland, Am Acad for Cerebral Palsy, 1965.

Phelps WM: Long-term results of orthopaedic surgery in cerebral palsy. J Bone Joint Surg [Am] 39:53–59, 1957.

Pletcher DFJ, Hoffer MM, Koffman DM: Non-traumatic dislocation of the radial head in cerebral palsy. J Bone Joint Surg [Am] 58:104, 1976.

Pollack GA: Surgical treatment of cerebral palsy. J Bone Joint Surg [Br] 44:68, 1962.

Sakellarides HT, Mital M: Treatment of the pronator contracture of the forearm in cerebral palsy. J Hand Surg 1:79, 1976.

Samilson RL: Principles of assessment of the upper limb in cerebral palsy. Clin Orthop Rel Res 47:105–125, 1966.

Samilson RL, Morris JM: Surgical improvement of the cerebral palsied upper limb: Electromyographic studies and results of 128 operations. J Bone Joint Surg [Am] 46:1203–1216, 1964.

Sherk HH: Treatment of the severe rigid contractures in cerebral palsied upper limbs. Clin Orthop Rel Res 125:151–155, 1977.

Steindler A: Pathokinetics of cerebral palsy. In AAOS Instructional Course Lectures, vol 9. St. Louis, Mosby, 1900, p 118.

Stelling FH, Meyer LC: Cerebral palsy: The upper extremity. Clin Orthop Rel Res 14:70, 1959.

Strecker WB, Emanuel JP, Dailey L, Manske PR: Comparison of pronator tenotomy and pronator rerouting in children with spastic cerebral palsy. J Hand Surg 13:540–543, 1988.

Swanson AB: Surgery of the hand in cerebral palsy and the swan-neck deformity. J Bone Joint Surg [Am] 42:951–964, 1960.

Swanson AB: Surgery of the hand in cerebral palsy and muscle origin release procedures. Surg Clin North Am 48:1129, 1968.

Tachdijian MO: Pediatric Orthopedics, vol 2. Philadelphia, WB Saunders, 1972, pp 830–857.

Tachdijian MO, Minear WL: Sensory disturbances in the hands of children with cerebral palsy. J Bone Joint Surg [Am] 40:85, 1958.

Tonkin M, Gschwind C: Surgery for cerebral palsy: Part 2—Flexion deformity of the wrist and fingers. J Hand Surg 17(B):396–400, 1992.

Van Heest AE, House J, Putman M: Sensibility deficiences in the hands of children with spastic hemiplagia. J Hand Surg 18:278–281, 1993.

Wenner SM, Johnson KA: Transfer of the flexor carpi ulnaris to the radial wrist extensors in cerebral palsy. J Hand Surg 13:231–233, 1988.

White WF: Flexor muscle slide in spastic hand. J Bone Joint Surg [Br] 54:453–459, 1972.

Zancolli EA: Structural and Dynamic Bases of Hand Surgery, ed 2. Philadelphia, JB Lippincott, 1979.

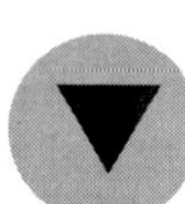

Chapter 64

• Asa J. Wilbourn
• Robert W. Shields, Jr

Generalized Polyneuropathies and Other Nonsurgical Peripheral Nervous System Disorders

The somatic components of the peripheral nervous system (PNS) consist of peripheral motor and sensory fibers and their cell bodies of origin. The motor PNS is composed of the anterior horn cells in the spinal cord and the axons extending distally from them, and the sensory PNS consists of the dorsal root ganglion (DRG) cells, located on the distal sensory roots, and the processes extending peripherally from them. For classification purposes, disorders of the PNS usually are grouped in two categories: (1) generalized sensorimotor disturbances and (2) focal, multifocal, or regional disturbances. These are based on the pattern of involvement that usually, in turn, is related to causation (Thomas and Ochoia, 1993).

There are several disorders in the category of generalized sensorimotor PNS disturbances. In the most common, generalized polyneuropathies, the clinical abnormalities typically are in a bilaterally symmetrical distribution. Most often the nerve fiber dysfunction is "length dependent," so the symptoms characteristically begin in the distal lower extremities (toes, feet) and tend to slowly ascend. The distal upper extremities (fingers, hands) usually are not involved until the lower extremity symptoms reach the knees. Polyradiculopathies and polyradiculoneuropathies are less commonly encountered diffuse PNS disorders. With polyradiculopathies, symptoms often are less severe distally in the limbs. Instead, they may be diffuse, indicating involvement of all the nerve fibers, proximal and distal, to the same degree, or they may be more severe proximally. When such changes coexist with findings of a distal symmetrical polyneuropathy, a polyradiculoneuropathy is present. In addition, in some patients, the peripheral nerve fiber disturbances are caused by abnormalities of the motor and sensory nerve cell bodies within the intraspinal canal and intervertebral foramen, respectively. These are called motor neuronopathies or motor neuron diseases and sensory ganglionopathies.

All the disorders included in this category of PNS disease result from diffusely acting injurious agents, such as systemic metabolic disorders, external toxins, various deficiency states, and immune dysfunction (Thomas and Ochoia, 1993).

Focal, multifocal, and regional PNS lesions, which are more restricted PNS disorders, typically result from processes that produce localized damage along one or more portions of the PNS. In the majority of instances, the injurious agent actually is focal in nature, such as entrapment or compression. Sometimes, however, the symptoms and signs are caused by a focal or multifocal presentation of a more diffuse PNS disorder, e.g., a vasculitis. The underlying pathological process with the latter often is focal ischemia (Thomas and Ochoia, 1993).

It must be appreciated that this classification is rather arbitrary, and many exceptions are encountered. Distal symmetrical polyneuropathies, for example, may initially cause symptoms in one, rather than both, distal lower extremities. Moreover, certain disorders labeled "peripheral polyneuropathies" sometimes begin in the upper extremities, and frequently are asymmetrical, e.g., "pure" sensory polyneuropathies (discussed below). Most of the motor neuronopathies also begin asymmetrically. Finally, many of the multifocal PNS disorders can become secondarily symmetrical because of sequential involvement of various peripheral nerves; this can cause substantial diagnostic difficulties.

In this chapter, the etiology, presentation, and evaluation of some of the disorders in these two categories will be described. The more common generalized symmetrical distal polyneuropathies will be discussed, as will several diverse focal or multifocal neuropathies that usually do not respond to surgical therapy or are often mistaken for focal lesions at other levels of the peripheral neuraxis.

Before specific disorders are reviewed, some information regarding the electrodiagnostic (EDX) examination, and the manner in which it is affected by the pathophysiology resulting from various PNS lesions, will be provided. This is pertinent, because the EDX examination is the optimal laboratory study for assessing most of the disorders in both categories. When properly performed and interpreted, it frequently can provide very useful data regarding the location, pathophysiology, extent, and severity of PNS lesions. For this reason, the EDX findings will be mentioned with the description of each entity.

THE ELECTRODIAGNOSTIC EXAMINATION

The EDX examination consists of, at minimum, nerve conduction studies (NCS) and a needle electrode examination (NEE). Both of these procedures assess only the largest,

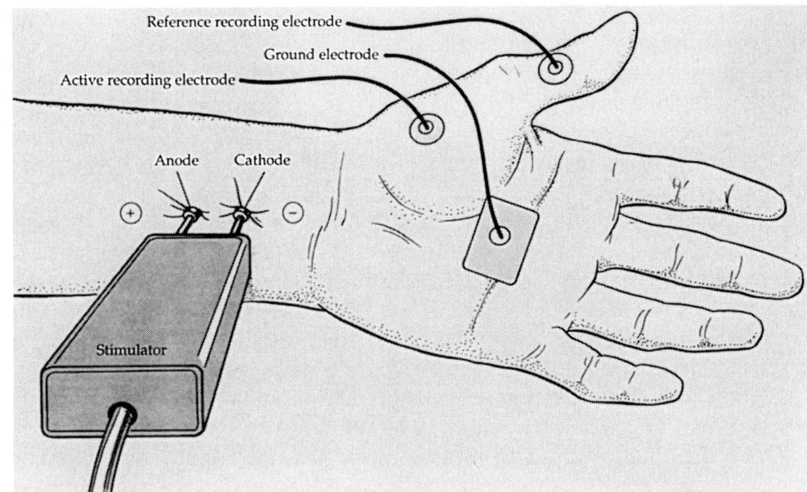

FIGURE 64–1. Electrode placement for performing a median motor nerve conduction study, distal stimulation. (From Isley MR, Krauss GL, Levin KH, Litt B, Shields RW, Wilbourn AJ: Electromyography/Electroencephalography. Redford, WA, Spacelabs Medical, Inc., 1993, p 38; used with permission.)

most heavily myelinated axons; the lightly myelinated and unmyelinated fibers that transmit pain are not directly evaluated in the electromyography (EMG) laboratory.

The NCS evaluate both motor and sensory components of the PNS. For technical reasons, the motor and sensory fibers are studied separately. During motor NCS, recording electrodes are placed over a muscle and its tendon, and the motor axons supplying that muscle then are stimulated at one or, more often, two points along their course (Fig. 64–1). The response recorded from the muscle is a compound muscle action potential (CMAP) (Fig. 64–2A). During sensory NCS, peripheral sensory axons are stimulated at some point, and the nerve action potentials invoked by that stimulus are then recorded, usually percutaneously, at some more distal or, less often, some more proximal site along the nerve. The sensory response obtained is a sensory nerve action potential (SNAP) (see Fig. 64–2B).

For each NCS performed, various measurements are recorded. These include amplitude, distal or peak latency, and, if the nerve has been stimulated at two points, a conduction velocity (CV). The amplitude of the response is its height, measured from baseline to negative (upward) peak and reported in millivolts (mv) for the CMAPs and microvolts (μv) for the SNAPs. The distal latency is the elapsed time between the instant the distal stimulus was applied to the motor axons and the onset of the CMAP; the peak latency is the elapsed time between the instant the stimulus was applied to the sensory axons and the peak of the SNAP. Both the distal and peak latencies are reported in milliseconds (see Fig. 64–2). If the nerve is stimulated at two points, e.g., the

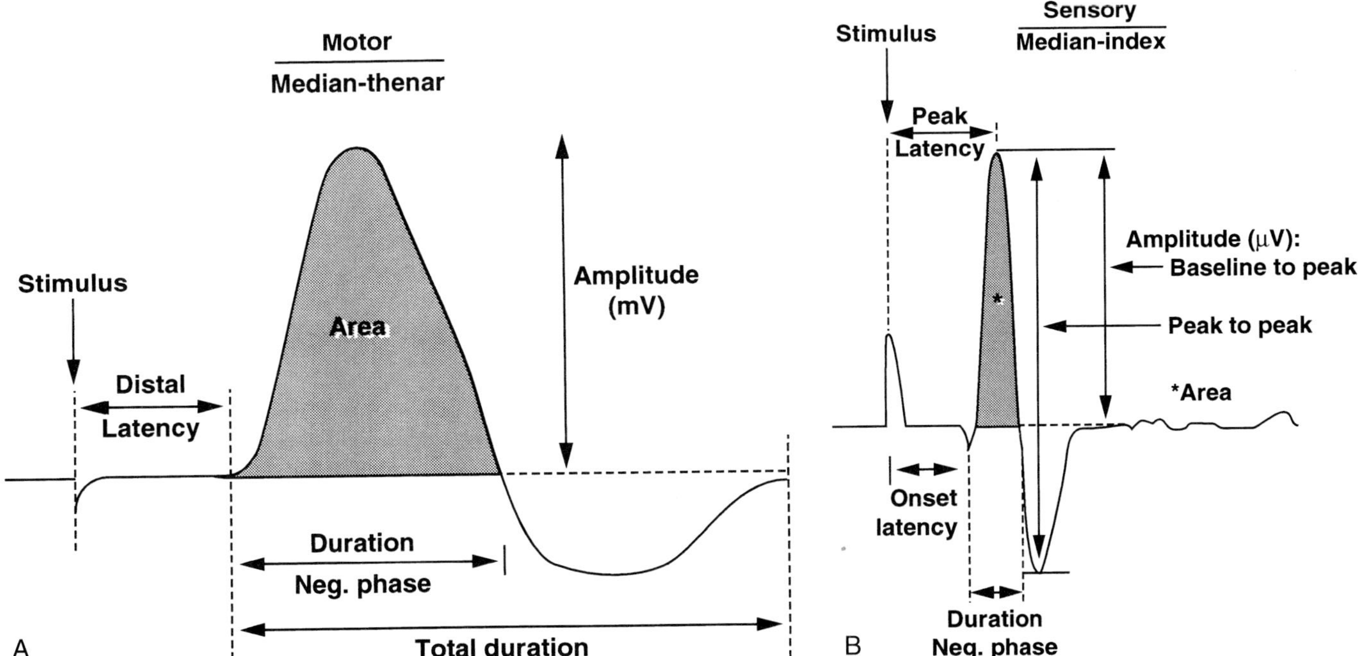

FIGURE 64–2. *A,* The components of the median motor nerve conduction response. *B,* The components of the sensory nerve conduction study response. (From Isley MR, Krauss GL, Levin KH, Litt B, Shields RW, Wilbourn AJ: Electromyography/Electroencephalography. Redford, WA, Spacelabs Medical, Inc., 1993, p 40; used with permission.)

median nerve at elbow and wrist, then a motor CV can be calculated. This is done by subtracting the distal latency from the proximal latency (the time interval between the proximal stimulus and the onset of the response), to determine the time, in milliseconds, that it took the nerve impulses to travel between the two stimulation points. This difference is then divided into the distance, in centimeters, between the two points, as ascertained by surface measurements. The resulting CV is reported in meters per second (m/sec). Both the latencies and CVs are measurements of the speed of impulse conduction along various segments of the nerves: the latencies along the distal segment, between the distal stimulation point and the recording point, and the CV along the segment between the stimulation points (Fig. 64–3) (Dumitru, 1995; Isley et al, 1993; Wilbourn, 1992).

The NEE, unlike the NCS, assesses only the motor component of the PNS. During the NEE, a small-needle recording electrode is inserted into various muscles, and the electrical activity present during various observation periods is analyzed. One such period is when the needle is held fixed in the relaxed muscle. Usually, no electrical activity is seen during this time. However, in many instances—the majority reflecting PNS abnormalities—various types of "spontaneous activity" appear. The most common (and the most important) of these are fibrillation potentials: spontaneous, regularly firing action potentials originating from individual muscle fibers that, in the context of PNS disease, have been denervated (i.e., without their nerve supply) for at least 3 weeks. Fibrillation potentials are the cardinal sign of muscle denervation. These potentials are also one of the most sensitive indicators of muscle denervation, because the death of a single motor axon causes all the muscle fibers that it innervates to fibrillate. The number of muscle fibers supplied by a single motor axon ranges from approximately 200 in the intrinsic hand muscles to more than 1900 in the gastrocnemius muscles. For this reason, unequivocal evidence of motor axon loss can be detected in a muscle by the presence of fibrillation potentials at a time when the overall amount of muscle denervation is insufficient to produce any detectable clinical weakness. Fibrillation potentials usually persist no longer than approximately 2 years after nerve injury; they disappear either because the denervated muscle fiber is reinnervated (and stops fibrillating) or because, lacking a nerve supply, it degenerates (and then becomes unable to fibrillate). Fasciculation potentials are another type of spontaneous activity. However, in contrast to fibrillation potentials, they characteristically fire in an irregular fashion and are the result of spontaneous activation of entire motor units. (A motor unit consists of an anterior horn cell, its axon, and all the muscle fibers it innervates.) Fasciculation potentials thus are evidence of motor unit "irritation," rather than denervation, as is sometimes mistakenly assumed (Dumitru, 1995; Isley et al, 1993; Wilbourn, 1992).

During the activation phase of the NEE, the patient is requested to contract the muscle being studied, and the voluntary motor unit potentials (MUPs) that appear are assessed in regard to their firing pattern, their external and internal configuration, and the stability of their configuration and amplitude on repetitive firing. On very minimal effort, only a single MUP fires in a semiregular manner, at approximately 5 to 10 times per second. With progressively greater patient effort, progressively more MUPs are recruited. Under normal circumstances, with maximal effort so many MUPs are firing simultaneously that the characteristics of the individual ones cannot be appreciated. However, if substantial dropout of motor units has occurred in the muscle being assessed, as a result of either conduction block or conduction failure affecting a significant number of the motor axons innervating it, then on maximal effort the MUPs firing are observed to do so in decreased numbers at a rapid rate. This neurogenic MUP firing pattern, or "reduced recruitment," is unequivocal evidence of a lower motor neuron lesion. In contrast, if submaximal activation of the MUPs results from an upper motor neuron lesion or incomplete voluntary effort, then the MUPs fire in decreased numbers, but at a slow-to-moderate rate.

A substantial change in the external configuration of the MUPs occurs whenever a muscle is partially denervated, and then some of the initially denervated muscle fibers are reinnervated by nerve branches from nearby, unaffected motor units. As a result of this collateral sprouting, fewer motor axons supply the muscle, and each of the functioning motor units now contains more muscle fibers than normal. On NEE, these motor units generate MUPs that are of increased duration and sometimes increased amplitude as well. Such alterations in the external configuration of the MUPs, which usually require at least 4 to 6 months to develop after motor axon loss has occurred, are called "chronic neurogenic MUP changes." Once they appear, they are usually permanent, in contrast to fibrillation potentials.

A few important points regarding EDX studies and PNS disorders will now be reviewed. One of the most fundamental but important of these is that, regardless of the etiology

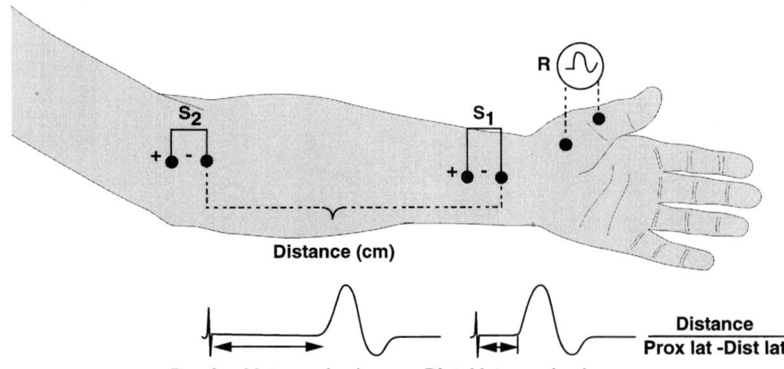

FIGURE 64–3. Method for calculating a motor conduction velocity (in this case, the median motor forearm conduction velocity). (From Isley MR, Krauss GL, Levin KH, Litt B, Shields RW, Wilbourn AJ: Electromyography/Electroencephalography. Redford, WA, Spacelabs Medical, Inc., 1993, p 40; used with permission.)

of a nerve injury, EDX studies essentially can detect only two types of pathophysiology affecting PNS fibers: axon loss and focal demyelination. The former is manifested as conduction failure, whereas the latter can cause either conduction slowing or conduction block, depending on the severity of the process. Concerning the NCS, axon loss (i.e., conduction failure) essentially affects only the amplitudes of the responses; the more axons that have been killed, the fewer that are available to conduct impulses and therefore the lower the amplitudes. Thus, the amplitudes are semiquantitative measures of the number of nerve fibers capable of being activated and of conducting impulses to the recording site. Obviously, if all, or nearly all, the axons being studied have degenerated, then no NCS responses are obtainable. With incomplete axon loss lesions, conduction along the surviving unaffected fibers remains normal. Consequently, the components of the NCS that assess the rate of conduction along a nerve, the latencies and CVs, typically are not materially affected by axon loss, even when it is substantial. (Obviously, when axon loss has been so severe that no NCS responses can be obtained, then the amplitudes are "zero," and neither latencies nor CVs can be determined.) On NEE, motor axon loss lesions cause the denervated muscle fibers to generate fibrillation potentials. Moreover, with rather severe lesions, reduced MUP recruitment is seen. Finally, when the lesions are of at least moderate severity and of at least 6 or more months' duration, chronic neurogenic MUP changes also are observed.

Even though an axon can be killed by a very focal injury, the degenerative process that inevitably follows never remains focal, because the nerve fiber undergoes wallerian degeneration from the site of injury distally. Consequently, the motor, and particularly the sensory, NCS amplitudes are affected by most symptomatic axon loss lesions, irrespective of where the nerve fibers are stimulated in regard to the level of the lesion. Thus, a median CMAP, obtained by recording from the lateral thenar muscles, will be equally low in amplitude, regardless of whether those muscles have been substantially denervated by a lesion at the C8/T1 anterior horn cell level (e.g., motor neuron disease), at the intraspinal C8/T1 root level (e.g., a compressive radiculopathy), at the proximal lower trunk of brachial plexus level (e.g., true neurogenic thoracic outlet syndrome [TOS]), at the medial cord of brachial plexus level (e.g., traumatic brachial plexopathy), at the arm or forearm median nerve level (e.g., traumatic median nerve lesion), or at the wrist level (e.g., very severe carpal tunnel syndrome [CTS]). The SNAPs, in contrast to the CMAPs, are not affected by axon loss lesions within the intraspinal canal; because the preganglionic sensory fibers are being injured, sensory axon degeneration occurs along the central, rather than the peripheral, pathway. In contrast, axon loss lesions that affect the postganglionic sensory fibers, in the plexuses or more distally, separate the peripheral sensory fibers from their cell bodies in the DRG and thereby reduce the SNAP amplitudes. Once the nerve fibers in the distal stump become incapable of conducting impulses, which requires • 7 to 10 days of healing after injury, the location of an axon loss lesion cannot be determined by the NCS amplitude changes it produces. This is because the NCS responses are all equally affected, i.e., low in amplitude or unelicitable, regardless of

whether the stimulation sites are proximal or distal to the lesion (Dumitru, 1995; Isley et al, 1993; Wilbourn, 1992).

Acute focal demyelinating lesions characteristically are manifested as conduction block, which is clinically referred to as "neurapraxia." Conduction block clinically and electrically resembles axon loss: whenever sufficient motor axons are involved, the weakness found on clinical examination and the reduced MUP recruitment seen on NEE are indistinguishable from that which occurs when axon loss affects the same number of motor fibers. Similarly, when sufficient sensory fibers have their transmission blocked at some point along their course, the large fiber sensory deficits that result are identical to those found with axon loss lesions of the same severity. Nonetheless, there are some major differences between axon loss and demyelinating conduction block lesions. First, focal demyelination affects only the large, heavily myelinated sensory fibers. Consequently, those sensory modalities transmitted over unmyelinated and lightly myelinated fibers, such as pain and temperature, are not altered by demyelinating conduction block lesions, as they are with axon loss lesions. Second, focal demyelinating conduction block lesions frequently are accompanied by positive sensory phenomena, such as paresthesias, whereas they are seldom associated with pain, which is mediated over small fibers. In contrast, pain, rather than paresthesias, typically accompanies axon loss. Third, on NCS, focal conduction block lesions are readily recognized if the nerve can be stimulated distal to the lesion site (while recording even more distally), because conduction along the segment of nerve distal to a focal demyelinating lesion is not impaired. Thus, demyelinating conduction block lesions can be localized readily if the nerve can be stimulated both proximal and distal to the lesion site, because low amplitude or unelicitable responses will be elicited on proximal stimulation, whereas much higher amplitude responses will be seen on distal stimulation. This is in contrast to axon loss lesions, in which the amplitudes of the NCS responses are equally low at all stimulation sites (Dumitru, 1995; Wilbourn, 1992). The NEE of muscles supplied by nerves that have sustained a conduction block lesion can yield findings very similar to those caused by axon loss. These include (1) MUP recruitment alterations identical to those seen with axon loss lesions of the same degree; (2) frequent fibrillation potentials, even though they generally are considered characteristic of axon loss. This latter, confusing aspect of demyelinating conduction block lesions occurs because any focal lesion that is severe enough to cause demyelinating conduction block along most axons almost always has been severe enough to kill a few of them; hence, the presence of fibrillation potentials (Fowler et al, 1972).

Only a few focal demyelinating lesions manifest as focal slowing. This fact is surprising to many physicians because of the very common misconception that all focal nerve lesions do so. Focal demyelinating conduction slowing is seen only with a few chronic entrapment syndromes, specifically with most cases of CTS until very late in their courses, at which time axon loss supervenes, and with many (approximately half) of the ulnar neuropathies along the elbow. Similarly, generalized demyelinating slowing is found with some of the demyelinating polyneuropathies and polyradiculoneuropathies, but these occur less commonly than axon loss polyneuropathies. Conduction slowing is rarely seen with any acute-onset PNS lesions, e.g., those due to trauma, and it is not detectable with many chronic PNS lesions, e.g., with true neurogenic TOS and with lesions caused by neoplasms. A pertinent point is that conduction slowing has no correlation with clinical symptoms, such as weakness or static large fiber sensory loss. Consequently, if these are present, then substantial amounts of either conduction block or axon loss, or a combination of both, must be present.

GENERALIZED POLYNEUROPATHIES

A wide variety of disorders can produce the clinical syndrome of a generalized polyneuropathy. The precise mode of evolution as well as the symptoms and signs that are encountered are a product of the pathophysiology of the disorder and the particular nerve fiber types that are affected. With most generalized polyneuropathies, a combination of sensory and motor changes occurs. Autonomic fibers may also be involved, leading to various types of autonomic dysfunction. Thus, the spectrum of clinical symptomatology that can result from a peripheral polyneuropathy may be quite extensive and variable.

As a rule, with generalized polyneuropathies, symptoms begin in the toes and feet and ascend as the condition progresses. Once they are at or above the level of the knees, then similar symptoms often appear in the fingertips and hands. The clinical features, therefore, conform to a "length dependent" pattern, with symptoms evolving in a distal to proximal gradient. This is an important clinical point to consider in the differential diagnosis of PNS symptoms in the upper extremities. Specifically, sensory symptoms involving the hands and fingers should not be attributed to a generalized polyneuropathy until the lower extremity symptoms are at or above knee level. Therefore, hand or finger paresthesias or pain in patients with lower extremity polyneuropathy symptoms restricted to the feet suggest the presence of another process, possibly superimposed entrapment neuropathies such as bilateral CTS, ulnar neuropathy at the elbow, or both. In addition, certain PNS disorders, e.g., those caused by vasculitis, may also cause disproportionate involvement of the upper extremities compared with the lower extremities (Dyck and Thomas, 1993).

Most generalized polyneuropathies are relatively symmetrical in their onset and evolution. However, on occasion they may begin focally, such as in the toes of one foot. Typically, however, they then will gradually spread to the other foot and subsequently ascend bilaterally in a relatively symmetrical fashion. Symptoms that begin and remain highly focal and asymmetrical suggest a focal lesion, such as a nerve infarction.

The sensory complaints with generalized polyneuropathies may include a variety of "positive" symptoms, such as pain, paresthesias, dysesthesias, and hyperpathia. Pain often is the predominant sensory symptom with polyneuropathy. It can range from being dull, diffuse aching, to highly focal, sharp piercing or jabbing sensations. "Negative" sensory complaints also occur. These consist of a "dead feeling," heaviness, or a diminution or lack of sensation in the affected areas. The sensory symptoms with polyneuropathy can range from mild to severe and incapacitating. Typically, when pain

or dysesthesias are prominent, they will be most severe, and therefore most disturbing, at night, interfering with sleep (Dyck and Thomas, 1993; Wilbourn and Shields, 1995).

Motor fiber dysfunction with generalized polyneuropathies may produce various degrees of symptomatic weakness. When only the very distal motor axons are affected—those supplying the intrinsic foot muscles—patients usually are not aware of weakness. However, when the motor fiber involvement ascends to the mid portion of the leg, patients note weakness of toe flexion and, in particular, ankle dorsiflexion, since that results in foot drop. Depending on the severity and chronicity of the process, muscle atrophy may also be observed by the patient. However, because this most often affects only the intrinsic foot muscles, it is rarely reported. Muscle cramps may occur in the distribution of weakened muscles, but generally they are not prominent.

A wide variety of symptoms may result if autonomic fibers are affected. Sudomotor fiber compromise may cause a reduction in sweating. The pattern of involvement tends to follow a distal to proximal gradient, similar to that seen with the sensory and motor fibers. Occasionally, however, patients will report excessive sweating of the face and upper torso. This usually represents hyperhidrosis in unaffected areas that compensates for anhidrosis involving the lower extremities and thorax. Other symptoms of autonomic dysfunction may involve the gastrointestinal tract. Most often patients complain of constipation or alternating constipation and diarrhea, early satiety, and postprandial bloating and belching. These latter symptoms are caused by reduced upper gastrointestinal motility. Urinary retention and incontinence are common symptoms of urinary bladder dysfunction. Erectile impotence in males is a very frequent early indicator of autonomic involvement in many generalized polyneuropathies. When the cardiovascular system is affected, patients may complain of orthostatic lightheadedness or faintness. Such symptoms usually signify rather advanced involvement of the cardiovascular sympathetic nervous system. Finally, various vasomotor symptoms may occur, such as coolness or alternating pale and cyanotic discoloration of the distal limbs (Dyck and Thomas, 1993; Wilbourn and Shields, 1995).

The neurological examination of patients with generalized polyneuropathies will often reveal some alteration of sensory perception, manifested in a distal to proximal gradient, with the lower extremities more involved than the upper extremities. Superficial modalities, i.e., pin prick, light touch, and temperature sense, most often are affected. In addition, vibratory sense and joint position sense may also be abnormal. A Romberg sign may be elicited: the patient is unable to stand with feet together and eyes closed because of dysfunction of the proprioceptive sensory fibers in the lower extremities. With severe involvement of limb proprioceptive fibers, sensory ataxia occurs; purposeful limb movements are severely hampered because of loss of sensory input.

The motor examination with generalized polyneuropathies may disclose mild to moderate degrees of atrophy, especially in the intrinsic foot muscles. In addition, weakness may be detected first in the intrinsic foot muscles by assessing extension and flexion of the toes. The deep tendon reflexes (DTRs) usually are reduced or absent, most often because of compromise of the sensory, rather than the motor, component of the reflex arc. Again, the distribution of these findings follows a distal to proximal gradient, so that the Achilles tendon reflexes are most often involved in the early phase of a generalized polyneuropathy. With severe widespread involvement, generalized areflexia may be found (Dyck and Thomas, 1993).

Assessing autonomic function during the clinical examination is difficult. Blood pressure and pulse may be measured in the reclining and upright positions to evaluate cardiovascular baroreceptor reflex activity. This test, however, is rather insensitive and is not likely to be abnormal until autonomic involvement is rather advanced. If dysautonomia is suspected clinically, patients should be referred for noninvasive cardiovascular reflex tests. These typically include assessing heart rate variability with deep breathing, Valsalva maneuver, and blood pressure and pulse rate responses to head-up tilting. In addition, quantitative assessment of sudomotor function can be performed. Significant gastrointestinal or genitourinary dysfunction should initiate specific investigations of gastrointestinal motility and cystometrics, respectively.

The evaluation of the patient with symptoms and signs of a generalized polyneuropathy must address the rather lengthy list of potential disorders that may produce this syndrome (Table 64–1). A very fundamental method of classifying the generalized polyneuropathies is to divide them according to their mode of evolution: acute versus chronic.

The most important of the acute generalized polyneuropathies (actually, in this case, polyradiculoneuropathy) is the Guillain-Barré syndrome (GBS), an inflammatory demyelinating immune-mediated disorder of the PNS. Guillain-Barré syndrome typically involves motor fibers to a greater extent than sensory fibers. Significant autonomic involvement also is often noted. The syndrome typically evolves over a period of several days to 1 or 2 weeks, in a generalized and relatively symmetrical fashion, with involvement of both distal and proximal muscles. Most often, it follows an infectious illness, especially a nonspecific viral infection. An infection with *Campylobacter jejuni,* a gram-negative rod that causes diarrhea, is the antecedent event in some patients and the pathophysiology typically is axon loss, rather than demyelination. Guillain-Barré syndrome may also be associated with infectious mononucleosis, viral hepatitis, and human immunodeficiency virus (HIV) infection. Guillain-Barré syndrome is a very distinctive clinical entity, and its diagnosis usually is not difficult. It should be suspected whenever a patient develops rather rapidly progressive symmetrical weakness, usually beginning in the lower extremities and frequently accompanied by intense paresthesias. Electrodiagnostic studies often will provide evidence of an acquired demyelinating polyneuropathy/polyradiculoneuropathy by showing conduction blocks or, much less often, focal slowing at various points along the motor nerves; in addition, the SNAPs often are low in amplitude or unelicitable. Examination of the cerebrospinal fluid (CSF) will reveal increased protein with acellular fluid, the so-called cytoalbuminologic dissociation. In most patients, GBS requires hospitalization, usually in an intensive care unit, for close monitoring of pulmonary and autonomic function. In addition, specific treatment against the immune-mediated process will often incorporate plasma exchange treatments or intravenous gammaglobulin therapy. Other disorders that can cause a GBS-like disorder include rare inherited disorders of hemoglobin synthesis, the porphyric neuropathies, and acute intoxication with heavy metals, principally arsenic. A key point concerning arsenic polyneuropathy is that it is virtually always accompanied, or immediately preceded, by gastrointestinal symptoms (Dyck and Thomas, 1993).

Chronic polyneuropathies, usually evolving rather slowly, are the most common type of generalized polyneuropathy. These often are secondary to underlying medical disorders. Consequently, the evaluation of a patient with a chronic generalized polyneuropathy always begins with a careful history that may immediately identify its potential cause, such as diabetes mellitus, alcoholism, nutritional deficiency, uremia, malignancy, exposure to drugs or toxins, endocrine disorders, systemic inflammatory disorders, and heredofamilial factors. For the same reason, it often is useful to perform general screening blood studies that may identify a potential cause. These include a complete blood count, chemical profiles of the blood, fasting blood sugar with 2-hour postprandial blood sugar, vitamin B12 and folic acid levels, serum and urine for protein immunoelectrophoresis, thyroid function studies, and sedimentation rate (Dyck and Thomas, 1993).

Electrodiagnostic studies are performed on all patients with significant symptoms and signs of a chronic generalized polyneuropathy. These are useful not only for documenting the presence of a polyneuropathy, but also in characterizing its underlying pathophysiology as being one of either axon loss or segmental demyelination. Detecting evidence on the NCS of an acquired demyelinative process is extremely valuable, because such EDX findings raise the possibility of chronic inflammatory demyelinating polyneuropathy (CIDP) and related disorders, i.e., polyneuropathy associated with myeloma, osteosclerotic myeloma, monoclonal gammopathy of uncertain significance (MGUS), or HIV infection. The diagnosis in these patients often is clarified by performing a skeletal survey, bone marrow examination, HIV serology, and protein immunoelectrophoresis of the serum and urine. Alternately, the EDX studies may indicate the presence of a multifocal, asymmetrical axon loss process that raises the possibility of a vasculitic neuropathy (discussed below). This possible diagnosis can be further explored by more comprehensive rheumatological screening studies, including antinuclear factor, rheumatoid factor, and other autoantibody assays.

▼ **TABLE 64–1**
Classification of Generalized Polyneuropathies

    Acute polyneuropathies
        Guillain-Barré syndrome
        Porphyric
        Metal
    Chronic polyneuropathies
        Diabetic
        Alcoholic/nutritional
        Uremic
        Paraneoplastic
        Myeloma/dysproteinemia
        Drugs/toxins
        Endocrine disorders
        Infectious disorders
        Sarcoidosis
        Vasculitis
        Amyloidosis
        Heredofamilial
        Chronic inflammatory demyelinating polyneuropathy (CIDP)

There are relatively few indications for lumbar puncture in the evaluation of a chronic generalized polyneuropathy. Usually this procedure is restricted to those patients suspected of having an immune-mediated process, such as CIDP and related disorders, or an inflammatory disorder, such as Lyme disease. With the immune-mediated disorders, CSF analysis often will disclose acellular fluid, elevation of protein, and indications of increased IgG synthesis. With inflammatory disorders, the CSF may show a lymphocytic pleocytosis consistent with a meningitis or meningoencephalitis.

Sural nerve biopsy is helpful in identifying immune-mediated polyneuropathy and vasculitic disorders when the EDX studies or CSF findings are atypical or inconclusive. It also aids in detecting systemic amyloidosis, although typically the diagnosis of that disorder may be confirmed by the biopsy of other tissues that may be affected, especially the rectal mucosa and abdominal fat pad. Occasionally, a nerve biopsy is obtained on a patient with a rather severe, evolving sensorimotor polyneuropathy of unknown cause in an effort, all-too-often futile, to find a treatable etiology. Nonetheless, with most chronic polyneuropathies, sural nerve biopsy is nondiagnostic and unhelpful. Consequently, it has limited applicability; unlike EDX studies, it definitely is not an indicated procedure in the routine assessment of patients with chronic polyneuropathy (Dyck and Thomas, 1993).

The most common chronic sensorimotor polyneuropathy of known cause encountered in North America is diabetic distal symmetrical polyneuropathy (DDSPN). This disorder accounts for approximately 75% of all "diabetic neuropathies"; the latter is an umbrella designation for all diabetes mellitus–related disorders of the somatic and autonomic nervous systems as well as some of the cranial nerves (Wilbourn and Shields, 1995). Approximately 90% of diabetics have type II, or mature-onset, diabetes, which usually begins after age 30 or 40 and increases substantially in incidence with each decade of life. Moreover, among the population with diabetes, the instance of DDSPN has a high correlation with the duration of the disease process. For these two reasons, most DDSPN occurs in the elderly (Wilbourn, 1993b).

The symptoms of DDSPN can vary markedly in their onset, course, and severity. Some patients are asymptomatic, although EDX studies often will show definite evidence of a mild polyneuropathy. Most patients, however, have symptoms, usually sensory in nature and most often consisting of various types of painful paresthesias or hyperpathia. These typically begin in the toes and are usually bilateral and symmetrical, but sometimes bilateral and asymmetrical and occasionally unilateral initially. They often develop insidiously and progress proximally in the limbs. Occasionally, DDSPN begins in a much more abrupt fashion and evolves much more rapidly, affecting the motor and sensory fibers, and often is accompanied by substantial weight loss. Symptoms of DDSPN may be the first manifestation of diabetes in a patient not known to have the disease; also, in known diabetics, DDSPN is sometimes triggered by stressful events, such as surgical procedures. Thus, diabetes mellitus and DDSPN should be considered in the differential diagnosis whenever a patient in the postoperative period (for example, after hip surgery), begins to complain of sensory symptoms in both feet.

The EDX features of DDSPN are rather nonspecific. They are indicative of an axon-loss polyneuropathy, often accompanied by some mild slowing that is suggestive but not severe enough to be diagnostic of a demyelinating component as well. The EDX findings with DDSPN, similar to the clinical findings, can range from mild, and when restricted to the lower extremities, to very severe and diffuse. One confounding feature regarding the EDX changes that occur with DDSPN is that frequently, on NEE, fibrillation potentials are found bilaterally in the lumbar paraspinal muscles. Thus, their value for detecting a compressive radiculopathy in these patients is seriously compromised. Electrodiagnostic studies should be performed on every patient with suspected DDSPN; the diagnosis can be confirmed in most cases and the severity of the process can be determined, if for no other reason than to obtain a baseline. Moreover, other disorders that may mimic DDSPN clinically can be excluded. It is important to remember that diabetic patients experience the same incidence of non–diabetes-related neurological diseases as do patients without diabetes. Consequently, it is important to exclude other disorders, particularly treatable ones, before concluding that polyneuropathy symptoms in a patient with diabetes are due to DDSPN. We have seen patients with diabetes who had their CIDP go untreated for years because their symptoms had been erroneously attributed to DDSPN, and EDX studies had not been considered necessary. The EDX features of DDSPN are rather nonspecific; they cannot confirm that a nonspecific generalized symmetrical polyneuropathy found in a diabetic patient represents DDSPN. However, in some instances the EDX studies can definitely exclude DDSPN as the cause, e.g., DDSPN is never manifested electrically as a demyelinating polyradiculopathy and only very rarely as a "pure" sensory polyneuropathy (Wilbourn, 1993b).

Examination of the CSF rarely is indicated in evaluating patients with suspected DDSPN because it will either be normal or show only a modest elevation in protein. Similarly, nerve biopsy is not indicated because it will reveal only evidence of a nonspecific process, primarily axon loss. Autonomic testing is sometimes helpful because it is now appreciated that dysfunction of the autonomic nervous system tends to parallel that of the PNS, and symptoms caused by the autonomic nervous system may dominate the clinical presentation.

Peripheral nerves affected by polyneuropathy often are more vulnerable to focal entrapment or compressive lesions. This is particularly the case with DDSPN. We have found in our EMG laboratory population that about half of patients younger than age 50 with DDSPN have superimposed CTS, whereas almost two thirds of those older than age 50 do so. Ulnar neuropathy at the elbow is also commonly encountered with DDSPN. In fact, in our experience, the majority of patients with bilateral CTS and bilateral ulnar neuropathy at the elbow are diabetic patients with DDSPN. In diabetic patients, focal lesions caused by compression or entrapment must be clearly separated from those that are a component of mononeuropathy multiplex (discussed in the next section). The latter, caused by focal axon loss resulting from vasculitic nerve infarcts, are nonoperative lesions. In contrast, the focal entrapment and compressive lesions that occur with DDSPN should respond well to operative intervention, as long as they are not end-stage. Thus, studies have demonstrated very satisfactory results after carpal tunnel release in patients who have a symptomatic CTS superimposed on a DDSPN (Clayburgh et al, 1987; Dobyns, 1991). Clinical clues to the presence of underlying entrapment or compression include focal or asymmetrical sensory and motor symptoms in the upper extremities and symmetrical upper extremity symptoms that occur in a patient whose DDSPN is so mild that the lower extremity complaints are limited to the feet. Confirming the presence of such a compressive or entrapment lesion by EDX studies is easily accomplished in patients with mild polyneuropathy but becomes increasingly difficult as the polyneuropathy becomes more severe (Wilbourn, 1993).

Although surgery is the mainstay of therapy for patients who have focal entrapment or compressive lesions superimposed on DDSPN, there is no convincing evidence, in spite of one report to the contrary (Dillon, 1988), that the sensorimotor disturbances in the lower extremities in patients with DDSPN are the products of multiple compressions or entrapments, rather than simply the generalized PNS dysfunction itself. Consequently, there appears to be no role for distal lower extremity surgical decompressions in these patients to treat their DDSPN symptoms. On the contrary, the fact that many of these patients have not only distal peripheral and autonomic nerve fiber deficits, but also impaired distal limb circulation, which often leads to poor wound healing, renders such surgical treatments ill-advised.

Patients in renal failure frequently develop a uremic polyneuropathy. Both the clinical and EDX features of this chronic, axon loss polyneuropathy are rather nonspecific. Confounding the situation is that often the renal failure is caused by end-stage diabetic nephropathy. Thus, there are two possible etiologies for the polyneuropathy changes, diabetic and uremic. These cannot be distinguished from one another by EDX studies (Dyck and Thomas, 1993).

The decision to investigate a patient for an occult malignancy as a cause for a chronic generalized polyneuropathy is usually prompted by the presence of a progressive polyneuropathy of uncertain or unknown cause. In these patients, a careful physical examination is followed by imaging of the chest, abdomen, and pelvis, frequently with the use of computed tomography (CT) or magnetic resonance imaging (MRI) scans. The yield for these "occult malignancy evaluations" typically is very low. On the other hand, patients with polyneuropathies highly characteristic of a paraneoplastic process should have very careful evaluation for an occult malignancy. One type of paraneoplastic polyneuropathy is the so-called pure sensory neuropathy syndrome that occurs in patients with small cell cancer of the lung. This disorder will be discussed in the next section.

Heredofamilial polyneuropathies are often diagnosed on the basis of a positive family history and characteristic clinical and EDX features. Some of the hereditary polyneuropathies can now also be diagnosed by genetic testing. This is the case for Charcot-Marie-Tooth disease or Hereditary Motor-Sensory Neuropathy, Type I.

Despite careful, methodical, and comprehensive evaluation of patients with chronic generalized polyneuropathy, in about 40% a definite etiology will not be established. It is prudent to continue to follow these patients very closely and observe the further evolution of their disease, because this may provide additional clues to the cause of their disorder. Such an approach sometimes requires reassessing them clinically at 6 to 12 month intervals and repeating various laboratory and clinical tests (Dyck and Thomas, 1993).

PNS SIMULATORS OF FOCAL COMPRESSIVE/ ENTRAPMENT LESIONS

Several disorders will now be discussed that can produce PNS findings readily mistaken for those caused by focal compressive or entrapment lesions, or for more common focal lesions. These can result not only in unnecessary operative procedures at the root, plexus, or peripheral nerve level, but also in delays in recognition of the actual etiology and in postponement of appropriate therapy. Some of these entities frequently develop under circumstances in which they are readily confused with iatrogenic PNS lesions. Hence, if unrecognized, they can serve as a nidus for initiation of unjustified medicolegal actions. Their underlying causes are variable, but the pathophysiology most often directly responsible for symptom production is axon loss. These disorders will be discussed according to the symptoms they produce: solely or predominantly motor, solely or predominantly sensory, and motor and sensory complaints.

Motor or Predominantly Motor Disorders

Amyotrophic Lateral Sclerosis (ALS). This fatal disorder is the most common form of motor neuron disease. Of unknown etiology, it results from progressive degeneration of the motor neurons of the cortex, brain stem, and spinal cord. It affects men somewhat more than women; the majority of patients are older than 50 years. The pathognomonic feature of ALS is simultaneous involvement of both the upper and lower motor neurons. In approximately 30% of patients, the initial symptoms are dysarthria and dysphagia, indicative of brain stem (bulbar) involvement. In the remaining 70%, the initial symptoms are weakness, muscle cramps, and wasting of various upper or lower extremity muscles. Characteristically, in the limbs the disorder begins focally or at least asymmetrically. Because sensory symptoms are lacking, lower motor neuron involvement can be rather marked, with prominent weakness and atrophy, before functional loss is apparent (Mulder, 1980).

Two very characteristic limb presentations of ALS are weakness and wasting of the intrinsic hand muscles, particularly the first dorsal interosseous (FDI), and weakness of the tibialis anterior muscle, resulting in foot drop. When ALS is not considered in the differential diagnosis of patients who have these early findings, the hand changes often are mistaken for C8 radiculopathies or, even more commonly, ulnar neuropathies at the elbow or in the hand, and the lower extremity symptoms commonly are attributed to L5 radiculopathies. Many unnecessary surgical procedures then are performed. Another misleading presentation we have encountered with some frequency is bilateral, multisegmental lower extremity involvement, usually asymmetrical, suggestive of a cauda equina lesion—a common syndrome in this age group, because of lumbar canal stenosis.

Whenever patients, particularly elderly men, have progressive, painless weakness, wasting, and often cramping of various limb muscles, but with retained or heightened DTRs,

ALS should be considered in the differential diagnosis. It should also be considered whenever a patient appears to have a very severe, progressive cauda equina lesion without back pain, sphincter dysfunction, or sensory loss.

The EDX examination can be very helpful in the diagnosis of ALS for several reasons. First, it can separate lower motor neuron from upper motor neuron involvement by demonstrating, with the former, evidence of active and chronic denervation (i.e., fibrillation potentials, chronic neurogenic MUP changes, and sometimes reduced MUP recruitment), as well as MUP irritation (i.e., fasciculation potentials). Second, it can show that the responsible lower motor neuron lesion is within the intraspinal canal. Third, it can reveal that the lower motor neuron involvement is more widespread than clinically suspected. Fourth, it can exclude other disorders that clinically may be confused with ALS, e.g., polymyositis, myasthenia gravis, and ulnar neuropathy in the hand (Mulder, 1980).

Benign focal motor neuron disease represents a small subgroup of motor neuron disease that is especially likely to be confused with a surgically treatable disorder. In contrast to typical ALS, this uncommon entity occurs in young adults, usually males, and has a marked tendency to involve the C8 and T1 segments. Often, it begins unilaterally and then becomes bilateral, usually asymmetrical, with the initial side persistently the more severe. These patients typically are considered to have C8/T1 cervical radiculopathies or ulnar neuropathies. The EDX examination can demonstrate that the motor abnormalities are caused by a cervical intraspinal canal lesion rather than an ulnar neuropathy, but it cannot distinguish this degenerative focal cervical spinal cord lesion from other focal intraspinal canal lesions at the same level, such as a syrinx, a neoplasm, or even root compression. Consequently, these other disorders must be excluded by neuroimaging studies.

True Neurogenic Thoracic Outlet Syndrome. This rare disorder is seen almost solely in young to middle-aged females. It is caused by a congenital anomaly: a radiolucent cervical band extending from the tip of a rudimentary cervical rib, or just an elongated C7 transverse process, to the normal first thoracic rib. The C8 and T1 anterior primary rami (APR), particularly the latter, sustain slowly progressive axon loss damage by being stretched and angulated around this congenital band. Clinically, all the intrinsic hand muscles are weak, and in the majority of patients they are all wasted as well. However, the lateral thenar muscles, i.e., those innervated by the median nerve, are always the most severely involved, and in approximately 25% of the patients they are the only intrinsic hand muscles that are obviously wasted. With severe involvement of the C8 APR, the medial forearm muscles are also weak and atrophic. The motor disturbance characteristically is much more severe than the sensory. Some patients have no sensory symptoms at all, whereas others experience intermittent paresthesias and aching along the medial forearm, sometimes extending into the medial aspect of the hand. These sensory complaints may be present for months to years, but seldom are they severe enough to cause the patients to seek medical attention. Instead, their disorder is first recognized when their hand wasting is noticed by themselves or by others.

The EDX findings with true neurogenic TOS are almost pathognomonic, revealing a very chronic axon-loss lesion involving the proximal lower trunk, particularly the T1 fibers. Thus, the amplitudes of the median motor and the medial antebrachial cutaneous NCS responses are severely affected, whereas the amplitude of the ulnar sensory NCS response is less involved; the ulnar motor response amplitudes usually are in the low-normal range. Radiographs of the neck show the bony abnormality; frequently, cervical ribs are present bilaterally, with the larger rib on the asymptomatic side. In contrast, the cervical band that is directly responsible for the injury to the APR fibers is not visible on radiographic examination and often cannot be demonstrated on MRI.

The appropriate treatment for this congenital disorder is sectioning of the band via a supraclavicular surgical approach. The transaxillary approach, which is the standard operative procedure used for removing the normal first thoracic rib, is not a satisfactory substitute. After resection of the cervical band, the hand and medial forearm wasting is arrested, the intermittent medial forearm aching disappears, and in some patients, the medial forearm bulk is at least partially restored. However, as with any very severe, chronic axon loss lower trunk brachial plexopathy, intrinsic hand muscle strength and bulk are not regained (Gilliatt, 1986; Wilbourn, 1993a).

Patients with true neurogenic TOS frequently undergo unnecessary cervical laminectomies, CTS surgery, and even ulnar nerve operations at the elbow before the actual cause for their symptoms is appreciated. It is ironic that TOS surgery—specifically transaxillary rib resection, anterior scalenectomy, or both—is performed so readily on so many patients to treat a highly debatable type of neurogenic TOS, whereas it typically is delayed, often for long periods, in this small group of patients with neurogenic TOS who will definitely benefit from operation.

True neurogenic TOS should be suspected whenever a young or middle-aged woman presents with hand weakness and wasting, especially if the lateral thenar eminence is the most affected and yet median nerve sensation in the hand is intact. Carpal tunnel syndrome substantial enough to cause marked lateral thenar wasting is rarely seen in young women, and strictly unilateral CTS of this severity is rarer still. Moreover, any CTS this severe invariably will have associated marked sensory loss in a median nerve hand and finger distribution. The diagnosis of a substantial axon loss ulnar neuropathy is not consistent with the lateral thenar muscles being the most severely involved. Finally, the possibility that a single cervical radiculopathy, either C8 or T1, is capable of causing this much atrophy is quite remote, particularly in view of the patient's age and the lack of neck complaints.

Multifocal Motor Neuropathy (MMN). This is an uncommon disorder that only recently has been recognized. It principally affects young adults and persists over many years. Clinically, it causes progressive weakness and atrophy with cramps, fasciculations and sometimes myokymia in the distribution of two or more peripheral nerves, most often in the upper extremities. The weakness often is caused by prolonged demyelinating conduction block, so muscle bulk may be retained; in other instances, however, it is caused by axon loss, and the muscle subsequently is quite atrophic. Nerve fiber enlargement is not generally detectable. Although the MMN implies that only motor fibers are involved, some sensory changes are usually present as well, although usually only minor in degree. These can consist of paresthesias in the distribution of the affected nerve(s) (often associated with severe weakness and atrophy in the same distribution) or simply loss of DTRs that cannot be explained by the degree of motor involvement. The etiology of this disorder continues to be debated. Although it has a superficial resemblance to ALS, most authorities consider it to be a variant of CIDP. Electrodiagnostic studies are vital for diagnosis because they demonstrate the prominent motor conduction blocks that are the hallmark of the disease. Nonetheless, sensory NCS involvement and evidence of motor axon loss usually are also present. High concentrations of both IgG and IgM antibodies to GM_1 ganglioside are seen in some, but not all, patients. However, similarly elevated levels can be seen with other PNS disorders. As a result, the presence or absence of these antibodies neither confirms nor excludes the diagnosis (Parry and Sumner, 1992).

The focal nerve lesions caused by MMN may be erroneously attributed to those caused by compression/entrapment. This is likely to occur early in the course of the disorder, when only one or two peripheral nerves are affected. However, decompressive nerve surgery not only does not relieve the symptoms, but it may also be performed on a nerve segment that does not contain the lesion because MMN typically affects nerves at other than the usual compressive/entrapment sites. Thus, a patient with a slowly progressive proximal median nerve lesion is considered to have pronator syndrome and has his or her nerve decompressed near the elbow. Only after it is obvious that this operation had no effect are extensive EDX studies performed, which reveal that the lesion is affecting the median nerve in the mid-arm. Later in its course, when several nerves are involved, MMN most often is mistaken for ALS (Parry and Sumner, 1992).

This disorder can trigger personal-injury lawsuits. We are aware of two patients who sued for damages, attributing their symptoms to coincidental injuries. A 19-year-old woman, for example, considered her marked static right hand weakness had resulted from an automobile accident, although her symptoms did not even begin until several months after the accident had occurred. Even though we could demonstrate that she had a prominent conduction block along her ulnar nerve in the midarm, and not a lower trunk brachial plexopathy caused by "traumatic" TOS, as was suspected by her physicians, she still underwent a transaxillary first rib resection; as would be expected, this operation had no effect on her symptoms.

Multifocal motor neuropathy should be suspected whenever a young to middle-aged person has one or more very slowly progressive PNS lesions, usually along major limb nerves, that are causing very disproportionately motor, as opposed to sensory, symptoms. The suspicion should be especially high if, on EDX studies, the lesion or lesions can be shown to be predominantly conduction block in nature and located at points along the nerves that only very rarely are the sites of entrapment, e.g., along the ulnar nerve in the mid-forearm or mid-arm, rather than at the elbow segment.

Predominantly Sensory Disorders

"Pure" Sensory Polyneuropathies. Approximately 2% of all polyneuropathies involve only sensory fibers. These have a great variety of causes, including hereditary, paraneoplastic, immune-mediated, metabolic, toxic (including vitamin B6 overdose), and HIV infection. Nearly half, however, are idiopathic in nature; patients in this latter group often are elderly women. With "pure" sensory polyneuropathies, pain and paresthesias may begin distally in the lower extremities in a symmetrical fashion, but they also may first appear in the upper extremities, either bilateral but asymmetrical or unilateral. On EDX studies, some or all of the SNAPs are low in amplitude or unelicitable, and both the motor NCS and the NEE are normal (Mitsumoto and Wilbourn, 1994).

Whenever upper extremity symptoms result from "pure" sensory polyneuropathies, they frequently are thought to be caused by focal compressive or entrapment lesions. Many unnecessary operations are performed in vain efforts to treat them. The most common misdiagnosis of this nature is to have sensory disturbances in one or more of the lateral four fingers be mistaken for CTS symptoms, even though both the clinical and EDX features are not typical for that disorder. Clinically, the complaint is persistent, nonfluctuating "numbness," and sometimes pain, which may have developed rather abruptly; nocturnal exaggeration of symptoms is conspicuously absent. On EDX studies, the median SNAPs recorded from the involved digits are not prolonged in peak latency, as typically is seen with CTS. Instead, they are low in amplitude with normal peak latencies or even unelicitable; these changes are suggestive of axon loss. When the median SNAPs are unelicitable, the fact that the median motor NCS, including the distal latencies, are normal virtually excludes CTS. Patients with "pure" sensory polyneuropathies require an extensive evaluation, preferably by a neurologist who specializes in peripheral nerve disorders; even some neurologists elect to refer these patients rather than attempting these assessments themselves.

Radiation-Induced Brachial Plexopathies. Some patients develop a progressive brachial plexopathy after receiving forequarter radiation therapy; most are women whose axillary lymph node chains were radiated in the course of their therapy for breast cancer. The latency period between radiation treatment and onset of symptoms is remarkably wide, ranging from almost immediately after completion of therapy to 34 years later. Paresthesias generally are the first symptom of radiation-induced brachial plexopathy, and often they are the only symptoms for years. The most typical presentation is the appearance of paresthesias and a fixed sensory deficit in one or more of the median nerve–innervated fingers. As time passes, other fingers are involved, and the sensory disturbance appears in other nerve distributions. At some point, motor weakness becomes apparent and tends to slowly spread throughout the limb. Although the clinical course is somewhat variable, the most common is slow progression, ultimately resulting, after many years, in a completely useless appendage, due to a combination of rather substantial motor deficits and marked sensory ataxia. The underlying pathophysiology with radiation-induced brachial plexopathy is an unusual type of demyelinating conduction block, similar to that seen with MMN but very different from that which occurs with many acute onset traumatic lesions. It is persistent, rather than short-lived, in nature; instead of ultimately resolving as the conduction blocks underlying neurapraxia always do, it simply persists indefinitely or converts to axon loss. There is no effective treatment. On EDX studies, the SNAPs recorded from the symptomatic fingers are of normal peak latency but low in amplitude. In all but its earliest stages, this disorder frequently has characteristic EDX features, seen on both NCS and NEE. On NCS, conduction blocks often can be demonstrated between the supraclavicular and axilla stimulation points, indicating the lesion is affecting the distal trunks, the divisions, or the proximal cords of the brachial plexus. On NEE, an unusual type of spontaneous activity, called myokymic discharges, is sometimes seen (Wilbourn, 1993a).

Many of the patients we have seen with radiation-induced brachial plexopathy have undergone operations to treat various focal compressive or entrapment lesions, particularly CTS. Some have been subjected to multiple fruitless surgical procedures; one of our patients had three CTS releases over several years, none of which proved beneficial.

Radiation-induced brachial plexopathy should always be considered in the differential diagnosis whenever limb paresthesias develop in a patient who had radiation therapy to the ipsilateral axilla or the supraclavicular regions, regardless of the number of years that have elapsed since the therapy was given. Electrodiagnostic studies always should be performed on these patients; if the SNAPs are low in amplitude with normal peak latencies, the findings are very likely caused by radiation and are not the result of a focal compression or entrapment lesion.

Predominantly Motor and Sensory Disorders

Neuralgic Amyotrophy (Brachial Neuritis; Parsonage-Turner Syndrome). This uncommon disorder affects mainly adults, often young adults. It is of unknown cause and produces axon loss. Neuralgic amyotrophy usually is considered a type of brachial plexopathy, although it most likely results from involvement of one or more nerves that supply the proximal upper extremity or shoulder girdle. It can be both familial and acquired, although the latter is far more common. In most patients it appears to be triggered by some nonspecific antecedent event, such as a nondescript upper respiratory infection, inoculation, trauma, and hospitalization for any reason, including childbirth, medical disorders, and surgical procedures. It has a striking tendency to begin at night, awakening the patient from sleep. Its characteristic presenting symptom is pain that most often is localized to the shoulder region, abrupt in onset, and very severe in degree. Weakness and subsequent atrophy of various shoulder girdle and upper extremity muscles soon are obvious, usually within a week of onset. In many patients, the abnormalities are limited to the distribution of one or two peripheral nerves, such as the suprascapular, long thoracic, axillary, or anterior interosseous. In other patients, however, multiple nerves are involved, and often all of them derive from the upper trunk of the brachial plexus. (Hence, the tendency to consider this disorder a brachial plexus lesion.) The main trunks of the more distal limb nerves—median, ulnar, and radial—seldom are affected. Occasionally, extraplexal nerves, such as the spinal accessory and phrenic, are involved. In part because neuralgic amyotrophy has a marked

propensity to affect motor nerves, sensory loss usually is undetectable or restricted to the lateral shoulder (if there is axillary nerve involvement). Most often only one limb is affected, but bilateral involvement, either simultaneously or sequentially, occurs with some frequency. When bilateral, asymmetry is the rule. Recurrent attacks also occur. Although the pain usually abates within a few weeks, and often even sooner, the weakness and wasting caused by axon loss typically persists for months to years. There is no effective treatment, although the pain may respond to high-dose steroid therapy (Parsonage and Turner, 1948; Wilbourn, 1993a).

The diagnosis of neuralgic amyotrophy depends on the clinical and EDX examinations; neuroimaging studies are unrevealing. On EDX examination there is evidence of one or more axon loss peripheral nerve lesions, often severe. One of the characteristic findings is dissociated involvement of the muscles innervated by an affected nerve. Thus, the infraspinatus muscle may be severely denervated while the supraspinatus shows only minimal, if any, changes. Another common finding is branch lesions; e.g., the pronator teres is severely denervated, but similar changes are not found in any other C6 or C7/median nerve–innervated muscles. The EDX study often demonstrates that the process is more extensive than it appears to be clinically.

Very few surgeons, including those who deal extensively with PNS lesions, possess a clear understanding of neuralgic amyotrophy. This is regrettable because, as a result of the incidence of this disorder, they are very likely to encounter several patients with it during their professional careers. Whenever it is not considered in the differential diagnosis, patients may undergo unneeded operations for cervical radiculopathies (especially C5 or C6), rotation cuff tears, and traumatic mononeuropathies. Moreover, neuralgic amyotrophy has great potential for being the initiating factor in unjustified medicolegal litigation. Whenever patients suddenly develop severe shoulder pain, followed rapidly by weakness and wasting of various upper limb muscles, within a few hours or days of childbirth, open heart surgery, a knee repair, a herniorrhaphy, or even an arteriogram, and yet none of the medical personnel attending them can provide reasonable explanations for their symptoms, lawsuits follow. Finally, many physicians readily testify in these instances that the pain and disability resulted from iatrogenic injuries, simply because, being unaware of neuralgic amyotrophy, they know of no other possible reason for their occurrence.

Neuralgic amyotrophy generally is not a diagnosis of exclusion. Instead, it should be considered the most likely etiology whenever someone, particularly a young person, suddenly develops severe pain about the shoulder and, soon after, weakness and wasting of various muscles, most often shoulder girdle muscles, especially if he or she were awakened from sleep by the pain, and if he or she has no neck stiffness or interscapular pain. The same admonition applies whenever someone is suspected of having sustained a traumatic or iatrogenic injury, e.g., while playing football or undergoing a surgical procedure, and yet detailed questioning reveals that several hours to a few days elapsed between the time of the reputed causal event and the abrupt onset of symptoms. Thus, a high school student who plays in a football game on Friday evening and is asymptomatic until 2 a.m. Sunday, when he is awakened from sleep by pain, does not have a traumatic nerve lesion sustained during the athletic contest; he has neuralgic amyotrophy. Detecting the "latent period" between the suspected antecedent event and the onset of symptoms is one of the most helpful clinical points in determining the correct diagnosis. The EDX examination can also be very beneficial. Not only may it demonstrate that the abnormalities are more extensive than clinically apparent, but also it often reveals one or more EDX features so typical of neuralgic amyotrophy (Wilbourn, 1993a).

Mononeuropathy Multiplex. This syndrome is defined as involvement of two or more peripheral nerves, usually sequentially and in different limbs. With few exceptions, these are axon loss lesions; generally, the pathogenesis is a necrotizing vasculitis producing partial or complete occlusion of principally small- to medium-sized arteries. Listing this disorder under "sensory-motor presentations" is somewhat arbitrary because, depending on the particular nerve fibers involved, the symptoms may be solely sensory or solely motor in nature as well as mixed. Moreover, sometimes only one lesion of the PNS occurs, rather than two or more, so this disorder can present as a single axon loss mononeuropathy. There are multiple causes for mononeuropathy multiplex, the most common being one of the vasculitides such as hypersensitivity vasculitis (which includes the collagen vascular subgroup) and the polyarteritis nodosa group. Mononeuropathy multiplex also can be seen with several disorders not customarily classified as vasculitides, including diabetes mellitus and HIV disease.

Mononeuropathy multiplex most often affects peripheral nerves, rather than roots or plexus elements. The nerve most frequently involved is the peroneal; the median and ulnar nerves are also commonly affected. The amount of nerve fiber involvement can be extremely variable, ranging from virtually complete and producing a severe, static deficit, to so mild that it is essentially asymptomatic and detectable only by it causing relatively minor EDX changes. Although vasculitis frequently presents as a mononeuropathy or mononeuropathy multiplex, it is important to remember that it can also present as a generalized polyneuropathy as a result of involvement of multiple distal lower extremity nerves bilaterally, with resulting confluence of symptoms (Kissel and Mendell, 1992; Wilbourn and Levin, 1993).

Mononeuropathy multiplex usually begins abruptly. However, sometimes the presentation is subacute, evolving over several hours to a few days. The lesions that result tend to be located along nerve trunks at points other than the usual compressive/entrapment sites, e.g., along the median and ulnar nerves in the arm and the peroneal nerve in the distal thigh. Pain, paresthesias, and weakness are the most common symptoms; once established, they characteristically are fixed and nonvariable (Kissel and Mendell, 1992; Kissel et al, 1985). Thus, one patient we studied was awakened from sleep by the sudden onset of painful paresthesias in one of her index fingers. These symptoms persisted, without change, for several months. Unfortunately, during this period they were attributed to CTS by one of her physicians, and she subsequently underwent a CTS release that proved to be of no benefit.

This syndrome should be suspected whenever a patient suddenly and spontaneously develops symptoms in the distribution of a single peripheral nerve, particularly if it is followed, after a variable period of time, by similar abrupt involvement of another peripheral nerve that is often, but not always, in a different limb. When this occurs in patients with certain medical disorders, such as diabetes mellitus or one of the collagen vascular diseases, the diagnosis usually is rather obvious. When there is no known underlying medical disorder, an extensive evaluation typically is required.

Both nerve and muscle biopsy can be helpful in establishing the presence of a vasculitic process. The EDX examination can readily separate median nerve lesions caused by nerve infarct from those caused by CTS; the former process causes solely axon loss, and this affects the amplitudes of the SNAPs and CMAPs, rather than their latencies or CVs. Moreover, because with median nerve infarcts the lesion is usually situated in the arm segment, the NEE shows active denervation and often MUP loss in all the median nerve-innervated muscles, including those innervated by the main trunk proximal to the carpal tunnel. Electrodiagnostic studies are of less help in determining the etiology of ulnar and peroneal mononeuropathies because these frequently present as axon loss lesions when caused by compression or entrapment. Nonetheless, the EDX examination in many cases reveals the lesion is focal demyelinating in nature, and therefore not only localizes it but excludes vasculitis as its cause. In all cases, it can demonstrate the extent of axon loss and its boundaries (Wilbourn et al, 1983).

Ischemic Monomelic Neuropathy (IMN). This entity could be considered a type of mononeuropathy multiplex because more than one peripheral nerve is always involved. However, with IMN the affected nerves are all in the same limb, and they all are injured simultaneously because of transient compromise of the arterial blood flow in the limb. Causes for this include occlusion of the major proximal limb artery or the shunting of blood from it. Although all the more distal limb structures are rendered ischemic by this temporary blood flow compromise, only the peripheral nerves apparently sustain structural damage. This entity can occur in both the upper and lower extremities; in either case the clinical and EDX presentations are remarkably stereotyped. Pain is the most prominent symptom; it is persistent and burning in character, and it is most severe in the palm and fingers with upper extremity IMN, and in the foot and toes with lower extremity IMN. Sensory and motor deficits are also present, which are significant only in the hands and feet. A distal to proximal gradient of change invariably is seen, with essentially no abnormalities present proximal to the mid-forearm or mid-leg. Within the affected portions of the limbs, the PNS findings are not limited to or distinctly more pronounced in the distribution of any single peripheral nerve; rather, they are fairly uniform circumferentially at any particular level, regardless of nerve supply (Wilbourn et al, 1983; Wilbourn and Levin, 1993).

Upper extremity IMN has, for practical purposes, only one cause: the construction of arteriovenous shunts, for dialysis purposes, in the arms of diabetic patients who are in renal failure. With lower extremity IMN, which occurs more frequently than does upper extremity IMN, the causes are more diverse, and the patients are, as a group, considerably older. Moreover, only a minority of the lesions are iatrogenic in nature; these are caused by cannulation of the superficial femoral artery, either for cardiopulmonary bypass or for use of an intra-aortic balloon pump. Noniatrogenic causes include thrombosis of the superficial femoral artery or iliofemoral artery and aortoiliac emboli.

On EDX studies, the striking distal to proximal gradient of abnormalities noted on the clinical examination is confirmed. Electrophysiologically, IMN presents as a rather severe axon loss polyneuropathy involving a single limb. On NCS, only the amplitudes are affected, and how severely involved they are depends almost solely on the segment of nerve studied; the more distal in the limb it is, the more affected the NCS amplitude is. Thus, the median SNAPs recorded from the various fingers often are unelicitable, whereas the radial SNAP, recorded somewhat more proximal, may be present, although low in amplitude. The distal to proximal gradient of axon degeneration is particularly obvious on the NEE. Fibrillation potentials and MUP loss are substantial in the intrinsic hand and foot muscles and equally severe in all of them, regardless of their particular nerve innervation. The changes are much less prominent in the distal forearm and leg muscles and are essentially undetectable in the proximal forearm and leg muscles (Wilbourn et al, 1983; Wilbourn and Levin, 1993).

Ischemic monomelic neuropathy must be distinguished from multiple compression and entrapment neuropathies, from infarction of major peripheral nerve trunks (such as the sciatic nerve in the lower extremity), and from plexus lesions. Because so many cases of IMN are iatrogenic, this disorder has significant medicolegal implications. In many instances, however, particularly when it follows placement of intra-aortic balloon pumps in critically ill patients, IMN is both unpredictable and unavoidable.

Upper extremity IMN should be suspected whenever a patient with diabetes in renal failure begins to complain of burning hand pain and weakness after placement of an arteriovenous shunt in the arm. Lower extremity IMN should be considered whenever a patient experiences severe burning foot pain after open heart surgery, the temporary use of an intra-aortic balloon pump, or spontaneous thrombosis of the femoral artery. Because the latter often is promptly followed by a vascular reconstructive procedure to restore blood flow, the symptoms produced by IMN may mistakenly be attributed, by both patients and physicians, to iatrogenic injury (Wilbourn et al, 1983; Wilbourn and Levin, 1993).

References

Clayburgh RH, Beckenbaugh RD, Dobyns JH: Carpal tunnel release in patients with diffuse peripheral neuropathies. J Hand Surg (Am) *12*:380–383, 1987.

Dillon AL: A cause for optimism in diabetic neuropathy. Ann Plast Surg *20*:103–105, 1988.

Dobyns JH: Carpal tunnel release in patients with peripheral neuropathy. *In* Gelberman RH (ed): Operative Nerve Repair and Reconstruction. Philadelphia, JB Lippincott, 1991, pp 963–965.

Dumitru D: Electrodiagnostic Medicine. Philadelphia, Hanley & Belfus, 1995.

Dyck PJ, Thomas PK (eds): Peripheral Neuropathy, ed 3. Philadelphia, WB Saunders, 1993.

Fowler TJ, Danta G, Gilliatt RW: Recovery of nerve conduction after a pneumatic tourniquet: Observations on the hind limb of the baboon. J Neurol Neurosurg Psychiatry *35*:638–647, 1972.

Gilliatt RW: Thoracic outlet syndromes. *In* Dyck PJ, Thomas PK, Lambert EH, Bunge R (eds): Peripheral Neuropathy, ed 2. Philadelphia, WB Saunders, 1986, pp 1409–1424.

Isley MR, Krauss GL, Levin KH, Litt B, Shields RW, Wilbourn AJ: Electromyography/Electroencephalography. Redford, WA, Spacelabs Medical Inc., 1993.

Kissel JT, Mendell JR: Vasculitic neuropathy. Neurol Clin *10*:761–781, 1992.

Kissel JT, Slivka AP, Warmotts JR, et al: The clinical spectrum of necrotizing angiography of the peripheral nervous system. Ann Neurol *18*:251–257, 1985.

Mitsumoto H, Wilbourn AJ: Causes and diagnosis of sensory neuropathies: A review. J Clin Neurophysiol *11*:553–567, 1994.

Mulder D (ed): The Diagnosis and Treatment of Amyotrophic Lateral Sclerosis. Boston, Houghton Mifflin, 1980.

Parry GJ, Sumner AJ: Multifocal motor neuropathy. Neuro Clin *10*:671–684, 1992.

Parsonage MJ, Turner AJW: Neuralgic amyotrophy: The shoulder-girdle syndrome. Lancet *1*:973–978, 1948.

Thomas PK, Ochoia J: Clinical features and differential diagnosis. *In* Dyck PJ, Thomas PK (eds): Peripheral Neuropathy, ed 3. Philadelphia, WB Saunders, 1993, pp 749–774.

Wilbourn JA: Electrodiagnosis: The electromyographic examination. *In* Rothman RH, Simeone FA: The Spine, ed 3. Philadelphia, WB Saunders, 155–172, 1992.

Wilbourn AJ: Brachial plexus disorders. *In* Dyck PJ, Thomas PK (eds): Peripheral Neurology, ed 3. Philadelphia, WB Saunders 1993a, pp 911–950.

Wilbourn AJ: Diabetic neuropathies. *In* Brown WF, Bolton CF (eds): Clinical Electromyography, ed 2. Boston, Butterworth-Heinemann 1993b, pp 477–515.

Wilbourn AJ, Furlan AJ, Hulley W, Ruschaupt W: Ischemic monomelic neuropathy. Neurology *33*:447–457, 1983.

Wilbourn AJ, Levin KH: Ischemic Neuropathy. *In* Brown WF, Bolton CF (eds): Clinical Electromyography, ed 2. Boston, Butterworth-Heinemann, 1993, pp 369–390.

Wilbourn AJ, Shields RW: Diabetic neuropathy. *In* Samuels (ed): Office Practice of Neurology. New York, Churchill-Livingstone, 1995, pp 506–510.

Part X

RECONSTRUCTION

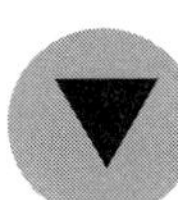

Chapter 65

• P.J. Guelinckx

• Nadia K. Sinsel

• René Dom

Contemporary Muscle Morphology as Related to Nerve Pathology

The trophic influence of the nervous system on the prenatal and postnatal development and maintenance of muscle tissue during life has been well described by many authors (Burke et al, 1971; Pette, 1984). It is established that the morphology, physiology, and biomechanical characteristics of muscle fiber are determined by the type of innervating motor neuron (Burke et al, 1971; Cote and Faulkner, 1986). The muscle as an organ displays variability and plasticity in fiber type distribution, fiber diameter, oxidative capacity, fatigability, velocity of contraction, and other parameters because of different types of motor units (Galvas and Gonyea, 1980; Pette, 1984; Lexell et al, 1984).

The trophic status of the muscle fibers is directly related to the integrety of the motor nerve, and it is obvious that nerve injury will produce changes in the physiological and histochemical characteristics of the involved striated muscle (Kugelberg et al, 1970). For example, type grouping after muscle denervation and subsequent reinnervation is well known (Brown 1984). However, the nerve-muscle relationship is not as clear, because many other factors, even with an intact nerve, may lead to the same pathological conditions as denervation atrophy. The histological and histochemical analyses of muscle biopsies have currently been restricted to differentiate and diagnose different types of neurogenic and myogenic muscle diseases. This chapter will define the value of muscle biopsies in modern surgery and discuss their value in the management of peripheral nerve lesions. Techniques of biopsy preservation, preparation for histology, histochemistry, and quantitative and qualitative analysis of the specimen are discussed. Eight biopsies obtained from a series of 50 muscles biopsies in diverse pathological circumstances are presented. The effect of muscle innervation, denervation, and reinnervation on muscle morphology will be discussed from three aspects:

1. Does the biopsy and the histological evaluation add to the understanding and treatment of the pathology? Does it aid in the prediction of prognosis for the individual lesion?

2. Studying the morphological results in retrospect, does the microsurgeon alter the management plan? What are the implications for muscle transposition and muscle transplantation surgery?

3. Is contemporary muscle histology and morphometry essential to understanding the results of nerve and muscle reconstruction?

MATERIALS AND METHODS

Harvesting the Biopsy and Histological Preparation

The muscle biopsies were nearly all harvested during the initial nerve surgery or during secondary interventions. Some elective biopsies were performed under local anesthesia. The involved muscle was exposed at the point where the nerve enters the muscle. A muscle strip, parallel to the direction of the muscle fibers and measuring 5 mm in length, 4 mm in width and 4mm in thickness, was elevated using microscissors. The fresh muscle biopsies were transported to the laboratory cooled on a wet gauze and quickly frozen in isopentane and dry ice. Thereafter, 10 µm-thick slices of a complete cross-section were cut in a cryostat, and histological slides were prepared for histochemical staining.

Histological and Histochemical Procedure

Several staining techniques were used such as hematoxylin-eosin (H&E), Gomori, Periodic Acid–Schiff (PAS) and stainings for enzyme activity such as ATPase stain at different pHs (9.4, 5.6, 4.6) and nicotinamide adenine dinucleotide (NADH) diaphorase stain. The most important was the ATPase stain, which visualized the reaction of myofibrillar actomyosine ATPase and enabled differentiation between type I (slow) and type II (fast) muscles fibers (Gollnick et al, 1983). Type II muscle fibers show a high activity of myosin and actomyosin ATPase, whereas type I fibers demonstrate a low activity. Type II fibers are mainly anaerobic and possess a large amount of glycogen. However, the concentration of mitochondral enzymes, such as succinic dehydrogenase, is low. Additional NADH staining of serial cross-sections can be performed to differentiate between type IIA and type IIB fibers. Type IIA fibers express a high NADH activity when compared with type IIB fibers. In summary, it can be stated that type I fibers are red, aerobic, contain mitochondria and myoglobin, have a diameter of ± 50 µm, and store fat as energy. Type II fibers are white, anaerobic, have a diameter of ± 80 to 100 µm, and store glycogen as energy. The most important staining techniques are based on different enzymatic reactions inherent to the biochemical reactions of anaerobic or aerobic metabolism.

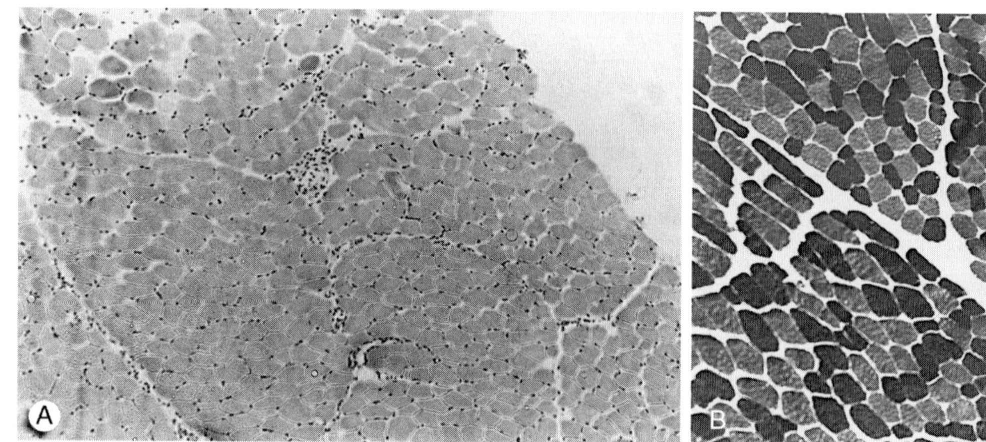

FIGURE 65–1. *A,* Muscle biopsy 3 hours after the transplantation illustrates the immediate polynuclear infiltration into the muscular septa. No edema is present. H & E staining, magnification 10 ×. *B,* Representative cross section of the gracilis muscle indicates a typical mosaic pattern of Type I and Type II fibers with a densely packed muscle pattern. ATP-ase staining at pH 9.4, magnification 10 ×.

After completing histochemical staining, a quantitative analysis of the muscle tissue was performed using a Leitz automatic video-analyzing system. This provides exact measurements of the diameters and circumference of the muscle fibers. Distribution histograms were plotted for all individual fibers when desired.

CASE STUDIES

▼ CASE 1:

NORMAL MUSCLE MORPHOLOGY: SELECTION CRITERIA FOR FUNCTIONAL MUSCLE TRANSPLANTATION AFTER NERVE PATHOL-OGY: A 10-year old boy had unilateral partial congenital facial paralysis with intact eye closure. A cross-facial nerve grafting procedure was performed. Eight months later, muscle substitution was done using a free gracilis muscle transfer to the face. The gracilis was reinnervated by the cross-face nerve graft. A biopsy from the gracilis muscle was harvested at the time of muscle transfer. A mosaic pattern of type I and type II fibers was seen (52%, type I; 43%, type IIA). Type II fibers showed a mild degree of fiber atrophy (Fig. 65–1*A* and *B*). One year after the transplantation, a good contraction of the muscle transplant was obtained. These data illustrate the biopsy findings of a normal intact active muscle. They also demonstrate that the gracilis muscle is an ideal donor muscle for facial reanimation because its fiber type distribution is compatible to normal facial muscles. This is ideal because muscle fiber conversion toward another fiber type is not required, and optimal reinnervation is then possible.

▼ CASE 2:

THE EFFECT OF GRADUALLY INCREASING THE RESTING LENGTH OF A MUSCLE, WITH INTACT NEUROVASCULAR STRUCTURES: A 20-year-old woman was evaluated after a third-degree burn injury of her left thoracic wall at the age of 5 years. Initial treatment had been conservative, resulting in scar contractures of the axilla and hypertrophic scars in the upper quadrants of her left breast. Scar excision and tissue expansion were performed. One expander was placed in the neck area beneath the platysma muscle, and the other was placed subcutaneously in the left flank. Tissue expansion was obtained within 4 months. The expanders were then removed; the scarred area was resected; and the defect was directly closed by tissue transposition. At the time of the operation, a muscle biopsy of the platysma muscle was harvested. Isolated small groups of necrotic muscle fibers were seen. A slight balance toward type II fibers was found. The endomysial tissue was increased, with increased cellularity of the interstitium. Around the arteries and veins, a mononuclear inflammatory reaction was seen (Fig. 65–2). These findings illustrate that slow expansion of skeletal muscle tissue and subsequent increased resting length does not dramatically alter muscle morphology, in contrast to dramatic alterations that are seen after disturbed neurovascular supply and long-standing muscle inactivation.

▼ CASE 3:

THE COMBINED EFFECT OF ALTERED MUSCLE RESTING LENGTH AND MUSCLE INACTIVITY ON MUSCLE MORPHOLOGY WITH IN-TACT NEUROVASCULAR STRUCTURES: A 59-year-old woman was seen for breast reconstruction after mastectomy. A myocuta-

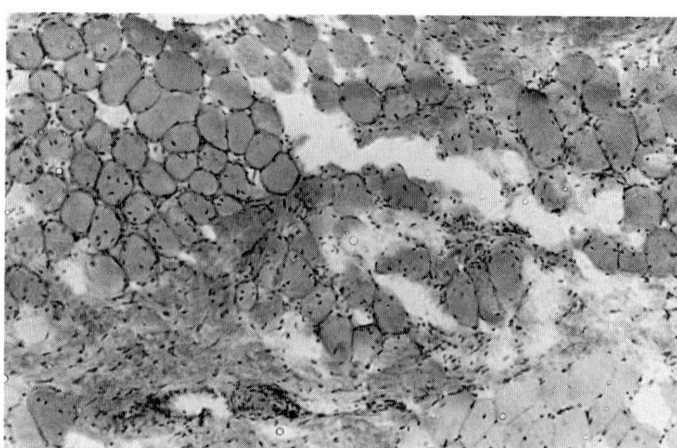

FIGURE 65–2. PAS staining demonstrates the glycogen storage in the muscle fibers after slow expansion of the platysma muscle. Reactive inflammation and fibrosis is seen between the muscle fibers, displaying signs of intracellular repair reaction. PAS staining, magnification 10 ×.

neous, neurovascular intact, latissimus dorsi transposition was performed. Six months later, a muscle biopsy was harvested during a secondary surgery. Muscle fibers were globally smaller than usual, and groups of atrophic fibers were interspersed. Type grouping revealed an excess of type II fibers. Muscle fibers were broadly infiltrated by large bands of fat tissue (Fig. 65–3). This muscle biopsy indicates that despite a neurovascular intact muscle transposition, significant muscle atrophy occurs when inactivity and poor excursion occur after unipolar muscle disinsertion (Guelinckx, 1991). Normal muscle fibers are largely replaced by fat cells, typical for inactivation atrophy.

▼ CASE 4:

THE EXCLUSIVE EFFECT OF MUSCLE DENERVATION WITH INTACT VASCULAR SUPPLY AND RESTING LENGTH: An 8-year-old boy was seen after a left brachial plexus injury, affecting C5, C6 and C7, caused by birth trauma with major weakness of the deltoid and biceps muscles. At the age of 3 years, a nerve graft repair of C5 and C6 combined with neurolysis of C7 was performed. Reinnervation of the biceps, extensor digitorum communis, and, to a lesser extent, the deltoid muscle was documented electromyographically. Because of a deficit of dorsal flexion of the wrist, a tendon transfer had been done at the age of 6 years. However, at the age of 8 years, deltoid function remained insufficient, and a neurovascular transposition of the latissimus dorsi muscle was planned. Intraoperatively, muscle biopsy of the deltoid muscle of the involved side was harvested. Neurogenic atrophy with signs of reinnervation were found. Muscle fibers were highly variable in diameter, and type grouping was seen (Fig. 65–4). The deltoid muscle was found to be atrophic despite good reinnervation of the other territories. This case demonstrates the irreversible muscle degradation after long-term denervation and highlights the necessity of muscle tissue replacement after long-standing nerve injury. This biopsy confirms clinical findings.

▼ CASE 5:

THE EFFECT OF DENERVATION OR INACTIVITY: A 20-year-old man sustained a brachial plexus injury 8 years before he was seen and had a complete palsy in the median, radial, axillary,

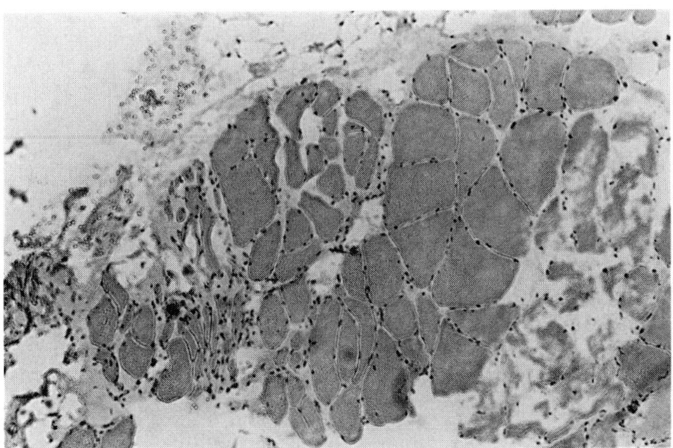

FIGURE 65–4. Cross section through the deltoid muscle shows the large variability with atrophic and hypertrophic muscle fibers. A poor architectonic organization with interfascicular fibrosis and hypercellularity is seen. H & E staining, magnification 10 ×.

and musculocutaneous nerve territories. To reconstruct biceps function a bipolar neurovascular transposition of the latissimus dorsi muscle was performed. Intraoperatively, muscle biopsies of the latissimus dorsi muscle and the biceps muscle were obtained. Histochemical and planimetrical data of the long-standing paralyzed biceps muscle revealed an atrophy variable between 40% and 60%, compared with control muscle fibers. The latissimus dorsi muscle demonstrated, despite a normal clinical evaluation, an increased variation in fiber diameter, with type grouping and groups of atrophic fibers, mostly type 1. These data show that it is difficult to differentiate between secondary disuse of a muscle or partial denervation based on biopsy findings. However, despite atrophy of the latissimus muscle seen morphometrically, a good biceps function was found postoperatively.

▼ CASE 6:

THE EFFECT OF PROLONGED ISCHEMIA WITH INTACT NERVE VERSUS TRANSCIENT ISCHEMIA: A 19-year-old man was seen for soft tissue reconstruction after an open tibia fracture and compartment syndrome treated by fasciotomy 1 year before. A muscle biopsy of the involved muscles was harvested at the time of the second operation. An almost complete, but persistent necrosis of muscle tissue was seen. Only few atrophic muscle fibers remained, and a strong myophagic reaction was seen with large zones of fibrosis. A free latissimus dorsi muscle was transplanted without nerve repair for reconstruction of the soft tissues. A latissimus dorsi muscle biopsy harvested 4 weeks after transplantation demonstrated perifascicular inflammation and few necrotic fibers (Fig. 65–5). These histologic data show the dramatic effect of prolonged interrupted blood supply on muscle morphology. Human muscles possess very little regeneration capacity, especially in ischemic conditions (Lehto et al, 1986). On the other hand, it becomes evident that muscle tissue is easily damaged after microvascular muscle transfer, as observed by signs of transient inflammation. However, alterations due to long-standing denervation are expected to occur later on.

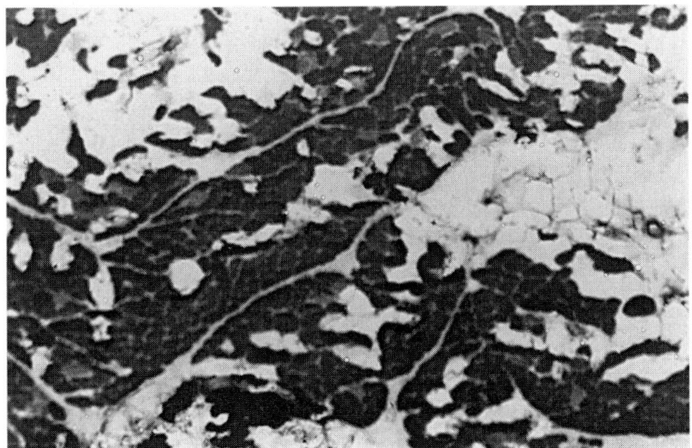

FIGURE 65–3. The small atrophic fibers after muscular disuse with intact neurovascular structures can be seen. A significant replacement by fat cells is diffusely spread all over the cross section. ATPase staining at pH 9.4, magnification 10 ×.

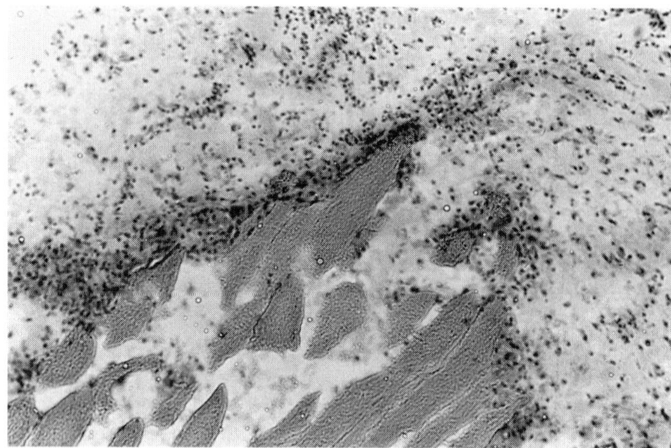

FIGURE 65–5. An intense zone of myophagic activity around desintegrated muscle fibers is seen in the lower part of the picture. In the upper part, all muscle fibers are replaced by scar tissue. H & E-staining, magnification 4 ×.

 **CASE 7:**

THE EFFECT OF A FEW HOURS ISCHEMIA AND LONG-STANDING DENERVATION ON MUSCLE MORPHOLOGY. A 22-year-old man sustained total traumatic amputation of his left arm 2 years before. Because of a persistent radial nerve palsy, re-exploration was performed and a large neuroma was found at the site of previous osteosynthesis of the humerus. The neuroma was resected and the resulting 20-cm defect was grafted using three sural nerve graft cables. A biopsy of the extensor muscles of the arm was obtained.

Some muscle fascicles showed only networks were muscle ghosts were present. Muscle atrophy and fiber loss were widely dispersed through the biopsy. Intense, dispersed, fibrotic infiltration of the muscle was observed (Fig. 65–6). These findings are compatible with irreversible muscle damage, and reinnervation will not be able to provide functional recovery because the receptor organ is damaged.

 **CASE 8:**

THE EFFECT OF TRANSIENT ISCHEMIA AND REINNERVATION: A 42-year-old man sustained a frostbite injury of both feet, requiring bilateral amputation after debridement of the left stump, soft tissue coverage was necessary, and a microneurovascular myocutaneous latissimus dorsi flap was performed. To restore sensibility, reinnervation of the flap was attempted by repair of the dorsalis pedis nerve to the thoracodorsal nerve. A muscle biopsy of the latissimus dorsi muscle was harvested 1 year after the transplantation. Zones of muscle with increase of fat cells into the interstitial space were seen. Extreme variation of muscle fiber diameters was found, with an excess of type II fibers. Signs of early regeneration were found (Fig. 65–7*A* and *B*). These findings indicate that sensory nerves fibers with an innervation pattern other than motor nerves may provide some trophic influence on the transplanted muscle with some signs of muscle regeneration.

DISCUSSION

 It is obvious from these histological data that muscle tissue is very dynamic and adapts continuously to different circumstances and pathologies. Alterations in neuronal input, vascular supply, resting length, and muscle activity will produce an alteration in muscle morphology. With an intact nerve, muscle tissue continuously adapts to external factors such as training and loading. This is expressed in reversible changes of muscle fiber diameter, length, and composition. The trophic status of the muscle should therefore be considered as multifactorially as illustrated by the several examples. It is known that after neurovascular muscle transfer, the restoration of resting length by means of tendon repair is the most important determinant of functional recovery (Guelinckx et al, 1988; Kadhiresan et al, 1993; Terzis et al, 1978). This was shown in Case 3 where, despite intact neurovascular structures, significant atrophy and fat infiltration were seen after unipolar muscle disinsertion. Unfortunately, these histological findings are not specific for muscle inactivity; they can also be seen after long-standing muscle denervation, as shown in Cases 4 and 5. It is very difficult to differentiate with biopsy findings between denervation and inactivation atrophy. However, compared with long-standing muscle denervation, more severe disrupture of muscle architecture will be seen after long-term ischemia (Guelinckx et al, 1984). Complete muscle fiber necrosis will occur despite intact neuronal input (Case 6). Transient ischemia, on the other hand, is more tolerated. Only temporary signs of inflammation will be seen. Biopsy findings after transient ischemia with long-standing denervation will, however, be dominated by neurogenic atrophy with intense fibrosis (Case 7). Re-establishment of some neuronal input will result in some regeneration (Case 8) (Guelinckx et al, 1992, Faukner et al, 1983). In general, it may be stated that interruption of the neuronal supply will result in atrophy in the initial phase and in fibrosis and fat cell replacement in the long-term (Frey et al, 1983). The lapse time between these periods is specimen dependant. Reinnervation in the final state will cause immature nerve regeneration and misdirection of many axons into scar tissue because of the absence of normal target organs for sprouting axons (Guelinckx et al, 1984).

In what has been mentioned above, it becomes evident that muscle biopsies do not entirely inform the surgeon about the innervation status of the muscle. They do provide information concerning the present trophic status of the muscle, and they enable one to differentiate between reversable atrophy and

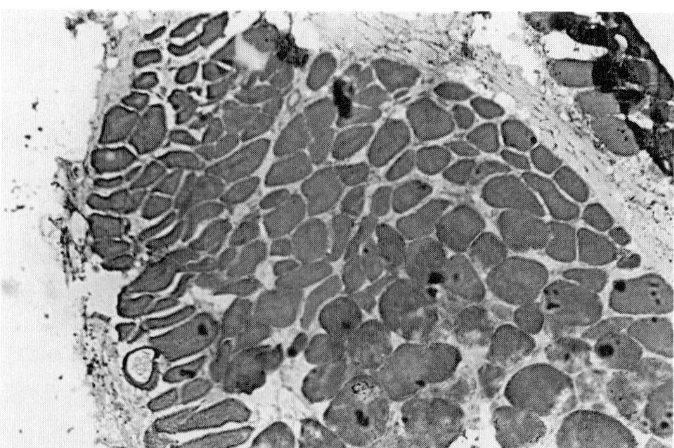

FIGURE 65–6. Despite a 2-year period of radial nerve palsy, moderate muscle fibers integrity can still be seen. Some atrophic fibers, vacuolization in the muscle fibers, and septal fibrosis are visible. ATPase staining pH 9.4, magnification 25 ×.

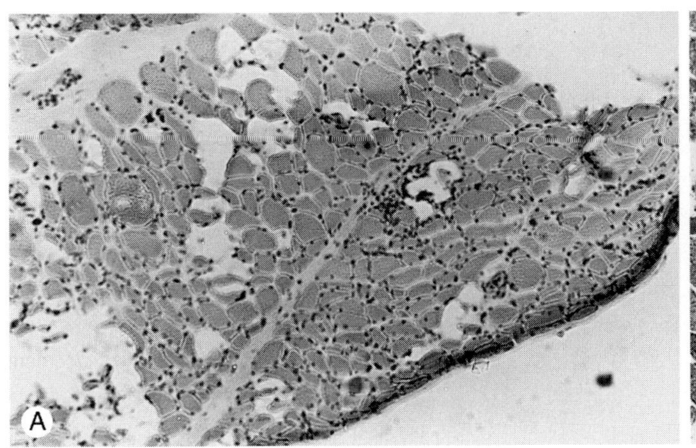 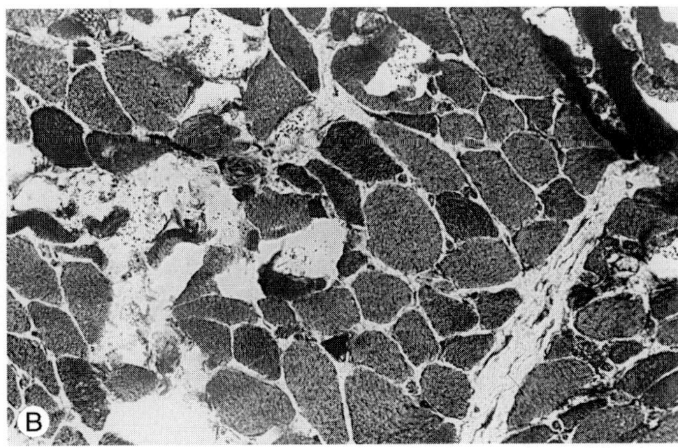

FIGURE 65–7. *A,* Replacement of muscle cells by fat cells is typical, and the atrophic fibers and the reactive hypercellularity around the muscle fibres are clearly seen. H & E-staining, magnification 10 ×. *B,* The NADH staining displays the nearly homogenic color intensity of the muscle fibers, indicating a loss of differentiation into several fiber types. NADH staining, magnification 25 ×.

irreversable muscle damage caused by nerve or other pathology such as vascular impairment (Doriguzzi et al, 1984). Unfortunately, extensive muscle regeneration as reported in many experimental studies, does not occur in humans (Carlson, 1973; Schultz et al, 1985).

Today, irreversability of muscle denervation is defined by the duration of denervation, and few data are available concerning human histology as related to the length of denervation period. Moreover, important interfering facts, such as age of the patient, alteration of vascular supply, or resting length after complex trauma, are often neglected or cannot be judged adequately. Harvesting a muscle biopsy in uncertain cases with denervation periods of 1 to 2 years may provide important information regarding management of a nerve lesion primarily or to perform other procedures. Muscle biopsies also provide valuable information about underlying transient or permanent physiopathological circumstances such as edema, necrosis, or regeneration signs that are inherent to the denervation or reinnervation process. This information, which cannot be obtained by electromyography, computed tomography, or clinical evaluation of the patient, enables us to predict to some extent the expected degree of functional recovery after nerve injuries or nerve repair.

Biopsies also give an estimation of type distribution within a muscle. This is important if an irreversably denervated muscle is to be reconstructed by means of functional muscle transplantation. Similarity in type distribution permits the most prompt muscle recruitment after reinnervation because no biochemical conversion within the muscle fibers has to take place. Biopsies reveal information about fiber type changes after simple muscle transposition with intact neurovascular structures resulting from altered workload. Interactions between the muscle tissue and altered neuronal recruitment caused by central neuroplasticity inherent to changed functional demands may be quantified (Salmons and Henriksson, 1981).

In circumstances where the results of nerve and muscle reconstruction need improved documentation on, harvesting of a muscle biopsy will provide valuable information about underlying physiological mechanisms of the recovery process and the quality of muscle reinnervation. If the biopsy is obtained preoperatively, some prediction of the final outcome of the nerve lesion can be made because the state of the target organ is one of the major determining facts in the efficiency and maturity of the nerve regeneration process, which is very important for the final functional outcome after the nerve repair (Frey et al, 1991; Hatano 1981).

References

Brown MC: Sprouting of motor nerves in adult muscles: A recapitulation of oncogeny. Tips in Neurological Science, Jan 10, 1984.

Burke, RE, Levine DN, Azjac FE III, Tsairis P, Engel WK: Mammalian motor units: Physiological-histochemical correlates in three types of cat gastrocnemius. Science *174:*709, 1971.

Carlson BM: The regeneration of skeletal muscle: A review. Am J Anat *137:*119, 1973.

Cote C, Faulkner JA: Characteristics of motor units in muscles of rats grafted with nerves intact. Cell Physiol *19:*C828, 1986.

Doriguzzi C, Mongini T, Palmucci L, Gagnor E, Schiffer D: Quantitative analysis of quadriceps muscle biopsy. J Neurol Sci *66:*319, 1984.

Faukner JA, Markley JM, McCully KK, Watters CR, White TP: Characteristics of cat skeletal muscles grafted with intact nerves or with anastomosed nerves. Exp Neurol *80:*682, 1983.

Frey M, Gruber H, Havel M, Steiner E, Freilnger G: Experimental free muscle transplantation with neurovascular anastomosis. Plast Reconstr Surg *71:*689, 1983.

Frey M, Happak W, Girsch W, Bittner RE, Gruber H: Histomorphometric studies in patients with facial palsy treated by functional muscle transplantation: New aspects for the surgical concept. Ann Plast Surg *26:*370, 1991.

Galvas PE, Gonyea WJ: Motor-end-plate and nerve distribution in a histochemically compartmentalized pennate muscle in the cat. Am J Anat *159:*147, 1980.

Gollnick PD, Parsons D, Oakley CR: Differentiation of fibre types in skeletal muscle from sequential inactivation of myofibrillar actomyosin ATP-ase during acid incubation. Histochemistry *77:*543, 1983.

Guelinckx PJ: Free microneurovascular muscle grafts: Deficits resulting from transplantation and speculations for myocardial repair. J Cardiac Surg *6:*190, 1991.

Guelinckx PJ, Carlson BM, Faulkner JA: Morphologic characteristics of muscles grafted in rabbits with neurovascular repair. J Reconstr Microsurg *6:*481, 1992.

Guelinckx PJ, Dom R, Bex M, Boeckx WD, Gruwez JA: Rectus femoris grafts performed with and without vascular anastomosis: An experimental study in the rabbit. Br J Plast Surg *37:*585, 1984.

Guelinckx PJ, Faulkner JA, Essig DA: Neurovascular-anastomosed muscle grafts in rabbits: Functional deficits result from tendon repair. Muscle Nerve *11:*745, 1988.

Hatano E: A comparative study on primary and secondary nerve repair. Plast Reconstr Surg *68:*760, 1981.

Kadhiresan VA, Guelinckx PJ, Faulkner JA: Tenotomy and rcpair of latissimus dorsi muscles in rats: Implications for transposed muscle grafts. J Appl Physiol *75:*1294, 1993.

Kugelberg E, Edström L, Abbruzzese M: Mapping of motor units in experimentally reinnervated rat muscle. J Neurol Neurosurg Psychiatry *33:*319, 1970.

Lehto M, Järvinen J, Nelimarkka O: Scar formation after skeletal muscle injury. Arch Orthop Trauma Surg *104:*366, 1986.

Lexell J, Downham D, Sjöström M: Distribution of different fibre types in human skeletal muscles. J Neurol Sci *65:*353, 1984.

Pette D: Activity induced fast and slow transition in mammalian muscle. Med Sci Sports Exerc *6:*517, 1984.

Salmons S, Henriksson J: The adaptive response of skeletal muscle to increased use. Muscle Nerve *4:*94, 1981.

Schultz E, Jaryszak DL, Vallaire CR: Response of satellite cells to focal skeletal muscle injury. Muscle Nerve *8:*217, 1985.

Terzis J, Sweet RC, Dykes RW, Williams HB: Recovery of function in free muscle transplants using microneurovascular anastomoses. J Hand Surg *3:*37, 1978.

Electrical Stimulation of Denervated Muscles

Thousands of patients with injuries to the peripheral nerves and many others with facial paralysis are treated each year in clinical practice. Despite the best of modern microsurgical skills, the functional motor result that is achieved following repair of a severed peripheral nerve is always less than complete due to muscle atrophy and loss of muscle end-plates. This muscle atrophy or wasting results in weakness, loss of size, or bulk and poor coordination, leading to a marked reduction in functional capacity. The permanent disability from these injuries can be debilitating for both the skilled and the heavy manual worker. The disability is particularly true in individuals who require advanced manual dexterity such as musicians, athletes, machine operators, typists, computer technicians, and many others. Nerve injuries in the workplace can be a life-long problem and often result in the loss or change in occupation. Patients with facial paralysis are also severely disfigured on a permanent basis, and most individuals are devastated with the change in their appearance and decreased functional capacity. Facial expression, both at rest and with such simple movements as talking or smiling, becomes impaired, and problems with drooling, chewing, and communication are constant reminders of the problem to the patients affected with this disorder.

THE PROBLEM

Electrical stimulation of denervated muscles continues to be a controversial subject, particularly in regard to its benefit for patients who have repaired peripheral motor nerve injuries. External stimulation requires excellent patient compliance, and the required voltage, frequency, duration, and length of treatments are extremely difficult to maintain. In fact, our information reveals that most centers have largely abandoned serious attempts at external muscle stimulation due to these difficulties. A completely implanted muscle-stimulating device has been developed in the author's laboratories that eliminates any problem related to patient compliance and allows continuous muscle stimulation around the clock for many weeks. Animal experiments using this device have been most encouraging, and this research has been expanded to include a controlled patient study for assessment of the efficacy of this modality.

LABORATORY STUDIES

Several experiments have been completed in the author's laboratory over the past 8 years for both peripheral nerve injuries and for facial paralysis in two animal species (rabbits and dogs). The results obtained are extremely encouraging, with a striking improvement in the return of functional capacity in those animals treated with continuous muscle stimulation following nerve injury and repair. This study has now been expanded to a controlled clinical pilot study on muscle stimulation following nerve injuries in the upper extremity, median, ulnar, radial, and mixed nerve lesions.

NORMAL SEQUENCE OF NEUROMUSCULAR TRANSMISSION AND MUSCLE CONTRACTION

1. Arrival of an impulse at the motor nerve terminal.
2. Release of acetylcholine from the presynaptic nerve terminal vesicles.
3. Binding of acetylcholine to the end-plate receptors with production of local end-plate potential charges (depolarization).
4. Depolarization of the muscle fibers and surface membranes, and production of a muscle action potential (in-wave).
5. Production of a muscle contraction.

The process by which a nerve impulse releases acetylcholine from synaptic vesicles at the terminal is promoted by calcium ions and inhibited by magnesium ions. A single stimulus of the nerve or muscle produces a single action potential. Repeated maximum stimulation produces a tetanic contraction. In denervated muscles, the muscle membrane becomes as sensitive as the motor end-plate to the depolarizing action of acetylcholine, causing increased fibrillation potentials and positive sharp waves to occur.

Direct stimulation of a muscle also produces muscle action potentials. Using this technique, it is probable that one can maintain full muscle length and strength, and lessen the degree of atrophy until nerve regeneration is complete. With continuous electrical stimulation, muscle activity is maintained and its functional capacity is preserved until neuromuscular communication is restored. This was the basis for our animal experiments.

CURRENT STATE OF KNOWLEDGE OF THE EFFECTS OF ELECTRICAL MUSCLE STIMULATION

Reports from recent investigations indicate that electrical stimulation of denervated muscles may lead to significant biochemical, electrophysiological, and biomechanical changes. Histochemically, animal and human skeletal muscle fibers are not homogeneous in their physiological, ultrastructural, or metabolic characteristics. Differences between fibers within a muscle fascicle have been denoted by various names depending on the techniques employed to demonstrate these differences; hence, the terms red and white, slow twitch, fast twitch, oxidative, and glycolytic muscle fibers. A compromised terminology has evolved designating muscle fibers as Type I or Type II, which satisfies their physiological morphological, and biochemical orientation. Type I muscle fibers correspond to the slow-twitch type because they contract more slowly than the Type II fibers. They also sustain their contracture for longer periods, whereas Type II fibers fatigue more rapidly. These different contractile properties are associated with differences in metabolic characteristics that can be identified with histochemical stains. Myofibrillar ATPase (adenosine triphosphatase) is a useful stain because it yields good contrast between the fiber types. With a pH of 7.4, Type II fibers stained darker than those of Type I, and the staining characteristics can be reversed with acidic preincubation at pH of 4.6 or 4.7 for brief periods. Type II muscles can also be subdivided into Type II-A and Type II-B fiber types. Lomo and associates (1980) reported that high-frequency electrical stimulation (100 pps) was most effective in preventing muscle atrophy and reduction in force output. Dewar and Chiu (1986) revealed that high-rate stimulation (120 trains per minute) was effective in decreasing muscle fatigability (conversion of Type II to Type I fibers). In our animal experiments, the analysis of the cross-sectional area of Type I and Type II fibers substantiates the finding that fiber size is maintained in the stimulated muscle group and is significantly greater in total fiber area than that found in the denervated but nonstimulated group.

Crush Nerve Injuries

Guttmann and Guttmann (1944) demonstrated the effect of galvanic exercise on denervated and reinnervated muscles in the rabbit, and they found that atrophy could be slowed but not completely prevented. Eberstein and co-workers (1981) demonstrated that stimulation significantly retarded the atrophy of both Type I and Type II muscle fibers in Wistar rats. Nix (1982) studied the effect of low-frequency electrical stimulation on the denervated extensor digitorum longus muscle of the rabbit. He concluded that the stimulation reduced the duration of the active state of denervated muscles. He also believed that the stimulation seemed to reduce the denervation effect so that the time course of contraction and relaxation of the stimulated muscle tended to be faster than that of nonstimulated denervated muscles and, thus, more similar to that of normal muscles. The nerve Nix studied was of the crush type. Girlanda and colleagues (1982) performed a similar study in rabbits. Their results were inconclusive without a statistically significant difference in the stimulated and nonstimulated groups. Harada (1983) showed that electrical stimulation with high-frequency cycles in rats significantly suppressed the increase in diameter of Type II muscle fibers. He also noted that electrical stimulation with low-frequency cycles significantly suppressed the decrease in diameter of Type I muscle fibers. Electrical stimulation also suppressed the weight loss of

the denervated muscle, and Harada believed that electrical stimulation could retard muscle atrophy. Pachter and associates (1982) repeated the experiments on the effect of electrical stimulation on denervated rat extensor digitorum muscles. They concluded that electrical stimulation retards denervation atrophy, but the experiment was completed before nerve regeneration. Cole and Gardiner (1984) again studied the crush nerve model in rats using the sciatic nerve gastrocnemius model. By 8 weeks after the crush injury, the nonstimulated muscles were significantly lighter in weight and they showed slower isometric contractile responses in situ than the controls. The denervated muscles that had been stimulated daily were heavier and tetanically stronger than those in the nonstimulated group.

Incomplete Nerve Injuries

Using a rat model, Kanaya (1985) showed that electrical stimulation reduced the degree of denervation atrophy. The electrical stimulation was given for 30 minutes daily through an external source, and his study included a comparison of Type I and Type II muscle fibers. Miyazawa (1986) published his histochemical studies on skeletal muscle atrophy and the changes produced with electrical stimulation. The nerve was neither crushed nor severed, and he found that electrical stimulation prevented the transformation of muscle fiber types from Type I to Type II. He believed that his results confirmed the importance of muscle tension, not only in the nutrition but also in the differentiation of muscle cells.

Nerve Injuries and Implanted Electrodes

Salmons and Henriksson (1981) demonstrated clearly that, when it is subjected to chronic low frequency electrical stimulation, a fast-twitch mammalian skeletal muscle will gradually transform to slow-twitch muscle in all of its characteristics. A detailed ultrastructural study of the muscle fiber transformation by Eisenberg and Salmons (1981) supports their earlier findings. In rabbits, they noted several changes using electromicroscopic techniques, including changes in mitochondrial volume, transformation of Z-band structures, and in the sarcotubular system. Their experiments were done in a rabbit model using implantable electrodes. Cooper and Salmons (1988) also described an improved implanted stimulator that was self-contoured for muscle stimulation. In the author's laboratory, the maintenance of skeletal muscle, as an end-organ target, followed by enhanced and functional reinnervation, appeared to be a unique and clinically useful adjunct to peripheral nerve repair.

EXPERIMENTAL MODELS FOR CONTINUOUS MUSCLE STIMULATION FOLLOWING NERVE INJURY AND REPAIR USING A COMPLETELY IMPLANTABLE SYSTEM

Three animal models have been studied in the author's laboratory for the objective assessment of the effects of continuous electrical stimulation on the preservation of muscle function following the reinnervation process after nerve repair.

Rectus Femoris Muscle Model in the Rabbit

In the rabbit model, the femoral nerve was severed at 4 cm from the neuromuscular junction and repaired using microsurgical techniques. The stimulating electrodes (Medtronic Model 7420 Itrel Pulse Generator) were placed in the rectus femoris muscle and connected to the pulse generator, which was also completely implanted. The rectus femoris muscle was then continuously stimulated until nerve regeneration had occurred and muscle contraction was evident through nerve stimulation. Stimulated and nonstimulated muscle groups were studied using force measurements for functional recovery; histological studies were performed with both light (H & E, Trichrome) and electron microscopy. ATPase stains were studied for muscle fiber type. Muscle weights were obtained to compare the stimulated and non-stimulated groups.

The results at 10 weeks following nerve repair showed a definite improvement in functional muscle recovery in the stimulated group. In this rabbit model, the wet muscle weight in the stimulated group remained at 80% of normal, whereas the nonstimulated group was only 40%. The maximum force of tetanic contraction was twice as strong as that in the stimulated group when studied at 8 weeks postoperatively. In addition, the cross-sectional area of Type II muscle fibers was maintained at a higher level with electrical stimulation when compared with the nonstimulated muscle group (Nemoto et al, 1988) (Figs. 66–1 to 66–3).

Histologically, there was a reduction in muscle fibrosis and atrophy and an improved histological appearance in the stimulated muscle group when compared with the nonstimulated animal group.

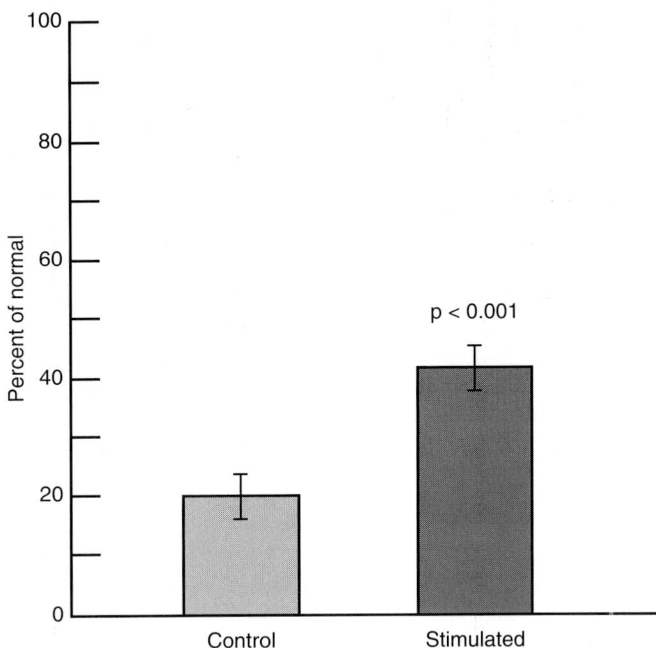

FIGURE 66–2. Maximum force of tetanic contraction.

Peroneus Longus and Tibialis Cranialis Muscle Study in the Dog Model

In this protocol, the common peroneal nerve was severed 10 cm from its neuromuscular junction (to compare with the shorter distance in the rabbit model of 4 cm). The long distance for nerve regeneration in this experimental group would compare similarly with nerve injuries in patients (for example, radial nerve severance above the elbow, high median and ulnar nerve injuries, and peroneal nerve injuries).

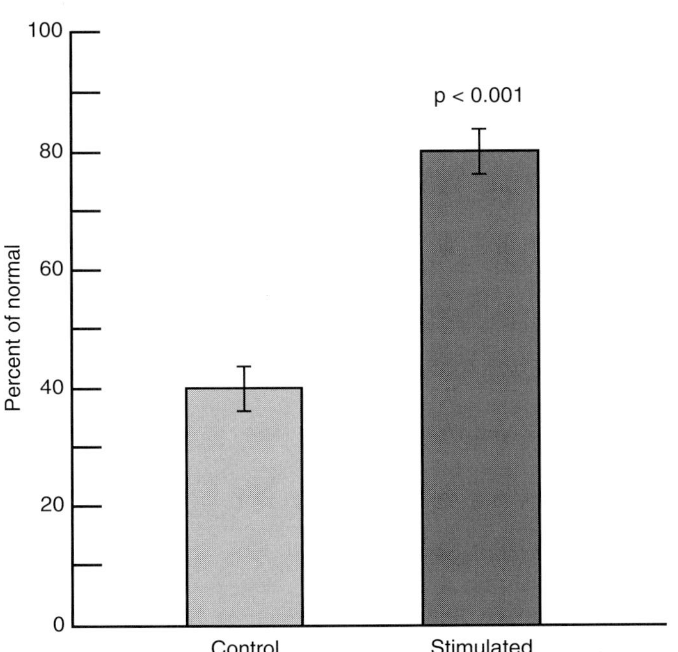

FIGURE 66–1. Muscle net weight.

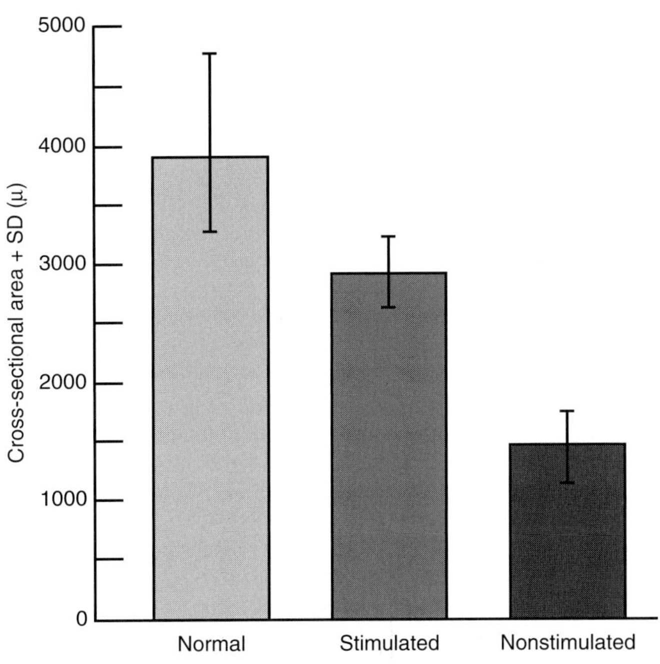

FIGURE 66–3. Type II fibers.

In this experiment, the muscle groups (peroneus longus and tibialis cranialis [anterior]) were stimulated for a period of 12 to 14 weeks until nerve regeneration had occurred. As in the rabbit model, there was marked improvement in the stimulated muscle when compared with the nonstimulated animal group. The animals were studied at 16 weeks following nerve repair, and muscle weight was maintained with a mean of 73% preservation in the stimulated muscles when compared with the nonstimulated group, which showed a mean of 39.25% preservation. Twitch tension in the stimulated group was three times that of the nonstimulated animal group (20.70 versus 7.31), and in a similar manner, electrical stimulation resulted in a greater than three-fold larger tetanic tension force compared with that of the nonstimulated group (23.04 versus 6.55). Direct electrical stimulation of the muscle resulted in a four-fold larger direct tetanic force in the stimulated group when compared with nonstimulated controls (42.98 versus 10.56). Resistance to fatigue was also better in the stimulated muscle group, as was the preservation of muscle fiber area in both Type I and Type II groups. As in the rabbit model, histology showed a relative increase in Type I (slow) muscle with preservation of muscle fiber size and uniformity in the stimulated group (Durand and Williams, 1990; Thomas et al, 1991).

Facial Muscle Protocol in Dogs

This experiment was formulated to study the effects of continuous facial muscle stimulation following cross-facial nerve grafts in an attempt to simulate the clinical condition of facial palsy. Facial paralysis in patients usually follows resection of brain tumors such as acoustic neuromas and facial nerve grafts from the normal side are usually necessary in order to restore muscle function on the paralyzed side. A true reanimation of the face following facial paralysis can be accomplished only through reconstruction of the facial nerve by means of direct nerve suture or, in the case of a nerve defect, through a nerve graft. Substitute motor innervation using the hypoglossal, spinal accessory, or glossopharyngeal cranial nerves can activate the paralyzed facial muscles and occasionally will achieve some facial symmetry. However, almost always, these methods result in an unnatural facial muscle action and loss of normal facial muscle expression. The basic principle underlying the cross facial nerve grafting procedure consists of redirecting a sufficient number of intact nerves from the healthy side toward the paralyzed side by way of nerve transplants (sural donor nerves). It is necessary to wait from 3 to 6 months after the primary anastomosis of the intact facial nerve branches to the sural nerve graft to allow regeneration of the axons across the length of the graft. In a second operation, the distal end of the nerve graft is then sutured to the remaining facial nerve fascicles on the paralyzed side. The main reason why cross-facial nerve grafts fail is the advanced muscle atrophy and fibrosis that takes place before and during the course of treatment. Salimbeni-Ughi (1982) reported on 36 patients of facial palsy who were treated with nerve grafting. Sixteen of these patients had cross-facial nerve grafts. She concluded that the major problem with this technique was that the regenerating nerve fibers must travel a long distance before they reach their motor end-plates, and atrophy has

already occurred. Ander (1976), Samii (1977), Ferreira (1984), and Gary-Bobo and Fuentes (1993) all agree with this conclusion. Facial muscle stimulation was continued for 10 months in our experimental animals, and a remarkable preservation of contractile activity remained.

METHOD

Ten dogs were used, with 5 animals assigned to two groups. The left facial nerve was transected, thus creating complete unilateral facial palsy. Electrodes were placed over the left frontalis muscle and connected to a pulse generator (Itrel Medtronic 7420), which was secured subcutaneously in the neck region, then activated. Two sural nerves (20 to 25 cm in length) were then anastomosed microsurgically to branches of the right facial nerve and tunneled subcutaneously to the left side. Six months later, the second stage of the cross-facial nerve graft procedure was completed with suture of the sural grafts to the frontal branch of the facial nerve. Four months later, once partial reinnervation had occurred, the left and right frontal muscles were tested and analyzed. This evaluation included muscle force measurements, muscle endurance, histology, histochemical studies, and electron microscopy. The frontalis muscle was thus continuously stimulated (8.5 to 10.0 volts; 85-Hz frequency, 0.45 millisecond pulse duration; 1.5 seconds on and 24 seconds off over a 10-month period from the initial operation). The control group received no stimulation.

As in the peripheral muscle groups in the rabbit and the dog, facial muscle integrity was maintained and the functional capacity improved when stimulation was applied. Muscle force in the stimulated group was significantly greater than that in the nonstimulated animals, and the muscles were less fatigable. Muscle fiber area with stimulation was close to twice that seen without stimulation and both light and electron microscopy revealed less atrophy, fibrosis, and morphological irregularities in the experimental group. Our experiments showed an improved preservation of both muscle fiber types in the stimulated group, which likely indicates a lesser degree of atrophy.

Selection of Stimulating Parameters in the Experimental Groups

Nerve stimulation results in activation of the neurilemma of the axon and not the sarcolemma of the muscle. In electrical stimulation of denervated muscles, it is the sarcolemma alone that is being excited. The parameters of electrical stimulation research have been extensively studied in both denervated and innervated conditions.

FREQUENCY

The frequency of a current is the number of waveforms per unit time; its unit of measurement is the Hertz (Hz) or pulses per second (pps). If the voltage is sufficient, a stimulus of 1 Hz results in a muscle twitch. Increasing the frequency results in summating the twitches and, to a point, decreases the voltage or current required to elicit a contraction.

Skeletal muscles consist of motor units that may differ

considerably in contractile properties and demands for function. Some units participate mainly in relatively rare quick movements and contract rapidly and are easily fatigued (Type II). Others contribute to the maintenance of posture and, hence, contract slowly and are fatigue resistant (Type I). Hennig and Lomo (1987) have studied the firing patterns of motor units in normal rats—wires were placed in both the extensor digitorum muscle (Type II) and the soleus muscle (Type I). The muscle action potentials were then recorded over a 24-hour period. In their study, the fast fatigable muscle (extensor digitorum longus [EDL]) was active for only 3 minutes per day, with a range of 2600 to 11,200 impulses per day. The frequency of contractions ranged from 67 to 91 Hz. In contrast, the slow muscle (soleus) was active for 5.3 to 8.4 hours per day with impulses ranging form 309,500 to 495,800 per day. The frequency of contractions range from 18 to 21 Hz. It was determined that high-frequency stimulation restored a normal fast twitch in denervated but fast muscles (EDL) and even the appearance of some fast twitch-fibers in slow muscles (soleus). With this background, the extremity and facial muscles were analyzed and typed in our laboratory. There is a predominance of Type II fibers or fast-twitch muscles compared with the Type I or slow-twitch fibers, with a ratio of 4:1. From this information, the frequency of muscle stimulation was established at 80 to 100 Hz (high frequency).

In a detailed experiment, the rectus femoris muscle in the rabbit (Type II), was stimulated at low-, medium-, and high-frequency pulses. It was noted that stimulation at all frequencies showed an improved maintenance of functional capacity and histological appearance when compared with the non-stimulated control group. However, it was clearly evident that stimulation at high frequency (100 Hz) gave a superior result in all animals when compared with medium- and low-frequency stimulation. This finding supported previous studies, which indicated that stimulation at low frequencies would maintain Type I muscle fibers while stimulation at high frequency would maintain the integrity of Type II or fast muscle fibers. It should be noted that electrical stimulation results in improved preservation of both fiber types at all frequencies but there is a preferential sparing effect with different stimulation parameters.

VOLTAGE

Initial voltage for stimulation of the denervated muscle groups was first set at 1.0 volts and usually an increase was necessary, which was likely due to fluid accumulation and, possibly, fibrosis at the level of the stimulating electrodes.

PULSE WIDTH

From the laboratory studies that have been performed over the past 5 years, the most satisfactory muscle contractile response was obtained at 210 microseconds in the early days following application of the stimulus. Later, this is usually increased up to a level of 450 microseconds in order to maintain a palpable and visible muscle contraction.

These stimulating parameters closely relate to the protocol established in the cardiomyoplasty clinical cases performed at McGill University and other worldwide centers involved in this control clinical investigative project. The latissimus

dorsi muscle is transferred to completely envelop the failing heart in this clinical trial and continuous stimulation is applied to the thoracodorsal nerve. On direct observation of the patients in the group at McGill University, there was no apparent pain or even discomfort in the patients under treatment.

Facial Paralysis Experiment in Dog Model Using Cross-Facial Sural Nerve Grafts

The facial nerve was completely transected causing a complete unilateral facial paralysis. Electrodes were placed over the paralyzed muscle groups (frontalis and orbicularis oculi) and connected to a pulse generator, which was secured subcutaneously in the neck region. Sural nerve grafts removed from the hind limbs were then anastomosed microsurgically to branches of the normal right facial nerve and tunneled subcutaneously to the left side. Six months later, the second stage of the cross-facial nerve graft procedure was completed and the nerve graft ends were anastomosed to the severed facial nerve branches supplying the frontalis and orbicularis oculi muscles. Four months later, once partial reinnervation had occurred, the left and right frontalis muscles were tested and analyzed. Evaluation of the frontalis muscles included measurements of muscle force, muscle endurance, histology, histochemical studies, and electron microscopy.

The parameters of stimulation with the continuous model are as follows: volts 8.5 to 10.0; frequency 85 Hz; pulse duration 0.45 microseconds; 1.5 seconds on, 24 seconds off. These parameters were used over the 10-month period from the initial operation. The control group of animals received no stimulation.

RESULTS

Muscle force measurements are expressed as a percentage of the force obtained from the normally innervated frontalis muscle. The stimulated muscle groups showed improvements in muscle forces that at 1 Hz were 33.3 versus 20.6; at 10 Hz, 31.4 versus 17.4; at 25 Hz, 37.6 versus 18.5; at 50 Hz, 30.4 versus 19.8; at 100 Hz (tetanic tension), 30.3 versus 19.3. Muscle endurance (fatigue test) showed the stimulated muscles at 78.5 versus 49.9 for the nonstimulated group, and the muscle fiber area in the stimulated group (both Type I and Type II) showed a 64.2 versus 34.3 in the nonstimulated group. Light and electron microscopy studies also revealed less atrophy, fibrosis, and morphological irregularities in the stimulated animals (Campanile, 1992).

SUMMARY

These experimental studies in both the rabbit and canine extremity model, as well as in the facial paralysis group, show a significant functional improvement in the electrically stimulated muscle groups.

The results obtained offer a strong possibility that similar results can be obtained in patients. A controlled clinical pilot study on a series of patients with median, ulnar, and radial nerve injuries is now close to completion. It is planned to extend these pilot studies to a facial paralysis model and to other peripheral nerve centers in order to test the author's hypothesis. Distinct advantages of the implantable system is that patient compliance is not required and muscle stimulation can be continued throughout each 24-hour period for several months. This type of stimulation would appear to offer improved muscle preservation in contrast to external muscle stimulation after nerve injury and repair. Previous trials in our center, as well as others using percutaneous techniques, has usually resulted in uncertainty as to the value of such a treatment modality.

Possible future applications of continuous electrical muscle stimulation using an implantable system include other peripheral nerve injuries, brachial plexus paralysis, free microvascular muscle transfers, and in rehabilitation following extremity injuries and possibly cerebrovascular accidents.

References

Ander H: Cross-face nerve transplantations in facial paralysis: Principles and further experience. *In* Marchac D Hueston J (ed): Transactions of the 6th International Congress of Plastic and Reconstructive Surgery. Paris, Masson, 1976, pp 337–340.

Campanile F: Personal Communication, 1992.

Cole BG, Gardiner PF: Does electrical stimulation of denervated muscle, continued after reinnervation, influence recovery of contractile function? Exp Neurol *85:*52, 1984.

Cooper JP, Salmons S: Simple three program implantable muscle stimulator with optical control. J Biomed Eng *10:*467, 1988.

Dewar ML, Chiu RJC: Cardiomyoplasty and the pulse-train stimulator. In Chiu RCJ (ed): Biomedical Cardiac Assistant: Cardiomyoplasty and Muscle-Powered Devices. New York, Future Publishing Co, 1986, pp 43–58.

Durand D, Williams HB: The prevention of muscle atrophy after peripheral motor nerve repair with an implantable electrical system. Surg Forum XLI: 661–664, 1990.

Eberstein A, Johnson R, Wolff T, Zimmer B, Spielholzx N: The effect of electrical stimulation on denervated muscle. New York University Medical Center, Progress Report NIHR. 16-P-58601/2-19, 1981, p 309.

Eisenberg BR, Salmons S: The reorganization of subcellular structure in muscle undergoing fast-to-slow type transformation. Cell Tissue Res *220:*449, 1981.

Ferreira MC: Cross-facial nerve grafting. Clin Plast Surg *11:*211–214, 1984.

Gary-Bobo A, Fuentes JM: Long term follow-up report on cross-facial nerve grafting in the treatment of facial paralysis. Br J Plast Surg *36:*48–50, 1993.

Girlanda P, Dattola R, Vita G, Oteri G, LoPresti R, Messina C: Effect of electrotherapy on denervated muscles in rabbits: An electrophysiological and morphological study. Exp Neurol *77:*483, 1982.

Gutmann E, Guttmann L: Effect of galvanic exercise on denervated and reinnervated muscles in rabbit. J Neurol Neurosurg Psychiatry *7:*7, 1944.

Harada Y: The effects of electrical stimulation on the denervated rat muscles. J Jpn Orthop Ass *57:*859, 1983.

Hennig R, Lomo T: Effects of chronic stimulation on the size and speed of long-term denervated and innervated rat fast and slow skeletal muscles. Acta Physiol Scand *130:*115, 1987.

Kanaya F: Experimental investigation of the effect of electrical stimulation on denervated muscle. J Jpn Surg Hand *2:*648, 1985.

Lomo T, Wesgaard RH, Engebretsen LK: Different Stimulation Patterns Affect Contractile Properties of Denervated Rat Soleus Muscles. Plasticity of Muscle Symposium. Berlin, Walter De Gruyter & Co, 1980.

Miyazawa H: Histochemical studies on skeletal muscle atrophy. J Jpn Orthop Assoc *60:*1003, 1986.

Nemoto K, Williams HB, Nemoto K, Lough J, Chiu RCJ: The effects of electrical stimulation on denervated muscle using implantable electrodes. J Reconstr Microsurg *4:*251, 1988.

Nix WA: The effect of low frequency electrical stimulation on the denervated extensor digitorum longus muscle of the rabbit. Acta Neurol Scand *66:*521, 1982.

Pachter BR, Eberstein A, Goodgold J: Electrical stimulation effect on denervated skeletal myofibers on rats: A light and electronmicroscopic study. Arch Phys Med Rehabil *63:*427, 1982.

Salimbeni-Ughi G: Evaluation of results in 36 cases of facial palsy treated with nerve grafts. Ann Plast Surg *9:* 36–41, 1982.

Salmons S, Henriksson J: The adaptive response of skeletal muscle to increased use. Muscle Nerve. *4:*94, 1981.

Samii M: Aspects modernes de la chirurgie des nerfs periferiques. Paris, Pierre Fabre, 1977, pp 67–77.

Thomas DS, Williams HB, Lough JO: Muscle preservation in peripheral nerve injury using continuous implantable electrical stimulation. Surg Forum XLII;601, 1991.

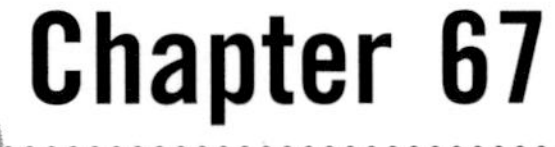

Chapter 67

• George E. Omer, Jr

Reconstruction of the Forearm and Hand After Peripheral Nerve Injuries

Reconstructive procedures after peripheral nerve injuries include tendon transfers to regain a lost basic function and varied surgical procedures to improve sensibility in tactile areas of the hand. Motor reconstruction should be done before sensory reconstruction because precise sensibility depends on precise muscle control as well as appropriate sensory end-organs.

The successful tendon transfer has one basic objective: to either eliminate a deforming force that will produce further imbalance or to replace a single motion that assists in grasp, pinch, or release. The anticipated result should be an achievement of limited, but balanced, functional performance by means of redistributing assets rather than creating new ones.

PATIENT EVALUATION

Homeostasis, or tissue equilibrium, must be regained before tendon transfers. Chronic wounds are contraindications to elective surgery. Soft tissues should be free of scar contracture. There should be stable skeletal alignment. Tendon transfers across a bony nonunion fail because the telescoping skeleton prevents adequate tension for functional power (Fig. 67–1). Joints should have normal motion, because the functional motion expected after tendon transfer should be easily demonstrated by passive motion before surgery (Fig. 67–2).

The involved neuromuscular mechanisms should be evaluated for the level and extent of injury. Return of good muscle power across two joints distal to the nerve injury is rare (Omer, 1974a). Ongoing assessment requires multiple quantitative tests that are repeated at regular intervals: a voluntary muscle test with recorded range of motion, a test for light touch two-point discrimination distance over autonomous zones for pertinent peripheral nerves, a wrinkle test for sudomotor function, gross grip and finger pinch strength tests, and a timed pick-up test for median or ulnar nerve lesions (Omer and Spinner, 1975).

The etiology of the neuromuscular imbalance is important. Muscle imbalance is usually static after trauma, but unusual functional loss may indicate progressive neuromuscular impairment. Many developmental conditions, such as Charcot-Marie-Tooth progressive muscular atrophy, are complicated by an unpredictable rate of involvement. Muscle imbalance related to vascular problems may be limited, as in an injection injury or Volkmann's ischemia, or may be progressive secondary to a series of cerebrovascular accidents. Tendon transfers can be done for a traumatic loss, but the

prognosis for a progressive functional impairment may make it obvious that the muscle imbalance will never be static.

Age and intelligence are pertinent because the patient must have developed the cerebral imprint for the proposed function to be reconstructed, the patient must comprehend what is to be done and accept the postoperative discipline for rehabilitation. Are there related conditions, such as chronic pain syndrome or emotional problems? It is important to determine whether the patient desires an increase in functional performance or only cosmetic improvement.

SELECTION OF THE MOTOR MUSCLE (Table 67–1)

In the normal forearm and hand there are 50 muscles to activate movement. Five control supination and pronation, 7

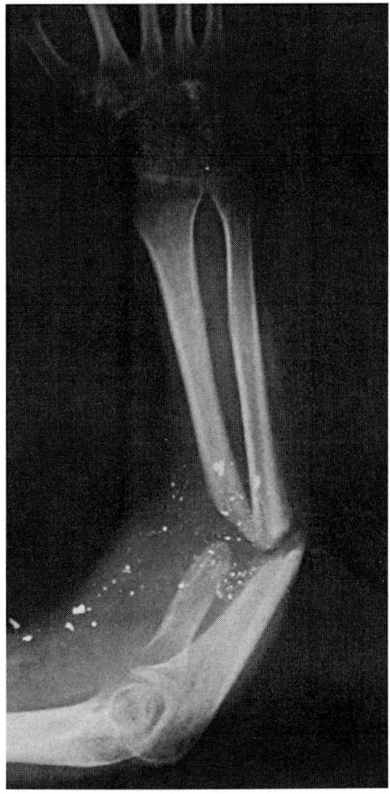

FIGURE 67–1. Tendon transfers across a site of bony nonunion fail because the telescoping skeleton prevents the development of adequate tension for functional muscle power.

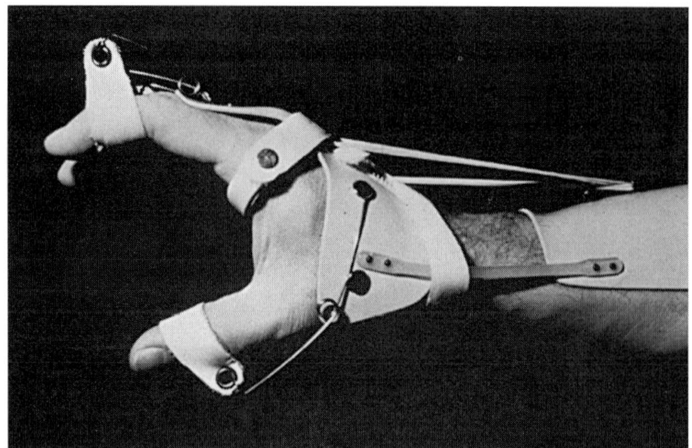

FIGURE 67–2. The functional motion expected after tendon transfer should be easily demonstrated by passive motion before surgery. The thumb is the most vulnerable digit following intrinsic muscle loss, and a combined median-ulnar palsy results in supination and adduction of the thumb, with a contracted thumb-index web. (From Omer GE Jr: Tendon transfers in radial nerve paralysis. *In* Hunter JM, Schneider LH, Mackin LPT [eds]: Tendon Surgery in the Hand. St. Louis, C.V. Mosby, 1987, p 425.)

move the hand at the wrist, 18 flex and extend the digits, and 20 small muscles of the hand contribute to precise motion. As few transfers as necessary are used to meet the basic objective, because all tendon transfers potentially complicate the basic imbalance.

The selected muscle-tendon unit should have amplitude adequate for the anticipated motion. Normal amplitude approximates 33 mm for wrist movers, 70 mm for finger flexors, and 50 mm for finger extensors and the thumb extrinsic muscles (Boyes, 1960). The amplitude expected after tendon transfer cannot exceed the passive amplitude present before surgery. Arthrodesis of the wrist is rare in reconstructive surgery because wrist motion often enhances tendon transfers through dynamic tenodesis.

The motor muscle selected must be strong enough for its new task, because it will have to pull itself free of the

▼ TABLE 67–1
Abbreviations Used in Reconstruction of the Forearm and Hand

ADQ	Abductor digiti quinti
AP	Adductor pollicis
APB	Abductor pollicis brevis
APL	Abductor pollicis longus
BR	Brachioradialis
ECRB	Extensor carpi radialis brevis
ECRL	Extensor carpi radialis longus
ECU	Extensor carpi ulnaris
EDC	Extensor digitorum communis
EDM	Extensor digiti minimi (quinti)
EIP	Extensor indicis proprius
EPB	Extensor pollicis brevis
EPL	Extensor pollicis longus
FCR	Flexor carpi radialis
FCU	Flexor carpi ulnaris
FDP	Flexor digitorum profundus
FDS	Flexor digitorum superficialis (sublimis)
FPL	Flexor pollicis longus
IP	Interphalangeal
MP	Metacarpophalangeal
PL	Palmaris longus
PT	Pronator teres

▼ TABLE 67–2
Work Chart for Tendon Transfers: Radial Palsy

Needed Function	Available Motor	Motor Retained for Balance
Wrist extension (ECRB)	PT to ECRB	Pronator quadratus
Finger and thumb extension (EDC and EPL)	FCU to EDC and EPL	FCR and PL
	or	
	FDS (long and ring) to EDC and EPL	FDP
	or	
	FCR to EDC and PL to EPL	FCU
Proximal thumb stability (APL)	FCR split insertion to APL and FCR	PL and FCU

Note: See Table 67–1 for abbreviations.

healing process after surgery and will usually lose one grade of strength on Lovett's clinical scale (Omer, 1968). A muscle's work capacity is calculated by multiplying strength times amplitude. The range of normal work capacity for forearm muscles can be illustrated: flexor carpi ulnaris (FCU), 2.0 kg; flexor digitorum profundus (FDP), 1.2 kg each or 4.8 kg for the entire muscle; extensor digitorum communis (EDC), 0.5 kg each or 2.0 kg for the whole muscle (Boyes, 1960). The muscle selected must have a work capacity equal to that of the antagonist of the reconstructed motion.

The present action of the selected motor muscle should be synergistic with the anticipated action or at least retrainable by conscious control (Littler, 1964). Muscles that have had temporary total denervation should not be transferred, even if they have regained function (Moneim and Omer, 1986). Paralyzed muscles that have regained function after nerve suture usually lack the individualized control and strength desirable for successful transfer. Even synergistic action muscles are not predictable in upper motor lesions such as cerebral palsy (Omer, 1974b).

The motor muscle for transfer is selected on the basis of its current clinical function. Selected muscles should be charted against retained motion to determine that secondary dysfunction will be avoided (Table 67–2).

OPERATIVE TECHNIQUES

Incisions are placed so that tendon junctures are beneath skin flaps and free of subcutaneous scars. Incisions should be transverse to the subcutaneous path of the transferred tendon. The subcutaneous pathway must glide with the transferred tendon. The motor muscle is mobilized to protect its neurovascular bundle, which usually enters the proximal third of the muscle. Amplitude is related to the length of the muscle fibers, and excursion can be increased by a more complete release of the muscle from the surrounding tissue (Boyes, 1960). The texture, vascularity, and excursion of the selected muscle should be re-evaluated under direct vision at the operating table.

The transferred tendon should not cross raw bone. Muscle-tendon units that must move through fascial planes, such as an interosseous membrane, should have as large an opening in the fascia as practicable. The muscle should be placed in the fascial window, because the exterior muscle fibers will "freeze," but the interior muscle fibers will retain motion; if the tendon is placed in the fascial window, it will bind fast and motion will be lost (Omer, 1974c).

An appropriate moment arm should be selected for the direction of muscle-tendon action (Cooney, 1988). Most muscles are parallel to bone, and the angle of approach between the transferred tendon and its insertion should be small. The greater the angle of approach for the tendon to its insertion point, the greater the force the muscle can exert, but this creates a bowstring. A pulley is required to increase the approach angle, and the result is actually a loss of force secondary to friction when the angle is greater than 45 degrees. Eventually, a bowstrung tendon will shift to a straight line and then become too slack for effective action. The more distal to the axis of motion of a joint the transfer is anchored, the more force the muscle can exert on the joint, but also the more excursion required of the tendon to provide a normal range of motion in the joint. If the insertion of a transferred tendon is split, the motor will act primarily on the slip under greater tension.

A tendon transfer is more effective when it crosses only one joint. If a tendon bowstrings across a proximal joint, its mechanical advantage at that joint will be so great that it may force that joint into unwanted movement or use up all its amplitude so that it cannot move the distal joint. An example is the transfer of the brachioradialis (BR) into the flexor pollicis longus (FPL): when the elbow and wrist are extended, the patient can hold an object tightly, but when the elbow is fully flexed the muscle-tendon power is dissipated at the elbow, and the patient drops the object. A second example is a bony nonunion; these fail because the telescoping skeleton prevents the development of adequate amplitude for functional power.

Suture material for tendon fixation should be synthetic material with minimal tissue reaction. The suture material can be relatively large, such as 3-0 for forearm transfers. Some tendon ischemia is prevented when the suture is inserted through the center of the tendon and then circles only half of the tendon; sutures along the length of the tendon should alternate the circle to be tied from side to side to further protect circulation. "Lacing" a transferred tendon into a group of paralyzed muscle-tendon units should be avoided because it creates bulk, twist, scar, and increases friction. A precise insertion point should be selected, but at that point a short length of paralyzed and transfer tendons should be sutured side-to-side to prevent "whipsawing." A second technique is leaving the initial tendon in its bed and passing the transferred tendon across it, as done with the FCU to the EDC. This is an oblique transfer, and there should be a double line of nonabsorbable sutures to prevent shifting in the tension to several slips. One may disconnect the paralyzed tendon from its fibrosed muscle and connect it directly to the transferred muscle. However, complete excision of the paralyzed muscle belly may bring unwelcome hemorrhage and should not be done unless the paralyzed muscle mass is causing deformity.

Appropriate tension for the transferred muscle-tendon unit depends on mean fiber length, cross-sectional area, and total muscle volume (Brand, 1987, 1988). Laser light diffraction has been used to measure muscle sarcomere length and thus determine optimal muscle tension during transfer (Fleeter et al, 1988); electrical stimulation has also been used to note the functional tension (Omer and Vogel, 1965). If there has been good evaluation of tissue homeostasis, tension can be evaluated and determined at operation (Omer and Pirela-Cruz, 1994). The tension of a tendon transfer is judged best while the hand is placed in the position it will assume when the new tendon contracts. For extensor transfers, resting tendon tension should be strong enough to passively hold the extremity in functional position against gravity; however, one should be sure that the wrist has the potential for a normal arc of flexion. Flexor tendons often cross more than one joint and should be fixed at somewhat greater than normal tension against gravity. Appropriate tension brings perception of the new muscle more readily into consciousness as stretch reflexes and other feedback mechanisms are stimulated when opposing muscles restore the neutral position of the extremity (Brand, 1991).

PREOPERATIVE CARE

The extremity must be immobilized in the appropriate position to maintain the desired result. After either median or ulnar palsy, the thumb-index web must be maintained to prevent contracture with thumb adduction and supination. Maintaining a mobile extremity without deforming contracture demands a planned and persistent rehabilitation program. The functional performance expected after tendon transfer should be possible to effect by passive movement before surgery.

TIMING OF TENDON TRANSFERS

The timing of tendon transfers is a debatable problem that varies with the level of the nerve injury. When a precise neurorrhaphy has been performed early in a patient with low (distal) nerve laceration, the prognosis for reinnervation of palsied muscles has improved during the past decade (Birch and Raji, 1991; Mailander et al, 1989; Millesi, 1990). In these patients, selected tendon transfers may be performed early as internal splints to support partial function and prevent deformity while awaiting the potential nerve recovery. Patients with a severe or extensive extremity injury, a long nerve graft, or a high (proximal) nerve lesion are all candidates for a complete reconstruction program. The potential for functional motor action is better than recovery of normal sensibility in the high (proximal) nerve palsy.

EARLY TENDON TRANSFERS AS INTERNAL SPLINTS
(Table 67–3)

The goal of reconstruction after peripheral nerve injury is to restore maximum function as rapidly as possible. This is difficult in more proximal nerve injuries secondary to the time required for axon regrowth to distal muscles and sensory end-organs. Selected early tendon transfers as internal splints enhance function while awaiting the return of nerve

Palsy	Functional Need	Available Motors
Low median	Thumb abduction (APB)	EIP to APB (and EPL) *or* EDM *or* PL *or* FDS (ring) to APB (and EPL)
Radial	Wrist extension (ECRB)	PT to ECRB
Low ulnar	Thumb adduction (AP) *and*	FDS (long) in 3 slips to AP *plus*
	Correct ring and little fingers' clawing	A2 pulley flexor sheath for flexion *or* Dorsal apparatus for extension

Note: See Table 67–1 for abbreviations.

control and total muscle activity. The objectives of early tendon transfers are to stimulate sensibility re-education and to improve the coordination of residual muscle-tendon units. The early tendon transfer may substitute function during nerve regrowth and allow the patient to be splint-free, with nearly full use during axon regrowth. Axon regrowth may be less than optimal for the denervated muscle, and the early tendon transfer may assist in function. The combined results of early tendon transfer plus the return from nerve repair often are better than those of either procedure separately. If there is no functional recovery from the neurorrhaphy, then the early tendon transfer becomes a complete substitute on a permanent basis (Burkhalter, 1993).

The muscle-tendon units used as internal splints should be synergistic with the muscle-tendon unit to be replaced, such as a wrist flexor in substitution for a finger extensor. A synergistic muscle-tendon unit will be able to use spinal reflex arcs and other autonomic feedback mechanisms to enhance re-education. Two points are important: (1) use as few muscle-tendon transfers as possible, because any active muscle-tendon unit used to restore a useful motion will weaken the strength of the residual function; and (2) the muscle-tendon transfer should not cause deformity when nerve function is recovered. For example, it would be foolish to transfer the FCU, the palmaris longus (PL), and the flexor carpi radialis (FCR) to varied wrist and digit extensors in a case of radial palsy. Subsequent recovery of radial nerve function would result in an inability to actively flex the wrist and would create a new deformity (Omer, 1982b) (see Table 67–2).

Radial Palsy: Extension of the Wrist

The most visible clinical activity of the muscles innervated by the radial nerve is extension of the fingers and thumb. However, the major function may be to stabilize the wrist for power grip. Power grip is impossible in radial palsy, even through there is no volar injury (Boyes, 1960). The pronator teres (PT) transferred to the extensor carpi radialis brevis (ECRB) will produce active wrist extension, encourage passive flexion of the metacarpophalangeal (MP) joint, and allow ulnar innervated intrinsic muscle interphalangeal (IP) extension. Increasing dorsal extension power of the wrist by an increment of one may increase power grip three to five times (Burkhalter, 1974).

Through a longitudinal incision over the radial aspect of

the middle third of the forearm, the PT is freed with a tongue of periosteum from the radius. The muscle belly is bluntly freed, avoiding neurovascular injury in the volar forearm. The freed muscle is passed subcutaneously over the BR and the extensor carpi radialis longus (ECRL) muscles to be attached to the muscle-tendon junction of the ECRB (Omer, 1987b) (Fig. 67–3). The PT should be inserted only into the ECRB (Fig. 67–4). If the PT is inserted into both the ECRB and ECRL, the usual result is radially deviated dorsal extension. After suture, the wrist should rest for 5 weeks in 20 degrees of extension against gravity.

Low Median Palsy: Abduction of the Thumb

Low median palsy results in a loss of functional abduction and pronation of the thumb. The functioning extensor pollicis longus (EPL), extensor pollicis brevis (EPB), and adductor pollicis (AP) will create a supination deformity of the thumb and eventually an adduction contracture of the first metacarpal. Reconstructive transfers will fail if there is contracture of the first web space (Burkhalter et al, 1973).

Opposition of the thumb is normally initiated by the abductor pollicis brevis (APB) (Omer, 1978b, 1987a). A transfer to only the tendon of the APB has the appropriate result except in patients with very mobile MP joints. In these patients, the transfer should include the tendon of the EPL (Omer, 1990). Thumb opposition is a complex function discussed in the section on isolated low median palsy.

The extensor indicis proprius (EIP) is the preferred transfer to achieve abduction of the thumb (Fig. 67–5). The tendon is identified through a longitudinal incision over the index MP joint and freed from the radial aspect of the extensor hood. The defect in the extensor hood is meticulously repaired with nonabsorbable sutures. Through short transverse incisions the EIP is freed from the index EDC tendon and isolated above the wrist. A short oblique incision is made distal to the pisiform, and a tendon passer is used to advance the tendon subcutaneously around the ulnar border of the forearm, using the pisiform and adjacent vertical fibrous tissue as a pulley. The tendon is passed subcutaneously across the wrist, through a muscle tunnel in the paralyzed APB, and on to the MP joint. This will prevent the transferred tendon from becoming a painful bowstring across the proximal palm (Omer, 1982b).

When the transfer is done for a isolated median palsy, the transfer can be attached to the tendon of the APB (Littler, 1949). In combined palsies with no intrinsic muscle activity in the thumb, the transfer should be attached to the APB tendon and the EPL tendon over the proximal phalanx (Riordan, 1953). By increasing the tension on the EPL, the FPL becomes a flexor of the MP joint as well as the IP joint. The transfer should be sutured with the wrist in 30 degrees flexion and the thumb in maximum abduction. If passive wrist dorsiflexion is restricted by the transfer, the tendon should be resutured a bit longer (White, 1960).

Transfer of the extensor digiti minimi (EDM) has the same technique and advantages as the EIP transfer (Schneider, 1969). If the median nerve is lacerated by an oblique injury that spares the PL tendon, this tendon can be lengthened into the palmar fascia and transferred to the insertion of the APB (Braun, 1978; Camitz, 1929).

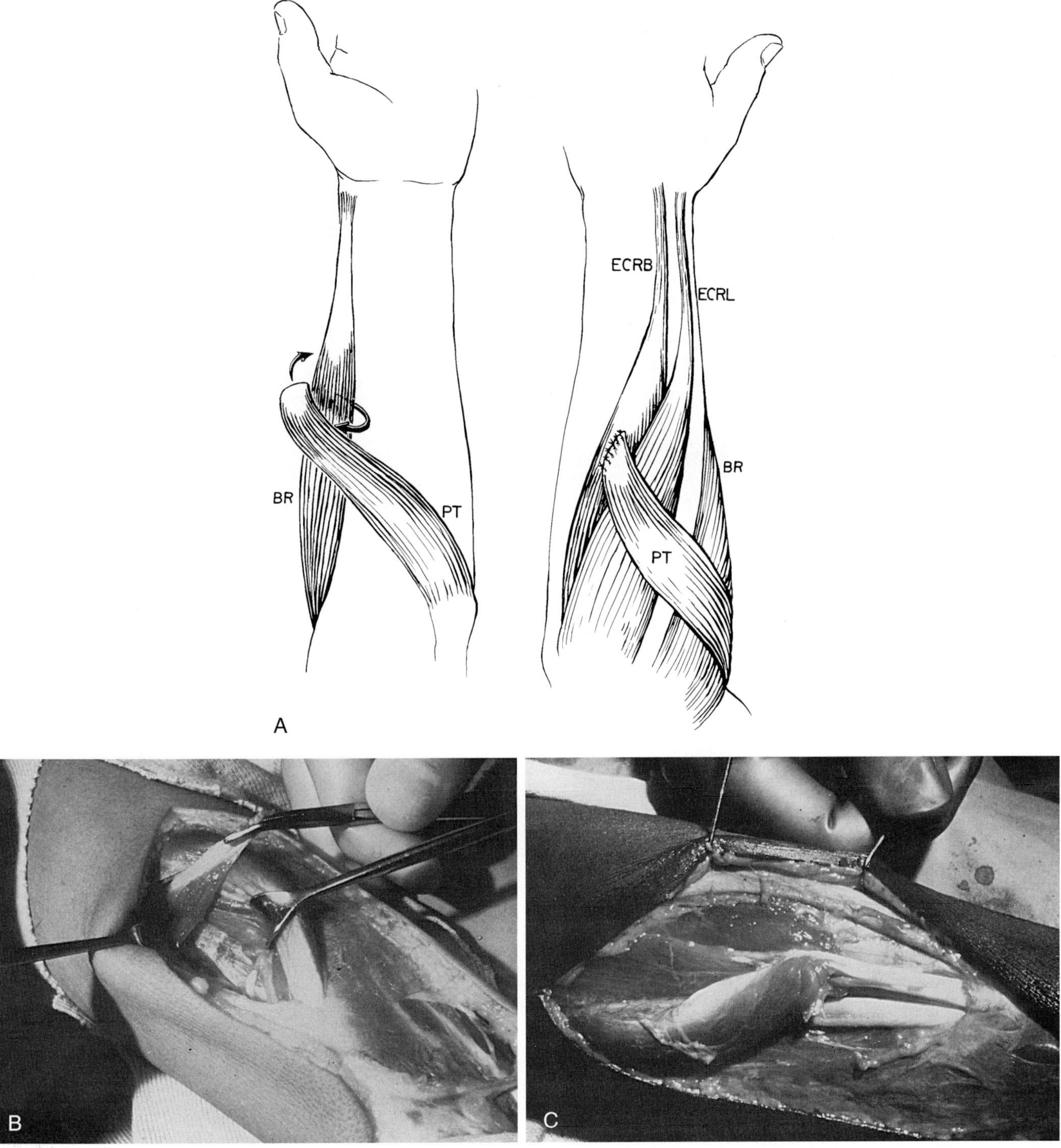

FIGURE 67–3. *A,* Transfer of the pronator teres (PT) tendon to the tendon of the extensor carpi radialis brevis (ECRB) for wrist extension. (From Omer GE Jr: J Bone Joint Surg *50(A)*:1454, 1968.) *B,* Release of PT insertion into the radius. *C,* Subcutaneous transfer of PT over the brachioradialis and extensor carpi radialis longus muscles into the tendon of ECRB. (From Omer GE Jr: Early tendon transfers as internal splints after nerve injury. *In* Hunter JM, Schneider LH, Mackin LPT [eds]: Tendon Surgery in the Hand. St. Louis, C.V. Mosby, 1987, p 414.)

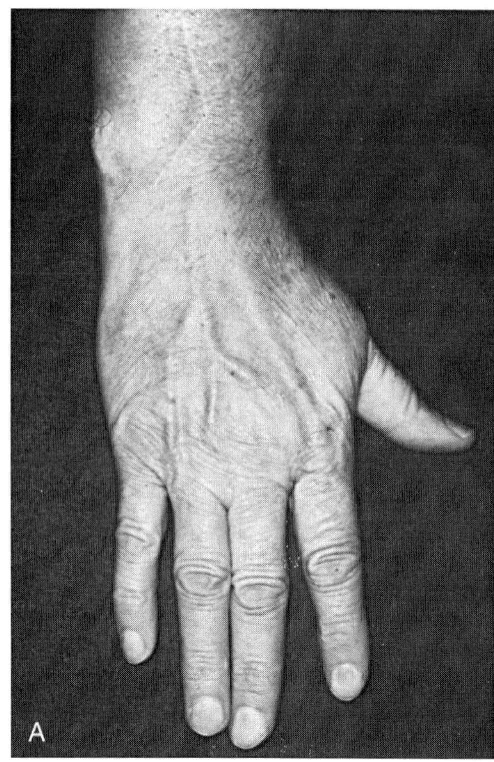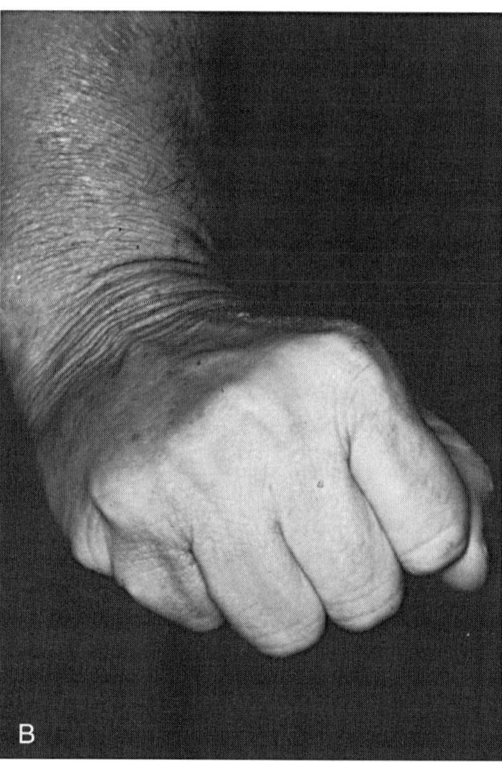

FIGURE 67–4. The pronator teres (PT) tendon should insert only into tendon of the extensor carpi radialis brevis (ECRB). In this case, the pronator teres was inserted into tendon of the extensor carpi radialis longus (ECRL) (*A*), resulting in radial deviation with functional extension (*B*).

Postoperatively, a short arm cast is applied, holding the thumb in full abduction. The cast is removed after 5 weeks, and the patient is taught to observe thumb abduction when the fingers are extended. If there is continued instability in the longitudinal arch of the thumb, the MP joint should be arthrodesed.

Low Ulnar Palsy: Adduction of Thumb, Clawed Fingers, and Metacarpal Arch

Ulnar nerve palsy results in a visibly awkward hand with profound functional weakness. An isolated tendon transfer cannot restore all the power requirements in a low ulnar palsy, but a single flexor digitorum superficialis (FDS) tendon can improve thumb adduction for key pinch, the clawed position of the ring and little fingers, and the flattened metacarpal arch (Omer, 1968, 1971a, 1987a). Arthrodesis of the MP joint of the thumb will improve stability for tip pinch (Littler, 1949, Omer, 1968).

The FDS tendon of the long finger is preferred; however, the ring FDS may be used if the ulnar innervated portion of the FDP is not paralyzed (Fig. 67–6). The superficialis tendon is exposed through a volar zigzag incision in the long finger that extends into the palm. The distal radial insertion of the superficialis tendon is released proximal to the proximal IP joint and tenodesed to prevent hyperextension of the joint after completion of the transfer. The distal ulnar insertion of the superficialis tendon is released at its terminal insertion. The flexor sheath should be retained, especially the proximal A1 and A2 pulleys. The FDS is first split longitudinally, then the ulnar half of the tendon is split again into two slips.

If the IP joints cannot be extended actively by the EDC

when the MP joint is stabilized in flexion, a procedure is done to improve finger extension power (Omer, 1971a, 1990). Short longitudinal incisions are made over the dorsal aspect of the proximal IP joints of the ring and little fingers. The two slips of the ulnar half of the transfer tendon are directed volar to the deep transverse metacarpal ligament and then dorsal to be sutured at the insertion of the central slip of the dorsal apparatus on the middle phalanx of the ring and little fingers. It is important that the dorsal apparatus is not injured. Traction on the transferred tendon slips should flex the MP joint and extend the proximal IP joint.

A different insertion is preferred for the two superficialis slips when increased power for grip is desirable, and the extrinsic extensor tendon can extend the proximal IP joints with the MP joints stabilized in flexion (Omer, 1993; Riordan, 1959). Longitudinal zigzag incisions are made on the volar side of the ring and little fingers in addition to the incision on the volar side of the long finger. The proximal edge of the flexor sheaths are exposed, and the transferred superficialis slips are passed distally through the flexor sheaths and volar around the distal edge of the A2 pulley and sutured in place. This insertion does not extend the proximal IP joint and is similar to dynamic transfers for proximal phalanx flexion (Zancolli, 1978).

A short longitudinal incision is made over the abductor tubercle of the first metacarpal. The radial half of the superficialis tendon is directed transversely over the volar surface of the AP, but dorsal to the flexor tendons and neurovascular structures, and is sutured into the insertion of the APB. The pulley for this transfer is the distal edge of the palmar fascia inserted into the third metacarpal (Edgerton and Brand, 1965).

The functional mechanism of this tendon transfer (Omer, 1974a) is similar to the Bunnell "tendon T" operation (Bun-

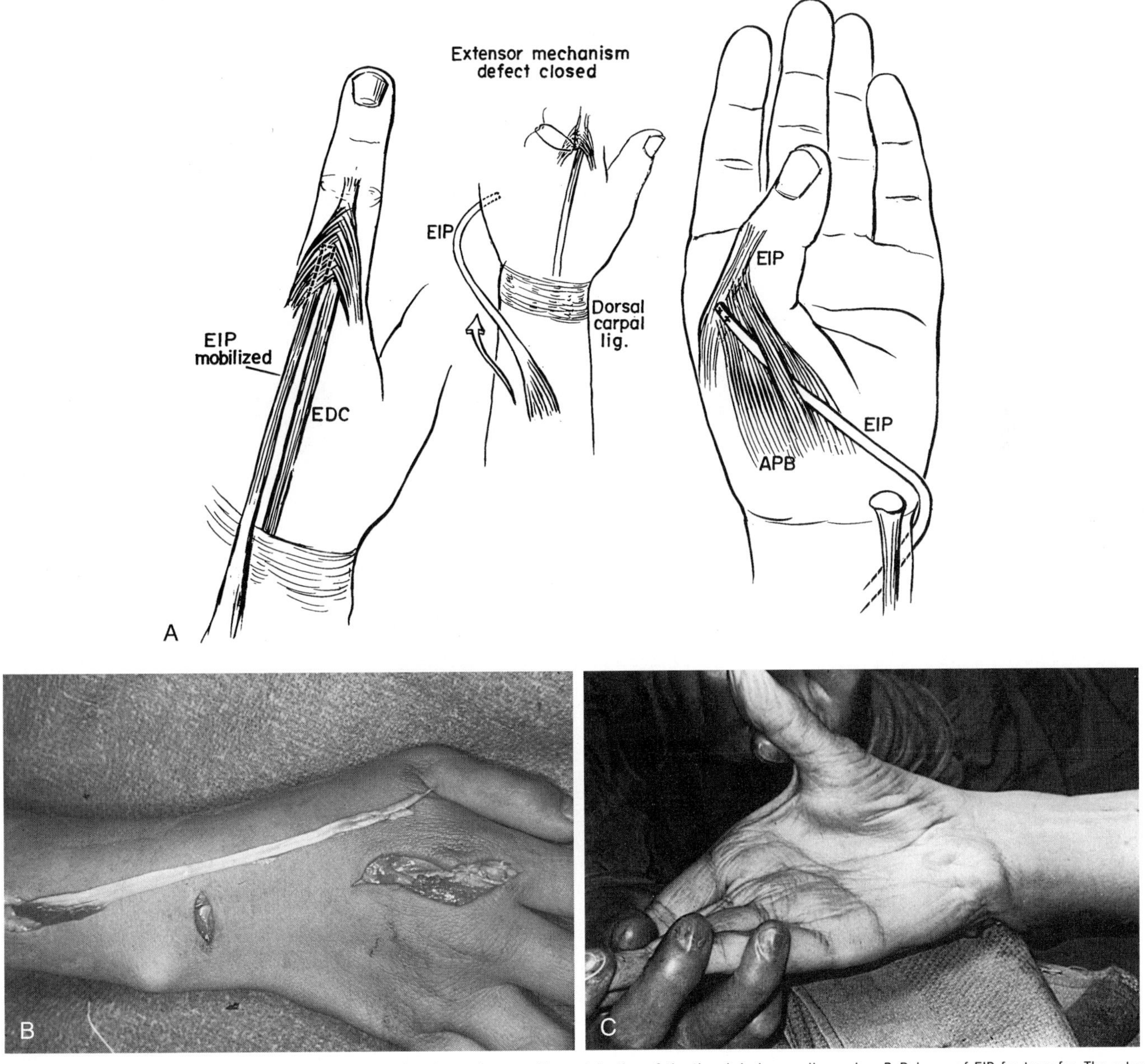

FIGURE 67–5. *A,* The extensor indicis proprius (EIP) is the preferred transfer to achieve abduction of the thumb in low median palsy. *B,* Release of EIP for transfer. The extensor apparatus over the index finger must be repaired if an incision has been made into the dorsal hood. *C,* Insertion of the EIP into tendon of abductor pollicis brevis (APB). The pulley for this transfer is the pisiform and adjacent vertical fibrous tissue. The transfer is passed beneath the APB to prevent "bowstring" of the transfer across the base of the palm. (*B* and *C* from Omer GE Jr: Early tendon transfers as internal splints after nerve injury. *In* Hunter JM, Schneider LH, Mackin LPT [eds]: Tendon Surgery in the Hand. St. Louis, C.V. Mosby 1987, p 414.)

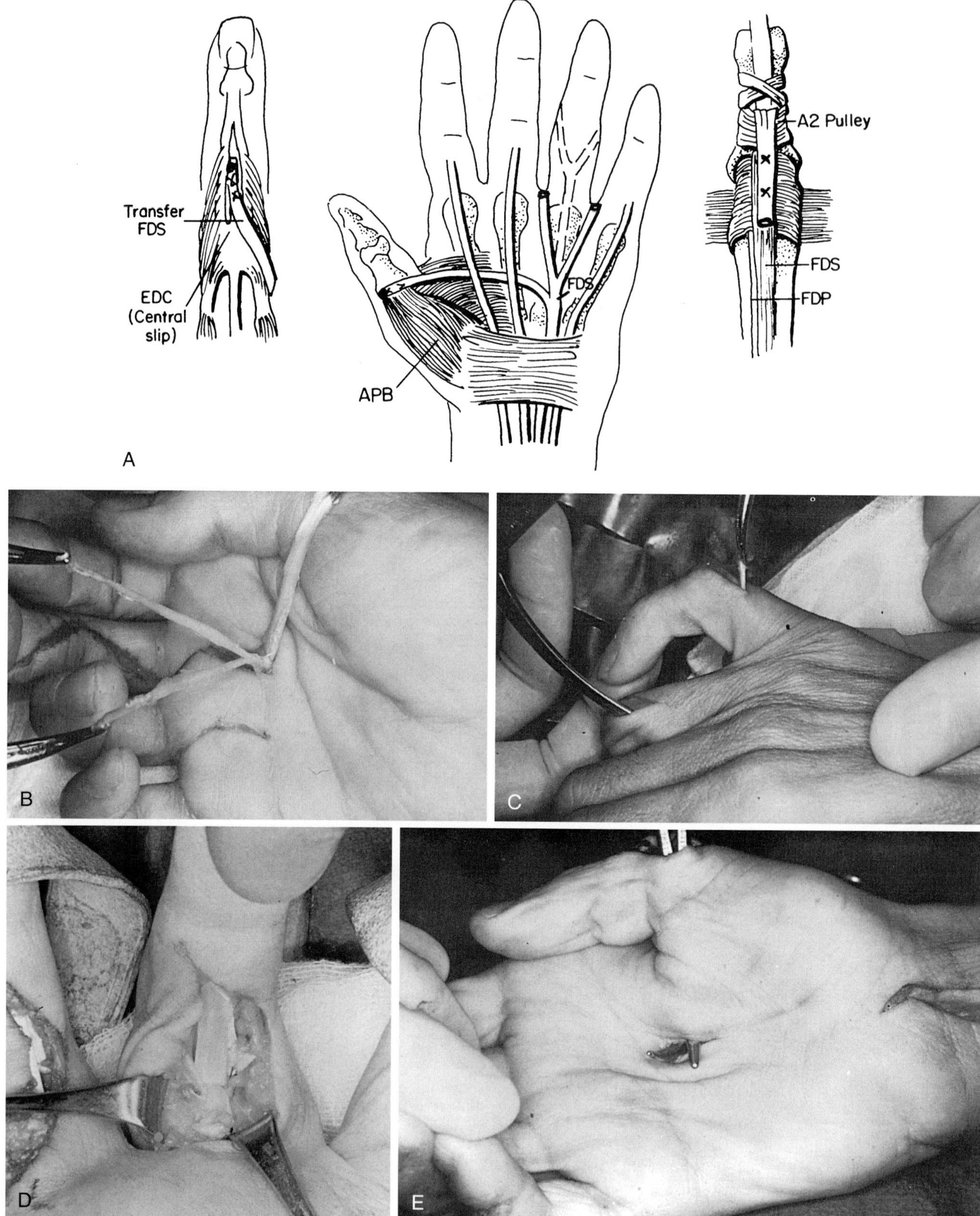

FIGURE 67–6. *A,* Transfer of the flexor digitorum superficialis (FDS) for thumb adduction and opposition power, and to prevent clawing of the ring and little fingers. The long FDS is preferred; however, the ring FDS may be used if the ulnar innervated portion of the flexor digitorum profundus is not paralyzed. *B,* The long FDS has been split longitudinally, and the ulnar half divided into two slips. *C,* The two ulnar slips may be transferred to insert on the central slip of the dorsal apparatus of the ring and little fingers, or, *D,* The two ulnar slips may be transferred to the A2 pulley of the flexor sheath of the ring and little fingers. (*B* to *D* from Omer GE Jr: Early tendon transfers as internal splints after nerve injury. *In* Hunter JM, Schneider LH, Mackin LPT [eds]: Tendon Surgery in the Hand. St. Louis, C.V. Mosby, 1987, p 416.) *E,* The radial half of the long FDS is inserted into tendon of the abductor pollicis brevis.

nell, 1944), except that the distal edge of the palmar fascia is the pulley rather than a free tendon graft between the first and fifth metacarpals. Tension of the transferred superficialis tendon should adduct and pronate the first metacarpal, increase the metacarpal (palmar) arch, and depress the clawed fingers.

The resting tension of the transferred superficialis tendon is adjusted at the insertion points while the wrist is in neutral flexion-extension and the hand is supinated into a palm-up position. The MP joints of the clawed fingers are placed in 45 degrees of flexion, and the proximal IP joints are placed in zero degrees of extension (10 degrees of flexion if tenodesed). The first metacarpal is adducted so that it is parallel with the plane of the second metacarpal. This intrinsic-plus position is maintained in plaster immobilization for 4 weeks before active extension is permitted.

After the tendon transfer to correct an intrinsic-minus thumb and the clawed fingers of ulnar palsy, the wrist should be in slight dorsiflexion, the thumb should be adducted and pronated, the MP joints of the fingers should be flexed, and the IP joints of the fingers should be extended—the "hoe-hand" position.

Median or Ulnar Palsy: Thumb Metacarpophalangeal Joint Arthrodesis

Distal stability for tip pinch between the thumb and index finger is improved by arthrodesis of the MP joint of the thumb (Omer, 1968) and is indicated when the patient develops a hyperextension deformity of the MP joint (Jeanne's sign) after tendon transfers (Fig. 67–7).

The MP joint surfaces are cut back to produce a chevron-shaped mortise, with the point of the chevron directed proximally. The apex of the phalangeal half of the chevron mortise is made perpendicular to the long axis of the phalanx, and the apex of the metacarpal half of the mortise is inclined (undercut) palmarward to obtain the desired flexion (0 to 10 degrees) and held in pronation (10 to 15 degrees) and abduction (5 degrees). The mortise is then stabilized with buried crossed Kirschner wires perpendicular to the joint surface.

The thumb is pronated to improve the pulp-to-pulp pinch and held in extension to decrease the supination effect on the thumb by the fingers. The thumb is placed in a spica cast for 6 weeks, and then active motion without power is continued until bone healing is recognized on radiographs.

COMPLETE LESIONS OF INDIVIDUAL NERVES

Reconstruction of a complete nerve lesion should be limited to essential function. The key to success for transfer procedures is simplicity, because complexity invites failure. Increased power for a given function must be introduced from another normal power train.

Radial Palsy (see Table 67–2)

The goals of preoperative management are maintenance of a full passive range of motion in all joints of the hand and wrist, with prevention of contractures, giving particular attention to the thumb-index web. The patient may prefer only a volar cock-up splint with a C-bar for the thumb-index web during the day; however, that splint should be supplemented with a nighttime splint that holds the wrist and fingers in full extension. If the wrist and fingers are not stabilized in full extension, there will be progressive loss of fiber length of the flexor muscles, making it difficult to achieve normal balance after reinnervation or reconstructive surgery (Brand, 1987).

The requirements for restoration of forearm and hand function after radial palsy are (1) wrist extension, (2) finger extension, (3) thumb extension, and (4) stability of the carpometacarpal joint of the thumb. Usually, there is loss of accessory elbow flexion and forearm supination, but these are not obvious if there is a normal biceps brachii. Disruption of sensibility on the radial side of the forearm is a major impairment if there is a painful neuroma; otherwise, it is not a clinical problem (Green, 1993). Trauma to the upper arm (high lesion) may include loss of elbow extension, and an injury to the forearm (low lesion) may spare radially deviated wrist extension (Schneider, 1991).

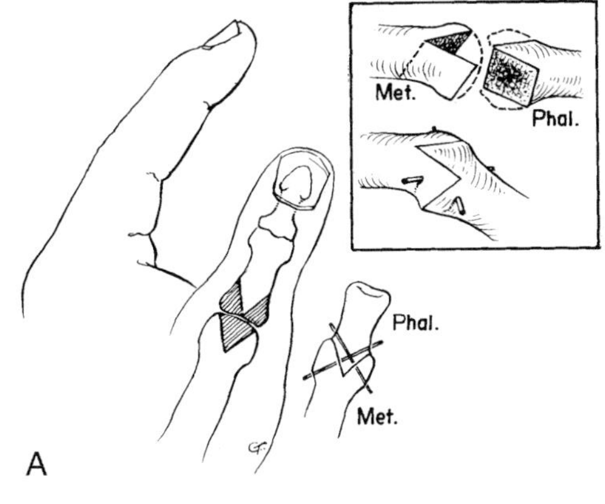

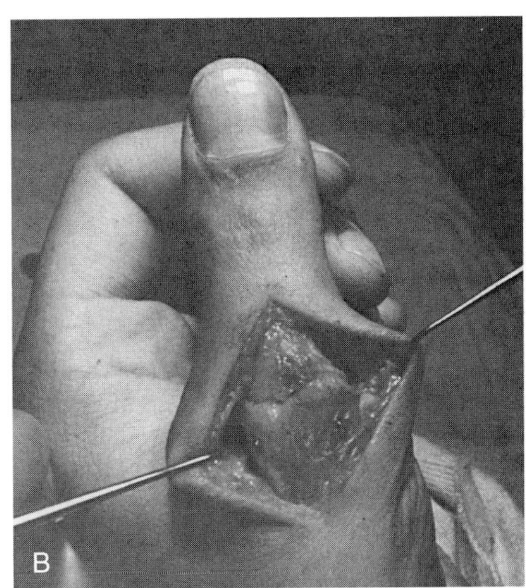

FIGURE 67–7. *A,* The chevron-shaped mortise cut for arthrodesis of the metacarpophalangeal and proximal interphalangeal joints. The metacarpal bone cut is inclined proximally from the dorsal to volar surface to obtain the desired flexion of the joint. *B,* Crossed Kirschner wires are used for fixation. (*B* from Omer GE Jr: Early tendon transfers as internal splints after nerve injury. *In* Hunter JM, Schneider LH, Mackin LPT [eds]: Tendon Surgery in the Hand. St. Louis C.V. Mosby, 1987,) p 417.)

Active wrist extension is obtained by transferring the median-innervated PT to the ECRB tendon (Omer, 1987a), as described in the section on early tendon transfers. The PT remains a pronator of the forearm after transfer.

DIGITAL EXTENSION

The oldest procedure for digital extension uses the ulnar-innervated FCU muscle (Boyes, 1960). A longitudinal incision is made over the muscle, and the FCU is freed from its fascial attachments. The limiting factor is the innervation of the FCU, which enters the muscle in its proximal 5 cm (Omer, 1993). A longitudinal incision is made on the dorsal surface of the forearm, and the FCU is directed subcutane-ously around the ulna and superficial to the tendons of the EDC, which remain in their normal compartment. The transferred tendon is attached in an oblique line of sutures proximal to the dorsal retinaculum (Omer, 1982a). If the transferred tendon is not attached proximally and distally at each EDC tendon, then motion will result in "whipsawing" between the tendons. The EDM is not included unless the EDC slip to the little finger is absent. Tension on individual EDC tendons should be adjusted to fit the appropriate finger pattern in extension.

After appropriate tension is set for the EDC, the EPL tendon can be included as the final insertion of the FCU transfer. Tension should be adjusted so that the thumb fits into the functional extension splay against gravity demon-

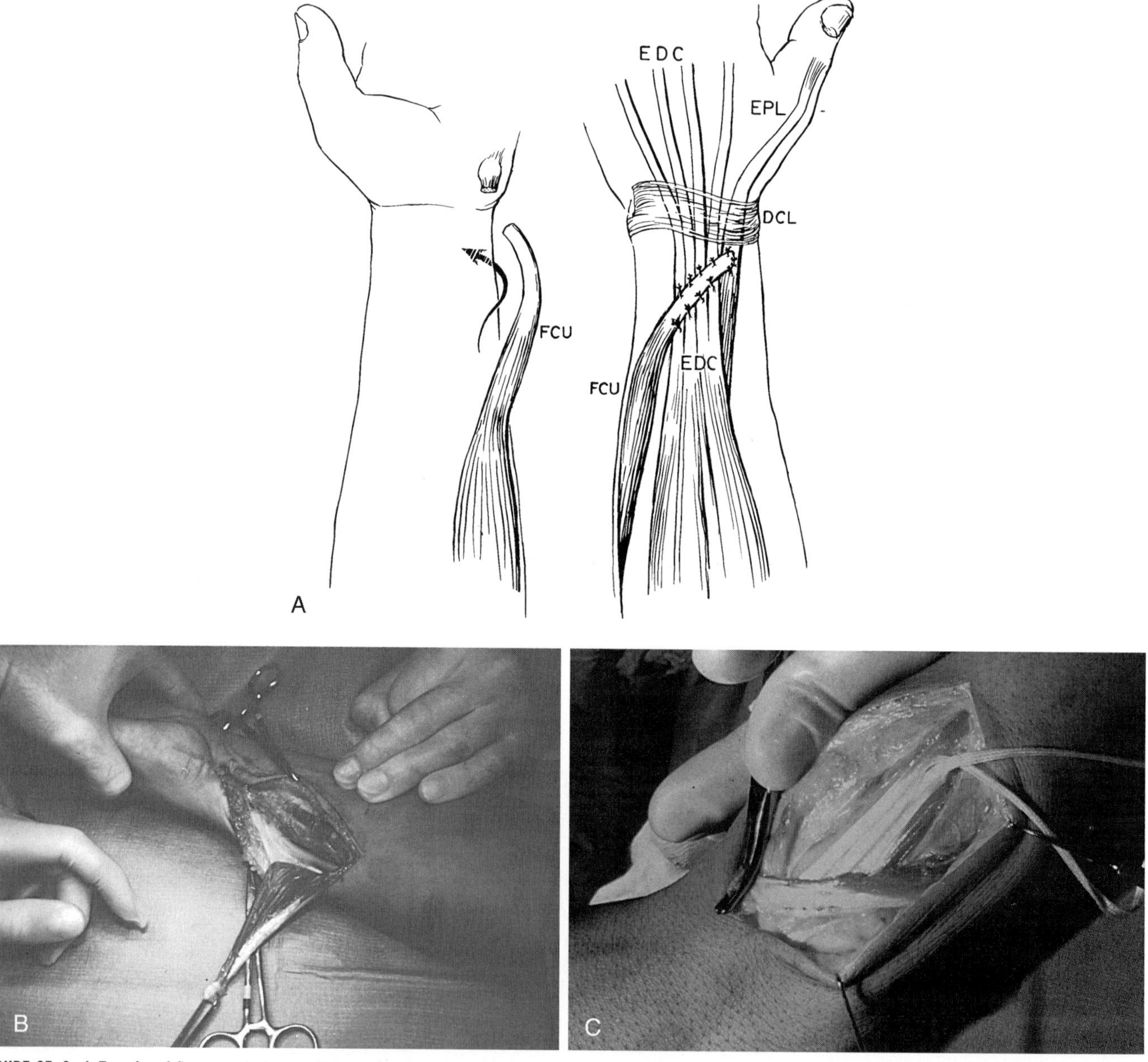

FIGURE 67–8. *A*, Transfer of flexor carpi ulnaris (FCU) for finger and thumb extension. *B*, Intraoperative photograph. *C*, The FCU should be subcutaneous and superficial to the tendons of the extensor digitorum communis (EDC) and the extensor pollicis longus (EPL). The oblique position enhances appropriate tension, but each tendon anastomosis should have a proximal and distal suture to prevent "whipsawing" of the tendons. The extensor pollicis longus (EPL) will be included in the same anastomosis.

strated by the digits. This full FCU transfer often results in a slight radial deviation of the hand at the wrist. If the patient has significant preoperative radial deviation of the hand at the wrist, either the FCU transfer should not be done or the insertion of the ECRL should be transferred to the extensor carpi ulnaris (ECU).

A few months after the FCU transfer, the patient usually can extend only the thumb, only the index finger, only the little finger, or all the fingers, or the patient may extend the wrist with the fingers open or closed in a fist (Fig. 67–8).

This is a "trick motion," because all digits are extended and then selectively flexed to leave only the appropriate one extended; both the mass extension and selective counter-flexion are done quickly, and the visual effect is one of independent single digit extension (Omer, 1968, 1992; Omer and Pirela-Cruz, 1994).

The fingers and thumb also can be extended by the median-innervated FDS tendons to the long and ring fingers (Boyes, 1960). The FDS tendons are exposed through a transverse incision in the distal palm and a longitudinal

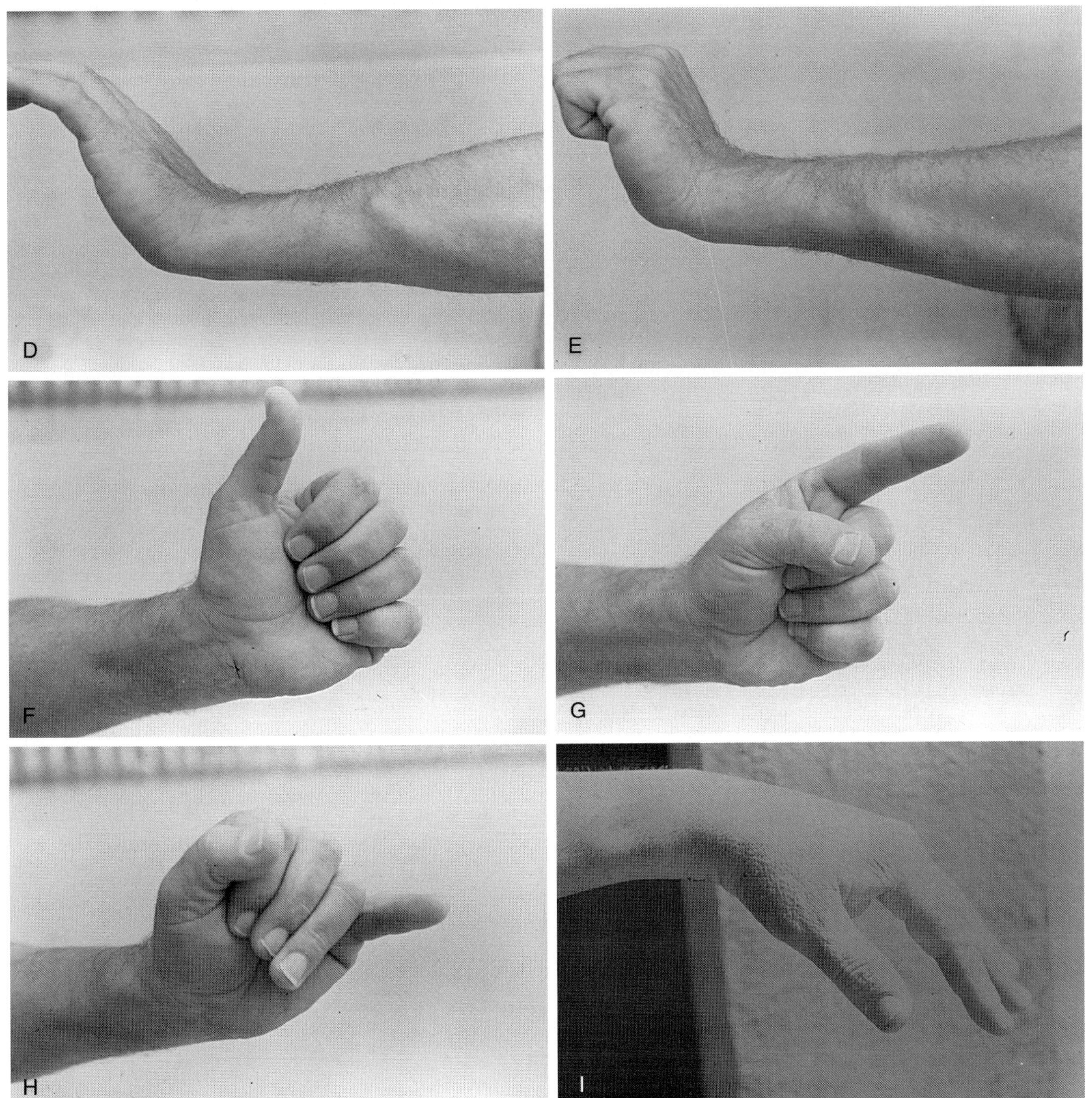

FIGURE 67–8 *Continued* Ten-year follow-up of a so-called mass action transfer of FCU to EDC and EPL. *D,* Wrist and finger extension. *E,* Wrist extension independent of finger extension. *F,* Independent thumb extension. *G,* Independent index extension. *H,* There is limitation of extension by tendon junctures, and the patient mass extends all the fingers and then selectively flexes all the fingers except the one to remain in extension. (*C* to *G* from Omer GE Jr: Tendon transfers in radial nerve paralysis. *In* Hunter JM, Schneider LH, Mackin LPT [eds]: Tendon Surgery in the Hand. St. Louis, C.V. Mosby, 1987, p 423 and 426.) *I,* Functional flexion of the wrist. The range of wrist motion is less than that of opposite wrist.

incision in the volar forearm. The tendons are then divided proximal to the chiasma, separated from the profundi tendons, and delivered into the forearm. Just proximal to the pronator quadratus, two windows are incised in the interosseous membrane, one on each side of the anterior interosseous artery (Fig. 67–9). The windows should be as large as practicable (Omer, 1987b). The two tendons are passed to the dorsum of the forearm through the windows in the interosseous membrane, with the long FDS to the radial side of the profundus muscle group and the ring FDS to the ulnar side. Bare FDS tendons without muscle cover will adhere to the membrane during healing, with resulting loss of motion. If there is potential injury to either the anterior or posterior interosseous vessels, the tourniquet should be deflated and hemostasis obtained. It is very difficult to stop bleeding after completion of the transfer. If it is not possible to pull the muscles of the FDS units through the windows in the interosseous membrane, then the FDS units are routed around both sides of the forearm in the subcutaneous tissues.

A passive fist is formed with the wrist held in 45 degrees of extension, and then the tendons are sutured at "normal" tension. The ring FDS is attached to the tendons of the EDC in a side-to-side oblique anastomosis similar to the FCU transfer. The long FDS tendon is attached to the EPL and the EIP. The anastomoses should be made well proximal to the dorsal retinaculum, and the recipient tendons are not divided proximal to the suture anastomoses. When the passive fist is released, the digits should posture in functional extension against gravity.

A third technique to extend the fingers uses the median-innervated FCR (Starr, 1922). The FCR is subcutaneously passed around the radial border of the forearm and obliquely across the EDC tendons. Tsuge and Adachi (1969) pass the FCR through the interosseous membrane to obtain a straight line for pull.

Thumb extension may be motored by the PL (Riordan, 1974). The EPL tendon is cut at its musculoskeletal junction and withdrawn distally, and then pulled proximally in line with the APB tendon. The PL tendon is released at its insertion and sutured into the EPL in the region of the anatomical snuffbox. An end-to-end anastomosis allows adjustment of tension for extension of the thumb.

In FCU, FDS, or FCR transfers, the tendons must be tight enough to provide functional extension of the wrist, thumb, and fingers, yet not so tight as to limit functional flexion of the wrist and fingers. Full flexion of the wrist is uncommon after reconstruction. If there is blocking of the suture lines against the dorsal retinaculum, this fascial band should be narrowed.

Boyes (1960) emphasized the importance of the FCU in ulnar deviation. Transfer of the FCU often results in radial deviation of the wrist and hand on the forearm. If the injury is distal to the division of the radial nerve into the posterior interosseous and superficial branches, then the BR and ECRL motors may be intact and enhance radial deviation of the wrist and hand. However, Brand (1991) has recommended using the PL for thumb extension if the FCR is used for finger extension. An advantage of the FDS tendons is

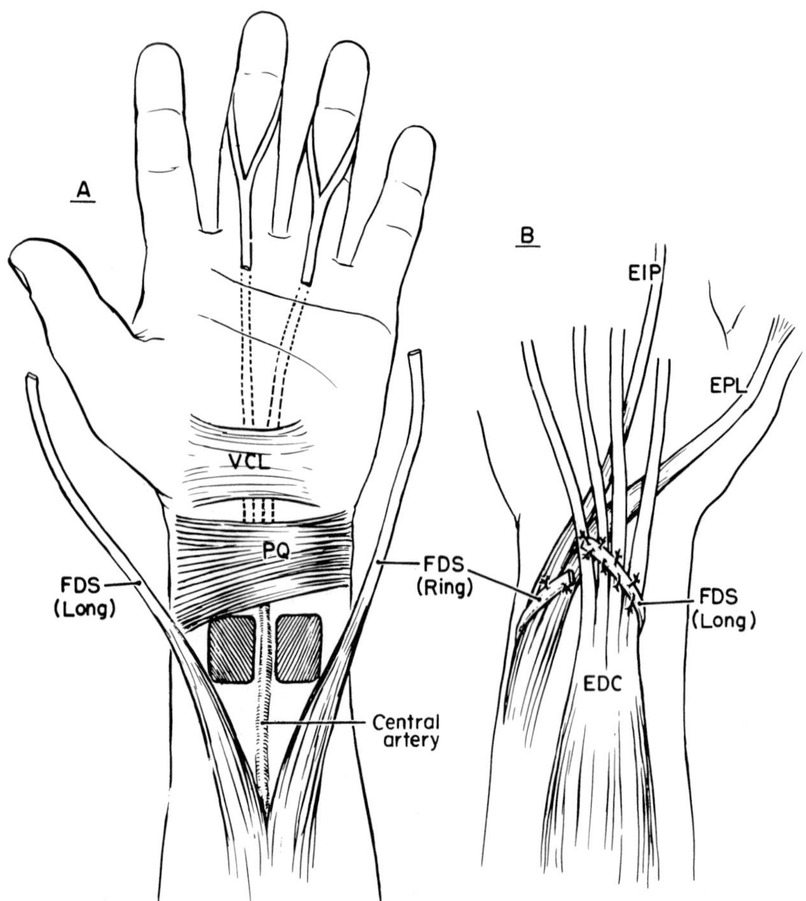

FIGURE 67–9. Transfer of the long and ring flexor digitorum superficialis tendons through the interosseous membrane for finger and thumb extension. The holes in the interosseous membrane must be large but must not damage the central artery on the volar side of the forearm. The long finger superficialis provides extension of the four fingers, whereas the ring finger superficialis provides extension of the thumb and index finger. (From Omer GE, Jr: Am Acad Orthop Surg Instructional Course Lectures *18* [J1]:93, 1962–1969.)

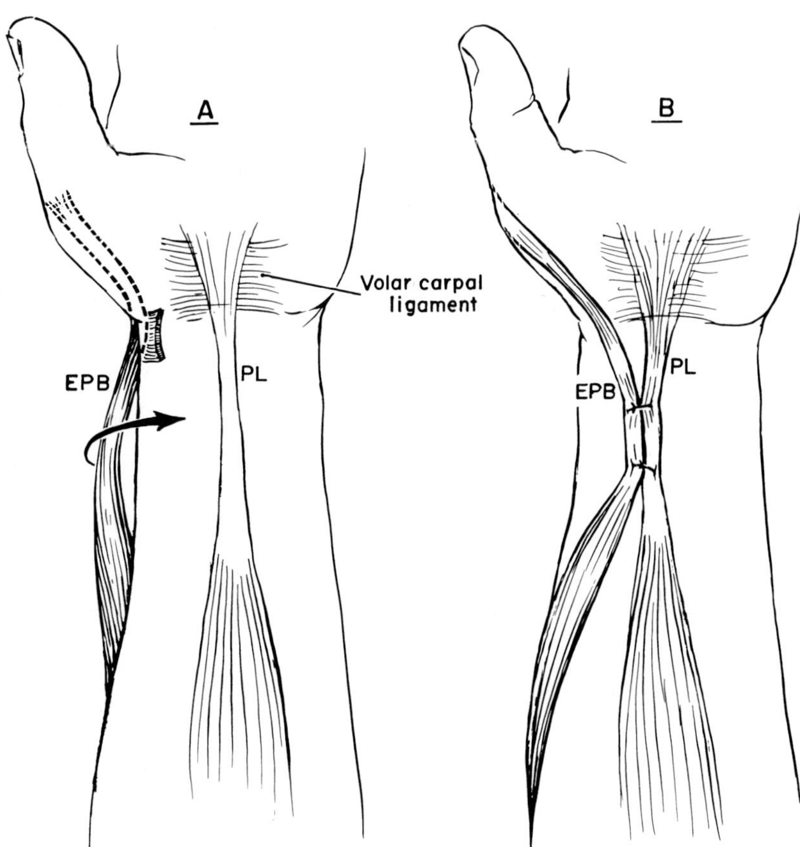

FIGURE 67–10. Tenodesis of the palmaris longus and the extensor pollicis brevis (EPB) for proximal stability of the thumb. The EPB is mobilized from the first dorsal compartment.

their greater excursion compared with the wrist flexors; in addition, wrist flexors are synergistic with finger extensors.

THUMB PROXIMAL STABILITY

Without a stable thumb, strong pinch is impaired. The FCR tendon can be split and the radial half of the tendon transferred into the abductor pollicis longus (APL) (Omer, 1982a). Boyes (1960) has recommended transferring the FCR to both the APL and the EPL tendons. An alternative is to suture the PL to the EPB (Fig. 67–10). Riordan (1974) has split the ECRB, and the radial half is transferred to the APL. However, with these techniques it is possible to create a painful neuroma.

ELBOW EXTENSION

Trauma to the upper extremity resulting in isolated radial palsy usually is distal to the branches to the triceps muscle in the upper arm. Moberg's (1990) posterior deltoid-to-triceps transfer is the preferred method for restoring elbow extension. Tendon grafts to connect the posterior deltoid to the triceps insertion can be obtained from several anatomical locations. Moberg prefers the toe extensors, whereas Hentz and associates (1983) recommend tubing a wide strip of fascia lata to lengthen the deltoid. The fascia lata is passed through drill holes in the proximal ulna.

POSTOPERATIVE MANAGEMENT

A double sugar-tong splint is applied in the operating room to immobilize the forearm in 30 degrees pronation, the wrist in 45 degrees of extension, the MP joints in zero degrees of extension, and the thumb in maximum extension and abduction. Usually the first splint extends distal to the proximal IP joints, supported in 45 degrees of flexion. In 48 hours a long arm cast is applied, the IP joints are freed, but all other joints are immobilized as before. Six weeks after surgery, the patient is placed in a dynamic splint to obtain independent action for wrist and finger extension. A planned exercise program will include synergistic movements. Usually there is good control of wrist extension and mass extension of fingers 3 months after surgery.

Sometimes the tendon transfer ruptures, attenuates, or becomes adherent secondary to poor healing after surgery. If a free tendon graft is considered to have the best reconstructive potential, it is possible to insert a silicone rod along the intended transfer path for 3 to 6 weeks, and then insert the free tendon graft by suturing it to one end of the silicone rod. Independent rehabilitation is guarded and slower in these cases.

Median Nerve Palsy (Table 67–4)

The goals of preoperative management are maintenance of a full passive range of motion in all joints of the forearm and hand, plus prevention of contractures. Adduction and supination of the thumb metacarpal are the principle deformities of the thumb-index web contracture. A two-point discrimination distance greater than 12 mm for the autonomous area of the median nerve provides only protective sensibility, and the patient will "divorce" the index finger for motor

▼ TABLE 67–4
Isolated Median Nerve Palsy

Needed Function	Preferred Motor	Alternate Motors
Thumb abduction (APB)	EIP to APB (and EPL)	EDM, PL, FDS (ring), ADQ
Thumb flexion (FPL)	BR to EPL (may need more distal origin for BR)	ECRL to EPL
Finger flexion (FDP) (index and long)	Tenodesis of FDP (ring and little) to FDP (index and long); may need tenodesis of distal IP joint (index)	ECRL to FDP (index) and tenodesis FDP (ring and little) to FDP (long)
Power flexion for proximal phalanges (usually ring and little clawed fingers)	ECRL, plus four-tailed free tendon graft transfer volar to deep tranverse metacarpal ligament to either the flexor sheath (A2 pulley) or the lateral band of the dorsal extensor apparatus	Free tendon graft between lateral bands of dorsal extensor apparatus around deep transverse metacarpal ligament to adjacent digits (index-long; ring-little)
Forearm pronation (rarely indicated)		Biceps brachii tendon rerouted around radius
Radial volar sensibility	Ulnar digital nerve translocation *or* superficial radial neurocutaneous flap	Neurovascular cutaneous island pedicle from ring finger *or* free neurovascular cutaneous island transfer

Note: See Table 67–1 for abbreviations.

activities. External splints may limit the patient's ability to use the hand, and tendon transfers are beneficial for overall rehabilitation.

The requirements for restoration of forearm and hand function after median palsy are (1) abduction/opposition of the thumb; (2) flexion of the index and long fingers (on examination, flexion of the index finger may be the only obvious functional defect because the long finger shares a common muscle belly with the ring and little fingers that is partially innervated by the ulnar nerve); (3) flexion of the thumb at the IP joint; (4) sensibility on the volar pulp surfaces of the thumb, index, and long fingers; and (5) there is loss of FDS power for flexion for the proximal phalanges. Loss of the FDS lessens the degree of flexor domination over the combined extensor intrinsic complex in the normal flexion of the fingers. Synchronism, the quality of grace and fluidity, involves the simultaneous flexion and extension of joints (Omer, 1994). In addition, there is loss of forearm pronation against resistance and loss of radial strength in wrist flexion.

Low Median Nerve Palsy

A low median palsy involves the intrinsic muscles of the hand and the cutaneous sensation of the hand and usually results from injuries in the distal third of the forearm or the wrist. Active thumb abduction is achieved by transfer of the EIP to the APB (Burkhalter et al, 1973), as described in the section on early tendon transfers.

Thumb opposition is a complex function that results in pulp-to-pulp pinch between the thumb and the index and long fingers. The thumb must abduct from the palm and extend at the MP joint, then rotate into position, and flex at the IP joint to achieve opposition (Cooney, 1988). Patients with normal sensibility use a pulp-to-pulp pinch; however, those with impaired sensibility use a thumb-pulp-to-index-side pinch (Eversmann, 1991). Elective reconstruction of thumb opposition should not be done if there is a thumb-index finger web contracture. A second prerequisite for a functional opponensplasty is active extension of the MP joint. Extension of the MP joint can be gained with partial insertion of the opponensplasty into the EPL tendon or be

ensured by arthrodesis of the joint (see Figs. 67–5 and 67–7). The patient's functional needs indicate the selection of an appropriate opponensplasty, but an important consideration is adequate thumb sensibility. Without both position sense, provided by the radial nerve, and volar sensibility provided by the median nerve, it is necessary to select an opponensplasty that requires minimal retraining.

In low median palsy, many motors are available for opponensplasty. The EDM may be used if preoperative evaluation has determined the presence of an independent muscle that extends the little finger. The transfer has the same techniques and advantages as the EIP transfer (Schneider, 1969). If the median nerve is lacerated by an oblique injury that spares the PL, the tendon can be lengthened into the palmar fascia and transferred to the APB (Camitz, 1929) (Fig. 67–11). The tendon of the AP can be transferred from the ulnar to the radial side of the proximal phalanx to reinforce thumb pronation (de Vicci procedure). The abductor digiti quinti (ADQ) muscle can be folded from the hypothenar to the thenar area on its neurovascular bundle to provide active thumb opposition (Cooney, 1988; Littler, 1949). This transfer has limited amplitude and reduces the power for sensible gross grip by its loss from the hypothenar area (Fig. 67–12). The ECU, FPL, and EPL have been used for opposition of the thumb (Burkhalter, 1993) and are more indicated in patients with progressive neurological deterioration.

High Median Nerve Palsy

A high median palsy involves intrinsic and extrinsic muscles of the hand as well as cutaneous sensation of the hand, thus contributing to the loss of power grasp as well as loss of pulp pinch.

FLEXION OF THE INDEX AND LONG FINGERS

A volar midline longitudinal incision is made from above the wrist crease to the mid third of the forearm. The index and long tendons of the FDP are identified by traction, and then individually freed and pulled proximally until all four finger pulps are in transverse alignment instead of normal oblique alignment. To maintain the transverse alignment, the

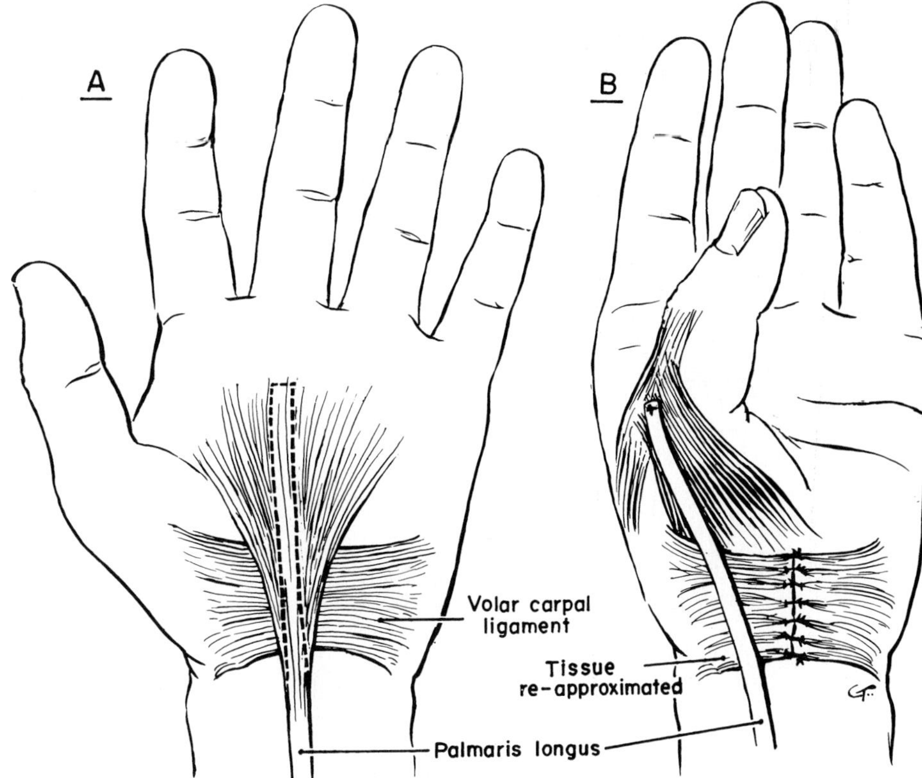

FIGURE 67–11. Release of the palmaris longus with palmar fascia for thumb opposition. The tendon must be lengthened by cutting a strip from the volar carpal ligament as well as palmar fascia.

tendons of the median innervated inactive index and long FDP are stitched (tenodesed) with nonabsorbable sutures to the tendons of the ring and little finger FDP ulnar innervated muscles (White, 1960). Sutures are adjusted to avoid excessive tension that would create a flexion contracture of the index or long fingers when the wrist is in 20 degrees of flexion. A double line of sutures is important to prevent "whipsawing" of the tendons during power grasp (Omer, 1982a, 1982b). If appropriate, the index FDP can be tenodesed in 10 degrees of flexion across the distal IP joint to increase the mechanical advantage at the proximal IP joint

(Fig. 67–13). The combination of ulnar innervated muscle motor, tendon tenodesis, and wrist extension will provide functional grasp.

For the patient who needs independent index finger pinch, the ECRL can be transferred to the index FDP (Eversmann, 1991). The ECRL is passed subcutaneously over the BR to the index FDP. If the ECRL is transferred to the index FDP, the long FDP is tenodesed to the ring and little finger FDP tendons.

FLEXION OF THE THUMB

The FPL and BR tendons are identified in the forearm. The BR should be extensively freed from all tissue attachments, so that it has approximately 5 cm of passive mobility (Eversmann, 1991) (Fig. 67–14). The FPL also must glide freely, especially distal to the wrist. The BR is released near its insertion and withdrawn to check its mobility. The BR tendon is then interwoven into the tendon of the FPL and held with nonabsorbable sutures (White, 1960). Tension is adjusted so that there is full extension of the thumb when the wrist is in 20 degrees of flexion. The tourniquet should be deflated when setting final tension for the transfers.

POSTOPERATIVE MANAGEMENT/REHABILITATION

The forearm and hand should be held in immobilization for 5 to 6 weeks after surgery. The elbow is supported in 90 degrees of flexion (Munster level), the wrist in 0 to 20 degrees of flexion, and the thumb in full abduction and extension. By the fifth postoperative week, static splints can support full thumb abduction, and elastic splinting can be used to support finger flexion. Gentle active motion, includ-

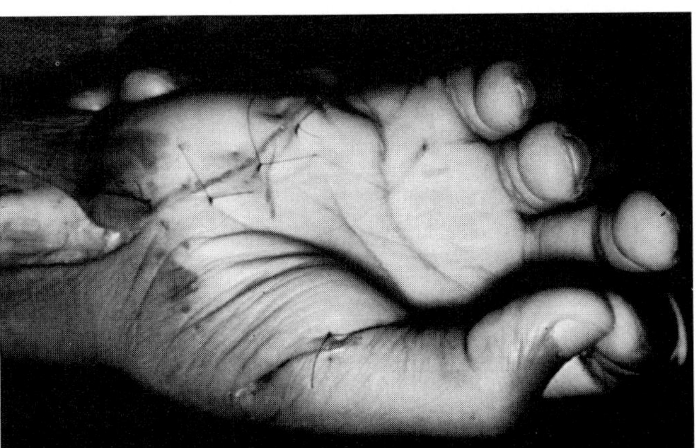

FIGURE 67–12. Transfer of the abductor digiti quinti (ADQ) from its hypothenar position to the thenar area for thumb abduction. The ADQ is freed from distal to proximal, and then folded radialward 170 degrees and passed subcutaneously, to be inserted into the tendon of the abductor pollicis brevis. (From Omer GE Jr: Combined nerve lesions. *In* Green DP [ed]: Operative Hand Surgery, 3rd ed. New York, Churchill Livingstone, 1993, p 1479.)

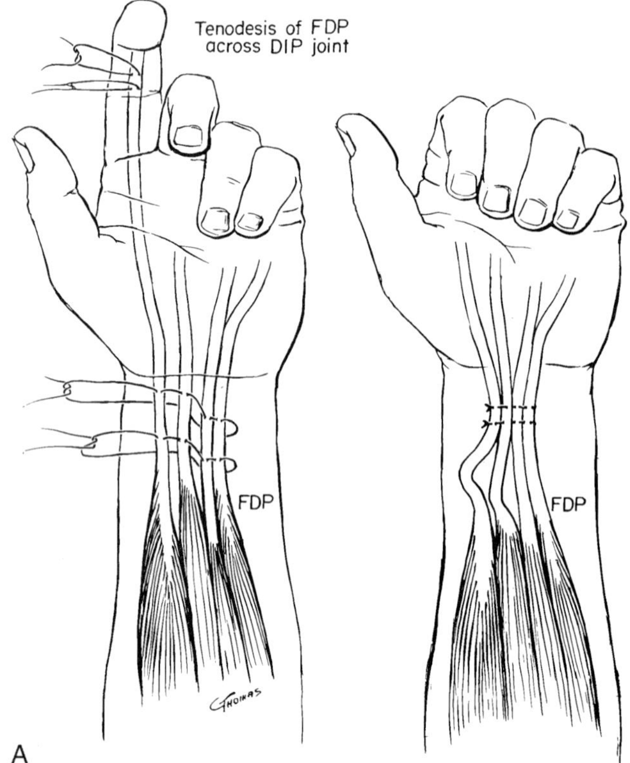

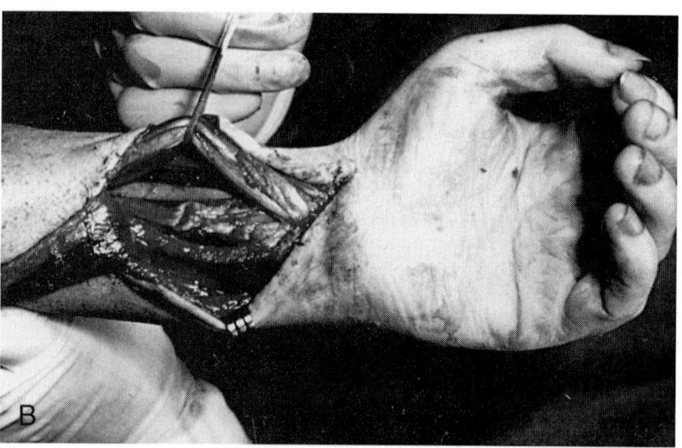

FIGURE 67–13. *A*, Tenodesis of the denervated index and long flexor digitorum profundus (FDP) tendons to the innervated ring and little tendons of the FDP for active flexion of all four fingers. The index profundus may be tenodesed across the distal interphalangeal joint (DIP) to establish more equal resistance for the ulnar innervated portion of the FDP. *B*, Intraoperative photograph. A double line of sutures is important to prevent "whipsawing" of the tendons with power grip. The DIP of the index finger has been tenodesed. The finger pulps are in a "straight" rather than oblique line, creating more passive tension in the index and long fingers. (*B* from Omer GE Jr: Combined nerve lesions. *In* Green DP [ed]: Operative Hand Surgery, 3rd ed. Churchill Livingstone, New York, 1993, p 142.)

ing finger extension, can be initiated under supervision. For the EIP transfer, the patient can facilitate rehabilitation by simply extending the index finger. Massage will soften the subcutaneous scar. By the sixth or seventh week, soft tissue healing is strong enough to withstand resistance, and full passive motion may be initiated.

Gradually, the emphasis changes to functional use of the hand. Sensibility re-education depends on movement as an important factor in the appropriate stimulation of sensory organs (Omer, 1974b) and is related to tactile, propriocep-

tive, and visual input. The patient will alter motor patterns to obtain the best available sensory function; an example is the patient with loss of index volar pulp sensibility secondary to median palsy and adapts by "divorcing" the index finger and extending it out of the pinch pattern, which will be altered to a chuck between the thumb and long finger. The Moberg pick-up test is a good check of functional motor patterns if one of the test objects is a short length of soft chalk. The chalk will rub against the fingers and leave a visible trail of functional surfaces (Omer, 1971b). The abnormal motor function that usually accompanies nerve loss enhances the distorted sensibility and contributes to dysesthesia. These functional problems are the basis for an aggressive motor re-education program. Emphasis can be placed on improving coordination. Finally, the patient concentrates on speed and accuracy. The Moberg pick-up test and the Jebson hand function test are good measurements of improvement.

These tendon transfer procedures should result in a hand that functions well as a "helper," assisting in grasp. It will not be strong for grip activities. One should not expect recovery of tactile gnosis with precise function for thumb-index pulp pinch. The young person will adapt visual and position senses with other feedback mechanisms to obtain better function than indicated by the surgical reconstruction.

Sensory Defects in Median Palsy

Methods for restoration of sensation include free nerve grafts, free vascularized nerve grafts, digital nerve translocation, neurocutaneous flaps, neurovascular cutaneous island pedicles, and free neurovascular cutaneous islands.

MICROSURGICAL DIGITAL NERVE TRANSLOCATION
(Lewis, 1984)

A volar zigzag incision is used to expose the ulnar proper digital nerve of the ring finger. Using microsurgery technique, the ulnar proper digital nerve of the ring finger is freed from the distal IP joint to the common digital nerve of the ring and little fingers. The radial proper digital nerve of the little finger is dissected free into the common digital nerve. The ulnar proper digital nerve of the thumb is identified with a second incision. The ulnar proper digital nerve to the ring finger is cut distally and passed subcutaneously into the thumb incision, and care is taken to ensure there is sufficient soft tissue protection both palmar and dorsal to the nerve. The ulnar proper digital nerve of the ring finger is sutured to the ulnar proper digital nerve of the thumb with 10-0 sutures, using microsurgical technique.

A similar technique may be used to translocate the superficial radial nerve found on the radial dorsal aspect of the index finger. The superficial radial nerve is exposed to the base of the thumb-index web. The ulnar proper digital nerve of the thumb is exposed with a volar zigzag incision. The superficial radial nerve is translocated to the ulnar proper digital nerve of the thumb, using microsurgical technique. If indicated, the nerve translocation procedures may be done at the same time as the tendon transfers for median palsy.

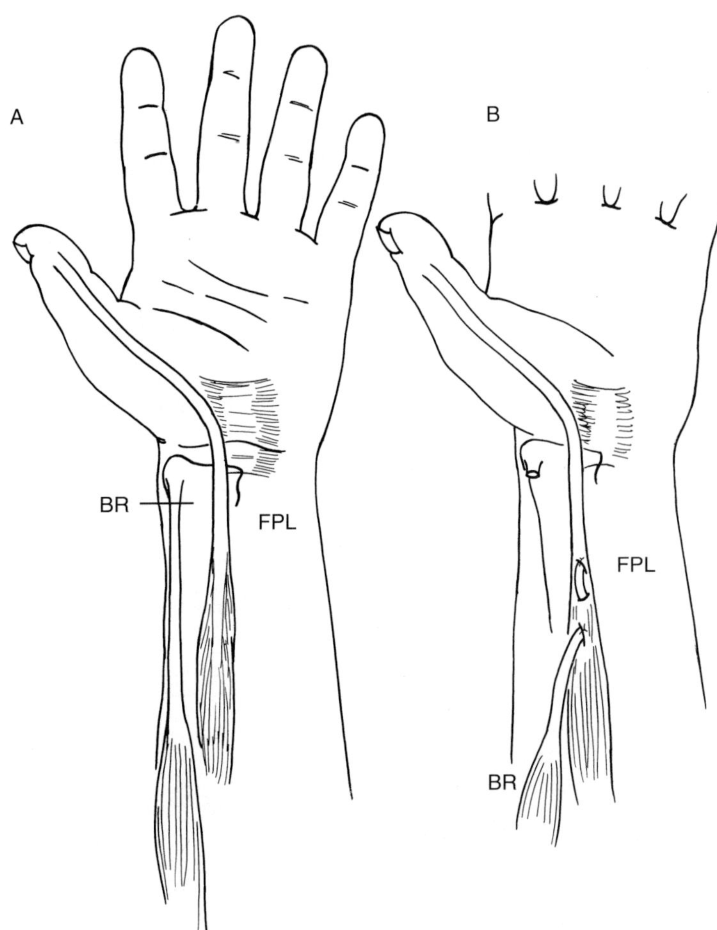

FIGURE 67–14. Transfer of the brachioradialis (BR) into the tendon of the flexor pollicis longus (FPL) for thumb flexion. The BR should be freed well into the mid-third of the forearm but avoid injury to the neurovascular bundle to the muscle. The FPL must glide freely, especially distal to the wrist. (From Omer GE Jr: J. Bone Joint Surg *50*A: 1454, 1968.)

NEUROVASCULAR CUTANEOUS ISLAND PEDICLE
(Omer, 1975, 1978a; Omer et al, 1970)

These procedures should not be done until all tendon transfers have been rehabilitated and there is a potential for the retention of precise sensibility in the cutaneous transfer.

A palmar longitudinal zigzag incision is made over the common digital nerve and vessels to the ring and little fingers, from the level of the volar superficial vascular arch to the distal edge of the palm. If there is abnormal vascular or nerve anatomy, the incision is closed.

Using microsurgical technique, a cutaneous island is developed that is centered over the ulnar proper digital nerve to the ring finger. The radial proper digital nerve to the little finger is identified and dissected free into the common digital nerve. The radial digital artery to the little finger is ligated. To retain physiological tension on the neurovascular pedicle, the cutaneous island is freed except for the most distal portion, which is left intact until actual transfer (Fig. 67–15).

A pattern of the cutaneous island is traced on sterile surgical glove paper. From the pattern, a cutaneous island is drawn over the ulnar volar aspect of the thumb, including the pulp tip. The more precise the reconstructed motor function, the more indication for thumb volar pulp coverage. The distance between the two cutaneous islands is measured to determine that the recipient site is easily reached by the ring finger island. A free full-thickness skin graft is removed from within the pattern at the recipient site on the thumb. This free graft fits into the cutaneous island donor site.

A transverse palmar incision is made distal to the superficial volar vascular arch from the ring incision to the selected thumb recipient site. If necessary for additional pedicle length, the vascular arch is interrupted on the ulnar side. Palmar fascia is incised so that the neurovascular pedicle is placed in a trough without tension, acute angulation, or constriction. The microsurgical procedure must be done with tourniquet ischemia, but when the dissections are complete, the tourniquet is released to obtain hemostasis.

NEUROCUTANEOUS FLAP (Holevich, 1963; Small and Brennan, 1988)

A superficial radial-innervated island flap can be transferred from the dorsal surface of the index proximal phalanx to the thumb pulp (Fig. 67–16). It is advisable to confirm innervation of the area by the superficial radial nerve before surgery. A V-shaped skin incision is made, with one limb at the level of the midlateral line on the radial side of the index finger and the other limb at the midlateral line on the ulnar side of the thumb. Microsurgical dissection will expose the longitudinal brances of the superficial radial nerve and vascular structures dorsal to the second metacarpal. A racket-shaped cutaneous island with a neurovascular pedicle is dissected from the dorsal-radial surface of the index finger and fitted into the volar-ulnar aspect of the thumb pulp. The arterial supply to the cutaneous island is not constant, and the procedure is often modified by developing a cross-finger

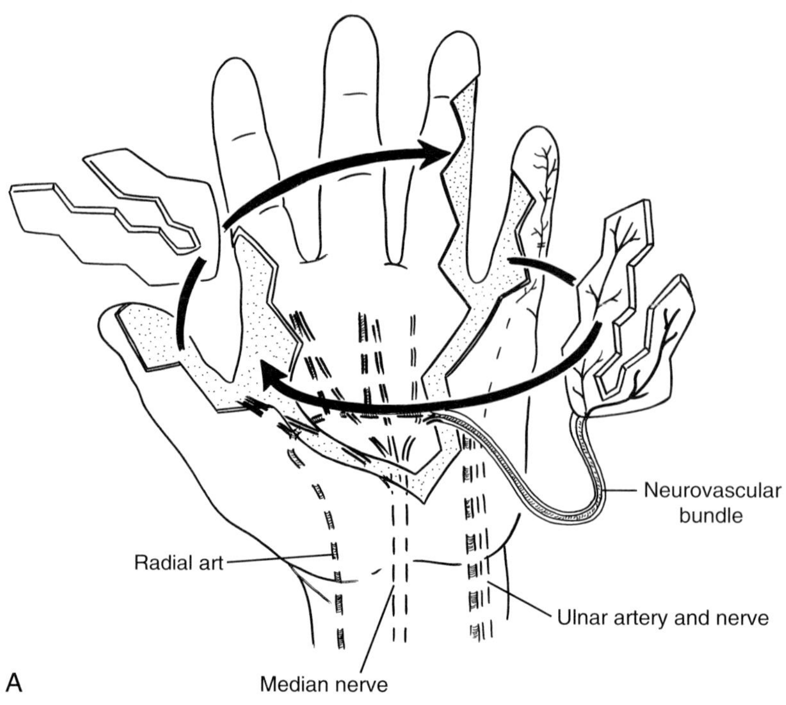

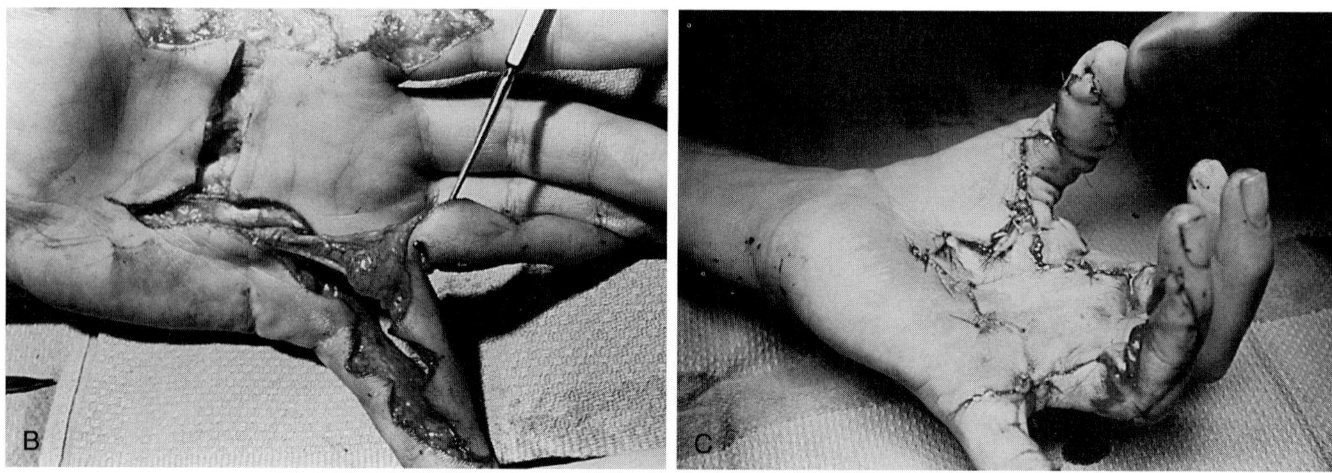

FIGURE 67–15. *A,* Double cutaneous island with neurovascular pedicle for high median nerve loss. It is designed to restore sensibility for gross grip, not precise pinch. *B,* The flaps on the ring and little fingers and the thumb and index finger should be patterned so that they are interchangeable, and skin flaps are not needed. The most distal portion of the cutaneous island is left intact until actual transfer to retain physiological tension. *C,* There is inadequate intrinsic motion and power for precise median innervated prehension, and precise sensibility will be lost. (*B* and *C* from Omer GE Jr: Tendon transfers for combined traumatic nerve palsies of the forearm and hand. J Hand Surg *17B:* 603–610, 1992.)

flap from the index to the thumb instead of the free cutaneous island flap (Gaul, 1969).

PROGNOSIS FOR PROCEDURES TO RESTORE SENSIBILITY

Moberg (1964) indicated that all neurovascular sensory island transplants will have three negative aspects: (1) a loss of sensibility at the donor site, (2) a margin of hyperesthesia around the edges of the cutaneous island, and (3) a loss of the quality of sensibility secondary to cortical disorientation. For several months after transplant, the patient recognizes stimulation over the island as coming from the original donor digit. Later, sensation is localized in both the recipient and donor sites. Finally, some patients learn to interpret the

sensibility to the recipient digit. If the extremity is immobilized and nonfunctional for a prolonged period of time, the interpretation process may need to be repeated. In an emergency, such as a burn, the patient usually loses his interpretation ability and moves the original digit.

Omer and associates (1970) reported their findings in 15 patients with high (proximal) median nerve loss who were followed with evaluation tests at 8 week intervals for 14 to 43 months after surgery. The two-point discrimination distance recognition and the von Frey light touch pressure tests demonstrated a gradual reduction from normal sensation to merely protective sensation. It was believed that this gradual loss of sensibility was directly related to the associated motor loss for the radial side of the hand, and without adequate motion and power for precise prehension, the sensi-

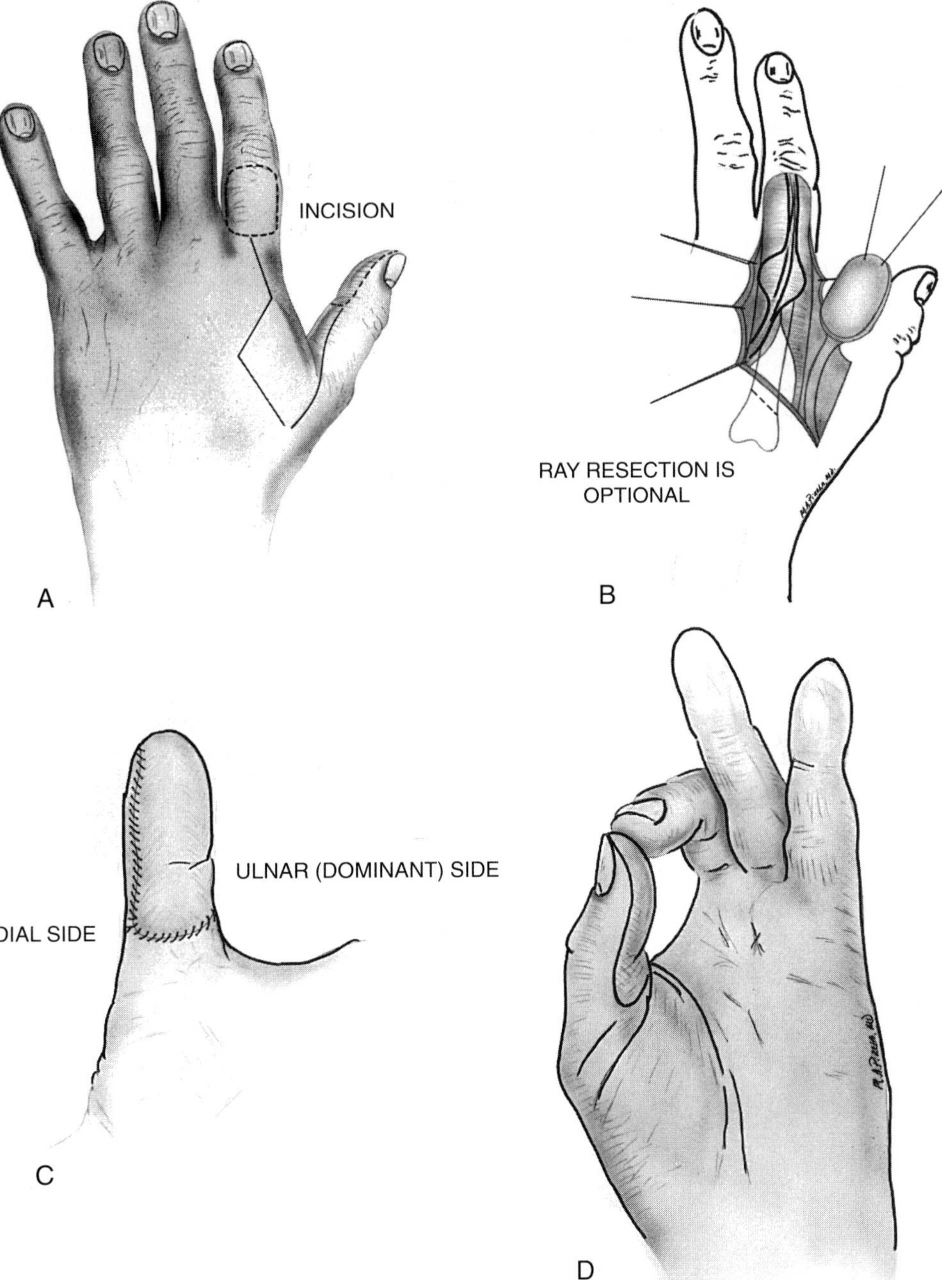

FIGURE 67–16. *A*, Incisions for a radial-innervated cutaneous island on the first dorsal metacarpal surface of the index finger between the metacarpal and the proximal interphalangeal joints. *B*, Completed dissection; the procedure is precarious because there is no constant vascular supply to the island. The technique can be modified so that a cross-finger flap is created from the index finger to the thumb. *C*, Flap in place on the ulnar-palmar surface of the thumb. If the index finger is filleted, a larger flap is available. *D*, Superficial radial innervated pinch can be obtained.

bility for precise prehension must be lost (Omer, 1975). Adani and associates (1994) reported 30 patients with an average follow-up of 75.5 months. These patients had thumb pulp reconstruction with neurovascular island flaps, but none had total median nerve loss that required motor reconstruction. In these patients, sensory acuity did not decrease with time. Murray and associates (1967) reported results in 16 patients with median nerve deficiency who were followed 1 to 10 years after surgery. Based on two-point discrimination distance and light touch, the sensibility in the neurovascular island was less than normal. Twelve patients had continued intolerance to cold and 7 had significant hyperesthesia at all times. In contrast, Tubiana and Duparc (1961) noted the gradual spread of protective sensibility into the tissue surrounding the transplanted cutaneous island.

Reconstruction of precise sensibility is the greatest functional need in median palsy, but all available techniques are likely to have complications. In addition, usually there is inadequate muscle function for precise sensibility. For isolated median nerve palsy, local nerve translocation procedures have the best potential function because the procedure can be done at the same time as the tendon transfers. The ulnar innervated neurovascular cutaneous island pedicle probably should be done only in special circumstances.

Ulnar Nerve Palsy (Table 67–5)

There are several anomalous neural patterns of the ulnar nerve in the forearm and hand that can lead to confusion concerning the level of the ulnar nerve lesion. The Martin-Gruber communication (Kaplan and Spinner, 1980, Omer, 1971a), occurs adjacent to the ulnar artery in the proximal forearm. Riche and Cannieu described a connection between the motor branch of the ulnar nerve and the recurrent branch of the median nerve in the hand (Kaplan and Spinner, 1980). The dorsal cutaneous sensory branch of the ulnar nerve perforates the fascia 6 to 8 cm proximal to the wrist and supplies the dorsoulnar surface of the hand and little finger. However, this area can be supplied by the superficial branch of the radial nerve. Diagnostic errors can be avoided with careful voluntary muscle testing, precise evaluation of sensibility and sudomotor activity, anesthetic blocks of intact nerves, and electrodiagnostic studies that include conduction times across selected segments of the ulnar nerve (Omer, 1971b).

An important aspect of initial treatment is the appropriate use of individualized splints, which should be fabricated for each patient (see Fig. 67–2). Problems in splinting the hand with ulnar palsy are the maintenance of the palmar arch, the thumb-index web space, and adequate lumbrical and thenar stops to maintain the functional position. External splints are always awkward and often interfere with sensory rehabilitation.

The requirements for restoration of forearm and hand function after ulnar palsy are as follows.

1. Thumb adduction power for key pinch. The thumb MP joint may hyperextend 10 to 15 degrees with key pinch or gross grip. The impairment for power grip is greater than the loss of power for precise grasp. The residual strength for key pinch may be diminished as much as 77% to 80% (Mannerfelt, 1966).

2. Power for flexion of the proximal phalanges of the fingers. An unconscious effort to extend the fingers by tenodesing the extensor tendons with palmar flexion of the wrist only increases the deformity. There is associated loss of integration (synchronism) of MP and IP joint flexion. Normal finger flexion is initiated at the MP joint, and then all three finger joints flex simultaneously. In ulnar intrinsic paralysis, the MP joint does not flex until all IP joint flexion has been completed. If extrinsic muscle function is intact (low ulnar palsy), the ring and little fingers will claw.

3. Distal stability for tip pinch between the thumb and index finger. There is inability to bring the tips of the

▼ **TABLE 67–5**
Isolated Unlar Nerve Palsy

Needed Function	Preferred Transfer	Alternate Transfer
Thumb adduction for key pinch (AP)	ECRB with free tendon graft to AP, with palmar fascia as pulley	FDS to APB tendon (FDS long is only candidate)
Proximal phalanx power flexion and integration of MP and IP motion (clawed fingers)	ECRL to all four fingers using four-tailed free graft volar to deep transverse metacarpal ligament to either A2 pulley of flexor sheath *or* lateral bands of dorsal extensor apparatus	FCR (if wrist flexion contracture) with four-tailed free graft to either flexor sheath (A2 pulley) or lateral bands of dorsal extensor apparatus
Thumb-index tip pinch	Accessory slip of APL to first dorsal interosseous tendon and arthrodesis of MP joint of thumb	EPB to first dorsal interosseous tendon (if thumb MP has been fused)
Metacarpal (palmar) transverse arch and adduction for little finger	EDM tendon split and ulnar half transferred volar to deep transverse metacarpal ligament to radial collateral ligament of proximal phalanx or lateral band of extensor apparatus (EDC to little finger must be effective)	If little finger is clawed as well as abducted, insert ulnar half of EDM into A2 pulley of flexor sheath
Finger flexion; ring and little distal IP joints	FDP (long) tenodesed to FDP (ring and little), with possible tenodesis across distal IP joints	
Wrist flexion; ulnar aspect	FCR to FCU	PL to FCU
Ullnar volar sensibility; ring and little fingers	Median digital nerve translocation	Free or vascularized nerve graft

Note: See Table 67–1 for abbreviations.

extended digits together in a cone. The thumb IP joint may flex 80 to 90 degrees as the FPL attempts to hold an object without the assistance of the first and second palmar interossei and the AP muscles.

4. Restore metacarpal arch and adduction power to the extended little finger. There is a loss of active lateral mobility in all fingers in extension.

5. Restore power to flex the distal phalanges of the ring and little fingers.

6. Restore sensibility over the volar side of the little finger and the ulnar aspect of the volar side of the ring finger.

7. Restore ulnar power for wrist flexion.

8. Restore additional sensibility over the dorsal-ulnar aspect of the palm and the dorsal side of the little finger.

Ulnar palsy results in a hand with so many functional problems that there is no "accepted program" for construction. Available tendon assets must be invested wisely. For example, the ubiquitous FDS has been overused—for proximal phalanx flexion, as a substitute for the lumbricals, as a thumb adductor, to restore the metacarpal arch, as an index abductor—yet, it provides the only flexor power in the ring and little fingers in a high (proximal) ulnar palsy!

Low Ulnar Nerve Palsy

A low ulnar palsy does not include the loss of extrinsic power for flexion of the ring and little fingers, ulnar power for wrist flexion, and the loss of sensibility over the dorsum of the palm and little finger.

THUMB ADDUCTION

Thumb adduction may be restored by using a strong wrist motor, the BR, or several digital tendons. Most transfers for thumb adduction provide power pinch only in the range of 25% to 50% of normal strength (Smith, 1983).

The ECRB is sharply released at its insertion and attached to a free tendon graft. The graft is brought into the palm through the third intermetacarpal space and tunneled superficial (volar) to the AP and deep (dorsal) to the flexor tendons and neurovascular structures (Omer, 1985). The tendon graft is attached to the tendon of the APB, which improves pronation for pinch (Edgerton and Brand, 1965). When the wrist is in palmar flexion, the thumb falls into abduction; when the wrist is in dorsiflexion, the thumb is drawn against the palm (Fig. 67–17).

Littler (1949) recommended a long or ring FDS transfer in those patients with hyperextension deformity of the MP joint of the thumb. The decussation of the superficialis is split to leave one limb; it is tenodesed across the proximal IP joint. The superficialis tendon is tunneled across the volar surface of the AP and sutured to the AP tendon at its insertion. The pulley for this procedure is the vertical septum of the palmar fascia attached to the third metacarpal (Edgerton and Brand, 1965; Omer, 1971a). The thumb and wrist

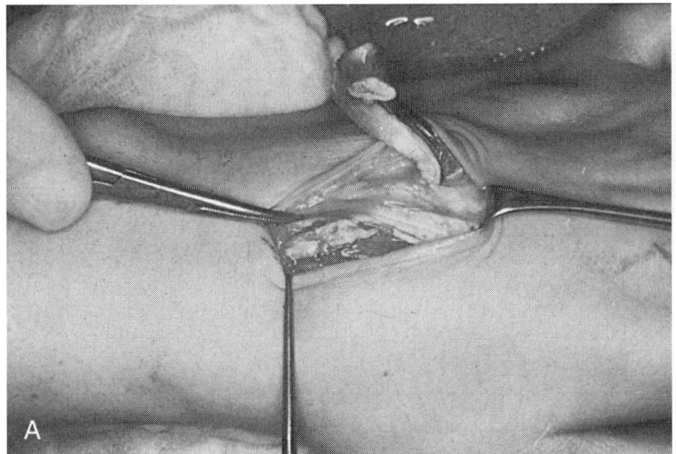

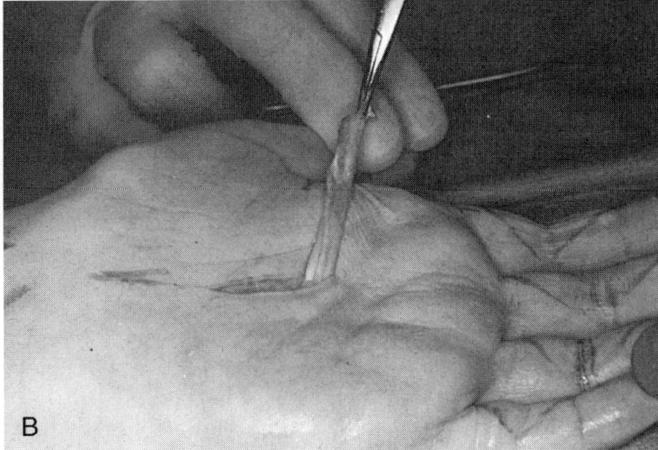

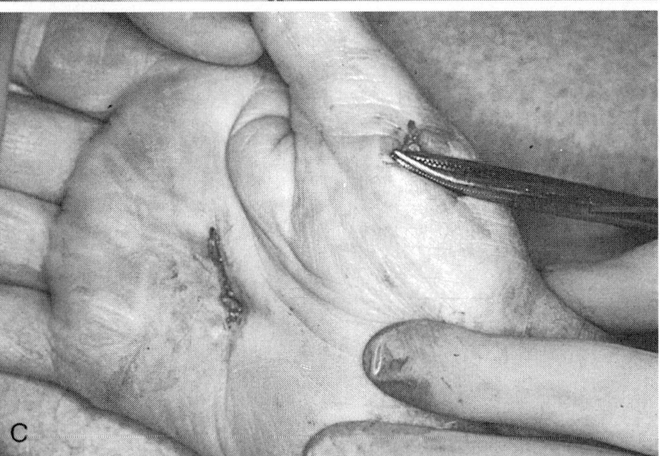

FIGURE 67–17. *A,* The extensor carpi radialis brevis (ECRB) can be used for thumb adduction and pronation. The ECRB is released from its insertion and elongated with a free tendon draft. *B,* The ECRB graft has been extended into the palm through the third metacarpal interspace. *C,* The ECRB graft has been passed dorsal to the flexor tendons and volar to the adductor pollicis muscle to reach the tendon of the abductor pollicis brevis. Wrist motion is not altered; when the wrist is in palmar flexion, the thumb falls into abduction; when the wrist is in dorsiflexion, the thumb is drawn against the palm. (*B* and *C* from Omer GE Jr: Tendon transfers for combined traumatic nerve palsies of the forearm and hand, J Hand Surg *17B*:603–610, 1992.)

are immobilized for 4 weeks, and then active motion is permitted. Hamlin and Littler (1979) recorded a return of pinch power to 70% of the uninvolved hand.

FLEXION OF THE PROXIMAL PHALANGES

The most reliable method to increase power for gross grip is to add an extra muscle-tendon unit to the power-train for flexion of the proximal phalanx. Burkhalter and Strait (1973) prolonged the ECRL with a free graft, usually PL or plantaris. The free graft is split into two slips, which are passed through the intermetacarpal spaces between the long and ring fingers and the ring and little fingers. The tendon slips pass volar to the deep transverse metacarpal ligament and are sutured either into the A2 pulley of the flexor sheath or into the lateral band of the extensor apparatus. The flexor pulley insertion does not assist in finger extension, and the extensor apparatus insertion is a potential "swan-neck" deformity. The same procedure might use the ECRB or the BR as the motor muscle. The FCR may be used as the motor in patients with palmar flexion deformity (Riordan, 1964). Brand (1970) noted that a stronger pinch can be obtained by stabilizing the index finger in adduction at the MP joint, and a four-tailed (slips) graft could be used. Postoperative immobilization is continued for 4 weeks, with the wrist maintained in 45 degrees dorsiflexion and the MP joints in 60 degrees flexion. The ECRL contracts during finger flexion and is easily retrained.

THUMB-INDEX TIP PINCH

Neviaser and associates (1980) transferred an accessory slip of the APL, elongated with a free tendon graft, palmaris or plantaris, into the tendon of the first dorsal interosseous. Only the slip of the APL that inserts on the first metacarpal is essential; if there are additional slips, one may be used for the first dorsal interosseous transfer. This transfer does not appreciably increase the force of tip pinch, but it stabilizes the index finger (Smith, 1987).

Bruner transferred the EPB to the tendon of the first dorsal interosseous, but Graham and Riordan (1947) stated that this transfer is lacking in strength. DeAbreu (1989) combined transfer of the EPB to the tendon insertion of the first dorsal interosseous with transfer of the EIP tendon to the tendon insertion of the AP muscle as a one-stage procedure. Postoperative immobilization includes holding the index finger in abduction and extension with the wrist slightly flexed or neutral. At the end of 3 weeks, active motion is permitted.

I recommend arthrodesis of the MP joint when there is instability in the longitudinal arch of the thumb (Omer, 1971a, 1974c, 1985) (see section on early tendon transfers).

METACARPAL TRANSVERSE ARCH AND LITTLE FINGER ADDUCTION

Paralysis of the four dorsal interossei, three volar interossei, and ADQ prevents active abduction and adduction of the fingers, with associated instability of the transverse metacarpal arch. Instability (flattening) of the transverse metacarpal arch may contribute to recurrent clawing after lumbrical replacement procedures. Ranney (1973) depressed the metacarpal arch with a volar transfer of the EDM to the neck of the fifth metacarpal. Blacker and colleagues (1976) found that the EDM had the potential to abduct the little finger through its indirect insertion into the abductor tubercle on the proximal phalanx. The balancing force is provided by the third palmar interosseous, which becomes inactive in ulnar palsy.

The ulnar half of the EDM is detached from the dorsal apparatus and dissected proximally to the distal edge of the dorsal carpal ligament (extensor retinaculum). A oblique palmar incision is made from the distal palmar crease to the proximal digital crease of the little finger to expose the deep transverse metacarpal ligament and the flexor sheath. The ulnar half of the EDM is passed between the fourth and fifth metacarpals into the palm. If the little finger is clawed as well as abducted, the tendon slip is passed beneath the deep transverse metacarpal ligament and inserted into a radially based flap of the flexor tendon sheath just distal to the proximal pulley (Brooks and Jones, 1975). If the little finger is not clawed, the tendon slip is passed beneath the deep transverse metacarpal ligament and inserted into the phalangeal attachments of the radial collateral ligament of the MP joint of the little finger (Omer, 1993).

High Ulnar Nerve Palsy

FLEXION OF THE RING AND LITTLE FINGERS AND ULNAR WRIST FLEXION

Brand (1991) does not consider the loss of the ulnar half of the FDP to be a functional problem unless there is also median or radial nerve loss. However, if there is marked weakness of the ring and little fingers in isolated ulnar paralysis, I attach (tenodese) the FDP of the ring and little fingers to the FDP of the long finger in the forearm (Omer, 1968; Omer and Pirela-Cruz, 1994). The index FDP should be left free. The surgeon should also consider tenodesis of the FDP across the distal IP joints of the ring and little fingers (Omer, 1990). Bunnell (1944) did not join the ring and little FDP to the long FDP because the additional flexors might increase clawing. This has not been my experience, but those patients with high ulnar palsy should have transfers for proximal phalanx flexion and integration of finger flexion as well as a procedure to restore the metacarpal arch.

Ulnar deviation is as important for wrist flexion as radial deviation is for wrist extension. It is useful to transfer the FCR tendon to the insertion of the FCU in a patient with high ulnar palsy who might perform activities requiring strong wrist flexion.

POSTOPERATIVE MANAGEMENT AND REHABILITATION

The extremity must be immobilized in the appropriate position to maintain the anticipated result. In either ulnar or median palsy, the thumb-index web must be maintained to prevent thumb adduction and supination. After procedures for clawed fingers, the hand should be positioned with the MP joints of the fingers flexed and the IP joints straight. Extremity fixation is more extensive when two joint lengths have been transferred. Children need immobilization longer than adults. Flexor tendon transfers should be immobilized for 3 to 4 weeks and protected with a splint for at least 1 more week. Extensor tendon transfers should be immobilized for 5 weeks and protected with a splint for at least 1 more week.

Surgical results should be assessed only after a minimum of 6 months of follow-up. Many elements of function should be considered: power on the voluntary clinical scale; range of motion; balance, or the passive equilibrium between opposing myotonic forces; stability, or the positive action between antagonist muscles; synergism, such as the action between wrist flexors and finger extensors, or wrist extensors and finger flexors; and coordination, the smooth transference of force from one synergistic muscle group to another.

SENSORY DEFECTS IN ULNAR PALSY

Loss of sensibility for the ulnar border of the hand and loss of proprioception for the little finger are significant functional limitations. Free nerve grafting, vascularized nerve grafts, and digital nerve translocation are technically demanding and clinically unpredictable.

Lewis and co-workers (Lewis et al, 1984; Stocks et al, 1991) performed digital nerve translocation: a functioning digital nerve of median origin is sutured into the nonfunctional distal ulnar digital nerve of the small finger. These authors reported that 85% of their patients obtained sensibility of S3+ or S4 after surgery. Patients who returned to work after surgery rated significantly better than those who did not work.

COMBINED NERVE PALSIES

Tendon transfers in combined nerve palsies are more complicated than those in isolated nerve palsy because of complex extremity injuries, poor proprioception, distorted sensibility, weakness of muscles for potential transfer, and the need for multiple operations. Specific composite tissue transplantation is useful in sensory-depleted glabrous skin areas required for precise pinch and grasp, provided precise motor function is available to manipulate the transplanted composite tissue. Reconstructive procedures should not be under-

taken until appropriate joint motion has been established and skeletal alignment is stable (Omer, 1974c, 1988). Tendon or tissue transfers in combined nerve palsies require longer follow-up than do isolated nerve palsies to make valid outcome decisions.

Low (Distal) Median and Ulnar Nerve Palsy
(Table 67–6)

Low (distal) median and ulnar nerve palsy is the most common combined nerve palsy. In chronic low median-ulnar palsy, the complete loss of palmar sensation and intrinsic motor muscles produces an almost useless claw hand (Fig. 67–18). Reconstruction of the thumb is the best investment of tendon transfers, and special effort should be made to prevent adduction contracture of the thumb-index web. Additional strength in a paralyzed power train requires a new muscle-tendon unit, and in combined median-ulnar palsy, additional strength must be added by radial innervated muscle-tendon units (Omer and Pirela-Cruz, 1994).

The loss of simultaneous MP flexion with either IP extension or flexion disrupts the rhythm necessary to grasp large and small objects. There are no available motors to provide dynamic integration of these extrinsic-intrinsic motions, so static techniques must be used. Parkes (1973) placed a free tendon graft between the radial lateral band of the dorsal apparatus of the finger and the deep transverse metacarpal ligament. It is more effective to attach a free tendon graft to the dorsal apparatus of one finger (index), and then pass the graft around the deep transverse metacarpal ligament to the dorsal apparatus of the adjacent finger (long); a second tendon graft is similarly placed in the ring and little fingers (Omer, 1971a). This technique allows adjustment of the static tension. Zancoli (1957) opens the proximal A1 pulley, and a distally based flap is removed from the volar plates (Fig. 67–19). Long-term follow-up of the capsulodesis procedure of Zancolli has demonstrated indifferent results in isolated ulnar palsy (Brown, 1974), but it has been effective in combined palsies (Omer, 1974c). After individualized tendon transfers, the residual loss of sensibility is likely to

▼ **TABLE 67–6**
Combined Low (Distal) Median and Ulnar Palsy

Needed Function	Preferred Transfer	Alternate Transfer
Thumb adduction, key pinch (AP)	ECRB with free tendon graft, between third and fourth metacarpals, to APB tendon	FDS (long) to APB, with palmar fascia and flexor tendons as pulleys
Thumb abduction (APB), for opposition	EIP around pisiform pulley to APB and EPL tendons	PL to APB *or* EDM to APB *or* FDS (ring) to APB
Thumb-index tip pinch	APL slip with free graft to first dorsal interosseous tendon and arthrodesis of MP joint of thumb	EPB to first dorsal interosseous tendon (if thumb MP joint has been fused)
Metacarpal (palmar) transverse arch and adduction for little finger	EDM tendon split and ulnar half transferred volar to deep transverse metacarpal to A2 pulley of flexor sheath *or* lateral band of dorsal extensor apparatus	FDS (little) to deep transverse metacarpal ligament between fourth and fifth metacarpals *or* combined with FDS (long) transfer for thumb adduction
Power flexion for proximal phalanges and integration of MP and IP motion (clawed fingers)	ECRL or BR to all four fingers using four-tailed free graft volar to deep transverse metacarpal ligament to A2 pulley of flexor sheath *or* lateral bands of dorsal extensor apparatus	FCR (if wrist flexion contracture) with four-tailed free graft to either flexor sheath (A2 pulley) or lateral bands of dorsal extensor apparatus
Radial and ulnar volar sensibility	Free neurovascular cutaneous island flap	Cross-finger index-to-thumb neurocutaneous flap

Note: See Table 67–1 for abbreviations.

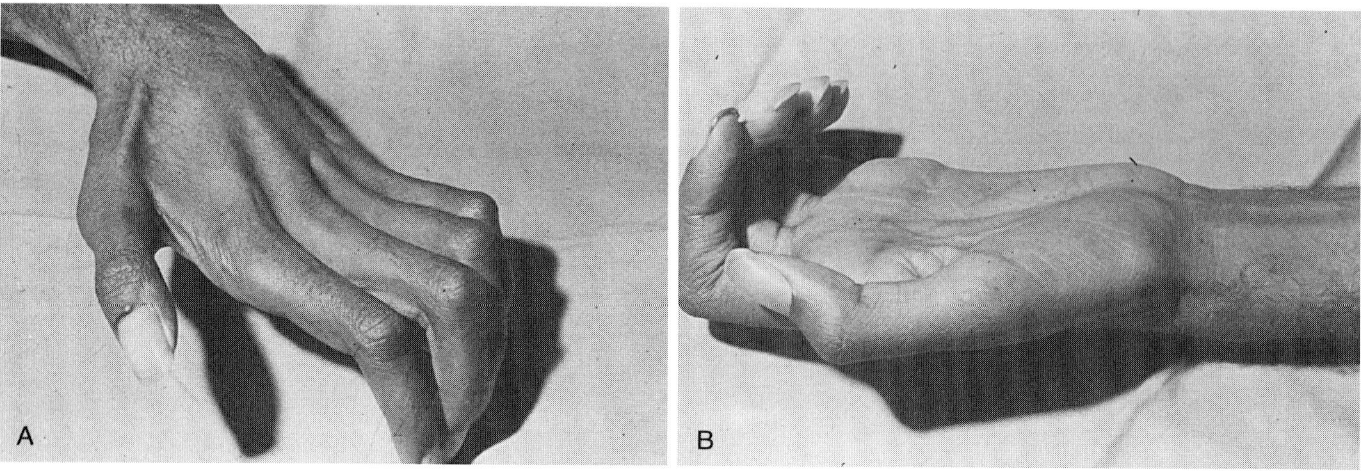

FIGURE 67–18. *A,* Combined median and ulnar nerve palsy with intrinsic motor atrophy. There is an adduction contracture of the thumb and atrophy of the pulp of the fingers. (From Omer GE Jr: *In* Gelberman RH [ed]: Operative Nerve Repair and Reconstruction. Philadelphia, J.B. Lippincott Company, 1991, p 753.) *B,* Combined median-ulnar palsy with atrophy of the thenar and hypothenar muscle masses. There is an extensor-driven rotation deformity of the thumb. (From Omer GE Jr: J Hand Surg *17B*:603–610, 1992.)

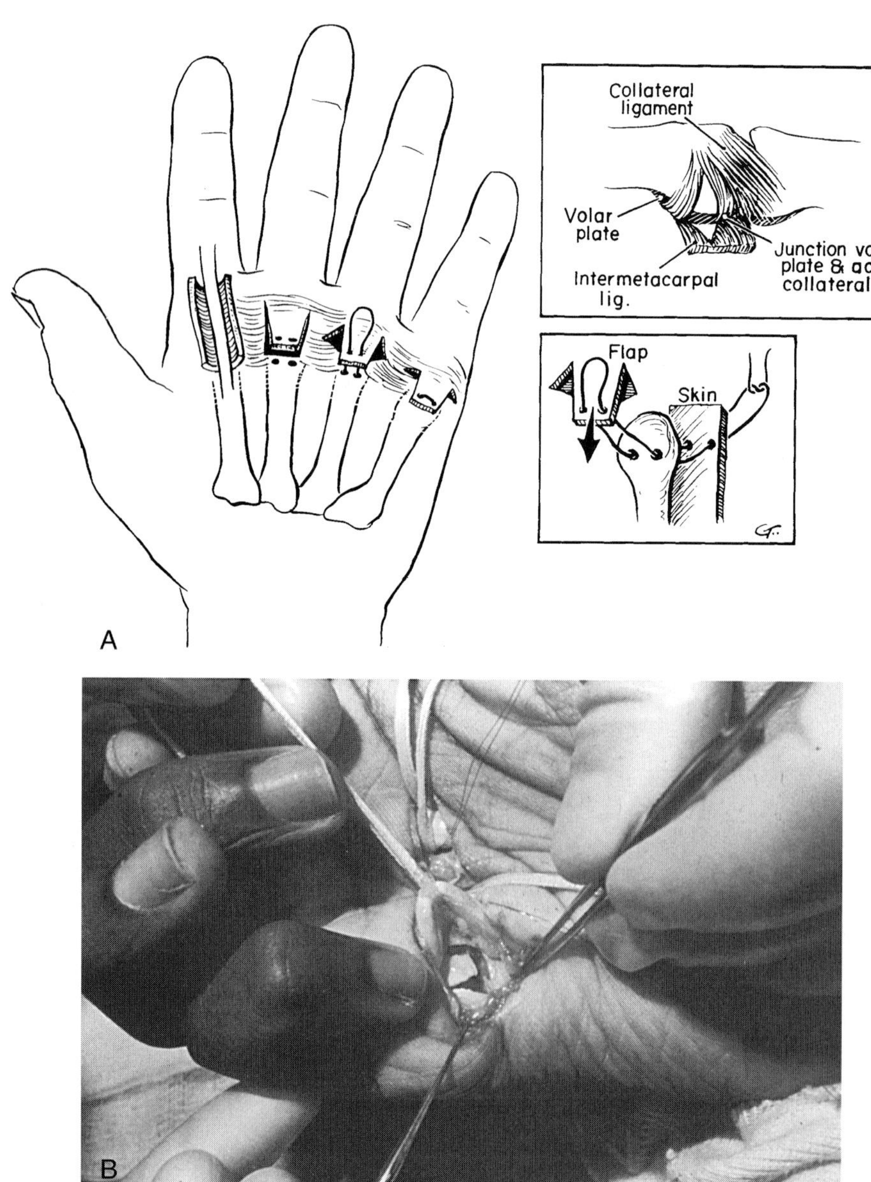

FIGURE 67–19. *A,* Zancolli capsulodesis of the metacarpophalangeal (MP) joint to correct finger clawing. The excised triangles adjacent to the volar plate flaps extend into the intermetacarpal (deep transverse metacarpal) ligament, and into the accessory collateral ligament on each side of the flap in the volar plate. *B,* Intraoperative photograph demonstrating the anticipated shortening of the volar side of the MP joint.

be a greater functional problem than motor patterns for grasp and pinch.

High (Proximal) Median and Ulnar Palsy
(Table 67–7)

The involved hand will rarely be used for precision activities after this severe injury, even if minimal muscle balance is restored. Atrophy of the finger pulps will discourage both power and precise grip. If the contralateral hand is normal, it is useful to direct surgical endeavours toward key pinch and simple grasp.

Before the initial surgical reconstruction, it may appear that restoration of intrinsic function in the hand will not be necessary. The fingers and the thumb may extend fully at the MP joints and may have full extension at the IP joints despite intrinsic paralysis. The extrinsic extensors can fully extend the IP joints if they have no antagonists (Omer, 1988, 1992; Smith, 1987). However, when flexion is surgically restored to the IP joints, the fingers gradually assume a clawed position.

As in low median-ulnar combined palsy, the ECRB is used to restore thumb adduction; the EIP is used to improve thumb abduction; and a slip of APL to the tendon of the first dorsal interosseous with arthrodesis of the MP joint of the thumb is used to strengthen thumb-index tip pinch. The BR to the FPL will result in active thumb flexion; however, this transfer crosses two joints and is most effective when the elbow is extended. On occasion, the BR will require fixation to bone distal to the elbow, thus eliminating that mechanical disadvantage. The ECRL is transferred around the radial side of the forearm to all four tendons of the FDP to provide finger flexion (Brand, 1970; Omer and Pirela-Cruz, 1994) (Fig. 67–20). There is some limitation of motion, and wrist movement is necessary to obtain an optimal range of motion. This mass action can be further balanced with selective tenodesis of the individual FDP tendons across the distal IP joints. If there is functional imbalance resulting in clawed fingers, one can use a multiple digit tenodesis through free tendon grafts from the extensor retinaculum, volar to the deep transverse metacarpal ligament, to the extensor apparatus of the fingers (Riordan, 1983).

Use of the ECRB, ECRL, EIP, and BR for functional insertion on the radial side of the hand, with no ulnar-innervated counterbalance, has resulted in ulnar translocation of the carpus with an associated decrease in the thumb-index web space after a decade of follow-up evaluation (Omer, 1992, 1993) (Fig. 67–21).

Sensibility can be transferred to the radial volar aspect of the hand, but this entails the sacrifice of the index finger (Bralliar and Horner, 1969; Omer, 1992) (Fig. 67–22). Careful testing of the superficial radial nerve will demonstrate the distal level of sensibility on the dorsum of the index finger. The skeleton of the index finger is removed distal to the proximal third of the second metacarpal. The insensitive distal skin is discarded. The filleted index finger flap is then fitted into an additional volar defect created for it in the insensitive palmar skin. This broad-based finger flap is innervated by the superficial radial nerve and will provide protective sensibility within the thumb-index web space, which seems to be of benefit in such activities as holding a steering wheel.

High (Proximal) Ulnar and Radial Nerve Palsy
(Table 67–8)

These patients retain radiovolar sensibility, and reconstruction is a useful surgical investment to improve function.

▼ **TABLE 67–7**
Combined High (Proximal) Median and Ulnar Palsy

Needed Function	Preferred Transfer	Alternate Transfer
Thumb adduction, key pinch (AP)	ECRB, with free tendon graft, between third and fourth metacarpals to APB tendon	EIP between third and fourth metacarpals to APB tendon
Thumb flexion (IP joint)	BR to FPL (in forearm)	Tenodesis of FPL across IP joint of thumb
Thumb abduction (APB) for opposition	EIP around pisiform pulley to APB and EPL tendons	ECU or EPL around pisiform to APB and EPL tendons (thumb MP is fused and no active flexion at IP)
Thumb-index tip pinch	APL slip with free tendon graft to first dorsal interosseous tendon and arthrodesis of MP joint of thumb	EPB to first dorsal interosseous tendon (if thumb MP joint has been fused)
Finger flexion (FDP)	ECRL to all four tendons of FDP with possible tenodesis of distal IP joints of ulnar three fingers	Biceps trachii extended with FCR tendon to tendons of FDP
Power flexion for proximal phalanges and integration of MP and IP motion (clawed fingers)	Four-tailed free tendon graft from dorsal carpal ligament transferred volar to deep transverse metacarpal ligament to lateral bands of dorsal extensor apparatus	Capsulodesis of MP volar capsule *or* free tendon grafts between dorsal extensor apparatus around deep transverse metacarpal ligament to adjacent digits (index-long; ring-little)
Metacarpal (palmar) transverse arch and adduction for little finger	EDM tendon split and ulnar half transferred volar to the deep transverse metacarpal ligament to the radial collateral ligament of the proximal phalanx or lateral band of dorsal extensor apparatus	EDM to deep transverse metacarpal ligament (EDC to little finger must be effective)
Wrist flexion, ulnar aspect		ECU to tendon of FCU
Radial and ulnar volar sensibility	Free vascularized nerve graft to distal cutaneous nerve or neurovascular cutaneous island flap	Superficial radial innervated index fillet flap to palm

Note: See Table 67–1 for abbreviations.

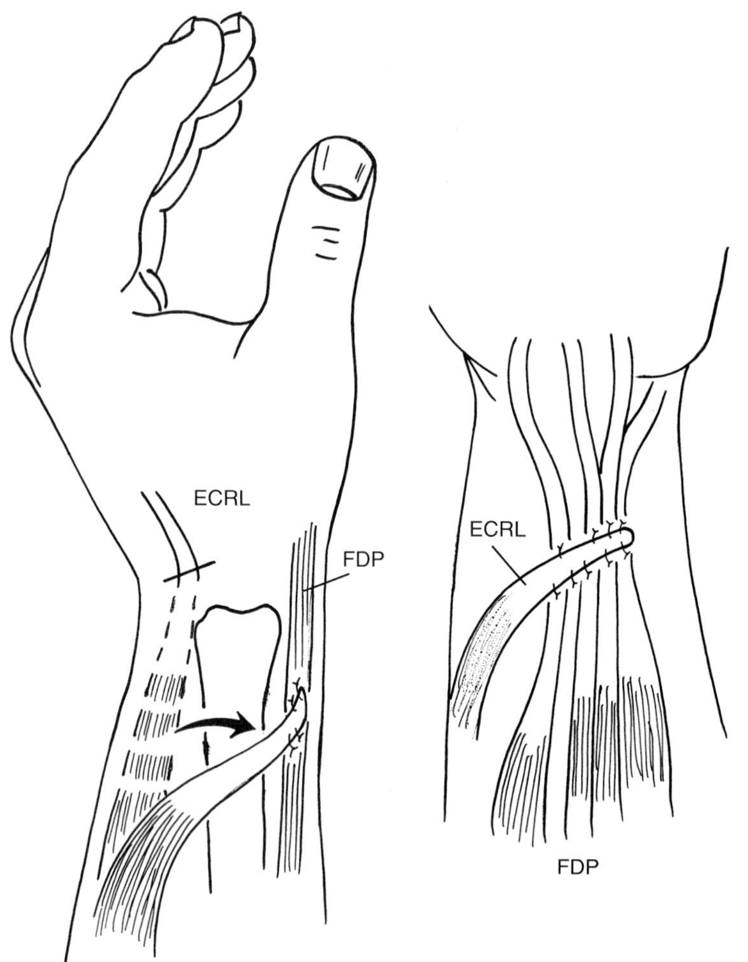

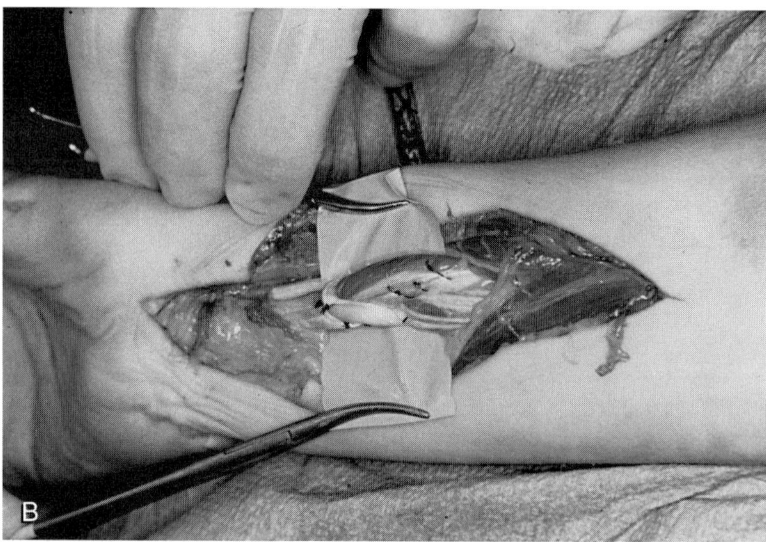

FIGURE 67–20. *A,* Transfer of the extensor carpi radialis longus (ECRL) around the radial aspect of the forearm to the tendons of the flexor digitorum profundus (FDP) for finger flexion. The range of finger motion is less than normal secondary to the comparable limited excursion of ECRL. *B,* Intraoperative photograph. The transfer has been sutured well proximal to the transverse carpal ligament. (*B* from Omer GE Jr: Combined nerve lesions. *In* Green DP [ed]: Operative Hand Surgery. New York, Churchill Livingstone, 1993, p 1470.)

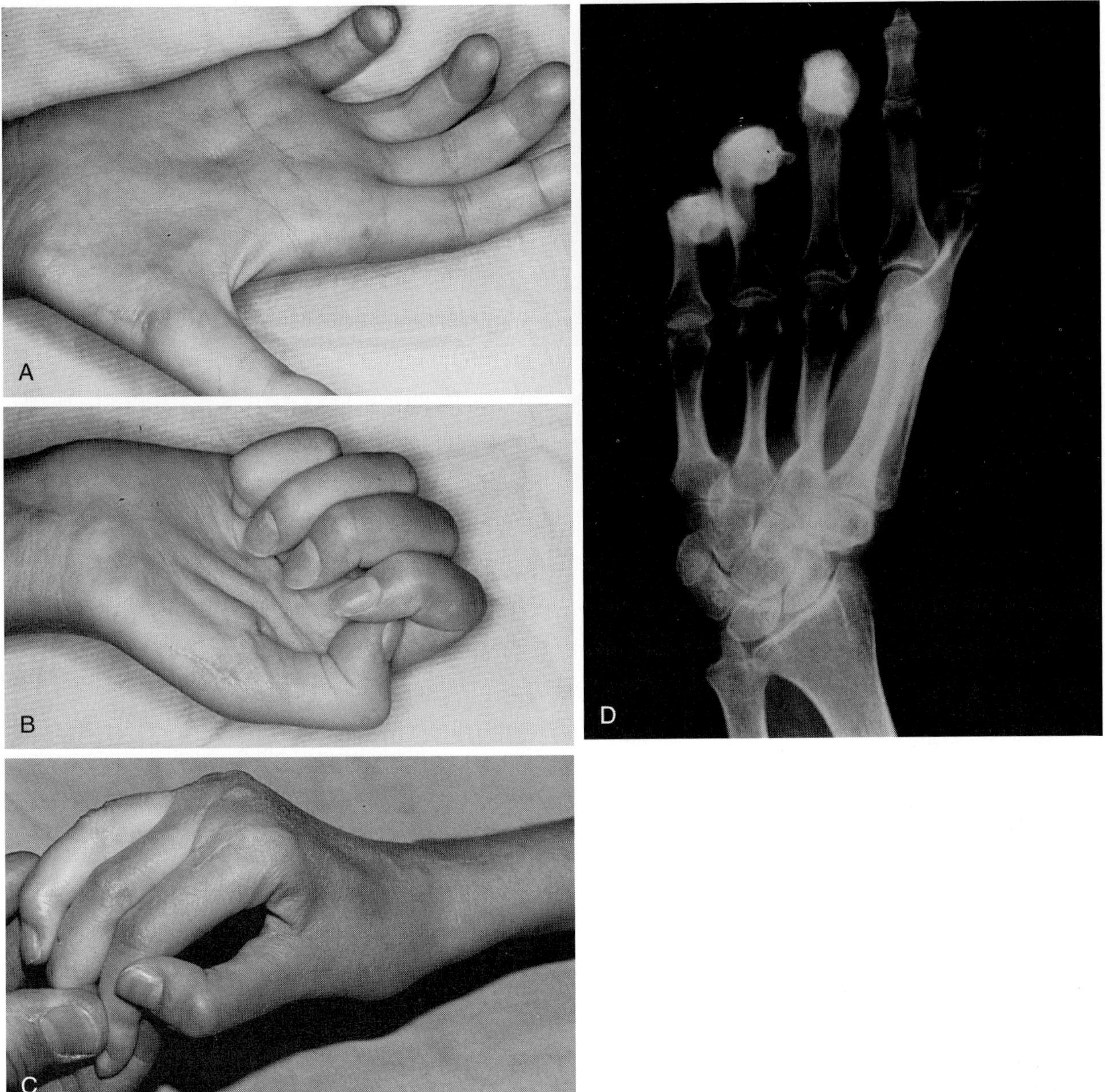

FIGURE 67–21. Time results in deformity if the transfers are not balanced. *A* and *B,* Range of active motion in a high median-ulnar palsy following reconstruction. The extensor carpi radialis brevis (ECRB), with free tendon graft, provided thumb adduction. The brachioradialis (BR) was transferred to the flexor pollicis longus (FPL) and provided thumb flexion. The extensor carpi radialis longus (ECRL) was passed around the radial aspect of the forearm to the flexor digitorum profundus (FDP) for finger flexion. The palmaris longus was tenodeses to the abductor pollicis brevis. *C,* Nine years after injury, intrinsic tenodesis of the index, long, fing, and little fingers was done, using free grafts from the foot. Finger clawing was corrected, but a wrist extension contracture developed with radial deviation of the hand on the wrist. *D,* Eleven years after injury, radiographs demonstrated ulnar translocation of the carpus on the radius, loss of thumb-index web space, and a notch in the third metacarpal related probably to the ECRB thumb adduction transfer. There was no improvement in the radial deviation deformity following release of the intrinsic tenodesis and tenolysis of the thumb adductorplasty 12 years after injury. (From Omer GE Jr: Combined nerve lesions. *In* Green DP [ed]: Operative Hand Surgery, 3rd ed. New York, Churchill-Livingstone, 1993, pp 1471 and 1772.)

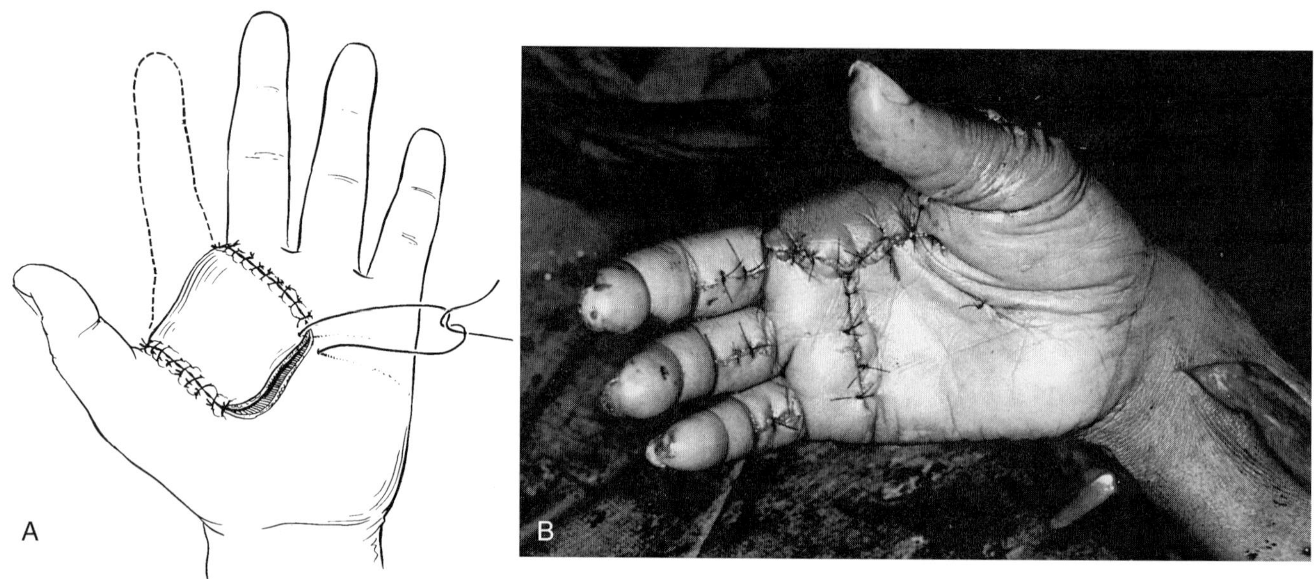

FIGURE 67–22. *A*, Radial innervated dorsal skin flap for combined high median—high ulnar palsy. The insensitive palmar skin is excised to create space for the fillet flap, which brings radial-innervated tissue into the radial side of the palm. (From Omer GE Jr: Orthop Clin North Am 5:377, 1974.) *B*, Intraoperative photograph. The extensor indicis proprius can be used for adduction of the thumb, but it is not an effective substitute. (*B* from Green DR (ed): Operative Hand Surgery. New York, Churchill Livingstone, 1993, p 1473.)

Transfer of the PT into the ECRB for wrist extension results in less radial deviation of the hand than does insertion into the ECRL. Either the long or ring FDS tendons may be used in low ulnar palsy to improve the coordination of MP and proximal IP joint flexion, but in a high ulnar palsy, the long FDS is preferred (Omer, 1971a, 1974c). The technique is the same as used for the early tendon transfer. The single transfer provides key pinch for the thumb, improves the integration of MP and IP joint motion, and the Y-configuration insertion assists the flattened metacarpal arch in grasp (Omer, 1971a; Omer and Elton, 1972).

Extension of the fingers and thumb is obtained by transfer-ring the index and ring FDS tendons through the interosseous membrane to the EDC and EPL (Boyes, 1960; Omer, 1987b). The transfers should be passed through a large hole in the interosseous membrane, and the muscles should be pulled into the plane of the interosseous membrane to maintain motion. The fibers on the circumference of the muscles will eventually adhere to the interosseous membrane, but the central fibers will remain mobile to provide function. The tourniquet should be released to check the anterior interosseous vessels before the muscle-tendon units fill the surgical opening. The patient usually develops the ability to "independently" extend the thumb, or the index finger, or

▼ **TABLE 67–8**
Combined High (Proximal) Ulnar and Radial Nerve Palsy

Needed Function	Preferred Transfer	Alternate Transfer
Wrist extension	PT to ECRB	
Thumb adduction, key pinch (AP)	One-half FDS (long) as split transfer, to APB tendon	
Clawed fingers: metacarpal (palmar transverse arch) and power flexion for proximal phalanx *and* integration of MP and IP motion	One-half FDS (long) in two slips to insert in A2 pulley of flexor sheath of ring and little fingers *and, later,* arthrodesis of proximal IP joints, ring and little fingers	Free tendon graft between lateral bands of dorsal extensor apparatus around deep transverse metacarpal ligament to adjacent digits (index-long; ring-little) *or* capsulodesis of MP volar capsule
Thumb-index tip pinch	Arthrodesis of thumb MP joint	
Proximal thumb abduction stability *and* wrist flexion (radial side)	FCR (yoke insertion) to APL and EPB	Tenodesis of APL to radius
Wrist flexion (ulnar side)		PL to FCU tendon
Finger and thumb extension	FDS (index and ring) through interosseous membrane to EDC and EPL	PL to EDC and EPL
Finger flexion (ring and little)	Tenodesis of FDP (long) (active motor) to ring and little FDP *and, later,* tenodesis of distal IP joint of ring and little fingers, using FDP	
Ulnar volar sensibility	Median digital nerve translocation	Free or vascularized nerve graft

Note: See Table 67–1 for abbreviations.

▼ **TABLE 67–9**
Combined High (Proximal) Median and Radial Palsy

Needed Function	Preferred Transfer	Alternate Transfer
Forearm pronation	Biceps brachii tendon rerouting around the radius	
Wrist extension and flexion	Radiocarpal arthrodesis	
Finger flexion	Tenodesis of FDP (ring and little) (active motors) to index and long FDP	
Finger and thumb extension	FCU to tendons of EDC and EPL	
Proximal thumb abduction stability	Arthrodesis of thumb MP joint *and* tenodesis of APL tendon to radius	
Thumb abduction (APB)		ADQ rotated to APB insertion *or* AP transfer to APB tendon origin
Thumb flexion (FPL)	Tenodesis of FPL tendon across across thumb IP joint	Biceps brachii extended with FCR tendon to tendon of FPL
Radial volar sensibility	Median digital nerve translocation	Neurovascular cutaneous island pedicle from ring finger *or* free or vascularized nerve graft

Note: See Table 67–1 for abbreviations.

the little finger; this is done through mass extension, followed by selective flexion of the digits.

The FDS tendon of the little finger is often congenitally absent, or not functionally independent, and should not be used for tendon transfers. Removal of the FDS may cause loss of balanced power across the proximal IP joint, but the resulting flexion contracture or a swan-neck deformity may take 10 years to develop (Omer, 1993). The swan-neck deformity will occur in some cases in spite of tenodesis of one slip of the FDS tendon proximal to the proximal IP joint. Because these deformities cannot be accurately predicted in an individual patient, it is preferable to await the onset of deformity before correcting it. The most predictable corrective procedure may be arthrodesis of the proximal IP joint.

Flexion of the ring and little fingers is obtained by tenodesis of the FDP of these fingers to the median innervated FDP tendon of the long finger (Omer, 1993). The finger alignment may eventually need improvement through tenodesis of the FDP tendon across the DIP joint of the little and ring finger.

These cases demand multiple steps in reconstruction, probably at 3-month intervals. The first phase might include wrist extension, finger and thumb extension, and thumb abduction. The second phase might include thumb adduction and finger flexion. The third phase might include sensation procedures. Splints need modification for each phase.

High (Proximal) Median and Radial Palsy

(Table 67–9)

All wrist motors are lost except FCU, and arthrodesis of the wrist is indicated. Tendon transfers in this combined palsy will result in a hand that functions only marginally more effective than a prosthesis.

For finger flexion, the FDP tendons of the index and long fingers are sutured side-to-side (tenodesis) to the ulnar innervated FDP of the ring and little fingers. The tendons to the index and long fingers must be under greater tension at the suture line to obtain appropriate balance. There is a better range of motion with a mobile wrist.

For finger and thumb extension, the FCU is freed up

the forearm, brought subcutaneously around the forearm proximal to the dorsal retinaculum, and sutured obliquely across the tendons of the EDC and EPL. The extensor tendons are left in their bed, and the FCU is placed superficially across each tendon with a double suture line for stability.

The ADQ has been transferred for abduction of the thumb (Burkhalter, 1974; Littler and Cooley, 1963; Omer, 1993). The neurovascular pedicle to the ADQ is proximally situated, and the muscle should be freed from distal to proximal, then turned like a page in a book to its new position as thumb abductor. However, it is questionable whether total hand function is improved, because the little finger, with sensibility intact, has now lost its ability for opposition. A more effective procedure is arthrodesis of the MP joint of the thumb (Omer, 1968).

Radial volar sensibility can be improved with a double neurovascular cutaneous island flap from the ring and little finger (Omer, 1978a). However, there is inadequate motor function for precise sensibility (4 mm or less two-point discrimination distance), and these transfers do not improve total function of the hand. A free vascularized nerve graft (Taylor, 1978) with distal neurovascular cutaneous island flap is more effective in this combined palsy.

SUMMARY

Surgeons concerned with reconstruction of the forearm and hand after nerve palsies should be experienced enough to select appropriate procedures based on the individual case. Procedures to restore motor function should be done before those to improve sensibility, such as a neurovascular island pedicle, because precise sensibility requires precise motor function. To add strength, a new muscle-tendon unit must be placed in the power train. The anticipated result should be a balanced simplification of functional performance, because surgery will redistribute the few remaining assets rather than create new ones. Skillful and motivated patients create successful surgeons, and the key to success for these surgical techniques is simplicity; complexity invites failure.

References

Adani R, Squarzina PB, Castagnetti A, Lagana A, Pancaldi G, Caroli A: A comparative study of the heterodigital neurovascular island flap in thumb reconstruction, with and without nerve reconnection. J Hand Surg *19B:*552–559, 1994.

Birch R, Raji ARM: Repair of median and ulnar nerves: Primary suture is best. J Bone Joint Surg *73B:*154–157, 1991.

Blacker GJ, Lister GD, Kleinert HE: The abducted little finger in low ulnar nerve palsy. J Hand Surg *1:*190–196, 1976.

Boyes JW: Tendon transfers for radial palsy. Bull Hosp Joint Dis *21:*97–105, 1960.

Bralliar F, Horner RL: Sensory cross-finger pedicle graft. J Bone Joint Surg *51A:*1264–1268, 1969.

Brand PW: Tendon transfers for median and ulnar nerve paralysis. Orthop Clin North Am *1:*447–454, 1970.

Brand PW: Biomechanics of tendon transfer. *In* Lamb DW, (ed): The Hand and Upper Limb. Vol 2: The Paralyzed Hand. Edinburgh, Churchill-Livingstone, 1987, pp 190–213.

Brand PW: Biomechanics of tendon transfer. Hand Clin *4:*137–154, 1988.

Brand PW: Tendon transfers in the forearm. *In* Jupiter JB (ed): Flynn's Hand Surgery, 4th ed. Baltimore, Williams & Wilkins, 1991, pp 490–506.

Braun RM: Palmaris longus tendon transfer for augmentation of the thenar musculature in low median palsy. J Hand Surg *3:*488–491, 1978.

Brooks AL, Jones DS: A new intrinsic tendon transfer for the paralytic hand. J Bone Joint Surg *57A:*730, 1975.

Brown PW: Reconstruction for pinch in ulnar intrinsic palsy. Orthop Clin North Am *5:*323–342, 1974.

Bunnell S: Surgery of the Hand. Philadelphia, JB Lippincott, 1944, pp 373–375.

Burkhalter WE: Early tendon transfers in upper extremity peripheral nerve injury. Clin Orthop *104:*68–79, 1974.

Burkhalter WE: Median nerve palsy. *In* Green DP (ed): Operative Hand Surgery, 3rd ed. New York, Churchill-Livingstone, 1993, pp 1419–1448.

Burkhalter WE, Christensen RC, Brown P: Extensor indicis proprius opponensplasty. J Bone Joint Surg *53A:*725–732, 1973.

Burkhalter WE, Strait JL: Metacarpophalangeal flexor replacement for intrinsic-muscle paralysis. J Bone Joint Surg *55A:*1656–1676, 1973.

Camitz H: Surgical treatment of paralysis of the opponens muscle of thumb. Acta Chir Scand *65:*77–81, 1929.

Cooney WP: Tendon trans for median nerve palsy. Hand Clin *4:*155–165, 1988.

DeAbreu LB: Early restoration of pinch grip after ulnar nerve repair and tendon transfer. J Hand Surg *14B:*309–314, 1989.

Edgerton MT, Brand PW: Restoration of abduction and adduction to the unstable thumb in median and ulnar paralysis. Plast Reconstr Surg *36:*150–164, 1965.

Eversmann WW: Median nerve palsy. *In* Gelberman RH (ed): Operative Nerve Repair and Reconstruction. Philadelphia, JB Lippincott, 1991, pp 711–728.

Fleeter TB, Adams JP, Brenner B, Podolsky RJ: A laser diffraction method for measuring muscle sarcomere length in vivo for application to tendon transfers. J Hand Surg *10A:*542–546, 1988.

Gaul JS: Radial-innervated cross-finger flap from index to provide sensory pulp to injured thumb. J Bone Joint Surg *51A:*1257–1263, 1969.

Graham WC, Riordan D: Sublimis transplant to restore abduction of index finger. Plast Reconstr Surg *2:*459–462, 1947.

Green DL: Radial nerve palsy. *In* Green DL (ed): Operative Hand Surgery, 3rd ed. New York, Churchill-Livingstone, 1993, pp 1401–1417.

Hamlin C, Littler JW: Restoration of power pinch. Orthop Trans *3:*319–320, 1979.

Hentz VR, Brown M, Keoshian LA: Upper limb reconstruction in quadriplegia: Functional assessment and proposed treatment modifications. J Hand Surg *8:*119–131, 1983.

Holevich J: A new method of restoring sensibility to the thumb. J Bone Joint Surg *45B:*496–502, 1963.

Kaplan EB, Spinner M: Normal and anomalous innervation patterns in the upper extremity. *In* Omer GE Jr, Spinner M (eds): Management of Peripheral Nerve Problems. Philadelphia, WB Saunders, 1980, pp 75–99.

Lewis RC Jr, Tenny J, Irvine D: The restoration of sensibility by nerve translocation. Bull Hosp Joint Dis Orthop Inst *44:*288–296, 1984.

Littler JW: Tendon transfers and arthrodeses in combined median and ulnar nerve paralysis. J Bone Joint Surg *31A:*225–234, 1949.

Littler JW: Principles of tendon transfer. *In* Converse JM (ed): Reconstructive Plastic Surgery. Philadelphia, WB Saunders, 1964, vol 4, pp 1678–1680.

Littler JW, Cooley SGE: Opposition of the thumb and its restoration by abductor digiti quinti transfer. J Bone Joint Surg *45A:*1389–1396, 1963.

Mailander P, Berger A, Schaler E, Ruhe K: Results of primary nerve repair in the upper extremity. Microsurgery *10:*147–150, 1989.

Mannerfelt L: Studies on the hand in ulnar nerve paralysis: A clinical experimental investigation in normal and anomalous innervation. Acta Orthop Scand (Suppl) *87:*89–97, 1966.

Millesi H: Peripheral nerve surgery today: Turning point or continuous development? J Hand Surg *15B:*281–287, 1990.

Moberg EA: Evaluation and management of nerve injuries in the hand. Surg Clin North Am *44:*1019–1029, 1964.

Moberg EA: Upper limb surgical rehabilitation in tetraplegia. *In* Evarts C Mc (ed): Surgery of the Musculoskeletal System, 2nd ed. New York, Churchill-Livingstone, 1990, pp 915–941.

Moneim MS, Omer GE Jr: Latissimus dorsi muscle transfer for restoration of elbow flexion after brachial plexus disruption. J Hand Surg *11A:*135–139, 1986.

Murray JF, Ord JVR, Gavelin GE: The neurovascular island flap: An assessment of late results in sixteen cases. J Bone Joint Surg *49A:*1285–1297, 1967.

Neviaser RJ, Wilson JN, Gardner MM: Abductor pollicis longus transfer for replacement of first dorsal interosseous. J Hand Surg *5:*53–57, 1980.

Omer GE Jr: Evaluation and reconstruction of the forearm and hand after traumatic peripheral nerve injuries. J Bone Joint Surg *50A:*1454–1478, 1968.

Omer GE Jr: Restoring power grip in ulnar palsy. J Bone Joint Surg *53A:*814, 1971a.

Omer GE Jr: Assessment of peripheral nerve injuries. *In* Cramer LM, Chase RA (eds): Symposium on the Hand (Foundation of the American Society of Plastic and Reconstructive Surgeons, Inc). Vol. 3, St Louis, Mosby, 1971b, pp 1–11.

Omer GE Jr: Injuries to nerves of the upper extremity. J Bone Joint Surg *56A:*1615–1624, 1974a.

Omer GE Jr: The technique and timing of tendon transfers. Orthop Clin North Am *5:*243–252, 1974b.

Omer GE Jr: Tendon transfers in combined nerve lesions. Orthop Clin North Am *5:*377–387, 1974c.

Omer GE Jr: Neurovascular island flaps and fillet of finger. *In* Grabb WC, Myers MB (eds): Skin Flaps. Boston, Little, Brown, 1975, pp 471–480.

Omer GE Jr: Neurovascular cutaneous island pedicle flaps. *In* Fredericks S, Brody GS (eds): Symposium on the Neurologic Aspects of Plastic Surgery. St Louis, Mosby, 1978a, pp 52–60.

Omer GE Jr: Tendon transfers as early internal splints following peripheral nerve injury in the upper extremity. *In* Hunter JM, Schneider LH, Mackin EJ, Bell JA (eds): Rehabilitation of the Hand. St Louis, Mosby, 1978b, pp 292–303.

Omer GE Jr: Reconstructive procedures for extremities with peripheral nerve defects. Clin Orthop *163:*80–91, 1982a.

Omer GE Jr: Early tendon transfers in the rehabilitation of the median, radial and ulnar palsies. Ann Chir Main *1:*187–190, 1982b.

Omer GE Jr: Reconstruction of a balanced thumb through tendon transfers. Clin Orthop *195:*104–116, 1985.

Omer GE Jr: Early tendon transfers as internal splints after nerve injury. *In* Hunter JM, Schneider LH, Mackin EJ (eds): Tendon Surgery in the Hand. St Louis, Mosby, 1987a, pp 413–418.

Omer GE Jr: Tendon transfers in radial nerve paralysis. *In* Hunter JM, Schneider LH, Mackin EJ (eds): Tendon Surgery in the Hand. St Louis, Mosby, 1987b, pp 425–431.

Omer GE Jr: Timing of tendon transfers in peripheral nerve injury. Hand Clin *4:*317–322, 1988.

Omer GE Jr: The palsied hand. *In* Evarts C Mc (ed): Surgery of the Musculoskeletal System, 2nd ed. New York, Churchill Livingstone, 1990, pp 849–878.

Omer GE Jr: Tendon transfers for combined traumatic nerve palsies of the forearm and hand. J Hand Surg *17B:*603–610, 1992.

Omer GE Jr: Ulnar nerve palsy. *In* Green DP (ed): Operative Hand Surgery, 3rd ed. New York, Churchill Livingstone, 1993, pp 1449–1466.

Omer GE Jr, Day DJ, Ratliff H, Lambert P: Neurovascular cutaneous island pedicles for deficient median-nerve sensibility. J Bone Joint Surg *52A:*1181–1192, 1970.

Omer GE Jr, Elton RC: Tendon transfers for the nerve injured upper extremity. Orthop Rev *1:*25–28, 1972.

Omer GE Jr, Pirela-Cruz M: Complications of peripheral nerve injuries. *In*

Epps CH Jr, (ed): Complications in Orthopaedic Surgery, 3rd ed. Philadelphia, JB Lippincott, 1994, pp 811–856.

Omer GE Jr, Spinner M: Peripheral nerve testing and suture techniques. Instr Course Lect Am Acad Orthop Surg 24:122–143, 1975.

Omer GE Jr, Vogel JA: Determination of physiological length of a reconstructed muscle-tendon unit through muscle stimulation. J Bone Joint Surg 47A:304–310, 1965.

Parkes A: Paralytic claw fingers: A graft tenodesis operation. Hand 5:192–199, 1973.

Ranney DA: Reconstruction of the transverse metacarpal arch in ulnar palsy by transfer of the extensor digiti minimi. Plast Reconstr Surg 52:406–412, 1973.

Riordan DC: Tendon transplantations in median nerve and ulnar nerve paralysis. J Bone Joint Surg 35A:312–320, 1953.

Riordan DC: Surgery of the paralytic hand. Instr Course Lect Am Acad Orthop Surg 16:59–90, 1959.

Riordan DC: Tendon transfers for nerve paralysis of the hand and wrist. Curr Pract Orthop Surg 2:17–40, 1964.

Riordan DC: Radial nerve paralysis. Orthop Clin North Am 5:283–287, 1974.

Riordan DC: Tendon transfers in hand surgery. J Hand Surg 8:748–753, 1983.

Schneider LH: Opponensplasty using the extensor digiti minimi. J Bone Joint Surg 51A:1297–1302, 1969.

Schneider LH: Tendon transfer for radial nerve palsy. In Gelberman RH (ed): Operative Nerve Repair and Reconstruction. Philadelphia, JB Lippincott, 1991, pp 697–709.

Small JO, Brennan MD: The first dorsal metacarpal artery neurovascular island flap. J Hand Surg 13B:136–145, 1988.

Smith RJ: Extensor carpi radialis brevis tendon transfer for thumb adduction: A study of power pinch. J Hand Surg 8:4–15, 1983.

Smith RJ: Tendon Transfers of the Hand and Forearm. Boston, Little, Brown, 1987, pp 35–133, 135–150.

Starr CL: Army experiences with tendon transference. J Bone Joint Surg 4:3–21, 1922.

Stocks GW, Cobb T, Lewis RC Jr: Transfer of sensibility in the hand: A new method to restore sensibility in ulnar nerve palsy with use of microsurgical digital nerve translocation. J Hand Surg 16A:219–226, 1991.

Taylor GI: Nerve grafting with simultaneous microvascular reconstruction. Clin Orthop 133:56–70, 1978.

Tsuge K, Adachi N: Tendon transfer for extensor palsy of the forearm. Hiroshima J Med Sci 18:219–232, 1969.

Tubiana R, Duparc J: Restoration of sensibility in the hand by neurovascular skin island transfer. J Bone Joint Surg 43A:474–480, 1961.

White WL: Restoration of function and balance of the wrist and hand by tendon transfers. Surg Clin North Am 40:427–459, 1960.

Zancolli EA: Claw hand caused by paralysis of intrinsic muscles. J Bone Joint Surg 39A:1076–1080, 1957.

Zancolli EA: Structural and Dynamic Bases of Hand Surgery, 2nd ed. Philadelphia, JB Lippincott, 1978, pp 168–174.

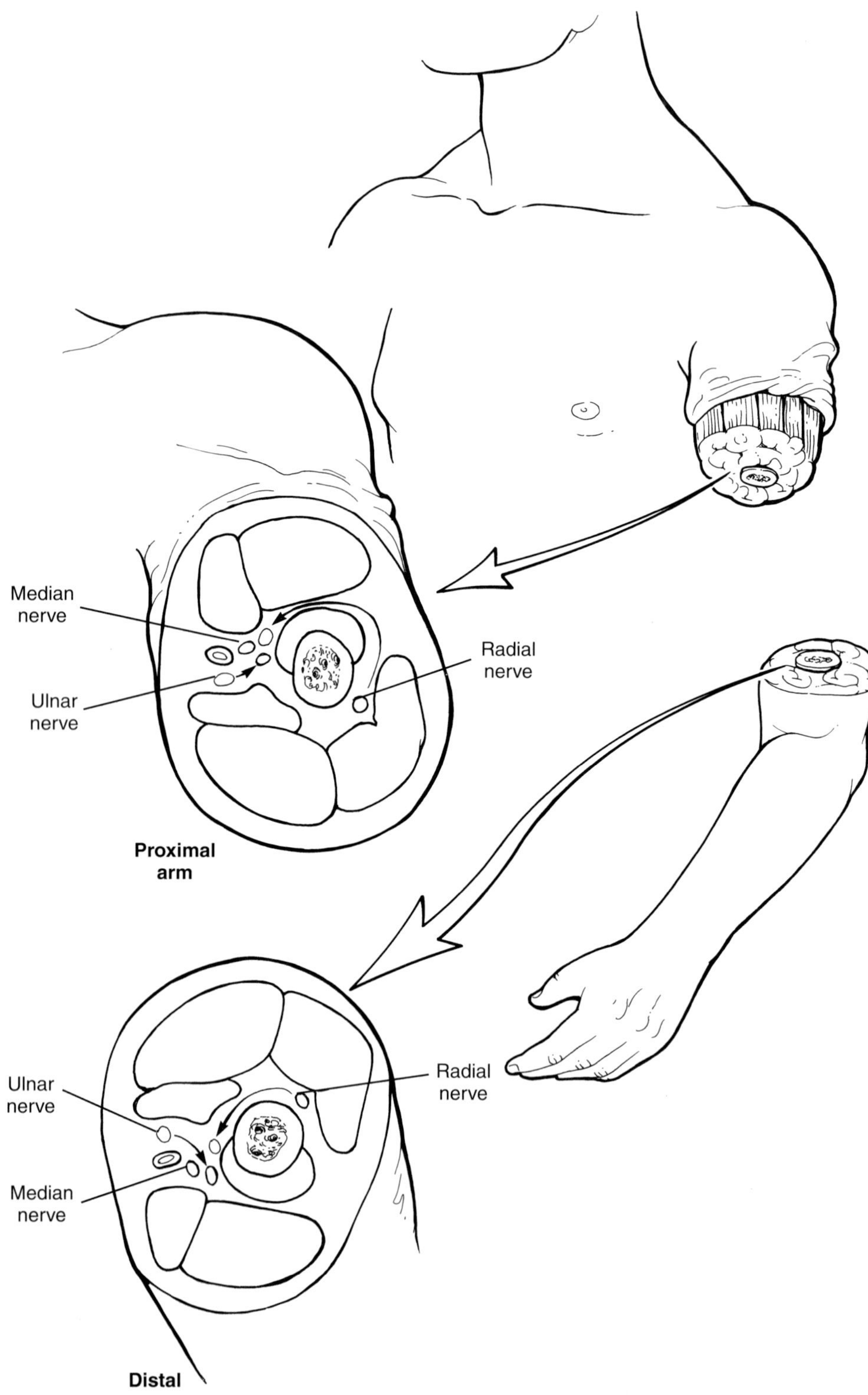

FIGURE 68–4. When skin cover is a problem, transposing the nerve and blood vessels in close proximity to each other provides limited amounts of reliable skin or flap coverage of the exposed vital structures. On the proximal side of the replant, the radial nerve is transposed, and on the distal side, the ulnar nerve is transposed.

being measured (motor vs. sensory). From a personal series of 12 successful above-elbow replants, the muscles of the forearm recovered M4 function in either flexor or extensor muscle groups in 10 replants. Muscle function to a level of M4 can be reliably expected to occur for the brachioradialis, extensor carpi radialis longus, supinator, palmaris longus, flexor carpi ulnaris, flexor carpi radialis, pronator, and some of the digital flexors. Although M3-M4 function can occur in the other forearm muscle units, it will not be as reliable as the large muscles of the proximal forearm. Direct muscle injury in the forearm will decrease muscle function. Useful intrinsic regeneration is not expected for either the ulnar or median innervated muscles of the hand, except in children, but intrinsic fasciotomies are still required. Neural regeneration to the digits will be protective or diminished; protective sensibility and two-point discrimination are not expected. Some sympathetic activity usually occurs after high-level replantation, but it is limited. The skin is usually dryer, overreacts to cold, and more prone to injury and delayed healing than normal extremity skin. In lower-level replantation, more pronounced sympathetic activity is likely to return, which seems related to vascular continuity rather than to neural regeneration.

It is well documented that reliable nerve regeneration occurs after arm replantation (Peacock and Tsai, 1987; Wood and Cooney, 1986; Zuker and Stevenson, 1988). However, the return of function is compromised because of diminished sensibility coupled with significant motor loss. The most common posture of the hand is for the interphalangeal joints of the digits to be flexed and for the metacarpophalangeal joints to be straight, with the thumb in a flat palm position (Fig. 68–5). This claw-hand deformity posture is associated with high ulnar and median palsy. Splinting is essential to prevent severe contracture of the interphalangeal joints because of nerve paralysis combined with ischemic muscle

contraction. Physical therapy is essential to keep range of motion and muscle length as normal as possible. Often, there is the ability to extend and flex the metacarpophalangeal joints. The proximal interphalangeal joints are flexed and can be extended passively but not actively. There is an ability to extend and flex the wrist, but the paralytic flexed-position deformity of the fingers blocks hand function, preventing the patient from opening the hand to grasp. The greatest problem facing the surgeon wishing to augment hand function after arm replantation is the mass action that occurs with muscle groups located distally to the nerve repairs in combination with muscle weakness and fibrosis (Fig. 68–6). In six of our patients, concomitant direct injuries occurred in the forearm. The patient cannot isolate individual muscles, distal to the site of reattachment. Activation of a major nerve's muscle distribution will result in all the muscles supplied being triggered to respond. With concerted effort to increase strength or effectiveness of contracture, the problem may be amplified by co-contraction of other muscle units. Co-contraction can be decreased by biofeedback and therapy, but isolating individual muscle function has not occurred in adults. Our experience with children with above-elbow replantation is more favorable than with adults because of improved regeneration after replantation. Whether this is regeneration or neuroplasticity is undetermined.

The surgeons reconstructing the amputated upper arm will be working with a patient who has three or fewer major nerves that are providing muscle function to the forearm. In our experience, because groups of muscle are innervated by different nerves, their individual group mass function can usually be separate based on different nerve reinnervation, but because of co-contraction, not even this is ensured. Isolation of individual muscle function within a nerve's distribution is not possible in adults. The separation of function by nerve distribution permits the use of mass action

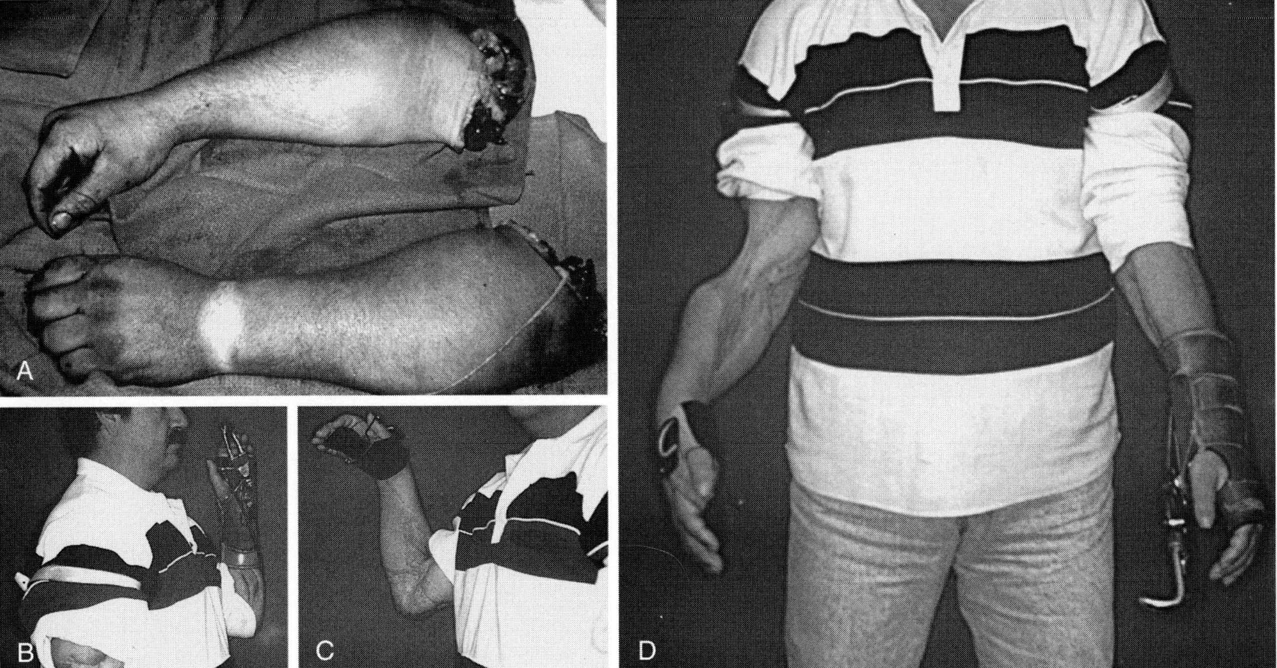

FIGURE 68–5. *A* to *D,* These arms were replanted. The position of the digits following replantation may block effective function, or paralysis may preclude function. This patient has excellent elbow function but uses orthotic devices to substitute for paralytic absence of digit function.

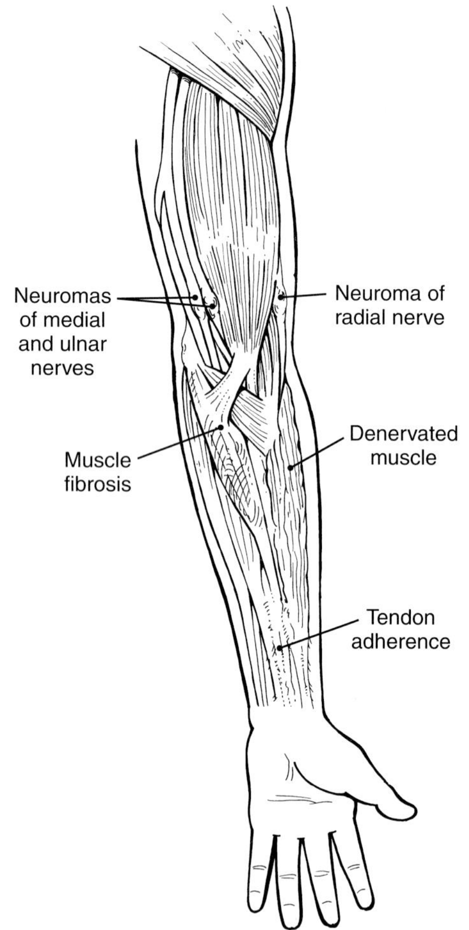

FIGURE 68–6. Replantation produces neuromas with distal muscle weakness from denervation and muscle fibrosis. This problem, combined with mass action contraction and co-contraction, makes the planning of a functional restoration a formidable task.

muscles to be used for very limited tendon transfers. Remember that after replantation, none of the muscle units have normal strength, none of them can be specifically isolated by the patient, and mass action with co-contraction occurs (see Fig. 68–6). For example, the replantation patient cannot usually separate pronator, flexor carpi radialis, thumb, index, and middle digital flexor function. The flexor carpi ulnaris can be separated from the flexor carpi radialis, and the ring and small flexors may be separated from the other digit flexors. This provides some potential for tendon transfer even though the muscle does not have normal strength and in a transferred location may be even less effective. The radial nerve's innervated muscles cannot be functionally isolated independently in the replanted arm, but they can be differentiated from flexor muscle function. Even this will take training, because mass action and co-contraction of flexor and extensor muscles occurs as the patient valiantly tries to use an extremity, firing all the muscle units simultaneously.

Because of the global but partial paralysis of all the muscles in all the nerves after arm replantation, planning tendon transfers is very difficult (Leffert and Pess, 1988; Omer, 1982), and transfer may not be possible in many circumstances. When co-contraction seems to make tendon transfers not advisable, biofeedback training started as soon

as muscle reinnervation begins may help the patient avoid or interrupt this counterproductive effort. Otherwise, joint stabilization, tenodesis, and orthotics may be required to augment function. Stabilization procedures should not be performed until the status of neural regeneration and muscle activity can be accurately assessed, usually 18 to 24 months after replantation. Patient and surgeon must have very defined needs and goals designed to provide improved specific functions for the patient. The assistive helper hands have limited function and will never be normal hands.

RECONSTRUCTION TECHNIQUES

Because above-elbow amputation is a rare injury, the reconstructive techniques discussed here have been performed in limited numbers but have helped hand function. The experiences of Berger and Brenner (1995), Doi et al (1995), Hoang et al (1989), Moneim and Omer (1982), Omer (1980), and Narakas (1993) for plexus injury give insight into management of replant patients.

Opening the Hand

After upper-arm replantation, it is usually not possible for the patient to actively open the interphalangeal joints because of ischemia-induced intramuscular fibrosis coupled with profound intrinsic paralysis and partial extrinsic paralysis involving all the muscle units. In most circumstances, it can be determined if profundus and sublimus functions are present. If the profundi have sufficient strength for flexing the digits, the sublimi of the fingers may be used to perform a Zancolli lasso procedure around the A2 pulley. If the sublimi muscles are M3 or less, secure the transfer where the metacarpophalangeal joint is positioned at 90 degrees of flexion while the wrist is in neutral position. Two lasso procedures in our patients failed to maintain metacarpophalangeal joint flexion after transfer, presumably because the sublimus activity was too weak to prevent the recurrent claw deformity. If the sublimi are not functioning at M4 level, this transfer may fail. If failure occurs, re-exploration and tenodesis with the proximal sublimus tendon attached to the metacarpal will prevent recurrent metacarpophalangeal extension. In one hand, fusion has been performed at the metacarpophalangeal level to assist opening the hand and gaining hook function. The goals are to prevent metacarpophalangeal hyperextension, assist the patient in opening the hand, and improve hook and grasp function. Grasp is very dependent on thumb position and function.

Thumb Control

The second part of getting the patient's hand to function is being able to position the thumb in an opposition position rather than flat palm position. Unless the thumb is readily available for pinching against weak flexors with limited amplitude, key pinch and tip pinch may not be possible (Fig. 68–7). When the extrinsic muscles are too weak and the intrinsic muscles are paralyzed, we have found a bone block or tenodesis has been most reliable in maintaining thumb

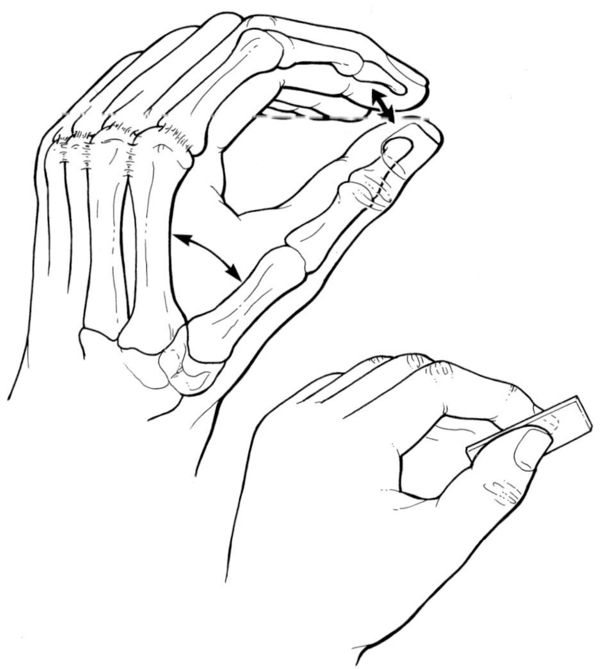

FIGURE 68–7. The thumb must be positioned to allow the index finger to key pinch against it, but the digits must also be able to clear the thumb tip during flexion.

position (Fig. 68–8). As an alternative to bone block, Omer (1982) reported that the extensor carpi radialis brevis can be lengthened with a tendon graft routed between the third and forth metacarpals passed under the flexor tendons and then attached to the abductor tubercle of the thumb. This transfer has a dynamic abduction effect on the thumb when the wrist is either flexed or extended if the transfer is positioned with the wrist in neutral position (Omer, 1982). One can also consider extensor indicis proprius tenodesis around the pisiform combined with metacarpophalangeal joint fusion. If the extrinsic flexor and extensor muscle units are strong, they may be used as transfers to abduct the thumb. This would be preferred to a bone block. Although keeping the thumb abducted in the face of partial paralysis of median, ulnar, and radial nerves; muscle contracture produced by ischemic changes in the muscle; and muscle fibrosis resulting from direct trauma is a difficult task, it has to be accomplished to

improve hand function. When the thumb is positioned properly, extrinsic muscle transfers and tenodesis can provide reliable key pinch. Extensor carpi radialis, brachioradialis, pronator teres, flexor carpi radialis, and flexor carpi ulnaris are usually the only muscles strong enough to consider for flexor or extensor tendon transfer (Figs. 68–9 and 68–10). If weak but useful function is present it must be ensured that important functional losses do not occur after their use for tenodesis. Because of its proximal location, the palmaris longus often is useful to transfer for thumb opposition, as described by Camitz (1929) (Fig. 68–11). Because of muscle weakness, tenodesis instead of transfer of extensor pollicis brevis, abductor pollicis longus, extensor digitorum communis, and extensor pollicis longus will provide useful functional adjuncts when active wrist function is strong. After above-elbow replantation, flexor strength usually exceeds extensor strength. Tenodesis on the flexor surface using the active extension has not been tried. Without sufficient wrist flexor strength, an extensor digitorum tenodesis is not effective in straightening the interphalangeal joints of the digits. A bone block makes a reliable base for the extrinsic muscles to work around, but it also creates some difficulties for

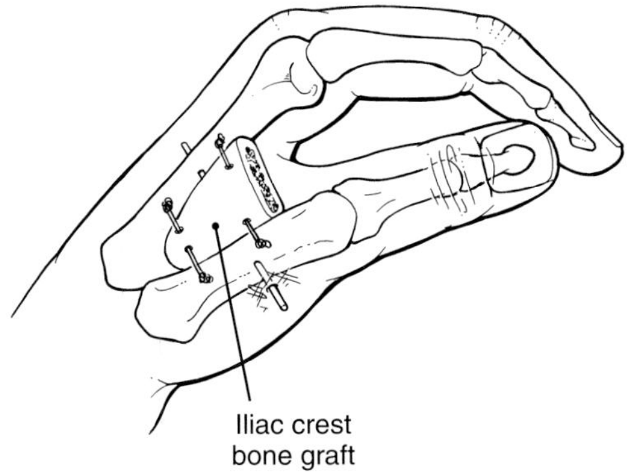

FIGURE 68–8. When complete intrinsic paralysis is combined with weak extrinsic muscle units, a bone block can position the thumb in a useful position. The bone harvest from the ilium is fixed in position with interosseous wires and pin fixation.

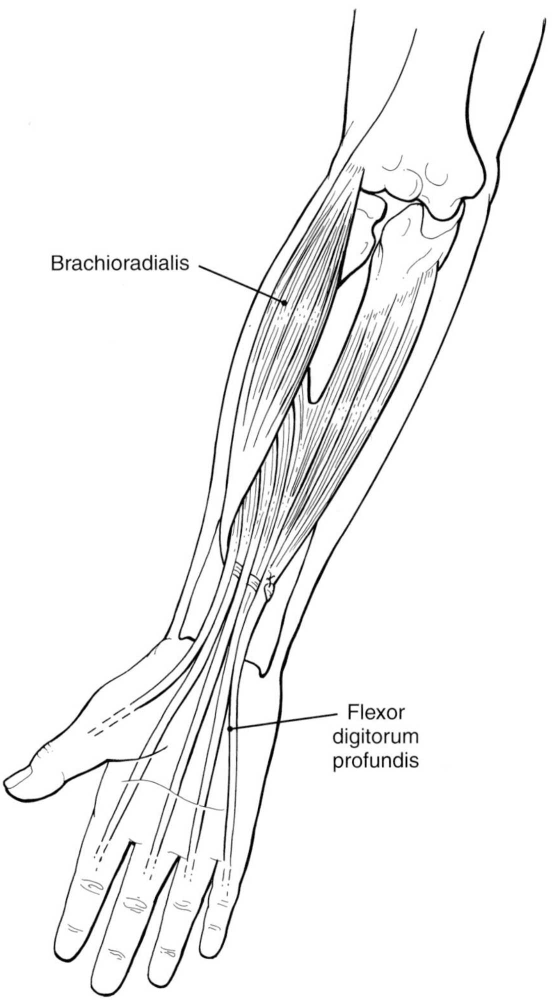

FIGURE 68–9. When the brachioradialis is innervated, it can be used to augment flexor strength or to provide flexion. Even with mass action, this transfer has provided effective digital flexion. Remember, the first goals of surgery are hook and grasp. If this transfer is adjusted for tight grip, it will prevent the fingers from extending.

concise separation of muscle function and strength grades in the replant patient is difficult because of muscle mass action.

Wrist fusion has not been attempted in this series of upper arm replantation because much of the function on which patients rely is centered on wrist movement. Orthotic devices are frequently used to augment limited hand function. Some orthotic devices rely on wrist flexion and extension. Before performing wrist fusion, consultation with an experienced occupational therapist is essential to ensure that use of such aids to daily living would not be limited by wrist fusion.

Even with the presence of mass action and weakness in forearm movement, elbow movement is often near normal and controlled. One of our patients with bilateral arm replantation has no muscle function below the elbow in either arm. He uses bilateral orthotic devices. A small wire hook on the palm of his right dominant hand and a shoulder harness–driven hook on his left forearm that is positioned volar to the digits permit a great deal of functional independence because of his elbow movement and wrist flexibility.

The combination of bilateral intrinsic and extrinsic paraly-

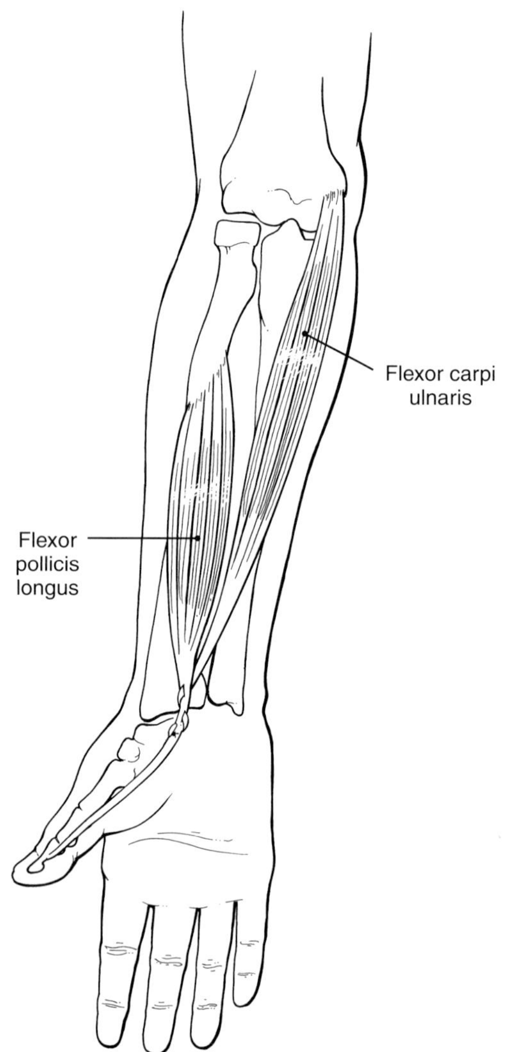

FIGURE 68–10. The flexor carpi ulnaris transferred to the flexor pollicis longus for thumb flexion combined with interphalangeal joint fusion will provide reasonable key pinch when opposition is established by other methods. The flexor carpi ulnaris can be used only when the flexor carpi radialis is able to flex the wrist.

patients because of the fixed position of the thumb. The bone block is created using a portion of the iliac crest and wire fixation to the first and second metacarpals (see Fig. 68–8). Proper placement of the block is crucial and must permit the thumb pulp to close against the index finger's pulp. In very active individuals, the bone fusion between the metacarpals could be limiting. Balancing the thumb and index function is crucial; it is one of the most desired and useful functions in a replanted arm, hook function by the fingers being the most important.

If the digital extensors do not function and the wrist flexors are graded at least M4, tenodesis of the finger extensors to the radius will help open the fingers, but only if the metacarpophalangeal joints are stabilized in flexion and cannot hyperextend. Muscle weakness and fibrosis of the forearm digital flexors usually precludes them as active transfers. If profundus and sublimus strength can be determined to be M4 or greater, then the sublimus tendons can be used in a more traditional method of transfer. Unfortunately,

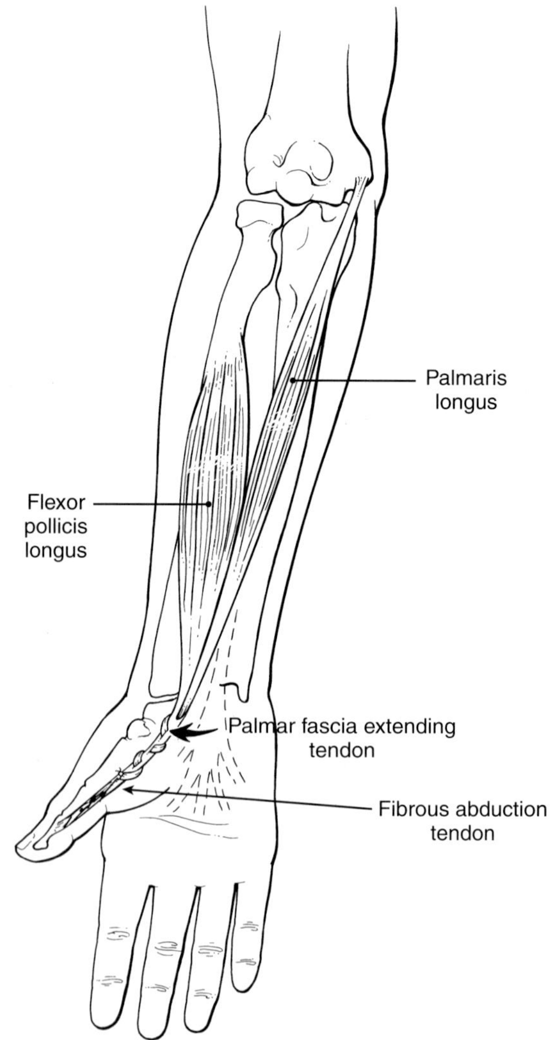

FIGURE 68–11. When it is functioning, the palmaris longus, which has been lengthened with palmar fascia, can be transferred to the thumb abductor tendon for thumb opposition. The palmaris longus may be strong enough following replantation for thumb opposition but not for multiple digit flexion.

sis or muscle loss makes hand function and the many reconstructions available in other circumstances more limited, because the distribution of all three nerves is affected with motor and sensory impairments.

ELBOW FUNCTION

Tendon or muscle transfers for elbow or shoulder function have been discussed by Beaton et al (1995), Brunelli et al (1995), Chuang et al (1993), Freund et al (1986), Hou and Tai (1991), and Liu et al (1993).

After some upper-arm replantations, the biceps, brachialis, and triceps muscles are destroyed or need to be débrided because of circulation loss. To extend the arm overhead the triceps is important, and to flex the elbow the biceps and brachialis are important. In this series of replantation, it has never been necessary to do transfers to substitute triceps and biceps muscle transfers. In this group of patients, the latissimus dorsi (Narakas, 1993) has been the ideal muscle to transfer for either biceps or triceps function in the perioperative period after replantation. In this setting, the latissimus is used to provide muscle function and to secure viable tissue cover for crucial nerve and vessel repairs. In the delayed setting, because the muscle is long enough to cross the shoulder and elbow joints, the patient can gain more potential use of the transfer, and it can provide some digit flexion. When the muscle is transferred for flexion of the elbow, a bipolar transfer is performed with the coracoid serving as origin and the forearm flexor mass or the biceps tendon as insertion points. The resting length of this muscle must be marked and maintained in the transferred position or else the transfer will be loose and not provide enough power for elbow flexion (Fig. 68–12) (Freund et al, 1986; Moneim and Omer, 1986; Zancolli and Mitre, 1973).

The pectoralis major muscle is another potential muscle transfer for elbow flexion or extension (Beaton et al, 1995; Hou and Tai, 1991; Leffert and Pess, 1988). The transfer is limited by its length and can be used for elbow function, but, compared with the latissimus, it would not provide reliable cover for the distal half of the humerus and would not be as useful for resurfacing exposed hardware or neurovascular bundles. Technically, the pectoralis transfer is the more difficult transfer to perform and adjust for tension.

When the triceps is available and in circumstances where the pectoralis major or latissimus dorsi transfer is not advisable, the triceps can be transferred to an anterior position for elbow flexion and coverage (Hoang et al, 1989). This transfer will require relearning of its function, but it can serve as a reliable method of providing useful elbow flexion transfer when the latissimus is not available for transfer or will be used for other functions (Fig. 68–13).

For triceps reconstruction, the proximal insertion of the latissimus is not disturbed, and the origin is sutured into the triceps and the extensor fascia of the forearm.

After muscle transfer, the transferred muscle must be

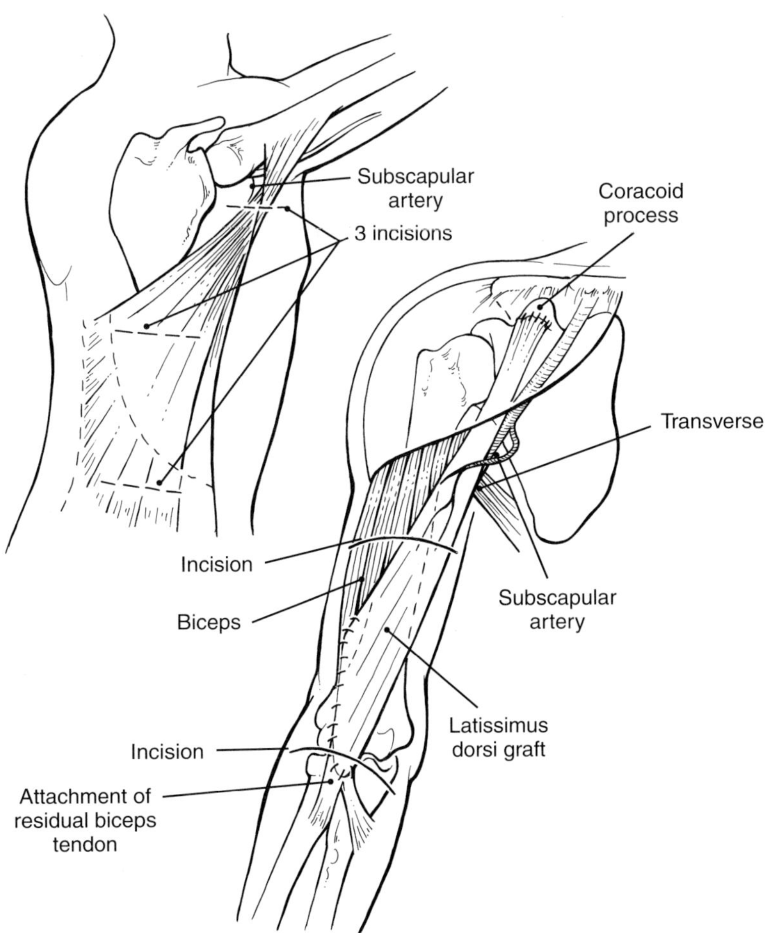

FIGURE 68–12. The latissimus dorsi muscle transfer is useful in emergent situations to resurface and help restore biceps function. It is also very successful in delayed reconstruction if biceps or triceps function needs to be restored. The muscle is mobilized on the supplying thoracodorsal artery, veins, and nerve. The pedicle leash is sufficiently long and mobile to permit a wide range of movement within the area of the axilla and shoulder. If the brachial plexus is injured, this transfer may not be advisable, emphasizing the need for brachial plexus assessment before beginning proximal replantation.

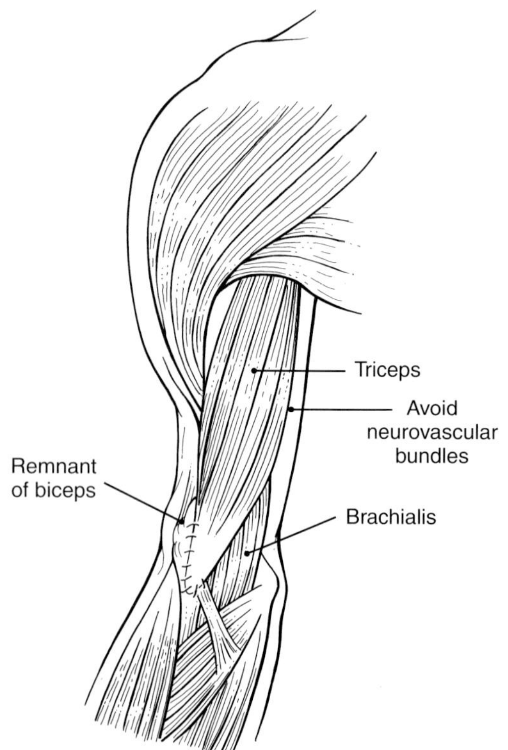

FIGURE 68–13. When the triceps is transferred following replantation, the distal tendon of the triceps is detached and then reattached to the distal fibrous matrix or tendon stump of the previous biceps. In our series, the distal biceps muscle mass in the amputated part is missing in all above-elbow replants. Because of the distal location, it is devascularized and débridement is essential. The shorter muscle units produce a shorter amplitude of excursion of the remaining proximal biceps and eventually result in a 20- to 40-degree-flexion contracture of the elbow.

protected from disruption from its new origin or insertion for 6 weeks. After an acute latissimus transfer, the elbow must be kept flexed to protect nerve, vessel, tendons, and the transferred muscle. When transferring the latissimus, it is helpful if the latissimus fascia is maintained because it helps secure the sutures when the muscle is being fixed in position. It is emphasized that the resting tension of the muscle should be established and marked before transecting the origin and insertion. The resting distance can then be reestablished when located in its new position. Sutures or staples every 3 to 5 cm mark resting tension for reference.

Considerable support, patient education, and supervised therapy are essential for these transfers to function. Strengthening a weak muscle can be the difference between a successful or unsuccessful transfer. Biofeedback using muscle-evoked potentials can assure the patient that the correct process is being used in activating a muscle or tendon transfer. If the muscle has just been reinnervated, galvanic muscle stimulation can increase muscle contraction and provide more visible evidence of muscle function in muscle that previously would not contract. Reconstruction is not a single operation or procedure, but a planned combination of elements designed to enhance the function of very impaired extremities.

In our patients and those of Wood and Cooney (1986), and Peacock and Tsai (1987), replantation and reconstruction for above-elbow amputation was superior to amputation and

above-elbow prosthesis. One of our patients with bilateral unsuccessful upper-arm replantation does not live independently because he is unable to perform all the functions required to live independenty using bilateral above-elbow prostheses. Our patients with successful bilateral upper-arm replants all live independently and are able to perform function's necessary for daily living. We are often asked why is replantation better than prosthetic fitting. We believe the patient's sense of being whole, sensory input from the extremity, immediate availability, avoiding the harness, avoiding mechanical breakdown, appearance, function of digits, and even orthotic function are improved when the elbow and wrist are present. When the elbow and wrist are functioning, the hand can be reconstructed to provide hook, grasp, and often pinch function. When coupled with some sensibility, the replant is superior to prosthetic alternatives.

References

Beaton DE, Dumont A, Mackay MB, Richards RR: Steindler and pectoralis major flexorplasty: A comparative analysis. J Hand Surg (Am) 20:747–56, 1995.

Berger A, Brenner P: Secondary surgery following brachial plexus injuries. Microsurgery 16:43–47, 1995.

Biemer E: Evaluation of the results of replantation. In Brunelli G (ed): Textbook of Microsurgery. Milano, Italy, Masson, 1988.

Brunelli GA, Vigasio A, Brunelli GR: Modified Steindler procedure for elbow flexion restoration. J Hand Surg (Am) 20:743–746, 1995.

Buncke HJ, Alpert BS, Johnson-Giebink R: Digital replantation. Surg Clin North Am 61:383–394, 1981.

Camitz H: Uber die be Handlung der Opposition-slahmung. Acta Chir Scand 65:77, 1929.

Chen ZW, Meyer VE, Kleinert HE, Beasley RW: Present indications and contraindications for replantation as reflected by long term functional results. Orthop Clin North Am 12:849, 1981.

Chuang DC: Functioning free muscle transplantation for brachial plexus injury. Clin Orthop 314:104–11, 1995.

Chuang DC, Epstein MD, Yeh MD, Wei FC: Functional restoration of elbow flexion in brachial plexus injuries: Results in 167 patients (excluding obstetric brachial plexus injury). J Hand Surg (Am) 18:285–291, 1993.

Daoutis NK, Gerostathopoulos N, Efstathopoulos D, Misitzis D, Bouchlis G, Anagnostou S: Major amputation of the upper extremity: Functional results after replantation/revascularization in 47 cases. Acta Orthop Scand Suppl 264:7–8, 1995.

Datiashvili RO, Lein AP: Restoration of lymph drainage after extremity replantation. J Reconstr Microsurg 6:325–329, 1990.

Doi K, Sakai K, Kuwata N, Ihara K, Kawai S: Double free-muscle transfer to restore prehension following complete brachial plexus avulsion. J Hand Surg (Am) 20:408–414, 1995.

Freund RK, Terzis JK, Jordan L, Taylor G: Modified latissimus dorsi and teres major transfer for external rotation deficit of the shoulder. Orthopedics 9:505–506, 1986.

Hales P, Pullen D: Hypotension and bleeding diathesis following attempted arm replantation. Anesth Intensive Care 10:359, 1982.

Harris WH, Malt RA: Late results of human limb replantation: Eleven year and six year follow-up of two cases with description of a new tendon transfer. J Trauma 14:44, 1974.

Hoang PH, Mills C, Burke FD: Triceps to biceps transfer for established brachial plexus palsy. J Bone Joint Surg (Br) 71:268–271, 1989.

Hou CL, Tai YH: Transfer of upper pectoralis major flap for functional reconstruction of deltoid muscle. Chin Med J (Engl) 104:753–757, 1991.

Kleinert HE, Juhala CA, Tsai TM, Van Beek AL: Digital replantation-selection, technique and results. Orthop Clin North Am 8:309–315, 1979.

Krarup C, Upton J, Creager MA: Nerve regeneration and reinnervation after limb amputation and replantation: Clinical and physiological findings. Muscle Nerve 13:291–304, 1990.

Leffert RD, Pess GM: Tendon transfers for brachial plexus injury. Hand Clin 4:273–288, 1988.

Liu TK, Yang RS, Sun JS: Long-term results of the Steindler flexorplasty. Clin Orthop 296:104–108, 1993.

Malt RA: Replantation of severed arms. JAMA 189:716–722, 1964.

Meyer VE: Replantation of the hand. General Considerations. *In* Brunnelli EG (ed): Textbook of Microsurgery. Milano, Italy, Masson Publishers, 1988, pp 481–490.

Meyer VE. Wound closure and decompression in upper limb replantation. Ann Chir Main Memb Super *9:*129–134, 1990.

Moneim MS, Omer GE: Latissimus dorsi muscle transfer for restoration of elbow flexion after brachial plexus disruption. J Hand Surg *11A:*135–139, 1986.

Omer GE: The technique and timing of tendon transfers. Orthop Clin North Am *5:*243–252, 1974.

Omer GE: Tendon transfers for reconstruction of the forearm and hand following peripheral nerve injuries. Management of Peripheral Nerve Problems. Philadelphia, WB Saunders, 1980, pp 817–846.

Omer GE: Combined Nerve Palsies: Operative Hand Surgery. New York, Churchill Livingstone, 1982, pp 1081–1089.

Narakas AO: Muscle transpositions in the shoulder and upper arm for sequelae of brachial plexus palsy. Clin Neurol Neurosurg *95(suppl):*S89–91, 1993.

Parry SW, Ward JW, Mathes SJ: Vascular anatomy of the upper extremity muscles. Plast Reconstr Surg *81:*358–365, 1988.

Patradul A, Ngarmukos C, Parkpian V: Major limb replantation: A Thai experience. Ann Acad Med Singapore *24(4 suppl).*82–88, 1995.

Peacock K, Tsai TM: Comparison of functional results of replantation versus prosthesis in a patient with bilateral arm amputation. Clin Orthop *214:*153–159, 1987.

Russell RC, O'Brien BM, Morrison WA, Pamamull G, MacLeod A: The late functional results of upper limb revascularization and replantation. J Hand Surg (Am) *9:*623–633, 1984.

Wood MB, Cooney WP III: Above elbow limb replantation: Functional results. J Hand Surg (Am) *11:*682–687, 1986.

Zancolli EA, Mitre H: Lattissimus dorsi transfer to restore elbow flexion. J Bone Joint Surg *55A:*1265–1275, 1973.

Zuker RM, Stevenson JH: Proximal upper limb replantation in children. J Trauma *28:*544–547, 1988.

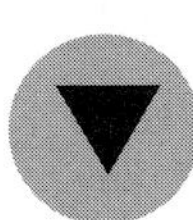

Chapter 69

• John S. Gould
• Eugene E. Curry

Tendon Transfers as Reconstructive Procedures in the Leg and Foot Following Peripheral Nerve Injuries

Tendon transfers in the lower extremity are performed for traumatic muscle loss; irreparable nerve injury; congenital muscle imbalance, as in clubfoot; muscle dysfunction (muscular dystrophy); flaccid paralysis due to lower motor neuron lesions at the spinal cord level, as in poliomyelitis and Guillain-Barré syndrome; progressive spinal cord disorders, such as Charcot-Marie-Tooth disease; and spastic upper motor neuron lesions, such as cerebral palsy, head injury, and stroke. Although mobility is particularly important in the proximal extremity (hip and knee), the need for stability with weightbearing in the distal extremity often mandates the use of bony stabilization procedures (arthrodeses) instead of or to supplement many tendon transfers. In addition, digital (toe) active mobility or dexterity is not particularly necessary for almost all normal function of the foot, in contrast with the hand and upper extremity. For the foot to function well, biomechanically, it should be flexible enough to dissipate the ground reaction force with a controlled braking action of the ankle dorsiflexors to avoid a slapping or foot-drop gait. At heel strike, the calcaneus must gently move into valgus through the subtalar joint and the mid-foot pronates through the mid-tarsal joints as the position of foot flat is reached. As the body weight moves forward and the toes begin to dorsiflex, the static windlass mechanism of the plantar fascia tightens and the flattened arch reforms. The mid-foot supinates as the heel goes into varus, and with this rigid configuration, the foot toes off with power. The flexible flatfoot, on the other hand, gives way too quickly with the stretched out medial structures and has no power in toe off; the cavus foot remains rigid throughout, and does not dissipate the ground reaction force at heel strike. Thus, the normal gait occurs due to normal joint alignment and flexibility, intact joint ligaments and plantar fascia, and functionally balanced extrinsic and intrinsic muscles. Muscle power cannot substitute for ligament dysfunction, which when it exists, necessitates ligament reconstruction or arthrodesis. Ligaments also fail when dynamic stabilizers no longer function (e.g., tibialis posterior tendon rupture). With inappropriate joint alignment, as with bunions, hallux varus, or clubfoot, muscles become unbalanced, accentuating the deformity. Finally, with muscle or nerve dysfunction, and subsequent ligament stretching or contracture, joint malalignments occur. This is particularly true with growing children, who may require osteotomies in order to re-establish a plantigrade foot before tendon transfer.

The initial requirement, before tendon transfer in the adult foot, is also to re-establish flexibility in the appropriate plane before considering a tendon transfer. Phase of gait requires special consideration or at least an understanding in the foot. During the swing phase of gait, the anterior muscles (tibialis anterior, extensor digitorum, and extensor hallucis longus) are active. They also play a role at heel strike, providing the braking action that prevents the slapping gait. During the stance phase, the posterior and lateral muscles come into play, controlling the forward movement of the tibia over the foot, followed by plantar flexion at the ankle joint. Although in-phase transfers seem to work easily and automatically, out-of-phase transfers are commonly performed but may require training.

The primary goals of tendon transfer are to re-establish motor balance and to replace lost motor functions, when necessary. The basic principles of joint flexibility, donor muscle power and excursion, integrity, straight lines of pull, appropriate bed, and adequate insertions all apply. As elsewhere in the body, if an adequate bed does not exist, it must be created by conventional or free flap coverage during or before the tendon transfer procedure. Some unique bone insertion methods have been described, including the use of a trephined plug, which is replaced after the tendon is pulled through a bone (Fig. 69–1A and B) (Gould, 1973); placement of a button under the foot after drilling through the mid-tarsus (Fig. 69–2); and various paired drill holes sometimes accompanied by trephined plugs (Fig. 69–3). Although a standard tendon interweave insertion ascribed to Pulvertaft is still used in many instances, studies (Ward et al, 1988) have suggested that the trephined plug technique affords the strongest fixation. Several modifications exist for protection of the plantar foot when using the pull-through technique with the button. Large rubber and metal discs have been used for such protection (Cheng et al, 1994). Silver has provided a relative strength of muscle table based on muscle mass and fiber length that is somewhat helpful in selecting appropriate transfers (Table 69–1) (Silver et al, 1993).

In the lower extremities, one must also differentiate between a true tendon transfer, in which a muscle tendon unit is transferred to provide motor function, and other uses of

N. Gould Technique
Bone Plug Fixation

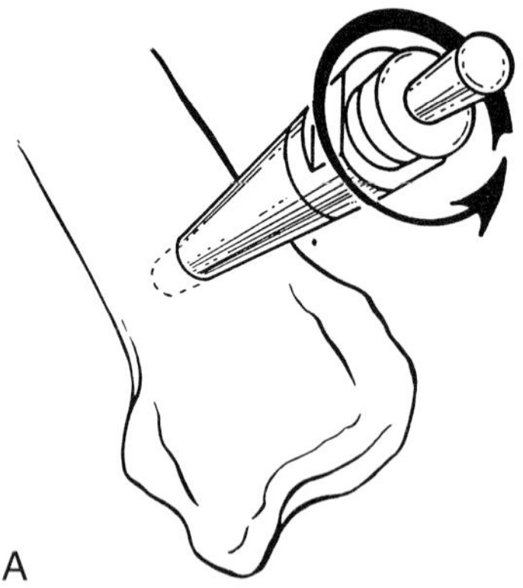

A

Bone Plug Fixation

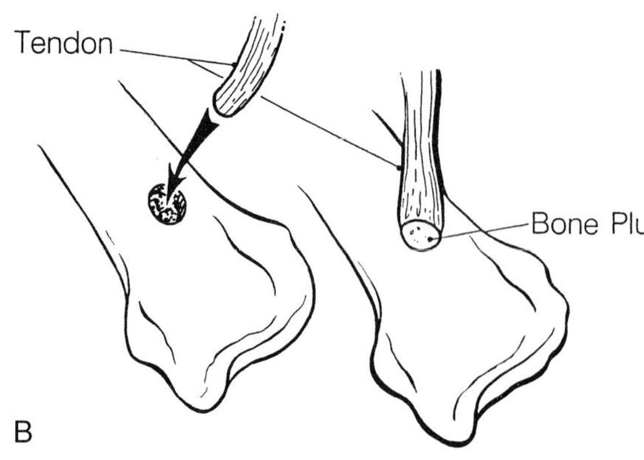

B

FIGURE 69–1. *A,* A plug of bone is removed with a trephine. *B,* The tendon is inserted into the hole in the cortex and the bone plug replaced.

muscle and particularly tendon units such as tenodeses, in which a tendon is placed under maximum tension and fixed proximally and distally, or when the side-to-side transfer essentially only substitutes for lost tendon tissue, with little if any transfer of motor power. Finally, distal tendon is commonly used as a ligament reconstruction for lateral ankle instability and in other areas. This chapter only discusses efforts to use the muscle tendon unit as an active motor.

Split tendon transfers are also used extensively to provide better balance in the foot, but they are used more often to correct congenital disorders, such as clubfoot or cavus foot, or spastic problems. One must also remember that in the foot, various muscles play several roles and use of such a muscle in a transfer could lead to secondary deformities of consequence. For example, the tibialis posterior muscle, which travels behind the medial malleolus, is a plantar flexor of the ankle and, lying medial to the axis of rotation of the subtalar joint, is an inverter of the foot. In addition, this muscle, with its multiple insertions along the medial and plantar aspect of the foot, also supports the arch. Consequently, loss of this muscle not only affects the first two active motions but also could lead to the development of a flatfoot deformity. The peroneus longus is also a flexor of the ankle and an evertor of the subtalar joint. In addition and most importantly, it acts as a plantar flexor of the first

metatarsal. When the tibialis anterior muscle, which inserts on the first metatarsal, is active and functional, loss of the peroneus longus leads to elevation of the first metatarsal with secondary imbalance at the metatarsophalangeal joint of the great toe and a dorsal bunion. If one is to use the peroneus longus as a transfer, the distal stump should be stabilized to the peroneus brevis and a first tarsometatarsal arthrodesis may be required later to reposition this ray. Attention to the complex action of each potential motor, given the particular circumstances in the involved foot, is essential and distal tenodeses or bony stabilizations, or both, may be necessary to supplement a transfer. If the antagonist muscle is not functional, this may not be a factor. Although the authors do not discuss spinal cord, central, congenital, or myogenic etiologies relative to the appropriate transfers, muscle transfers used for these conditions, as well as those for pure nerve palsies, are discussed and reference to uses in these conditions are made. Although lacerations to individual nerves in the lower extremity do occur, traction injuries and severe compressions occur more commonly with both blunt closed and open trauma to the lower limb. Below the knee, both extrinsic and intrinsic muscles are innervated by distal branches of the sciatic nerve. The peroneal branch enters the lateral compartment innervating the peroneal musculature and then splits into the deep and superficial peroneal nerves. The deep branch supplies innervation of the muscles of the anterior compartment and finally passes under the extensor retinaculum to supply the extensor hallucis brevis and exten-

Bone Pull-Through with Plantar Button

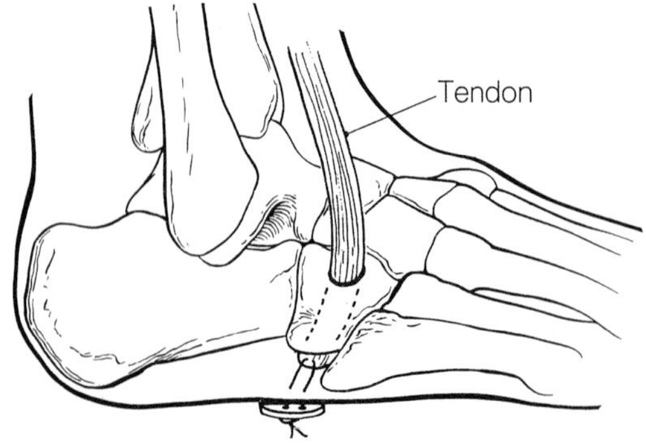

FIGURE 69–2. The tendon is pulled through the hole in the bone, with the sutures tied over a button.

Bone Pull-Through Fixation

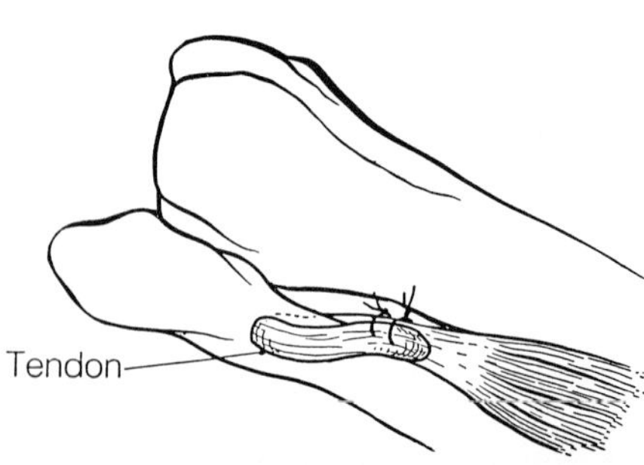

FIGURE 69–3. The tendon is pulled through two holes in the cortex and tied onto itself.

▼ **TABLE 69–1**
Relative Strengths of Muscles

Plantar Flexion		Dorsiflexion	
Soleus	29.9	Tibialis anterior	5.6
Gastrocnemius—medial	13.7	EDL	1.7
Gastrocnemius—lateral	5.5	EHL	1.2
FHL	3.6	Peroneus tertius	0.9
FDL	1.8	Total	9.4
Tibialis posterior	6.4		
Peroneus longus	5.5		
Peroneus brevis	2.6		
Total	69.0		
Inversion		**Eversion**	
Tibialis posterior	6.4	Peroneus longus	5.5
FHL	3.6	Peroneus brevis	2.6
FDL	1.8	EDL	1.7
G-S	49.1	EHL	1.2
Total	60.9	Peroneus tertius	0.9
		Total	11.9

EDL, extensor digitorum longus; EHL, extensor hallucis longus; FDL, flexor digitorum longus; FHL, flexor hallucis longus; G-S, gastrocnemius-soleus.

From Silver RL, DeLa Garza J, Rang M: The myth of muscle balance: A study of relative strengths and excursions of normal muscles about the foot and ankle. In Mann RA, Coughlin MJ (eds): Surgery of the Foot and Ankle, 6th edition. St. Louis, Mosby–Year Book, 1993, pp. 826–827.

sor digitorum, finally ending in a sensory branch to the first web space. The superficial peroneal nerve pierces the crural fascia in the distal third of the leg before dividing into the medial and intermediate sensory branches on the dorsum of the foot. The tibial nerve supplies the posterior compartment musculature, passes behind the medial malleolus with the tibialis posterior artery and veins, splitting into the medial and lateral plantar nerves before passing under the fascia of the abductor hallucis and then supplying the plantar intrinsic motors as well as the sensibility on the plantar aspect of the mid-foot and forefoot. Calcaneal branches from the tibial nerve supply medial and plantar heel skin, whereas the sural nerve and its various branches provide sensibility to the lateral heel, lateral border of the foot, and dorsolateral aspect of the foot as the lateral cutaneous nerve of the foot. The saphenous nerve, which emerges through the heads of the pes anserinus, provides the sensory infrapatellar branch and then continues down the medial aspect of the anterior leg to terminate in the sensory branch to the anteromedial ankle. Thus, motor loss occurs from injuries to the sciatic, common peroneal, deep peroneal and tibial nerves, and distal branches. With traction and crush injuries, various degrees of nerve injury occur with both complete and incomplete palsies. Consequently, although complete motor transfers are indicated on many occasions, split transfers provide the opportunity to rebalance the foot without creating a reverse deformity from overpull and, in some occasions, to prevent complete loss of a donor muscle action.

ANTERIOR TRANSFERS

Although the motor loss to the anterior compartment typically includes the tibialis anterior, extensor hallucis longus, and extensor digitorum muscles, the main functional problem is the foot-drop gait from the loss of the tibialis anterior muscle. Consequently, attention is primarily directed toward

restoring its action. On the rare occasion that the toe extensors retain normal power and the tibialis anterior alone is lost, the extensor digitorum longus tendons may be transferred into the second and third cuneiforms as an in-phase transfer. Despite the accessibility of this muscle, however, its power is about a third of the tibialis anterior. Although voluntary dorsiflexion is possible, the muscle fatigues easily and the use of a foot-drop orthosis still is required. The more commonly utilized muscle transfers are the tibialis posterior, peroneus brevis, and peroneus longus. With a long-standing deformity, a tendo Achillis lengthening and posterior capsulotomy may be necessary. In addition, if one uses the tibialis posterior or the peroneus brevis alone, an inversion or eversion imbalance may occur. When these muscles are used in combination, a triple arthrodesis is also considered, which not only stabilizes the subtalar joint but also allows one, with a modified procedure, to bring the navicular dorsal to the talar head, thus decreasing excursion needed to bring the foot into dorsiflexion.

Tibialis Posterior Tendon Transfer Through the Interosseous Membrane

This classic transfer (Watkins and Jones, 1954) is used for foot drop secondary to nerve injury and also for loss of musculature secondary to poliomyelitis, in Charcot-Marie-Tooth, and in Duchenne muscular dystrophy (Greene, 1992; Jaivin, 1992).

Technique. The tibialis posterior tendon is exposed distally just proximal to its insertion in the tarsal navicular and, posteromedially, through another short incision in the distal third of the leg. Once the muscle is identified proximally, umbilical tape is placed around its tendon component in each incision. The release is performed distally and the tendon extracted into the proximal wound. Also, the authors detach the flexor digitorum longus (FDL) tendon a little more distally and place the FDL through a drill hole in the tarsal navicular made from dorsal to plantar, routing the tendon from plantar to dorsal and back onto itself to re-establish the stability of the arch. Dissecting bluntly through the proximal incision, the posterior aspect of the tibia is followed around to the interosseous membrane. A window is sharply cut out from the interosseous membrane, staying close to the tibia and carefully avoiding damage to the adjacent vessels. A large Kelly clamp is then passed from posterior to anterior, and a counter incision is made anteriorly to expose the Kelly clamp. A second Kelly clamp is used to grasp the first clamp and is passed from anterior to posterior to grasp the tendon of the tibialis posterior and bring it into the anterior wound. It is very important to pull a portion of muscle of the tibialis posterior through the interosseous window. If the window is not large enough or muscle is not pulled into the window, the likelihood of tenodesis at this point is very high. A Bunnell-type suture weave using a monofilament suture, such as a 2-0 polypropylene, is placed in the end of the tendon, and the needles are removed. Exposure is then made over the middle cuneiform just proximal to the base of the second metatarsal. Subcutaneous tunneling is then performed with a tendon passer superficial to the extensor retinaculum and deep to the superficial peroneal nerve. The tendon is grasped in the anterior proximal wound and brought into the distal wound. A drill hole or a trephine core is made through the middle cuneiform to the plantar aspect of the foot. Keith needles are placed on the sutures, and the needles are passed through the hole and through the plantar aspect of the foot. Tension is established by placing the ankle in the neutral position and applying longitudinal traction to the muscle tendon unit. Once the resting and maximum elastic length of the tendon are established, the tension is set at about 60% of the maximum excursion (or elasticity). The tendon should be tight enough to maintain the ankle in the neutral position. A 1/8 inch drill bit is usually used to drill the appropriate hole but occasionally it needs enlargement. An equivalent trephine is also used. If a trephine plug is used, it is replaced in the defect after the tension on the muscle tendon unit is established. Otherwise, the tendon is sutured to the overlying periosteum adjacent to the drill hole. The suture is then placed over a large rubber shield and tied over a plastic button. The two-hole method of tendon insertion into the cuneiform may also be used (Fig. 69–4). Tendon-anchoring devices, inserted within the drill hole, are under investigation to replace plantar buttons. The foot is immobilized for 6 weeks, after which time the button is removed and the foot mobilized. An ankle-foot orthosis is used for at least the first 3 months and often up to 9 months after the surgery is carried out when the patient anticipates prolonged walking before re-establishment of adequate muscle strength.

Peroneus Brevis and Tibialis Posterior Into the Dorsum of the Foot

The peroneus brevis and tibialis posterior may be used for the foot-drop deformity, and the transfer is often accompa-

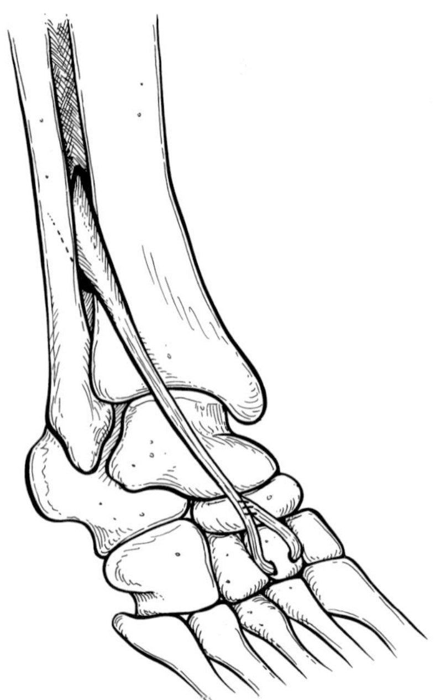

FIGURE 69–4. Tibialis posterior tendon transfer through the interosseous membrane to the dorsum of the foot (middle cuneiform).

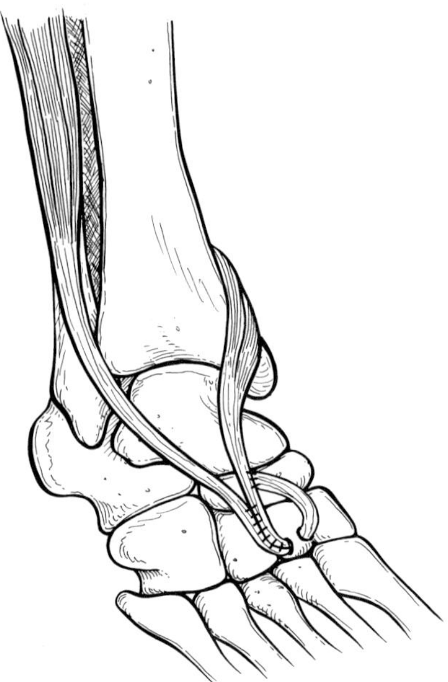

FIGURE 69–5. Peroneus brevis and tibialis posterior transferred to the middle cuneiform.

nied by subtalar arthrodeses in the child and a triple arthrodesis in adults.

Technique. The peroneus brevis and tibialis posterior are both exposed at their insertions and released. The eversion of the foot is left to the peroneus longus, and the tibialis posterior is stabilized by using the FDL as a replacement transfer through a drill hole in the tarsal navicular, placing the tendon from plantar to dorsal and back onto itself. The donor tendons are then exposed more proximally in the distal third of the leg and rerouted subcutaneously and superficial to the extensor retinaculum to the second cuneiform. A drill hole is placed through the middle cuneiform or a trephine plug is taken, the tendons inserted into the hole and the sutures passed through the middle of the foot and secured with a plantar button. Tension and balance are established in the same manner as with the tibialis posterior transfer alone through the interosseous membrane. Alternative and equally popular insertions are created by using paired drill holes through the second and sometimes third cuneiform, which are connected by curettage. The bony bridge must be fairly broad, and the technique is ill advised in osteoporotic bone. The ankle should rest in the neutral position following setting the tension for these transfers. Rehabilitation is carried out as with the tibialis posterior transfer (Fig. 69–5).

Peroneus Longus Transferred Into the Dorsum of the Foot

The use of the peroneus longus as well as the peroneus brevis is often obviated by the fact that both are paralyzed along with the tibialis anterior. The advantage of this transfer, however, is that the strength of the peroneus longus, although less than that of the tibialis posterior, is at least twice that of the peroneus brevis. The potential disadvantage, however, is the risk of creating, with a too distal an insertion, an unopposed dorsiflexion force on the first metatarsal. The distal stump of the peroneus longus is attached to the peroneus brevis, just proximal to its insertion on the base of the fifth metatarsal, to stabilize the first ray.

Technique. The peroneus longus is divided proximal to its passage under the groove in the cuboid. The distal component is transferred laterally and dorsally, and passed through a slit in the tendon of the peroneus brevis. It is secured in this position to the peroneus brevis. The peroneus longus is exposed in the distal third of the leg and then transferred subcutaneously to the level of the middle cuneiform. If length is sufficient, it is passed either through a drill hole with a plantar button attachment, through paired drill holes in the middle cuneiform, or if length is a problem and the peroneus brevis is active, the distal nonfunctional tibialis anterior tendon is divided proximally and the peroneus longus woven through the distal component of the tibialis anterior. Alternatively, the peroneus longus can be lengthened using a tendon graft from the tibialis anterior tendon, which is then inserted into bone at the level of the middle cuneiform. Rehabilitation is carried out as described in the previously mentioned transfers.

Flexor Digitorum Longus and Flexor Hallucis Longus Transfer Through the Interosseous Membrane to the Dorsum of the Foot

Loss of the FDL is well tolerated owing to the action of the short flexors, the residual attachment of the quadratus plantae to the distal flexor tendons, and the interconnections between the flexor hallucis longus and the residual digital flexors. Similarly, loss of the flexor hallucis longus may have significant drawbacks in toe off in the normal foot but is well tolerated, particularly if the flexor digitorum is left intact, due to the interconnection of these two distal tendons. When both motors are taken for a transfer, the loss is still tolerated in the compromised foot, with the residual short flexors and the quadratus plantae providing some flexion power to the lesser toes. Given the deficiency of loss of dorsiflexion, and particularly without the availability of the stronger tibialis posterior, the flexor hallucis provides about half the strength and the flexor digitorum about a third of the strength of the tibialis anterior. The combination can be satisfactory, however, and the excursion is greater than that of the other potentially stronger and commonly used muscle transfers.

Technique. The exposure of the flexor hallucis and flexor digitorum is carried out in the longitudinal arch just distal to the master knot of Henry. A plantar medial incision is made in the longitudinal arch, and the dissection carried just plantar and slightly lateral to the inferior edge of the abductor hallucis. The interval between the lower border of the abductor hallucis and the plantar fascia is located and divided, with the medial plantar nerve exposed and carefully retracted. The tendons of the flexor hallucis and flexor digitorum are exposed and umbilical tapes placed around them. A posteromedial incision is made in the distal third of the leg to expose the flexor digitorum and flexor hallucis. To more easily see the flexor hallucis tendon, the dissection may need to be carried more distally toward the medial malleolus. With umbilical tapes placed around the tendons proximally as well as distally, and the interconnections between the flexor hallucis and flexor digitorum divided, the tendons are individually extracted from the distal wound into the proximal one. A window is then made in the posteromedial edge of the interosseous membrane adjacent to the tibia, protecting the overlying vessels, and a Kelly clamp is placed through this wound to the anterior component. A counter incision is made and a counter clamp is placed into the posterior incision. Both tendons are then drawn through an adequately sized window and the muscles pulled into the window as well. As with the tibialis posterior transfer, the subcutaneous route is then used superficial to the extensor retinaculum to the proposed insertion site at the middle cuneiform. The insertion is carried out as is described for the earlier transfers. Both the tensioning of the tendons and the rehabilitation program are similar to those used for the other transfers as well.

Split Tibialis Posterior Tendon Transfer Into Second Cuneiform with Rerouting of Peroneus Longus Anterior to Lateral Malleolus

In essence, this procedure (Rodriguez, 1992), creates a split transfer on the dorsal medial side balanced against a functional alignment on the lateral side to improve dorsiflexion and maintain balance.

Technique. The tibialis posterior tendon is released proximal to its insertion and passed subcutaneously through a split in the tibialis anterior tendon to be inserted in the middle cuneiform through paired drill holes or a plantar button. When the tension is properly set, sutures are placed between the transfer motor and the tibialis anterior tendon to create a yoke effect on the dorsomedial side. Although not described originally, the authors still reconstruct the loss of the tibialis posterior with the flexor digitorum, as described in the previously mentioned transfers. Second, the peroneus longus is exposed from the distal third of the leg through its sheath to the point where it passes under the cuboid. The sheath is repaired, leaving the peroneus brevis behind the lateral malleolus, but the peroneus longus is replaced subcutaneously anterior to the malleolus to provide a dorsiflexion moment. In addition, the tendon is reefed or shortened above the malleolus to create better tendon balance. The authors carry out a long coronal diagonal cut in the tendon, overlap, and repair under some tension using horizontal mattress sutures of 3-0 braided polyester. The excess tendon is excised proximally and distally. Tendon balancing is important, and the transfer and shortening of the peroneus longus should maintain the foot in a balanced neutral position at the completion of the procedure. Immobilization and rehabilitation is similar to the previously described transfers.

Tibialis Anterior Balancing Procedures

When eversion strength has been lost owing to loss of function in the peroneal tendons and, in particular, to the peroneus brevis, repositioning of the tibialis anterior may be desirable to correct a tendency toward hindfoot varus. The need for this procedure is also seen in other neurologic problems, such as stroke. The classic procedure (Garceau and Manning, 1947) for balancing the tibialis anterior is to completely detach it from its insertion on the medial cuneiform and first metatarsal, and to reinsert it into the middle cuneiform.

Technique. A short incision is made over the medial cuneiform and first metatarsal, and the tendon of the tibialis anterior is identified and umbilical tape placed around it. A second incision is made in the distal third of the leg just lateral to the crest of the tibia, and the proximal muscle and tendon are identified. The tendon is completely dissected away from the bone and pulled into the proximal incision. A second dorsal incision is made over the middle cuneiform at the base of the second metatarsal. The tendon is rerouted subcutaneously with a tendon passer into this incision after a Bunnell weave using 3-0 polypropylene is made through the distal tendon. A trephine plug or drill hole is made in the second cuneiform or paired drill holes with a wide cortical window. The tendon is inserted and the tension set as previously described to maintain the foot in the neutral position (Fig. 69–6A).

Split Dorsal Insertion of Tibialis Anterior

Although rarely used for nerve palsy lesions, a simplified form of repositioning of the insertion is also used in correcting club foot (Gould, 1986). At the completion of reconstructive procedures to eliminate the deformities of the club foot, including a posterior medial and lateral release, the distal half of the tibialis anterior insertion on the medial side is released from its attachment and rolled over the lateral side to be reattached to the dorsum of the first metatarsal

(see Fig. 69–6B). It is sutured in place with 3-0 permanent suture to the overlying periosteum. This simple maneuver creates a more dorsal pull to the tibialis anterior tendon to help balance the peroneal-deficient foot (see Fig. 69–6C).

Split Tibialis Anterior Tendon Transfer

The split tibialis anterior tendon transfer (SPLATT) is most commonly used in cerebral palsy when dynamic electromyography identifies spastic overactivity of the tibialis anterior in mid-stance with decreased peroneus brevis activity (Barnes, 1991; Edwards, 1993; Hoffer et al, 1974). Earlier soleus contraction is also noted in this condition. The SPLATT procedure may also be used in the cavus foot, which also features deficiency in the peroneus brevis. When a foot-drop problem in Charcot-Marie-Tooth also accompanies this condition, other transfers may be considered.

Technique. The insertion of the tibialis anterior is exposed distally and umbilical tape placed around it. In the distal third of the leg, an anterolateral incision is made to again identify the tibialis anterior muscle and tendon. From the distal incision, a long split in the tendon is made, which involves a half to two thirds of the tibialis anterior tendon. Umbilical tape is placed through the split and around the lateral component. The sheath is split proximally as far as possible from the distal incision. Similarly, the sheath is opened from proximal to distal down to the extensor retinaculum. A long tendon passer is placed through the proximal incision along the course of the tibialis anterior muscle and tendon within the sheath into the distal wound, and the two ends of the umbilical tape are grasped and pulled into the proximal wound. If the split follows the natural fibers of the tendon, the tendon will be neatly divided from distal to the proximal wound. If the tape does not adequately divide the tendon and working under the flaps is not successful in

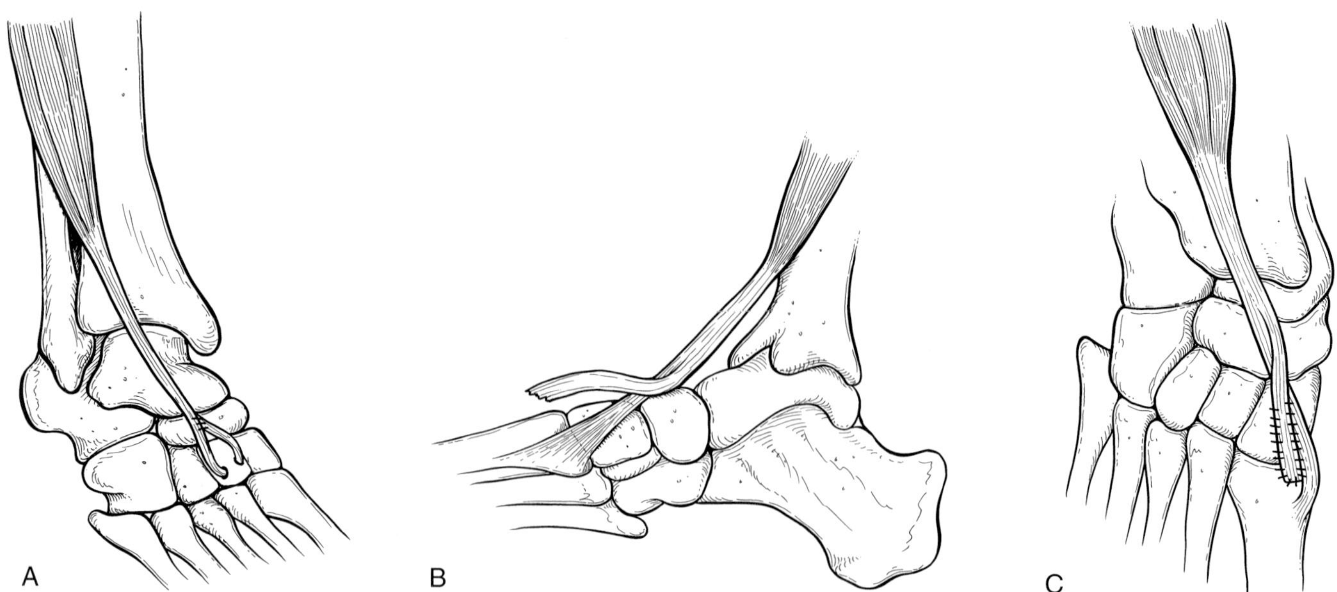

FIGURE 69–6. *A,* Tibialis anterior inserted into the middle cuneiform. *B,* The medial half of the anterior tibial insertion is released from its attachment and rolled over the lateral side. *C,* The detached portion of the tibialis anterior tendon is reattached to the dorsum of the first metatarsal and sutured into the overlying periosteum and to the medial half of the tendon.

releasing interconnecting fibers, an additional incision between the proximal and distal incisions is sometimes necessary to complete the split. We have not had particular success using tendon strippers, which risk premature division of the tendon; an initial release distally in an attempt to peel the lateral half back into the proximal incision also has not been particularly successful. Overall, the technique described is a satisfactory method of creating the split tendon. Once the umbilical tape is brought into the proximal wound, the distal half to two thirds of the lateral tendon is released, and the split tendon is delivered into the proximal incision. A second curvilinear incision is made over the cuboid, and two paired drill holes are made in this structure. The authors have sometimes found that the lateral limb is not of sufficient length to be placed through the cuboid drill holes, and the plantar button technique may be preferable. On other occasions, the authors have simply prolonged the lateral limb with a free tendon graft. This has included the use of plantaris or a strip of the tendo Achillis. The tendon graft is connected to the lateral component of the split tibialis anterior tendon through an interweave technique. The lateral component is then passed subcutaneously from the proximal incision to the more distal one after a straight line subcutaneous channel is created. After the lateral tendon is placed through the drill hole, umbilical tape or a hemostat is placed under both proximal limbs of the transfer and the tension is compared. If one or the other limb is tighter, imbalance will occur. Applying traction to the tendon proximal to the split should bring the foot into neutral dorsiflexion. The drill holes in the cuboid are made using either a 1/8 or 7/64 inch drill. The tendon is secured using 3-0 braided polyester suture (Fig. 69–7A).

Microsurgical Approach to Peroneal Nerve Palsy

A unique approach using neurotization of the transposed lateral head of the gastrocnemius transferred into the tibialis

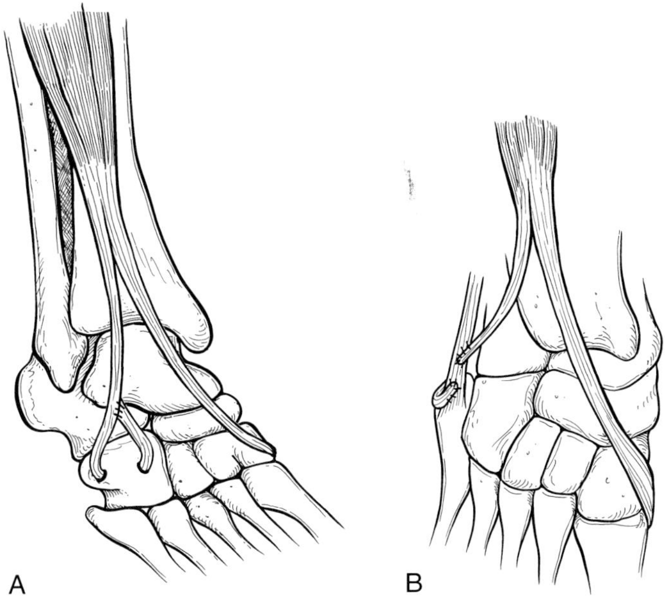

FIGURE 69–7. *A,* Split anterior tibial tendon transfer with insertion of the lateral limb into the cuboid. *B,* Split anterior tibial tendon transfer with insertion of the lateral limb into the tendon of peroneus brevis.

anterior muscle tendon unit has been used in six clinical cases (Ninkovic et al, 1994). With this interesting Austrian technique, the undamaged proximal end of the deep branch of the peroneal nerve is sutured to the motor branch of the tibial nerve, innervating the lateral head of the gastrocnemius. The lateral head of the gastrocnemius is transposed and inserted into the tibialis anterior. With reinnervation, an in-phase muscle now activates the anterior musculature. With minimal clinical results obtained to date, the ultimate fate of this approach is uncertain. The authors have no experience with this technique.

POSTERIOR TRANSFERS

Transfers into the posterior calcaneus or tendo Achillis are applicable for paralysis of the triceps surae but are also used for weakness of this muscle in the postpolio syndrome and for injuries to the tendo Achillis. For the paralytic problem, the most commonly used transfer is the tibialis anterior passed through the interosseous membrane into the tendo Achillis or calcaneus, which, although out of phase, has proved to be a successful maneuver (Close, 1959; Fernandez-Feliberti, 1992; Georgiadis, 1990). The tibialis posterior or the peroneus longus, or both, have also been transferred into the tendo Achillis or calcaneus, particularly in the postpolio scenario. For reconstruction of a tendo Achilles rupture, transfers have included the flexor hallucis longus, peroneus brevis, and FDL.

Tibialis Anterior Through the Interosseous Membrane Into Tendo Achillis or Calcaneus

The use of important motors such as the tibialis anterior to restore plantar flexion strength is only understood when one realizes that management of a calcaneus deformity is far more difficult than that of foot-drop or dorsiflexion weakness. The patients tolerate loss of dorsiflexion far better than in the calcaneus deformity, and bracing is significantly easier. If there is no posterior musculature available for transfer, the tibialis anterior may be placed through the interosseous membrane into the tendo Achillis or calcaneus. This maneuver may overcome the calcaneus deformity, create balance, and bring the foot to the neutral position. In the event that talipes equinus results, the extensor digitorum longus could be transferred into the second cuneiform.

Technique. The tibialis anterior tendon is exposed at its insertion on the first metatarsal and proximally in the distal third of the leg. After identification, it is released distally and withdrawn into the proximal wound. The interosseous membrane is identified adjacent to the tibia, and an adequate window is created in this structure. A Kelly clamp is placed through the window, and a counter incision is made on the posterolateral aspect of the leg with a counter clamp brought into the anterior wound. The tibialis anterior tendon is then passed posteriorly and either woven through the distal insertion of the tendo Achillis or placed through a drill hole in the calcaneus just distal to the tendo Achillis insertion. The incision in the tendo Achillis is typically made just proximal to the insertion, transversely through the tendon from lateral to medial, bringing the donor tendon back onto itself for suturing. Enough tension is applied to the tendon to maintain the foot in a neutral position. The desired tension is typically 60% of the elastic length of the muscle tendon unit of the donor as compared with the positions of no tension and the maximally stretched out or elastic length (Fig. 69–8). Immobilization is carried out for 6 weeks, followed by an exercise program using a dorsiflexion stop at neutral brace, which allows free plantar flexion but dorsiflexion only to the neutral position. Such bracing is typically needed at least through the end of the first year postoperatively.

Tibialis Posterior and Peroneus Longus Into the Tendo Achillis or Calcaneus

The tibialis posterior or peroneus longus transfer (Di-Cesare et al, 1995) achieves significant improvement for weakness of the triceps surae experienced by postpolio patients. The results have been encouraging to date in 14 feet in 12 patients.

Technique. The tibialis posterior and peroneus longus tendons are exposed at their insertions and more proximally at the insertion of the tendo Achillis medially and laterally. The distal stump of the peroneus longus is sutured into a split in the peroneus brevis, with reconstruction of the tibialis posterior considered optional. The authors use the FDL reconstruction with a drill hole through the tarsal navicular. Paired drill holes are made in the calcaneus on either side of the tendo Achillis insertion, and the transferred tendons are passed through these drill holes and back onto themselves (Fig. 69–9). An alternative insertion into the tendo

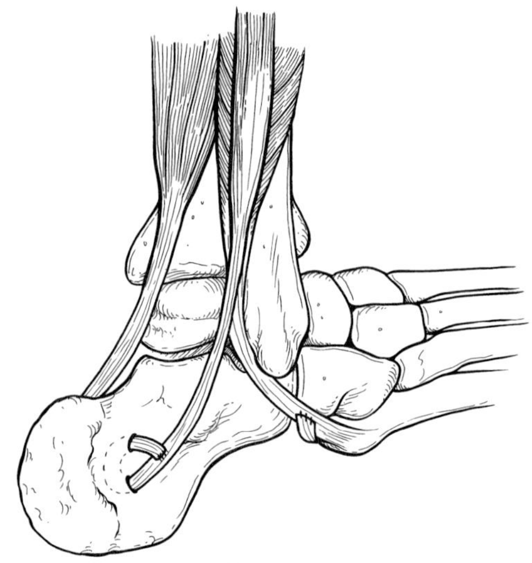

FIGURE 69–9. Tibialis posterior and peroneus longus transferred into the calcaneus. Note the attachment of the distal stump of peroneus longus into the peroneus brevis.

Achillis just proximal to the insertion is also acceptable. After 6 weeks of immobilization, rehabilitation is initiated.

Flexor Hallucis Longus Transfer Into the Tendo Achillis or Calcaneus

The flexor hallucis longus is used to reinforce a direct repair of the tendo Achillis by detaching the tendon in the longitudinal arch and suturing the stump to the flexor digitorum. The flexor hallucis is withdrawn into the operative repair site of the tendo Achillis and woven through the distal insertion of the tendo Achillis, across the repair site and back to itself (Wapner et al, 1993, 1994, 1995) (Fig. 69–10). The advantages of using the flexor hallucis longus include its immediate accessibility, length, and in-phase characteristic.

Peroneus Brevis Transfer Into the Tendo Achillis

The peroneus brevis has classically been used to reinforce tendo Achillis repairs with reports of excellent results (Gallant et al, 1995; Turco and Spinella, 1987). The argument in favor of the use of the peroneus brevis suggests that this muscle is expendable due to the eversion power of the peroneus longus. Although this concept may be questionable, from a practical point of view, the results are reported to be very satisfactory with long-term follow-up. The muscle is also not as strong as the flexor hallucis longus.

Technique. The peroneus brevis is harvested at its insertion on the base of the fifth metatarsal. Following a release, it is extracted into the proximal wound, where the repair of the tendo Achillis has been initiated. The tendon is woven through the distal segment of the tendo Achillis or through the bone, under moderate tension. The immobilization and management is the same as that for the tendo Achillis with 6 weeks of immobilization, followed by the use of a heel lift to create equinus and decrease the stress on the repair.

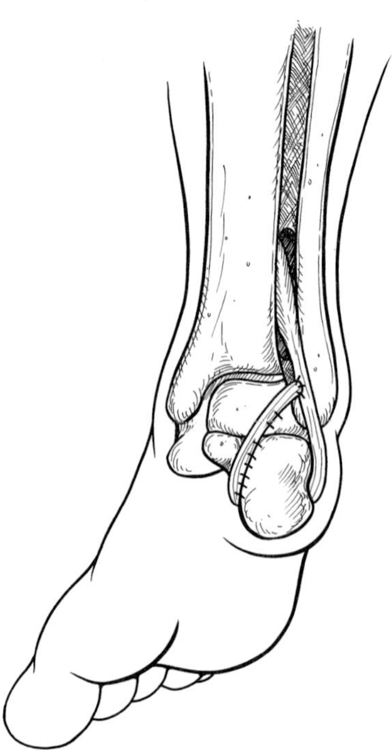

FIGURE 69–8. Tibialis anterior transferred into the calcaneus through the interosseous membrane.

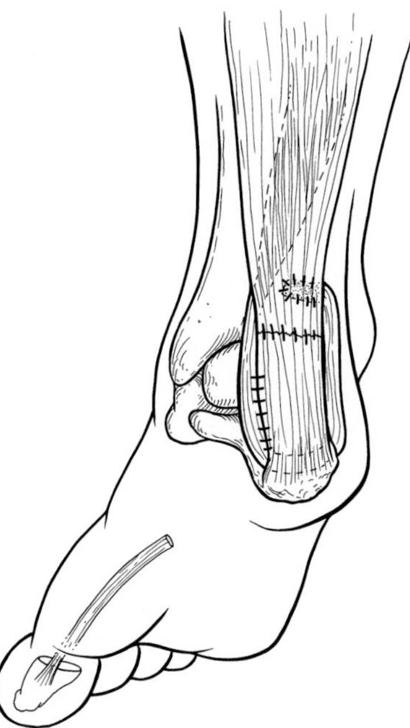

FIGURE 69–10. Flexor hallucis longus transferred to the calcaneus to reinforce the repair of the Achilles tendon rupture.

The patient's ankle is gradually brought to the neutral position as strength of the tendo Achillis is achieved (Fig. 69–11).

Flexor Digitorum Longus Tendon Transfer Into the Calcaneus

The technique of using the FDL is essentially identical to that of the flexor hallucis longus, with strength comparable to that of the peroneus brevis. The motor functions of the FDL are still maintained by the flexor brevis and the quadratus plantae. The longus tendon is harvested in the longtitudinal arch and drawn into the repair wound for the tendo Achillis. The tendon may be inserted into bone or the stump of the tendo Achillis (Mann et al, 1991).

LATERAL TRANSFERS

Lateral transfers are carried out when peroneal muscle paralysis or significant weakness has occurred. For the most part, this is achieved by balancing the dorsiflexion vector of the anterior tibial muscle. As described previously, this may be achieved by use of the SPLATT procedure into the cuboid or on occasion into the tendon of the peroneus brevis (see Fig. 69–7A and B). The split posterior tibial tendon may also be transferred to the cuboid or peroneus brevis, especially when the dynamic electromyogram demonstrates overactivity of the posterior tibial tendon, creating equinovarus in cerebral palsy (Green et al, 1983).

Technique. A posteromedial incision is made to expose the posterior tibial insertion. The lateral half is released from the insertion and split up the tendon to just distal to the musculotendinous junction. The peroneus brevis is exposed near its insertion on the fifth metatarsal base, and tunneling is carried out anterior to the tendo Achillis to retrieve the lateral end of the split posterior tibial. The lateral component is woven through the insertion of the peroneus brevis, distributing equal tension to both limbs. This transfer may require further rebalancing of the anterior tibial, but a full evaluation of the outcome of the first procedure should be considered before moving on to other transfers (Fig. 69–12).

Peroneus Longus Into the Peroneus Brevis

This transfer is typically used for isolated denervation of the peroneus brevis or in the cavus foot, in which overactiv-

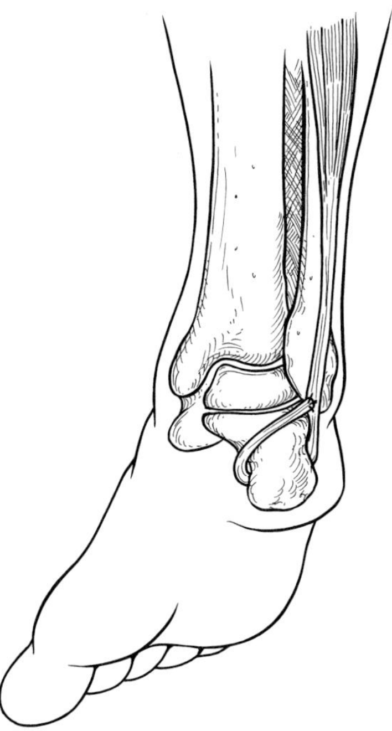

FIGURE 69–11. Peroneus brevis transferred to the calcaneus.

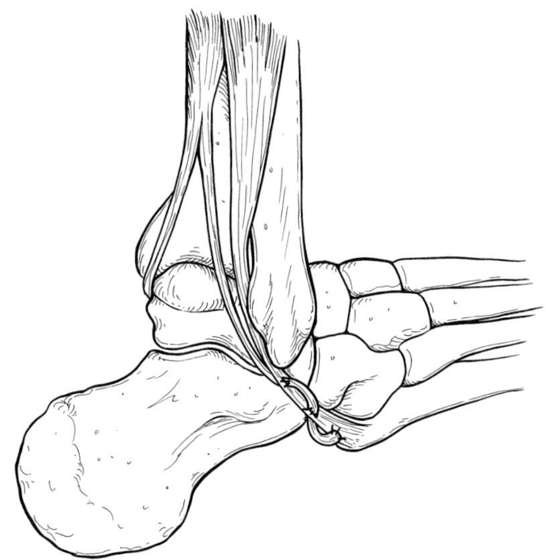

FIGURE 69–12. Split tibialis posterior transfer with lateral half inserted into peroneus brevis.

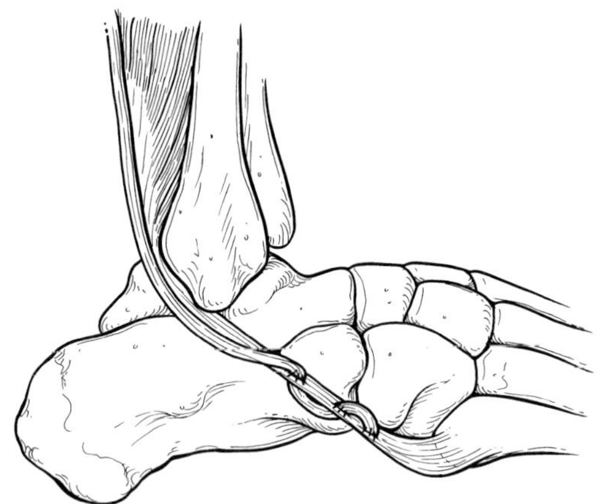

FIGURE 69–13. Peroneus longus transferred into peroneus brevis.

ity of the peroneus longus may be seen in Charcot-Marie-Tooth disease, resulting in a plantar flexed first metatarsal with significant weakness in eversion due to denervation of the peroneus brevis. The transfer of the peroneus longus can be made either proximal or distal to the lateral malleolus, whereas the common sheath is left intact to maintain the position of the tendons. The procedure is usually carried out proximal to the retinaculum, using a tendon interweave (Fig. 69–13).

MEDIAL TRANSFERS

Posterior tibial dysfunction results in the development of a unilateral flatfoot deformity. This is typically a muscular phenomenon resulting from deterioration of the tendon with attenuation or rupture. In addition, reconstruction for this muscle may be required if the tibialis posterior is used as a transfer, as described previously. Either the FDL or flexor hallucis longus may be used for the reconstruction (Masterson, 1994). As indicated earlier, each can compensate for the other as a partial replacement for distal function. The insertion can be made as a tendon weave through the distal portion of the posterior tibial or preferably through a drill hole in the tarsal navicular (Fig. 69–14). If good proximal

muscle excursion is available but there is a loss of distal tendon substance, use of the Cobb technique (Fig. 69–15) (Helal, 1990; Lindell and Carroll, 1994) can be used. This technique consists of splitting the anterior tibial tendon and, while leaving the insertion intact, the medial half of the tendon is divided proximally and rerouted along the course of the tibialis posterior for a tendon interweave attachment to the proximal motor. This procedure obviates the need for a tendon transfer when there is good proximal muscle function.

FOREFOOT TENDON TRANSFERS

Extensor Tendon Transfers

A variety of extensor tendon transfers have been devised to deal primarily with intrinsic paralysis and other etiologies of claw-toe deformities. The best known of these is the Jones transfer, in which the extensor hallucis longus is released distally on the great toe and transferred to the neck of the first metatarsal with a concomitant interphalangeal joint arthrodesis (Fig. 69–16) (Jones, 1908; Tynan and Klenerman, 1994).

Technique. A curvilinear incision is made from the dorsum of the great toe to proximal to the neck of the first metatarsal. The extensor hallucis longus is dissected from the extensor hood to proximal to the neck of the first metatarsal. The distal extensor mechanism is repaired with care to preserve the underlying bed over the dorsum of the bone. The hood repair maintains integrity of the extensor hallucis brevis. An arthrodesis is carried out of the interphalangeal (IP) joint, the neck of the first metatarsal is exposed medially and laterally, and a drill hole is placed transversely across the neck. The initial hole is made with a 5/64-inch drill bit and is enlarged if necessary. A Hewson suture passer is placed across the hole from medial to lateral. The suture attached to the end of the tendon is passed through the loop of this device, and the tendon is threaded from lateral to medial and then back onto itself. The procedure relieves the clawing tendency of the great toe but generally does little to elevate

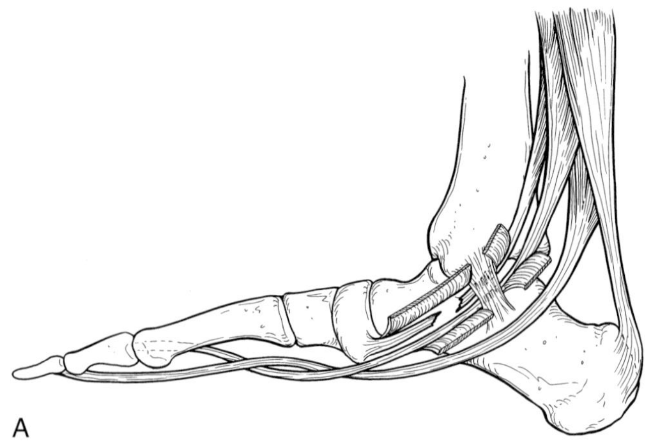

A

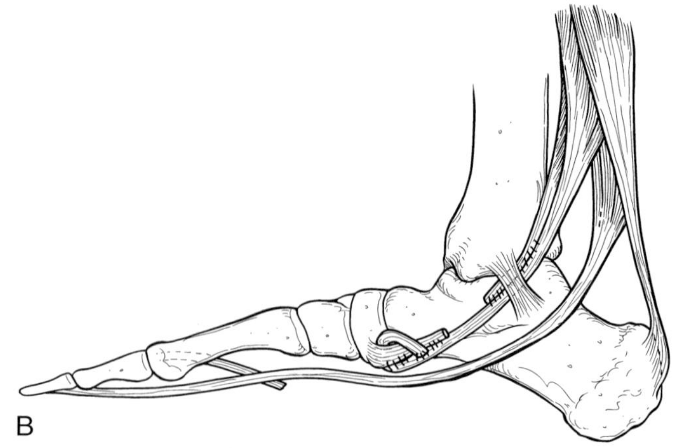

B

FIGURE 69–14. *A,* Rupture of tibialis posterior tendon near the insertion into the navicular. *B,* Transfer of flexor digitorum longus into the navicular. Note proximal and distal suture to the tendon of tibialis posterior, when it is available.

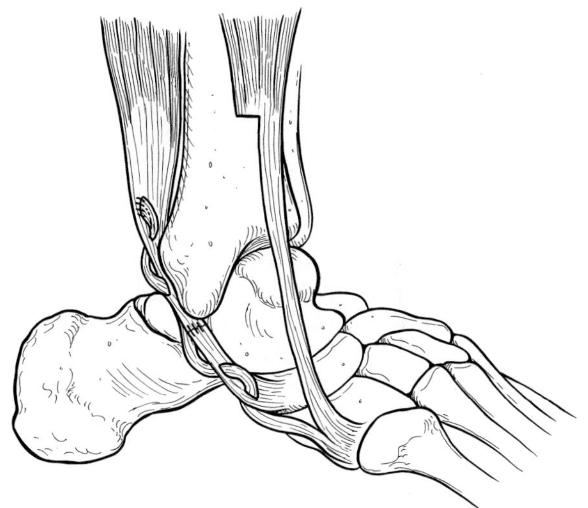

FIGURE 69–15. The Cobb repair. The medial one half of the anterior tibial tendon is transferred to the repaired tibialis posterior tendon or to the proximal posterior tibial component when there is a segmental loss.

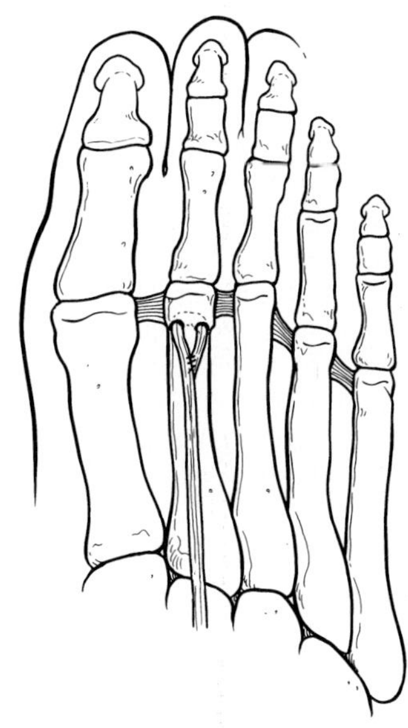

FIGURE 69–17. The Jones transfer in the lesser toes.

the first metatarsal. In addition, a lag in extension of the toe is a common complication.

Jones Transfer for the Lesser Toes-Extensor Digitorum Longus Into Metatarsal Necks

This procedure for the flexible paralytic deformity has been reasonably successful for management of the paralytic deformity of the intrinsics, resulting in claw toes and for metatarsalgia secondary to prominent middle metatarsal heads in the so-called spread-foot deformity (Fig. 69–17) (Mulier et al, 1994).

Second or Third Extensor Digitorum Longus Transfer to Distal Extensor Hallucis Longus

The problem with extensor lag in the great toe may be resolved by transferring the common extensor of the second or third toe into the extensor hood at the metatarsophalangeal (MTP) joint of the great toe (Fig. 69–18). The stump of the extensor digitorum longus of the donor toe is sutured to the extensor digitorum brevis. Extensor digitorum longus from the donor toe is mobilized and transferred subcutaneously to the great toe MTP extensor hood and repaired with a tendon weave at that site. This is an in-phase transfer and tends to be very successful in relieving this minor but annoying deformity.

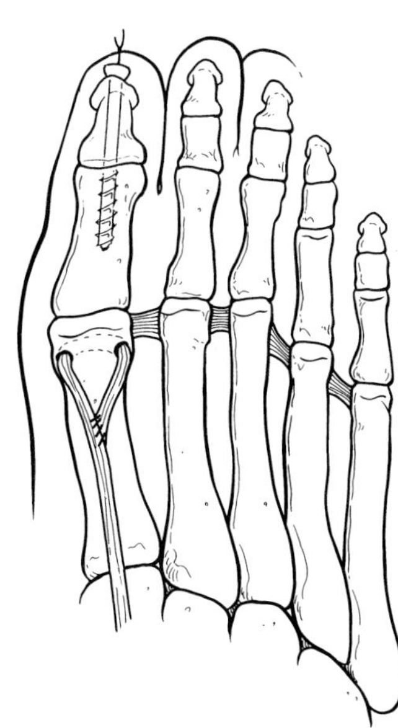

FIGURE 69–16. The Jones transfer. The interphalangeal joint is arthrodesed.

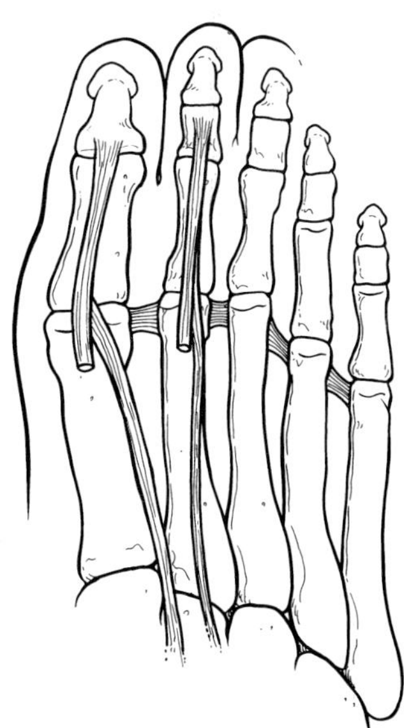

FIGURE 69–18. The extensor digitorum longus is transferred to the extensor of the hallux, while the distal stump of extensor digitorum longus is attached to the extensor brevis.

Extensor Hallucis Longus Transfer to Correct Hallux Varus

Spontaneous or iatrogenic hallux varus secondary to bunion corrections, when flexible, can be treated by transfer of the extensor hallucis longus (Goldman et al, 1993; Johnson and Spiegel, 1994; Skalley and Myerson, 1994). After appropriate medial structure lengthening or releases, which include the abductor hallucis and joint capsule, the extensor hallucis is released just proximal to the IP joint and an arthrodesis is carried out at this level. A drill hole is made in the base of the proximal phalanx on the lateral aspect from dorsal to plantar. Beginning in the first web space, a hemostat is used to tunnel below the axis of rotation of the MTP joint under the intermetatarsal ligament or the scar that has replaced the structure. The tip of the hemostat is then brought up proximally and more dorsally, and the distal end of the extensor hallucis tendon is grasped and brought distally to the plantar position. The Hewson suture passer is placed from dorsal to plantar through the drill hole. The suture on the end of the extensor hallucis is placed through the loop of the suture passer, and the tendon is delivered from plantar to dorsal. As the tendon is tightened, the toe is brought into the corrected position and the tendon is sutured upon itself. In the flexible hallux varus deformity, or one that can be easily reduced with medial releases, this tendon transfer is effective in maintaining the stability and alignment of the toe. Correction brings the toe to neutral in the medial-lateral plane and eliminates the tendency for dorsiflexion at the MTP joint (Fig. 69–19*A* and *B*).

Flexor Tendon Transfers for Claw Toes

Claw or hammer toes may be secondary to intrinsic paralysis, which may be caused by damage to the medial or lateral plantar nerves or in conditions such as the cavovarus foot, with particular reference to Charcot-Marie-Tooth disease. The classic approach is the Girdlestone-Taylor transfer with various modifications (Barbari, 1984; Biyani et al,

1992; Coughlin, 1987; Cyphers and Feiwell, 1988; Taylor, 1940, 1951; Thompson and Deland, 1993).

Technique (Classic). A curvilinear incision is made on the dorsum of the MTP joint of the involved toe. If the skin is markedly shortened, a Z-plasty of the skin is carried out. The extensor tendon is either Z-lengthened or cut; a dorsal capsulectomy is also carried out to reduce the MTP joint. On the plantar side of the toe, a transverse incision is made at the insertion of the long flexor tendon and a second one is made at the base of the toe, which is at about the level of the middle of the proximal phalanx (Fig. 69–20*A*). The tendon is released distally and extracted through the proximal incision. A zigzag incision on the plantar aspect of the toe is also an alternative. The tendon is then divided longitudinally from distal to proximal (see Fig. 69–20*B*). A hemostat is used to tunnel from plantar to dorsal on both sides of the phalanx, between the proximal phalanx and the neurovascular bundles. A second hemostat is passed through the dorsal incision on the toe on either side from dorsal to plantar, grasping each half of the tendon and bringing it to the dorsum. A slit is made in the extensor mechanism on either side of the phalanx, and the tendons are brought through. Maintaining the toe in the neutral position at the MTP joint and the ankle also in the neutral position, the two tendon slips are brought together at the dorsum, inserted one into the other, and into the extensor tendon at mid-range tension (see Fig. 69–20*C*). Absorbable suture is used on a noncutting needle. At the completion of the procedure, the toe should rest in the neutral position, with the clawing tendency resolved. Attachment to the extensor tendon mechanism at about the mid-proximal phalanx level is usually satisfactory. The closer to the proximal interphalangeal (PIP) joint the attachment is made, the better the extension of the toe, but an increased flexion moment is created at the MTP joint, which is also less desirable. PIP joint flexibility is mandatory if this procedure is used alone. In some cases, release of the plantar plate and the accessory collateral ligaments at the PIP joint, as a concomitant procedure with the transfer, allows passive correction.

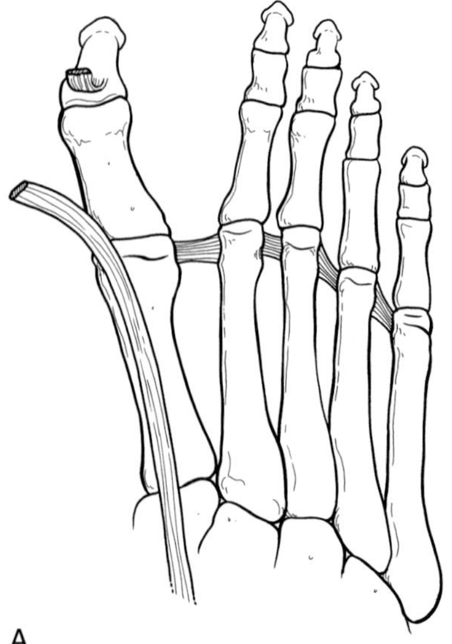
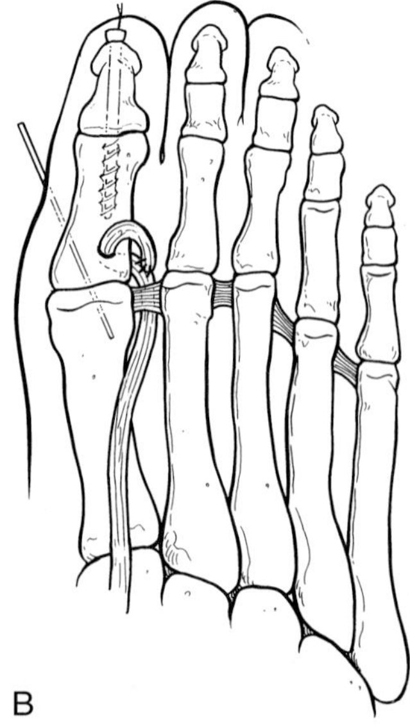

A

B

FIGURE 69–19. *A*, The Johnson extensor hallucis longus transfer for hallux varus: the long extensor to the hallux is detached at its insertion. *B*, Insertion into the lateral aspect of the proximal phalanx and arthrodesis of the interphalangeal joint.

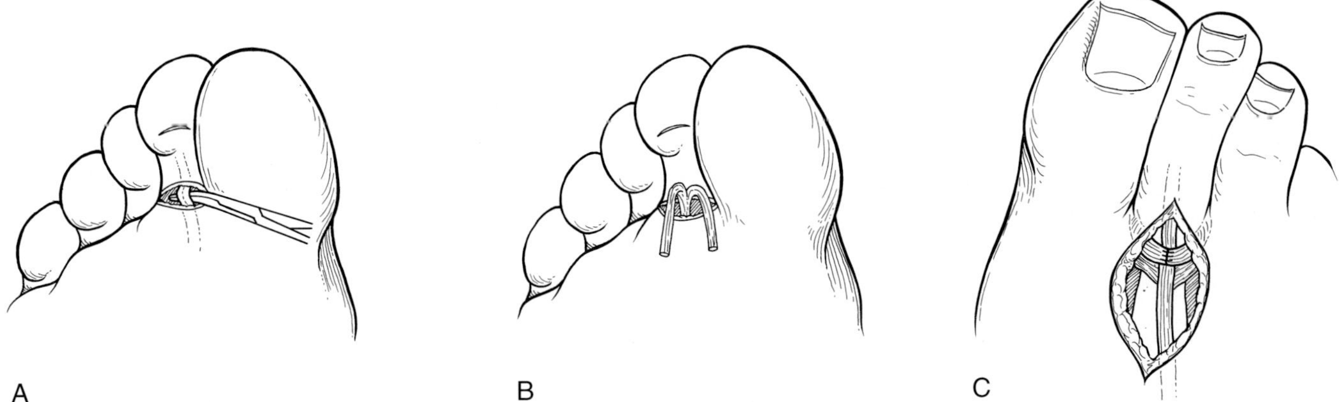

FIGURE 69–20. *A,* The Girdlestone-Taylor transfer: The long flexor is identified and detached at its insertion. *B,* The tendon is split longitudinally. *C,* The two limbs of the tendon are sutured into the extensor hood and to each other.

With a fixed deformity at the PIP joint, the resection arthroplasty at the joint may be combined with a flexor transfer. The same basic technique is carried out, but from the dorsum, the head of the proximal phalanx is excised at the metaphyseal flare. The flexor tendon is not divided; the plantar plate is separated distally from the middle phalanx, but the attachment of the flexor brevis tendon is maintained. The long flexor tendon is brought between the two slips of the flexor brevis, through the resection site at the joint, and inserted into the extensor mechanism. Curvilinear mid-line incisions on the dorsal and plantar aspects of the toe are usually preferable for achieving adequate exposure. The tendon not only provides a flexion moment on the proximal phalanx at the MTP joint but also acts as an interposition tissue to allow at least a passive flexibility of the PIP joint (Fig. 69–21*A*).

In some situations, the tendency for dorsal subluxation or hyperextension at the MTP joint is more of a problem than the flexion deformity at the PIP joint. In these cases, the technique is modified by placing a drill hole from dorsal to plantar through the mid-proximal phalanx. This is typically done with a 1/8-inch drill bit through a tendon-splitting incision on the dorsum. The Hewson suture passer is placed

from dorsal to plantar, and the flexor tendon is brought through the drill hole in the bone to the dorsum of the proximal phalanx. This provides a very strong plantar flexion moment and is very useful in both paralytic and congenital dislocations at the MTP joint (see Fig. 69–21*B*).

Complications of tendon transfers in the leg and foot occur for the obvious reasons seen elsewhere in the extremities. Most complications can be avoided with adequate surgical planning, appropriate choice of the donor muscle, maintenance of adequate stability and mobility, knowledge of the basic principles of tendon transfers, and meticulous attention to detail. Postoperative management and therapy are also relevant factors.

References

Barbari SG, Brevig K: Correction of clawtoes by Girdlestone-Taylor flexor-extensor transfer procedure. Foot Ankle 5:67–73, 1984.

Barnes MJ, Herring JA: Combined split anterior tibial-tendon transfer and intramuscular lengthening of the posterior tibial tendon. Results in patients who have a varus deformity of the foot due to spastic cerebral palsy. J Bone Joint Surg 73A:734–738, 1991.

Biyani A, Jones DA, Murray JM: Flexor to extensor tendon transfer for curly toes. Forty-three children reviewed after 8 (1–25) years. Acta Orthop Scand 63:451–454, 1992.

Cheng YM, Chien SH, Chou PH, et al: A fixation method of tendon transfer in foot surgery. Kao Hsiung I Hsueh Ko Hsueh Tsa Chih 10:97–99, 1994.

Close JR, Todd FN: The phasic activity of muscles of the lower extremity and the effect of tendon transfer. J Bone Joint Surg 41A:189–208, 222, 1959.

Coughlin MJ: Lesser toe deformities. Orthopedics 10:63–75, 1987.

Cyphers SM, Feiwell E: Review of the Girdlestone-Taylor procedure or clawtoes in myelodysplasia. Foot Ankle 8:229–233, 1988.

DiCesare PE, Young S, Perry J, Baumgarten M: Perimalleolar tendon transfer to the os calcis for triceps surae insufficiency in patients with postpolio syndrome. Clin Orthop 310:111–119, 1995.

Edwards P, Hsu J: SPLATT combined with tendo achilles lengthening for spastic equinovarus in adults: Results and predictors of surgical outcome. Foot Ankle 14:335–338, 1993.

Fernandez-Feliberti R, Fernandez SA, Colon C, Ramirez N, Alegria M, Cintron K: Transfer of the tibialis anterior for the calcaneus deformity in myelodysplasia. J Bone Joint Surg 74A:1038–1041, 1992.

Gallant GG, Massie C, Turco VJ: Assessment of eversion and plantar flexion strength after repair of Achilles tendon rupture using peroneus brevis tendon transfer. Am J Orthop 24:257–261, 1995.

Garceau GJ, Manning KR: The anterior tibial tendon transfer. J Bone Joint Surg 29:1044, 1947.

Georgiadis GM, Aronson DD: Posterior transfer of the anterior tibial tendon

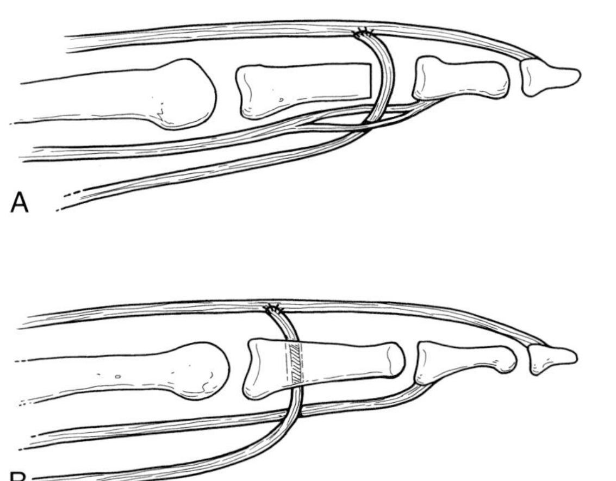

FIGURE 69–21. *A,* Flexor to extensor transfer, with resection of the distal proximal phalanx. *B,* Flexor to extensor transfer: the entire tendon is transferred through a drill hole in the proximal phalanx.

in children who have a myelomeningocele. J Bone Joint Surg *72A*:392–398, 1990.

Goldman FD, Siegel J, Barton E: Extensor hallucis longus tendon transfer for correction of hallux varus. J Foot Surg *32*:126–131, 1993.

Gould JS: Clubfoot. *In* Gould JS (ed): The Foot Book. Baltimore, Williams & Wilkins, 1986, pp 153–172.

Gould N: Trephining your way. Orthop Clin North Am *4*:157–164, 1973.

Green NE, Griffin PP, Shiavi R: Split posterior tibial tendon transfer in spastic cerebral palsy. J Bone Joint Surg *65A*:748–754, 1983.

Greene WB: Transfer versus lengthening of the posterior tibial tendon in Duchenne's muscular dystrophy. Foot Ankle *13*:526–531, 1992.

Helal B: Cobb repair for the tibialis posterior tendon rupture. J Foot Surg *29*:349–352, 1990.

Hoffer M, Reiswig J, Garrett A, Perry J: Split anterior tibial tendon transfer in cerebral palsy. Orthop Clin North Am *5*:31–38, 1974.

Jaivin JS, Bishop JO, Braly WG, Tullos HS: Management of acquired adult dropfoot. Foot Ankle *13*:98–104, 1992.

Johnson KA, Spiegel PV: Extensor hallucis longus transfer for hallux varus deformity. J Bone Joint Surg *66A*:681–686, 1984.

Jones R: An operation for paralytic calcaneocavus. Am J Orthop Surg *5*:371–376, 1908.

Lindell EB, Carroll NC: Longitudinal tendon splitting: A simple technique. J Pediatr Orthop *14*:385–386, 1994.

Mann RA, Holmes GB Jr, Seale KS, et al: Chronic rupture of the Achilles tendon: A new technique of repair. J Bone Joint Surg *73A*:214–219, 1991.

Masterson E, Jagannathan S, Borton D, Stephens MM: Pes planus in childhood due to tibialis posterior tendon injuries. Treatment by flexor hallucis longus tendon transfer. J Bone Joint Surg *76B*:444–446, 1994.

Mulier T, Dereymaeker G, Fabry G: Jones transfer to the lesser rays in metatarsalgia: technique and long-term follow-up. Foot Ankle Int *15*:523–530, 1994.

Ninkovic M, Sucur D, Starovic B, Miarkovic S: A new approach to persistent traumatic peroneal nerve palsy. Br J Plast Surg *47*:185–189, 1994.

Rodriquez RP: The Bridle procedure in the treatment of paralysis of the foot. Foot Ankle *13*:63–69, 1992.

Silver RL, DeLa Garza J, Rang M: The myth of muscle balance: A study of relative strengths and excursions of normal muscles about the foot and ankle. *In* Mann RA and Coughlin MJ (ed): Surgery of the Foot and Ankle, 6th ed. St. Louis, Mosby–Year Book, 1993, pp 826–827.

Skalley TC, Myerson MS: The operative treatment of acquired hallux varus. Clin Orthop *306*:183–191, 1994.

Taylor RG: An operative procedure for the treatment of hammertoe and claw-toe, J Bone Joint Surg *22A*:608–609, 1940.

Taylor RG: The treatment of clawtoes by multiple transfers of flexor into extensor tendons. J Bone Joint Surg *33B*:539–542, 1951.

Thompson FM, Deland JT: Flexor tendon transfer for metatarsophalangeal instability of the second toe. Foot Ankle *14*:385–388, 1993.

Turco VJ, Spinella AJ: Achilles tendon ruptures: Peroneus brevis transfer. Foot Ankle *7*:253–259, 1987.

Tynan MC, Klenerman L: The modified Robert Jones tendon transfer in cases of pes cavus and clawed hallux. Foot Ankle Int *15*:68–71, 1994.

Wapner KL, Hecht PJ, Mills RH Jr: Reconstruction of neglected Achilles tendon injury. Orthop Clin North Am *26*:249–263, 1995.

Wapner KL, Hecht PJ, Shea JR, Allardyce TJ: Anatomy of second muscular layer of the foot: Considerations for tendon selection in transfer for Achilles and posterior tibial tendon reconstruction. Foot Ankle Int *15*:420–423, 1994.

Wapner KL, Pavlock GS, Hecht PJ, Naselli F, Walther R: Repair of chronic Achilles tendon rupture with flexor hallucis longus tendon transfer. Foot Ankle *14*:443–449, 1993.

Ward JJ, Meyer, RD, Lemmons JE: Tensile strength comparison of dowel plug technique to standard techniques of tendon-bone attachment. Foot Ankle *8*:248–253, 1988.

Watkins MB, Jones JB: Transplantation of the posterior tibial tendon. J Bone Joint Surg *36A*:1181–1189, 1954.

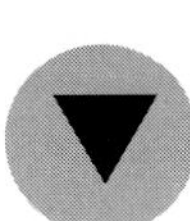

Chapter 70

Microneurovascular Free Muscle Transfer

BACKGROUND AND CLINICAL APPLICATION
Ralph T. Manktelow

By using microneurovascular techniques, skeletal muscle can be transferred from one site to another. This allows the placement of functioning muscles in an area that is deficient due to muscle loss. A critical factor is the provision of a healthy motor nerve to innervate the transfer. In irreparable nerve injuries, which result in a loss of functioning muscle, it is necessary to get above the level of the injury in order to innervate the muscle that is being transferred. Alternately, a different nerve that is not the primary nerve for the function intended can be used in some situations. An example of this situation in facial paralysis is the use of the opposite facial nerve through a cross-facial nerve graft. An example in extremity reconstruction is the use of intercostal nerves to provide innervation to a free functioning muscle transfer used for reconstruction of biceps function.

The quality of muscle function following microneurovascular transfer depends on the muscle selected, the adequacy of reinnervation, the placement of the muscle at optimum tension, and the quality of the muscle bed. Finally and of particular importance is the postoperative exercise program, which is necessary to develop maximum contractile strength.

HISTORY

The first clinical case was carried out in the early 1970s in Shanghai when the lateral portion of the pectoralis major muscle was transplanted to the forearm to replace flexor musculature in a patient who had Volkmann's ischemic contracture (Shanghai Sixth People's Hospital, 1976). The application of functioning free muscle transfer to the upper extremity continues to be the major area of extremity reconstruction today. The authors have had clinical experience with over 50 functioning muscle transfers in Toronto for extremity reconstruction (Manktelow et al, 1984). Interestingly, the application of microneurovascular transfer for facial paralysis has now eclipsed that of the extremities, with the author's experience with more than 160 patients.

INDICATIONS FOR FREE MUSCLE TRANSFER TO THE FOREARM

The forearm is the single most important area for functioning muscle transfer. Muscle can be transferred to replace the long finger flexors or the long finger extensors. The most common applications for this procedure are not in nerve injury but in major loss of skeletal musculature subsequent to trauma, Volkmann's ischemic paralysis, electrical burns, and following tumor excision. In addition to long finger flexor reconstruction, muscle transplantation has been used for long finger extensor function and for biceps, deltoid, and triceps reconstruction. The most useful muscle is the gracilis muscle because it is readily available, has reliable neurovascular pedicles, and is easy to elevate, and there is insignificant functional loss following removal from the leg.

Muscle transplantation is a particularly complex procedure, with a long period before maximum rehabilitation is accomplished. It should not be used when simpler satisfactory techniques, such as tendon transfer, are available.

Muscle transplantation has been used in brachial plexus injuries. This procedure has been primarily for long-standing brachial plexus injuries for biceps reconstruction. There has been a major effort by Doi and others to use muscle transplantation to provide finger flexion and wrist extension, and this research is in the early stage of development (Doi et al, 1996).

MUSCLES AVAILABLE FOR FREE FUNCTIONING MUSCLE TRANSFER

The muscles that are most commonly used are the gracilis, the latissimus dorsi, the tensor fascia lata, the pectoralis major, the gastrocnemius, and the serratus anterior.

The anatomical structures of the muscle must fit the recipient site. The length of the muscle and the location of the vascular nerve pedicles must be appropriate to the recipient area. The origin and insertion of the muscle should have sufficient tendon structure to allow strong attachment to recipient structures. For the extremities, the gracilis muscle is particularly suitable and is discussed in detail.

GRACILIS ANATOMY

The gracilis muscle is found on the medial aspect of the thigh in a superficial location. It is a strap muscle proximally and tapers distally with a pennate type of insertion to the tendon. There is a thin aponeurosis at the origin of the muscle that is the body of the pubis and the adjacent ramus of the ischium. The belly of the muscle is just posterior to the adductor longus and ends in a long, thin tendon that inserts into the medial shaft of the tibia just below the tibial tubercle.

There are at least two or three vascular pedicles; however, the proximal pedicle is the dominant one and will reliably perfuse the entire muscle. This pedicle lies under the adductor longus and takes its origin from the profunda femoris artery. The artery is usually 1 to 2 mm in diameter and at least 6 cm in length and there are two venae comitantes, one or both of which is slightly larger than the artery. The pedicle enters the muscle 8 to 12 cm from the muscle's origin, and a larger perforator is given off from the muscle to supply the overlying skin at the same level as the dominant pedicle. The single motor nerve is a branch of the obturator and is composed of two to seven fascicles. It enters the muscle just proximal to the dominant vascular pedicle. The muscle may frequently be separated into separate neuromuscular territories on the basis of separate fascicle stimulation of the motor nerve. Ninety percent of the time, there is a single fascicle that controls the anterior 20 to 50 percent of the muscle, and the remaining portion of the muscle is controlled by the remaining fascicles. This functional separation is occasionally useful as in the provision of separate thumb and finger flexion.

PREOPERATIVE PLANNING

Preoperative planning involves an assessment of the patient's needs and a review of the possible options for reconstruction. If a simpler procedure, such as a tendon transfer, is available, it should be carried out. When assessing the donor site, it is important to identify the intended origin and insertion of the muscle, its innervation, and the vascular supply. From the history and physical examination, it is usually possible to make a good guess as to which motor nerve branch is likely to be present and undamaged. If there is a significant concern about the availability of a motor nerve, a preliminary exploration and nerve biopsy should be performed. Neurohistological evaluation is used to assess the availability of an undamaged motor nerve. The recipient site is assessed for its ability to accept the free flap in terms of skin coverage. It is very important to have skin coverage over the muscle to allow good muscle and tendon gliding. If local skin is not available, then a skin flap may be transferred with the muscle or may be constructed as an adjacent local or distant flap. Flap coverage is critical, especially for the distal half of the muscle and tendon, where good gliding is essential.

The gracilis muscle can be raised as a myocutaneous flap. Unfortunately, the subcutaneous fat of the medial thigh is often much thicker than it is in the upper extremity and the skin paddle is aesthetically bulky. The skin paddle over the gracilis is reliable over the proximal 40 percent of the muscle but is unreliable distally to this. The critical area for skin coverage is usually the distal portion of the muscle. Thus, local skin flaps are usually necessary if adequate skin is not available to house the muscle.

OPERATIVE TECHNIQUE

Preparation of the recipient site following trauma is often tedious because the small neurovascular structures are encased in scar tissue and are difficult to dissect without damaging them.

Preparation of the recipient site includes the identification and repair of all structures that will be involved in the transfer. In the scarred tissue bed, dissection from proximal to distal usually identifies undamaged tissues and allows dissection into the damaged area without injuring the critical neurovascular structures.

Following the muscle dissection in the leg, the muscle is left attached to its dominant pedicle and allowed to perfuse to assess the adequacy of the circulation. This can be evaluated most readily by examining the color of the muscle. Occasionally, there will be a few centimeters of distal muscle that turns blue. This section can be resected with reinsertion of the proximal viable muscle into the tendon with a few sutures. The muscle is then separated from the leg, positioned at its recipient site, and tacked loosely in place, and neurovascular repairs are carried out. In placing the muscle in the forearm, it is important that it be positioned at the site that is going to represent its normal excursion in a functional position so that the positioning of the pedicle can be carried out without traction on the pedicle by muscle movement.

REHABILITATION

The rehabilitation program begins 2 to 4 weeks following the operation and consists initially of stretching the muscle by manipulating the limb. This program is designed to obtain full passive muscle extension and to prevent adhesions of the muscle in its bed. This approach will reduce the need for subsequent tenolysis. When spontaneous contraction of the muscle occurs, the patient is then encouraged to attempt to contract the muscles as frequently as possible. Once a good range of motion develops, a program of graduated resisted grip exercises commences, and this program assists in developing maximum muscle strength. The authors have not used electrical stimulation to develop muscle strength but believe that active resisted exercises are the most useful way to develop the muscle's maximum capability. The exercise program should be pursued for approximately 1 year following the development of a useful range of muscle movement. If patients incorporate the extremity into their daily activities and work activities, it is easier to maintain their interest and enthusiasm, and this approach usually provides a useful resisted exercise program.

CLINICAL RESULTS

The authors have used this technique to provide motor function to the upper extremity in more than 50 patients. The majority of these procedures have been performed to provide finger flexion. Microvascular muscle transfers have also been useful for finger extension, elbow flexion, and deltoid replacement.

Because this procedure is relatively complex and there are many areas where errors can be made that would affect functioning, it is important to limit the application of the procedure. Patients who can be adequately managed by simpler, less complex procedures such as tendon transfers should be offered the simpler approach as a preferred reconstructive technique.

The return of muscle function is markedly improved by a resistive exercise program, which is given to the patient once reinnervation develops.

The experimental work with microneurovascular transfer has shown that it is possible to have a contractile strength that is up to 100 percent of the pretransfer strength of the muscle. However the muscle strength that is obtained in clinical practice is variable and depends on many factors, particularly the adequacy of the muscle, tension of the nerve, and the quality of the nerve repair.

Of these factors, the most important technical considerations are

(1) revascularization
(2) nerve repair
(3) placing the muscle at the appropriate tension
(4) adequate flap coverage

Revascularization

A microvascular anastomosis depends on a technically good repair in a normal vessel. Vessels that have to be used in the zone of injury are less prone to spasm if an end-to-side repair is carried out. A good spurt from the cut artery must be present before performing the microvascular anastomosis if good perfusion is to be expected. The muscle will become pink and bleed from all cut areas on completion of the arterial anastomosis. In the gracilis muscle, the distal few centimeters of the muscle usually take about 5 minutes or more to become pink. Any distal musculature that does not become pink should be resected and reattached to the intramuscular portion of the gracilis tendon.

Nerve Repair

The nerve repair should be as close as possible to the neurovascular hilum of the muscle. It is critical that the repair involves undamaged motor nerves, and if possible, a motor nerve should be used that is synchronous with the desired function of the muscle. A fascicular repair is important because the motor nerve of the gracilis muscle has a large fatty component and about 40 percent of the nerve is actually fascicular tissue.

Placing the Muscle at Optimum Tension

The placement of the muscle depends on the assumption that the muscle's most powerful contraction begins near its maximum range of excursion and that the muscle has a normal physiological range of excursion that is greater than that required at the recipient site. This will provide a full range of motion of the joints that the muscle is powering.

The technique of muscle tension adjustment begins when the muscle is still in the leg. At this time, it is stretched to its maximum physiological extended length by positioning the extremity appropriately, with the knee extended and the thigh abducted, and then markers are placed along the surface of the muscle every 5 cm. Usually a small suture in the upper epimysium is a good way of accomplishing this.

When the muscle is revascularized, the origin is firmly attached proximally and the muscle is stretched distally so that the markers are spaced 5 cm apart when the extremity is at its maximum extended position, that is, fingers and wrist are fully extended. This allows planning for the tension of the muscle in its attachment to its insertion. Another important factor if the muscle is providing finger flexion or extension is that the finger flexor or extensor tendons be sutured side to side to each other in a balanced position so that when the transfer muscle contracts, all fingers come into flexion or extension in unison and provide a balanced grip or extension. With the extremity and the muscle in their stretched positions, adjacent positions are marked on the flexor tendons and on the tendon of the transplanted muscle. This marks the position of the tendon, and the attachment can be performed with the fingers and wrist flexed and the muscle relaxed.

Flap Coverage

Skin flap coverage must be obtained over the distal half of the muscle so that the tendon can glide. If a myocutaneous flap is chosen, it may need to be debulked at a later time. Occasionally, a distal flap, such as an abdominal or groin flap, may be used to cover the forearm or the forearm skin may be expanded by tissue expanders before the muscle is transferred. A split-thickness skin graft may be applied directly to the proximal half of the muscle; this method will not affect its function and provides a better aesthetic result.

POSTOPERATIVE CARE

Adequate circulation to the extremity must be maintained by providing an adequate volume of fluids, maintaining the patient's temperature, and maintaining his or her blood pressure. If thrombosis does occur, it is more difficult to recognize in a muscle than in a skin flap. The patient must be returned to the operating room rapidly and the anastomosis revised. If the ischemia lasts longer than 4 hours, then it is likely that the muscle will suffer irreversible ischemic damage and will not obtain a good function. For this reason, it is important that the anastomosis be performed with maximum care to minimize any postoperative thrombosis.

The author's experience with muscle transplantation of the forearm has revealed that the gracilis muscle can provide a functional grip strength of up to 50 percent of normal. Owing to the great excursion of the gracilis muscle, full finger flexion and extension can be expected in all wrist positions.

The successful application of functioning muscle transfers depends on careful patient selection, correct operative technique, and an appropriate postoperative therapy program. Once reinnervation has developed, muscle power can be developed by a resisted exercise program, which is modeled along the same principles as any strength training program used in athletics.

References

Doi K, Sakai K, Fuchigami Y, Kawai S: Reconstruction of irreparable brachial plexus injuries with reinnervated free muscle transfer. J Neurosurg 85:174–177, 1996.

Manktelow RT, Zuker RM, McKee, NH: Functioning free muscle transplantation. J Hand Surg 9A:32, 1984.

Shaghai Sixth People's Hospital: Free muscle transplantation by microsurgical neurovascular anastomoses: Report of a Case. Chin Med J 2:47, 1976.

MICROVASCULAR FINE MUSCLE TRANSFER TECHNIQUE
Allen L. van Beek • Aamir Siddiqui

After the introduction of the binocular operating microscope as a clinical tool by Nylan (1954) and Holmgren (1923) in the 1920s, only otolaryngology and ophthalmology specialists worked with structures small enough and delicate enough to require magnification for repair. Perhaps it was a lack of understanding or reticence to incorporate new technology that delayed the application of microsurgery to the nerve and blood vessel until 40 years later. Yasargil (1969), Jacobson and Suarez (1973), Cobbett (1967), and Smith (1964) then became advocates of the binocular operating microscope in certain clinical settings in neurosurgery, hand surgery, and peripheral nerve surgery. Malt reported an arm replantation (1964). Kleinert and colleagues (1963) advocated very small vessel repair using loupes in the digit and revascularized fingers. Microscopic replantation of digits produced higher success rates and was first reported by Komatsu and Tamai (1968). However, one of the most significant impacts of microsurgery had to await for the knowledge known by Tansini (1896) and Shaw (1944) but explained and implemented by McCraw and associates (1977), Mathes (1974), Dibbell (1974), O'Brien (1980), Nahai (1980), and others.

The physiology and anatomy of axial, musculocutaneous, muscle, fasciocutaneous, and over-random flaps were clarified by Mathes (1981), McGregor and Morgan (1973), McCraw and associates (1977), and O'Brien (1982b). This information was vital. Armed with this knowledge, reconstructive surgeons throughout the world (Akasaka et al, 1990; Doi et al, 1995; Gilbert, 1981; O'Brien 1982a; Jones, 1995) began to perform free muscle transfers for problems that in the past had seemed almost insurmountable, at the worse; at the best, solutions were grim or multistaged. From information learned from clinical free flap musculocutaneous transfers and from basic science labs, separating a muscle from its native bed, moving it to another remote recipient bed, revascularizing and reinnervating it became a reality.

The technology of free flap transfer, including free microneurovascular muscle transfer, became the centerpiece of reconstructive surgery in the late 1980s. Harii (1988), O'Brien (1990), Logan and colleagues (1988), Manktelow (1988), Gilbert (1981), Van Beek (1983), and Terzis (1989) began to report successful experiences with reanimation of the face and upper extremities using free muscle transfers.

Reports by Ueda and colleagues (1998), Oldfors and associates (1989), O'Brien (1990), Manktelow (1989), and Harii (1988) have all reported definitive techniques and uses for microneurovascular muscle transfer.

MUSCLE ANATOMY

As reported by Frey and associates (1983), Manktelow (1989), and Van Beek and associates (1983), there are notable anatomical features of muscle that must be incorporated into the planning of a free muscle transfer. Muscle fiber length; direction; vascular distribution; nerve distribution; vascular pedicle length; muscle length, width, and thickness; nature of origin (Fig. 70–1) and insertion; and location of nerve and vascular pedicle along the length of the muscles are crucial to the planning and performance of one of the most difficult, sophisticated, and elegant reconstructive procedures available to reconstructive surgeons.

Fiber Length

A muscle fiber has an amplitude of contraction that is approximately one half of its fiber length (Brand et al, 1981). Therefore, a muscle such as the gracilis, with a muscle

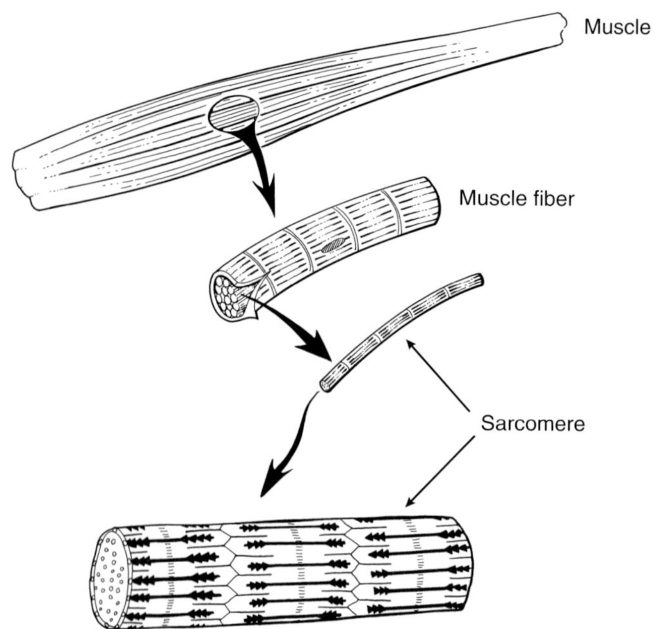

FIGURE 70–1. The sarcomere is the basic building block of muscle. End-to-end stacking of sarcomeres creates a very long cellular structure—the muscle fiber. Muscle fibers are bundled into groups of fascicles, completing the structured organization of muscle.

length before its transition to a tendon of approximately 30 cm, has muscle fibers 30 to 40 cm in length. These fibers, if maximally contracted, could produce an amplitude of excursion of approximately 15 cm. This excursion is beyond what is required in most reconstructive procedures. For flexor tendon reconstruction, an amplitude of 8 cm is sufficient, and in facial reconstruction, an amplitude of 1.5 to 2 cm is sufficient to give excellent oral commissure movement. Excessively long muscle length in the face will produce excessive pull on the oral commissure, as reported by Harii (1988) in his early series of facial reanimation using the gracilis muscle. Excessive pull by transferred muscles in the face was solved by using shorter segments of the gracilis and serratus for facial reanimation. Terzis (1989) introduced use of the pectoralis minor because of its shorter muscle length, shape, and thickness.

MUSCLE VASCULARITY

Muscle vascularity has been divided into five general types by Mathes and Nahai (1981) (Fig. 70–2). Linear and segmental blood supply are the dominant features of this classification.

Segmental blood supply means the muscle has more than one vascular pedicle supplying circulation along the length of the muscle. Survival of the entire muscle after separation of the blood supply will usually occur, particularly if the dominant pedicle has been identified and is used as the supplying vessel. In the gracilis muscle, the second segmental vessel to the gracilis is usually the dominant pedicle and will reliably revascularize the entire muscle. The same cannot be said for the overlying skin when it is included. Including an island of skin that lies over the muscle's supplying pedicle will provide reliable circulation to the skin flap, unless the paddle of skin length exceeds a radius of about 8 cm from the site where the muscle's vascular pedicle enters the muscle and sends cutaneous perforators to the overlying island of skin.

Muscles with a dominant linear blood supply, such as the latissimus supplied by the thoracodorsal artery and vein, rely on a dominant vascular pedicle to provide circulation to the muscle in contrast to the segmental supply of some muscles. Even the latissimus dorsi muscle has a secondary system of circulation from paraspinous perforators to the muscle.

Once researchers determined the vascular supply of muscles, the patterns of innervation soon followed. Muscle flaps with skin grafts and musculocutaneous flaps were initially used for coverage of cutaneous deficits. A small series of microvascular transfer of muscle for purposes of restoring animation was first reported by Harii and colleagues in 1976. The nerve supply to the gracilis, serratus anterior, latissimus dorsi, pectoralis minor, and rectus femoris were well established, and because of microvascular surgery, they could

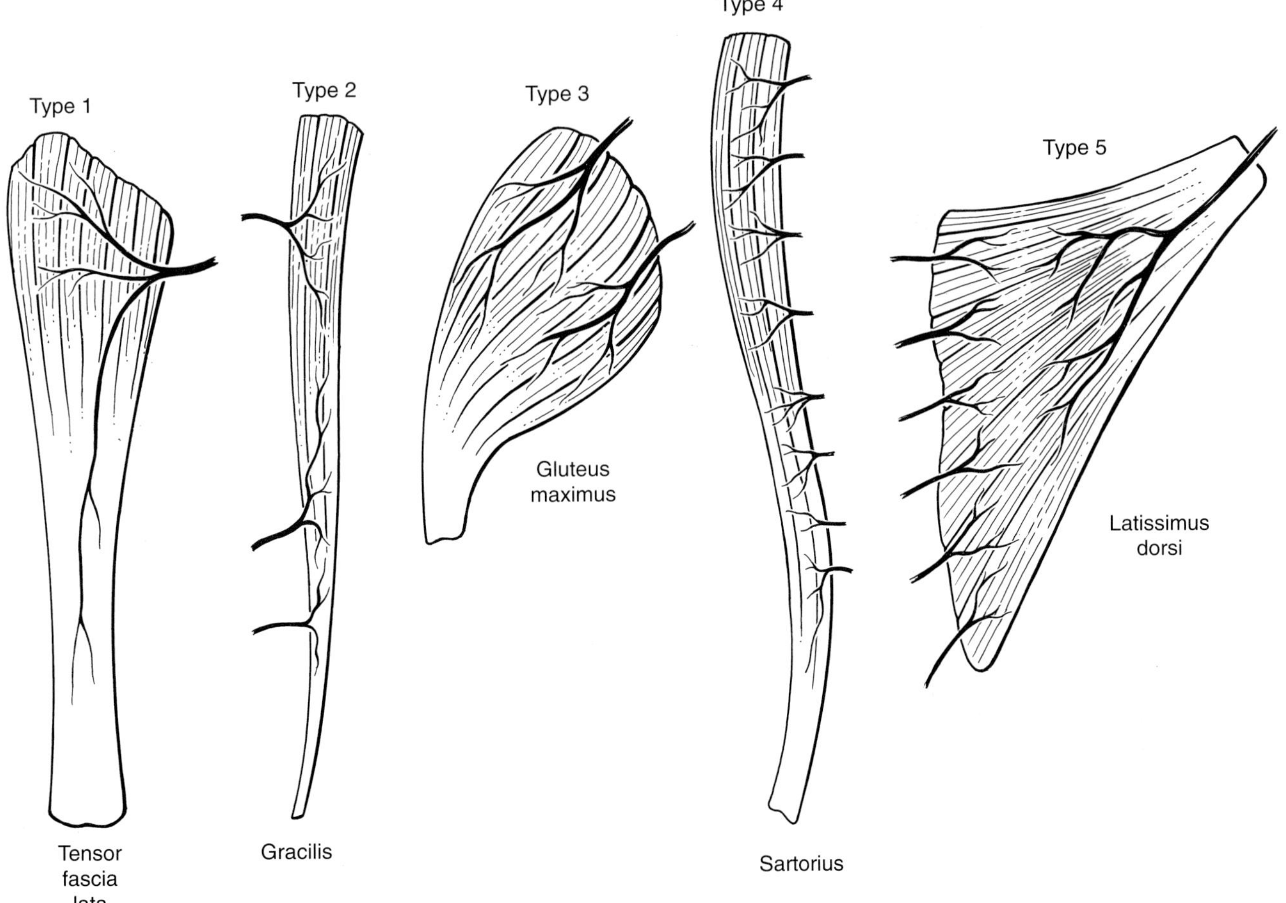

FIGURE 70–2. The vascularity of muscle varies with location. Understanding the types of circulation present in muscle identifies its suitability for pedicle or microvascular transfer. Type 1: Single pedicle supplies entire muscle. Type 2: One dominant pedicle with other minor pedicles. Type 3: Two dominant pedicles, either of which can supply the entire muscle. Type 4: Segmental supply. Type 5: Dominant pedicle with secondary pedicles.

▼ **TABLE 70–1**
Characteristics of Selected Muscle Flaps

Factor	Gracilis	Latissimus	Serratus	Pectoralis Minor
Fiber length	30 cm	20 cm	110 cm	12 cm
Muscle length	30 cm	35 cm	12 cm	12 cm
Muscle width	5 cm	8–25 cm tapered	2 cm/slip	3–8 cm
Muscle thickness	1.5–2.5 cm	1–2.5 cm	1–2 cm	1–1.5 cm
Blood supply	Medial femoral artery	Thoracodorsal artery	Thoracodorsal artery	Thoracoacromial artery
Pedicle length	4–7 cm	8–10 cm	8–10 cm	3 cm
Type of circulation	Type II	Type V	Type III	Type V
Origin	Muscle	Muscle	Muscle	Muscle
Insertion	10 cm tendon	3 cm tendon	Muscle	4 cm tendon
Pedicle location	Side entrance	End entrance	Side entrance	Side entrance
Innervation	Obturator	Thoracodorsal	Long thoracic	Medial pectoral
Face animation	Excellent	Fair	Excellent	Excellent
Extremity animation	Excellent	Excellent	Poor	Poor

now be used to restore function of the paralyzed face and the severely devastated extremity. Defined motor fascicle territories within a muscle were demonstrated by Van Beek and colleagues (1983) and Manktelow (1984). Two isolated functions from one transferred muscle became possible.

Many muscles have been transferred by microsurgical technique for animation. However, the majority of procedures performed to restore motor function involve transferring the gracilis, serratus, latissimus, or pectoralis minor muscles. Table 70–1 demonstrates many of the attributes and difficulties we have found associated with each of these flaps. Figures 70–3 to 70–6 demonstrate the anatomy and technique of elevation of each of the flaps.

The myriad of reanimations possible using free muscle

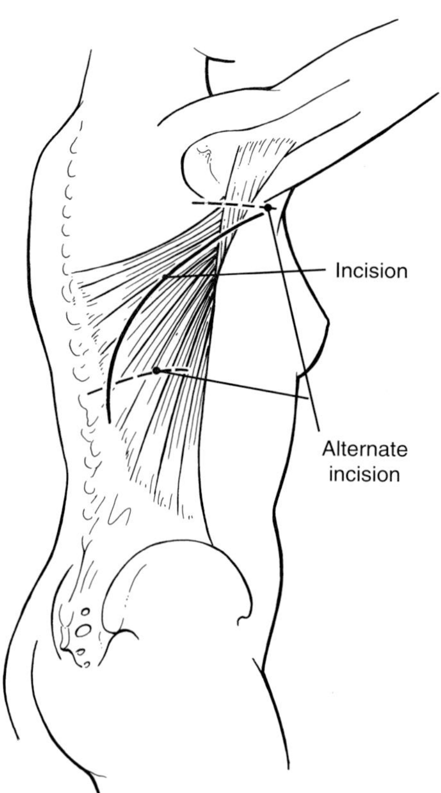

FIGURE 70–3. When removing the gracilis muscle, the incision should be marked with the leg extended. The incision should be along a line extending from the pubic tubercle to the medial condyle. The gracilis muscle originates from the pubis immediately posterior to the pubic tubercle and the adductor longus. The branch of the medial femoral circumflex artery to the gracilis enters the muscle 10 cm below the inguinal ligament. A linear incision aids removal and marking of resting tension. The obturator nerve supplies innervation and enters the muscle superior to the second dominate perforator.

FIGURE 70–4. The latissimus dorsi muscle is readily removed using a curvilinear incision. Multiple transverse incisions will provide improved cosmesis at the price of more difficulty. The thoracodorsal artery, veins, and nerve enter the muscle approximately 8 cm below the axilla. This provides a nice length of pedicle for microsurgical transfers. The muscle is thin and flat. If it seems thick and short after removal, restoring the resting tension to the muscle will restore its size.

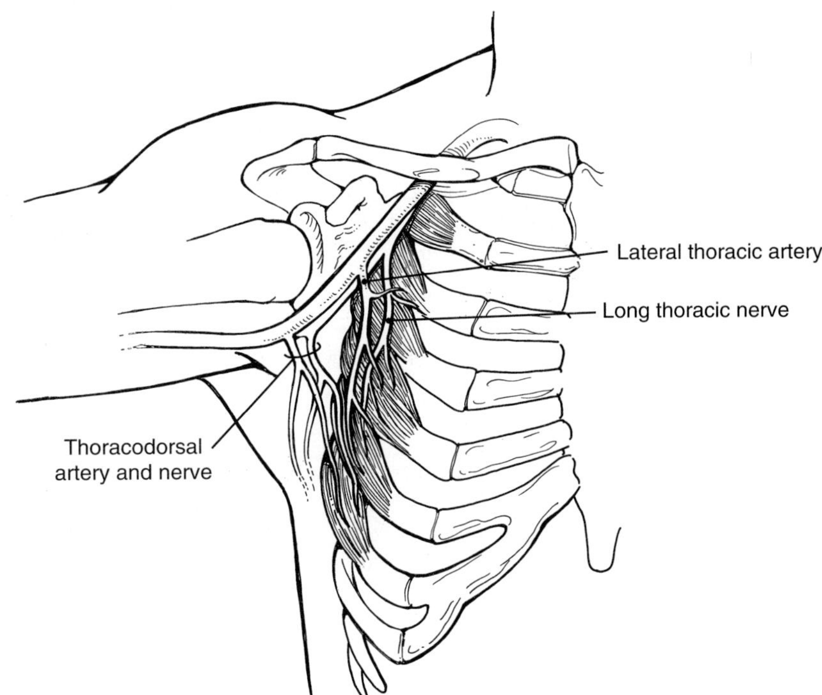

FIGURE 70–5. The serratus anterior is removed through a curvilinear incision similar to that used for latissimus removal. When microsurgical transfer is anticipated, it is necessary to preserve the thoracodorsal vessel and its communicating branch to the serratus. The lateral thoracic artery supplies backup circulation to the muscle but would be difficult to use for revascularization of the muscle.

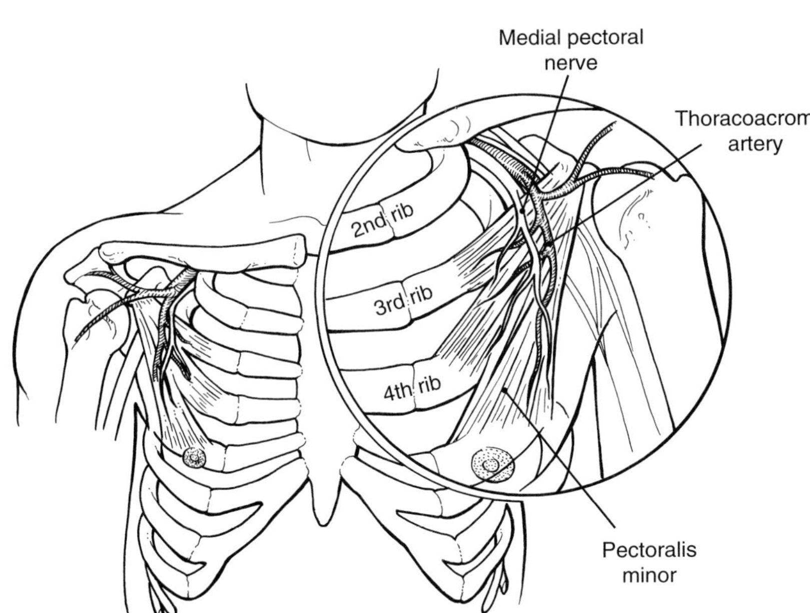

FIGURE 70–6. The pectoralis minor muscle is suitable for facial reconstructions but will not provide sufficient strength or size for most extremity reconstructions. To remove the muscle, an incision parallel to the clavicle and 3 cm below it provides access. This incision provides access for identification of the innervation and blood supply for both the pectoralis major and minor muscles. Avoid injury to the short pedicle of the thoracoacromial system and the medial pectoral nerve during early phases of dissection. Division of the pectoralis major insertion with later reattachment is essential for exposure and access for the surgeon wishing to use the pectoralis minor.

transfer makes specific details for every circumstance impossible to delineate in this chapter. This chapter will outline general guidelines for planning a free muscle transfer and then provide the detail for performing a transfer to the forearm for flexor function and to the face for facial reanimation. These are the two most common reasons for free microneurovascular transfer of muscle.

PREOPERATIVE PLANNING

Planning one of the most complex reconstructive procedures available requires a checklist of items to consider.

Where are recipient vessels and nerves located?
Will vessel or nerve grafts be required?
What animation function is needed?
What amplitude of muscle excursion will accomplish that function?
Where can the muscle be anchored to provide both origin and insertion?
What methods of muscle/tendon fixation will work?
How will resting tension be established?
How will the patient be positioned?
What type of vessel repairs are anticipated?
What type of nerve repairs are likely?
How will ischemic time be minimized?
How will cold ischemia be provided?
How will postoperative protection be provided?
How will muscle circulation and viability be monitored?

The answers to these questions will ensure that the surgeon is thoroughly addressing the problem and has planned what muscle and vessels, the surgical steps, and from what side of the patient should the muscle be removed. Because orientation of the vessel as it enters the flap can be crucial to placement and securing the muscle, selection of from which side to remove the flap is often a crucial decision.

INTRAOPERATIVE TECHNICAL STEPS

Prepare recipient bed.
Explore recipient bed to ascertain status.
Identify potential recipient veins, arteries, and nerves.
Identify potential alternative vessels.
Identify where the flap will be positioned and how recipient and flap vessels will be positioned and be repaired.
What technique of vessel and nerve repairs is likely?
What positioning of the flap will be required to see and perform neurovascular repairs?
How can resting length of the muscle be determined and re-established in the recipient bed?

FLAP EXPLORATION AND PREPARATION

Expose the surface of muscle.
Identify the dominant vascular supply.
Identify the innervating nerve.
Mark resting length muscle interval with sutures (Fig. 70–7).

Transect nerve and establish fascicle territories, if needed.
Determine what area of the muscle best fits the recipient bed.
Determine the length and width of muscle required (sutured origins and insertion do not contract).
Divide muscle; protect vessels.
Divide vessels only when recipient vessels are completely prepared.
Ice the muscle with cardiac saline slush.
Move muscle to recipient bed.
Suture muscle into recipient bed; establish resting length.
Revascularize flap.
Repair nerves.

Although this extensive series of steps will aid the surgeon, obviously not all the variable criteria that one can encounter are listed. Adjust the detail to fit the circumstance.

In circumstances in which a severe Volkmann's contracture is present, a transferred muscle such as the gracilis may be used to provide two functions (Fig. 70–8 and 70–9). If this is desired, it is necessary to determine the motor nerve distribution within the muscle. This is easiest to determine before the muscle is removed from its native bed. Once determined, the muscle is split along the planes of innervation, and the two separate components are connected

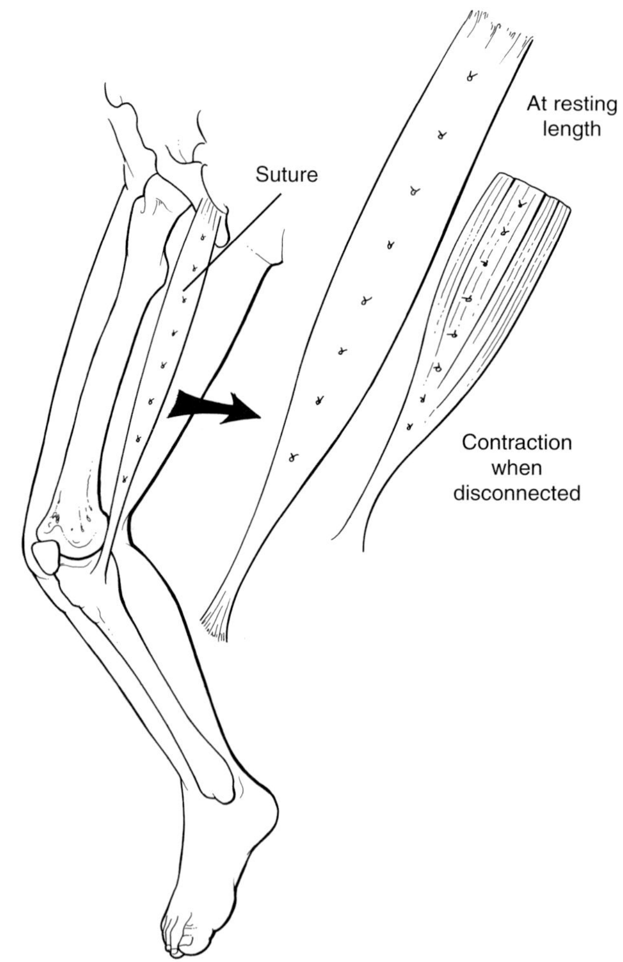

FIGURE 70–7. Just before dividing origin and insertion, and before removing the muscle from its native bed, the resting tension of the muscle should be established using marking sutures, stain, or clips. When the muscle is free, the marked interval decreases in length and the muscle becomes bulky.

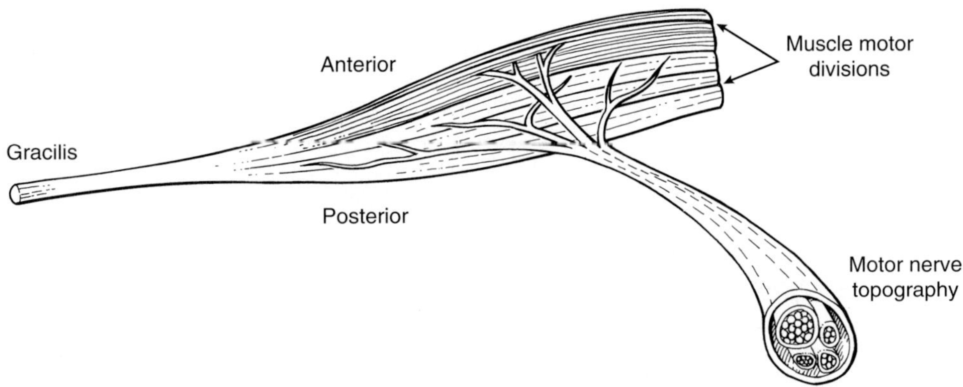

FIGURE 70–8. The gracilis can be split linearly into two muscle territories, with each territory supplied by a specific group of nerve fascicles. When connected to appropriate recipient nerves, the split muscle will provide two functions. Assessing muscle function should be accomplished after muscle paralyzing agents have been reversed or metabolized.

to different tendon units that need to be functional. The recipient bed must have two different motor nerves available for the nerve repairs; an example would be to use a branch of the anterior interosseous nerve and the branch that supplies the flexor carpi radialis or a motor branch from the ulnar nerve. When split into two components to provide dual functions, the muscle will have less strength at each function compared with not splitting the muscle.

NERVE REPAIR

Accurate vessel repairs will be judged immediately by patency. Accurate nerve repair is essential for motor reinnervation, but unfortunately, it cannot be assessed for months. Because the patterns of fascicular topography will be completely different and because the size and grouping of fascicles will be dissimilar, a single fascicle alignment and repair is advocated. Often, the recipient bed fascicles are large, and the motor nerve of the transferred muscle will be small by comparison.

It is often asked, How does one repair muscle? Don't the sutures pull out? When suturing muscle alone to an insertion point or point of origin, the suture is woven within the muscle substance and into the epimysium of the muscle, and then secured to the anchoring point. Permanent sutures of 0 size are used for the connection. This repair technique has sufficient strength to maintain resting tension in the muscle. Unless the resting length is accurately established and joint positioning is appropriate, it may be necessary to readjust the muscle length at a later date to establish the desired amount and arc of joint motion.

Once the muscle has been inset, the repairs must be protected from inadvertent stress during surgery and after surgery. Without protection, disruption of the muscle repairs or its crucial nerve and vessel supply could occur. Long-arm splinting of the reconstructed elements of an extremity to prevent disruption is prudent. Preoperative education of the facial patient is the best protection and consists of restricted facial activity, diet restrictions, avoiding inadvertent sleeping on the flap, and restricted neck activity.

Monitoring of circulation to the transferred muscle can be difficult. If the surface of the muscle is visible, monitoring can be done with ultrasound Doppler, laser Doppler, or evoked muscle activity. When completely covered, monitoring the muscles is more formidable, and evoked muscle

activity and evoked muscle action potentials are very useful techniques (Van Beek et al, 1983).

FOREARM TRANSFER

The most commonly used muscle for forearm reanimation is the gracilis muscle. It can be used for flexor, extensor, or simultaneous reconstruction in the forearm for reanimation.

The muscles' entire length is used. The origin from just posterior to the pubic tubercle is used to establish a new origin in the arm. The resting length of the muscle is established before removal, as advocated by Manktelow (1973, 1989) (see Fig. 70–7). The medial or lateral epicondyle of the humerus makes an excellent point of fixation, using permanent 2-0 suture. The gracilis tendon is interwoven into a common tendon formed by plication of the profundus tendons to each other (Fig. 70–10). This weave is secured with 4-0 permanent sutures. The profundus plication sutures are 2-0 permanent sutures. Final resting tension is provided

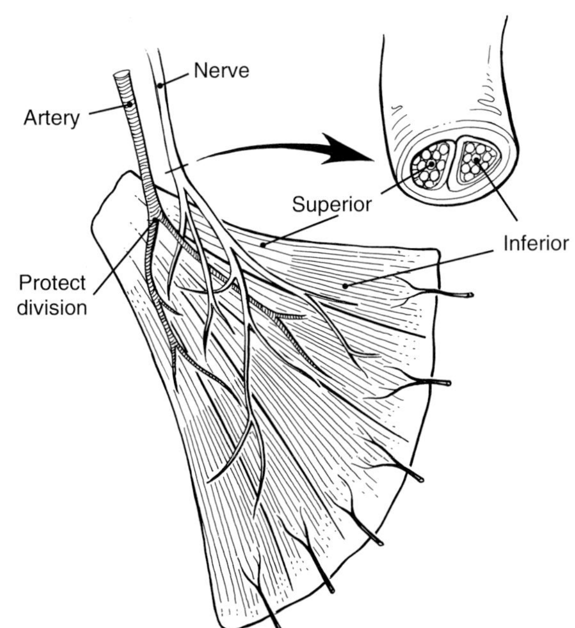

FIGURE 70–9. The latissimus dorsi muscle can be divided into an anterior and posterior segment. Differential stimulation of the thoracodorsal nerve fascicles helps identify their distribution within the muscle.

by adjusting the origin of the transplanted tendon, avoiding complex adjustments in the distal tendon's weave (Fig. 70–10). Adjusting the muscle tension is very important, or the full effect of muscle use will not be in the desired motion arc of the hand.

Once the origin and insertion points are established, the vessels and nerves are repaired. End-to-side arterial, end-to-end vein, and fascicular nerve repairs are common in the recipient bed. Grafts can be avoided in most circumstances by careful planning.

When the muscle is securely inserted and vascularized, positioning the wrist in extension gracilis tension will provide a finger posture that would permit hook function and gripping with the fingers. When the wrist is placed in flexion, the fingers should extend to allow release of objects that are grasped or hooked by the hand.

FACIAL REANIMATION

Facial reanimation is more complex than extremity reanimation. Fixed points of origin and insertion are less defined.

The transferred muscle origin can be attached to the zygomatic arch, temporal fascia, or preauricular fascia, but the insertion is attached to that most plastic of structures: the skin (Fig. 70–11). The functioning muscle unit does not have to be longer then 6 cm to provide adequate animation of the mouth. Attachment to the zygomatic arch is accomplished with 3-0 permanent sutures, and pull-out sutures are used to anchor to the corner of the mouth. Pull-out sutures over buttresses help secure the insertion into the skin and provide some flexibility in final tension adjustments. It is difficult to ascertain exact resting tension because of the mobility of the circumoral skin and a limited length of muscle.

The vessel repairs are usually end to end. Both temporal and facial arteries and veins have been used successfully. The temporal veins are branched and difficult to harvest. Loupe magnification is essential to finding and preventing injury to the recipient vein. Often, the temporal artery in front of the ear may be tortuous. Careful adventitia removal will help with the vessel's tortuous anatomy. Planning is crucial because the vessels can leave the inferior flap if the facial vessels are used to avoid the use of grafts. In this use,

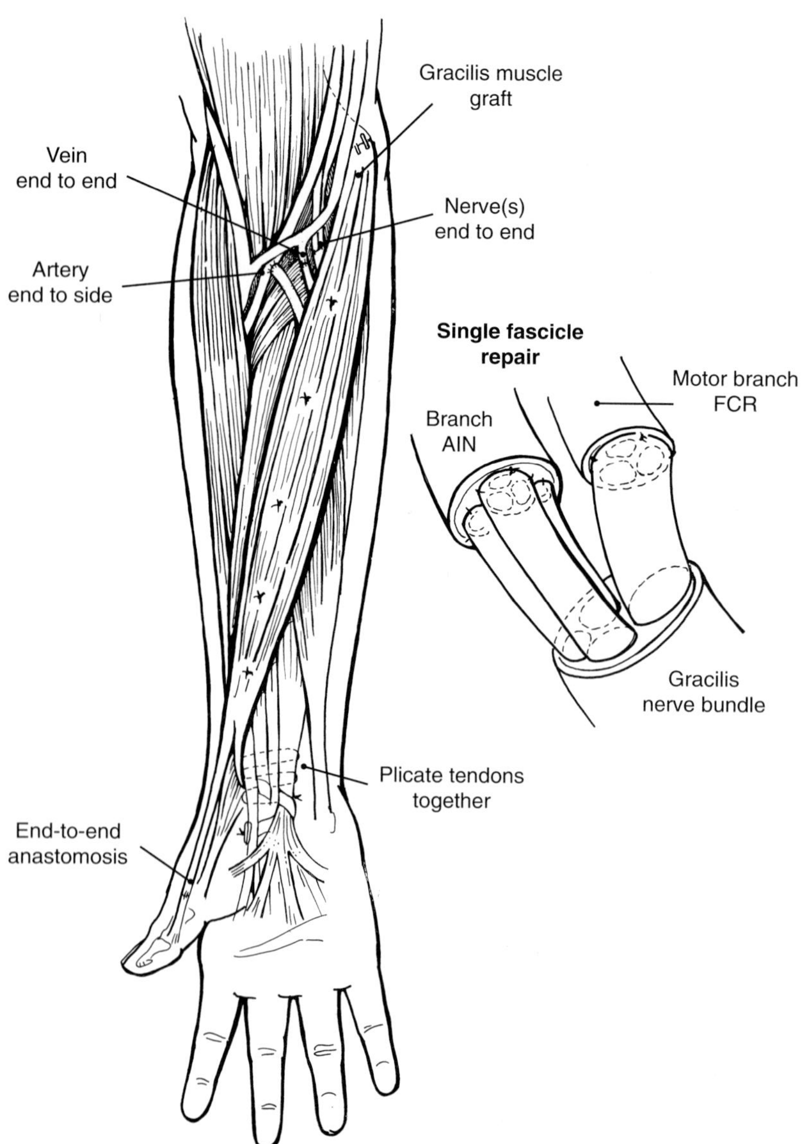

FIGURE 70–10. The gracilis muscle has been divided into two components. The posterior two thirds of the muscle and its tendon are woven into the plicated flexor digitorum profundus. The anterior one third is attached to the flexor pollicis longus. The resting length of the muscle is established by fixing the origin of the muscle. End-to-side arterial repairs and end-to-end venous repairs are most common. Single fascicle nerve repairs are recommended because of fascicle size and pattern differences.

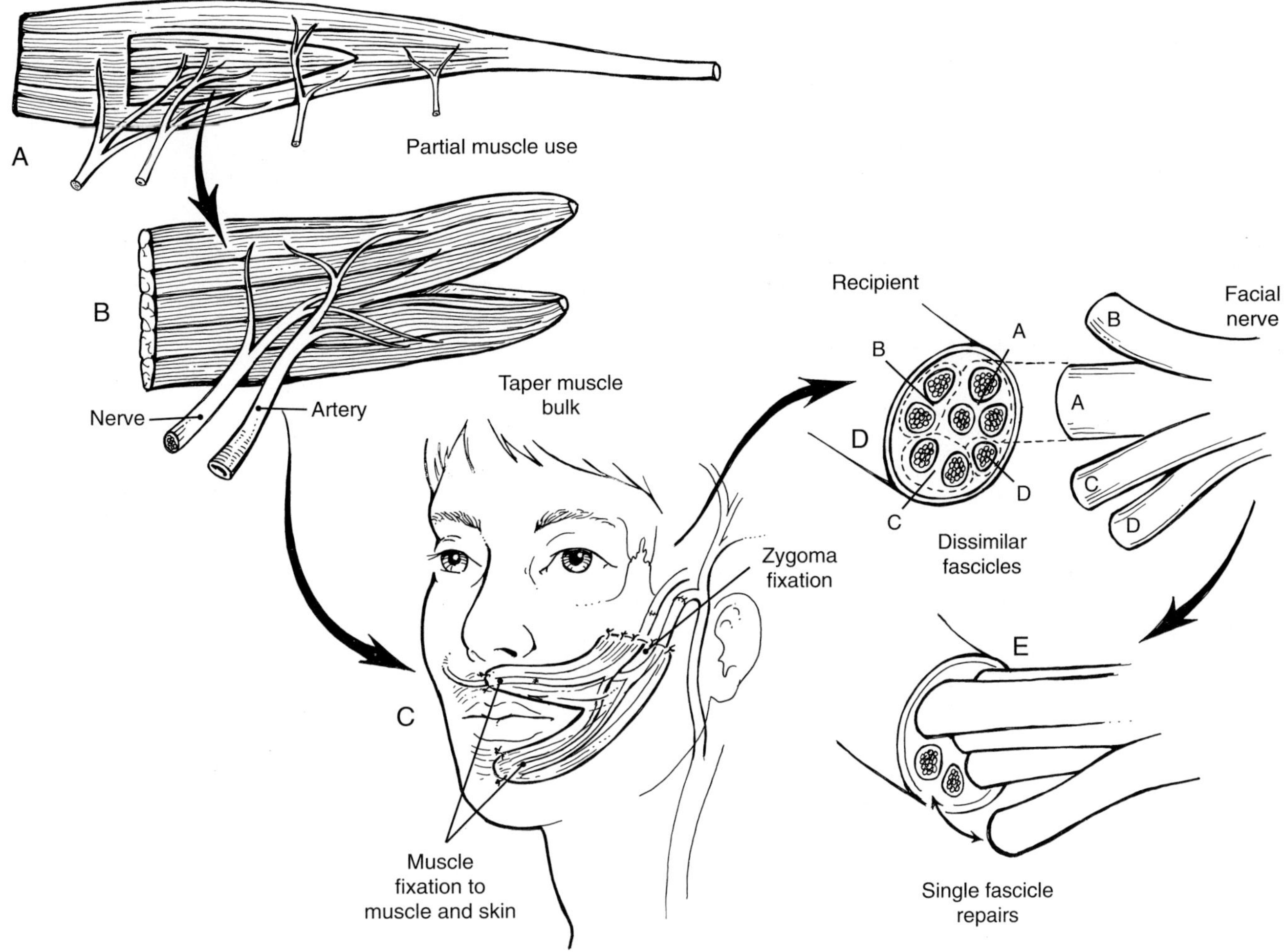

FIGURE 70–11. A predetermined portion of the gracilis is removed along with vessels and nerves. It is split into two linear components. The upper slip will be attached by pullout sutures to the upper lip and the lower slip to the lower lip. The pullout sutures will bring a narrow slip of muscle at least 1.5 cm medial to the oral commissure. Single fascicle nerve repairs are essential to preserve nerve fiber contact with the transferred muscle. If available differential innervation of the transferred muscle is preferred. This is accomplished by connecting the buccal branch to the upper slip and mandibular branches to the lower slip of transferred muscle's supplying nerve.

the muscle is reversed in position within the face. The gracilis origin is distal and insertion is proximal. This places the vessels closer to the mandibular border location of the facial artery and vein. A 2.0-cm incision directly over the vessel and below the inferior edge of the mandible allows the vessel to be tunneled to this site for repair. When using subcutaneous tunnels, make sure the vessel does not inadvertently rotate in the tunnel. The use of metal ligature clips is often the culprit in undesirable rotation of the vascular leash. The vessel repairs can be monitored in the completely covered flap with the ultrasound flow probe when the vessel course is known under the facial skin and is carefully marked on the skin's surface.

Because of the different topography that will be encountered, single-fascicle coaptation repair with 11-0 suture is performed. It is possible to have adequate nerve length in some ipsilateral reconstructions. Direct repair is possible and selective muscle function can be attempted. Crossed facial nerve grafting seldom provides that option because of limited supplying axons in the graft and because mixing of fibers within the course of the graft occurs.

Diet restrictions, edema control, and flap monitoring are crucial issues during the postoperative period.

LONG-TERM CONSIDERATIONS

Recovery of function in transferred muscle occurred in all but one patient in the authors' experience with 32 transferred muscles. Failure to contract occurred in a patient with a shotgun blast to his face reconstructed with a gracilis muscle and direct facial nerve repair. Monitoring ensured that the muscle survived. It is presumed that the proximal facial nerve was not connected to the central nervous system because of facial nerve damage in the mastoid portion of its course. One transfer in a child's extremity produces function but the muscle is weaker then desired.

Recovery of function in the face can be too dramatic. In that circumstance, the muscle can be surgically debulked to decrease strength of the muscle. One patient in this series had excessive debulking with loss of too much of the function of the muscle.

The use of *Botulinum* exotoxin A has not been tried in this series of patients. Theoretically, repeated use could retrain the patient's conscious effort in using the muscle to smile excessively.

One patient in this series has excessive resting tone of the transferred muscle. The transfer was a direct connection to

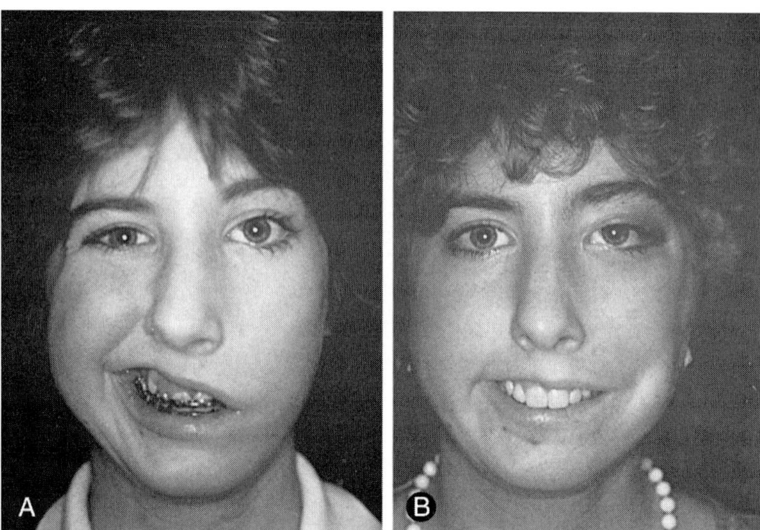

FIGURE 70–12. *A*, Congenital unilateral paralysis *B*, Following reanimation with a partial gracilis muscle transfer. Transferring a portion of the muscle to the eyelid is not recommended.

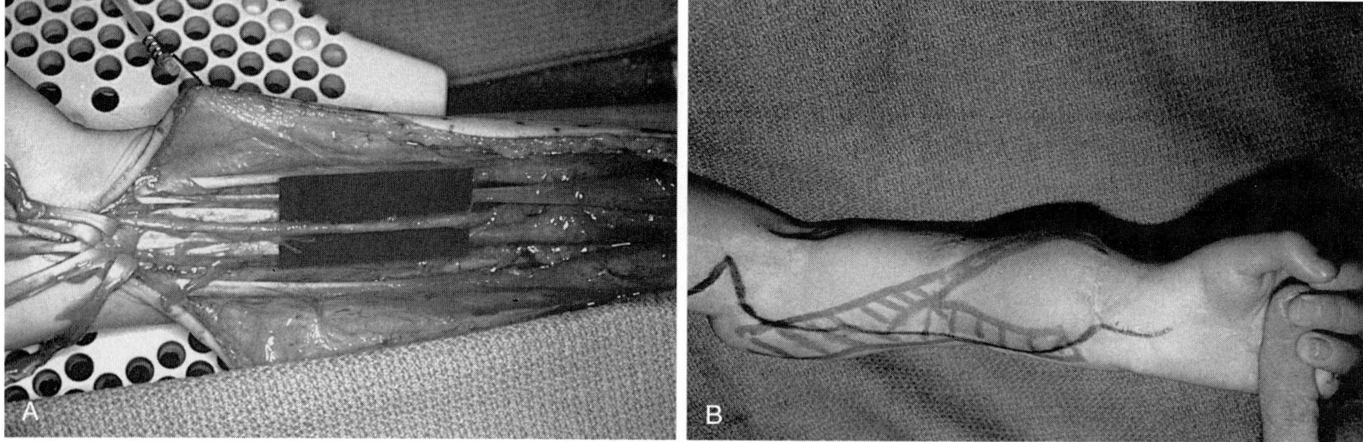

FIGURE 70–13. Total loss of extrinsic muscles occurred in dorsal and volar compartments of the forearm because of ischemia. The intact nerves are noted. *B*, When splitting function in a transferred gracilis muscle, careful planning of tendon routes and strength needs are essential.

the ipsilateral facial nerve after a sarcoma excision from the cheek. This is a problem in the facial area when the tone is excessive and produces a smile on the paralyzed side that is excessive compared to the normal side (Fig. 70–12). Similar problems would probably not be noted in extremity reconstruction. The tension in this transferred muscle could be the result of having a greater than normal resting tension established in the transferred muscle, or it could be related to the reinnervation process of the muscle. Treatment for this condition is poorly delineated.

The reconstruction of extremities with animating muscles is difficult because a large number of motor functions that have been compromised (Fig. 70–13). This mandates that the surgeon use this resource in extremity reconstruction wisely and in conjunction with other procedures as tenodesis and fusion.

Reconstruction of the face with an animating muscle is difficult because of the bulk of the transferred muscle, limited directions of contraction, contralateral synchronization, and the potential problems of excessive or inadequate excursion of contraction.

Despite these problems, the technique of microneurovascular transfer of muscle from a remote site to restore animation is a major milestone in reconstructive surgery.

References

Acland RD: Microvascular anastomosis: A device for holding stay sutures and a new vascular clamp. Surgery 75:185, 1974.

Akasaka Y, Hara T, Takahashi M: Restoration of elbow flexion and wrist extension in brachial plexus paralysis by means of free muscle transplantation innervated by intercostal nerve. Ann Chir Main Memb Super 9:341–350, 1990.

Brand P, Peach RB, Thompson DE: Relative tension and potential excursion of muscles in the forearm and hand. J Hand Surg 6:209–219, 1981.

Buncke HF Jr., Schulz WP: Experimental digital amputation and reimplantation. Plast Reconst Surg 36:62, 1965.

Cobbett JR: Microvascular surgery. Surg Clin North Am 47:521, 1967.

Dibbell DG: Use of a long island flap to bring sensation to the sacral area in young paraplegics. Plast Reconst Surg 54:220, 1974.

Doi K, Sakai K, Kuwata N, Ihara K, Kawai S: Double free-muscle transfer to restore prehension following complete brachial plexus avulsion. J Hand Surg (Am) 20:408–414, 1995.

Frey M, Gruber H, Freilinger G: The importance of the correct resting tension in muscle transplantation: Experimental and clinical aspects. Plast Reconstr Surg 71:510–518, 1983.

Gilbert A: Free muscle transfer. Int Surg 66:33–35, 1981.

Goodstein WA, Buncke HJ: Patterns of vascular anastomoses vs. success of free groin flap transfers. Plast Reconst Surg 64:37–110, 1979.

Harii K: Microneurovascular free muscle transplantation for reanimation of facial paralysis. Clin Plast Surg 6:361–375, 1979.

Harii K: Refined microneurovascular free muscle transplantation for reanimation of paralyzed face. Microsurgery 9:169–176, 1988.

Harii K, Ohmori K, Torii S: Free gracilis muscle transplantation, with microneurovascular anastomoses for the treatment of facial paralysis: A preliminary report. Plast Reconstr Surg 57:133–143, 1976.

Holmgren G: Some experiences in surgery of otosclerosis. Acta Otolaryngol 5:460–466, 1923.

Ikuta Y, Kubo T, Tsuge K: Free muscle transplantation by microsurgical technique to treat severe Volkmann's contracture. Plast Reconstr Surg 58:407–411, 1976.

Ikuta Y, Yoshioka K, Tsuge K: Free muscle transfer. Aust NZJ Surg 50:401–405, 1980.

Jacobson JH, Suarez EL: Microsurgery in anastomosis of small vessels. Surg Forum 11:243–245, 1973.

Jones BM: Cross-face reanimation of the paralysed face, with single stage microneurovascular gracilis transfer without nerve graft (letter). Br J Plast Surg 48:519–520, 1995.

Kleinert HE, Kasdan ML, Romero JL: Small blood vessel anastomosis for salvage of severely injured upper extremity. J Bone Joint Surg (Am) 45A:788–796, 1963.

Komatsu S, Tamai S: Successful replantation of a completely cut-off thumb: Case report. Plast Reconstr Surg 42:374–377, 1968.

Logan SE, Alpert BS, Buncke HJ: Free serratus anterior muscle transplantation for hand reconstruction. Br J Plast Surg 41:639–643, 1988.

Malt RA: Replantation of severed arms. JAMA 189:716–722, 1964.

Manktelow RT: Functioning microsurgical muscle transfer. Hand Clin 4:289–296, 1988.

Manktelow RT, McKee NH: Free muscle transplantation to provide active finger flexion. J Hand Surg (Am) 3:416–426, 1978.

Manktelow RT, Zuker RM: Muscle transplantation by fascicular territory. Plast Reconstr Surg 73:751–757, 1984.

Manktelow RT, Zuker RM: The principles of functioning muscle transplantation: Applications to the upper arm. Ann Plast Surg 22:275–282, 1989.

Mathes SJ, McCraw JB, Vasconez LO: Muscle transposition flaps for coverage of lower extremity defects: Anatomical considerations. Surg Clin North Am 54:1337, 1974.

Mathes SJ, Nahai F: Classification of the vascular anatomy muscles: Experimental and clinical correlation. Plast Reconst Surg 67:177, 1981.

McCraw JB, Dibell DG, Carraway JH: Clinical definition of independent myocutaneous vascular territories. Plast Reconstr Surg 60:341, 1977.

McGregor IA, Morgan G: Axial and random pattern flaps. Br J Plast Surg 26:202, 1973.

Nahai F: The tensor fascia lata flap. Clin Plast Surg 7:51, 1980.

Nylen CO: The microscope in aural surgery, its first use and later development. Acta Otolaryngol 116:226, 1954.

O'Brien BM, Franklin JD, Morrison WA: Cross-facial nerve grafts and microneurovascular free muscle transfer for long established facial palsy. Br J Plast Surg 33:202–215, 1980.

O'Brien BM, Lawlor DL, Morrison WA: Microneurovascular free muscle reconstruction for long established facial paralysis. Ann Chir Gynaecol 71:65–69, 1982a.

O'Brien BM, Morrison WA, MacLeod AM, Weiglein O: Free microneurovascular muscle transfer in limbs to provide motor power. Ann Plast Surg 9:381–391, 1982b.

O'Brien BM, Pederson WC, Khazanchi RK, Morrison WA, MacLeod AM, Kumar V: Results of management of facial palsy with microvascular free-muscle transfer. Plast Reconst Surg 86:12–22; 23–24, 1990.

Oldfors A, Mair WG, Fogdestam I: The morphological sequences in man of de- and reinnervation in free muscle transfer with microneurovascular anastomoses. Scand J Plast Reconstr Surg Hand Surg 23:35–42, 1989.

Paletz JL, Manktelow RT, Chaban R: The shape of a normal smile: Implications for facial paralysis reconstruction. Plast Reconstr Surg 93:784, 1994.

Serafin D, Smith PJ: Vascularized transplantation of skeletal muscle: A case report. J Microsurg 1:259–266, 1980.

Shaw DT: Open abdominal flaps for repair of surface defects of upper extremity. Surg Clin North Am 24:293–308, 1944.

Smith SW: Microsurgery of peripheral nerves. Plast Reconst Surg 33:317–329, 1964.

Tansini I: Sopra il niro nuovo progresso di amputazione della mammella. Riforma Med 12:757, 1896.

Taylor GL, Watson N: One-stage repair of compound leg defects with free, revascularized flaps of groin skin and iliac bone. Plast Reconst Surg 61:494–506, 1978.

Terzis JK: Pectoralis minor: A unique muscle for correction of facial palsy. Plast Reconst Surg 83:767–776, 1989.

Ueda K, Harii K, Yamada A: Free neurovascular muscle transplantation for the treatment of facial paralysis using the hypoglossal nerve as a recipient motor source. Plast Reconst Surg 94:808–817, 1994.

Van Beek AL, Hubble B, Kinkead L, Tomos S, Suchy H: Clinical use of nerve stimulation and recording technique. Plast Reconst Surg 71:225–238, 1983.

Whitney TM, Buncke HJ, Alpert BS, Buncke GM, Lineaweaver WC: The serratus anterior free-muscle flap: Experience with 100 consecutive cases. Plast Reconst Surg 86:481, 1990.

Yasargil MG: Anastomosis between the superficial temporal and a branch of the middle cerebral artery. Microsurgery Applied to Neurosurgery. Stuttgart, Thieme Verlag, 1969, pp 105–155.

Sensation-Bearing Flaps

PRINCIPLES AND TERMINOLOGY

The ability of skin grafts and flaps to bear sensation has long been a subject of interest to the reconstructive surgeon. Skin grafts and random pedicle flaps, by their very nature, must rely either on some pre-existing deep pressure receptors in the recipient bed (whose acuity may or may not increase with time) or neural ingrowth from the bed or adjacent skin.

Return of sensation in nonsensate skin grafts and flaps has been documented in a number of classical publications (Davis, 1934; Hoppenreijs et al, 1990; Kredel and Evans, 1933). Suffice it to say that this sensation starts peripherally, takes years to develop, and never approaches the quality of sensation in adjacent, normal tissue. Hermanson and colleagues (1987) found both the function and morphologic reinnervation in a mixed bag of nonsensate free flaps to be poor at between 2 months and 3 years. We can anticipate protective sensation at best.

However, sensation may be carried with a flap. An example of this is the digital neurovascular island flap (Littler, 1960; Moberg, 1955). Here, a small digital skin island from the ulnar aspect of the long or ring fingers is mobilized on the ulnar neurovascular bundle of the digit. This is then pedicled from the origin of the digital artery in the palm and transposed to provide sensate cover to a damaged or partially amputated thumb. This kind of flap may be termed an "innervated" flap. The sensation felt in the reconstructed thumb will be referred to the digit from which the flap came and, in the absence of cortical relearning—difficult to achieve in the adult (Murray et al, 1967)—this may present a functional problem. The Karapandzic flap (1974) for lip reconstruction is a circumoral rotation lip-sharing flap in which motor as well as sensory innervation is preserved by careful dissection at its periphery. The functional unity, as well as the proximity of donor and recipient sites, obviates the need for sensory relearning.

In other cases, sensation may be maintained by carrying out a repair between the sensory nerve of the flap and an appropriate nerve in the recipient site. This always occurs with sensate free flaps, but may also take place with pedicled tissue transfer. These "reinnervated" flaps allow sensation to be perceived orthotopically but are dependent on the quality of the anastomosis, the regenerative capacity of the recipient nerve, and the extent of its cortical representation (discussed below). Furthermore, sensory return is subject to the delay necessitated by the regeneration process. Sometimes, the nerve passes through the flap and, perhaps after supplying it with sensory twigs, emerges at its distal end. This "vascularized nerve graft" may be used to reinnervate a more distant part, and helps constitute a "sensory flow-through flap."

What, then, of the quality of sensation produced in rein-nervated flaps? It has long been assumed that the quality of sensory return was limited by the sensory acuity in the tissue being transferred. Imperfections in the technique of nerve repair might be expected to make the resulting sensation inferior to that of the donor tissue in its native location. However, recent work indicates that the limiting factor is the sensory acuity in the recipient rather than the donor site (Boyd et al, 1994). The sensory acuity in forearm skin is rather poor, two-point discrimination being measured in centimeters rather than millimeters (Weinstein, 1968). Nevertheless, when a forearm flap is used for intraoral reconstruction and reinnervated by anastomosing the lateral antebrachial cutaneous nerve to the lingual, the resulting two-point discrimination is often less than 5 mm—normal for the mouth (Fig. 71–1). This phenomenon will be referred to as "sensory upgrading."

It appears, then, that the sensory return in reinnervated forearm flaps (used for intraoral reconstruction) approaches normal intraoral sensation and that this level is vastly superior to that of normal forearm skin. To attempt an explanation of these findings, it is necessary to consider the cutaneous and mucosal sensory receptors, the cortical representation of the sensory areas involved, and the process of collateral and distant inhibition that modify and differentiate the sensory signals reaching the brain.

It is widely quoted that the density and type of sensory receptors vary over the surface of the body and that their density is proportional to the cortical representation of the cutaneous areas they subserve (Weinstein, 1968). Cutaneous receptors may be specialized or nonspecialized. The former are usually encapsulated and easily visible under light microscopy. The latter consist of "free nerve endings" that are unmyelinated and extend via extensive arborization into superficial dermis and even epidermis (Fig. 71–2). They are equivalent to the "nerve net" of more primitive animals. Because of difficulties in visualization, free nerve endings have not been quantified to the same extent as encapsulated ones (Cauna, 1968; Iggo and Andres, 1982), yet they may hold the key to the reinnervation potential of sensate flaps.

None of the expanded or encapsulated endings appear to be necessary for cutaneous sensation. It has repeatedly been demonstrated that all four cutaneous sensory modalities can be elicited from areas that on histological examination contain only naked nerve endings (Ganong, 1991). The specialized receptors, on the other hand, have a more subtle purpose. The combination of slowly adapting and rapidly adapting receptors at different levels in the skin allows the determination of the shape and size of objects moving over it (Martin and Jessell, 1991). This is of great importance in the fingertips, where encapsulated receptors are common. It is not so important in the forearm (where they are rare), but the ability of the mouth to determine the size and shape of a food bolus has definite significance in terms of the quality

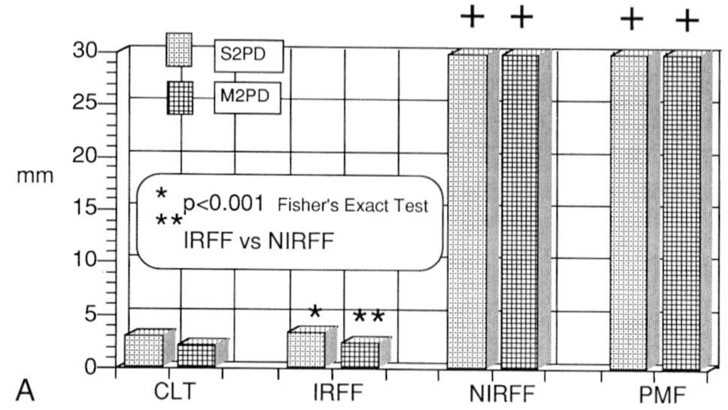

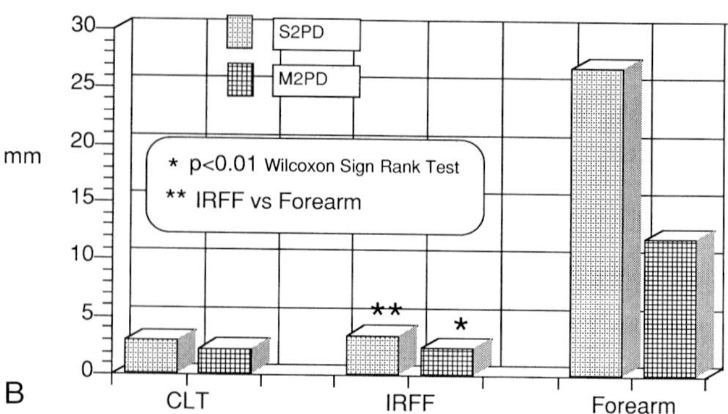

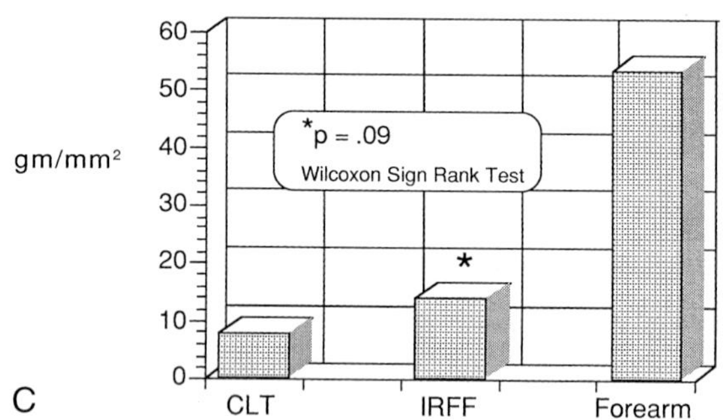

FIGURE 71–1. In a controlled prospective study of patients undergoing anterior floor of mouth reconstruction, 8 received innervated radial forearm flaps (IRFF) and 10 received noninnervated radial forearm flaps (NIRFF). A further matched control group of 10 patients undergoing pectoralis flap (PMF) repair was also considered. CLT signifies contralateral, normal tongue. Detailed, blinded, sensory testing was performed at least 6 months later. Both static and moving two-point discrimination (S2PD, M2PD) were superior in the innervated radial forearm flaps compared to the non-innervated flaps *(A)* as well as to the forearm donor sites *(B)*. Semmes-Weinstein pressure testing was also superior in the innervated flaps showing an upgrading over the tissue in its native site *(C)*. Measurements of hot/cold sensibility, pinprick, and the subjective ability to sense the presence of food showed similar findings. (From Boyd B, Mulholland S, Gullane P, Irish J, Kelly L, Rotstein L, Brown D: Lateral antebrachial cutaneous neurosome flaps in oral reconstruction: Are we making sense? Plast Reconstr Surg *93*:1350, 1994. © Williams & Wilkins, 1994.)

of oral function. If tactile stereognosis could easily be tested, we would anticipate a poor response in reinnervated forearm skin, because the density of encapsulated receptors there is poor.

It appears that the density of receptors (uncounted free nerve endings or otherwise) in forearm skin is adequate for an extremely high degree of sensory discrimination *even though that degree of discrimination is not normally present in the forearm.* By free neurovascular transfer, we can elevate one of the least sensate areas of the body to the level of the most highly sensate. It follows that sensory acuity is not simply proportional to the numbers of, for example, Meissner's corpuscles in a given area, and that the explanation of this phenomenon must lie elsewhere.

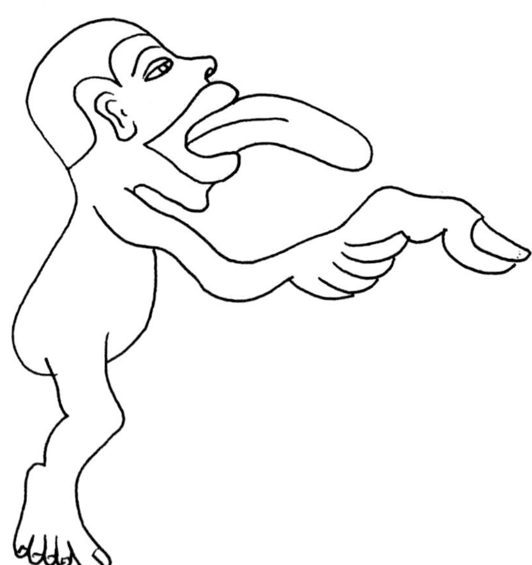

FIGURE 71–2. Diagram of sensory receptors in the skin. Specialized receptors are rare in non-glabrous skin, but are not required for two point discrimination, pain, temperature and pressure sensation. "Bare nerve endings" form a nerve net over the surface of the body and are probably responsible for the return of sensation in reinnervated flaps. (From Martin JH: Sensory systems of the brain. *In* Kandel ER, Schwartz TC, Jessell FM [eds]: Principles of Neural Science, 3rd ed. New York, Elsevier Science Publishing Company, Inc., 1991, p 343. © Appleton & Lange, 1991.)

FIGURE 71–3. Diagram of a man, drawn in proportion to the representation of body parts on his sensory cortex. The sensory homunculus illustrates the disproportionately large sensory cortical representation given to the lips, tongue, and hands.

The representation of the body on the sensory cortex is termed the "sensory homunculus." Topographically, this takes the form of a distorted human with all anatomical areas represented in proportion to their sensory acuity. The resulting figure has huge hands, lips, and tongue and diminutive thorax and limbs. The area representing the tongue is much larger than that representing the whole arm (Fig. 71–3). Clearly, sensory signals from an innervated flap now travel from the flap via the lingual nerve to the sensory cortex where they project to a larger area of the brain than previously. A given stimulus thus has a greater potential for reaching the conscious level than when the cortical area is smaller. If the interneuronal connections at each of the central nervous system (CNS) relay stations serve to amplify the signal by projecting onto successively more and more cell bodies, the effect is compounded (Fig. 71–4A). Less important nerves (e.g., the lateral antebrachial cutaneous nerve) normally project to smaller cortical areas, perhaps undergoing less amplification in the dorsal horns, dorsal

column nuclei, thalamus, etc. This would explain the superior results of Semmes-Weinstein monofilament testing in the innervated flap over the forearm, but it would not explain the superior two-point discrimination.

Two-point discrimination is the ability of the brain to distinguish two closely applied stimuli as separate entities. The amplification process illustrated in Figure 71–4A serves only to activate a greater number of cells in the cerebral cortex—a process akin to turning up the volume on a cheap transistor radio. It would not, in itself, increase the discriminatory power (fidelity) of the system. For this to happen, the architecture of the sensory tract must allow for peripheral inhibition (see Fig. 71–4B). This process is one of fine-tuning and, like amplification, occurs at the relay stations but usually involves inhibitory interneurons that are activated when a sensory neuron is stimulated. The interneurons inhibit the surrounding neurons—spatially isolating one stimulus from another—and, by preventing the fusion of two excitations, preserve two distinct peaks of activity at the

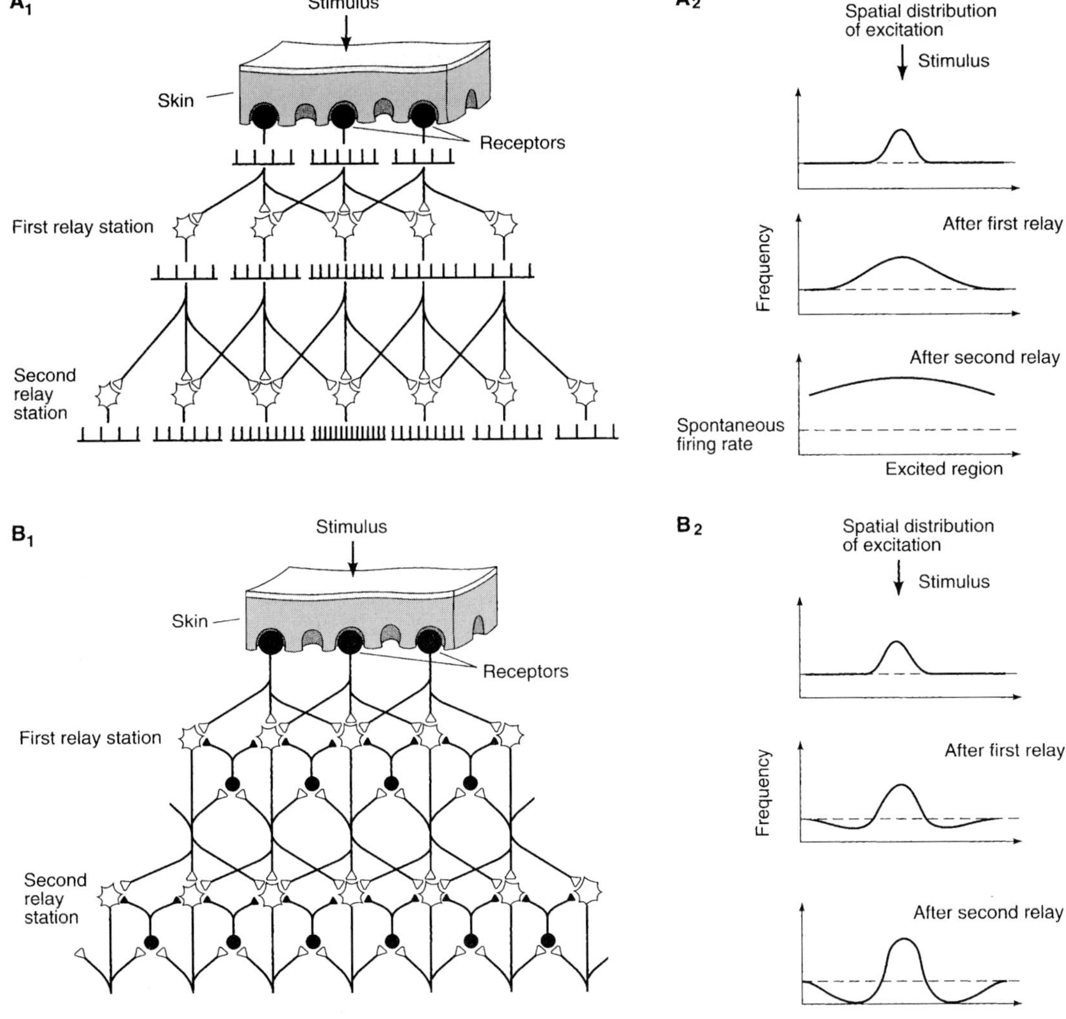

FIGURE 71–4. A_1, Diagram of the excitatory synaptic connections among three receptors and the interneurons at the next two relays in the absence of inhibitory interneurons. The inset over each axon shows its relative rate of discharge during stimulation. A_2, In the absence of inhibitory interneurons there is a large discharge zone at each of the relays in response to a stimulus in the excitatory region of the receptive field. This process of unrestricted amplification tends to obliterate the troughs between two distinct but close signals impairing two-point discrimination. B_1 and B_2, The addition of inhibitory interneurons (*black*) narrows the discharge zone. On either side of the excitatory region, the discharge rate is driven below resting level by feedback inhibition. This process helps distinguish two close stimuli, facilitating two-point discrimination. (From Martin JH: Sensory systems of the brain. *In* Kandel ER, Schwartz JA, Jessell TM [eds]: Principles of Neural Science, 3rd ed. New York, Elsevier Science Publishing Company, Inc., 1991, p 376. © Appleton & Lange, 1991.)

cortical level. In other words, they facilitate two-point discrimination. Descending fibers from the cerebral cortex can also act on inhibitory interneurons and modify the discriminatory power of the sensory input (Fig. 71–5). In sensory re-education this facilitates the sharpening of digital two-point discrimination to as little as 1.5 mm, enabling the blind to read Braille.

If we assume that the lingual nerve and its CNS connections in the gasserian ganglion, the trigeminal nuclei, and the thalamus represent a far more complex neurosensory unit with greater cortical representation, more inhibitory interneurons, and more capacity for descending inhibition (a feature of greater cortical representation?) than the lateral antebrachial cutaneous nerve, we would have an explanation for sensory upgrading. The reason that the sensory discrimination is so poor in the forearm is not because of a lack of receptors, but more likely because of a comparative lack of sophistication in the lateral antebrachial cutaneous nerve's neurosensory unit. Sensory re-education of the forearm skin in situ (Brown et al, 1989) may improve sensory perception, thereby maximizing whatever descending inhibition is available. However, the architecture of the subcortical relay stations of any given neurosensory unit could easily limit the amount of improvement possible. When the flap is transferred, the lingual nerve, by means of its central connections, is able to make maximal use of the input it receives and give two-point figures approaching normal. It is dubious

whether similar results would be possible if the recipient was one of the supraclavicular nerves, for example. Because these nerves innervate an area of skin with poor sensory acuity (Weinstein, 1968), it seems unlikely that the results would ever match those obtained with either the lingual or the inferior alveolar nerve, sensory re-education notwithstanding. Investigation of the "sensory potential" of free flap donor sites should probably consist of precise mapping of the neurosomes of the body together with analysis of recipient nerves for their sensory acuity and fidelity. Sensory testing in situ is unlikely to be of any predictive importance.

Some mention should be made of "surrogate reinnervation." Here, sensory receptors of one modality may substitute for those of another and provide some degree of useful function. Dellon (1991) has argued that the muscle spindles within free muscle transfers may become reinnervated when the "pure" motor nerve of the transferred muscle is anastomosed to a sensory nerve in the recipient site. Forces that produce deformation of the muscle spindles would then stimulate the sensory nerve, producing feelings of pressure, pain, or paresthesia referred to the neurosome of the recipient nerve. A pathological form of surrogate reinnervation occurs in Frey's syndrome (1923). This is common after parotidectomy and involves secretomotor rather than sensory nerve fibers. It is caused by regeneration of the secretory fibers of the parotid gland (which are contained in the auriculotemporal nerve) to sweat glands in its area of distribution. Thus,

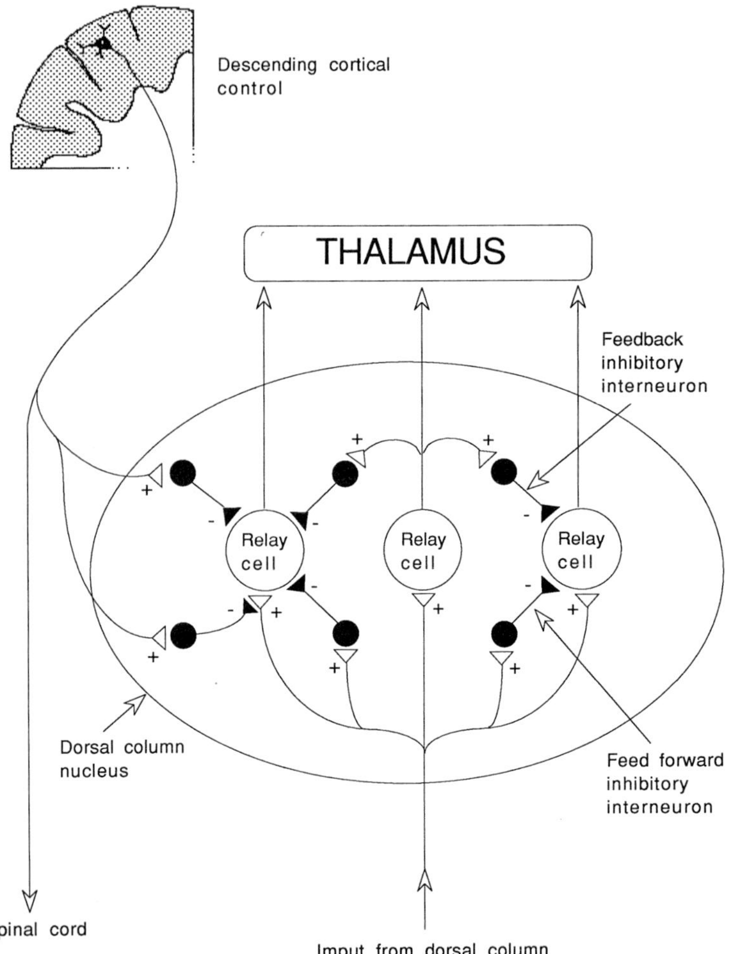

FIGURE 71–5. A typical sensory relay station (here, the dorsal column nucleus) in the central nervous system. Two-point discrimination is facilitated and enhanced by a process of peripheral inhibition. Here, the normal process of amplification (the projection of the signal onto increasing numbers of cell bodies as it travels to the sensory cortex) is suppressed by collateral and descending inhibition so that two distinct stimuli do not summate and continue to be perceived separately. Inhibition is mediated by inhibitory interneurons. Collateral inhibition is derived from collateral branches of the main conducting fiber and may feed forward or feed back as shown. Descending or *distant* inhibition originates from the sensory cortex and can also modify the signal. It may be presynaptic or postsynaptic, and it probably plays a major role in sensory relearning, as well as selective perception. The complexity of these interconnections at such relay stations determines the discriminatory power of a sensory nerve.

the sweat glands respond to the nerve impulses that should provoke reflex parotid secretion.

ANATOMY OF THE NEUROSOME

The outstanding work of Taylor and colleagues (1994) constitutes a timely reference to the anatomical theory underlying the transfer of sensate flaps. It is compulsory reading for basic scientists as well as clinicians working in this area. At the heart of this monograph is the concept of the territorial supply of tissues by arteries, veins, and nerves, and their inter-relationship. Taylor defined the angiosome as a composite vascular territory supplied by a single artery. For the purposes of the present discussion, a neurosome will be considered exactly the same way: an innervated territory supplied by a single nerve. It should be noted that the word "neurotome," refers to a composite nerve root territory just as the word "dermatome" refers to the skin territory of a specific nerve root. Consequently, both neurotomes and dermatomes are associated with individual spinal levels such as L1, S5, etc. This is impractical when the transfer of sensate tissue is being planned. A sensory nerve may contain fibers derived from multiple spinal levels, and it is of more practical value to know the extent of its own cutaneous territory rather than root values that may be shared with other neurosomes.

Many sensory nerves supply twigs to the ligaments and joints over which they pass. Technically, these structures belong to the neurosome of the sensory nerve in question. However, unless a joint or ligament is being transferred together with the skin (as in a toe to thumb transfer), these components of the neurosome are not usually considered in its description. Practically speaking, sensory neurosomes consist of skin or mucosa, and those of motor nerves consist only of muscle (setting aside the issue of the muscle spindles!). Clearly, then, the neurosome of a mixed nerve will include both skin and muscle (as in the case of the segmental nerves supplying the rectus abdominis).

Because a reliable blood supply is required for flap survival and predictable innervation essential for sensation, some relationship between angiosome and neurosome is desirable. Many of the long axial skin flaps that have appeared in the literature over the past three decades are in fact neurovascular flaps. Taylor's work (1994) has shown that the neurosome often overlaps several vascular territories. This correlates with his finding that a cutaneous nerve is often associated with a chain-linked system of vessels that may be derived from the same or adjacent angiosomes. In practical terms, known flaps are frequently assessed for their sensation-bearing potential either by anatomical dissections or by selective nerve blocks. The design of flaps may be modified to incorporate the desired neurosome; occasionally, ways are sought to vascularize a specific nerve territory. Care should be taken in interpreting the results of anatomical dissections: frequently, large nerves pass through subcutaneous tissue without supplying the overlying skin ("neurosensory flow-through flap"). The fibers supplying a particular patch of dermis are probably too fine to dissect in its immediate vicinity. The notion of a "dual nerve supply" is often an erroneous assumption based on the anatomical findings of two nerves in close proximity. It is more likely that each has its own individual neurosome, one nerve merely "passing through" on its way elsewhere.

Finally, it should be noted that there is frequently a significant overlap between adjacent neurosomes just as there is between adjacent angiosomes. As with angiosomes, there is a certain amount of plasticity in the arrangement: when one neurosome is denervated by division of its nerve (or harvesting of a flap) there is initially a large area of sensory loss that shrinks with time. Part of the neurosome is "captured" by adjacent intact nerve territories. The mechanism by which this occurs is unclear, but it is probably related to an anatomical overlap together with some degree of cortical relearning. Some degree of neural ingrowth cannot be excluded.

SENSATE FLAPS

Digital Flaps

Many variants of sensate digital flaps have been described for hand reconstruction. Basically, there are seven types: type 1, neurovascular island flap used as an advancement flap for fingertip injuries in the same digit; type 2, neurovascular island flap (Fig. 71–6) with a rerouted, intact, neurovascular pedicle (innervated neurovascular island flap); type 3, neurovascular island flap with a rerouted, intact vascular pedicle and neuroanastomosis to a recipient digital nerve (reinnervated neurovascular island flap); type 4, reversed neurovascular island flap (Fig. 71–7) with retrograde flow through a rerouted, distal, intact vascular pedicle and neuroanastomosis to a recipient digital nerve (reversed reinnervated neurovascular island flap); type 5, staged cross-finger flap with rerouting of neural pedicle (innervated cross finger flap); type 6, staged cross-finger flap with neuroanastomosis to a recipient digital nerve (reinnervated cross finger flap); and type 7, neurovascular island flap transplanted using vascular and neuroanastomosis (reinnervated free flap).

NEUROVASCULAR ISLAND FLAPS

Anatomy. Neurovascular island flaps are based on the digital artery, vein, and nerve of a finger. Although not recognized as such, their simplest form is represented by the V-Y advancements of Kutler (1947) and Kleinert (1959) used for fingertip reconstruction. Moberg (1964) and Snow (1967, 1973) extended the principle by mobilizing and advancing almost the entire volar skin of the thumb (Moberg) and fingers (Snow) and relying on flexion of the denuded digit to facilitate distal closure. Venkataswami and Subramanian (1980) elevated a large oblique neurovascular island flap that they advanced in V-Y manner by stretching the pedicle.

However, the classical neurovascular island flap (Littler, 1960; Moberg, 1955) usually consists of the corresponding hemi-pulp of the finger extending proximally as far as is necessary on the digit (see Fig. 71–6). The donor site is repaired with a skin graft and the flap is transferred to where sensation and cover are more vitally required, usually the thumb. To overcome difficulties with spatial relearning, the nerve can be transected proximally in the finger and its distal stump anastomosed to the recipient digital nerve in the thumb.

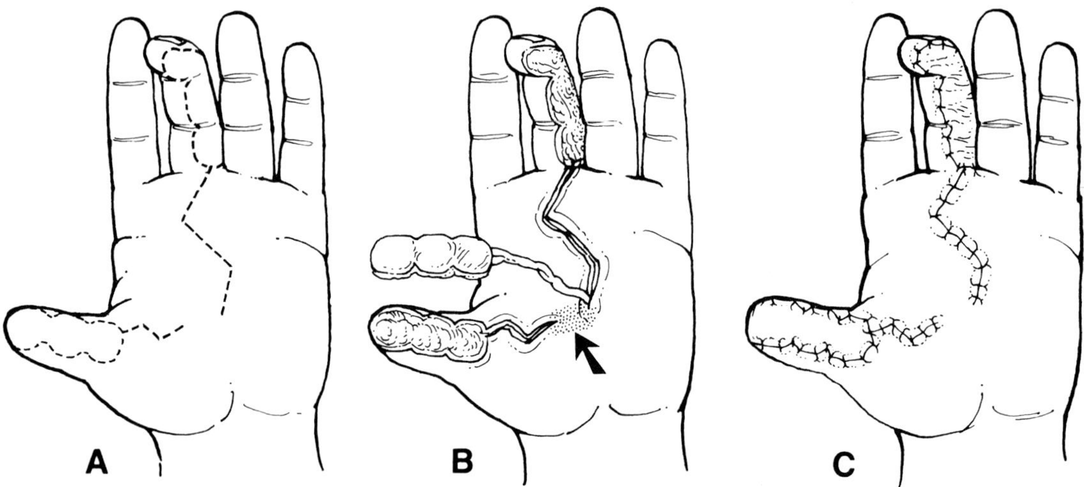

FIGURE 71–6. Diagram of a neurovascular island transfer from the long finger to the thumb. The entire ulnar side of the long finger is taken to resurface the volar aspect of the thumb. The pedicle is dissected into the palm and then tunneled a short distance. The donor defect is skin grafted. Longitudinal scars are avoided there by making zig-zag incisions. (From Strickland JW: Thumb reconstruction. *In* Green DP [ed]: Operative Hand Surgery. New York, Churchill Livingstone, 1982, p 1571.)

Reverse neurovascular island flaps have also been described (Lai et al, 1995). These flaps rely on a retrograde flow via the contralateral digital vessels, but their donor sites have the advantage of being situated inconspicuously at the side of the proximal phalanx (Fig. 71–7). A long pedicle allows a wide arc of rotation, allowing the flap to be used for repair of either the same or an adjacent digit. The former depends on intact anastomoses between the two digital arteries at the finger pulp. The latter involves its use as a staged cross-finger flap. The digital nerve is not taken, but its dorsal branch may be included either as a flow-through graft or as a means of reinnervating the flap itself. It may be used to bridge a digital nerve defect in an adjacent finger or provide it with a sensate tip.

Indications. The most common use of the innervated neurovascular island flap is for thumb reconstruction when there has been extensive loss of the pulp. It may also be used secondarily to provide sensation to a thumb reconstructed by noninnervated means. The reversed reinnervated neurovascular island flap may be used for adjacent fingertip repair when there has been a loss of pulp, but its main indication lies in defects of nerve and skin on the side of that digit.

Elevation and Closure. The conventional neurovascular flap is designed in the ulnar side of the long or ring finger. A reverse template is used to define the size and shape of the flap that will extend proximally from the distal pulp. A zigzag incision then connects the flap to the distal palmer crease and then to the thumb defect. Using loupe magnification, the neurovascular bundle is identified at the base of the finger. It is traced distally into the flap, the plane of dissection remaining deep to it. The flap and bundle are elevated from the finger. Dissection then proceeds into the palm toward the origin of the digital vessels from the palmer arch. The flap is pedicled at this point and transposed to fill the thumb defect. A skin graft is used to repair the donor defect and is held in place by a meticulous tie-over dressing.

Elevation of the reverse neurovascular flap involves the separation of the digital nerve from the artery. At the same time, a large quantity of fatty tissue is included with the vessel to ensure adequate venous drainage. The skin flap is designed over the radial or ulnar aspect of the proximal phalanx. A fine Doppler probe can be used to locate the digital artery. The proximal incision is made first and the vessel is identified and ligated. The digital nerve is left intact, but its dorsal branch is divided at its origin on a level with the proximal volar digital crease. The flap is elevated with artery and dorsal branch of the nerve as far distally as required. As with the conventional neurovascular flap, the donor site is skin grafted.

Comments. Although sensory return is excellent after conventional neurovascular transfer, there is a severe problem with cortical representation (Murray et al, 1967). The patient perceives the sensory return as emanating from the donor digit. So severely does this reduce the usefulness of the transfer that some have described dividing the nerve and anastomosing it to the stumps of the thenar digital nerves.

STAGED CROSS-FINGER FLAPS

Like neurovascular island flaps, sensate cross-finger flaps have mostly—but not entirely—been described for thumb reconstruction. Conventionally, a cross-finger flap is derived from the dorsal skin of an adjacent finger and pedicled, like a page of a book, along its radial or ulnar border, dorsal to its digital vessels. The flap is elevated superficially to the extensor paratenon, which is then skin grafted. The skin pedicle is divided at a second stage 2 to 3 weeks later. The radial innervated cross-finger flap to the thumb (Adamson et al, 1967; Brailler and Horner, 1969; Gaul, 1969; Miura, 1973; Wilkinson, 1972) is based on the skin over the dorsum of the proximal phalanx of the index and the dorsal branch of the radial nerve. It can be used to provide the thumb with tactile pulp. At the first operation, the nerve is identified in the dorsum of the hand, traced into the flap; and, via connecting incisions, rerouted into the thumb. The innervated flap is then elevated and attached to the defect. The flap may be reinnervated by dividing the nerve and anastomosing it to

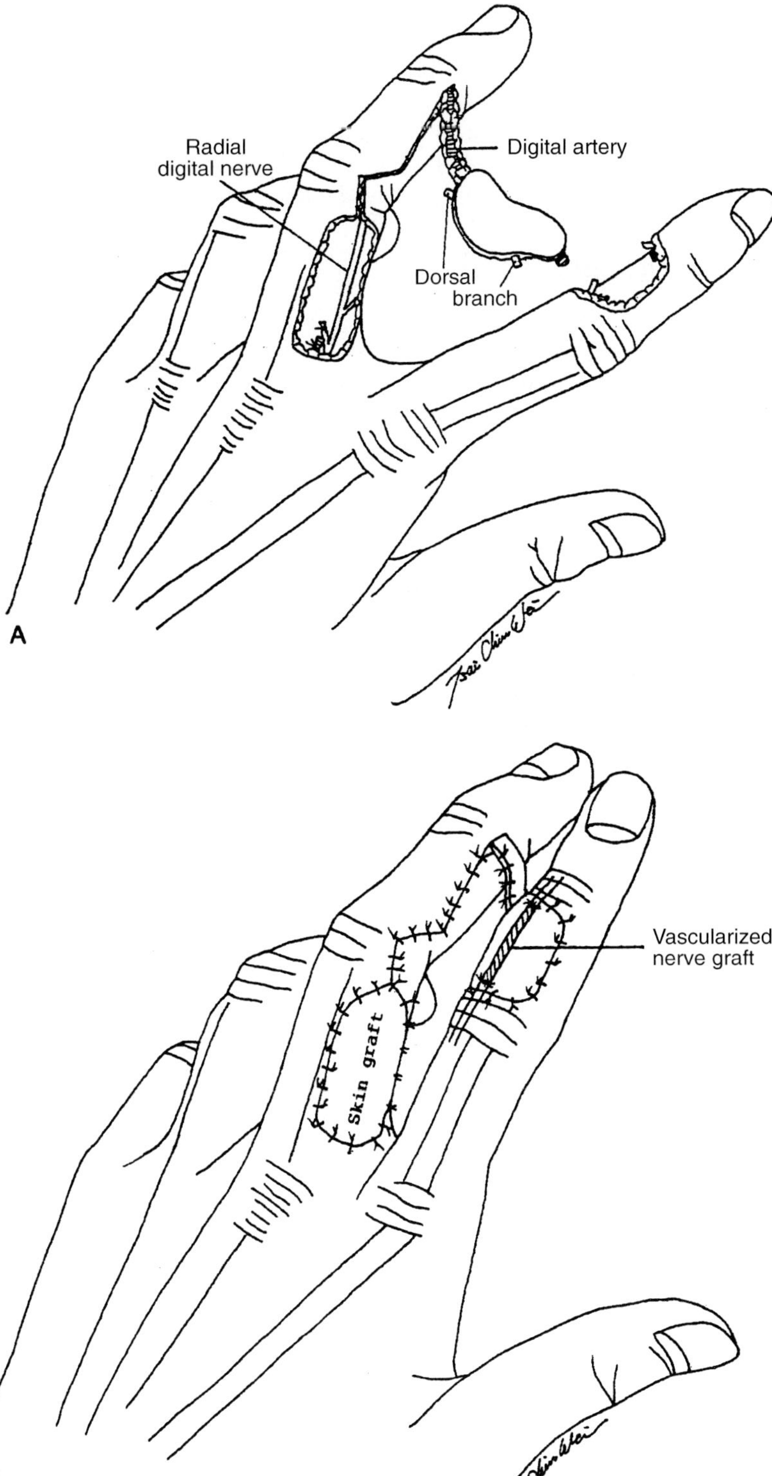

FIGURE 71–7. The reverse digital artery flap contains a segment of the digital nerve's dorsal branch. The digital nerve proper is left undisturbed. The vascularized nerve graft makes this a "neurosensory flow-through flap" which may be used for nerve and skin repairs in the same or an adjacent digit. (From Lai C-S, Lin S-D, Tsai C-C, Tsai C-W: Reverse digital artery neurovascular and cross-finger flap. J Hand Surg 20:397, 1995. © Churchill Livingstone, New York.)

one or both digital nerves, if available. This would not only provide better spatial recognition, but would theoretically provide superior sensory acuity.

Sensate cross-finger flaps based on skin overlying the middle phalanx are innervated via the dorsal branch of the digital nerve. Such flaps are useful in resurfacing more distal defects on the volar aspect of adjacent digits. Once again,

the flap may be either innervated by nerve rerouting (Joshi, 1976) or reinnervated by neuroanastomosis (Cohen and Cronin, 1983). The former option involves interconnecting incisions, fascicular stripping, and transposition of the dorsal sensory nerve from the donor to the damaged digit. Reinnervation carries the same advantages as previously stated.

Reinnervated staged pedicle flaps to the thumb and fingers

may also be derived from other areas of the body that are comfortably accessible to the hand, have thin and supple skin, and have an easily identifiable yet expendable nerve supply. Such flaps include the cross-forearm neurocutaneous flap based on the dorsal branch of the radial nerve (Dolich et al, 1978) and the supraclavicular innervated flap based on the supraclavicular nerves (Sommerlad and Boorman, 1981).

REINNERVATED DIGITAL FREE FLAPS

Digital replantation (Komatsu and Tamai, 1968), toe to thumb transfers (Cobbett, 1969; Ohmori and Harii, 1975), and wraparound procedures (Morrison et al, 1980) are all examples of reinnervated digital free flaps. The details of these procedures lie beyond the scope of this chapter, but, setting aside orthotopic replantation, it should be emphasized that the anticipated sensory return matches that of the recipient site more closely than that of the donor (Boyd et al, 1994; Dykes et al, 1979). These flaps also have the advantage of replacing specialized tissue with like tissue. Their ability to carry specialized sensory receptors means that sensory return may involve stereognosis in addition to two-point discrimination. Although it has never been proved, this would represent a qualitative improvement in sensory return over that achieved by other sensate flaps. Reinnervated partial toe transfers for hand reconstruction include the free pulp flap and the first web space flap.

PARTIAL TOE FLAPS

Anatomy. The toes have a dual system of arterial vascularization via dorsal and plantar metatarsal arteries and their paired digital branches. There is a communicating vessel at the distal end of the intermetacarpal space that allows the toe or part thereof to be taken on the dorsalis pedis artery while incorporating both the plantar and the dorsal digital vessels. The anatomy of the dorsalis pedis–first dorsal metatarsal artery is discussed under the dorsalis pedis flap (see below). The first web space flap is based on the same vascular system as the partial toe pulp flap. A single digital nerve supplies the pulp, whereas, in the case of the first web space flap, the nerve supply is derived from the deep peroneal nerve (supplies apex of first web space) and the plantar digital nerves (supply sides of toes).

Indications. Free pulp transfer can replace traumatic or surgical loss of a fingertip or be used to secondarily reconstruct an atrophic, painful, or insensate pulp on a damaged finger. Generally, it is only used when cross-finger alternatives are not possible; however, this may be changing because the cosmetic results are superior and the functional return excellent (Gilbert, 1976). The flap may be customized by including part of the nail bed, the web space, or even the terminal phalanx. The inclusion of any more tissue would render it a toe transfer. The first web space flap provides a surprisingly large amount of glabrous skin for reinnervated hand reconstruction. When opened up, the flap can have dimensions of 7 × 15 cm in the adult. This tissue has the ideal quality for innervated hand reconstruction, particularly in extensive degloving injuries when a sensate opposition pad is required.

Elevation and Closure. The flaps are mapped out on the skin using a reverse template procedure. Venous drainage is provided by means of the superficial venous system that may be identified and marked out preoperatively with the aid of a tourniquet. A longitudinal incision over the dorsalis pedis artery is then used to dissect a suitable vein and trace it into the proximal margin of the flap. The dorsalis pedis–first metatarsal axis is dissected out as described under the dorsalis pedis flap (see below). The deep branch of the peroneal nerve can be seen passing into the web. It is dissected proximally to obtain maximal pedicle length and distally into the proximal margin of the flap. At the distant level of the intermetatarsal space, the communicating branch of the artery is dissected through to the sole to include both the dorsal and plantar arterial systems in the flap. In the case of the web-space flap, the vessels to both sides of the web are included, whereas only those passing to the lateral side of the great toe are taken with the toe pulp flap. The digital nerves are identified running with the plantar arteries and may be dissected proximally to obtain greater length. Once all the relevant structures have been dissected into the flap, the flap is elevated together with the soft tissue that envelops them. The defect is meticulously repaired using a split-thickness skin graft held in place with a bolus tie-over dressing.

Comments. In finger and thumb reconstruction, the pulp flap replaces like tissue with like and, because of its specialized nature, looks extremely natural and functions superbly. It is the best cosmetic substitute for digital pulp and, unlike cross-finger flaps, limits the scarring to the finger being reconstructed. However, in this era of managed care, it is difficult to justify such a complex and expensive operation for something that can be handled almost as well by much simpler and cheaper means. The operation is popular in the Orient, where the appearance of the female hand is valued more highly than the function of her foot.

With the proliferation of innervated flaps, the web-space flap is used less often than formerly. However, with its specialized glabrous nature, it remains an outstanding flap for resurfacing parts of severely injured hands.

Forearm Flaps

Radial (Yang et al, 1981) and ulnar (Lovie et al, 1984) forearm flaps are fasciocutaneous flaps based on each of the major forearm arteries.

RADIAL FOREARM

Anatomy. The skin of the anterior forearm is supplied by the radial artery via septocutaneous vessels passing along the septum between the brachioradialis and the flexor carpi radialis muscles. After emerging from the septum, the vessels branch laterally and medially, piercing the deep fascia and quickly passing to the subdermal plexus to supply the skin. These vessels do not travel on the surface of the deep fascia for any significant distance; therefore, very little of the deep fascia needs to be taken when a skin flap based on the radial artery is raised.

Practically the whole anterior and anterolateral forearm

skin may be safely harvested. Raising a flap of such dimensions would require the entire vascular septum to be preserved. The "base" of any radial forearm skin flap is that portion in direct contact with the vascular septum. Like any flap, if the base is made shorter, the surviving length is reduced.

In the distal third of the forearm, the radial artery first overlies the flexor pollicis longus and then the pronator quadratus. These two muscles intimately clothe the flat anterior surface of the distal radius. Muscular branches from the radial artery give periosteal twigs to the underlying bone and are the basis for the osseous component of the flap if one is required (Berger and Meissl, 1975; Soutar et al, 1983).

In the region of the bifurcation of the brachial artery, there is a confluence of veins. Here the venae comitantes of both ulnar and radial arteries communicate with each other as well as with one or more of the large subcutaneous veins of the forearm. Either the deep or superficial system can be used for venous drainage. The superficial veins are often preferred because of their greater diameter and their independence from the arterial pedicle.

The medial antebrachial cutaneous nerve (C8, T1) enters the forearm in the company of the basilic vein (Fig. 71–8). It soon gives a number of large anterior branches that pass

down the radial side of the basilic vein and supply the ulnar half of the anterior forearm as far as the wrist. An ulnar branch supplies the ulnar border of the forearm. The lateral antebrachial cutaneous nerve (C5, C6) is the forearm continuation of the musculocutaneous nerve. It enters the forearm on the ulnar side of the cephalic vein (Fig. 71–8) and, via multiple branches, supplies the radial half of the forearm as far as the wrist as well as the dorsoradial aspect of the forearm.

Operative Technique. The radial artery and cephalic vein are marked on the skin surface, and the flap is positioned to straddle them in the distal forearm. The watershed between the neurosomes of the lateral and medial antebrachial cutaneous nerves lies down the midline of the anterior forearm. Flaps positioned over the cephalic vein and extending to the midline need only the lateral antebrachial cutaneous nerve for full reinnervation. Those positioned centrally—and occupying two neurosomes—require both superficial nerves for optimal sensory return (Boyd et al, 1994).

Under tourniquet control the skin flap is incised, and dissection is carried down to the muscle fascia. Proximally, the cephalic vein is identified and preserved. An incision passing from the flap to the antecubital fossa permits dissection of this vessel. The sensory nerves lie immediately superficial to the deep fascia. Precise identification of the nerves is best made in the proximal forearm, where they are large and located next to the cephalic and basilic veins. These nerves and their delicate branches are traced into the proximal margin of the flap, encased in a protective mesentery of deep subcutaneous tissue.

The ulnar dissection is performed just superficial to the deep fascia, working toward the intermuscular septum between the brachioradialis and the flexor carpi radialis. One centimeter from the septum, dissection passes beneath the deep fascia, remaining superficial to the paratenon of the flexor carpi radialis. It then extends around the radial edge of the tendon into the space beneath. The radial dissection also passes immediately superficial to the deep fascia until 1 centimeter lateral to the intermuscular septum, where the deep fascia is incised. The brachioradialis tendon is seen and the dissection hugs the paratenon of this tendon. Once around its ulnar border, the radial artery becomes visible. This is ligated and divided at the distal margin of the flap. The superficial branch of the radial nerve passes through the deep portion of the flap and is visible during the radial dissection. It can be easily dissected from the undersurface of the flap, and *it is virtually never necessary to sacrifice it.*

The flap, together with its vascular leash, is elevated from its bed and stripped proximally. The superficial venous system communicates with the deep system of veins just distal to the origin of the radial artery. Both cephalic vein and superficial nerves may be dissected into the upper arm to obtain greater length. Perfusion of the hand is assessed after tourniquet release: the surgeon should be prepared to graft the radial artery in the face of obvious arterial insufficiency.

To facilitate wound closure, the palmaris longus tendon is usually removed and discarded. The paratenons are approximated to provide a flat, well-vascularized bed to receive an unmeshed skin graft.

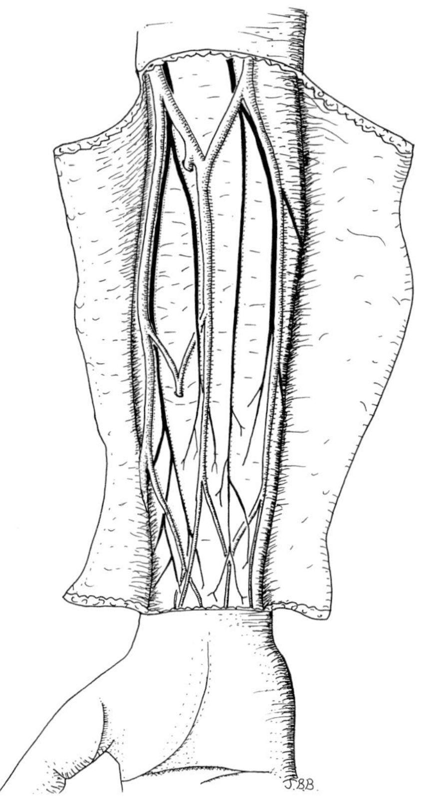

FIGURE 71–8. The lateral antebrachial cutaneous (LABC) neurosome flap is centered over a longitudinal line running between the radial artery and the cephalic vein in the distal forearm. This appears to be the area of maximal cutaneous innervation (neurosome) of the LABC nerve. The watershed between LABC and medial antebrachial cutaneous (MABC) neurosomes lies down the midline of the anterior forearm. The main trunks of the LABC and MABC nerves are located internal to their associated veins in the proximal forearm. This is where they should be identified because their peripheral branches are tiny. The donor nerve or nerves harvested during elevation of a radial or ulnar innervated forearm flap depends on the location of the skin paddle with respect to the two neurosomes.

Indications. The innervated radial forearm flap finds its most frequent indication in oromandibular reconstruction, where a thin, pliable flap is required for oral lining (Soutar et al, 1983), bone is available if needed, and sensory return can restore oral function (Boyd et al, 1994; Dubner and Heller, 1992; Urken et al, 1990). Defects where sensory return is most important include the lower lip, anterior floor of mouth, and tongue.

Resurfacing of weightbearing amputation stumps, the sole of foot, and the heel are less frequent indications (Chicarilli and Price, 1986). The use of the radial forearm flap in hand and thumb reconstruction has also been described (Biemer and Stock, 1983).

Comments. The reinnervated radial forearm flap is likely to remain the most frequently used sensate flap because of its large potential surface area, its constant anatomy, its thinness and versatility, its ease of elevation, and its well-tolerated donor site. The donor defect becomes more significant when radial bone is taken for composite reconstruction, but this is often an acceptable trade-off when its unique advantages are taken into consideration.

ULNAR FOREARM

Anatomy. The ulnar artery, like the radial, commences at the bifurcation of the brachial artery in the proximal forearm. It passes under the pronator teres, the median nerve, the flexor carpi radialis, the palmaris longus, and the flexor digitorum superficialis. It reaches the flexor carpi ulnaris at the mid-forearm and then runs distally between this and the flexor digitorum superficialis. The ulnar nerve lies on its medial side in its distal two thirds. The vessel leaves the forearm, passing superficial to the flexor retinaculum and lateral to the pisiform bone. Via fasciocutaneous branches that pass between the flexor carpi ulnaris and the flexor digitorum superficialis muscles, it contributes to the blood supply of the overlying skin. The distribution of the superficial cutaneous nerves and veins has already been discussed.

Indications. The ulnar forearm flap has the same indications as the radial forearm flap.

Elevation and Closure. A line joining the medial epicondyle to the lateral edge of the pisiform bone traces the course of the ulnar nerve and artery in the distal two thirds of the forearm. The skin flap is designed to straddle this line distally. A more proximal location would position it over the superficial flexors that cross anterior to the artery obstructing the passage of perforators in that zone.

Under tourniquet control, the distal incision is made, and the ulnar artery and nerve are located between the flexor carpi ulnaris and the flexor digitorum superficialis. The artery is carefully separated from the nerve. Proximally, the basilic vein is identified and the wound extended toward the antecubital fossa. In that region, the medial cutaneous nerve of the forearm is easily identified as one or two main trunks lying alongside the vein. To avoid damage to the smaller branching filaments of this nerve, it is best to include them and the basilic vein in a "mesentery" of protective subcutaneous tissue that may be traced into the proximal margin of the flap.

The medial and lateral portions of the dissection are then carried out as with the radial forearm flap. The major difference is the presence of the ulnar nerve, which is carefully separated from the vascular bundle during the medial dissection. This, in turn, is greatly facilitated by medial retraction of the flexor carpi ulnaris. Completion of the lateral dissection allows the vascular pedicle to be divided distal to the flap and dissected out of its bed. Proximally, the pedicle is divided just distal to the common interosseous artery. Distal placement of the skin paddle increases pedicle length.

Comments. Although the ulnar forearm flap has the same indications as the radial forearm flap, there are certain advantages. First, it is situated on the ulnar border of the anterior forearm, so the donor scar is less conspicuous. Second, and for the same reason, it is less likely to be hairbearing. On the down side, its pedicle is shorter than that of the radial forearm flap because of the desirability of maintaining the integrity the common interosseous artery. This vessel comes off the ulnar artery shortly after its origin.

Lateral Arm Flap

Anatomy. The deep brachial artery (profunda brachii) divides into its two terminal branches while traveling along the groove for the radial nerve. The middle collateral artery descends within the medial head of the triceps while the radial collateral artery continues to accompany the nerve. On the lateral aspect of the humerus, this artery itself divides into two: an anterior branch that accompanies the radial nerve between the brachialis and brachioradialis and a posterior branch that enters the lateral intermuscular septum between the brachioradialis and triceps, passing down toward the lateral epicondyle. This posterior branch of the radial collateral artery gives off fasciocutaneous branches to supply the skin of the lower lateral arm. The first of these is closely related to the posterior cutaneous nerve of the forearm. Venous drainage is provided by the venae comitantes of the radial collateral artery or the cephalic vein. The flap is innervated, not by the posterior cutaneous nerve of the forearm, which passes through, but by the lower lateral cutaneous nerve of the arm, a branch of the radial. This perforates the lateral head of the triceps just behind the deltoid insertion.

Indications. This flap has been described for head and neck reconstruction (Matloub et al, 1989) as well as resurfacing the hand (Katsaros et al, 1984; Song et al, 1982). The size of the skin paddle may be very large, and it may safely be extended from the lower lateral arm down onto the lateral aspect of the adjacent forearm. For this reason, large sensate reconstructions may be contemplated, including the sole of foot and the penis (Shenaq and Dinh, 1989).

Elevation and Closure. The axis of the flap is a line drawn from the insertion of the deltoid to the lateral epicondyle of the humerus. The distal half of the lateral aspect of the arm can be taken along with the lateral aspect of the proximal fifth of the forearm. Flaps of up to 15×20 cm of skin may be harvested.

The sensory nerve to the flap, the lower lateral cutaneous

nerve of the arm, is located in the soft tissues at the posterior proximal edge of the flap and preserved. The posterior dissection is then carried out subfascially until the lateral intermuscular septum is reached. Dissection then proceeds inward, keeping outside the septum. Small branches to the triceps are ligated, and this muscle is retracted posteriorly. The posterior branch of the radial collateral artery and the posterior cutaneous nerve of forearm are identified within the septum. Next, the anterior dissection is performed as a mirror image of the posterior dissection. When the posterior branch of the radial collateral artery and the posterior cutaneous nerve of forearm are identified, the nerve is sacrificed and the artery divided distally. The septum is then detached from the humerus and the flap lifted outward. Dissection of the vascular pedicle proceeds proximally (the skin incision may need to be lengthened) and the anterior branch of the artery is divided. The radial collateral vessels are dissected for extra pedicle length, which can vary according to flap design (4 to 8 cm).

Comments. This is a reliable and versatile flap. It is usually hairless and almost as thin as a radial forearm flap. The donor-site deficit is mild if primary closure can be achieved, and this is much more likely than in the case of the forearm. However, the dissection is a little more difficult and the vessels a little smaller. Furthermore, tourniquet control is difficult to use.

Lateral Thigh Flap

Anatomy. The innervated or reinnervated lateral thigh flap (Baek, 1983; Hayden, 1994) is based on the lateral cutaneous nerve of the thigh (Fig. 71–9). As a free tissue transfer, its vascular pedicle is the third cutaneous perforator of the profunda femoris artery together with its venae comitantes. (The dominant supply is rarely from the second or the fourth perforators.) This vessel exits the lateral thigh between the biceps femoris and the vastus lateralis (the lateral intermuscular septum) halfway between the greater trochanter and the lateral condyle of the femur. It supplies a large area of lateral thigh skin, permitting a longitudinal ellipse, centered on this perforator and oriented along the intermuscular septum, to be safely harvested.

The third perforator branches off the profunda femoris artery just distal to the insertion of the adductor brevis into the linea aspera (Fig. 71–9). It passes round the posterior aspect of the femur close to the bone, perforating various muscles to which it sends branches. Its terminal cutaneous branch reaches the lateral intermuscular septum by penetrating the femoral head of the biceps femoris or simply passing behind it. The length of the vascular pedicle measured from the origin of the third perforator is 8 to 12 cm.

The lateral femoral cutaneous nerve enters the thigh under the lateral extremity of the inguinal ligament just medial to the anterior superior iliac spine (Fig 71–9). It passes distally and laterally either anterior to, through, or posterior to the sartorius muscle. It bifurcates, sending branches down into the anterior and lateral thighs. These nerves then branch extensively before entering the dermis.

Indications. The sensate lateral thigh flap could be used as a superiorly based, innervated, random flap to resurface

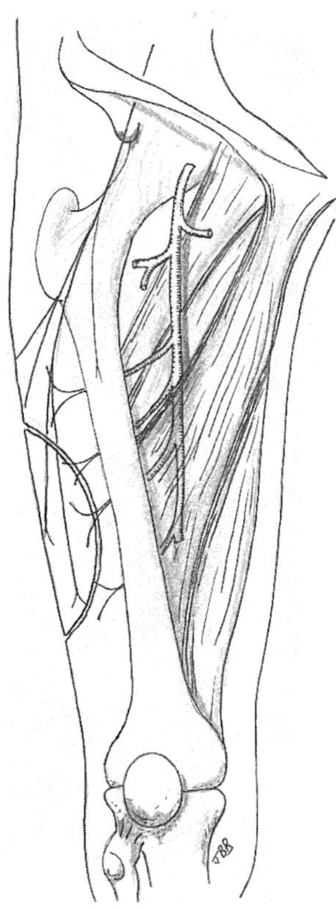

FIGURE 71–9. The lateral thigh flap is supplied by the third perforator of the profunda femoris artery. It passes to the skin via the lateral intermuscular septum. Innervation is by the lateral cutaneous nerve of the thigh, which emerges from the abdomen under the lateral extremity of the inguinal ligament. As with other innervated flaps, the sensory nerve should be identified proximally and traced toward the flap swaddling the terminal branches in a cloak of connective tissue.

trochanteric ulcers. Here, delay procedures would be helpful to obtain sufficient length. However, it is more commonly used as a free flap in the reconstruction of large postablative head and neck and burn defects (Hayden, 1994). Although bulkier than the forearm flap, it may be used for intraoral lining, particularly when that extra bulk would be useful, such as in tongue reconstruction. Severe anterior neck burn contractures have been excised and replaced by this flap, which is one of the few large enough to do the job.

Elevation and Closure. The patient is supine with hip flexed, adducted, and internally rotated. The knee is flexed and secured over a pillow with a cushion under the heel. A line is drawn between the greater trochanter and the lateral femoral condyle. The flap is oriented along this line and centered at its midpoint. The exact position of the third perforator may be identified by Doppler probe and the position of the flap adjusted to suit the siting requirements of the vascular pedicle.

The anterior part of the flap is elevated toward the lateral intermuscular septum. The fascia lata may be included or excluded as required. When the lateral intermuscular septum is reached, the third perforator is identified within its substance. The second and fourth should also come into view about 5 cm cephalic and 5 cm caudal, respectively. The vastus lateralis is retracted anteriorly and dissection proceeds inwards toward the linea aspera. Muscular branches to the vastus lateralis and biceps femoris are ligated and divided, as are the fasciocutaneous branches of the second and fourth perforators.

The posterior part of the flap is then raised with dissection proceeding inward along the posterior surface of the lateral intermuscular septum. To preserve the pedicle, part of the origin of the short head of the biceps may be detached from the femur. Mobilizing the long head of biceps then allows its retraction. The third perforator is traced to the deep femoral vessels by windowing the adductor magnus.

Branches of the lateral femoral cutaneous nerve enter the flap from its anterior and superior aspects. However, at this level they are extremely fine, difficult to identify, and easy to damage. It is better to make a separate incision over the sartorius muscle, identify the main trunk of the nerve, and trace it distally until it gives off the branch to the anterior thigh (see Fig. 71–9). This may then be severed. Nerve filaments are then traced into the flap within a protective mesentery of subcutaneous tissue.

Comments. Like the radial forearm flap, the lateral thigh flap is capable of supplying a vast amount of potentially sensate skin to the reconstructive surgeon. Although dependent on the patient's body habitus, the tissue is generally thin, hairless, and pliable. In most cases, however, radial forearm skin would be thinner. The remote donor site facilitates two-team head and neck surgery and is reasonably well tolerated.

Tensor Fascia Lata Flap

Anatomy. The tensor fascia lata (TFL) takes origin from the anterior superior iliac spine and the outer lip of the adjacent 5 cm of iliac crest. It inserts via the iliotibial band into the lateral condyle of the tibia. The muscle measures approximately 18 cm in length, 5 cm in width, and 1.5 cm in thickness; it gives way to fascia just below the level of the greater trochanter. It acts as an accessory flexor and medial rotator of the thigh.

The main blood supply of the muscle is derived from the lateral circumflex femoral artery and its two venae comitantes. This usually originates from the lateral side of the profunda femoris artery. It passes laterally between the branches of the femoral nerve, behind the sartorius and rectus femoris muscles, and divides into three major branches. The ascending branch is the major vessel to the TFL. It reaches its target 8 cm below the anterior superior iliac spine after passing upward and laterally between the rectus femoris and the vastus lateralis. Before entering the muscle, the artery divides into three branches: superior, middle, and inferior. There are between five and seven musculocutaneous perforators from the muscle to the overlying skin and the iliac crest. The lowest perforator runs down over the iliotibial tract to supply skin over the lower lateral thigh.

The motor nerve of the TFL muscle is the inferior branch of the superior gluteal nerve. This nerve courses between gluteus medius and minimus, entering the underside of TFL near its vascular pedicle. Sensation to the lateral thigh skin is dual: T12 to the upper third and the lateral femoral cutaneous nerve to the rest; T12 pierces the external oblique just above the iliac crest in the anterior axillary line. The lateral femoral cutaneous nerve emerges from under the lateral border of the inguinal ligament and runs downward and laterally, piercing the deep fascia over the sartorius.

Indications. Although not widely advocated as a functional muscle flap, it has great potential for use in the total glossectomy defect (Haughey, 1993). Here, a functioning tongue reconstruction may be rendered sensate by appropriate nerve anastomoses. As a pedicled flap, the TFL has been used for the repair of trochanteric ulcers (Mathes and Nahai, 1979). However, the lateral femoral cutaneous nerve would be severed during its mobilization. To preserve sensation in the distal portion of the flap, the nerve would have to be elongated with a graft. Where there is a significant amount of tissue loss, the relative bulkiness of this flap can prove a great advantage. The strong fascia it contains can also come in useful in the repair of dense retaining structures like the abdominal wall and the Achilles tendon.

Elevation and Closure. The anterior border of the muscle is surface-marked by a line connecting the anterior iliac spine with the lateral border of the patella. A parallel line, 5 cm behind the first, passing through the anterior edge of the greater trochanter and the lateral condyle of the femur, marks its posterior border. A safe skin paddle would reach the iliac crest and extend only a few centimeters anterior or posterior to the muscle. Inferiorly, the flap should be at least 15 cm from the knee.

The vascular pedicle is also surface-marked on the anterior border of the muscle 8 cm below the anterior superior iliac spine.

The flap is raised distal to proximal in the subfascial plane. The dermis is tacked to the fascia lata to protect the perforators. On the undersurface of the TFL, the vascular pedicle should be seen entering the muscle at a point corresponding to its surface-marking.

If a sensory flap is required, the cutaneous branch of T12 is identified above the iliac crest in the anterior axillary line, and the lateral femoral cutaneous nerve is dissected 1 to 2 cm inferomedial to the anterior superior iliac spine. For a functioning muscle transfer, the inferior branch of the superior gluteal nerve is located at the posterior border of the muscle 4 to 5 cm below the crest.

Comments. This flap is very reliable except for the distal 15 to 20 cm of skin overlying the iliotibial tract. Only the smallest of skin paddles would permit primary closure, and a skin graft is usually necessary. There is hardly any functional loss as a result of harvesting this skin-muscle unit, but the donor scar can be very conspicuous.

Fibula Flap

Anatomy. The fibula flap is based on the peroneal artery, which originates from the posterior tibial artery 7 cm distal to the head of the fibula. This vessel passes inferolaterally toward the fibula between the tibialis posterior and soleus muscles. It then runs down the medial crest of the fibula either within the substance of the flexor hallucis muscle or on its posterior surface. At the ankle it divides into its calcaneal branches. Although it gives off a large nutrient artery to the middle third of the fibula, it is also responsible for a significant periosteal supply via segmental vessels that encircle the fibular shaft. In the mid to lower third of the leg, these give rise to sizable skin perforators capable of sustaining a large skin paddle.

Some perforators emerge at the posterior crural septum; others emerge slightly behind, after passing through the lateral fibers of the soleus muscle.

The cutaneous nerve supply to the lateral leg (Fig. 71–10) is derived from the common fibular (peroneal) nerve, which, shortly before winding round the neck of the fibula, gives off the lateral sural cutaneous nerve (LSCN). This, in turn, gives off the communicating fibular cutaneous nerve (CFCN) that angles posteriorly to join the medial sural cutaneous (sural) nerve. The LSCN then passes down the lateral aspect of the leg that it supplies. Inferiorly, there is a variable area of overlap with the superficial fibular (peroneal) nerve neurosome extending upward for a variable distance via a fascia-piercing "recurrent" branch.

Indications. The innervated fibula flap has been almost exclusively used for oromandibular reconstruction (Mulholland et al, 1995). Here, the fibula may be osteotomized and ultimately osseointegrated to reconstruct the ablated

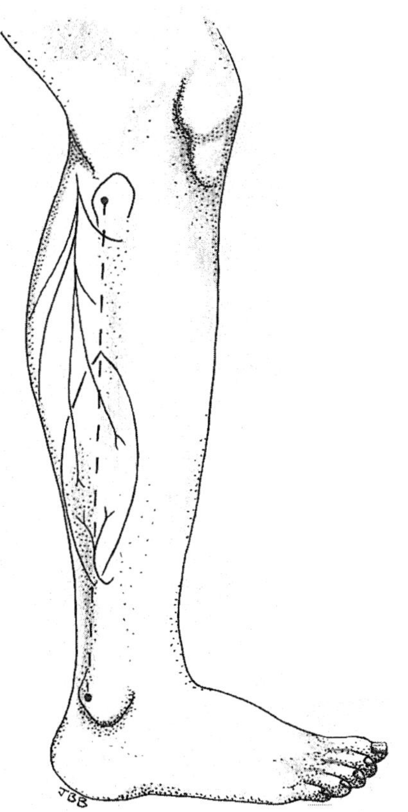

FIGURE 71–10. The skin paddle for the osteocutaneous, innervated fibula flap lies at the junction of the middle and lower thirds of the leg. It is centered over perforators emerging from behind the posterior border of the fibula. These are identified by Doppler probe or angiogram. Sensation is derived from the lateral sural cutaneous nerve (LSCN). The nerve lies in subcutaneous tissue, passing distally through a point 3 to 5 cm behind the center of the fibular head. As in other cases, it is most readily identified proximally and traced into the flap. A recurrent branch from the superficial peroneal nerve supplies a variable amount of the lower lateral leg from below. A significant overlap may be responsible for less than expected sensory acuity when this flap is reinnervated on the LSCN.

mandible complete with dentition. The innervated skin paddle is useful in restoring function to the lip, the anterior floor of mouth, and the tongue. Other, rarer applications may be envisioned such as hand, foot, and penile reconstruction.

Elevation and Closure. The fibula is surface-marked on the overlying skin. A 3-cm horizontal line is drawn backward from a point 2-cm behind the fibula head. The main trunk of the LSCN will lie in the soft tissues deep to this line. A Doppler probe is then used to locate the skin perforators of the peroneal artery emerging along the posterior border of the fibula. The major ones will lie near the junction between the middle and lower thirds of the bone. Their presence can often be confirmed by inspection of the preoperative angiogram. The skin island is centered on the major perforators using the posterior border of the fibula as its axis.

The anterior dissection is performed subfascially. The skin flap is elevated toward the septum between the peronei and soleus. As dissection turns inward toward the fibula, the perforators, which lie posterior to the intermuscular septum, are visible through it. Final up-down adjustments to skin paddle position can be made at this stage. When the fibula is reached, sharp extraperiosteal dissection is used to elevate the peronei and the extensor digitalis and hallucis longus muscles from the anterolateral aspect of the fibula. The bone is left clothed with a minimal muscle cuff all the way to the interosseous membrane.

Before the posterior dissection is begun, the LSCN is identified proximally behind the head of the fibula and via a longitudinal incision traced distally toward the skin paddle. As with other sensory nerve dissections, it is wise to incorporate a mesentery of fatty subcutaneous tissue to protect the fine branching nerve filaments into which the LSCN rapidly degenerates. The nerve is finally divided behind the head of the fibula and protected during the remainder of the dissection.

The posterior dissection proceeds subfascially. The position of the perforators should have been obvious at the time of the anterior dissection. After locating and protecting the perforators, the fascial band that unites the soleus to the posterolateral fibula is divided. Where perforators pass through the soleus muscle, a cuff of soleus may be left attached to the fibula. Some perforators may need to be dissected through the soleus muscle fibers. Once the soleus has been divided, blunt dissection will open up the posterior compartment.

To facilitate further exposure, the fibula is osteotomized no less than 8 cm from the lateral malleolus. At the superior end of the posterior dissection, below the common fibular (peroneal) nerve, the peroneal artery is visualized as it passes laterally from its origin toward the fibula. This vessel is carefully isolated from the fibula, and the superior osteotomy is performed.

The fascia of the flexor hallucis longus is incised and elevated medially until the posterior tibial artery and nerve are visualized. A space is cleared lateral to them to facilitate safe division of the tibialis posterior origin.

The flexor hallucis longus muscle belly is then divided at the lower end of the proposed fibula resection. This muscle is taken to simplify the dissection; prevent ischemic contracture and a claw toe; and provide vascularized bulk if needed in the reconstruction. The peroneal artery is usually within the substance of the muscle or just deep to it. It is ligated at this point.

Back in the anterior dissection, the interosseous membrane is divided to expose the tibialis posterior muscle. As the bones are pulled apart, the fibers of the tibialis posterior, which are attached to both sides of the incised interosseous membrane, take on an artificially bipennate appearance. Proceeding from inferior to superior, the muscle is divided along its midline raphe. A finger can be inserted beneath the raphe from behind to protect the vessels. At the superior portion of this dissection, the peroneal artery can be felt crossing to the fibula from its origin from the common popliteal artery. The posterior tibial artery passes distally on the medial side of the posterior tibial nerve.

With the use of loupe magnification and the application of gentle traction to the fibula, the peroneal artery pedicle is dissected back to its origin from the posterior tibial artery.

Comments. Because of anatomical anomalies and acquired vascular disorders, it is sometimes dangerous to harvest a fibula. The patient should have a thorough preoperative vascular evaluation, including an angiogram, to rule out potential problems such as an absent posterior tibial artery (8%) or severe atherosclerotic disease. The flap is otherwise safe and easy to elevate. The skin paddle is a little bulkier than the radial forearm flap, and the defect caused by its removal usually requires skin grafting. If there is a significant contribution from the superficial fibular nerve to the cutaneous sensation of the skin island, then the resulting sensory acuity will be diminished rather than absent. It appears that the LSCN and the SFN frequently share the territory, implying that it is a watershed area between two neurosomes.

Dorsalis Pedis

Anatomy. The skin of the dorsum of the foot may be elevated at a level superficial to the paratenons of the extensor tendons, the elevation including the dorsalis pedis artery, a superficial network of veins and the terminal branches of the superficial peroneal nerve. The donor site is closed by skin grafting. The innervated flap may be pedicled on its vessels and nerve and rotated to cover the malleoli or the sides of the heel (McCraw and Furlow, 1975). Alternatively, when used as a reinnervated flap, it may be transferred to the undersurface of the heel or a more distant site using microvascular and microneuronal anastomoses (Daniel et al, 1975, 1976; Gilbert, 1976; May et al, 1977; Man and Acland, 1980; Sharzer, 1990).

The anterior tibial artery lies between the tendons of the extensor digitorum longus and the extensor hallucis longus muscles as it passes under the inferior extensor retinaculum of the ankle. The dorsalis pedis artery is the continuation of the anterior tibial artery: it begins at the level of the ankle joint and passes distally on the dorsum of the foot to end over the base of the second metatarsal, where it divides into its terminal branches, the laterally directed arcuate artery and the deep plantar artery. The first dorsal metatarsal artery is an early branch of the latter. It is given off at a variable depth between the bases of the first and second metatarsals just as its parent vessel dives between them (to communicate

with the first plantar metatarsal artery). Its origin is crossed superficially by the extensor hallucis brevis, which it soon leaves behind as it passes distally on the interosseous membrane medial to the deep peroneal nerve and between the first and second metatarsals. It terminates at the base of the first web by dividing into the dorsal digital arteries supplying that cleft. At the same level, it again communicates with the plantar system via a small branch passing distal to the transverse metatarsal ligament.

The superficial fibular (peroneal) nerve is one of the terminal branches of the common peroneal. It pierces the deep fascia at the junction between the upper two thirds and lower third of the leg. Via a recurrent branch, it supplies a variable area on the lower lateral leg, partially overlapping the territory of the lateral femoral cutaneous nerve (see above). It usually crosses the anterior aspect of the ankle joint superficial to the extensor retinaculum as two branches: medial and lateral. These branches supply the dorsum of the foot except for the first web space (deep peroneal) and the lateral border (sural). The first web space is supplied by the deep peroneal nerve, which passes distally with the first dorsal metatarsal artery.

Indications. Local transfer of this innervated flap for coverage of heel and ankle defects has a limited but definite application (McCraw and Furlow, 1995). To fully cover the weightbearing portion of the heel or forefoot, it has to be used as a free flap (Sharzer, 1990). In cases of toe transfer, part of the flap can be taken to provide sensate cover for adjacent parts of the hand (Moberg, 1955; Murray et al, 1967). As a noninnervated free flap, it has been used extensively in mucosal replacement after head and neck resection (Franklin et al, 1979). This remains a leading indication, although alternatives with less donor site morbidity are available. Areas benefiting most from sensate reconstruction include the lower lip, the anterior floor of the mouth, the tongue, and the hypopharynx.

Elevation and Closure. Elevation of the flap involves isolation of the vascular trunk from deeper structures and the preservation of its attachments to the overlying skin. The vascular trunk is composed of the anterior tibial, deep plantar, and first dorsal metatarsal arteries. The skin flap is designed to lie over this axis and may include most of the dorsal skin of the foot from the mid-extensor retinaculum proximally to the web spaces distally. Medially and laterally, the boundaries lie just beyond the margins of the dorsal venous arch. The flap is elevated at the level of the paratenons toward the interval separating the extensor digitorum longus from the extensor hallucis longus. This vascular septum is then preserved as the arterial trunk is identified proximally and elevated from its bed. The terminal portion of the first dorsal metatarsal artery (together with the deep peroneal nerve) is identified quite superficially in the first web space at the distal end of the flap. Venous drainage is maintained by preserving a large superficial vein that, like the artery, may be dissected proximally to obtain a long vascular pedicle. Branches of the superficial fibular nerve are easily identified at the proximal margin of the flap and, for extra length, they may be dissected superiorly toward their common trunk.

Elevation of the artery from its bed involves resection of

that part of the extensor hallucis brevis that passes between it and the overlying skin. Care must be taken when dissecting the origin of the first dorsal metatarsal artery from the doralis pedis: sometimes the take-off lies deep within the interosseous musculature. Failure to recognize this may lead to its inadvertent ligation.

The paratenons of the extensor digitorum longus and the extensor hallucis longus are then sutured together to produce a flat bed to receive a skin graft.

Comments. The dorsalis pedis flap offers thin pliable skin with excellent reinnervation potential. For composite reconstruction, the second metatarsal can be included. Unfortunately, the size of the flap is small, and the donor defect is potentially disabling. Frequently, delayed healing over the extensor tendons can delay ambulation and prolong convalescence. This flap may not be safe in the presence of peripheral arterial disease or vascular anomalies, when the loss of the dorsalis pedis artery can result in an ischemic foot. As a pedicled innervated flap for local cover, the dorsalis pedis flap is disappointing. Only the most peripheral portions of the heel are within reach. For complete resurfacing, the flap usually needs to be detached and used as a reinnervated flap.

Muscle Flaps

Anatomy. To minimize the bulk associated with musculocutaneous flaps, it has become commonplace to resurface certain limb defects by the use of free muscle flaps covered by partial-thickness skin grafts. With maturation, the muscle atrophies to about 30% of its former bulk, and the skin forms a durable, nonwobbly surface well suited for sole of foot repair. Unfortunately, "time wounds all heels," and in the absence of protective sensation and meticulous skin care, there is a tendency for recurrent breakdown over weightbearing prominences. Recently, Dellon (1991) has exposed the notion of surrogate reinnervation in relation to sensory return in free muscle transfers. By connecting the motor nerve of a free muscle transfer to a recipient sensory nerve, protective sensation in the flap is achieved. He theorizes that the muscle spindles become the sensory receptors for pain and touch fibers running in the recipient nerve. Pressure on the muscle flap distorts the muscle spindles producing impulses in the sensory nerve that are, in turn, interpreted as pain or touch by the brain.

Any free muscle flap has the potential for surrogate reinnervation. The commonest muscle transfers are latissimus dorsi, gracilis, and rectus abdominis. Unfortunately, the rectus abdominis has a segmental nerve supply, which puts it at a technical disadvantage for neuroanastomosis. A muscle flap with a single motor nerve is preferable. Descriptions of the anatomy and elevation of free muscle transfers lie beyond the scope of this chapter, but they are well described in comprehensive texts on the subject (Strauch et al, 1990; Strauch and Yu, 1993).

Indications and Comments. Resurfacing the sole of the foot or weightbearing amputation stumps are the main indications for this technique. With the lack of controlled studies, it remains uncertain whether the method is superior to the use of innervated cutaneous flaps. Perhaps superior sensation in the latter is offset by the "wobbliness" of skin and

▼ **TABLE 71–1**
Other Sensate Flaps

Flap	Nerve	Vessel	Comments and References
Deltoid	Upper lateral cutaneous nerve of arm	Posterior circumflex humoral artery	Thin, hairless; color matches face; poor donor site (Serafin and Voci, 1983)
Medial arm	Medial cutaneous nerve of arm	Superior ulnar collateral artery	Medial cutaneous nerve of forearm sacrificed; small, hairless (Dolmans et al, 1979; Kaplan and Pearl, 1980)
Posterior arm	Posterior cutaneous nerve of arm	Branch of brachial	Questionable reliability; small, hairless (Masquelete et al, 1985)
Lateral intercostal	Lateral cutaneous branch of T10 or T11	Intercostal artery	Venous congestion common (Kerrigan and Daniel, 1979)
Gluteus maximus	Inferior gluteal nerve + posterior femoral cutaneous nerve	Superior and inferior gluteal arteries	Short pedicle; innervated breast reconstruction? (Fujino et al, 1975; Hurwitz et al, 1981)
Gracilis flap	Anterior branch of obturator	Profunda femoris artery	Unreliable skin paddle; functioning muscle transfer (Strauch and Yu, 1993)
Medial thigh	Medial femoral cutaneous nerve	Branch of femoral artery	Limited experience (Baek, 1983)
Anterolateral thigh	Anterior + lateral femoral cutaneous nerve	Branch of lateral femoral circumflex artery	Limited experience (Press et al, 1988; Strauch and Yu, 1993)
Anteromedial thigh	Medial femoral cutaneous nerve	Branch of lateral femoral circumflex artery	Limited experience (Koshima et al, 1988)
Posterior thigh	Posterior cutaneous nerve of thigh	Descending branch inferior gluteal artery	Decubitus ulcers (Hurwitz et al, 1981)
Saphenous	Medial femoral cutaneous nerve + saphenous nerve	Saphenous artery	Artery absent in 5%; thin, hairless (Acland et al, 1981)
Posterior calf	Posterior cutaneous nerve of thigh + sural	Lateral popliteal cutaneous artery	Variable anatomy; small vessels; pedicle flap best (Walton and Bunkis, 1984)
Medial plantar	Medial plantar nerve	Medial plantar artery	Pedicled flap for heel cover (Shanahan and Gingrass, 1978)
Lateral calcaneal	Sural nerve	Lateral calcaneal artery	Pedicled flap for heel cover (Grabb and Argenta, 1981)
Plantar artery flap	Lateral plantar nerve	Lateral plantar artery	Pedicled flap for heel cover (Reiffel and McCarthy, 1980)
Toe transfers	Digital nerves	Dorsal pedis + metatarsal arteries	Not discussed here (Cobbett, 1969)
Karapandzic	Trigeminal nerve (V2, V3)	Facial artery	Theoretically motorized and sensate; microstomia (Karapandzic, 1974)

subcutaneous tissue lacking the fibrous septa responsible for stabilizing the glabrous skin on the sole of the foot.

Other Sensate Flaps

Some of the other sensate flaps are listed in Table 71–1.

CONCLUSION

1. Sensate flaps are an integral part of reconstructive surgery and, in different forms, have been used for many years. Their repertoire has been increased by the advent of microvascular surgery and the realization that the quality of reinnervation parallels the recipient rather than the donor site.

2. Areas of the body benefiting most from sensate flap reconstruction include weightbearing areas, the hand, the penis, the female breast, the mouth, and the lips.

3. With most innervated free tissue transfers, it is advisable to identify the sensory nerve proximally (where its size is large, its position is known, and where a preliminary nerve block may have revealed the extent of its primary neurosome) and then trace it distally into the flap. As it breaks up into fine filamentous branches, these may be preserved by raising with them a mesentary of protective subcutaneous tissue that then becomes part of the neural pedicle.

4. Many common flaps are capable of innervation or reinnervation. The provision of sensation usually requires little extra operating time and generally does not increase the donor defect. When flap closure is required—whether local, pedicled, or free—it is therefore appropriate to use sensate flaps whenever feasible.

5. A thorough knowledge of the neurosensory anatomy of the flaps in common usage is essential to offer the patient optimal reconstruction and give the surgeon the means of providing it.

References

Acland RD, Shusterman M, Godina M, et al: The saphenous neurovascular free flap. Plast Reconstr Surg 67:763, 1981.

Adamson JE, Horton CE, Crawford HH: Sensory rehabilitation of the injured thumb. Plast Reconstr Surg 40:53, 1967.

Baek SM: Two new cutaneous free flaps: The medial and lateral thigh flaps. Plast Reconst Surg 71:354, 1983.

Berger A, Meissl G: Innervated skin grafts and flaps for restoration of sensation to anesthetic areas. Chir Plast (Berlin) 3:33, 1975.

Biemer E, Stock W: Total thumb reconstruction: A one-stage reconstruction using an osteocutaneous forearm flap. Br J Plast Surg 36:52, 1983.

Boyd B, Mulholland S, Gullane P, Irish J, Kelly L, Rotstein L, Brown D: Lateral antebrachial cutaneous neurosome flaps in oral reconstruction: Are we making sense? Plast Reconstr Surg 93:1350, 1994.

Brailler F, Horner RH: Sensory cross-finger pedicle graft. J Bone Joint Surg 51:1264, 1969.

Brown CJ, MacKinnon SE, Dellon AL, et al: The sensory potential of free flap donor sites. Ann Plast Surg 23:135, 1989.

Cauna N: Light and electron microscopical structure of the sensory end-organs in human skin. *In* Kenshalo DR (ed): The Skin Senses. Springfield, Il, C.C. Thomas, 1968, p 15.

Chicarilli ZN, Price GJ: Complete plantar foot coverage with the free neurosensory radial forearm flap. Plast Reconstr Surg 78:94, 1986.

Cobbett JR: Free digital transfer. J Bone Joint Surg 518:677, 1969.

Cohen BE, Cronin ED: An innervated cross-finger flap for finger-tip reconstruction. Plast Reconstr Surg 72:688, 1983.

Daniel R, Terzis J, Midgley R: Restoration of sensation to an anesthetic hand by free neurovascular flap from the foot. Plast Reconstr Surg 57:275, 1976.

Daniel R, Terzis J, Schwartz G: Neurovascular free flaps: A preliminary report. Plast Reconstr Surg 56:13, 1975.

Davis L: The return of sensation to transplanted skin. Surg Gynecol Obstet 59:533, 1934.

Dellon AL: Muscle sense or nonsense? Ann Plast Surg 26:444, 1991.

Dolich BH, Olshansky KJ, Barbar AH: Use of a cross-forearm neurocutaneous flap to provide sensation and coverage in hand reconstructions. Plast Reconstr Surg 62:550, 1978.

Dolmans S, Guimberteau JC, Baudet J: The upper arm flap. Microsurgery 1:162, 1979.

Dubner S, Heller KS: Re-innervated radial forearm free flaps in head and neck reconstruction. J Reconstr Microsurg 8:467, 1992.

Dykes RW, Terzis JK, Strauch B: Sensations from surgically transferred glabrous skin; central versus peripheral factors. J Can Sci Neurol 6:437, 1979.

Franklin J, Withers E, Madden J, et al: Use of a free dorsalis pedis flap in head and neck repairs. Plast Reconstr Surg 63:195, 1979.

Frey L: Le syndrome du nerf auriculotemporal. Rev Neurol 2:97–104, 1923.

Fujino T, Harashina T, Aoyagi F: Reconstruction for aplasia of the breast and pectoral region by microvascular transfer of a free flap from the buttock. Plast Reconstr Surg 56:178, 1975.

Ganong WF: Initiation of impulses in sense organs. *In* Ganong WF (ed): Review of Medical Physiology, ed 15. Norwalk, CT, Lange, 1991, p 106.

Gaul JS: Radial innervated cross-finger flap from index to provide sensory pulp to injured thumb. J Bone Joint Surg 51:1257, 1969.

Gilbert A: Composite tissue transfers from the foot: Anatomic basis and surgical technique. *In* Daniller A, Strauch B (eds): Symposium on Microsurgery. St. Louis, Mosby, 1976.

Grabb WC, Argenta LC: The lateral calcaneal artery skin flap (the lateral calcaneal artery, lesser saphenous vein, and sural nerve skin flap). Plast Reconstr Surg 68:723, 1981.

Haughey BH: Tongue reconstruction: Concepts and practice. Laryngoscope 103:1132, 1993.

Hayden RE: Lateral thigh flap. Otolaryngol Clin North Am 27:1171, 1994.

Hermanson A, Dalsgaard CJ, Arnander C, et al: Sensibility and cutaneous reinnervation in free flaps. Plast Reconstr Surg 79:422, 1987.

Hoppenreijs TJM, Freihofer HPM, Brouns JJA, et al: Sensibility and cutaneous re-innervation of pectoralis major myocutaneous island flaps. J Craniomaxillofac Surg 18:237, 1990.

Hurwitz DJ, Swartz WM, Mathes SJ: The gluteal thigh flap: A reliable, sensate flap for the closure of buttock and perineal wounds. Plast Reconstr Surg 68:521, 1981.

Iggo A, Andres KH: Morphology of cutaneous receptors. Ann Rev Neurosci 5:1, 1982.

Joshi BB: A sensory cross-finger flap for use on the index finger. Plast Reconstr Surg 58:210, 1976.

Kaplan EN, Pearl RM: An arterial medial arm flap: Vascular anatomy and clinical applications. Ann Plast Surg 4:205, 1980.

Karapandzic M: Reconstruction of lip defects by local arterialized flaps. Br J Plast Surg 27:93, 1974.

Katsaros J, Shusterman M, Beppu M, et al: The lateral arm flap: Anatomy and clinical applications. Ann Plast Surg 12:489, 1984.

Kerrigan CL, Daniel RK: The intercostal flap: An anatomical and hemodynamic approach. Ann Plast Surg 2:411, 1979.

Kleinert HE: Fingertip injuries and their management. Am Surg 25:41, 1959.

Komatsu S, Tamai S: Successful replantation of a completely cut-off thumb: Case report. Plast Reconstr Surg 42:374–377, 1968.

Koshima I, Soeda S, Yamasaki M, Kyou J: The free or predicled anteromedial thigh flap. Ann Plast Surg 21:480, 1988.

Kredel FE, Evans JP: Recovery of sensation in denervated pedicle and free skin grafts. J Neurol Neurosurg Psychiatry 29:1203, 1933.

Kutler W: New method for fingertip amputation. JAMA 133:29, 1947.

Lai C-S, Lin S-D, Tsai C-C, Tsai C-W: Reverse digital artery neurovascular cross-finger flap. J Hand Surg 20:397, 1995.

Littler JW: Neurovascular island transfer in reconstructive hand surgery. *In* Wallace AB (ed): International Congress of Plastic Surgery, 2nd ed. Edinburgh, Churchill-Livingstone, 1960, pp 175–178.

Lovie MJ, Duncan GM, Glasson DW: The ulnar artery forearm free flap. Br J Plast Surg 37:486, 1984.

Man D, Acland R: The microanatomy of the dorsalis pedis flap and its clinical implications. Plast Reconstr Surg *64:*419, 1980.

Martin JH, Jessell TM: Modality coding in the somatic sensory system. *In* Kandel ER, Schwartz JH, Jessel TM (eds): Neural Science, ed 3. New York, Elsevier, 1991, p 341.

Masquelet AC, Rinaldi S, Mouchet A, Gilbert A: The posterior arm free flap. Plast Reconstr Surg *76:*908, 1985.

Matloub HS, Larsen DL, Kuhn JC, et al: Lateral arm free flap in oral cavity reconstruction: A functional evaluation. Head Neck Surg *11:*205, 1989.

Mathes SJ, Nahai F: Clinical atlas of muscle and musculocutaneous flaps. St. Louis, CV Mosby, 1979.

May JW, Chait LA, Cohen BE, O'Brien BM: Free neurovascular flap from the first web of the foot in hand reconstruction. J Hand Surg *2:*387, 1977.

McCraw JB, Furlow LT, Jr: The dorsalis pedis arterialized flap. Plast Reconstr Surg *55:*177, 1975.

Miura T: Thumb reconstruction using radial innervated cross-finger pedicle. J Bone Joint Surg *55:*563, 1973.

Moberg E: Transfer of sensation. J Bone Joint Surg *37:*305, 1955.

Moberg E: Aspects of sensation in reconstructive surgery of the upper limb. J Bone Joint Surg *46:*817, 1964.

Morrison W, O'Brien B, MacLeod A, et al: Neurovascular free flaps from the foot for innervation of the hand. J Hand Surg *3:*235, 1978.

Morrison WA, O'Brien BM, MacLeod AM: Thumb reconstruction with a free neurovascular wraparound flap from the big toe. J Hand Surg *5:*575, 1980.

Mulholland RS, Neligan PC, Kelly J, Tong L, Gullane PJ, Boyd JB, Thoma A: The sensate fibular flap for oromandibular reconstruction. First Conjoint Symposium on Contemporary Head and Neck Reconstruction (PSEF/AAOHNSF). Chicago, July 29, 1995.

Murray JF, Ord JVR, Gavelin GF: The neurovascular island pedicle flap. J Bone Joint Surg *49:*1285, 1967.

Ohmori K, Harii K: Transplantation of a toe to an amputated finger. Hand *7:*134, 1975.

Ohmori K, Harii K: Free dorsalis pedis sensory flap to the hand, with microneurovascular anastomosis. Plast Reconstr Surg *58:*546, 1976.

Press BHJ, Cohen SR, Boyd A, Golomb F: Reconstruction of a large chest wall defect with a musculocutaneous free flap using anterolateral thigh musculature. Ann Plast Surg *20:*238, 1988.

Reiffel RS, McCarthy JG: Coverage of heel and sole defects: A new subfascial arterialized flap. Plast Reconstr Surg *66:*250, 1980.

Serafin D, Voci VE: Reconstruction of the lower extremity: Microsurgical composite tissue transplantation. Clin Plast Surg *10:*55, 1983.

Shanahan RE, Gingrass RP: Medial plantar sensory flap for the coverage of heel defects. Plast Reconstr Surg *64:*295, 1979.

Sharzer LA: Microneurovascular transfer of the dorsalis pedis flap to the heel. *In* Strauch B, Vasconez LO, Hall-Findlay E (eds): Grabb's Encyclopedia of Flaps, vol 3. Boston, Little, Brown, 1990, pp 1797–1800.

Shenaq SM, Dinh TA: Total penile reconstruction with an expanded sensate lateral arm flap. J Reconstr Microsurg *5:*245, 1989.

Snow JW: The use of a volar flap for fingertip amputations. Plast Reconstr Surg *40:*163, 1967.

Snow JW: Follow-up clinic: The use of a volar flap for the repair of fingertip injuries—preliminary report. Plast Reconstr Surg *52:*299, 1973.

Sommerlad BC, Boorman JG: An innervated flap incorporating supraclavicular nerves for reconstruction of major hand injuries. Hand *13:*5, 1981.

Song R, Song Y, Yu Y, Song Y: The upper arm free flap. Clin Plast Surg *9:*27, 1982.

Soutar DS, Scheker LR, Tanner NSB, McGregor IA: The radial forearm flap: A versatile method for intraoral reconstruction. B J Plast Surg *36:*1, 1983.

Strauch B, Vasconez LO, Hall-Findlay EJ (eds): Grabb's Encyclopedia of Flaps. Boston, Little, Brown, 1990.

Strauch B, Yu H-L: Atlas of Microvascular Surgery. New York, Thieme Medical Publishers, 1993.

Taylor GI, Gianoutsos MP, Morris SF: The neurovascular territories of the skin and muscles: Anatomic study and clinical implications. Plast Reconstr Surg *94:*1–36, 1994.

Urken ML, Weinberg H, Vickery C, et al: The neurofasciocutaneous radial forearm flap in head and neck reconstruction: A preliminary report. Laryngoscope *100:*161, 1990.

Venkataswami R, Subramanian N: Oblique triangular flap: A new method of repair for oblique amputations of the finger tip and thumb. Plast Reconstr Surg *66:*296, 1980.

Walton RL, Bunkis J: The posterior calf fasciocutaneous free flap. Plast Reconstr Surg *74:*76, 1984.

Weinstein S: Intensive and extensive aspects of tactile sensitivity as a function of body part, sex, and laterality. *In* Kenshalo DR (Ed): The Skin Senses. Springfield, Il, C.C. Thomas, 1968, p 195.

Wilkinson TS: Reconstruction of the thumb by radial nerve innervated cross-finger flap. South Med J *65:*992, 1972.

Yang G, Chen B, Gao Y: Forearm free skin flap transplantation. From National Medical Journal of China *61:*139, 1981. Abstracted in Plast Reconstr Surg *69:*1041, 1982.

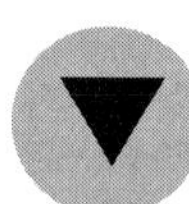

Chapter 72

• Paul W. Brand

Management of Sensory Loss in the Extremities

A few decades ago, the word trophic dominated any discussion of the management of insensitive limbs. Charcot, the great French scientist, said that when a limb becomes denervated, it loses a trophic factor (literally, a nourishing factor), and is thereby less able to resist trauma and less able to heal.

There is some truth in this concept. The author has studied it in the footpads of rats, comparing normal footpads with those in which the limb has been made insensitive by cutting the dorsal roots. When equal stress is applied to both, it is true that there is just a little more fragility in those that are denervated. The differences are small, as are the differences in rates of healing of wounds if both are kept in plaster casts. However, if the rats are allowed to run free, the denervated footpads not only break down, they are sometimes eaten by the rat that owns them. Thus, it is *the loss of restraints imposed by pain* rather than any so-called trophic change that causes severe damage and that hinders healing after denervation.

This chapter is not about pathology but about practical ways of managing insensitive limbs. The reason the author begins the chapter by talking about trophic change is that the concept is a hindrance in the management of insensitive limbs. If the patient or the doctor gets the idea that there is a basic fragility within a limb and a deficiency of healing, a sort of fatalism is likely to develop. The author observed that kind of fatalism in India while trying to help patients with leprosy. Doctors and patients told the author that leprosy resulted in nonhealing flesh. The stigma of leprosy was based on the concept of rotting flesh. It turned out that the only real problem was lack of pain sensation. The same fatalism is the basis for the high rate of amputation among diabetics, whose surgeons have been likely to offer surgical ablation as an alternative to inevitable and progressive trophic ulceration.

Instead of looking inward, to identify incompetence in the limb, we need to look outward and identify the mechanical factors or sources of heat that, in the absence of pain, may impinge on the limb and destroy it. Protection of a limb is not difficult if one knows the dangers.

First, two changes within the limb are considered that may accompany sensory denervation: loss of vasomotor control and loss of sweating. Then, the external forces that cause damage are identified and quantified.

LOSS OF VASOMOTOR CONTROL

In many peripheral neuropathies, the sympathetic nerves are lost along with sensation. The immediate result is vasodi-latation, and the limb becomes warmer than normal. Then gradually, the limb becomes cooler than normal, as humeral control takes over. Vasoconstriction becomes the normal condition of the resting limb.

Because the limb feels cold, and the pulses and Doppler readouts are reduced, the denervated limb is often thought to have a reduced vascular capability. In fact, such a limb responds very well to the demand for extra blood supply. In the event of trauma or infection, inflammation causes the vessels to open up and the limb becomes warm. The author has found that the cool baseline temperature allows the examiner to observe the progress of inflammation very easily by thermometry. A normal warm limb does not get much warmer when it is mildly inflamed. However a limb that is cool at rest has a wide range of temperature that can be used to alert the patient and the doctor when some unnoticed problem has called for extra local blood supply, producing a so-called hot spot.

LOSS OF SWEATING

Most denervated extremities are very dry, owing to loss of sweating and sebaceous secretion. A serious result of dryness is a change in the physical qualities of keratin in the cuticle of the skin. Hydrated keratin is soft and compliant; it can be folded and stretched like a rubber membrane. Dry cuticle is hard and brittle. It will not stretch, and it cracks when folded. The cuticle layer of the skin cracks and exposes the dermis. Continued movement opens and closes the cuticular crack until it becomes inflamed and infected. Keratin builds up into a thick callus along the margins of the crack. Finally, the crack deepens through the dermis and becomes a true ulcer and a source of infection for the whole limb.

Treatment

The patient must learn a routine of skin care. The dry limb is soaked in water for 15 minutes once or twice every day and then blotted lightly with a towel. The whole skin area is then rubbed with petroleum jelly to prevent evaporation of the water that has now hydrated the keratin. If cracks have already occurred, the thickened cuticle around the edges may be pared down and the floor of the crack painted with gentian violet. If the crack is in a finger flexure, the finger should be splinted in extension so that it may heal without causing a contracture.

PRESSURE SORES

This term is sometimes used to lump together a variety of conditions that need to be understood separately. I have found it best to divide these ulcers into four groups, each of which is associated with a different level of mechanical force and a different time factor.

Pathology	Typical Force	Time Factor
Ischemic necrosis	1/2–5 pounds per square inch	Several hours *continuously*
Direct mechanical injury	600 pounds per square inch and over	Immediate
Inflammatory autolysis	20–75 pounds per square inch	Thousands of repetitions over several days
Spreading infection	Any localized pressures	A few repetitions on an already infected hand or foot

Pressure Sores from Ischemia

In active people, it is rare for the limbs to be subjected to continuous pressure for long enough to cause necrosis from ischemia. No one stands still on his or her feet long enough to cause ischemic ulcers on the sole. The only common cause of continuous pressure on a foot is from a tight shoe. The ulcers occur most often at the edges of the foot (Fig. 72–1), where the radius of curvature of the shoe is smallest. These ulcers can be prevented by making sure that new shoes are carefully fitted, and that no new shoe is worn for a long time on the first day. I have found it impractical to measure the small pressures around the edges of the foot inside a shoe. The best way to prevent ischemic necrosis is to measure time rather than pressure. The following routine works well if the patient accepts it.

Buy shoes with leather uppers. They adapt to the shape of the foot over time. Never wear new shoes for more than 2 hours on the first day. Look carefully at the foot when the shoe is first removed to see the danger signs of recent ischemia, such as a red flush (or hot spot). If in doubt, let the shoemaker put a stretcher inside the tight place. In the absence of signs of reaction to pressure, wear the shoe for longer periods of time but always change shoes at mid-day and on return home in the evening. The ideal situation is to have three 5-hour shoe periods each day—morning, afternoon, and evening—with a different pair of shoes or slippers for each period. To simplify the routine, one pair of shoes can be kept at the workplace.

In the upper limb, pressure sores from ischemia are rare, except sometimes from poorly fitted splints.

Direct Damage from Mechanical or Thermal Energy

It takes about a thousand times more pressure to cause direct mechanical disruption of the skin than it does to cause ischemic necrosis. Because pressure is force divided by area, the pressure can be high either because of very high force or, more often, because moderate force is applied through a very small area.

This type of damage is rare on the foot in people who wear shoes. Barefoot walkers suffer injury by stepping on objects such as thumbtacks, broken glass, or sharp stones. All of these injuries can be prevented by a simple rule. People with insensitive feet should never walk barefoot, and they should shake out their shoes before putting them on to remove any small object that may have fallen in.

Direct mechanical damage is much more common on the hand. People without skin sensation sometimes become efficient at estimating force, perhaps from muscle sensors, but they find it very hard to judge pressure. Thus, a good rule is to beware of small handles. The occupational therapist should go to the workbench or home of a person with insensitive hands and remove all small handles and replace them with larger ones. The edges of the handles of small keys often cause damage, so key handles should be covered in a leather sandwich (Fig. 72–2). Some of the worst offenders are the little metal knobs on drawers or cupboards; they look pretty but have sharp edges on their rims. If a drawer sticks, a patient can tear the skin off of his or her finger just trying to open it. Patients should keep a pair of pliers in their pockets to manipulate small handles.

Heat is a constant hazard. Feet may rest on a hot floor of a pickup truck. Steam heating coils may have handles that are too close to the heater, causing burns during adjustment. The kitchen is full of hazards. All cooking implements must have long wooden or plastic handles. Cigarettes are a hazard from every point of view; they cause vasoconstriction of the

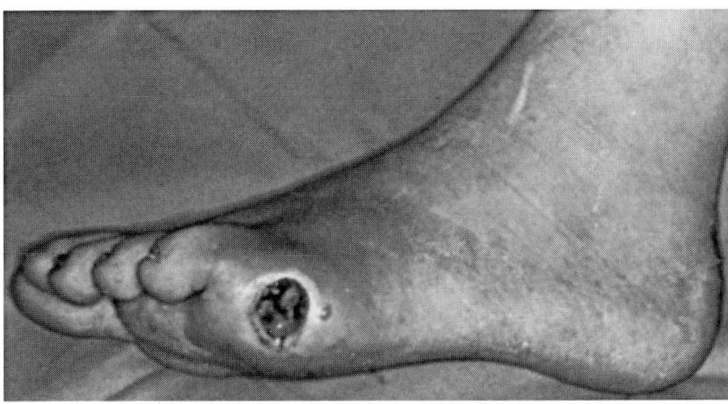

FIGURE 72–1. Ischemic ulcer caused by a tight shoe being worn all day.

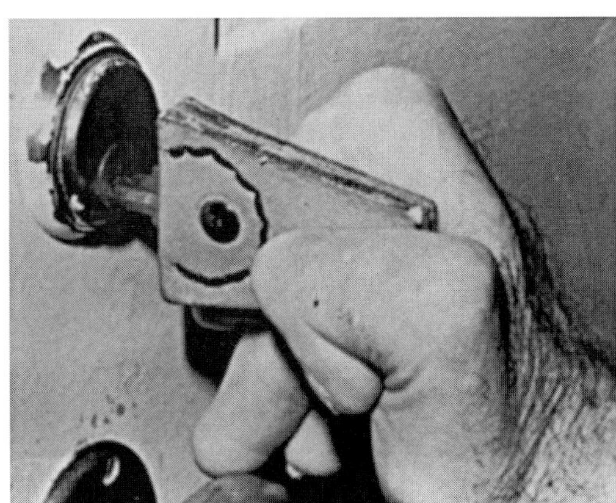

FIGURE 72–2. Low ulnar and median paralysis with insensitivity, injured by edge of small key. The hand is now protected by a leather sandwich.

hands and feet when the patient inhales, and they burn the fingers when the patient forgets that he or she is holding a cigarette. We give cigarette holders to patients who cannot quit smoking. Gloves should be worn in the kitchen and for some types of manual work.

Tissue Autolysis from Repetitive Stress

This is by far the most common cause of damage to active but insensitive limbs. Almost all plantar ulcers in patients who wear shoes are caused by thousands of repetitions of moderate local stress at every step they take. The breakdown commonly occurs in response to a range of pressures between 20 and 75 pounds per square inch. These pressures are harmless for a few repetitions and are painless to people with normal sensation.

Our own extensive studies with the footpads of rats have shown that at the pressure level of 20 pounds per square inch over 10,000 repetitions a day resulted in an inflammatory change in the tissues. This is about equivalent to a brisk 7-mile walk. Hyperemia developed, and a large number of inflammatory cells migrated into the tissue spaces, along with edema fluid. Tests on normal young people have shown that before this distance, they begin to feel just enough soreness at some point on the foot to make them alter their gait. They shift pressure to other parts of the sole. They may shorten their stride or limp a little. The person who is insensitive may have the same or a little more inflammatory change, but he or she does not limp because no discomfort is felt. *This failure to adapt the gait to changes in the internal state of the tissues is probably more significant than failure to perceive external forces.* The inflammatory state of the tissues that follows the frequent repetition of moderate stresses can be observed by noting localized redness and swelling, and the inflammation can be observed even better by noting an area of increased temperature (a so-called hot spot), which is easily distinguished by a sensitive hand.

This inflammation develops slowly and persists for hours or days. If the repetitive stress is continued on the same area day after day, necrosis develops at the center of the inflammation. Further stress from more walking increases the amount of necrosis, which then breaks through the skin as an ulcer.

When the ulcer appears, patients are at a loss to explain it. They do not recall any gross trauma or stress, so they say "It just happened by itself." At this time, the physician must explain the whole process. The ulcer that he or she sees is only the end point of a process that has probably taken days and weeks to develop. The patient has either been walking too much during the past few days (or weeks), or he or she has been wearing shoes that concentrate too much stress on just one or two parts of the foot. In many cases, both of these factors have been present. The pressure in the shoe might have been acceptable if there had been less walking. The amount of walking might have been acceptable if the local pressure had been less.

To prevent recurrence, both factors should be changed. The patient must learn to walk less, to take shorter steps, and to walk more slowly. Also, the shoe should be changed or modified to spread the stress of weightbearing more evenly over the foot. Spreading the stress of weightbearing

can often be accomplished by obtaining an extra-depth shoe, such as those by P. Minor (Treadeasy), Alden, or Scholls and putting a molded insole in place of the removable insole that comes with the shoe. For insensitive feet, standard, preformed insoles should not be used. Insoles must be made individually, molded on the patient's own foot or on a plaster model of the foot.

If ulceration under the metatarsal heads recurs or the area heats up while walking in spite of molded insoles, then a more radical change of footwear is needed.

The forefoot is very vulnerable to breakdown both because it takes the whole thrust of body weight at the push-off phase of gait and because shear stresses occur as the heel is lifted and the metatarsal heads roll while the toes remain flat on the shoe. These shear stresses occur between the metatarsal heads and the skin and soft tissues beneath them. They are much more severe if there has been previous ulceration and scar formation. To prevent these shear stresses, the foot must be prevented from bending at the metatarsophalangeal joints during walking. This is accomplished by walking in rigid-soled shoes.

If a regular flat shoe is made inflexible, it forces the patient to push off on the tip end of his shoe. This is uncomfortable and unnecessary. It is much better to have the rigid shoe tilt on the floor at the place that the metatarsophalangeal (MTP) joint previously flexed in the shoe. This is called a rocker shoe (Fig. 72–3). This is excellent from the point of view of mechanics. However, patients sometimes object that it is ugly and it forces them to shorten their stride. We may explain that short strides are better for the foot. However, because their dislike of the rocker shoe may result in failure to use it, we usually advise the roller shoe (Fig. 72–4). This is nearly as good for reducing shear stresses and is much more acceptable to patients. Their feet roll over rather than rock over, and the shoe looks more like regular Oxford shoes. These special shoes can usually be adapted from a commercial extra-depth shoe by bending and then stiffening the sole, and adding the rocking or rolling feature underneath. Only a few patients need custom-made shoes.

Physicians cannot win the battle to save insensitive limbs unless patients fully understand their problem and take responsibility for their own feet (Assal et al, 1985). They or

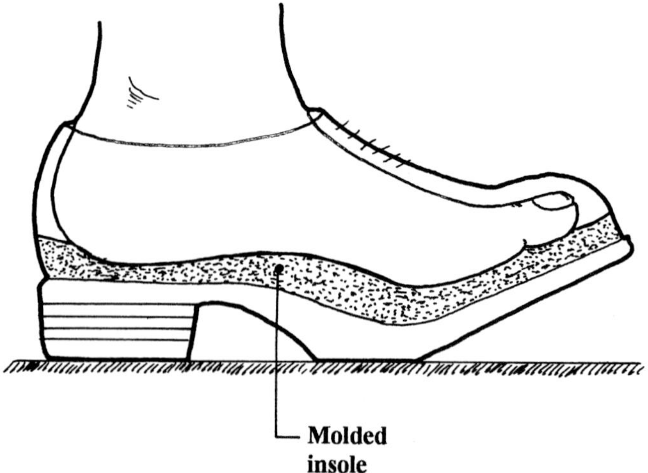

FIGURE 72–3. Diagram of a rigid-soled rocker shoe. The slope, from the rocker forwards, is steep enough to allow the heel to lift without any toe pressure.

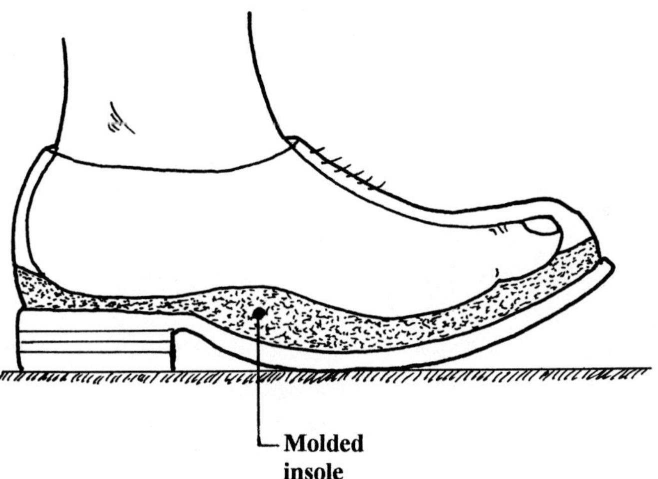

FIGURE 72–4. Diagram of a rigid-soled roller shoe. When the heel lifts, the ground contact rolls forward but without shear stress.

their spouses must feel their feet every evening when going to bed. They must learn to find hot spots and know what they mean. Then they may modify their program and note how the hot spot becomes cooler. Some of the author's patients keep a skin thermometer beside the bed and keep a graph of the temperature of their risk area compared with a neutral area. They quickly learn how much walking their feet can stand.

Spreading Infection

Ulceration is bad but reversible. It will heal. The real disaster for a foot is spreading infection. It starts from an ulcer and then involves bone, joint, and tendon sheath. Soon, the whole foot may be hot, swollen, and septic, and bones may be destroyed. This is the sort of problem that results in amputation. Also, this is what has given rise to the idea that insensitive feet and diabetic feet cannot deal with infection. The problem is mechanical. Most neuropathic feet would heal about as well as normal feet if the patients did not walk on them. No person with normal sensation could put a wounded, ulcerated foot to the ground and walk on it. That is why normal feet heal. Pain forces them to rest, and the patient's own cells are able to localize the infection and heal the wound.

For insensitive feet, the physician may have to force a reluctant patient to do what pain would do if he or she had sensation. Many doctors tend to rely on medication for healing wounds and controlling infection. They forget that this is only an ancillary approach to the real essential of rest to the part. For most patients, every acute ulcer or infection of the foot should be treated with complete rest in bed until the infection has localized. When the fever has subsided and the swelling has reduced, a plaster cast may be applied and the patient allowed to walk. For very careful and cooperative patients who prefer not to have a cast, the use of crutches is permitted. However, the cast is the surest method.

Total-Contact Casting

The special value of a total-contact plaster cast is that it takes the weight evenly all over the foot and up the leg (Coleman et al, 1984). No part of the foot takes more than about 5 pounds per square inch. A padded cast cannot spread the weight up the calf because cast padding is compressible and the cast therefore tends to move (the so-called piston effect) up and down on the leg. Doctors need not be afraid that the foot may swell in the cast and cause pressure. The opposite is a danger. The foot begins to shrink in the cast as soon as immobilization takes effect. A loose cast should be replaced to avoid the effects of friction. It is unnecessary to inspect or dress a wound after it has been immobilized. It is harmful to leave a window in a cast because it results in localized swelling in the window and thus shear stresses occur at the edge of the opening, causing wounds.

The technique of cast application is important. The inner layer must be smooth and wrinkle free. The following routine has proved safe and effective (Fig. 72–5).

1. The foot should be elevated for a long enough period to allow major swelling to subside before the cast is applied. If time does not allow this, the first cast must be removed and reapplied after a very few days. A loose cast is the most common cause of friction blisters or secondary ulcers.

2. The patient lies face down on a plinth with the knee flexed and the foot horizontal.

3. A saddle of felt is applied to cover the malleoli and the angle between the foot and the leg. A strip of felt is laid along the anterior margin of the leg and foot, and is fixed with strips of adhesive. This felt facilitates removal of the cast with a saw. The toes may be covered with a strip of foam because they tend to move instinctively with gait.

4. The leg is covered with a tube of stockinet. The foot is kept at right angles to the leg, with the toes slightly angled into extension.

5. One single plaster bandage is applied loosely around the foot and lower part of the leg.

6. Before any more plaster is wetted, this first bandage is rubbed continuously into all hollows and around prominences of the limb until the plaster has started to set.

7. The rest of the plaster can be applied rapidly. Slabs of plaster may be applied under the sole and up the back of the leg, and from side to side under the heel; the cast is held in position by circular bandages.

8. Finally, a sole plate of 4-mm plywood is applied under the sole, as far forward as the metatarsal heads. This is to avoid the danger to an insensitive foot of a rubber heel pressing through a plaster sole softened by discharge. Plaster is tucked into the hollows between the plywood and the cast. A rubber heel is placed on the plywood at about the center of the foot and fixed with a few turns of plaster bandage. The toes may be enclosed in their cover of polyurethane foam.

9. No weightbearing is allowed for the first 24 hours. After this, reasonable activity is permitted, including return to work in many cases. Patients are warned to return at once if the plaster gets soft or cracks, or if any pain or fever is experienced.

10. The cast should be changed when it becomes a little loose, but the second cast may be kept on for 2 or 3 weeks or more and, in many cases, is all that is needed for healing of the ulcer. The first few days after healing are critical. Only a little walking is advised, preferably in a special molded sandal and using short steps.

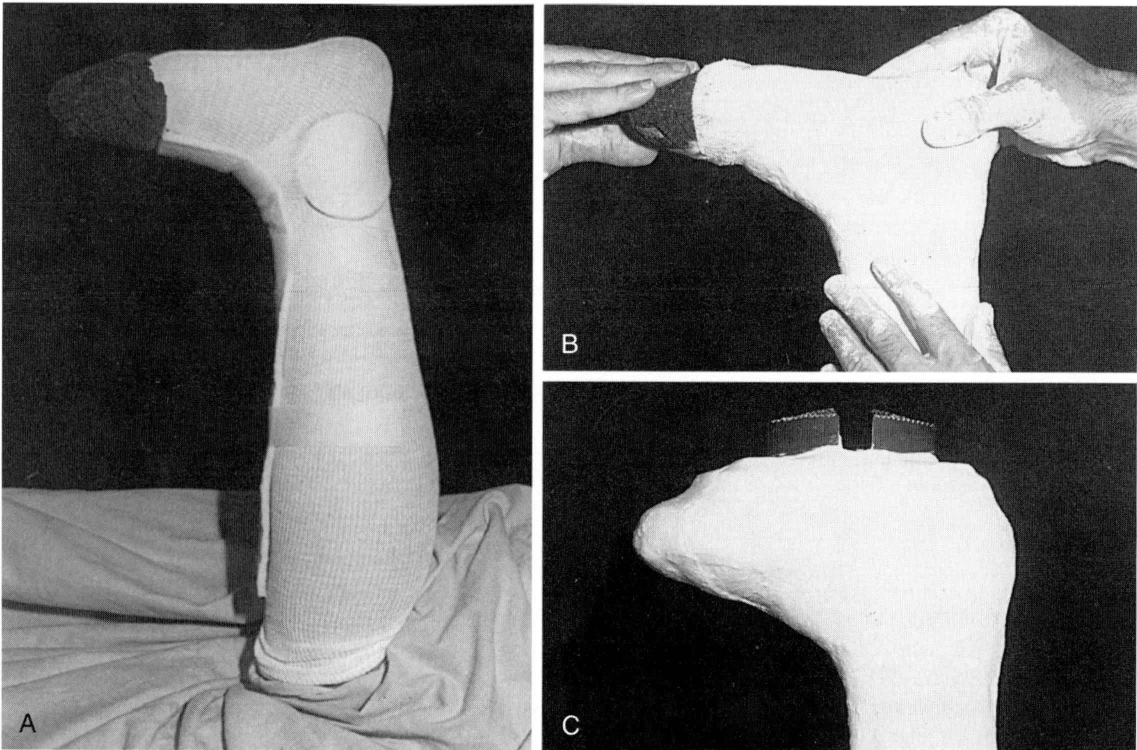

FIGURE 72–5. Total contact plaster cast. *A,* Patient prone, knee flexed. Felt strips covering front of tibia and dorsum of foot. Felt patch over each malleolus. Polyurethrane foam around toes. *B,* Assistant holds toes extended while inner layer of plaster is molded into every contour of foot, leg. *C,* Rubber heel on a plywood sole plate to serve as rocker. (From Birke JA, Novick A, Graham SL, Coleman WC, Brasseaux DM: Methods of treating plantar ulcers. Phys Ther *71:*116, 1991.)

NEUROPATHIC BONE AND JOINT DAMAGE

In the foot, most neuropathic bone and joint damage follows previous infection (Hodgson, 1948). The infection results in osteoporosis, which may persist long after the ulcer has healed. The actual bony collapse may begin as a small crack in a bone that results from a sudden strain or twist of the foot, or it may begin as a fatigue fracture. Such small cracks are much more common in normal feet than is realized. However, in normal feet, where these cracks are often diagnosed as a sprain, the pain that accompanies them forces the patient to limp until the condition resolves. The insensitive person walks on the foot without a limp, and the small crack extends to become a major fracture. Harris and Brand (1966) have described typical patterns of neuropathic collapse, based on the starting point of the first crack: (1) os calcis, (2) talus, (3) navicular, (4) cuneiform, and (5) metatarsal. Common to all of these types is the clinical feature of localized heat and some swelling. If an insensitive patient presents with a persistent hot spot on the dorsum of the foot or the side of the mid-foot or heel, the surgeon should consider damage to the bone and perform an x-ray study. Even if the x-ray study is negative but the hot spot remains, it is wise to immobilize the foot pending a further x-ray study 10 days later, by which time the crack will be apparent.

Early neuropathic damage usually heals by immobilization in a plaster cast. Late cases with more extensive damage may be better treated by surgical intervention and arthrodesis. Neuropathic joints have a bad reputation for nonunion after surgery. However, we have had good success by insisting upon two rules—(1) the bone must be excised back until good bleeding bone is exposed; (2) internal fixation must be reinforced by external plaster cast immobilization, and both must be maintained for 50% longer than would be expected for normal bones. This measure is required because neuropathic bones heal slowly. However, the main reason is that whereas normal people spare their operated limbs and limp when first free from their plaster cast, patients with insensitive limbs walk with full uninhibited stride as soon as restraint is removed.

References

Assal JP, Mulhauser I, Pernat A, Gfeller R, Jorgens V, Berger M: Patient education as the basis for diabetes care in clinical practice. Diabetalogia 28:602–613, 1985.

Coleman WC, Brand PW, Birke JA: The total contact cast: A therapy for plantar ulceration on insensitive feet. J Am Podiatr Med Assoc 74:548–552, 1984.

Harris JR, Brand PW: Patterns of disintegration of the tarsus in the anesthetic foot. J Bone Joint Surg (Br) *48B:*4, 1966.

Hodgson JR, Pugh DG, Young HH: Roentgenologic aspect of certain lesions of bone: Neuropathic or infectious? Radiology *50:*65, 1948.

Chapter 73

- Alfred B. Swanson
- Geneviève de Groot Swanson

Impairment Evaluation of the Peripheral Nerve System of the Upper Extremity

An evaluation method of physical impairment of the hand and upper extremity was developed (Swanson 1964), tested by many hand surgeons around the world, and approved for international application by the International Federation of Societies for Surgery of the Hand at its first Congress, held in Rotterdam in 1980. The system has been endorsed by the American Society for Surgery of the Hand, the American Academy of Orthopaedic Surgeons, and the American Medical Association for national usage and has been included in the AMA's *Guide to the Evaluation of Permanent Impairment of the Extremities and Back,* third and fourth editions.

PRINCIPLES AND METHODS OF IMPAIRMENT EVALUATION

This method rates permanent anatomical impairment and is based on a detailed physical examination after appropriate medical, surgical, or rehabilitation methods have been applied and an optimal time of recovery has elapsed. The regional evaluation rates impairments caused by amputation, sensory loss, and abnormal motion of the digits, wrist, elbow, and shoulder. Techniques to rate impairments of the upper extremity caused by lesions of the peripheral vascular, peripheral nerve, and musculoskeletal systems and loss of strength have been defined. However, this chapter is more specifically focused on evaluation of permanent impairment after peripheral nerve problems. The reader is referred to previous publications to learn the entire scope of this method (Swanson and de Groot Swanson, 1993; Swanson et al, 1995).

The most practical and useful approach to evaluate digit impairment is to compare it with the loss of function resulting from an amputation at various levels. Impairment resulting from total transverse sensory loss is considered to be 50% of that caused by amputation. Impairment values for sensory deficits caused by lesions proximal to digital nerves, symptomatic neuromas, and motor deficits of the upper extremity are based on the anatomical distribution and function of the nerve structures involved. A brief presentation of the principles of amputation impairment evaluation and of a method to combine two or more impairments of a specific unit or of the entire upper extremity is fundamental.

Amputation Impairment Evaluation

The upper limb is considered a unit of the whole person and is divided into hand, wrist, elbow, and shoulder. The hand is further separated into digits and their parts. Amputation of the entire extremity or 100% loss of the limb is considered 60% impairment of the whole person. Amputations distal to the biceps insertion and proximal to the metacarpophalangeal (MP) level are considered a 95% loss of the limb. Amputation of the fingers and thumb through the MP joint removes the most essential parts and is considered 100% impairment of the hand or 90% impairment of the upper extremity, and equals 90% × 60%, or 54% impairment of the whole person (Fig. 73–1A). The digits represent five coordinated units into which all hand function is unequally divided. Each digit is given a relative value to the entire hand as follows: thumb, 40%; index and middle fingers, 20% each; and ring and little fingers, 10% each (Fig. 73–1B). Each portion of a digit is given a relative value as follows: digit MP joint, 100%; finger proximal interphalangeal (PIP) joint, 80%; finger distal interphalangeal (DIP) joint, 45%; and thumb IP, 50%. The value of each portion of a digit can be related to the entire hand by multiplying it by the digit's relative value to the hand.

Example: Amputation through the PIP joint of the index finger represents 80% finger impairment; the index finger's relative hand value is 20%; therefore, this amputation represents 80% × 20%, or 16% hand impairment.

When multiple digits are involved, the hand impairment values for each digit are added directly together to obtain the total hand impairment, which is multiplied by 90% to obtain the upper extremity impairment and then by 60% to obtain impairment of the whole person. Using this principle of progressive multiplication of percentage values, one can relate the impairment of each digit or portion thereof to the hand, the upper limb, and eventually to the whole person (Tables 73–1, 73–2, and 73–3).

Example: Amputation of the entire thumb (40% hand impairment) with amputation through the DIP joint of the index finger (45% × 20% = 9% hand impairment) equals 49% impairment of the hand; 49% × 90% = 44% impairment of the upper extremity, and 44% × 60% = 26% impairment of the whole person.

Impairment Estimation for Combined Values

The method to *combine* various impairments is based on the principle that each impairment acts not on the whole part (for example, the whole finger) but on the portion that

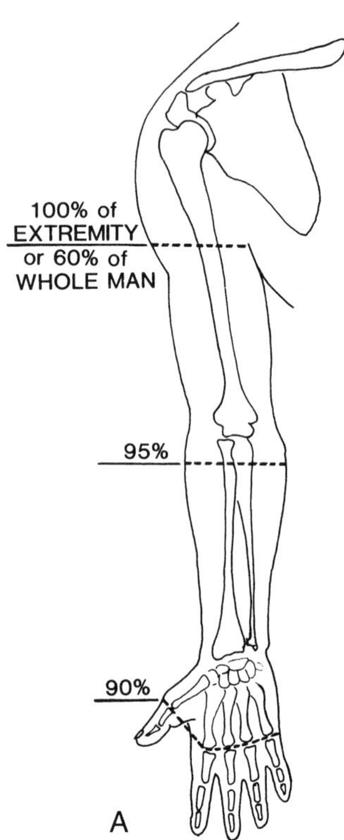

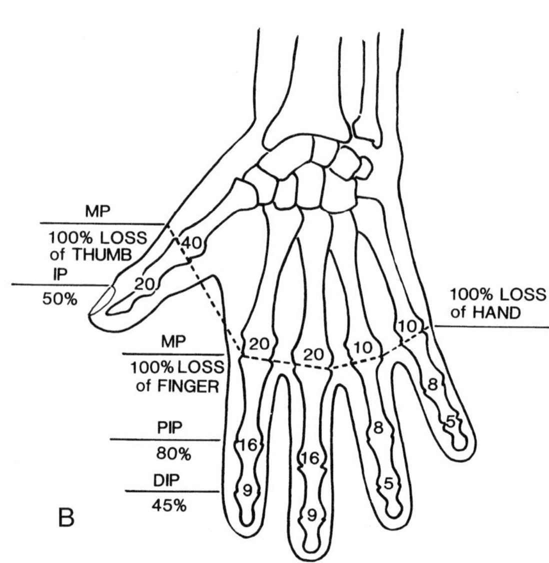

FIGURE 73–1. Amputation impairments related to the whole person, extremity, hand, or digits: *A,* impairments of the upper extremity. *B,* digit impairments *(numbers outside drawing)* and hand *(numbers inside drawing)* for amputation at various levels (MP, metacarpophalangeal; IP, interphalangeal; PIP, proximal interphalangeal; DIP, distal interphalangeal). (From Swanson AB: Evaluation of impairment of function in the hand. Surg Clin North Am *44:*925–940, 1964.)

remains (for example, the PIP joint and proximally) after the preceding impairment has acted (for example, on the DIP joint). When there is more than one impairment to a given part, these impairments must be *combined* before the conversion to a larger part is made. The *combined* values determination is based on the formula:

$$A\% + B\% (100\% - A\%) =$$
$$\text{the combined values of } A\% + B\%.$$

All percentages to be *combined* must be expressed on a common denominator. When multiple impairments of a digit are present, such as abnormal motion, sensory loss, or amputation, these are *combined* as expressed on the 100% relative value of the digit. The combined value is converted to the next larger part, for example, the hand. If three or more values are to be *combined,* two may be selected and their combined value found. This combined value and the third value are *combined* to give the total value. This procedure can be repeated indefinitely, with the value obtained in each being a *combination* of all the previous values.

Example: Index finger amputation impairment is 45%; sensory impairment, 20%; and abnormal motion impairment, 50%. The combined impairment value of the index finger is

45% + 20% (100% − 45%) = 45% + 11% = 56%
56% + 50% (100% − 50%) = 56% + 25% = 81%

The index finger represents 20% to the hand, and the above impairment would represent a 20% × 81% hand impairment, or 16%. This corresponds to a 14% impairment of the upper extremity, and 8% impairment of the whole person (Tables 73–2 and 73–3).

Similarly, when both sensory and motor functions of a mixed nerve are involved, the impairment percent derived for each function is *combined.* Multiple regional impairments such as those of the hand, wrist, elbow, and shoulder are expressed individually in terms of the upper extremity before being *combined* together. Note that when more than one digit is involved, the hand impairments contributed by each digit are *added* directly together before relating the hand impairment to upper extremity impairment.

NEUROLOGICAL EXAMINATION

The neurological examination includes a complete motor and sensory evaluation of the hand and upper extremity to determine the presence and location of peripheral nerve disorders, including those of the nerve roots, brachial plexus, and major peripheral nerves. Digital nerve loss and the presence and location of neuromas are evaluated. Tenderness, sensitivity, and painful states such as causalgias and other sympathetic dystrophies are appraised.

Sensory Evaluation

The classic Weber static two-point discrimination test is most practical (Omer, 1980). With the patient's eyes closed, the device tips are lightly touched to the digit in the longitudinal axis, without blanching or indenting the skin. A series of one or two points is applied, and the subject indicates whether he or she feels one or two points. The distance of the tips is first set at 15 mm and is decreased with accurate responses. Testing is started distally and proceeds proximally

▼ **TABLE 73–1**
Relationship of Impairment of the Digits to Impairment of the Hand

% Impairment of		% Impairment of		% Impairment of	
		Index or Middle		*Ring or Little*	
Thumb	*Hand*	*Finger*	*Hand*	*Finger*	*Hand*
0–1	= 0	0–2	= 0	0–4	= 0
2–3	= 1	3–7	= 1	5–14	= 1
4–6	= 2	8–12	= 2	15–24	= 2
7–8	= 3	13–17	= 3	25–34	= 3
9–11	= 4	18–22	= 4	35–44	= 4
12–13	= 5	23–27	= 5	45–54	= 5
14–16	= 6	28–32	= 6	55–64	= 6
17–18	= 7	33–37	= 7	65–74	= 7
19–21	= 8	38–42	= 8	75–84	= 8
22–23	= 9	43–47	= 9	85–94	= 9
24–26	= 10	48–52	= 10	95–100	= 10
27–28	= 11	53–57	= 11		
29–31	= 12	58–62	= 12		
32–33	= 13	63–67	= 13		
34–36	= 14	68–72	= 14		
37–38	= 15	73–77	= 15		
39–41	= 16	78–82	= 16		
42–43	= 17	83–87	= 17		
44–46	= 18	88–92	= 18		
47–48	= 19	93–97	= 19		
49–51	= 20	98–100	= 20		
52–53	= 21				
54–56	= 22				
57–58	= 23				
59–61	= 24				
62–63	= 25				
64–66	= 26				
67–68	= 27				
69–71	= 28				
72–73	= 29				
74–76	= 30				
77–78	= 31				
79–81	= 32				
82–83	= 33				
84–86	= 34				
87–88	= 35				
89–91	= 36				
92–93	= 37				
94–96	= 38				
97–98	= 39				
99–100	= 40				

From Doege TC, Houston TP: Guides to the Evaluation of Permanent Impairment, 4th ed. Chicago, American Medical Association, 1993.

to determine the longitudinal level of involvement. The minimum distance at which the patient can discriminate between one-point and two-point applications in two out of three trials is recorded. Two-point discrimination values greater than 15 mm represent a total sensory loss; values between 15 and 7 mm represent a partial sensory loss; and values equal to or less than 6 mm are considered normal. The distribution of the sensory loss is noted according to the involvement of one or both digital nerves and to the percentage of digit length involved. The digit sensory impairment is rated according to Tables 73–4, 73–5, and 73–6 as detailed later.

Objective tests for sensory impairment are limited, and one must rely on the patient's honesty. When malingering is suspected, more objective methods include the Ninhydrin test for sudomotor function and antegrade or orthograde electrodiagnostic testing. It also may be possible to prick the patient's fingertip to see whether the finger is withdrawn from this painful stimulus. Functional isolation of the finger,

as noted in the blindfolded pick-up test, will aid the examiner in determining the presence or absence of any useful sensation in the digit.

The Ninhydrin test for sudomotor function can be a useful method for documenting the interruption of the digital nerves (Moberg, 1958). However, it has limitations in evaluating the "recovering" nerve, because there is not a direct relationship between return of sudomotor function and return of tactile gnosis. The moving two-point discrimination test can help assess the regenerating nerve, because this function recovers before the static two-point discrimination.

Muscle Power Testing

Muscle power testing is important to evaluate the upper extremity disabled by paralysis or paresis resulting from nervous system disorders. It is based on the ability of the muscle to contract, move a joint through its range of motion against gravity, and hold that motion against resistance. Motor impairments can be classified according to the severity of motor power loss as described later in Table 73–9.

▼ **TABLE 73–2**
Relationship of Impairment of the Hand to Impairment of the Upper Extremity

% Impairment of		% Impairment of		% Impairment of	
Hand	*Upper Extremity*	*Hand*	*Upper Extremity*	*Hand*	*Upper Extremity*
0	= 0	35	= 32	70	= 63
1	= 1	36	= 32	71	= 64
2	= 2	37	= 33	72	= 65
3	= 3	38	= 34	73	= 66
4	= 4	39	= 35	74	= 67
5	= 5	40	= 36	75	= 68
6	= 5	41	= 37	76	= 68
7	= 6	42	= 38	77	= 69
8	= 7	43	= 39	78	= 70
9	= 8	44	= 40	79	= 71
10	= 9	45	= 41	80	= 72
11	= 10	46	= 41	81	= 73
12	= 11	47	= 42	82	= 74
13	= 12	48	= 43	83	= 75
14	= 13	49	= 44	84	= 76
15	= 14	50	= 45	85	= 77
16	= 14	51	= 46	86	= 77
17	= 15	52	= 47	87	= 78
18	= 16	53	= 48	88	= 79
19	= 17	54	= 49	89	= 80
20	= 18	55	= 50	90	= 81
21	= 19	56	= 50	91	= 82
22	= 20	57	= 51	92	= 83
23	= 21	58	= 52	93	= 84
24	= 22	59	= 53	94	= 85
25	= 23	60	= 54	95	= 86
26	= 23	61	= 55	96	= 86
27	= 24	62	= 56	97	= 87
28	= 25	63	= 57	98	= 88
29	= 26	64	= 58	99	= 89
30	= 27	65	= 59	100	= 90
31	= 28	66	= 59		
32	= 29	67	= 60		
33	= 30	68	= 61		
34	= 31	69	= 62		

From Doege TC, Houston TP: Guides to the Evaluation of Permanent Impairment, 4th ed. Chicago, American Medical Association, 1993.

▼ TABLE 73–3
Relationship of Impairment of the Upper Extremity to Impairment of the Whole Person

% Impairment of		% Impairment of		% Impairment of	
Upper Extremity	Whole Person	Upper Extremity	Whole Person	Upper Extremity	Whole Person
0 = 0		35 = 21		70 = 42	
1 = 1		36 = 22		71 = 43	
2 = 1		37 = 22		72 = 43	
3 = 2		38 = 23		73 = 44	
4 = 2		39 = 23		74 = 44	
5 = 3		40 = 24		75 = 45	
6 = 4		41 = 25		76 = 46	
7 = 4		42 = 25		77 = 46	
8 = 5		43 = 26		78 = 47	
9 = 5		44 = 26		79 = 47	
10 = 6		45 = 27		80 = 48	
11 = 7		46 = 28		81 = 49	
12 = 7		47 = 28		82 = 49	
13 = 8		48 = 29		83 = 50	
14 = 8		49 = 29		84 = 50	
15 = 9		50 = 30		85 = 51	
16 = 10		51 = 31		86 = 52	
17 = 10		52 = 31		87 = 52	
18 = 11		53 = 32		88 = 53	
19 = 11		54 = 32		89 = 53	
20 = 12		55 = 33		90 = 54	
21 = 13		56 = 34		91 = 55	
22 = 13		57 = 34		92 = 55	
23 = 14		58 = 35		93 = 56	
24 = 14		59 = 35		94 = 56	
25 = 15		60 = 36		95 = 57	
26 = 16		61 = 37		96 = 58	
27 = 16		62 = 37		97 = 58	
28 = 17		63 = 38		98 = 59	
29 = 17		64 = 38		99 = 59	
30 = 18		65 = 39		100 = 60	
31 = 19		66 = 40			
32 = 19		67 = 40			
33 = 20		68 = 41			
34 = 20		69 = 41			

From Doege TC, Houston TP: Guides to the Evaluation of Permanent Impairment, 4th ed. Chicago, American Medical Association, 1993.

Pain Evaluation

Pain is difficult to evaluate because it is a subjective symptom. Pain can be defined as a disagreeable sensation that has as its basis a highly variable complex made up of afferent nerve stimuli interacting with the emotional state of the individual and modified by his or her experience, motivation, and state of mind (Swanson, 1964). Pain may be verified and the intensity of pain may be evaluated in a thorough physical examination. Pretended pain may be detected by tests that confuse the patient into responding with signs that are contradictory to the usual clinical examination. Examination can further demonstrate whether the pain has an anatomical background or whether it is associated with other signs of nerve dysfunction. Impairment caused by abnormal sensations or pain associated with peripheral nerve disorders can be classified according to how the pain interferes with performance of activities (as shown later in Table 73–8) (Swanson, 1964).

SENSORY IMPAIRMENT EVALUATION OF THE DIGITS
Principles

Sensory deficits must be unequivocal and permanent to rate for permanent impairment. Sensibility on the distal

▼ TABLE 73–4
Sensory Impairment Classification

Sensory Loss	Two-Point Discrimination	Sensory Impairment
Total	> 15 mm	100%
Partial	15 to 7 mm	50%
None	6 mm or less	0%

palmar surface contributes to the function of the digit. Sensory loss on the least-often opposed surfaces of the fingers and thumb is given less value than the more important surfaces used in the pinch and grasp activities. Loss of sensibility on the dorsal surface of the digits is not considered disabling. Sensory deficits proximal to the level of the digits, and symptomatic neuromas are considered in the peripheral nerve section. The sensory impairment is based on the results of the two-point discrimination test over the distal palmar area of the digit or over the most distal area of the digital stump in the presence of a partial amputation. The sensory impairment is rated according to the *sensory quality* and the *distribution of the sensory loss*.

The *sensory quality* is classified based on the results of the two-point discrimination test, and the impairment is rated according to Table 73–4.

The *distribution of the sensory loss* is determined by the level of involvement of one or both digital nerves and is classified as follows:

1. *Transverse sensory loss:* both digital nerves involved.
2. *Longitudinal sensory loss:* one digital nerve involved on either the radial or ulnar side of the digit.

The *level of involvement* corresponds to the percentage of digit length presenting a sensory loss.

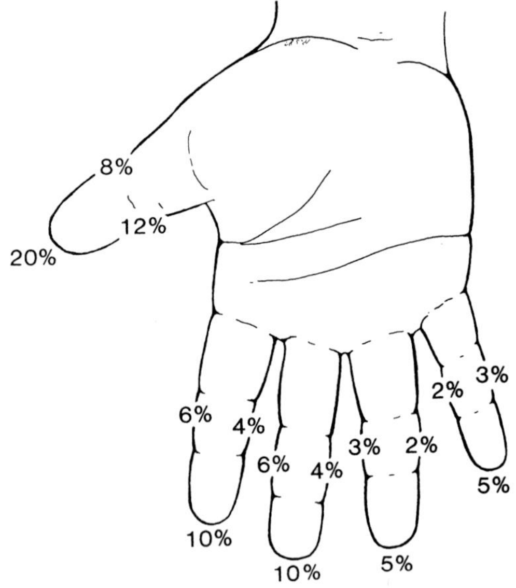

FIGURE 73–2. Hand impairments for total transverse sensory loss of entire length of digit *(numbers at tips of digits)* and total longitudinal sensory loss of entire radial and ulnar sides *(numbers at sides of digits)*. Total transverse sensory loss is calculated as 50% that of amputation. (From Swanson AB: Evaluation of impairment of function in the hand. Surg Clin North Am *44*:925–940, 1964.)

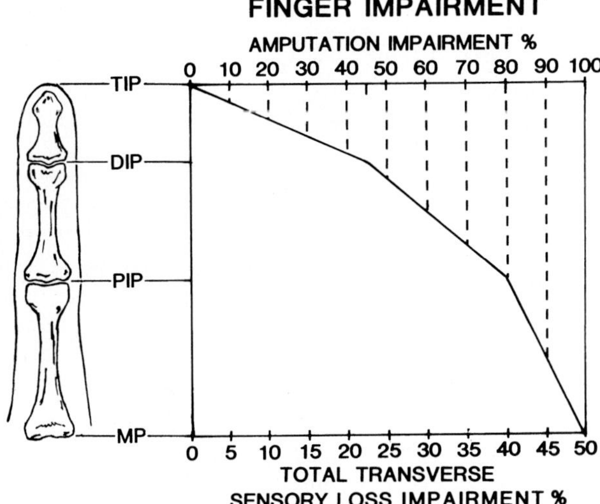

FIGURE 73–3. Finger impairments for amputation at various lengths *(top scale)* and total transverse sensory loss *(bottom scale)*, which corresponds to 50% of amputation values. (From Swanson AB: Evaluation of impairment of function in the hand. Surg Clin North Am *44*:925–940, 1964.)

Total transverse sensory loss (>15 mm) represents a 100% sensory loss involving both digital nerves and receives 50% of the amputation impairment value for that level of involvement (see Figs. 73–1 to 73–4 and Tables 73–5 and 73–6). Complete loss of both digital nerves at the level of the MP joint therefore receives the following hand impairment values: thumb, 20%; index and middle fingers, 10%; ring and little fingers, 5% (see Fig. 73–2).

Partial transverse sensory loss (15 to 7 mm) represents a 50% sensory loss involving both digital nerves and receives 25% of the amputation impairment value for that level of involvement (see Tables 73–5 to 73–6).

Longitudinal sensory loss impairments are calculated according to the relative importance of the side of the digit for sensory function as follows: thumb and little finger, radial side 40% and ulnar side 60%; index, middle, and ring fingers, radial side 60% and ulnar side 40%. The corresponding hand impairment values for total longitudinal sensory

loss of the entire length of each side of each digit are shown in Figure 73–2.

Impairment values for total and partial transverse and longitudinal sensory losses are calculated according to the level of involvement, or percentage of digit length affected by the sensory loss. Consult Table 73–5 for the index, middle, and ring fingers and Table 73–6 for the thumb and little finger. In the presence of amputation, the sensory impairment is similarly rated according to the length of the digital stump.

Example: Total sensory loss (50% amputation impairment) along the distribution of the ulnar nerve of the thumb starting at the level of the IP joint represents a 60% sensory loss of 50% of the thumb length, or 50% × 60% × 50% = 15% thumb impairment and 6% hand impairment (see Tables 73–1 and 73–6).

Sensibility on the ulnar aspect of the border finger is rated more highly. Therefore, if the little finger has been amputated, the relative value of the ulnar side of the ring finger becomes 60%, and that of the radial side 40%. Loss

▼ TABLE 73–5

Finger Impairment for Transverse and Longitudinal Sensory Loss of Index, Middle, and Ring Fingers Based on Percentage of Digit Length Involved

| | Transverse Loss | | Longitudinal Loss | | | |
| | | | Ulnar | | Radial | |
% Digit Length	Total	Partial	Total	Partial	Total	Partial
100	50	25	20	10	30	15
90	45	23	18	9	27	14
80	40	20	16	8	24	12
70	35	18	14	7	21	11
60	30	15	12	6	18	9
50	25	13	10	5	15	8
40	20	10	8	4	12	6
30	15	8	6	3	9	5
20	10	5	4	2	6	3
10	5	3	2	1	3	2

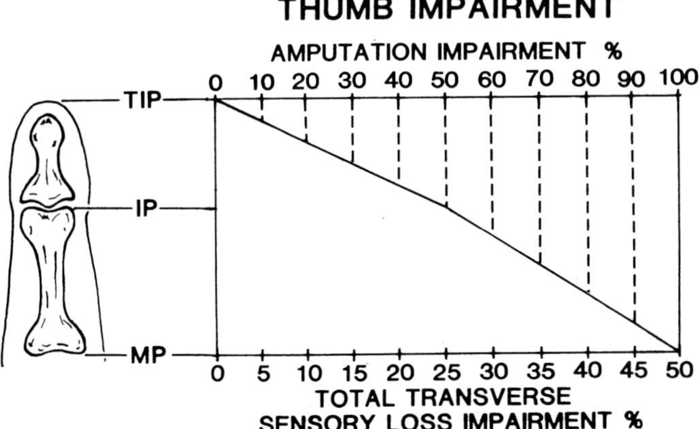

FIGURE 73–4. Thumb impairments for amputation at various lengths *(top scale)* and total transverse sensory loss *(bottom scale)*, which corresponds to 50% of amputation values. (From Swanson AB: Evaluation of impairment of function in the hand. Surg Clin North Am *44*:925–940, 1964.)

▼ TABLE 73–6

Digit Impairments for Transverse and Longitudinal Sensory Loss of Thumb and Little Finger Based on Percentage of Digit Length Involved

| | Transverse Loss | | Longitudinal Loss | | | |
| | | | Ulnar | | Radial | |
% Digit Length	Total	Partial	Total	Partial	Total	Partial
100	50	25	30	15	20	10
90	45	23	27	14	18	9
80	40	20	24	12	16	8
70	35	18	21	11	14	7
60	30	15	18	9	12	6
50	25	13	15	8	10	5
40	20	10	12	6	8	4
30	15	8	9	5	6	3
20	10	5	6	3	4	2
10	5	3	3	2	2	1

of palmar cutaneous nerve sensibility is considered to be a 5% impairment of the hand. Zero to 10% impairment of the upper extremity may be given for loss of sensibility of the palmar or dorsal ulnar cutaneous nerve, the palmar branch of the medial nerve, or the superficial branch of the radial nerve.

Method

1. Use the two-point discrimination test to identify the type of sensory loss as total (>15 mm) or partial (7 to 15 mm).

2. Determine whether one (longitudinal sensory loss) or both (transverse sensory loss) digital nerves are involved.

3. Identify the level of involvement or percentage of digit length involved (see the top scale of Fig. 73–3 for fingers and Fig. 73–4 for thumb).

4. Consult Table 73–5 for the index, middle, and ring fingers, and Table 73–6 for the thumb and little finger to determine the digit impairment for total or partial, transverse, and longitudinal (ulnar or radial) sensory loss according to the percentage of digit length involved.

5. *Convert* the digit impairment to hand, upper extremity, and whole person impairment.

Examples: A total transverse sensory loss (>15 mm) over the index finger palmar surface starting at the level of the PIP joint (80% finger length) is equivalent to a 40% finger impairment (see Table 73–5) and 8% hand impairment (see Table 73–1).

A partial transverse sensory loss (7 to 15 mm) involving the full length of the palmar surface of the little finger starting at the level of the MP joint (100% length) gives a 25% impairment of the finger (see Table 73–6) and 3% hand impairment (Table 73–1).

A total longitudinal sensory loss (>15 mm) over the distribution of the thumb ulnar digital nerve starting at the level of the IP joint (50% thumb length) is equivalent to a 15% thumb impairment (see Table 73–6) or a 6% hand impairment.

A partial longitudinal sensory loss (7 to 15 mm) over the distribution of the thumb radial nerve starting at the level of the MP joint (100% length) is equivalent to 10% thumb impairment (see Table 73–6) or 4% hand impairment.

IMPAIRMENT EVALUATION OF PERIPHERAL NERVE DISORDERS

Principles

This section presents criteria for evaluation of permanent impairment of the upper extremity resulting from disorders of the spinal nerves, C5 to C8 and T1, of the brachial plexus, and of major peripheral nerves. Permanent impairment of the upper extremity from peripheral nerve disorders results from abnormalities of the motor and/or sensory function that remain after appropriate treatment and a sufficient length of time to allow optimal regeneration and the appearance of signs of physiological recovery. The impairment determination is based on the extent of loss of function resulting from

(1) sensory deficits or pain and (2) motor deficits. It is not necessary to rate separately certain characteristic deformities and manifestations of peripheral nerve lesions such as restricted motion; atrophy; vasomotor, trophic, reflex changes; and decreased strength, because these deficits have been reflected in the sensory and/or motor impairment values presented.

Accurate diagnosis is based on a complete medical history, a thorough medical and neurological examination, and appropriate laboratory testing. The anatomical distribution and severity of the motor and/or sensory loss must be verified and related to dysfunction of specific peripheral nerves, spinal nerves, or the brachial plexus. The origins and functions of the peripheral nerves of the upper extremity are summarized in Table 73–7. The motor and sensory innervation and cutaneous dermatomes of the upper extremity are illustrated in Figures 73–5 through 73–7. A schematic diagram of the brachial plexus is shown in Figure 73–8.

Methods

The impairment evaluation is based on the anatomical distribution of the motor and/or sensory loss and its severity. The severity of loss of function caused by sensory deficits or pain (Table 73–8) and/or motor deficits (Table 73–9) is appropriately graded and related to the anatomical structure(s) involved. Maximum percentages of upper extremity impairment caused by sensory and motor deficits have been derived for the spinal nerves (Table 73–10), brachial plexus (Table 73–11), and major peripheral nerves (Table 73–12). For each structure involved, impairment percentages are calculated by *multiplying* the maximum impairment value for sensory or motor deficit (see Tables 73–10 to 73–12) by the grade of severity of sensory or motor loss (see Tables 73–8 and 73–9). When both functions are involved, the impairment percentages derived for each are *combined*.

SENSORY DEFICITS AND PAIN

A wide range of abnormal sensations can be associated with peripheral nerve lesions and can include anesthesia, dysesthesia, paresthesia, hyperesthesia, cold intolerance, and an intense burning pain. Pain and sensory deficits associated with peripheral nerve disorders must be evaluated according to the following criteria: (1) degree of interference with performance of activities; (2) distribution along defined anatomical pathways; (3) description consistent with characteristics of peripheral nerve involvement; and (4) consistent correspondence with other disturbances of the involved nerve structure. Permanent loss of function because of pain or sensory abnormalities are described as a condition that exists after optimum physiological adjustment and maximum medical rehabilitation have been administered. Subjective complaints of pain that cannot be substantiated along these lines should not be considered for impairment.

The upper extremity impairment caused by sensory deficits or pain is calculated as follows:

1. Localize the distribution of cutaneous sensory deficits using Figures 73–6 and 73–7.

2. Determine the severity of sensory deficit or pain according to the classification shown in Table 73–8.

Origins and Functions of the Peripheral Nerves of the Upper Extremity Emanating from the Brachial Plexus*

Nerves of Plexus	Primary branches	Secondary Branches	Function
Muscular branches Dorsal scapular (C5) Long thoracic (C5, C6, C7) Suprascapular (C5, C6) Lateral pectoral (C5, C6, C7) Medial pectoral (C8, T1) Upper subscapular (C5, C6) Lower subscapular (C5, C6) Thoracodorsal (±C6, C7, C8)	Unnamed		Motor to longus colli, scalenes, and subclavius Motor to rhomboideus major and minor, levator scapulae Motor to serratus anterior Motor to supraspinatus and infraspinatus Motor to pectoralis major Motor to pectoralis major and minor Motor to subscapularis Motor to teres major and subscapularis Motor to latissimus dorsi
Medial brachial cutaneous (T1)			Sensory to anteromedial surface of arm (with intercostobrachial)
Medial antebrachial cutaneous (C8, T1)			Sensory to anteromedial surface of arm and ulnar surface of forearm
Musculocutaneous (C5, C6, C7)	Unnamed Lateral antebrachial cutaneous		Motor to coracobrachialis, biceps brachii, brachialis Sensory to radial surface of forearm
Axillary (C5, C6)	Posterior	Teres minor branch	Motor to teres minor Motor to posterior part of deltoid
		Superior lateral brachial-cutaneous	Sensory to skin over lower two thirds of deltoid
	Anterior		Motor to central and anterior parts of deltoid
Radial (C5, C6, C7, C8, ±T1)	Unnamed Ulnar collateral Posterior brachial cutaneous Inferior lateral brachial cutaneous Posterior antebrachial cutaneous Superficial and dorsal digitals		Motor to triceps brachii, anconeus, brachioradialis, extensor carpi radialis longus, brachialis (lateral part only) Motor to medial head of triceps brachii Sensory to posteromedial surface of arm (with intercostobrachial) as far as olecranon Sensory to distal posterolateral surface of arm Sensory to dorsal surface of arm and forearm and distal posterolateral one third of arm Sensory to dorsum of radial one half of wrist and hand; thumb, index, middle and radial one half of ring finger to middle phalanx
	Posterior interosseous	Unnamed branch	Motor to extensor carpi radialis brevis, supinator
		Superficial branch	Motor to extensor digitorum conmunis, extensor digiti quinti proprius, extensor carpi ulnaris
		Deep branch	Motor to extensor pollicis longus, extensor pollicis brevis, abductor pollicis longus, extensor indicis proprius
		Terminal branch	Sensory to wrist joint capsule
Median (±C5, C6, C7, C8, T1)	Unnamed	Cubital fossa and forearm branches	Motor to pronator teres, flexor carpi radialis, palmaris longus, flexor digitorum superficialis
	Anterior interosseus Palmar cutaneous		Motor to radial half of flexor digitorum profundus of the index and middle fingers, flexor pollicis longus, pronator quadratus Sensory to radial surface of palm
	Common palmar radial digital	Thenar muscular branch	Motor to abductor pollicis brevis, flexor pollicis brevis and opponens pollicis
		Proper palmar digitals (1st, 2nd, 3rd)	Motor to first lumbrical; sensory to first web space, to palmar and distal dorsal surfaces of thumb, and to index palmar surface and distal dorsal surface on radial side
	Common palmar central digital	Proper palmar digital (4th)	Motor to second lumbrical; sensory to 2nd web space and to palmar surfaces and distal dorsal surfaces of contiguous sides of index and middle fingers
	Common palmar ulnar digital	Proper palmar digital (5th)	Sensory to 3rd web space and to palmar surfaces and distal dorsal surfaces of contiguous sides of middle and ring fingers
Ulnar (±C7, C8, T1)	Unnamed Palmar and dorsal cutaneous Superficial palmar Deep palmar		Motor to flexor carpi ulnaris, ulnar half of flexor digitorum profundus of ring and little fingers Sensory to ulnar half of hand, little finger and ulnar half of ring finger Motor to palmaris brevis Motor to abductor pollicis, deep head of flexor pollicis brevis, abductor digiti quinti, flexor digiti quinti brevis, opponens digiti quinti, third and fourth lumbricals, all interossei

*Modified from Doege TC, Houston TP: Principles and methods of impairment evaluation in the hand and upper extremity. In Guides to the Evaluation of Permanent Impairment, 4th ed. Chicago, American Medical Association, 1993, pp 13–74.

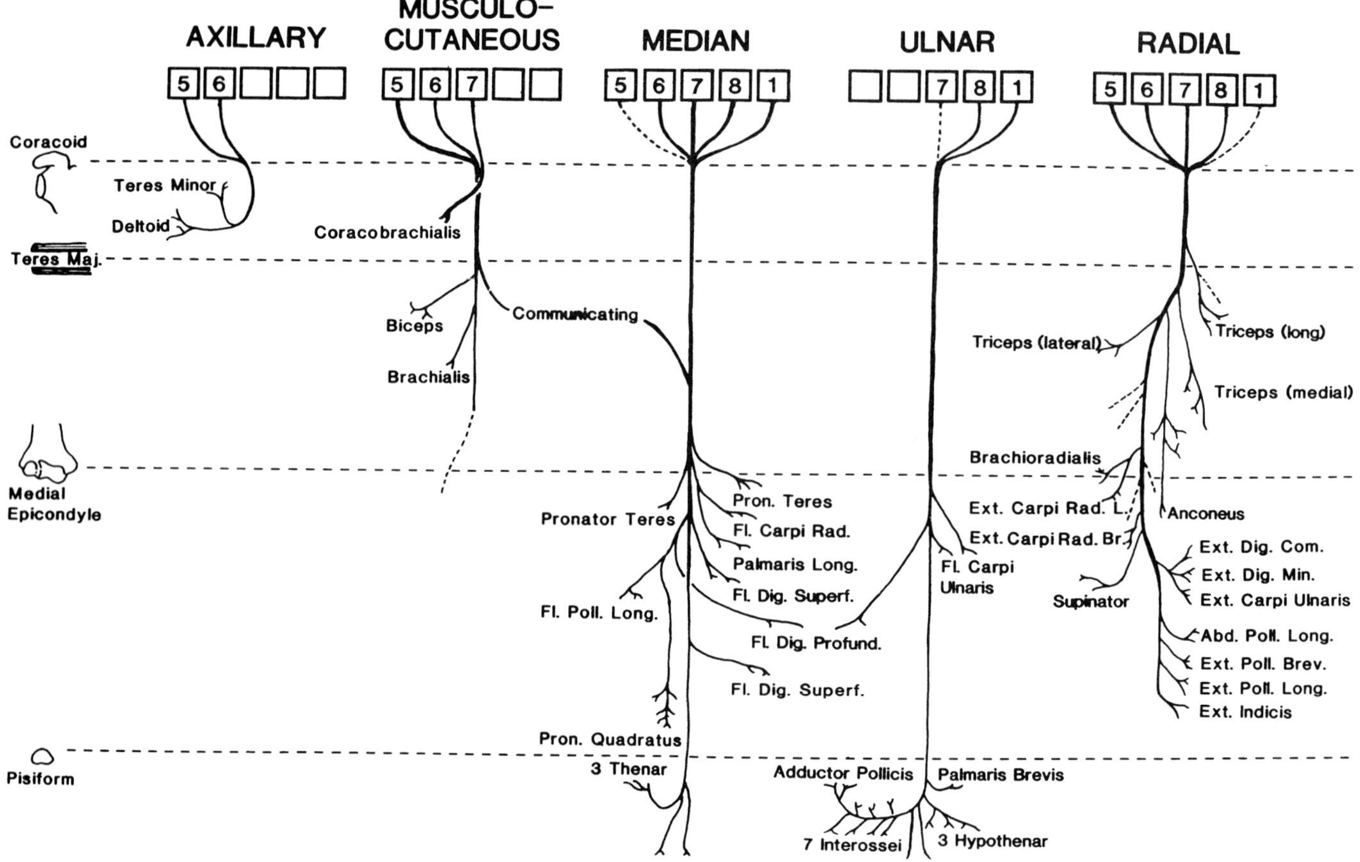

FIGURE 73–5. Motor innervation of the upper extremity. (From Doege TC, Houston TP: Principles and methods of impairment evaluation in the hand and upper extremity. In Guides to the Evaluation of Permanent Impairment, 4th ed., Chicago, the American Medical Association, 1993, pp 13–74.)

3. Identify the nerve structure(s) involved (Table 73–7 and Figs. 73–6 to 73–8).

4. Find the maximum impairment of the upper extremity caused by sensory deficit for each structure involved: spinal nerves (see Table 73–10), brachial plexus (see Table 73–11), and major peripheral nerves (see Table 73–12).

5. *Multiply* the severity of sensory deficit by the maximum impairment value to obtain the upper extremity impairment for each structure involved.

Sensibility losses caused by digital nerve lesions are rated according to the method described earlier in the text. Symptomatic neuromas are evaluated with the criteria presented in this section (see Tables 73–8, and 73–12). Both methods should not be used in the same patient.

MOTOR DEFICITS

Muscle testing can help evaluate the motor function of specific nerves. Muscle testing rates the ability of a muscle unit to contract, move a joint through its full range of motion against gravity, and hold the part against resistance. Both upper extremities should be tested and the results compared. The upper extremity impairment caused by motor deficits is calculated as follows:

1. Identify the motion and muscles involved.
2. Determine the severity of motor deficit according to the classification shown in Table 73–9.

3. Identify the nerve structure(s) involved (see Table 73–7 and Figs. 73–5 and 73–8).

4. Find the maximum impairment of the upper extremity caused by motor deficit for each structure involved: spinal nerves (see Table 73–10), brachial plexus (see Table 73–11), and major peripheral nerves (see Table 73–12).

5. *Multiply* the severity of motor deficit by the maximum impairment value to obtain the upper extremity impairment for each structure involved.

Note that decreased strength should not be rated separately because this factor has been taken into consideration in the motor impairment values presented.

Peripheral Nerve System Impairment Determination

The determination of impairment of the peripheral nerve system includes the following:

1. Spinal nerves, C5 to C8 and T1.
2. Brachial plexus.
3. Major peripheral nerves.
4. Entrapment neuropathies.
5. Causalgia and reflex sympathetic dystrophy (RSD).

SPINAL NERVES

The impairment caused by spinal nerve disorders is based on the severity of loss of function of the peripheral nerves

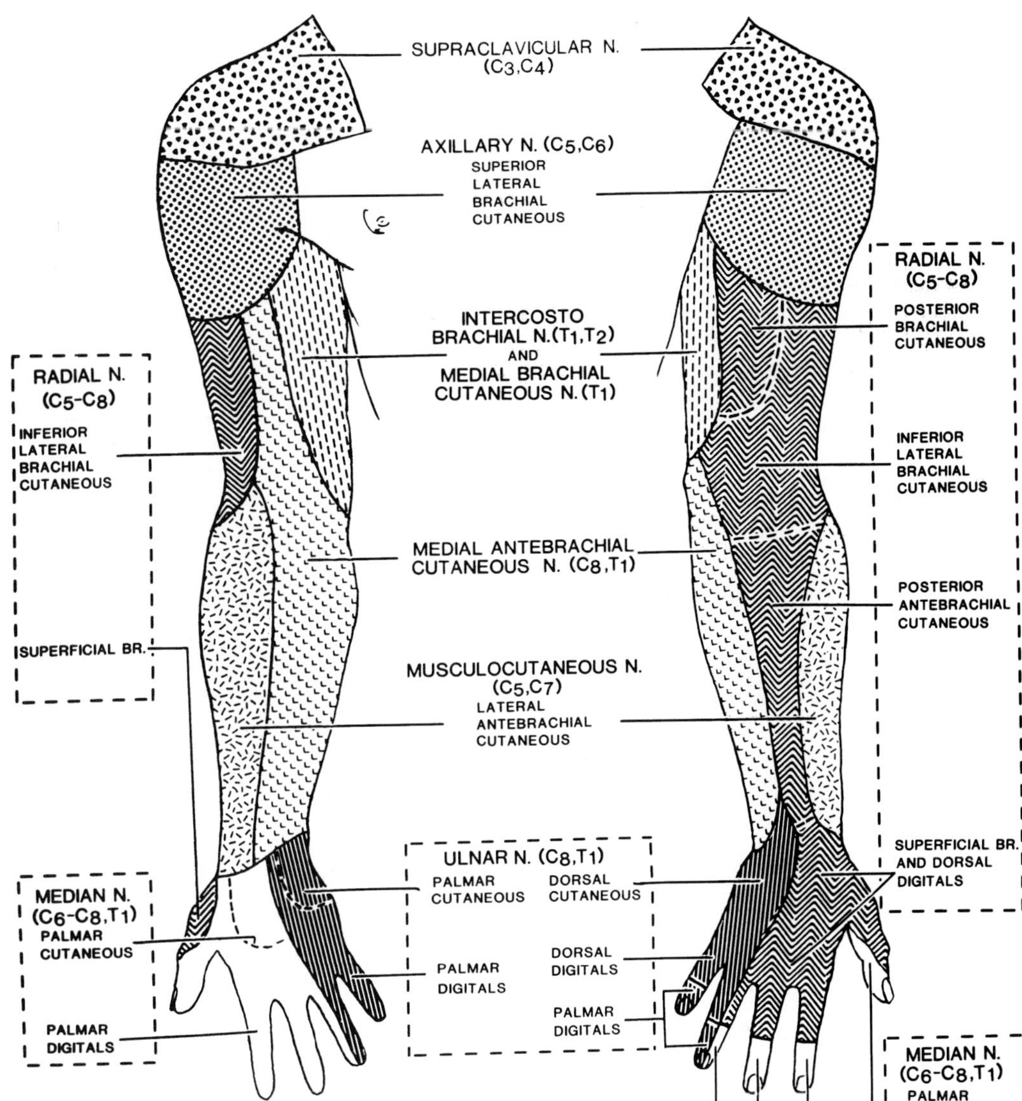

FIGURE 73–6. Cutaneous nerves of the upper limb. (Adapted with permission from Netter FH: The Atlas of Human Anatomy. Summit, NJ, CIBA-GEIGY Corp. 1989.)

FIGURE 73–7. Dermatomes of the upper limb. (Adapted with permission from Netter FH: The Atlas of Human Anatomy. Summit, NJ, CIBA-GEIGY Corp, 1989.)

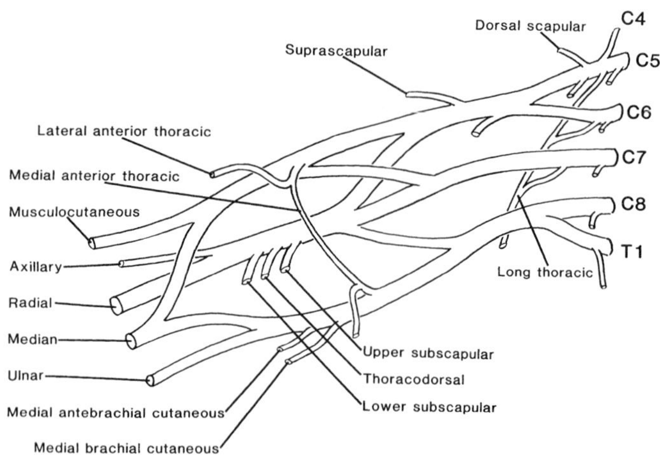

FIGURE 73–8. The brachial plexus.

receiving fibers from a specific spinal nerve. Because peripheral nerves receive fibers from more than one spinal root, involvement of two or more spinal nerves giving fibers to the same peripheral nerve produces a greater loss of function of a specific nerve, and the impairment is then rated according to the brachial plexus values (see Table 73–11) rather than *combining* individual spinal nerve values (see Table 73–10). For example, the maximum upper extremity impairment caused by *combined* motor and sensory deficits resulting from a lesion of the lower trunk (C8 and T1) is 76% (see Table 73–11); the combination of the impairment values for C8 (48%) and T1 (24%), as shown on Table 73–10, gives a 60% upper extremity impairment and does not reflect the severity of loss of function.

The spinal nerve–related impairment is derived as follows:

1. Localize the distribution of the cutaneous sensory deficit according to the dermatome involved (see Figs. 73–6 and 73–7). Evaluate the motor deficit and identify the muscles involved (see Table 73–12 and Fig. 73–5).

Classification of Severity of Sensory Deficits or Pain Caused by Peripheral Nerve Disorders*

Grade	Description of Sensory Deficit or Pain	% Sensory Deficit
1	No loss of sensibility, abnormal sensations, or pain	0
2	Decreased sensibility with or without abnormal sensations or pain that is forgotten during activity	1–25
3	Decreased to absent sensibility, with or without abnormal sensations or pain, that interferes with activity	26–60
4	Decreased to absent sensibility, with or without abnormal sensations or pain, that may prevent activity and/or minor causalgia	61–80
5	Decreased to absent sensibility with abnormal sensations or severe pain that prevents activity, and/or major causalgia	81–100

*Modified from Swanson AB: Evaluation of impairment of function in the hand. Surg Clin North Am *44*:925–940, 1964.

2. Identify the spinal nerve involved.

3. Rate the severity of sensory (see Table 73–8) and motor (see Table 73–9) deficits.

4. Find the values for maximum impairment of the upper extremity caused by motor and/or sensory deficits of individual spinal nerves (see Table 73–10).

5. Multiply the severity of sensory (see Table 73–8) and/or motor (see Table 73–9) deficits by the appropriate values from Table 73–10 to obtain upper extremity impairment value for each function.

6. *Combine* the impairment values for motor and sensory deficits to obtain the total upper extremity impairment value and multiply this value by 60% to convert to whole person impairment (Table 73–3).

Example: After a neck injury, a 50-year old man has neck pain radiating down the right arm. The examination shows a 25% sensory deficit of the C5 dermatome and a 25% motor deficit of the muscles innervated by C5. The loss of function is determined as a permanent impairment.

1. Sensory impairment: 25% × 5% (see Table 73–10) = 1% of upper extremity.

2. Motor impairment: 25% × 30% (see Table 73–10) = 8% of upper extremity.

3. 1% combined with 8% equals 9% impairment of the upper extremity, or 5% of the whole person (Table 73–3).

Classification of Severity of Motor Deficits Caused by Peripheral Nerve Disorders*

Grade	Description of Muscle Function	% Motor Deficit
5	Active movement against gravity with full resistance	0
4	Active movement against gravity with some resistance	1–25
3	Active movement against gravity only, without resistance	26–50
2	Active movement with gravity eliminated	51–75
1	Slight contraction and no movement	76–99
0	No contraction	100

*Modified from Swanson AB: Evaluation of impairment of function in the hand. Surg Clin North Am *44*:925–940, 1964.

Maximum Upper Extremity Impairments Caused by Unilateral Sensory and/or Motor Deficits of Individual Spinal Nerves*

Spinal Nerve	Sensory Deficit or Pain	Motor Deficit	Combined Motor and Sensory Deficits
C5	5	30	34
C6	8	35	40
C7	5	35	38
C8	5	45	48
T1	5	20	24

See Table 73–8 for grading sensory deficit or pain.
See Table 73–9 for grading motor deficit.
*From Doege TC, Houston TP: Principles and methods of impairment evaluation in the hand and upper extremity. In Guides to the Evaluation of Permanent Impairment. Chicago, American Medical Association, 1993, pp 13–74.

BRACHIAL PLEXUS

The brachial plexus innervates the shoulder girdle and upper extremity and is formed by the anterior primary divisions of the fifth through eighth cervical roots and the first thoracic root. These roots anastomose to form three primary trunks: upper trunk (C5 and C6), middle trunk (C7), and lower trunk (C8 and T1) (see Fig. 73–8). Specific findings result from the involvement of these structures.

Total brachial plexus paralysis is seen as flail arm, paralysis of all muscles of the hand, and no sensibility. Sudorific function is intact when lesion is preganglionic.

Upper trunk paralysis (C5, C6), Erb-Duchenne type, is seen as paralysis of biceps, deltoid, brachialis, supraspinatus, infraspinatus, and rhomboids; weakness of triceps, pectoralis major, and extensor carpi radialis brevis and longus; most finger movements are intact; biceps reflex is absent; and sensory deficit in C5 and C6 dermatomes (see Fig. 73–7).

Lower trunk paralysis (C8, T1), Déjerine-Klumpke type, is seen as paralysis of all intrinsic muscles of the hand; weakness of the flexor carpi ulnaris and flexor digitorum profundus of the little finger; Horner syndrome (ptosis, mitosis, enophthalmos) if T1 root is avulsed from spinal cord; and sensory deficit of C8 and T1 dermatomes (see Fig. 73–7).

The brachial plexus–related impairment is derived as follows:

1. Localize the distribution of the sensory deficit according to the dermatomes involved (see Figs. 73–6 and 73–7). Evaluate the motor deficit and identify the muscles involved (see Table 73–12 and Fig. 73–5).

2. Identify the brachial plexus trunk involved.

3. Rate the severity of sensory (see Table 73–8) and motor (see Table 73–9) deficits.

4. Find the values for maximum impairment of the upper extremity caused by motor and sensory deficits of the brachial plexus and its trunks for the level of involvement (see Table 73–11).

5. Multiply the severity of sensory (see Table 73–8) and motor (see Table 73–9) deficits by the appropriate values from Table 73–11 to obtain upper extremity impairment values for each function.

6. *Combine* the impairment values for motor and sensory

deficits to obtain the total upper extremity impairment value and multiply this value by 60% to convert to the whole-person impairment (see Table 73–3).

MAJOR PERIPHERAL NERVES

Impairment of major peripheral nerves is derived as follows:

1. Identify the nerve(s) involved and determine the level of the lesion.

2. Rate the severity of sensory (see Table 73–8) and motor (see Table 73–9) deficits.

3. Find the value(s) for maximum impairment of the upper extremity caused by motor and/or sensory deficits of each major peripheral nerve involved (see Table 73–12).

4. Multiply the degree of sensory (see Table 73–8) and/or motor (see Table 73–9) deficit by the appropriate values from Table 73–12 to obtain upper extremity impairment values for each function of each nerve involved.

5. For mixed nerves, *combine* the impairment values for motor and sensory deficits to obtain the total upper extremity impairment value.

6. If more than one nerve is involved, *combine* the upper extremity impairment derived for each nerve. Multiply by 60% to convert the upper extremity impairment to whole-person impairment (Table 73–3).

Example: A patient had a subluxation of the right shoulder that was reduced anatomically. After an appropriate course of treatment, the patient, while standing, had full shoulder abduction against gravity and some resistance, starting with the arm alongside the body. There was some hypesthesia of the skin over the lower two thirds of the deltoid, which did not interfere with activity. The impairment was classified as permanent. The impairment evaluation is based on the sensory and motor deficits.

The sensory deficit is determined as follows:

1. Cutaneous sensory defect distribution involves the axillary nerve (see Fig. 73–6).

2. Maximum upper extremity impairment caused by sensory deficit of axillary nerve is 5% (see Table 73–12).

3. Gradation of severity of sensory deficit is 25% (see Table 73–8).

4. Impairment of the upper extremity caused by sensory deficit of the axillary nerve is 25% × 5% = 1%.

The motor deficit is determined as follows:

1. Muscle involved is deltoid.

2. Nerve involved is axillary (see Table 73–7 and Fig. 73–5).

3. Maximum upper extremity impairment caused by motor deficit of the axillary nerve is 35% (see Table 73–12).

4. Gradation of loss of muscle strength is 25% (see Table 73–9).

5. Impairment of the upper extremity caused by motor deficit of the axillary nerve: 25% × 35% = 9%.

Combined motor and sensory deficit caused by involvement of the axillary nerve: 9% combined with 1% = 10% upper extremity impairment, or 6% whole-person impairment (see Table 73–3).

▼ TABLE 73–11
Maximum Upper Extremity Impairments Caused by Unilateral Sensory and/or Motor Deficits of Brachial Plexus*

Brachial Plexus Trunks	Sensory Deficit or Pain	Motor Deficit	Combined Motor and Sensory Deficits
Brachial plexus (C5-C8, T1)	100	100	100
Upper trunk (C5, C6) (Erb-Duchenne)	25	75	81
Middle trunk (C7)	5	35	38
Lower trunk (C8, T1) (Déjerine-Klumpke)	20	70	76

See Table 73–8 for grading sensory deficit or pain.
See Table 73–9 for grading motor deficit.
*From Doege TC, Houston TP: Principles and methods of impairment evaluation in the hand and upper extremity. In Guides to the Evaluation of Permanent Impairment, 4th ed. Chicago, American Medical Association, 1993, pp 13–74.

▼ **TABLE 73–12**
Maximum Upper Extremity Impairments Caused by Unilateral Sensory and/or Motor Deficits of the Major Peripheral Nerves*

Nerves	Maximum % Upper Extremity Impairment		
	From Sensory Deficit or Pain	*From Motor Deficit*	*From Combined Motor and Sensory Deficits*
Pectorals (medial and lateral)	0	5	5
Axillary	5	35	38
Dorsal scapular	0	5	5
Long thoracic	0	15	15
Medial antebrachial cutaneous	5	0	5
Medial brachial cutaneous	5	0	5
Median (above midforearm)	39	44	66
Median (anterior interosseous branch)	0	15	15
Median (below midforearm)	39	10	45
Radial palmar digital of thumb	7	0	7
Ulnar palmar digital of thumb	11	0	11
Radial palmar digital of index finger	5	0	5
Ulnar palmar digital of index finger	4	0	4
Radial palmar digital of middle finger	5	0	5
Ulnar palmar digital of middle finger	4	0	4
Radial palmar digital of ring finger	3	0	3
Musculocutaneous	5	25	29
Radial (upper arm with loss of triceps)	5	42	45
Radial (elbow with sparing of triceps)	5	35	38
Subscapulars (upper and lower)	0	5	5
Suprascapular	5	16	20
Thoracodorsal	0	10	10
Ulnar (above midforearm)	7	46	50
Ulnar (below midforearm)	7	35	40
Ulnar palmar digital of ring finger	2	0	2
Radial palmar digital of little finger	2	0	2
Ulnar palmar digital of little finger	3	0	3

See Table 73–8 for grading sensory deficit or pain.
See Table 73–9 for grading motor deficit.
*From Doege TC, Houston TP: Principles and methods of impairment evaluation in the hand and upper extremity. In Guides to the Evaluation of Permanent Impairment, 4th ed. Chicago, American Medical Association, 1993, pp 13–74.

ENTRAPMENT NEUROPATHY

Only cases of permanent damage not responding to treatment qualify for impairment ratings. Impairment values caused by entrapment neuropathy can be calculated from the motor and/or sensory deficits of each nerve involved as described earlier. For ease of determination, Table 73–13 provides upper extremity impairments values for each major nerve and site of entrapment according to its degree of severity. Do not use both methods.

Example: A 40-year old landscaper had a 1-year history of median nerve compression in the right dominant hand with abnormal median nerve conduction studies and an abnormal electromyogram. Six months after surgical decompression of the median nerve in the right carpal tunnel, followed by a change of occupation to salesman, his only symptoms were infrequent transient episodes of numbness in the thumb and index finger after 40 minutes of driving. Examination showed a full range of movement of all joints and a normal two-point discrimination sensory testing. The grip strength was 45 kg in the left hand and 30 kg in the right hand. The upper extremity impairment caused by a mild residual carpal tunnel syndrome was rated at 10% (see Table 73–10) or 6% of the whole person. No additional rating was given for decreased grip strength.

CAUSALGIA AND REFLEX SYMPATHETIC DYSTROPHY

Causalgia is a term that describes the constant and intense burning pain usually seen with RSD when the causative painful lesion involves injury to a nerve. The term "major causalgia" designates an extremely serious form of RSD produced by a partial injury to a major mixed nerve in the proximal portion of the extremity. The term "minor causalgia" designates a more common form of RSD produced by an injury to the distal part of the extremity involving a purely sensory nerve. Other clinical forms of RSD not associated with injury of a peripheral nerve include minor traumatic dystrophy, shoulder-hand syndrome, and major traumatic dystrophy. The four cardinal symptoms of RSD are pain, swelling, stiffness, and discoloration. The diagnosis of RSD can be supported with a three-phase nucleotide flow study, cold-stress testing, recurrence of pain after previously successful stellate ganglion (Horner's syndrome must be present) or Bier blocks.

The impairment secondary to RSD is usually calculated by first separately rating:

1. The upper extremity impairment caused by loss of motion of each joint involved (Swanson & deGroot Swanson, 1995).

2. The sensory deficit or pain impairment according to the guidelines of this section (see Table 73–8).

▼ TABLE 73–13
Upper Extremity Impairment Caused by Entrapment Neuropathy*

Entrapped Nerve	Entrapment Site	Severity and % Upper Extremity Impairment		
		Mild	*Moderate*	*Severe*
Suprascapular		5	10	20
Axillary		10	20	38
Radial	Upper Arm	15	25	45
Posterior interosseous	Forearm	10	20	35
Median	Elbow	15	35	55
Anterior interosseous	Proximal forearm	5	10	15
Median	Wrist	10	20	40
Ulnar	Elbow	10	30	50
Ulnar	Wrist	10	30	40

See Table 73–8 for grading sensory deficit or pain.
See Table 73–9 for grading motor deficit.
*From Swanson AB, de Groot Swanson G: Principles and methods of impairment evaluation in the hand and upper extremity. In Guides to the Evaluation of Permanent Impairment. Chicago, American Medical Association, 1993, pp 13–74.

3. The motor deficit impairment of the injured peripheral nerve, if it applies (see Table 73–9).

The appropriate impairment values for loss of motion, pain and sensory deficits, and motor deficits (if applicable) are then *combined* to obtain the impairment of the upper extremity. Major causalgia that persists despite appropriate treatment can result in a complete loss of function of the upper extremity or an impairment as great as 100%.

Combining Impairments Caused by Multiple Deficits of the Peripheral Nerve System

When a structure with mixed sensory and motor fibers is involved, the sensory impairment is *combined* with the motor impairment. When more than one peripheral nerve system structure is involved, their respective upper extremity impairments are *combined*. When multiple impairments of the extremity are present (e.g., amputation, loss of motion, vascular disorders, or other conditions), the peripheral nerve system impairment is *combined* with the other impairments to obtain the total upper extremity impairment. When both upper extremities are involved, the respective upper extremity impairments are converted to wholeperson impairments and then *combined*.

SPECIAL CONSIDERATIONS

Cumulative trauma disorders, also known as repetition strain injury and a long list of various pseudonyms, have reached epidemic proportions and have become a prevalent problem in the practice of hand surgery and in our society. It is only reasonable to consider the vast accumulated experience of Ireland (1995), Kasdan and Stutts (1995) to differen-

tiate these less understood, nonphysical psychological conditions from well-recognized physical conditions.

In his report on the Australian repetitive strain injury experience, Ireland has made critical observations relating the symptoms, clinical and laboratory findings, patient's socioeconomic profile, and response to physical treatment. He noted that the condition commonly affected young to middle-aged employees engaged in low-paying, monotonous, repetitious, and low-prestige occupations. In the array of symptoms presented, pain was the most prominent. Although pain was consistent in a given patient, the pain was not consistent among patients and did not conform to any known neurological pathway, anatomical structure, or physiological pattern. There were no primary objective findings in the upper limb other than tenderness, which was frequently of equal severity at any randomly selected point on the upper limb. Clinical and laboratory investigations were negative. The symptoms failed to respond to any form of physical treatment and usually deteriorated following hand therapy, physiotherapy, and anti-inflammatory medication.

Commonly accepted overuse conditions include rotator cuff tendinitis, bicipital tendinitis, tennis elbow, golfer's elbow, ulnar neuritis, olecranon bursitis, radial tunnel syndrome, intersection syndrome, de Quervain's stenosing tenosynovitis, flexor tenosynovitis causing median nerve compression, and digital flexor tenosynovitis, to mention a few. All of these ubiquitous syndromes differ from CTD and RSI in meeting the criteria for physical conditions, namely:

1. Clearly defined and reproducible subjective symptoms.
2. Consistent objective clinical findings.
3. Macroscopic and microscopic histological pathology or abnormal laboratory or other investigational findings.
4. A predictable response to appropriate forms of recognized physical treatment.

It is essential to differentiate both groups of patients properly in order to provide appropriate forms of treatment to each. Similarly, an individual who does not meet the criteria for the physical conditions listed earlier is not considered permanently impaired.

References

Ireland CR: Repetition strain injury: The Australian experience—1992 update. J Hand Surg *20A(Part2):*553–556, 1995.
Kasdan L, Stutts T: Factitious injuries of the upper extremity. J Hand Surg *20A(Part2):*557–560, 1995.
Moberg E: Objective methods for determining the functional value of sensibility in the hand. J Bone Joint Surg *40B:*454–476, 1958.
Omer GE Jr: Sensibility testing. *In* Omer GE, Spinner M (eds) Management of Peripheral Nerve Problems. Philadelphia, WB Saunders, 1980, pp 3–15.
Stutts JT, Kasdan ML: Disability: A new psychosocial perspective. J Med *35:*825–827, 1993.
Swanson AB: Evaluation of impairment of function in the hand. Surg Clin North Am *44:*925–940, 1964.
Swanson AB, de Groot Swanson G: Principles and methods of impairment evaluation in the hand and upper extremity. *In* Guides to the Evaluation of Permanent Impairment. Chicago, American Medical Association, 1993, pp 13–74.
Swanson AB, de Groot Swanson G, Göran-Hagert C: Evaluations of impairment of hand function. *In* Hunter JM, Schneider LH, Mackin EJ, and Callahan AD (eds): Rehabilitation of the Hand: Surgery and Therapy, 4th ed. St. Louis, Mosby, 1995, pp 1839–1896.

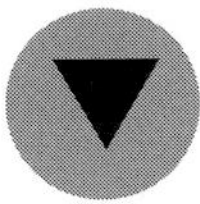

Index

Note: Page numbers in *italics* refer to illustrations; page numbers followed by (t) refer to tables.

A fibers, 11–12, 12(t), *108*
  diagnostic differential block of, 128
  pain transmission by, 121, 128
Abscesses, leprous, 615, *616*, 618, *619*
Acetylcholinesterase, histochemical methods and, 244, *245*
Achilles tendon, tendon transfer to, 723–725, *725*
Action potential, compound muscle, *649*, 649–652
  nerve fiber stimulation evoking, 251–258, *252–255*
  neurolysis correlated with, 326, *326*, 326(t)
  neuroma in continuity and, *255*, 321–326, *323–326*, 326(t)
  recording of, 251–258, *252–255*
  sciatic nerve, 421–422, *422*
  sensory nerve polyneuropathy and, *649*, 649–652
Adhesives, 311–313
  blood used in, *315*, *316*
  fibrinogen-derived, 311–313, *312*, *313*
  historical aspects of, 311–313
  nerve repair using, 311–313, *312*, *313*
Adjuncts, 311–317
  fibrin glue and, 311–313, *312*, *313*
  historical aspects of, 311–313
  laser use and, 313–317, 314(t), *315*, *316*
  suturing and, 311–313, *312*
Adson's maneuver, 496, *496*
Adventitia, innervation of, 158, 166–167
  ischemia related to, *166*, 166–167, *167*
  removal of, *166*, 166–167, *167*
  sympathectomy of, *166*, 166–167, *167*
Age, carpal tunnel syndrome and, 502–503, *503*
  cerebral palsy and, 630, 633
Allen test, 78
Allodynia, 554
  definition of, 124
ALS (amyotrophic lateral sclerosis), 655–656
Amaurosis, head injury with, *371*
  ophthalmic nerve keratitis causing, *374*
Amputation, 767–768
  impairment evaluation role of, 767–768, *768*, *771*
  replantation following, digital, 706
    upper extremity, 706–714, *706–714*
Amyotrophic lateral sclerosis (ALS), 655–656
Amyotrophy, neuralgic, 658–659
Anastomosis, arteriovenous, *107*, 107–108
  crossover cross-face, 381–383, *383*
  faciofacial, 381–383, *383*
  Martin-Gruber, arm with, 49
  Riche-Cannieu, hand with, 49
Anesthesia. See also *Nerve block.*
  epineural infusion of, 116–119, *117*, *118*
  local, 67–68, 130
  nerve block using, 67–68
  systemic lidocaine as, 128
  trigger point infusion with, 116–119, *117*, *118*

Aneurysm, carotid artery with, 372, *373*
Ankle, 52
  motor function testing across, 52, *52*, *53*
Anterior horn, pain pathways in, 121–123, *122*, *123*
Antidepressants, 132
Antiepileptics, 132
Antoni A areas, 602, *603*
Arcade of Frohse, radial tunnel syndrome and, 521–524
Arcade of Struthers, ulnar nerve entrapment and, *518*, *520*
Argon laser, 314(t), 314–315, *315*
Arm. See *Extremities, upper; Forearm.*
Arterioles, *107*
Arteriovenous anastomosis, *107*, 107–108
Artery(ies), Allen test applied to, 78
  brachial, *181*, *184*, *190*
    vascularized graft and, 303, *303*
  carotid, *160*, *161*
    aneurysm of, 372, *373*
  digital, sympathectomy of, *166*, 166–167, *167*
  facial, *32*, *33*, 231, *232*
  sympathetic innervation of, 109, *110*
  vascularized nerve graft role of, 295(t), 295–299, 298(t), *300–303*
  vertebral, nerve block near, *69*
Arthritis, 587–595
  compression syndromes due to, 587–594
    Guyon's canal in, 590
    interdigital nerve in, 593–594
    lower extremity with, 591–594, *593*
    median nerve in, 587–589, *588*, *589*
    peroneal nerve in, 592
    popliteal cyst and, 592, *593*
    posterior interosseous nerve in, 590–591, *591*
    posterior tibial nerve in, 592–593
    sciatic nerve in, 592
    tarsal tunnel and, 592–593
    ulnar nerve in, 589–590, *590*
Arthrodesis, Johnson transfer with, 728, *728*
  Jones transfer with, 727, *727*
  metacarpophalangeal joint in, 683, *683*
  thumb in, 645, 683, *683*
  toe with, 727, *727*, *728*
  wrist in, 641
Athletics, compression neuropathy associated with, 487–488
Auditory canal, acoustic neuroma of, 376–379, *377–381*
  fracture affecting, 380–381, *381*, *382*
Autonomic nervous system, 157–159, *158*. See also *Sympathetic nervous system.*
  anatomic centers of, 157–159, *158*
Awake stimulation, sensory vs. motor components in, 335
Axilla, nerve entrapment related to, 515, *517*, *519*, 524–525, *525*
  sympathectomy through, *162*, *163*, 163–165

Axon, 11–12
  anatomy of, microscopic, *353*, 353–355, *354*
  balloon expander effect on, 290, *291*
  cell matter transported by, *354*, 354–355
  compression pathology in, 475–482, *476–482*, 555–559, *556*
  degeneration of, 357–358, *358*
  diameter of, 11
  grafting and, 280–281, *281*, 289
  histochemical examination of, 243–246, *243–246*
  leprosy effect on, 615, *617*
  morphology of, 11–12, *265*, *274*
  regeneration of, 280–281, *281*, 289, 358, *358–359*
    neurotrophism in, 235–239
    neurotropism in, 238–239
  Schwann cell complex with, *353*, *354*, 354–355
  signal transmission by, 11–12
  types of, 11–12
Axonotmesis, brachial plexus affected by, *446*
  compression syndrome with, 501–502, *502*
  injury extent in, 356
Axoplasm, transport of, 243–244

Baker's (popliteal) cyst, nerve compression due to, 592, *593*
Balance, extremity coordination affecting, 343–344
  motor-sensory evaluation and, 343–344
Balloon, nerve expansion using, *290–292*, 290–293
Basement membrane, nerve fiber with, *274*
Beck Depression Inventory, 129
Bell's palsy, etiology of, 375–376, 384
  facial nerve and, 375–376, 384
  neuroanatomy of, 29–30
  surgical treatment of, 384
Bicycling, compression neuropathy associated with, 487, 570
  pudendal syndrome due to, 570
Biofeedback, therapy using, 131
Blood, nerve repair technique using, 313, 315, *315*
Blood flow, 107–114
  diagnostic testing of, 78–80, 109–113, *111–113*
    noninvasive, 78–80, 110–111, *111*, *112*
  extremities affected by, *107–113*, 107–114
    cold sensitivity in, *107*, 107–109, 113–114
    diagnostic testing in, 109–113, *111–113*
    pain related to, 107–114, *108*, 110(t)
    pathologies related to, 110(t), 113–114
    sympathectomy for, 157–170
  nerve trunk with, *353*, 353–355, *354*
  sympathetic control of, 109, *110*, *122*, *123*, 157–159, 166–167

Blood pressure, diagnostic use of, 79–80
Blood-nerve barrier, 354
Bodies, Verocay, 602, *603*
Body building, case report related to, 85–86, *86, 87*
Body position, receptors for, 11–12, 12(t)
  sensibility testing and, 16(t), 24
Body temperature, blood flow regulation of, *107,* 107–109, *108*
  sensibility testing related to, 25
  thermoreceptors and, 11–12, 12(t)
Bone(s). See also named bone, e.g., *Humerus.*
  leg and foot tendon transfer and, 717–729, *718, 720, 722–729*
  neuropathic damage to, 766
  tendon fixation in, 717–719
    button used for, 717, *718*
    plug used for, 717, *718*
Bowler's thumb, 149, 487, *528,* 528–529
Brachial plexus, 82–85, 175–178, 445–471
  anatomy of, 82–85, *83, 160,* 175–178, *176, 776*
  body building effects in, 82–86, *86, 87*
  MRI studies of, 82–86, *86, 87*
  nerve block of, 70
  nerve expander use and, 290, *292*
  nerve gap affecting, *328,* 336, *336*
  nerves of, 175–177, *176*
    impairment evaluation related to, 773(t), *776,* 777, 777(t)
    origins and functions of, 773(t)
  neuralgic amyotrophy affecting, 658–659
  neuroma in continuity affecting, 326(t)
  obstetric injury to, 454–458
    evaluation of, *454,* 454–455, *455*
    prognosis for, 454, 458
    surgical treatment of, 455–458, *456–458*
  radiation injury to, 657–658
  surgical exposure of, *177,* 177–178
  traumatic injury to, 433–443, 445–453
    donor nerves for, 441–442, 451–453, 460–463, *463*
    elbow reconstruction following, *469,* 469–471, *470*
    graft repair of, *450–452,* 450–453, 451(t), 453(t), 460–463
    nerve transfer in, 451, *451,* 453, 453(t)
    neurotization in, 451, 453, 453(t), 459–464, *460, 463, 464*
    pathology of, 445, 445(t), *446*
    patient evaluation in, 445(t), 445–446, *446, 449, 452*
    repair priorities for, 450
    shoulder reconstruction following, 465–469, *466–470*
    spontaneous recovery prognosis for, 366–367
    surgical treatment of, 437–443, 447–453, *448–452,* 451(t), 453(t)
    tendon transfer for, 465–467, *466, 467*
Brain, pain perception by, 121–123, *122,* 125
  pain signal transmission to, 107–109, *108*
British Medical Research Council Grading System, 340, 342, 416, 416(t)
  muscle recovery and, 340(t), 347(t), 416(t)
  sensory recovery and, 342, 342(t), 346(t), 416(t)
  vs. Moberg System, 346(t)
Bupivacaine, nerve block using, 67–68
Burn injury, 623–628
  chemical causing, 624, 625(t)
  electrical, *624,* 624–626, *627*
  radiation causing, 626–628, *628*
  thermal, *623,* 623–624, *624*
Button, tendon fixation in bone using, 717, *718*

C fibers, 11–12, 12(t), *108*

C fibers *(Continued)*
  diagnostic differential block of, 128
  pain transmission by, 121–123, 128
Café-au-lait spots, neurofibroma associated with, 600
Calcaneus, tendon transfer to, 723–725, *724, 725*
Cancer. See *Neoplasia.*
Capillaries, nailfold capillaroscopy of, 112–113, *113*
  nerve blood supply and, *353,* 353–354, *354*
  thermoregulation role of, *107,* 107–109
Capsulorrhaphy, proximal interphalangeal joint volar, 646
Carbon dioxide laser, 314(t), *315,* 315–316, *316*
Carbonic anhydrase, histochemical use of, 245–246, *246*
Carpal tunnel, 190, *191*
  leprosy affecting, 615, *617*
Carpal tunnel syndrome, 511–512, 534–541
  compression injury causing, 356
  economic impact of, 489–490
  epidemiology of, 485(t), 485–489
  etiology of, 486–489
  occupation related to, 484, 488–489, 546–549
  older patient with, 502–503, *503*
  pathology in, 478–481, *479, 480*
  rheumatoid, 587–589, *588, 589*
  signs and symptoms of, 511–512
  stages of, 356
  surgical release in, 534–541
    complications of, 536, 541
    conventional (open), *534–536,* 534–537
    endoscopic, 538–541, *539*
    hand function testing following, 543–545, *544, 545*
    outcome of, 535–536, 540–541, 543–549
    recovery curve for, 544–549, *546–548*
  testing for, 13–14
Case reports, 85–93
  bilateral cervical ribs in, 86–90, *88–90*
  body building effects in, 85–86, *86, 87*
  injection injury in, 409(t), 409–413
  median nerve neurolemmoma in, 90, *91*
  MRI studies in, 85–93
  old rib fracture in, 90–91, *92*
Casting, total contact, 765–766, *766*
Catheters, epineural anesthesia infusion using, 116–119, *117, 118*
Cauda equina, *561*
Causalgia, 581
  definition of, 554
  gunshot injury causing, 402
  impairment evaluation for, 778–779
  pain of, 124–125
  tibial, 581
Cerebellopontine angle, facial nerve and, 376–379, *377–380*
  neuroma of, 376–379, *377–381, 384*
Cerebral cortex, hand trauma reorganization of, 359–360, *360*
  pain pathways to, 121, *122*
  sensory function representation in, 745–749, *746–748*
Cerebral palsy, 630–646
  age and, 630, 633
  classification method for, 630, 633(t)
    functional level in, 633(t), 633–634
    operative results used in, 633(t), 633–634
    symptom-based, 630
  clinical features of, 630–633, *633*
  described types of, 630
  general management principles for, 634
  incidence and epidemiology of, 630
  motor evaluation in, 631–632
  patient motivation related to, 631
  sensibility evaluation in, 632–633, *633*

Cerebral palsy *(Continued)*
  surgical approach to, 634–646
    digital deformity in, *635,* 638–646, *642, 646*
    elbow flexion deformity in, *635,* 636–637, *637*
    forearm pronation in, *635,* 637–638
    shoulder deformity in, 634–636, *635*
    swan-neck deformity in, 645–646, *646*
    thumb-in-palm deformity in, *635,* 642–645, *642–645*
    wrist flexion deformity in, 638–642, *639, 640, 642*
Cervical nerves, brachial plexus supplied by, 175–177, *176*
Cervical plexus, anatomy of, *233,* 233–234, *234*
  brachial plexus repair related to, 462, 463
  nerve branches of, *233,* 233–234, *234*
Chalk, picking-up test using, 344, *345*
Chassaignac's tubercle, *69,* 69–70, *159,* 159–160, *160*
Chemical burn injury, 624, 625(t)
Chemotropism, 235, 238–239
Chloroprocaine, nerve block using, 67
Cholesteatoma, facial nerve affected by, *385*
Choline acetyltransferase assay, 244–245
Ciliary neurotrophic factor (CNTF), 236–237
  acid, 236–237
  basic, 236–237
Circulation, control mechanisms of, 109
  extremity affected by, *107,* 107–114, *109–113*
  loss of sensation affecting, 762
Claudication, pain due to, 113
CNTF (ciliary neurotrophic factor), acid, 236–237
  basic, 236–237
Coccygeal plexus, anatomy of, 195–196, *196*
Cognitive function. See also *Cerebral cortex.*
  cerebral palsy affecting, 630–631
Cold, 11–12, 98–99
  intolerance to, 98–99, 113–114
    blood flow role in, *107,* 107–109, 113–114
    therapeutic approach to, 98–99
  receptors for, 11–12, 12(t)
  stress testing and, 113
Collagen, nerve morphology role of, 353
Compression syndrome(s), 355–357, 475–582.
  See also *Entrapment syndrome(s).*
  acute, 475–478, *476–479*
  arthritis association with, 587–594, *588, 589, 593*
  carpal tunnel. See *Carpal tunnel syndrome.*
  chronic, 478–482, *479–482*
  classification of lesion in, 501–503, *502, 556, 556–557*
  cranial nerves affected by, 371–388
  cubital tunnel, 518
  double crush in, 582
  economic impact of, 489–490
  epidemiology of, 484–492, 485(t)
  etiology of, 484, 486–489, 555–557
  evaluation principles for, *503,* 503–505, *504, 506,* 557–559
  evoked potentials in, 506–510, *509, 510*
  Guyon's tunnel, 189, *190,* 590
  interdigital (foot), rheumatoid compression of, 593–594
  low back region and, 559–564
  lower extremity, 554–582, 591–594, *593*
  lumbosacral region with, 561–563, *561–563*
  management of, 505–529, *506–510*
  occupation related to, 484, 488–489, 543–549
  pathophysiology of, nerve fiber in, 475–482, *476–482,* 501–503, *502,* 555–559, *556*
  popliteal cyst and, 592, *593*
  prevention of, 490–492

Compression syndrome(s) *(Continued)*
   radial tunnel, 521–524
   rehabilitation factors for, 551–552
   risk factors for, 486–489
   surgical approaches to, 505–529, *506–523,*
      528
      hand function testing following, 543–544,
         544, 544(t), *545*
      internervous planes for, 506, *507–509*
      recovery curve for, 544–549, *546–548*
      tarsal tunnel, *579,* 579–580
      rheumatoid, 592–593
      thoracic outlet affected by, 494–499
   types of, 501–505, *502,* 511–529, 556, 556–
     557
   upper extremity, 501–529
   vibration causing, 356–357
Conditioning lesion effect, 359
Conduction block. See also *Nerve block.*
   compression causing, 356–357
   ischemic, 355–356
Conduction studies, 650, *650.* See also *Action*
   potential; Electrophysiologic studies.
   polyneuropathy diagnosis by, 648–652, *649,*
     650
   signal transmission and, 11–12
   velocity measurement in, 650, *650*
Conduits, 305–309, 335
   autogenous venous, 306–308, *307,* 335
   historical aspects of, 305–306
   muscle-derived, 308, 335
   perineurial tube, 308
   synthetic, 308–309, 335–336
Coordination, 344
   cerebral palsy affecting, 630–633, *633*
   hand tested for, 344, *344, 345*
   motor-sensory evaluation and, 343–348, *344,*
     345
   postsurgical testing of, 343–344, *344, 345*
Costoclavicular maneuver, 496, *496*
Cricoid cartilage, *159–161*
   stellate ganglion block and, *159–161,* 160
"Cross-talk," nerve fiber in, 124–126
Cubital tunnel, leprosy affecting, 615, *617*
   nerve compression in, 518
      rheumatoid, 589
Cumulative trauma disorders. See *Compression*
   syndromes.

DDS (diaminodiphenylsulfone), leprosy
   treatment with, 616–617
Debridement, of gunshot wound, 400, *401*
Decision pathways, 94–104
   assessment tools for, 94–96, *95*
   cold intolerance affecting, 98–99
   gunshot wounds and, 97–98
   multilevel injury and, 97–98
   nerve injury management using, 94–104
   postsurgical therapies in, 95–97
Degeneration, injury followed by, 357–358, *358*
Déjerine-Klumpke paralysis, 49
Dellon's two-point discrimination test, 22, *22*
Delta fibers, 108. See also *A fibers; C fibers.*
Demyelination, compression pathology and,
   476–481, *477–480,* 555–557, *556*
Dendrite, morphology of, *265*
Denervation, extremities affected by, 762–766,
   763(t), *763–766*
      muscle affected by, electrical stimulation of,
       669–674
      sympathetic. See *Sympathectomy.*
Depolarization, 252. See also *Action potential.*
Depression, 126
   Beck Inventory for, 129

Depression *(Continued)*
   diagnostic criteria for, 126
Dermatomes, nerve sensitivity in, 558
   upper extremity, *775*
Devices, electrical nerve stimulation by, *138,*
   138–139, *139*
   implantable, drug delivery by, 130
Diabetes mellitus, neuropathy caused by, 14,
   654–655
Diagnostic studies. See also *Electrophysiological*
   studies.
   electrodiagnostic, 648–652
   historical aspects of, 4
   polyneuropathies in, 648–652, *649, 650*
Diagrams, hand and foot test results on, *26,*
   26–27
   neuropathy assessment using, 94–95, *95*
   pain assessment using, 94–95, *95*
Diaminodiphenylsulfone (DDS), leprosy
   treatment with, 616–617
Diffusion, axon role in, 354
Disability evaluation, 767–779. See also
   Impairment evaluation.
Disc (intervertebral), anatomy of, *560–563*
   entrapment syndromes related to, 559–563,
     560–563
   protrusion of, 559–563, *562, 563*
Dislocation, arm, 367
   elbow, 367–368
   glenohumeral, 367
   hip, 368
   knee, 368
   management approach in, 368–369
   shoulder, 366–367
   spontaneous recovery prognosis for, 366–368
Doppler studies, 78–79
   blood flood testing in, 110–112, *112*
   equation for, 79
Dorsal horn, pain pathways in, 121–123, *122,*
   123
Double crush compression syndrome, 582
Drugs. See also *Anesthesia.*
   implantable device delivery of, 130
Dysesthesia, therapeutic modalities for, 102
Dyskinesia, cerebral palsy with, 630

Elbow, *43*
   anatomy of, *43*
   brachial plexus injury affecting, *452, 454,*
     458, 464
      reconstruction and, *469,* 469–471, *470*
   cerebral palsy flexion deformity in, *635,* 636–
     637
      surgical approach to, 636–637, *637*
   flail, *468*
   gunshot wound of, *402, 403*
   muscles of, 40(t), *42, 43*
   nerve supply through, 40(t), *42, 43*
      surgical exposure of, *179–181,* 185, 189,
      190, 191
   replantation of arm and, *709,* 709–710, *713,*
     713–714, *714*
   Steindler effect in, 469, *469, 471*
   traumatic nerve injury related to, 367–368
Electrical burn injury, *624,* 624–626, *627*
Electrical nerve stimulation, 131, 669–674
   complications of, 142
   denervated muscle treated with, 669–674
   experimental models for, 670–673
   following nerve repair, *671,* 671–672
   frequency, voltage and pulse width in, 672–
     673
   leads and devices used in, *138,* 138–139, *139*
   neuroma treated with, 152

Electrical nerve stimulation *(Continued)*
   pain pathways affected by, 135–137
   patient selection for, 131, 137–138
   peripheral nerve in, *143,* 143–144
   spinal cord, 135–143, *136, 137, 141, 142*
   surgical procedures and, 139–142, *141, 142*
Electrodes, electromyographic, *323,* 323–324
   needle, 648–652
   nerve potential evoked with, 251–258, *252–*
     256
   nerve stimulation using, *138,* 138–140, *139,*
     141, 142
Electrodiagnostic testing, 648–652
   polyneuropathies in, 648–652, *649, 650*
Electromyography, equipment for, *323,* 323–324
   neuroma in continuity in, 321–326, *323–326*
   technique for, 324–325, *325*
Electrophysiologic studies, 251–258, *252–257*
   facial nerve in, 34
   intraoperative use of, 251–258, *252–257*
   nerve stimulation in, 251–258, *252–257*
   neuroma in continuity in, 321–326, *323–326*
   recording of, 251–258, *252–255*
Endoneurium, *124*
   compression injury of, 355
   diffusion role of, 354
   fluid pressure in, 354–355
   microanatomy of, *353,* 353–354, *354*
   morphology of, *265, 274*
   MRI studies of, *84*
Endophthalmus, Horner's syndrome with, 161,
   161
Endorphins, electrical stimulation therapy and,
   135–136
Endoscopy, carpal tunnel release using, 538–541,
   539
Entrapment syndrome(s). See also *Compression*
   syndrome(s).
   arthritis association with, 587–594, *588, 589,*
     593
   axillary, *526,* 526–527
   carpal tunnel, 511–512, 534–541
   cubital tunnel, 518
      rheumatoid, 589
   cutaneous nerve in, of gluteal region, 563–564
     of thigh, 563–568, *565, 567, 571*
   diagnosis of, 503–505, 557–559
   digital nerve of toe in, *579,* 580–581
   dorsal scapular nerve in, 528
   epidemiology of, 485(t), 485–489
   etiology of, 486–489
   femoral nerve in, 568–569, *569*
   genitofemoral nerve in, *565, 566, 567*
   Guyon's tunnel, 189, *190,* 590
   hand function testing following, 543–545,
     544, 545
   iliohypogastric nerve in, 564–566, *565, 567*
   ilioinguinal nerve in, *565, 566, 567*
   impairment evaluation and, 778, 779(t)
   infraclavicular nerve, 514–516, *517*
   lateral femoral cutaneous nerve in, 429,
     429(t), 566–568, *567*
   leprosy with, 615–616
   ligament of Struthers in, 514, *516*
   long thoracic in, *526,* 527–528
   median anterior interosseous nerve in, *512,*
     512–513, *513*
   median nerve in, 511–516, *514–517*
   median palmar cutaneous nerve in, 512
   median recurrent motor branch in, 511–512
   multiple, 529
   nerve root in, 559–563, *560–563*
   obturator in, *567,* 568
   pathology in, 478–482, *479–482,* 555–559,
     556
   peroneal nerve in, *574,* 574–577, *576*

Entrapment syndrome(s) *(Continued)*
 plantar in, *577, 579,* 580
 pronator teres in, 513–514, *514*
 pseudoanterior interosseous in, 513, *513*
 pudendal in, 564, *565, 569,* 569–570, *570*
 radial nerve in, 519–525, *524, 525*
 radial posterior interosseous in, 519–524, *522, 523*
 radial tunnel, 521–524
 recovery curve for, 544–549, *546–548*
 saphenous nerve in, 568, *579*
 sciatic nerve in, 570–573, *571–573*
 suprascapular nerve in, *183,* 183–184, *526, 527*
 sural nerve in, 573–574, *576*
 tarsal tunnel, *579,* 579–580
  rheumatoid, 592–593
 testing for, 503–505, 558–559
 tibial nerve in, *577,* 577–580, *579*
 ulnar dorsal cutaneous in, 518
 ulnar nerve in, 516–519, *518–521,* 590
 vs. polyneuropathy, 655–660
Ephapse, injury causing, 481
Epicondylectomy, leprous neuritis treated with, 620
Epidural space, electrical stimulation therapy in, 135–143, *136, 137, 141, 142*
Epinephrine, nerve block prolongation with, 67–68
Epineurium, *124*
 anatomy of, microscopic, *353,* 353–354, *354*
 anesthesia infusion to, 116–119, *117, 118*
 graft proliferation of, 281, *281*
 morphology of, *265, 274*
 suturing of, *264, 266,* 266–267, 271–273, *335, 415*
 sympathectomy and, *167*
 sympathetic nerve fibers in, *167*
Equilibrium, motor-sensory evaluation and, 343–344
Equipment, microsurgical, 261–269, *262–264*
 nerve approximator, *264*
 nerve stimulator, *138,* 138–139, *139*
 operating table, *263*
Erb-Duchenne paralysis, 49
Erb's palsy, 454
Etidocaine, nerve block using, 68
Evoked potentials, brachial plexus injury evaluation with, 448–450, *449*
 compression syndrome evaluation by, 506–510, *509, 510*
 intraoperative use of, 251–258, *252–255*
Examination. See also *Impairment evaluation.*
 impairment evaluation based on, 768–770, 769(t), *770,* 771(t)
 neurological, 768–770
Excimer laser, 314(t)
Expander, balloon, nerve gap repair using, 290–292, *290–293*
Extremities, 39–55
 blood flow in, *107–113,* 107–114
  cold tolerance affected by, *107,* 107–109, 113–114
  diagnostic testing of, 109–113, *111–113*
  pain affected by, 107–114, *108,* 110(t)
  pathologies affecting, 110(t), 113–114
 denervation effects in, 762–766
  management of, 762–766, 763(t), *763–766*
 fracture, dislocation and traction injury of, 366–369
 lower, 50–55, 217–227
  compression syndromes of, 554–582
   rheumatoid, 591–594, *593*
  gait patterns of, 50–51
  motor function testing of, 50–55, 341–342
  muscles of, 50–55, *53, 54*

Extremities *(Continued)*
  relative strengths of, 719(t)
 nerves of, 195–208. See also specific nerve.
  anatomy of, 195–208, *196–202, 204–207,* 217–227
  block of, *72,* 72–73, *73*
  injury of, *56–58,* 56–62, *60, 61*
  innervation and, 50–55, *51–54*
  sensibility grading for, 341(t), 341–348, 346(t)–348(t)
  surgical exposure of, 195–208, *197–202, 204–207*
  surgical repair of, 56–62, 420–429
  topography (cross section) of, 217–227, *218, 222–224, 226*
  neuroma of, 151–155, *153, 154, 155*
  parasympathetic centers for, 157–159, *158*
  reconstruction techniques for, 717–729
  sensation-bearing flaps in, *755,* 755–759, *757,* 759(t)
  short, 51
  sympathetic centers for, 157–159, *158*
 muscle-nerve associations of, 346(t)
 nerves of, 346(t)
 paravertebral ganglia chain and, 157–159, *158*
 postsurgical functionality testing of, 343–348, *344, 345,* 346(t)–348(t)
 upper, 39–49, 328–339
  cerebral palsy affecting, 634–646. See also *Cerebral palsy.*
  compression syndromes of, 501–529
  dermatomes of, *775*
  impairment evaluation for, 767–779. See also *Impairment evaluation.*
  internervous planes for, *507–509*
  motor function testing of, 39–49, 341–342
  motor innervation of, 773(t), *774, 775*
  muscles of, 39–49, 40(t), *43–49,* 46(t)
   reinnervation in, 393–396, *394–396*
   transfer affecting, *713,* 713–714, *714*
  nerves of, 39–49, 40(t), *41–43,* 175–195
   anatomy of, 175–195, *176–188, 190–195*
   block of, *70,* 70–71, *71*
   gap repair in, *328–338,* 328–339
   sensibility grading for, 341(t), 341–348, 346(t)–348(t)
   surgical exposure of, 175–195, *177, 179–188, 190–195*
   topography (cross-section) of, *210,* 210–214, 211(t), *212–214*
   trauma to, 367–368
  neuroma of, 146–149, *148*
  parasympathetic centers for, 157–159, *158*
  reconstruction techniques for, 634–636, 675–714
  replantation procedures for, 706–714, *706–714*
  sensation-bearing flaps in, 745–755, *750, 751, 753*
  sensory deficit in, 767–779, *768,* 769(t), *770,* 770(t), *771*
  sympathetic centers for, 157–159, *158*
  tendon transfer in, 639–646, 675–703. See also *Tendon transfer.*
Eye, muscles of, *32,* 35–36
 nerve supply to, *30, 32,* 35–36

Face, *30, 230–232*
 expression of, 29–34, *32*
 muscle transfer to, 740–743, *741, 742*
 muscles of, 29–34, *32, 33, 230, 232*
 nerve supply to, 29–36, *30, 32, 33*
  innervation patterns of, 228–232, *229–232*

Face *(Continued)*
 pain pathways from, 121, *122*
Fascicles, 274–279, 330
 anatomy of, 274, *274, 275,* 282–284, *283–285,* 330, *330–335*
  microscopic, *353,* 353–355, *354*
 blood supply to, *353,* 353–354, *354*
 coaptation of, 281–282, *281–284,* 288, *288*
 grafting technique for, 275–278, *276,* 281–289, *282–284, 288*
 median nerve with, *275, 277,* 330, *330–335*
 microsurgical technique and, 261–269, *264–268*
 morphology of, *265, 274, 274, 275,* 282–284, *283–285,* 330, *330–335*
 motor and sensory, 256–257, *257*
 plexus formation by, *330*
 stimulation of, *256,* 256–258, *257*
 surgical repair of, 274–278, *275–278,* 281–289, 330–333, *332–335*
Femoral stretch test, nerve sensitivity in, 558
Fibrin, nerve repair using, 311–313, *312, 313*
Fibroblast growth factor (FGF), 237–238
Fibrosis, graft proliferation of, 281, *281,* 289
Filament test(s), 11–27
 Moberg, 19–22, *20–23,* 22(t)
 Semmes-Weinstein, 17(t), 17–19, *20–23*
 von Frey, 16, 16(t), *17*
Fingers, 675–703
 blood flow in, *112,* 112–113, *113,* 166–167
 cerebral palsy flexion deformity in, 631–632, *635,* 638–646
  surgical approach to, 638–646, *642, 646*
 clawed, 678(t), 697–699, *698*
  capsulodesis for, 697–699, *698*
  flexor digitorum superficialis prevention of, 680–683, *682*
 coordination testing of, picking-up test in, 23–24, *23–25,* 344
  postsurgical, 344, *344, 345*
 diagnostic nerve block in, 71
 impairment evaluation of, 767–772, *768,* 769(t), *770, 771,* 771(t)
 ischemia affecting, *166,* 166–167, *167*
 muscles of, 40(t), *42, 43, 48,* 48–49
 nailfold capillaroscopy of, 112–113, *113*
 nerves of, 40(t), *42, 43*
  surgical exposure of, 189–194, *192–194*
 replantation of arm and, 706–712, *706–713*
 sensate flaps used on, 691–694, *692, 693,* 750, 750–752, *751*
 sensory loss evaluation for, 767–772, 770(t), *771,* 771(t)
 sympathectomy in, *166,* 166–167, *167*
 tendon transfer for, 638–646, 675–703. See also *Tendon transfer.*
 wrinkle test for, 25–26, *26*
Fingertips, neuropathy causing loss of, 14, *14*
 pinch strength test of, *18*
Fist, 685, *685*
Flap(s), 691–694, 745–760. See also *Graft(s); Muscle transfer; Tendon transfer.*
 hand reconstruction using, 691–694, *692, 693, 702, 750, 751*
 Karapandzic, 745
 muscle. See *Muscle transfer.*
 neurocutaneous, 691–692, *693*
 neurovascular, 691, *692*
 palmar, 699, *702*
 sensation-bearing, 745–760, 759(t)
  biological principles of, 745–749, *746, 747*
  digital (finger), 749–752, *750, 751*
   cross-finger, 750–752, *751*
   neurovascular island, 749–750, *750, 751*
   reinnervated, 752
  digital (toe), 752

Flap(s) *(Continued)*
  dorsal foot, 758–759
  fibular, 756–758, *757*
  forearm, 752–754, *753*
    radial, 752–754, *753*
    ulnar, 754
  hand with, 691–694, *692, 693, 702, 750, 751*
  lateral arm, 754–755
  lateral thigh, *755*, 755–756
  tensor fascia lata, 756
Flexor-pronator slide technique, 636–637, *637*
Fluids, endoneurial pressure and, 354–355
Foot, 52
  bones of, *718, 720, 722–729*
  denervation effect on, *764*, 764–765, *765*
  dorsiflexion test for, 558
  elevation test for, 558
  examination form for, *26*, 26–27
  gunshot wound of, *401*
  hot spot on, 764–765
  motor function testing of, 52, *52, 53*
  nerve entrapment affecting, 573–582, *574, 576, 577, 579*
  nerve supply to, 52, *52–54*
  neuroma affecting, *151*, 151–155, *153–155*
  repetitive stress injury affecting, *764*, 764–765, *765*
  rigid-soled shoes for, *764*, 764–765, *765*
  sensation-bearing flaps and, 752, 758–759
  tendon transfers in, 717–729
  tissue autolysis in, *764*, 764–765, *765*
Foramen (foramina), infraorbital, *68*, 69
  mental, *68*, 69
Forearm, 675–703
  cerebral palsy pronation of, 631–632, *635, 637–638*
    surgical approach to, 637–638
  muscle reinnervation in, *395*
  muscle transfer in, 731, 739–740, *740, 742*
  sensation-bearing flaps from, 752–754, *753*, 759(t)
  surgical internervous planes of, *507–509*
  tendon transfer and, 636–638, 675–703. See also *Tendon transfer.*
Forehead, nerve branching patterns in, 230, *230, 232*
Forms, hand and foot tests results on, *26*, 26–27
Fracture(s), arm, 367
  elbow, 367–368
  hip, 368
  knee, 368
  management approach to, 368–369
  rib callus due to, 90–91, *92*
  shoulder, 366–367
  skull, facial nerve affected by, 379–381, *381, 382*
  spontaneous recovery prognosis for, 366–368
  tendon transfer affected by, 675, *675*
Free nerve endings, 12(t), *746*
Frostbite, ischemia related to, 166

Gait, adductor lurch pattern of, 51
  denervated foot and, 764
  hip affecting, 50–51, *51*
  leg and foot reconstruction and, 717–719, *718*
  short leg pattern in, 51
  Trendelenburg, 50–51
Ganglion(a), geniculate, 30, *30*
  nerve sheath with, 607–608
    clinical presentation of, 607
    treatment of, 608
  pterygopalatine, 30, *30*
  stellate, *69, 70, 161*

Ganglion(a) *(Continued)*
  anesthetic block of, *69, 70, 70*, 127–128, 159–161, *161*
  sympathetic chain of, 157–159, *158*
    cervical, *159*, 159–165, *160*
    lumbar, 73–74, *74, 158*, 167–168, *168*
    nerve block in, 73–74, *74*, 159–161, *161*, 167–168, *168*
    resection of, 157–170, *162–165, 167–170*
    thoracic, *158*, 161–165, *162–165*
Gate control theory, 135–136
Genitalia, nerve supply to, *570*
Gigantic clubs, nerve regeneration and, 475, *476*
Girdlestone-Taylor transfer, toe with, 728–729, *729*
Glenohumeral joint, dislocation of, 367
  suprascapular nerve near, *183*
Glial cell neurotrophic factor, 238
Gliding, 96–97, 271–272, 328–329
  excursion in, 271–272, 328–329
  length of, 353
  median nerve, 353
  nerve sensitivity test and, 558–559
  ulnar nerve, 353
Glomus bodies, sympathetic innervation of, *158*
Glue, 311–313
  fibrinogen-derived, 311–313, *312, 313*
  historical aspects of, 311–313
Golgi-Mazzoni corpuscle, 12(t)
Gonalgia paresthetica, 568
Gould technique, tendon insertion using, 717, *718*
Grading system(s), 341–348
  nerve sensibility, 341–348
    British Medical Research Council, 340, 340(t), 342
    Louisiana State University Medical Center, 347, 348(t)
    Lovett method in, 341(t)
    Moberg's Scale, 342, 342(t), 346(t)
    United States Veterans Administration, 341(t), 347(t)
Graft(s), 261–269, 280–289, 295–303, 305–309, 333–339. See also *Flap(s); Muscle transfer; Tendon transfer.*
  allograft, 306–307, *328*, 339
  blood supply of, 295(t), 295–303, *299, 300*
  brachial plexus repair using, *450–452, 450–453*, 451(t), 453(t)
  cable, *402, 416*
  clinical outcome following, 414–418, 416(t), *417, 418*
  coaptation of, 281–282, *281–284*, 288, *288*
  donor sites for, 286–287, *333*, 333–334, *334*
  end-to-end suture vs., 416–418, *417, 418*
  facial nerve treated with, *380–383*, 381–383
  gunshot injury treated with, 401–403, *402, 403*
  indications for, 282
  length of, 285–286
  leprosy treatment and, 620
  median nerve repair with, 415–418, *415–418*
  microsurgical technique for, 261–269, *262–268*
  nerve gap repair using, 306–308, *328*, 333–338, *333–339*
  nerve transfer in, 280–289, *281–284, 287, 288, 336, 336*
  postoperative care for, 288–289
  preparation of, 280–287, *282–284, 287, 288*
  skin, 745–760
  St. Clair Strange pedicle for, 403, *403*
  stump preparation for, 283
  sural nerve source of, *396, 402, 416*
  surgical outcome analysis for, lower extremity, 423(t), *424*, 424(t), *425*, 425(t), 426(t), 428(t)

Graft(s) *(Continued)*
  surgical techniques for, 280–289, *281–284, 288*
    blood supply and, 295(t), 295–303, *299–303*
    microscope used in, 261 269, *262–268*
  survival factors for, 280–283, 289, 295
  ulnar nerve repair with, 415–418, *416–418*
  vascularized, 285, 295–303
    cable formation in, *299*, 299–300, *300*
    cadaver dissection for, 297–299, 298(t)
    clinical studies on, 296(t)–298(t), 296–297
    indications for, 297
    monitoring of, 300–301
    operative techniques for, 299–303, *299–303*
    sural, 297(t), 298(t), *301*, 301–302, *302*
    types of, 295(t)–298(t), 295–299, *299*, 299–300, *300*
    ulnar, 297(t), 298(t), 302–303, *303*
Granular cell tumor, 602–603
  clinical presentation of, 602
  pathology of, 602–603
Grasp strength test, hand in, *18*
Gunshot wounds, 398–404
  ballistics and, 398–399
  clinical outcomes of, 402–404, 423(t)–426(t)
  incidence and prevalence of, 365
  management principles for, 399–402, *400–403*
  neurorrhaphy of, 347(t)
  penetration of, 398–399
  shotgun, 398–399, *399*
  spontaneous nerve recovery prognosis for, 365–366
  surgical nerve repair in, 401–402, *401–403, 423*
  tissue disruption due to, 398–399
Guyon's tunnel, 189, 190, *191*
  ulnar nerve entrapment in, 590

Hallux varus, correction of, 728, *728*
  Johnson transfer for, 728, *728*
Hamartoma, 608–609
  lipofibromatous, 608
  neuromuscular, 608–609
  peripheral nerve with, 608–609
Hand, 107–114, 675–703
  blood flow in, 78–80, 107–109, *109, 112*
  cerebral palsy affecting, 630–633, *633, 635, 640, 642–646*
  clawing of, 503–504, *504, 506*
  coordination testing for, 344, *344, 345*
  examination form for, *26*, 26–27
  function measurement of, 543–549
    assembly testing in, 544, *545*
    pinch, grasp, twist, and hold in, 543–544, *544*
    recovery curves related to, 544–549, *546–548*
    return to work and, 546(t), 546–547, *547, 548*
    sensory testing in, 544, 544(t), *545*
    technological devices for, 543–544, *544, 545*
    volumetric testing in, 544, *545*
    work simulator in, 543–544, *544, 545*
  grasp strength test of, *18*
  impairment evaluation for, 767–772, *768*, 769(t), *770, 771*
  ischemia affecting, *166*, 166–167, *167*
  muscles of, 346(t)
  nerves of, 189–194, *192–194*, 346(t)
    fasciculation and, 330, *330–332*, 336
    surgical exposure of, 189–194, *192–194*
    transfer graft of, 336, *336, 339*

Hand *(Continued)*
traumatic transection affecting, 359–360, *360*
neuroma affecting, *148, 338*
periarterial sympathectomy in, *166,* 166–167, *167*
picking-up test and, 23–24, 344, *344, 345*
postsurgical pain affecting, 342–343, *343*
replantation of arm and, *706–712,* 706–713
sensate flap used in, 691–694, *692, 693, 750,* 750–753, *751*
tendon transfer and, 641–646, 675–703. See also *Tendon transfer.*
topographical lines of, *193*
Hansen's disease. See *Leprosy.*
Harkin and Reed classification, 598, 598(t)
Head. See also *Face; Neck.*
flexion test for, nerve sensitivity in, 558
pain pathways from, 121, *122*
Heat receptors, 11–12, 12(t)
Heel (calcaneus), gait and, 717
Hemangioma, peripheral nerve with, 609
Hemoglobin, laser energy absorbed by, 315, *315*
nerve repair technique using, 315, *315*
Henry approach, *508, 522*
Highet Scale of Sensory Recovery, 342(t)
Hip, 50–51
abnormal gaits due to, 50–51
motor function testing across, 50–51, *51*
stiff, 51
trauma to, nerve injury related to, 368
Histochemical techniques, 243–246
axons demonstrated in, 243–246, *243–246*
nerve repair examined with, 243–246, *243–246*
Homunculus, *746, 747*
Horner's sign, brachial plexus injury with, 445
Horner's syndrome, 128, 161, *161*
nerve block causing, 128, 157, 161, *161*
signs of, 128, 161, *161*
stellate ganglion and, 128, 157, 161, *161*
Humerus, fracture affecting, radial nerve and, 367–368
supracondylar process of, 514, *516*
Hunter's canal, saphenous nerve entrapment in, 568
Hyoid bone, *161*
Hyperalgesia, 121–123
primary vs. secondary, 121–123
Hyperesthesia, 554, 555
lateral femoral cutaneous, 429
Hyperpathia, 554
Hypnosis, therapy using, 131
Hypochondriasis, 126
diagnostic criteria for, 126
Hypothalamus, pain pathways to, 121, *122,* 125
Hypothenar hammer syndrome, 113–114

Iatrogenic nerve injury, lower extremity, 424(t), 425(t), 426(t), 427(t)
ILGs (insulin-like growth factors), 237
Ilium, sciatic nerve block near, 72, *72*
IMN (ischemic monomelic neuropathy), 659–660
Impairment evaluation, 767–779
amputation vs. neuropathy in, 767–768, *768, 771*
brachial plexus and, 773(t), *776, 777,* 777(t)
digits (fingers) in, 767–772, *768,* 769(t), *770, 771,* 771(t)
motor loss and, 769
sensory loss and, 767–772, 770(t), *771,* 771(t)
entrapment syndromes and, 778, 779(t)

Impairment evaluation *(Continued)*
hand in, 767–772, *768,* 769(t), *770, 771*
neurological examination in, 768–770, 769(t), *770,* 771(t)
peripheral nerve disorders in, 772–779, 773(t), *774–776,* 776(t), 777(t)–779(t)
motor loss in, 774, 776(t), 778(t)
pain in, 772–774, 776(t), 778(t)
sensory loss in, 772–774, 776(t), 778(t)
principles and methods for, 767–768, *768,* 772–774
spinal nerves and, 774–776, 776(t)
thumb in, 767–772, *768,* 769(t), *770, 771,* 771(t)
upper extremity in, 767–779
whole person in, 767, *768,* 770(t)
Implantable devices, drug delivery by, 130
Infants, obstetric brachial plexus injury in, 454–458, *454–458*
Inflammation, neurogenic, 121–123
pain physiology related to, 121–123
Inhibition, interneuronal, 745–749, *747*
Injection injury, 406–413
case histories of, 409(t), 409–413
pathology in, *407,* 407–408
patient management for, 408–409
Injury. See *Trauma.*
Insulin-like growth factors (ILGs), 237
Intervertebral disc, anatomy of, *560–563*
entrapment syndromes related to, 559–563, *560–563*
protrusion of, 559–563, *562, 563*
Intima, innervation of, 158
Ischemia, arterial denervation for, *166,* 166–167, *167*
conduction block due to, 355–356
hands and fingers affected by, *166,* 166–167, *167*
pain due to, 113
pressure sores caused by, 763, *763,* 763(t), *764*
transient nerve block due to, 475–476
Ischemic monomelic neuropathy (IMN), 659–660

Jeanne's sign, 683, *683*
Johnson transfer, toe with, 728, *728*
Jones transfer, lesser toe with, 727, *727*
Jugular foramen, cranial nerves in, 385, *386*

Kaplan's cardinal line, *193*
Karapandzic flap, 745
Knee, 51–52
motor function testing across, 51, *52*
surgical nerve exposure in, *199, 200, 202*
trauma to, nerve injury related to, 368
Krypton laser, 314(t), 316
Kuntz' nerve, 160

Lacerations, 365
Lacrimal gland, nerve supply to, *30*
Laminotomy, electrode implantation by, 140–141, *141, 142*
Lasers, 313–317
characteristics of, 314(t), *315*
low-energy, 316–317
nerve repair using, 313–317, 314(t), *315, 316*
types of, 313–317, 314(t), *315*
Leads, electrical nerve stimulation using, *138,* 138–139, *139*

Leg. See *Extremities, lower.*
Leprosy, 615–621
deformities associated with, prevention of, 616
reconstruction of, 620
lepromatous (multibacillary), 615, *617, 619*
neuritis of, *615–620,* 615–621
localized sites of, 615–616, *617*
medical treatment of, 616–621
pathogenesis of, 615, *615, 616*
surgical approach in, 618–621, *618–621*
neuropathy caused by, 14
tuberculoid (paucibacillary), 615, *616*
Lhermitte's sign, 595
Lidocaine, challenge test using, 128
nerve block using, 67
systemic use of, 128, 132
Ligament(s), carpal, nerve entrapment by, *534–536,* 534–541
of Struthers, 514, *516*
Lip, muscles of, 31, *32, 230, 741, 742*
Lipoma, radial nerve entrapment related to, 521, *523*
Lisch nodules, neurofibromatosis with, 600
Louisiana State University Medical Center Grading System, 347, 348(t)
whole nerve in, 347, 348(t)
Lovett grading method, 341(t)
Lumbosacral plexus, 52–53, 56–62
anatomy of, 56, *56*
mechanism of injury to, 56
motor testing related to, 52–53
surgical exploration of, 56–58, *57, 58*
Lumbosacralcoccygeal plexus, anatomy of, 195–196, *196*

MacGill Pain Questionnaire, 129
MacKinnon and Dellon classification, 598, 598(t)
Macrophages, degenerative process role of, *358, 359*
Magnetic resonance imaging. See *MRI (magnetic resonance imaging).*
Malingering, 126
diagnostic criteria for, 126
Mandible, fracture of, 374
neoplasia of, *374,* 374–375, *375*
nerve branching patterns in, 228–232, *229–232*
nerve supply to, 31–34, *32, 33, 36*
Mannerfelt's syndrome, 588
Martin-Gruber anastomosis, arm with, 49
Maxilla, nerve branching patterns in, *229, 230, 230, 232*
Mechanical injury, denervated extremity due to, *763,* 763(t), 763–764
Mechanical receptors, 11–12, 12(t)
Media, innervation of, 158
Medulla, pain pathways in, 121, *122*
parasympathetic role of, *158*
Meissner's corpuscle, 12(t), *746*
Meningioma, optic nerve sheath with, 372, *373*
Mepivacaine, nerve block using, 67
Meralgia paresthetica, 429
Merkel's receptor, 12(t), *746*
Mesencephalon, pain pathways in, 121, *122*
Microscopy, axon histochemistry in, 243–246, *243–246*
surgical techniques using, 5, 261–269, *262, 263*
Midbrain, parasympathetic role of, *158*
Military brace maneuver, 496, *496*
Minnesota Multiphasic Personality Inventory (MMPI), 129
MMN (multifocal motor neuropathy), 656–657

MMPI (Minnesota Multiphasic Personality Inventory), 129
Moberg test, 19–22, *20–23*, 22(t). See also *Two-point discrimination test.*
Moberg's Rating Scale of Sensibility, 342, 342(t), 346(t)
Molluscum fibrosum, neurofibroma associated with, 600, *600*
Monofilaments, 16–22
    hand function measurement using, 544, 544(t), *545*
    scale of interpretation for, 17(t), *20*
    tests using, 16–22, 17(t), *19–23*
Mononeuropathy multiplex, 594, 659
Morton's neuroma, 153–155, *155*, 557
    interdigital nerve entrapment by, 593–594
Motor end-plate, muscle reinnervation role of, 393–395, *394*
Motor function, 675–714. See also *Cerebral palsy; Palsy.*
    intraoperative awake stimulation of, 335
    loss of, grading of, 774, 776(t)
        impairment evaluation related to, 774, 776(t), 778(t)
    reconstructive restoration of, 675–714. See also *Palsy; Reconstruction techniques; Tendon transfer.*
    testing of, postsurgical evaluation using, 340(t), 340–341, 341(t), 346(t)–348(t)
Motor function testing, 39–55
    cerebral palsy in, 631–632
    end-to-end suture vs. grafting in, 416–418, *417, 418*
    facial region, 29–35
    historical aspects of, 4
    lower extremity, 50–55
    rating scales for, 340(t), 340–341, 341(t), 346(t)–348(t)
    upper extremity, 39–49
Motorcycle accidents, brachial plexus injury in, 445(t), 445–453, *448–452*
Movement disorders, cerebral palsy and, 630–634
MRI (magnetic resonance imaging), 82–85
    case reports related to, 85–93
        bilateral cervical ribs in, 86–90, *88–90*
        body building effects in, 85–86, *86, 87*
        median nerve neurolemmoma in, 90, *91*
        old rib fracture in, 90–91, *92*
    procedure for, 85
Multifocal motor neuropathy (MMN), 656–657
Muscle(s), 39–55, 675–714. See also *Cerebral palsy; Tendon transfer.*
    adductor brevis, motor function testing of, 53, *53*
    adductor longus, motor function testing of, 53, *53*
    adductor magnus, motor function testing of, 53, *53, 54*
    adductor pollicis, 48, *48*
    arrector pili, sympathetic innervation of, *158*
    biceps, 45, *47*
        median nerve entrapment by, 514, *514*
        surgical reinnervation of, 330, *333*
    biceps femoris, motor function testing of, 54, *54*
    brachialis, 45, *47*
    brachioradialis, 46, *47*
    deltoid, 40(t), 44, *45*, 46t
    elbow flexor-pronator slide and, 636–637, *637*
    extensor digitorum longus, motor function testing of, 52, 55
    extensor hallucis longus, motor function testing of, 52, *53*, 55
    facial, 29–34, *32, 33, 230, 741, 742*
    first dorsal interosseous, 48, 49, *49*

Muscle(s) *(Continued)*
    flexor digitorum longus, motor function testing of, 52, 54, *54*
    flexor digitorum superficialis, median nerve entrapment by, 514, *515*
    flexor hallucis longus, motor function testing of, 52, 54
    flexor pollicis longus, 48
        median nerve affected by, 587–589, *588, 589*
        nerve compression affecting, 504, 504–505
    forearm, *395*
    frontalis, 31, *32*
    gastrocnemius, motor function testing of, 54, *54*
    gastrocnemius soleus, peroneal nerve compressed by, 577, *577*
    gluteus, motor function testing of, 51
        surgical nerve exposure and, 196–197, *197, 198*
    gracilis, anatomy of, *735, 736, 738, 739*
        motor function testing of, 53, *53*
        physical characteristics of, 736(t)
        reconstructive transfer using, 731–743, *735, 736*, 736(t), *738–742*
    hamstring, motor function testing of, 51, *52*
    iliopsoas, *168*
        motor function testing of, 51, *51*
    infraspinatus, 44, *46*
    Langer's, median nerve entrapment by, 515
    latissimus, anatomy of, *735, 739*
        physical characteristics of, 736(t)
        reconstructive transfer using, *735, 736*, 736(t), *739*, 739–740
    levator scapulae, *43*
    lip depressor, 31, *32*
    lower extremity, 50–55, *51–54*, 217–220
        relative strengths of, 719(t)
    nerve repair conduit of, 308
    orbicularis oculi, 31, *32*
    orbicularis oris, 31, *32*
    pectoralis, 44, *45*
        anatomy of, *735, 737*
        contracture release incision of, 635, *635*
        physical characteristics of, 736(t)
        reconstructive transfer using, 731, 736, 736(t), *737*
        transfer of, elbow flexion due to, *470*, 470–471
    peroneus brevis, motor function testing of, 52, *53*, 55
    peroneus longus, motor function testing of, 52, *53*, 55
    piriformis, *72*
        sciatic nerve compressed by, *572*, 572–573
    platysma, auricular nerve and, *234*
    profundus, 48, *48*
    pronator teres, contracture release technique for, 638
    psoas major, *168*
    quadriceps, 51, *51, 53*
        femoral nerve repair and, 427, *427*
        motor function testing of, 51, *51*, 53–54
        nerve supply to, 51, *51, 53*
    reconstruction procedures and, 675–714. See also *Muscle transfer; Reconstruction techniques; Tendon transfer.*
    reinnervation of, direct, 393–396, *394–396*, 396(t)
    rhomboid major, *43*
    sacrospinalis, *168*
    sartorius, motor function testing of, *53*, 54
    scalene, thoracic outlet syndrome and, 494–495, *495*
    semimembranosus, motor function testing of, 52, 54, *54*

Muscle(s) *(Continued)*
    semitendinosus, motor function testing of, 52, 54, *54*
    serratus, anatomy of, *735, 737*
        physical characteristics of, 736(t)
        reconstructive transfer using, 731, 736, 736(t), *737*
        transfer graft reinnervation of, 336, *337*
    soleus, motor function testing of, 54, *54*
    sternocleidomastoid, 69, 70, *70, 161*
        accessory nerve and, *386, 387*
        anatomy of, *230, 233, 234*
    strength grading of, 39, 39(t), 50, 50(t)
    subscapularis, *45*
    supraspinatus, 41, *44*
    teres minor, 44, *46*
    testing of, 52, 54, *54*, 55
        postsurgical evaluation using, 340(t), 340–348, 341(t), 346(t)–348(t)
    thenar, *343, 395, 418*
    tibialis, motor function examination of, 52, 54, *54*, 55
    trapezius, *395*
    triceps, 46, *47*
    upper extremity, 39–49, 40(t), *43–49*, 46(t)
    zygomatic, 31, *32*
Muscle fibers, *734, 734–735*
    anatomy and morphology of, *734*, 734–735
    cerebral palsy affecting, 630–646
    denervation affecting, 665, *665*, 666, *666*
        electrical stimulation in, 669–674
    disuse effect on, 665, *665*
    histology of, 663–667, *664–667*
    ischemia effect on, 665–666, *666, 667*
    length alteration effect on, *664*, 664–665, *665*
    nerve pathology effect on, 663–667, *664–667*
    reinnervation effect on, 666, *667*
Muscle transfer, 731–743. See also *Tendon transfer.*
    blood supply in, 733, *735*, 735–738, 736(t), *739, 741*
    elbow reconstruction using, pectoral in, *470*, 470–471, *471*
    facial reanimation using, 740–743, *741, 742*
    forearm in, 731, 739–740, *740, 742*
    gracilis used in, 731–743, *735, 736*, 736(t), *738–742*
    latissimus used in, *735, 736*, 736(t), *739*, 739–740
    nerve supply in, 733, 736(t), *739*, 739–741
    pectoralis used in, 731, 736, 736(t), *737*
    serratus used in, 731, 736, 736(t), *737*
    upper extremity replantation and, *713*, 713–714, *714*
Musicians, compression neuropathy in, 487
Myelin sheath, *274*
    microanatomy of, *353*, 353–355, *354*
Myelination, *124*
    compression affecting, 476–481, *477–480*
Myelopathy, rheumatoid, 595
Myopathy, rheumatoid, 594–595
Myxoma, nerve sheath, 603–604
    clinical presentation of, 603–604
    pathology of, 604

NAP (nerve action potential). See *Action potential.*
Nd:YAG laser, 314(t), *315, 316*
Neck. See also *Face; Head.*
    innervation anatomy of, 228–234, *229–234*
    posterior triangle of, 195, *195*
    spinal accessory nerve in, 195, *195*
Needle electrode examination, 648–652
Neoplasia, 597–611

Neoplasia *(Continued)*
  benign, *598–603, 598–604*
  cerebellopontine angle with, 376–379, *377–380*
  classification of, 598, 598(t)
  facial nerve affected by, 376–379, *377–381, 385*
  floor of mouth, 375, *375*
  ganglionic, 607–608
  hamartoma as, 608–609
  hemangioma as, 609
  malignant, 604–607, *605–607*
  mandibular, 374, *374, 375*
  median nerve with, *78*
  myxomatous, 603–604
  nerve sheath with, 603–604
  neurolemmoma as, 90, *91*
  optic nerve affected by, 371–373, *372, 373*
  oral, *374*, 374–375, *375*
  peripheral nerve, 597–611, 598(t)
  pituitary gland with, 371, *372*
  radial nerve entrapment related to, 521, *523*
  reactive, *609*, 609–611, *610*. See also *Neuroma.*
Nerve(s), abducent, 372–373
  accessory, *386, 387–388*
  acoustic, 384
  alveolar, *374*, 374–375
  anatomy of, microscopic, *263, 264, 353*, 353–355, *354*
  anococcygeal, 195–196, *196*
  antebrachial cutaneous, *41, 42*
    fascicular morphology of, 330, *333*
    graft prepared from, 286
    reinnervation using, 330, *333*
    vascularized graft using, 298(t)
  anterior cutaneous, 233, *233*
  anterior tibial, 298(t)
  axillary, *41–43*, 42–44, *175, 176*
    anatomy of, 181, *182*
    dermatomes and, *775*
    entrapment of, *526*, 526–527
    surgical exposure of, 181–183, *182*
  balloon expansion of, *290–292, 290–293*
  blood supply to, capillary, *353*, 353–354, *354*
  brachial, dermatomes and, *775*
  brachial cutaneous, *41, 42*
  buccal, 31, *32, 33*
  capping of, 153
  chemical lysis of, 152–153, *153*
  chorda tympani, anatomy of, 30, *30*
  common peroneal, fascicular anatomy of, 220, *222–224*
    origin of, 195–196, *196*
    surgical exposure of, *202, 203, 204*
  cranial, 371–388
    lesions of, 371–388
    surgical treatment of, 371–388
  cross sectional morphology of, *265, 271, 274, 275*
  cutaneous, of gluteal region, compression of, 563–564
    of thigh, compression of, 563–568, *565, 567, 571*
    of upper extremity dermatomes and, *775*
  deep peroneal, anatomy of, 220, 221, *222–224*
    surgical exposure of, 203, *204*
    vascularized graft using, 297(t)
  digital, 189–194
    nerve gap affecting, *328*, 328–333, *329*
    neuroma of, *276*
    postsurgical sensibility of, 346(t), 347(t)
    surgical exposure of, 189–194, *192–194*
    surgical repair of, 274–278, *276*
    vascular penetration of, *528*
  digital (of toe), entrapment of, *579*, 580–581

Nerve(s) *(Continued)*
  dorsal scapular, 39, *41, 43, 175, 176*
    entrapment of, 528
  electrical stimulation therapy of, 131, 135–144. See also *Electrical nerve stimulation.*
  electron microscopy of, *124*
  epineural anesthesia infusion of, 116–119, *117, 118*
  face region supplied with, 29–36, *30, 32, 33*
  facial, 29–36, 375–384
    anatomy of, 29–36, *30, 32, 33*, 228–232, *229–232*
    Bell's palsy and, 375–376, 384
    branching patterns of, 228–232, *229–232*
    caudal, 384–388, *385–387*
    cerebellopontine compression of, 376–379, *377–380*
    electrophysiologic testing of, 34
    faciofacial anastomosis of, 381–383, *383*
    leprosy affecting, 616
    neoplasia affecting, 376–379, *377–381, 385*
    paresis related to, 375–376, *381, 382*, 384
    skull fracture affecting, 379–381, *381, 382*
    surgical repair of, 34–36
    surgical treatment of, 376–384, *378–383*
    symptoms related to, 29–30
  femoral, 221–227, *565*
    anatomy of, *53*, 53–54, 58, *58*, 221–227, *226*
    branches of, 225
    cross section of, 221–227, *226*
    diagnostic block of, 72
    entrapment of, 568–569, *569*
    fascicular topography of, 221–227, *226*
    injection injury of, 409(t), 412–413
    injury to, 58–59
    motor testing related to, *51, 53*, 53–54
    muscles innervated by, 225
    origin of, 195–196, *196*
    surgical exploration of, *58*, 58–59
    surgical exposure of, 197–198, *201*
    surgical repair outcome analysis for, *427*, 427–429, *428*, 428(t)
  frontal, *32, 33*
    anatomy of, 31, *32, 33, 35*, 228–230, *230, 232*, 232–233
    danger zone for, 230, *230*
  genitofemoral, *168, 170, 565*
    compression of, *565, 566, 567*
    origin of, 195–196, *196*
  gliding of, 96–97, 271–272, 328–329
  glossopharyngeal, *386–387*
  gluteal, *565, 569, 572*
  great auricular, anatomy of, 233, *233, 234*
  greater petrosal, 30, *30*
  hypoglossal, *385, 387*, 388
  iliohypogastric, *565*
    entrapment of, 564–566, *565, 567*
  ilioinguinal, *170, 565*
    compression of, *565, 566, 567*
  inferior gluteal, anatomic origin of, 195–196, *196*
  infraorbital, *232*, 232–233
    anatomy of, 35–36
    diagnostic block of, *68*, 68–69
  infrapatellar, 225
  intercostal, axon donation by, 287
    brachial plexus repair using, *451, 452*, 453(t), 461
    diagnostic block of, 72–73, *73*
  Kuntz', 160
  lateral antebrachial cutaneous, anatomy of, 179, *179*
    surgical exposure of, 179, *179*
  lateral cutaneous of forearm, 525–526

Nerve(s) *(Continued)*
  lateral femoral cutaneous, *202, 203, 565*
    compression of, 566–568, *567*
    diagnostic block of, 72, *73*
    graft prepared from, 286
    neuropathies of, 429, 429(t)
    origin of, 195–196, *196*
    resection of, 429, 429(t)
    surgical exposure of, *202, 203*
  lesser occipital, 233, *233*
  lingual, surgical treatment of, 375, *375*
  long thoracic, *41, 83*
    brachial plexus repair using, 462–463
    entrapment of, *526*, 527–528
    transfer graft repair of, 336, *337*
  lower extremity, 50–55, *51–54*, 217–227
  mandibular, 31–34, *32, 33*
  marginal mandibular, 230, *231*
    danger zone for, 230, *232*
  medial antebrachial cutaneous, 175, *176*, 179, *179*
  medial brachial, 175, *176*
  median, *41–43*, 47–48, *48*
    anatomy of, *176*, 179–180, *180, 181*, 192–194
    anterior interosseous branch of, *512*, 512–513, *513*
    brachial plexus and, 175, *176, 181*
    branching patterns of, 212–213, *213, 214*
    cadaver dissection of, *331*
    dermatomes and, *775*
    diagnostic block of, 71, *72*
    elbow injury affecting, 367–368
    entrapment of, 511–516, *514–517*, 534–541
    expander use on, 290, *292*
    fascicular morphology of, *262*, 274–275, *275, 277*, 330, *330–334*
    graft repair of, 415–418, *415–418*
    gunshot injury to, 401–403, *403*
    injection injury of, 409(t), 410–411, *411*
    leprosy affecting, 615, *617, 620*
    nerve gap affecting, *328*, 328–333, *330–334*
    nerve transfer procedure and, 336, *336*
    neurilemoma of, 90, *91*
      MRI studies of, 90, *91*
    neuroma in continuity of, 326(t)
    palmar cutaneous branch of, 512
    palsy affecting. See under *Palsy.*
    postsurgical sensibility of, *343–345*, 344, 346(t), 347(t)
    recurrent motor branch of, 511–512
    replantation of arm and, 706–710, *708–710*
    rheumatoid compression of, 587–589, *588, 589*
    surgical exposure of, 180, *180, 181*, 192–194
    surgical internervous planes and, *507–509*
    surgical repair of, 274–277, *275, 277*, 328, 330, 332, 333
    transection affecting, 359–360, *360*
    tumor affecting, *77, 78*
    vascular penetration of, 515, *517*
  median cutaneous of forearm, graft prepared from, 286
  mental, anatomy of, 35–36, 233
    diagnostic block of, *68*, 69
  metacarpal, diagnostic block of, 71
  metatarsal, *205*
  musculocutaneous, *41–43*, 44–45, *47*
    anatomy of, surgical exposure and, 175, *176, 178*, 178–179
    brachial plexus repair and, *451, 452, 460*, 460–461, *464*
    branching patterns of, *257*
    compression of, 525
    dermatomes and, *775*

Nerve(s) *(Continued)*
  elbow contracture release and, 636
  obturator, *565*
    anatomy of, 53, *53*, 198
    diagnostic block of, 72, *73*
    entrapment of, *567*, 568
    motor testing related to, 53, *53*
    origin of, 195–196, *196*
    surgical exposure of, 198–203
  oculomotor, compression of, 372–373, *373*
    surgical treatment of, 372–373, *373*
  olfactory, 371
  ophthalmic, surgical treatment of, 374, *374*
  optic, compression of, 371–372, *371–373*
    surgical treatment of, 371–372, *371–373*
  pectoral, 41, *41*, *44*, *45*, 175, *176*
  perineal, *570*
  peripheral, 127, 127(t)
    diagnostic block of, 127, 127(t)
    electrostimulation of, *143*, 143–144
  peroneal, *571*, *574*
    anatomy of, *53*, *54*, 54–55, *56*, *61*
    common, *56*, *61*, 346(t), *574*, 574–575
    compression of, *574*, 574–577, *576*
    deep, *574*, *576*, 577
    graft prepared from, 287
    injury of, 61–62
    leprosy affecting, 615
    motor testing related to, *52–54*, 54–55
    muscular reinnervation role of, 393, *394*
    postsurgical sensibility of, 346(t), 347(t)
    rheumatoid compression of, 592
    superficial, *574*, 575–576, *576*
    surgical exposure of, 61–62
    surgical outcome analysis for, 423(t), *424*,
      424(t), *425*, 426(t), 426–427, *427*
    traction injury to, 368
  phrenic, brachial plexus repair using, 461–
    462, *464*
  physiology of, *353*, 353–355, *354*
  plantar, *54*
    anatomy of, 219–220
    entrapment of, *577*, *579*, 580
    lateral, *577*, *579*, 580
    medial, *577*, *579*, 580
  posterior femoral cutaneous, 195–196, *196*
  posterior interosseous, 185–189
    anatomy of, 185–187, *187*, *188*
    rheumatoid compression of, 590–591, *591*
    surgical exposure of, *187*, 187–189, *188*
  posterior tibial, rheumatoid compression of,
    592–593
  pudendal, *569*
    compression of, 564, *565*
    entrapment of, 569–570, *570*
    origin of, 195–196, *196*
  radial, 41–43, 45–47, *47*, *48*
    anatomy of, *176*, *181*, 184, *184*, *186*, *188*
    brachial plexus and, 175, *176*, *181*, *184*
    branching patterns of, 214
    dermatomes and, *775*
    diagnostic block of, 71, *71*
    entrapment of, 519–525, *522–525*
    fascicular morphology of, *277*, 330, *332*
    humeral fracture affecting, 367–368
    injection injury of, 409(t), 409–410, *410*
    leprosy affecting, 616
    nerve transfer procedure and, 336, *336*
    neuroma in continuity of, 326(t)
    palsy affecting. See under *Palsy.*
    posterior antebrachial cutaneous branch of,
      524
    posterior interosseous branch of, entrapment
      of, 519–524, *522–523*
    postsurgical sensibility of, 346(t), 347(t)
    replantation of arm and, 706–710, *708–710*

Nerve(s) *(Continued)*
  superficial, 524, *524*
  surgical exposure of, 184–185, *184–188*,
    189
  surgical internervous planes and, *507–509*
  surgical repair of, *332*
  recurrent, 387
  saphenous, 225
    entrapment of, 568, *579*
    graft prepared from, 286–287, 298(t)
    surgical exposure of, 198
  sciatic, 217–221, *569*
    action potential of, 421–422, *422*
    anatomy of, *54*, *56*, *60*, *61*, 218, 222–224,
      226
    balloon expander use in, 290, *291*
    branches of, 218–221
    cadaver dissection of, 217–221, *218*, 222–
      224
    cross section of, 217–221, *218*, 222–224
    diagnostic block of, 72, *72*
    entrapment of, 570–573, *571–573*
    fascicular topography of, 217–221, *218*,
      222–224, 262
    hip injury affecting, 368
    injection injury of, 409(t), *411*, 411–412,
      412
    motor testing related to, *52*, *54*, *54*
    muscles innervated by, 218–221
    neuroma in continuity of, *324*, *326*
    rheumatoid compression of, 592
    surgical exposure of, 59–60, 196–197, *197–*
      199
    surgical repair outcome analysis for, 420–
      424, 423(t), *424*, 424(t)
    tethering of, 572–573, *573*
  sensitivity testing for, 558–559
  spinal accessory, 194–195
    anatomy of, 195, *195*
    brachial plexus repair using, 452, 453(t),
      460, 460–461, *464*
    surgical exposure of, 195, *195*
  subscapular, *41*, 41–42, *45*, 175, *176*
  superficial peroneal, fascicular anatomy of,
    220, *222–224*
    vascularized graft using, 298(t)
  superficial radial, graft prepared from, 286
    vascularized, 297(t), 298(t)
    neuroma of, *307*
  superior gluteal, origin of, 195–196, *196*
  supraclavicular, 233, *233*
    dermatomes and, *775*
  supraorbital, anatomy of, 35, 232, *232*
    diagnostic block of, 68, 69
  suprascapular, 41, *41*, *44*, 175, *176*
    entrapment of, 526, 527
    surgical exposure of, *183*, 183–184
  supratrochlear, diagnostic block of, 68, 69
  sural, 286, *576*
    entrapment of, 573–574, *576*
    graft prepared from, *276*, *278*, 286, *396*,
      416
      fascicular, *276*, 278
      gunshot injury treated with, 401–403,
        402, *403*
      vascularized, 297(t), 298(t), *301*, 301–
        302, *302*
    surgical exposure of, 203–208, *204*, 286
  temporal, 31, *32*, *33*
  thoracodorsal, *41*, 42, *45*, 175, *176*
  tibial, *571*, *577*
    anatomy of, 54, *54*, *60*
    entrapment of, *577*, 577–580, *579*
    expander use on, 290, *291*
    fascicular anatomy of, 219–220, 221, *222–*
      224, 330

Nerve(s) *(Continued)*
  graft repair of, 330, *338*
  leprosy affecting, 615
  motor testing related to, *52*, 54, *54*
  muscular reinnervation role of, 393, *394*
  nerve gap affecting, 330, *338*
  origin of, 195–196, *196*
  posterior, *60*, 60–61, *61*
  postsurgical sensibility of, 346(t), 347(t)
  surgical exposure of, *60*, *61*, *199*, *200*, 203,
    206, *207*
  surgical repair outcome analysis for, 420–
    424, *424*, 424(t), *425*, 425(t), 426(t)
  toes supplied with, 52, *53*
  trigeminal, 373–375
    anatomy of, 35–36, *232*, 232–233
    branches of, *232*, 232–233
    lesions of, 373–375, *374*, *375*
    surgical treatment of, 373–375, *374*, *375*
  trochlear, surgical treatment of, 372–373
  ulnar, 41–43, *48*, 48–49
    anatomy of, 189, *190–194*
    brachial plexus and, 175, *176*, *181*, *184*
    branching patterns of, 213–214
    dermatomes and, *775*
    diagnostic block of, 71, *71*
    donor graft from, 463, *463*
    dorsal cutaneous branch of, 518
    elbow injury affecting, 367–368
    electrode stimulation of, *143*, 143–144
    entrapment of, 516–519, *518–521*, 590
    fascicular morphology of, 274–275, *276*,
      330, *332*
    graft repair to, 415–418, *416–418*
    graft taken from, 287
      vascularized, 297(t), 298(t), 302–303, *303*
    gunshot injury to, 401–403, *402*, *403*
    injection injury of, 409(t), 411
    leprosy affecting, 615, *616*, *617*, 618–619,
      619, *620*
    nerve gap affecting, *328*, 328–333, *332*
    nerve transfer procedure and, 336, *336*
    neuroma in continuity of, 326(t)
    palsy affecting. See under *Palsy.*
    postsurgical sensibility of, 344, *344*, *345*,
      346(t)
    proper digital, microsurgical translocation
      of, 690
    replantation of arm and, 706–710, *708–710*
    rheumatoid compression of, 589–590, *590*
    surgical exposure of, 189–193, *190–194*
    surgical internervous planes and, *507–509*
    surgical repair of, 274–278, *276*, *332*
    tendinous penetration of, 505, *506*
    transection affecting, 359–360, *360*
    transposition of, *518–520*, 519
  upper extremity, 39–49, 40(t), *41–43*, 46(t),
    175–195
  venous intima wrapping of, 153, *154*
  vestibular, *384*
  zygomatic, 230, *230*
    anatomy of, 31, *32*, *33*
Nerve block, 65–75, 127(t), 127–128
  cervical plexus with, 69, 69–70
  cervicothoracic, *159*, 159–165, *160*
  diagnostic use of, 65–75, *68–74*, 127(t), 127–
    128
  epineural infusion for, 116–119, *117*, *118*
  head and neck region, 68–70, *68–70*, 127–128
  intercostal, 72–73, *73*
  local anesthetic drugs used in, 67–68
  lower extremity, 72, 72–73, *73*
  lumbar, 73, 73–75, *74*, 128, 167–168, *168*
  pain relief assessment of, 66
  paravertebral, *69*, *70*, *73*, *74*, 157–170, *161*,
    168

Nerve block (*Continued*)
  patient preparation for, 65–66
  peripheral nerves with, 127, 127(t)
  sympathetic ganglion, 157–170
    cervical, *69, 70, 159,* 159–165, *160*
    lumbar, *73, 74,* 128, 167–168, *168*
    sensorimotor vs., 66–67
    stellate, *69, 70, 70,* 127–128, 159–161, *161*
  techniques for use of, *68–74, 68–75, 161, 168*
  transient ischemic, 475–476
  upper extremity, *70,* 70–71, *71*
Nerve fibers, 11–12, *108*
  anatomy of, microscopic, *353,* 353–355, *354*
  balloon expansion of, *290–292,* 290–293
  branching patterns of, *210,* 210–214, *212–214,* 217–221, *218*
  burn injury to, *623,* 623–628, *624,* 625(t), *626–628*
    chemical, 624, 625(t)
    electrical, *624,* 624–626, *627*
    radiation causing, 626–628, *628*
  compression injury of, 355–357
    pathology in, 475–482, *476–482,* 501–503, *502,* 555–559, *556*
  conduction studies of, 650, *650*
    polyneuropathy diagnosis by, 648–652, *649, 650*
    signal transmission and, 11–12
    velocity measurement in, 650, *650*
  "cross-talk" between, 124–126
  degeneration of, 357–358, *358*
  diameter of, 11
  electron microscopy of, *124*
  electrophysiologic studies of, 251–258, *252– 257*
  end-organ complex of, *265*
  evoked potentials of, 251–258, *252–255*
  fascicles of. See *Fascicles.*
  histochemical examination of, 243–246, *243– 246*
  historical aspects of, 1–6, *210,* 210–212
  injection injury of, 406–413, 409(t), *409–412*
  lengthening techniques for, *290–292,* 290–293
  morphology of, *265, 274, 274, 353,* 353–354, *354*
  MRI studies of, 82–85, *84*
  myelinated, *124, 353,* 353–355, *354*
    vs. unmyelinated, *243, 244*
  neoplasia affecting. See *Neoplasia.*
  plexus formation by, *210*
  reconstruction and, 675–714. See *Nerve repair techniques; Reconstruction techniques; Tendon transfer.*
  regeneration of, *281, 281,* 305–309, *358,* 358– 359. See also *Nerve repair techniques.*
    blood supply and, 295–297, 298(t)
    compression syndromes followed by, 475– 482, *476–482*
    crush injury followed by, *556*
    low-energy laser stimulation in, 316–317
    neurotrophism in, 235–239
    replantation and, 706–710, *708, 710*
    trauma injury followed by, 357–359, *358*
  stimulation and recording of, 251–258, *252– 257*
  stretch injury to, 97
  surgery effects on, therapeutic decisions and, 95–97
  tension affecting, 329–330
  trauma injury to. See *Trauma.*
  types of, 11–12, 12(t)
  unmyelinated, *124, 353,* 353–355, *354*
    vs. myelinated, 11–12
Nerve gap, 328–339
  balloon nerve expander in, *290–292,* 290–293
  definition of, 328

Nerve gap (*Continued*)
  grafting of, 306–308, *328, 333–338,* 333–339
  nerve deficit vs., 328, *329*
  repair principles for, 306–308, *328–338,* 329– 339
  surgical technique related to, *333–338,* 334– 339
Nerve growth factor (NGF), 235–239
  axonal transport of, *354,* 354–355
  ciliary neurotrophic factor as, 236–237
  fibroblast, 237–238
  insulin-like, 237
  physiology of, 235–238
  receptors for, 235
Nerve repair techniques, 251–348
  adjunct use in, 311–317
    fibrin glue and, 311–313, *312, 313*
    historical aspects of, 311–313
    laser and, 313–317, 314(t), *315, 316*
    suturing and, 311–313, *312*
  balloon nerve expander used in, *290–292,* 290–293
  clinical evaluation following, 340–348
    extremity coordination in, 343–344, *344, 345*
    motor strength in, 340(t), 340–341, 341(t)
    rating scales used in, 340(t)–343(t), 345– 348, 346(t)–348(t)
    recovery time and, 344–345
    sensory function in, 341(t)–343(t), 341–343, *343*
  conduits used in, 305–309, 335
    autogenous venous, 306–308, *307,* 335
    history of, 305–306
    muscle-derived, 308, 335
    perineurial tube, 308
    synthetic, 308–309, 335–336
  electrostimulation in, 669–674
  epineurial, *264, 266,* 266–267, 271–273, 335
  evaluation following, 414–418, 420–429
    lower extremity, 420–429
    motor function in, 416–418, *417, 418*
    operative results analysis for, 420–429, 423(t)–429(t), *424, 425*
    sensory function in, 416–418, *417, 418*
    suture vs. grafting in, 416–418, *417, 418*
  facial muscle transfer and, 740–743, *741*
  fascicular, 261–269, 274–279, 280–289, 330– 333. See also *Fascicles.*
  grafts used in, 267–269, 280–289, 295–303, 305–309, 333–338. See also *Graft(s).*
  historical aspects of, 1–6, 305–306, 311–313
  microscope used in, 261–269, *262–268*
  nerve gap treatment using, *290–292,* 290–292, 328–339, *333–338*
  nerve transfer in, 280–289, *281–284, 287, 288, 336, 336*
  postsurgical functionality testing of, 341–348, 342(t), 343(t), *343–345,* 346(t)–348(t)
  replantation using, upper extremity in, 706– 710, *708, 710*
  sensibility grading following, 341–348, 342(t), 343(t), *343–345,* 346(t)–348(t)
  surgical techniques used in. See *Reconstruction techniques; Surgical techniques.*
  suturing for. See *Suture technique(s).*
Nerve roots, anatomy of, *555,* 560–563
  brachial plexus and, 82, *83,* 445(t), 445–453, *448–451*
    injury and, 445(t), 445–453, *448–451*
    innervation of, *41, 83,* 175–177, *176*
  cervical, *41, 83,* 175–177, *176*
  entrapment syndromes of, 559–563, *560–563*
  lumbosacral, *560–563, 573*
  sciatic nerve and, 570–573, *571, 573*
Nerve sheath, ganglion of, 607–608

Nerve sheath (*Continued*)
  clinical presentation of, 607
  treatment of, 608
  myxoma affecting, 603–604
    clinical presentation of, 603–604
    pathology of, 604
Nerve transfer, gap repair using, 306–308, *328, 333–338,* 333–339
  grafts in, 280–289, *281–284, 287, 288, 336, 336*
Neuralgic amyotrophy, 658–659
Neurapraxia, 356, 402
  brachial plexus affected by, *446*
  compression syndrome with, 501–503, *502*
  conduction block as, 356
  pathology in, 475–482, *476–482*
Neurectomy, musculocutaneous, elbow contracture treated with, 636
Neurilemoma (schwannoma), 601–602
  clinical presentation of, 601–602
  histology of, 602, *603*
  malignant, 604–606, *605, 606*
  median nerve with, 90, *91*
  MRI of, 90, *91*
  pathology of, 602, *602, 603*
  treatment of, 602
Neuritis, leprous, 615–620, *615–621*
  sensibility testing in, 13–14
  therapeutic modalities for, 102
Neuroablation, 129–130
Neurofibroma, 598–601
  clinical presentation of, 598, 599–600, *600*
  histology of, *599, 601*
  malignant transformation of, 598, 599–600, *600,* 601
  multiple, 599–601, *600, 601*
  pathology of, 598, *598, 599,* 600–601, *601*
  plexiform, 601, *601*
  solitary, 598, 598–599
  treatment of, 598–599, 601
Neurofibromatosis, 599–601
  central, 600
  clinical presentation of, 599–600, *600*
  pathology in, 600–601, *601*
  peripheral, 600
  treatment of, 601
Neurolemmoma. See *Neurilemoma (schwannoma).*
Neurolysis, gunshot injury treated with, 402–403
  intraoperative, 510, *511*
  neuroma treated with, 152–153, *153*
Neuroma, 146–149, 151–155, 319–326, 336–339
  acoustic, 376–379, *377–381*
  amputation associated with, 146, 147, 148– 149
    stump affected by, 609, *609*
  bulb, 557
  cerebellopontine angle and, 376–379, *377– 381, 384*
  chemical injection of, 152–153, *153*
  digital, *276*
  examination of, 147–148, 151–152
  facial nerve affected by, 376–379, *377–381*
  in continuity, 149, 319–326, 336–339
    action potential correlated with, 321–326, *323–326,* 326(t)
    electrophysiologic studies of, 254, *255,* 321–326, *323–326*
    evaluation of, *319,* 319–326, *323–326,* 509, 510, *510*
    evoked potential and, 510, *510*
    fiber count related to, 482, *482*
    interdigital, 609–610, *610*
    neuropathology of, *319,* 319–320
    palpation of, *509*
    preoperative assessment of, 320–322

Neuroma *(Continued)*
surgical assessment of, 322, 337–339, *338*
lower extremity with, 151–155, *153, 154, 155, 338*
Morton's, 153 155, *155*, 557
interdigital nerve entrapment by, 593–594
nerve block for, 152
nonsurgical approaches to, 148, 152–155
pain due to, 148, 151
therapeutic modalities for, 102
plantar, 153–155, *155*
pseudoneuroma vs., 557
reactive neoplasia of, *609*, 609–611, *610*
superficial radial, *307*
surgical approach to, 147–149, *148*, 152–155, *153–155*, 336–339, *337, 338*
terminal branch, 147, 149
translocation of, 148, *148*, 152–153
treatment of, 148–149, 152–155, 336–339
true, 557
ulnar, surgical repair of, 337–339, *338*
upper extremity with, 146–149, *148*
venous conduit repair for, 306–308, *307*
Neuromuscular junction, morphology of, *265*
Neuron(s), arterial wall with, *110*
cell matter transport in, *354*, 354–355
degeneration of, 357–358, *358*
morphological components of, *265*
pain transmission by, 120–123, *122, 123*
postganglionic (central), 157–159, *158*
preganglionic (central), *122, 123*, 157–159, *158*
regeneration of, *358*, 358–359
Neuropathy, 13–15. See also *Compression syndrome(s)*; *Entrapment syndrome(s)*; specific nerve.
edema with, 101
etiologies of, 13–15
fingertip loss due to, 14, *14*
impairment evaluation in, 772–779, 773(t), *774–776*, 776(t), 777(t)–779(t)
ischemic monomelic, 659–660
radicular, hereditary sensory, 14, *14*
Neuroplasticity, pain induction of, 123
Neurosis, pain as focus of, 125–126
Neurosomes, 749
Neurothekeoma, 603–604
clinical presentation of, 603–604
pathology of, 604
Neurotization, basic principles of, 459–460
brachial plexus, 459–464
donor nerves for, *460*, 460–463, *463, 464*
neglected injury and, 451, 453, 453(t)
muscular, clinical results of, *395*, 395–396, *396*, 396(t)
surgical techniques for, 393–396, *394–396*
Neurotmesis, compression syndrome with, 501–502, *502*
injury extent in, 356
Neurotomes, 749
Neurotrophism, 235–238
biochemistry of, 235–238
definition of, 235
future directions in, 238
growth factors in, 235–238
Neurotropism, 235, 238–239
definition of, 238–239
specificity of target in, 238–239
NGF. See *Nerve growth factor (NGF)*.
Nitric oxide, neuroplasticity stimulated by, 123
Nociception, 121–123. See also *Pain*.
definition of, 121
nerve pathways for, 107, *108*
ongoing beyond healing, 123
signal transmission for, 107–109, *108*, 120–123, *122, 123*

Node of Ranvier, *477*, 477–478, *478, 480*
Nonsteroidal anti-inflammatory drugs (NSAIDs), 132
Norepinephrine, arterial wall receptors for, 109, *110*
Notch(es), sciatic, *72*
supraorbital, *68, 69*
Nucleus, facial, *30, 30*

Occupation, compression syndromes related to, 486–489, 543–549
disease vs. disorder associated with, 551
work simulator for, 543–544, *544*
Olfactory function, nerve compression affecting, 371
Omer's picking-up test, 23–24, *23–25*
Operating table, *263*
Opioids, therapy using, 131–132
Optic chiasm, 372, *372*
Overhead test maneuver, 496, *496*

Pacinian corpuscle, 12(t), *746*
Pain, 107–170
acute vs. chronic, 121–126
anatomic diagram for, 94–95, *95*, 129
assessment of, 100–101, 126–129
blood flow effects on, 107–109, *108*, 110(t), 113–114
extremity with, 107–114
central, 125
deafferentation causing, 125
definition of, 120–121
first vs. second, 121
gunshot injury causing, 402
historical aspects of, 120, *120*
inflammation mediators in, 121–123
neural pathways for, 107, *108*, 121–123, *122, 123*, 135–137
neuroma causing, 102, 148, 151
neuropathic, 123–124
pathophysiology of, 121–126, *122*
peripheral nerve disorders with, impairment evaluation related to, 772–774, 776(t), 778(t)
persistence of beyond healing, 123–126
phantom limb, 125
postsurgical recovery affected by, 342–343, *343*, 343(t)
psychogenic, 125–126, 128–129
questionnaire about, 129
receptors for, 11–12, 12(t)
transmission of, 11–12, 65, 107, *108*, 121–123, *122, 123*
treatment of, 129–132
electrical nerve stimulation in, 131, 135–137
epineural (peripheral) anesthesia infusion in, 116–119, *117, 118*
medicinal approach to, 131–132
neuroablation in, 129–130
systemic lidocaine in, 128, 132
visual analog scales for, 94–95, *95*
Pain Severity Scale, 342–343, 343(t)
Palm, nerves of, 189–194, *192–194*
surgical exposure of, 189–194, *192–194*
topographical lines of, *193*
Palsy, 675–703. See also *Cerebral palsy*; *Paralysis*.
Bell's, neuroanatomy of, 29–30
brachial plexus injury causing, 445(t), 445–453, *448–452*
Erb's, 454

Palsy *(Continued)*
median nerve, 678(t), 678–680, *681*, 683, 687–694, *689–693*
combined (with radial and ulnar), 697(t), 697–699, *698*, 699(t), 703, 703(t)
complete, 687–694, 688(t), *689–693*
early treatment of, 678(t), 678–680, *681*
high, 688–690, *690, 691*, 699, 699(t), *700–702*, 703, 703(t)
low, 678–680, *681*, 688, *689*
reconstruction for, 678(t), 678–680, *681*, 683, 687–694, *689–693*
sensation restoration for, 690–694, *692, 693*
radial nerve, 676(t), 678, 678(t), *679, 680*, 683–687, *684–687*
combined (with median and ulnar), 699–702, 702(t), 703, 703(t)
complete, 676(t), 683–687, *684–687*
early treatment of, 678, 678(t), *679, 680*
high, 524–525, *525*
reconstruction for, 676(t), 678, 678(t), *679, 680*, 683–687, *684–687*
Saturday night, 524
ulnar nerve, 678(t), 680–683, *682*, 694(t), 694–697, *695*
combined (with median and radial), 697(t), 697–703, *698*, 699(t), *700–702*, 702(t)
early treatment of, 678(t), 680–683, *682*
high, 696–697, 699–702, 702(t)
low, 680–683, *682, 695*, 695–696
reconstruction for, 678(t), 680–683, *682*, 694(t), 694–697, *695*
sensory defects in, 697
Paralysis, cerebral palsy with, 630
Déjerine-Klumpke, 49
Erb-Duchenne, 49
facial, 29–35
muscle transfer for, 740–743, *741, 742*
hypoglossal, *387*, 388
lower plexus, 49
tourniquet induction of, 476
transient ischemic, 475–476
upper plexus, 49
vocal cords affected by, 387
Parasympathetic nervous system, 157–159, *158*
anatomic centers of, 157–159, *158*
Paresis, facial nerve related to, 375–376, *381, 382, 384*
Paresthesia, 554
electrical nerve stimulation with, 135–137
Parsonage-Turner syndrome, *504, 505*, 658–659
Patient evaluation. See *Impairment evaluation*.
Pediatric patient, cerebral palsy affecting, 630, 633
Penetrating wounds. See *Gunshot wounds*.
Percussion test, nerve sensitivity in, 558
Perfusion. See *Blood flow*.
Perineurium, anatomy of, microscopic, *353*, 353–354, *354*
empty tube graft from, 308
morphology of, *265, 274*
MRI studies of, *84*
nerve repair using, 308
Peripheral nervous system. See also *Nerve(s)*; *Neuropathy*; *Polyneuropathy*.
impairment evaluation related to, 772–779, 773(t), *774–776*, 776(t), 777(t)–779(t)
Phantom limb, 125
Picking-up test, 23–24, *23–25*
postsurgical coordination and, 343–344, *344, 345*
Pinch test, arm replantation and, 710–712, *711, 712*
fingertip strength in, *18*
hand function measurement using, 543–544, *544*

Pinch test *(Continued)*
  square, *513*
Piriformis syndrome, sciatic nerve in, *572*, *572–573*
Plethysmography, 80
  blood flow testing with, 111, *111*
Plexus(i), axillary, nerve block of, 70–71
  brachial. See *Brachial plexus.*
  cervical, *69*, 69–70
    nerve block of, *69*, 69–70
  cervicobrachial, 40(t), *41*
  coccygeal, 195–196, *196*
  formation of, median nerve fascicles in, 330, *330–332*
  historical aspects of, *210*
  lumbar, nerve block of, 75
  lumbosacral, 52–53, 56–62
  lumbosacralcoccygeal, 195–196, *196*
  pelvic, surgical repair of, 429
Pneumatic cuff, anesthesia induced by, 476
Policeman's tip position, *454*
Polyglactin mesh tube, nerve repair using, 308–309
Polyglycolic acid tube, nerve repair using, 309
Polymyositis, 594–595
Polyneuropathy, 648–660
  electrodiagnostic examination of, 648–652, *649, 650*
  etiology of, 652–655, 653(t)
  generalized, 652–655, 653(t)
  motor-predominant, 655–657, 658–660
  sensory, 594
  sensory-predominant, 657–660
  symptoms and signs of, 652–655
  vs. entrapment lesions, 655–660
Pons, pain pathways in, 121, *122*
  parasympathetic role of, *158*
Popliteal (Baker's) cyst, compression due to, 592, *593*
Porter's letter test, 344
Potential. See *Action potential.*
Pressure, blood, 79–80
  endoneurial fluid, 354–355
  receptors for, 11–12, 12(t)
  sensibility to, 11–27
    testing and mapping of, *15*, 16(t), 17(t), 17–27, *19*
Pressure sores, 763–765
  infection of, 763(t), 765
  ischemia causing, 763, *763*, 763(t)
  management of, 762–766
  mechanical injury causing, 763, 763(t), 763–764
  neuropathic bone damage and, 766
  repetitive stress causing, 763(t), 764, 764–765, *765*
  tissue autolysis in, *764*, 764–765, *765*
  total contact cast and, 765–766, *766*
Procaine, nerve block using, 67
Projectile injuries. See also *Gunshot wounds.*
  spontaneous recovery prognosis for, 365–366
Pronator syndrome, 513–514, *514, 515*
  diagnostic testing for, 513–514, *514*
Proprioceptors, 11–12
Protective sensibility, loss of, 13–15, *14, 15*
Pseudo-nodes, *477*
Pseudosynovial tube, nerve repair using, 308
Psychological factors, pain perception related to, 125–126
  screening tests for, 128–129
Psychometric screening tests, 128–129
Pulvertaft side-weave technique, *640*, 640–641

Quadriplegia, spastic, *635*

Radial tunnel syndrome, 521–524
  diagnosis of, 521–524
Radiation injury, brachial plexus affected by, 657–658
  burn due to, 626–628, *628*
Radiculopathy, rheumatoid, 595
Radius, fracture of, nerve entrapment related to, 521, *523*
Raynaud's disease, 114
Receptors, arterial wall with, *110*
  nerve growth factor and, 235–236
  sensory, skin with, *746*
    types of, 745, *746*
  structure of, 11–13, 12(t)
    adaptability of, 11–13, 12(t)
    protective function of, 13–15, *14, 15*
    sensibility testing and, 11–27
    types of, 11–13, 12(t), 745, *746*
Reconstruction techniques. See also *Nerve repair techniques; Tendon transfer;* specific anatomic sites.
  arm and hand, 630–646, 675–703, 710–714
    upper arm replantation in, 706–714, *706–714*
  brachial plexus trauma and, 433–443
  cerebral palsy management using, 630–646. See also *Cerebral palsy.*
  leg and foot, 717–729
  operative principles in, 676–677
Recording. See also *Electrophysiologic studies.*
  nerve potential in, 252–255, *252–256*
Rectum, nerve supply to, *570*
Reflex sympathetic dystrophy, pain of, 124–125
  therapeutic modalities for, 102–104
Regeneration. See *Nerve fibers, regeneration of.*
Reinnervation. See also *Graft(s); Nerve transfer.*
  muscular, clinical results of, 395, 395–396, *396*, 396(t)
    surgical techniques for, 393–396, *394–396*
Relaxation therapy, 131
Remyelination, compression syndromes followed by, 475–480, *476–480*
Repetitive stress injury, 484. See also *Compression syndrome(s).*
  foot tissue autolysis due to, 763(t), *764*, 764–765, *765*
Rib(s), cervical bilateral, case report related to, 86–90, *88–90*
  diagnostic nerve block near, 72–73, *73*
  old fracture of, case report related to, 90–91, *92*
  resection of, thoracic outlet syndrome treated with, 495, *498*, 498–499
Riche-Cannieu anastomosis, hand with, 49
Ropivacaine, nerve block using, 68
Rosenberg classification, 598, 598(t)
Ruffini's corpuscle, 12(t), *746*

Sacral plexus, anatomy of, 195–196, *196*
Sacrum, *563*
St. Clair Strange pedicle, 403, *403*
Salivary glands, nerve supply to, *30*
Sarcomere, *734*
Saturday night palsy, 524
Scapula, thoracic outlet syndrome and, 494, *499*
Schizophrenia, 126
  diagnostic criteria for, 126
Schwann cell, *124*
  axonal complex with, *353, 354*, 354–355
  balloon expander effect on, 290, *290, 291*
  blood supply affecting, 295
  compression syndromes affecting, *477*, 477–478
  nerve fiber with, *274*

Schwann cell *(Continued)*
  nerve grafting role of, 295
  physiology of, 353–355
  regenerative proliferation of, 358, *358*
  vascularized graft and, 295
Schwannoma, clinical presentation of, 601–602, 604
  histology of, 602, *603, 606*
  malignant, 604–606, *605, 606*
  pathology of, 602, *602, 603*, 604–605, *605*
  treatment of, 602, 605–606
Sciatica, 570–573, *571–573*
  "credit card," 571
  piriformis muscle in, *572*, 572–573
Scoliosis, radiography of, *88*
Sebacious gland, sympathetic innervation of, *158*
Seckel's danger zone, 230, *232*
Seddon's classification, 356, 365
  compression lesion in, 501–502, *502*
Semmes-Weinstein test, 17–19, *19*, 342, 342(t)
  procedure for, 18–19, *19*
  threshold mapping with, *15*, 17(t), 17–19, *19*
Sensation-bearing flaps. See under *Flap(s).*
Sensibility testing, 11–27, 558–559
  historical aspects of, 4
  patterns of loss and recovery in, 13–15, *14, 15*
  protective sensation in, 13–15, *14, 15*
  receptor structures in, 11–13, 12(t)
  test selection for, 13–15, *14, 15*
  threshold factors for, 12(t), 12–13
Sensory function, 341–343
  cortical representation of, 745–749, *746–748*
  flaps and grafts with, 745–760. See also *Flap(s), sensation-bearing.*
  grading scales for, 341–343, 342(t), 343(t), 346(t)–348(t)
  intraoperative awake stimulation of, 335
  losses in, impairment evaluation for, 772–774, 776(t), 778(t)
    in extremities, 762–766, 763(t), *763–766*
    management of, 762–766, 763(t), *763–766*
  pain intensity in, 342–343, *343*, 343(t)
  postsurgical evaluation of, 341–343, 342(t), *343*, 343(t), 346(t)–348(t)
  receptors for, 745, *746*
  testing of, 341–343, 342(t), 343(t), 346(t)–348(t), 416–418. See also *Sensibility testing.*
    cerebral palsy in, 632–633, *633*
    end-to-end suture vs. grafting in, 416–418, *417, 418*
    facial trauma effects and, 35–36
    hand function measurement in, 544, 544(t), *545*
    regional nerve sensitivity in, 558–559
    sensation-bearing flaps and, 745–749, *746–748*
Shoes, rigid-soled, *764*, 764–765, *765*
  rocker, 764, *764*
  roller, 764, *765*
Shoulder, arm replantation and, *713*, 713–714, *714*
  arthrodesis of, 467–469, *468, 469*
  axillary nerve in, *182*
  brachial plexus and, 175–178, *176, 177*
    injury affecting, 445–453, *448, 451, 452, 454, 464*
    muscle transfer to, 470, *470*
    reconstruction in, 465–469, *466–470*
  cerebral palsy contracture of, 634–636, *635*
    surgical approach to, 634–636, *635*
  flail, *468*
  muscles of, 39, 40(t), *42, 43*
  nerve compression in, *526*, 526–528
  nerve supply through, 39, 40(t), *41–43*
  trauma injury to, spontaneous recovery prognosis for, 366–367

Skin, blood flow in, *107*, 107–109, 113–114
   dry, 762
      loss of sweating in, 762
      nerve sensitivity in, 558
      pressure sores affecting, 762–766, 763(t),
         763–766
      sensory receptors of, types of, *746*
      surface temperature of, blood flow and, 111,
         113
Snapping, ulnar nerve surgery followed by, 519,
   521
Somatoform pain disorder, 125–126
Sores, pressure. See *Pressure sores.*
Spasticity, cerebral palsy with, 630–632
Spillane-Parsonage-Turner syndrome, 569
Spinal cord, 157–159, *158*
   cross section of, *555*
   differential nerve block in, 128
   electrode stimulation therapy in, 130, 135–
      143, *136*, *137*, *141*, *142*
   nerve compression and, *555*
   nerve roots of, *555*
   pain pathways in, *108*, 121–123, *122*, *123*
   pain windup of, 123
   parasympathetic centers and, 157–159, *158*
   sensory relay by, *748*
   sympathetic centers and, 157–159, *158*
Spinal nerves, brachial plexus supplied by,
      175–177, *176*, 776, 776(t), *777*
   cervical, 175–177, *176*, 776, 776(t)
      graft taken from, 463
      stump neurotization of, 462
   facial pain pathways in, *122*
   impairment evaluation related to, 774–776,
      776(t)
Spinal reflexes, pain response and, 121–123, *123*
   splinting (muscle spasm) due to, 121, *123*
Spine, 157–159, *158*
   autonomic ganglia chain beside, *122*, 157–
      159, *158*
   cervical, 157–159, *158*
      MRI studies of, *89*, *90*
      nerve block in, *159*, 159–161, *160*
   coccygeal, *168*
   lower, compression syndromes and, 559–564
   lumbar, 128, *158*, 167–170, *168*, *169*
      nerve block in, 73–74, *74*, 128, 167–170,
         168
      sympathectomy of, 167–170, *168*, *169*
   lumbosacral, 559–563, *561–563*
   rheumatoid processes affecting, 595
   sacral, *168*
   somatic nerve block near, 75, 127(t), 127–128
   thoracic, 161–165, *162–165*
      sympathectomy of, 161–165, *162–165*
Spinomesencephalic tract, 121, *122*
Spinoreticular tract, 121, *122*
Spinothalamic tract, 121, *122*
SPLATT procedure, *723*, 725, *725*
Splinting, 121
Sports, compression neuropathy associated with,
      487–488
Spots, café-au-lait, neurofibroma associated with,
      600
Steindler effect, 469, *469*, *471*
Stereognosis, cerebral palsy affecting, 632–633,
   633
Steroids, leprosy treated with, 617–618
Stimulator, 252–256, *254*. See also *Electrical
   nerve stimulation; Electrophysiologic
   studies.*
Straight leg raising test, 558
Stretch test, nerve sensitivity in, 558
Struthers' ligament, *516*
   median nerve entrapment by, 514, *516*
Succinylcholine, compression syndrome
      evaluation using, 505

Sunderland classification, 356, 365
   brachial plexus injury and, 435–436
   compression lesion in, 501–503, *502*
Sunderland Society, 5
Surgical techniques. See also *Nerve repair
   techniques; Reconstruction techniques;
   Tendon transfer;* specific anatomic structure.
   awake stimulation during, 335
   balloon nerve expander use in, *290–292*, 290–
      293
   brachial plexus in, obstetric injury repair for,
      455–458, *456–458*
      trauma repair for, 447–453, *448–452*,
         451(t), 453(t)
   carpal tunnel release, *534–536*, 534–541, *538*
   cerebral palsy management with. See *Cerebral
      palsy.*
   clinical evaluation following, 269, 340(t)–
      343(t), 340–348, 346(t)–348(t)
   cranial nerves in, 371–388
   fascicular, 261–269, *265–268*, 274–279, *275–
      278*, 330–333, *332–335*
   grafts in, *281–284*, 282–289, *288*. See also
      Graft(s).
      cable formation for, *299*, 299–300, *300*
      vascularized, 299–303, *299–303*
   gunshot injury treated with, *401–403*, 401–404
   laser use in, 313–317, 314(t), *315*, *316*
   microsurgical, 5, 261–269, *262–268*
   muscle reinnervation in, 393–396, *394–396*.
      See also *Muscle transfer.*
   nerve exposure using, 175–208. See also spe-
      cific nerve.
   nerve gap repair in, *333–338*, 334–339. See
      also *Nerve transfer.*
   pain following, 342–343, *343*, 343(t)
   postoperative care for, 288–289
   Pulvertaft side-weave, *640*, 640–641
   reconstructive, arm and hand, 630–646, 675–
      703, 710–714
      cerebral palsy management with, 630–646
      leg and foot, 717–729
      operative principles in, 676–677
      upper arm replantation in, 706–714
   sensibility grading following, 269, 340(t)–
      343(t), 340–348, 346(t)–348(t)
Suture technique(s), 251–348
   adjunct use with, 311–313, *312*
   end-to-end nerve repair, *415*, 415–418, *417*,
      418
   fascicular, 264, *266–268*, 275–278, *276–278*,
      334, 334–335, *335*
   grafting and, 268, 284, 288, *334*, 334–335,
      335
   historical aspects of, 311–313, *312*
   microsurgical, 261–269, *262–268*
Swan-neck deformity, surgical approach to,
      645–646, *646*
Sweat glands, loss of function of, 762
   sympathetic innervation of, *158*
Sympathectomy, 157–170
   cervical region, 161–162
   digital, *166*, 166–167, *167*
   lumbar region, 168–170, *168–170*
   periarterial (adventitial), *166*, 166–167, *167*
   thoracic region, 161–166, *162–165*
   thoracoscopic, *165*, 165–166
   transaxillary, *162*, *163*, 163–165
Sympathetic nervous system, 157–159, *158*
   anatomic centers of, 157–159, *158*
   blood flow controlled by, 109, *110*, 158–159,
      166–167
   ganglia of, cervical, *159*, 159–165, *160*
      lumbar, 73–74, *74*, *158*, 167–168, *168*
      nerve block of, 73–74, *74*, 159–161, *161*,
         167–168, *168*

Sympathetic nervous system *(Continued)*
   resection of, 157–170, *162–165*, *167–170*
   stellate, *69*, 70, *70*, 127–128, 159–161, *161*
   thoracic, *158*, 161–165, *162–165*
   reflex dystrophy of, pain of, 124–125

Table, operating, *263*
Tarsal tunnel, arthritis effect on, 592–593
   entrapment syndrome of, *579*, 579–580, 592–
      593
   leprosy affecting, *618*
Teeth, extraction of, nerve damage due to, 375,
   375
Temperature, blood flow regulation of, *107*,
      107–109, *108*
   receptors for, 11–12, 12(t)
   sensibility testing related to, 25
Tendon(s), reflexes of, nerve sensitivity in, 558
   ulnar nerve penetration by, 505, *506*
Tendon transfer, 630–646, 675–703
   arm and hand reconstruction by, 675–703,
      710–714
      digital extensor in, 676(t), 678(t), 702(t),
         703(t)
         flexor carpi ulnaris transfer to, *684*, 684–
            687, *685*
         flexor digitorum superficialis transfer to,
            685–687, *686*
      digital flexor in, 688(t), 694(t), 697(t),
         699(t), 702(t), 703(t)
         brachioradialis transfer to, 711, *711*
         extensor carpi radialis longus transfer to,
            699, *700*, *701*
         flexor digitorum profundis transfer to,
            688–689, *690*
      replantation of upper arm followed by, 710–
         714, *711–714*
      thumb extensor in, 676(t), 678(t), 694(t),
         697(t), 699(t), 702(t), 703(t)
         extensor carpi radialis transfer to, *695*,
            695–696, *701*
         flexor carpi ulnaris transfer to, 711, *712*
         flexor digitorum transfer to, *672*, 680–
            683, *684–686*
         palmaris longus transfer to, 711, *712*
         pronator teres transfer to, 678, *679*, *680*
      thumb flexor in, 678(t), 688(t), 694(t),
         697(t), 699(t), 702(t), 703(t)
         abductor digiti quinti transfer to, 688,
            689
         brachioradialis transfer to, 689, *691*, *701*
         extensor indicis proprius transfer to, 678–
            680, *681*
         palmaris longus transfer to, 688, *689*
      wrist extensor in, 676(t), 678(t), 702(t),
         703(t)
      wrist flexor in, 694(t), 699(t), 702(t), 703(t)
   brachial plexus injury and, 465–471, *466–470*
   cerebral palsy management and, 630–646
      digital extensor in, flexor carpi ulnaris trans-
         fer to, 641–642, *642*
      digital flexor in, surgical lengthening of,
         638–639, *639*
      thumb extensor in, 641–643
         adductor pollicis and, *643*, 643–644, *644*
         first dorsal interosseous release and, 644,
            644
         flexor digitorum superficialis transfer to,
            641–642, *642*
         flexor pollicis lengthening and, 644, *644*
      wrist extensor in, extensor carpi ulnaris
         transfer to, 641
         flexor carpi ulnaris transfer to, *639*, 639,
            640

Tendon transfer *(Continued)*
  pronator teres transfer to, 640, *640*
  wrist flexor in, surgical lengthening of, 638–639, *639*
 elbow reconstruction using, *469*, 469–470, *471*
  flexors in, 469–471, *470*
 leg and foot reconstruction by, 717–729
  anterior approach in, 719–723
   flexor digitorum longus in, 721
   flexor hallucis longus in, 721
   peroneus brevis in, 720, *720*
   peroneus longus in, 720–721
   tibialis anterior in, 721–723, *722, 723*
   tibialis posterior in, 719–720, *720*, 721
  bone attachment techniques for, 717–719, *718*
  forefoot in, 726–729
   digital extensors and, 726–728, *727, 728*
   digital flexors and, 728–729, *729*
  lateral approach in, 725–726
   peroneus longus in, 725–726, *726*
   tibialis anterior in, 725, *725*
  medial approach in, 726
   flexor digitorum longus in, 726, *726*
   tibialis posterior in, 726, *726, 727*
  posterior approach in, 723–726
   flexor digitorum longus in, 725
   flexor hallucis longus in, 724, *725*
   peroneus brevis in, 724–725, *725*
   tibialis anterior in, 723–724, *724*
   tibialis posterior in, 724, *724*
 shoulder reconstruction using, 465–467, *466–468*
  latissimus dorsi in, 466, *466, 467*
  teres major in, 466, *466, 467*
Tenodesis, flexor digitorum profundus in, *690*
 leg and foot reconstruction and, 718
 proximal interphalangeal, 646, *646*
Tenosynovitis, median nerve affected by, 587–589, *588, 589*
Tethering, sciatic nerve with, 572–573, *573*
Thalamus, pain pathways to, *108*, 121, *122*, 125
Thermoregulation, blood flow role in, *107*, 107–109, 113–114
 receptors in, 11–12, 12(t)
Thoracic outlet, 494–499
 anatomy of, 494, *495*
Thoracic outlet syndrome, 494–499
 anatomy related to, 494, *495*
 diagnosis of, *496*, 496–497
 pathogenesis of, 494–495, *495, 499*
 symptoms and signs of, 495–496
 treatment of, 497–498, *498, 499*
 true neurogenic, 656
Thoracoscopy, thoracic sympathectomy by, *165*, 165–166
Thrombosis, thoracic outlet syndrome causing, 495
 ulnar artery with, 113–114
Thumb, 675–703
 arthrodesis of, 645
  metacarpophalangeal joint in, 683, *683*
 bone block for, 710–711, *711*
 Bowler's, 149
 cerebral palsy deformity of, 632, *633, 635*, 642–645
  surgical approach to, 642–645, *642–645*
 impairment evaluation of, 767–772, *768*, 769(t), *770, 771*, 771(t)
 muscles of, 40(t), *42, 43*
 nerve supply through, 40(t), *42, 43*
 replantation of arm and, 710–713, *711, 712*
 sensation-bearing flap on, *750*
 tendon transfers for, 642–643, 675–703, 711–712. See also *Tendon transfer.*

Thumb *(Continued)*
 volar plate advancement for, 644–645
 web space deepening for, 644, *645*
Thyroid cartilage, anatomy of, *234*
Tibia, neuroma affecting, *154*
Tinel's sign, 25, 559
 brachial plexus injury with, 447
 percussion test vs., 558, *559*
 test procedure for, 25, *26*
Tinnel-Hoffman sign, fibrosis affecting, 289
Tissue autolysis, 763(t)
 denervated extremity with, *764*, 764–765, *765*
 foot affected by, *764*, 764–765, *765*
 ischemia causing, *763, 763*
 pressure causing, 763(t), 763–765
 repetitive stress injury causing, 763(t), *764*, 764–765, *765*
 sensory loss causing, 13–15, *14, 15*
Toes, 52
 claw (hammer), *728*, 728–729, *729*
 Girdlestone-Taylor transfer in, 728–729, *729*
 Johnson transfer in, 728, *728*
 Jones transfer in, 727, *727*
 motor function testing of, 52, *53*
 nerve entrapment affecting, 573–582, *574, 576, 577, 579*
 nerves in, 52, *53*, 205
 sensation-bearing flaps and, 752
 tendon transfer in, 726–729, *726–729*
Tongue, hypoglossal paralysis of, *387*, 388
 nerve supply to, *30*
Tooth, extraction of, nerve damage due to, 375, *375*
Touch, 11–27. See also *Pressure, sensibility to; Sensibility testing.*
 postsurgical evaluation of, 341–348, 342(t), *343, 344*, 346(t), 348(t)
Tourniquet, paralysis induced by, 476
Traction injury, knee and, 366–368
 spontaneous recovery prognosis for, 366–368
Transport, neuron cell matter in, *354*, 354–355
Trauma, 353–471. See also specific trauma, e.g., *Fracture(s).*
 brachial plexus affected by, 433–453. See also *Brachial plexus, traumatic injury to.*
 classification and types of, 355–357
 cold intolerance following, 114
 degeneration following, 357–358, *358*
 facial function affected by, 29–36
 gunshot injury as, 398–404, *399–403*. See also *Gunshot wounds.*
 injection, 406–413. See also *Injection injury.*
 management approach to, 368–369
 muscle reinnervation following, 393–396, *394–396*, 396(t)
 pathophysiology of, *353*, 353–360, *354, 358, 360*
 regeneration following, 357–359, *358*
 sensibility testing in, 15, *15*
 spontaneous recovery prognosis for, 365–369
 untreated, 365–369
Trendelenburg gait, 50–51
Trigger points, anesthesia infusion near, 116–119, *117, 118*
Trophic factors, 359
Tropic factors, 359
Tubercle(s), Chassaignac's, *69*, 69–70, *159*, 159–160, *160*
 pubic, *73*
Tube(s), empty perineurial, 308
 polyglactin mesh, 308–309
 polyglycolic acid, 309
 pseudosynovial, 308
 synthetic, 308–309
Tumors. See *Neoplasia*; specific tumor, e.g., *Hamartoma.*

Tunnels. See under *Entrapment syndrome(s)*; specific tunnel.
Two-point discrimination test, 19–22, *20–23*
 cerebral palsy affecting, 632–633
 impairment evaluation using, 768–769, 770(t)
 Moberg, 19–22, *20–23*, 22(t)
 moving, 22, *22*
 procedure for, 19–22, *19–23*, 768–769
 sensation-bearing flaps and, 745–749, *746–748*
 Weber, 16(t), *21*
Tyrosine kinase, nerve growth factor receptor and, 235

Ulcers, ischemia pressure sore causing, 763, *763*, 763(t), 764. See also *Pressure sores.*
Ultrasonography, 78–79
United States Veterans Administration Grading System, 341(t), 347(t)

Vasa nervorum, vascularized graft and, *299*
Vascular system, 107–109, 113–114
 cold intolerance and, 107–109, 113–114
 constriction affecting, 109, *110, 123*, 159
 sympathetic innervation of, *122*, 157–159, *158*
 testing related to, 78–80
Vein(s), intima of, nerve wrapped with, 153, *154*
 nerve repair conduit made from, 306–308, *307*, 335
 vascularized nerve graft role of, 295(t), 295–299, 298(t), *301, 302*
Venules, *107*
Verocay bodies, 602, *603*
Vertebrae. See *Spine.*
Veterans Administration Grading System, 341(t), 347(t)
Vibration, compression syndromes related to, 489
 injury due to, 356–357, 489
 sensibility testing with, 16(t), 24
Vision, nerve compression affecting, 371–372, *371–373*
Visual analog scales, 94–95, *95*
Vocal cords, paralysis affecting, 387
 recurrent nerve and, 387
Von Frey nylon filament test, 16, 16(t)
Von Recklinghausen's disease, 599–601
 clinical presentation of, 599–600, *600*
 pathology in, 600–601, *601*
 treatment of, 601

Waiter's tip position, *454*
Wallerian degeneration, *556*
War, gunshot wounds of, 365–366
 neurorraphy related to, 347, 347(t)
 periperal nerve injuries due to, 1–6
Wartenberg's syndrome, 524
Weber test, 16(t), *21*. See also *Two-point discrimination test.*
Whipsawing, prevention of, *684, 689, 690*
Work simulator, hand function measurement using, 543–544, *544, 545*
Wounds, gunshot. See *Gunshot wounds.*
Wright's maneuver, 496, *496*
Wrinkled finger test, 25–26, *26*
Wrist, *192, 193*
 arthrodesis of, 641
 brachial plexus injury affecting, *452, 454, 455, 458, 464*
 cerebral palsy flexion deformity in, 631, *635*, 638–642

Wrist *(Continued)*
  surgical approach to, *635*, 638–642, *639, 640, 642*
  diagnostic nerve blocks in, *71*, 71–72, *72*
  graft nerve repair in, 415–418, *415–418*
  muscles of, 40(t), *42, 43*
  nerve supply through, 40(t), *42, 43*

Wrist *(Continued)*
  surgical nerve exposure in, 189–193
  tendon transfer and, 638–641, 675–703. See also *Tendon transfer.*

YAG laser, 314(t), *315*, 316

Zancolli capsulodesis, clawed fingers and, 697–699, *698*
Z-plasty, thumb web deepening with, 644, *645*
Zygomatic arch, anatomy of, 230, *230*
  nerve branching patterns in, 230, *230*